TEXTBOOK OF

NEUROANESTHESIA

WITH

NEUROSURGICAL AND
NEUROSCIENCE
PERSPECTIVES

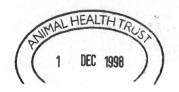

T E X T B O O K   O F

NEUROANESTHESIA

W I T H

NEUROSURGICAL AND NEUROSCIENCE PERSPECTIVES

MAURICE S. ALBIN, M.D., M.Sc., (Anes.)

Professor of Anesthesiology and Neurological Surgery
The University of Texas Health Science Center at San Antonio
Department of Anesthesiology
San Antonio, Texas

The McGraw-Hill Companies
HEALTH PROFESSIONS DIVISION

New York   St. Louis   San Francisco   Auckland   Bogotá   Caracus   Lisbon   London   Madrid
Mexico City   Milan   Montreal   New Delhi   San Juan   Singapore   Sydney   Tokyo   Toronto

McGraw-Hill

A Division of The **McGraw·Hill** Companies

TEXTBOOK OF NEUROANESTHESIA: With Neurosurgical and Neuroscience Perspectives

Copyright © 1997 by *The McGraw-Hill Companies* Inc. All rights reserved. Printed in the United States of America. Except as permitted under the United States Copyright Act of 1976, no part of this publication may be reproduced or distributed in any form or by any means, or stored in a data base or retrieval system, without prior written permission of the publisher.

1234567890 KGPKGP 9876

ISBN 0-07-000966-X

This book was set in Palatino by Bi-Comp, Inc.
The editors were Martin J. Wonsiewicz and Steven Melvin;
the production supervisor was Richard Ruzycka;
the cover designer was Marsha Cohen/Parallelogram.

Quebecor Printing/Kingsport, was the printer and binder.

Library of Congress Cataloging-in-Publication Data
Textbook of neuroanesthesia with neurosurgical and neuroscience
    perspectives / Maurice S. Albin, editor.
        p. cm.
    Includes bibliographical references and index.
    ISBN 0-07-000966-X
    1. Anesthesia in neurology.   I. Albin, Maurice S.
    [DNLM: 1. Anesthesia—methods.   2. Central Nervous System—drug
effects.   3. Neurosurgery.   WO 200 T3554 1997]
RD87.3.N47T49 1997
617.9'6748—dc20
DNLM/DLC
for Library of Congress   96-24790

To Marguerite
. . . who was always there . . .

Contents

vii

FOREWORDS

The subspecialty of neuroanesthesiology has been recognized for about 30 years. In its simplest form, it involves the care of patients undergoing a wide variety of neurosurgical procedures, from lumbar laminectomies to the most complex intracranial vascular operations. Almost every academic department and large group practice now has individuals who devote a large portion of their time to this clinical area. I think we have clearly improved the lot of our patients; while scientific data are hard to produce, I know of many "older" anesthesiologists and neurosurgeons—by which I mean those who started practice before the emergence of neuroanesthesia—who firmly believe that operative neurosurgery is now a much less harrowing venture than before. However, this improvement is not simply the product of devoted clinicians; it is also the product of a dramatic increase in our understanding of just what happens to the brain, lungs, and circulation during surgery and anesthesia.

In the early decades of this specialty, most investigative work was focused on one major area: the effects of anesthetics and adjuvants on cerebral blood flow (CBF), cerebral metabolism (CMR), and intracranial pressure (ICP). Inevitably, as more inquisitive people began to enter the field, more questions were raised, and the field began to broaden. Once upon a time, a patient awoke with a new focal neurologic deficit and an anesthesiologist asked himself "why did that happen, and how could it be prevented." This lead us into the broad field of cerebral ischemic physiology. This in turn demanded that we increase our understanding of cerebral electrophysiology, which gave rise to our deep involvement in perioperative electroencephalographic and evoked response monitoring. This almost certainly played a role in our interest in single-cell electrophysiology. The advent of "seizure surgery" and the unusual excitatory effects of some anesthetics drew some individuals into studies of epilepsy. The desire to prevent new injury resulted in innumerable studies on the protective effects of anesthetics and other drugs. When we realized that these effects could not be explained simply by changes in cerebral metabolic demand, neurochemistry was mastered. More recently, the molecular biology of ischemia has become a popular field. All of these interests combined to increase interest in basic mechanisms of anesthesia, a field that had heretofore been largely the province of chemists. It was also only a matter of time before the tools we had developed to study the brain were used to study the spinal cord.

These ideas indicate that, in 1996, it is almost impossible to easily define the field of knowledge encompassed by "neuroanesthesiology." It ranges from the most practical of clinical issues (e.g., the effects of different body positions on intraoperative blood loss or on ICP), to areas that would once have been considered extremely esoteric (e.g., the impact of anesthetics on c-*fos* gene expression during and after brain injury). Even the lines between neuroanesthesia and other anesthetic disciplines has blurred, as individuals study the effects of cardiopulmonary bypass on the cerebral circulation, the neurochemical changes occurring during fetal hypoxia, the role of the NMDA, AMPA, and glycine receptors in pain, among others. Other neuroanesthesiologists spend as much time working in neuroradiology and brain imaging as they do in the operating room.

The current text is an effort to present neuroanesthesia in this broader light. It includes the "traditional" chapters on the CBF effects of anesthetics, ICP dynamics, EEG and EP monitoring, as well as chapters on the practical clinical care of patients undergoing craniotomies, intracranial vascular surgery, carotid endarterectomies, posterior fossa surgery, and others. However, it also devotes a great deal of attention to the newer areas noted above, including neurotransmitters, excitotoxicity, epilepsy, brain protection, and spinal cord physiology and injury. I believe that this is both significant and critically important. I seriously doubt that progress in the care of neurosurgical patients will come from more work in older areas (e.g., the effects of desflurane on ICP), but will instead result from anesthesiologists becoming much more sophisticated neuroscientists. This book is a wonderful step in that direction.

Michael M. Todd, M.D.
Professor and Vice Chairman
Department of Anesthesia
University of Iowa College of Medicine
Iowa City, Iowa

On July 9, 1960, in Antwerp, Belgium, a group of anesthesiologists from nine countries gathered to form a commission of neuroanesthesia to advance teaching and research in this field. In that same year, a young, curious, and enthusiastic NIH trainee in anesthesia at the Mayo Clinic, Dr. Maurice Albin, began his fellowship in physiology and surgical research. As neuroanesthesia evolved over the ensuring 30 years to become a unique discipline within anesthesia, virtually no field included in this special area evaded the critical and creative mind of that young trainee.

From his earliest years, the neuroscience of anesthesia was Dr. Albin's passion. Together with Dr. Robert White, a brilliant and pioneering neurologic surgeon in Cleveland, a neuroanesthesia/neurosurgical team, unlimited in imagination and innovation, was formed. In the early 1960s, they were the first to completely isolate a simian brain, keep it alive with mechanical support, and study the metabolic parameters of cerebral blood flow and ischemia. This feat led to the study of spinal cord injury models and the protection afforded by perfusion of the subarachnoid space with hypothermic solutions. Subsequently, a cerebral ischemia model from ligation of the basilar artery was developed, which led to new studies, using evoked potentials, electroencephalography, neurobehavioral evaluations, and resuscitative measures—all covered in this text.

As a clinician scientist, the operating room was Dr. Albin's laboratory; nothing escaped his curous mind. Each anesthetized patient represented a potential for new scientific information. Various agents were evaluated for their effect on intracranial pressure, hypotension, cerebral metabolic activity, monitoring techniques, and postanesthetic neurocognitive sequelae. The anesthetized patients placed in the sitting position for neurosurgical procedures ultimately led to many seminal papers on the diagnosis and prevention of venous air emboli. The subsequent effects of these emboli on the lungs, brain, and various physiologic parameters were all dutifully documented and disseminated to colleagues.

In this same clinical laboratory, the potentially lethal effect of surgical brain retraction and subsequent cerebral edema and increased intracranial pressure were observed, and a pressure-sensitive device was constructed and patented to warn the surgeon of his potential "heavy handedness." Similarly, a pneumoelectric epidural intracranial pressure transducer was patented for the monitoring of brain-injured patients.

Somewhat like Harvey Cushing, who introduced the sphygmomanometer and blood pressure record, Dr. Albin in the 1960s was the prototype intensivist who emphasized the importance of tracking patients through monitoring of blood gases and various biochemical studies, and the significance of the patient's nutritional status—all things that are taken for granted today.

This text represents the summation of a teacher/mentor par excellence. One of Dr. Albin's students best characterized his influence as follows: "He imbued in all of us a single standard of excellence in the laboratory and in the clinic. There was no room for compromise where scientific integrity and the safety and welfare of patients were concerned. An understanding of the neurosciences, including neurosurgery, are elemental to our profession." He asked nothing of his students, residents, fellows, or neurosurgical collaborators that he did not demand of himself.

As a neurosurgeon fortunate enough to work and collaborate with Dr. Albin daily, I am well prepared to speak of his contributions as a clinician/scientist and as a teacher/mentor. But beyond the science, so ably and lucidly presented in this text, the editor is a humanist, historian, and practitioner of the art of medicine, which allows him to practice the science of his profession without "hardening the human heart by which we live." He possesses that "coolness and presence of mind under all circumstances, calmness amid storm, clearness of judgement in moments of great peril, immobility and impassiveness . . ." and is, indeed, the epitome of Osler's aequanimitas.

What has all this to do with a book on neuroanesthesia? Like an invisible thread woven through the tapestry of this book, the authors were selected for the same qualities exemplified by the editor: clinician investigators, teachers, mentors, and humanists, who have their patient as their highest concern. This textbook of neuroanesthesia is really best described as a text on the neuroscience of neuroanesthesia. From the molecular biology of excitatory and amino acid receptors and the cellular mechanisms of excitotoxicity to the cerebral metabolic effects of subarachnoid hemorrhage, all subjects are covered in a lucid and laconic style.

Although this is a multi-authored book, the depth and breadth of knowledge of its editor assures its place as a classic on the subject. Dr. Albin and his collaborators provide the reader a definitive text and a superb educational experience.

Joseph C. Maroon, M.D.
Professor and Chairman
Department of Surgery
Allegheny General Hospital and the Medical
  College of Pennsylvania and Hahnemann
  University
Pittsburgh, Pennsylvania

CONTRIBUTORS

James W. Albers, M.D., Ph.D. [13]
Department of Neurology
University of Michigan Medical Center
Ann Arbor, Michigan

Roger L. Albin, M.D. [15]
Department of Neurology
University of Michigan Medical Center
Ann Arbor, Michigan

Maurice S. Albin, M.D., M.Sc. (Anes.) [12, 30]
Department of Anesthesiology
University of Texas Health Science Center at San Antonio
San Antonio, Texas

Michael S. Aldrich, M.D. [11]
Department of Neurology
University of Michigan Medical Center
Ann Arbor, Michigan

Derek C. Armstrong, M.D. [35]
Department of Radiology
University of Toronto
Hospital for Sick Children
Toronto, Ontario
Canada

Alan A. Artru, M.D. [3]
Department of Anesthesiology
University of Washington School of Medicine
Seattle, Washington

Anthony M. Avellino, M.D. [34]
Department of Neurosurgery
University of Washington School of Medicine
Harborview Medical Center
Seattle, Washington

Claudio Bassetti, M.D. [11]
Department of Neurology
University of Michigan Medical Center
Ann Arbor, Michigan

M. Flint Beal, M.D. [16]
Department of Neurology
Massachusetts General Hospital
Harvard University School of Medicine
Boston, Massachusetts

Bruno Bissonnette, M.D. [35]
Department of Anesthesiology
University of Toronto
Hospital for Sick Children
Toronto, Ontario
Canada

Bradley S. Boop, M.D. [14]
Neurology Department
University of Arkansas For Medical Sciences
Little Rock, Arkansas

Cecil O. Borel, M.D. [24]
Department of Anesthesiology
Duke University Medical Center
Durham, North Carolina

Samuel R. Bowen, M.D. [28]
Division of Neurosurgery
Department of Surgical Sciences
Bowman Gray School of Medicine
Winston-Salem, North Carolina

Michelle Bowman-Howard, M.D. [32]
Department of Anesthesiology
University of Texas Health Science Center at Houston
Houston, Texas

Charles L. Branch, M.D. [28]
Division of Neurosurgery
Department of Surgical Sciences
Bowman Gray School of Medicine
Winston-Salem, North Carolina

Lois L. Bready, M.D. [23]
Department of Anesthesiology
University of Texas Health Science Center at San Antonio
San Antonio, Texas

Numbers in brackets refer to chapters written or cowritten by the contributors.

Leonid Bunegin, B.S. [8]
Department of Anesthesiology
University of Texas Health Science Center at San Antonio
San Antonio, Texas

Raymond M. Costello, Ph.D. [9]
Department of Psychiatry
University of Texas Health Science Center at San Antonio
San Antonio, Texas

Ignatius DiStefano, M.D. [22]
Greater Houston Anesthesiology
Houston, Texas

Francois Dubeau, M.D. [21]
Department of Neurology
McGill University
Montreal Neurological Institute
Montreal, Quebec
Canada

Leon S. Dure IV, M.D. [19]
Division of Pediatric Neurology
Department of Pediatrics
University of Alabama-Children's Hospital
Birmingham, Alabama

Kirk A. Frey, M.D., Ph.D. [15]
Department of Medicine
University of Michigan Medical Center
Ann Arbor, Michigan

Elizabeth A. M. Frost, M.D. [1]
Department of Anesthesiology
New York Medical College
Westchester County Medical Center
Valhalla, New York

Fred H. Geisler, M.D. [33]
Comprehensive Spinal Care Center
Chicago Institute Neurosurgery/Neuroresearch
Chicago, Illinois

Phillip L. Gildenberg, M.D., Ph.D. [22]
Department of Neurosurgery
Baylor University College of Medicine
Houston, Texas

Ake Grenvik, M.D., Ph.D. [38]
Department of Anesthesiology/Critical Care Medicine
University of Pittsburgh School of Medicine
Pittsburgh, Pennsylvania

Carin A. Hagberg, M.D. [32]
Department of Anesthesiology
University of Texas Health Science Center at Houston
Houston, Texas

Rukaiya K. A. Hamid, M.D. [26]
Department of Anesthesiology
Los Angeles Children's Hospital—University of Southern California
Los Angeles, California

E. Ralph Heinz, M.D. [24]
Department of Radiology
Duke University Medical Center
Durham, North Carolina

Ian A. Herrick, M.D. [20]
Department of Anesthesia
University Hospital
London, Ontario
Canada

Rosemary Hickey, M.D. [27, 31, 37]
Department of Anesthesiology
University of Texas Health Science Center at San Antonio
San Antonio, Texas

William E. Hoffman, Ph.D. [2]
Department of Anesthesiology
University of Illinois School of Medicine
Chicago, Illinois

Carswell H. Jackson, M.D. [28]
Department of Anesthesiology
Bowman Gray School of Medicine
Winston-Salem, North Carolina

M. Jones-Gotman, Ph.D. [21]
Department of Neurology
McGill University
Montreal Neurological Institute
Montreal, Quebec
Canada

David L. Kelly, Jr., M.D. [28]
Division of Neurosurgery
Department of Surgical Sciences
Bowman Gray School of Medicine
Winston-Salem, North Carolina

Eberhard Kochs, M.D., Ph.D. [2]
Department of Anesthesiology
Technische Universitat München
Munich, Germany

W. Andrew Kofke, M.D. [36]
Department of Anesthesiology
University of Pittsburgh School of Medicine
Pittsburgh, Pennsylvania

Arthur M. Lam, M.D. [26, 34]
Department of Anesthesiology
Harborview Medical Center
Seattle, Washington

Thomas W. Lew, M.B.B.S. [38]
Department of Anesthesiology
Tan Tock Seng Hospital
Singapore

Colin F. Mackenzie, M.D. [33]
Department of Anesthesiology
University of Maryland School of Medicine
Baltimore, Maryland

Christopher K. McQuitty, M.D. [4]
Department of Anesthesiology
The University of Texas Medical Branch—Galveston
Galveston, Texas

Howard C. Mitzel, Ph.D. [9]
Department of Anesthesiology
University of Texas Health Science Center
San Antonio, Texas

Mary B. Neal, M.D. [22]
Greater Houston Anesthesiology
Houston, Texas

Phillipa Newfield, M.D. [26]
Department of Anesthesiology
California Pacific Medical Center
University of California-San Francisco
San Francisco, California

Mark F. Newman, M.D. [10]
Department of Anesthesiology
Duke University Medical Center
Durham, North Carolina

Andre Olivier, M.D. [21]
Department of Neurosurgery
McGill University
Montreal Neurological Institute
Montreal, Quebec
Canada

Patricia H. Petrozza, M.D. [28]
Department of Anesthesiology
Bowman Gray School of Medicine
Winston-Salem, North Carolina

John Pile-Spellman, M.D. [25]
Department of Radiology
Columbia–Presbyterian Medical Center
New York, New York

Susan S. Porter, M.D. [29]
Department of Anesthesiology
St. Luke's Hospital–University of Missouri
Kansas City, Missouri

Donald S. Prough, M.D. [4]
Department of Anesthesiology
University of Texas Medical Branch—Galveston
Galveston, Texas

Viswanathan Rajaramen, M.D. [28]
Division of Neurosurgery
Department of Surgical Sciences
Bowman Gray School of Medicine
Winston-Salem, North Carolina

Ira J. Rampil, M.D., M.S. [6]
Department of Anesthesiology
University of California, San Francisco
San Francisco, California

Setti S. Rengachary, M.D. [29]
Department of Neurological Surgery
University of Minnesota School of Medicine
Minneapolis, Minnesota

James Rogers, M.D. [31]
Department of Anesthesiology
University of Texas Health Science Center at San Antonio
San Antonio, Texas

Harlan David Root, M.D., Ph.D. [27]
Department of Surgery
University of Texas Health Science Center at San Antonio
San Antonio, Texas

James T. Rutka, M.D. [35]
Department of Neurosurgery
University of Toronto
Hospital for Sick Children
Toronto, Ontario
Canada

Peter Safar, M.D. [17]
Department of Anesthesiology
International Resuscitation Research Center
University of Pittsburgh School of Medicine
Pittsburgh, Pennsylvania

Satwant K. Tiwana Samra, M.D. [5]
Department of Anesthesiology
University of Michigan Medical Center
Ann Arbor, Michigan

Abhay Sanan, M.D. [29]
Department of Neurological Surgery
University of Minnesota School of Medicine
Minneapolis, Minnesota

Sandra L. Schneider, Ph.D. [9]
Department of Radiology
University of Texas Health Science Center at San Antonio
San Antonio, Texas

David G. Sherman, M.D. [14]
Division of Neurology
Department of Medicine
University of Texas Health Science Center at San Antonio
San Antonio, Texas

Tod B. Sloan, M.D., Ph.D. [7, 31, 37]
Department of Anesthesiology
University of Texas Health Science Center at San Antonio
San Antonio, Texas

Dale E. Solomon, M.D. [12]
Department of Anesthesiology
University of Texas Health Science Center at San Antonio
San Antonio, Texas

Diane H. Solomon, M.D. [12]
Division of Neurology
Department of Medicine
University of Texas Health Science Center at San Antonio
San Antonio, Texas

Davy Trop, M.D. [21]
Department of Anesthesia
McGill University
Montreal Neurological Institute
Montreal, Quebec
Canada

Debra S. Tyler, M.D. [23]
Department of Anesthesiology
University of Texas Health Science Center at San Antonio
San Antonio, Texas

John J. Wald, M.D. [13]
Department of Neurology
University of Michigan Medical Center
Ann Arbor, Michigan

David S. Warner, M.D. [18]
Department of Anesthesiology
Duke University Medical Center
Durham, North Carolina

Lawrence Wechsler, M.D. [36]
Department of Neurology
University of Pittsburgh School of Medicine
Pittsburgh, Pennsylvania

Bryce D. A. Weir, M.D.C.M. [26]
Department of Neurosurgery
Univeristy of Chicago School of Medicine
Chicago, Illinois

William C. Welch, M.D. [32]
Department of Neurosurgery
University of Pittsburgh School of Medicine
Pittsburgh, Pennsylvania

Christian Werner, M.D. [2]
Department of Anesthesiology
Technische Universität Munchen
Munich, Germany

H. Richard Winn, M.D. [34]
Department of Neurosurgery
University of Washington School of Medicine
Seattle, Washington

Howard Yonas, M.D. [36]
Department of Neurosurgery
University of Pittsburgh School of Medicine
Pittsburgh, Pennsylvania

William L. Young, M.D. [25]
Department of Anesthesiology
Columbia–Presbyterian Medical Center
New York, New York

Fernando M. Zalduondo, M.D. [24]
Department of Radiology
Duke University Medical Center
Durham, North Carolina

Mark H. Zornow, M.D. [4]
Department of Anesthesiology
University of Texas Medical Branch—Galveston
Galveston, Texas

PREFACE

A number of years ago, two apparently unrelated events took place. Being a neuroscience bibliophile for many years, I was going through some old files for historical information on one of the early American neurologists, Weir Mitchell. As I peered through these alphabetized folders, my thumb stuck at the letter "H" and on opening a file I noted a letter from Professor Andrew Hunter, a pioneer British neuroanesthesiologist and author of the first published book on neuroanesthesia (1964). Underneath this letter was a mistakenly filed paper that Loyal Davis and Harvey Cushing had written in 1925 on blood scavenging. The other event took place at the Audie Murphy Veteran's Administration Hospital in San Antonio. We were placing EEG electrodes and a transcranial Doppler transducer on a patient for an aortic valve repair as part of a study we were carrying out concerning neurobehavioral and embolic responses during and after cardiopulmonary bypass. As we were finishing the monitoring applications, one of our residents came into the recovery room and wanted to know my thoughts concerning responses to anesthetic agents and adjuvants in an elective case where the patient was suspected of having multiple sclerosis.

In many ways the two events symbolize the rationale for putting together this book. They emphasize our debt to those who, in the past, have toiled so hard for us giving us a historical perspective. The initial chapter by Professor Elizabeth Frost burrows deep down into our origins and allows us to understand the scientific traditions that have significantly influenced the development of neuroanesthesia as a subspecialty. The book by the late Professor Hunter was followed two years later by a Canadian text edited by Drs. Gilbert, Galindo, and Brindle, all from the Montreal Neurological Institute and McGill University School of Medicine. Professor Gilbert was indeed an important early pioneer in neuroanesthesia as well as Chairman of the Department of Anaesthetics at McGill University School of Medicine and Anaesthetist-in-Chief at the Montreal Neurological Institute. These two books, published in the 1960s, seem to herald the beginning of an explosion that took place in the clinical neurosciences and neuroanesthesia with extraordinary progress taking place in the physiopathology of head and spinal cord trauma, intracranial hypertension, air embolism, and effects of anesthetics on cerebral blood flow and metabolism, to name only a few. This interest, coupled with incredible advances in electronic technology and monitoring, propelled us into the 1970s which saw the formalized development of clinicians dedicated to neuroanesthesia.

With membership coming from the United States and Canada, the organization of the Society of Neurosurgical Anesthesia and Neurological Supportive Care (SNANSC) was formed in 1972 to "improve the art and science of neurological anesthesia and care of the critically ill neurosurgical and neurological patient." The initial organizers of SNANSC in 1972 were Maurice S. Albin, M.D. (Pittsburgh), James Harp, M.D. (Philadelphia), and Harvey Shapiro, M.D. (Philadelphia). They were assisted by Brian Marshall, M.D. (Toronto), John D. Michenfelder, M.D. (Rochester), and Thomas J. Langfitt, M.D. (Philadelphia). Langfitt was Chairman of the Department of Neurosurgery at the University of Pennsylvania. Interestingly, the first meeting of this neuroanesthesia group took place in Philadelphia on June 15, 1973 (during the International CBF Meeting). The proposed name, Neurosurgical Anesthesia Society, was subsequently changed to SNANSC. The three neurosurgeons present at this meeting, Drs. Langfitt, Becker, and White were all known for their work in the areas of head and spinal cord injury, intracranial hypertension, hypothermia, and cerebrovascular dynamics. It has always been the custom of our neuroanesthesia society to include all varieties of neuroscientists into the membership. The original 1973 membership list can be seen in Fig. 1 and a list of presidents from 1974 to 1991 is noted in Table 1.

The challenges posed to the concept of "neuroanesthesia" as a clinical entity were succinctly stated in an editorial published in the *British Journal of Anaesthesia* in 1965 (vol 37) and brought to my attention by Dr. Jean Horton, another pioneering British neuroanesthetist: "However, if the contribution of anaesthesia to neurosurgery is firmly established, its basis remains largely empirical. There is little precise knowledge of the numerous and interrelated ways in which anaesthetic agents influence surgical exposure of the brain. To extend this knowledge, and to participate in (initiate, even) the circumvention of those formidable anatomical and physiological obstacles which appear to bar the way to radical new progress in neurosurgery, is the challenge for the future." Concomitant with the organizational development of neuroanesthesia, the late 1960s and 1970s marked the beginning of the application of concepts drawn from molecular biology and genetics, which announced advances on an almost daily basis. Ideas involving autonomic blockade, receptor binding, pharmacodynamics and pharmcokinetics, genetic mapping of diseases and disease traits, neurotransmitters, imaging techniques, and extraordinarily sensitive on-line measurement capability of physiologic variables,

Members of the
"Neurosurgical Anesthesia Society"
(June 15, 1973)

most of which were relatively unknown but 25 years ago, have revolutionized our methods of evaluating and treating the patient with neurologic dysfunction and impacted enormously on our practice of neuroanesthesia.

The mention of a resident asking about the anesthetic management of a patient with possible multiple sclerosis while I was applying the EEG electrodes and transducers for the transcranial Doppler to another patient again emphasizes the paradoxical bind we find ourselves. On the one hand we must be competent to use (and to teach the use of) the latest techniques of neuromonitoring, while on the other preserving, and perhaps "polishing," our acumen in the clinical neurosciences. With all this, the overwhelming nature of the information explosion has made it difficult for us to thread our way along the pathway of safe and efficacious patient care. The thrust of managed care and cost containment with its insistence on minimizing the amount of professional time spent in preoperative and postoperative care because of our increased work load, can also be a factor making diligent evaluations difficult. This has become especially true in cases relating to the central nervous system. I can well remember the concern of a resident who was faced with the problem of anesthetizing a patient for an emergent head injury who also had a history of von Hippel-Lindau disease, or the bewilderment of another having to anesthetize a patient with the Hand-Schuler-Christian Syndrome (histiocytosis X). While the information on these rare neurologic syndromes is available, it is indeed difficult to find this information quickly and often the anesthetic consequences are not touched on. For this reason, we are dedicating a significant amount of

TABLE 1
Presidents
Society of Neurosurgical Anesthesia and Critical Care

Dates of Office	Specialty	Name
1991–1992	Anesthesiologist	David S. Smith, M.D., Ph.D.
1990–1991	Neurosurgeon	Lawrence H. Pitts, M.D.
1989–1990	Anesthesiologist	Wayne K. Marshall, M.D.
1988–1989	Neurosurgeon	Neal Kassell, M.D.
1987–1988	Anesthesiologist	Philippa Newfield, M.D.
1986–1987	Neurosurgeon	Lawrence Marshall, M.D.
1985–1986	Anesthesiologist	Robert F. Bedford, M.D.
1984–1985	Neurosurgeon	Derek Bruce, M.D.
1983–1984	Anesthesiologist	Jane Matjasko, M.D.
1982–1983	Neurosurgeon	Peter J. Jannetta, M.D.
1981–1982	Anesthesiologist	James E. Cottrell, M.D.
1980–1981	Anesthesiologist	S. Craighead Alexander, M.D.
1979–1980	Anesthesiologist	James R. Harp, M.D.
1978–1979	Neurosurgeon	Donald P. Becker, M.D.
1977–1978	Anesthesiologist	Harvey M. Shapiro, M.D.
1976–1977	Anesthesiologist	Brian M. Marshall, M.D.
1975–1976	Anesthesiologist	Maurice S. Albin, M.D.
1974–1975	Anesthesiologist	John D. Michenfelder, M.D.

space to covering these neurologic states and syndromes and indicating any anesthetic interactions.

Like neuroanesthesia, neurosurgery itself has advanced remarkably since the early 1960s with the introduction of the operating microscope, the new neuroimaging techniques, the use of the computer to enhance surgical manipulation, the development of new instrumentation for tissue-tumor removal, innovations in microcatheter design and adjuvants for neurovascular procedures (interventional neuroradiology), and the introduction of a host of new chemotherapeutic agents. These exciting developments place the neuroanesthesiologist in the center of all these activities. It becomes important for the neuroanesthesiologist to have more than a passing understanding of the steps involved in the neurosurgical or neuroradiologic procedure. Essentially, he/she must become a knowledgeable "cognoscente," so that potential problems that may develop can be anticipated.

So far, I have tried to address how neuroanesthesia came into being; our extraordinary development since the early 1960s; our need to have a better understanding of the clinical neurosciences; and the necessity to appreciate the complexity of the neurosurgical and neuroradiologic procedures. The final ingredient characterizing our practice of neuroanesthesia involves our determination to understand new knowledge that has come from the basic neurosciences and that has accelerated remarkably in the 1980s and 1990s (now being called "the decade of the brain"). These advances have affected all aspects of neuroanesthesia—from our understanding of CSF–CBF dynamics to our appreciation of the role of blood glucose concentrations as a factor in spinal cord and cerebral ischemia. The terms "neuroprotection" and "neuro-

toxicity" have taken on new meaning because of our appreciation of the role of excitotoxic amino acids, receptor binding and inhibition, free-radical formation, and ionic intra- and extracellular neuronal fluxes.

In developing this *Textbook of Neuroanesthesia*, I was drawn to the critical aspects mentioned above and thought how to reconcile these needs with the practicality of producing a manageable and coherent book. As one who has contributed many chapters in books on neuroanesthesia, critical care medicine, and neurosurgery, I had always been concerned that I could never completely get my message across because of space limitations relating to the text and bibliography. Interviews with many dozens of those with expertise in the various basic and applied neuroscience disciplines confirmed my feeling that the question of space limitations was an important critical factor in producing a text that would allow the writer to adequately present a viewpoint with a high degree of intellectuality.

The essential strategy of this book is to present the reader with an understanding of the fundamental considerations relating to neuroanesthesia and neurosurgery in terms of both the anesthetic and the surgical techniques used during these procedures in the adult and pediatric age groups. Interposed with these chapters you will find chapters giving the basic science, neurologic, neurobehavioral, and neuroradiologic substrate in order to achieve a better understanding of problems relating to neurosurgery and to neurologic dysfunction. We have not neglected the problem of seizures and seizure surgery, nor have we forgotten about the spine and spinal cord trauma, as well as those of head injury. The increase in the geriatric population made it important to address the problems of aging and neurologic syndromes and to give us a perspective on electroconvulsive therapy. Conversely, the pediatric population has been addressed in an ample chapter on pediatric neuroanesthesia. Because of their importance and the many issues involved, the reader will find chapters of considerable length when we discuss cerebral blood flow and metabolism, cerebral edema and the CSF, cerebral ischemia, and neuro-intensive care. A significant amount of space has been dedicated to the chapter on neuroradiology since I think it is so critical to define the imagery of the anatomic pathology. The radiologic anatomy of a hemispheric shift, enlarged ventricles, and epidural hematoma, or a C6-C7 fracture dislocation with spinal cord involvement should be understood by the anesthesiologist, as well as by the neurosurgeon, since so much of our neuroanesthesia management will be influenced by these findings.

We hope that this text will be used as a reference source because we have not stinted in allowing our authors to include all the references they thought important. We have tried hard to reduce the amount of redundancy among these chapters, but in order to achieve a sense of coherency and completeness, some overlap was necessary. The authors contributing to this book were chosen because of their expertise in their selected areas. I am sure that many controversial statements are present in the text that may provoke disagreement among readers. In reviewing each of the chapters, I made no attempt to change any of the concepts or opinions held by the authors, for I feel that controversy is a valuable approach to distilling the truth.

Acknowledgments

There are indeed many people to thank in putting together this type of book. Above all, I want to thank R. Brian Smith, M.D., the Professor and Chairman of the Department of Anesthesiology at the University of Texas Health Science Center at San Antonio. Without the continuous support and encouragement of this friend and colleague, scientist and superb clinician, this book would have never seen the printer's ink.

Mrs. Olivia Pape mounted the original secretarial effort to get this book off the ground for which I am grateful. To Mrs. Linda Gonzales go all the kudos for doing the yeowoman's work in getting out the correspondence, helping me in the manuscript review, keeping track of the illustrations, sending the chapters back to the publishers, and even correcting my mistakes. Thank you Linda! I am also most appreciative of the help given by Ann Hix, Ann Franklin, and Louise Raymond. Finally, without the initial encouragement of Michael Houston and the efforts of my editor, Jamie Kircher, I don't know how this book would have been possible.

Maurice S. Albin, M.D., M.Sc. (Anes.)

TEXTBOOK OF

NEUROANESTHESIA

WITH

NEUROSURGICAL AND NEUROSCIENCE PERSPECTIVES

HISTORY OF NEUROANESTHESIA

ELIZABETH A. M. FROST

While the greatest advances in neurosurgery are linked to developments in anesthesia, archaeologic excavations and history indicate a long course of intracranial intervention with and without anesthetic assistance.

Prehistoric Times

Operations upon the skull are among the oldest of human surgical endeavors (Fig. 1-1). Cranial remains as far back as the late Paleolithic period indicate that humans knew several methods of opening the skull. Only in Australia (but not in New Zealand), the Malay peninsula, Japan, China, and among African black nations has no evidence of skull surgery been documented.[1] Many individuals survived the initial procedure long enough not only for healing processes to be identified but even for reoperation. The ancients appeared to have had a certain familiarity with anatomy, as suture lines and large venous sinuses were rarely violated. Openings were also not made in the mastoid region, and the dura was usually left intact.

Speculation has been made on the purpose of these holes.[2] Although some perforations may be related to injury, the presence of multiple openings in the absence of other injuries in young and old of both sexes suggests, among other things, prophylactic action. It has been supposed that the skull was opened to relieve pain, drain pus, allow evil spirits to depart, or prevent inflammation. On the other hand, holes may have been made as a rite of passage to manhood or postmortem for cannibalism or to obtain amulets or allow suspension of the corpse for embalming.[3] Also, bony defects were occasionally filled with gold, suggesting a ceremonial role or indicating the belief that the presence of an inert metal would retard infection.

Two principal means of opening the skull have been identified. Simple boring of a hole was done with a perforator (terebra or exfoliator). A central drill or terebra was whirled by a thong (Fig. 1-2). A more elaborate and larger hole was made by removal of a piece of bone by cutting around it with a sawlike instrument (trepanation or trephination). From instruments dating to about 500 B.C. found in burial caves in Peru it may be deduced that trephining was done with an obsidian, triangular, knifelike instrument fixed in a wooden handle (Fig. 1-3). Bronze knives (tumis) made rectangular holes by crisscross cuts (Fig. 1-4).

Trepanation was continued by some primitive peoples up to the beginning of the twentieth century, particularly in North Africa, South America, and the Pacific Islands.[4] To prevent illness in children, mothers did not hesitate to make a prophylactic trephination using fragments of obsidian, sharks' teeth, or sharp shells.

How the patient was controlled during what must have been at least a 30-min procedure is unknown. There is no evidence that anesthesia or narcotics were available to Neolithic man in Europe. Coca leaves were available in Peru, and their ability to deaden pain has been known since early times. Indeed, perhaps a very early anesthetist was an assistant employed to chew leaves and spit into the wound—a technique that has been used and described through the centuries in South America.[5]

Babylon and Egypt

Despite the high degree of social culture in Babylon and Assyria, little evidence of medical and surgical knowledge has survived. Surgical practice was regulated by law. The Code of Hammurabi (twenty-first century B.C.) noted that a physician who made a wound and cured a freeman was to receive 10 pieces of silver; if the patient was the son of a plebeian, he would receive 5 pieces, which sum was reduced to 2 pieces if the patient was a slave.[6] Nevertheless, if the physician treated a patient with a metal knife for a severe wound

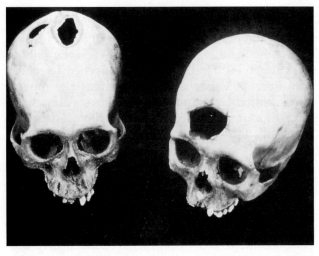

Figure 1-1   Trephined skulls. Large holes in the crania have been made by hand tools.

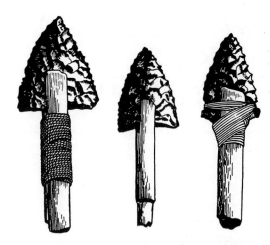

Figure 1-3   Trephines of obsidian found in burial caves in Peru, South America.

and the patient died, the physician's hands were to be cut off.

Several medical records have survived from ancient Egypt. The Ebers manuscript (University of Leipzig) is a collection of medical recipes and incantations, as

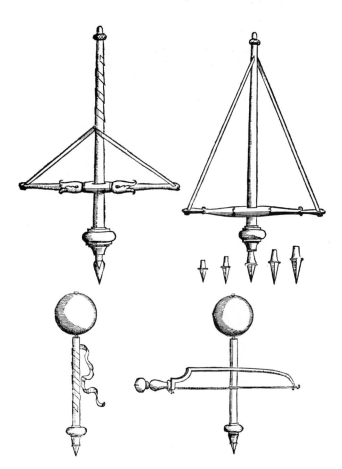

Figure 1-2   Several types of terebra and the means whereby they are used.

are the Berlin Medical Papyrus (Berlin), the London Medical Papyrus (British Museum), and the Papyrus Hearst (University of California). The Edwin Smith Papyrus is the earliest written record of surgical practice. It is named after an American Egyptologist who purchased the document from Mustapha Aga in Luxor in 1862. The papyrus is an incomplete copy of an earlier treatise composed about 3000 B.C. It describes 48 cases from what may originally have been the records of patients of Imhotep, Egypt's great architect-physician and advisor to Pharaoh Yoser. This text may well represent the original neurosurgical practice manual, and of the 48 cases, 15 concern head injury, 12 facial wounds and fractures, and 7 vertebral injuries. The other 14 cases involve pathology of the upper thorax. Although pain is recognized as a sensation caused by the injury and by movements made by the patient on instruction from the physician, the latter is exhorted to "palpate his wound, although he shudders exceedingly . . . cause him to lift his face; if it is painful for him to open his mouth, his heart beats feebly" (from case 7, a depressed skull fracture).[7] It is suggested that pain, associated only with the injury, cannot be intensified by anything the physician does, and therefore cannot be alleviated by him.

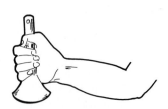

Figure 1-4   A hand-held tumi and how it was used.

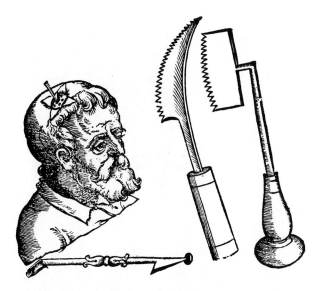

Figure 1-5   The lenticular saw preferred by Hippocrates and Galen and how it was used.

However, wine making was a highly developed skill in ancient Egypt and the soporific effects of alcohol have been well documented by hieroglyphics. Perhaps some analgesic effects were obtained from this source.

Greek and Roman Times

Several treatises written about 400 B.C., probably by several authors, have been ascribed to Hippocrates. One text, "On Injuries of the head," described trephining for skull fractures, epilepsy, blindness, and headaches. The practitioner was advised to avoid suture lines and the temporal areas because of fear of damaging the (middle meningeal?) artery that would lead to contralateral convulsions.[8] It was also noted that the inner table should be preserved to protect the dura and that this bone fragment would later be extruded by suppuration.

Celsus (first century A.D.) further described the signs and symptoms of head injuries, noting that fractures of the base of the skull were usually fatal.[9] He associated bleeding from the nose and ears, bilious vomiting, coma, stupor, roving eyes, and convulsions with a poor outcome and recommended incinerated egg yolk as a styptic powder for meningeal hemorrhage.

Galen (A.D. 130–201), an eminent neurophysiologist, added little to neurosurgical technique and repeated much of the Hippocratic teachings.[10] He preferred the lenticular saw, a knifelike instrument with a button edge, over the trephine. It was noted that the dura mater could not be perforated even if the operator fell asleep (but no mention is made of the patient's sensorium) (Fig. 1-5).

Aretaeus, a Cappadocian monk who lived in Rome,

outlined the treatment of seizures in the second century A.D. He recommended perforating the skull with a trepan "when the meninx there is found black," combined with surface cooling, sedation, and catharsis.[11] If the putrefaction could be cleansed (i.e., subdural clot could be released), cure was to be expected. Apparently, he recognized little need for anesthesia, as "the habit of such persons renders them tolerant of pains and their goodness of spirits and good hopes render them strong in endurance."

During these times neurosurgical instruments were developed and scalpels were made with blades of steel and handles of bronze. Probes, directors, guards, and elevators were available. Tissue and bone forceps, chisels, and gouges were all described. However, few advances in intracranial surgery were made because of the lack of anesthesia. The narcotic effects of mandrake, henbane, and opium were known, as were the effects of alcohol,[12] and had been described extensively by Dioscorides, a Greek surgeon in Nero's army in the first century A.D. His work, *De materia medica*, was the source of almost all botanical knowledge for some 1500 years. On at least two occasions Dioscorides recommended that mandrake be used for surgery.[13] Incidentally, although tradition credits Oliver Wendell Holmes with the term *anesthesia*, Dioscorides actually used it first. The word was revived by Quistorp in 1719 and used by John Elliotson and others in association with mesmerism in the nineteenth century, before Holmes finally applied it definitively to Morton's use of ether in 1846.[13] The Greek word for sleep, *Karoun*, may be connected to the carotid artery. Perhaps the ancients realized that pressure on the neck could cause unconsciousness, or perhaps it was evident that laceration of the carotid arteries resulted in permanent coma. The implication is that if pressure was a measure of causing anesthesia, surgeons would have to work quickly.

The Middle Ages

Medical advancement stopped with the decline of the Roman Empire. The Roman Catholic Church became most influential in medical and surgical care, and monasteries were the seats of science and culture. The art of surgery deteriorated, and with the edict of 1163, "Ecclesia abhoret a sanguine," surgery became a lay trade.

During the Byzantine period, Paul of Aegina (625–690) mainly reiterated the teachings of Hippocrates and Galen. He did, however, suggest some refinements—for example, stuffing the patients' "ears with wool in order to avoid the noise of the perforation."[14] Of interest, too, because it implies some experimentation of the mechanisms of head injury, is the explanation put forward by Paul for the cause of contrecoup fracture. In writing of types of skull fractures, he noted disagreement with others of the time:

> Some also add that by repercussion, which happens, say they, when a fracture of the cranium takes place opposite to the part which received the blow. But they are in mistake, for what happens to glass vessels does not, as they say, happen here; for, this happens to them from their being empty, but the skull is full and otherwise strong. But when many other parts of the head have been struck, as in a fall, and a fissure of the skull takes place without a solution or continuity of the skin, an abscess afterwards forms in it, and being opened, this fissure is discovered.[15]

The groundwork was laid for the Arab physicians who followed to accumulate, store and, in some instances, distill the work of the ancient masters. Rhazes (850–923), the most famous doctor of the tenth century, compiled a *Liber Continens* of all the knowledge of the Arab world.[16] His philosophy, stated in an aphorism, was, "If Galen and Aristotle are of one mind on a subject, then surely their opinion is true. If divided, it is extremely difficult to decide which opinion should be accepted."[16] Rhazes realized that pressure on the brain, rather than skull fracture itself, is the more important factor in head injury.

During the ninth century, a medical school had been founded at Salerno. There, during the tenth century, Constantinus Africanus translated the Arabian medical manuscripts to Latin, reviving the knowledge of the old masters. The techniques described were far ahead of those practiced at the time and were transmitted quickly to France, Britain, and elsewhere in Europe as the Renaissance was initiated.

Still, however, few references are made to anesthesia, perhaps because pain is mentioned so frequently in religious teachings and is envisioned rather as a "noble" state (Fig. 1-6). Rather, theological doctrine held that pain serves God's purpose and therefore was not to be alleviated. Usually European surgeons used mandrake, cannabis indica, henbane, opium, and wine, much as described 1000 years before. Theodoric, a pioneer surgeon from the school of Bologna in the thirteenth century, described a soporific sponge:

> Take of opium, of the juice of the unripe mulberry, of hyoscyamus, of the juice of hemlock, of the juice of the leaves of the mandragora, of the juice of the wood ivy, of the seeds of dock which has large round apples and of the water-hemlock, each an ounce. Mix all these in a brazen vessel and then place in it a new sponge; let the whole boil as long as the sun lasts on the dog-day until the sponge consumes it all. Place this sponge in hot water for a hour and let it be applied to the

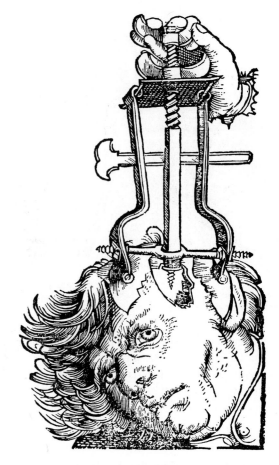

Figure 1-6 Pain relief was not considered necessary during trephination.

nostrils of him who is to be operated on until he has fallen asleep and so let the surgery be performed.[17]

Recent attempts to fill this recipe found it had little soporific effect. Apparently Theodoric himself did not have complete confidence in the anesthetic effects of his sponge as he advised that the patients also be securely tied down.[18] Mandrake (mandragora) (Fig. 1-7) belongs to the potato family but contains belladonna alkaloids from which atropine is obtained. At best it is a very mild narcotic. Probably the addition of wine during boiling enhanced its effects. A variation of Theodoric's sponge contained cannabis indica (i.e., hemp grown in India). This drug was swallowed in a wine solution, smoked, or burned in bonfires. It is now more commonly known as marijuana.

Henbane (or hyoscyamus) is a mild narcotic, also belonging to the belladonna family of drugs. It was usually included in the somniferous mixtures. A more modern version is scopolamine.

Yet another refinement of Theodoric's prescription was described in "The Physicians of Myddvai" (thirteenth century). Directions are: "when you are pre-

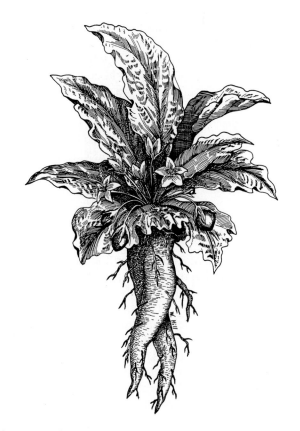

Figure 1-7 The mandrake plant. Its roots have been likened to the legs of man.

pared to operate upon the patient, direct that he shall avoid sleep as long as he can, and then let some of the potion be poured into his nostrils, and he will sleep without fail"[19]

One interesting account of anesthetic use is found in Hindu writings. In A.D. 927, two surgeon brothers operated on the king of Dhasi. They induced anesthesia with a drug named "samohine," trephined the skull, removed a tumor, and stitched the wound closed.[20] As a reversal agent (i.e., to arouse the patient), an onion compounded with vinegar, was poured into the mouth. Soporific sponges were in widespread use up until the seventeenth century.

Renaissance

During the early Middle Ages, with the exception perhaps of Avicenna in Isfahan, anatomical dissection of the dead was forbidden, and few advances were made in understanding the physiology of the central nervous system.

In the fourteenth century, Roland de Parme gave a detailed description of the use of the trephine in his book *La Chirurgia*. An elderly patient, head shaven, is shown sitting placidly, hands crossed in his lap,

while a man of the Church drills a hole in his head (Fig. 1-8). A tumi, dating from A.D. 1300, was also used for trephination (Fig. 1-9). The figures on the handle depict its use: while one man holds the patient, the other trephines the skull. A century later, Charaf-ed Din in his book *La Chirurgie des Ilkhani* (A.D. 1465) shows the treatment of a child with hydrocephalus (Fig. 1-10). The child is held by an assistant while the surgeon, using a bistoury, cuts off the excess head.

About the middle of the fourteenth century, the ban on human dissection was eased. Shortly, thereafter, great advances were made in the understanding of the anatomy of the central nervous system by Vesalius (the internal anatomy of the brain and ventricular system), Falloppias (the trigeminal, auditory, glossopharyngeal, and chorda tympani nerves), Eustachius (the abducens and optic nerves), Willis (the spinal accessory nerve), Sylvius, and Morgagni.[21]

That neurosurgery was practiced widely in the sixteenth century is evidenced by the surgeon's case of Ambroise Paré, who was the surgeon to the king of France during the 1560s. Of 13 surgical instruments, 5 were trephines (Fig. 1-11).

In 1639, one of the first medical texts in English was written,[22] *The Physician's Practice*, "wherein are con-

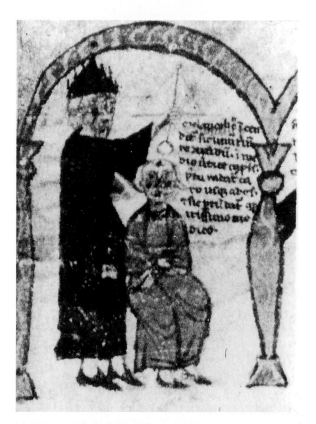

Figure 1-8 Illustration of skull operation performed by trephination. From *La Chirurgia*, by Roland de Parme, fourteenth century.

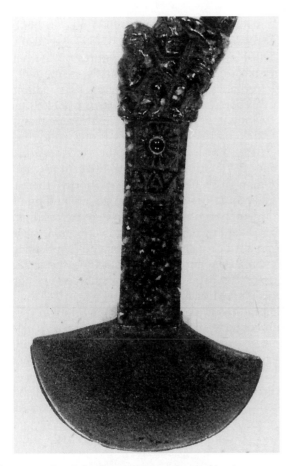

Figure 1-9   Pre-Columbian tumi used for trephination, recovered from the northern coast of Peru, Chimu period circa A.D. 1300–1500. Sculpture on the handle depicts its use. The tumi is made of champi, an alloy of copper, gold, and silver.

tained all inward diseases from the head to the foot by that famous and worthy Physician, Walter Bruel.'' Bruel had an interesting view of the afflictions of the head. He noted

> that the head is more tormented with paine than any other part of the body, which is partly caused by the location of the head; for sharpe vapors and swelling humours ascending from the lower parts, doe assault the head, partly because the braine is of a cold and moyst temperature, superfluidity of excrements are there in generated, which if they increase and be not avoyded by the expulsive faculty in their due season are wont to disturb the head with aches.

This book describes in detail headaches, palsies, paralyses, brain inflammations, and all the causes thereof. Surgery was not recommended. Rather, "if a chirurgeon, there also you may bee furnished with Powders, Oyntments and Emplasters, without which a man cannot excel in the art of Chirurgery." The practitioner was advised to bleed the nose to let the evil out and

to use rosemary flowers and the roots of elecampane as an opiate. Further, bathing the patient in water prepared from flayed foxes and their whelps was sure to produce results. Of course, horse leeches to the temporal artery must never be omitted. Diuretics were also strongly recommended.

But great discoveries were also being made in neurophysiology. In 1765, Cotugno described the cerebrospinal fluid.[23] Magendie and his pupil Claude Bernard laid down the principles of experimental cerebral physiology.[24,25]

Nineteenth Century

The most important influence on the development of neurosurgery in the nineteenth century was the introduction of anesthesia. Toward the end of the eighteenth century, the discovery of carbon dioxide, hydrogen, and nitrogen by Black, Cavendish, and Rutherford, respectively, and the experimentation by Joseph Priestley on several other gases, including oxygen and nitrous oxide, created an interest in exploring possible uses for these agents.[26] Inhalation of both nitrous oxide and ether was used for pleasure in the early nineteenth century. Sir Humphrey Davy, one of the founders of the Pneumatic Institute in Bristol, England, in 1799, suggested that nitrous oxide be used to relieve the pain of surgical operations.[27]

On March 30, 1842, Dr. Crawford Long anesthetized James M. Venable at Jefferson, Georgia, for removal of a small tumor from the back of his neck. Long suggested that Venable be given ether as he, himself, had noticed that when under the influence of ether, falls and bruises were not painful.[28] Also, Venable was already well used to ether. Long did not initially publi-

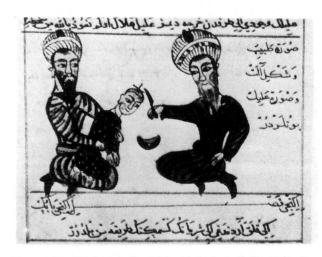

Figure 1-10   Treatment of a child with hydrocephalus. From *La Chirurgie des Ilkhani,* by Charaf-ed Din, Bibliothèque Nationale, Paris.

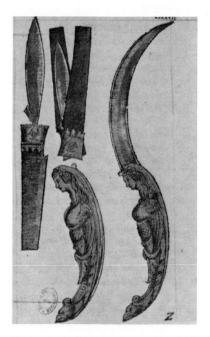
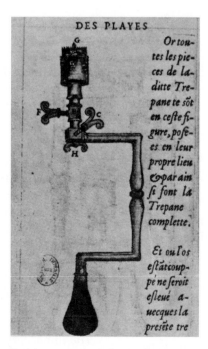
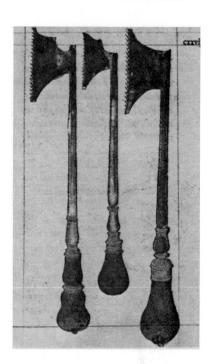

Figure 1-11   Instruments used by Ambroise Paré for neurosurgical procedures.

cize his work and it was not until Morton gave the first public demonstration of ether anesthesia at the Massachusetts General Hospital on October 16, 1846, that modern-day anesthesia started. The news of the anesthetic properties of ether and, within a year, also of chloroform spread quickly around the world. Many types of procedures, especially orthopedic surgery involving the extremities, were soon performed on anesthetized subjects. However, little presentation of this new invention to the neurosurgical arena was evidenced immediately.

In 1829 Sir Astley Cooper, consulting surgeon to Guy's Hospital in London, had published a series of lectures he had delivered in the operating theater at St. Thomas's Hospital on the principles and practice of surgery. He noted that "trephining in concussion is now so completely abandoned that in the last four years I do not know that I have performed it once, whilst 35 years ago I would have performed it five or six times a year." He recommended frequent bleeding, calomel purges, and leeches to be applied to the temporal arteries.[29] The many successes recounted in his lectures may have been due to a premorbid reduction of intracranial pressure by hypovolemia. Anesthesia was achieved with liberal doses of wine if it was needed at all. The surgeon noted that wine was rarely necessary, as either the patients were already in an obtunded state or the surgery was not painful enough.

Almost 30 years later, in 1846, Dr. J. F. Malgaigne from the Faculté de Médicine in Paris wrote a *Manual of Operative Surgery*, which included descriptions of puncture operations for hydrocephalus and various types of nerve divisions for pain relief (frontal, infraorbital, facial, inferior dental, and sciatic).[30] Some small advances had been made in relieving surgical pain. A chapter on the means of diminishing pain suggested the use of narcotics, animal magnetism (or mesmerism), cutting the nerve supply to the area, or excessive venesection. Malgaigne also outlined James Moore, an English surgeon's experiments using a Dupuytren compressor to exert sufficient pressure to damage a nerve and render the incised area anesthetic.[30]

In 1869, after more than 20 years of experience with the use of general anesthesia, Dr. John Erichsen of University College Hospital in London wrote:

> The employment of anaesthetics in surgery is undoubtedly one of the greatest boons ever conferred upon mankind. To the patient it is invaluable in preventing the occurrences of pain and to the surgeon in relieving him of the stress of inflicting it. Anaesthesia is not, however, an unmixed good. Every agent by which it can be induced produces a powerful impression on the system and may occasion dangerous consequences when too freely or carelessly given; and even with every possible care, it appears certain that the inhalation of any anaesthetic agent is in some cases almost inevitably fatal. We cannot purchase immunity from suffering without incurring a certain degree of danger. There can, however, be little doubt that many of the deaths that have followed the inhalation of anaesthetics have resulted from want of knowledge or of due care on the part of the administrators. Yet, what-

ever precautions be taken, there is reason to fear that a fatal result must occasionally happen. This immediate result, which is but very small, is more than counterbalanced by the immunity from other dangers during operations which used formerly to occur.[31]

On the treatment of cerebral injuries, Dr. Erichsen wrote that "the safest practice (for concussion) is to wrap the patient up warmly in blankets; to put hot bottles around him. Alcoholic stimulants of all kinds should be avoided." Should deterioration in the general condition occur, however, purging, bleeding, and leeches were still the principal therapy.[31] Active treatment for acute inflammation included shaving the head and applying an ice-bladder.[32] He did note a beneficial effect of opiates in general cerebral irritation to quiet the patient and induce sleep, although great care was to be taken, especially if tachycardia was apparent. In summary, he wrote:

> In the treatment of injuries of the brain, little can be done after the system has rallied from the shock, beyond attention to strict antiphlogistic treatment, though this need not be of a very active kind. As much should be left to nature as possible, the surgeon merely removing all sources of irritation and excitement from his patient and applying simple local dressings.

He described trephining as important but not used much. Indications were compression and inflammation. Results were not favorable: of 45 patients described by Lente at New York Hospital, 11 recovered. Of 17 patients that Erichsen himself, along with Cooper and Liston, had treated at University College Hospital, only 6 recovered.[33]

A new, but not very successful attempt at neurosurgical intervention is recorded in Lumberton, New Jersey.[34] Mary Catherine Anderson, age 17, was shot in the head on February 7, 1887. On February 22, four notable physicians—Pancoast, Spitzka, Girdner, and Spiller—crowded together in a tiny cottage and used a telephonic probe in an unsuccessful attempt to locate the bullet. Under ether anesthesia and spontaneous ventilation the girl's condition rapidly deteriorated, and the procedure was abandoned. Unfortunately, she died some two weeks later without regaining consciousness, and the case was referred to the judicial system where the thwarted lover was accused, convicted, and executed for murder.

The realization that anesthetic drugs and techniques could be adapted to improve neurosurgical outcome was established by the founders and leaders of today's neurosurgery. From these pioneers came not only a better understanding of the specific needs of the patient with cranial disease, but advances of lasting importance to the whole field of anesthesiology.

SIR WILLIAM MACEWEN

William Macewen, a Scot, born on the Port Bannantyre side of Skeach Wood on the Island of Bute in 1848 and acknowledged as the chief pioneer of neurologic surgery, made significant advances in the development of anesthesia in general, and emphasized the importance of specialty training and quality assurance (Fig. 1-12).[34]

Shortly after he graduated in 1869, he was appointed medical superintendent of the Glasgow Fever Hospital at Belvedere. Prompted by the many deaths due to upper respiratory obstruction in patients with diphtheria, he began intensive cadaveric investigations of peroral intubation. A French surgeon, Pierre Desault, had observed in the late eighteenth century that foreign bodies such as tubes could be tolerated by the larynx in conscious individuals.[35] On July 5, 1878, Macewen passed a tube into the trachea of a patient prior to the induction of chloroform anesthesia for removal of an epithelioma from the pharynx and base of the tongue. The upper laryngeal opening was packed with gauze which encircled the metal tube and prevented blood entering the trachea. "The assured patency of the air passage was a source of comfort to everyone concerned and the respiratory currents were both felt and heard as they traversed the tube. The after result of the operation was admirable."[35]

At a meeting of the Glasgow Medico-Chirurgical Society in 1879 he reported on this and three other cases—one of which died, but only after the patient had removed the tube himself and insisted that he would "prefer to take the chloroform without it."[36,37] The cases were published in the *Glasgow Medical Journal* that year and recycled to the *British Medical Journal* in 1880.

The flexible tubes were made of brass, about nine inches long and three-eighths inch in diameter (Fig. 1-13). Macewen also described the use of gum elastic catheters, especially in acute situations.[38] The tube was guided into the larynx by the finger, which was used as a tongue depressor. He also described nasotracheal placement of a metal tube through which a catheter could be passed, which was then guided digitally into the larynx. Tube placement was practiced several times prior to surgery until the patient was comfortable with the situation and could hold the tube himself.

Professor Macewen was dedicated to training in anesthesia. His predecessor in the Surgical Chair at the University of Glasgow, Lord Lister (the pioneer of antiseptic surgery), had published a paper in 1861 on chloroform anesthesia. He was vehemently opposed to the introduction of any anesthetic apparatus and to the emergence of specialist anesthesia—believing that his own clerks were superior to other chloroformists.[39]

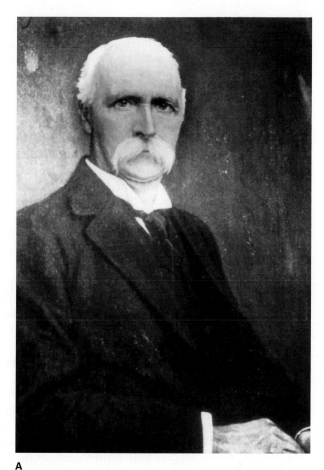

A

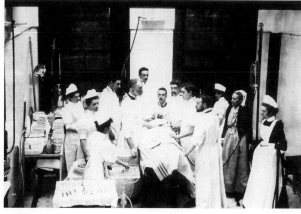

B

Figure 1-12   *A.* Sir William Macewen. *B.* Sir William Macewen in OR at Glasgow infirmary around 1900.

Macewen at first continued in Lister's tradition by mandating practical instruction and certification in anesthetics for students and residents who worked in his wards. After the death of an elderly patient during chloroform anesthesia early in 1883, a bitter debate ensued—mainly in the local press (*The Glasgow Herald*)—between the hospital administrator, supported by Macewen, and two staff members (Mr. James Morton and Dr. Leishman). The former wished to ban administration of anesthetics by all untrained personnel; the latter argued that surgeons should not be held up by petty, unproven rules and paperwork. A national questionnaire regarding the degree of proficiency and complication rate of anesthetia administration resulted in the adoption of a resolution on March 7, 1883, that required organized training in anesthetics for all medical students and clerks.[40]

Macewen was noted for his clinical acumen and tenacity in reporting physical signs. He mapped out pupillary changes in response to anesthetics, cerebral injuries, and intoxication. His preference was for chloroform. He based his dislike of ether on the drug's stimulant effect on the heart and salivary glands.[41] He felt that the cardiac depressant effect of chloroform was of little importance and even advantageous and could be reversed by ether if necessary. He noted that in acute inflammatory cerebral disease, anesthetic use should be minimized, as deeper planes could increase edema in an already edematous brain. He suggested

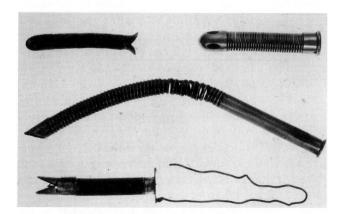

Figure 1-13   Sir William Macewen's brass endotracheal tubes.

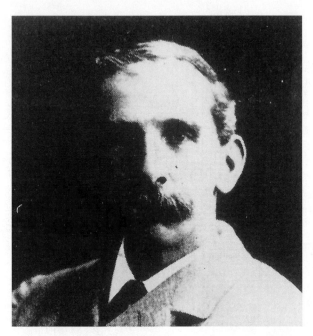

Figure 1-14 Sir Victor Horsley.

supplementation of chloroform with morphine (7.5 mg) by suppository.

SIR VICTOR HORSLEY

Quite a contrast from the poor Scottish family of William Macewen, was the London family of Victor Horsley (Fig. 1-14). His first two names, Victor Alexander, were given by Queen Victoria.[42] Thwarted in his childhood ambition to become a cavalry officer, he chose the profession of physician and surgeon and went on to become the acknowledged father of neurosurgery in England.[43]

As a house surgeon to Mr. John Marshall at University College Hospital, London, he started a long series of self-experimentation. He and his friends anesthetized him some 50 times. He devised several ways to monitor and read his sensations. The hospital authorities even reported on increased use of gas during his apprenticeship—an association that might well prompt suspension and/or mandate drug rehabilitation today.[44]

Of special interest are his observations on nitrous oxide anesthesia, published in 1883: "experimenting on myself . . . the anaesthesia was complete and pushed until rigidity and sometimes cyanosis resulted. The recovery of consciousness was very frequently attended with considerable muscular spasm and semi-coordinated convulsive struggles and excitement."[45]

Many years passed before these potentially detrimental effects of nitrous oxide on the central nervous system were again realized and emphasized.[46] From

1883 to 1885, Horsley investigated the intracranial effects during surgery of chloroform, ether, and morphine sulfate. He noted that ether caused blood pressure to rise, increased blood viscosity, and prompted excessive bleeding, dangerous postoperative vomiting, and excitement. He concluded that it should not be used in neurosurgery.[47] Morphine was valuable because of the apparent increase in cerebral blood flow and more readily controlled hemorrhage in the surgical field.[47] His preference was also for chloroform, but he also advised the "judicious use of chloroform to control hemorrhage."

During an operation at Queen Square Hospital on May 25, 1886, under chloroform anesthesia, Horsley removed a cortical scar and surrounding brain tissue from a 22-year-old who suffered from intermittent status epilepticus due to a childhood injury.[48] Dr. Hughlings Jackson, the physician of record, noted that the outcome was most successful except for one fault: "Here's the first operation of this kind that we ever had at the Hospital; the patient is a Scotsman. We had the chance of getting a joke into his head and we failed to take advantage of it."[49]

Horsley preferred to undertake major vascular surgery in two stages to minimize shock. He recognized the value of hypotension, which he achieved by increasing the depth of anesthesia.[49] Although he favored combining morphine and chloroform early in his career, he subsequently abandoned morphine because of its respiratory depressant effects.[50]

But death related to administration of chloroform anesthesia was not uncommon, and between 1864 and 1912 eight committees and commissions were convened to study the effects of the drug. In 1901, the British Medical Association appointed a "Special Chloroform Committee," including Doctors Wallers, Sherrington, Harcourt, Buxton, and Horsley. It was known that rather less than 2% chloroform vapor in air was sufficient to induce anesthesia, and much less was required for maintenance. But was there a need for an apparatus to determine the percentage of vapor exactly, as opposed to simply sprinkling the drug on a fold of cloth? The issue was between science and practice. Horsley insisted that the percentage should be controlled. He used a vaporizer designed by Vernon Harcourt, a physical chemist, which delivered chloroform 2% maximum (Fig. 1-15). During craniotomy, Horsley felt that chloroform administration should be reduced to 0.5% or less after removal of the bone (Fig. 1-16).[51] Exact determination of the percentage delivered was particularly important in patients with raised intracranial pressure, as a concentration safe under normal circumstances might be fatal in these patients. A cylinder of oxygen was adjusted to the inhaler in the belief that giving oxygen instead of chlo-

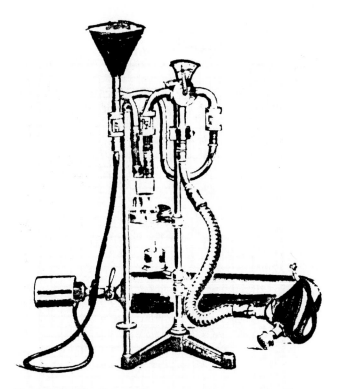

Figure 1-15   The Vernon Harcourt vaporizer arranged with a cylinder of compressed oxygen.

vivisection. The National Antivivisection Society had organized the British Union for the Abolition of Vivisection in 1884.[49] Miss Frances Cobbe, a militant spokesperson, had published a book, *The Nine Circles from Dante's Inferno*, in 1892 in which English scientists were attacked as inhumane animal experimenters. At a church congress in Folkestone in October 1892, Horsley replied that all 26 of his experiments had been performed under ether or chloroform anesthesia.[49] From the beginning of his career, he had recorded the effects of all anesthetics in his animal work. He noted that the present (1892) state of neurosurgery could not have been achieved had animal work not laid the foundations. In giving evidence before the Royal Commission in 1907 on animal experimentation, he argued the necessity of vivisection based on (1) the need to teach students how to operate, (2) the need to teach students how to give anesthetics, and (3) the development of new methods in surgery.[49] His statement, covering 31 pages, was incorporated in the final act and remains pertinent in Great Britain today.

roform would reduce capillary bleed. Dr. Mannell, his anesthetist from 1904 to 1914, noted that Horsley's insistence on low concentrations often required that the patient be restrained on the table toward the end of the case.

Yet another contribution, albeit somewhat oblique, that Sir Victor Horsley made to the neurosciences was in his active political involvement in the laws related to

DR. HARVEY CUSHING

The pioneer North American neurosurgeon, Dr. Harvey Cushing, was less successful as an anesthetist (Fig. 1-17). When Cushing was a second-year medical student at Harvard Medical School, Dr. Frank Lynan, anesthetist at Massachusetts General Hospital, asked him to serve as his substitute. Dr. Lynan noted that Cushing "was not as anxious for the position as I had expected, said that he had anaesthetized only a couple of times but consented to try it."[53]

His diary entry for Tuesday, January 10, 1893, records: "Have promised to substitute at MGH for Lynan

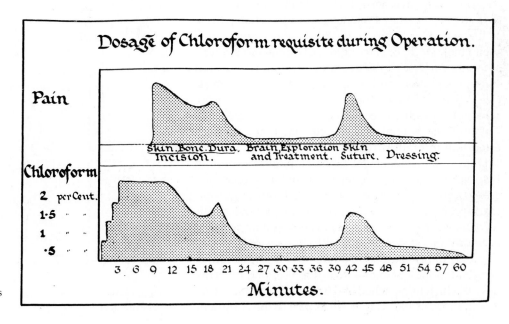

Figure 1-16   Sir Victor Horsley's "pain graph."

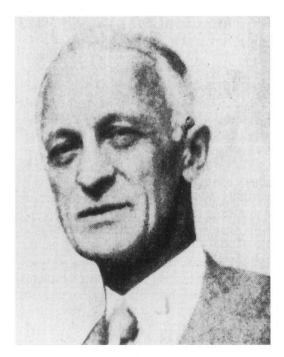

Figure 1-17 Dr. Harvey Cushing.

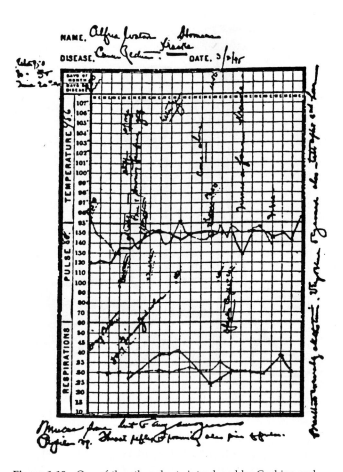

Figure 1-18 One of the ether charts introduced by Cushing and Codman in 1895 to increase safety in surgical procedures.

for a week. Strangulated hernia case—woman died on table before the Class. Had had Strych G1/60, Atropine 1/60, Brandy sub. eu and Nitro Glyc. 1/100gr. Am pretty low in mind."[53]

Apparently the patient died after a few minutes of ether anesthesia. The surgeon, Dr. C. B. Porter, reported that he had found a sac of gangrenous black intestines floating in pus. Dr. Lynan reassured Cushing that death was the usual outcome in such cases and encouraged him to continue as his substitute for two weeks. Durng that time, Cushing recorded rather limited success as an etherizer. He remained unconvinced that adverse reactions to anesthesia were due entirely to the patient's condition. In 1894, at the suggestion of their chief, Dr. F. B. Harrington, Cushing and a fellow student, Amory Codman, devised charts to record pulse, respiration, and temperature during anesthesia (Fig. 1-18).[54,55] These ether charts were soon incorporated into anesthetic records. Codman later noted that Cushing's early fatal case was the one that first interested him in brain surgery.[56]

During his residency at Johns Hopkins Hospital in Baltimore, Cushing's interest in neurosurgery increased. In 1900 he began an extended tour of Europe. During a visit to Professor Theodore Kocher in Bern, he recognized the association between raised intracranial pressure and systemic arterial hypertension.[57] At the Ospidale di St. Matteo in Padua, he was impressed by an adaptation of Scipione Riva-Rocci's blood pressure device which he sketched and introduced on his return to Baltimore in 1901 (Fig. 1-19) as part of the anesthetic

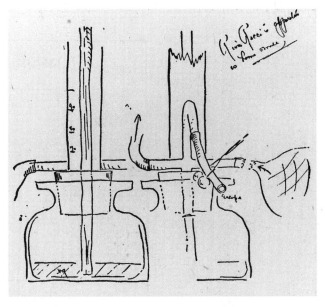

Figure 1-19 Dr. Harvey Cushing's sketch of Riva-Rocci's blood pressure device.

record.[58,59] He also attached great importance to continuous auscultation of the heart and lungs, a technique that he learned from his anesthesiologist, Dr. S. Griffith Davis.[59]

In 1903, in the United States, the Gaertner tonometer was in use in Cleveland, mainly because of the work of George Crile. Perhaps the first meeting on blood pressure, "Considerations of Blood Pressure," was held in the Boston Medical Library on January 19, 1903.[60] Because of the papers presented by Crile and Cushing advocating the intraoperative routine use of blood pressure recording, a committee was formed by Harvard Medical School. After long deliberation, it was decided that the skilled finger was of much greater value clinically for determination of the state of the circulation than any pneumatic device. The work of Crile and Cushing was to be put aside as of no significance.[61] In years to come, the rest of the country did not concur with the Harvard decision, and in 1930, in a letter to Ralph Major in Kansas City, Cushing remarked:

> I am sure that the general use of a blood pressure apparatus in clinical work has done more than harm. Just as Floyer's pulse watch led to two previously unknown diseases, tachycardia and bradycardia, so the sphygmomanometer has led to the uncovering of the diseases (God save the world) of hypertension and hypotension, which have vastly added to the numbers of neuroanesthenics in the world.[62]

Cushing remained skeptical about general anesthesia for neurosurgery—mainly because of continued intraoperative mortality with ether. Students at Johns Hopkins Hospital were permitted to administer anesthesia with little or no training, much as had been the case at Harvard. Under Professor William Halsted, Cushing could do little to change the situation, so he experimented on work started by Halsted with block anesthesia by circumferential cocaine infiltration.[63] He popularized the use of several local anesthetic techniques and coined the term *regional anesthesia*. In 1929, a patient from whom he had removed a large intracranial cyst noted: "One of the secrets of Dr. Cushing's success is that he uses nothing except a local anesthetic, which permits the normal functioning of the heart and other organs during the operation."[64]

PROFESSOR FEDOR KRAUSE

The founder of German neurosurgery, Dr. Fedor Krause, was born in Friedland in 1857 (Fig. 1-20). As an assistant to Professor Richard Volkman, he was exposed to a morphine-chloroform combination but was unconvinced of its advantages for neurosurgical procedures. Rather he, too, preferred chloroform

alone.[65] He did, however, recognize the value of small doses of morphine for postoperative pain relief. He felt that the safety of ether was offset by venous bleeding and reserved its use for patients with failing hearts.

He advocated controlled hypotension by increasing chloroform concentration. He noted that in cases of intracranial tumors, sudden death might occur if respiration ceased. He preferred to use the Roth-Dräger oxygen-chloroform apparatus, which permitted the administration of 100% oxygen (Fig. 1-21). He also emphasized that the brain was insensitive to pain and only very light planes of anesthesia were necessary.[65] But he questioned the technique of local anesthesia advocated by many surgeons, noting that pain was not the only problem and, in preparation for surgery, a positive attitude and psychological status must exist. In particular, he realized that severe anxiety could cause or contribute to death preoperatively.

He concluded that a good outcome in neurosurgical procedures required a rapid, aseptic technique, minimal blood loss, normothermia, and general narcosis. Krause did, however, use local anesthesia for spinal surgery. He injected 0.5% procaine with adrenaline (15 drops 1% in 100 ml) above and below the spinous processes in 4 aliquots of 5 ml. The method had been recommended by H. Braun.[66] Anesthesia was satisfactory until the dura had to be detached from the inner surface of the vertebral arch. The laminectome caused less pain; however, the technique "is only effective in patients who can exercise a certain degree of self

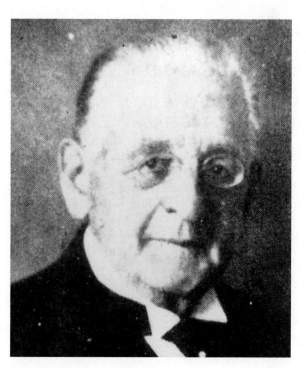

Figure 1-20 Professor Fedor Krause.

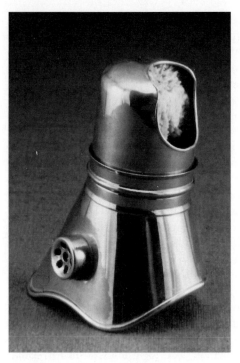

Figure 1-21 Roth-Dräger oxygen-chloroform apparatus.

control."[67] Krause felt that spinal anesthesia as described by Augustus Bier was unnecessary, especially if the cord was not compressed.[68]

Early Twentieth Century

Many advances in the beginning of the twentieth century contributed to the development of neuroanesthesia.

DELIVERY SYSTEMS

At the beginning of the twentieth century, anesthesia was still administered by an open drop method. A tourniquet was tied around the head to decrease bleeding (Fig. 1-22). The Vernon Harcourt system, popularized by Victor Horsley has already been mentioned. Pumping devices were attached with tubes between the patient and the inhaler, moving the source of anesthesia away from the head. The Junker bottle (air blown through a vaporizer with hand bellows) was another device. The Ombrédanne ether inhaler could also be used in the prone position (Fig. 1-23).

AIRWAY MANAGEMENT

Although Macewen had first used endotracheal intubation in neurosurgery, it was not immediately universally accepted. The anesthetist still usually positioned himself at the side of the table, supporting the jaw or pulling the tongue forward with a suture or clip. Hewitt designed a pharyngeal airway in 1908 that helped to relieve obstruction but required a greater depth of anesthesia.

Meltzer and Auer described endotracheal insufflation to maintain oxygenation without respiratory movement in 1909.[69] Charles Elsberg advocated intratracheal insufflation anesthesia with ether and oxygen or ether and air—a technique that had been used satisfactorily in neurosurgery by Charles Frazier in Philadelphia.[70] Credit for the practical development and introduction of endotracheal intubation goes to Sir Ivan Magill and Dr. Edgar Rowbotham, anesthetists at Queens Hospital for Maxillo-Facial Injuries.[71] They used a piece of rubber tubing with one end beveled from a Boyle anesthesia machine. By the 1930s, endotracheal anesthesia was recommended for neurosurgical anesthesia.

OTHER AGENTS

Willstaetter and Duisburg synthesized tribromethanol in 1923. Butzengeiger and Eichholtz used it that same year as the sole anesthetic agent for neurosurgical procedures.[72] At the Johns Hopkins Hospital in 1931, the neurosurgeon Walter Dandy administered tribromethanol rectally to reduce elevated intracranial pressure.[73] Professor Leo Davidoff at Montefiore Hospital in New York, finding that the effects wore off too quickly, used tribromethanol in combination with local infiltration.[74]

Trichlorethylene with nitrous oxide as a neuroanesthetic technique, described by D. E. Jackson in 1934, gained considerable popularity in the British Commonwealth.[75] Hershenson used low concentrations of closed-circuit cyclopropane and reported on his

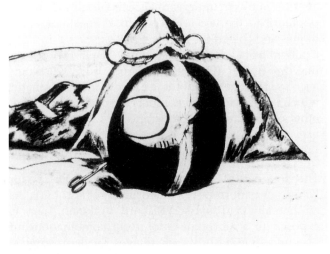

Figure 1-22 Open drop ether craniotomy—tourniquet around the head to decrease bleeding.

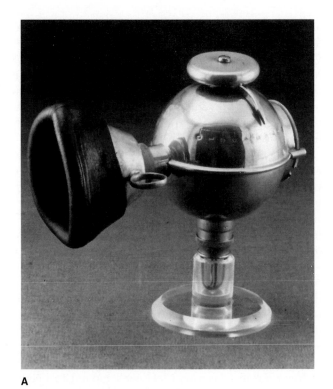

A

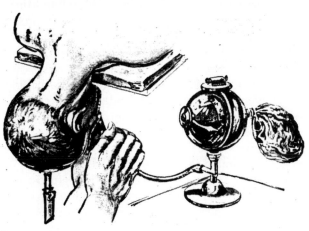

B

Figure 1-23   *A.* Ombrédanne inhaler. *B.* Ombrédanne inhaler in use.

method in 1942.[76] The cyclopropane technique never became popular, however, undoubtedly because of the danger of explosion.

Volwiler and Tabern synthesized thiopental in 1930, and Lundy and Waters introduced it into clinical practice four years later.[77] A report by Shannon and Gardner in 1946 describes the use of thiopental for all types of neurosurgery,[78] but its popularity as sole agent was short-lived in this arena. Halothane was synthesized by Raventos and Suckling in 1956 and introduced into clinical anesthesia by Johnstone in the same year.[79,80] It became a popular anesthetic in neurosurgery but its propensity to increase intracranial pressure by cerebrovasodilation concerned many anesthetists and neurosurgeons.

The number of agents used between 1920 and 1950 suggested that no technique was satisfactory for neurosurgery. In 1932 Wood reported on 550 brain operations at the University of California.[81] Nitrous oxide/ether anesthesia was most commonly used with a pharyngeal airway. Fluids were given rectally (proctoclysis). Livingstone and colleagues reviewed over 1000 neurosurgical procedures in 1936.[82] A wide variety of techniques were used, including ether, basal anesthesia with local anesthetics, rectal ether in oil, ethylene, and nitrous oxide.

Techniques used at the Montreal Neurologic Institute showed that of 1000 cases, 700 were performed under general anesthesia and 300 under local anesthesia.[83] The major concerns remained airway management and fluid replacement. Again a wide variety of agents were used, although by 1949, pentothal, oral intubation, vaseline throat packing, and use of a nonrebreathing valve to prevent buildup of carbon dioxide were increasingly commonplace. Mortality was quoted as 6.7 percent. Seventeen perioperative deaths occurred in patients undergoing surgery under local anesthesia.

Neuroanesthetic Principles

Most of the major neuroanesthetic principles have been established over the past 60 years. Controlled ventilation using ether was introduced by Guedel and Treweek in 1934.[84] By 1942 Lundy noted that in the presence of hypoxia and hypoventilation "it is difficult to reduce ICP unless resort is made to artificial respiration."[85] Kety and Schmidt in 1945 identified the effects of hyperventilation on intracranial and systemic dynamics.[86] In the same year they also described a method to measure cerebral blood flow (CBF) using nitrous oxide inhalation.[87] Ingvar and Lassen used the intraarterial injection of krypton and measured the washout.[88] An inhalation technique to measure flow was added by Obrist and colleagues in 1967.[89] A more scientific measure was now available to assess the effects of anesthetic agents on the cerebral vasculature. Intracranial pressure had been measured much earlier—probably as early as 1901 by Walter B. Cannon—but it was not until 1960 that Lundberg clearly described the continuous measurement of ventricular fluid pressure waves.[90] He further described and quantified means to reduce intracranial pressure by altering ventilation. He summarized the dependency of cerebral blood flow on carbon dioxide and oxygen tension.[91] Professor Thomas Langfitt further defined intracranial dynamics, based in part on the classical work of Weed and McKibben published in 1919.[92] He also described the pressure-volume curve.[93]

Neuroanesthesia Today

With the introduction of electrocautery and the operating microscope, many more intracranial procedures became possible. Greatly improved neurodiagnostic techniques were able to pinpoint pathology. The introduction of short-acting barbiturates, the routine use of endotracheal intubation, ready availability of muscle relaxants and a host of other pharmaceutical agents all contributed to the ability of the anesthesiologist to adjust to the needs of the patient.

Performance of neurosurgical procedures outside of the operating room required that the anesthesiologist be aware not only of different pathologies but of how anesthetic drugs act on altered intracranial dynamics under differing circumstances.

Neuroanesthesia as a Specialty

By 1960, a few anesthesiologists, including A. R. Hunter in England and R. G. B. Gilbert in Montreal, began to define a specialty of neuroanesthesia. The first book devoted exclusively to anesthesia for neurosurgery was published by Hunter in 1964, to be followed by the second neuroanesthesia book by Gilbert in 1966.

Modern research in neuroanesthesia was initially centered in three centers—Philadelphia, Glasgow, and Rochester, Minnesota. In the early 1960s, at the University of Pennsylvania, Wollman, Pierce, Alexander, Cohen, Smith, and Dripps, among others, formed a nucleus of investigators that set out to study the cerebral effects of nitrous oxide, cyclopropane, halothane, enflurane, neuroleptic agents, hypotension, and hyperventilation.[94–102] Although most of these early studies were conducted on healthy volunteers (i.e., medical students), subsequent work has shown that many of the findings could be equally applied to neurosurgical patients.

Dr. Gordon McDowall, a prominent British anesthetist working with Dr. Murray Harper, a physiologist at the University of Glasgow, began intense studies of anesthetic effects on intracranial dynamics. Two clinical neuroanesthetists, Drs. John Barker and William Fitch, joined the basic investigators and took into the operating room the findings from the laboratory. They were among the first to confirm, during the 1960s, that anesthetic agents did indeed exert measurable effects on cerebral blood flow and metabolism in patients with intracranial mass lesions.[103–107] They were later joined by a neurosurgeon, Professor W. B. Jennett who later became very well known for, among other things, his work on central nervous system trauma.[108,109] One result of the interdisciplinary collaborations may have been

an editorial, published anonymously, in the *British Journal of Anesthesia* in 1969 condemning the use of all volatile anesthetics.[110] The author used the work of McDowall to justify the abandonment of halothane particularly and even stated that hyperventilation was insufficient to prevent the devastating effects of inhaled agents on intracranial pressure in patients with mass lesions.

At the Mayo Clinic, in Rochester, Minnesota, the early emphasis of research by Michenfelder and Theye was on means of providing cerebral protection, using initially hypothermic techniques during clipping of cerebral aneurysms. As part of their work they studied means to measure cerebral blood flow and metabolism on line.[111–114]

During the 1970s, the three original institutions of research continued to flourish. At the University of Pennsylvania, Shapiro expanded the role of the neuroanesthesiologist to the intensive care unit. He later moved to San Diego and established another neuroanesthetic center with Todd, Drummond, and others. Later still, Todd joined with Warner at the University of Iowa. From Glasgow, McDowall moved to Leeds, while Barker, Fitch, and Harper continued. In Minnesota, Michenfelder continued productive research in brain protection and resuscitation and was joined for varying periods by Gronert, Tinker, Artru, Steen, Takeshita, Lacier, Milde, and Cucchiara. Two other major centers that developed during this time included the University of Pittsburgh under the direction of Safar, whose research centered on cerebral-cardiopulmonary resuscitation, and the Albert Einstein College of Medicine, where Shulman, Marmarou, Shapiro, and Frost collaborated in studies on head injuries.

During the 1980s, research centered on glucose control and yet again on the effects of modest hypothermia. A wide range of drugs emerged as possible cerebral protective agents. A much clearer understanding of the pathways involved in cell damage was achieved. Research on trauma, especially as it involves so many young people with such devastating effects, commanded many research dollars but, as yet, has provided few answers for how to reestablish neuronal connections and prevent secondary cerebral damage.

Monitoring has seen major advances in the past 20 years. Air embolism can be easily detected by use of a precordial Doppler,[115] end-tidal CO_2 monitor,[116] central venous[117] or pulmonary artery catheter.[118] Transesophageal Doppler[119] and transesophageal echocardiography[120] further increase the sensitivity of detecting small amounts of embolized air.

Although EEG monitoring had been advocated as early as 1937, it was not until Stockard and Bickford described compressed spectral assay in 1972 that EEG patterns became more comprehensible to the anesthesiologist.[121] Sensory-evoked potentials monitoring has seen major advances since Dawson first described a mechanical method of averaging evoked potentials from background EEG recordings in 1947.[122] Clinical applications were considered in the 1970s,[123] when Jewett described the characteristic deflections of brainstem auditory evoked potentials. Wilson first monitored visual evoked potentials in 1976,[124] while Nash and Brown had used somatosensory evoked potential monitoring in 1953.[125]

Motor evoked potentials, still not routine, were investigated first by Raudzens in 1982.[126] This research continues.

Communication

This past quarter century has seen enormous developments in communication between basic scientists and clinicians, between neurosurgeons and neuroanesthesiologists. Many textbooks devoted to neuroanesthesia have followed since Hunter's first book published in 1964. Authors include Michenfelder, Neufield, Cottrell, and Frost among others.

Studies related to neuroanesthesia are frequent in anesthesia journals. For example, *Anesthesiology* publishes scientific work that is 11 percent neuro-related.[127] Other major journals such as *Anesthesia & Analgesia*, the *Canadian Journal of Anesthesia*, and the *British Journal of Anesthesia* devote about 5 percent of space to neuroanesthesia. At annual meetings of the American Society of Anesthesiologists, again about 11 percent of papers are neuro-related.[127] In 1922 approximately 20 percent of Young Investigator Award Applications dealt with neuroanesthesia.[127] Sadly, at this point (1995), NIH funding has been greatly decreased, as has the ability of clinical practice to support basic research. It seems that the plethora of laboratory studies that characterized the 1970s and 1980s may fade.

Over the past few years, several major anesthesia journals such as *Anesthesiology* and *Anesthesia & Analgesia* have established sections related to neuroanesthesia with recognized specialists as section editors.

In 1989 the *Journal of Neurosurgical Anesthesiology* grew out of and eventually replaced the *Newsletter of the Society of Neurosurgical Anesthesia and Critical Care*. By 1993, the *Journal* was recognized and listed in the *Index Medicus* and *Current Contents*. Currently it is the official journal not only of the United States society but also of the neuroanesthesia societies of France and Great Britain.

To initiate research and teaching in the field of neuroanesthesia, the Commission of Neuroanesthesia, comprising anesthesiologists from nine countries, was founded on July 9, 1960, in Antwerp, Belgium.[72] Since then, societies have been established throughout the world. Among them was founded the Society of Neuroanesthesia and Neurologic Supportive Care, now known as the Society of Neurosurgical Anesthesia and Critical Care, in the United States in 1973. The society is recognized by the American Society of Anesthesiologists and the American Association of Neurological Surgeons, and participates actively in their annual meetings as well as sponsoring meetings of its own.

Other societies include the Arbeits in Linz, Austria; the Association de Neuroanesthésie-Réanimation de Langue Française in Bordeaux, France; the Neuroanesthesia and Intensive Care Section, Association of Baltic Anesthesiologists in Tartu, Estonia; the Neuroanesthesia Chapter, Indian Society of Anesthesiologists in New Delhi, India; the Neuroanesthesia Society of Great Britain and Ireland in Glasgow, Scotland; and the Subcommittee of Neurosciences, European Society of Anesthesiologists in Leuven, Belgium.

Concluding Comments

The history of the development of neuroanesthesia within neurosurgery is long. The age of skulls trephined with little or no anesthesia has, over the centuries, been replaced by techniques of precise diagnostic placement of lesions allowing small craniotomies under closely monitored, complete anesthesia. These developments have evolved only by close cooperation among basic scientists, neurosurgeons, and anesthesiologists. As a tribute to the anesthetic contribution, Professor Wilson, Chair of Neurosurgery at the University of California at San Francisco, noted ". . . among surgeons no group has greater respect for, or greater dependence on, its counterparts in anesthesia than neurosurgeons."[128]

References

1. Mettler FA, Mettler CC: Historic development of knowledge relating to cranial trauma in trauma of the central nervous system. In: *Proceedings of the Association for Research in Nervous and Mental Disease*. Baltimore, Williams & Wilkins, 1945:1.
2. Wakefield EG, Dellinger SC: Possible reasons for trephining the skull in the past. *Ciba Symp* 1939; 1:166.
3. Broca P: Sur les trèpanations prehistoriques. *Bull et Mens Soc d'Anthropol de Paris* 1874; (S2)9:542.
4. Wölfel J: Die Trepanation. Studien über Ursprung Zusammenhänge und kulturelle Zugehärigkeit der Trepanation. *Antropos* 1925; 20:1.
5. Lastres JB, Cabiese F: *La trepanacion del craneo en el antiiguo Peru*. Lima, Universidad Nacional Mayor de San Marcos, 1960:146.
6. Edwards C: *The Hammurabi Code and the Sinatic Legislation*. London, Watts & Co, 1921:39.
7. The Edwin Smith Surgical Papyrus: In Breasted JH (trans, ed): *University of Chicago Oriental Institute Pub*. Chicago, University of Chicago Press, 1930:177.

8. Hippocrates on Injuries of the Head: Adams F (trans): *The Genuine Works of Hippocrates,* in 2 vols. London, 1849.

9. Celsus, AC: *De Medicina,* Spencer WG (trans). Cambridge, Mass, 1935, 3 vols.

10. Galen: *Oeuvres Anatomiques, physiologiques et mèdicales de Galien,* Davenberg C (trans). Paris, Baillière JB, 1854, 2 vols.

11. Aretaeus, the Cappadocian: Extant works. Adams, F (trans). London, Sydenham Society, 1856:469.

12. Gunther RT: *The Greek Herbal of Dioscorides.* Oxford, University Press, 1934:701.

13. Nuland SB: *The Origins of Anesthesia.* Birmingham, Gryphon Editions, 1983:8.

14. Paul of Aegina: Book 6, Sect 90. *The Seven Books of Paulus Aegineta,* vol 2, Adams F (trans). London, 1844:431.

15. Paul of Aegina: Book 6, Sect 90. *The Seven Books of Paulus Aegineta,* vol 2, Adams F (trans). London, 1844:430.

16. Rhazes: *Continens Lugduni.* J. de Ferraiirus, 1511.

17. Raper HR: *Man Against Pain.* New York, Prentice-Hall, 1945:7.

18. Robinson V: *Victory over Pain.* New York, Henry Schumann, 1946:29.

19. Raper HR: *Man Against Pain.* New York, Prentice-Hall, 1945:8.

20. Walker AE: *A History of Neurological Surgery.* New York, Hafner, 1967:17.

21. Walker AE: *A History of Neurological Surgery.* New York, Hafner, 1967:19.

22. Bruel W: *Physician's Practice.* Printed by John North for William Sheares, London, 1639:A2, B2–3.

23. Cotugno D: *De ischiade nervosa commentarius.* Naples, Simoniana, 1762.

24. Magendie F: *Anatomie des systèmes nerveux des animaux à vertèbes.* Paris, J. B. Bailliere et fils, 1825, 2 volumes.

25. Bernard C: *Leçons sur la physiologie et la pathologie du système nerveux.* Paris, J. B. Bailliere et fils, 1858, 2 volumes.

26. Priestley J: *Experiments and Observations on Different Kinds of Air.* Birmingham, England, Thomas Pearson, 1790.

27. Davy H: *Researches, Chemical and Philosophical, Chiefly Concerning Nitrous Oxide.* Bristol, Biggs & Cottle, 1800:333.

28. Tayler FL: *Crawford W Long and the Discovery of Ether Anesthesia.* New York, Paul B. Hoehe, Inc, 1928:43.

29. Cooper A: *Lectures in the Principles and Practice of Surgery.* London, Westley, 1829:119.

30. Malgaigne JF: *Manual of Operative Surgery.* London, Henry Renshaw, 1846:42, 109.

31. Erichsen JE: *Science and Art of Surgery.* Philadelphia, Henry C Lea, 1869:41.

32. Erichsen JE: *Science and Art of Surgery.* Philadelphia, Henry C Lea, 1869:335.

33. Erichsen JE: *Science and Art of Surgery.* Philadelphia, Henry C Lea, 1869:356.

34. Jefferson G: Sir William Macewen's contributions to neurosurgery and its sequels. In: *Sir Geoffrey Jefferson: Selected Papers.* Springfield, IL, Charles C Thomas, 1960:527.

35. Bowman AK: *The Life and Teaching of Sir William Macewen.* London, William Hodge & Co, 1942:527.

36. Macewen W: The introduction of tubes into the larynx through the mouth instead of tracheotomy and laryngotomy. *Glasgow Med J* 1879; 9:72 and 12:218.

37. Macewen W: Clinical observations on the introduction of tracheal tubes by the mouth instead of performing tracheotomy and laryngotomy. *Br Med J* 1880; 2:122, 2:163.

38. Watt OM: *Glasgow Anaesthetics 1846–1946.* Clydebank, James Pender, 1962:19.

39. Watt OM: *Glasgow Anaesthetics 1846–1946.* Clydebank, James Pender, 1962, p 15.

40. Board of Managers Reports, Glasgow Royal Infirmary 1882–1883, Archives, University of Glasgow.

41. Macewen W: Introduction to a discussion on anesthetics. *Glasgow Med J* 1890; 34:321.

42. McNalty A: Sir Victor Horsley: His life and work. *Br Med J* 1957; 2:911.

43. Green JR: Sir Victor Horsley. A Centennial Recognition of his impact on neuroscience and on neurological surgery. *Barrow Neurol Instit Quat* 1987; 3:2.

44. Paget S: *Sir Victor Horsley. A Study of His Life and Work.* London, Constable, 1919:40.

45. Paget S: *Sir Victor Horsley. A Study of His Life and Work.* London, Constable, 1919:41.

46. Frost E: Central nervous system effects of nitrous oxide. In: Eger EI, II (ed): *Nitrous Oxide, N₂O.* New York, Elsevier, 1985:157.

47. Horsley V: On the technique of operations on the central nervous system. *Br Med J* 1906; 2:411.

48. Horsley V: Brain surgery. *Br Med J* 1886; 2:670.

49. Lyons JB: *Citizen Surgeon.* London, Peter Downay, 1966.

50. Paget S: *Sir Victor Horsley. A Study of His Life and Work.* London, Constable, 1919:184.

51. Horsley V: On the technique of operations on the central nervous system. Address in Surgery. *Toronto Lancet* 1906; 2:484.

52. Mennell Z: Anaesthesia in intracranial surgery. *Am J Surg* 1924; 38:44.

53. Fulton JF: *Harvey Cushing: A Biography.* Oxford, Blackwell, 1946:69.

54. Beecher HK: The first anesthesia records (Codman Cushing). *Surg Gynecol Obstet* 1940; 71:689.

55. Shepard DAE: Harvey Cushing and anaesthesia. *Can Anaesth Soc J* 1965; 12:431.

56. Fulton JF: *Harvey Cushing: A Biography.* Oxford, Blackwell, 1946:95.

57. Cushing HW: Concerning a definitive regulatory mechanism of the vasomotor center which controls blood pressure during cerebral compression. *Bull Johns Hopkins Hosp* 1901; 12:290.

58. Cushing HW: On the avoidance of shock in major amputations by cocainization of large nerve trunks preliminary to their division. With observations on blood pressure changes in surgical cases. *Ann Surg* 1902; 36:321.

59. Cushing HW: Some principles of cerebral surgery. *JAMA* 1909; 52:184.

60. Cushing HW: On routine determinations of arterial tension in operating room and clinic. *Boston Med Surg J* 1903; 148:250.

61. Division of Surgery of the Medical School of Harvard University: *Report of Research Work, 1903–4.* Bulletin 11, March 1904:1.

62. Fulton JF: *Harvey Cushing: A Biography.* Oxford, Blackwell, 1946:115.

63. Halsted WS: *Surgical Papers.* Baltimore, Johns Hopkins Press, 1924:167.

64. Fulton JF: *Harvey Cushing: A Biography.* Oxford, Blackwell, 1946:578.

65. Krause F: *Surgery of the Brain and Spinal Cord Based on Personal Experiences,* vol 1, Haubold H, Thorek M (trans). New York, Rebman & Co, 1912:137.

66. Braun H: Über die Lokalanästhesie im Krankenhaus nebst Bemerkung über die Technik der örtlichen Anästhesierung. *Beitr Klin Chir* 1909; 62:641.

67. Krause F: *Surgery of the Brain and Spinal Cord Based on Personal Experiences,* vol 3, Haubold H, Thorek M (trans). New York: Rebman & Co, 1912:957.

68. Bier A: Versuche über cocainisirung des Rückenmarkes. *Deutsche Zeitschrift für Chirurgie* 1899; 51:361.

69. Meltzer SJ, Auer J: Continuous respiration without respiratory movements. *J Exp Med* 1909; 11:622.

70. Elsberg CA: Experiences in thoracic surgery under anaesthesia by the intratracheal insufflation of air and ether with remarks

on the value of the method for general anaesthesia. *Ann Surg* 1910; 53:23.

71. Rowbotham ES, Magill IW: Anaesthetics in the plastic surgery of the face and jaws. *Proc Resp Soc Med* 1921; 14:17.

72. Schapira M: Evolution of anesthesia for neurosurgery. *NY State J Med* 1964; 64:1302.

73. Dandy WE: Avertin anesthesia in neurologic surgery. *JAMA* 1931; 96:1860.

74. Davidoff LM: Avertin as a basal anesthetic for craniotomy. *Bull Neurol Inst* 1934; 3:544.

75. Jackson DE: A study of analgesia and anesthesia with special reference to such substances as trichlorethylene and vinesthene together with apparatus for their administration. *Anesth Analg (Current Researches)* 1934; 13:198.

76. Hershenson BB: Some observations on anesthesia for neurosurgery. *NY State J Med* 1942; 42:2111.

77. Lundy JS: Intravenous anesthesia. Preliminary report of the use of two new thiobarbiturates. *Mayo Clin Proc* 1935; 10:536.

78. Shannon EW, Gardner WJ: Pentothal sodium anesthesia in neurological surgery. *N Engl J Med* 1946; 234:15.

79. Raventos J: 20th International Physiological Congress, Brussels. Abstracts of Communications, 1956:754.

80. Johnstone M: The human cardiovascular response to flurothane anaesthesia. *Br J Anesth* 1956; 28:392.

81. Wood DA: Survey of the anesthesias given in 550 brain operations in the years 1921–1930 inclusive. *Anesth Analg* 1932; 11:201.

82. Livingstone H, et al: Anesthesia in neurosurgical operations. *Anesth Analg* 1936; 15:169.

83. Stephen CR, Pasquet A: Anesthesia for neurosurgical procedures. Analysis of 1000 cases. *Anesth Analg* 1949; 28:77.

84. Guedel AE, Treweek DN: Ether apnoeas. *Anesth Analg* 1934; 13:263.

85. Lundy JS: *Clinical Anesthesia.* Philadelphia, WB Saunders, 1942:3.

86. Kety SS, Schmidt CF: The effects of active and passive hyperventilation on cerebral blood flow, cerebral oxygen consumption, output and blood pressure of normal young men. *Ann Soc Clin Invest* 1945; 25:107.

87. Kety SS, Schmidt CF: Determination of cerebral blood flow in man by the use of nitrous oxide in low concentrations. *Am J Physiol* 1945; 143:53.

88. Lassen NA, Ingvar DH: The blood flow of the cerebral cortex determined by radioactive krypton. *Experientia* 1961; 17:42.

89. Obrist WD, et al: Determination of regional cerebral blood flow by inhalation of 133-xenon. *Circ Res* 1967; 20:124.

90. Lundberg N: Continuous recording and control of ventricular fluid pressure in neurosurgical practice. *Acta Psychiat Neurol Scand* 36(Suppl 149), 1960.

91. Lundberg N, et al: Reduction of increased intracranial pressure by hyperventilation. *Acta Psychiat Neurol Scand* 34 (Suppl 139), 1959.

92. Weed LH, McKibben PS: Experimental alteration of brain bulk. *Am J Physiol* 1919; 48:531.

93. Langfitt TW: Increased intracranial pressure. *Clin Neurosurg* 1969; 16:438.

94. Cohen PJ, et al: Effects of hypoxia and normocarbia on cerebral blood flow and metabolism in conscious man. *J Appl Physiol* 1967; 23:183.

95. Alexander SC, et al: Cerebral vascular responses to $PaCO_2$ during halothane anesthesia in man. *J Appl Physiol* 1964; 19:561.

96. Wollman H, et al: Cerebral circulation in man during halothane anesthesia. *Anesthesiology* 1964; 25:180.

97. Smith AL, Wollman H: Cerebral blood flow and metabolism: Effects of anesthetic drugs and techniques. *Anesthesiology* 1972; 36:378.

98. Wollman H, et al: Cerebral circulation during general anesthesia and hyperventilation in man. *Anesthesiology* 1965; 26: 329.

99. Smith AL: Dependence of cerebral venous oxygen tension on anesthetic depth. *Anesthesiology* 1973; 39:291.

100. Smith AL, Wollman H: Cerebral blood flow and metabolism: Effects of anesthetic drugs and techniques. *Anesthesiology* 1972; 36:378.

101. Wollman H, et al: Cerebral blood flow and oxygen consumption in man during electroencephalographic seizure patterns induced by anesthesia with Ethrane. *Fed Proc* 1969; 28:356.

102. Pierce EC Jr, et al: Cerebral circulation and metabolism during thiopental anesthesia and hyperventilation in man. *J Clin Invest* 1962; 41:1664.

103. Fitch W, et al: The influence of neurolept analgesic drugs on cerebrospinal fluid pressure. *Br J Anaesth* 1969; 41:800.

104. Moss E, McDowall DG: ICP increases with 50 percent nitrous oxide in oxygen in severe head injuries during controlled ventilation. *Br J Anaesth* 1979; 51:757.

105. Okuda Y, et al: Changes in CO_2 responsiveness and in autoregulation of the cerebral circulation during and after halothane induced hypotension. *J Neurol Neurosurg Psychiatry* 1976; 39: 221.

106. Harper AM, Bell RA: The effect of metabolic acidosis and alkalosis on the blood flow through the cerebral cortex. *J Neurol Neurosurg Psychiatry* 1963; 26:341.

107. Fitch W, et al: The influence of neurolept analgesic drugs on cerebrospinal fluid pressure. *Br J Anaesth* 1969; 41:800.

108. Jennett WB, McDowall DG: Effect of anesthesia on intracranial pressure (abstract). *J Neurol Neurosurg Psychiatry* 1964; 27: 582.

109. Jennett WB, et al: Effect of anesthesia on intracranial pressure in patients with space occupying lesions. *Lancet* 1969; 1:61.

110. Anonymous: Halothane and neurosurgery (editorial). *Br J Anaesth* 1969; 41:277.

111. Michenfelder JD, et al: Simultaneous cerebral blood flow measured by direct and indirect methods. *J Surg Res* 1968; 8: 475.

112. Michenfelder JD, Theye RA: The effects of profound hypocapnia and dilutional anemia on canine cerebral metabolism and blood flow. *Anesthesiology* 1969; 31:449.

113. Theye RA, Michenfelder JD: Effect of nitrous oxide on canine cerebral metabolism. *Anesthesiology* 1968; 29:1119.

114. Theye RA, Michenfelder JD: Effect of halothane on canine cerebral metabolism. *Anesthesiology* 1968; 29:1113.

115. Maroon JC, et al: An ultrasonic method for detecting air embolism. *J Neurosurg* 1969; 31:196.

116. Bethune RWM, Brechner VL: Detection of venous air embolism by carbon dioxide monitoring (abstract). *Anesthesiology* 1968; 29:178.

117. Michenfelder JD, et al: Air embolism during neurosurgery: An evaluation of right-atrial catheters for diagnosis and treatment. *JAMA* 1969; 208:1353.

118. Munson ES, et al: Early detection of venous air embolism using a Swan-Ganz catheter. *Anesthesiology* 1975; 42:228.

119. Martin RW, Colby PS: Evaluation of transesophageal Doppler detection of air embolism in dogs. *Anesthesiology* 1983; 58:117.

120. Furuya H, et al: Detection of air embolism by transesophageal echocardiography. *Anesthesiology* 1983; 58:124.

121. Bickford RG, et al: The compressed spectral array (CSA)—a pictorial EG. *Proceedings of the San Diego Biomedical Symposium,* San Diego, CA, 1972; 2:365.

122. Dawson GD: Cerebral responses to electrical stimulation of peripheral nerve in man. *J Neurol Neurosurg Psychiatry* 1947; 10:137.

123. Jewett DL, et al: Human auditory evoked potentials: Possible brain stem components detected on the scalp. *Science* 1970; 167:1517.

124. Wilson WB, et al: Monitoring of visual function during parasellar surgery. *Surg Neurol* 1976; 5:323.

125. Nash CC, et al: Spinal cord monitoring during operative treatment of the spine. *Clin Orthop* 1977; 126:100.

126. Raudzens PA: Intraoperative monitoring of evoked potentials. *Ann NY Acad Sci* 1982; 388:308.

127. Michenfelder JD: The past, present and future of research in neuroanesthesia. *J Neurosurg Anesthesiol* 1993; 5:22.

128. Wilson CB: Foreword. In Newfield P, Cottrell JE (eds): *Handbook of Neuroanesthesia, Clinical and Physiologic Essentials.* Boston, Little Brown & Company, 1983:11.

Chapter 2

CEREBRAL BLOOD FLOW AND METABOLISM

CHRISTIAN WERNER

EBERHARD KOCHS

WILLIAM E. HOFFMAN

Cerebral Metabolism

The central nervous system (CNS) includes the brain and the spinal cord. At the cellular level, the CNS comprises nerve cells and glial cells. The nerve cells (neurons) are specialized to transmit impulses by changing their membrane permeability. These signaling functions are the basis of processing sensory information, the programming of motor and emotional responses, learning, and memory. Neurons are surrounded by the glial cells (astrocytes, oligodendrocytes, Schwann cells, and microglia). Glial cells most likely are not involved in the processing of information, but serve as supporting elements. They provide the firmness and the structure of the CNS and insulate the large neuronal axons by forming myelin sheaths. Glial cells also contribute to the formation of the blood-brain barrier, provide nutrition to neurons, re-uptake neurotransmitters and potassium ions, and serve as scavengers of cellular debris following CNS injury. The complex functions of the CNS are related to the generation of membrane potentials and their synaptic transmission.[1,2]

MEMBRANE POTENTIALS AND SYNAPTIC TRANSMISSION

Neurons have electrical potential across their membranes which is related to differences between the intracellular and extracellular ion concentration. The intracellular concentration of potassium ions ($[K^+]$) is higher compared to the surrounding interstitial fluid, while the intracellular sodium ion concentration ($[Na^+]$) is substantially lower compared to the extracellular space. This imbalance in ion concentration is actively maintained by membrane pumps (Na^+/K^+-ATPase) and creates a charge separation (i.e., an opposing voltage potential/electrical field) across the cell membrane (resting potential). The pump transports sodium and potassium against their net electrochemical gradients while hydrolysis of ATP provides energy to drive these active transport fluxes.[3] In unexcited neurons the conductance for potassium is much higher compared to the sodium conductance. At rest this results in an excess of positive charges on the outside of the membrane and an excess of negative charges on the inside. This charge separation produces the resting membrane potential of -70 mV. The gates of membrane-bound protein ion channels regulate a selective passage of ions across the neuronal membrane. The position of the ion channel gates (i.e., open vs. closed) controls the conductance of the cell membrane for the individual ion. During resting conditions most of the sodium channel gates are in a closed position, while the potassium channels keep their gates in a semi-open position.[3]

When membranes are exposed to an adequate stimulus, changes in the membrane permeability for ions occur. The action potential is generated by the sequen-

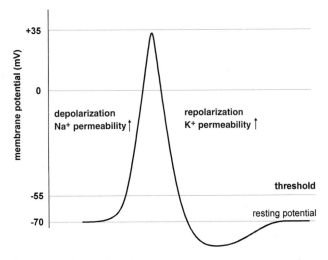

Figure 2-1   Generation of an action potential.

tial opening of sodium and potassium channels and is conducted along the axon. The first stage of the action potential is the opening of sodium channel gates, which in turn rapidly increases the intracellular sodium concentration. This depolarization elevates the membrane potential from −70 mV to +30 mV and generates an action potential. At the peak of sodium conductance the membrane changes its selective permeability and the repolarization process starts as the second stage of the action potential. The sodium conductance decreases owing to the closing of sodium channel gates, and the potassium conductance increases with opening of the potassium channel gates. The decrease of the intracellular potassium concentration and the increase of the extracellular potassium concentration reverses the positive membrane potential back to resting potential conditions[1-3] (Fig. 2-1).

Two signaling mechanisms enable rapid and precise communication between neurons: electrical and chemical synapses. Both types of synapse differ in their morphology and function. Electrical synapses show cytoplasmatic continuity between the pre- and postsynaptic cells, form gap junction channels, use ionic currents as their mode of transmission, and their direction of transmission may be uni- or bidirectional. Transmission across electrical synapses is generated by voltage-gated channels in the presynaptic neuron and is extremely rapid owing to the direct flow of current into the postsynaptic membrane. Electrical synapses participate in communications that require speed and synchrony. They are also important in developmental and regulatory signals between cells. In contrast, chemical synapses have no cytoplasmatic continuity between the pre- and postsynaptic cells, consist of presynaptic active zones and vesicles and postsynaptic receptors, use chemicals as transmitters, and their

direction of transmission is unidirectional. Following an action potential along the presynaptic neuron, voltage-gated channels of the presynaptic membrane open to allow calcium influx into the axonal terminal from the extracellular space. This calcium influx triggers the fusion of vesicles with the terminal membrane, and the neurotransmitter is released in quantal units from the vesicles into the synaptic cleft. Following release, the neurotransmitter diffuses and binds to receptors within the postsynaptic cell membrane. The binding of neurotransmitter to specific receptor sites produces changes in the receptor conformation which in turn alter postsynaptic membrane conductance and membrane potential. However, the effect of any synaptic transmission is not a function of the chemical nature of the transmitter but is related to the characteristics of the receptor and second messenger pathways. Synaptic transmission may occur directly via ion receptor channels, multisubunit transmembrane proteins [i.e., receptors for gamma-aminobutyric acid (GABA), glycine, or glutamate], and transmitter-gated ion channels, or indirectly via second messengers. Both of these transmission modalities may cause excitatory as well as inhibitory receptor effects.[1,2]

Various substances such as amino acids, amines, purines, and polypeptides may serve as neurotransmitters.[4] The amino acid glutamate is the major excitatory neurotransmitter. Glutamate stimulates N-methyl-D-aspartate (NMDA), kainate, and quisqualate receptors. Stimulation of the NMDA receptor complex induces the influx of calcium, sodium, and potassium. This process is facilitated by glycine. NMDA receptors can be blocked by magnesium, phencyclidine, and ketamine. Antagonism of NMDA receptors is part of the therapeutical concept of antiexcitatoxicity following cerebral ischemia and head injury. GABA is a presynaptic inhibitory amino acid that stabilizes membrane potentials via an increased permeability of chloride ions. This reduces the sensitivity of membranes to depolarize. The effects of benzodiazepines, barbiturates, propofol, and phenytoin are related to the potentiation of GABA at the receptor sites. The amino acid glycine is a direct inhibitor of spinal cord synapses; it stabilizes membranes by increasing the conductance for chloride ions. Acetylcholine increases the conductance for sodium ions at nicotinic receptors and increases calcium influx at muscarinic receptors. Acetylcholine is the neurotransmitter of motor neurons of the spinal cord and of all preganglionic and parasympathetic postganglionic neurons. Norepinephrine is a biogenic amine used by neurons located in the locus coeruleus of the brain stem. These cells diffusely spread throughout the cortex, cerebellum, and spinal cord. The biogenic amine serotonin mediates indirect neuronal inhibition in subcortical structures and the spinal cord. Norepinephrine and serotonin are inactivated by active reuptake and monoamine oxidase (MAO).[1,2,4,5]

Membrane potentials and synaptic transmission are based on effective ion pumps within cellular membranes, the metabolism of proteins, lipids, and carbohydrates, and the intracellular transport of molecules. All these cellular processes require the generation, consumption, and conservation of energy. In general, the CNS converts glucose and oxygen into usable forms of energy, such as adenosine triphosphate (ATP). The consumption of these energetic molecules of the CNS is substantial. This is indicated by the fact that the brain constitutes only 2 percent of body weight, yet it receives 15 percent of the resting cardiac output and it is responsible for 20 percent of the total body oxygen utilization. High rates of oxidative metabolism are essential for the survival of the CNS. Neuronal tissue cannot compensate for inadequate supply of energy, and glucose or oxygen deprivation for more than 10 min will irreversibly damage the cells. Although the compensatory potential of the neuronal energy stores is low, conservation of energy is possible using the mechanism of coupling between neuronal activity and energy consumption.

GENERATION OF ENERGY

Under physiologic conditions, the entire metabolic requirement of the CNS is provided by degradation of glycogen from the liver and muscle into glucose, which is oxidized to carbon dioxide and water in an energy generating process.[6] The high oxidative metabolism is reflected in the consumption of 35 to 70 ml O_2/min. The range of cerebral oxygen consumption is related to the different activation states of the CNS. Since the delivery of oxygen (cerebral blood flow × arterial oxygen content) is higher than cerebral oxygen demand, decreases in O_2 delivery can be compensated to a certain extent by increases in O_2 extraction. Although there are some alternatives in the generation of energy (e.g., utilization of phosphocreatine, ketone bodies, dicarboxylic acids), the metabolism of these substances does not provide sufficient energy to maintain cellular function and integrity during oxygen or glucose deprivation. Glucose enters the cells of the CNS by facilitated diffusion due to membrane-based carrier mechanisms. The oxidation of glucose starts with the process of glycolysis within the cytoplasm where the glucose molecule (six-carbon) is converted into two molecules of pyruvate (three-carbon). The net gain of this reaction is two molecules of ATP for each molecule of glucose. The metabolism of the pyruvate molecules may follow two different pathways, based on the availability of oxygen. In the absence of oxygen, pyruvate is reduced to lactic acid by the addition of two hydrogen atoms.

This process is associated with a net hydrogen ion production, which lowers intracellular pH. Anaerobic glycolysis forms only two molecules of ATP for each molecule of glucose. Unfortunately, this amount of ATP generation is not sufficient to meet the energy demands of the CNS. In the presence of oxygen, pyruvate enters the mitochondria and is oxidized to carbon dioxide and water following conversion into acetyl coenzyme A (acetyl CoA). This molecule enters the citric acid (Krebs) cycle and passes through a series of oxidations and reductions that provide a large amount of energy. The citric acid cycle transfers electrons to coenzymes. This process generates four molecules of carbon dioxide per two molecules of acetyl CoA, reduced coenzymes (NADH[+], H[+], FADH$_2$) containing stored energy and two molecules of guanosine triphosphate (GTP) for later formation of ATP. Following the passage of the electron transport chain, a total of 38 molecules of ATP are generated per molecule of glucose by the transfer of the energy stored in NADH[+], H[+], and FADH$_2$ to adenosine diphosphate (ADP) and inorganic phosphate. ATP is transported into the cytoplasm in exchange of ADP by membrane proteins. Hydrolysis of ATP releases the effective (nonstored) energy constantly utilized by the CNS.[1,6,7]

CONSUMPTION OF ENERGY

What is the purpose for this intense and continuous generation of energy? Neurons are specialized to process consciousness, sensory information, motor and emotional responses, learning, and memory. These multiple neuronal network functions are based on the maintenance of transmembrane electrical and ionic gradients provided by active transport (Na[+]/K[+]-ATPase) against net electrochemical gradients to provide depolarization and synaptic transmission. The continuous activity of membrane-bound ionic pump systems to restore sodium and potassium concentrations requires most of the energy derived from hydrolysis of ATP. Calcium ions are very important for most of the transmembrane (synaptic) and intracellular processes, and the preservation of normal calcium gradients requires energy-dependent pump mechanisms within the membrane of cells and organelles. Synthesis, storage, release, and reuptake of the neurotransmitters are energy-dependent intracellular processes immediately related to proper CNS function. The dynamic structure of the phospholipid bilayer of membranes of cells and organelles and physiologic cytoplasmatic conditions are essential prerequisites for intact cellular functions. Membrane and cytoplasmatic homeostasis involves the energy-consuming synthesis of protein, amines, lipids, and carbohydrates and the intracellular transport of molecules. Astrocytes, oligodendrocytes,

Schwann cells, and microglia serve as supporting elements and mediate neuronal metabolism. Glial cells insulate the large neuronal axons by forming myelin sheaths, contribute to the formation of the blood-brain barrier, provide nutrition to neurons (storage of glycogen), reuptake neurotransmitters and potassium ions, and serve as scavengers of cellular debris following CNS injury. All of these glial functions are associated with the consumption of energy. In summary, the high rate of oxidative metabolism (generation of ATP) within the CNS is related to: (1) the continuous activity of ionic pump systems to maintain transmembrane and electrochemical gradients; (2) synthesis of proteins, amines, lipids, and carbohydrates; (3) the intracellular transport, storage, release and reuptake of molecules; and (4) the structural and metabolic functions of the glial cells.[2,3,5]

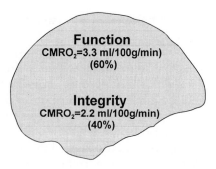

Figure 2-2 Functional and basal activity: 60 percent of the expenditure of energy is based on the functional activity of the CNS; the other 40 percent is related to the basal metabolism that maintains cellular integrity. (Adapted from Cucchiara RF, Michenfelder JD: *Clinical Neuroanesthesia, Churchill Neuroanesthesia.* New York, Churchill-Livingstone, 1990, with permission.)

CONSERVATION OF ENERGY

The CNS has the ability to adjust the expenditure of energy to the level of cellular activity in order to conserve energy.[7] The parallel behavior of cellular activation and metabolic turnover is based on the tight coupling between cerebral metabolic demand and cerebral substrate supply.[6,7] Cerebral functional activation (e.g., mental or physical activation, seizures) is associated with a raise in cerebral energy demand due to the increased activity of ionic pump systems and the synthesis, transport, and release of molecules. The need for a rise in energy supply is met by increases in cerebral blood flow (CBF) to provide adequate oxygen and glucose delivery.[8,9] In contrast, cerebral energy demands are reduced during cerebral functional depression (e.g., at rest, physiologic sleep, coma) along with a decrease in cerebral energy supply. The coupling between energy demand and energy supply is regulated in a regionally specific fashion. Under physiologic conditions the various functional units and subunits of the CNS exhibit different activation states. These differences in the basal activity of the resting CNS produce a heterogeneous metabolic pattern with units of low metabolic activity and substrate supply next to tissues with high metabolic activity and substrate supply. Another mechanism in the process of energy conservation is the concept of the separation between functional and basal activity (Fig. 2-2). According to this concept, 60 percent of the expenditure of energy is based on the functional activity of the CNS (which is reflected by the brain electrical activity), while the other 40 percent is related to the basal metabolism that maintains cellular integrity. During critical reductions in cerebral substrate supply, neurons can reduce or shut off their cellular function (EEG isoelectricity), which in turn may save up to 60 percent of

energy expenditure. This may be potentially invested in favor of the basal metabolism and integrity of the cell.[10,11]

In summary, the complex functions of the CNS are based on the generation of membrane potentials and their synaptic transmission. Membrane potentials and synaptic transmission require effective ion pumps within cellular membranes, the metabolism of proteins, lipids, and carbohydrates, and the intracellular transport of molecules. All of these cellular processes depend on the generation, consumption, and conservation of energy. High rates of oxidative metabolism generate ATP to fuel the cells of the CNS for their functional activity and integrity. Conservation of energy is realized by the coupling between neuronal activity and energy consumption in a regionally specific fashion. However, the neuronal threshold to compensate for inadequate substrate supply is low. The utilization of phosphocreatine, ketone bodies, and dicarboxylic acids and the cessation of functional activity appear to be the only cellular mechanisms by which energy can be saved in favor of the cellular integrity.

Cerebral Blood Flow

ANATOMY

ARTERIAL CIRCULATION
In humans, CBF is almost completely supplied by two pairs of arterial trunks, the internal carotid arteries and the vertebral arteries.[12] The internal carotid arteries supply the anterior portion of the circle of Willis (Fig. 2-3). The vertebral arteries join to form the basilar artery, which supplies the posterior portion of the circle of Willis.[13] The circle of Willis is located within the subarachnoid space, but varies in 48 percent of the population because the different segments of the circle

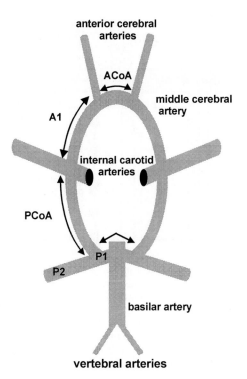

Figure 2-3   Brain supplying arteries and the Circle of Willis (ACoA, anterior communicating artery; PCoA, posterior communicating artery).

rior cerebellar artery originates from the rostral part of the basilar artery. The anterior inferior cerebellar artery originates from the trunk of the basilar artery and perfuses the lateral part of the pons, the upper part of the medulla, and the cerebellar hemisphere. The posterior inferior cerebellar arteries originate from the vertebral arteries. The external carotid arteries supply leptomeningeal arteries, which terminate in cortical brain regions (Fig. 2-4). Despite this network of arteries and anatomic anastomoses, the watershed areas of the cerebral cortex are extremely vulnerable to critical reductions in CBF via the circle of Willis because the contribution of leptomeningeal arteries to cortical blood flow is very low.

VENOUS CIRCULATION
Superficial cerebral veins may be divided into the ascending superficial veins, the superficial sylvian veins,

of Willis are inconsistently connected with each other.[14] Most frequently, blood flow may be shunted between both internal carotid territories via the single anterior communicating artery and between the anterior and posterior circulation via two posterior communicating arteries. Under physiologic conditions, blood flow within the communicating arteries is low. However, in the presence of a functional stenosis of one of the carotid or vertebral arteries, arterial flow will be shunted along the pressure gradient via the communicating arteries. The circle of Willis consists of three pairs of cerebral endarteries: the anterior, middle, and posterior cerebral arteries. The anterior cerebral artery runs in a medial and anterior direction above the optic nerve and chiasm. The areas of supply of these six major cerebral arteries shows a considerable variation in distribution.[15] The anterior communicating artery is an inconsistent link between the two anterior cerebral arteries. The middle cerebral arteries run in a lateral direction to the sylvian fissure and the insula, where they divide into frontal, parietal, and temporal branches. The posterior cerebral arteries derive from the rostral end of the basilar artery and inconsistently communicate at the level of the midportion of the peduncular segment via the posterior communicating artery. The posterior cerebral arteries divide into four branches: the anterior temporal, posterior temporal, parieto-occipital, and the calcarine arteries. The supe-

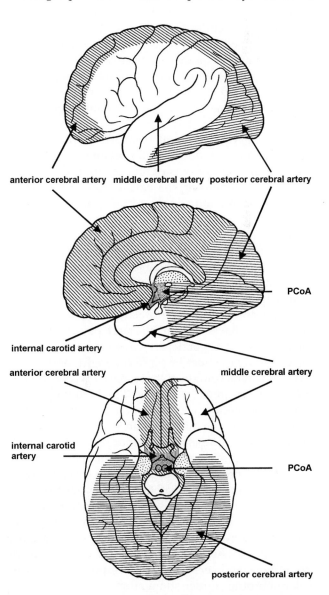

Figure 2-4   Territories of perfusion of the basal cerebral arteries.

and the inferior cerebral veins. Most of the ascending cerebral veins drain into the sagittal sinus. The internal cerebral and basal veins drain into the great vein of Galen. The Galenic group of veins receives most of the venous return from the midbrain and from medial and paravermal regions of the superior cerebellar surface. The petrosal vein collects blood from the veins of the horizontal fissure, the transverse pontine vein, the brachial vein, and the vein of the lateral recess of the fourth ventricle and then drains into the superior petrosal sinus. The superior veins of the cerebellum drain into the transverse sinus. The inferior hemispheric cerebellar veins open into the transverse sinus.[12]

The superior sagittal sinus receives venous outflow from the lateral lacunae and from the ascending superficial veins. The inferior sagittal sinus receives venous outflow from the roof of the corpus callosum, the cingulate gyrus, and the adjacent hemisphere. The straight sinus receives blood from the inferior sagittal sinus and from the vein of Galen and communicates with the transverse sinus and the superior sagittal sinus. From the superior petrosal sinus, blood flows into the transverse sinus which communicates with the sigmoid sinus and drains blood into the jugular vein. Following passage of the sinuses, about 85 percent of the cerebral venous blood is drained to the jugular bulb without contamination from extracranial sources. This anatomic situation is an important prerequisite in the measurement of oxygen saturation in the jugular bulb when monitoring the balance between cerebral oxygen demand and supply.

INNERVATION OF CEREBRAL VESSELS
Nerve fibers have been demonstrated on cerebral blood vessels since the time of Thomas Willis in 1664.[13] Willis' observation of cerebrovascular innervation was confirmed and extended by light microscopy, electron microscopy, and fluorescent histochemical studies. Cerebral vessels have sympathetic and parasympathetic innervation.[16-19] Several pathways originating in the locus coeruleus, superior cervical ganglia, and the intermediolateral column of the spinal cord contribute to the adrenergic innervation (Fig. 2-5). Parasympathetic innervation occurs via the sphenopalatine ganglion and likely from the otic ganglion.[20,21] Sympathetic and parasympathetic innervation is more dense in the anterior circulation than in the posterior circulation. Several amines and neuropeptides may serve as neurotransmitters within the sympathetic and parasympathetic innervation of cerebral vessels: norepinephrine; acetylcholine; neuropeptide Y; vasoactive intestinal polypeptide; calcitonin gene-related peptide; and substance P.[4,21,22] Table 2-1 summarizes the origin of nerve fibers, vessel type, and cerebrovascular response to perivascular neurotransmitter stimulation.

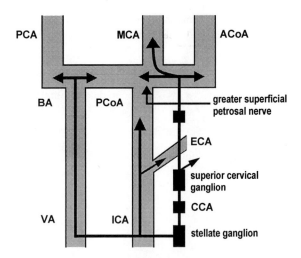

Figure 2-5 Schematic representation of the perivascular innervation (PCA, posterior cerebral artery; MCA, middle cerebral artery; ACoA, anterior communicating artery; BA, basilar artery; PCoA, posterior communicating artery; ECA, external carotid artery; VA, vertebral artery; ICA, internal carotid artery; CCA, common carotid artery). (Adapted from Edvinsson L, MacKenzie ET, McCulloch J: *Cerebral Blood Flow and Metabolism.* New York, Raven Press, 1993, with permission.)

PHYSIOLOGY

METABOLIC REGULATION
The energy requirements of the brain are substantial. During resting conditions, approximately 15 percent of the cardiac output is directed to the brain to match cerebral oxygen consumption, which is about 20 percent of the total body oxygen consumption. Both cerebral oxygen and cerebral glucose consumption are indirect measures of the rate at which ATP is utilized. The energy stored in ATP is utilized to fuel biochemical reactions in cells. Unfortunately, the energy storing capacity of the CNS is very low, and regulatory mechanisms are necessary to maintain continuous substrate supply. There is a wide range of metabolic rates within the CNS tissues, and resting CBF and metabolism are higher in cortical compared with subcortical tissues. Studies of functional imaging of the brain have shown that motor, visual, or cognitive activation is associated with regionally specific increases in metabolism. The energy requirements of the brain during activation are instantaneously met by increases in substrate delivery to the activated functional subunits (i.e., increases in CBF).[9,23-25] This mechanism of flow-metabolism coupling has an almost identical spatial distribution and blood flow increases as quickly as 1 s following neuronal excitation.[26,27] The increase in local CBF is limited to 250 μm from the site of increased neuronal activity.[27] These data demonstrate the rapid and regionally specific adjustment of cerebral metabolic demand and substrate supply at the microvascular level. However, cou-

TABLE 2-1
Origin of Nerve Fibers, Vessel Type, and Cerebrovascular Responses to Perivascular Neurotransmitter Stimulation

Neurotransmitter	Origin	Vessel	Response	Putative Role
Norepinephrine	Sympathetic ganglia	A, V	Constriction Dilation	Attenuates increased CBF in severe hypertension.
	Locus coeruleus	C, A	Controversial	Intracranial blood volume regulation? Modifies permeability of blood-brain barrier to water?
Neuropeptide Y	Sympathetic ganglia	A, V	Constriction	Similar to norepinephrine, which is colocalized with, but with more sustained effects.
Acetylcholine	Seventh cranial nerve	A	Vasodilation	Unknown. Involved in vasodilatory responses.
	Sphenopalatine ganglion	A, V		
	Otic ganglion	A, V		
	Cortical perikarya	A		
	Endothelium	C		
5-Hydroxytryptamine	Raphé nuclei	A, C	Dilation (high tone)	Unknown. Involved in vascular phenomena associated with classical migraine?
	Sympathetic ganglia		Constriction (low tone)	
Substance P/neurokinin A	Fifth cranial nerve	A, V, C	Dilation	Sensory afferent conveying nociceptive information of vascular origin inflammatory response
Calcitonin gene-related peptide	Fifth cranial nerve	A, V	Dilation	The restoration of normal caliber in excessive vasoconstriction
Somatostatin	Fifth cranial nerve?	A	Unknown	
Gastrin-releasing peptide	Fifth cranial nerve?	A	None	
Vasoactive intestinal polypeptide/peptide HI	Cortical perikarya	A, V	Dilation	Unknown
	Sphenopalatine ganglion	A, V		Thermoregulation
	Otic ganglion	A, V		
	Microganglion	A, V		
Cholecystokinin	Cortical perikarya	A, V, C	None	Unknown
Neurotensin	Intracerebral (?)		None	Unknown
Met-Enkephalin	Unknown	C	None	Unknown

NOTE: A, arterial; V, venous; C, capillary.
SOURCE: Adapted from Edvinsson L, MacKenzie ET, McCulloch J: *Cerebral Blood Flow and Metabolism*. New York, Raven, 1993, with permission.

pling of metabolic activity and CBF may not always be of identical magnitude. In human volunteers, sensory stimulation produced 29 percent increases in CBF but only 5 percent increases in oxidative metabolism, both of which were regionally specific.[28] Several mechanisms are involved in the rapid coupling between cerebral metabolism and CBF.

Chemical Regulation of Flow-Metabolism Coupling

Neurons within the active subunits release vasodilating substances that diffuse directly to the smooth muscle cells of the vascular wall or indirectly change vascular tone via endothelial mediators. Adenosine, nitric oxide, and hydrogen and potassium ions appear to be the most important mediators of flow-metabolism coupling.

ADENOSINE   Adenosine is a potent dilator of the major cerebral arteries and pial arterioles. The smooth muscle relaxation seen with adenosine is related to an increase in cyclic AMP production, and CBF increases with adenosine administration. The view that adenosine may be an important mediator of the flow-metabolism coupling is based on the fact that adenosine is the product of metabolic activity that accumulates as a result of dephosphorylation of adenosine nucleotides. Rising adenosine concentrations within the cells and extracellular space consecutively induce cerebral vasodilation.[29,30] This concept is supported by two factors: (1) Perivascular concentrations of adenosine increase in response to neuronal activation. (2) In rats, CBF increases with whisker stimulation, and this response can be reduced or abolished in the presence of adenosine antagonists.[31] However, the temporal resolution of adenosine accumulation is too low to accept this mechanism as the major regulating factor of flow-metabolism coupling.

NITRIC OXIDE   Nitric oxide (NO) is a molecular messenger involved in a variety of biologic processes.[32,33] There is increasing evidence that NO plays an important role in the regulation of the cerebral circulation. NO is synthesized from L-arginine by the enzyme nitric oxide synthase (NOS). There are three isoforms of NOS: two constitutive NO synthases that derive from neurons, astrocytes, perivascular nerves, and the endothelium; and one inducible NOS that derives from macrophages. NO is a diffusible, short-lived, and highly reactive molecule. Most investigations have therefore used inhibitors of NOS activity to study the CNS effects of NO. Numerous experiments using different species of laboratory animals have shown that the topical or intravenous inhibition of NOS decreases CBF in a dose-dependent fashion. However, the decreases in CBF seen with inhibition of NOS were not related to changes in cerebral oxygen consumption or cerebral glucose consumption.[34–37] This suggests that NO is an important mediator of resting CBF while suppression of cerebral energy metabolism is not related to NO pathways.

Several studies have investigated the effects of focal and global neuronal activation on CBF with and without inhibition of NOS. The results from these studies are inconsistent. While the increase in CBF to functional stimulation was attenuated in some experiments, others failed to demonstrate a reduction of CBF responses to increased neuronal activity.[31,37–40] The discrepancy of these results may be related to the dose and route of administration of the NOS inhibitor (i.e., intravenous vs. topical) and to the degree of NOS inhibition. Additionally, while participation of NO pathways in the coupling between neuronal activation and cerebral vasodilation have been clearly demonstrated, this effect appears to be restricted to certain activation paradigms.[32] In conclusion, the available data indicate that NO pathways are involved in mediating increases in CBF following metabolic activation. However, NOS inhibition attenuates rather than abolishes cerebrovascular responses to functional activation. This suggests that other mediators have to be involved in the coupling of CBF and metabolism.

HYDROGEN AND POTASSIUM IONS   The perivascular concentration of hydrogen ions is a direct function of the local energy metabolism. Increases in the perivascular concentration of potassium ions is not directly related to energy metabolism but accumulates as a consequence of its prominent role in membrane function in neurons, astrocytes, and smooth muscle cells. Hydrogen and potassium ions are mediators of the flow-metabolism coupling. Extracellular hydrogen ions decrease cerebrovascular resistance and increase CBF. This effect is not related to a direct effect of hydrogen ions on vascular smooth muscle cells or endothelial derived factors rather than indirectly by changing the perivascular pH. Increases in neuronal activity are associated with the production of CO_2, which may be converted to HCO_3^- and hydrogen ions in the presence of water. Based on the inverse relationship between the hydrogen ion concentration and the perivascular pH, the decrease in pH mediates increases in arteriolar diameter.[41,42] Extracellular potassium ions have pronounced effects on cerebrovascular tone. Potassium ions are released by active neurons, transported through astrocytes, and released onto cerebral vessels. Moderate elevations of the local potassium concentration during neuronal activation induce pial arteriolar dilation, which in turn increases local CBF.[4,43] The vasodilation in response to potassium release shows a latency of 5 to 10 s,[4] which may be due to the mediating effects of NO on potassium ion release.[44] However, the time lag of cerebrovascular response to increases in perivascular potassium indicates that other mechanisms induce the immediate cerebrovascular response seen following functional activation. This is in line with the evidence that CBF is substantially increased following amphetamine-induced neuronal activation while the extracellular concentrations of hydrogen or potassium ions remain unchanged.

In summary, adenosine, NO, and hydrogen and potassium ions are important in the process of coupling cerebral energy metabolism and flow. However, the temporal response of these mechanisms is too slow to explain the explosive increases in CBF following functional activation. It is possible that some rapid initiator evokes the immediate first step of CBF increase. In a second step, this activated level could be maintained by the mechanisms related to adenosine, NO, and hydrogen and potassium ions.[4]

Neurogenic Regulation of Flow-Metabolism Coupling

Cerebral vessels have sympathetic and parasympathetic innervation.[16–19] Table 2-1 summarizes the origin of nerve fibers, vessel type, and cerebrovascular response to perivascular neurotransmitter stimulation. Several pathways originating in the locus coeruleus, superior cervical ganglia, and the intermediolateral column of the spinal cord contribute to the adrenergic innervation (Fig. 2-5). These fibers contain norepinephrine, ATP, and neuropeptide Y. The effects of catecholamines on the cerebral circulation are diverse. Catecholamines may produce increases as well as decreases in cerebrovascular resistance and CBF. The individual response of the cerebral vasculature is related to the origin of the neurotransmitter (i.e., circulating catecholamines from the adrenal gland vs. norepinephrine released from perivascular nerve fibers vs. intrathecal administration), catecholamine concentration, and the status of the blood-brain barrier. Norepinephrine is a vasoconstrictor of isolated cerebral arteries. This alpha-adrenergic vasoconstrictor response to adrenergic agents can be blocked by alpha-adrenoceptor antagonists. However, the effects of norepinephrine appear to be related to the baseline cerebrovascular tone. In preconstricted cerebral arteries catecholamines may induce vasodilation.[4] Stimulation of sympathetic perivascular nerves or the adrenoceptor stimulation by catecholamines released from the adrenal medulla can be considered as mechanisms of the extrinsic nerve system. In vivo studies with intact blood brain barrier have shown that circulating catecholamines as well as cervical nerve stimulation produce modest increases in cerebrovascular resistance, which in turn decreases CBF.[16,43–46] In contrast, circulating catecholamines in the presence of blood-brain barrier disruption as well as intraventricular injection of norepinephrine produce substantial increases in CBF, cerebral oxygen consumption, and cerebral glucose consumption.[47] These effects are consistent with experiments where stimulation of the dorsal medullary reticular formation or the locus coeruleus was associated with increases in plasma catecholamines and CBF.[48,49] In contrast to the perivascular sympathetic fibers of peripheral origin (extrinsic nerves), the responses of the cerebral circulation to stimulation of central sympathetic subunits are related to the signaling via intrinsic sympathetic pathways. Intrinsic neurogenic control originates from sympathetic or serotonergic neurons and neuronal subunits that directly innervate cerebral microvessels or release neurotransmitters, which per se modulate cerebrovascular tone. The stimulation of the dorsal medullary reticular formation is closely coupled with increased metabolic activity in certain cortical regions.[50,51] The intrinsic innervation of cerebral microvessels and temporal relation between increases in intrinsic sympathetic activity and increases in metabolism and flow demonstrates that the brain can control its own circulation. In humans, resting CBF appears to be unaffected by baseline sympathetic tone.[52] The available data indicate that circulating catecholamines and stimulation of sympathetic perivascular nerve fibers produces mild cerebrovascular constriction (extrinsic system). In contrast, stimulation of central sympathetic units induces substantial increases in CBF and metabolism (intrinsic system).

Parasympathetic innervation occurs via the sphenopalatine ganglion and likely from the otic ganglion.[20,21] The fibers contain acetylcholine, vasoactive intestinal peptide, and peptide histidine isoleucine as tentative neurotransmitters. Parasympathetic sensory fibers originate in the trigeminal ganglion and at the level of C2. Sensory fibers contain calcitonin gene-related peptide, substance P, and neuroleukin A. The parasympathetic innervation supplies the large cerebral arteries at the basis of the skull, pial arteries, arterioles, and cerebral veins. Studies in laboratory animals have shown that the infusion of acetylcholine as well as the stimulation of extracerebral parasympathetic units like the major petrosal nerve (i.e., stimulation of the extrinsic pathways of innervation) produce a dose- or frequency-dependent increase in cerebrovascular diameter and CBF.[53,54] The cerebrovascular dilation in response to parasympathetic activation is mediated by the stimulation of nicotinic and muscarinic receptors. Microapplication of acetylcholine to cerebral vessels produces a dose-dependent dilation that can be inhibited by atropine or scopolamine. Similar to the intrinsic system of sympathetic cerebrovascular control, there is evidence for the presence of central parasympathetic subunits. Stimulation of the cerebellar fastigial nucleus produces increases in cortical CBF which persists even following transection of the spinal cord at the level of C1.[55,56] The increases in regional CBF were not related to increased oxidative metabolism. The ventromedial globus pallidus is the primary source of cortical cholinergic innervation in rodent brains. The stimulation of these parasympathetic units increases acetylcholine release and blood flow in the parietal cortex in rats.[57] These studies indicate that the stimulation of central parasympathetic units is mediated by intrinsic pathways that depend on the integrity of cholinergic neurons.

In conclusion, the metabolic regulation of CBF is synergistically mediated by chemical and neurogenic factors. Neurons within the active subunits release vasodilating substances that diffuse directly to the smooth muscle cells of the vascular wall or act indirectly to change vascular tone via endothelial mediators. Adenosine, NO, and hydrogen and potassium ions are important in the chemical regulation of coupling cerebral energy metabolism and flow. Neurogenic control is mediated by extrinsic and instrinsic regulation. Extrinsic neurogenic regulation describes the sympathetic and parasympathetic perivascular nerve fibers of extracerebral origin that innervate arteries of the CNS as well as circulating vasoactive chemicals (e.g., catecholamines). The cerebrovascular effects of perivascular neurotransmitters or circulating vasoactive substances are diverse, dose-dependent, and related to the status of the blood-brain barrier and include vasoconstriction and vasodilation. Intrinsic neurogenic regulation describes sympathetic or serotonergic neurons and neuronal subunits that directly

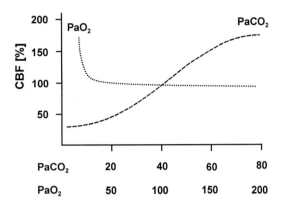

Figure 2-6 Changes in cerebral blood flow as a function of arterial carbon dioxide (Pa$_{CO_2}$) and oxygen tension (Pa$_{O_2}$). (Adapted and redrawn from: Harper AM, Glass HI: Effect of alterations in the arterial carbon dioxide tension on the blood flow through the cerebral cortex at normal and low arterial pressures. *J Neurol Neurosurg Psychiatry* 1965; 28:449, and Sakabe T, Siesjö BK: The effect of indomethacin on the blood-flow-metabolism couple in the brain under normal, hypercapnic, and hypoxic conditions. *Acta Physiol Scand* 1979; 107:283.)

innervate cerebral microvessels or release neurotransmitters, which per se modulate cerebrovascular tone.

ARTERIAL GAS TENSIONS

Carbon Dioxide

CO_2 is a potent modulator of cerebrovascular resistance and CBF.[41] Arterial hypercapnia dilates cerebral blood vessels, decreases cerebrovascular resistance, and increases CBF. In contrast, arterial hypocapnia constricts cerebral vessels, increases cerebrovascular resistance, and decreases CBF[58,59] (Fig. 2-6). The changes in CBF during changes in Pa$_{CO_2}$ are associated with a nonlinear change in cerebral blood volume.[60,61] The dynamic changes in the diameter of the cerebral vessels occur at the level of the small cortical and tissue-penetrating arteries and arterioles. However, larger arteries are also involved in the regulation of cerebrovascular resistance.[62] Since CO_2 is one of the major products of oxidative metabolism, cerebrovascular CO_2-reactivity was traditionally considered the most important mechanism to control flow-metabolism coupling. Cerebrovascular CO_2-reactivity is defined as the change in CBF per unit change Pa$_{CO_2}$. In normotensive individuals, the change in CBF is nearly linear to the change in carbon dioxide within the Pa$_{CO_2}$ range of 20 to 75 mmHg. Within this linear range, CBF changes 3 to 5 percent per mmHg change in Pa$_{CO_2}$. At the upper and lower end of the Pa$_{CO_2}$, the CO_2-reactivity curve plateaus to an extent where further increases or decreases in Pa$_{CO_2}$ produce no further change in CBF. This effect is due to the maximal vasodilation or vasoconstriction that occurs at extreme hypercapnic or hypocapnic values. Baseline arteriolar tone is an important variable

in the individual CBF response to changes in CO_2. As a consequence, the magnitude of cerebrovascular CO_2-reactivity may be modulated by the level of arterial blood pressure. Decreases in arterial blood pressure induce autoregulatory cerebrovascular dilation. In the presence of hypotension, the preexisting autoregulatory decrease in cerebrovascular tone reduces or abolishes the potential of cerebral vessels to further dilate in response to hypercapnia[59,63] (Fig. 2-7). Profound hyperventilation may decrease CBF below the ischemic threshold. Studies in cats have shown that hyperventilation below 25 mmHg Pa$_{CO_2}$ decreases cerebral venous oxygen saturation and increases cerebral oxygen extraction and the concentration of lactic acid in cerebral tissue and cerebrospinal fluid.[64,65] In a rat model of focal cerebral ischemia, hypocapnic cerebrovascular constriction may even increase the ischemic area compared to normocapnia.[66]

Numerous studies have investigated the mechanisms of cerebrovascular CO_2-reactivity. Topical application of low-pH solutions to the surface of the brain produce cerebrovascular dilation. In contrast, topical application of high-pH solutions produces cerebrovascular constriction.[67,68] These reproducible responses were observed with solutions of varying P$_{CO_2}$ but constant bicarbonate concentration, as well as with solutions containing varying concentrations of bicarbonate but constant P$_{CO_2}$. These experiments indicate that the mechanism by which CO_2 modulates cerebrovascular resistance is related to changes in the extracellular/intracellular pH next to the vascular smooth muscle cells. Molecular CO_2 and bicarbonate ions do not ap-

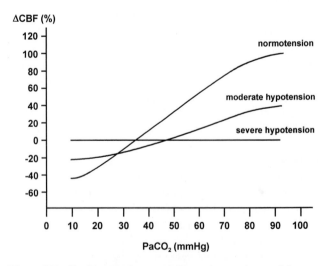

Figure 2-7 Cerebrovascular reactivity to changes in arterial carbon dioxide tension (Pa$_{CO_2}$) at different levels of arterial blood pressure. (Adapted from: Harper AM, Glass HI: Effect of alterations in the arterial carbon dioxide tension on the blood flow through the cerebral cortex at normal and low arterial pressures. *J Neurol Neurosurg Psychiatry* 1965; 28:449.)

pear to have intrinsic vasoactivity. The modulation of perivascular pH by changes in arterial Pa_{CO_2} and the extracellular bicarbonate concentration is based on the chemical reaction between CO_2 and water:

$$CO_2 + H_2O \leftrightarrow H_2CO_3 \leftrightarrow HCO_3^- + H^+$$

CO_2 is a diffusible molecule that easily passes the blood-brain barrier and penetrates the vascular smooth muscle cell. In contrast, the permeability of the blood-brain barrier and smooth muscle cell membranes for hydrogen ions is low. This explains why respiratory acidosis substantially decreases the cerebrovascular resistance while metabolic acidosis does not.[67] As a consequence, increases in the interstitial and cerebrospinal fluid concentration of hydrogen ions induce vasodilation, but increases in arterial hydrogen ion concentration leaves cerebrovascular tone almost unaffected.

Although the major mechanism of cerebrovascular dilation is the decrease in perivascular pH induced by the increase in tissue P_{CO_2}, NO and cyclooxygenase pathways appear to be involved in this regulatory process. Experiments in rats, cats, dogs, monkeys, and rabbits have shown that the infusion or topical application of NOS inhibitors attenuates the increases in CBF evoked by hypercapnia.[32,69–74] The magnitude of the reduction ranges from 35 to 95 percent. This attenuation is not related to an unspecific mechanism, since vasodilation due to nitroprusside, hypotension, and/or hypoxia is not affected by NOS inhibition.[32] Thus, synthesis of NO is a necessary step for the hypercapnic vasodilation to occur. However, the incomplete blockade of hypercapnic cerebrovascular dilation by NOS inhibitors indicates that NO is not the universal mediator in the CBF response to changes in Pa_{CO_2}.

The cyclooxygenase inhibitor indomethacin potently blocks increases in CBF induced by hypercapnia in laboratory animals and humans.[75,76] The indomethacin-induced decreases in cerebrovascular CO_2 reactivity are not associated with changes in oxidative metabolism: cerebral oxygen consumption and cerebral glucose consumption remain unaffected. However, the decreases in CBF seen with indomethacin infusion may produce increases in cerebral oxygen extraction and ischemic changes of the EEG.[77] Decreases in cerebrovascular CO_2 reactivity seen with indomethacin are highly specific as this agent has no effect on CBF autoregulation or hypoxic hyperemia.[78,79] This suggests that hypercapnic cerebrovascular dilation is related to cyclooxygenase inhibition or to the release of eicosanoids.[80]

Oxygen

Changes in the arterial oxygen tension (Pa_{O_2}) are associated with changes in CBF. In unanesthetized animals

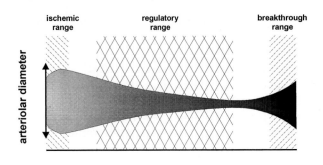

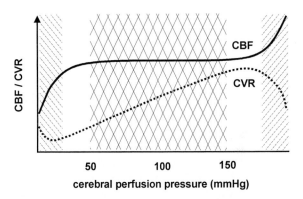

Figure 2-8   Dynamic changes or arteriolar diameter and cerebrovascular resistance (CVR) in the regulation of CBF during changes in cerebral perfusion pressure. (Adapted and redrawn from Young WL, Columbia University.)

subjected to hypoxia, CBF increases, thereby maintaining cerebral oxygen transport.[81] The cerebrovascular responses to hypoxia are maintained regardless of the baseline cerebral metabolic status. In animals anesthetized with barbiturates or isoflurane, hypoxic hypoxia increases CBF as well.[82,83] The cerebrovascular dilation during reduced arterial oxygen content is not related to the activation of chemoreceptors, NO-pathways, or alpha-2-adrenergic receptors.[83,84] This suggests that molecular oxygen affects vascular smooth muscle directly (Fig. 2-6).

AUTOREGULATION

One of the most important regulatory mechanisms of CBF is the potential of the cerebral vasculature to maintain CBF constant (autoregulation) over a wide range of cerebral perfusion pressure (Fig. 2-8). Within the physiologic range of cerebral perfusion pressure, autoregulation protects the neuronal tissue against hypoxia when cerebral perfusion pressure decreases, and against hyperemia, capillary damage, and edema when cerebral perfusion pressure increases.[4,85]

CBF autoregulation is a function of changes in cerebrovascular resistance in response to changes in cerebral perfusion pressure. This relation is expressed by the following formula: CBF = CPP/CVR, where CPP is cerebral perfusion pressure and CVR is cerebrovascular resistance. Cerebral perfusion pressure is defined as the difference between mean arterial blood pressure minus intracranial pressure ($CPP = MAP - ICP$). Since cerebral perfusion pressure is a function of mean arterial blood pressure and intracranial pressure, any change in these variables will induce autoregulatory responses.[86] Effective autoregulation implies that decreases in cerebral perfusion pressure induce concomitant decreases in cerebrovascular resistance. Likewise, any increase in cerebral perfusion pressure is associated with a proportional increase in cerebrovascular resistance to maintain CBF constant. In anatomic terms, CBF autoregulation predominantly occurs at the level of the small arteries and arterioles. However, even the larger cerebral arteries have some potential to contribute to vasodilation and vasoconstriction during changes in cerebral perfusion pressure.[62,87] The lower and upper limit of CBF autoregulation is not a fixed point on the autoregulatory curve. The individual response of the cerebral vasculature to changes in CPP is related to the preexisting cerebrovascular tone, which is modulated by sympathetic activity, cerebral metabolism, the level of Pa_{CO_2}, and vasoactive substances (e.g., anesthetics). In contrast, abolished autoregulation implies that CBF decreases or increases proportionally to decreases or increases in CPP while cerebrovascular resistance remains constant.

Range of CBF Autoregulation

Autoregulation of CBF is effective within the range of cerebral perfusion pressure of ~50 to 140 mmHg. The autoregulatory range is similar for changes in blood pressure and intracranial pressure (Fig. 2-8).

Lower Limit of CBF Autoregulation

Progressive decreases in blood pressure or increases in intracranial pressure induce proportional cerebrovascular dilation to maintain constant CBF and neurologic function. Autoregulatory vasodilation increases cerebral blood volume and may further elevate intracranial pressure in patients with pathologic intracranial pressure volume relation.[88–91] The lower limit of CBF autoregulation is defined as the level of cerebral perfusion pressure which induces maximal cerebrovascular dilation. Decreases in cerebral perfusion pressure below this level produce decreases in CBF in a pressure-passive fashion and oxygen extraction increases to compensate for the decrease in oxygen delivery (Fig. 2-8). Neurologic complications (dizziness, confusion, coma) occur as soon as compensatory O_2 extraction is exhausted and cerebral perfusion pressure is too low to maintain CBF above the ischemic threshold.[92]

Upper Limit of CBF Autoregulation

During increases in CPP, the autoregulatory responses of the cerebral vasculature operate in an inverse fashion. Progressive increases in blood pressure or decreases in intracranial pressure induce proportional cerebrovascular constriction to maintain constant CBF and neurologic function. Autoregulatory vasoconstriction is associated with a decrease in cerebral blood volume. However, this does not necessarily decrease intracranial pressure.[91] The upper limit of CBF autoregulation is defined as the level of cerebral perfusion pressure that induces maximal cerebrovascular constriction. Further increases of cerebral perfusion pressure beyond this level dilate the cerebral vasculature in a pressure-passive fashion and in turn raises CBF (Fig. 2-8). Vascular distension above the upper limit of autoregulation induces cerebral hyperemia, increases cerebral blood volume, and produces disruption of the blood brain barrier and vasogenic edema. The consequences of pathologic transmural pressure are associated with neurologic complications such as headache, confusion, and coma.

Several mechanisms modulate the rapid cerebrovascular response to changes in cerebral perfusion pressure, including myogenic regulation, metabolism, neurogenic regulation, and NO.

Myogenic Control of Autoregulation

The myogenic mechanism of CBF autoregulation is related to the intrinsic vasoreactivity of the cerebrovascular smooth muscle cells to changes in transmural pressure.[93] Reduced vascular distension due to decreases in transmural pressure induces dilation of the small arteries and arterioles. In contrast, increases in vascular distension due to raised transmural pressure induces arterial and arteriolar constriction. This regulatory process is related to a conformation change of the actin-myosin complex and is completed within seconds. The mechanism of myogenic regulation is likely related to changes in ionic conductance across the membrane of smooth muscle cells, which in turn adjusts membrane potentials according to the individual status of transmural pressure.[94]

Metabolic Control of Autoregulation

The concept of metabolic regulation of the pressure-flow relation suggests the release of a chemical factor in response to decreases in CBF. Consistent with the view of a metabolic mechanism, adenosine and hydrogen and potassium ions may potentially mediate CBF autoregulation. Adenosine is a potent cerebral vasodilator, and there is experimental evidence that the brain adenosine concentration increases as cerebral perfusion pressure gradually decreases.[95,96] However, CBF autoregulation was not impaired following adminis-

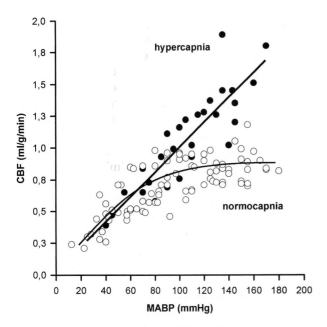

Figure 2-9   CBF autoregulation at different levels of arterial carbon dioxide tension (Pa$_{CO_2}$). (Adapted from Harper AM, Glass HI: Effect of alterations in the arterial carbon dioxide tension on the blood flow through the cerebral cortex at normal and low arterial pressures. *J Neurol Neurosurg Psychiatry* 1965; 28:449.)

oxygen concentration.[98] Arteriolar di[...] with increases in venous pressure an[...] with the induction of local hyperoxia. The[...] gest that decreases in cerebral perfusion pres[...] duce immediate decreases in CBF. The consecut[...] crease in tissue oxygen may stimulate cerebrovasc[...] dilation to compensate for the reduction in flow.

Neurogenic Control of Autoregulation

As indicated earlier in this chapter there is increasing evidence that the CNS is influenced by extrinsic neural pathways which originate from cranial autonomic ganglia.[101] These fibers form a perivascular plexus and innervate cerebral arteries and veins. The innervation is dense in the larger and smaller cerebral vessels but is less developed at the arteriolar and parenchymal levels of the cerebral circulation. Stimulation of sympathetic nerves produces cerebrovascular constriction, the magnitude of which is species-dependent.[43–45] The contribution of perivascular sympathetic nerve activity to basal cerebrovascular tone is still controversial, but the balance of the available data suggests that it is limited. Stimulation of baroreceptors, chemoreceptors, or denervation of these structures changes resting cerebrovascular tone or CBF insignificantly. However, sympathetic tone modulates the autoregulatory responses of the vasculature. With higher sympathetic tone, the consecutive cerebrovascular constriction increases the capacity of the cerebral vasculature to compensate for high cerebral perfusion pressure, i.e., the autoregulatory curve shifts to the right. In consequence, decreases in cerebral perfusion pressure are less well tolerated with the lower limit of CBF autoregulation being shifted towards higher pressures (Fig. 2-10). Acute sympathetic denervation shifts the autoregulatory curve toward lower pressures, while chronic sympathetic denervation leaves the curve unaffected.[4,102] Infusion of acetylcholine as well as the stimulation of extra-

tration of adenosine antagonists. This suggests that adenosine is not the primary mediator of CBF autoregulation but may be released secondary to hypotensive challenges. The perivascular accumulation of hydrogen and potassium ions is a consequence of increased membrane function in neurons, astrocytes, and smooth muscle cells. Hydrogen and potassium ions are mediators of the flow-metabolism coupling, and it is possible that this mechanism is also effective during CBF autoregulation. However, decreases in perivascular pH or increases in the potassium ion concentration do not occur during graded hypotension.[97] It is thus unlikely that changes in the hydrogen and potassium ion concentration are primary factors in the metabolic regulation of CBF autoregulation. In this context, changes in Pa$_{CO_2}$ may substantially modify the autoregulatory curve.[59,63] During hypercapnia, cerebral vessels are dilated, CBF is increased and there is reduced vasodilatory capacity to decreases in cerebral perfusion pressure (Fig. 2-9). In contrast, cerebral vessels are preconstricted during hypocapnia, and CBF is reduced. This augments the vasodilatory capacity to decreases in cerebral perfusion pressure. It is more likely that the metabolic component of CBF autoregulation is related to an oxygen-sensitive mechanism.[98–100] Experiments in laboratory animals have shown that decreases in arterial blood pressure induce pial arteriolar dilation secondary to a reduction in the brain tissue

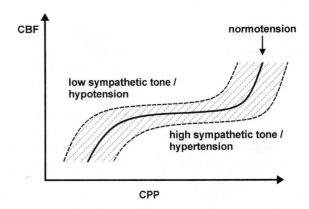

Figure 2-10   Modulation of the autoregulatory range. (Adapted from Edvinsson L, MacKenzie ET, McCulloch J: *Cerebral Blood Flow and Metabolism.* New York, Raven Press, 1993.)

...ike the major petrosal ...ilation.[53,54] While stim- ...erves elicits increases ...tion of several extrin- ...F and autoregulation. ...pathetic innervation ...cerebrovascular tone

...ation also occurs ...is reversible ...e data sug- ...sure pro- ...ve de- ...ular

only in the presence or intact endothelial cell layers.[104] This suggests that cerebrovascular dilation to decreases in cerebral perfusion pressure might be related to the activity of NO. However, CBF was maintained constant during decreases in arterial blood pressure and inhibition of NOS did not shift the lower limit of CBF autoregulation.[70] Although the available data do not support that CBF autoregulation is related to NO-sensitive mechanisms, further investigations need to study the entire autoregulatory range using different species as well as different NOS inhibitors.

Autoregulatory Failure

CBF autoregulation is a sensitive and vulnerable mechanism that can be altered, impaired, or abolished by a variety of pathologic processes. In patients with chronic systemic arterial hypertension, the autoregulatory curve is shifted toward higher pressure. This protects the brain from the hyperemia associated with elevated arterial blood pressure but decreases the tolerance of the brain to compensate for arterial hypotension.[85] The shift of the lower limit of CBF autoregulation may produce cerebral ischemia at arterial blood pressure levels within the autoregulatory range in normotensive individuals.[105] This is of clinical importance in patients with chronic hypertension who suffer from hemorrhage, shock, or during antihypertensive treatment (Fig. 2-10).

CBF autoregulation may be impaired or lost in acute ischemic lesions, following trauma, inflammation, or with diabetes mellitus and neoplasms.[106–108] Dissociation between CBF autoregulation and CO_2 reactivity is frequently observed in patients with severe head injury or cerebral ischemia. Following experimental subarachnoid hemorrhage, CBF autoregulation was lost during normocapnia but was maintained following induction of hypocapnic vasoconstriction.[109] This is consistent with the view that cerebrovascular autoregulation is a function of the preexisting cerebrovascular tone induced by the perivascular pH. Studies in patients with severe head injury have shown that CBF autoregulation was lost in 40 to 60 percent of the patients while CO_2 reactivity was maintained in most of them.[110] Loss of autoregulation is characterized by cerebral vasomotor paralysis likely due to tissue acidosis and potassium release in the area of the lesion.[85,109] Disturbed CBF autoregulation is not always restricted to the immediate vicinity of the focus. CBF autoregulation may be also impaired or abolished in areas remote from the lesion (e.g., in the hemisphere contralateral to a brain tumor or infarction). This phenomenon may be related to spreading edema or increased intracranial pressure which induces compression of contralateral cerebrovascular tissues.[85]

The status of CBF autoregulation is of clinical importance in the management of cerebral perfusion pressure following head injury. In patients with intact CBF autoregulation, maintenance of cerebral perfusion pressure > 80 mmHg downregulates cerebral blood volume while CBF is adequate.[91,100] In patients with abolished CBF autoregulation, cerebral perfusion pressures exceeding 90 mmHg will increase cerebral blood volume and intracranial pressure. High levels of cerebral perfusion pressure also promote vasogenic edema and cerebral hemorrhage. These patients may benefit from lower cerebral perfusion pressures and reduced cerebral venous blood volume. This approach was recently introduced as the "Lund concept" and combines the administration of alpha 2 adrenergic agonists, beta$_1$ antagonists, and dihydroergotamine.[111,112]

RHEOLOGY

CBF is a function of cerebral perfusion pressure and cerebrovascular resistance. Physiologic or pharmacologic challenges exert their effects on CBF by either changing pressure and/or resistance. According to the law of Hagen-Poiseuille, resistance is related to viscosity. Hematocrit is the major determinant of blood viscosity, and changes in hematocrit will change CBF as long as other determining variables of CBF remain constant. These theoretical considerations have been confirmed by most of the available studies where decreases in hematocrit were associated with an increase in CBF and cerebral blood volume.[113] The parallel rise in cerebral blood volume seen with hemodilution suggests that increases in CBF are related to active cerebrovascular dilation in response to reduced oxygen delivery and improved rheology.[114] However, hemodilution does not always change CBF. Studies in rats have shown that CBF remains constant following mannitol infusion. The maintenance of CBF is related to decreases in pial arteriolar diameter as viscosity decreases.[115,116] These data suggest that cerebral perfusion pressure changes and blood viscosity changes share the same autoregulatory mechanism.[117]

Effects of Temperature on Cerebral Blood Flow and Metabolism

In the last few years, increasing interest has developed concerning the cerebral effects of moderate hypother-

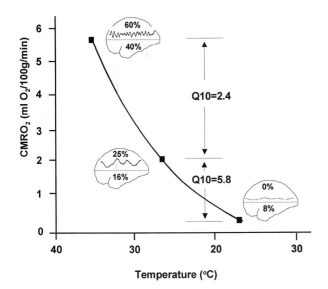

Figure 2-11   The relationship of temperature to cerebral metabolism as described by the temperature coefficient Q_{10}. (Adapted from Cucchiara RF, Michenfelder JD: *Clinical Neuroanesthesia*. Churchill-Livingstone, New York, 1990, with permission.)

mia. This is due to observations in laboratory animals and humans showing brain protection with small reductions in brain temperature during increased intracranial pressure and cerebral ischemia.[118–120] It has been suggested that hypothermic protection is related to suppression of major biochemical processes such as decreases in cerebral metabolism, reduction of excitatory neurotransmitter release,[121] and inhibition of accumulation of lipid peroxidation products and free radical generation.[122] Other studies indicate that the cerebral protective effects of hypothermia are a function of economizing CBF with the prevention of postischemic hyper- and hypoperfusion and formation of brain edema.[123] However, the mechanisms by which hypothermia changes CBF are still controversial, as is the concept of acid-base management during mild, moderate, or deep hypothermia.

CEREBRAL METABOLISM AND CBF

Hypothermia decreases cerebral metabolism in a temperature-dependent fashion. The relationship of temperature to cerebral metabolism can be described by the temperature coefficient Q_{10}. The Q_{10} value defines the ratio of two metabolic rates separated by 10°C (Fig. 2-11). For example, a Q_{10} value of 2.0 indicates that a decrease of 10°C in temperature produces a 50 percent decrease in cerebral metabolism. Q_{10} values are related to the functional status of the brain and may vary between 2.0 and 5.0.[124] The Q_{10} value is close to 2.0 within the temperature range of 37°C and 27°C as long as the EEG is active. With EEG isoelectricity at tempera-

tures less than 27°C, the substantial decrease in active and basal metabolic rate increases the Q_{10} value to 5.0. This indicates that the Q_{10} for cerebral oxygen consumption is integrally related to basal cerebral activity.[10,11] In contrast, the Q_{10} value remains around 2.0 over the entire temperature range when EEG isoelectricity is produced by barbiturate anesthesia.

Several experimental and clinical studies have investigated the effect of different levels of hypothermia on CBF in normal and ischemic subjects. Under normal conditions, 60 percent of the expenditure of energy is based on the functional activity of the CNS (which is reflected by the brain electrical activity), while the other 40 percent of energy expenditure is related to the basal metabolism that maintains cellular integrity. Barbiturates potently suppress functional metabolism with only minor or no effects on basal metabolism. In contrast, hypothermia decreases both the functional and the basal metabolic rate. This may explain why hypothermia appears to be more neuroprotective during critical reductions in cerebral substrate supply.[10,11] Rosomoff and Holaday[125] were among the first to measure CBF and cerebral oxygen consumption during hypothermia. In their dog studies, progressive hypothermia (35 to 26°C) resulted in decreases in CBF secondary to decreases in cerebral oxygen consumption. This is consistent with data from isoflurane anesthetized dogs[126] and pentobarbital anesthetized monkeys[127] (37 to 22°C) showing hypothermia-induced decreases in CBF and cerebral oxygen consumption. In patients undergoing hypothermic cardiopulmonary bypass, CBF decreased with time, while cerebral oxygen consumption remained constant.[128] Since the relationship between cerebral oxygen consumption-reduction and CBF changes was not always linear during hypothermia,[126–128] other factors appear to be involved. In support of this, Hägerdal and coworkers[129] found decreases in CBF and cerebral oxygen consumption to a similar extent in N_2O/O_2 anesthetized rats, but there was a substantial scatter in the individual CBF values between 32 and 27°C. In dogs and monkeys subjected to 48 h of hypothermia (28°C), the pattern of cerebral perfusion was regionally specific with areas of complete nonperfusion next to well-perfused territories.[130,131] This specific CBF pattern was not associated with the cerebral metabolic state and may be consistent with the observation that hypothermic brain protection is related to areas with high excitatory neurotransmitter turnover.[120]

CEREBRAL BLOOD FLOW AUTOREGULATION

Does hypothermia influence regulatory mechanisms of CBF? Experiments in halothane anesthetized rats indicate that CBF autoregulation is maintained during hypothermia (30.5°C).[132] This is consistent with studies in rabbits[133] and patients[134,135] during hypothermic cardiopulmonary bypass, where changes in pump flow and/or mean arterial blood pressure did not change CBF. However, CBF autoregulation in experimental animals and patients with or without cardiopulmonary bypass was directly dependent on the management of arterial carbon dioxide tension (Pa_{CO_2}) and arterial pH (pHa). While hypothermia decreases cerebral oxygen consumption in a fairly predictable fashion, the variability of hypothermic CBF is likely due to the nonuniformity of acid-base management during hypothermia.

ACID-BASE MANAGEMENT

The choice of the acid-base management critically determines dynamic CBF. Using the pH-stat approach, Pa_{CO_2} and pHa are maintained at 40 mmHg and 7.4 respectively, as corrected for the actual temperature of the patient. Owing to the increased plasma solubility of CO_2 during hypothermia, pH-stat management produces relative hypercapnia and acidemia. With alpha-stat management (referring to the alpha-imidazole ring of the histidine amino acid moiety of hemoglobin), Pa_{CO_2} and pHa are measured at 37°C and maintained at 40 mmHg and 7.4, respectively, uncorrected for the actual temperature of the patient. This technique is believed to maintain intracellular pH close to the temperature-dependent electrochemical neutrality, thus preserving protein charge state, structure, and function.[136]

In hypothermic animals and humans, CBF did not change with decreases in arterial blood pressure during alpha-stat conditions.[132–135] This indicates preserved CBF autoregulation. In contrast, CBF was linearly decreased with graded hypotension when blood gases were managed according to pH-stat conditions.[137,138] In patients undergoing hypothermic cardiopulmonary bypass and alpha-stat conditions, CBF was independent of cerebral perfusion pressure but linearly related to cerebral oxygen consumption.[22,23] In contrast, CBF was correlated with cerebral perfusion pressure while flow/metabolism coupling was not maintained during pH-stat management. This is likely due to the nonphysiologic hypercapnia induced by the pH-stat technique. During hypercapnia, cerebral resistance vessels are dilated, CBF is increased, and the autoregulatory plateau narrowed because of reduced dilatory capacity to keep CBF constant with hypotension.[85] This shows that experimental and clinical CBF dynamics during hypothermia are dependent on the preexisting cerebrovascular tone induced by the individual acid-base management.

CO₂-REACTIVITY

Differences in CBF between pH-stat and alpha-stat management depend on preserved responsiveness of the cerebral vasculature to changes in Pa_{CO_2}. Because CO_2-reactivity varies with baseline CBF, it has been hypothesized that hypothermia-induced reductions in CBF would decrease CO_2-reactivity. In rats subjected to hypothermia (22°C), changes in CBF were of the same relative magnitude compared to normothermia within the Pa_{CO_2} range of 35 to 60 mmHg. However, decreases in CBF were much more pronounced with Pa_{CO_2} values of less than 30 mmHg during hypothermia.[139] Hindman and coworkers[140] tested the effects of different Pa_{CO_2} levels (20, 40, 60 mmHg Pa_{CO_2} temperature corrected) on CBF in rabbits with cardiopulmonary bypass. They found hypothermia-induced reductions in CBF but without differences in the CO_2-reactivity between the normothermic and hypothermic animals. This suggests that hypothermia either increased the sensitivity of the cerebral vasculature to CO_2, or increased the effective level of cerebral spinal fluid respiratory acidosis produced by each increment of temperature corrected Pa_{CO_2}. Maintenance of CO_2-reactivity has also been shown in patients undergoing hypothermic cardiopulmonary bypass[134,141,142] as long as the alpha-stat management of blood gases is used.

Effects of Anesthetics and Anesthetic Adjuvants on Cerebral Blood Flow, Metabolism and Intracranial Pressure

Neurosurgical patients require specific anesthetic regimens that will maintain coupling between cerebral metabolism and CBF while achieving hypnosis, analgesia, and low central sympathetic tone. Anesthetic and narcotic agents substantially change CBF, cerebral oxygen consumption, and intracranial pressure. Since all of the anesthetic agents and adjuvants currently available for neuroanesthetic practice present advantages and disadvantages, any narrow anesthetic concept may potentiate neurologic damage. Instead, anesthetic treatment of neurosurgical patients must be based on knowledge of how the selected agents affect CBF, metabolism, and intracranial pressure in order to titrate care according to individual pathophysiology.

INHALATIONAL ANESTHETICS

The inhalational anesthetics halothane, isoflurane, sevoflurane, and desflurane depress cerebral metabolism in a dose-dependent fashion while producing direct cerebral vasodilation with increasing concentrations of the volatile agent. This results in increases in cerebral blood volume and intracranial pressure, which are most pronounced in the presence of nitrous oxide. In contrast to halothane, isoflurane, sevoflurane, or desflurane, cerebral metabolism appears to be stimulated

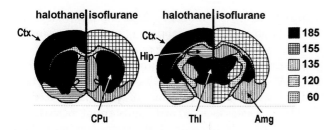

Figure 2-12 Distribution of regional CBF in rats anesthetized with halothane or isoflurane. (Adapted from Hansen TD, et al: Distribution of cerebral blood flow during halothane versus isoflurane anesthesia in rats. *Anesthesiology* 1988; 69:332.)

with N₂O, which in turn increases CBF and intracranial pressure.

HALOTHANE, ISOFLURANE
Halothane and isoflurane decrease cerebrovascular resistance and increase CBF.[143,144] This increase in CBF is not related to cerebral metabolic stimulation rather than to direct cerebrovascular dilation. Studies in N₂O-anesthetized cats have shown that incremental concentrations of isoflurane (0.5 to 1.5 MAC) depress cerebral oxygen consumption in a dose-dependent fashion without changing cortical CBF.[145] In contrast, both isoflurane and halothane increased CBF in barbiturate-anesthetized rabbits.[144] These results suggest that the cerebrovascular effects of isoflurane and halothane are related to the cerebral metabolic state before the agents are administered.

Inconsistencies in regional CBF among the numerous animal studies may be also related to differences in the spatial resolution of the measurement techniques used in these investigations. Measurements of cortical CBF using the xenon-133 injection technique have shown that CBF was increased with halothane while cortical CBF was unchanged with isoflurane despite decreases in cerebrovascular resistance.[145] This suggests that isoflurane and halothane produce regionally specific changes in CBF. In support of this, autoradiographic CBF measurements found substantial differences in regional CBF between isoflurane and halothane. While hemispheric CBF was similar with the two agents, neocortical CBF was higher with halothane and subcortical CBF was higher with isoflurane[146] (Fig. 2-12).

Increasing concentrations of isoflurane reduce cerebral metabolism until EEG isoelectricity.[143,144,147] The cerebral metabolic depression appears to be greater with isoflurane than with halothane.[145] With EEG isoelectricity, further increases in the isoflurane concentrations had no effect on cerebral metabolism. At high isoflurane concentrations (4 MAC), brain biopsy analyses revealed normal concentrations of ATP, phosphocreatine and normal energy charges.[147] This indicates

that isoflurane does not abolish cerebral cortical activity at the price of toxic effects on cerebral metabolic pathways.

Inhalational anesthetics depress cerebral metabolism in a dose-dependent fashion. However, the decreases in global cerebral metabolism are associated with increases in global CBF due to direct cerebral vasodilation with increasing concentrations of the volatile agent. It was therefore generally concluded that CBF and metabolism are uncoupled with increasing concentrations of volatile anesthetic agents. However, autoradiographic measurements of CBF and cerebral glucose consumption have shown that local coupling of flow and metabolism is well maintained[148] (Fig. 2-13). Territories with high metabolic rates presented the highest flow values at each respective MAC level; areas with low metabolic rates presented the lowest flows.[148]

In general, cerebrovascular CO₂ reactivity is maintained with halothane and isoflurane but there may be quantitative differences between the two agents. In cats, the CO₂ reactivity was greater during 1 MAC isoflurane compared with 1 MAC halothane.[149] This is consistent with studies in dogs showing cerebral vasoconstriction to hypocapnia with 1 and 2 MAC isoflurane.[150] However, CO₂ reactivity to hypercapnia may be impaired or abolished at anesthetic concentrations > 2 MAC owing to the preexisting cerebral vasodilation. During 3 h of isoflurane anesthesia, cerebral

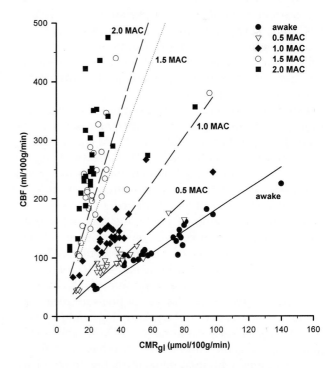

Figure 2-13 Relation between CBF and cerebral glucose consumption at different levels of isoflurane anesthesia. (Modified with permission from Warner DL, Duke University, and Maekawa T, et al. *Anesthesiology* 1986; 65:144, with permission.)

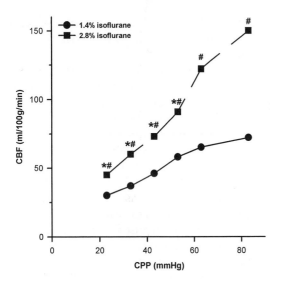

Figure 2-14 CBF autoregulation at 1 MAC and 2 MAC isoflurane anesthesia. (Redrawn from McPherson RW, Traystman RJ: Effects of isoflurane on cerebral autoregulation in dogs. *Anesthesiology* 1988; 69:493, with permission.)

CO_2 reactivity decreases over time, as does normocapnic CBF.[151] CBF autoregulation is modulated by the concentration of the inhalational anesthetic. In cats and dogs, CBF autoregulation was maintained within the mean arterial blood pressure range of 85 to 120 mmHg with 1 MAC isoflurane but was impaired with 1 MAC halothane. However, increases in CBF occurred with increases in cerebral perfusion pressure during 2 MAC isoflurane, indicating impaired CBF autoregulation with higher concentrations of isoflurane[152] (Fig. 2-14). This is likely related to decreases in baseline cerebrovascular tone as the concentration of the inhalational anesthetic agent increases.

In animal experimentation, isoflurane produces less brain surface protrusion and smaller increases in intracranial pressure at 0.5, 1.0, and 1.5 MAC isoflurane compared with halothane.[145,153] This effect appears to be consistent with the substantial increases in cortical CBF seen with halothane but not isoflurane anesthesia. In fentanyl/droperidol-anesthetized hypocapnic baboons, administration of isoflurane did not significantly change CBF or cerebral blood volume.[154] However, the combination of isoflurane with N_2O may increase cerebral blood volume and intracranial pressure even in the presence of hypocapnia.[155,156] This suggests that increases in intracranial pressure seen with isoflurane are related to the preexisting cerebrovascular tone induced by isocapnia or N_2O. In rabbits subjected to cryogenic brain injury, halothane anesthesia was associated with less edema formation in the vicinity of the insult compared with isoflurane, although the animals may have differed in the severity of the lesion and intracranial hypertension.[157]

In humans, the effects of isoflurane and halothane on CBF and cerebral metabolism appear to be similar to the results from studies in laboratory animals. In neurosurgical patients, isoflurane anesthesia (0.65 to 1.5 MAC) produced only minor changes in cortical CBF, whereas administration of halothane (0.65 to 1.5 MAC) was associated with substantial increases in cortical CBF.[158-160] In contrast, the reduction in cerebral metabolism was more pronounced with isoflurane compared to halothane at any given MAC level.[159,160] Measurements of the regional distribution of CBF during 1 MAC isoflurane versus 1 MAC halothane anesthesia have confirmed autoradiographic studies in rats where subcortical CBF was higher with isoflurane while cortical CBF was higher with halothane anesthesia.[161] Cerebrovascular CO_2 reactivity was also maintained with isoflurane and halothane anesthesia in clinically relevant concentrations.[161]

Intracranial pressure increases during isoflurane anesthesia in normocapnic neurosurgical patients, but this effect is reversible with hyperventilation or infusion of barbiturates.[162,163] Available data suggest that inhalation of isoflurane in concentrations lower than 1 MAC and in combination with hypocapnia is not associated with clinically relevant increases in intracranial pressure.

SEVOFLURANE, DESFLURANE

Sevoflurane and desflurane are inhalational anesthetic agents with lower blood/gas partition coefficients than halothane or isoflurane. The low solubility of these inhalational anesthetics is associated with more rapid pharmacokinetics, promising fast induction and emergence from anesthesia.

Sevoflurane has effects on CBF, cerebral metabolism, and intracranial pressure similar to isoflurane. In 1 MAC sevoflurane-anesthetized rats without controlled ventilation, CBF was increased 35 percent compared with the awake state.[164] However, increases in CBF with sevoflurane may have been due to the hypercapnic effect induced by the anesthetic state. Sevoflurane decreases cerebral metabolic rate. In morphine/N_2O-anesthetized rabbits, 1 MAC sevoflurane or isoflurane produced a 50 percent reduction in cerebral oxygen consumption in parallel to EEG burst-suppression with no evidence of spike or seizure activity, while global and cortical CBF did not change.[165] Intracranial pressure was increased despite the fact that CBF did not change. This indicates dilation of cerebral capacitance vessels and a nonlinear relation between CBF and cerebral blood volume with the administration of sevoflurane and isoflurane.[165]

Desflurane (0.5 to 2.0 MAC) produces a dose-related decrease in canine cerebral oxygen consumption.[166] The cerebral metabolic suppression seen with desflurane was associated with suppression of cortical electrical activity. The cerebrovascular responses to desflurane are related to the status of cerebral perfusion pressure. CBF was unchanged when cerebral perfusion pressure decreased with increasing concentrations of desflurane. In contrast, CBF increased when cerebral perfusion pressure was maintained using phenylephrine infusion. This suggests that CBF autoregulation is impaired during desflurane in concentrations >1 MAC. This is consistent with results in dogs, where desflurane-induced systemic hypotension (mean arterial blood pressure: 40 mmHg) decreased CBF 60 percent and cerebral oxygen consumption 21 percent.[167] However, normal cerebral metabolite concentrations of high-energy phosphates taken at the end of the hypotensive challenge suggest that CBF was still adequate to meet cerebral metabolic demands. In desflurane-anesthetized dogs (0.5–1.5 MAC) with and without systemic hypotension, cerebrovascular CO_2 reactivity to hypocapnia (Pa_{CO_2}: 20 mmHg) was maintained, although attenuation occurs at higher MAC levels.[168] In dogs, desflurane increases intracranial pressure due to general cerebrovascular dilation, but this effect appears not to be dose-related.[166]

In hyperventilated neurosurgical patients, CBF was similar with 1.0 MAC desflurane compared with 1.0 MAC isoflurane.[169] CBF did not change when desflurane or isoflurane concentrations were increased to 1.5 MAC. Cerebrovascular reactivity to CO_2 was maintained with both anesthetics within the Pa_{CO_2} range of 25 to 35 mmHg. This is consistent with results from patients with ischemic cerebrovascular disease and 0.88 MAC sevoflurane anesthesia, where cerebrovascular CO_2 reactivity was maintained within a Pa_{CO_2} range of 35 to 45 mmHg.[170] In these patients, CBF remained unchanged within the mean arterial blood pressure range of 89 to 113 mmHg, indicating preserved CBF autoregulation. In patients with supratentorial mass lesions, cerebrospinal fluid pressure measured in the lumbar subarachnoid space may increase during 1 MAC desflurane anesthesia but not during 1 MAC isoflurane anesthesia.[171] Experiments in dogs suggest that the increases in cerebrospinal fluid pressure seen during desflurane anesthesia are related to an imbalance between the formation and reabsorption of cerebrospinal fluid.[172]

NITROUS OXIDE
Administration of N_2O is associated with substantial changes in CBF and cerebral metabolism. N_2O increases CBF, cerebral blood volume, and intracranial pressure and there is considerable controversy whether N_2O should be avoided as a supplemental anesthetic/analgetic in neurosurgical patients.

In unanesthetized laboratory animals, inhalation of 70 percent N_2O increased CBF and cerebral oxygen consumption in a regionally specific fashion.[173,174] However, the background anesthetic state changes the metabolic responses to N_2O. Experiments in rabbits anesthetized with halothane, isoflurane, or fentanyl/pentobarbital have shown that 70 percent N_2O increases CBF during normocapnia and hypocapnia without affecting cerebral metabolism.[175] This is consistent with experiments in halothane- or isoflurane-anesthetized normocapnic rats where 0.5 MAC N_2O increased CBF with both background anesthetics while cerebral glucose consumption remained unchanged.[176,177] N_2O appears to be a stimulator of cortical functional activity. In dogs, isoflurane-induced isoelectricity was reversed with the addition of N_2O, although cerebral metabolism did not change.[178] In humans anesthetized with propofol sufficient to induce EEG isoelectricity, N_2O stimulates neuronal activity and cerebral metabolism as indicated by recurrence of EEG activity and increased cerebral oxygen extraction.[179] Together, these data indicate that N_2O is a potent cerebral vasodilator that increases CBF by mechanisms other than cerebral metabolic activation. However, the vasodilation induced by N_2O is related to the baseline cerebrovascular tone induced by the background anesthetic. N_2O increases cerebral blood volume, which in turn raises intracranial pressure, and this effect occurs regardless of differences in baseline cerebrovascular tone. In rabbits anesthetized with either halothane, isoflurane, or fentanyl/pentobarbital, the administration of 70 percent N_2O was associated with increases in intracranial pressure during normocapnia and even hypocapnia.[175] This is consistent with studies in dogs showing increases in cerebral blood volume when 50 percent N_2O was given in fentanyl-background anesthesia.[160]

The cerebrovascular effects of N_2O in man are similar to animal data. In awake, normocapnic humans, inhalation of 30, 50, or 60 percent N_2O increased regional and global CBF during normocapnia and hypocapnia.[180,181] In contrast, CBF increased 43 percent during normocapnia but was unchanged during hypocapnia in isoflurane-anesthetized patients.[182] In this study, cerebral oxygen consumption was unchanged while spontaneous brain electrical activity increased with the administration of N_2O. These data support results from animal studies suggesting some interaction between the cerebrovascular responses to N_2O and the background anesthetic technique. While cerebrovascular CO_2 reactivity may be reduced during N_2O inhalation, the regional distribution of CBF is related to the level of Pa_{CO_2}.[181] During hypocapnia, inhalation of 50 percent N_2O increased CBF to frontal, parietal, and temporal brain structures as well as to the thalamus and basal ganglia compared with hypocapnic CBF without

N_2O.[181] Several clinical reports indicate that N_2O increases intracranial pressure.[183,184] The rise in intracranial pressure seen with the administration of N_2O appears to be reduced with the induction of hypocapnia or the infusion of cerebral vasoconstrictors. This suggests that the increase in intracranial pressure is related to increases in CBF and cerebral blood volume as suggested by animal experiments. However, clinical studies have shown that inhalation of N_2O was not associated with increases in intracranial pressure following dural closure in neurosurgical patients.[185] This suggests that it is not necessary to discontinue N_2O for reasons of avoiding expansion of intracranial air.

INTRAVENOUS ANESTHETICS

Intravenous anesthetic agents are considered as cerebral vasoconstrictors, an effect which appears to be secondary to the suppression of cerebral metabolic rate. Cerebrovascular constriction with intravenous anesthetics reduces cerebral blood volume and intracranial pressure as long as ventilation is controlled to prevent hypercapnia. Experimental studies indicate decreases in infarct size following cerebral ischemia as long as the anesthetic agents are infused prior to the ischemic challenge. Despite speculation concerning potential brain protective effects, total intravenous anesthesia may prolong emergence from anesthesia and critically decrease cerebral perfusion pressure.

BARBITURATES

In laboratory animals, infusion of thiopental produced dose-dependent decreases of cerebral oxygen consumption and suppression of the spontaneous EEG until EEG burst-suppression.[186] A similar reduction in CBF and cerebral oxygen consumption has been reported with phenobarbital and pentobarbital.[187,188] This cerebral metabolic and functional depression was paralleled by increases in cerebrovascular resistance and concomitant decreases in CBF. With maximal suppression of cortical functional activity (EEG isoelectricity), cerebral oxygen consumption or CBF remain constant despite further increases in barbiturate plasma concentration. This indicates coupling of cerebral functional activity, cerebral oxygen consumption, and CBF during barbiturate infusion. Cerebrovascular reactivity to CO_2 is qualitatively maintained but quantitatively reduced as a function of increases in cerebrovascular resistance due to the barbiturate. In contrast to time-dependent changes in the cerebrovascular responses to CO_2 during isoflurane anesthesia, CO_2 reactivity does not change with barbiturates over time.[151]

In volunteers, infusion of thiopental (10 to 55 mg/kg total dose) was associated with 50 to 55 percent decreases in cerebral oxygen consumption and CBF

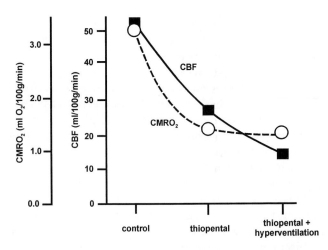

Figure 2-15 Effect of thiopental and hyperventilation on human CBF and cerebral oxygen consumption. (Adapted from original data in Pierce EC, et al: Cerebral circulation and metabolism during thiopental anesthesia and hyperventilation in man. *J Clin Invest* 1962; 41:1664, and Kety SS, Schmidt CF: The determination of cerebral blood flow in man by the use of nitrous oxide in low concentrations. *Am J Physiol* 1945; 143:53.)

compared to values reported in previous studies[58,189] (Fig. 2-15). Cerebrovascular CO_2 reactivity was also maintained. Patients with increased intracranial pressure may thus benefit from bolus applications of barbiturates as well as from transient hyperventilation during barbiturate background anesthesia since the reduction in intracranial blood volume can reduce intracranial pressure.[190] However, barbiturate infusion may lead to cerebral ischemia in patients with elevated intracranial pressure whenever the administration produces concomitant decreases in mean arterial blood pressure and therefore cerebral perfusion pressure.

ETOMIDATE

Studies in laboratory animals indicate that etomidate produces a dose-dependent reduction in cerebral oxygen consumption (maximal suppression of functional metabolism is indicated by EEG burst-suppression) and CBF.[191] In contrast to the barbiturates, CBF and cerebral oxygen consumption were decreased in a nonlinear fashion. Near maximal reduction of CBF was induced by low doses of etomidate (0.02 mg/kg per min), while increasing concentrations of etomidate (0.3 mg/kg per min) produced progressive suppression of cerebral oxygen consumption until EEG burst-suppression without further decreases in CBF. This suggests that etomidate decreases canine CBF by two mechanisms: (1) direct cerebrovascular constriction; (2) suppression of functional metabolism. Unlike barbiturates, etomidate changes cerebral metabolism in a regionally specific fashion. Etomidate decreases cerebral glucose consumption predominantly in frontal and parietal brain areas, while metabolic suppression is less pronounced in occipital tissue.[192]

In humans, clinically relevant concentrations of etomidate (0.02 to 0.06 mg/kg per min) produced concomitant decreases in cerebral oxygen consumption and CBF.[193] The cerebrovascular reactivity to CO_2 was maintained with etomidate. Systemic hemodynamic depression was less pronounced with etomidate than with barbiturate infusion. Studies in head-injured patients have shown that etomidate administration decreases intracranial pressure with only minor reductions in mean arterial blood pressure or cerebral perfusion pressure.[194] In this regard, etomidate appears to be superior to barbiturates or propofol.

PROPOFOL

The cerebrovascular effects of propofol are similar to those reported for barbiturates or etomidate. Propofol produces a dose-dependent reduction of cerebral oxygen consumption and CBF.[195,196] With the induction of EEG isoelectricity, further increases in the propofol plasma concentration did not change cerebral oxygen consumption or CBF. In vitro studies indicate that propofol is a cerebral vasodilator by mechanisms which reduce Ca^{2+}-influx via voltage-dependent Ca^{2+}-channels. The fact that propofol decreases CBF in animals suggests that in vivo cerebrovascular constriction occurs secondary to metabolic suppression. Studies in laboratory animals have shown that the cerebrovascular reactivity to CO_2 is maintained even with high doses of propofol (48 mg/kg per h).[195] The effects of propofol on CBF autoregulation are controversial. In dogs, propofol infusion of 48 mg/kg per h was associated with impaired CBF autoregulation when cerebral perfusion pressure was decreased from 76 ± 14 mmHg to 42 ± 11 mmHg.[195] In contrast, studies in rats found CBF autoregulation maintained within a mean arterial blood pressure range of 50 to 140 mmHg with doses as high as 120 mg/kg per h[197] (Fig. 2-16).

In cardiac patients, propofol infusion (12 mg/kg per h) was associated with parallel decreases in cerebral oxygen consumption and CBF.[198] However, cerebral metabolic depression was more pronounced in cortical than in subcortical tissue.[199] Cerebrovascular reactivity to CO_2 was also maintained with propofol (3 to 12 mg/kg per h).[198] Propofol reduces intracranial pressure in a fashion comparable to barbiturates or etomidate.[200,201] However, propofol may critically reduce cerebral perfusion pressure, although the extent of this response is related to the propofol dose, speed of infusion, and preexisting volume status of the patients. Recent data suggest that infusion of propofol may be associated with the occurrence of convulsions or EEG abnormalities. Although propofol has been associated with grand-mal seizures and has been used for cortical mapping of epileptogenic foci, no controlled study has proved any intrinsic epileptogenic effects of propofol.[202]

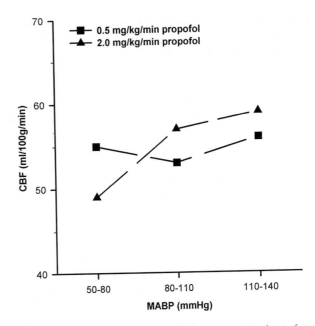

Figure 2-16 CBF autoregulation at different concentrations of propofol. (Redrawn from Werner C, et al: The effects of propofol on cerebral and spinal cord blood flow in rats. *Anesth Analg* 1993; 76:971.)

BENZODIAZEPINES

The benzodiazepines produce hypnosis, sedation, anxiolysis, amnesia, and anticonvulsive activity. The clinical effects and side effects of benzodiazepines can be reversed by a specific antagonist, as recovery from sedation or anesthesia following benzodiazepine infusion may be prolonged.

Benzodiazepines reduce CBF in a dose-dependent fashion in laboratory animals. This effect occurs secondary to cerebral metabolic suppression.[203] However, benzodiazepines appear to have some direct vasoconstrictor effects on cerebral vessels within the low-dose range. Studies in dogs have shown that the infusion of midazolam (0.2 mg/kg) produces decreases in CBF without changing cerebral oxygen consumption.[204] This "uncoupling" between CBF and cerebral oxygen consumption was not associated with electrophysiologic or biochemical evidence of cerebral ischemia. The infusion of higher doses of midazolam (2 to 10 mg/kg) was associated with a parallel reduction of CBF and cerebral oxygen consumption.[205]

In patients, midazolam produced concomitant decreases in cerebral oxygen consumption and CBF when fentanyl was given as a background narcotic agent.[206] CBF autoregulation and cerebrovascular CO_2-reactivity are maintained with benzodiazepines. Decreases in

CBF following benzodiazepine infusion are not associated with substantial changes in cerebral blood volume. This suggests that benzodiazepines should be less effective in decreasing intracranial pressure in patients with low intracranial elastance but may be effective in patients with high intracranial elastance. In support of this hypothesis, intracranial pressure remained unaffected in patients with a normal intracranial elastance following midazolam.[207] In contrast, intracranial pressure was decreased following midazolam in patients with intracranial hypertension.

NARCOTICS

Over the last few years there has been an interesting and controversial discussion concerning the cerebrovascular effects of narcotic agents. In vivo experiments using the cranial window technique have shown that fentanyl, alfentanil, and sufentanil produce dose-dependent pial arteriolar vasoconstriction. These results are in line with data from experiments in N_2O-anesthetized laboratory animals and humans showing decreases in CBF secondary to cerebral metabolic suppression following fentanyl (6 to 400 g/kg) or sufentanil (<20 g/kg). CBF autoregulation as well as cerebrovascular reactivity to changes in arterial CO_2 were maintained in these studies.[208-211] In contrast, sufentanil (10 to 200 g/kg) may increase CBF when infused to paralyzed, mechanically ventilated dogs (no N_2O) without background anesthesia. However, this response is completely abolished in the presence of N_2O.[212] This is consistent with the view that the responses of CBF to opioid infusion are related to the baseline cerebrovascular tone induced by N_2O.[173]

Several studies indicate that infusion of opioids may affect intracranial pressure in response to decreases in cerebral perfusion pressure. Intracranial pressure was increased following fentanyl (3.0 g/kg) or sufentanil (0.6 to 1.0 g/kg) in patients with head injury and normal or elevated intracranial pressure.[213,214] In these patients, the administration of opioids was consistently associated with decreases in mean arterial blood pressure, and increases in intracranial pressure are likely related to autoregulatory vasodilation of cerebral vessels secondary to systemic hypotension. This autoregulatory response will decrease cerebrovascular resistance, raise cerebral blood volume, and in turn increase intracranial pressure. In support of this, studies in piritramide-anesthetized dogs with and without intracranial hypertension and controlled mean arterial blood pressure have shown that intracranial pressure was constant following 2 g/kg sufentanil.[215] This is consistent with studies in midazolam-sedated, head-injured patients where sufentanil (0.5 to 2.0 g/kg) did not change intracranial pressure as long as mean arterial blood pressure was maintained constant.[216,217] The

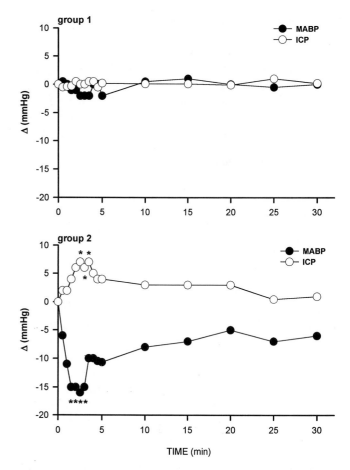

Figure 2-17 The effects of sufentanil on intracranial pressure in head-injured patients: Relation to mean arterial blood pressure (MABP). (Redrawn from Werner C, et al: The effects of sufentanil on cerebral hemodynamics and intracranial pressure in patients with brain injury. *Anesthesiology* 1995, 83:721.)

available data indicate that narcotic agents can be used in hyperventilated patients with intracranial hypertension and controlled mean arterial blood pressure[217] (Fig. 2-17).

KETAMINE

The phencyclidine derivative, ketamine, is a noncompetitive *N*-methyl-D-aspartate (NMDA) receptor antagonist with the thalamo-neocortical projection system as the primary site of action. Ketamine induces regional neuronal excitation and produces a cataleptoid state with dose-related unconsciousness and analgesia. Ketamine has hardly ever been considered as an adequate anesthetic agent in neurosurgical patients since it produces regionally specific stimulation of cerebral metabolism and increases CBF and intracranial pressure. However, recent experiments suggest that ketamine may reduce infarct size in animal models of incomplete cerebral ischemia and brain injury. This experimental protective effect appears to be related to decreases in Ca^{2+}-influx and maintenance of brain tissue magnesium due to the NMDA and quisqualate receptor blockade of ketamine.

Studies in dogs and patients have shown that ketamine (1.1 to 2.0 mg/kg) reduces CBF in the presence of cerebral vasodilators like halothane or N_2O.[218,219] In contrast, studies in awake animals (100 mg/kg IP) and humans (2 to 3 mg/kg) found increases in CBF with ketamine.[200-222] This suggests that the cerebrovascular effects of ketamine are related to the preexisting cerebrovascular tone induced by background anesthetics. Cerebrovascular CO_2 reactivity was maintained regardless of the baseline cerebrovascular resistance. There are several mechanisms by which ketamine may increase CBF. Ketamine induces a dose-dependent respiratory depression with consecutive mild hypercapnia in spontaneously ventilating subjects. This produces vasodilation based on the intact cerebrovascular CO_2 reactivity. Ketamine also induces regional neuroexcitation. This leads to stimulation of cerebral glucose consumption in the limbic, extrapyramidal, auditory, and sensory-motor systems.[220,222] This regional neuroexcitation with consecutive increases in cerebral metabolism produces increases in CBF which can be blocked with the infusion of barbiturates or benzodiazepines. However, increases in CBF with ketamine (1 mg/kg) may also occur during isocapnia and without changes in cerebral metabolism.[223] This indicates some additional direct cerebral vasodilating potency of ketamine.[224]

Infusion of ketamine alters intracranial volume and intracranial pressure. Studies in spontaneously ventilating pigs with and without intracranial hypertension have shown that ketamine (0.5 to 5.0 mg/kg) produced increases in Pa_{CO_2} and intracranial pressure.[225] In contrast, identical experiments with mechanical ventilation and controlled Pa_{CO_2} found no changes in intracranial pressure following ketamine infusion. This shows that increases in intracranial pressure are related to inadequate ventilation with consecutive hypercapnia and increases in intracranial blood volume.[226] However, mechanical ventilation may not be sufficient to control intracranial pressure following ketamine. Experiments in mechanically ventilated dogs indicate that ketamine (2 mg/kg) increases cerebral blood volume and intracranial pressure even in the presence of normoventilation, a response that is reversible with hyperventilation or the administration of diazepam. Studies in humans with and without intracranial pathology confirm the data from animal experiments. In patients, increases in intracranial pressure appear to be most pronounced when baseline intracranial pressure is elevated and when the infusion of ketamine induces hypercapnia with consecutive increases in cerebral blood volume.[225,227] This is consistent with the

view that infusion of ketamine is not indicated in patients with intracranial hypertension.

ALPHA-2-ADRENERGIC AGONISTS

Clonidine and dexmedetomidine are alpha-2-adrenergic agonists. The clinical effects of these anesthetic adjuvants are related to stimulation of alpha-2-adrenergic receptors, which reduces secretion of norepinephrine from presynaptic sympathetic nerve terminals. The reduction in central and peripheral sympathetic tone produces systemic hypotension, sedation, and analgesia. In laboratory animals, stimulation of alpha-2-receptors was associated with a reduction of the minimal alveolar concentration (MAC) for halothane of 48 percent with clonidine and of almost 100 percent with dexmedetomidine.[228,229] These results are consistent with clinical studies showing a reduction in the requirements of barbiturates and isoflurane with perioperative administration of dexmedetomidine.[230,231] The increasing clinical interest in alpha-2-adrenergic agonists is due to experimental and clinical observations showing excellent hemodynamic stability associated with substantial reductions in the concentrations and side effects of intravenous and volatile anesthetics as well as an increased tolerance of the brain during ischemic challenges.

Infusion of clonidine (20 g/kg) produced a 37 percent reduction in CBF in barbiturate-anesthetized cats.[232] In the same experiments, CBF autoregulation was maintained within a mean arterial blood pressure range of 60 to 180 mmHg. This is in contrast to studies in dogs, where infusion of the more potent alpha-2-adrenergic agonist dexmedetomidine (10 g/kg) decreased CBF only in the presence of isoflurane and halothane but not barbiturates. However, cerebral oxygen consumption did not change regardless of the background anesthetic.[233,234] The "uncoupling" between cerebral metabolism and CBF did not induce cerebral ischemia. This indicates that the changes in CBF induced by alpha-2-adrenergic agonists are related to the baseline cerebrovascular dilation induced by volatile anesthetics. The qualitative cerebrovascular reactivity to CO_2 is maintained with clonidine[232] or dexmedetomidine[233] but may be reduced by >50 percent compared with subjects without alpha-2-adrenergic stimulation. This is likely related to the increased cerebrovascular tone induced by clonidine or dexmedetomidine which in part antagonizes the vasodilating stimulation of CO_2. The cerebral vasoconstriction of alpha-2-adrenergic agonists affects both the arterial and the capacitance vessels with consecutive reductions in cerebral blood volume. This is suggested by studies in dogs with subarachnoid hemorrhage showing dose-related decreases in intracranial pressure with the alpha-2-adrenergic agonist xylazine.[235] In contrast, experiments in rabbits with low and high elastance states found no decreases in intracranial pressure following dexmedetomidine (20 to 320 g/kg).[236]

In summary, the inhalational anesthetics isoflurane, sevoflurane, and desflurane depress cerebral metabolism in a dose-dependent fashion. However, the decreases in cerebral metabolism are not associated with a linear decrease in CBF. Inhalational anesthetics produce direct cerebral vasodilation with increasing concentrations of the volatile agent. This uncoupling between CBF and cerebral metabolism may result in increases in cerebral blood volume and intracranial pressure that are most pronounced in the presence of N_2O. In contrast, cerebral metabolism appears to be unaffected or stimulated with N_2O. As with the other inhalational anesthetics, CBF is increased with N_2O. The administration of hypnotics, benzodiazepines, opioids, and alpha-2-agonists is associated with a reduction in CBF. With these agents, the reduction in CBF occurs secondary to cerebral metabolic suppression, except for alpha-2-agonists, where decreases in CBF appear to be related to decreases in central sympathetic tone. Ketamine infusion induces regionally-specific changes in CBF and cerebral metabolism, with areas of the brain showing stimulation and areas showing suppression in CBF and cerebral metabolism. Hypnotic agents reduce intracranial pressure, while benzodiazepines may reduce intracranial pressure only in the presence of intracranial hypertension but not during normal intracranial pressure. However, all hypnotic agents may reduce mean arterial blood pressure. This decreases cerebral perfusion pressure despite the reduction in intracranial pressure. Narcotic agents may increase intracranial pressure in parallel to decreases in cerebral perfusion pressure. This response appears to be due to autoregulatory cerebral vasodilation. Ketamine may increase intracranial pressure, particularly in normocapnic subjects. However, the induction of hypocapnia attenuates the rise in intracranial pressure seen with ketamine. The infusion of alpha-2-adrenergic agonists produces a transient reduction in intracranial pressure.

Measurement of CBF and Metabolism

Several pathologic conditions are associated with an imbalance of cerebral substrate delivery and demand. Cerebral ischemia or metabolic pathology occur during neurosurgical procedures and following head trauma due to retractor pressure, temporary or permanent ligation of intracranial vessels, release of vasoconstrictor substances, or increases in intracranial pressure. Measurements of CBF and metabolism are useful during anesthesia and critical care, where the clinical diagnosis of cerebral ischemia is impossible in most instances. Unfortunately, traditional cerebral monitoring techniques such as measurements of intracranial pressure or brain electrical activity provide only indirect information concerning CBF and metabolism since there is no linear relation between changes in intracranial volume or cerebral function and CBF. Experimental and clinical measurements of CBF and metabolism using microspheres, inert gases, SPECT, PET scanning, or flow probes directly placed around arteries are either discontinuous or invasive and require complex collimation or scanning devices. Additionally, there are substantial differences in the temporal and spatial resolution among the various measurement techniques. More recently, invasive laser Doppler flow and fiberoptic measurements of jugular bulb venous oxygen saturation have been introduced as continuous cerebral monitoring techniques in patients with intracranial pathology. However, these techniques are restricted to either local or global measurements, and absolute flow or metabolism values cannot be inferred from these monitoring techniques.

DIRECT CBF MEASUREMENT

Direct measurements of CBF require the exposure of brain-supplying arteries or cerebral tissues and use electromagnetic or Doppler flow techniques. Attempts have been made to directly measure CBF in animals by taking advantage of the unique cerebral circulation of the goat[237] and by surgically isolating the brain circulation of the monkey or dog.[238,239] However, these attempts and direct measurements in man are complicated by the fact that the brain receives multiple arterial inflow from the carotid and vertebral arteries and by the presence of venous communications between the venous sinuses of the brain and extracerebral tissue by emissary veins.

Direct measurements of arterial blood flow are possible in patients following craniotomy or exposure of brain-supplying arteries. Nornes and Wikeby[240] measured blood flow in several arteries, including the internal carotid artery (ICA), middle cerebral artery (MCA), and anterior cerebral artery (ACA) using electromagnetic flow probes during aneurysm surgery. They reported an average flow of 144 ml/min for the ICA, 97 ml/min for the MCA, and 65 ml/min for the ACA. In addition, these continuous measures could be used to evaluate collateral circulation and re-establishment of CBF after temporary occlusion. Using transit time flow probe technology, Hoffman et al[241] also measured brain arterial blood flow in neurosurgical patients following craniotomy. Flow measures were MCA = 58 ml/min; ACA = 36 ml/min; posterior cerebral artery = 33 ml/min; posterior inferior cerebellar ar-

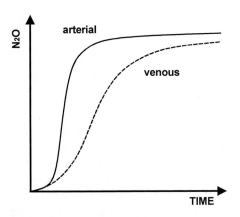

Figure 2-18   Graphic presentation of the Kety-Schmidt technique: The area between the curves represents CBF.

tery = 18 ml/min. Using continuous measures of CBF they also showed that nitrous oxide increased arterial blood flow 39 percent during normocapnia but not during hypocapnia.

KETY-SCHMIDT TECHNIQUE

The development of the inert gas method for measuring global CBF was reported by Kety and Schmidt 50 years ago.[242] Most of the current CBF measurements have been derived from the Kety-Schmidt technique. Catheters are placed into one peripheral artery and the jugular bulb for intermittent blood sampling and later analysis of tracer concentrations. In laboratory animals, catheters may alternatively be placed into cerebral sinuses. The measurement and calculation of CBF is based on a non-steady state application of the Fick principle, which states that the amount of a substance metabolized over time (Qm) is equal to the arterial minus the venous concentration of that substance times the flow:

$$Qm/t = F(Ca - Cv)$$

Since the metabolism of an inert gas such as N_2O is zero, the amount of the substance (dQi) taken up by the brain at any instant is equal to:

$$dQi/dt = F(Ca - Cv)$$

If we measure the arteriovenous concentration of N_2O over time after administration of N_2O to the inspired gases, we see the concentration curves shown in Fig. 2-18.

If we assume that flow is constant during the time of N_2O administration, then CBF can be calculated by the integral of the arteriovenous difference, corrected for the weight of the brain (Wb).

$$CBF = \frac{Qi(T)/Wb}{(Ca - Cv)dt}$$

Kety and Schmidt[243] assumed that N_2O was in equilibrium between blood and brain when time (T) was 10 min. The ratio of tissue and venous N_2O concentration in equilibrium is represented by the partition coefficient (λ),

$$\lambda_{N_2O} = \frac{Qi(T)/Wb}{Cv(T)}$$

Substituting for lambda,

$$CBF = \frac{\lambda Cv(T)}{(Ca - Cv)dt}$$

If arterial and venous oxygen content are measured, cerebral oxygen or glucose consumption can be calculated by CBF times the arterial and cerebral venous oxygen or glucose concentration difference. This equation is applicable to any substance that passes the blood-brain barrier with sufficient speed. The substance must not be a gas. The assumptions made by these calculations are based on: (1) Constant CBF during the calculation (this may not be a valid assumption since N_2O has been shown to increase CBF).[241] (2) It is assumed that blood is the only source of inflow and outflow for N_2O. In this regard, cerebrospinal fluid produces a small error by serving as a sink for N_2O absorption. (3) The site of venous sampling must represent a mixed cerebral venous sample of the tissue being analyzed. In the case of the internal jugular vein, this may not always be true, owing to extracerebral contamination and inadequate mixing of venous blood draining the assumed region.[244]

In later studies, Lassen and Munck[245] substituted krypton-85 for N_2O and increased the arterial and venous sampling period to 14 min. They interpreted earlier studies with shorter sampling periods as not allowing for complete equilibration within brain tissue, particularly in regions with low blood flow such as the white matter. When the period of data integration was extended to 14 min, CBF was approximately 10 percent lower. Another modification of the original method of Kety and Schmidt was to sample arterial and venous blood during desaturation rather than the saturation phase.[246] This ameliorated the problem of maintaining a constant step increase in gases by mask administration and improved the ability to detect differences in arterial and venous blood samples in the latter part of the sampling period.

In order to measure regional CBF, the tissue concentration of the tracer (Ci) is substituted for venous measures by assuming that the tracer instantly equilibrates across the blood-tissue barrier and that venous concentration is equal to tissue concentration divided by the partition coefficient (λ):

$$\frac{dCi}{dt} = \frac{Fi(Ca - Ci)}{\lambda}$$

Fi is the flow of the tissue measured as a function of weight. Solving for Ci:

$$Ci(T) = Ki\, Cae^{-Ki*T} * dt$$

Ki is the blood flow per unit weight times $1/\lambda$.

The tissue method has been applied with intravenous radioactive tracers in rats.[247] Arterial concentrations of the tracer is sampled during the integration period. Brain tissue is collected at the end of the period and regional concentrations determined autoradiographically. Regional CBF is then determined by solving for Ki.

INTRAARTERIAL XENON-133

According to Kety,[248] a monoexponential curve can describe the clearance of inert gas from tissue:

$$C(T) = C(0)e^{-Ki*T}$$

Where C(T) is the concentration at time T and C(0) is the concentration at time 0.

This principle has been used to evaluate the clearance of xenon-133 and krypton-85 following intraarterial injection of the tracers.[249,250] 133-xenon is the preferred tracer because its higher gamma activity can be more easily evaluated with external detectors than the lower beta energy of krypton-85. The desaturation curves produced by these methods show a biexponential washout curve. The two components of this curve can be related to gray and white matter blood flow, with values approximating 80 ml/100 g per min and 20 ml/100 g per min, respectively.[251] The initial slope of the logarithmically displayed clearance curve provides a close relationship to gray matter flow, although flow values are 20 to 30 percent lower.[252] In contrast, the second component of the bicompartment model shows a relatively constant blood flow of 20 ml/100 g per min. Thus, only flow of gray matter changed between patients. It was concluded that the CBF initial slope index was superior to compartmental and stochastic (height over area) analysis with respect to reproducibility and variation for the calculation of CBF.[252] Territories without perfusion remain undetected during CBF measurements using isotope clearance techniques. Thus, ischemic areas of the brain remain invisible, since the scintillation detectors record no washout from the ischemic area while normal washout is detected from adjacent territories.

INHALED AND INTRAVENOUS XENON-133

Understanding the need for an atraumatic technique for measuring regional CBF, investigators developed methods for evaluating regional CBF by inhaling xenon-133 for 1 min. A major drawback of the method was contamination of clearance curves by radioactivity from extracerebral sources. This was overcome by using a three-compartment analysis of the washout curves, in which the first two compartments represented gray and white matter and the third components indicated the slower extracerebral tissues.[253] However, initially this procedure required a 40-min recording. The low perfusion rate of extracerebral tissue is revealed by the prolonged washout of xenon-133 following inhalation. The overlap of these flows with white matter CBF suggests that these may be considered as one compartment. In this case, the washout of the combined white matter and extracerebral components can be approximated by a single exponential when the observation period is short relative to their half-times.

In an evaluation of these procedures, Obrist et al[253] tested regional CBF using collimated scintillation detectors following 1-min xenon-133 inhalation. The arterial input curve was estimated by measuring end tidal xenon-133 concentrations during the washout period. They determined that the start time for curve fitting should begin after the end tidal xenon-133 concentration was decreased to 20 percent of maximum levels. This was done to decrease the error of radiation scatter associated with high ventilatory levels. This necessitated that the start curve fit time be approximately 0.4 min after xenon-133 inhalation was terminated. An end fit time of 11 min was chosen, based on its ability to provide accurate estimates of gray and white matter flow with limited variation in curve fitting. Synthetic curves which were compared using two- and three-compartment models showed that the two-compartment model gave a lower estimate of white matter blood flow because of the extracerebral component. When the fractional flows of the gray matter compartment were compared with estimates using intracarotid xenon-133 injection, values of 0.76 versus 0.80 were observed. This difference may be attributed to the extracerebral component with inhalational xenon-133.

Rapid intraoperative monitoring of regional CBF has been also reported using intravenous xenon-133 injections.[254] The initial slope index was derived from bicompartment models which required 11 min of clearance and a monocompartment model which required only 3 min. Each respective model used the clearance curves to solve for unknowns which represent separate compartment sizes and clearance rates. The initial slope index, which provided a measure of CBF, was determined from the deconvoluted clearance curves as the monoexponential slope between 0.5 and 1.5 min, assuming a xenon-133 blood-brain partition coefficient of 1. The results show that the bicompartment models generated by the methods of Obrist and coworkers[253] and Prohovnik and associates[255] provide similar CBF measures. In addition, the monocompartment model, which was generated with 3 min washout times, provided CBF values not different from the two-compartment models. This suggests that a monitoring setup with intravenous xenon-133 injections and multiple extracranial detectors can be used to evaluate regional CBF over relatively short (3 min) intraoperative intervals. When the intravenous xenon-133 method was compared to the intracarotid injection technique, excellent agreement was found.[250] This indicates that intravenous xenon-133 injection methods are a reasonable and safe alternative method for regional CBF measurement compared to intracarotid injection.

A modification of the intravenous method has been used to evaluate CBF during hypothermic cardiopulmonary bypass.[128] The method involves injection of xenon-133 into the arterial inflow cannula of the pump oxygenator. The technique of clearance curve analysis for CBF determination is similar to those described above. The authors conclude that the method provides reproducible measures of CBF during bypass procedures, provided that flow estimates are separated by 15 to 25 min.

Limitations of xenon-133 CBF measurement include lack of anatomic correlation, which prevents comparison of the same region from one study to the next and poor resolution due to isotope scatter. There is also a problem of look-through with this technique which can obscure the observation of low flow regions.[256] Because xenon-133 produces a weak signal, it provides little information concerning flow within deep brain regions, even when SPECT is the imaging modality.

XENON-ENHANCED COMPUTED TOMOGRAPHY (sXE-CT)

Nonradioactive or stable xenon is radiodense. Subanesthetic concentrations of xenon (33 percent) have been used with rapid sequence CT to measure quantitative regional CBF.[257] Xenon is inhaled for 4 to 5 min and delivers contrast adequate for imaging by sequential CT scans (two before and six during xenon inhalation) for each level of brain examined. CBF is quantitated by integrating the build-up of xenon within the tissue and within the arterial blood by CT enhancement. The key equation is then solved for each of 20,000 voxels per CT level. The technique allows the measurement of high-resolution CBF images that can be correlated directly with anatomic location. A local partition coefficient (λ) is calculated and integrated into each flow measurement, increasing the accuracy of regional measurements. Because of the fast clearance of xenon following each study, repeated measurements can be performed 20 min apart. This allows one to measure sequential changes such as reactivity to CO_2.

The problems with sXE-CT are signal resolution and absolute CBF measures associated with an unfavorable signal-to-noise ratio, possible anesthetic and CBF changes produced by xenon alone, and the requirement that the patient remain motionless for several minutes during the scan. Sources of error also include CT noise, tissue heterogeneity, and estimation of arterial xenon concentration.[258] Xenon has several characteristics similar to nitrous oxide and it is possible that xenon, like nitrous oxide, increases CBF in higher doses. It is unclear whether this occurs with 33 percent xenon.

SINGLE PHOTON EMISSION COMPUTED TOMOGRAPHY (SPECT)

Single photon emission computed tomography dates from the early 1960s when the idea of emission transverse section tomography was presented by Kuhl and Edwards.[259] They used a rectilinear scanner and analogue backprojection methods to detect emissions from a series of sequential positions transverse to the cephalad-caudad axis of the body. The data collection from several angles was facilitated by employing several banks of detectors. Later, computers were used to compensate for the blurring caused by the process of superposition. These are the same basic approaches used today. Projections of emission data made at angular intervals around 360° are detected using moving detectors and then backprojected to form the superposition image. Blurring is removed by computed methods similar to x-ray CT.

SPECT measures regional CBF as well as cerebral blood volume by labeling plasma or red blood cells. Two methods are used to measure brain blood flow using SPECT. The first approach involves rapidly sampling the change in activity using xenon-133. This has been evaluated using a rotating four-detector system termed a dynamic SPECT[260] and a ring detector.[261] Regional CBF calculations are based on the Kety-Schmidt model for single compartment tissue perfusion. In tomographic systems, the tissue evaluated is the voxel determined by the reconstruction process. For the inhalational xenon-133 method, the arterial input function is measured by placing a scintillation detector over the chest and observing the lung activity curve. Resolution for the SPECT exam in the range of 2 cm has been indicated. Modifications in the calculations are made for voxels which receive little activity, enhancing the resolution of ischemic areas. In the future, xenon-127 may be used because of its higher energy and dose advantage. A lipophilic technetium [99mTc] labeled compound that is initially extracted by brain and later washes out also has been used with dynamic SPECT.[262]

The second approach has become available with the development of iodinated phenylalkylamines, which accumulate in the brain and [99mTc] labeled lipophilic compounds which accumulate in the brain and do not wash out. The static measurement of the relative accumulation of these compounds has been used to infer local cerebral metabolism.[263] New labeled compounds and methods using SPECT suggest that this technique can be used to measure brain perfusion, metabolism, permeability, and blood volume with a resolution in a range similar to positron emission tomography (PET). Loss of resolution is produced with SPECT with xenon-133 due to large scatter fraction and modest energy discrimination of the instrument. The trade-off is a gain in sensitivity to tracer activity and decreased accumulation time.

Whereas typical values of gray matter blood flow are 70 to 90 ml/100 g per min and 20 to 30 ml/100 g per min for white matter as seen using a two-dimensional array of probes and Xe-CT,[264] white matter blood flow is erroneously higher with SPECT technique, due in part to inappropriate choice of partition coefficients.[265] Because the incidence of stroke following transient ischemic attacks (TIA) may be as high as 60 percent, endarterectomy or bypass procedures have evolved to treat TIAs that are hemodynamic in nature.[266] The use of rCBF studies with SPECT has contributed little in the management of TIAs, but follow-up studies have proved to be valuable in determining the success of the surgery.[267]

SPECT may have the potential of evaluating strokes earlier than other noninvasive techniques. Although reduced rCBF is seen initially in areas of stroke, normal flow may be seen in and around the stroke site within 7 to 10 days, which represents luxury perfusion. Reduced perfusion states may be present within stroke regions 2 to 4 weeks after the insult, which may or may not be matched by anatomic defects seen by CT. In patients with chronic stroke, rCBF defects are seen in a majority of cases. Regional CBF and CT images show a similar defect when the infarct results in dissolution of brain tissue. The rCBF defect was larger than the CT defect in two-thirds of the cases, suggesting the presence of a penumbra area that is intact physiologically but inactive electrically. In these cases, clinicians are interested in identifying methods that can improve perfusion of the penumbral region and decrease the sign of neurological stroke.

POSITRON EMISSION TOMOGRAPHY (PET)

The PET technique can be used to measure regional CBF, cerebral blood volume, pH, and cerebral oxygen and glucose consumption. A class of unstable nuclei, predominantly proton-rich isotopes of low atomic number elements, decay by the emission of a positron and electron neutrino. When such a nucleus decays, the energetic positron scatters off the nuclei and electrons and comes to rest, annihilates with an atomic electron, and yields two 511-KeV gamma rays emitted at 180°. Two detectors located on opposite sides of the head are connected in coincidence and will record an event only when simultaneous gamma rays are detected. Circular or polygonal ring detectors confine the detected events to the volume within the detectors. Coincidence detection is self-collimating and scattered radiation can be effectively suppressed. Intrinsic limitations in resolution occur due to irregularities in the range of the positron path and lack of colinearity of the two annihilation gamma rays due to intrinsic motion of the participating atomic electron. These errors can be of significance for the high resolution tomograph. As the ring diameter increases the sensitivity decreases, accidental rejection becomes more efficient, resolution becomes more uniform, and angular sampling improves. An optimized ring is twice the diameter of the evaluated object, and is typically 60 cm for the head. Computed methods for image reconstruction produce a resolution (7 to 9 mm), which is better than SPECT, but a sensitivity that is poorer. This increases the acquisition time requirements of PET with respect to SPECT.

Several tracers are available for PET studies to evaluate physiologic processes. These positron emitting isotopes of carbon, oxygen, nitrogen, and fluorine can be measured in trace amounts. They are hypothesized to be indistinguishable from their unlabeled counterparts and are used to evaluate such physiologic functions as blood flow, metabolism, vascular permeability, and blood volume. Because of the short half-life of these tracers, it is necessary to have a cyclotron in the facility to manufacture the isotopes.

Local blood flow can be measured by microsphere or trapping technique or by freely diffusible tracers. An ideal tracer for trapping would be extracted from the blood with high efficiency and irreversibly held in the tissue, which would allow high count rate images. If the extraction fraction was equal to 1, blood flow or metabolism would be proportional to local tissue activity. Actual tracers commonly have an extraction fraction less than one, and this may vary with blood flow, leading to nonlinearity. The tracer N-13 ammonia has a long retention time in tissue and has been used to measure blood flow in the brain. However, the permeability-surface area product (PS) falls with flow in the brain, producing a significant nonlinear response. Freely diffusible tracers can be used to measure regional CBF by evaluating the clearance of the tracer from the brain, which should occur in an exponential fashion. [77]Kr, ^{18}F fluoromethane, and [15]O water have been used for regional CBF studies. [15]O may be most suitable and can be delivered in an intravenous bolus of [15]O water or by inhalation of [15]O carbon dioxide. However, there are difficulties with [15]O water flow, which include effects of recirculation, decrease in extraction with high rates, and logistic problems with the 2-min half-life. This may result in lower regional CBF using this technique.[267]

Local blood volume is measured using a single breath of ^{11}C carbon monoxide or [15]O carbon monoxide. Regional glucose consumption may be evaluated using ^{11}C glucose or ^{18}F flouro-deoxyglucose (FDG). With ^{11}C glucose, measurement of regional activity must be made shortly after injection of the tracer. The unmetabolized tracer in the blood must be substracted by estimating blood volume. Corrections must also be made for unmetabolized tracer in the tissue and for regress of labeled metabolite from the region of interest. Repeated measures are possible with this technique because of the short half-life of ^{11}C glucose as opposed to the decay half-life of ^{18}F, which is longer, and because trapping of FDG is more efficient in the cells. This allows for delayed scanning until blood levels of the compound are negligible. High count rates may be obtained with this procedure in order to improve resolution and sensitivity.

Evaluation of regional oxygen metabolism is difficult because of the rapid regress of the [15]O metabolite from brain tissue. Newer methods take recirculation into account and are based on continuous inhalation of [15]O oxygen as well as continuous regional CBF measurement using inhalation of [15]O carbon dioxide.[268] This allows the calculation of oxygen extraction fraction, regional cerebral oxygen consumption, and regional CBF. The model assumes unit partition coefficients for water and oxygen between blood and cerebral tissue. The combination of regional cerebral oxygen consumption and regional cerebral glucose consumption can assess ischemia by evaluating aerobic versus anaerobic metabolism.

MAGNETIC RESONANCE FLOW ANALYSIS (MRA)

The ability to quantify flow velocity and volume flow rate has added a new dimension to the use of MRA to image vascular morphology. The most widely used methods of velocity measurement rely on phase contrast acquisitions, which can be extracted from a gated cine exam, a two-dimension phase contrast slice, or a three-dimension acquisition.

The cine phase contrast method has been implemented clinically by many authors.[269] A single MR brain slice is oriented perpendicularly to the vessel of interest. Flow is detected as it passes through the slice by using a bipolar flow encoding gradient applied along the axis of flow. In the cine phase contrast sequence the gradient generates a phase shift for moving spins proportional to their velocity. Two interleaved acquisitions are obtained with opposite polarities of the bipolar gradient, and the difference between these two acquisitions is then calculated. For a single pixel, the phase difference between the two acquisitions is directly proportional to the velocity of flow along the applied axis. Typically, 16 or 32 velocity and flow measurements are calculated at sequential points in the cardiac cycle, providing time resolved flow information. The resultant velocity waveform provides assessment of pulsatility and flow dynamics during the cardiac cycle.[270] The cine exam can be triggered by cardiac or peripheral gating. Peripheral gating is easier to set up and is generally more reliable than cardiac gating, although the systolic waveform may be displaced in time and difficult to identify in pathologic situations.

It is important that the vessel orientation be perpendicular to the slice in order to minimize errors in flow measurement due to overestimation of vessel cross section area. The small size of intracranial vessels requires that thin slices be used to reduce partial volume effects at the vessel edge. New techniques for automated vessel detection decrease the variability of flow measurements from 19 to 6 percent compared with manual methods.[271] These automated methods hold promise to improve the precision of cine phase contrast flow measurements.

Average flow can be measured from a nongated two-dimensional phase contrast slice with flow encoding perpendicular from the slice. The intravascular signal intensity is summed, allowing measurement of average flow across the slice over several cardiac cycles.[272] This technique is useful for measuring nonpulsatile flow, as in venous vessels. Average velocity can also be obtained from a three-dimensional phase contrast technique.[273] In this technique thin slices can be obtained, reducing partial volume averaging and images can be reformatted with the vessel flow perpendicular to the slice to reduce flow artifact.

Cerebral blood flow measures are technically difficult at present, and normal absolute values have not been established. An alternative is to evaluate relative changes in flow in comparison to analogous contralateral vessels. Possible errors in the signal may occur with incorrect velocity encoding, partial loss of signal due to turbulent flow, excessive obliqueness of the vessel with respect to the slice plane, and poor resolution of the vessel edge. The advantages of the MR PC technique is that it provides a high resolution flow signal that evaluates flow dynamics in brain vessels noninvasively. This will be useful in evaluating cerebral ischemia and cerebrovascular pathology.

MICROSPHERES

Radioactive and color-labeled micropheres have been used extensively to measure regional CBF and metabolism, but this technique is restricted to animal experimentation.[274] Fifteen-μm microspheres have been shown to be the optimal size in regional tissue measurements. Larger microspheres produce axial streaming, which misrepresents blood flow by allowing shunting of the microspheres. Smaller sized microspheres underestimate CBF.[275,276] The technique requires catheterization of two arteries for blood withdrawal and the left atrium for microsphere injections. This allows adequate mixing of the microspheres within the heart before they are distributed in the blood according to the cardiac output. Injection of microspheres into the left ventricle may not allow adequate mixing, and withdrawing from only one artery during the microsphere injection does not allow verification of adequate mixing. During the microsphere injection into the heart, arterial blood samples are withdrawn using pumps operating at a fixed rate. Since the microspheres are trapped in one pass through the tissue, a specific tracer can only be used once. However, several tracers can be used in one study, allowing for sequential measurements of CBF and metabolism. At the end of the study, the brain is removed and regional tissue samples obtained. The activity of radiolabeled microspheres is measured in tissue and blood samples using a gamma counter. The analysis of the distribution of color-labeled microspheres in tissue and blood samples is performed using color chromatography. Regional CBF is calculated by considering the blood as a sample in which the withdrawal of flow rate is known. The tissue flow rate can then be determined by calculating for one unknown. Regional CBF/tissue activity = blood withdrawal rate/blood activity. Catheterization of cerebral sinuses for simultaneous cerebral venous blood sampling allows for calculation of cerebral metabolism.

Radioactive or color-labeled microspheres are a reliable method for measuring CBF and, if performed correctly, are subject to only a few technical problems. The mixing of microspheres must be complete within the heart before they are distributed throughout the body. As stated above, this should be validated by multiple arterial blood withdrawals. If the blood flow to a tissue is low, random inaccuracies in flow measurements may occur due to inadequate microsphere accumulation. Studies evaluating the measurement error as a function of sample size have determined that a minimum of 400 microspheres per sample is necessary for adequate flow measurement.[274] If an ischemic region is measured, the sample size must be large enough to maximize microsphere collection.

LASER DOPPLER FLOWMETRY (LDF)

LDF has been used for tissue blood flow measurements in such extracranial territories as the skin, renal cortex, and intestinal mucosa and in models of tissue microcirculation. Following craniotomy, LDF measures local CBF of the cortex and subcortex. LDF measures the movement of red blood cells within the microcirculation by using the Doppler shift of a laser light source. Monochromatic coherent laser light, delivered via a transmitting fiber optic, is scattered by biologic tissues. Light scattered from moving red blood cells experiences a Doppler shift in frequency while stationary structures remain constant (reference light). The shifted and reference light are collected by a receiving afferent optical fiber and detected by the surface of a photodetector. The interference of the two signals produces optical beating (heterodyning), the frequency of which is equal to the Doppler shifted frequency. A spectrum of shifted frequencies is generated from variations in red cell velocities and variations in the angle or incidence of light on red cell surfaces. The spectral density of the shifted frequencies is determined by the red cell concentration and velocity. Algorithms have been generated to convert the varying photodetector current to values of red cell flux.

In the microcirculation, the velocity of red blood cells varies from zero to several millimeters per second. The major portion of this energy is detected by a Doppler shift within a band-width of 12 kHz to 20 kHz.[277] Several time constants are available for evaluating the flow signal and it is advised to use a fast time constant to evaluate the rhythmic components of the laser Doppler signal. Variations in the signal have been attributed to the cardiac cycle, respiration, normal vasomotion, and Brownian motion.[278] Normal vasomotion is seen in a frequency range of 4 to 20 cycles/min, and it has been found that this component is lost with large space-occupying lesions.[277] Further, recovery of vasomotion is a good indication for recovery of the patient. The laser Doppler flow signal has been shown to be linearly related to changes in blood flow.[279] Although attempts have been made to convert the laser Doppler flow signals to absolute blood flow, these conversions are controversial.[279,280]

The laser light source can be placed on the cortical surface or fixed within the tissue. However, movement artifact can be a problem, particularly with tissue implantation, if the probe is fixed to the skull and the brain is moving due to ventilation.[277] The sampled "volume" of the laser Doppler has been estimated to be

1 mm or slightly greater, and these volumes may depend on the laser light source. Within the sampled tissue, the laser Doppler measures the movement of red blood cells within capillaries, arterioles, and venules with diameters ranging from 5 to 500 μm. The flow signal is generated by measuring the volume or concentration of red blood cells within the sample area and their velocity and multiplying the two components. All three components of the signal, volume, velocity, and flow, can provide important information concerning the microcirculation, and their values are available from current instruments.

Clinical studies have demonstrated the use of LDF as a continuous cerebral blood flow measurement technique for the perioperative period and during neurocritical care.[281-284] In patients undergoing craniotomy for resection of arteriovenous malformations, tumor, and occlusion of aneurysms, LDF reflected changes in CBF during manipulations of arterial CO_2 and mean arterial blood pressure.[283-285] The application of LDF to measure CO_2 reactivity may guide early therapeutic intervention with decreases in the cerebral vascular response to CO_2, or the level of hyperventilation necessary to improve CBF. Laser Doppler flowmetry can be used to assess CBF autoregulation,[286] which may be impaired or abolished with the use of anesthetics, in patients with intracranial mass lesions or following head injury. However, the status of CBF autoregulation varies between patients and insults. Manipulations to increase cerebral perfusion pressure may be of advantage[287] but may as well be detrimental to the brain, depending on the autoregulatory status.[91] The application of LDF to measure changes in CBF during changes in arterial blood pressure permits adjustment of cerebral perfusion pressure to maintain adequate CBF levels.[288] There is potential use for LDF in monitoring in the clinical evaluation of cerebral ischemia.[277,281] Dirnnagl and coworkers[280] have correlated changes in CBF with changes in laser Doppler flow in a rat model of cerebral ischemia. The authors have shown a close correlation between relative changes in cerebral blood flow and laser Doppler flow, but they did not define or identify specific laser Doppler flow patterns that indicate cerebral ischemia. Although the ischemic threshold level of laser Doppler signals is still unclear, this technique may significantly improve the quality of treatment in patients with intracranial pathology, particularly when combined with measurements of intracranial pressure, brain electrical activity, or jugular bulb venous oxygen saturation.

THERMAL DIFFUSION

Based on the concept that thermal conductivity varies proportionally to CBF, thermal diffusion devices have been constructed that measure cortical CBF following exposure of the cortical surface. The mathematical formula for calculation of CBF states that flow is equal to a constant times the reciprocal of the difference of voltage at flow X minus the reciprocal of the voltage at flow zero[289]:

$$CBF = \frac{1}{V_X} - \frac{1}{V_0}$$

Two types of thermal sensors are available. An isothermal sensor maintains a constant temperature between the two contact points. The determination of power needed to maintain the temperature gradient constant is proportional to CBF. An isocaloric sensor maintains a constant power input, and the change in the temperature gradient is correlated with a change in CBF. These measures have been proposed to provide absolute CBF values. This is based on the assumption that thermal conductivity is constant. This is true in general in man and several other species, but changes in tissue fluid composition may alter thermal conduction. Absolute calibration of the instrument requires a measurement at zero flow (see above), which has been done in animals. However, zero calibration cannot be performed in patients. Therefore, assumptions of calibration without this measure may lead to inaccuracies. Wei and coworkers[290] have validated the responses of thermal measurement systems to rapid changes in mean arterial blood pressure in rats. Using microthermistor probes, their results[290] indicate that the thermal measurement system can quantitate changes in CBF. These results are consistent with experiments by Voorhees and associates,[291] who found a linear relationship between nitroprusside-induced changes in CBF measured with microspheres and cerebral blood flow data from thermal clearance measurements. In patients undergoing craniotomy for cerebral aneurysm clipping following subarachnoid hemorrhage, Abe and coworkers[292,293] employed thermal gradient CBF measurements to monitor the effects of nicardipine and prostaglandin on CBF and CO_2-reactivity. The results from these clinical studies show that thermal measurement systems assess dynamic cerebral blood flow during neurosurgical procedures. During cerebral aneurysm surgery with temporary clipping of a brain artery, it has been shown that neurologic deficits are related to the length of time and the magnitude of decrease in CBF.[294] During surgery for AVMs, a decrease in CBF in tissue adjacent to the AVM has been found and increases in these flows are consistently shown during AVM resection.[295] Pathologies in which regional ischemia may be present provide potential uses for this CBF technique. These would include epilepsy, cerebral mass lesions, and cerebral revascularization.[289]

JUGULAR BULB VENOUS OXYGEN SATURATION (SjO$_2$)

Measurements of SjO$_2$ have been employed as a monitoring technique to estimate changes in CBF and cerebral oxygen consumption in patients at risk of developing perioperative cerebral ischemia or hypoxia.[296] SjO$_2$ can be measured continuously using a fiberoptic catheter or intermittently by drawing blood samples through the catheter. In patients with focal or diffuse intracranial pathology, the catheter should be placed on the side with the dominant venous drainage. This side may be identified by manual compression of each internal jugular vein and the observation of concomitant changes in intracranial pressure. Following cannulation of the internal jugular vein at the level of the thyroid cartilage in a retrograde fashion, a catheter is inserted through the introducer with the tip positioned at the level of the base of the skull.[297] Under normal conditions, CBF is regulated by oxygen demand. Arterial-jugular bulb oxygen saturation AjVDO$_2$ can be related to CBF and cerebral oxygen consumption by the Fick principle: AjVDO$_2$ = CMRO$_2$/CBF. Physiologically, AjVDO$_2$ is between 1.8 and 3.9 mol/ml.[298] Assuming that cerebral oxygen consumption is constant for a given period, changes in AjVDO$_2$ will reflect changes in CBF. If a change in cerebral oxygen consumption occurs due to anesthesia, hypothermia, seizures, or other causes, and if CBF is coupled to changes in cerebral oxygen consumption, then AjVDO$_2$ will remain constant. Therefore, it is hypothesized that variations of AjVDO$_2$ reflect changes in CBF and that large increases or decreases in AjVDO$_2$ indicate cerebral hypoperfusion or hyperemia, respectively. However, in order for these monitoring techniques to be valid, cerebral oxygen consumption must be constant and must be within a normal range for adequate CBF coupling because changes in arterial blood gases (Pa$_{O_2}$, Pa$_{CO_2}$ and pH), body temperature, hemoglobin concentration, intracranial pressure, and the administration of drugs will modulate the relationship between CBF and SjO$_2$. Robertson and coworkers[298] have shown that this is not always true in patients with ischemia, and as a result changes in AjVDO$_2$ and CBF are poorly correlated. However, if a correction is made for the presence of ischemia, based on low CBF or increased venous lactate concentration, then the correlation between CBF and AjVDO$_2$ improved to r = 0.74. They suggested that a cerebral lactate-oxygen index less than 0.08 may serve as a reliable indicator of ischemia. This is supported by others who have shown that the lactate-oxygen index provides a significant indication of outcome in patients with cerebral aneurysms.[299] However, this has been questioned by the results of Cruz and coworkers,[300] who showed that in patients with head injury, the presence of anemia leads to an artificially low lactate-oxygen index and an indication of ischemia when it is not present. Therefore, this index was abandoned in patients with acute head injury because most of these patients sustain anemia in the first few days of the injury. Instead, measures of AjVDO$_2$ and arterial-jugular bulb lactate content are evaluated separately.

With constant arterial oxygen saturation and hemoglobin concentration, changes in SjO$_2$ reflect dynamic CBF. Robertson and coworkers[298] have shown in head-injured patients that changes in CBF can be reliably estimated based on the calculation of AjVDO$_2$ and the arteriovenous difference of lactate content. Several studies indicate that desaturation of jugular venous blood (SjO$_2$ < 40%) is associated with development of EEG abnormalities, neurologic deterioration, unconsciousness, and depletion of cerebral energy stores, indicating cerebral ischemia.[301-303] This is consistent with data from head-injured patients showing desaturation of jugular venous blood as a function of intracranial hypertension, hypotension, hypocapnia, and hypoxia.[304] In patients undergoing carotid endarterectomy, neurologic dysfunction was associated with lateral sinus oxygen saturation below 50 percent, while no neurologic complication occurred in patients with lateral sinus oxygen saturation above 60 percent.[305] These results confirm that monitoring of SjO$_2$ indicates critical cerebral perfusion (and cerebral oxygen consumption) associated with vascular engorgement or decreases in cerebral perfusion pressure. In patients with intracranial hypertension, prolonged hyperventilation may be associated with worsened outcome. Cruz and coworkers[300] suggested that the level of hyperventilation necessary to reduce acute increases in intracranial pressure should be geared according to the optimal O$_2$-extraction ratio (as derived from the AjVDO$_2$ and arterial O$_2$-content) of the patients. Brain tumors, arteriovenous malformations, head injury, or stroke may be associated with impaired or abolished cerebral blood flow autoregulation.[300] In these patients, monitoring SjO$_2$ can identify the level of cerebral perfusion pressure necessary to maintain cerebral blood flow and cerebral oxygen consumption above the individual ischemic threshold.[306]

References

1. Aidley DJ: *The Physiology of Excitable Cells.* New York, Cambridge University Press, 1989.
2. Kandel ER, et al: *Principles of Neural Science.* Norwalk, CT, Appleton and Lange, 1991.
3. Siegel GJ, et al: Ion transport. In Siegel GJ, et al (eds): *Basic Neurochemistry,* 3d ed. Boston, Little, Brown, 1981:107–143.
4. Edvinsson L, et al: *Cerebral Blood Flow and Metabolism.* New York, Raven Press, 1993.
5. Lajtha AL, et al: Metabolism and transport of carbohydrates

and aminoacids. In Siegel GJ, et al (eds): *Basic Neurochemistry*, 3d ed. Boston, Little, Brown, 1981:329–353.

6. Siesjö BK: *Brain Energy Metabolism*. New York, John Wiley and Sons, 1978.

7. Lowry OH: Energy metabolism in brain and its control. In Ingvar DH, Lassen NA (eds): *Brain Work. The Coupling of Function, Metabolism and Blood Flow in the Brain*. Copenhagen, Munksgaard, 1975:48–64.

8. Roy CS, Sherrington CS: On the regulation of the blood-supply of the brain. *J Physiol* 1890; 11:5.

9. Siesjö BK: Cerebral circulation and metabolism. *J Neurosurg* 1984; 60:883.

10. Nemoto EM, et al: Compartmentation of whole brain blood flow and oxygen and glucose metabolism in monkeys. *J Neurosurg Anesth* 1994; 6:170.

11. Nemoto EM, et al: Suppression of cerebral metabolic rate for oxygen ($CMRO_2$) by mild hypothermia compared with thiopental. *J Neurosurg Anesth* 1996; 8:52.

12. Carpenter MB: *Human Neuroanatomy*. Baltimore, Williams & Wilkins, 1976.

13. Willis T: Cerebri Anatome, cui accessit nervorum descriptio et usus. Londini, Flesher J, 1664; as quoted by Mitchell GAG in *Cardiovascular Innervation*. Edinburgh, E & S Livingstone, 1956.

14. Alpers BJ, et al: Anatomical studies of the circle of Willis in normal brains. *Arch Neurol Psychiatry* 1959; 81:409.

15. Van der Zwan A, et al: Variability of the territories of the major cerebral arteries. *J Neurosurg* 1992; 77:927.

16. DÁlecy LG, Feigl EO: Sympathetic control of cerebral blood flow in dogs. *Circ Res* 1972; 31:267.

17. Busija DW, Heistad DD: Effects of cholinergic nerves on cerebral blood flow in cats. *Circ Res* 1981; 48:62.

18. Iwayama T, et al: Dual adrenergic and cholinergic innervation of the cerebral arteries of the rat. *Circ Res* 1970; 26:635.

19. Nielsen KC, Owman CH: Adrenergic innervation of pial arteries related to the circle of Willis in the cat. *Brain Res* 1967; 6:773.

20. Vasquez J, Purves MJ: The cholinergic pathway to cerebral blood vessels. I: Morphological studies. *Pflügers Arch* 1979; 379:157.

21. Hara H, et al: Origin of cholinergic nerves to the rat major cerebral arteries: Coexistence with vasoactive intestinal polypeptide. *Brain Res* 1985; 14:179.

22. Lundberg JM, et al: Vasoactive intestinal polypeptide in cholinergic neurons of exocrine glands: Functional significance of coexisting transmitters for vasodilation and secretion. *Proc Natl Acad Sci USA* 1980;77:1651.

23. Plum F, Duffy TE: The couple between cerebral metabolism and blood flow during seizures. In Ingvar DH, Lassen NA (eds): *Brain Work. The Coupling of Function, Metabolism and Blood Flow in the Brain*. Copenhagen, Munksgaard, 1975:197–214.

24. Kennedy C, et al: Mapping of functional neural pathways by autoradiographic survey of local metabolic rate with 14C-deoxyglucose. *Science* 1975; 187:850.

25. Raichle ME, et al: Correlation between regional cerebral blood flow and oxidative metabolism. In vivo studies in man. *Arch Neurol* 1976; 33:523.

26. Greenberg J, et al: Localized metabolic-flow couple during functional activity. *Acta Neurol Scand* 1979; 60(suppl 72):12.

27. Silver IA: Cellular microenvironment in relation to local blood flow. In Elliott K, O'Connor M (eds): *Cerebral Vascular Smooth Muscle and its Control*. New York, Elsevier, 1978:49–61.

28. Fox PT, Raichle ME: Focal physiological uncoupling of cerebral blood flow and oxidative metabolism during somatosensory stimulation in human subjects. *Proc Natl Acad Sci USA* 1986; 83:1140.

29. Wahl M, Kuschinsky W: Dependency of the dilatory action

of adenosine on the perivascular H^+ and K^+ at pial arteries of cats. *Acta Neurol Scand* 1977; 56:218.

30. Wahl M, Kuschinsky W: The dilatory action of adenosine on pial vessels of cats and its inhibition by theophylline. *Pflugers Arch* 1976; 362:55.

31. Dirnagl U, et al: Coupling of cerebral blood flow to neuronal activation: Role of adenosine and nitric oxide. *Am J Physiol* 1994; 267:H296.

32. Iadecola C, et al: Nitric oxide synthase inhibition and cerebrovascular regulation. *J Cereb Blood Flow Metab* 1994; 14:175.

33. Garthwaite J, Boulton CL: Nitric oxide signaling in the central nervous system. *Annu Rev Physiol* 1995; 57:683.

34. Iadecola C: Does nitric oxide mediate the increases in cerebral blood flow elicited by hypercapnia? *Proc Natl Acad Sci USA* 1992; 89:3913.

35. Iadecola C, Xu X: Nitro-L-arginine attenuates hypercapnic cerebrovasodilation without affecting cerebral metabolism. *Am J Physiol* 1994; 266:R518.

36. McPherson RW, et al: Hypoxia, alpha-2-adrenergic, and nitric oxide dependent interactions on canine cerebral blood flow. *Am J Physiol* 1994; 266:H476.

37. Wang Q, et al: Nitric oxide does not act as a mediator coupling cerebral blood flow to neural activity following somatosensory stimuli in rats. *Neurol Res* 1993; 15:33.

38. Dirnagl U, et al: Role of nitric oxide in the coupling of cerebral blood flow to neural activation in rats. *Neurosci Lett* 1993; 149:43.

39. Irikura K, et al: Importance of nitric oxide synthase inhibition to the attenuated vascular responses induced by topical L-nitroarginine during vibrissae stimulation. *J Cereb Blood Flow Metab* 1994; 14:45.

40. Faraci FM: Nitric oxide mediates vasodilation in response to activation of N-methyl-D-aspartate receptors in brain. *Circ Res* 1993; 72:476.

41. Madden JA: The effect of carbon dioxide on cerebral arteries. *Pharmacol Ther* 1993; 59:229.

42. Lassen NA: Luxury-perfusion syndrome and its possible relations to acute metabolic acidosis localised within the brain. *Lancet* 1966; 2:1113.

43. Iadecola C, Kraig RP: Focal elevations in neocortical interstitial K^+ produced by stimulation of the fastigial nucleus in rat. *Brain Res* 1991; 563:273.

44. Dreier JP, et al: Nitric oxide modulates the CBF response to increased extracellular potassium. *J Cereb Blood Flow Metab* 1995; 15:914.

45. DÁlecy LG, et al: Sympathetic modulation of hypercapnic cerebral vasodilation in dogs. *Circ Res* 1979; 45:771.

46. Busija DW, Heistad DD: Effects of activation of sympathetic nerves on cerebral blood flow during hypercapnia in cats and rabbits. *J Physiol* 1984; 347:35.

47. MacKenzie ET, et al: Cerebral circulation and norepinephrine: Relevance of the blood brain barrier. *Am J Physiol* 1976; 231:483.

48. Lacombe PM, et al: Plasma epinephrine modulates the cerebrovasodilation evoked by electrical stimulation of dorsal medulla. *Brain Res* 1990; 506:93.

49. Iadecola C, et al: Role of adrenal catecholamines in cerebrovasodilation evoked from brain stem. *Am J Physiol* 1987; 252:H1183.

50. Iadecola C, et al: Global cerebral vasodilation elicited by focal electrical stimulation within the dorsal medullary reticular formation in anesthetized rat. *J Cereb Blood Flow Metab* 1983; 3:270.

51. Iadecola C, et al: Global increase in cerebral metabolism and blood flow produced by focal electrical stimulation of dorsal medullary reticular formation in rat. *Brain Res* 1983; 372:101.

52. Ohta S, et al: Effect of stellate ganglion block on cerebral

blood flow in normoxemic and hyperoxemic states. *J Neurosurg Anesth* 1990; 2:272.

53. DÁlecy LG, Rose CJ: Parasympathetic cholinergic control of cerebral blood flow in dogs. *Circ Res* 1977; 41:324.

54. Busija DW, Heistad DD: Effects of cholinergic nerves on cerebral blood flow in cats. *Circ Res* 1981; 48:62.

55. Nakai M, et al: Global cerebral vasodilation by stimulation of rat fastigial cerebellar nucleus. *Am J Physiol* 1982; 243:H226.

56. Nakai M, et al: Electrical stimulation of cerebellar fastigial nucleus increases cerebral cortical blood flow without change in local metabolism: Evidence for an intrinsic system in brain for primary vasodilation. *Brain Res* 1983; 260:35.

57. Kurosawa M, et al: Stimulation of the nucleus basilaris of Meynert increases acetylcholine release in the cerebral cortex in rats. *Neurosci Lett* 1989; 98:198.

58. Kety SS, Schmidt CF: The effects of altered arterial tensions of carbon dioxide and oxygen on cerebral blood flow and cerebral oxygen consumption of normal young men. *J Clin Invest* 1948; 27:484.

59. Harper AM, Glass HI: Effect of alterations in the arterial carbon dioxide tension on the blood flow through the cerebral cortex at normal and low arterial pressures. *J Neurol Neurosurg Psychiatry* 1965; 28:449.

60. Greenberg JH, et al: Local cerebral blood volume response to carbon dioxide in man. *Circ Res* 1978; 43:324.

61. Keyeux A, et al: Induced response to hypercapnia in the two-compartment total cerebral blood volume: Influence on brain vascular reserve and flow efficiency. *J Cereb Blood Flow Metab* 1995; 15:1121.

62. Heistad DD, et al: Role of large arteries in regulation of cerebral blood flow in dogs. *J Clin Invest* 1978; 62:761.

63. Harper AM: Autoregulation of cerebral blood flow: Influence of the arterial blood pressure on the blood flow through the cerebral cortex. *J Neurol Neurosurg Psychiatry* 1966; 29:398.

64. Granholm L, Siesjö BK: The effects of hypercapnia and hypocapnia upon the cerebrospinal fluid lactate and pyruvate concentration and upon lactate, pyruvate, ATP, phosphocreatine and creatine concentrations of cat brain tissue. *Acta Physiol Scand* 1969; 75:257.

65. Sutton LN, et al: Cerebral venous oxygen content as a measure of brain energy metabolism with increased intracranial pressure and hyperventilation. *J Neurosurg* 1990; 73:927.

66. Ruta TS, et al: The effect of acute hypocapnia on local cerebral blood flow during middle cerebral artery occlusion in isoflurane anesthetized rats. *Anesthesiology* 1993; 78:134.

67. Kontos HA, et al: Analysis of vasoactivity of local pH, PCO_2, and bicarbonate on pial vessels. *Stroke* 1977; 8:358.

68. Kontos HA, et al: Local mechanism of CO_2 action on cat pial arterioles. *Stroke* 1977; 8:226.

69. Wang Q, et al: Effect of nitric oxide blockade by N-nitro-L-arginine on cerebral blood flow response to changes in carbon dioxide tension. *J Cereb Blood Flow Metab* 1992; 12:947.

70. Wang Q, et al: Is autoregulation of cerebral blood flow in rats influenced by nitro-L-arginine, a blocker of the synthesis of nitric oxide. *Acta Physiol Scand* 1992a; 145:297.

71. Bonvento G, et al: Widespread attenuation of cerebrovascular reactivity to hypercapnia following inhibition of nitric oxide synthase in the conscious rat. *J Cereb Blood Flow Metab* 1994; 14:699.

72. McPherson RW, et al: Effect of nitric oxide synthase inhibition on the cerebral vascular response to hypercapnia in primates. *Stroke* 1995; 26:682.

73. Wang Q, et al: The role of neuronal nitric oxide synthase in regulation of cerebral blood flow in normocapnia and hypercapnia in rats. *J Cereb Blood Flow Metab* 1995; 15:774.

74. Pelligrino DA, et al: Nitric oxide synthesis and regional cerebral blood flow responses to hypercapnia and hypoxia in the rat. *J Cereb Blood Flow Metab* 1993; 13:80.

75. Pickard JD, MacKenzie ET: Inhibition of prostaglandin synthesis and the response of baboon cerebral circulation to carbon dioxide. *Nature New Biol* 1979; 245:187.

76. Wennmalm Å, et al: Effect of indomethacin on basal and carbon dioxide-stimulated cerebral blood flow in man. *Clin Physiol* 1981; 1:227.

77. Nilsson F, et al: Cerebral vasoconstriction by indomethacin in intracranial hypertension. *Anesthesiology* 1995; 83:1283.

78. Pickard JD, et al: Response of the cerebral circulation in baboons to changing perfusion pressure after indomethacin. *Circ Res* 1977; 40:198.

79. Sakabe, T, Siesjö BK: The effect of indomethacin on the blood-flow-metabolism couple in the brain under normal, hypercapnic and hypoxic conditions. *Acta Physiol Scand* 1979; 107:283.

80. Wang Q, et al: Indomethacin abolishes cerebral blood flow increases in response to acetazolamide-induced extracellular acidosis: A mechanism for its effect on hypercapnia. *J Cereb Blood Flow Metab* 1993; 13:724.

81. Koehler RC, et al: Influence of reduced oxyhemoglobin affinity on cerebrovascular response to hypoxic hypoxia. *Am J Physiol* 1986; 251:H756.

82. Donegan JH, et al: Cerebrovascular hypoxic and autoregulatory responses during reduced brain metabolism. *Am J Physiol* 1985; 249:H421.

83. Häggendal E, Johansson B: Effect of arterial carbon dioxide tension and oxygen saturation on cerebral blood flow autoregulation in dogs. *Acta Physiol Scand* 1965; 66(suppl 258):27.

84. Traystman RJ, et al: Cerebral circulatory responses to arterial hypoxia in normal and chemodenervated dogs. *Circ Res* 1978; 42:649.

85. Paulson OB, et al: Cerebral autoregulation. *Cerebrovasc Brain Metab Rev* 1990; 2:161.

86. McPherson RW, et al: Effect of jugular venous pressure on cerebral autoregulation in dogs. *Am J Physiol* 1988; 255:H1516.

87. MacKenzie ET, et al: Effects of hemorrhagic hypotension on the cerebral circulation. I. Cerebral blood flow and pial arteriolar caliber. *Stroke* 1979; 10:711.

88. Risberg J, et al: Correlation between cerebral blood volume and cerebral blood flow in the cat. *Exp Brain Res* 1969; 8:321.

89. Gray WJ, Rosner MJ: Pressure-volume index as a function of cerebral perfusion pressure. *J Neurosurg* 1987; 67:377.

90. Ferrari M, et al: Effects of graded hypotension on cerebral blood flow, blood volume, and mean transit time in dogs. *Am J Physiol* 1992; 262:H1908.

91. Bouma GJ, et al: Blood pressure and intracranial pressure-volume dynamics in severe head injury: Relationship with cerebral blood flow. *J Neurosurg* 1992; 77:15.

92. Kovach AGB, Sandor P: Cerebral blood flow and brain function during hypotension and shock. *Ann Rev Physiol* 1976; 38:571.

93. Folkow B: Description of the myogenic hypothesis. *Cric Res* 1964; 15(suppl 1):279.

94. Harder DR: Pressure-dependent membrane depolarization in cat middle cerebral artery. *Circ Res* 1984; 55:197.

95. Winn HR, et al: Brain adenosine production in rat during sustained alteration in systemic blood pressure. *Am J Physiol* 1980; 239:H636.

96. Winn HR, Morii S: The role of adenosine in autoregulation of cerebral blood flow. *Ann Biomed Eng* 1985; 13:321.

97. Kuschinsky W, Wahl M: Local chemical and neurogenic regulation of cerebral vascular resistance. *Physiol Rev* 1978; 58:656.

98. Kontos HA, et al: Responses of cerebral arteries and arterioles to acute hypotension and hypertension. *Am J Physiol* 1978; 234:H371.

99. Kontos HA, et al: Role of tissue hypoxia in local regulation of cerebral microcirculation. *Am J Physiol* 1978; 234:H582.

100. Wei EP, Kontos HA: Responses of cerebral arterioles to increased venous pressure. *Am J Physiol* 1982; 243:H442.

101. Kontos HA: Regulation of the cerebral circulation. *Ann Rev Physiol* 1981; 43:397.

102. Fitch W, et al: Effects of decreasing arterial blood pressure on cerebral blood flow in the baboon. *Circ Res* 1975; 37:550.

103. Hoff JT, et al: Responses of the cerebral circulation to hypercapnia and hypoxia after VIIth cranial nerve transsection in baboons. *Circ Res* 1977; 40:258.

104. Harder DR: Pressure-induced myogenic activation of cat cerebral arteries is dependent on intact endothelium. *Circ Res* 1987; 60:102.

105. Barry DI, et al: Cerebral blood flow in rats with renal and spontaneous hypertension: Resetting of the lower limit of autoregulation. *J Cereb Blood Flow Metab* 1982; 2:347.

106. Enevoldsen EM, Jensen FT: Autoregulation and CO_2 responses of cerebral blood flow in patients with acute severe head injury. *J Neurosurg* 1978; 48:689.

107. Dirnagl U, Pulsinelli W: Autoregulation of cerebral blood flow in experimental focal brain ischemia. *J Cereb Blood Flow Metab* 1990; 10:327.

108. Tranmer BI, et al: Loss of cerebral regulation during cardiac output variations in focal cerebral ischemia. *J Neurosurg* 1992; 77:253.

109. Hauerberg J, et al: Cerebral blood flow autoregulation after experimental subarachnoid hemorrhage during hyperventilation in rats. *J Neurosurg Anesth* 1993; 5:258.

110. Bouma GJ, Muizelaar JP: Cerebral blood flow, cerebral blood volume, and cerebrovascular reactivity after severe head injury. *J Neurotrauma* 1992; 9:S333.

111. Asgeirsson B, et al: Cerebral haemodynamic effects of dihydroergotamine in patients with severe traumatic brain lesions. *Acta Anaesthesiol Scand* 1995; 39:922.

112. Asgeirsson B, et al: Effects of hypotensive treatment with alpha 2 agonist and beta 1 antagonist on cerebral haemodynamics in severely head injured patients. *Acta Anaesthesiol Scand* 1995; 39:347.

113. Todd MM, et al: Cerebral blood flow, blood volume, and brain tissue hematocrit during isovolemic hemodilution with hetastarch in rats. *Am J Physiol* 1992; 263:H75.

114. Cole DJ, et al: Effects of viscosity and oxygen content on cerebral blood flow in ischemic and normal rat brain. *J Neurol Sci* 1994; 124:15.

115. Muizelaar JP, et al: Cerebral blood flow is regulated by changes in blood pressure and in blood viscosity alike. *Stroke* 1986; 17:44.

116. Muizelaar JP, et al: Mannitol causes compensatory cerebral vasoconstriction and vasodilation in response to blood viscosity changes. *J Neurosurg* 1983; 59:822.

117. Harrison MJG: Influence of haematocrit in the cerebral circulation. *Cerebrovasc Brain Metab Rev* 1989; 1:55.

118. Shiozaki T, et al: Effect of mild hypothermia on uncontrollable intracranial hypertension after severe head injury. *J Neurosurg* 1993; 79:363.

119. Marion DW, et al: The use of moderate therapeutic hypothermia for patients with severe head injuries: A preliminary report. *J Neurosurg* 1993; 79:354.

120. Minamisawa H, et al: The influence of mild body and brain hypothermia on ischemic damage. *J Cereb Blood Flow Metab* 1990; 10:365.

121. Illievich UM, et al: Effects of hypothermia or anesthetics on hippocampus glutamate and glycine concentrations after repeated transient global cerebral ischemia. *Anesthesiology* 1994; 80:177.

122. Baiping L, et al: Effect of moderate hypothermia on lipid peroxidation in canine brain tissue after cardiac arrest and resuscitation. *Stroke* 1994; 25:147.

123. Karibe H, et al: Mild intraischemic hypothermia reduces postischemic hyperperfusion, delayed hypoperfusion, blood-brain barrier disruption, brain edema, and neuronal damage after temporary focal cerebral ischemia in rats. *J Cereb Blood Flow Metab* 1994; 14:620.

124. Steen PA, et al: Hypothermia and barbiturates: Individual and combined effects on canine cerebral oxygen consumption. *Anesthesiology* 1983; 58:527.

125. Rosomoff HL, Holaday DA: Cerebral blood flow and cerebral oxygen consumption during hypothermia. *Am J Physiol* 1954; 179:85.

126. Frizzell RT, et al: Effects of etomidate and hypothermia on cerebral metabolism and blood flow in a canine model of hypoperfusion. *J Neurosurg Anesth* 1993; 5:104.

127. Behring EA, et al: The effect of hypothermia on the cerebral physiology and cerebral metabolism of monkeys in the hypothermic state. *Surg Gynecol Obstet* 1956; 102:134.

128. Prough DS, et al: Cerebral blood flow decreases with time whereas cerebral oxygen consumption remains stable during hypothermic cardiopulmonary bypass in humans. *Anesth Analg* 1991; 72:161.

129. Hägerdal M, et al: The effect of induced hypothermia upon oxygen consumption in the rat brain. *J Neurochem* 1975; 24:311.

130. Steen PA, et al: The detrimental effects of prolonged hypothermia and rewarming in the dog. *Anesthesiology* 1980; 52:224.

131. Steen PA, et al: Detrimental effect of prolonged hypothermia in cats and monkeys with and without regional cerebral ischemia. *Stroke* 1979; 10:522.

132. Verhaegen MJJ, et al: Cerebral autoregulation during moderate hypothermia in rats. *Stroke* 1993; 24:407.

133. Hindman BJ, et al: Differences in cerebral blood flow between alpha-stat and pH-stat management are eliminated during periods of decreased systemic flow and pressure. *Anesthesiology* 1991; 74:1096.

134. McNeill BR, et al: Autoregulation and the CO_2 responsiveness of cerebral blood flow after cardiopulmonary bypass. *Can J Anaesth* 1990; 37:313.

135. Rogers AT, et al: Response of cerebral blood flow to phenylephrine infusion during hypothermic cardiopulmonary bypass: Influence of $PaCO_2$ management. *Anesthesiology* 1988; 69:547.

136. Nattie EE: The alpha-stat hypothesis in respiratory control and acid-base balance. *J Appl Physiol* 1990; 69:120.

137. Murkin JM, et al: Cerebral autoregulation and flow/metabolism coupling during cardiopulmonary bypass: The influence of $PaCO_2$. *Anesth Analg* 1987; 66:825.

138. Stephan H, et al: Acid-base management during hypothermic cardiopulmonary bypass does not affect cerebral metabolism but does affect blood flow and neurological outcome. *Br J Anaesth* 1992; 69:51.

139. Hägerdal M, et al: Influence of changes in arterial PCO_2 on cerebral blood flow and cerebral energy state during hypothermia in the rat. *Acta Anaesth Scand* 1975; suppl 57:25.

140. Hindman BJ, et al: Cerebral blood flow response to $PaCO_2$ during hypothermic cardiopulmonary bypass in rabbits. *Anesthesiology* 1991; 75:662.

141. Johnsson P, et al: Cerebral vasoreactivity to carbon dioxide during cardiopulmonary perfusion at normothermia and hypothermia. *Ann Thorac Surg* 1989; 48:769.

142. Prough DS, et al: Response of cerebral blood flow to changes in carbon dioxide tension during hypothermic cardiopulmonary bypass. *Anesthesiology* 1986; 64:576.

143. Stullken EH, et al: The nonlinear responses of cerebral metabo-

lism to low concentrations of halothane, enflurane, isoflurane and thiopental. *Anesthesiology* 1977; 46:28.

144. Drummond JC, et al: A comparison of the direct vasodilating potencies of halothane and isoflurane in the New Zealand white rabbit. *Anesthesiology* 1986; 65:462.

145. Todd MM, Drummond JC: A comparison of the cerebrovascular and metabolic effects of halothane and isoflurane in the cat. *Anesthesiology* 1984; 60:276.

146. Hansen TD, et al: Distribution of cerebral blood flow during halothane versus isoflurane anesthesia in rats. *Anesthesiology* 1988; 69:332.

147. Newberg LA, et al: The cerebral metabolic effects of isoflurane at and above concentrations that suppress cortical electrical activity. *Anesthesiology* 1983; 59:23.

148. Maekawa T, et al: Local cerebral blood flow and glucose utilization during isoflurane anesthesia in the rat. *Anesthesiology* 1986; 65:144.

149. Drummond JC, Todd MM: The response of the feline circulation to $PaCO_2$ during anesthesia with isoflurane and halothane and during sedation with nitrous oxide. *Anesthesiology* 1985; 62:268.

150. McPherson RW, et al: Cerebrovascular responsiveness to carbon dioxide in dogs with 1.4% and 2.8% isoflurane. *Anesthesiology* 1989; 70:843.

151. McPherson RW, et al: Changes in cerebral CO_2 reactivity over time during isoflurane anesthesia in the dog. *J Neurosurg Anesth* 1991; 3:12.

152. McPherson RW, Traystman RJ: Effects of isoflurane on cerebral autoregulation in dogs. *Anesthesiology* 1988; 69:493.

153. Drummond JC, et al: Brain surface protrusion during enflurane, halothane, and isoflurane anesthesia in cats. *Anesthesiology* 1983; 59:288.

154. Archer DP, et al: Measurement of cerebral blood flow and volume with positron emission tomography during isoflurane administration in the hypocapnic baboon. *Anesthesiology* 1990; 72:1031.

155. Archer DP, et al: Cerebral blood volume is increased in dogs during administration of nitrous oxide or isoflurane. *Anesthesiology* 1987; 67:642.

156. Artru AA: Relationship between cerebral blood volume and CSF pressure during anesthesia with isoflurane or fentanyl in dogs. *Anesthesiology* 1984; 60:575.

157. Kaieda R, et al: A comparison of the effects of halothane, isoflurane, and pentobarbital anesthesia on intracranial pressure and cerebral edema formation following brain injury in rabbits. *Anesthesiology* 1989; 71:571.

158. Entrei C, et al: Local application of 133-xenon for measurement of regional cerebral blood flow (rCBF) during halothane, enflurane, and isoflurane anesthesia in humans. *Anesthesiology* 1985; 63:391.

159. Madsen JB, et al: The effect of isoflurane on cerebral blood flow and metabolism in humans during craniotomy for small supratentorial tumors. *Anesthesiology* 1987; 66:332.

160. Algotsson L, et al: Cerebral blood flow and oxygen consumption during isoflurane and halothane anesthesia in man. *Acta Anaesthesiol Scand* 1988; 32:15.

161. Reinstrup P, et al: Distribution of cerebral blood flow during anesthesia with isoflurane or halothane in humans. *Anesthesiology* 1995; 82:359.

162. Gordon E, et al: The effect of isoflurane on cerebrospinal fluid pressure in patients undergoing neurosurgery. *Acta Anaesthesiol Scand* 1988; 32:108.

163. Adams RW, et al: Isoflurane and cerebrospinal fluid pressure in neurosurgical patients. *Anesthesiology* 1981; 54:97.

164. Crawford MW, et al: Hemodynamic and organ blood flow

165. Scheller MS, et al: The effects of sevoflurane on cerebral blood flow, cerebral metabolic rate for oxygen, intracranial pressure, and the electroencephalogram are similar to those of isoflurane in the rabbit. *Anesthesiology* 1988; 68:548.

166. Lutz LJ, et al: The cerebral functional, metabolic, and hemodynamic effects of desflurane in dogs. *Anesthesiology* 1990; 73:125.

167. Newberg Milde L, Milde JH: The cerebral and systemic hemodynamic effects of desflurane-induced hypotension in dogs. *Anesthesiology* 1991; 74:513.

168. Lutz LJ, Milde JH, Newberg Milde L: The response of the canine cerebral circulation to hyperventilation during anesthesia with desflurane. *Anesthesiology* 1991; 74:504.

169. Ornstein E, et al: Desflurane and isoflurane have similar effects on cerebral blood flow in patients with intracranial mass lesions. *Anesthesiology* 1993; 79:498.

170. Kitaguchi K, et al: Effects of sevoflurane on cerebral circulation and metabolism in patients with ischemic cerebrovascular disease. *Anesthesiology* 1993; 79:704.

171. Muzzi DA, et al: The effect of desflurane and isoflurane on cerebrospinal fluid pressure in humans with supratentorial mass lesions. *Anesthesiology* 1992; 76:720.

172. Artru AA: Rate of cerebrospinal fluid formation, resistance to reabsorption of cerebrospinal fluid, brain tissue water content, and electroencephalogram during desflurane anesthesia in dogs. *J Neurosurg Anesth* 1993; 5:178.

173. Pelligrino DA, et al: Nitrous oxide markedly increases cerebral cortical metabolic rate and blood flow in the goat. *Anesthesiology* 1984; 60:405.

174. Baughman VL, et al: Cerebrovascular and metabolic effects of N_2O in unrestrained rats. *Anesthesiology* 1990; 73:269.

175. Kaieda R, et al: The effects of anesthetics and $PaCO_2$ on the cerebrovascular, metabolic, and electroencephalographic responses to nitrous oxide in the rabbit. *Anesth Analg* 1989; 68:135.

176. Hansen TD, et al: Effects of nitrous oxide and volatile anaesthetics on cerebral blood flow. *Br J Anaesth* 1989; 63:290.

177. Reasoner DK, et al: Effects of nitrous oxide on cerebral metabolic rate in rats anesthetized with isoflurane. *Br J Anaesth* 1990; 65:210.

178. Roald OK, et al: Cerebral effects of nitrous oxide when added to low and high concentrations of isoflurane in the dog. *Anesth Analg* 1991; 72:75.

179. Matta BF, Lam AM: Nitrous oxide increases cerebral blood flow velocity during pharmacologically induced EEG silence in humans. *J Neurosurg Anesth* 1995; 7:89.

180. Field LM, et al: Effect of nitrous oxide on cerebral blood flow in normal humans. *Br J Anaesth* 1993; 70:154.

181. Reinstrup P, et al: Effects of nitrous oxide on human regional cerebral blood flow and isolated pial arteries. *Anesthesiology* 1994; 81:396.

182. Algotsson L, et al: Effects of nitrous oxide on cerebral haemodynamics and metabolism during isoflurane anaesthesia in man. *Acta Anaesthesiol Scand* 1992; 36:46.

183. Phirman JR, Shapiro HM: Modification of nitrous oxide-induced intracranial hypertension by prior induction of anesthesia. *Anesthesiology* 1977; 46:150.

184. Moss E, McDowall DG: ICP increases with 50% nitrous oxide in oxygen in severe head injuries during controlled ventilation. *Br J Anaesth* 1979; 51:757.

185. Domino KB, et al: Effect of nitrous oxide on intracranial pressure after cranial-dural closure in patients undergoing craniotomy. *Anesthesiology* 1992; 77:421.

186. Kassell NF, et al: Influence of changes in arterial pCO_2 on

cerebral blood flow and metabolism during high-dose barbiturate therapy in dogs. *J Neurosurg* 1981; 54:615.

187. Hodes JE, et al: Selective changes in local cerebral glucose utilization induced by phenobarbital in the art. *Anesthesiology* 1985; 63:633.

188. Nilsson L, Siesjö BK: The effect of phenobarbitone anaesthesia on blood flow and oxygen consumption in the rat brain. *Acta Anaesthesiol Scand* 1975; (suppl 5):18.

189. Pierce EC, et al: Cerebral circulation and metabolism during thiopental anesthesia and hyperventilation in man. *J Clin Invest* 1962; 41:1664.

190. Shapiro HM, et al: Rapid intraoperative reduction of intracranial pressure with thiopentone. *Br J Anaesth* 1973; 45:1057.

191. Newberg Milde L, et al: Cerebral functional, metabolic, and hemodynamic effects of etomidate in dogs. *Anesthesiology* 1985; 63:371.

192. Davis DW, et al: Regional brain glucose utilization in rats during etomidate anesthesia. *Anesthesiology* 1986; 64:751.

193. Cold GE, et al: CBF and $CMRO_2$ during continuous etomidate infusion supplemented with N_2O and fentanyl in patients with supratentorial cerebral tumour. *Acta Anaesthesiol Scand* 1985; 29:490.

194. Dearden NM, McDowell DG: Comparison of etomidate and althesin in the reduction of increased intracranial pressure after head injury. *Br J Anaesth* 1985; 57:361.

195. Artru AA, et al: Electroencephalogram, cerebral metabolic, and vascular responses to propofol anesthesia in dogs. *J Neurosurg Anesth* 1992; 4:99.

196. Ramani R, et al: A dose-response study of the influence of propofol on cerebral blood flow, metabolism and the electroencephalogram in the rabbit. *J Neurosurg Anesth* 1992; 4:110.

197. Werner C, et al: The effects of propofol on cerebral and spinal cord blood flow in rats. *Anesth Analg* 1993; 76:971.

198. Stephan H, et al: Effects of disoprivan on cerebral blood flow, cerebral oxygen consumption, and cerebral vascular reactivity. *Anaesthesist* 1987; 36:60.

199. Alkire MT, et al: Cerebral metabolism during propofol anesthesia in humans studied with positron emission tomography. *Anesthesiology* 1995; 82:393.

200. Pinaud M, et al: Effects of propofol on cerebral hemodynamics and metabolism in patients with brain trauma. *Anesthesiology* 1990; 73:404.

201. Ravussin P, et al: Effect of propofol on cerbrospinal fluid pressure and cerebral perfusion pressure in patients undergoing craniotomy. *Anaesthesia* 1988; 43:37.

202. Ebrahim ZY, et al: The effect of propofol on the electroencephalogram of patients with epilepsy. *Anesth Analg* 1994; 78:275.

203. Fleischer JE, et al: Cerebral effects of high-dose midazolam and subsequent reversal with Ro 15-1788 in dogs. *Anesthesiology* 1988; 68:234.

204. Nugent M, et al: Cerebral metabolic, vascular and protective effects of midazolam maleate. *Anesthesiology* 1982; 56:172.

205. Hoffman WE, et al: The effects of midazolam on cerebral blood flow and oxygen consumption and its interaction with nitrous oxide. *Anesth Analg* 1986; 65:729.

206. Forster A, et al: Effects of midazolam on cerebral blood flow in human volunteers. *Anesthesiology* 1982; 56:453.

207. Griffin JP, et al: Intracranial pressure, mean arterial pressure, and heart rate following midazolam or thiopental in humans with brain tumors. *Anesthesiology* 1984; 60:491.

208. Keykhah MM, et al: Influence of sufentanil on cerebral metabolism and circulation in the rat. *Anesthesiology* 1985; 63:274.

209. Mayer N, et al: Sufentanil does not increase cerebral blood flow in healthy human volunteers. *Anesthesiology* 1990; 73:240.

210. Stephan H, et al: Effects of high-dose sufentanil-O_2 anesthesia

211. McPherson RW, Traystman RJ: Fentanyl and cerebral vascular responsivity in dogs. *Anesthesiology* 1984; 60:180.

212. Newberg Milde L, et al: Effects of sufentanil on cerebral circulation and metabolism in dogs. *Anesth Analg* 1990; 70:138.

213. Albanese J, et al: Sufentanil increases intracranial pressure in patients with head trauma. *Anesthesiology* 1993; 79:493.

214. Sperry RJ, et al: Fentanyl and sufentanil increase intracranial pressure in head trauma patients. *Anesthesiology* 1992; 77:416.

215. Van Hemelrijck J, et al: The effect of sufentanil on intracranial pressure (ICP) in anesthetized dogs. *Acta Anaesthesiol Belg* 1989; 40:239.

216. Weinstabl C, et al: Effect of sufentanil on intracranial pressure in neurosurgical patients. *Anaesthesia* 1991; 46:837.

217. Werner C, et al: The effects of sufentanil on cerebral hemodynamics and intracranial pressure in patients with brain injury. *Anesthesiology* 1995; 83:721.

218. Kreuscher H, Grote J: The effect of the phencyclinidine derivative ketamine (CI 581) on cerebral blood flow and cerebral oxygen uptake in dogs. *Anaesthesist* 1967; 16:304.

219. Herrschaft H, Schmidt H: Changes in the global and regional cerebral blood flow under the influence of propanidid, ketamine and sodium thiopental. *Anaesthesist* 1973; 22:486.

220. Cavazzuti M, et al: Ketamine effects on local cerebral blood flow and metabolism in the rat. *J Cereb Blood Flow Metab* 1987; 7:806.

221. Hougaard K, et al: The effect of ketamine on regional cerebral blood flow in man. *Anesthesiology* 1974; 41:562.

222. Takeshita H, et al: The effects of ketamine on cerebral circulation and metabolism in man. *Anesthesiology* 1972; 36:69.

223. Oren RE, et al: Effect of ketamine on cerebral cortical blood flow and metabolism in rabbits. *Stroke* 1987; 18:441.

224. Wendling WW, et al: Ketamine directly dilates bovine cerebral arteries by acting as a calcium entry blocker. *J Neurosurg Anesth* 1994; 6:186.

225. Pfenninger E, Reith A: Ketamine and intracranial pressure. In Domino EF (ed): *Status of Ketamine in Anesthesiology.* NPP Books, 1990:109.

226. Artru AA, Katz RA: Cerebral blood volume and CSF pressure following administration of ketamine in dogs; modification by pre- or posttreatment with hypocapnia or diazepam. *J Neurosurg Anesth* 1989; 1:8.

227. Gibbs JM: The effect of intravenous ketamine on cerebrospinal fluid pressure. *Br J Anaesth* 1972; 44:1298.

228. Bloor BC, Flacke WE: Reduction in halothane anesthetic requirement by clonidine, an alpha-adrenergic agonist. *Anesth Analg* 1982; 61:741.

229. Segal IS, et al: Dexmedetomidine diminishes halothane anesthetic requirements in rats through a postsynaptic alpha 2 adrenergic receptor. *Anesthesiology* 1988; 69:818.

230. Aantaa R, et al: Dexmedetomidine, an alpha 2 adrenoceptor agonist, reduces anesthetic requirements for patients undergoing minor gynecologic surgery. *Anesthesiology* 1990; 73:230.

231. Aho M, et al: The effect of intravenously administered dexmedetomidine on perioperative hemodynamics and isoflurane requirements in patients undergoing abdominal hysterectomy. *Anesthesiology* 1991; 74:997.

232. Kanawati I, et al: Effects of clonidine on cerebral blood flow and the response to arterial CO_2. *J Cereb Blood Flow Metab* 1986; 6:358.

233. Fale A, et al: Alpha-2-adrenergic agonist effects on normocapnic and hypercapnic cerebral blood flow in the dog are anesthetic dependent. *Anesth Analg* 1994; 79:892.

234. Zornow MH, et al: Dexmedetomidine, an alpha-2-adrenergic

agonist, decreases cerebral blood flow in the isoflurane-anesthetized dog. *Anesth Analg* 1990; 70:624.

235. McCormick JM, et al: Intracranial pressure reduction by a central alpha-2-adrenoceptor agonist after subarachnoid hemorrhage. *Neurosurgery* 1993; 32:974.

236. Zornow MH, et al: Intracranial pressure effects of dexmedetomidine in rabbits. *Anesth Analg* 1992; 75:232.

237. Miletich DJ, et al: Cerebral hemodynamics following internal maxillary ligation in the goat. *J Appl Physiol* 1975; 38:942.

238. Michenfelder JD, et al: Simultaneous cerebral blood flow measured by direct and indirect methods. *J Surg Res* 1968; 8:475.

239. Schmidt CF, et al: The gaseous metabolism of the brain of the monkey. *Am J Physiol* 1945; 143:33.

240. Nornes H, Wikeby P: Cerebral arterial blood flow and aneurysm surgery. *J Neurosurg* 1977; 47:810.

241. Hoffmann WE, et al: Nitrous oxide added to isoflurane increases brain artery blood flow and low frequency brain electrical activity. *J Neurosurg Anesth* 1995; 7:82.

242. Kety SS, Schmidt CF: The determination of cerebral blood flow in man by the use of nitrous oxide in low concentrations. *Am J Physiol* 1945; 143:53.

243. Kety SS, Schmidt CF: The nitrous oxide method for the quantitative determination of cerebral blood flow in man: Theory, procedure and normal values. *J Clin Invest* 1948; 27:476.

244. Shenkin HA, et al: Dynamic anatomy of the cerebral circulation. *Arch Neurol* 1948; 60:240.

245. Lassen NA, Munck O: The cerebral blood flow in man determined by the use of radioactive krypton. *Acta Physiol Scand* 1955; 33:30.

246. McHenry LC Jr: Determination of cerebral blood flow by a krypton-85 desaturation method. *Nature* 1963; 200:1297.

247. Freygang WH, Sokoloff L: Quantitative measurement of regional circulation in the central nervous system by the use of radioactive inert gas. In Tobias CA, JH Lawrence (eds): *Advances in Biological and Medical Physics*, vol 6. New York, Academic Press, 1958:263.

248. Kety SS: Theory and applications of exchange of inert gas at lungs and tissues. *Pharmacol Rev* 1951; 3:1.

249. Lassen NA, Ingvar DH: Blood flow of the cerebral cortex determined by radioactive Krypton 85. *Experientia (Basel)* 1961; 17:42.

250. Young WL, et al: Cerebral blood flow and metabolism in patients undergoing anesthesia cardiopulmonary bypass in humans. *Anesth Analg* 1991; 72:161.

251. Ingvar DH, et al: Normal values of regional cerebral blood flow in man, including flow and weight estimates of grey and white matter. *Acta Neurol Scand* (suppl)1965; 14:72.

252. Obrist WD, et al: Determination of regional cerebral blood flow by inhalation of 133-xenon. *Circ Res* 1967; 20:124.

253. Obrist WD, et al: Regional cerebral blood flow estimated by 133-xenon inhalation. *Stroke* 1975; 6:245.

254. Young WL, et al: Rapid monitoring of intraoperative cerebral blood flow using 133 Xe. *J Cereb Blood FLow Metab* 1988; 8:691.

255. Prohovnik I, et al: Accuracy of models and algorithms for determination of fast compartment flow by non-invasive 133 Xe clearance. In Magistretti PL (ed): *Functional Radionuclide Imaging of the Brain*. New York, Raven Press, 1983:87.

256. Halsey JH Jr, et al: Sensitivity of rCBF to focal lesions. *Stroke* 1981; 12:631.

257. Yonas H, et al: Mapping cerebral blood flow by xenon-enhanced computerized tomography: Clinical experience. *Radiology* 1984; 152:435.

258. Good WF, Gur D: Errors in cerebral blood flow determination by xenon-enhanced computed tomography due to estimation of arterial xenon concentrations. *Med Phys* 1987; 14:377.

259. Kuhl DE, Edwards RQ: Image separation radioisotope scanning. *Radiology* 1963; 80:653.

260. Stokely EM, et al: A single photon dynamic computer assisted tomograph (DVAT) for imaging brain function in multiple cross sections. *J Comput Assist Tomogr* 1980; 4:230.

261. Kanno I, et al: A hybrid emission tomograph for single photon and positron emission imaging of the brain. *J Comput Assist Tomogr* 1981; 5:216.

262. Holm S, et al: Dynamic SPECT of the brain using a lipophilic technetium-99m complex, PnAO. *J Nucl Med* 1985; 26:1129.

263. Neirinckx RD, et al: Technetium-99m d,1-HM-PAO. A new radiopharmaceutical for SPECT imaging of regional cerebral blood perfusion. *J Nucl Med* 1987; 28:191.

264. Brust JCM: Transient ischemic attacks: Natural history and anticoagulation. *Neurology* 1977; 27:701.

265. Crom W, Guinto FC Jr: Limitations of CT in the evaluation of transient ischemic attacks. *Tex Med J* 1982; 78:65.

266. Lassen NA: The luxury-perfusion syndrome and its possible relation to metabolic acidosis located with the brain. *Lancet* 1966; 2:113.

267. Bonte FJ, et al: Single-photon tomographic study of regional cerebral blood flow in patients with arteriovenous malformations. *J Nucl Med* 1983; 24:105.

268. Jones T, et al: The continuous inhalation of oxygen-15 for assessing regional oxygen extraction in the brain of man. *Br J Radiol* 1976; 49:339.

269. Firmin D, et al: In vivo validation of MR velocity imaging. *J Comput Assist Tomogr* 1987; 11:751.

270. Dumoulin C, et al: Time resolved magnetic resonance angiography. *Magn Reson Med* 1988; 6:275.

271. Burkart DJ, et al: Cine phase-contrast MR measurements: Improved precision using an automated method of vessel detection. *J Comput Assist Tomogr* 1993; 18:469.

272. Sommer G, et al: Normal renal blood flow measurement using phase contrast cine magnetic resonance imaging. *Invest Radiol* 1992; 27:465.

273. Pernicone J, et al: Three dimensional phase contrast MR angiography in the head and neck. Preliminary report. *AJNR* 1990; 11:457.

274. Heymann M, et al: Blood flow measurements with radionuclide-labelled particles. *Prog Cardiovasc Dis* 1977; 20:55.

275. Phibbs RH, et al: Rheology of microspheres injected into circulation of rabbits. *Nature* 1967; 216:1339.

276. Phibbs RH, Dong L: Nonuniform distribution of microspheres in blood flowing through a medium-size artery. *Can J Physiol Pharmacol* 1970; 48:415.

277. Bolognese P, et al: Laser-Doppler flowmetry in neurosurgery. *J Neurosurg Anesth* 1993; 5:151.

278. Caspary L, et al: Biological zero in laser Doppler flowmetry. *Int J Microcirc Clin Exp* 1988; 7:367.

279. Skarphedinsson JO, et al: Repeated measurements of cerebral blood flow in rats. Comparison between the hydrogen clearance method and laser Doppler flowmetry. *Acta Physiol Scand* 1988; 134:133.

280. Dirnagl U, et al: Continuous measurement of cerebral cortical blood flow by laser-Doppler flowmetry in a rat stroke model. *J Cereb Blood Flow Metab* 1989; 9:589.

281. Meyerson BA, et al: Bedside monitoring of regional cortical blood flow in comatose patients using laser Doppler flowmetry. *Neurosurgery* 1991; 29:750.

282. Haberl RL, et al: Applicability of laser-Doppler flowmetry for cerebral blood flow monitoring in neurological intensive care. *Acta Neurochir* (suppl) 1993; 59:64.

283. Rosenblum BR, et al: Intraoperative measurement of cortical blood flow adjacent to cerebral AVM using laser Doppler velocimetry. *J Neurosurg* 1987; 66:396.

284. Fasano VA, et al: Intraoperative use of laser Doppler in the study of cerebral microvascular circulation. *Acta Neurochir (Wien)* 1988; 95:40.

285. Arbit E, et al: Intraoperative measurement of cerebral and tumor blood flow with laser-Doppler flowmetry. *Neurosurgery* 1989; 24:166.

286. Florence G, Seylaz J: Rapid autoregulation of cerebral blood flow: A laser-Doppler flowmetry study. *J Cereb Blood Flow Metab* 1992; 12:674.

287. Rosner MJ: Cerebral perfusion pressure: Link between intracranial pressure and systemic circulation. In Wood JH (ed): *Cerebral Blood Flow.* New York, McGraw-Hill, 1987:425.

288. Kirkpatrick PJ, et al: Continuous monitoring of cortical perfusion by laser Doppler flowmetry in ventilated patients with head injury. *J Neurol Neursurg Psychiatry* 1994; 57:1382.

289. Carter LP, et al: Cortical blood flow: Thermal diffusion vs isotope clearance. *Stroke* 1981; 23:513.

290. Wei D, et al: Validation of continuous thermal measurement of cerebral blood flow by arterial pressure change. *J Cereb Blood Flow Metab* 1993; 13:693.

291. Voorhees WD, et al: Continuous monitoring of cerebral perfusion by thermal clearance. *Neurol Res* 1993; 15:75.

292. Abe K, et al: Effect of prostaglandin E1 induced hypotension on carbon dioxide reactivity and local cerebral blood flow after subarachnoid hemorrhage. *Br J Anaesth* 1992; 68:268.

293. Abe K, et al: The effect of nicardipine on blood flow velocity, local cerebral blood flow, and carbon dioxide reactivity during cerebral aneurysm surgery. *Anesth Analg* 1993; 76:1227.

294. Ogama A, et al: Limitation of temporary vascular occlusion during aneurysm surgery. *Surg Neurol* 1991; 36:453.

295. Barnett GH, et al: Cerebral circulation during arteriovenous malformation operation. *Neurosurgery* 1987; 20:836.

296. Matta BF, et al: A critique of the intraoperative use of jugular venous bulb catheters during neurosurgical procedures. *Anesth Analg* 1994; 79:745.

297. Andrews PJD, et al: Jugular bulb cannulation: Description of a cannulation technique and validation of a new continuous monitor. *Br J Anaesth* 1991; 67:553.

298. Robertson CD, et al: Cerebral arteriovenous oxygen difference as an estimate of cerebral blood flow in comatose patients. *J Neurosurg* 1989; 70:222.

299. Moss E, et al: Effects of changes in mean arterial pressure on SjO$_2$ during cerebral aneurysm surgery. *Br J Anaesth* 1995; 75:527.

300. Cruz J, et al: Cerebral lactate-oxygen index in acute brain injury with acute anemia: Assessment of false versus true ischemia. *Crit Care Med* 1994; 22:1465.

301. Meyer JS, et al: Effects of anoxia on cerebral metabolism and electrolytes in man. *Neurology* 1965; 115:892.

302. Lennox WG, et al: Relationship of unconsciousness to cerebral blood flow and to anoxemia. *Arch Neurol* 1935; 34:1001.

303. Cruz J: On-line monitoring of global cerebral hypoxia in acute brain injury: Relationship to intracranial hypertension. *J Neurosurg* 1993; 79:228.

304. Sheinberg M, et al: Continuous monitoring of jugular venous oxygen saturation in head-injured patients. *J Neurosurg* 1992; 76:212.

305. Lyons C, et al: Cerebral venous oxygen content during carotid thrombintimectomy. *Ann Surg* 1964; 160:561.

306. Dearden NM: Jugular bulb venous oxygen saturation in the management of severe head injury. *Curr Opinion Anaesth* 1991; 4:279.

Chapter 3

CSF DYNAMICS, CEREBRAL EDEMA, AND INTRACRANIAL PRESSURE

ALAN A. ARTRU

By definition, cerebral edema is a condition in which increased brain tissue water content results in increased brain tissue volume. At the microscopic level, brain tissue water is in the intracellular fluid (ICF) and extracellular fluid (ECF) spaces. Intracerebral water is also located in macroscopic spaces, as in the cerebrospinal fluid (CSF). Water in the ICF space equilibrates with water in the ECF space, and both spaces equilibrate with CSF (Figure 3-1). Several types of cerebral edema are recognized. For some types, the increase of brain tissue water may be precipitated by increased water content in either the ICF or ECF space, or both. For other types, increase of CSF volume is the precipitating cause.

Water enters the ECF by passage from the vasculature across the "blood-brain barrier" (BBB), and the CSF by passage from the vasculature across the "blood-CSF barrier" at the choroid plexus. Water is created within the ICF as a result of metabolism of glucose. The ventricular ependyma separates the CSF space from the ECF space. Because the ependymal cells are not contiguous (i.e., there are gaps between ependymal cells), the ependyma does not constitute a barrier to free movement of water between the CSF and the ECF spaces. The "barrier" to exchange of water between the ICF and ECF spaces is the cell membrane of neurons and glial cells.

The first two parts of this chapter review the routes of intracerebral water formation—CSF, ICF, and ECF. The section on CSF also reviews CSF reabsorption because that is a principal route of egress of water from the intracerebral space. In the section on ICF and ECF, special attention is given to BBB functions that are in addition to ECF formation. The third part of this chapter reviews the several types of cerebral edema that have been recognized and, as well, presents approaches to treatment for each type of edema. The fourth part of this chapter reviews intracranial pressure (ICP), techniques to monitor ICP, and approaches to treatment of intracranial hypertension.

Cerebrospinal Fluid

ANATOMY OF THE CSF SPACES AND PROPERTIES OF CSF

CSF is formed in the brain. CSF circulates through macroscopic spaces and freely exchanges between these and the adjacent microscopic ECF spaces that are in continuity. The macroscopic CSF spaces include two lateral ventricles, the third (cerebral) ventricle, the aqueduct of Sylvius, the fourth (cerebellar) ventricle, the central canal of the spinal cord, and the subarachnoid space. The total volume of these spaces ranges from 50 ml in infants to 140 to 150 ml in adults (Table 3-1).

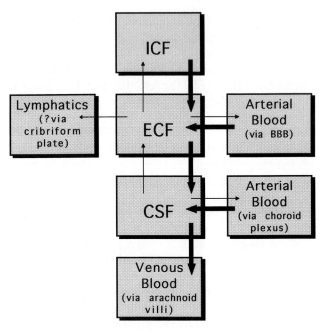

Figure 3-1   Paths of fluid movement between cerebral intracellular fluid (ICF), extracellular fluid (ECF), cerebrospinal fluid (CSF), blood and lymphatics. Large arrows represent major paths of fluid movement under normal conditions such as from arterial blood, across the blood-brain barrier (BBB), and into the ECF space. Small arrows represent minor paths of fluid movement under normal conditions. Under pathologic conditions, the major path of fluid movement may change. For example, during the formation of ischemic edema, there is substantial fluid movement from the ECF to the ICF space. During the formation of hydrocephalic edema, there is substantial fluid movement from the CSF to the ECF space.

Ventricular volume composes about 16 to 17 percent of macroscopic CSF volume in adults.[1]

MACROSCOPIC SPACES

The choroid plexuses (CPs) of the lateral ventricles extend from the inferior horn to the central part of the ventricle. The CPs of the two lateral ventricles and the

TABLE 3-1
CSF Pressure and Volume in Humans

	Range of CSF Values*
CSF Pressure (mmHg)	
Children	3.0–7.5
Adults	4.5–13.5
Volume (ml)	
Infants	40–60
Young children	60–100
Older children	80–120
Adult	100–160

* Values based on Artru.[38]

third ventricle become continuous with each other at the interventricular foramina. Tela choroidea are vascular invaginations of the pia mater which form the support structure for each CP. The CPs in the body of the lateral and third ventricles receive their blood supply from the posterior and anterior choroidal arteries, respectively. The CPs in the temporal horns and the fourth ventricle are supplied by the superior and posterior inferior cerebellar arteries, respectively.[2] The nervous supply to the CPs includes branches of the vagus, glossopharyngeal, and sympathetic nerves.

A single layer of epithelial cells lines most of the macroscopic CSF spaces. However, the ventricles and central canal of the spinal cord are lined by ependyma, a ciliated, low-columnar epithelium. There are no tight junctions between the ependymal cells covering most of the surface area of the ventricles and central canal. In contrast, there are tight junctions between the ependymal cells covering the CP. An "open" mesothelium, formed inwardly by the pia and outwardly by a loose investment of arachnoid cells, covers the cisterns and sulci of the subarachnoid space.

COMPOSITION OF CSF

CSF is a clear aqueous solution that, compared with plasma, contains higher concentrations of sodium, chloride, and magnesium and lower concentrations of glucose, proteins, amino acids, uric acid, potassium, bicarbonate, calcium, and phosphate (Table 3-2). The concentration of these and other substances in the macroscopic spaces varies according to the sampling site due to exchange of water and other substances between CSF and ECF as CSF passes through the ventricles and subarachnoid spaces.[1] That the composition of CSF differs from an ultrafiltrate of plasma is cited as evidence that active secretion occurs during CSF formation. Regional variations in potassium, urea, albumin, globulin, and amino acids is cited as evidence that transport of solutes into and out of the CSF occurs at sites other than the CP.[3] For example, calcium movement out of CSF is reported to occur by a transport mechanism and to be concentration-independent.[4] The higher concentration of protein in lumbar CSF relative to cisternal CSF probably reflects net addition of central nervous system (CNS) metabolites to CSF as it drains toward sites of absorption.[5]

CSF FORMATION

The rate of CSF formation is about 0.35 to 0.40 ml/min or 500 to 600 ml/day in humans. Approximately 0.25 percent of total adult CSF volume is replaced by freshly formed CSF each minute. The turnover time for total CSF volume is about 5 to 7 hours, yielding a

TABLE 3-2
Composition of CSF and Plasma in Humans

	Mean CSF Concentration*	Mean Plasma Concentration*
Specific gravity	1.007	1.025
Osmolality (mosm/kg H_2O)	289	289
pH	7.31	7.41
P_{CO_2} (mmHg)	50.5	41.1
Sodium (meq/liter)	141	140
Potassium (meq/liter)	2.9	4.6
Calcium (meq/liter)	2.5	5.0
Magnesium (meq/liter)	2.4	1.7
Chloride (meq/liter)	124	101
Bicarbonate (meq/liter)	21	23
Glucose (mg/100 ml)	61	92
Protein (mg/liter)		
Albumin	192	42,150
Globulin	50	22,700
Alpha-2-macroglobulin	4.6	3000
Beta-2-microglobulin	1.1	2
Haptoglobulin	2.24	4800
Thyroxine-binding globulin	0.132	9.9
Fibrinogen	0.6	2800
Plasminogen	0.25	700
Transferrin	14	2600
Cystatin C	7.3	1.4
Transthyretin	14.7	176
Alpha-1-acid glycoprotein	3.5	980
Alpha-2-HS glycoprotein	1.7	600
Ceruloplasmin	0.9	370
Alpha-1-antitrypsin	7	3000

* Average values based on Artru[38] and Schreiber and Aldred.[311]

turnover rate of about four times per day.[6] Roughly 40 to 70 percent of CSF enters the macroscopic spaces via the CP, whereas 30 to 60 percent of CSF enters the macroscopic spaces from extrachoroidal sites.[7]

CSF FORMATION AT THE CHOROID PLEXUS

Unlike the capillary endothelium of other cerebral vessels, the capillary endothelium of the CP and seven other small, specialized areas do not possess tight junctions between its cells. Instead, the capillary endothelium of the CP and these other areas is fenestrated. Blood entering CP capillaries is filtered across this endothelium and forms a protein-rich fluid within the CP stroma that is similar in composition to interstitial fluid in other tissues of the body. The CP stroma is separated from the macroscopic CSF spaces by the CP epithelial cells. These contain apical tight junctions that restrict passive solute exchange and constitute a "blood-CSF barrier" at the CP.[8] Epithelial-cell enzymes that are involved with the active, bidirectional trans-

port of substances between plasma and CSF,[5,9] and pinocytotic vesicles and lysosomes also contribute to this "barrier."[10] The small, specialized areas which, in addition to the CP, lack capillary endothelial tight junctions are the area postrema, median eminence, neural lobe of the hypophysis, organum vasculosum lamina terminalis, pineal gland, subcommissural organ, and subfornical organ. These areas, along with the CP, border the cerebral ventricles and are termed the circumventricular organs.

Substances in the CP stromal fluid are transported across the relatively impermeable CP epithelium by the combined processes of ultrafiltration and secretion.[5,9] Stroma fluid enters clefts between the CP epithelial cells due to hydrostatic pressure and bulk flow (Fig. 3-2). Adenosine triphosphate (ATP)-dependent membrane pumps on the abdominal surface move sodium ions into the epithelial cell and potassium and hydrogen ions into the stroma as counter ions.[11] Water moves into the cell along the resultant osmolar gradient. Chloride ions move into the cell as a result of coupling with sodium ions. Bicarbonate and hydrogen ions are formed within the epithelial cell by the action of carbonic anhydrase on carbon dioxide created within the cell as a result of cellular metabolism or diffusing into the cell from capillary blood. On the secretory surface of the cell, ATP-dependent membrane pumps move sodium ions into the CSF and potassium ions in the direction of the stroma. Water entering the epithelial cell along the osmotic gradient established by active sodium secretion continues along that gradient and passes into the ventricle. Water may also move from the stroma into the CSF via "leaky" tight junctions. Chloride and bicarbonate anions in the epithelial cell move passively into the CSF along an electrochemical gradient. Some chloride anions and the ions found in low concentrations in the CSF (such as calcium and magnesium) also pass through "leaky" tight junctions.

EXTRACHOROIDAL CSF FORMATION

Oxidation of glucose within brain cells continually adds water to the ICF space. Ultrafiltration of water out of the brain vasculature across the BBB continually adds water to the ECF. Sixty percent of extrachoroidal CSF formation results from oxidation of glucose by the brain, and 40 percent results from ultrafiltration from cerebral capillaries.[12] In most of the cerebral vasculature, passage of large and polar molecules across the BBB is restricted by capillary tight junctions and specialized heterolytic vesicles within endothelial cells. Water, electrolytes, glucose, amino acids, urea, lipid-soluble materials, and a number of small non-electrolytes pass more freely across this interface.[13] Some of these substances may be actively transported by the astrocyte layer that envelops the capillary endothe-

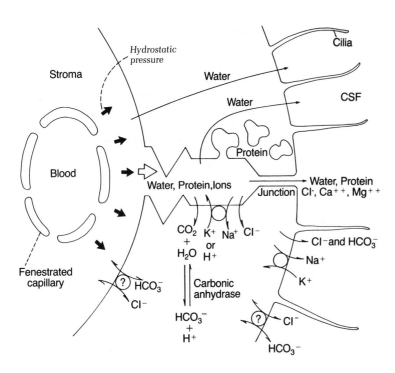

Figure 3-2 Some of the processes involved in CSF formation at the choroid plexus are shown in schematic form. ATP-dependent membrane "pumps" transport Na^+ across the abluminal surface to within the choroid plexus cell and across the secretory surface, into the macroscopic CSF space, in exchange for K^+ and H^+. Water moves from the stroma into CSF as it follows the concentration gradient produced by the ionic "pumps." (From Cucchiara RF, Michenfelder, JD, eds: *Clinical Neuroanesthesia.* New York, Churchill-Livingstone, 1990, with permission.)

lium; others move into the brain ECF by diffusion. This glucose-rich and protein-poor "lymph" moves through the ECF space toward the macroscopic CSF spaces. As it moves, transport systems further modify the chemical composition of substances entering the macroscopic CSF spaces. These systems include not only sodium and potassium pumps associated with neurons, but also specialized transport mechanisms possessed by the ventricular ependyma.[13,14]

MOVEMENT OF GLUCOSE
The concentration of glucose in CSF at the CP or in mixed samples is approximately 60 percent of that in blood. This ratio remains constant unless blood glucose increases to above 15 to 20 mM (270 to 360 mg/dl). Glucose in blood enters CSF by facilitated transport, so that glucose crosses the "blood-CSF barrier" more quickly than would be predicted on the basis of its lipid solubility.[15] Transport follows saturable kinetics, with the rate being directly related to serum glucose concentration and independent of the serum-to-CSF glucose concentration gradient.[16] Diffusion of glucose from blood is insignificant under conditions of normoglycemia. Glucose moves into CSF along the downhill blood-CSF glucose concentration gradient needed for facilitated diffusion and independently of the rate of CSF formation ($\dot{V}_f$).

Movement of glucose in the opposite direction, from the cerebral ventricles into the surrounding brain and blood, occurs via oubain-sensitive -insensitive fluxes and diffusion. One transport site may be located at the CP. Periventricular tissue clears and metabolizes

50 percent of the glucose in CSF.[16] As glucose is cleared from the CSF, it is replaced by glucose from serum in an amount that is about 25 percent of the serum glucose concentration.

MOVEMENT OF PROTEIN
Movement of protein from blood into CSF at the CP and extrachoroidal sites is limited, so that CSF protein concentrations are normally 0.5 percent or less of the respective plasma or serum concentrations. Entry rates at CP and extrachoroidal sites for many proteins remain to be determined.[1,8,17] Proteins entering the brain ECF drain into the macroscopic CSF space by bulk flow, so long as no structural barrier between the brain ECF and the macroscopic CSF space is present. Once in CSF, proteins are transported along with CSF through the macroscopic pathways and are cleared from the CSF space into dural venous sinuses. This "sink effect" of flowing CSF keeps the CSF and brain protein concentration low and far from equilibrium with blood.[1,12] In normal infants and adults, CSF protein concentrations are lowest in the ventricles (about 26 mg/100 ml), intermediate in the cisterna magna (about 32 mg/100 ml), and highest in the lumbar sac (42 mg/100 ml). The lumbar : ventricle CSF concentration ratio for albumin is 2.2 : 1; for immunoglobulin (Ig)G, it is 2.6 : 1; and for prealbumin, it is 0.7 : 1. Albumin and IgG in CSF derive from blood, whereas prealbumin is produced in part by nervous tissue or is transported actively into CSF. The increased concentration of protein is the lumbar subarachnoid compartment (56 percent of total CSF compartment volume),

as compared with the ventricular and cisternal compartments (26 and 18 percent of total volume, respectively), presumably is related to decreased CSF flow and washout rate in the lumbar space.

Under normal conditions, 60 percent of protein entry into CSF occurs at the CP and 40 percent occurs at extrachoroidal sites. Proteins within the CP stroma may, like water, enter into the CSF via "leaky" tight junctions.[18,19] Proteins within the CP stroma may also enter the CSF by vesicular transport across the CP epithelium.[20] Further, stromal proteins may diffuse into CSF at the edge of the CP, where a functional leak exists at the border between CP epithelium and ventricular ependyma.[20] Models have been proposed to explain the reported negative relationship between the steady state CSF : blood concentration ratio and the hydrodynamic ratio of blood-derived proteins. The most likely model is one comprised of both aqueous pores with a 117 Å radius and transfer by pinocytotic vesicles with an assumed radius of 25 Å.[21]

EFFECTS OF INCREASED ICP
ON CSF FORMATION

There is a weak, negative correlation between $\dot{V}_f$ and ICP, and a stronger, positive correlation between $\dot{V}_f$ and cerebral perfusion pressure (CPP).[22] Increase of ICP to 20 mmHg produces no change in $\dot{V}_f$, so long as CPP remains above ~70 mmHg.[23] $\dot{V}_f$ decreases when CPP is reduced below ~70 mmHg, whether by arterial hypotension or by combining arterial hypotension with increased ICP.

These $\dot{V}_f$ results are consistent with reported effects of changes in CPP on cerebral blood flow (CBF), lateral ventricle CP blood flow (CPBF), and fourth ventricle CPBF.[22] A decrease of CPP to 70 mmHg by arterial hypotension, combined with increased ICP, reduces CBF and CPBF. A decrease of CPP to 50 mmHg causes a further decline in CPBF when CPP is reduced by an even greater increase of ICP, but not when CPP is reduced solely by arterial hypotension. Lower CPBF with increased ICP than when CPP is decreased solely by arterial hypotension may be due to increased CP vascular resistance (due to CP compression), as well as to changes in hydrostatic forces within the CP vascular bed.[22] Both factors reduce ultrafiltration across CP capillaries.

CIRCULATION OF CSF

CSF moves from sites of formation, through the macroscopic spaces, to sites of reabsorption. Several factors contribute to CSF movement and reabsorption. The hydrostatic pressure of CSF formation, 15 cmH$_2$O, produces CSF flow where it is freshly formed.[1] Cilia on ependymal cells generate currents that propel CSF to-

ward the fourth ventricle and its foramina. Respiratory variations and vascular pulsations of the cerebral arteries and CP cause ventricular excursions, supplying additional momentum for CSF movement. A pressure gradient for passage of CSF across the arachnoid villi is supplied by the difference between mean CSF pressure, 15 cmH$_2$O, and superior sagittal sinus pressure 9 cmH$_2$O.[5] The high velocity of blood flow through the fixed diameter of the sinuses and the low intraluminal pressure that develops at the circumference of the sinus wall where the arachnoid villi enter causes a "suction-pump" action that may explain how the circulation of the CSF continues through a wide range of postural pressures.[24]

The path of CSF movement is well described. CSF passes through the paired interventricular foramina of Monro into the midline third ventricle, then flows caudally through the aqueduct of Sylvius and fourth ventricle and into the subarachnoid space by one of three exits. Two are the paired lateral foramina of Luschka, from which CSF flows around the brain stem into the cerebellopontine angle and prepontine cisterns. The third exit is the midline foramen of Magendie, from which CSF flows through the valecular into the cisterna magna. A small portion of CSF may also leave the fourth ventricle through the central canal of the spinal cord.

CSF follows three paths out of the cisterna magna. CSF may pass superiorly into the subarachnoid space surrounding the cerebellar hemisphere. CSF may pass inferiorly into the spinal subarachnoid space. Here CSF flows in a caudal direction dorsal to the cord (posterior to the dentate ligaments) to the lumbar theca and then in a cephalad direction ventral to the cord to the basilar cisterns.[24] A third path is for cisternal CSF to move cephalad, into the premedullary, pontine, and interpeduncular cisterns. CSF flows in two directions out of these basilar cisterns. One course is inferiorly, through the interpeduncular cistern, sylvian fissure, and prechiasmatic cisterns, to the subarachnoid space of the lateral and frontal cerebral cortex. A second course is dorsomedially, through the ambient cisterns and cisterna venae magnae cerebri, to the subarachnoid space of the medial and posterior aspects of the cerebral cortex. CSF circulation concludes with reabsorption across arachnoid villi into the superior sagittal sinus and spinal dural sinusoids located on dorsal nerve roots (Fig. 3-3).

Radioisotope studies indicate that labeled CSF flows from the ventricles to the basal cisterns within a few min, low cervical-high thoracic region at 10 to 20 min, thoracolumbar area at 30 to 40 min, lumbosacral cul de sac at 60 to 90 min, and basal cisterns at 2 to 2.5 h.[25] About 20 to 33 percent of the labeled CSF reaches the intracranial cavity within 12 h. Labeled

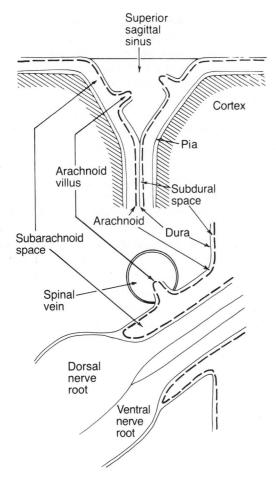

Figure 3-3 CSF is reabsorbed via arachnoid villi at the sagittal sinus and at spinal veins on dorsal nerve roots. (From Cucchiara RF, Michenfelder JD, eds: *Clinical Neuroanesthesia.* New York, Churchill-Livingstone, 1990, with permission.)

CSF collects along the superior sagittal sinus area at 12 to 24 h. Circulation of CSF is not substantially altered by posture or ambulation, although physical activity disturbs CSF concentration gradients by promoting CSF mixing[26] and coughing causes spinal CSF to flow toward the cisterna magna.[27]

REABSORPTION OF CSF

CSF passes from the subarachnoid space into venous blood through microscopic arachnoid villi and macroscopic arachnoid granulations (collections of villi). Intracranial arachnoid villi are located within the dural wall bordering the superior sagittal sinus and venous lacunae, and spinal arachnoid villi are located within the dural wall bordering dural sinusoids on dorsal nerve roots. Under usual conditions, 85 to 90 percent of CSF is reabsorbed at intracranial sites and 10 to 15 percent is reabsorbed at spinal sites.

The arachnoid villus is composed of arachnoid cells protruding from the subarachnoid space into and through the wall of an adjacent venous sinus[28] (Fig. 3-4). At sites other than the villus, the arachnoid membrane that covers the subarachnoid space is made up of several layers of arachnoid cells. Tight junctions between these cell layers form a barrier that prevents the transfer of CSF from the subarachnoid space into the dura.[29] In contrast, at the arachnoid villus, large spaces are present between the inner layers of arachnoid cells. This loose arrangement does not constitute an effective barrier. CSF in the subarachnoid space passes readily into the villus, the center of which contains a maze of loosely arranged arachnoid cells and intercellular spaces. Apart from their lack of tight junctions, the arachnoid cells within the villus are structurally similar to those of the rest of the subarachnoid space.[29] Collagen fibers—either singly or, more frequently, in bundles—are located in the open spaces within the villus. In addition, occasional myelinated and unmyelinated nerves are present. Under normal conditions, an endothelium composed of arachnoid

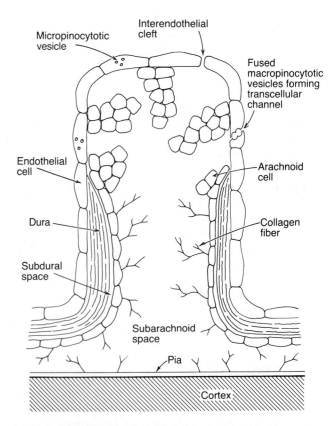

Figure 3-4 Schematic drawing of the microscopic anatomy of an arachnoid villus. (From Cucchiara RF, Michenfelder JD, ed: *Clinical Neuroanesthesia,* New York, Churchill-Livingstone, 1990, with permission.)

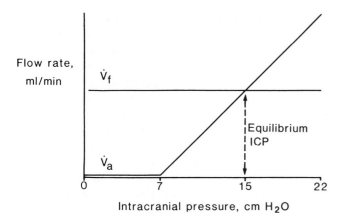

Figure 3-5 $\dot{V}_f$ and $\dot{V}_a$ are plotted as a function of ICP. So long as CPP remains above ~70 mm Hg, $\dot{V}_f$ is unaffected by ICP. At ICP <7 cm H_2O, $\dot{V}_a$ is minimal. At 7 cm H_2O <ICP <25 to 30 cm H_2O, R_a is relatively constant and $\dot{V}_a$ is linearly related to ICP. ICP stabilizes at a value where $\dot{V}_f$ equals $\dot{V}_a$. (From Cucchiara RF, Michenfelder JD, eds: *Clinical Neuroanesthesia*. New York, Churchill-Livingstone, 1990, with permission.)

cells joined by tight junctions covers the villus. In adults, this endothelial covering may be multilayered.

REABSORPTION WHEN ICP IS NORMAL
The endothelium covering the villus acts as a CSF-blood "barrier" that limits the rate of passage of CSF and solute into venous blood. The rate of CSF passage through the subarachnoid space and arachnoid villi and across the endothelium is determined by: (1) the transvillus hydrostatic pressure gradient (CSF pressure minus venous sinus pressure); and (2) a pressure-sensitive resistance to CSF outflow at the arachnoid villus. Transvillous osmotic differences probably do not play a major role in determining CSF movement through arachnoid villi because the endothelium is highly permeable.

CSF may exit the villus by passing between or through endothelial cells. While most endothelial cells are connected by tight junctions, some cell junctions have no areas of membrane fusion or significant focal narrowing of the intercellular space. These intercellular spaces form open channels extending from the abluminal to the luminal surface of the cell, allowing CSF to move from the subarachnoid space into blood. CSF may pass through endothelial cells via micropinocytotic vesicles and transcellular openings formed by chains of fused vesicles extending from one surface of the epithelium to the other.[30] These vesicles transport macromolecular tracers, as well as fluid, from CSF to blood.

REABSORPTION WHEN ICP IS INCREASED
The rate of reabsorption of CSF ($\dot{V}_a$) increases as the pressure gradient across the villus (CSF pressure minus venous pressure) increases (Fig. 3-5). Resistance

to reabsorption of CSF (R_a) remains close to "normal" as CSF pressure increases to about 30 cmH_2O. R_a declines with further increases in CSF pressure.[31] An increase in the size and number of endothelial vesicles was reported when CSF pressure was increased from 9 to 30 cmH_2O.[32] At CSF pressures greater than 30 cmH_2O, increasing numbers of transcellular channels were present concurrent with progressive increases in steady-state pressures, and R_a decreased. Comparison of the outflow-resistance curve (as a function of increasing CSF pressure) with these structural changes suggests that the decrease in R_a at the arachnoid villus is primarily related to the formation of open transcellular channels. Presumably, this transition from micropinocytotic vesicles to larger pinocytotic vesicles and transendothelial channels permits transfer of a proportionately greater volume of fluid across the endothelium with progressively increased steady state CSF pressure.[33] In addition, increased CSF pressure may increase CSF outflow from the villus by facilitating passage through existing intercellular clefts and by opening closed intercellular spaces that, at resting CSF pressure, appear occluded by tight junctions.

FUNCTION OF CSF

The varied and complex functions of CSF include protection, support, and chemical regulation of the brain. The low specific gravity of CSF (1.007) relative to that of the brain (1.040) reduces the effective mass of a 1400-g brain to only 47 g.[34] CSF, in continuity with the brain ECF, provides a stable supply of substrates, primarily glucose, even though concentrations of substrates in plasma are continuously changing. CSF maintains the chemically precise environment required for neurotransmission and removes metabolic products, unwanted drugs, and harmful substances resulting from CNS injury.

PROTECTION OF BRAIN AND SPINAL CORD
CSF cushions neural tissue from external forces applied to the rigid skull and spinal column. The buoyancy provided by CSF prevents the brain's full weight from producing traction on emerging nerve roots, blood vessels, and delicate membranes.[34] When CSF is replaced by air, the reduction of brain effective mass provided by CSF is lost, and most patients experience pain.

CONTROL OF THE CHEMICAL ENVIRONMENT
Exchange between CSF and neural tissue ECF occurs readily because the maximum distance for diffusion between CSF and any brain area in humans is 15 mm, and the ECF space of the brain and spinal cord is continuous with the macroscopic CSF spaces.[34] The acid-base characteristics of CSF influence respiration,

CBF, autoregulation of CBF, and cerebral metabolism.[35] CSF calcium, potassium, and magnesium influence heart rate, blood pressure, vasomotor and other autonomic reflexes, respiration, muscle tone, and emotional states. Calcium, potassium, magnesium, and bicarbonate ions are actively transported by "primary pumps," whereas hydrogen and chloride ions are passively transferred by "secondary pumps."[36] Within limits, CSF composition of large molecules is regulated by the BBB with the almost total exclusion of toxic or potentially toxic large, polar, and lipid-insoluble drugs, humoral agents, and metabolites.

EXCRETION

Passage of metabolites and substances from brain ECF into CSF, cerebral veins, or cervical lymphatics prevents their accumulation in ECF. While passage into CSF may occur by two mechanisms, net diffusion and bulk flow of ECF, bulk flow accounts for the majority of passage of many substrates of different molecular weight.[34,37] Bulk flow is reported to account for clearance of substances entering the brain, as well as substances synthesized by the brain. Bulk flow is particularly important for clearing lipid-insoluble substances such as inulin, mannitol, sulfanilic acid, urea, albumin, globulin, dopamine, homovanillic acid, serotonin, and norepinephrine.[38] For other substances, less than 20 percent of solute clearance from the ECF is accounted for by drainage into CSF.[37] Many of these substances—such as penicillin, methotrexate, and neurotransmitter acid metabolites—are absorbed into the veins of the CP via a probenecid-sensitive transport mechanism.[39] Prolactin is taken up and bound by the CP. This may reflect a role for prolactin in regulating CSF composition, or the CP may serve to transport prolactin from blood to CSF, permitting prolonged delivery of prolactin to hypothalamic receptor neurons.[40] Other substances, such as valproic acid, are absorbed into the cerebral vasculature across the BBB (and not via CP veins) via a probenocid-sensitive transport mechanism.[41-43]

INTRACEREBRAL TRANSPORT

CSF circulates to regions of the brain known to participate in neuroendocrine activity. In so doing, it serves as a convenient vehicle for intracerebral transport of neurotransmitters. Neurohormone-releasing factors are synthesized in the hypothalamus and released into the brain ECF and CSF by neurons having axonal contact with specialized cells of the ependyma.[44] These factors are carried by the CSF to the median eminence, where they stimulate the dendrites of receptor neurons.[44] Median eminence factors may also be taken up by certain ependymal cells, tanycytes; pass to the abluminal surface; and be released into the pituitary-hypothalmic portal system to stimulate hormone release from the pituitary gland.[12] Injection of dopamine into the third ventricle is reported to also stimulate release of pituitary hormones.[45] Electrical stimulation of the medial thalamus or periaqueductal gray increases the level of beta-endorphins in ventricular CSF, suggesting that opioid effects, such as analgesia and respiratory depression, may be mediated by third-ventricle cellular elements in contact with CSF.[46] Adenohypophyseal hormones are present in CSF in quantities suggesting that they reach CSF by a saturable active transport system rather than by simple diffusion.[47] Antidiuretic activity in CSF is increased by conditions that release vasopressin from the neurohypophysis. Release of antidiuretic hormone during perfusion of the cerebral ventricles with hypertonic saline suggests that CSF alterations may affect CNS osmoreceptors.[47] CSF vasopressin may also influence memory and learning or regulate the formation of CSF.[48] CSF melanin concentration exhibits a diurnal rhythm. It also increases in response to stimuli that increase blood melanin and may mediate reproductive function via hypothalamic receptors bathed in CSF.[49] Patients with pituitary tumors may have symptoms of hormone imbalance when hormone concentrations in CSF are elevated but concentrations in plasma are normal.[50]

EFFECTS OF ANESTHETICS AND OTHER INFLUENCES ON FORMATION AND REABSORPTION OF CSF

ANESTHETIC AND DRUG-INDUCED CHANGES IN $\dot{V}_f$ AND R_a

Anesthetics

Increase of $\dot{V}_f$ tends to increase CSF volume, thereby favoring an increase of ICP. When R_a is increased, a higher than "normal" CSF pressure must be present before "normal" amounts of CSF are reabsorbed. Thus, increase of R_a also favors an increase of ICP. Conversely, decrease of $\dot{V}_f$ or R_a tends to decrease ICP. Enflurane tends to increase ICP due to increased R_a at low concentrations and increased $\dot{V}_f$ at high concentrations[51] (Table 3-3). Halothane tends to increase ICP because halothane increases R_a to a greater extent than it decreases $\dot{V}_f$.[52,53] At normocapnia and normal or increased CSF pressure, and at hypocapnia and normal CSF pressure, desflurane causes no change in $\dot{V}_f$ or R_a.[54] However, at hypocapnia and increased CSF pressure, desflurane increases $\dot{V}_f$, favoring increased ICP. Isoflurane causes no change in $\dot{V}_f$, and no change or increased R_a at low concentrations and decreased R_a at high concentrations.[51] Sevoflurane decreases $\dot{V}_f$ and increases R_a.[55] Addition or withdrawal of nitrous oxide to halothane or enflurane causes no change of $\dot{V}_f$ or R_a.[52,56]

TABLE 3-3
Effects of Inhaled Anesthetics on CSF Dynamics

Inhaled Anesthetics	$\dot{V}_f$	R_a	Predicted Effect on ICP
Desflurane	0,+[#]	0	0,+[#]
Enflurane			
Low concentration	0	+	+
High concentration	+	0	+
Halothane	−	+	+
Isoflurane			
Low concentration	0	0,+*	0,+*
High concentration	0	−	−
Nitrous oxide	0	0	0
Sevoflurane	−	+	?

NOTE: $\dot{V}_f$, rate of CSF formation; R_a, resistance to reabsorption of CSF; +, increase; 0, no change; −, decrease; #, effect occurs only during hypocapnia combined with increased CSF pressure; *, effect dependent on dose; ?, uncertain.

Effects of midazolam on ICP are uncertain because midazolam causes no change of $\dot{V}_f$ at low doses and decreases $\dot{V}_f$ at high doses, but causes no change or increased R_a[57] (Table 3-4). Flumazenil, a benzodiazepine antagonist, causes no change of $\dot{V}_f$ and no change or a decrease of R_a when given to dogs not receiving benzodiazepines.[58] Partial reversal of midazolam with flumazenil results in "normal" $\dot{V}_f$ and increased R_a, while complete reversal of midazolam with flumazenil results in $\dot{V}_f$ and R_a similar to pre-midazolam (control)

TABLE 3-4
Effects of Sedative-Hypnotic and Related Intravenous Drugs on CSF Dynamics

Sedative-Hypnotic and Related Intravenous Drugs	$\dot{V}_f$	R_a	Predicted Effect on ICP
Etomidate			
Low dose	0	0	0
High dose	−	0,−*	−
Flumazenil			
Low dose	0	0	0
High dose	0	−	−
Midazolam#			
Low dose	0	+,0*	+,0*
High dose	−	0,+*	−,?*
Pentobarbital	0	0	0
Propofol	0	0	0
Thiopental			
Low dose	0	+,0*	+,0*
High dose	−	0,−*	−

NOTE: $\dot{V}_f$, rate of CSF formation; R_a, resistance to reabsorption of CSF; +, increase; 0, no change; −, decrease; *, effect dependent on dose; #, partial reversal with flumazenil causes CSF dynamics similar to lowest dose of midazolam; complete reversal with flumazenil causes CSF dynamics similar to pre-medazolam (control) values; ?, uncertain.

values. Low doses of thiopental cause no change of $\dot{V}_f$ and no change or increase of R_a, favoring no change or increase of ICP.[57] High doses of thiopental cause a decrease of $\dot{V}_f$ and no change or a decrease of R_a, favoring decrease of ICP. Pentobarbital and propofol cause no change of $\dot{V}_f$ or R_a,[59,60] while etomidate causes no change or a decrease of $\dot{V}_f$ and R_a.[57]

At low doses the opioids alfentanil, fentanyl, and sufentanil cause no change of $\dot{V}_f$ and decrease R_a, favoring decrease of ICP[61] (Table 3-5). At high doses alfentanil causes no change of $\dot{V}_f$ or R_a, fentanyl decreases $\dot{V}_f$ and causes no change or increase of R_a, and sufentanil causes no change of $\dot{V}_f$ and no change or increase of R_a. Ketamine increases R_a and causes no change of $\dot{V}_f$, favoring increase of ICP.[59] The local anesthetic lidocaine causes a dose/time-related decrease of $\dot{V}_f$ and causes no change of R_a.[62] Cocaine causes no change of $\dot{V}_f$ or R_a.[62]

The mechanism(s) by which inhalational and intravenous anesthetics alter CSF dynamics is uncertain. Increase of $\dot{V}_f$ with enflurane may result from an enflurane-induced increase of CP metabolism.[63] Decrease of $\dot{V}_f$ with halothane may result from halothane-induced stimulation of vasopressin receptors.[64]

Diuretics

Although diuretics differ in their mechanism of action, most are reported to decrease $\dot{V}_f$. Acetazolamide reduces $\dot{V}_f$ by up to 50 percent. Acetazolamide inhibits carbonic anhydrase (the enzyme that catalyzes the hydration of intracellular carbon dioxide), thereby decreasing the amount of hydrogen ions available for exchange with sodium on the abluminal border of the

TABLE 3-5
Effects of Opioids and Other Intravenous Drugs on CSF Dynamics

Opioids and Other Intravenous Drugs	$\dot{V}_f$	R_a	Predicted Effect on ICP
Alfentanil			
Low dose	0	−	−
High dose	0	0	0
Fentanyl			
Low dose	0	−	−
High dose	−	0,+*	−,?*
Sufentanil			
Low dose	0	−	−
High dose	0	+,0*	+,0*
Ketamine	0	+	+
Lidocaine	−*	0	−
Cocaine	0	0	0

NOTE: $\dot{V}_f$, rate of CSF formation; R_a, resistance to reabsorption of CSF; +, increase; 0, no change; −, decrease; *, effect dependent on dose; ?, uncertain.

epithelial cell. Acetozolamide may also decrease $\dot{V}_f$ by an indirect action on ion transport mediated by an effect on bicarbonate.[65] Another view is that acetazolamide constricts CP arterioles, reducing CPBF. Methazolamide, another carbonic anhydrase inhibitor, also is reported to reduce $\dot{V}_f$ by up to 50 percent. The effects of carbonic anhydrase inhibitors are additive with those produced by drugs that work by other mechanisms. For example, the combination of acetazolamide and oubain decreases $\dot{V}_f$ by 95 percent.[66]

Ethacrynic acid decreases $\dot{V}_f$, presumably by inhibiting the exchange of sodium ions for potassium or hydrogen at the abluminal border of the cell.[66] Spironolactone and amiloride decrease $\dot{V}_f$, probably by minimizing the entry of sodium into cells at the abluminal transport site. Furosemide decreases $\dot{V}_f$, either by reducing the transport of sodium or reducing the transport of chloride, which is linked to sodium transport on the abluminal surface but follows an electrochemical gradient on the luminal surface.[67] Mannitol decreases $\dot{V}_f$ because of reduced CP output and reduced ECF flow from cerebral tissue to the macroscopic CSF compartment.[68]

Steroids

Numerous steroids are reported to alter R_a and $\dot{V}_f$. With increased R_a secondary to pneumococcal meningitis, methylprednisolone reduced R_a to a value that was intermediate between control and untreated animals,[69] presumably by improving CSF flow in the supracortical subarachnoid space and/or arachnoid villi. When R_a was increased due to pseudotumor cerebri, prednisone decreased R_a to a value that was intermediate between pretreatment and normal values for patients,[70] presumably because impaired transport across arachnoid epithelial cells was improved or because metabolically induced changes in the structure of the villi were reversed. Cortisone was reported to decrease $\dot{V}_f$. Rapid uptake of radioactive-labeled hydrocortisone into the CP suggests that cortisone exerts its action at the CP rather than at extrachoroidal sites.[71] Dexamethosone decreases $\dot{V}_f$ by up to 50 percent,[72] probably because it inhibits sodium-potassium-ATPase, thereby reducing the activity of the sodium-potassium pump at the CP epithelial membrane.

Other Drugs

A number of other drugs are reported to alter $\dot{V}_f$ and R_a. Theophylline increases $\dot{V}_f$, presumably because inhibition of phosphodiesterase elevates CP cyclic adenosine monophosphate levels, stimulating the CP epithelial sodium-potassium pump.[73] Cholera toxin is also reported to increase $\dot{V}_f$.[74] Vasopressin decreases $\dot{V}_f$, perhaps by constricting CP blood vessels. Others contend that physiologic doses of vasopressin provide insufficient CP vascular effect to explain the observed decrease of $\dot{V}_f$.[73] Vasopressin also decreases R_a.[74] Hypertonic saline (3%) decreases $\dot{V}_f$, presumably by reducing the osmolality gradient for movement of fluid out of plasma and into the CP stroma or across brain tissue and into CSF.[75] Hypertonic saline increases R_a at some doses but not others. Dinitrophenol decreases $\dot{V}_f$, probably as a result of its action to uncouple oxidative phosphorylation, thereby reducing the energy available for active secretory and transport processes, such as the membrane pumps. Atrial natriuretic peptides decrease $\dot{V}_f$ by stimulating production of cyclic guanine monophosphate.[74] Digoxin and oubain decrease $\dot{V}_f$ by inhibition of the sodium-potassium-ATPase of the CP epithelial sodium-potassium pump.[66]

In contrast to the aforementioned drugs, both succinylcholine (continuous infusion) and vecuronium (continuous infusion) produce no change in $\dot{V}_f$ or R_a.[76]

NEUROGENIC REGULATION OF $\dot{V}_f$ AND R_a

Structural Aspects

Adrenergic nerves form networks around the small arteries and veins of the CP, and their nerve terminals are located between the CP epithelium and the underlying fenestrated capillaries.[77] Adrenergic nerve density is greatest in the third ventricle, least in the fourth ventricle, and intermediate in the lateral ventricles. For the most part these adrenergic nerves originate in the superior cervical ganglia, though some fibers in the CP of the fourth ventricle derive from lower ganglia.[78] Innervation of the lateral ventricles is unilateral, whereas innervation of the midline ventricles is bilateral.[79]

Cholinergic nerves also form networks around the small arteries and veins of the CP, with terminals located between the epithelium and adjacent capillaries.[80] The CP of the third ventricle is richly supplied by cholinergic nerves, whereas the fourth ventricle is almost devoid of cholinergic innervation. The origin of the cholinergic nerve supply to the CP is uncertain. Adrenergic and cholinergic terminals have been identified at the base of choroid epithelial cells, in the clefts between cells, and near the smooth muscle cells of the choroid arterioles.

Peptidergic nerves are also found in the CP, but the density of these nerves is less than that of adrenergic and cholinergic nerves.[81] Similar to the former networks, peptidergic nerves are located between the small blood vessels of the CP and the overlying CP epithelium.[82] Peptidergic nerves contain vasoactive intestinal peptide or substance P, both potent dilators of cerebral vessels.

Functional Aspects

Constriction of isolated anterior CP arteries with norepinephrine, phenylephrine, and isoproterenol (in that order of potency) was blocked by phentolamine and so presumably occurs via alpha-adrenergic receptors. In vessels in which active tone was first induced by prostaglandin F_{2a}, relaxation with isoproterenol, norepinephrine, epinephrine, and terbutaline (in that order of potency) was blocked with propranolol, and so presumably occurs via beta-adrenergic receptors. The adrenergic system also appears to exert a functional influence on CP epithelial cells. Carbonic anhydrase activity increased by 125 to 150 percent in CP homogenate after sympathectomy achieved by surgical removal of the superior cervical ganglion or injection of reserpine.[4] In another study, sympathetic denervation altered epithelial cell transport of organic acids and bases in isolated CP.[83]

Changes in adrenergic nerve activity alter $\dot{V}_f$. Cervical sympathetic stimulation decreased $\dot{V}_f$ by 32 percent,[78,84,85] and bilateral excision of the superior cervical ganglia increased $\dot{V}_f$ by 33 percent.[79] Intraventricular perfusion with norepinephrine caused a dose-related decrease of $\dot{V}_f$ that was reversed by intraventricular perfusion of phentolamine or propranolol or intravenous infusion of phentolamine.[85] In contrast, intravenous infusion of propranolol potentiated the reduction of $\dot{V}_f$. Norepinephrine-induced decrease of $\dot{V}_f$ may occur by a beta-adrenoreceptor-mediated effect on the secretory epithelium at low concentrations of norepinephrine, and by alpha-adrenoreceptor-mediated CP vasoconstriction at high concentrations of norepinephrine. The beta-induced decrease of $\dot{V}_f$ appears to derive from a direct, inhibitory action on the CP epithelium via $beta_1$ and not $beta_2$ adrenoreceptors.

The cholinergic system is also reported to alter $\dot{V}_f$. Intraventricular perfusion with carbacholine or with acetylcholine in the presence of the cholinesterase inhibitor neostigmine reduced $\dot{V}_f$ by 25 percent to 55 percent.[86] Cholinergic receptors presumably are muscarinic, because the effect of carbachol is blocked by atropine but is not altered by hexamethonium. The site of action of cholinergic agonists or antagonists is uncertain. It is believed that they act on the CP epithelium, rather than on the CP vasculature, because carbacholine has no vasomotor effect on isolated anterior choroidal arteries.[87]

There are no reports on the effects of nitric oxide on $\dot{V}_f$ or R_a. However, intravenous injection of NG-nitro-L-arginine, an inhibitor of the enzymatic formation of nitric oxide, at doses that caused no change in CBF, decreased CPBF by 36 to 51 percent.[88] A decline in CPBF of that magnitude may result in a decrease of $\dot{V}_f$.

METABOLIC REGULATION OF $\dot{V}_f$ AND R_a

Hypothermia decreases $\dot{V}_f$, probably by reducing the activity of active secretory and transport processes and by reducing CBF.[1] Each 1°C reduction in temperature between 41°C and 31°C decreases $\dot{V}_f$ by 11 percent.[89] Hypercapnia increases $\dot{V}_f$ to normal values if $\dot{V}_f$ was decreased at normocapnia, but does not change $\dot{V}_f$ if it was normal at normocapnia.[90] Normalization of $\dot{V}_f$ by hypercapnia presumably occurs as a result of improved CPBF. In contrast, hypocapnia acutely decreases $\dot{V}_f$, either due to reduced CPBF or reduced hydrogen ion availability for exchange with sodium at the abluminal surface of the CP epithelial cells. After several hours of hypocapnia, $\dot{V}_f$ returns to normal values.[91] Prolonged hypercapnia or hypocapnia does not significantly change $\dot{V}_f$.[90,91] Metabolic acidosis does not change $\dot{V}_f$, but metabolic alkalosis decreases $\dot{V}_f$, presumably due to a pH effect unrelated to ion or substrate availability.

Reduced osmolarity of ventricular CSF or increased osmolarity of serum decreases $\dot{V}_f$.[92] Similarly, increased osmolarity of ventricular CSF or reduced osmolarity of serum increases $\dot{V}_f$.[92,93] The increase or decrease of $\dot{V}_f$ caused by change in serum osmolarity was four times greater than that caused by a comparable change in ventricular fluid osmolarity. It was suggested that the changes in $\dot{V}_f$ resulting from altered ventricular fluid osmolarity occurred at the CP, whereas the changes resulting from altered serum osmolarity occurred at extrachoroid sites.

Intracellular and Extracellular Fluid

ANATOMY OF THE EXTRACELLULAR SPACES

Water and certain other ECF constituents enter the ECF by passage from the vascular space across the BBB (Fig. 3-6). Water and certain other ICF constituents are created within the ICF by metabolism of glucose. The total volume of water in the ICF and ECF spaces may range from 1000 to 1200 ml in adults. ICF and ECF compositions are similar to those elsewhere in the body, with the exception that brain ICF and ECF contain constituents unique to the brain, such as CNS neurotransmitters, chemicals, and metabolites[74,94] (Table 3-6).

The ECF spaces of the cortex, gray matter nuclei, brain stem, and spinal cord, unlike those of other organs in the body, are small in diameter. Spaces measuring 150 to 200 Å exist between the membranes of cell bodies, cellular processes (i.e., dendrites, axons, and astrocytic foot processes) and the cells of lining epithelia (ependyma and pia) as well as around the basement membrane of cerebral capillaries. These narrow, interconnecting channels are anatomically continuous with the adjoining macroscopic CSF spaces. In less dense areas of the white matter, the intercellular clefts tend to be larger, and vary from characteristic 150 to 200 Å gaps to those with a diameter of 1000 to 2000 Å.[6] Exchange between cerebral capillaries and the ECF is limited by the BBB. The BBB architecture is unique to cerebral blood vessels and is found in all areas of the

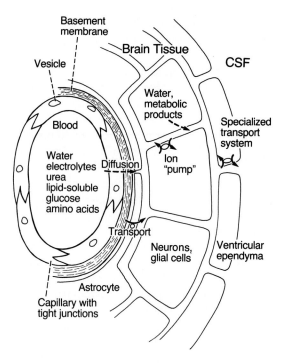

Figure 3-6 Water and other constituents of plasma cross the BBB (capillary endothelial cells, basement membrane, and astrocyte foot processes) into the brain ECF space by diffusion or transport. This fluid diffuses toward the macroscopic CSF space and subarachnoid space. Water and other cellular metabolites are added to the ECF from neurons and glial cells. (From Cottrell JE, Smith DS, eds: *Anesthesia and Neurosurgery.* St. Louis, Mosby-Year Book, Inc., 1994, with permission.)

brain except at the CP (and the other circumventricular organs).

There is evidence that the ECF spaces communicate with lymphatic channels. Up to 30 percent of labeled CSF or tracers injected into the brain can be recovered in the deep cervical lymph system.[37,95,96] ECF and CSF may reach these lymphatics via the cribriform plate. The arachnoid of the plate joins with olfactory perineu-

rium composed of fibroblasts and large intercellular spaces.[97] ECF and CSF may thus enter the nasal submucosa and from there pass into the deep cervical lymph nodes via afferent ducts.

THE BLOOD-BRAIN BARRIER

Two morphologically distinct barriers prevent the free passage of plasma constituents into the cerebral ECF: (1) the capillary endothelium, and (2) the specialized ependyma of the circumventricular organs[98] (Fig. 3-7). The principal surface across which blood-tissue exchanges take place is the capillary endothelium. The distinctive features of the BBB are: (1) the absence of fenestrae and presence of tight junctions (zonulae occludentes) between adjacent capillary endothelial cells; (2) a paucity of plasmalemmal pits and vesicles and abundance of mitochondria and enzymes within endothelial cells; and (3) the investment of endothelial cells by closely applied astrocytic foot processes[99] (Table 3-7).

A number of characteristics of the cerebral endothelial cell contribute to its "barrier" function. The endothelium is comprised of a sheet of cells on a basement membrane; the cells are connected by tight junctions; there is low permeability to ions and hydrophilic nonelectrolytes, and low hydraulic conductance; passive solute permeability is mainly via intercellular junctions; there is facilitated transport of certain organic solutes; saturation kinetics, stereospecificity, and competitive interactions occur; induction mechanisms are present; there is high electrical resistance; high osmolality increases permeability; and sodium-potassium pumps are located in the abluminal endothelial membrane.[100] Some of the enzymes and receptors in endothelial plasma membranes in brain include sodium-potassium-ATPase, adenylate cyclase, guanylate cyclase, glucose "transporter," serotonin receptor, γ-glutamyl transpeptidase (GGTP), DOPA decarboxylase,

TABLE 3-6
Composition of Brain ICF, ECF, and "Tissue"[a]

	Mean ICF Concentration	Mean ECF Concentration	Mean Tissue Concentration
Sodium (meq/liter)	48	146	250 ± 6*
Potassium (meq/liter)	145	4.1	415 ± 8*
Chloride (meq/liter)	65	118	176 ± 5*
Bicarbonate (meq/liter)	9.5	22	—
pH	7.05	7.44	—
water	—	—	3.506 ± 0.059#

[a] Averaged values based on Rosenberg[74] and Bradbury.[95]

NOTE: *, units are mmol · kg^{-1} dry weight; #, units are ml · g^{-1} dry weight.

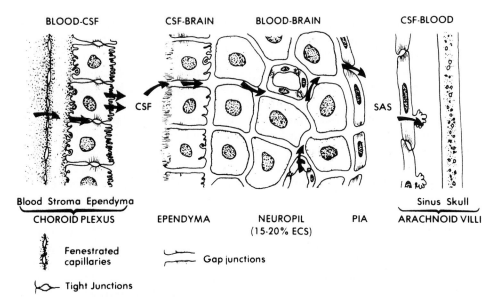

Figure 3-7   Fluid moves across the brain parenchymal capillary endothelium (two capillaries are shown here in the neuropil as circular structures; a black arrow is located in the lower of the two parenchymal capillaries), and across the capillary endothelium (shown here as a single longitudinal structure) and ependyma of the circumventricular organs such as the choroid plexus (black arrows in the CHOROID PLEXUS portion of the figure). Fluid originating from the parenchymal capillaries passes through the ECF and into the subarachnoid space (SAS) via the pia (black arrow next to the upper two parenchymal capillaries and in the PIA portion of the figure) or into the macroscopic CSF space (CSF) via the ventricular ependyma. Fluid originating from choroid plexus capillaries passes into the macroscopic CSF space (CSF) and thence along macroscopic CSF pathways to the SAS. Under pathologic conditions, such as hydrocephalic edema, fluid may pass from the macroscopic CSF space (CSF) across the ventricular ependyma (black arrows in CSF and CSF-BRAIN portions of the figure) and into the ECF. (From Rosenberg GA: *Brain Fluids and Metabolism.* New York, Oxford University Press, 1990, with permission.)

and alkaline phosphatase. The permeability coefficients of most hydrophilic non-electrolytes are about one-hundredth of that found in muscle capillaries.[101]

ENDOTHELIAL CELLS
Tight Junctions
Numerous studies have examined the "tightness" of the cerebral capillary endothelium. While the cerebral capillary endothelium is impermeable to large or polar molecules, it is highly permeable to most lipid soluble

TABLE 3-7
Features of the BBB That Contribute to Its "Barrier" Function

Endothelial cells connected by tight junctions

Paucity of plasmalemmal pits and vesicles

Abundance of mitochondria and lytic enzymes

Facilitated transport of selected substances

Investment of endothelial cells by astrocyte foot processes

Astrocyte-endothelial cell interactions

Low permeability and hydraulic conductance

High electrical resistance

substances and exhibits variable permeability to ions, small nonelectrolytes, and urea.[102] Intraarterial injection of hyperosmotic agents, such as urea or mannitol, causes shrinkage of cerebral endothelial cells and a "reversible opening" of the tight junctions.[12] Other conditions that probably produce junctional uncoupling are hyperthermia, prolonged hypercarbia, and vasodilation associated with the loss of autoregulation of CBF.[12,103] Current data suggest that the tight junctions of the cerebral endothelium are perforated by aqueous channels having a diameter of 6 to 8 Å.[104] Channels of this size permit the passage of only water and sodium and chloride ions. Functionally, the tight junctions of the cerebral endothelium appear to restrict the intercellular movement of molecules having a diameter of 20 Å or more.

Permeability and Conductance
Ion permeability is low as reflected in the high electrical resistance of these membranes. The low potassium concentration in brain ECF is regulated by means of an ATP-dependent sodium-potassium pump system located at the antiluminal side of the brain endothelium.

The difference in hydraulic conductance between brain and muscle capillaries is similar to the difference in permeability between the two; that is, the brain capillary has a filtration coefficient that is 100 times lower than that in muscle capillaries.[101] Owing to low hydraulic conductance and near impermeability to plasma colloids, the cerebral vessels model the "ideal" Starling capillary. Here the Starling forces operate to their full extent, not being blunted by reflection coefficients below unity. Because cerebral capillaries are nearly impermeable to the ions in plasma, the osmotic contribution of ions must be included in the formulation of the Starling equation for brain capillaries—in contrast to other organs where the reflection coefficients to ions are as low as 0.1.[105]

The Starling equation for the fluid balance across the cerebral capillary has the following form:

$$J_v = L_p S \left[(P_c - P_T) - \left(C_{coll} + \sum_i RTc_i \right) \right]$$

where J_v is the volume flow when the balance is disturbed, L_p is the hydraulic conductance (filtration coefficient), S is the surface area, P_c is the average capillary pressure, P_T is tissue pressure, C_{coll} is the colloid osmotic pressure in plasma, R is the gas constant, T is the absolute temperature, and c_i is the difference in ion concentrations across the capillary wall. The final term plays a major role in halting net fluid shifts between blood and brain, as any filtration of water rapidly creates a counter force that stops the filtration.

Passive Permeability

Passive ion movement occurs mainly through weakly charged, well hydrated pores in the BBB, much as occurs in other capillaries. What generates the small transcapillary DC-potential in the brain—and its strong dependence upon the pH of plasma—is not known. The entire system of blood-brain interphases (the CP and the arachnoid membrane as well as the capillary membrane) may contribute as sources and sinks.

Facilitated Transport, Saturation Kinetics, and Induction

Facilitated transport of organic non-electrolytes is indicated by a nonlinear relation between transport rate and plasma concentration. The permeability-surface area produce (PS) in facilitated transport systems is described by the equation:

$$PS = \frac{V_{max}}{K_m + C_s}$$

where V_{max} is the maximal transport rate, K_m is an affinity of the "transporter" to the solute, and C_s is the average intracapillary concentration of the solute in question.

Saturation kinetics, stereospecificity, and competitive interaction are reflections of the mechanisms dealt with above. Induction mechanisms refer to the ability to change transport parameters with changes in "environment." Brain capillary endothelial cells adapt to changes in the plasma concentration of substrates such as ketone bodies during fasting. In neonates, induction and repression of the monocarboxylic acid carrier takes place during the suckling period.[106] Amino acid transport is claimed to be induced by the changes in hepatic metabolism that takes place after portocaval anastomosis.[107] Finally, with lasting increases in plasma glucose concentration, down regulation of glucose transport occurs, a mechanism that tends to stabilize the interstitial glucose concentration.[108]

Electrical Resistance

The cerebral endothelium has an electrical resistance of about 2000 Ω cm^2. Other capillary membranes have much lower electrical resistance. The mesenteric capillary has a resistance of 1 to 2 Ω cm^2, and the muscle capillary endothelium has a resistance about 20 Ω cm^2.[109] Electrical resistance reflects ionic permeability. The relation between electrical conductance (the reciprocal of resistance) and ionic conductance is given by:

$$G_m = F^2/RT \sum_i z_i P_i C_i,$$

where G_m is the membrane conductance, z_i is the valency of the ion in question, P_i is permeability, C_i is the concentration in plasma, R, T and F are the usual numbers for thermodynamics and molecular physics, that is, the molar gas constant, temperature, and the Helmholtz function.

Pumps

There is compelling evidence that a sodium-potassium pump is located in the abluminal endothelial membrane of the BBB (Fig. 3-8). Epithelial cells in the CP also contain sodium-potassium-stimulated ATPase in the cell membrane that faces the CSF.[110] Thus, both the ATPase in the endothelial cells in the CP epithelial cells face the "brain" side, that is, they pump potassium "away" from the brain or its fluids. CP epithelial cells pump sodium in the opposite direction as a counter ion, and capillary endothelial cells probably do the same.

VESICLES, MITOCHONDRIA, AND ENZYMES

The cells of the cerebral endothelium contain comparatively few pinocytotic pits and vesicles. These structures are believed to be responsible for transcellular

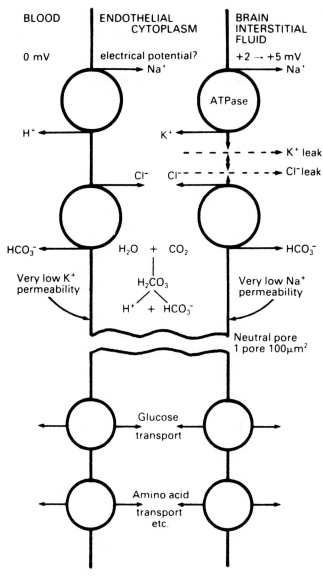

Figure 3-8   The figure shows possible transport systems in cerebral endothelium. The luminal membrane is believed to contain a coupled Na^+-H^+ antiport system and a Cl^--HCO_3^- exchanger. The abluminal membrane is believed to contain a coupled Na^+-K^+ pump driven by energy from ATP hydrolysis, pumping K^+ ions out of, and Na^+ ions into, the interstitium. This membrane also contains a Cl^--HCO_3^- exchanger. Cl^- (that follows the net Na^+ transport) leaves the cell by electrodiffusion. The junction between two endothelial cells represents the very low conductance passive pathway that is present in all tight epithelial membranes and presumably also in the BBB. Only two of the many equilibrating transport systems for organic solutes are indicated, the glucose transporter and the amino acid transporter (of which there are various types). It is suggested that the luminal cell membrane has an extremely low permeability to K^+, while the abluminal membrane has a very low permeability to Na^+. (From Suckling AJ, Rumsby MG, Bradbury MWB, eds: *The Blood-Brain Barrier in Health and Disease.* Chichester, Ellis Horwood Limited, 1986, with permission.)

vesicular transport in cardiac and skeletal endothelia, and their paucity in normal cerebral endothelium is an important feature of the BBB.[104] In vasogenic edema, greatly stimulated pinocytotic activity appears to be an important mechanism in the transport of serum proteins into the ECF spaces.[111] Increased vesicular transport of proteins also is reported with cerebral hypoxia, stroke, head injuries, infections, inflammatory and autoimmune reactions, intoxications, brain tumors, cold injury lesions, hyperthermia, prolonged hypercapnia, vasodilatation associated with the loss of CBF autoregulation, and acute arterial hypertension.[103,111]

It is estimated that in regions of the brain where tight junctions exist between endothelial cells, mitochondria account for 8 to 11 percent of the endothelial cell volume, as compared with 2 to 5 percent in all other organs of the body.[112] Mitochondria are known to be involved with a variety of complex metabolic activities and appear to act within the endothelial cells of the BBB as a means for trapping certain substrates and for facilitating the transcapillary transport of others.[113] Mitochondria of cerebral capillaries contain large amounts of gamma aminobutyric acid (GABA) transaminase which is thought to exclude the passage from blood to brain of systemically administered GABA. Mitochondria also contain dopa decarboxylase (an enzyme that converts L-DOPA into the highly impermeable solute dopamine) which probably contributes to the exclusion of this biologically active neurotransmitter. Other endothelial enzymes that probably contribute to the permeability characteristics of the BBB, either by restricting or by facilitating transcellular transport, include GGTP, ATP, monoamine oxidase, acid phosphatase, alkaline phosphatase, nicotinamide adenine dinucleotide, and various glucose, glutamate, lactate, and succinate dehydrogenases.[103]

ASTROCYTE FOOT PROCESSES
The astrocyte foot processes are closely applied to the basement membrane of the capillary endothelial cells. These processes create an incomplete casing around the circumference of the vessel. The pericapillary space and the intercellular clefts between astrocytic foot processes are open, and channels measuring approximately 150 to 200 Å in diameter communicate with the ECF space. Astrocytes contain high concentrations of certain enzymes, including carbonic anhydrase (involved in water and sodium transport) and nucleoside phosphatase (necessary for ATP-driven energy systems). Nucleoside phosphatase is not found in endothelial cells, but is found in astrocyte foot processes and the pericapillary basement membrane. An enzyme involved with amino acid and peptide exchange, GGTP, is not found in pure cultures of endothelial cells

but is produced in significant concentrations when the endothelial cells and glial cells are grown together.[114] Astrocytic foot processes are reported to make rapid and sensitive adjustments in the microchemical environment of ECF and thus contribute indirectly to the permeability characteristics of the BBB.[104]

BRAIN ENDOTHELIAL-ASTROCYTE INTERACTIONS

Recent studies suggest that interactions between astrocytes and endothelial cells influence many of the BBB functions expressed by the endothelial cell in the microvasculature of the CNS.[115]

TIGHT JUNCTIONS AND ELECTRICAL RESISTANCE

Electrical resistance is a measure of tight junction formation in endothelial and epithelial cells. In bovine brain microvessel endothelial cells grown in the absence of astrocytes or astrocyte-conditional media, resistance values in the range of 157.4 ± 4.5 to 783.2 ± 7 ohms/cm^2 were obtained.[116] Similarly prepared bovine aortic endothelial cells and endothelial cells derived from epidydimal fat pads showed values of 13.5 ± 0.2 and 0.45 ± 0.03 ohms/cm^2 respectively.[117] Rat brain endothelial cells grown on a commercially available cell matrix-coated substrate cultured with 50 percent rat brain astrocyte-conditioned medium and 50 percent α-minimal essential medium 10 percent horse serum developed numerous, elaborate, complex tight junctions.[118] The same medium used with cells grown on bare plastic or fibronectin-coated surfaces resulted in no junction formation. It was concluded that tight junction formation was due to a factor produced by the astrocyte acting with a competent (cell-produced) extracellular matrix. Part of the action of the astrocyte on the endothelial cell may thus be mediated through factors bound to their shared basal lamina.

ENZYMES AND TRANSPORT

The presence of GGTP has been used to identify brain-derived microvasculature and endothelial cells from the CNS.[119,120] GGTP was found in endothelial cells derived from mouse brain microvascular isolates and in cells migrating from them.[118] However, endothelial cells lost the enzyme as they migrated away from the vessel. The endothelial cells no longer had contact with astrocytes, and it was postulated that contact with astrocytes is required for the expression of GGTP by endothelial cells. Another study used an in vivo system of injury and repair to study the relationship of astrocytes to endothelial cells and the expression of GGTP.[121] Only microvessels associated with astrocytes expressed GGTP. It was suggested that endothelial re-

generation and new vessel formation resulted in a chemotactic effect that attracted the astrocyte to the endothelial cells or its basal lamina.

In a two-chamber model, when astrocytes were present on the side of the membrane opposite the endothelium, enhanced transport was detected from the astrocytic side to the endothelial side, that is, the abluminal to the luminal side.[122] These results were interpreted to indicate a glial influence on the polarity of uptake and transport of A-system neutral amino acids by the endothelium in isolated microvessels. [The A-system transporter prefers neutral amino acids with short polar or linear side chains (see below).]

It is well known that glucose is transported through the endothelium of the CNS by specific, carrier-mediated transport systems or by facilitated diffusion. In tissue culture systems, media conditioned by normal or neoplastic astrocytes secreted a product that stimulated glucose uptake by brain-derived endothelial cells by 23 and 50 percent respectively.[123] There was no effect of media conditioned by smooth muscle cells or oligodendrogial cells. The astrocytic effect was time-dependent and required the constant presence of the product for continued effect. The astrocytic effect was abolished by protein synthesis inhibitors during the phase of conditioning and by protease. It was concluded that a protein or peptide released by the astrocyte contributed to the glucose transport expression of the brain-derived endothelium.

Biochemical and enzyme histochemical studies at the ultrastructural level indicate that sodium-postassium-ATPase and alkaline phosphatase are located on brain endothelial cell membranes. Sodium-potassium-ATPase localizes on the abluminal surface, while alkaline phosphatase is distributed on both the luminal and abluminal membranes.[115] In a two-chamber model, endothelial cells not expressing the enzyme could be induced to express it when astrocytes or C6 glioma cells were cultured on the side of the membrane opposite the endothelium.[124] When human umbilical vein endothelium and astrocytes derived from the rat were cocultured in a system using a porous membrane to separate the two cell types, alkaline phosphatase activity was induced in the endothelial cells after 3 days.[125]

CELL GROWTH AND GENE EXPRESSION

Astrocytes appear to exert both stimulatory and inhibitory effects on endothelial cells. Some CNS neoplasms of astrocytic origin (e.g., malignant astrocytoma, glioblastoma multiforme) are often accompanied by hyperplasia of endothelial cells in vessels within or adjacent to the neoplasm. Recent studies indicate that astrocytes are the source of the factor producing the endothelial response.[126] In contrast, medium conditioned by normal (i.e., nonneoplastic) astrocytes has been shown to be inhibitory to endothelial cell growth.[123] Exposure of brain-derived endothelial cells to astrocyte-conditioned medium for 21 h resulted in a 75 percent decrease in [³H]thymidine incorporation in the treated compared to the control cells.

In vivo studies of microvascular regeneration after injury have shown that there is an orderly series of events leading to repair and regeneration of the vasculature and reestablishment of the BBB.[115] In a model of freeze injury and repair, endothelial cells moved into the area of injury and formed new blood vessels before the astrocyte established contact with the vessel.[121] Chemotactic signaling of the astrocyte by the endothelial cell was proposed. In vitro, astrocytes seeded randomly on vitrogen preferentially migrated to endothelial cells and established an anatomic relationship similar to that seen in vivo. Whereas 10 percent of astrocytes were in contact with the endothelial tube-like structures at 5 h, 71.5 percent of the astrocytes had established contact by 24 h. Migration assays containing either dispersed endothelial cells or fully developed tube-like structures indicated that the chemotactic effect of the endothelial cell on the astrocyte was operational only with the endothelial tube-like structures. An in vivo model, in which astrocytes migrated to newly formed vessels, suggested that a degree of differentiation of the endothelial cell must be present before the chemotactic factor is released.[121] In the in vivo model, BBB properties were established in the endothelial cell after the astrocyte had contacted the endothelium.

The astrocyte content of glial fibrillary acidic protein (GFAP) has been examined in vivo and in vitro. In models of brain injury, GFAP mRNA increased quickly beginning at 6 h after injury.[127,128] Astrocytes expressed GFAP mRNA at or near the site of the lesion or at sites away from the lesion including the contralateral hemisphere. Expression of GFAP mRNA followed exactly the distribution of cerebral swelling and edema as outlined by a protein tracer, horseradish peroxidase.[127] GFAP immunoreactivity and GFAP mRNA expression persisted for up to 14 days, mainly in association with areas of vessel regeneration.

MOVEMENT ACROSS THE BBB

UPTAKE INTO THE BRAIN

Lipid solubility of the un-ionized and unbound fraction of a substance influences its rate of uptake into the brain. Attempts have been made to make this relationship more quantitative by defining a partition parameter that contains the product of partition coefficient and fraction of un-ionized unbound substance.[12] As the partition coefficient (and hence permeability of the capillary) increases, the entry of a solute into brain

will be progressively more dependent on blood flow until, at the highest lipid solubility, uptake is linear with flow. At high values of the partition coefficient, entry of the compound into brain is so fast that the capillary blood is depleted of the solute during a single pass. Uptake into brain is calculated from the equation

$$PS = Q \cdot \ln(1 - E)$$

where PS is the permeability-surface area product, Q the blood flow, and E the extraction.[129] The equation assumes a linear uniform capillary with no back diffusion from the tissue compartment.

Water

Water movement across membranes can be described in two ways. First, net flux or bulk flow of water occurs in response to either a hydrostatic or an electrochemical gradient, or both. Since the activity of water varies inversely with increasing solute concentration, this net flow will occur toward the side having the greater concentration of osmotically active particles. Second, self-diffusion of water occurs without bulk flow and can be estimated from the movement of isotopically labeled water, just as self-diffusion of a solute can be measured in absence of a concentration gradient. In membranes lacking water-filled channels or pores, osmotic permeability of the membrane (P_f, the filtration coefficient) equals diffusional permeability to water, P_d.[129] In membranes containing channels, P_f may be anticipated to be greater than P_d.

The reflection coefficient of the normal BBB for ions and polar compounds is close to unity because the BBB permeability to ions and to polar compounds of even low molecular weight is very low. As a result, potential gradients of osmotic pressure across the BBB are much greater than any likely gradient of hydrostatic pressure. In the event of filtration due to hydrostatic pressure, an osmotic gradient in the opposite direction will immediately limit such filtration. If, however, the BBB is pathologically opened, filtration of fluid from plasma with or without protein becomes possible.[129] Such a mechanism is probably responsible for so-called vasogenic cerebral edema.

Protein Binding

Until recently it was believed that flux into brain of a compound that is partially protein bound should be proportional to the unbound concentration. For this reason, the unbound concentration was considered to be the correct value to use when calculating the PS product. However, development of the intracarotid injection technique has permitted direct measurement of the brain uptake of labeled compounds in the absence or in the presence of different concentrations of protein, usually albumin.[130] Results of such studies suggest that the above view may be an oversimplification.

For example, tryptophan, an important determinant of the content of the neurotransmitter serotonin in brain, is about 90 percent bound to plasma albumin in blood. Yet the presence of albumin had little effect on brain uptake of [^{14}C]tryptophan following an intracarotid bolus.[131] It was concluded that bound tryptophan was stripped from albumin during a single capillary pass. Suggested mechanisms include rapid dissociation due to uptake into brain, local physiologic pH changes, or metabolite displacements that would alter the association constant of the trytophan-albumin complex. Similarly, most steroid hormones are nearly completely bound in plasma to either albumin or to a specific binding globulin, with only a small percentage existing in the unbound form. The brain uptake index was 80 to 100 percent under normal conditions and was not significantly decreased by the presence of even large amounts of albumin, [^{3}H]progesterone, and [^{3}H]testosterone.[132] Again it was concluded that the steroid-albumin complex dissociated during passage through the capillary. Thyroid hormones, unlike the steroid hormones that are generally highly lipid-soluble, are polar and enter brain by a specific transport system.[133] However, thyroid hormones, like the tryptophan and the steroid hormones, appear to be stripped from albumin during passage through the brain capillary.

In contrast, for some substances there is convincing evidence that entry into brain is related to the unbound fraction of the substance in blood. For example, in dogs given rifampin to increase the serum concentration of alpha 1-acid glycoprotein (the major binding protein for lidocaine), the free lidocaine concentration was lower than in untreated dogs following intravenous infusion of lidocaine, 3 mg/kg. The partition ratio of lidocaine between brain and serum or between CSF and serum was lower in rifampin treated dogs, and there was a strong and positive correlation between time-averaged brain to serum or CSF to serum ratios and serum free fractions. Moreover, partition ratios expressed on the basis of serum free drug concentrations did not differ betweeen control and rifampin treated dogs. These results indicated that the distribution of lidocaine between serum and the CNS after intravenous administration is governed by the free drug concentration in the circulation.[134]

Movement in ECF

In extracerebral tissues, large-molecular-weight compounds or particles in suspension, which cannot readily cross the capillary wall from ECF to blood, are removed by drainage with the lymph. Clearance from brain of even small polar solutes presents a similar problem, since these cannot easily pass across the BBB from ECF to blood, unless there is a specific transport mechanism in the endothelium. The presence of a non-specific clearance mechanism is indicated by the fact that many slowly penetrating polar solutes, for example, [^{35}S]sulfate and [^{14}C]inulin, have a low CSF-plasma ratio in the steady state and have brain spaces much lower than the 20 percent ECF space of cerebral cortex. Historically, these findings have been attributed to the sink action of CSF.[1] As a polar solute slowly enters cerebral ECF from blood, there will be a steady slow removal because of its diffusion into adjacent CSF in the ventricular or subarachnoid spaces. Since CSF, deficient in the solute, is continually being renewed by secretion of bulk fluid, the concentrations of the solute in ECF and CSF are maintained below that in blood plasma—the smaller the permeability of the solute at the BBB and blood-CSF barrier, the lower the steady-state concentrations in cerebral ECF.

In addition, there is evidence for convective flow of cerebral ECF. This motion has been studied by observing the distribution of large-molecular-weight tracers in brain sections at set times after microinjection in vivo.[37] Tracers such as colored dextrans, Evans blue albumin, and horseradish peroxidase initially appear to diffuse concentrically out from the injection site, but soon become concentrated in the perivascular spaces, seeeming to move centrifugally in these channels.

SPECIFIC TRANSPORT ACROSS THE BBB

The aforementioned intracarotid tissue-sampling technique provides a simple, rapid, reproducible method for characterizing specific transport at the endothelium.[130] Results of studies using this technique indicate specific mechanisms facilitating the transport of certain compounds within several groups: monosaccharides; monocarboxylic acids; neutral amino acids; basic amino acids; dicarboxylic amino acids; and certain amines, of which coline is the main representative (Table 3-8). In each case, the transport is stereospecific, saturable, and subject to competitive inhibition.

Monosaccharides

The monosaccharide transporter is highly stereospecific, the D-sugar being selected. Affinity to D-glucose is high whereas the uptake of L-glucose is barely measurable.[135] The rank order of affinities of the transporter for D-hexoses, based on either the Michaelis constant for uptake of the sugar or its inhibition of glucose uptake is 6-chloro-6-deoxyglucose > 2-fluoro-2-deoxyglucose > 2-deoxyglucose > glucose > 3-O-methylglucose > mannose > galactose. The transport is sodium-independent and is not influenced by insulin.

TABLE 3-8
Transport Systems at the BBB[a]

System	Substrate	V_{max} (μmol · g^{-1} · min^{-1})	K_m (mM)
Monosaccharides	D-glucose	1.42–4	7–11
Monocarboxylic acids	β-hydroxybutyrate	0.16	2.5
	L-lactate	0.091–2	1.8–2
Neutral amino acids	Phenylalanine	0.022–0.03	.026–0.11
	L-dopa	0.063	0.43
	L-leucine	0.022–60	0.025–0.1
	Tryptophan	–	0.009
	Tryosine	–	0.050
	Isoleucine	–	0.051
	Methionine	–	0.075
	Melphalan	–	0.150
Basic amino acids	Ornithine	0.01	0.2
	Lysine	0.008	0.11
	L-arginine	0.005–8	0.04–0.09
Dicarboxylic amino acids	L-glutamate	low	–
Amine	Choline	11	0.34
Nucleosides	Adenosine	0.01–0.75	0.025–0.03
Purines	Adenine	0.05	0.01–0.011

[a] Values based on Crone,[100] Bradbury,[129] Pardridge and Boado,[312] Greig,[313] and Rosenberg.[314]

NOTE: V_{max}, maximum transport capacity; K_m, apparent Michaelis constant.

Monocarboxylic Acids

L-Lactate is preferentially transported into brain (as compared with D-lactate) via a transporter at the BBB that is active for a number of monocarboxylic acids.[136] The rank order of affinities appears to be α-ketomethiobutyrate (the ketoacid of methionine) > α-keto-isocaproate (the ketoacid of leucine) > butyrate > pyruvate > lactate > β-hydroxybutyrate.[137] Important functions of this transporter are that it permits escape of lactate from brain and allows the entry of ketone bodies. Its capacity is subject to a high degree of modulation in relationship to the availability of certain metabolic substrates.

Amino Acids

The transport of most neutral amino acids across cell membranes is accounted for by three distinct transport systems, designated the L system, the A system, and the ACS system.[138] Characteristic pattens of amino acid transport and/or selective sensitivity to specific amino acid analogues distinguish these transport systems. The L system prefers neutral amino acids with branched or ringed side chains (e.g., leucine, valine), is sodium-independent, and is competitively inhibited by 2-aminobicycloheptane-2-carboxylic acid. The A system prefers neutral amino acids with short polar or linear side chains (e.g., alanine, serine), is sodium-dependent, and is inhibited by α-methylaminoisobutyric acid. The ASC system prefers alanine, serine, and cysteine, is sodium-dependent, and is insensitive to both of the above-mentioned inhibitors.

Transport of the three basic amino acids, arginine, lysine, and ornithine, is accounted for by a transport system that is completely separate from the transport of neutral amino acids. These basic amino acids have K_m values that are of similar magnitude to the K_m of the L-group amino acids for their specific transporter. However, the estimated V_{max} values of the basic amino acids are about 0.2 of those for the large neutral amino acids.[137]

Finally, a third system, yielding low uptakes, has been described for the dicarboxylic amino acids, aspartate and glutamate.[139]

Other Substances

A number of polar compounds other than metabolic substrates and neurotransmitter precursors themselves are needed by the brain. These include the precursors of DNA and RNA, as well as cofactors derived from vitamins. The presence of specific saturable transport at the BBB has been demonstrated for certain purines, including adenine, guanine, and hypoxanthine, for certain nucleosides, including adenosine, inosine, guanosine, and uridine, and for thiamine.[140,141]

Certain essential polar compounds may reach the brain via the CSF after prior transport through the CP. This mechanism allows for regulating and distributing certain substances required in only small amounts by the brain. In vitro, the CP is able to accumulate actively and specifically ascorbic acid, folates, thymidine, and probably certain other deoxynucleosides, riboflavin and vitamin B_6.[142]

When extraction during a single capillary pass has been measured and hydrolysis before barrier transport has been excluded, the uptake of enkephalins, thyrotropin-releasing hormone, angiotensin II, and insulin is close to the value of sucrose, that is, the blood background.[129] Movement of peptides of low molecular weight might be facilitated by combination with membrane transporters of the general type involved in transport of metabolic substrates. Possible transporters include specific carriers for certain di-, tri-, or larger peptides, and L-amino acid transporter, carrying a small peptide with an L-system amino acid in a terminal position. It is also possible that endocytosis/exocytosis in the endothelium function as a system for transferring smaller amounts of larger peptides or proteins from blood to brain. For example, insulin binds specifically and avidly to the luminal membrane of the cerebral endothelium (dissociation constant of 1.2 nM), with roughly 75 percent becoming internalized.[143] This internalized and largely intact insulin was re-exported into a radiotracer-free medium with a half-time of about 70 min. The findings are consistent with, but do not prove, the hypothesis that insulin may be translocated from blood into ECF by specific binding to the luminal membrane of the endothelium, followed by endocytosis and finally exocytosis through the abluminal membrane.

Anesthetics and Other Factors
Modifying Permeability

A PS product, rather than a permeability coefficient, is often used to characterize apparent BBB permeability because the precise area of endothelium per unit weight of brain is not generally known. There are two ways in which this apparent permeability might vary for a given solute concentration in plasma. First, changes in the distribution of cerebral perfusion might alter the effective area of endothelium available for transport or, in the case of specific transport, alter the access to transport sites. Second, again in the case of specific transport, there might be a modulation of the transporter itself with a change in either V_{max} or K_m, or both. An increased V_{max} suggests the presence of more transport sites. Which of these two mechanisms is the primary one leading to an altered PS product

may be difficult to determine. If the transport of several independent solutes is changed by the same amount, an alteration in endothelial area is suggested, whereas if the change in transport is restricted to a single solute or to a group of chemical analogues, modulation of the specific transporter is indicated.[129]

If a PS product has been calculated by the use of an equation that takes account of the fall in solute concentration along the length of the capillary, the PS should be independent of the magnitude of flow in a perfused capillary. If the apparent permeability increases with increasing blood flow, it is suggestive of the recruitment of more capillaries from a pool of unperfused microvessels, therby providing a larger endothelial surface area. While recruitment takes place in tissues such as skeletal muscle, it was believed that there are normally no unperfused capillaries in brain, and thus no scope for recruitment. However, the apparent permeability of several solutes not subject to specific transport increases when blood flow is raised by hypercapnia or electrically induced convulsions, and decreases when flow is reduced by hypocapnia.[144–146] These results suggest that, if recruitment does not occur, redistribution of blood flow takes place in such a way that, at higher total flows, a greater fraction of the blood must be exposed to higher surface areas of endothelium or to more transport sites.

Pentobarbital anesthesia was reported in one study to cause no significant change of V_{max}, K_m, and unidirectional influx into brain for glucose,[147] and in another study to decrease V_{max}, K_m, influx, and utilization by 35 to 50 percent[148] (Table 3-9). Pentobarbital also increased the brain uptake index of the amino acids L-lucine, L-phenylalanine, L-tyrosine, and L-tryptophan but not of L-lysine, L-arginine or L-glutamate.[149] Pentobarbital decreased the K_i for the small hydrophilic neutral amino acid α-aminoisobutyric acid,[150] but caused no change in the movement into brain of water,[151] the small hydrophilic molecule technetium-99m, or proteins (albumin) or large nonspecific molecules (Evans Blue dye)[152] or horseradish peroxidase.[153] However, pentobarbital combined with ethanol increased BBB permeability to horseradish peroxidase.[53] Thiopental caused no change in movement into brain of water, sodium, or potassium,[154] and decreased BBB permeability to Evans Blue dye during hypertension as compared to that during halothane anesthesia combined with hypocapnia.[155] In an in vitro study, thiopental did not change the permeability of a brain endothelial cell monolayer to ions, sucrose, or proteins (albumin), but did increase permeability to the small hydrophilic neutral amino acid α-aminoisobutyric acid.[156] In the same in vitro study, methohexital did not alter permeability to any of the aforementioned substances. Sufentanil combined with thiopental decreased the rate of move-

TABLE 3-9
Effects of Anesthetics on BBB Dynamics

Anesthetic	GLUCOSE TRANSPORT			Brain Uptake Index for Amino Acids (*)	Movement of Water	Movement of Electrolytes	Ki for Small Hydrophilic Amino Acids (μl/g per m)	Movement of Proteins or Large Nonspecific Molecules (% of Index Used)
	V_{max} (μmol/g per m)	K_m (mM)	Unidirectional Glucose Influx (μmol/g per m)					
Control	1.0–4.09	8.8–15.9	0.48–1.02	28.8–41.8	(0)	(0)	1.8–8.9	100
Pentobarbital	2.3–2.35(0/−)	4.9–14.0(0/−)	0.52–0.65(0/−)	36.7–57.7(0/+)	(0)	X	1.0–3.4(−)	100(0)
Pentobarbital/ ethanol	X	X	X	X	X	X	X	762(+)
Thiopental	X	X	X	X	(0)	(0)	(0)	15(−)
Thiopental/ sufentanil	X	X	X	X	X	X	X	30–45(−)
Ketamine	X	X	X	X	X	X	1.1–4.4(0/−)	100–108(0)
Isoflurane	X	X	X	X	(0)	(0)	4.6–5.1(−)	100(0)
Enflurane	X	X	X	X	(0)	(0)	X	X
Halothane	0.4–0.8(0/−)	2.0–11.7(0/−)	0.54(0)	X	(0/+)	(0/+)	(−)	25–216(0/+/−)
Nitrous oxide	0.61(−)	4.3(−)	X	X	X	X	X	X
Fentanyl	X	X	X	X	(0)	(0)	5.2–5.7(−)	13–33(−)

NOTE: +, increase; 0, no change; −, decrease; *, brain uptake index defined as $\dfrac{\text{dpm (test substance)/brain sample}}{\text{dpm (reference substance)/brain sample}} \div \dfrac{\text{dpm (test substance)/injectate}}{\text{dpm (reference substance)/injectate}}$

ment of albumin or IgG into CSF.[157] Ketamine was reported in one study to decrease the transport of the small hydrophilic neutral amino acid α-aminoisobutyric acid across the BBB.[150] However, in other studies ketamine was reported to cause no significant change in the movement into brain of the small hydrophilic molecule technetium-99m, or proteins (albumin) or large nonspecific molecules (Evans Blue dye[152] or horseradish peroxidase.)[153] Isoflurane decreased the K_i for the small hydrophilic neutral amino acid α-aminoisobutyric acid and, as well, decreased E (from 0.4 to 2.6 percent to 0.3 to 1.3 percent) and PS (from 4.6 to 21.5 to 2.2 to 12.8 μl/g/min).[158] Isoflurane also caused no change in movement into brain of water, sodium, potassium,[154] the small hydrophilic molecule technetium-99m, or proteins (albumin) or large nonspecific molecules (Evans Blue dye).[152] Enflurane caused no change in movement into brain of water, sodium, or potassium.[154] Halothane was reported in one study to cause no significant change of V_{max} and K_m for glucose influx into or efflux out of brain.[159] In another study halothane was reported to decrease V_{max} and K_m for glucose influx but to increase the diffusional permeability for glucose into brain (to 22% compared with an awake value of 7%), with the result of no net change in overall brain glucose influx.[147] Halothane was reported in one study to increase movement into brain of sodium, but not water or potassium,[154] and in another study to increase movement into brain of sodium, chloride, and water.[151] Movement into brain of the small

hydrophilic molecule technetium-99m during halothane/normocapnia was 8 to 10 percent of that during halothane/hypocapnia, while diffusion of the lipophilic molecule cortisol was not significantly changed.[160] Finally, in one study halothane appears to have caused no significant change in movement into brain of proteins (albumin and IgG),[157] whereas a second study reported movement of albumin during halothane/normocapnia was 11 to 25 percent of that during halothane/hypocapnia,[160] and a third study reported that movement of Evans Blue dye during halothane/normocapnia was 216 percent of that during halothane/hypocapnia.[155] Nitrous oxide decreases V_{max} and K_m for brain glucose influx and efflux.[159] Fentanyl caused no change in movement into brain of water, sodium, or potassium,[154] and decreased movement into brain of the small hydrophilic molecule technetium-99m, the small hydrophilic neutral amino acid α-aminoisobutyric acid, and proteins (albumin) and large nonspecific molecules (Evans Blue dye).[152,161] In an in vitro study, fentanyl did not change the permeability of a brain endothelial cell monolayer to ions, sucrose, proteins (albumin), or the small hydrophilic neutral amino acid α-aminoisobutyric acid.[156] Treatment of rats with the tremor-inducing stimulant of cerebral metabolism, cismethrin, not only stimulated regional glucose utilization and blood flow, but also markedly increased unidirectional influx of glucose into brain; that is, there was an increase in the apparent permeability.[162]

The greatly increased utilization of ketone bodies

by brain in starvation is cited as an example of true adaptation of a transporter.[163] This adaptive process is accompanied by a large increase in the V_{max} and to some extent in the K_m for the system that transports β-hydroxybutyrate and other monocarboxylic acids into brain. The activity of the transporter is enhanced during suckling in the baby rat, whose diet is rich in fat and lactose, and suppressed after portacaval anastomosis when the ability of the liver to produce ketone bodies is severely impaired.[164,165] Portacaval anastomosis produces other changes in transport at the BBB, presumably in response to some aspect of the metabolic disturbance. The pattern of increased influx of the large neutral amino acids phenylalanine, tryptophan, and leucine into brain indicates greater capacity of the transporter.[166,167] This enhancement of transport can also be induced by prolonged infusion of ammonium salts and seems to depend on the ability of the brain to synthesize glutamine.[168,169]

RECEPTOR MEDIATED TRANSPORT

In terms of peptide and protein ligands, a number of receptor systems have been identified on brain capillary endothelial cells, including those for transferrin, insulin and insulin-like growth factors (IGF)-I and -II. The results of both in vitro and in vivo experiments suggest that these receptors may be involved in the transport of their respective ligands across the BBB.[170] Receptors for low-density lipoproteins and atrial natriuretic peptide also are present on the BBB endothelium.

Transferrin

As a cofactor for heme and nonheme iron-containing enzymes, iron plays an essential role in cellular metabolism. The involvement of iron in the mitochrondrial respiratory pathway and the ATP requirements of neuronal cells necessitates high levels of iron in the brain. Transferrin is a monomeric glycoprotein with a molecular weight of 80,000 daltons whose function is the transport of iron from sites of storage and absorption to tissues throughout the body. The transferrin receptor, an integral membrane glycoprotein consisting of two identical 95,000-dalton subunits linked by a disulfide bridge, mediates the uptake of iron by individual cells.

The first step of iron delivery into cells is the binding of diferric ferrotransferrin to the receptor with a dissociation constant (K_d) in the nanomolar range. Endocytic vesicles rapidly internalize (half-time of about 3 min) the surface-bound ligand. Once inside the cell, the receptor-ligand complex enters a vesicle termed CURL (compartment of uncoupling of receptor from ligand), which has a pH < 5.5. The receptor-apotransferrin complex enters tubular vesicles, which are associated

with the CURL, and is then recycled back to the cell surface. Binding of aprotransferrin to the receptor is poor (KD > 7×10^{-7} M) at the neutral pH of ECF, leading to the rapid dissociation of the ligand (the half-time for dissociation of the apotransferrin-receptor complex is approximately 30 times faster than that for diferric transferrin).

While this cellular pathway for transferrin internalization has been well established in a number of different cell types, brain capillary endothelia appear to diverge considerably in the processing of this ligand. In vivo, antibodies that recognize the transferrin receptor are transported across the BBB due to their interaction with the receptor protein, suggesting that the iron-transferrin complex also is transported across the BBB.[171,172] While it is clear that iron is transported into the brain across the BBB, and there is evidence both in vitro and in vivo that transferrin is also transported across the BBB, the exact cellular pathway involved in this transport process has yet to be elucidated.

Insulin

Because the brain posesses insulin receptors, it has been speculated that insulin may play a role in brain function, possibly in regulating appetite, or as a growth factor during development. Before insulin could be considered to play such a role, however, entry of insulin into the CNS first had to be shown. Specific binding of radiolabeled insulin to isolated bovine cerebral capillaries has been demonstrated in vitro. Two classes of insulin binding sites were identified on isolated microvessels: a high-affinity, low-capacity site with an affinity constant (K_a) of 22.29 nM^{-1} and a low-affinity, high-capacity site with a K_a of 0.05 nM^{-1}.

The uptake of insulin into the brain after a single pass was eight-, five- and threefold higher than inulin, a vascular space marker, in newborn, 3-week-old, and 11-week-old rabbits, respectively.[173] Reduced uptake of the labeled insulin when excess unlabeled insulin was present in the infusate indicated that a saturable receptor was involved in the brain uptake process. Autoradiography localized labeled insulin beyond the capillary endothelium and within the brain parenchyma. Carotid infusion of [^{125}I]insulin confirmed transport of insulin across the BBB.[174]

Insulin-Like Growth Factors

Like the physiologic role of insulin within the CNS, that of IGF-I and IGF-II remains to be determined. These peptides are present in the CNS and have been reported to be involved in a diverse array of CNS functions, from regulation of glucose uptake by glial cells to effects on food intake and body weight maintenance.[175] IGF-II mRNA concentrations in the brain are higher than in any other major organ, and as much as 50-fold greater than that in liver, due to active synthesis of IGF-II by CP.

Receptors for both IGF-I and -II have been identified.[176–178] In cross-linking studies using either rat or bovine capillaries, an α-receptor subunit with a molecular weight of 138 kDa was identified with IGF-I, and a band with a molecular weight of 250 kDa was identified with IGF-II. Thus, bovine and rat brain microvessel endothelial cells appear to contain classic type I and type II IGF receptors with properties similar to those found in peripheral tissues. In contrast, cross-linking studies using human brain microvessels have suggested that only a type I receptor with a slightly higher affinity for IGF-II over IGF-I is present at the human BBB.[178]

Low-Density Lipoprotein

A receptor for low-density lipoprotein (LDL), which is distinct from the scavenger pathway responsible for the uptake of chemically modified forms of LDL (such as acetylated LDL), has recently been identified on brain capillary endothelial cells.[179] Dot blots and ligand binding studies were used to examine the characteristics of the endothelial cell LDL receptor. It was reported that the endothelial cell receptor binds human LDL, LDL binding to the receptor is not completed by high-density lipoprotein 3 or methyl-LDL, and LDL binding is dependent on the presence of divalent cations. It was further reported that the receptor is sensitive to enzymatic proteolysis, and the receptor has a molecular weight of 132 kD.

PHARMACOLOGY OF THE BLOOD-BRAIN BARRIER

MEASUREMENT OF DRUG TRANSFER

Mathematical description of drug transfer across the BBB requires measurement of the amounts of the test material in plasma and brain samples, and of the sampling times. With these values, a transfer constant can be computed, that is, the extraction fraction (E), the influx constant (K_i), or the efflux constant (K_o).[180] None of these constants is a membrane permeability coefficient per se. However, PS, defined above in the section entitled "facilitated transport, saturation kinetics and induction," can be derived from these transfer constants (see "transport models" below).[181,182] PS combines the two unknown variables that set the flux rate across the BBB, that is, the permeability coefficient and the effective capillary surface area. E is determined by injecting a bolus containing both a test substance plus a reference material into one carotid artery and measuring brain uptake during the next several seconds. E can be described by the equation:

$$E = B/A$$

where B is the amount of test substance taken up by brain tissue and A is the total amount of extractable test material that has flowed into brain capillaries during the experimental period, as indicated by the reference material. Methods used to measure E include indicator diffusion, the brain-uptake index, and external registration.[180] Useful values of E are obtained by these three techniques when the capillary is moderately to highly permeable to the test material, the experimental duration is very short (usually less than 5 s), and the backflux of test material from brain to blood is minute compared with the influx.[181,182] E is the transfer constant, which should be measured in most instances when dealing with a rapidly transformed drug or substrate.

K_i is determined by either bolus injection or continuous infusion of a test substance intravenously, and sampling plasma and CNS tissue at various times thereafter.[180] K_i is defined as:

$$K_i = B/\int_0^T C_a(t)dt$$

where T is the experimental duration, and $C_a(t)$ is the activity or concentration of free and exchangeable test material in arterial plasma during the experiment (i.e., from zero time to T).[182,183] In this equation the denominator is comparable to A in the equation $E = B/A$ and represents the exposure, that is, the amount of test material available for transfer across the BBB during the experiment.

K_o is determined either by intracarotid injection or ventriculocisternal perfusion to "load" the brain with a test substance, measuring the tissue washout or clearance of that substance. K_o is determined from the tissue concentration which changes as a function of time when the brain is loaded by intracarotid injection, and as a function of distance from the ventricular surface when the brain is loaded by ventriculocisternal perfusion.[181,182] K_i and K_o are related by the equation:

$$K_i = K_o V_b$$

where V_b is the space in the brain in which the test material distributes during loading and from which it washes out as it clears from the tissue.

Usually, BBB transfer is measured by either bolus injection or continuous infusion of the test material intravenously, and sampling blood and CNS tissue at various times thereafter, with subsequent calculation of the transfer constants by compartmental analysis rather than by the above equation. A large number of experiments which vary widely in duration (e.g., from several minutes to several hours) must be performed in order to produce sufficient data for compartmental analysis. The transfer constants are then obtained by assuming a blood-tissue distribution model of two or more compartments and of specific configuration (e.g., serially arranged), combining all the experimental data and processing the grouped data according to the appropriate format. The simplest system is the two-compartment model (one blood plus one tissue compartment), which yields estimates of K_o, V_b, and K_i.

TRANSPORT MODELS

E, K_i, or K_o are used to derive a PS by assuming a particular capillary-tissue exchange model and knowing or approximating the rate of intracapillary fluid flow (F) and the effective volume of distribution of the exchangeable test substance in intracapillary fluid (V_c). Ligand-protein dissociation, and plasma protein and red blood cell flows determine V_c. Generally, the following assumptions are made: (1) the velocity of F is constant during the time of the experiment; (2) changes in F are produced by changes in flow velocity; (3) the capillary is a tube of fixed diameter and uniform permeability surrounded by a cylinder of tissue; and (4) the transfer constants indicate unidirectional flux. With these assumptions the transfer constants can be expressed as:

$$E = 1 - \exp(-PS/FV_c)$$
$$K_i = FV_c[1 - \exp(-PS/FV_c)]$$
$$K_o = (FV_c/V_b)[1 - \exp(-PS/FV_c)]$$

where exp symbolizes exponentiation of the term $(-PS/FV_c)$, and the PS and FV_c products are expressed in the same units, (e.g., ms/g/min).

TRANSPORT MECHANISMS

Numerous drugs, hormones, and other substances bind to plasma proteins and are delivered to sites of BBB transfer.[184] When little dissociation of the substance from plasma proteins occurs relative to the rate of protein passage through the capillaries (the mean capillary transit time of protein is about 1 s for most brain areas), V_c need only account for the free concentration of the substance in plasma and red blood cell water. When substantial dissociation of the substance from plasma proteins occurs relative to the velocity of flow within the capillary, then V_c must reflect both the free and the protein-dissociable concentrations of the substance.

In order for solutes to pass between blood and CNS parenchyma, they generally must move through the endothelial cell. The capacity for substances to dissolve in and diffuse through the endothelial cell, and carrier-mediated transfer are two accepted transcellular mech-

anisms of passage across the BBB. Vesicular transport has been proposed (but not proved) as another mechanism of material transfer through cerebral endothelial cells.[185]

The passage of some substances through the cerebral endothelial cell is facilitated by specific carrier systems. These BBB systems are stereospecific, saturable, and competitively inhibited by structurally similar compounds, like carrier systems in other membranes. The PS of substrates transported by BBB carriers are larger than would be expected with respect to their lipid solubility and diffusivity.[186] Some of these carrier systems were presented in the above section entitled "specific transport across the BBB." The transfer of some neuroactive compounds such as dopamine, acetylcholine, and encephalins is impaired by endothelial cell enzyme systems, which convert them to inactive and/or less permeable metabolites. These enzyme systems play an integral role in overall function of the BBB.

The capillaries within certain structures that are adjacent to the ventricles of the brain are markedly more permeable than typical BBB capillaries. These structures, discussed earlier, are known as the circumventricular organs and include the CP, the median eminence, the organum vasculosum of the lamina terminalis, the pineal gland, the subcommissural organ, the subfornical organ, the neural lobe of the pituitary, and the area postrema. Because their capillaries tend to leak, these structures also may serve as points of entry into adjacent brain areas for other blood-borne materials, such as drugs, antibodies, and neurotoxins. It is reported that aspartate moves from blood into structures such as the median eminence and subfornical organ, and then subsequently spreads into adjacent areas of the brain with typical BBB capillaries.[187] Additional quantitative evidence of such transfer is needed to prove that significant penetration of substances into brain tissue occurs via this route.

Substances may enter the CNS not only directly from the blood across the BBB but also by transport from the blood to CSF, and then to brain. The major site of blood-CSF exchange is the CP. Other sites of blood-CSF exchange could be microvessels in the pia-arachnoid and dura-arachnoid membranes and the circumventricular organs.

Blood flow varies widely throughout the CNS. Under normal conditions, blood flow in gray matter structures is several-fold greater than in white matter areas. Regardless of the cause of local and regional differences in blood flow (i.e., differences in flow velocity or differences in numbers of perfused capillaries), these blood flow patterns suggest that highly permeable drugs such as thiopental and nicotine will distribute during the first-pass period (<10 s) mainly to high-flow areas of the CNS.[188]

TABLE 3-10
Cerebral Edema

Type of Edema	Precipitating Cause	Initial Changes During Edema Formation
Vasogenic edema	Increased permeability of BBB	Fluid and substances move from blood into brain ECF space
Ischemic edema	Cellular energy failure	ECF and electrolytes move from ECF into ICF space
Osmotic edema	Osmolality of brain tissue greater than that of blood	Fluid moves from blood into brain ECF space
Hydrocephalic (or interstitial) edema	CSF or lymphatic drainage channels are blocked	Fluid and substances move from CSF into brain ECF space
Cytotoxic edema	Cellular energy failure	ECF and electrolytes move from ECF into ICF space
Metabolic storage	Intracellular sequestration of metabolites	Increased ICF volume
Increased cerebral blood volume	Venous obstruction or arterial dilation	Increased CBV

Cerebral Edema

DEFINITION OF EDEMA

Cerebral edema is said to be present when brain ICF and/or ECF volume increases. Such an increase of brain fluid content increases total intracranial volume and, hence, ICP.[189] Increased ICP may be due not only to cerebral edema, but also to increased cerebral blood volume (CBV), increased CSF volume, or a combination of the three (Table 3-10). The likelihood of successful treatment of increased ICP is enhanced if the underlying mechanism(s) responsible for increased ICP is identified. When the mechanism(s) responsible for increased ICP is not identified, some prefer to use the term "brain swelling" rather than "cerebral edema."

VASOGENIC EDEMA

The most frequently occurring variety of cerebral edema characterized by increased ECF volume is vasogenic edema. Vasogenic edema results from increased permeability of brain capillaries and hence is a frequent complication of clinically important disorders, such as head injury, tumor, infection, inflammation, and certain types of cerebrovascular accidents. There are several causes for increased brain capillary permeability. Causes of increased permeability include: (1) metabolic impairment of endothelial transport systems; (2) neovascularization by vessels lacking BBB characteristics; and (3) structural injury of the cerebral endothelium leading to opening of tight junctions, increased pinocytosis, or disruption of cells.[190]

Regardless of the cause of BBB dysfunction, increased brain capillary permeability results in the formation of ECF edema. The chemical composition of the edema fluid is influenced by the magnitude of BBB dysfunction, so that with significant loss of normal BBB characteristics a protein-rich fluid is likely to be formed, representing a mixture of plasma, normal ECF, and the products of tissue damage.

The major characteristics of vasogenic edema are BBB dysfunction (or its absence in the case of tumors), extravasation of a plasma-like fluid that penetrates the tissue under the force of systemic pressure, and spread of that fluid driven by pressure gradients that develop within the tissue. The extravasated fluid accumulates mainly in white matter.

FORMATION OF VASOGENIC EDEMA

Local disruption of normal brain capillary permeability at the site of disorder, commonly referred to as a breakdown of the BBB, initiates a cascade that leads to the development of vasogenic edema.[191] In the case of tumors, the vessels within the tumor are the main site of focal leakage. Dysfunction of the BBB is localized to the site of disorder, with brain capillary pemeability characteristics of the edematous tissue distant from the lesion remaining unchanged.

The precise cause for local BBB dysfunction at the site of disorder is uncertain.[192] Extravasation of fluid through ruptured endothelial cell membranes in the damaged tissue has been reported, but this mechanism appears to be only a part of the overall process. In the periphery of the injured area, BBB markers move through apparently intact, but obviously damaged, endothelial cells as well as through leaky interendothelial clefts. Pinocytosis also is suggested as a mechanism of fluid passage across the BBB.

Results of certain recent studies indicate that the kallikrein-kinin system may contribute to the formation of vasogenic edema.[193] Although oxygen-derived free radicals generated from an exogenous xanthine oxidase/hypoxanthine/ADP-Fe^{3+} system have been shown to induce brain injury and edema, involvement of endogenously formed free radicals has not been demonstrated.[194] In contrast, hydroxy-free radicals were reported following pressure-induced focal cerebral ischemia with and without ethanol pretreatment.[195,196]

EXTRAVASATION OF EDEMA FLUID

Increased capillary-hydraulic conductance resulting from BBB dysfunction leads to extravasation of plasma derived fluid, while tissue hydrostatic and oncotic pressure is the force that drives the extravasated fluid through the tissue.[197] That edema fluid moves by bulk flow is indicated by the observation that substances of diverse molecular weights, ranging from sucrose to protein molecules, spread from the site of injury at the same speed.[198] Brain tissue pressure is increased at the site of injury, and decreases with increasing distance away from the site of injury.[199] These data indicate that tissue pressure gradients exist that could account for the bulk movement of fluid within the edematous brain from the site of injury and toward the cerebral ventricles. Labeled plasma proteins and other markers in the CSF are recovered when the edema front reaches the ventricles, suggesting that this may be an important route of removal of extravasated fluid.[200]

SPREAD OF EDEMA FLUID

The extent of spread of vasogenic edema away from the site of injury is influenced by a number of factors. One factor is the actual surface area of barrier damage. The larger the area affected, the greater will be the volume of extravasated fluid. A second factor is arterial blood pressure. Arterial blood pressure provides the hydrostatic pressure that drives fluid into brain tissue. Drug-induced hypertension increased both the speed and extent of edema formation, while in animals made hypotensive by use of appropriate drugs, the rate of spread and the extent of edema decreased.[189] In addition, movement of edema fluid into CSF was reported to be directly related to the hydrostatic pressure gradient between edematous tissue and the CSF. Increasing the gradient enhanced the clearance of edema fluid, while decreasing it had the opposite effect.[201]

Edema fluid spreads along the normal pathways of ECF bulk flow. Fluid moves from the site of injury through the pericapillary spaces, the intercellular clefts between astrocytic foot processes, and the 150- to 200-Å ECF spaces that are anatomically continuous with the CSF spaces. Brain ECF volume reportedly increases by nearly 50 percent at sites of BBB dysfunction.[13]

DISTRIBUTION OF EDEMA FLUID

Following cerebral insult, most vasogenic edema fluid localizes in the white matter ECF space of the lesioned hemisphere.[189] Edema fluid spreads preferentially through the white matter, whose meager cellularity and straighter ECF clefts create a resistance to flow that is less than that of gray matter. In addition, the parallel arrangement of fibers in white matter presumably allows opening up of potential ECF spaces, while interwoven cell processes in the cortex present considerable mechanical resistance to expansion of ECF volume and accumulation of the extravasated fluid.

EQUILIBRIUM OF EDEMA FLUID

After a certain time fluid equilibration occurs, that is, the volume of fluid extravasated in the area of lesion is balanced by the clearance of water from the area of edema.[191] The timing of this equilibrium phase is influenced by numerous factors, including the size of the lesion and the level of arterial blood pressure.[202] BBB permeability remains increased during this equilibration phase. The ECF spaces become enlarged and, as a result, pressure gradients within brain tissue are minimized.[200] Fluid continues to move into the edematous areas, but this is matched by clearance of edema fluid, so no further spread of edema takes place. As pressure gradients within brain tissue progressively decrease, movement of edema fluid into the CSF also decreases, with fluid moving by diffusion rather than by bulk flow.[202] Ions and molecules may be transferred across intact capillaries from the edematous tissue into the blood, although total clearance by cerebral capillaries appears to be quantitatively relatively small.[203] Protein clearance from the ECF space by astrocytes may contribute to redistribution of water according to the Starling hypothesis.[204] Removal of large molecules across the capillary wall by pinocytosis has also been proposed as one mechanism involved in removal of edema fluid, but the significance of this process remains a subject of controversy.[205]

RESOLUTION OF VASOGENIC EDEMA

Eventually, normal BBB function is restored, either by regeneration of normally impermeable microvessels in an area of injury or excision of abnormally permeable capillaries in a tumor.[206] Once normal BBB function is restored, no further extravasation of fluid occurs. Clearance of edema fluid continues until all the edema is resolved, presumably by the various mechanisms operating during the equilibrium phase. These may include transport processes for ions and small molecules, protein clearance by astrocytes, redistribution of water in accordance with the Starling hypothesis, and possible pinocytosis of large molecules.

CHARACTERISTICS OF VASOGENIC EDEMA

Measurement of edema fluid composition has aided the characterization of types of edema and the processes resulting in edema formation. Determination of water content defines the presence of edema. Chemical analysis of edematous tissue provides data on the nature of the edema fluid, such as its electrolyte and protein content. This is vital to establishing the source of fluid taken up by the tissue, for example, whether it is derived from plasma, is a plasma ultrafiltrate, or is not related to plasma at all. Attempts at isolating and analyzing edema fluid itself have also been made.[207]

The lesion resulting from cerebral cold injury has been used as a model of vasogenic edema. The sodium concentration (143 mEq/liters) and a colloid osmotic pressure (14 mmHg) of the edema fluid produced by such an injury are more similar to plasma values (146 mEq/liter and 20 mmHg), than to CSF values (158 mEq/liter and 0.6 mmHg). The extent of movement of plasma into vasogenic edema fluid is indicated by these data. These findings reflect the direct contribution of the plasma extravasate. The potassium concentration of vasogenic edema fluid (4.75 mEq/liter) is greater than that in plasma (3.94 mEq/liter) or CSF (3.40 mEq/liter) indicating that potassium moves from the ICF space into vasogenic edema fluid.[208]

PATHOPHYSIOLOGY OF VASOGENIC EDEMA

Extravasation of plasma into the cerebral ECF from the site of injury causes a decrease of regional CBF in those areas. Expansion of the ECF space by edema fluid increases local tissue pressure and leads to a compromise of the regional microcirculation. Thus, a primary effect of vasogenic edema is focal ischemia.[209]

Vasogenic edema also causes a number of secondary effects. Local glucose utilization is significantly decreased in the ipsilateral cerebral cortex, and is decreased to a lesser extent in the contralateral cortex, and the bilateral ipsi- and contralateral subcortical structures and white matter. Escape of biologically active substances, such as prostaglandins and catecholamines, from injured cerebral capillaries has been proposed as the cause for decreased cerebral metabolism of glucose. Glial cell swelling has been attributed to leakage of free radicals, lysosomal enzymes, and fatty acids from injured cerebral capillaries.[103] Toxic substances also may contribute to the formation and spread of vasogenic edema by increasing capillary permeability.[210]

The formation and spread of edema fluid also increases ICP. Increase of intracranial volume and ICP causes compartmental shifts of cerebral structures, which can lead to brain stem compression and signs of rostral-caudal deterioration, characterized by arterial hypertension, bradycardia, and cardiorespiratory collapse. Cerebral edema invariably results in mechanical damage to and compressive ischemia of brain tissue when the "mass effect" created by the edema fluid is large and rapidly expanding.

ISCHEMIC EDEMA

A completely different type of cerebral edema occurs as a consequence of ischemia.[211] Unlike vasogenic edema, ischemic edema forms primarily in the cerebral cortex, not in white matter. In the early stages, formation of ischemic edema is characterized by intracellular accumulation of water and sodium. Outward movement of potassium from ICF occurs at later stages. Initially the BBB remains intact. However, continuing decrease of CBF leads to cellular damage (including damage to the capillary endothelium), increased BBB permeability, extravasation of serum proteins, and the development of vasogenic edema. Generally, the bulk of ischemic edema formation is the result of processes associated with ischemia, not a consequence of changes at the BBB. It is reported that hypoxia per se does not lead to the formation of cerebral edema.[13]

The principal cause for the formation of ischemic edema appears to be a disturbance of the energy-dependent sodium-potassium pump of the cell membrane. Continuous pumping of sodium out of the intracellular compartment opposes movement of water from the ECF to the ICF. When energy deficit causes these pumps to fail, water moves from the ECF to the ICF and the affected cells swell.[111] The size of the ECF space decreases, and the concentration of solutes in the ECF increases.[208] Alone, redistribution of water to the ICF space from the ECF space causes no increase in brain mass. However, as water leaves the ECF space it is replaced by influx of water from the cerebral vasculature. The net effect, therefore, is a substantial increase of brain tissue water content due to significantly increased ICF water content and relatively unchanged ECF water content. Movement of water from the cerebral vasculature into the ECF space may occur by passive diffusion across the cerebral endothelium. There is also evidence that, as water moves from the ECF space to the ICF space, some of the restoration of ECF water content results from reverse bulk flow of ECF, that is, by movement of water from the CSF into the ECF.[212]

ISCHEMIC CHANGES

The magnitude and duration of CBF decrease must exceed critical values before depletion of cerebral energy supply is so severe that membrane sodium-potassium pumps fail.[213] Decreased cortical electrical activity and movement of water and sodium into the ICF space are the first changes seen following significant decrease of CBF. These changes are followed by loss of potassium and uptake of calcium into the ICF space, and eventually cell death.

After CBF decreases to the critical threshold for edema formation, further decrease in CBF correlates with decrease in the specific gravity of brain tissue, a frequently used method of determining brain water content.[214,215] With complete ischemia, ischemic edema does not develop, as under conditions of no CBF no extra fluid can enter the ischemic tissue.[216] However, under conditions of complete ischemia, water moves quickly from the ECF space into the ICF space, indicating that severe disturbances in ion and water homeostasis have occurred.[217]

POSTISCHEMIC EDEMA

Edema also is formed when CBF is restored to a previously completely ischemic area. Edema formed under these circumstances is referred to as postischemic brain edema.[216] Postischemic edema also may form when CBF is restored to an area of prolonged, incomplete ischemia.[217] During the time that CBF is decreased below the critical value needed to sustain cerebral energy stores, there is a severe disturbance of water and ion homeostasis and movement of water into ICF spaces, but no edema develops. When CBF is restored, water moves into the ECF from the vascular compartment, and edema develops.[216]

Subsequent events depend on the duration of ischemia and the quality of reoxygenation achieved during the postischemic period. The longer the period of ischemia, the less likely the reversal of changes that accompanied it. Reversal of ischemic changes also is influenced by the extent to which CBF is resumed. When CBF is resumed within a period of time compatible with recovery of metabolic activity, ion homeostasis is normalized and edema is resolved in a matter of hours, so long as no focal, postischemic flow disturbances exist.[218]

DELAYED BREAKDOWN OF BBB

When either the ischemic period is prolonged or postischemic recirculation remains deficient, there is progression of edema even during the postischemic period. The changes that occur are similar to those seen when CBF decreases below the critical value needed to maintain cerebral energy stores. ICP increases and can be fatal. With time, irreversable cellular injury occurs and normal BBB function is lost. The time course of development of various parameters of ischemic injury, including BBB damage, is inversely related to the intensity and/or duration of the ischemic insult. Some uncertainty remains regarding the mechanisms of delayed BBB breakdown.

In summary, the processes leading to ischemic edema are quite complex, consisting initially of shifts of water and sodium into the cortical ICF space, while the BBB remains intact. These sequelae are reversible, provided ischemia is not prolonged and CBF is restored to normal values postischemia. Prolonged ischemia and poor recirculation lead to permanent injury, loss of normal BBB function, and uncontrolled development of vasogenic edema.

OSMOTIC EDEMA

This type of edema forms when plasma osmolarity is less than brain tissue osmolarity.[219] Water moves along this osmotic gradient resulting in increased brain ECF water content. The BBB must be intact in order for osmotic edema to form. When normal BBB function is lost, no effective osmotic gradient exists. Drugs such as hypertonic saline and diuretics cause the reverse situation, that is, plasma osmolarity is greater than brain tissue osmolarity, resulting in decreased brain ECF water content.

DECREASED PLASMA OSMOLARITY

Circumstances or conditions causing plasma hypoosmolarity may lead to the formation of osmotic edema. Decreased plasma osmolarity may result from inappropriate secretion of the antidiuretic hormone, administration of excessive volume of hypoosmolar intravenous fluid, pseudotumor cerebri, excessive hemodialysis of uremic patients, and compulsive drinking by psychiatric patients.[190,220] When plasma osmolarity is substantially decreased, water moves from the cerebral vasculature into the brain ECF. This water distributes evenly within the gray and white matter ECF spaces.[103] The concentration of electrolytes in the ECF reflects the consequences of dilution, as modified by solvent drag. If this type of osmotic gradient is maintained for some time, brain tissue potassium content decreases, presumably as a consequence of cellular adaptation.[219]

Osmotic edema fluid moves by bulk flow through gray and white matter ECF spaces following the usual ECF pathways. A significant increase of ECF volume flow occurs when plasma osmolarity decreases by 10 percent or more. At the same time, movement of ECF and ECF tracers into the CSF increases.[221] This movement of osmotic edema fluid may increase extrachoroidal $\dot{V}_f$ and thus total $\dot{V}_f$ with no change of $\dot{V}_f$ at the CP.[222] With osmotic edema, brain bulk enlargement generally is less than with vasogenic edema or ischemic edema because osmotic edema fluid is readily cleared from the ECF space.

INCREASED TISSUE OSMOLARITY

Increase in tissue osmolarity at a time when plasma osmolarity is normal may also lead to the formation of osmotic edema. For example, intracerebral hematomas release proteins into the brain ECF space during the time of dissolution of the hematoma. Increased protein concentration in the ECF space increases brain tissue osmolarity, which in turn attracts fluid to the periphery of the hemorrhage area across the intact BBB.[190] Peritumoral edema may form via a similar mechanism, although this type of edema more often results from vasogenic or compressive edema processes.

HYDROCEPHALIC (OR INTERSTITIAL) EDEMA

Hydrocephalic edema differs from the aforementioned type of cerebral edema because of its similarity to lymphedema in the general body tissues. Both hydrocephalic edema and lymphedema occur when drainage channels are blocked, resulting in expansion of the tissue proximal to the obstruction with retrograde fluid accumulation in the ECF space. In acute hydrocephalus, the earliest finding involving the brain parenchyma is periventricular edema. The normally narrow ECF channels between glial cells and axons become distended, a finding typical of ECF edema. Astrocytes are particularly susceptible to hydrocephalic edema and undergo selective swelling, followed by gradual atrophy and cell loss. In patients with chronic hydrocephalus, destruction of axon collaterals, a gradual unraveling of the myelin sheath, and phagocytosis of lipid by the microglia are characteristic hisopathologic features.

Two factors contribute to hydrocephalic edema formation. One contributing factor is stasis of brain ECF. Stasis probably occurs secondary to the decreased gradient for bulk flow from the cerebral ECF space into the cerebral ventricles. A second contributing factor is backflow of CSF into the periventricular tissues. Increased intraventricular pressure is the presumed cause for backflow.[190] In patients with communicating hydrocephalus, isotope ventriculography typically reveals retrograde filling of the ventricular system. In addition, a "double-density" halo typically appears around the cerebral ventricles, indicating migration of the radiopharmaceutical into the periventricular tissues.[223] Decreased regional CBF occurs in areas of chronic or worsening periventricular edema.[68] It is likely that the functional disturbances of hydrocephalus are due in part to decreased regional CBF.[224]

CYTOTOXIC EDEMA

At one time this term was applied to ischemic edema. Currently it is recommended that the term cytotoxic edema should be applied only when intracellular swelling is the result of noxious factors, such as triethyltin and hexachlorophene poisoning, or when mechanisms underlying the cellular swelling are not clear. There are many sources of cytotoxic injury. Methionine sulfoximine, cuprizone, and isoniazid generally cause selective swelling of astrocytes. Astrocyte swelling also is reported in Reye's syndrome and after infections with transmissible viruses. With triethyltin and hexachlorophene, increased water content occurs principally in the intramyelinic clefts. With exposure to hydrogen cyanide, increased water content occurs principally in axons. Other agents known to produce cytotoxic injury include 2,4-dinitrophenol, 6-aminonicatinamide, and lead.[190]

COMPRESSIVE EDEMA

This type of edema forms when an intracranial space-occupying lesion or mass effect distorts the pathways for or completely blocks the bulk flow of brain ECF.[154,225] In its early stages compressive edema is characterized by increased brain ECF volume without the BBB breakdown seen in vasogenic edema, increased ICF volume seen in ischemic edema, or backflow of CSF into periventricular tissues seen in hydrocephalic edema. Compressive edema frequently occurs as an accompanying feature of benign tumors that do not alter BBB permeability (e.g., meningioma) and likely is present to a certain degree with most large intracranial masses. Shift or herniation of brain tissue is another cause for this type of edema. In this case, incarcerated tissue expands due to obstructed flow of brain ECF, impaired venous drainage, or both.

METABOLIC STORAGE

This form of brain tissue swelling results from the intracellular uptake of abnormal metabolites. Sequestration of progressively greater quantities of metabolites within neurons increases intracellular volume without necessarily increasing ICF volume. Increased intracellular volume is most pronounced in the early stages, leading eventually to neuronal atrophy and death. This rare group of inherited disorders is known collectively as the storage diseases. Some of the better known examples include the intracellular storage of glycosyl ceramide (Gaucher's disease), mucopolysaccharides (Hurler's disease), sphingomyelin (Niemann-Pick disease), glycogen (Pompe's disease), and GM2 ganglioside (Tay-Sachs disease).

INCREASED CEREBRAL BLOOD VOLUME

This form of cerebral enlargement is precipitated by increased cerebral vascular volume rather than increased volume of the cerebral ICF or ECF space. Commonly, cerebral vascular volume increases as a result of: (1) dilation of capacitance vessels due to obstruction of venous outflow; or (2) relaxation of resistance vessels. In the latter case, arterial dilation leads to increased capillary blood flow and volume. Venous volume may increase as outflow channels expand to accommodate increased CBF. Whether due to venous or arterial dilation, brain bulk increases solely as a function of increased CBV. In response to increased CBV, fluid shifts out of the CSF compartment, as evidenced by the small size of the cerebral ventricles. Initially CSF volume decreases offset the increase of CBV so that ICP increases only minimally. However, with severe or prolonged increase of CBV, compliance is lost, the ICP rises, and there is usually an alteration of brain capillary permeability that can lead to the formation of edema and hemorrhages.

VENOUS OBSTRUCTION

When cerebral veins are abruptly blocked, the brain becomes congested. As cerebral venous blood volume increases, CSF is reabsorbed and/or translocated to the spinal subarachnoid space causing the size of the ventricles to decrease. There is an effort to restore normal cerebral venous blood volume and pressure by rerouting blood through collateral vessels. Rerouting is less effective in cases of acute occlusion than with slowly evolving thromboses (e.g., sagittal sinus invasion by meningiomas) or with extracranial obstructions that can take advantage of alternative routes to the heart (e.g., Batson's plexus). With severe cerebral venous occlusion, the brain is congested and there is evidence of widespread venous stasis, interstitial edema, and hemorrhagic infarction. Conditions leading to obstruction of the cerebral veins or dural sinuses include parasagittal tumors, head trauma, head and neck tumors, radical neck dissection, strangulation, bacterial meningitis, subdural abscess, polycythemia, severe dehydration, pregnancy, superior vena cava syndrome, failure of the right side of the heart, and cor pulmonale.

ARTERIAL DILATION

Under normal conditions, brain mechanisms that regulate CBF match regional CBF to local metabolic needs.[226] These regulatory mechanisms act on smooth muscle cells in the cerebral arteries and arterioles. Participating in cerebrovascular regulation are endothelial, myogenic, neurogenic, chemical and metabolic systems. Any of these systems can be affected by pathologic processes that alter metabolic needs or directly disturb arterial tone and caliber. Conditions resulting in profound arterial dilation and increased CBV and ICP include: (1) hypoxia (hypoxic, anemic, poisoning, hemoglobinopathies, etc.); (2) global ischemia; (3) malignant hypertension; (4) severe, prolonged hypercapnia; (5) hypermetabolic states (seizures, hyperthermia, stimulant overdose, etc.); (6) sepsis and febrile infections; (7) uremia; and (8) other causes for loss of cerebral autoregulation.[227]

TREATMENT OF CEREBRAL EDEMA

STEROIDS

Glucocorticoids are not uniformly effective for the treatment of all types of cerebral edema (Table 3-11).

It is generally agreed that steroids exert a beneficial effect on the perifocal edema occurring with mass lesions.[103] When given a dexamethasone loading dose of 8 to 32 mg, patients with malignant brain tumors and an associated decreased level of consciousness and neurologic deficits often become conscious and free of focal neurologic signs within 24 h after treatment. Improvement in neurologic status has also been reported in certain cases where glucocorticoids were used to treat perifocal edema associated with cerebral abscesses, subdural hematoma, bacterial meningitis, tuberculous infections, and postoperative cerebral swelling. Decreased cerebral edema and neurologic deficit has been reported in some patients given steroids to treat pseudotumor cerebri. Glucocorticoid-induced improvement is especially likely in patients with vasogenically induced causes, such as Addison's disease, intoxications, and allergic reactions.[190]

In contrast, neurologic status often is not improved when steroids are used to treat cerebral edema associated with conditions in which cerebral autoregulation is impaired, such as severe closed head trauma and acute hemorrhagic conditions (e.g., intracerebral hematoma).[214,228] In fact, worsening neurologic outcome has been reported following administration of glucocorticoids to patients with traumatic brain injuries or hypoxic brain damage.[229,230] It was speculated that steroid treatment contributed to neurologic deterioration because steroids increased cerebral metabolic needs in excess of oxygen/substrate supply (i.e., ischemia occurred) and/or because steroids caused hyperglycemia and increased concentrations of lactate. Glucocorticoid therapy is also of little benefit in the management of osmotic, compressive, hydrocephalic, or ischemic edema, or of increased CBV.

Glucocorticoids may improve vasogenic edema by several mechanisms including: (1) endothelial cell membrane stabilization, which reduces plasma filtration across the cerebral endothelium; (2) decreased release of potentially toxic substances, such as fatty acids, free radicals, and prostaglandins; (3) electrolyte shifts favoring transcapillary efflux of fluid; (4) enhanced lysosomal activity of cerebral capillaries; and (5) increased focal and global cerebral glucose use, which improves neuronal function.[190] Steroids were reported not to inhibit the arachidonic acid-prostaglandin cascade in experimental cold injury edema. It was speculated that steroid-inducing modification of catecholamine metabolism may play a role in the improvement of vasogenic edema seen with glucocorticoids.[231]

Like the glucocorticoids, 21-aminosteroids also are not uniformly effective for the treatment of all types of cerebral edema. In a cold-lesion model of vasogenic edema, dexamethasone produced a small, insignificant decrease of edema, whereas treatment with a 21-

TABLE 3-11
Treatment of Cerebral Edema

Treatment	Effects	Possible Complications/Disadvantages
Steroids	Endothelial cell membrane stabilization Decreased release of toxins Favorable electrolyte, lysozyme and glucose effects	Gastrointestinal bleeding, electrolyte disturbances, reduced immunocompetence, hyperglycemia, mental disturbances
Anti-inflammatory drugs	Decreased capillary leak and toxin release	Little clinical experience
Hyperventilation	Decreased CBV and capillary leak Improved CSF outflow and ECF bulk flow	Cerebral ischemia
Head elevation	Decreased CBV and capillary leak Translocation of CSF to spinal subarachnoid space	Decreased CPP
Osmotherapy	Decreased brain tissue water content and CSF formation Decreased blood viscosity causing decreased CBV	Hypovolemia and hypotension Electrolyte disturbances and renal failure
Barbiturates	Decreased capillary leak and CBV	Unable to follow clinical signs May need life support, monitoring, etc.
CSF drainage	Decreased CSF volume Improved ECF bulk flow	Herniation, infection, obstruction
Antihypertensive drugs	Decreased capillary leak	Decreased CPP
Surgical excision	Decreased brain tissue volume Removal of areas of capillary leak and toxin release	Brain tissue damage/loss
Operative decompression	Decreased brain tissue volume	Brain tissue damage/loss

aminosteroid (U74389F) caused no reduction in swelling.[232] In experimental pneumococcal meningitis, treatment with a 21-aminosteroid (U74389F) reduced brain water content and the increase in ICP, but had no effect on the increase of regional CBF.[233]

ANTI-INFLAMMATORY AGENTS

Glucocorticoids also produce effects that may worsen neurologic outcome, such as hypeglycemia and impaired immune response. For that reason, the efficacy of nonsteroidal anti-flammatory drugs (e.g., indomethacin, probenecid, ibuprofen) for the management of vasogenic edema has been examined. Nonsteroidal anti-inflammatory drugs are effective in the treatment of systemic inflammations and are comparatively safe and well tolerated by most patients. In a model of carrageenan-induced brain inflammation, probenecid reduced cerebrovascular permeability.[234] Similarly, with experimental gliomas, indomethacin and ibuprofen decreased vascular permeability.[235] Although it is not certain by which mechanisms nonsteroidal anti-inflammatory drugs reduce capillary leakage, it has been speculated that they directly inhibit the arachidonic acid-prostaglandin cascade.[231,234] In experimental gliomas, the magnitude of decrease in cerebrovascular permeability following treatment with anti-inflammatory drugs was similar to the decrease in permeability seen with dexamethasone therapy.[235]

HYPERVENTILATION

One of the principal chemical-metabolic regulators of the state of contraction-relaxation of cerebrovascular smooth muscle is perivascular hydrogen ion concentration. CO_2 in cerebral vessels freely equilbrates with brain ECF CO_2 across the BBB. Brain ECF CO_2, in turn, equilibrates with brain ECF hydrogen ion concentration. When hyperventilation is used to decrease Pa_{CO_2}, brain ECF hydrogen ion concentration also decreases. With removal of the potent vasodilating influence of brain ECF hydrogen ion, regulators causing cerebrovasoconstriction are left unopposed and cerebral arteries and arterioles constrict resulting in decreased CBF and CBV.[226] The reduction in cerebral perfusion that accompanies hypocapnia-induced cerebral vasoconstriction potentially may decrease edema formation by reducing filtration forces. Prolonged or excessive hyperventilation may produce cerebral ischemia and the accumulation of lactic acid within brain tissue.[13]

HEAD ELEVATION

The intent of positioning patients with the head elevated relative to the rest of the body is to improve the outflow of cerebral venous blood from within the cranium and thus to decrease CBV and ICP. However, elevation of the head above the heart also reduces the hydrostatic force of the systemic arterial circulation, thereby decreasing CPP.[236] While elevation of the head may be desirable as a means for reducing "filtration edema," head elevation that decreases CPP so far that CBF falls to ischemic levels, triggers the release of "compensatory" cerebral vasodilators. The increase of CBV caused by these vasodilators may result in a paradoxical rise of ICP and abrupt deterioration of clinical status despite unchanged or reduced levels of ICP.[237] Clearly, the relative benefits and risks of head elevation must be weighed. Monitoring ICP and/or intracranial compliance/elastance and assessing clinical responses should assist the selection of the optimal degree of head elevation.

OSMOTHERAPY

Intravenous infusion of hyperosmolar solutions or drugs that cause the blood to become hyperosmolar produce a rapid reduction of brain water content. Mannitol (20% solution) probably remains the most commonly used hyperosmolar solution. It is generally administered intravenously in doses of 0.25 to 1.0 g/kg body weight over an interval of 60 to 90 min.[103] One mechanism by which hyperosmolar solutions decrease cerebral edema and ICP is by creating an osmolar gradient between brain tissue and blood that favors movement of water out of brain tissue. It is believed that creation of this osmolar gradient is a more important effect than the diuretic effect of hyperosmolar solutions, although the duration of action of osmotherapy can be prolonged by the use of loop diuretics (e.g., furosemide, ethacrynic acid), which preferentially excrete water as compared with solute.[103]

Hyperosmolar solutions and drugs that cause the blood to become hyperosmolar have little direct effect on edematous tissues and do not remove edema fluid per se. As noted above in the section on permeability and conductance of the BBB, efflux of fluid from brain tissue depends on the osmotic gradient that is established between the vascular and ECF compartments at the distal end of capillaries (Starling's hypothesis). Such a gradient can exist only in areas where the cerebral capillary membrane is intact. In edematous areas with intact capillaries, some efflux of fluid probably occurs.[238]

A second mechanism by which hyperosmolar solutions decrease cerebral edema and ICP is by reducing the CSF volume. One cause for decreased CSF volume is decreased $\dot{V}_f$.[239] Another cause for decreased CSF volume is retrograde drainage of CSF into the ECF compartment and subsequent efflux across cerebral capillaries.

A third mechanism by which hyperosmolar solutions decrease cerebral edema and ICP is by reducing blood viscosity.[239] For a given vascular diameter, decreased blood viscosity results in increased CBF. This state of local hyperemia triggers vasoconstricting regulators (so long as they are intact) to restore CBF to normal values. As a result of cerebral vasoconstriction, CBV decreases, with an accompanying decrease of ICP. Cerebral vasoconstriction may also lead to reduced "filtration edema" as mentioned above. A third means by which cerebral vasoconstriction may decrease ICP is that reduced CBV may reduce brain "bulk" to improve access of CSF to pathways of reabsorption, or to pathways for translocation from the cranial to the spinal subarachnoid space.[154,225] The administration of hypertonic agents must be carefully monitored because severe or prolonged hyperosmolarity can produce a number of systemic complications, such as metabolic acidosis, hypokalemia, oliguria, and permanent renal damage.[240]

A fourth mechanism by which mannitol may decrease cerebral edema is by free radical scavenging.[241] Focal co-injection of mannitol was reported to decrease hippocampal damage following focal injection of the neurotoxin beta-N-oxalylamino-L-alanine but not following focal injection of alpha-amino-3-hydroxyg-5-methyl-isoxazole-4-propionate, kainate, or N-methyl-D-asparate.[242] In vitro, mannitol prevented most of the oxidizing actions of N-methyl-D-aspartate receptors by xanthine/xanthine oxidase (but not by the thiol oxidizing agent 5,5′-dithio-bis-nitrobenzoic acid), but not the amounts of superoxide anion and peroxide produced by xanthine/xanthine oxidase.[243]

When plasma hypoosmolarity is the cause for osmotic edema, fluid restriction and correction of the electrolyte imbalance generally are effective treatments. When inappropriate secretion of antidiuretic hormone or imbalance of reproductive hormones (pregnancy, the use of oral contraceptives, etc.) are causes for pseudotumor cerebri, specific hormone replacement therapy or water intake coupled with restricted salt intake are appropriate therapies. Severe or refractory elevations of ICP can sometimes be treated effectively by acetazolamide or oral isosorbide.

BARBITURATES

Barbiturates are reported to decrease the cerebral metabolic rate of the brain, and to reverse the formation of vasogenic edema.[103] It was speculated that the improvement of vasogenic edema seen with barbiturates resulted from their effectiveness in reducing systemic arterial pressure and, hence, decreasing the filtration of fluid across leaky capillaries. A loading dose of pentobarbital (3 to 5 mg/kg) or thiopental (20 mg/kg) has been recommended, followed by constant intravenous infusion to achieve the desired effect on one or more measures such as ICP, electroencephalogram (EEG), neurologic exam, cerebral metabolism, and others. The "cost" of using barbiturates in doses causing near or complete suppression of the EEG include: (1) the reduction or elimination of neurologic responses, which are often crucial in following the patient's progress; and (2) the need for continuous physiologic monitoring (e.g., ICP, blood gas tensions, and pulmonary artery or central venous and arterial pressures), tracheal intubation and mechanical ventilation, and intravenous nutrition in a critical care unit.[99]

CSF DRAINAGE

CSF shunts are routinely placed in patients with hydrocephalic (or interstitial) edema. CSF shunting also may be attempted in patients with refractory pseudotumor cerebri. Resolution of periventricular edema is reported following shunt placement in patients with hydrocephalic edema. Studies of the effects of CSF drainage on brain water movement indicate that enhanced clearance of ECF edema occurs as a result of an increased gradient for ECF bulk flow into the cerebral ventricles.[244] The efficacy of using CSF drainage to treat patients with severe head injuries remains uncertain.[244,245]

ANTIHYPERTENSIVE DRUGS

Increase of cerebral vascular transmural pressure increases the rate of formation and spread of vasogenic edema. Reduction of arterial blood pressure is an effective method of reducing vascular transmural pressure.[13,103] A number of hypotensive treatments are available, including calcium channel blockers, "direct acting" vasodilators, sympatholytics, and drugs that minimize the renin-angiotension system. In patients with severe spreading edema, it is recommended that mean arterial blood pressure should be adjusted to within the normal physiologic range. In patients without other complicating risk factors, mean arterial blood pressures below the normal range may be acceptable. However, reduction of blood pressure to such levels must be done carefully and with appropriate monitoring in patients who are elderly or who have hypertension because of the risk of impairing cerebral perfusion.[99]

SURGICAL EXCISION

Compressive edema and the vasogenic edema associated with neovascularization or increased capillary permeability are improved by surgical removal of the mass lesions (e.g., tumors, abscesses, subdural hematoma) responsible for the edema. One of the causes for reduction of edema following surgical excision is that areas of capillary leak are removed. Other causes for reduction of edema include decreased release of potentially toxic substances (such as free radicals and prostaglandins) and improved local cerebral perfusion due to decreased mass effect.

OPERATIVE DECOMPRESSION

In certain cases of swelling it may be necessary to resort to removing a portion of the cranial vault (external decompression), with or without the resection of brain tissue (internal decompression). Operative decompression may be helpful in managing unilateral hemispheric swelling when there is evidence of progressive transtentorial herniation. Decompressive measures include opening the dura, excision of necrotic tissue, and resection of the temporal lobe tip to relieve compression of the brain stem. Operative decompression, even extreme measures such as bilateral hemicalvarectomy or circumferential craniotomy, are reported to be more effective in the treatment of focal swelling than in the treatment of diffuse swelling.[246]

Intracranial Pressure

CONTENTS OF THE INTRACRANIAL SPACE

Under normal conditions the intracranial space comprises three volumes—brain tissue volume, CSF volume, and CBV. Brain tissue accounts for 80 to 85 percent of total intracranial volume, CSF volume accounts for 7 to 10 percent, and CBV accounts for 5 to 8 percent. The cranium containing this volume is poorly distensible. ICP is the pressure created by the total volume within the intracranial space. Because of the poor distensibility of the cranial vault, even small increases in intracranial volume may cause large increases in ICP. Pathologic conditions may introduce a fourth volume component, the mass lesion. Causes for a mass lesion include tumor, hematoma, abscess, foreign body, pneumocephalus, and contusion. For ICP to remain normal, an increase in brain tissue volume, CSF volume, or CBV must be matched by a comparable decrease in the other volumes. This principle has been termed the Monro-Kellie hypothesis.[247] A mass lesion not matched by a comparable decrease in the other volumes, or an increase in brain tissue volume, CSF volume, or CBV not matched by a decrease in the other volumes results in increased ICP. This increase in ICP often is termed intracranial hypertension.

BRAIN TISSUE VOLUME

Brain tissue volume has been described as being comprised of cellular and extracellular compartments. Alternatively, brain tissue volume can be described as being comprised of brain tissue and brain water contents. Regarding the cellular compartment or brain tissue content, the volume of cell membranes and myelin changes very little. In contrast, ICF volume equilibrates with the ECF volume by passive movement of water along osmotic gradients established across semipermeable cell membranes. Changes in ICF and/or ECF volume frequently occur during pathologic conditions.[248] Vasogenic edema results from increased BBB permeability and is characterized by increased ECF volume. Ischemic edema results from failure of energy requiring processes that maintain cellular integrity and is characterized by increased ICF volume. Osmotic edema results when the osmolarity of the brain ECF space is increased compared to the osmolarity of the blood and is characterized by increased ECF volume. Hydrocephalic edema results from retrograde movement of fluid from the CSF space and also is characterized by increased ECF volume. While approaches to treatment may be quite different depending on the cause of the edema, the overall contribution of brain tissue volume to changes in total intracranial volume is determined by the sum of the ICF and ECF volume changes.

CSF VOLUME

CSF volume is determined by $\dot{V}_f$ relative to $\dot{V}_a$. $\dot{V}_f$ remains relatively constant despite change of ICP. $\dot{V}_f$ may decrease at substantially increased ICP, with decrease of blood pressure below the lower limit of CBV autoregulation, and under conditions of acute hypocapnia, ventriculitis and hypothermia. In contrast, $\dot{V}_a$ is directly related to change of ICP, being negligible at very low ICP and substantially increased at elevated ICP. $\dot{V}_a$ may be decreased by conditions that: (1) restrict the rate of CSF flow through the interventricular and subarachnoid spaces to arachnoid villi; (2) impair the formation of macropinocytotic vesicles and trans- and intercellular channels at the arachnoid cell layer covering the arachnoid villa; and (3) decrease the hydrostatic pressure gradient across the arachnoid villus (i.e., the CSF to venous blood pressure gradient). Conditions where $\dot{V}_f$ exceeds $\dot{V}_a$ results in increased CSF volume (hydrocephalus). In chronic situations this may be well tolerated for long periods, but severe acute hydrocephalus may be rapidly fatal.

CBV

CBV is the sum of cerebral arterial and venous blood volumes. Cerebral arterial blood volume is determined by the caliber of cerebral arteries and arterioles, whereas cerebral venous blood volume is determined chiefly by blood volume in the venous sinuses. The caliber of cerebral arteries and arterioles is regulated by numerous factors—endothelium derived factors, blood viscosity, myogenic responses, vasoactive chemicals and metabolites, and neurogenic influences.[226] Change in cerebral artery and arteriolar caliber in response to change in arterial blood pressure is termed autoregulation. Under normal circumstances, autoregulation serves to maintain a constant CBF over a wide range of systemic arterial blood pressures through

compensatory changes in cerebral vascular resistance. This is accomplished efficiently by changes in vessel tone or caliber because resistance to flow is inversely proportional to the fourth power of vessel radius (Poiseuille's law).[249] Changes in the caliber of cerebral arteries and arterioles also influences CBV because CBV is directly proportional to the square of vessel radius. Hypoxia and hypocapnia dilate cerebral arteries and arterioles, increasing CBV, and impair autoregulation. Failure of normal autoregulation may lead to significant alterations in CBV and perfusion; such changes may include the "breakthrough" phenomenon after resection of certain arteriovenous malformations and the hyperemia often seen after head injury, especially in children.[250-253] Because it affects not only CBV (and therefore ICP), but also CPP directly, autoregulation may play a critical role in intracranial pathophysiology.[251-253]

INTRACRANIAL MASS LESIONS

Intracranial mass lesions generally are comprised of relatively noncompressible materials. No natural mechanisms exist that permit intracranial mass lesions to expand or contract in response to decrease or increase in brain tissue volume, CSF volume, or CBV. As mentioned above, because the intracranial space is poorly distensible, even small mass lesions may produce substantial increases in ICP. Mass lesions also may increase ICP due to their position, such as by distorting or blocking CSF outflow pathways.

COMPARTMENTALIZATION WITHIN THE INTRACRANIAL SPACE

The arrangement of the intracranial contents is complex. The three principal contents, brain tissue volume, CSF volume, and CBV are separated from one another by bony, dural, and arachnoid barriers. Similar barriers exist within each of the three principal volume contents. Further complexity occurs when a mass lesion is present.

Some of these barriers are so extensive that they cause areas of the intracranial space to behave as though isolated from the remainder of the intracranial space. This effect is termed compartmentalization. The two cerebral hemispheres are separated from one another by a semirigid barrier, the falx cerebri, which allows only limited lateral displacement. Limited connection between hemispheres exists through an opening in the base of the falx at the level of the corpus callosum. The anterior and middle fossae are separated from the posterior fossa by a semirigid barrier, the tentorium cerebelli, which allows only limited craniocaudal displacement. Beneath the tentorium, the infratentorial space may behave like a single, isolated compartment. A limited connection between the infratentorial and the supratentorial spaces exists via the tentorial notch, and between the infratentorial space and the spinal subarachnoid space via the foramen magnum. The anterior temporal lobes are effectively surrounded by the sphenoid wing superiorly and anteriorly, the temporal bone laterally and inferiorly, and the tentorium medially, so that they may be considered as belonging to yet another partially isolated compartment.

Within each of these anatomic compartments brain tissue contains varying amounts of gray and white matter, the compliance of which may differ. The viscoelasticity of the brain substance exerts tangential forces that also diminish radial transmission of pressure inequalities. Cerebral blood also exerts shear forces that may alter transmission of pressure inequalities. Connections within the CSF space are made by numerous ventricles, aqueducts, and foramina. Under normal conditions, communication of pressure between the various compartments occurs via the CSF channels, both within and outside the brain substance. In the presence of a pathologic condition, communication of pressure between compartments may be impaired.

Localized pathologic conditions may cause obstruction of CSF flow and blockage of CSF egress from one portion of the ventricular system but not from another. Such asymmetric obstruction may produce conditions known as "trapped ventricle" or "trapped temporal horn," which often result from hemispheric lesions in different locations, or supratentorial "noncommunicating" hydrocephalus, which may occur when the aqueduct of Sylvius is affected. Under these conditions, a catheter inserted to measure pressure in one area of the CSF space (such as one of the lateral cerebral ventricles), may not accurately reflect pressure in another area.[254] Localized pathologic lesions may not only raise pressure within the affected compartment by a direct volume effect, but may alter the visoelastic properties of the injured brain as well. In addition, separate compartments within the intracranial space may be dissimilar with respect to capacitance. As a result, these compartments may respond at different rates to changes in volume and/or pressure.[255]

Displacement of intracranial contents from one compartment to another takes place when pressure gradients increase sufficiently to overcome the resistance of brain tissue to distortion. This phenomenon is termed as herniation (Fig. 3-9). Brain tissue may herniate outward through defects in the skull (surgical, traumatic, etc.), the cerebral hemispheres may herniate laterally under the falx (subfalcine herniation), the supratentorial contents may herniate inferiorly through the tentorial notch (transtentorial herniation), or the cerebellar tonsils may herniate inferiorly through the foramen

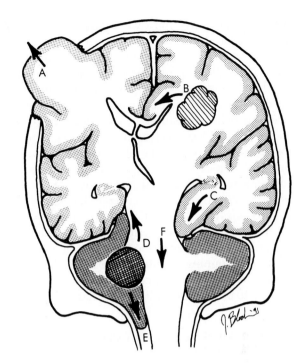

Figure 3-9 Herniation syndromes. *A,* transcalvarial; *B,* subfalcine; *C,* transtentorial (uncal); *D,* transtentorial ("Upward"); *E,* tonsillar; and *F,* transtentorial (central, or "coning"). (From Cottrell JE, Smith DS, eds: *Anesthesia and Neurosurgery.* St. Louis, Mosby-Year Book, Inc., 1994, with permission.)

magnum. Displacement of brain tissue continues until the pressure gradient is no longer present, or until the physical properties of the herniating tissue prevent further shift, despite the continued presence of a pressure gradient. Pressures on the two sides of the falx may differ following subfalcine herniation in the presence of a cerebral hemispheric lesion (sometimes accompanied by ventricular trapping). Pressures inferior and superior to the tentorium may become unequal when a small posterior fossa hematoma obstructs the aqueduct of Sylvius, expanding the posterior fossa volume. Intracranial and spinal subarachnoid pressures may become unequal following cerebellar tonsillar herniation. In many cases, the mechanical shear stress on brain tissue and vascular compression that accompanies herniation may be more harmful than the increase of ICP.[256,257] In addition, the pressures measured by an ICP monitor in a single compartment may not accurately reflect conditions in other compartments.[254,255] For example, an expanding temporal lobe mass lesion may lead to disastrous uncal herniation, despite a "normal" ICP measured in the frontal horn of the lateral ventricle.

Techniques designed to measure ICP or intracranial elastance/compliance routinely placed in only one compartment may provide limited and/or misleading information. Consider the case where a ventricular catheter is placed in the frontal horn of the lateral ventricle. Data from such a catheter provide information on the elastance/compliance of this ventricular compartment. Obstruction of CSF outflow anywhere along the intraventricular course decreases the effective volume being measured, yielding a calculation of increased elastance or decreased compliance whether or not a mass lesion is present. Conversely, a mass lesion located in a separate compartment some distance away from the frontal horn may not cause a measurable effect on elastance/compliance calculations based on frontal horn ICP values. Techniques to detect herniation and mass lesions, such as computed tomography and magnetic resonance imaging, may be useful in determining a suitable site for ICP monitor placement and the correct conclusions to draw and treatments to plan to follow based on that information.

RELATIONSHIPS BETWEEN INTRACRANIAL VOLUME AND ICP

ICP is determined by the sum of the volumes contained in the intracranial space—brain tissue volume, CSF volume, and CBV. Under pathologic conditions an intracranial mass lesion may exist that occupies space within the cranium and, therefore, also contributes to ICP. The relationship between volume and pressure in the intracranial space is termed the intracranial pressure-volume curve.[258,259] Numerous studies have collected data on the change of ICP that occurs with an increase or decrease of intracranial volume. Data from experimental animals generally have been obtained by increasing and decreasing the volume of an intracranial balloon-tipped catheter or by addition or removal of fluid from the CSF space. Data from patients more often are obtained by addition or withdrawal of fluid from the CSF space or by measuring ICP changes associated with the change in CBV that accompanies each heart beat. ICP is measured either by a CSF catheter or epidural pressure transducer. Typically the plot of ICP versus intracranial volume yields an exponential curve showing small increase in ICP for a given increase in intracranial volume when ICP is low, and increasingly larger increases in ICP for the same given increase in intracranial volume as ICP rises (Fig. 3-3 to 3-10).

INTRACRANIAL ELASTANCE, COMPLIANCE, AND CAPACITANCE

The slope at any given point on this pressure-volume curve characterizes the intracranial volume-pressure relationship. Two terms are used to describe this relationship. The first term and the one that currently enjoys the most popularity is cerebral or intracranial elas-

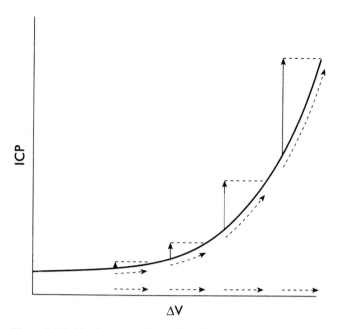

Figure 3-10 The intracranial pressure-volume relationship. The curves illustrates concepts derived from the experiments of Langfit and colleagues.[258,259] Each horizontal dashed line with arrowhead represents an increase in intracranial volume (ΔV). Each vertical solid line with arrowhead represents the increase of ICP caused by the increase in intracranial volume. Each curved dashed line with arrowhead indicates the point to which these volume additions shift the system along the single pressure-volume curve. Results from clinical studies suggest that for each individual this curve does not remain immutable, but instead undergoes minor changes in response to therapeutic measures or physiologic changes. Despite undergoing minor changes, the general exponential nature of the curve is retained. (From Cottrell JE, Smith DS, eds: *Anesthesia and Neurosurgery.* St. Louis, Mosby-Year Book, Inc., 1994, with permission.)

tance.[249] Cerebral or intracranial elastance is defined as change in ICP (ΔP) divided by change in intracranial volume (ΔV). The second term and the one more commonly used previously is cerebral or intracranial compliance. Cerebral or intracranial compliance is defined as $\Delta V/\Delta P$. Regardless of whether the relationship between intracranial volume and ICP is expressed as elastance or compliance, the relationship between ΔP and ΔV reflects both the viscoelastic properties, or stiffness, of the intracranial contents and the functioning of compensatory mechanisms available to reduce ICP at any given point on the curve. A third term applied to the relationship between intracranial volume and ICP is cerebral or intracranial capacitance. These terms refer to the rate at which the brain can accommodate intracranial volume, and are determined by time-dependent derivatives of the same variables determining cerebral or intracranial compliance. The concept of capacitance may be useful in predicitng the clinical impact of intracranial space-occupying lesions. For example, a slowly expanding tumor such as a meningioma may produce few symptoms even though it eventually increases to significant size. In contrast, a quickly expanding intracerebral hemorrhage likely causes acute, substantial elevation of ICP and, possibly, irreversible brain damage due to compression or herniation of brain tissue.

Certain aspects of brain tissue volume, CSF volume, CBV, and mass lesion volume change relatively slowly (i.e., over minutes to hours). These aspects include the initial size of the intracranial content, factors affecting the change in size, and the location of the intracranial content relative to important structures. Factors affecting the change in size of the intracranial content include: (1) rate of edema formation (for brain tissue volume); (2) $\dot{V}_f$, $\dot{V}_a$, head position, and translocation of CSF (for CSF volume); (3) mean arterial blood pressure, Pa_{CO_2}, head position, and anesthetic and other drug effects (for CBV); and (4) rate of expansion (for mass lesion volume). Because these aspects change relatively slowly, their contribution to the intracranial volume-pressure relationship is more static in nature. The contribution of CBV is made more complex by an additional highly dynamic component—that of local regulation of CBF and CBV. These changes take place over a period of seconds to minutes. Local regulation of CBF and CBV initiates vasoconstriction or vasodilation in response to changes in cerebral metabolism, mean arterial blood pressure, and blood rheology. Such vasodilating and vasoconstricting influences are thought to be reflected as transient increases in ICP. These transient ICP increases are termed plateau waves, and have been interpreted as being indicators of low cerebral compliance.[260] Regional and global CBF and CBV have been measured during plateau waves. It was reported that at the same time plateau waves were present, regional CBV increased and CBF decreased. This suggested that the pathologic plateau waves might be triggered by regional increases in CBV during the low compliance state. It was speculated that cerebral vasodilation causes a rapid rise in ICP with concomitant obstruction of cerebral venous drainage, thus resulting in increased regional CBV and decreased CBF. Plateau waves also may result when CBF is not adequate to meet cerebral metabolic needs. Focal ischemia triggers the release of metabolites and chemicals that possess cerebral vasodilating properties. Vasodilation increases CBF and CBV, and, hence, ICP. When CBF increases become adequate to meet brain metabolic needs, vasodilating metabolites and chemicals no longer are released, CBF and CBV decrease, and the transient elevation of ICP resolves. Increases in CBF and CBV also are caused by failure of cerebral autoregulation. For example, autoregulation frequently is impaired following head trauma. In such cases, the cerebral vasculature is not able to constrict

in response to sudden increases in mean arterial blood pressure. As a result, the increase in mean arterial blood pressure causes passive distension of cerebral blood vessels with accompanying increase of CBV and ICP. When normal mean arterial pressure is restored, the transient increase of ICP again resolves. Other causes for impaired autoregulation include diffuse brain tissue acidosis, certain "direct acting" antihypertensive drugs, inhalational anesthetics, hypoxia, and hypercapnia. Changes in blood rheology may alter ICP by causing CBV changes that do not parallel changes in CBF. In patients with severe head injuries who have intact autoregulation, administration of mannitol was reported to decrease ICP by 27 percent, while CBF remained unchanged.[261] The improved blood rheology provided by the mannitol permitted autoregulatory vasoconstriction while maintaining blood flow and tissue oxygenation at this reduced CBV. In patients with defective autoregulation, the decrease in ICP with mannitol administration was limited to 5 percent, while CBF actually increased 18 percent because no reflexive vasoconstriction was possible.

If the state of the contents of the intracranial space permits, expansion of the volume of any one of the contents (brain tissue, CSF, or CBV) initiates contraction of the volume of the other contents. The contraction of these contents has been termed compensation, and the individual components of the collective ability for contraction are termed the compensatory mechanisms. When intracranial volume is low, the compensatory mechanisms nearly completely offset an increase in one of the intracranial contents, resulting in a minimal increase of total intracranial volume and, hence, ICP. As the compensatory mechanisms become exhausted, there is less capacity to offset each incremental increase in volume of one of the intracranial contents resulting in progressively larger increases in ICP for a given increase in volume of one of the intracranial contents. Generally, the principal compensatory mechanisms are changes in CSF distribution and bulk flow.[262] CSF may be translocated into the spinal subarachnoid space, or $\dot{V}_a$ may increase. Reductions in CBV and brain tissue volume may follow but are obviously more limited. In the presence of autoregulatory dysfunction, changes in systemic arterial blood pressure or other factors affecting CBV may have significant effects on cerebral compliance and ICP.[252,261,263] The size and rate of expansion of intracranial masses and degree of cerebral edema influence cerebral compliance and capacitance and therefore the effectiveness of other compensatory mechanisms.

QUANTIFICATION OF INTRACRANIAL ELASTANCE/COMPLIANCE

Several approaches to quantification of the state of patients' intracranial elastance/compliance have been proposed. The goals of quantification are to provide a body of data describing normal values and variability so as to detect values indicating cerebral pathology, and to correlate values with neurologic status so as to provide: (1) guidelines for initiation of treatments; and (2) predictors of outcome. The first major attempt at quantifying intracranial elastance/compliance was made by Miller and colleagues approximately 20 years ago.[264,265] Small volumes of sterile fluid were injected into or small volumes of CSF were withdrawn from an intraventricular catheter and the increase or decrease of CSF pressure relative to baseline CSF pressure was noted. This approach to quantifying elastance/compliance was termed the volume-pressure response (VPR). Specifically, the VPR is defined as the change in ICP measured after injection or withdrawal of 1 ml of CSF over 1 s. VPR is calculated from the equation VPR = $\Delta P/\Delta V$ and is expressed as mmHg/ml. Being in the general form of $\Delta P/\Delta V$, the VPR is a measure of intracranial elastance. A normal VPR was found to be less than 2 mmHg/ml, whereas a VPR of greater than 5 mm/ml indicated a critical reduction in the volume-buffering capacity of the brain.[266] It was found that VPR could change independently of the baseline ICP. In clinical terms, the combination of a normal ICP and an elevated VPR almost always indicated the presence of a previously unexpected intracranial mass lesion.[267] Thus, the VPR served as a sensitive indicator of increased intracranial elastance or impaired cerebral compliance. In several studies of the effects of anesthetics and other drugs and treatments on the intracranial volume-pressure relationship, VPR reliably correlated inversely with changes in intracranial compliance and directly with changes in ICP. In contrast, other studies have documented limits to the usefulness of VPR as an indicator for initiating treatment and as a predictor of neurologic outcome. For example, 17 percent of 160 patients studied by Miller went on to die of malignant intracranial hypertension, despite a low VPR.[267]

The second major attempt at quantifying intracranial elastance/compliance was made by Marmarou and colleagues, also approximately 20 years ago.[268,269] Again, small volumes of sterile fluid were injected into or small volumes of CSF were withdrawn from an intraventricular catheter, and the log of the quantity peak CSF pressure divided by baseline CSF pressure was related to the volume injected or withdrawn. This approach to quantifying elastance/compliance was termed the pressure-volume index (PVI). Specifically the PVI calculates the volume which, when added to the intracranial space, increases ICP tenfold or, when withdrawn from the intracranial space, decreases ICP tenfold. PVI is calculated from the equation PVI = $\Delta V/[\log(P_p/P_o)]$, where P_p is the peak increase or decrease of ICP following volume change and P_o is the ICP prior to volume change, expressed as ml. Being in the general form of V/P, PVI is more a measure of intracranial compliance than intracranial elastance. Over the pressure range of 0 to 50 mmHg and the volume range of 3 percent of intracranial volume, the CSF pressure-CSF volume relationship was exponential.[270] A PVI of 22 to 30 ml was considered normal, below 18 ml was pathologic, and 13 ml or less indicated a critically low cerebral compliance.[271] Studies on the clinical usefulness of PVI have been ongoing since its introduction approximately 20 years ago. Many studies have concluded that PVI is useful for a variety of clinical purposes. For example, recent studies examined PVI as a means of assessing change in intracranial volume tolerance produced by hyperventilation, detecting patients likely to develop elevated ICP during weaning from sedation combined with mechanical ventilation, and assessing change in intracranial volume tolerance with various degrees of head elevation. In contrast, other studies have concluded that PVI may be of limited use. For example, in recent studies on the effects of anesthetics on measures of the intracranial volume-pressure relationship, PVI frequently increased (indicating improved intracranial volume tolerance) while intracranial compliance decreased and VPR increased (both indicating a worsening of the intracranial volume-pressure relationship). In another study, PVI was no more sensitive than ICP itself in indicating the presence of an experimental mass lesions (epidural balloon). At ICP values higher than the exponential range mentioned above, PVI increased (again, indicating improved intracranial volume tolerance) with increasing balloon volumes (which should worsen the intracranial volume-pressure relationship).[270,272]

The third major attempt at quantifying intracranial elastance/compliance has been to use the beat-to-beat changes in ICP produced as each systolic blood pressure pulse is transmitted to the cerebral arteries and the breath-to-breath changes in ICP produced as each respiration and attendant change in intrathoracic pressure is transmitted to the cerebral veins.[249] Use of these natural occurring changes in CBV avoids the need to add or withdraw fluid through a catheter in the subarachnoid space, thereby decreasing the risk of infection or unintentional excess volume addition or withdrawal. This new approach can be less labor-intensive than its predecessors because it does not require an individual's time to make multiple additons and/or withdrawals of sterile fluid. This new approach also offers the advantage of being continuous. On the other hand, the amount of data obtained with this approach and the many calculations that must be done generally necessitate a computer dedicated to data acquisition and processing.

A number of systems to quantify intracranial elastance/compliance have been developed based on the above approach. Most of these systems use the cerebral arterial pressure signal as the input and the ICP signal as the output. In some systems, because respiratory effects on cerebral venous pressure and arterial P_{CO_2} affect ICP with a frequency nearly an order of magnitude slower than arterial pulse pressure, the contribution of respiratory changes is not considered important.[273] The relationship between the arterial pressure input signal and the ICP output signal has been termed the intracranial transfer function. The intracranial transfer function is an expression of the frequency response of the intracranial space and is determined by the physiologic and hydrodynamic properties of the intracranial contents. This expression is based on the property that physical matter exhibits a frequency response when energy is applied. This frequency response is a function of the density and geometric shape of the matter, and the external forces being applied. The fundamental frequency of matter and its accompanying harmonic frequencies will change in response to alterations in density (such as formation of edema fluid within brain tissue), geometric shape (such as tumor growth within brain tissue, and distortion and compression of CSF spaces by mass lesions), and external forces (such as decreased intracranial compliance and increased ICP). As a result of changes in fundamental and harmonic frequencies, the ICP waveform output to the arterial pressure waveform input is altered, causing an altered intracranial transfer function.

Increased mean ICP and ICP pulse pressure and changes in the upward and downward slopes and other pressure deflection characteristics of the ICP waveform occur under pathologic states. Such alterations in the ICP waveform occur within the time frame of each waveform (i.e., generally within a period of 0.5 to 2.0 s), quite different from the Lundberg type A, B, and C patterns, which describe trends in mean ICP occurring over many seconds to several minutes.[274,275] Shifts in the fundamental and harmonic frequencies of the intracranial contents will cause corresponding, predictable shifts in the frequency components of the ICP waveform. Accordingly, measures of the intracranial pressure-volume relationship can be estimated from changes in the intracranial transfer function. One technique is to determine the power-weighted average frequency of the ICP waveform by computer-assisted fast Fourier transform (similar to the transform process used in computer-assisted analysis of the EEG).[276,277] The predominant frequency component has been termed the high frequency centroid (HFC). A number of studies have examined the correlation between the HFC and other measures of the intracranial volume-pressure relationship. In one study, HFC showed the expected inverse relationship to PVI, with a normal HFC of 6.5 to 7 Hz, and a HFC of 9 Hz corresponding to a reduction in PVI to 13 ml, indicative of critically low compliance. Other studies have examined the correlation between HFC or other similar measures with ICP, PVI, or intracranial compliance, or as a predictor of outcome in patients with head injury, subarachnoid hemorrhage and vasospasm, intracranial hypertension, and hydrocephalus and traumatic intracerebral hematoma. Most of these studies reported positive results.[278-282] In contrast, other studies have reported that HFC or other similar measures correlated poorly and/or did not predict outcome. For example, no prognostic value was observed in patients with traumatic intracerebral hematoma.[283] Another study reported that while in some patients the presence of a mass lesion was heralded by a shift in the HFC to 9 Hz before a rise in ICP, the method showed poor sensitivity, specificity, and positive or negative predictive values. HFC and ICP were not statistically related overall. It appears as though additional studies are needed to determine the usefulness of ICP waveform analysis as a continuous, low-risk method for early detection of impending intracranial decompensation.[284]

ICP MONITORING TECHNIQUES

It is said that the modern era of ICP monitoring began with the work of Lundberg and colleagues over 30 years ago, with their description of the complex ICP waveform and A-, B-, and C-type waves.[285,286] At that time the principal technique for monitoring ICP was the intraventricular catheter. A number of devices for ICP monitoring have been introduced since that time. Each is associated with certain risks (infection, herniation, trauma, etc.) and benefits (ease of placement, accuracy, reliability, longevity, etc). Further, they differ with respect to size and where they may appropriately be located (Fig. 3-11).

INTRAVENTRICULAR MONITORS

One of the two devices most commonly used today to measure ICP continues to be the intraventricular catheter. Because of its straightforward hydrodynamics, it is often used as a standard to which other devices are compared.[274,285,287] In its simplest form, the intraventricular catheter is a hollow, flexible tube with multiple orifices at the ventricular end. With the aid of a rigid stylet it is inserted through the brain parenchyma and into the frontal horn of a lateral cerebral ventricle near the foramen of Monro. In addition to providing a high fidelity ICP waveform, such catheters permit withdrawal of CSF for therapeutic or diagnostic purposes. When indicated, intrathecal antibiotics or other drugs

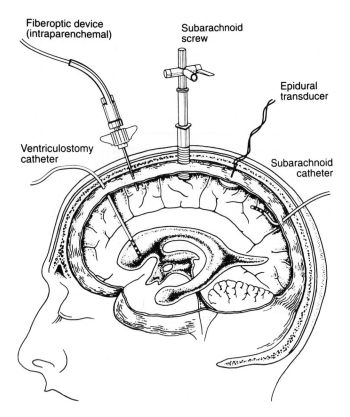

Figure 3-11 Ventricular, intraparenchymal, subarachnoid, and epidural pressure monitoring systems. Systems which are fluid-filled and whose fluid is in contact with CSF often are "zeroed" following insertion by placing the transducer at the same height as the distal end of the catheter or screw. The intraparenchymal and epidural monitors often are "zeroed" before insertion. With these latter monitors, the position of the device that displays the pressure readings does not affect the measurement.

can be introduced into the CSF space, and ventricular air contrast radiographic studies or cisternograms can be performed. Hemorrhage or neurologic sequelae due to parenchymal damage rarely occur, perhaps because of the soft, blunt, flexible nature of the catheter tip that divides rather than incises brain tissue.[288] Infection rates of less than 6 percent have been reported. The infection rate is substantially lower when the catheter is not retained for more than several days.[288,289] Disadvantages include the fact that this technique is invasive and that the catheter can only be inserted in areas where injury to brain areas subserving critical functions or damage of the cerebral vasculature is unlikely. More experience and skill is needed to place this monitor compared with other devices. Ventriculitis is a serious complication associated with a high incidence of mortality.

The catheter may be attached via a length of flexible tubing to a pressure transducer. The transducer generally is set to read zero when the transducer is located at the level of the patient's external auditory canal (usually the same level as the lateral cerebral ventricle). Securing the tubing and transducer and periodically zeroing the transducer can pose problems in a patient who is uncontrollable or for other reasons is constantly changing position. ICP cannot be measured during the time that the catheter is being used to withdraw CSF.[290] Observation of a triphasic ICP waveform indicates sat-

isfactory catheter placement. The presence of intraventricular air, incomplete obstruction of the catheter, or unsatisfactory location of the catheter tip are possible causes for a dampened waveform. Removal of air and relief of certain sources of obstruction may be achieved by irrigation with preservative-free sterile saline.

Newer intraventricular monitors contain the pressure sensor within the catheter. These devices offer the advantages of elimination of much of the external hardware needed with traditional ventriculostomy catheters, providing greater freedom of movement for the patient. Disadvantages include difficulty in checking the calibration of the sensor once the monitor is in place.

SUBDURAL-SUBARACHNOID MONITORS
The second of the two devices most commonly used today to measure ICP is the subdural-subarachnoid "bolt." In its simplest form, the subdural-subarachnoid bolt is a hollow, rigid cylinder with exterior threads that allow it to be screwed through the calvaria. Like the intraventricular catheter, pressure measurement is hydraulic. The tip of the fluid-filled bolt is located either in the subdural space or in the subarachnoid space. Because bolts are generally blunt-tipped, an additional instrument is needed to incise the dura if placement is desired in the subarachnoid space. Whether located in the subdural or subarachnoid space, bolts

provide a moderate to high fidelity ICP waveform, but do not permit withdrawal of CSF for therapeutic or diagnostic purposes. Under certain pathologic conditions, the intracranial volume-pressure relationships of the subdural and subarachnoid spaces may differ substantially.[291] In comparison to the intraventricular catheter, the bolt requires less experience and skill to place. In addition, the risk of infection and trauma to brain tissue is lower.

Like the intraventricular catheter, the bolt may be attached to a pressure transducer via a length of flexible tubing. In such cases, considerations for zeroing and calibrating the device, and causes for dampening of the ICP waveform, are much like those for the intraventricular catheter. More commonly than with intraventricular catheters, newer bolt designs incorporate the pressure sensor within the bolt.

ANTERIOR FONTANELLE MONITOR

Unlike other ICP monitors, this device is noninvasive. The device is applied to the anterior fontanelle and contains a pneumoelectric switch.[292] The switch closes when external pressure is exerted. Switch closure activates a pneumatic system, permitting internal pressurization of the switch. When external and internal pressures equalize, the switch opens, allowing an internal transducer to measure and display the pressure. The output of this system is linear to 100 mmHg and drift is less than 0.3 mmHg/h. The device is useful in infants up to 6 months of age.

INTRAPARENCHYMAL MONITORS

While intraventricular catheters have been used for over 30 years and subdural-subarachnoid bolts have been used for nearly 20 years, intraparenchymal monitoring devices have become available only recently.[293,294] Intraparenchymal monitors generally are comprised of a fine fiberoptic cable with a miniature transducer at the tip.[294,295] ICP is measured by determining the degree of phase shift of an externally generated laser beam reflected off a tiny deformable membrane in the transducer tip. Intraparenchymal ICP monitors are simpler to insert, may be of smaller diameter, and cause less trauma to brain tissue than ventriculostomies. An advantage of these devices is that they do not require access to the ventricular system, which may be extremely difficult to enter in the presence of edema and ventricular compression. Because intraparenchymal monitors do not utilize hydraulics to measure ICP, the risk of infection is lower than with intraventricular catheters. Disadvantages of intraparenchymal monitors include the need for calibration before insertion and the inability for subsequent recalibration, making it difficult to check for the occurrence of "drift" in the mechanism. Fiberoptic cable is more prone to damage

than is fluid-filled tubing or a fluid-filled bolt. Extremely high ICP values (e.g., 40 mmHg) are generally thought to be due to measurement error. Negative ICPs as low as −30 mmHg have been measured and are thought to be real, especially in patients with shunts for hydrocephalus. Withdrawal of CSF for therapeutic or diagnostic purposes or infusion of antibiotics or other drugs is not possible.

LUMBAR SUBARACHNOID MONITORS

A number of approaches have been used to measure spinal CSF pressure, including rigid needles, malleable needles, and a variety of through-the-needle catheters.[296] The lumbar region is the most commonly used site for insertion of a needle or catheter into the spinal CSF space, owing to the lower risk of spinal cord or nerve root damage as compared to thoracic or cervical sites of insertion. CSF pressure data from lumbar subarachnoid monitors was of limited clinical usefulness before it was recognized that substantial CSF pressure gradients could exist between the intracranial and lumbar CSF spaces, and that brain tissue could be damaged as a result of herniation. Today, lumbar subarachnoid monitors enjoy a number of clinical applications in addition to CSF pressure measurements.

A commonly used lumbar subarachnoid monitor is one consisting of a hollow, flexible tube with multiple orifices at the subarachnoid end. Perhaps more so than with intraventricular catheters, multiple orifices are necessary on subarachnoid catheters to prevent obstruction.[296] Catheters are placed through needles and may be equipped with a flexible stylet to assist with passage of the catheter through the needle. Like the intraventricular catheter, lumbar subarachnoid monitors provide a high fidelity CSF pressure waveform and permit CSF withdrawal for therapeutic or diagnostic purposes, antibiotic and other drug administration, and air contrast or liquid radiographic studies. Infection rates less than 1 percent have been reported. The disadvantage of most concern is herniation when an intracranial mass lesion is present. Herniation generally is the result of rapid and excessive CSF loss through the introducer needle, or rapid removal of CSF via the catheter. Measures can be taken to reduce CSF loss at the time of needle placement, and it has been reported that herniation is unlikely if the rate of withdrawal of CSF from the catheter does not exceed 0.4 ml/min.[296] For CSF pressure monitoring, the catheter is attached via a length of flexible, fluid-filled tubing to a pressure transducer. Considerations for zeroing and calibrating the system, and causes for dampening of the CSF pressure waveform, are similar to those for intraventricular catheters and subdural-subarachnoid bolts.

In addition to, or in some cases, independent from

the use of lumbar subarachnoid devices to monitor CSF pressure, such catheters may be used to drain CSF either intraoperatively (to improve operative conditions) or postoperatively (to reduce the incidence and severity of CSF leak from the operative site). In conditions where there is little risk for herniation, such as communicating hydrocephalus, benign intracranial hypertension, and meningitis, lumbar CSF pressure measurement continues to be a common technique to estimate ICP. Because of the difficulties in preventing dislodgment of a device upon which the patient may be lying a great deal of the time and which is subject to frictional forces each time the patient's position is altered, long-term lumbar subarachnoid monitoring is not frequently attempted.

INFRATENTORIAL SUBARACHNOID MONITORS

There are reports that ICP monitors can safely be placed in the posterior fossa to measure infratentorial pressure postoperatively. It was observed that pressures below the tentorium may be substantially different from those above the tentorium.[254] Despite these reports, posterior fossa pressures are not routinely monitored, presumably because of concerns regarding difficulties in identifying suitable access sites for placement and how easily critical neural and vascular structures could be injured. An additional concern is the likelihood for such sequelae as pseudomeningocele. Future reports of safe monitoring of the infratentorial space may stimulate common use of this technique in clinical practice.

INDICATIONS FOR ICP MONITORING

Clinical studies continue to document the circumstances for which ICP monitoring is clinically useful. Studies generally have focused on accuracy and reliability of monitoring to indicate when therapy should be instituted, the efficacy of therapy, and prediction of neurologic status and/or outcome. The success of ICP monitoring in these areas has increased as technology, safety features, and our understanding of intracranial pathophysiology has improved. The success of ICP monitoring also may be enhanced by computer-assisted processing of the ICP waveform. Based on the above, the range of situations in which knowledge of ICP serves a useful therapeutic role has expanded. Currently, the decision on whether or not to monitor ICP generally is based on clinical signs combined with diagnostic imaging studies. The radiologic imaging studies should confirm the clinical indications, and indicate that the proposed monitor can be placed safely. With the availability of high-resolution, noninvasive imaging techniques, such as computed tomog-

raphy and magnetic resonance imaging, these studies themselves may be the principal factor indicating the need for ICP monitoring and determining the efficacy of treatments to control ICP. Noninvasive imaging techniques also permit detection of conditions, such as mass lesions of the temporal lobes, in which ICP measurement may fail to reflect the progression of pathologic events.

HEAD INJURY

Many of the first clinical applications of ICP monitoring as an aid in deciding when therapies to control ICP should be initiated, and to assess the effectiveness of those therapies, were made in patients with head injury.[297-299] In these early attempts, ICP as monitored by lumbar CSF needles or catheters correlated poorly with clinical signs, presumably because herniation often was not recognized. With a better understanding of herniation and the existence of ICP or CSF pressure gradients, as well as the introduction of improved methods to measure ICP, the usefulness of ICP monitoring in this group of patients has improved substantially.[300] It is now recognized that a cycle of brain tissue damage, edema, increase of ICP, decrease of CPP, and further tissue damage contributes significantly to worsening neurological status and poor outcome. There are numerous reports that contemporary methods of monitoring ICP and processing ICP waveform data permit improved neurologic status and outcome by indicating when (and in some cases which) medical or surgical therapy should be instituted, and when treatment should be altered or discontinued. As mentioned above, intraventricular catheters are particularly helpful as they permit not only measurement of ICP and calculated indicators of intracranial volume-pressure relationships, but also withdrawal of CSF for therapeutic or diagnostic purposes, and administration of antibiotics and other drugs.

An accepted indication for ICP monitoring of head injured patients is a Glasgow coma scale score of 8 or less.[301] With prompt and proper treatment, the neurologic status and outcome of patients in this group can be improved. Owing to the substantial impairment of neurologic status in this group, alteration of neurologic status generally is not available as an indicator of deterioration within the intracranial space. In patients with higher Glasgow coma scale scores, ICP monitoring may be unnecessary because neurologic signs and symptoms may suffice. In patients with low Glasgow coma scale scores and indications of rapid, progressive deterioration, ICP monitoring may be futile. In patients with Glasgow coma scale score 8 or less but no indication of impending death, initial and subsequent noninvasive imaging studies are combined with ICP monitoring to guide clinical care. There are numerous reports that, under such conditions, neurologic outcome is worse when ICP is 20 mmHg or greater and remains untreated than when ICP is 20 mmHg or greater and treatment decreases ICP below 20 mmHg.[263,302,303]

BRAIN TUMORS

Another cause of increased brain tissue volume is tumors. Indications for ICP monitoring in this group of patients may be less clear than in patients with head injury because of differences in the pathophysiology of the conditions. The damage caused by severe head injury leads to easily recognizable neurologic deficits, decreased mental status, seizures, and other disorders that can be classified in a quantitative scoring system. Patients with tumors often present with less obvious, focal signs and symptoms, such as papilledema, sixth nerve palsy, headache, and nausea. Such signs and symptoms may be less amenable to classification. The signs and symptoms of increased ICP that occur in patients with brain tumors may result from compression by the mass or from increased CSF volume due to partial or complete blockage of CSF outflow pathways. Slowly expanding brain tumors may cause signs and symptoms of increased ICP only after the tumor reaches substantial size. During slow growth, compensatory mechanisms such as decreased intracranial CSF volume, decreased brain tissue water content, and compression of cerebral veins and venous sinuses minimize the impact of the tumor on ICP. With progressive recruitment of these compensatory processes, the volume tolerance of the intracranial space decreases, that is, compliance is reduced and elastance is increased. The onset of symptoms indicates that all available compensatory mechanisms have been exhausted and that any further increase of intracranial volume increase is likely to be tolerated poorly. In comparison, when there is a sudden blockage of CSF outflow pathways, even small increases of CSF volume may cause major increases of ICP.

Complete or partial blockage of CSF outflow pathways is especially common with posterior fossa tumors that compress the aqueduct of Sylvius. CSF shunting or ventriculostomy generally is employed to reestablish CSF outflow. When ICP is increased by the mass effect of the tumor rather than by obstruction of CSF outflow pathways, reduction of tumor size may be accomplished by surgery or drug or radiation therapy. As in cases of head injury, an intraventricular catheter may be used to monitor ICP, withdraw CSF for therapeutic or diagnostic purposes, or to administer antibiotics or other drugs. For patients with tumors, an intraventricular catheter may also assist in deciding when and if a CSF shunt is needed, and in monitoring and treating ICP prior to and during induction of anesthe-

sia, and intra- and postoperatively. The use of ICP monitoring in the presence of large intraparenchymal tumors without hydrocephalus has diminished with increased availability of computed tomography and magnetic resonance imaging. Intraventricular or intraparenchymal catheters may be used to monitor ICP during induction of anesthesia or postoperatively in patients who are comatose preoperatively or remain comatose after surgery because of their underlying pathologic condition. ICP monitoring may be used in patients whose level of consciousness is depressed as a result of treatments designed to improve neurologic outcome, such as hypothermia, barbiturates, excitatory amino acid antagonists, and others.

CEREBRAL ANEURYSMS
AND ARTERIOVENOUS MALFORMATIONS

In patients with these cerebral vascular disorders, ICP has been used for specific purposes pre-, intra-, and postoperatively. Preoperatively, ICP monitoring indicates the degree of blockage of CSF outflow caused by intracranial hemorrhage. Cellular debris or clot may obstruct access of CSF to arachnoid villi or movement of CSF within the villi or across the arachnoid endothelium. Larger intraventricular or intraparenchymal clots may compress or obstruct macroscopic CSF pathways, resulting in increased CSF volume. Preoperative ventriculostomy permits detection of these conditions and withdrawal of CSF pre- and intraoperatively to provide improved operative conditions. Preoperatively and intraoperatively, regulation of ICP is crucial. When ICP falls, the pressure gradient from inside to outside the wall of the aneurysm or arteriovenous malformation increases. This pressure gradient is termed the transmural pressure. Increase of this gradient increases the likelihood of rupture of the wall and resultant intracranial hemorrhage.[304] In contrast, when ICP rises, CPP decreases. Decrease of CPP increases the likelihood of focal cerebral ischemia. Intraoperatively, a ventriculostomy or lumbar subarachnoid catheter permits withdrawal of CSF to improve operating conditions. Postoperatively, communicating hydrocephalus may result from a preceding subarachnoid hemorrhage, and a CSF shunt or temporary intraventricular catheter may be needed. With arteriovenous malformations, alterations of CBF distribution and CBV, or postoperative changes in CSF volume caused by surgery, may be causes for increased ICP. Detection and management of such ICP increases may be enhanced by ICP monitoring.

HYDROCEPHALUS WITH OR WITHOUT
INCREASED CSF PRESSURE, AND BENIGN
INTRACRANIAL HYPERTENSION

$\dot{V}_f$ is remarkably unchanged over a wide range of CSF pressures. Thus, blockage of CSF movement from the arachnoid villi into cerebral venous channels, or through the macroscopic spaces or subarachnoid space, causes a decrease of $\dot{V}_a$ and, consequently, an increase of CSF volume. Expansion of CSF volume results in contraction of brain tissue volume and CBV. There are numerous causes for increased CSF volume. The condition of increased CSF volume is termed hydrocephalus. This term is a collective one and is applied irrespective of the cause for increased CSF volume. Increased CSF volume accompanied by increased CSF pressure is termed true hydrocephalus. Increased CSF volume without increased CSF pressure is termed normal pressure hydrocephalus.[249] A third term, benign intracranial hypertension, or pseudotumor cerebri, is characterized by increased CSF pressure without increased CSF volume. Benign intracranial hypertension occurs with hypercoagulable states, obesity, vitaminoses, and certain disorders of hormone release or metabolism. The etiology is thought to be thrombosis of cerebral veins and venous sinuses, which frequently is seen on noninvasive imaging studies.[305] Patients' chief complaint often is severe headache.

Generally, true hydrocephalus is corrected surgically by insertion of a CSF shunt. Complications of CSF shunt placement include shunt failure (i.e., too little CSF is drained) and "overshunting" (i.e., too much CSF is drained). Patients' presenting complaints may not differentiate between these two conditions. Noninvasive imaging studies often are diagnostic, but occasionally also fail to differentiate excessive drainage from inadequate drainage. In such cases, ICP monitoring may become necessary. ICP monitoring also may be useful in assessing whether drainage is excessive, satisfactory, or inadequate in patients with persistent severe headache following shunt insertion for benign intracranial hypertension. For both of the above circumstances intraparenchymal ICP monitoring has been recommended. In contrast, use of an ICP monitor that permits CSF drainage is recommended for evaluation of normal pressure hydrocephalus. Such monitoring aids in diagnosis by distinguishing normal ICP from increased ICP, and in treatment by determining the efficacy of permanent CSF drainage.

OTHER INDICATIONS

ICP monitoring with or without CSF drainage may be useful for a variety of conditions on a selected basis, in contrast to the conditions mentioned above where ICP monitoring and CSF drainage may be more routine. ICP monitoring with or without CSF drainage may be useful in conditions of substantial brain swelling from causes other than head injury or tumor, when ischemia or loss of structural integrity might be caused by failure to maintain ICP within tight limits, or for repeated withdrawal of CSF for diagnostic purposes or to improve operative conditions. Monitoring with or without drainage may be necessary in any cases where neurologic examination and noninvasive imaging studies are not sufficient to diagnose or to follow the progress of intracranial pathology. Specific conditions in which ICP monitoring with or without CSF drainage may be helpful include hepatic encephalopathy, hypothermic or barbiturate (or other drug-induced) coma for treatment of Reye's syndrome, status epilepticus, near-drowning, metabolic coma with cerebral edema, and viral hepatitis.[249]

TREATMENT OF INCREASED ICP AND INTRACRANIAL VOLUME

Small increases of intracranial volume and ICP may have little impact on neurologic status, operative conditions, or neurologic outcome. In contrast, larger increases in intracranial volume and ICP generally increase the risk for poor outcome. The increase of intracranial volume and/or ICP to critical values is often referred to as intracranial hypertension. As mentioned earlier in this chapter, intracranial hypertension may increase the risk for cerebral ischemia, herniation, structural damage due to shear forces and compression, and impaired operative conditions. Treatment of intracranial hypertension generally is classified according to the intracranial contents targeted by the treatment, that is, brain tissue volume, CSF volume, CBV, or mass lesion.

BRAIN TISSUE VOLUME

Treatments that decrease brain tissue volume are presented above in greater detail in the section entitled "Treatment of Cerebral Edema." The treatments discussed in that section include steroids; anti-inflammatory agents; hyperventilation, antihypertensive drugs, and barbiturates (all of which reduce "filtration edema"); head elevation; osmotherapy; CSF drainage; surgical excision; and operative decompression. Several of those treatments are discussed again in the following section as they apply to the treatment of intracranial hypertension.

Because brain tissue water content is approximately 75 to 80 percent, treatments to decrease brain tissue volume often attempt to do so by decreasing brain tissue water. Hyperosmolar agents such as mannitol decrease brain tissue water by creating an osmolar gradient between cerebral blood and brain tissue favoring movement of water from the tissue space into the vascular space.[261] This mechanism is effective only if the BBB is intact. When the BBB is impaired, mannitol is not limited to the vascular space and, being free to enter the tissue space, causes an increase of osmolarity in brain ECF similar to that in blood. Under these conditions, no gradient exists to favor movement of water out of brain tissue and into the vascular space.

Even with an intact BBB, prolonged (>48 h) administration of mannitol results in passage of sufficient amounts of mannitol into brain ECF that an osmolar gradient between brain tissue and cerebral blood no longer exists. Furosemide and other diuretics are also capable of decreasing brain tissue water via a similar mechanism. The loss of free water from the blood that accompanies diuresis results in increased blood osmolarity. As when hyperosmolar agents are present in the blood, an osmolar gradient between blood and brain tissue is created that favors movement of water from the brain tissue space into the cerebral vascular space. With both hyperosmolar agents and diuretics, therapy, if prolonged, must be discontinued slowly. Acute restoration of normal blood osmolality at a time when the osmolality of brain tissue remains increased, creates an osmolar gradient favoring movement of water from the blood into brain tissue. Because both hyperosmolar agents and diuretics act on the kidneys to cause substantial loss of free water from blood, hypovolemia and hypotension may occur. Hypotension, in turn, decreases CPP and increases the risk for cerebral ischemic damage. For that reason, it is generally recommended that intravenous fluids should be administered concurrently with hyperosmolar agents and/or diuretics with the aim of achieving a normovolemic, hyperosmolar state.

Corticosteroids are reported to decrease brain tissue water content when vasogenic edema is the chief cause for increased brain tissue water. Corticosteroids have not been consistently reported to be beneficial for other forms of cerebral edema or for conditions where both vasogenic edema and other forms of edema are present, such as head injury.[306] Steroids produce other effects that may worsen outcome in certain conditions such as head injury. These other effects include decrease of the immune response in areas of the body other than the brain, suppression of intrinsic steroid production, and hyperglycemia. There are numerous reports that hyperglycemia worsens mortality and neurologic outcome from ischemia and head injury.[307]

Clearance of increased brain tissue water occurs via the CSF, brain tissue lymphatics, and cerebral vasculature. Reduction of CSF volume and pressure is reported to increase clearance of brain tissue water from edematous areas. CSF volume and pressure can be decreased either by CSF drainage or by drugs or other treatments that decrease $\dot{V}_f$ and R_a. CSF volume and pressure also can be decreased by relieving obstruction to CSF flow through the macroscopic pathways.

CSF VOLUME

Treatments that decrease CSF volume are presented above in greater detail in the sections entitled "Anesthetic and Drug-Induced Changes in $\dot{V}_f$ and R_a", "Neurogenic Regulation of $\dot{V}_f$ and R_a" and "Metabolic Regulation of $\dot{V}_f$ and R_a". The treatments discussed in those sections include anesthetics, diuretics, steroids, phosphodiesterase inhibitors, vasopressin, hypertonic saline, atrial natriuretic peptide, adrenergic and cholinergic drugs, and hypothermia. Several of those treatments are discussed again in the following section as they apply to the treatment of intracranial hypertension.

The most direct means of decreasing CSF volume is by CSF drainage. Removal of CSF generally is accomplished by intraventricular catheter or lumbar subarachnoid catheter. A ventriculostomy catheter may provide better ICP waveform data and is more likely to reflect ICP in the area of intracranial pathology in the event of ICP or CSF pressure gradients between the pathologic area and other areas of the CNS. CSF drainage via ventriculostomy carries a greater infection risk and the possibility of herniation laterally under the falx cerebri in the presence of a large mass in one hemisphere or herniation superiorly through the tentorium cerebelli in the presence of a large infratentorial mass. CSF drainage via lumbar subarachnoid catheter carries a greater risk for herniation inferiorly through the tentorium cerebelli in the presence of a large supratentorial mass or inferiorly into the foramen magnum.

Intracranial CSF volume can also be decreased by translocation of CSF from the intracranial space to the spinal subarachnoid space. Positioning the patient with the head elevated relative to the spinal region favors such translocation. Drugs and other treatments can be used to decrease $\dot{V}_f$ and R_a. Mannitol, furosemide, and corticosteroids are reported to decrease $\dot{V}_f$ and/or R_a, as are other drugs and treatments commonly used during anesthesia for neurosurgical procedures, including etomidate, barbiturates, fentanyl, hypothermia, and, acutely, hypocapnia.[1,57,67,72,91,239]

CBV

Hypocapnia is an effective means of decreasing CBF and CBV when the brain is intact and under many conditions of brain stress or injury. In contrast, autoregulation of CBF is impaired by many conditions of brain stress or injury. Hypocapnia to Pa_{CO_2} of 20 to 25 mmHg generally decreases CBF to about 50 percent of normocapnic values.[308] The initial cerebral vasoconstriction that accompanies hypocapnia results from the acute increase of perivascular pH. With prolonged hypocapnia, perivascular pH is adjusted toward normal, in part by decreased bicarbonate concentration in freshly formed CSF, and the diameter of the cerebral vessels also returns toward normal. As a result, in the absence of ongoing acid production in the brain, the decrease of CBV, and hence ICP, produced by hypocapnia does not persist during prolonged hypocapnia. The half-time of this response is in the order of 4 to 8 h. In contrast, hypocapnia may continue to be effective for

ICP control for up to several weeks by preventing cerebral acidosis in the presence of ongoing acid formation within the brain.[226] Recent studies have re-emphasized the dangers associated with hypocapnia such as cerebral ischemia resulting from mild cerebral vasoconstriction in already stenotic vessels, decreased collateral circulation into ischemic areas where collateral vessels remain reactive to Pa_{CO_2}, and substantial cerebral vasoconstriction in apparently normal vessels caused by excessive reduction of Pa_{CO_2}. Recently, it was reported that neurologic outcome was worse in patients with initial Glasgow motor scale scores of 4 to 5 who were hyperventilated than in those in whom hyperventilation was not used.[309]

Autoregulation of CBF is easily disturbed by conditions of brain stress or injury such as head injury, hypoxia, and ischemia. Autoregulation is also impaired by drugs such as inhalational anesthetics and "direct acting" vasodilators (e.g., sodium nitroprusside, nitroglycerin, calcium channel blockers, prostacyclin, and adenosine).[226] Under such conditions, increase of arterial blood pressure causes increase of CBV and ICP. Control of blood pressure with "indirect acting" agents (e.g., labetalol, osmolol, and trimethaphan) prevents the increase of CBV and ICP.

There are also effects of drugs on CBV and ICP unrelated to autoregulation per se. Sedative hypnotic drugs such as barbiturates, etomidate, and propofol are cerebral vasoconstrictors and decrease ICP.[226] In extreme cases barbiturate-induced coma may be necessary to control ICP. In contrast, inhalational anesthetics cause a concentration-related increase of CBF and CBV. The vasodilation and/or ICP elevation seen with inhalational anesthetics may be offset by prior or concurrent use of hypocapnia and/or sedative hypnotic drugs.

Improved hemorheology may decrease CBV and ICP. This effect may contribute to the early decrease of ICP that occurs following administration of mannitol.[261] Intravenous infusion of mannitol increases blood osmolarity, creating a gradient for water to move from the systemic ECF space into blood. The increased water content of blood decreases blood viscosity. When the viscosity of blood is decreased, the rate of CBF through vessels of a given size increases. Local factors that regulate CBF react to this state of hyperemia by initiating vasoconstriction. Vessels continue to constrict until CBF returns to the pretreatment values necessary to meet metabolic demands. Because decrease of blood viscosity permits increased CBF, CBF adequate for metabolic needs is carried by vessels of smaller diameter post-mannitol (low viscosity) than pre-mannitol (high viscosity). The end result is restoration of CBF to normal values with accompanying decrease of CBV and ICP.

Like CSF volume, CBV can be reduced by elevation of the head. Positioning the head above the level of the heart decreases CBV primarily by improving cerebral venous outflow, which reduces cerebral venous blood volume. During cerebral ischemia, CBV with the head elevated 45° above horizontal was only 30 percent of CBV with the head lowered 10° below horizontal.[310] Cerebral venous outflow is also impaired by jugular venous compression. Thus ICP can be decreased by removing positional causes for jugular venous compression such as rotation or lateral flexion of the neck, and external causes of jugular venous compression such as neck stabilizing devices used in cases of head or cervical spine injury, or clothing, necklaces, and others.

Local perivascular regulatory mechanisms in the brain act to match CBF to cerebral metabolic needs. Conditions of excessive metabolic demand trigger increase of CBF that may increase CBV and ICP. Examples of such conditions are epileptic activity, intoxication with CNS stimulants, hyperthermia, and metabolic disorders causing brain hyperactivity.[226] In each case specific treatment of the underlying process may reverse the associated increase of CBV and ICP. Cerebral metabolism also may be intentionally depressed as a means of decreasing CBV and ICP. Means of elective suppression of cerebral metabolism include hypothermia and barbiturate-induced coma.

Finally, increased intrathoracic pressure reduces the hydrostatic pressure gradient favoring flow of venous blood from the cerebral venous sinuses to the internal jugular veins and then to the intrathoracic venous circulation. During mechanical ventilation, muscle relaxation minimizes the likelihood that patients will contract the muscles of respiration at the same time the ventilator delivers a tidal volume. Also during mechanical ventilation, ventilatory rate, inspiratory and expiratory times, and inspiratory flow rate may be adjusted to provide the desired minute ventilation with optimal time of no positive intrathoracic pressure (allowing maximum time for cerebral venous drainage) and minimal inspiratory pressure. Adequate anesthesia and muscle relaxation during endotracheal intubation also minimize the likelihood that patients will contract the muscles of respiration (which, if contraction occurs, increases intrathoracic pressure and hence cerebral venous blood volume and ICP). Appropriate doses of opioids, sedative-hypnotics, and local anesthetics intravenously, as well as topical anesthetics, may be used to achieve the same goals during endotracheal tube suctioning or other stimulating procedures, and at the time of removal of the endotracheal tube.

INTRACEREBRAL MASS LESIONS
Space-occupying masses increase total intracerebral volume thereby increasing ICP. Even when the volume

occupied by such masses is offset by contraction of the volume of one or more of the other intracranial contents (brain tissue volume, CSF volume, and CBV), intracranial compliance and volume tolerance is reduced, and intracranial elastance is increased. Thus, small increases of brain tissue volume, CSF volume, or CBV that might otherwise cause little change in ICP may cause significant increases of ICP. Treatments for mass lesions include removal (in cases of tumor, abscess, foreign body, hematoma, etc.), chemotherapy or radiation therapy (in cases of tumor), or creation of additional space for the normal intracranial contents (such as by subtemporal decompression or craniectomy).

Summary

Intracranial water exists in ICF, ECF, and CSF spaces. Cerebral edema occurs when increased brain tissue water content results in increased brain tissue volume. The precipitating event in cerebral edema formation is an increase in either ICF, ECF, or CSF volume. Resolution of edema occurs by egress of fluid through ECF and/or CSF spaces.

Intracranial hypertension occurs when cerebral edema causes a significant increase of ICP. Intracranial hypertension may also result from increased CSF volume or CBV. Adverse effects of intracranial hypertension include ischemic brain damage due to decreased CPP, and mechanical damage to brain tissue secondary to herniation. Diagnosis of intracranial hypertension and assessment of responses to treatment are facilitated by measurement of ICP. Methods of measuring ICP include intraventricular, subdural-subarachnoid, and intraparenchymal devices. In addition to measurement of ICP, attempts have been made to assess intracranial elastance/compliance. These attempts include determination of PVI and VPR, and computer-assisted approaches such as determination of HFC. Treatments to improve ICP or intracranial elastance/compliance include steroids, anti-inflammatory drugs, hyperventilation, head elevation, osmotic/diuretic drugs, barbiturates, CSF drainage, antihypertensive drugs, and surgery. Most clinical studies report improved neurologic outcome with treatments to control ICP and/or intracranial elastance/compliance.

Abbreviations

ATP	adenosine triphosphate
BBB	blood-brain barrier
CBF	cerebral blood flow
CBV	cerebral blood volume
CNS	central nervous system
CP	choroid plexus
CPBF	choroid plexus blood flow
CPP	cerebral perfusion pressure
CSF	cerebrospinal fluid
CURL	compartment of uncoupling of receptor from ligand
E	extraction fraction
ECF	extracellular fluid
EEG	electroencephalogram
GABA	gamma aminobutyric acid
GFAP	glial fibrillary acid protein
GGTP	gamma glutamyl transpeptidase
HFC	high frequency centroid
ICF	intracellular fluid
ICP	intracranial pressure
IGF	insulin-like growth factor
Ig G	immunoglobulin G
K_a	affinity constant
K_d	dissociation constant
K_i	influx constant
K_m	affinity of transporter system for substance transported
K_o	efflux constant
LDL	low density lipoprotein
P_d	diffusional permeability to water
P_f	filtration coefficient
PS	permeability-surface area product
PVI	pressure-volume index
R_a	resistance to reabsorption of cerebrospinal fluid
V_a	rate of reabsorption of cerebrospinal fluid
V_c	volume of distribution in intracapillary fluid
V_f	rate of formation of cerebrospinal fluid
V_{max}	maximum transport rate
VPR	volume-pressure response

References

1. Davson H: *Physiology of Cerebrospinal Fluid.* London, Churchill-Livingstone, 1967.
2. Milhorat TH: Pediatric neurosurgery. In Plum F, McDowell FH (eds): *Contemporary Neurology Series,* vol 16. Philadelphia, FA Davis, 1978:91–135.
3. Franklin GM, et al: Amino acid transport into the cerebrospinal fluid of the rat. *J Neurochem* 1975; 24:367.
4. Edvinsson L, et al: Ultrastructural and biochemical evidence for a sympathetic neural influence on the choroid plexus. *Exp Neurol* 1975; 48:241.
5. Milhorat TH: The third circulation revisited. *J Neurosurg* 1975; 42:628.
6. Milhorat TH, Hammock MK: Cerebrospinal fluid as reflection

of internal milieu of brain. In Wood JH (ed): *Neurobiology of Cerebrospinal Fluid*, vol 2. New York, Plenum Press, 1983:1–23.

7. Sahar A: Choroidal origin of cerbrospinal fluid. *Isr J Med Sci* 1972; 8:594.

8. Brightman MW, et al: Assessment with the electron microscope of the permeability of peroxidase of cerebral endothelium and epithelium in mice and sharks. In Crone C, Lassen NA (eds): *Capillary Permeability.* New York, Academic Press, 1970:468–476.

9. Milhorat TH, et al: Localization of ouabain-sensitive NaD-K-ATPase in frog, rabbit, and rat choroid plexus. *Brain Res* 1975; 99:170.

10. Davis DA, Milhorat TH: The blood-brain barrier of the rat choroid plexus. *Anat Rec* 1975; 181:779.

11. Johanson CE: The choroid plexus-arachnoid membrane-cerebrospinal fluid system. In Boulton AA, Baker GB, Walz W (eds): *Neuromethods: The Neuronal Microenvironment*, vol 9. Clifton, NJ, The Humana Press, 1988:33–104.

12. Rapoport SI: *The Blood-Brain Barrier in Physiology and Medicine.* New York, Raven Press, 1976:43–86.

13. Katzman R, Pappius HM: *Brain Electrolytes and Fluid Metabolism.* Baltimore, Williams & Wilkins, 1973.

14. Milhorat TH: Structure and function of the choroid plexus and other sites of cerebrospinal fluid formation. *Int Rev Cytol* 1976; 47:225.

15. Hochwald GM, et al: Transport of glucose from blood to cerebrospinal fluid in the cat. *Neuroscience* 1983; 10:1035.

16. Hochwald GM, et al: Cerebrospinal fluid glucose: Turnover and metabolism. *J Neurochem* 1985; 44:1832.

17. Rapoport SI: A mathematical model for vasogenic brain edema. *J Theor Biol* 1978: 74:439.

18. Bouldin TW, Krigman MR: Differential permeability of cerebral capillary and choroid plexus to lanthanum ion. *Brain Res* 1975; 99:444.

19. Castel M, et al: The movement of lanthanum across diffusion barriers in the choroid plexus of the cat. *Brain Res* 1974; 67:178.

20. Brightman MW: Ultrastructural characteristics of adult choroid plexus: Relation to the blood-cerebrospinal fluid barrier to proteins. In Netsky MG, Shuangshoti S (eds): *The Choroid Plexus in Health and Disease.* Charlottesville, VA, University Press of Virginia, 1975:86.

21. Rapoport SI: Passage of proteins from blood to cerebrospinal fluid: Model for transfer by pores and vesicles. In Wood JH (ed): *Neurobiology of Cerebrospinal Fluid*, vol 2. New York, Plenum Press, 1983:233–245.

22. Pollay M, et al: Alteration in choroid-plexus blood flow and cerebrospinal fluid formation by increased ventricular pressure. In Wood JH (ed): *Neurobiology of Cerebrospinal Fluid*, vol 2. New York, Plenum Press, 1983:687–695.

23. Weiss MH, Wertman N: Modulation of CSF production by alterations in cerebral perfusion pressure. *Arch Neurol* 1978; 35:527.

24. Milhorat TH: *Hydrocephalus and the Cerebrospinal Fluid.* Baltimore, Williams & Wilkins, 1972.

25. DiChiro G, et al: Spinal descent of cerebrospinal fluid in man. *Neurology* 1976; 26:1.

26. Post RM, et al: Cerebrospinal fluid flow and iodide[131] transport in the spinal subarachnoid space. *Life Sci* 1974; 14:1885.

27. Williams B: Cerebrospinal fluid pressure changes in response to coughing. *Brain* 1976; 99:331.

28. Upton ML, Weller RO: The morphology of cerebrospinal fluid drainage pathways in human arachnoid granulations. *J Neurosurg* 1985; 63:867.

29. Nabeshima S, et al: Junctions in the meninges and marginal glia. *J Comp Neurol* 1975; 164:127.

30. Simionescu N, et al: Structural basis of permeability in sequential segments of the microvasculature of the diaphragm. II. Pathways followed by microperoxidase across the endothelium. *Microvasc Res.* 1978; 15:177.

31. Johnson RN, et al: Intracranial hypertension in experimental animals and man: Quantitative approach to system dynamics of circulatory cerebrospinal fluid. In Wood JH (ed): *Neurobiology of Cerebrospinal Fluid*, vol 2. New York, Plenum Press, 1983:697–706.

32. Butler AB, et al: Mechanisms of cerebrospinal fluid absorption in normal and pathologically altered arachnoid villi. In Wood JH (ed): *Neurobiology of Cerebrospinal Fluid*, vol 2. New York, Plenum Press, 1983:707–726.

33. Wolff JR: Ultrastructure of the terminal vascular bed as related to function. In Kaley G, Altura BM (eds): *Microvascular Circulation*, vol I. Baltimore, University Park Press, 1977:95.

34. Cserr HF: Physiology of the choroid plexus. *Physiol Rev* 1971; 51:273.

35. Leusen IR, et al: Regulation of acid-base equilibrium of cerebrospinal fluid. In Wood JH (ed): *Neurobiology of Cerebrospinal Fluid*, vol 2. New York, Plenum Press, 1983:25–42.

36. Fenstermacher JD, Rall DP: Physiology and pharmacology of cerebrospinal fluid. In Capri A (ed): *Pharmacology of the Cerebral Circulation.* New York, Pergamon Press, 1972:41–72.

37. Cseer HF, et al: Flow of cerebral interstitial fluid as indicated by the removal of extracellular markers from rat caudate nucleus. *Exp Eye Res* 1977; 25(suppl)461.

38. Artru AA: Cerebrospinal fluid. In Cottrell JE, Smith DS (eds): *Anesthesia and Neurosurgery*, 3rd ed. St. Louis, CV Mosby, 1994:93–116.

39. Baramy EH: Inhibition by hippurate and probenicid of in vitro uptake of iodipamide and O-iodohippurate: A composite uptake system for iodipamide in choroid plexus, kidney cortex and anterior uvea of several species. *Acta Physiol Scand* 1972; 86:12.

40. Firemark HM: Choroid-plexus transport of enkephalins and other neuropeptides. In Wood JH (ed): *Neurobiology of Cerebrospinal Fluid*, vol 2. New York, Plenum Press, 1983:77–81.

41. Adkinson KDK, et al: Contribution of probenecid-sensitive anion transport processes at the brain capillary endothelium and choroid plexus to the efficient efflux of valproic acid from the central nervous system. *J Pharmacol Exp Ther* 1994; 268:797.

42. Artru AA, et al: Clearance of valproic acid from cerebrospinal fluid in anesthetized rabbits. *J Neurosurg Anesth* 1994; 6:193.

43. Adkinson KDK, et al: Role of choroid plexus epithelium in the removal of valproic acid from the central nervous system. *Epilepsy Res* 1995; 20:185.

44. Vigh B, Vigh-Teichman I: Comparative ultrastructure of the cerebrospinal fluid contacting neurons. In Bourne GH, Danielli JF (eds): *International Review of Cytology*, vol 35. New York, Academic Press, 1973:189–251.

45. Porter JC, et al: Role of biogenic amines and cerebrospinal fluid in the neurovascular transmittal and hypophysiotrophic substances. In Knigge KM, Scott DE, Weindl A (eds): *Brain-Endocrine Interaction, Median Eminence: Structure and Function* (*Proceedings of the International Symposium on Brain-Endocrine Interaction, Munich, 1971*). Basel, S. Karger, 1972:245–253.

46. Hosobuchi Y, et al: Stimulation of human periaqueductal gray for pain relief increases immunoreactive β-endorphin in ventricular fluid. *Science* 1979; 203:279.

47. Rodriguez EM, et al: Evidence for the periventricular localization of the hypothalamic osmoreceptors. In Knowles F, Vollrath L (eds): *Neurosecretion—The Final Neuroendocrine Pathway.* New York, Springer-Verlag, 1973:319–320.

48. Leurssen TG, Robertson GL: Cerebrospinal fluid vasopressin and vasotocin in health and disease. In Wood JH (ed): *Neurobiology of Cerebrospinal Fluid*, vol 1. New York, Plenum Press, 1980:613–623.

49. Reppert SM, et al: Cerebrospinal fluid melanin. In Wood JH (ed): *Neurobiology of Cerebrospinal Fluid*, vol 1. New York, Plenum Press, 1980:579–589.

50. Post KD, et al: Cerebrospinal fluid pituitary hormone concentrations in patients with pituitary tumors. In Wood JH (ed): *Neurobiology of Cerebrospinal Fluid*, vol 1. New York, Plenum Press, 1980:591–604.

51. Artru AA: Concentration-related changes in the rate of CSF formation and resistance to reabsorption of CSF during enflurane and isoflurane anesthesia in dogs receiving nitrous oxide. *J Neurosurg Anesth* 1989; 1:256.

52. Artru AA: Effects of halothane and fentanyl on the rate of CSF production in dogs. *Anesth Analg* 1983; 62:581.

53. Artru AA: Effects of halothane and fantanyl anesthesia on resistance to reabsorption of CSF. *J Neurosurg* 1984; 60:252.

54. Artru AA: Rate of cerebrospinal fluid formation, resistance to reabsorption of cerebrospinal fluid, brain tissue water content, and electroencephalogram during desflurane anesthesia in dogs. *J Neurosurg Anesth* 1993; 5:178.

55. Sugioka S: Effects of sevoflurane on intracranial pressure and formation and absorption of cerebrospinal fluid in cats. *Masui (Jap J Anesth)* 1992; 41:1434.

56. Artru AA, et al: Enflurane causes a prolonged and reversible increase in the rate of CSF production in the dog. *Anesthesiology* 1982; 57:255.

57. Artru AA: Dose-related changes in rate of cerebrospinal fluid formation and resistance to reabsorption of cerebrospinal fluid following administration of thiopental, midazolam, and etomidate in dogs. *Anesthesiology* 1988; 69:541.

58. Artru AA: The rate of CSF formation, resistance to reabsorption of CSF, and a periodic analysis of the EEG following administration of flumazenil to dogs. *Anesthesiology* 1990; 72:111.

59. Mann JD, et al: Differential effect of pentobarbital, ketamine hydrochloride, and enflurane anesthesia on CSF formation rate and outflow resistance in the rat. In Miller JD, et al. (eds): *Intracranial Pressure IV*. New York, Springer-Verlag, 1980:466.

60. Artru AA: Propofol combined with halothane or with fentanyl/halothane does not alter the rate of CSF formation or resistance to reabsorption of CSF in rabbits. *J Neurosurg Anesth* 1993; 5:250.

61. Artru AA: Dose-related changes in the rate of CSF formation and resistance to reabsorption of CSF during administration of fentanyl, sufentanil, or alfentanil in dogs. *J Neurosurg Anesth* 1991; 3:283.

62. Artru AA et al: Intravenous lidocaine decreases but cocaine does not alter rate of CSF formation in anesthetized rabbits. In Nagai H, Kamiya K, Ishii S (eds): *Intracranial Pressure IX*. Tokyo, Springe-Verlag, 1994:397–400.

63. Meyer RR, Shapiro HM: Paradoxical effect of enflurane on choroid plexus metabolism: Clinical implications (abstract). *American Society of Anesthesiologists*. 1978:489–490.

64. Maktabi MA, et al: Effect of halothane anesthesia on production of cerebrospinal fluid: Possible role of vasopressin V_1 receptors. *J Cereb Blood Flow Metab* 1991; 11:S268 (abst).

65. Vogh BP, Maren TH: Sodium, chloride and bicarbonate movement from plasma to cerebrospinal fluid in cats. *Am J Physiol* 1975; 228:673.

66. Smith RV, et al: Alteration of cerebrospinal fluid production in the dog. *Surg Neurol* 1974; 2:267.

67. Buhrley LE, Reed DJ: The effect of furosemide on sodium-22 uptake into cerebrospinal fluid and brain. *Exp Brain Res* 1972; 14:503.

68. Rosenberg GA, Kyner WT: Effect of mannitol-induced hyperosmolarity on transport between brain interstitial fluid and cerebrospinal fluid. In Wood JH (ed): *Neurobiology of Cerebrospinal Fluid*, vol 2. New York, Plenum Press, 1983:765–775.

69. Dacey RG Jr, et al: Bacterial meningitis: Selected aspects of cerebrospinal fluid pathophysiology. In Wood JH (ed): *Neurobiology of Cerebrospinal Fluid*, vol 2. New York, Plenum Press, 1983:727–738.

70. Mann JD, et al: Cerebrospinal fluid circulatory dynamics in pseudotumor cerebri and response to steroid therapy. In Wood JH (ed): *Neurobiology of Cerebrospinal Fluid*, vol 2. New York, Plenum Press, 1983:739–751.

71. Schwartz ML, et al: The uptake of hydrocortisone in mouse brain and ependymoblastoma. *J Neurosurg* 1972; 36:178.

72. Sato O, Hara M, et al: The effect of dexamethasone phosphate on the production rate of cerebrospinal fluid in the subarachnoid space of dogs. *J Neurosurg* 1973; 39:480.

73. Wright EM: Transport processes in the formation of cerebrospinal fluid. *Rev Physiol Biochem Pharmacol* 1978; 83:1.

74. Rosenberg GA: Physiology of cerebrospinal and interstitial fluids. In Rosenberg GA (ed): *Brain Fluids and Metabolism*. New York, Oxford University Press, 1990:36–57.

75. Foxworthy JC IV, Artru AA: Cerebrospinal fluid dynamics and brain tissue composition following intravenous infusion of hypertonic saline in anesthetized rabbits. *J Neurosurg Anesth* 1990; 2:256.

76. Artru AA: Muscle relaxation with succinylcholine or vecuronium does not alter the rate of CSF production or resistance to reabsorption of CSF in dogs. *Anesthesiology* 1988; 68:392.

77. Lindvall M: Fluorescence histochemical study on regional differences in the sympathetic nerve supply of the choroid plexus from various laboratory animals. *Cell Tissue Res* 1979; 198:261.

78. Lindvall M, et al: Sympathetic nervous control of cerebrospinal fluid production from the choroid plexus. *Science* 1978; 201:176.

79. Edvinsson L, et al: Adrenergic innervation of the mammalian choroid plexus. *Am J Anat* 1974; 139:299.

80. Lindvall M, et al: Histochemical study on regional differences in the cholinergic nerve supply of the choroid plexus from various laboratory animals. *Exp Neurol* 1977; 55:152.

81. Larsson LI, et al: Immunohistochemical localization of a vasodilatory peptide (VIP) in cerebrovascular nerves. *Brain Res* 1976; 113:400.

82. Lindvall M, et al: Peptidergic (VIP) nerves in the mammalian choroid plexus. *Neurosci Lett* 1978; 9:77.

83. Winbladh B, et al: Effect of sympathectomy on active transport mechanisms in choroid plexus in vitro. *Acta Physiol Scand* 1978; 102:85A.

84. Haywood JR, Vogh BP: Some measurements of autonomic nervous system influence on production of cerebrospinal fluid in the cat. *J Pharmacol Exp Ther* 1979; 208:341.

85. Lindvall M, et al: Effect of sympathomimetic drugs and corresponding receptor antagonists on the rate of cerebrospinal fluid production. *Exp Neuro* 1979; 64:132.

86. Lindvall M, et al: Reduced cerebrospinal fluid formation through cholinergic mechanisms. *Neurosci Lett* 1978; 10:311.

87. Edvinsson L, et al: Changes in continuously recorded intracranial pressure of conscious rabbits at different time-periods after superior cervical sympathectomy. *Acta Physiol Scand* 1971; 83:42.

88. Faraci FM, Helstad DD: Does basal production of nitric oxide

contribute to regulation of brain-fluid balance? *Am J Physiol* 1992; 262:PH340.

89. Snodgrass SR, Lorenzo AV: Temperature and cerebrospinal fluid production rate. *Am J Physiol* 1972; 222:1524.

90. Heisey SR, et al: Effect of hypercapnia and cerebral perfusion pressure on cerebrospinal fluid production in cat. *Am J Physiol* 1983; 244:R224.

91. Artru AA, Hornbein TF: Prolonged hypocapnia does not alter the rate of CSF production in dogs during halothane anesthesia or sedation with nitrous oxide. *Anesthesiology* 1987; 67:66.

92. Hochwald GM, et al: The effects of serum osmolarity on cerebrospinal fluid volume flow. *Life Sci* 1974; 15:1309.

93. Wald A, et al: Evidence for the movement of fluid, macromolecules and ions from the brain extracellular space to the CSF. *Brain Res* 1978; 151:283.

94. Bradbury M: Transport and homeostasis of ions in cerebral fluids. In Bradbury M (ed): *The Concept of a Blood-Brain Barrier.* Chichester, John Wiley & Sons, 1979:214–259.

95. Bradbury MWB: Lymphatic and the central nervous system. *Trends Neurosci* 1981; 4:100.

96. Cserr HF, et al: Efflux of radiolabeled polyethylene glycols and albumin from rat brain. *Am J Physiol* 1981; 240:F319.

97. Maren TH: Ion secretion into cerebrospinal fluid. *Exp Eye Res* 1977; 25(suppl):157.

98. Milhorat TH, et al: Two morphologically distinct blood-brain barriers preventing entry of cytochrome c into cerebrospinal fluid. *Science* 1973; 180:76.

99. Milhorat TH: The blood-brain barrier and cerebral edema. In Cottrell JE, Smith DS (eds): *Anesthesia and Neurosurgery,* 3d ed. St. Louis, CV Mosby, 1994:136–148.

100. Crone C: The blood-brain barrier: A modified tight epithelium. In Suckling AJ, Rumsby MG, Bradbury MWB (eds): *The Blood-Brain Barrier in Health and Disease.* Chichester, Ellis Horwood, 1986:17–40.

101. Crone C: The function of capillaries. In Baker PF (ed): *Recent Advances in Physiology,* vol 10. London, Churchill-Livingstone, 1984:125–162.

102. Oldendorf WH: Blood-brain barrier. In Himwich HE (ed): *Brain Metabolism and Cerebral Disorders,* 2d ed. New York, Spectrum Publications, 1976:163–180.

103. Pollay M: Blood-brain barrier; cerebral edema. In Wilkins RH, Rengachary SS (eds): *Neurosurgery,* vol 1. New York, McGraw-Hill, 1985:322–331.

104. Fenstermacher JD, et al: Structural and functional variations in capillary systems within the brain. In Strand FL (ed): *Fourth Colloquium in Biological Sciences: Blood-Brain Transfer. Ann NY Acad Sci* 1988; 529:21.

105. Crone C, Levitt DG: Capillary permeability to small solutes. In Renkin EM, Michel CC (eds): *Handbook of Physiology,* Section 2, Microcirculation, IV. Bethesda, American Physiology Society, 1984:411–466.

106. Cremer JE, Cunningham VJ: Effects of some chlorinated sugar derivatives on the hexose transport system of the blood-brain barrier. *Biochem J* 1979; 180:677.

107. Marrs AM, et al: Tryptophan transport across the blood-brain barrier during acute hepatic failure. *J Neurochem* 1979; 33:409.

108. Gjedde A, Crone C: Repression of blood-brain glucose transfer in chronic hyperglycemia. *Science* 1981; 214:456.

109. Oelsen SP, Crone C: Electrical resistance of muscle capillary endothelium. *Biophys J* 1983; 42:31.

110. Zeuthen T, Wright EM: Epithelial potassium transport: Tracer and electrophysiological studies in choroid plexus. *J Memb Biol* 1981; 60:105.

111. Klatzo I, et al: Aspects of the blood-brain barrier in brain edema. In de Vlieger M, de Lange SA, Beks JWF (eds): *Brain Edema.* New York, John Wiley, 1981:11–18.

112. Oldendorf WH, et al: The large apparent work capability of the blood-brain barrier: A study of the mitochondrial content of capillary endothelial cells in brain and other tissues of the rat. *Ann Neurol* 1977; 1:409.

113. Cutler RWP: Neurochemical aspects of blood-brain-cerebrospinal fluid barriers. In Wood JH (ed): *Neurobiology of Cerebrospinal Fluid,* vol 1. New York, Plenum Press, 1980:41–51.

114. Goldstein GW: Endothial cell-astrocyte interactions. A cellular model of the blood-brain barrier. In Strand FL (ed): *Fourth Colloquium in Biological Sciences: Blood-Brain Transfer. Ann NY Acad Sci* 1988; 529:31.

115. Cancilla PA, et al: Brain endothelial-astrocyte interactions. In Pardridge WM (ed): *The Blood-Brain Barrier.* New York, Raven Press, 1993:25–46.

116. Crone C, Olesen SP: Electrical resistance of brain microvascular endothelium. *Brain Res* 1982; 241:49.

117. Rutten MJ, et al: Electrical resistance and macromolecular permeability of brain endothelial monolayer cultures. *Brain Res* 1987; 425:301.

118. Arthur FE, et al: Astrocyte mediated induction of tight junctions in brain capillary endothelium: An efficient in vitro model. *Dev Brain Res* 1987; 36:155.

119. DeBault LE, Cancilla PA: γ-Glutamyl transpeptidase in isolated brain endothelial cells: Induction by glial cells in vitro. *Science* 1980; 207:635.

120. DeBault L: γ-Glutamyl transpeptidase induction mediated by glial foot process to endothelium contact in culture. *Brain Res* 1981; 220:432.

121. Cancilla PA, et al: Astrocytes and the blood-brain barrier. Kinetics of astrocyte activation after injury and induction effects on endothelium. In Johansson BB, Owman C, Widner J (eds): *Pathophysiology of the Blood-Brain Barrier.* Amsterdam, Elsevier, 1990:31–39.

122. Beck DW, et al: Glial cells influence polarity of the blood-brain barrier. *J Neuropathol Exp Neurol* 1984; 43:219.

123. Maxwell K, et al: Stimulation of glucose analogue uptake by cerebral microvessel endothelial cells by a product released by astrocytes. *J Neuropathol Exp Neurol* 1989; 48:69.

124. Beck DW, et al: Glial cells influence membrane associated enzyme activity at the blood-brain barrier. *Brain Res* 1986; 381:131.

125. Tio S, et al: Astrocyte-mediated induction of alkaline phosphatase activity in human umbilical cord vein endothelium: An in vitro model. *Eur J Morphol* 1990; 28:289.

126. Folkman J: How is blood vessel growth regulated in normal and neoplastic tissue? *Cancer Res* 1986; 46:467.

127. Cancilla PA, et al: Expression of mRNA for glial fibrillary acidic protein after experimental cerebral injury. *J Neuropathol Exp Neurol* 1992; 51:560.

128. Condorelli DF, et al: Glial fibrillary acidic protein messenger RNA and glutamine synthetase activity after nervous system injury. *J Neurosci Res* 1990; 26:251.

129. Bradbury MW: Transport across the blood-brain barrier. In Neuwelt EA (ed): *Implications of the Blood-Brain Barrier and Its Manipulation,* vol 1, Basic Science Aspects. New York, Plenum Medical Book Company, 1989:119–136.

130. Oldendorf WH: Measurement of brain uptake of radiolabeled substances using a tritiated water internal standard. *Brain Res* 1970; 24:372.

131. Yuwiler A, et al: Effect of albumin binding and amino acid competition on tryptophan uptake into brain. *J Neurochem* 1977; 28:1015.

132. Pardridge WM, Mietus LJ: Transport of steroid hormones through the rat blood-brain barrier. Primary role of albumin bound hormone. *J Clin Invest* 1979; 64:145.

133. Pardridge WM: Carrier-mediated transport of thyroid hormones through the rat blood-brain barrier. Primary role of albumin-bound hormone. *Endocrinology* 1979; 105:605.

134. Marathe PH, et al: Effect of serum protein binding on the entry of lidocaine into brain and cerebrospinal fluid in dogs. *Anesthesiology* 1991; 75:804.

135. Oldendorf WH: Brain uptake of radiolabelled amino acids, amines and hexoses after arterial injection. *Am J Physiol* 1971; 221:1629.

136. Oldendorf WH: Carrier-mediated blood-brain barrier transport of short chain monocarboxylic organic acids. *Am J Physiol* 1973; 224:1450.

137. Pardridge WM: Brain metabolism: A perspective from the blood-brain barrier. *Physiol Rev* 1983; 63:1481.

138. Laterra J, Goldstein GW: Brain microvessels and microvascular cells in vitro. In Pardridge WM (ed): *The Blood-Brain Barrier; Cellular and Molecualr Biology.* New York, Raven Press, 1993:1–24.

139. Oldendorf WH, Szabo J: Amino acid assignment to one of three blood-brain barrier amino acid carriers. *Am J Physiol* 1976; 230:941.

140. Cornford EM, Oldendorf WH: Independent blood-brain barrier transport systems for nucleic acid precursors. *Biochim Biophys Acta* 1975; 394:211.

141. Greenwood J, et al: Kinetics of thiamine transport across the blood-brain barrier in the rat. *J Physiol (Lond)* 1982; 327:95.

142. Spector R, Eells J: Deoxynucleoside and vitamin transport into the central nervous system. *Fed Proc* 1984; 43:196.

143. Pardridge WM, et al: Human blood-brain barrier insulin receptor. *J Neurochem* 1985; 44:1771.

144. Bolwig TG, et al: The permeability of the blood-brain barrier during electrically induced seizures in man. *Eur J Clin Invest* 1977; 7:87.

145. Hertz MM, Paulson OB: Transfer across the human blood-brain barrier. Evidence for capillary recruitment and for a paradox glucose permeability increase in hypocapnia. *Microvasc Res* 1982; 24:364.

146. Phelps ME, et al: Cerebral extraction of N-13 ammonia: Its dependence on cerebral blood flow and capillary permeability-surface area product. *Stroke* 1981; 12:607.

147. Nemoto EM, et al: Glucose transport across the rat blood-brain barrier during anesthesia. *Anesthesiology* 1978; 49:170.

148. Gjedde A, Rasmussen M: Pentobarbital anesthesia reduces blood-brain glucose transfer in the rat. *J Neurochem* 1980; 35:1382.

149. Sage JI, Duffy TE: Pentobarbital anesthesia: Influence on amino acid transport across the blood-brain barrier. *J Neurochem* 1979; 33:963.

150. Saija A, et al: Modifications of the permeability of the blood-brain barrier and local cerebral metabolism in pentobarbital- and ketamine-anaesthetized rats. *Neuropharmacology* 1989; 28:997.

151. Schettini A, Furniss WW: Brain water and electrolyte distribution during the inhalation of halothane. *Br J Anaesth* 1979; 51:1117.

152. Gumerlock MK, Neuwelt EA: The effects of anesthesia on osmotic blood-brain barrier disruption. *Neurosurgery* 1990; 26:268.

153. Stewart PA, et al: Ethanol and pentobarbital in combination increase blood-brain barrier permeability to horseradish peroxidase. *Brain Research* 1988; 443:12.

154. Artru AA: Reduction of cerebrospinal fluid pressure by hypocapnia: Changes in cerebral blood volume, cerebrospinal fluid volume and brain tissue water and electrolytes. II. Effects of anesthetics. *J Cereb Blood Flow Metabol* 1988; 8:750.

155. Forster A, et al: Anesthetic effects on blood-brain barrier function during acute arterial hypertension. *Anesthesiology* 1978; 49:26.

156. Fischer S, et al: In vitro effects of fentanyl, methohexital, and thiopental on brain endothelial permeability. *Anesthesiology* 1995; 82:451.

157. Pashayan AG, et al: Blood-CSF barrier function during general anesthesia in children undergoing ventriculoperitoneal shunt placement. *Anesth Rev* 1988; 15:30 (abstr).

158. Chi OZ, et al: Effects of isoflurane on transport across the blood-brain barrier. *Anesthesiology* 1992; 76:426.

159. Alexander SC, et al: Effects of general anesthesia on canine blood-brain barrier glucose transport. In Harper M, Jennett B, Miller O, et al. (eds): *Blood Flow and Metabolism in the Brain.* Edinburgh, Churchill-Livingstone, 1975:9.37–9.47.

160. Hannan CJ Jr, et al: Blood-brain barrier permeability during hypocapnia in halothane-anesthetized monkeys. In Strandl FL (ed): *Fourth Colloquium in Biological Sciences: Blood-Brain Transfer. Ann NY Acad Sci,* 1988; 529:172.

161. Chi OZ, et al: Effects of fentanyl on α-aminoisobutyric acid transfer across the blood-brain barrier. *Anesth Analg* 1992; 75:31.

162. Cremer JE, et al: Relationships between extraction and metabolism of glucose, blood flow and tissue blood volume in regions of rat brain. *J Cereb Blood Flow Metab* 1983; 3:291.

163. Gjedde A, Crone C: Induction processes in blood-brain transfer of ketone bodies during starvation. *Am J Physiol* 1975; 229:1165.

164. Cremer JE, et al: Changes during development in transport processes of the blood-brain barrier. *Biochim Biophys Acta* 1976; 448:633.

165. Sarna GS, et al: Brain metabolism and specific transport at the blood-brain barrier after portacaval anastomosis in the rat. *Brain Res* 1979; 160:69.

166. James JH, et al: Blood-brain neutral amino acid transport activity is increased after portacaval anastomosis. *Science* 1978; 200:1395.

167. Mans AM, et al: Regional blood-brain barrier permeability to amino acids after portacaval anastomosis. *J Neurochem* 1982; 38:705.

168. Jonung T, et al: Effect of hyperammonaemia and methionine sulfoxime on the kinetic parameters of blood-brain transport of leucine and phenylalanine. *J Neurochem* 1985; 45:308.

169. Mans AM, et al: Ammonia selectively stimulates neutral amino acid transport across blood-brain barrier. *Am J Physiol* 1983; 245:C74.

170. Friden PM: Receptor-mediated transport of peptides and proteins across the blood-brain barrier. In Pardridge WM (ed): *The Blood-Brain Barrier.* New York, Raven Press, 1993:229–247.

171. Friden PM, et al: Anti-transferrin receptor antibody and antibody-drug conjugates cross the blood-brain barrier. *Proc Natl Acad Sci USA* 1991; 88:4771.

172. Pardridge WM, et al: Selective transport of an antitransferrin receptor antibody through the blood-brain barrier in vivo. *J Pharmacol Exp Ther* 1991; 259:66.

173. Frank HJL, et al: Enhanced insulin binding to blood-brain barrier in vivo and to brain microvessels in vitro in newborn rabbits. *Diabetes* 1985; 34:728.

174. Duffy KR, Pardridge WM: Blood-brain barrier transcytosis of insulin in developing rabbits. *Brain Res* 1987; 420:32.

175. Baskin DG, et al: Insulin and insulin-like growth factors in the CNS. *TINS* 1988; 11:107.

176. Frank HJL, et al: Binding and internalization of insulin and insulin-like growth factors by isolated brain microvessels. *Diabetes* 1986; 35:654.

177. Rosenfeld RG, et al: Demonstration and structural comparison of receptors for insulin-like growth factor-I and -II (IGF-I and -II) in brain and blood-brain barrier. *Biochem Biophys Res Commun* 1987; 149:159.

178. Duffy DR, et al: Human blood-brain barrier insulin-like growth factor receptor. *Metabolism* 1988; 37:136.

179. Meresse S, et al: Low-density lipoprotein receptor on endothelium of brain capillaries. *J Neurochem* 1989; 53:340.

180. Fenstermacher JD: Pharmacology of the blood-brain barrier. In Neuwelt EA (ed): *Implications of the Blood-Brain Barrier and Its Manipulation*, vol. 1, Basic Science Aspects. New York, Plenum Medical Book Company, 1989:137–155.

181. Fenstermacher JD, Rapoport SI: Blood-brain barrier. In Renkin EM, Michel CC (eds): *Handbook of Physiology*, Section 2: *The Cardiovascular System*, vol IV, *Microcirculation*, Part 1. Bethesda, American Physiological Society, 1984:969–1000.

182. Fenstermacher JD, et al: Methods for quantifying the transport of drugs across brain barrier systems. *Pharmacol Ther* 1981; 14:217.

183. Fenstermacher JD, Patlak CS: CNS, CSF, and extradural fluid uptake of various hydrophilic materials in the dogfish. *Am J Physiol* 1977; 232:R45.

184. Cornford EM, et al: Increased blood-brain barrier transport of protein-bound anticonvulsant drugs in the newborn. *J Cereb Blood Flow Metab* 1983; 3:280.

185. Van Deurs B: Structural aspects of brain barriers, with special reference to the permeability of the cerebral endothelium and choroidal epithelium. *Int Rev Cytol* 1980; 65:117.

186. Fenstermacher JD: Drug transfer across the blood-brain barrier. In Breimer DD, Speiser P (eds): *Topics in Pharmaceutical Sciences*. Amsterdam, Elsevier, 1983:143–154.

187. Price MT, et al: Uptake of exogenous aspartate into circumventricular organs but not other regions of adult mouse brain. *J Neurochem* 1984; 42:740.

188. Oldendorf WH: Lipid solubility and drug penetration of the blood-brain barrier. *Proc Soc Exp Biol Med* 1974; 147:813.

189. Pappius HM: Cerebral edema and the blood-brain barrier. In Neuwelt EA (ed): *Implications of the Blood-Brain Barrier and Its Manipulation*, vol. 1, *Basic Science Aspects*. New York, Plenum Medical Book Company, 1989:293–309.

190. Milhorat TH: *Cerebrospinal Fluid and the Brain Edemas*. New York, Neuroscience Society of New York, 1987.

191. Rapoport SI: Roles of cerebrovascular permeability, brain compliance and brain hydraulic conductivity in vasogenic brain edema. In Popp AJ, Bourke RS et al (eds): *Seminars in Neurological Surgery*, vol. 4, *Neural Trauma*. New York, Raven Press, 1979:51–61.

192. Long DM: Microvascular changes in cold injury edema. In Go KG, Baethmann A (eds): *Recent Progress in the Study and Therapy of Brain Edema*. New York, Plenum Press, 1984:45–54.

193. Unterberg A, et al: Inhibition of the kalikrein-kinin system in vasogenic brain edema. In Inaba Y, Klatzo I, Spatz M (eds): *Brain Edema, Proceedings of the Sixth International Symposium*. New York, Springer-Verlag, 1985:294–298.

194. Chan PH, et al: Oxygen-free radicals: Potential edema mediators in brain injury. In Inaba Y, Klatzo I, Spatz M (eds): *Brain Edema. Proceedings of the Sixth International Symposium*. New York, Springer-Verlag, 1985:317–323.

195. Bunegin L, et al: Increased free radical formation following alcohol intoxication in dogs. *Crit Care Med* 1986; 14:387.

196. Albin MS, Bunegin L: An experimental study of craniocerebral trauma during ethanol intoxication. *Crit Care Med* 1986; 14:841.

197. Fenstermacher JD: Volume regulation of the central nervous system. In Staub NC, Taylor AE (eds): *Edema*. New York, Raven Press, 1984:383–404.

198. Blasberg RG, et al: Quantitative autoradiographic studies of brain edema and a comparison of multi-isotope autoradiographic techniques. In Cervos-Navarro J, Ferszt R (eds): *Advances in Neurology*, vol. 28. *Brain Edema*. New York, Raven Press, 1980:255–270.

199. Reulen HJ, et al: Role of pressure gradients and bulk flow in dynamics of vasogenic edema.. *J Neurosurg* 1977; 46:24.

200. Marmarou A, et al: The time course and distribution of water in the resolution phase of infusion edema. In Go KG, Baethmann A (eds): *Recent Progress in the Study and Therapy of Brain Edema*. New York, Plenum Press, 1984:37–44.

201. Reulen JH, et al: Clearance of edema fluid into cerebrospinal fluid. A mechanism for resolution of vasogenic brain edema. *J Neurosurg* 1978; 48:754.

202. Bruce DA, et al: Mechanisms and time course for clearance of vasogenic cerebral edema. In Popp AJ, Bourke RS, Nelson LR (eds): *Seminars in Neurological Surgery*, vol. 4, *Neural Trauma*. New York, Raven Press, 1979:155–172.

203. Marmarou A, et al: The time course of brain tissue pressure and local CBF in vasogenic edema. In Pappius HM, Feindel W (eds): *Dynamics of Brain Edema*. New York, Springer-Verlag, 1976:113–121.

204. Klatzo I, et al: Resolution of vasogenic brain edema. In Cervos Navarro J, Ferszt R (eds): *Advances in Neurology*, vol 28, *Brain Edema*. New York, Raven Press, 1980:359–373.

205. Vorbrodt AW, et al: Ultrastructural observations on the transvascular route of protein removal in vasogenic brain edema. *Acta Neuropath (Berl)* 1985; 66:265.

206. Cancilla PA, et al: Regeneration of cerebral microvessels: A morphologic and histochemical study after local freeze-injury. *Lab Invest* 1979; 40:74.

207. Gazendam KM, et al: Composition of isolated edema fluid in cold-induced brain edema. *J Neurosurg* 1979; 51:70.

208. Go KG, et al: The influence of hypoxia on the composition of isolated edema fluid in cold-induced brain edema. *J Neurosurg* 1979; 51:78.

209. Milhorat TH, et al: Relationship between oedema, blood pressure, and blood flow following local brain injury. *Neurol Res* 1989; 11:29.

210. Baethmann A, et al: Brain edema factors: Current state with particular reference to plasma constituents and glutamate. *Adv Neurol* 1980; 28:171.

211. Katzman R, et al: Report of the Joint Committee for Stroke Resources. IV. Brain edema in stroke. Study group of brain edema in stroke. *Stroke* 1977; 8:512.

212. Bradbury MWB: *The Concept of a Blood-Brain Barrier*. Chichester, Wiley, 1979.

213. Bell BA, et al: CBF and time thresholds for the formation of ischemic cerebral edema, and effect of reperfusion in baboons. *J Neurosurg* 1985; 62:31.

214. Shapira Y, et al: Methylprednisolone does not decrease eicosanoid levels or edema in brain tissue or improve neurological outcome following head trauma in rats. *Anesth Analg* 1992; 75:238.

215. Shapira Y, et al: Brain edema and neurological status following head trauma in the rat; no effect from large volumes of isotonic or hypertonic intravenous fluids, with or without glucose. *Anesthesiology* 1992; 77:79.

216. Hossman K-A: The pathophysiology of ischemic brain swelling. In Inaba Y, Klatzo I, Spatz M (eds): *Brain Edema, Proceedings*

of the Sixth International Symposium. New York, Springer-Verlag, 1985:367–384.

217. Hossman K-A: Treatment of experimental cerebral ischemia. *J Cereb Blood Flow Metab* 1982; 2:275.

218. Shapira Y, et al: Blood brain barrier permeability, cerebral edema and neurological function following closed head injury in rats. *Anesth Analg* 1993; 77:141.

219. Go KG: The classification of brain edema. In de Vlieger M, de Lange SA, Beks JWF (eds): *Brain Edema.* New York, John Wiley, 1981:3–10.

220. Stern J, et al: Visualization of brain interstitial fluid movement during osmotic disequilibrium. *Exp Eye Res* 1977; 25:475.

221. Doczi T, et al: Brain water accumulation after the central administration of vasopressin. *Neurosurgery* 1982; 11:402.

222. DiMattio J, et al: Effects of changes in serum osmolarity on bulk flow of fluid into cerebral ventricles and on brain water content. *Plfugers Arch* 1975; 359:253.

223. Milhorat TH, Hammock MK: Isotope ventriculography. Interpretation of ventricular size and configuration in hydrocephalus. *Arch Neurol* 1971; 25:1.

224. Vorstrup S, et al: Cerebral blood flow in patients with normal pressure hydrocephalus before and after shunting. *J Neurosurg* 1987; 66:379.

225. Artru AA: Reduction of cerebrospinal fluid pressure by hypocapnia: Changes in cerebral blood volume, cerebrospinal fluid volume and brain tissue water and electrolytes. *J Cereb Blood Flow Metabol* 1987; 7:471.

226. Artru AA: Influence of anesthetic agents and techniques on intracranial hemodynamics and cerebral metabolism. In Lam AM (ed): *Anesthetic Management of Acute Head Injury.* New York, McGraw-Hill, 1995:143–179.

227. Milhorat TH: Classification of cerebral edema with reference to hydrocephalus. *Child's Nerv Sys* 1992; 8:301.

228. Saul TG, et al: Steroids in severe head injury. A prospecive randomized clinical trial. *J Neurosurg* 1981; 54:596.

229. Deutschman CS, et al: Physiological and metabolic response to isolated closed head injury. II. Effects of steroids on metabolism. *J Neurosurg* 1987; 66:388.

230. Koide T, et al: Chronic dexamethasone pretreatment aggravates ischemic neuronal necrosis. *J Cere Blood Flow Metab* 1986; 6:395.

231. Pappius HM, Wolfe LS: Functional disturbances in brain following injury: Search for underlying mechanisms. *Neurochem Res* 1983; 8:63.

232. Schilling L, Wahl M: Effects of antihistaminics on experimental brain edema. *Acta Neurochir* 1994; 60(suppl):79.

233. Lorenzl S, et al: Protective effect of a 21-aminosteroid during experimental pneumococcal meningitis. *J Infect Dis* 1995; 172:113.

234. Gamache DA, Ellis EF: Effect of dexamethasone, indomethacin, ibuprofen, and probenecid on carrageenan-induced brain inflammation. *J Neurosurg* 1986; 65:686.

235. Reichman RH, et al: Effects of steroids and nonsteroid anti-inflammatory agents on vascular permeability in a rat glioma model. *J Neurosurg* 1986; 65:233.

236. Rosner MJ, Coley IB: Cerebral perfusion pressure, intracranial pressure, and head elevation. *J Neurosurg* 1986; 65:636.

237. Rosner MJ: The vasodilatory cascade and intracranial pressure. In Miller JD, Teasdale GM, Rowan JO, Gralbraith SL, Mendelow AD (eds): *Intracranial Pressure,* vol. 6. New York, Springer-Verlag, 1986:137–141.

238. Takagi H, et al: The mechanism of ICP reducing effect of mannitol. In Ishii S, Nagai H, Brock M (eds):*Intracranial Pressure,* vol 5, New York, Springer-Verlag, 1983:729–733.

239. Donato T, et al: Effect of mannitol on cerebrospinal fluid dynamics and brain tissue edema. *Anesth Analg* 1994; 78:58.

240. Langfitt TW: Increased intracranial pressure and the cerebral circulation. In Youmans JR (ed) *Neurological Surgery,* vol 2, Philadelphia, WB Saunders, 1982:846–930.

241. Archer DP, et al: Use of mannitol in neuroanesthesia and neurointensive care. *Ann Fr Anesth Ranim* 1995; 14:77.

242. Willis CL, et al: Neuroprotective effect of free radical scavengers on beta-N-oxalyamino-L-alanine (BOAA)-induced neuronal damage in rat hippocampus. *Neurosci Lett* 1994; 182:159.

243. Alzenman E: Modulation of N-methyl-D-aspartate receptors by hydroxyl radicals in rat cortical neurons in vitro. *Neurosci Lett* 1995; 189:57.

244. Cao M, et al: Resolution of brain edema in severe brain injury at controlled high and low intra-cranial pressures. *J Neurosurg* 1984; 61:707.

245. Jennett B, Teasdale G: *Management of Head Injuries.* Philadelphia, FA Davis, 1981.

246. Milhorat TH: *Pediatric Neurosurgery.* Philadelphia, FA Davis, 1978.

247. Lundberg N: The saga of the Monro-Kellie doctrine. In Ishii S, Nagai H, Brock M (eds): *Intracranial Pressure V.* Berlin, Springer-Verlag, 1983:68–76.

248. Fishman RA: Brain edema. *N Engl J Med* 1975; 293:706.

249. Schweitzer JS, et al: Intracranial pressure monitoring. In Cottrell JE, Smith DS (eds): *Anesthesia and Neurosurgery.* St. Louis, CV Mosby, 1994:117–135.

250. Sptezler RF, et al: Normal perfusion pressure breakthrough theory. *Clin Neurosurg* 1978; 25:651.

251. Kelly JP, et al: Concussion in sports. Guidelines for the prevention of catastrophic outcome. *JAMA* 1991; 266:2867.

252. Muizelaar JP, et al: Cerebral blood flow and metabolism in severely head injured children. I. Relationship with GCS score, outcome, ICP, and PVI. *J Neurosurg* 1989; 71:63.

253. Muizelaar, JP, et al: Cerebral blood flow and metabolism in severely head injured children. II. Autoregulation. *J Neurosurg* 1989; 71:72.

254. Rosenwasser RH, et al: Intracranial pressure monitoring in the posterior fossa. A preliminary report. *J Neurosurg* 1989; 71:503.

255. Piek J, Bock WJ: Continuous monitoring of cerebral tissue pressure in neurosurgical practice—experience with 100 patients. *Int Care Med* 1990; 16:184.

256. Finney LA, Walker EA: *Transtentorial Herniation.* Springfield, IL, Charles C Thomas, 1992.

257. Ropper AH: A preliminary study of the geometry of brain displacement and level of consciousness in patients with acute intracranial masses. *Neurology* 1989; 39:622.

258. Langfitt TW, et al: Cerebral vasomotor paralysis produced by intracranial hypertension. *Neurology* 1965; 15:622.

259. Langfitt TW, et al: Transmission of increased intracranial pressure. I. Within the craniospinal axis. *J Neurosurg* 1964; 21:989.

260. Risberg J, et al: Regional cerebral blood volume during acute rises of the intracranial pressure (plateau waves). *J Neurosurg* 1969; 31:303.

261. Muizelaar JP, et al: Effect of mannitol on ICP and CBF and correlation with pressure autoregulation in severely head-injured patients. *J Neurosurg* 1984; 61:700.

262. Cutler RWP, et al: Formation and absorption of cerebrospinal fluid in man. *Brain* 1968; 91:707.

263. Maramarou A, et al: Impact of ICP instability and hypotension on outcome in patients with severe head trauma. *J Neurosurg* 1991; 75 (suppl):S59.

264. Miller JD: Volume and pressure in the craniospinal axis. In Wilkins RH (ed): *Clinical Neurosurgery,* vol 22. Baltimore, Williams & Wilkins, 1975:76–105.

265. Miller JD: Intracranial volume-pressure relationships in pathological conditions. *J Neurosurg Sci* 1976; 20:203.

266. Miller JD, Pickard JD: Intracranial volume-pressure studies in patients with head injury. *Injury* 1974; 5:265.
267. Miller JD, et al: Significance of intracranial hypertension in severe head injury. *J Neurosurg* 1977; 47:503.
268. Maramarou A, et al: A compartmental analysis of compliance and outflow resistance and the effects of elevated blood pressure. In Lundberg N, Ponten U, Brock M (eds): *Intracranial Pressure II.* Berlin, Springer-Verlag, 1975:86–88.
269. Marmarou A, et al: Compartmental analysis of compliance and outflow resistance of the cerebrospinal fluid system. *J Neurosurg* 1976; 43:523.
270. Sullivan HG, et al: CSF pressure transients in response to epidural and ventricular volume loading. *Am J Physiol* 1978; 234:R167.
271. Shapiro K, et al: Characterization of clinical CSF dynamics and neural axis compliance using the pressure-volume index. I. The normal pressure-volume index. *Ann Neurol* 1980; 7:508.
272. Sullivan HG, et al: The physiological basis of ICP change with progressive epidural brain compression: An experimental evaluation in cats. *J Neurosurg* 1977; 45:532.
273. Lin ES, et al: Systems analysis applied to intracranial pressure waveforms and correlation with clinical status in head injured patients. *Br J Anaesth* 1991; 66:476.
274. Lundberg N: Continuous recording and monitoring of ventricular fluid pressure in neurosurgical practice. *Acta Psychiatr Neurol Scand* 1960; 36(suppl 149):1.
275. Lundberg N, et al: Clinical investigations on interrelations between intracranial pressure and intracranial hemodynamics. In Luyendijk W (ed): *Progress in Brain Research,* vol 30. Amsterdam, Elsevier, 1968:69–75.
276. Bray RS, et al: Development of a clinical monitoring system by means of ICP waveform analysis. In Miller JD, Teasdale GM, Rowan JO, et al (eds): *Intracranial Pressure VI.* Berlin, Springer-Verlag, 1986:260–264.
277. Robertson C, et al: Clinical experience with a continuous monitor of intracranial pressure. *J Neurosurg* 1989; 71:673.
278. Wong FC, et al: Waveform analysis of blood pressure, intracranial pressure and transcranial doppler signals and their relationship to cerebral perfusion pressure in head injured patients. In Nagai H, Kamiya K, Ishii S (eds): *Intracranial Pressure IX.* Tokyo, Springer-Verlag, 1994:144–145.
279. Lemaire J-J, et al: Statistical analysis of ICP and frequency analysis of slow waves during the course of subarachnoid haemorrhage following arterial aneurysm rupture: Effects of vasospasm. In Nagai H, Kamiya K, Ishii S (eds): *Intracranial Pressure IX.* Tokyo, Springer-Verlag, 1994:184–188.
280. Matsumoto T, et al: Analysis of intracranial pressure pulse wave in experimental hydrocephalus. In Nagai H, Kamiya K, Ishii S (eds): *Intracranial Pressure IX.* Tokyo, Springer-Verlag, 1994:196–199.
281. Czosnyka M, et al: Prognostic significance of the ICP pulse waveform analysis after severe head injury. In Hagai H, Kamiya K, Ishii S (eds): *Intracranial Pressure IX.* Tokyo, Springer-Verlag, 1994:200–203.
282. Roabe A, Schöche J: Epidural measurement of intracranial compliance by means of high frequency centroid: Comparison to intraventricular or intraparenchymal recordings. In Nagai H, Kamiya K, Ishii S (eds): *Intracranial Pressure IX.* Tokyo, Springer-Verlag, 1994:472–474.
283. Kobayashi S, et al: Does ICP monitoring indicated delayed appearance of traumatic intracerebral hematoma? In Nagai H, Kamiya K, Ishii S (eds): *Intracranial Pressure IX.* Tokyo, Springer-Verlag, 1994:462–463.
284. Hara K, et al: Detection of B waves in the oscillation of intracranial pressure by fast Fourier transform. *Med Inform* 1990; 15:125.

285. Allen R: Intracranial pressure: A review of clinical problems, measurement techniques and monitoring methods. *J Med Eng Technol* 1986; 10:299.
286. Jennett B, Teasdale G: *Epidural, Subdural and Ventricular Monitors for Management of Head Injuries.* Philadelphia, FA Davis, 1989.
287. North B, Reilly P: Comparison among three methods of intracranial pressure recording. *Neurosurgery* 1986; 18:730.
288. Aucoin PJ, et al: Intracranial pressure monitors. Epidemiologic study of risk factors and infections. *Am J Med* 1986; 80:369.
289. Mayhall CG, et al: Ventriculostomy-related infections. A prospective epidemiologic study. *N Engl J Med* 1984; 310:553.
290. Wilkinson HA, et al: Erroneous measurement of intracranial pressure caused by simultaneous ventricular drainage: A hydrodynamic model study. *Neurosurgery* 1989; 24:348.
291. Mollman HD, et al: A clinical comparison of subarachnoid catheters to ventriculostomy and subarachnoid bolt: A prospective study. *J Neurosurg* 1988; 68:737.
292. Bunegin L, et al: Intracranial pressure measurement from the anterior fontanelle utilizing a pneumoelectronic switch. *Neurosurgery* 1987; 20:726.
293. Chambers IR, et al: A clinical evaluation of the Camino subdural screw and ventricular monitoring kits. *Neurosurgery* 1990; 6:421.
294. Crutchfield JS, et al: Evaluation of a fiberoptic intracranial pressure monitor. *J Neurosurg* 1990; 72:482.
295. Ostrup RC, et al: Continuous monitoring of intracranial pressure with a miniaturized fiberoptic device. *J Neurosurg* 1987; 67:206.
296. Artru AA, Katz RA: Comparison of spinal needles, epidural catheters and Cordis/lumbar catheters for intraoperative removal of CSF. *Neurosurgery* 1988; 22:101.
297. Jackson H: The management of acute cranial injuries by the early exact determination of intracranial pressure and its relief by lumbar drainage. *Surg Gynecol Obstet* 1922; 34:494.
298. McCreery JA, Berry FB: A study of 520 cases of fracture of the skull. *Ann Surg* 1928; 88:890.
299. Browder J, Meyers R: Observations on behavior of the systemic blood pressure, pulse and spinal fluid pressure following craniocerebral injury. *Am J Surg* 1936; 31:403.
300. Lundberg N, et al: Continuous recording of ventricular fluid pressure in patients with severe acute traumatic brain injury: A preliminary report. *J Neurosurg* 1965; 22:581.
301. Marmarou A, et al: NINDS traumatic coma data bank: Intracranial pressure monitoring methodology. *J Neurosurg* 1991; 75(suppl):S21.
302. Marshall LF, et al: A new classification of head injury based on computerized tomography. *J Neurosurg* 1991; 75(suppl):S14.
303. Nordby HK, Gunnerod N: Epidural monitoring of the intracranial pressure in severe head injury characterized by nonlocalizing motor responses. *Acta Neurochir* 1985; 74:21.
304. Bailes JE, et al: Management morbidity and mortality of poor-grade aneurysm patients. *J Neurosurg* 1990; 72:559.
305. Adams RD, Victor M: Disturbances of cerebrospinal fluid circulation, including hydrocephalus and meningeal reactions. In Adams RD, Victor M (eds): *Principles of Neurology,* ed 3. New York, McGraw-Hill, 1985:461–473.
306. Dearden NM, et al: Effect of high-dose dexamethasone on outcome from severe head injury. *J Neurosurg* 1986; 64:81.
307. Lam AM, et al: Hyperglycemia and neurological outcome in patients with head injury. *J Neurosurg* 1991; 75:545.
308. Obrist WD, et al: Cerebral blood flow and metabolism in comatose patients with acute head injury: Relationship to intracranial hypertension. *J Neurosurg* 1984; 61:241.
309. Muizelaar JP, et al: Adverse effects of prolonged hyperventila-

tion in patients with severe head injury: A randomized clinical trial. *J Neurosurg* 1991; 75:731.

310. Stangland KJ, et al: Canine cerebral function and blood flow after complete cerebral ischemia: Effect of head position. *Anesthesiology* 1986; 64:430.

311. Schreiber G, Aldred AR: Molecular cloning of choroid plexus-specific transport proteins. In Pardridge WM (ed): *The Blood-Brain Barrier; Cellular and Molecular Biology.* New York, Raven Press, 1993:441–459.

312. Pardridge WM, Boado RJ: Molecular cloning and regulation of gene expression of blood-brain barrier glucose transporter.

In Pardridge WM (ed): *The Blood-Brain Barrier; Cellular and Molecular Biology.* New York, Raven Press, 1993:395–440.

313. Greig NH: Drug delivery to the brain by blood-brain barrier circumvention and drug modification. In Neuwalt EA (ed): *Implications of the Blood-Brain Barrier and Its Manipulation,* vol 1. *Basic Science Aspects.* New York, Plenum Medical Book Company, 1989:311–367.

314. Rosenberg GA: Glucose, amino acids, and lipids. In Rosenberg GA (ed): *Brain Fluids and Metabolism.* New York, Oxford University Press, 1990:119–144.

Chapter 4 _____

PERIOPERATIVE FLUID MANAGEMENT OF THE NEUROSURGICAL PATIENT

MARK H. ZORNOW

CHRISTOPHER MCQUITTY

DONALD S. PROUGH

The perioperative fluid management of patients with neurologic dysfunction presents many challenges. Optimizing intravascular volume, improving cerebral blood flow (CBF), and minimizing cerebral edema are just a few of the sometimes conflicting goals. This chapter reviews the basic physiologic principles that determine the movement of water between the intra- and extracellular spaces, both in peripheral tissues and the brain, before addressing specific pathologic conditions.

Physical Principles Governing Fluid Movement between the Intra- and Extravascular Spaces

Total body water is partitioned between the intracellular volume (ICV) and extracellular volume (ECV) by the cell membrane, which is semipermeable to water but poorly permeable to most ions and all proteins. Under certain circumstances, water can be redistributed between the ICV and ECV by the creation of osmotic gradients, usually accomplished by changing the serum sodium concentration ($[Na^+]$). In peripheral tissues, fluid distribution between the intravascular and interstitial compartments is governed by gradients of oncotic pressure, that is, the proportion of osmotic pressure attributable to colloid. With the notable exception of those located in the brain and spinal cord, capillaries are highly permeable to water, ions, and other low molecular weight (MW) compounds, but limit the movement of high MW substances, including albumin, globulins, and synthetic colloids such as hetastarch and dextrans.

OSMOLALITY

Osmolality is one of the four colligative properties of a solution (the others being vapor pressure, freezing point depression, and boiling point elevation). The addition of one osmole of any solute to 1 kg water will cause the vapor pressure to fall by 0.3 mmHg, the

TABLE 4-1
Osmolarities and Oncotic Pressures of Common Intravenous Fluids

Fluid	Solute(s) Primarily Responsible for Osmolarity	Osmolarity (mosm/liter)	Osmotic Pressure (mmHg)	Solutes Contributing to Oncotic Pressure	Oncotic Pressure (mmHg)[a]
Lactated Ringer's	Na+, Cl−	273	5269		0
D5 lactated Ringer's	Glu, Na+, Cl−	525	10,133		0
0.9% saline	Na+, Cl−	308	5944		0
D5 0.45% saline	Glu, Na+, Cl−	406	7836		0
0.45% saline	Na+, Cl−	154	2972		0
20% mannitol		1098	21,191		0
Hydroxyethyl starch (6%)	Na+, Cl−	310	5983	HES	312
Dextran 40 (10%)[b]	Na+, Cl−	≈300	5790	DEX	1693
Dextran 70 (6%)	Na+, Cl−	≈300	5790	DEX	193
Albumin (5%)	Na+, Cl−	290	5597	Alb	19
Plasma	Na+, Cl−	295	5694	Prot	21

[a]Colloid osmotic pressure

[b]Low molecular weight dextran

NOTE: Alb, albumin; D5, 5% dextrose (glucose); DEX, dextran; glu, glucose; HES, hydroxyethyl starch; Prot, serum protein

freezing point to decrease by 1.85°C, and the boiling point to increase by 0.52°C.[1] These colligative properties are determined solely by the *number* of particles in solution and are independent of the chemical structure, ionization, and MW of the solute. Equimolar concentrations of glucose, urea, or mannitol equally influence the colligative properties of a solution.

For physiologic solutions, *osmolality* is commonly expressed as milliosmoles (mosm) *per kg of solvent*, whereas the units of measure for *osmolarity* are mOsm *per liter of solution*. For dilute solutions (including most of physiologic importance), the two terms may be used interchangeably. The osmolarities of some commonly used intravenous fluids are shown in Table 4-1.

Osmolarity can be easily calculated if the MW of the solute is known. A 0.9% solution of sodium chloride (NaCl) contains 9 g/liter. Since the gram-MW of NaCl is 58.43, the 0.9% concentration provides a 0.154 molar or 154 millimolar solution.

$$9\text{ g/liter} \div 58.43\text{ g/mole} = 0.154\text{ mole/liter} \quad \text{(Eq. 1)}$$

Because, at this concentration, each molecule of NaCl disassociates into a Na+ and a Cl− ion, multiplying the molar value by 2 yields an osmolarity of 308 mosm/liter.

Osmolarity is important in determining fluid movement between various physiologic compartments because of the osmotic pressure generated when solutions of unequal osmolarity are separated by a membrane permeable to water but not the solutes. According to the second law of thermodynamics, which

states that all systems spontaneously change in a manner to maximize entropy, there will be a tendency for water to move from the solution of lower osmolality, across the membrane, and dilute the solution of higher osmolality. This movement of water continues until the osmolalities on both sides of the membrane equalize. The force driving the movement of water across the semipermeable membrane can be calculated from the following equation:

$$\pi = CRT \quad \text{(Eq. 2)}$$

where π is the osmotic pressure in atmospheres, C is the difference in the concentration of the solute in moles per liter, R is the gas constant (0.08206 liter-atm/mole-degree), and T is temperature in degrees Kelvin. Using this equation, we can calculate the osmotic pressure produced by two solutions that differ by 1 mosm separated by a semipermeable membrane at body temperature.

$C = 0.001$ moles (i.e., 1 mosm), $R = 0.08206$,
$T = 273° + 36° = 309°$ (body temperature in °K).

Therefore,

$$\begin{aligned} \pi &= 0.001 \times 0.08206 \times 309° \\ &= 0.02535\text{ atm or } 19.27\text{ mmHg} \end{aligned} \quad \text{(Eq. 3)}$$

Using the above formula, one can calculate that for each mosm difference across a semipermeable membrane, a pressure of approximately 19.3 mmHg will be generated (see Table 4-1). Thus, osmolar differences can provide a potent driving force for the movement of water between the ICV and ECV, and, as we shall discuss later, across the blood-brain barrier (BBB). Although transient osmolar gradients can be produced by the administration of hypo- or hyperosmolar fluids, these gradients are fleeting and water will move from one compartment to another so that all body fluids once again are of equal osmolarity.

OSMOTIC PRESSURE VERSUS ONCOTIC PRESSURE

Oncotic pressure is simply the osmotic pressure generated by solutes larger than an arbitrary limit (usually 30,000 MW). Albumin (approximate MW 69,000), hetastarch (mean MW 480,000), dextran 40 (mean MW 40,000), and dextran 70 (mean MW 70,000) are clinically important compounds that exert oncotic pressure. Osmotic and oncotic pressures of plasma and solutions of mannitol, hydroxyethyl starch, dextran, and albumin are shown in Table 4-1. Because colloids are particles suspended in solution, they will contribute to the total osmolality and osmotic pressure of the fluid. However, because they are present in such small numbers compared to the ionic components of the solution, their contribution is small. The oncotic pressure produced by all plasma proteins (albumin, globulins, fibrinogen, etc.) accounts for less than 0.5 percent of total plasma osmotic pressure.

THE STARLING EQUATION

Nearly 100 years ago, Starling described the forces that determine the movement of water between the tissues and the intravascular space.[2] This description was subsequently formalized as what is now known as the Starling equation:

$$Q_f = K_f S[(P_c - P_i) - \sigma(\pi_c - \pi_i)] \qquad \text{(Eq. 4)}$$

where Q_f represents the net amount of fluid that moves between the capillary lumen and the surrounding interstitial space; K_f is the filtration coefficient for the membrane; S is the surface area of the capillary membrane; P_c is the hydrostatic pressure in the capillary lumen; P_i is the hydrostatic pressure (usually negative) in the interstitium of the surrounding tissue; and σ is the reflection coefficient. This number, which can range from 0 (no movement of the solute across the membrane) to 1 (free diffusion of the solute across the membrane), quantifies the "leakiness" of the capillary and will be different for vessels in the brain versus peripheral tissues; π_c is the colloid osmotic pressure in the capillary plasma; and π_i is the colloid osmotic pressure of the fluid in the interstitium.[3]

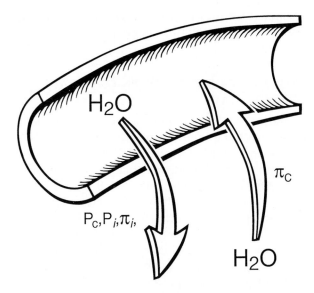

Figure 4-1 The Starling equation identifies the three forces favoring the movement of water from the intravascular space into the interstitium. These three forces are the capillary hydrostatic pressure (P_c), the interstitial hydrostatic pressure (P_i), and the interstitial oncotic pressure (π_i). The only force acting to maintain water in the capillary lumen is π_c, the plasma oncotic pressure.

P_c, P_i (which is negative in nonedematous tissues), and π_i act together to draw fluid from the capillaries and into the interstitial space of the tissue. The only factor that maintains intravascular volume is π_c, which is produced predominantly by albumin and to a lesser extent by immunoglobulins, fibrinogen, and other high MW plasma proteins (Fig. 4-1).

Under most circumstances, the summation of the forces results in a value for Q_f slightly greater than zero, indicating a net outward flux of fluid from the vessels and into the tissue interstitial space. This fluid is cleared from the tissue by the lymphatic system, thereby preventing the development of edema.

The clinical effects of altering one or more of the variables in the Starling equation may frequently be observed in surgical patients. Many patients who have been resuscitated from hemorrhagic hypovolemia with large volumes of crystalloid solutions develop pitting edema owing to dilution of plasma proteins, resulting in a decrease in π_c. In the face of relatively unchanged P_c, fluid movement from the vasculature into the tissues will increase. When this fluid flux exceeds the drainage capacity of the lymphatics, clinically apparent edema is the result. Another example of the Starling equation is profound facial edema, which is frequently seen in patients who have been placed in the prone, head-down position for extensive lumbar surgery. In these patients, the edema does not result from a decrease in π_c, but rather from a regional increase in P_c favoring increased transudation of fluid into facial tissue. In either case, the amount of edema tends to be self-limited because P_i increases as the fluid accumulates in the interstitium, thereby limiting further fluid transudation.

FLUID MOVEMENT BETWEEN CAPILLARIES AND THE BRAIN

The Starling equilibrium most accurately describes the factors governing fluid movement between the intravascular and peripheral interstitial spaces (e.g., the interstitium of lung, bowel, or muscle). In cerebral capillaries, σ for most solutes is nearly 1.0. The brain and spinal cord, unlike most other tissues, are isolated from the intravascular compartment by the BBB. Morphologically, this barrier is now thought to be composed of endothelial cells that form tight junctions in the capillaries supplying the brain and spinal cord. In normal brain, these tight junctions severely restrict the diffusion of molecules between the intravascular space and the brain. By measuring the movement of water out of the central nervous system (CNS) after abrupt changes in plasma osmolality, Fenstermacher and Johnson calculated the effective pore radius for the BBB to be only 7 to 9 Å.[4] This small pore size of the BBB thereby prevents the movement not only of plasma proteins, but also of sodium, chloride, and potassium ions between the intravascular compartment and the brain's interstitial space. In effect, the BBB functions in a fashion similar to the solute-impermeable membrane on an osmometer, that is, transmembrane movement of water is determined by the relative concentrations of impermeant solutes.

In contrast, in systemic capillary beds in which endothelial cells do not form tight junctions, the pore sizes may be a thousandfold larger. Although larger pores may preclude free movement of most protein components of plasma, electrolytes pass freely from the capillary lumen into the interstitial space. Hence, in peripheral tissues, movement of water is governed by the transcapillary concentration difference of large macromolecules ($\pi_c - \pi_i$), as predicted by the Starling equation. In contrast, fluid movement in and out of brain capillaries is primarily determined by the *osmolar* gradient (which is determined by relative concentrations of *all* osmotically active particles, including most electrolytes) between the plasma and the interstitium. This difference in the determinants of fluid flux explains why the administration of large volumes of iso-osmolar crystalloid will result in peripheral edema owing to dilutional reduction of plasma protein content, but does not increase brain water content or intracranial pressure (ICP).

IMPLICATIONS FOR PATIENT CARE

Because osmolality is the primary determinant of water movement across the intact BBB,[5] the administration of excess free water (i.e., in parenteral or enteral fluids in which the [Na^+] is less than or the [H_2O] is greater than plasma concentrations) can increase ICP and result in an edematous brain.[6] Conversely, the intravenous administration of markedly hyperosmolar crystalloids (e.g., mannitol) to increase plasma osmolarity will decrease brain water content and ICP. Use of hyperosmolar solutions, a routine part of neurosurgical practice, represents a standard therapy for the treatment of intracranial hypertension. Increasing plasma osmolality creates an osmotic gradient favoring the movement of water into plasma from both the brain interstitial space and the brain intracellular compartment.

Despite convincing experimental evidence that isotonic crystalloid solutions (those in which [Na^+] approximates serum [Na^+]) exert minimal effects on brain water or ICP, conventional clinical practice has restricted the use of crystalloids in patients at risk for intracranial hypertension.[7] The infusion of colloids has often been recommended to maintain plasma volume (PV) in such patients, with the inference by clinicians that maintaining or increasing π_c will decrease cerebral edema. However, if the BBB is intact, neither theory nor experimental evidence would suggest a benefit of colloids. More recently, the crystalloid-colloid question has been addressed in animal models of cerebral injury with varying and sometimes conflicting results. Warner and Boehland[8] studied the effects of hemodilution with either 0.9% saline or 6% hydroxyethyl starch (dissolved in 0.9% saline) in rats subjected to 10 minutes of severe forebrain ischemia. Despite approximately a 50 percent reduction in π_c in the saline group (from 17.2 ± 0.8 to 9.0 ± 0.6 mmHg), hetastarch produced no beneficial effect on cerebral edema formation. Similarly, in a study using cryogenic cerebral injury, Zornow and colleagues[9] found no differences in regional water content or ICP in animals that received 0.9% saline, 6% hetastarch (in 0.9% saline), or 5% albumin (in 0.9% saline). In contrast, Korosue and coworkers[10] found a smaller infarct volume and improved neurologic status in dogs hemodiluted with a colloid (low MW dextran) when compared with animals hemodiluted with lactated Ringer's solution after ligation of the middle cerebral artery (MCA). The authors speculated, but did not provide direct evidence, that this beneficial effect was attributable to decreased edema formation in the ischemic zone because of an ischemia-induced increase in the permeability of the BBB to ions with preservation of impermeability to high MW colloids. If this were correct, capillaries in ischemic brain tissue would function as peripheral capillaries (i.e., decreases in π_c would result in increased water movement into the tissue).[10] Unfortunately, this speculation remains in question as most other experimental studies of stroke have failed to show a benefit of colloid infusions.[11]

In contrast, hyperosmolar (hypertonic) solutions, in circumstances of localized brain injury with disruption of the BBB, appear to readily cause fluid flux out of brain tissue in which the BBB remains intact. In effect, "dehydration" of normal brain compensates for edema in injured brain. In experimental cryogenic brain injury, infusion of a hypertonic solution attenuated the increase in ICP associated with the lesion but did not change the water content of brain tissue at the lesion site or in its immediate vicinity.[12] The most likely mechanism for the reduced ICP is a decrease in brain water content in regions remote from the lesion.

Regulation of Extracellular Fluid Volume

Renal adaptation to hypovolemia (and decreased cardiac output) occurs through three primary mechanisms: reduction of renal blood flow (RBF), reduction of glomerular filtration rate (GFR), and increased tubular reabsorption of sodium and water.[13] Initially, RBF is maintained (i.e., RBF is autoregulated) as perfusion pressure decreases by reductions in renal afferent arteriolar resistance. Further decreases in cardiac output may decrease the fraction of cardiac output delivered to the kidneys. Increases in renal vascular resistance redistribute blood flow from the kidneys in an attempt to preserve perfusion of other tissues.

Renal perfusion during acute hypovolemia is determined by the balance between renal vasoconstrictive factors (the renal sympathetic nerves, angiotensin II, and catecholamines) and vasodilatory mechanisms (intrinsic renal autoregulation and the renal vasodilatory effects of prostaglandins).[14] Autoregulation of RBF (maintenance of relatively constant RBF over a wide range of perfusion pressures) may be impaired or lost during severe, acute hypovolemia.[15] Renal sympathetic stimulation with secretion of α-adrenergic catecholamines and angiotensin II increases renal vascular resistance.

To preserve PV, reabsorption of filtered water and sodium is enhanced by changes mediated by the hormonal factors antidiuretic hormone (ADH), atrial natriuretic peptide (ANP), and aldosterone. A 10 to 20 percent decrease in blood volume is necessary before ADH secretion from the posterior pituitary increases.[16] ADH acts primarily on the medullary collecting ducts to increase water reabsorption and cause excretion of smaller volumes of more highly concentrated urine. ANP secretion is decreased during hypovolemia. ANP, released from the cardiac atria in response to increased atrial stretch, exerts vasodilatory effects and increases the renal excretion of sodium and water.[17,18]

In volume-depleted states, sodium conservation results both from decreased filtration of sodium (decreased GFR) and from increased tubular reabsorption of sodium, mediated by aldosterone. Hypoperfusion stimulates the granular cells of the renal juxtaglomerular apparatus to release renin, which catalyzes the conversion of angiotensinogen to angiotensin I. Angiotensin-converting enzyme converts angiotensin I to angiotensin II, which stimulates the adrenal cortex to synthesize and release aldosterone.[19] Acting primarily in the distal tubules, high concentrations of aldosterone may reduce urinary excretion of sodium nearly to zero.

The kidney also contains large quantities of vasodilator prostaglandins that may play a crucial role in protecting the kidney from vasoconstrictor hormones and in maintaining RBF during hypovolemia. The protective effect of endogenous renal prostaglandins may be lost if renal circulatory compromise develops in patients receiving nonsteroidal anti-inflammatory drugs (NSAIDs).[20]

Characteristics of Intravenous Fluids

Most solutions used for intravenous administration are categorized as crystalloids or colloids. Crystalloid solutions are subdivided into hypotonic, isotonic, and hypertonic solutions.

CRYSTALLOIDS

Crystalloids are solutions composed solely of low MW solutes (MW < 30,000), which may be charged (e.g., Na^+, Cl^-) or uncharged (e.g., mannitol). Because these solutions by definition lack high MW solutes, the oncotic (colloid osmotic) pressure is zero. Colloquially, the terms *hypotonic, isotonic, and hypertonic* refer to fluids in which the total osmolarity is less than, roughly equal to, or greater than serum osmolality. However, as is evident from the discussion of the impermeability of the BBB to sodium, the more important consideration is whether the fluid has a [Na^+] less than, approximately equal to, or greater than plasma. Unless another osmole, such as dextrose or mannitol, is present in large quantities, the proportion of water in excess of that necessary to provide an isonatremic solution is the variable of greatest interest.

Solutions containing free water ([Na^+] substantially less than that of serum), when infused rapidly in large volumes, lower plasma osmolality, drive water across the BBB into the brain, and increase cerebral water content and ICP. The dextrose in solutions may temporarily increase serum glucose concentration, holding water intravascularly. However, as the serum glucose concentration decreases, changes in serum [Na^+] induced by the ratio of sodium to water in the infused fluid again become critical.

TABLE 4-2
Characteristics of Hetastarch, Pentastarch, and Pentafraction

Characteristic	Hetastarch	Pentastarch	Pentafraction
No. avg. molecular weight	70,000	63,000	120,000
Wt. avg. molecular weight	450,000	264,000	280,000
Colloid osmotic pressure (mmHg)(6% solution)	35	30	28

NOTE: No. avg. molecular weight, number average molecular weight, i.e., the arithmetic mean of all molecules; wt. avg. molecular weight, weight average molecular weight, i.e., the sum of the number of hydroxyethyl starch molecules at each number average molecular weight ÷ the total weight of all molecules. The removal of molecules < 100,000 explains the higher no. avg. molecular weight of pentafraction.

The most commonly used "isotonic" fluids are lactated Ringer's solution and 0.9% saline. Lactated Ringer's solution actually is mildly hyponatremic when compared to plasma (see Table 4-1). When large volumes of lactated Ringer's solution are infused rapidly, the free water (approximately 114 ml/liter) may decrease serum [Na^+] and plasma osmolality and increase brain water and ICP.

For many years, hypertonic mannitol, a six-carbon sugar (MW 182), has been the primary agent used for therapeutic brain dehydration. Excreted unchanged in the urine, mannitol is available as 20% and 25% solutions (osmolarities of 1098 and 1372 mosm/liter). Usually given in doses of 0.25 to 1.5 g/kg, mannitol cannot pass through the intact BBB; hence, intravenous administration acutely increases plasma osmolality and establishes an osmotic gradient favoring the movement of water from the brain's interstitial space into the vasculature. Rapid administration of large doses of mannitol may have a biphasic effect on ICP. Initially, ICP may increase owing to an increased cerebral blood volume as a consequence of the cerebral vasodilatory effects of the acute increase in plasma osmolarity. Subsequently, ICP will decrease owing to the movement of water from the brain interstitial space into the vasculature.

COLLOIDS

A variety of colloidal solutions are available for clinical use. Each gram of intravascular colloid holds approximately 20 ml of water in the circulation (14 to 15 ml/g of albumin; 16 to 17 ml/g of hetastarch; 20 to 25 ml/g of dextran 70).[21] After equilibration, PV expansion is determined primarily by the number of grams of colloid infused, not by the original volume or concentration of the infusate.[21] Concentrated colloid-containing solutions (e.g., 25% albumin) may exert sufficient oncotic pressure to translocate substantial volumes of interstitial fluid into the PV.

Hydroxyethyl starch or hetastarch (Hespan) is a 6% solution of hydrolyzed amylopectin dissolved in 0.9% saline (Table 4-2). Eighty percent of the molecules range in size from 30,000 to 2,400,000 daltons. The weight average MW for hetastarch is approximately 480,000 daltons. The low MW fraction of an administered dose of hetastarch (those hetastarch molecules weighing less than 50,000 daltons) is excreted by renal filtration within 24 h. Although the incidence of allergic reactions to hetastarch is extremely low, the compound can induce a coagulopathy when given in large doses. The mechanism by which hetastarch affects coagulation is multifactorial, including hemodilution of clotting factors, inhibition of platelet function and reduction of the activity of factor VIII.[22] Sporadic case reports of prolonged clotting times after administration of hetastarch have prompted many neurosurgeons and neurointensivists to use hetastarch with caution or to avoid it altogether in patients at risk for intracranial hemorrhage. In an uncontrolled series, 14 patients treated with hetastarch for volume expansion to treat cerebral vasospasm developed a significant increase in partial thromboplastin time; six developed clinically significant bleeding.[23] In contrast, 12 patients receiving plasma protein fraction had no increase in partial thromboplastin time and no clinical coagulopathy.

Pentastarch (Pentaspan), a new formulation of hydrolyzed amylopectin approved for use during leukopheresis, may have a role as a PV expander. Pentastarch differs from hetastarch in that it has a lower mean weight average MW (264,000 versus 480,000 for hetastarch), which results in more rapid and complete renal clearance of the compound. Seventy percent of pentastarch versus 30 percent of hetastarch is excreted in the urine within 24 h. Preliminary studies also suggest that pentastarch may have fewer adverse effects on coagulation than hetastarch.

Pentafraction is a diafiltered solution of hydrolyzed amylopectin similar to pentastarch but with a more narrow range of MW (see Table 4-2). Because both the high and low MW molecules have been eliminated from pentafraction, the weight average MW remains unchanged from that of pentastarch. One interesting hypothesis is that colloids with a MW near that of pentafraction may "plug leaks" that develop in the BBB after a variety of ischemic or traumatic insults. Several studies suggest that pentafraction decreases permeability in the vascular beds of tissues damaged by ischemia or thermal injury.[24–28] Pentafraction may be superior to hetastarch in the capillary leak syndrome that occurs in sepsis.[29] Pentafraction is not commercially available at this time.

Dextran solutions (dextran 40 and dextran 70) are colloids composed of glucose polymers with mean MWs, respectively, of 40,000 and 70,000. Whereas the oncotic pressure of dextran 70 approximates that of plasma, resulting in volume-expanding capabilities similar to albumin, dextran 40 is hyperoncotic and can transiently expand PV by more than the amount infused by recruiting interstitial water into the vascular space. About 50 percent of dextran 40 (low MW dextran) and dextran 70 is renally excreted within 24 to 48 h of administration. A variety of adverse effects have limited the clinical use of dextrans. Occasional anaphylactoid reactions, occurring in approximately 0.032 percent of patients, can be prevented by the prior administration of 20 ml of very low MW dextran (dextran 1) immediately before giving either dextran 40 or 70. Dextran 1 binds to circulating IgG, preventing it from cross linking with larger dextran molecules and activating complement. An additional problem with dextran solutions is that administration of volumes exceeding 20 percent of blood volume may interfere with blood typing and cross matching.

Available in either 5% or 25% concentrations, human serum albumin is an effective volume expander that has not been associated with allergic-type reactions and has no intrinsic effects on clotting. However, because albumin solutions are devoid of clotting factors found in whole blood or fresh plasma, large doses may produce a dilutional coagulopathy. Although derived from pooled human plasma, the risk of disease transmission is nearly eliminated by heat-treating and ultrafiltration. Albumin can be given without regard to the recipient's blood type because all of the isoagglutinins have been removed during processing. Although safe and effective as a volume expander, albumin solutions, volume for volume, are approximately three times more expensive than hetastarch.

Fresh frozen plasma (FFP) should be reserved for use only when there is an acute need to replace clotting factors and there is evidence of a dilutional coagulopathy. Volume expansion and nutritional support are no longer considered valid uses for fresh plasma or FFP. Although all plasma is derived from volunteer blood

donors and careful screening procedures have been implemented, the risk of disease transmission remains a reality. The risk of transmitting hepatitis C is estimated at 1 in 3300 units, hepatitis B at 1 in 200,000 units, and human immunodeficiency virus at 1 in 225,000 units.[30]

CRYSTALLOID VERSUS COLLOID CONTROVERSY

If membrane permeability is intact, colloids such as albumin or hydroxyethyl starch preferentially expand PV rather than interstitial fluid volume (IFV). Concentrated colloid-containing solutions (e.g., 25% albumin) may exert sufficient oncotic pressure to translocate substantial volumes of IFV into the PV. PV expansion unaccompanied by IFV expansion offers apparent advantages: lower fluid requirements, less peripheral and pulmonary edema accumulation, and reduced concern about the cardiopulmonary consequences of later fluid mobilization.

However, exhaustive research has failed to establish the superiority of either colloid-containing or crystalloid-containing fluids (Table 4-3). Much of the debate has centered on the relative risks of pulmonary edema and cerebral edema. Crystalloid solutions are associated with pulmonary edema, usually as a result of increased P_c, perhaps in combination with a reduction in π_c. Colloid may also produce increases, often sustained, in P_c. Moreover, in disease states associated with increased alveolar capillary permeability (i.e., sepsis or the adult respiratory distress syndrome), infusion of colloid may aggravate pulmonary edema. Increased microvascular permeability abolishes the gradient between π_c and π_i. In the absence of an oncotic pressure gradient, mimimal increases in the hydraulic gradient can generate clinically important pulmonary edema.

Hypoproteinemia in critically ill patients has been associated with the development of pulmonary edema[31] and with increased mortality.[32] Either crystalloid or colloid administration may precipitate pulmonary edema in patients who have valvular heart disease, decreased left ventricular compliance, or decreased left ventricular contractility (i.e., heart failure). However, physiologic defenses must be overwhelmed before the accumulation of interstitial fluid results in clinically apparent pulmonary edema. After experimentally increasing microvascular permeability, Pearl and colleagues found no differences between increases in extravascular lung water induced by colloid or crystalloid administration.[33]

In surgical patients at risk for the development of pulmonary edema, pulmonary artery catheterization may facilitate management. Pulmonary artery occlu-

TABLE 4-3
Colloid versus Crystalloid Intravenous Fluids

Solution	Advantages	Disadvantages
Colloid	Smaller infused volume	Greater cost
	Prolonged increase in plasma volume	Coagulopathy (dextran > HES)
	Less peripheral edema	Pulmonary edema (capillary leak states)
		Decreased GFR
		Osmotic diuresis (low molecular weight dextran)
Crystalloid	Lower cost	Transient hemodynamic improvement
	Greater urinary flow	Peripheral edema (protein dilution)
	Replaces interstitial fluid	Pulmonary edema (protein dilution plus high PAOP)

NOTE: GFR, glomerular filtration rate; HES, hydroxyethyl starch; PAOP, pulmonary artery occlusion pressure

sion pressure (PAOP) should be maintained at the lowest level compatible with adequate systemic perfusion. Theoretically, hemodynamic monitoring coupled with volume expansion with colloid (to preserve π_c) should minimize edema formation. However, Virgilio and coworkers found no correlation in surgical patients between intrapulmonary shunt fraction (Q_s / Q_t) and the π_c–PAOP gradient.[34]

Part of the difficulty in defining the superiority of crystalloid or colloid fluids is directly attributable to the difficulty of defining comparable end points in clinically relevant experimental models.[35] More recently developed models replicate clinical situations, permitting a more clinically useful comparison of crystalloid and colloid solutions. In animals infused with *Escherichia coli* lipopolysaccharide, which mimics some aspects of clinical sepsis, equivalent doses (defined in terms of PV) of lactated Ringer's solution of 6.0% hydroxyethyl starch produced comparable effects on the critical end point of oxygen delivery while producing the expected differences in extravascular fluid accumulation.[36] In a more complex porcine model, consisting of temporary exteriorization of the small intestine accompanied by incremental hemorrhage and replacement, colloid solutions, in contrast to Ringer's acetate solution, produced superior restoration of cardiac output, oxygen delivery, and oxygen consumption.[37] Further investigation is required.

HYPERTONIC SALINE SOLUTIONS

Recently, hypertonic saline solutions have been proposed for the treatment of hemorrhagic shock and control of intracranial hypertension. Although investigators have studied various hypertonic resuscitation solutions for much of this century,[38-45] current enthusiasm results from the work of Velasco and colleagues.[40]

In lightly anesthetized dogs that had been subjected to sufficient hemorrhage to reduce mean arterial pressure (MAP) to 45 to 50 mmHg for 30 min, small volumes (4.0 to 6.0 ml/kg) of 7.5% hypertonic saline restored systolic blood pressure and cardiac output and increased mesenteric blood flow to greater than control values for 6 h after resuscitation.[40] In experimental animals, hypertonic solutions decrease ICP by "dehydrating" brain tissue in which the BBB is intact. Intravenous infusions of small volumes of hypertonic saline solutions have been reported to rapidly restore blood pressure, improve urinary output, and decrease ICP in patients who have failed to respond to large doses of mannitol.[46] Three percent saline has been used to decrease ICP in hemodynamically stable, head-injured children.[47] These solutions should be administered in judicious amounts and with frequent monitoring of plasma osmolality and sodium concentrations (Table 4-4).

The primary mechanism by which hyperosmotic saline increases venous return is by expansion of PV.[48] Hypernatremic fluids acutely increase PV both by osmotic attraction of water from the ICV into the ECV and by transient translocation of IFV into the PV. The immediate effect is, in part, attributable to the fact that permeability of the systemic capillaries to sodium is not complete ($\sigma = 0.1$); therefore, IFV is translocated into the PV until equilibration occurs.

The effects after equilibration on ECV and ICV of adding hyperosmotic saline can be calculated as follows:[49]

$$\frac{\text{new total extracellular solute}}{\text{new ECV}} = \frac{\text{total intracellular solute}}{\text{new ICV}} \quad \text{(Eq. 5)}$$

For instance, assume that a healthy 70-kg patient ($[Na^+] = 140$ meq/liter) were to receive 2.0 ml/kg

TABLE 4-4
Advantages and Disadvantages of Hypertonic Resuscitation Fluids

Solution	Advantages	Disadvantages
Hypertonic crystalloid	Inexpensive Promotes urinary flow Small initial volume Improved myocardial contractility? Arteriolar dilation Reduced peripheral edema Lower intracranial pressure	Hypertonicity Subdural hemorrhage Transient effect
Hypertonic crystalloid plus colloid (in comparison to hypertonic crystalloid alone)	Sustained hemodynamic response Reduced subsequent volume requirements	Added expense Coagulopathy (dextran > HES) Osmotic diuresis Impaired crossmatch (dextran)

NOTE: HES, hydroxyethyl starch
SOURCE: Reproduced with permission from Prough and Johnston.[35]

of 7.5% saline (~1283 meq/liter); 179 meq of sodium would be added as new extracellular solute. Before infusion, total extracellular sodium would be 1960 meq (140 meq/liter × 14 liters) and total intracellular potassium, the predominant intracellular solute, would be 3920 meq (140 meq/liter × 28 liters). The equation would then be calculated as:

$$\frac{1960 \text{ meq} + 179 \text{ meq}}{141 + x} = \frac{3920 \text{ meq}}{281 - x} \quad \text{(Eq. 6)}$$

where x = the increase in ECV. The new total ECV would equal 14.8 liters (14 liters + 0.8 liter), and the new total ICV would equal 27.2 (28 liters − 0.8 liter). Assuming that the increase in ECV = 0.8 liter, the increase in PV would be approximately 160 ml, that is, one-fifth of the total increase in ECV.

Hypertonic saline has been associated, as has high-volume resuscitation using 0.9% saline, with hyperchloremic acidosis (Table 4-5). The gradual change in neuroanesthesia practice from the use of lactated Ringer's solution to 0.9% saline has resulted in the more common postoperative occurrence of hyperchloremic metabolic acidosis. Metabolic acidosis is usually characterized by a reduced pH (< 7.35) and reduced $[HCO_3^-]$ (Table 4-6). Metabolic acidosis associated with a high anion gap (> 13 meq/liter) occurs due to excess production of lactic acid or ketoacids, increased retention of waste products (such as sulfate and phosphate) that are inadequately excreted in uremic states, and ingestion of toxic quantities of substances such as aspirin, ethylene glycol, and methanol.

The treatment of metabolic acidosis consists of treatment of the primary pathophysiologic process, for example, hypoperfusion or hypoxia, and, if pH is severely decreased, administration of $NaHCO_3^-$. One continuing controversy is the use of $NaHCO_3$ to treat acidemia induced by lactic acidosis. Certainly, the best treatment is restoration of adequate tissue oxygenation. Although bicarbonate therapy is safe in critically ill patients and in perioperative patients,[51-53] no study has demonstrated that bicarbonate improves outcome.

TABLE 4-5
Production of Hyperchloremic Metabolic Acidosis by Rapid Administration of 0.9% Saline or Hypertonic Saline

Blood gases	pH	7.40	7.29
	$PaCO_2$	40 mmHg	29 mmHg
	$[HCO_3^-]$	24 meq/liter	14 meq/liter
Electrolytes	Na^+	140 meq/liter	140 meq/liter
	Cl^-	105 meq/liter	115 meq/liter
	"CO_2"	25 meq/liter	15 meq/liter
	Anion gap	10 meq/liter	10 meq/liter

TABLE 4-6
Differential Diagnosis of Metabolic Acidosis

Elevated Anion Gap	Normal Anion Gap
Diseases	Renal tubular acidosis
Uremia	Diarrhea
Ketoacidosis	Carbonic anhydrase inhibition
Lactic acidosis	Ureteral diversions
Toxins	Early renal failure
Methanol	Hydronephrosis
Ethylene glycol	HCl administration
Salicylates	NaCl administration
Paraldehyde	Hypertonic saline administration

Of specific concern in neurosurgical patients is the concept of paradoxical CNS acidosis. Administration of HCO_3^-, which does not cross the BBB, will, if alveolar ventilation remains unchanged, increase Pa_{CO_2}. Carbon dioxide will diffuse fluid into the brain, decreasing pH and worsening existing intracranial hypertension. Treatment of hyperchloremic acidosis associated with infusion of hypertonic saline is usually not required.

A greater obstacle to wider clinical application of hypertonic saline solutions is the transient nature of the PV expansion produced by hypertonic saline administration. To prolong the therapeutic effects beyond 30 to 60 min, investigators have infused additional hypertonic saline, blood, or conventional fluids, or added colloid to hypertonic fluids. Immediately after infusion, the combination of 7.5% saline and 6% dextran 70 increases PV by approximately seven times the original infused volume.[48] In hemorrhaged animals, adding 6.0% dextran 70 to 7.5% saline increased the duration of hemodynamic improvement when compared with equal volumes of hypertonic saline, sodium bicarbonate, or sodium chloride/sodium acetate.[54]

Because small volumes (relative to shed blood volume) of hypertonic saline, with or without added colloid, rapidly increase blood pressure and cardiac output, clinical trials have evaluated whether rapid infusion of hypertonic solutions might improve outcome when used for prehospital resuscitation. In the largest clinical study of prehospital hypertonic saline resuscitation, Mattox and colleagues randomized 422 patients, half of whom required surgery, to receive 250 ml of either conventional crystalloid fluid or 7.5% saline in 6% dextran.[55] Although overall survival was unaffected, survival *was* improved in those patients who required surgery. Vassar and coworkers compared 250 ml lactated Ringer's solution to an equal volume of 7.5% saline in 6.0% dextran 70 for prehospital resuscitation of trauma patients in whom systolic blood pressure was 100 mmHg or less.[56] Although there was no overall difference in mortality, in the subset of patients with severe head injury (53 of 186 patients), 32 percent of those who received hypertonic saline dextran survived, versus only 16 percent of the patients who received lactated Ringer's solution ($p = .04$).[56] In a subsequent randomized multicenter study, Vassar and colleagues evaluated the effects of 250 ml 7.5% sodium chloride with and without 6% and 12% dextran 70 for the prehospital resuscitation of hypotensive trauma patients.[56,57] A small subgroup of patients with Glasgow Coma Scale scores less than 8 but without severe anatomic injury seemed to benefit most from resuscitation with one of the hypertonic solutions.[57] One might speculate that the hypertonic fluids restored MAP while reducing ICP, therefore improving cerebral perfusion pressure.

To address concerns about CNS dysfunction caused by hypertonicity and hypernatremia associated with hypertonic saline solutions, Wisner and associates demonstrated, using high-energy phosphate nuclear magnetic resonance spectroscopy, a decreased intracellular pH after hypertonic saline resuscitation compared with lactated Ringer's solution.[58] However, this decrease was not attributable to anaerobic glycolysis, but to concentration of intracellular hydrogen ions in volume-contracted cells.[58] The effects of small volume, hypertonic saline resuscitation on regional CBF and metabolism have been examined in rats. Animals resuscitated from controlled hemorrhage with 7.5% saline in 10% hetastarch demonstrated a sufficient increase in regional blood flow to restore cerebral oxygen delivery to baseline levels. Administration of the hypertonic solution had no effect on the cerebral metabolic rate for glucose.[59] In humans resuscitated with hypertonic saline, acute increases in serum sodium to 155 to 160 meq/liter produced no apparent harm.[55,57] Central pontine myelinolysis, which follows rapid correction of severe, chronic hyponatremia,[60] has not been observed in clinical trials of hypertonic resuscitation.

The least encouraging observations regarding hyperosmotic resuscitation involve experimental models of uncontrolled hemorrhage,[61] in which hyperosmotic solutions increase bleeding and may adversely affect mortality. In urban patients with penetrating trauma, Bickell and coworkers have reported that immediate, prehospital resuscitation with conventional fluids does not improve mortality in comparison to resuscitation delayed until arrival in the operating room.[62]

BLOOD SUBSTITUTES

Because of the risk of disease transmissoin and the costs associated with maintaining an adequate supply of blood products, there has been an intensive search for blood substitutes. These blood substitutes can be classified as either perfluorochemical emulsions or modified hemoglobin (Hgb) solutions. Although these agents are not ready for widespread clinical use, it appears that modified Hgb solutions may be more suitable than perfluorochemicals for use in patients requiring volume resuscitation during and after hemorrhage. Cross linking of Hgb molecules has eliminated most of the renal toxicity of free Hgb. Problems that remain to be addressed include the low P50s of some of these compounds and their potential to produce vasoconstriction because of Hgb's propensity to scavenge endothelial nitric oxide.[63] Whether these problems are truly significant or can be overcome by additional molecular engineering awaits the results of ongoing clinical trials.

General Principles of Perioperative Fluid Administration

FLUID COMPARTMENTS

Rational decisions regarding intravenous fluid therapy require an understanding of how total body water (TBW) is partitioned. Accounting for approximately 60 percent of body weight (42 liters in a 70-kg person), TBW includes ICV (40 percent of TBW) and ECV (20 percent of TBW). ECV is further partitioned into PV, which equals about 20 percent of ECV and IFV, which accounts for the remaining 80 percent of ECV. Red cell volume, approximately 2 liters in a 70-kg person, is considered a subdivision of ICV. Blood volume in lean young individuals can be estimated by adding red cell volume (2 liters) to PV (2.8 liters) to arrive at 4.8 liters, or approximately 7 percent of adult body weight.

The ECV contains most of total body sodium, with [Na$^+$], approximately 140 meq/liter, in both the PV and IFV. The predominant intracellular cation, potassium, has an intracellular concentration ([K$^+$]) approximating 150 meq/liter. Albumin, the most important oncotically active constituent of ECV, is unequally distributed in PV (~4 g/dl) and IFV (~1 g/dl). The IFV concentration of albumin varies greatly among tissues. ECV is the distribution volume both for most crystalloid solutions, depending on [Na$^+$], and colloids, although the final concentrations of infused colloids may vary between PV and IFV.

DISTRIBUTION OF INFUSED FLUIDS

The formula describing the effects on PV of the infusion of 5% dextrose in water (D5W), lactated Ringer's solution, or 5% or 25% human serum albumin is as follows:

$$\text{Expected } \Delta\, PV = \frac{Vi \times \text{normal PV}}{Vd} \qquad \text{(Eq. 7)}$$

where Vi = volume infused and Vd = distribution volume of the fluid.

Rearranging the equation yields the following:

$$Vi = \frac{\text{expected } \Delta\, PV \times Vd}{\text{normal PV}} \qquad \text{(Eq. 8)}$$

Since D5W is distributed throughout TBW, 30 liters of D5W must be infused to replace a 2-liter blood loss:

$$30 \text{ liters} = \frac{2 \text{ liters} \times 42 \text{ liters}}{2.8 \text{ liters}} \qquad \text{(Eq. 9)}$$

where 2 liters is the desired Δ PV, 42 liters = TBW in a 70-kg person, and 2.8 liters is the normal estimated PV.

TABLE 4-7
Maintenance Water Requirements

Weight (kg)	ml/kg per h	ml/kg per day
1–10	4	100
11–20	2	50
>21	1	20

In comparison, to replace a 2-liter blood loss using lactated Ringer's solution, which distributes throughout ECV, requires the infusion of 10 liters:

$$10 \text{ liters} = \frac{2 \text{ liters} \times 14 \text{ liters}}{2.8 \text{ liters}} \qquad \text{(Eq. 10)}$$

where 14 liters = ECV in a 70-kg person.

If 5% albumin, which exerts colloid osmotic pressure similar to plasma, were infused, the infused volume initially would remain in the PV, perhaps attracting additional interstitial fluid intravascularly. Twenty-five percent human serum albumin, a concentrated colloid, expands PV by approximately 400 ml for each 100 ml infused.

MAINTENANCE REQUIREMENTS FOR WATER, SODIUM, AND POTASSIUM

In healthy adults, sufficient water is required to balance gastrointestinal losses of 100 to 200 ml/day, insensible losses of 500 to 1000 ml/day (half of which is respiratory and half cutaneous), and urinary losses of 1000 ml/day. Two simple formulas are used interchangeably to estimate maintenance water requirements based on the patient's weight (Table 4-7). Urinary losses exceeding 1000 ml/day may represent an appropriate physiologic response to ECV expansion or an inability to conserve salt or water.

Both renal sodium conservation and renal sodium excretion are highly efficient. During chronic sodium depletion, sodium excretion can decrease to less than 10 meq/day. Conversely, patients with normal cardiac and renal reserve tolerate sodium intake far in excess of normal daily requirements (~75 meq). Renal conservation and excretion of potassium is less efficient. Daily potassium requirements slightly exceed 40 meq.

Combining the above, the predicted daily maintenance fluid requirements for healthy, 70-kg adults is 2500 ml/day of a solution with a [Na$^+$] of 30 meq/liter and a [K$^+$] of 15 to 20 meq/liter. Intraoperatively, fluids containing sodium-free water (i.e., [Na$^+$] < 130 meq/liter) are rarely used in adults, because of the necessity for replacing isotonic losses.

DEXTROSE

Traditionally, glucose-containing intravenous fluids have been given in an effort to prevent hypoglycemia and limit protein catabolism. However, because of the hyperglycemic response associated with surgical stress, only infants and patients receiving insulin, oral hypoglycemics, or drugs that interfere with glucose synthesis are at risk for hypoglycemia. Iatrogenic hyperglycemia can limit the effectiveness of fluid resuscitation by inducing an osmotic diuresis and, in animals, may aggravate ischemic neurologic injury.[64] Although associated with worse outcome in both ischemic[65] and traumatic[66] brain injury in humans, hyperglycemia is a hormonally mediated response to severe injury.[65] Sieber and colleagues have concisely summarized the issue of intraoperative glucose administration by stating, "Glucose administration is indicated during clinical situations where hypoglycemia is likely to occur."[67]

WATER AND ELECTROLYTE COMPOSITION OF FLUID LOSSES

Surgical patients require replacement of PV and ECV losses secondary to wound or burn edema, ascites, and gastrointestinal secretions. Wound and burn edema and ascitic fluid are protein rich and contain electrolytes in concentrations similar to plasma. If ECV is adequate and renal and cardiovascular function are normal, all gastrointestinal secretions can be replaced using lactated Ringer's solution or 0.9% ("normal") saline. Substantial loss of gastrointestinal fluids requires replacement of other electrolytes (i.e., potassium, magnesium, phosphate). However, if cardiovascular or renal function is impaired, more precise replacement may require frequent assessment of serum electrolytes. Chronic gastric losses may produce a hypochloremic metabolic alkalosis that can be corrected with 0.9% saline; chronic diarrhea may produce a hyperchloremic metabolic acidosis that may be prevented or corrected by infusion of fluid containing bicarbonate or bicarbonate substrate (e.g., lactate).

FLUID SHIFTS DURING SURGERY

Replacement of intraoperative fluid losses must compensate for the acute reduction of functional IFV that accompanies trauma, hemorrhage, and tissue manipulation. For example, otherwise healthy patients who received no intraoperative sodium while undergoing gastric or gallbladder surgery demonstrated a decline in ECV of nearly 2 liters and a 13 percent decline in GFR.[68] In contrast, patients who received lactated Ringer's solution maintained ECV and increased GFR by 10 percent. No data describe changes in PV, IFV, and ICV during acute, unresuscitated shock in humans.

TABLE 4-8
Guidelines for Intraoperative Fluid Infusion Rates

Minimal trauma	4 ml/kg per h
Moderate trauma	6–8 ml/kg per h
Severe trauma	10–15 ml/kg per h

During prolonged experimental hemorrhagic shock, both sodium and water accumulate intracellularly,[69] in part due to impaired cellular membrane function.[70] Shock-induced alterations in cellular membrane function and intracellular concentrations of sodium appear to return to normal once systemic hemodynamic stability is restored. Patients studied during the first 10 days after resuscitation from massive trauma demonstrated a 55 percent increase in IFV.[71] Because of the reduction of colloid osmotic pressure in traumatized patients, the ratio of IFV to blood volume was increased, in some patients exceeding 5 : 1.[71] Therefore, the ratio of IFV to PV could be greater than 8 : 1 (versus the normal ratio of 4 : 1), thereby increasing the volume of infused fluid necessary to obtain any given increment in PV.

Based on the above considerations, guidelines have been developed for replacement of fluid losses during surgical procedures. The simplest formula provides, in addition to maintenance fluids and replacement of estimated blood loss, 4 ml/kg per h for procedures involving minimal trauma, 6 ml/kg per h for those involving moderate trauma, and 10 ml/kg per h for those involving extreme trauma (Table 4-8).

Fluid Administration for Craniotomy

Recommendations for fluid therapy can be formulated based on the preceding principles. As a general rule, isotonic crystalloid solutions should be used to replace preexisting deficits and blood loss. As the patient's Hgb approaches 8 g/dl, consideration should be given to transfusing red blood cells. Transfusion may be indicated at a higher Hgb if there is evidence of tissue hypoxia or ongoing uncontrolled hemorrhage. Solutions containing dextrose are to be avoided unless there is a specific indication for use (i.e., hypoglycemia). To reduce brain volume and improve operating conditions, the administration of hypertonic mannitol is considered standard practice. Hypertonic solutions, by creating osmotic gradients between the intracellular and extracellular spaces, cause fluid to move across the cell membrane and decrease brain tissue volume. Hypertonic saline solutions may be useful in the rapid volume resuscitation of hypovolemic trauma victims with brain injury and intracranial hypertension. FFP may be infused if hemorrhage persists despite adequate surgical hemostasis. There are few indications for the administration of synthetic colloids to neurosurgical patients. Colloids do not prevent the formation of brain edema, and some evidence indicates that dextran and hetastarch may be associated with coagulopathies.

Monitoring Fluid Administration

Two contrasting methods are used to assess the adequacy of intravascular volume. The first, conventional clinical assessment, is appropriate for most patients; the second, goal-directed hemodynamic management, may be superior for high-risk surgical patients. Recently, transesophageal echocardiography (TEE) has shown promise as a means of estimating cardiac dimensions and preload.

CONVENTIONAL CLINICAL ASSESSMENT

Clinical quantification of blood volume and ECV is difficult. The clinician must first recognize settings in which deficits are likely, such as protracted gastrointestinal losses, bowel obstruction, bowel perforation, preoperative bowel preparation, chronic hypertension, chronic diuretic use, sepsis, burns, pancreatitis, and trauma. The physical signs of hypovolemia are insensitive and nonspecific. Suggestive evidence includes oliguria, supine hypotension, tachycardia, and a positive tilt test. Oliguria implies hypovolemia although hypovolemic patients may be nonoliguric and normovolemic patients may be oliguric because of renal failure or stress-induced endocrine responses.[72] Supine hypotension implies a blood volume deficit exceeding 30 percent. However, arterial blood pressure within the normal range could represent relative hypotension in an elderly or chronically hypertensive patient. Substantial depletion of blood volume and organ hypoperfusion may occur despite an apparently normal blood pressure and heart rate.

In the tilt test, one of the traditional methods of assessing intravascular volume depletion, a positive response is defined as an increase in heart rate of at least 20 beats per minute and a decrease in systolic blood pressure of at least 20 mmHg when the subject assumes the upright position. However, a high incidence of false-positive and false-negative findings limits the value of the test. Young, healthy subjects can withstand acute loss of 20 percent of blood volume while exhibiting only postural tachycardia and variable postural hypotension. In contrast, 20 to 30 percent of elderly patients may demonstrate orthostatic changes in blood pressure despite normal blood volume.[73] In volunteers, withdrawal of 500 ml blood[74] was associated with a greater increase in heart rate on standing than before blood withdrawal but no significant difference in the response of blood pressure or cardiac index. Orthostatic changes in filling pressure, assessed before and after fluid infusion, may represent a more sensitive test of the adequacy of circulating blood volume.[75] In patients with chronic renal failure, infusion of fluid slightly increased the mean supine central venous pressure (CVP), but eliminated the marked postural decline in CVP.[75]

Laboratory evidence that suggests hypovolemia or ECV depletion includes hemoconcentration, azotemia, low urinary sodium, metabolic acidosis, and metabolic alkalosis (Table 4-9). Hematocrit, a poor indicator of intravascular volume, is virtually unchanged by acute hemorrhage; later, hemodilution occurs as fluids are administered or as fluid shifts from the interstitial to the intravascular space. If intravascular volume has been restored, hematocrit measurement will more accurately reflect current red cell mass and the extent of previous hemorrhage.

Measurements of blood urea nitrogen (BUN) and serum creatinine (SCr) require careful interpretation. BUN, normally 8.0 to 20 mg/dl, is increased by hypovolemia, high protein intake, gastrointestinal bleeding, or accelerated catabolism and decreased by severe hepatic dysfunction. SCr, a product of muscle catabolism, may be misleadingly low in elderly adults, in women, and in debilitated or malnourished patients. In contrast, in muscular or acutely catabolic patients, SCr may exceed the normal range (0.5 to 1.5 mg/dl) because of more rapid muscle breakdown. A ratio of BUN/SCr exceeding the normal range (10 to 20) suggests dehydration or other factors that alter the serum concentrations of BUN or SCr. In prerenal oliguria, enhanced sodium reabsorption should reduce urinary [Na$^+$] to 20 meq/liter or less and enhanced water reabsorption should increase urinary concentration (i.e., urinary osmolality >400; urine/plasma creatinine ratio >40:1). However, the sensitivity and specificity of measurements of urinary [Na$^+$], osmolality, and creatinine ratios may be misleading in acute situations. Severe hypovolemia may result in systemic hypoperfusion and lactic acidosis.

Although hypovolemia does not generate metabolic alkalosis, ECV depletion is a potent stimulus for the maintenance of metabolic alkalosis. Metabolic alkalosis, usually characterized by an alkalemic pH (> 7.45) and hyperbicarbonatemia (> 27.0 meq/liter), occurs frequently in neurosurgical patients who have been given diuretics and glucocorticoids, who have had prolonged nasogastric suction, or who have been fluid restricted. Total CO_2 content (usually abbreviated on electrolyte reports as CO_2) should exceed the normal value (~25 meq/liter) by 4.0 meq/liter or greater. The maintenance of metabolic alkalosis depends on a con-

TABLE 4-9
Laboratory Evidence of Hypovolemia

Test	Normal Range	Suggests Hypovolemia	False Positives
BUN (mg/dl)	8–20	>20	High protein intake Gastrointestinal bleeding Catabolic state Renal compromise
SCr (mg/dl)	0.5–1.2	>1.2	Advanced age Increased muscle mass Catabolism Renal compromise
BUN/Cr ratio	>20	>20	All of the above
U_{NA} (meq/liter)	>30	<20	Renal compromise
U_{OSM} (mosm/kg)	<800	>400	Renal compromise
Lactic acidosis (serum lactate; mmol/l)	<2.0	>3.0	Hypoperfusion from any cause
Metabolic alkalosis (serum bicarbonate; meq/l)	22–26	>26 (pH alkalemic)	

NOTE: BUN, blood urea nitrogen; SCr, serum creatinine; U_{NA}, urinary sodium concentration; U_{OSM}, urinary osmolality

tinued stimulus for the reabsorption of $[HCO_3^-]$ from the distal renal tubules. Renal hypoperfusion (often due to hypovolemia) and hypokalemia are major maintenance factors.

Metabolic alkalosis is associated with hypokalemia, ionized hypocalcemia,[76] cardiac arrhythmias, and digoxin toxicity. Metabolic alkalosis may also generate compensatory hypoventilation (hypercarbia) (Table 4-10).[77] Alkalemia also increases bronchial tone and, through a combination of increased bronchial tone and decreased ventilatory effort, may help to produce atelectasis. A leftward shift in the oxyhemoglobin dissociation curve may make oxygen less available to the tissues, as may cardiac output induced by alkalemia.

Recognition of an elevated total CO_2 on the preoperative serum electrolytes justifies arterial blood gas analysis and should alert the anesthesiologist to the possibility that the patient is hypovolemic. Confirmation of metabolic alkalosis should serve as a warning to avoid adding iatrogenic respiratory alkalosis to

metabolic alkalosis because that may produce cardiovascular depression, arrhythmias, and the other complications of severe alkalemia. Table 4-10 illustrates the effects of hyperventilation superimposed on metabolic alkalosis.

At times, it may be necessary to treat metabolic alkalosis in advance of surgery or to modify intraoperative fluid management. For a patient with metabolic alkalosis, 0.9% saline might be preferable to lactated Ringer's solution for intraoperative fluid administration because lactate provides additional substrate for generation of $[HCO_3^-]$. In general, treatment of metabolic alkalosis can be divided into etiologic and nonetiologic therapy. Etiologic therapy consists of measures such as expansion of intravascular volume to increase renal perfusion or the administration of potassium to reverse hypokalemia. Generic therapy includes the administration of $[H^+]$ (in the form of ammonium chloride, arginine hydrochloride, or 0.1 N hydrochloric acid), the administration of acetazolamide (a carbonic anhydrase inhibitor that causes renal $[HCO_3^-]$ wasting) or acid dialysis.[78] Of the above, in an acute situation associated with high risk secondary to metabolic alkalosis, 0.1 N hydrochloric acid most rapidly corrects metabolic alkalosis. However, dilute hydrochloric acid must be given into a central vein; peripheral infusion will cause severe tissue damage.

Visual estimation, the simplest technique for quantifying intraoperative blood loss, assesses the amount of blood absorbed by gauze sponges and laparotomy pads and modifies the estimate depending on whether or not the sponges have been prerinsed in saline. An estimate of blood accumulation on the floor and surgical drapes and in the suction containers is then added.

TABLE 4-10
Metabolic Alkalosis Plus Hyperventilation

		Intraoperative Hyperventilation	
Blood gases	pH	7.47	7.62
	$PaCO_2$	45 mmHg (compensatory hypercarbia)	30 mmHg
	$[HCO_3^-]$	32 meq/liter	29 meq/liter
Electrolytes	"CO_2"	33 meq/liter	30 meq/liter

NOTE: Respiratory alkalosis, produced by an inappropriately high minute ventilation, has been added to the previously compensated metabolic alkalosis.

Both surgeons and anesthesiologists tend to underestimate losses, the magnitude of the error being directly proportional to the actual blood loss.

The adequacy of intraoperative fluid resuscitation must be ascertained by evaluating multiple clinical variables, including heart rate, arterial blood pressure, urinary output, arterial oxygenation, and pH. Tachycardia is an insensitive, nonspecific indicator of hypovolemia. In patients receiving potent inhalational agents, maintenance of a satisfactory blood pressure implies adequate intravascular volume. Preservation of blood pressure, accompanied by a CVP of 6 to 12 mmHg, more strongly suggests adequate replacement. During profound hypovolemia, indirect measurements of blood pressure may significantly underestimate true blood pressure. In patients undergoing extensive procedures, direct arterial pressure measurements are more accurate than indirect techniques and provide convenient access for obtaining arterial blood samples. Decreases in arterial pressure during the inspiratory phase of positive-pressure ventilation are interpreted by many to be a sign of intravascular volume depletion.

Urinary output usually declines precipitously during moderate to severe hypovolemia. Therefore, in the absence of glycosuria or diuretic administration, a urinary output of 0.5 to 1.0 ml/kg per h during anesthesia suggests adequate renal perfusion. Arterial pH may decrease only when tissue hypoperfusion becomes severe. Cardiac output can be normal despite severely reduced regional blood flow. Mixed venous Hgb desaturation, a specific indicator of poor systemic perfusion, reflects average perfusion in multiple organs and cannot supplant regional monitors such as urinary output.

ECHOCARDIOGRAPHIC ASSESSMENT OF INTRAVASCULAR VOLUME

The limitations of traditional monitoring in estimating ventricular volume have been well documented.[79–82] Preload can also be estimated with TEE by using two-dimensional imaging and Doppler measurement of blood flow velocities.

Two methods by which two-dimensional echocardiography can be used to evaluate ventricular preload are measurement of ventricular end-diastolic volume (semiquantitative) and disappearance of the left ventricular cavity at end-systole (qualitative). The use of two-dimensional echocardiography to evaluate ventricular volume depends on obtaining end-diastolic measurements. The use of multiple tomographic slices through the ventricle at different levels allows a three-dimensional reconstruction of the ventricular cavity and enhances accuracy but requires extensive computer processing of the images and is not currently practical for on-line interpretation. Although the number of slices necessary to obtain an accurate reflection of end-diastolic volume is the subject of an ongoing debate,[83] the fewer the number that are required, the easier it will be to adapt this technology for intraoperative use.

Two-dimensional echocardiographic measurement of left ventricular end-diastolic volume (LVEDV) has been found to be a better measure of preload than traditional hemodynamic measures, but it is less than optimal when compared to radionuclide quantitation of LVEDV. Because the most frequently used view for evaluating left ventricular function is the transgastric view at the midpapillary muscle level, evaluation of end-diastolic volume in this single slice has been compared to evaluation of preload using PAOP (Fig. 4-2). In one study, changes in LVEDV correlated well with changes in cardiac index, whereas changes in PAOP did not.[84] End-diastolic volumes obtained at the midpapillary transgastric level have been sensitive enough to detect acute changes in preload, even in patients with ventricular wall motion abnormalities.[85–87] There are mixed findings, however, when comparing end-diastolic volumes obtained at a single level by TEE with radionuclide quantitation. Both good correlations[88,89] and poor correlations[90] between the two modalities have been reported.

End-systolic cavity obliteration visualized at the midpapillary transgastric level on TEE has been used clinically as an index of hypovolemia. There are few studies to validate this practice. One recent study comparing the presence of end-systolic cavity obliteration to decreases in LVEDV reported high sensitivity but poor specificity because of the complex interaction of ventricular contractility and afterload with changes in preload,[91] suggesting that this variable should be correlated with other echocardiographic or hemodynamic measures of preload.

Another echocardiographic modality that can be used as a qualitative index of changes in preload is the Doppler measurement of left ventricular inflow velocity. When measured by pulsed-wave Doppler, the diastolic flow across the mitral valve after mitral opening is biphasic, with an early, rapid acceleration of blood flow from the left atrium to the left ventricle (E velocity) followed by a period of diastasis (no flow) and a second filling period due to atrial contraction (A velocity) (Fig. 4-3). In normal hearts, the E velocity is greater than the A velocity because of the much greater contribution of early diastolic filling to the total LVEDV. With a decrease in preload, the E velocity decreases because of the decreased pressure gradient between the left atrium and left ventricle. The A velocity does not change or is slightly increased because a reduced preload does not influence atrial contraction.

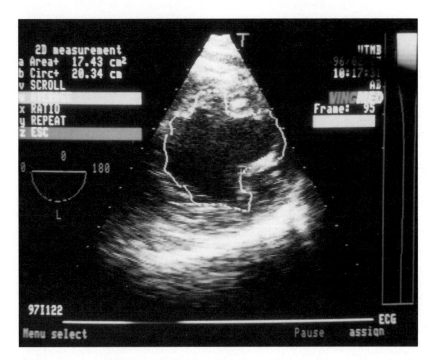

Figure 4-2 Two-dimensional image of a transverse slice of the left ventricle at the midpapillary muscle level demonstrating endocardial tracing used to determine the end-diastolic volume. Measurement of end-diastolic volume at this single level has been shown to accurately reflect acute changes in preload.

Increased preload results in an increase in the E velocity and a decrease in the A velocity as the rapid filling in early diastole results in an increased left ventricular diastolic pressure and left atrial contraction adds only a small pressure gradient.[92] These velocity changes allow a qualitative approach to monitoring changes in preload but give no quantitative data. They should be considered only in concert with other echocardiographic or hemodynamic measurements.

Diastolic mitral inflow velocities can give a quantitative measure of the transmitral stroke volume, which may be useful in assessing changes in left ventricular filling. The measurement of transmitral stroke volume is obtained by multiplying the integral of the diastolic transmitral flow velocities by the cross-sectional area (CSA) of the mitral valve (obtained by measuring the radius of the mitral annulus, $CSA = \pi r^2$). The calculation of the transmitral stroke volume is included in

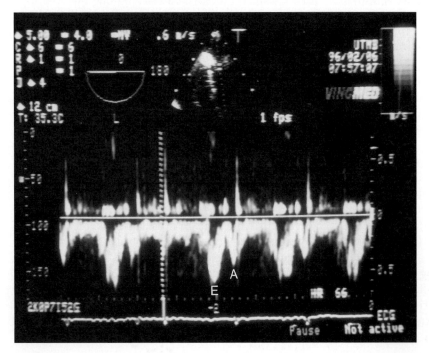

Figure 4-3 Spectral tracing from pulsed-wave Doppler measurement of mitral valve inflow velocities. E indicates the early, rapid acceleration of blood flow from the left atrium to the left ventricle (E velocity), and A indicates the blood flow across the mitral valve from atrial contraction (A velocity).

most echocardiographic software packages and can be obtained relatively rapidly. The use of the transmitral stroke volume as an assessment of preload has not been clinically studied but may afford a quantitative volumetric method for determining preload without relying on transmitted pressures. There are disadvantages to using Doppler left ventricular filling in that it requires an experienced echocardiographer. Moreover, normal variations occur with respiration, heart rate, and age. In addition, the presence of mitral regurgitation, arrhythmias, and diastolic dysfunction may interfere with accurate measurements.[93]

The use of TEE adds to our ability to accurately assess intravascular volume status or ventricular preload. There are several quantitative and qualitative methods by which this assessment can be performed, as outlined above. The use of left ventricular end-diastolic area measurement has been proven to be a more accurate measure of preload than conventional measurement of transmitted pressures in several studies. TEE is also associated with fewer adverse events than placement of a central venous or pulmonary artery catheter. The greatest disadvantages are the cost of the equipment and the need for experienced, well-trained echocardiographers to obtain and interpret the images. Echocardiographic measures can, however, be an important adjunct to traditional hemodynamic measurements and allow a more accurate clinical assessment of intravascular volume status.

SYSTEMIC OXYGEN DELIVERY AS A GOAL OF MANAGEMENT

No intraoperative monitor is sufficiently sensitive or specific to detect hypoperfusion in all patients. Moreover, acute renal failure, hepatic failure, and sepsis may result from unrecognized, subclinical tissue hypoperfusion. In critically ill surgical patients, average cardiac output and systemic oxygen delivery (D_{O_2}) are greater in those who survive than in those who succumb.[94,95] One key variable that has been associated with survival is a D_{O_2} of 600 ml O_2/m^2 per min or more (equivalent to a cardiac index of 3.0 liter/m^2 per min, a Hgb concentration of 14 g/dl, and 98% oxyhemoglobin saturation). In comparison to control groups receiving conventional monitoring, with or without pulmonary arterial catheterization, a group of high-risk surgical patients treated to achieve specific goals, including a D_{O_2} of at least 600 ml O_2/m^2 per min, had greater survival and decreased complications.[94] These data suggest that goal-directed hemodynamic support in high-risk surgical patients limits mortality and morbidity secondary to clinically inapparent hypoperfusion. Similar management also appears to improve outcome in septic patients[95] and in multiply traumatized patients.[96] However, recent clinical trials continue to generate controversy. Boyd and colleagues randomized 107 patients to conventional treatment or D_{O_2} of 600 ml O_2/m^2 per min or greater and demonstrated a decrease in mortality and in the number of complications in the patients managed at the higher level of D_{O_2}.[97] In contrast, Hayes and coworkers, who randomized 109 patients to conventional treatment or D_{O_2} above 600 ml O_2/m^2 per min using a combination of volume and dobutamine, demonstrated an increase in mortality in the treatment group maintained at the higher levels and speculated that aggressive elevations in D_{O_2} actually may have been harmful.[98] Gattinoni and associates, in a multicenter study of critically ill patients, also failed to demonstrate any beneficial effect of enhancing D_{O_2}.[99]

Normally, D_{O_2} is regulated through dilation and constriction of vascular beds in response to changes in regional and systemic oxygen consumption. In normal, anesthetized animals, oxygen consumption becomes D_{O_2} dependent if D_{O_2} is reduced to critical levels by progressive acute anemia.[100] When O_2 extraction reaches a maximum, oxygen consumption falls in proportion to further decrements in D_{O_2}. In anesthetized humans, the critical level of D_{O_2} appears to be approximately 330 ml O_2/m^2 per min.[101] In certain patients with the adult respiratory distress syndrome, hypovolemic shock, and septic shock, oxygen consumption can vary, depending on D_{O_2}, at levels that substantially exceed the normal critical level of D_{O_2}.[102,103] In critically ill humans, it is controversial whether D_{O_2} can be increased until oxygen consumption is no longer dependent on D_{O_2}.[104,105] Mohsenifar and coworkers noted that oxygen consumption was dependent on D_{O_2} until the latter exceeded 790 ml/m^2 per min.[104] In some patients, oxygen consumption was not supply independent even if D_{O_2} exceeded 1500 ml/m^2 per min.[105] However, in experimental endotoxemia, volume resuscitation using dextran improved oxygen extraction and reduced the dependency of oxygen consumption on D_{O_2}.[106]

Experimental design must always be considered when evaluating studies of the relationship between D_{O_2} and oxygen consumption. Correlations between calculated oxygen consumption and D_{O_2} have been questioned because they are mathematically coupled, that is, both are calculated using common variables.[107] More importantly, D_{O_2} under normal circumstances is the dependent variable and physiologically is controlled by oxygen consumption unless D_{O_2} is severely reduced.[100] In humans, assessment of supply dependency is more challenging. Multiple, uncontrolled calculations in individual patients should demonstrate highly correlated variations of oxygen consumption and D_{O_2}.[108] Studies in humans that purport to primarily change D_{O_2} may be suspect if they also alter oxygen consumption as a consequence of pharmacologic manipulation, for example, by catecholamine infusion,[109,110] which directly affects cardiac work and systemic metabolism.[111]

Improvement of systemic D_{O_2} may be less important than restoration of perfusion in individual organ systems. As reviewed recently by Fink, gastrointestinal mucosal ischemia and dysfunction, resulting from a variety of vasoconstrictive metabolites released in response to severe systemic stress, may increase mucosal permeability to bacteria and may produce late morbidity after shock, trauma, and sepsis.[112] In experimental porcine hemorrhagic shock, changes in intestinal perfusion are the most rapid, sensitive indicators of acute blood volume loss.[113] Consequently, prompt, effective restoration of gut mucosal perfusion is an important goal of resuscitation.

MONITORING THE CEREBRAL CIRCULATION

Theoretically, cerebral circulatory variables could reflect the adequacy of fluid resuscitation. Although clinical experience suggests that morbidity and mortality can be altered by therapeutic alteration of CBF and cerebral metabolism in some neurologically injured patients, no data confirm the general clinical utility of neurologic monitoring. Three questions are central to the question of utility of monitoring cerebral variables:

1. Under what circumstances do blood pressure, Pa_{CO_2}, Pa_{O_2}, and body temperature provide insufficient information about the adequacy of cerebral oxygen delivery (CD_{O_2} = [CBF] × Ca_{O_2})?
2. Under what circumstances does more precise information about the adequacy of CD_{O_2} permit therapeutic interventions that improve outcome?
3. Is the proportion of patients within a specific diagnostic category who will develop avoidable injury sufficiently large to justify extensive (and potentially expensive) application of neurologic monitoring devices?

Few data quantify the relationship between monitored variables and the risk of preventable neurologic injury. Virtually all neurologic monitors are intended to detect actual or possible cerebral ischemia. Cerebral ischemia, defined as CD_{O_2} insufficient to meet metabolic needs, can result from a critical reduction of any of the components of CD_{O_2}, including CBF, Hgb concentration, and arterial Hgb saturation (Sa_{O_2}). The brain constitutes only 2 percent of total body weight, but receives 15 percent of cardiac output and accounts for 15 to 20 percent of total oxygen consumption. Certain regions of the brain, such as the cerebellum, the basal ganglia, the CA-1 layer of the hippocampus, and the arterial boundary zones between major branches of the intracranial vessels, appear to be selectively vulnerable to ischemic injury.[114]

Practical use of brain monitors requires definition of critical thresholds at which therapeutic interventions should be undertaken. Thresholds of CBF that correlate with various clinical outcomes, physiologic changes, and changes in monitored variables have been defined based on animal experiments,[115–118] and to a lesser extent on clinical data.[119] If a monitor of brain function detects cerebral ischemia, the actual severity is not established. All that is known is that cerebral oxygenation in a region of brain that contributes to that function has fallen below a critical threshold. The shortfall could be slight or severe. Because more severe ischemia will produce neurologic injury in less time, it is impossible to predict with certainty if changes in function will be followed by cerebral infarction. In addition, if regional ischemia involves structures that do not participate in the monitored function, infarction could develop without warning. This predictable relationship no doubt explains the failure of monitors to detect cerebral ischemia in patients who subsequently develop clinical evidence of brain infarction as well as reports of profound changes in monitored variables that are followed by no apparent change in clinical condition. The complexity and heterogeneity of brain tissue virtually preclude development of a single, perfectly predictive brain monitor.

The first quantitative clinical method of measurement of CBF, the Kety-Schmidt technique,[120] calculated global CBF from the difference between the arterial and jugular bulb saturation curves of an inhaled, inert gas. Later techniques used extracranial gamma detectors to measure regional cortical CBF from washout curves after intracarotid injection of a radioisotope such as xenon-133 (^{133}Xe).[121] Carotid puncture was avoided by techniques that measured cortical CBF after inhaled[122] or intravenous administration of ^{133}Xe, using gamma counting of exhaled gas to correct clearance curves for recirculation of ^{133}Xe. Among the obstacles to wider use of ^{133}Xe clearance are technical complexity, cumbersome regulations governing radionuclides, and the sustained stable conditions (5 to 15 min) required to perform a single measurement.

In most patients, arterial flow velocity can be readily measured in intracranial vessels, especially the MCA, using transcranial Doppler ultrasonography. Doppler flow velocity uses the frequency shift, proportional to velocity, observed when sound waves are reflected by moving red blood cells. Blood moving toward the transducer shifts the transmitted frequency to higher frequencies; blood moving away, to lower frequencies. Blood flow is a function both of velocity and vessel diameter. If diameter remains constant, changes in velocity are proportional to changes in CBF; however, intersubject differences in flow velocity correlate poorly with intersubject differences in CBF.[123] Entirely noninvasive, transcranial Doppler measurements can be repeated at frequent intervals or even applied continuously. Intracranial Doppler ultrasonography has been used to monitor vasospasm after subarachnoid hemorrhage (SAH) and in patients with head trauma.

Measurements of jugular venous bulb oxygenation reflect the adequacy of CBF as systemic "mixed venous" oxygenation reflects the adequacy of cardiac output. CBF, the cerebral metabolic rate for oxygen (CMR_{O_2}), Ca_{O_2}, and jugular venous oxygen content (Cjv_{O_2}) are related according to the following equation:

$$CMR_{O_2} = CBF \times (Ca_{O_2} - Cjv_{O_2}) \qquad \text{(Eq. 11)}$$

Mixed cerebral venous blood, like mixed systemic blood, is a global average and may not reflect marked regional hypoperfusion. Therefore, abnormally low jugular venous saturation suggests the possibility of cerebral ischemia; but normal or elevated jugular venous saturation does not indicate adequate cerebral perfusion. The internal jugular vein can be located by external anatomic landmarks and the catheter is directed toward the mastoid process, above which lies the jugular venous bulb. In clinical use, jugular venous blood gas sampling or continuous monitoring has detected unexpected cerebral desaturation. Considerable data have been accumulated to evaluate jugular venous saturation after head injury.[124,125]

Near-infrared spectroscopy may eventually offer the opportunity to assess the adequacy of brain oxygenation continuously. Near-infrared light penetrates the skull and, during transmission through or reflection from brain tissue, undergoes changes in intensity that are proportional to the relative concentrations of oxygenated and deoxygenated Hgb in the tissue beneath the field.[126] The absorption (*A*) of light by a chromophore, that is, Hgb, is defined by Beer's law:

$$A = abc \qquad \text{(Eq. 12)}$$

where a = the absorption constant, *b* = path length of the light, and *c* = concentration of the chromophore.

Extensive preclinical and clinical data demonstrate the sensitivity of the technique for the detection of qualitative changes in brain oxygenation.[126–128] Technical challenges to quantification of the signal include difficulty in determining the path lengths of reflected lights of different wavelengths and estimating the relative proportions of arterial, venous, and capillary blood in the field.

For practical purposes, 75 percent of the blood is assumed to be venous and 25 percent arterial for calcu-

lation of mixed brain oxygen saturation. Recent data suggest that quantification of the signal may be practical.[129,130] Although near-infrared spectroscopy appears to reflect changes in cerebral Hgb oxygen saturation induced by breathing a hypoxic gas mixture (Fig. 4-4),[131] performance is adversely affected by changes in position (i.e., Trendelenburg or reverse Trendelenburg).[132] Further work is necessary to determine whether near-infrared spectroscopy represents a technologically feasible method for continuously monitoring brain oxygenation.

Currently, no noninvasive, continuous monitor of cerebral circulatory adequacy is available. A brain monitor that could be used for goal-directed therapy would provide the opportunity to manage the cerebral circulation as comprehensively as the systemic circulation can now be managed. The challenge then would be to demonstrate that improved therapy based on enhanced monitoring will improve outcome.

Fluid Administration in Specific Pathologic Syndromes

HEAD INJURY

Patients who sustain traumatic brain injury (TBI) often have multiple concurrent injuries and may hemorrhage substantially before arrival in the operating room or intensive care unit. In the absence of a history of myocardial injury or dysfunction, hypotension in traumatized patients should raise the suspicion of inadequate volume resuscitation after other treatable causes (e.g., tension pneumothorax, tamponade) have been excluded. Physicians caring for these patients must achieve adequate volume resuscitation while considering intracranial hemodynamics and ICP.

Isotonic crystalloid solutions (preferably 0.9% saline) are often the first solutions to be infused in hypotensive trauma patients because they are readily available and inexpensive. If the initial evaluation suggests intracranial hypertension, mannitol (0.5 g/kg) may also be appropriate. Fresh whole blood, arguably the ideal fluid for patients in hemorrhagic shock, is not available in most centers owing to the need to test all donated blood for infectious agents and the commitment that blood banks have made to fractionating donated units into their various components (platelets, plasma, red cells). Packed red blood cells resuspended in 0.9% saline or thawed plasma are suitable alternatives. Unfortunately, this increases the recipient's exposure to multiple donors and the attendant risks of transfusion reactions and infectious complications.

Although not yet considered a standard of care, hypertonic saline solutions may be useful in certain situations. In the presence of hypovolemia accompanied by

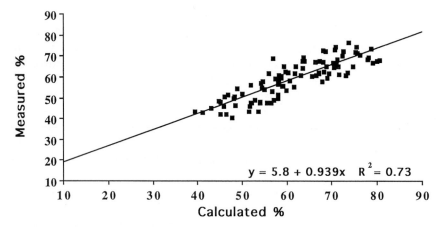

$$y = 5.8 + 0.939x \quad R^2 = 0.73$$

Figure 4-4 Correlation between calculated and measured brain tissue oxygen saturations in ten volunteers breathing hypoxic gas mixtures (fraction inspired O_2 between 0.13 and 0.06). Reproduced with permission from Pollard and coworkers.[131]

intracranial hypertension or when large volumes of isotonic crystalloid solutions are not available or cannot be rapidly infused, the use of hypertonic saline appears to be an attractive option. Extensive animal experience supports the efficacy of hypertonic solutions in reversing shock and, usually, decreasing ICP (Table 4-11). In those few studies in which hypertonic saline did not reduce ICP,[133,134] it is likely that the BBB was diffusely damaged by trauma or ischemia. In such cases, it is also unlikely that mannitol will be efficacious in reducing ICP. The value of small-volume hypertonic resuscitation may be greatest when dealing with mass or combat casualties; however, hypertonic saline solutions have been extensively studied for prehospital

TABLE 4-11
Cerebral Effects of Hemorrhage and Hypertonic Saline (with and without Brain Injury)

First Author	Reference Number	Species (Lesion(s))	Interventions	Observations
Prough	185	Dogs (no lesion)	LRS; 7.5% saline	↓ ICP with 7.5% saline; CBF no different
Prough	186	Dogs (no lesion)	7.5% saline (4 ml/kg); LRS (45 ml/kg)	↓ ICP after 7.5% saline
Gunnar	187	Dogs (no lesion)	Resuscitation with shed blood plus 0.9% saline; 3% saline; 10% dextran 40	↓ ICP with 3% saline
Schmoker	188	Swine (no lesion)	4 ml/kg HSL or LRS as bolus, then HSL or LRS to restore MAP to baseline for 24 h	↓ ICP; ↓ brain water; CDO_2 greater in HSL animals
Prough	189	Dogs (SB)	0.8% saline (54 ml/kg); 7.2% saline (6 ml/kg)	7.2% saline decreased ICP, ↑ CBF in the lesioned hemisphere
Gunnar	190	Dogs (EB)	0.9% saline; 3.0% saline; 10% dextran 40 for 2 h after resuscitation	↓ ICP with 3.0% saline; CBF similar in all groups
Gunnar	191	Dogs (EB)	0.9% saline; 3.0% saline; 10% dextran 40 for 2 h after resuscitation	↓ ICP, cerebral edema less with 3.0% saline; no difference in blood-brain barrier function
Ducey	192	Swine (EB)	Blood; 0.9% saline; 6.0% saline; 6.0% HES to normalize DO_2	↓ ICP with 6% saline, improved intracranial elastance
Walsh	193	Swine (cryo)	4 ml/kg bolus of LRS or 7.5% saline in 6.5% dextran 70, then LRS or HSL	↓ ICP with 7.5% saline + dextran 70, increased CBF
Battistella	194	Sheep (cryo)	LRS or 7.5% saline after shock to keep MAP ≥80 mmHg for 1 h	↓ ICP with 7.5% saline, brain water (uninjured hemisphere)
Whitley	133	Dogs (SB)	0.73% saline or 1.46% saline, each with and without 10% pentastarch to maintain cardiac output	No effect of fluid choices on ICP or CBF
Wisner	195	Rats (FPI)	LRS versus 6.5% saline	6.5% saline decreased brain water in uninjured, not injured brain
Prough	134	Cats (FPI)	Resuscitation with 3.0% saline or 10% HES	3.0% saline increased ICP, but not CBF

NOTE: CBF, cerebral blood flow; cryo, cryogenic injury; DO_2, systemic oxygen delivery; EB, epidural balloon; EEG, electroencephalogram; FPI, fluid percussion injury; HES, hydroxyethyl starch; HSL, hypertonic sodium lactate; ICP, intracranial pressure; LRS, lactated Ringer's solution; MAP, mean arterial pressure; SB, subdural balloon.

resuscitation in the United States,[55-57] and are currently being used in the prehospital transport of hypovolemic brain-injured patients in Europe. Whether this approach will gain popularity in the United States remains to be seen.

DIABETES INSIPIDUS

Neurogenic diabetes insipidus may occur in patients with lesions in the vicinity of the hypothalamus, after pituitary surgery, or after TBI. This syndrome is characterized by a failure of the neurons located in the supraoptic nuclei of the hypothalamus to release sufficient quantities of ADH (vasopressin) into the systemic circulation. Diabetes insipidus is characterized by the production of large volumes of dilute urine in the face of a normal or elevated plasma osmolality. In severe cases, urinary output can exceed 1 liter/h. Left untreated or unrecognized, diabetes insipidus can quickly result in severe hypernatremia, hypovolemia, and hypotension. To promptly make the diagnosis of diabetes insipidus, it is important to have a high index of suspicion when dealing with patients at risk. Confirmation may be obtained by documenting elevated serum osmolality and $[Na^+]$ in conjunction with a low urinary specific gravity or osmolality. Vigorous volume expansion should be accomplished. Because of the preexisting hyperosmolar/hypernatremic state, 0.9% saline may actually reduce serum $[Na^+]$. As a caution, rapid increases in serum $[Na^+]$ are rapidly compensated for by generation of intracellular idiogenic osmoles that preserve cerebral intracellular volume; if therapy too rapidly reduces serum $[Na^+]$, cerebral edema will result. Concomitantly, replacement of endogenous ADH should be initiated with either aqueous vasopressin (5 to 10 units by intravenous or intramuscular injection) or desmopressin (DDAVP) 1 to 4 μg subcutaneously or 5 to 20 μg intranasally every 12 to 24 h. DDAVP lacks the vasoconstrictor effects of vasopressin and is less likely to produce abdominal cramping.[135-138] Incomplete ADH deficits (partial diabetes insipidus) often are effectively managed with pharmacologic agents that stimulate ADH release or enhance the renal response to ADH. The combination of chlorpropamide (100 to 250 mg/day) and clofibrate or a thiazide diuretic has proven effective in patients who respond inadequately to either drug alone.

PATIENTS AT RISK FOR CEREBRAL ISCHEMIA

In patients at risk for cerebral ischemia, the most important concept related to fluid administration is hemodilution. Cerebral perfusion can be improved by reducing blood viscosity with hemodilution. Hypervolemic hemodilution with dextran produces small, statistically insignificant increases in CBF in animals with normal cerebral vasculature.[139] However, in brain tissue distal to an experimental MCA occlusion, dextran significantly improves CBF.[140,141] If CD_{O_2} increases, tissue with borderline viability may be preserved. Moderate hemodilution has been extensively studied in patients with stroke. In patients with acute stroke, normovolemic hemodilution increases CBF and improves electroencephalographic (EEG) activity.[142] Although moderate hemodilution is beneficial, marked decreases in hematocrit may be deleterious. In a recent study that measured cerebral infarct volumes in rabbits hemodiluted to a Hgb of 6 or 11 g/dl after embolization of the MCA, the authors found that profound hemodilution (Hgb of 6 g/dl) resulted in larger infarcts in both the cortex and subcortex.[143]

However, widespread clinical application of hemodilution has been impeded by concern regarding two physiologic risks. First, hypervolemia may produce cardiac failure or myocardial ischemia in patients who have coexisting cerebrovascular and coronary occlusive disease. Second, although flow may be slightly improved by moderate hemodilution, the reduction in Ca_{O_2} may prevent any improvement in local oxygen delivery. The Scandinavian Stroke Study Group, which randomized 373 patients to receive either conventional therapy or normovolemic hemodilution after stroke, demonstrated an increased incidence of cardiovascular complications and an increased early mortality among hemodiluted patients.[144] The Italian Acute Stroke Study Group randomized 1267 patients to receive conventional therapy or normovolemic hemodilution and found no difference in outcome.[145] However, both studies were constrained by the cardiovascular risk of volume expansion. In contrast, the Hemodilution in Stroke Study Group used invasive cardiovascular monitoring to guide hypervolemic hemodilution with pentastarch and increase cardiac output in patients with acute ischemic stroke.[146] Although overall mortality and neurologic outcome were not superior in the hemodilution group, neurologic outcome was apparently improved in patients who were entered into the trial within 12 h of the onset of stroke and in whom cardiac output increased by 10 percent or more.

Although no firm recommendation can be attached to the use of hemodilution in patients at risk for cerebral ischemia, it is certainly reasonable to avoid hypovolemia and the attendant risks of hypotension and hemoconcentration.

CEREBRAL ANEURYSMS AND VASOSPASM

Patients who present for surgery after rupture of a cerebral aneurysm require careful consideration of fluid management. Cerebral vasospasm is a leading cause of morbidity in these patients, producing death or severe disability in approximately 14 percent of patients who survive rupture of their aneurysm.[147] Angiographic evidence of vasospasm occurs in as many as 60 to 80 percent of patients after SAH.[147] Arteriography in patients who have vasospasm demonstrates luminal irregularities in large conducting vessels, although these are not the major site of precapillary resistance. CBF is not reduced until the angiographic diameter of the cerebral arteries is decreased by 50 percent or more compared to normal.[148] The intraparenchymal cerebral resistance vessels tend to dilate after the onset of spasm of the larger vessels, thus partially compensating for increased upstream resistance. ICP and cerebral blood volume may actually increase during vasospasm owing to dilation of cerebral capacitance vessels (veins) and accumulation of tissue edema resulting from cerebral ischemia.[149]

Recent positron emission tomography data indicate that in patients with focal deficits, CBF values are within the 10 to 20 ml/100 g per min range (50 ml/100 g per min being normal). In patients with sustained regional CBF values less than 12 ml/100 g per min, clinical deficits are not reversible.[150] Global CBF is markedly reduced (10 to 30 ml/100 g per min) in patients who are stuporous because of severe diffuse vasospasm.[150] The mediators by which blood in the subarachnoid space provokes large cerebral arteries to spasm are the subject of intense investigation and debate. What is known is that vasospasm after aneurysmal rupture can be so severe as to cause cerebral ischemia and infarction.

The incidence of vasospasm reaches a peak between the fourth and tenth days after the rupture of the aneurysm. Three to 9 days after SAH, the patient with symptomatic vasospasm will characteristically become disoriented and drowsy over a period of hours. Focal deficits may follow. Vasospasm is presumed to be the cause if recurrent hemorrhage, mass lesions, intracranial hypertension, meningitis, or metabolic encephalopathy can be excluded through proper diagnostic studies. The diagnosis may be confirmed by angiography or documentation of high-velocity flow patterns by Doppler examination of the cerebral vessels.

Two currently accepted therapeutic interventions may decrease the incidence or severity of vasospasm. The first of these is hypervolemic-hyperdynamic therapy. Theoretical evidence supporting the need for volume expansion includes the observation that 10 to 33 percent of patients after SAH develop hyponatremia, associated with negative sodium balance and intravascular volume contraction.[151] Hyponatremic patients are more likely to develop vasospasm.

In patients suffering from neurologic impairment secondary to vasospasm, volume loading in conjunc-

tion with inotropic support can reverse or reduce neurologic morbidity. In one series, prophylactic volume expansion was associated with outcomes as good as those achieved with prophylaxis with calcium channel blockers.[152] Although no large clinical trials have used a controlled randomized design to compare volume expansion to other therapies for symptomatic vasospasm, clinical reports provide circumstantial evidence of the efficacy of hypervolemia and induced hypertension to treat vasospasm. One algorithm for producing hypervolemia and increasing cerebral perfusion pressure consists of pulmonary artery catheterization and infusion of fluid, either saline or colloid, to increase the PAOP to 15 ± 3 mmHg. Associated therapeutic goals include a CVP of 10 ± 2 mmHg, a systolic blood pressure of 180 ± 10 mmHg (a MAP of 130 ± 10 mmHg), and adequate Ca_{O_2}, defined as a Hgb of 11 g/dl and an oxyhemoglobin saturation of 95%.[153] If volume expansion does not achieve these hemodynamic goals, vasopressors such as phenylephrine, 10 to 14 μg/min, or dopamine, 5 to 10 μg/kg per min, are added. Using this protocol, most neurologic deficits attributed to vasospasm improve within 1 to 4 h.[154] Although the use of pulmonary artery catheterization permits more precise quantification of systemic responses to hypervolemic therapy, central venous catheterization may provide adequate monitoring information in patients who have normal cardiovascular function.

Occasionally, hypertensive hypervolemic therapy is required for up to 3 weeks until neurologic status remains stable as treatment is tapered. A suggested protocol for weaning therapy involves 48 h of intensive volume expansion and then gradual discontinuation of therapy while carefully monitoring clinical neurologic signs.[153] Recurrent evidence of ischemic symptoms necessitates rapid return to previously effective hemodynamic goals. Needless to say, hypertensive hypervolemic therapy must be avoided in those patients who have not undergone aneurysm clipping and are at risk of rerupture.

Cardiac, hematologic, and pulmonary sequelae have been reported as consequences of volume expansion and induced hypertension. Institution of hypervolemic-hyperdynamic therapy can be guided by hemodynamic data provided by a pulmonary artery catheter. In patients with no history of heart disease, a PAOP of 14 mmHg is associated with maximum cardiac performance.[155] Volume expansion beyond this point will increase PAOP, but probably will not increase cardiac index.[155] Volume loading may be accomplished by infusion of red blood cells or isotonic crystalloids or colloids, with the goal of hemodiluting the patient to a hematocrit of approximately 30 percent. Frequent assessment of pulmonary function with arterial blood gases, chest radiographs, and physical examination is essential because the onset of pulmonary edema with hypoxemia will negate any possible beneficial effects of increased flow to ischemic brain tissue.

The second therapy for vasospasm is the use of the calcium channel blocker nimodipine. Nimodipine has been shown in numerous studies to reduce the morbidity and mortality associated with cerebral vasospasm. Nimodipine is an L-type calcium channel blocker that has superior penetration of the BBB and is administered orally or by nasograstric tube. It is a cerebral vasodilator that improves CBF after transient global cerebral ischemia without improvement in neurologic outcome. Although nimodipine does improve outcome in patients who have suffered a SAH, most studies have failed to demonstrate a reduction in the incidence of large vessel vasospasm. Thus, whether nimodipine's beneficial effects are due to improvements in the cerebral microcirculation or secondary to inhibition of calcium entry into the cell is unknown. Nimodipine (60 mg every 4 h) should be administered starting within 96 h of the hemorrhage and continued for a total of 21 days. Theoretically, volume expansion plus nimodipine should improve CD_{O_2} more than either intervention alone.

Common Electrolyte Abnormalities Important to Planning Fluid Therapy

SODIUM

Increases or decreases in total body sodium, the principal extracellular cation and solute, tend to increase or decrease ECV and PV. Disorders of sodium concentration (i.e., hyponatremia and hypernatremia) usually result from relative excesses or deficits, respectively, of water. Neurologic surgery, however, is associated with disorders of both total body sodium and [Na+].

Regulation of the quantity and concentration of sodium is accomplished primarily by the endocrine and renal systems. Aldosterone regulates total body sodium by controlling renal sodium reabsorption in exchange for potassium and hydrogen.[19] Secretion of ANP, in response to increased atrial stretch, increases renal sodium excretion and decreases PV.[17,18] *Sodium concentration* is primarily regulated by ADH, which is secreted in response to increased osmolality or decreased blood pressure. ADH stimulates renal reabsorption of water, diluting plasma [Na+]; inadequate ADH secretion results in renal free water excretion, which, in the absence of adequate water intake, results in hypernatremia. In response to changes in plasma [Na+], changes in secretion of ADH can vary urinary osmolality from 50 to 1400 mosm/kg and urinary volume from 0.4 to 20 liter/day.

The signs and symptoms of hyponatremia depend on both the rate and severity of the decrease in plasma [Na+]. Symptoms usually accompany [Na+] of 120 meq/liter or less. Because the BBB is poorly permeable to sodium but freely permeable to water, a decrease in plasma [Na+] promptly increases both extracellular and intracellular brain water. Acute CNS manifestations relate to increases in brain water content. Compensatory responses to cerebral edema include bulk movement of interstitial fluid into the cerebrospinal fluid and loss of intracellular solutes,[156] including potassium and organic osmolytes (previously termed "idiogenic osmoles").[157] Because the brain rapidly compensates for changes in osmolality, the symptoms are considerably more severe in acute than in chronic hyponatremia. In chronic hyponatremia, rapid correction may lead to abrupt decreases in brain water content and volume.

Hyponatremia is classified as true hyponatremia or pseudohyponatremia. Pseudohyponatremia is the term applied when hyperproteinemia or hyperlipidemia displaces water from plasma, thereby producing an apparently low plasma [Na+]. True hyponatremia may be associated with normal, high, or low serum osmolality. In turn, hyponatremia with hyposmolality is associated with a high, low, or normal total body sodium and PV. Hyponatremia ([Na+] < 135 meq/liter) with a normal or high serum osmolality results from the presence of a nonsodium solute, such as glucose or mannitol, which does not diffuse freely across cell membranes. The resulting osmotic gradient results in dilutional hyponatremia. A discrepancy exceeding 10 mosm/kg between measured and calculated osmolality suggests either factitious hyponatremia or the presence of a nonsodium solute. In the practice of neurosurgical anesthesiology, hyponatremia with a normal osmolality could be seen in patients after administration of mannitol but before urinary excretion had occurred.

Hyponatremia with hyposmolality, which may occur with high or low total body sodium, is evaluated by assessing BUN, SCr, total body sodium content, urinary osmolality, and urinary [Na+]. Increased total body sodium characteristically accompanies hyponatremia in edematous states, such as congestive heart failure, cirrhosis, nephrosis, and renal failure. Reduced urinary diluting capacity in patients with renal insufficiency can lead to hyponatremia if excess free water is given, as may occur with perioperative administration of hypotonic fluids. In hyponatremia with low total body sodium content (hypovolemia), volume-responsive ADH secretion sacrifices tonicity to preserve intravascular volume.

Euvolemic hyponatremia associated with a relatively normal total body sodium and ECV is almost

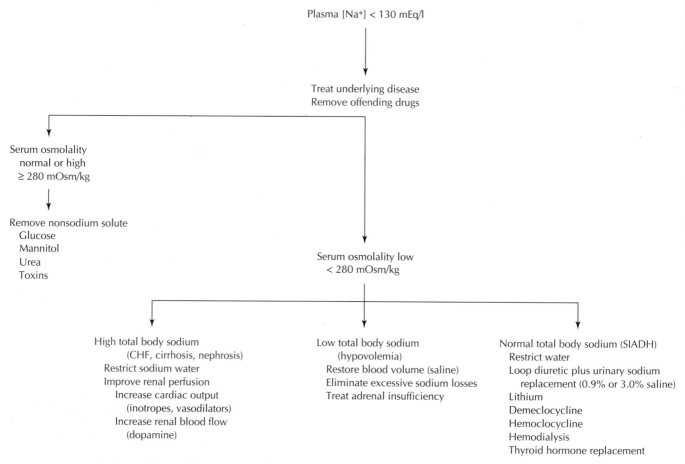

Plasma [Na⁺] < 130 mEq/l

Treat underlying disease
Remove offending drugs

Serum osmolality
normal or high
≥ 280 mOsm/kg

Remove nonsodium solute
Glucose
Mannitol
Urea
Toxins

Serum osmolality low
< 280 mOsm/kg

High total body sodium
(CHF, cirrhosis, nephrosis)
Restrict sodium water
Improve renal perfusion
Increase cardiac output
(inotropes, vasodilators)
Increase renal blood flow
(dopamine)

Low total body sodium
(hypovolemia)
Restore blood volume (saline)
Eliminate excessive sodium losses
Treat adrenal insufficiency

Normal total body sodium (SIADH)
Restrict water
Loop diuretic plus urinary sodium
replacement (0.9% or 3.0% saline)
Lithium
Demeclocycline
Hemoclocycline
Hemodialysis
Thyroid hormone replacement

Figure 4-5 Flow chart for treatment of hyponatremia. CHF, congestive heart failure; SIADH, syndrome of inappropriate antidiuretic hormone secretion.

invariably due to the syndrome of inappropriate ADH secretion (SIADH). Euvolemic hyponatremia is usually associated with excessive ectopic ADH secretion (as occurs with certain neoplasms), excessive hypothalamic-pituitary release of ADH (secondary to intracranial pathology, stress, pulmonary disease, or endocrine abnormalities), exogenous ADH administration, pharmacologic potentiation of ADH action, or drugs that mimic the action of ADH in the renal tubules.

Treatment of hyponatremia associated with a normal or high serum osmolality requires reduction of the elevated concentrations of the responsible solute (Fig. 4-5). Treatment of edematous (hypervolemic) patients necessitates restriction of sodium and water and is directed toward improving cardiac output and renal perfusion and using diuretics to inhibit sodium reabsorption. In hypovolemic, hyponatremic patients, blood volume must be restored, usually by infusion of 0.9% saline, and excessive sodium losses must be curtailed. Correction of hypovolemia usually results in removal of the stimulus of ADH release, accompanied by a rapid water diuresis.

The cornerstone of SIADH management is free water restriction and elimination of precipitating causes. Water restriction, sufficient to decrease TBW by 0.5 to 1.0 liter/day, decreases ECV even if excessive ADH secretion continues. The resultant reduction in GFR enhances proximal tubular reabsorption of salt and water, thereby decreasing free water generation, and stimulates aldosterone secretion. If renal, cutaneous, and gastrointestinal losses exceed free water intake, serum [Na⁺] will increase. Free water excretion can be increased by administering furosemide.

Acute neurologic symptoms of profound hyponatremia ([Na⁺] < 115 to 120 meq/liter) require more aggressive therapy. In patients who have seizures or who acutely develop symptoms of water intoxication, 3% saline can be administered at a rate of 1 to 2 ml/kg per h to increase plasma [Na⁺] by 1 to 2 meq/liter per h; however, this treatment should not continue for more than a few hours. Three percent saline may only transiently increase plasma [Na⁺] because ECV expansion also increases urinary sodium excretion. Intravenous furosemide, combined with quantitative replacement of urinary sodium losses with 0.9% or 3.0% saline, can rapidly increase plasma [Na$^+$], in part by increasing free water clearance.

Even symptomatic hyponatremia should be corrected cautiously. Although delayed correction may result in neurologic injury, inappropriately rapid correction may result in abrupt brain dehydration, central pontine myelinolysis,[60,158,159] cerebral hemorrhage, or congestive heart failure.

The symptoms of the osmotic demyelination syndrome vary from mild to severe (including pseudobulbar palsy and quadriparesis).[156,159] Within 3 to 4 weeks of the clinical onset of the syndrome, areas of demyelination are apparent on magnetic resonance imaging scans.[160] Rapid correction of hyponatremia to normal levels clearly plays a central role in the development of central demyelinating lesions. Although the magnitude of correction may also contribute to the development of demyelinating lesions,[156] experimental myelinolysis is not observed if the rate of correction is less than 2.5 meq/liter per h or if the magnitude of correction is limited to less than 25 meq in 24 h.[161] In rats, rapid correction of severe hyponatremia to normonatremic or hypernatremic levels results in severe demyelinating brain lesions; in contrast, rapid correction to mildly hyponatremic levels is associated with less severe pathology.[162] Greater chronicity of hyponatremia predisposes experimental animals to more severe demyelination.[60] Most patients in whom the osmotic demyelination syndrome is fatal have undergone correction of plasma [Na$^+$] of more than 20 meq/liter per day.[159] The rate at which plasma [Na$^+$] will increase during therapy is not predictable, varying based on both the composition of the infused fluid and the rate of renal water excretion.[163]

To limit the risk of myelinolysis, plasma [Na$^+$] may be increased by 1 to 2 meq/liter per h; however, plasma [Na$^+$] should not be increased more than 12 meq/liter in 24 h or 25 meq/liter in 48 h.[164–169] Hypernatremia should be avoided. Once the plasma [Na$^+$] exceeds 120 to 125 meq/liter, water restriction alone is usually sufficient to normalize [Na$^+$]. As acute hyponatremia is corrected, neurologic signs and symptoms usually improve within 24 h, although 96 h may be necessary for maximal recovery.

Demeclocycline and lithium, though potentially toxic, have been used effectively to reverse SIADH in patients in whom the primary disease process is irreversible. Although better tolerated than lithium, demeclocycline may induce nephrotoxicity, a particular concern in patients with hepatic dysfunction. In severely hyponatremic patients who cannot be adequately managed with drugs or hypertonic saline, hemodialysis is occasionally necessary. Once hyponatremia has improved, careful fluid restriction is necessary to avoid recurrence of hyponatremia.

Hypernatremia also produces neurologic symptoms (including stupor, coma, and seizures), hypovolemia, renal insufficiency and decreased urinary concentrating ability.[16,170] Because hypernatremia frequently results from diabetes insipidus or osmotically induced losses of sodium and water, many patients are hypovolemic or azotemic. Postoperative neurosurgical patients who have undergone pituitary surgery are at particular risk of developing transient or prolonged diabetes insipidus.[171] Polyuria may be present for only a few days within the first week of surgery, may be permanent, or may demonstrate a triphasic sequence: early diabetes insipidus, return of urinary concentrating ability, then recurrent diabetes insipidus. The clinical consequences of hypernatremia are most serious at the extremes of age and when hypernatremia develops abruptly. Brain shrinkage may damage delicate cerebral vessels, leading to subdural hematoma, subcortical parenchymal hemorrhage, SAH, and venous thrombosis. Polyuria may cause bladder distension, hydronephrosis, and permanent renal damage. At the cellular level, restoration of cell volume occurs remarkably quickly after tonicity is altered.[172]

By definition, hypernatremia ([Na$^+$] > 150 meq/liter) indicates an absolute or relative water deficit and is always associated with hypertonicity. Because hypovolemia accompanies most pathologic water loss, signs of hypoperfusion also may be present. In many patients, before the development of hypernatremia, an increased volume of hypotonic urine suggests an abnormality in water balance.[173] The TBW deficit can be estimated from the plasma [Na$^+$] using the equation:

$$\text{TBW deficit} = (0.6)(\text{weight in kg})$$
$$- \left(\frac{140}{\text{actual [Na}^+\text{]}} \right)(0.6)(\text{weight in kg}) \quad \text{(Eq. 13)}$$

Treatment of hypernatremia produced by water loss consists of repletion of water as well as associated deficits in total body sodium and other electrolytes. Hypernatremia must be corrected slowly because of the risk of neurologic sequelae such as seizures or cerebral edema.[174] The water deficit should be replaced over 24 to 48 h, and the plasma [Na$^+$] should not be reduced by more than 1 to 2 meq/liter per h. Reversible underlying causes should be treated. Hypovolemia should be corrected promptly with 0.9% saline. Once hypovolemia is corrected, water can be replaced orally or with intravenous hypotonic fluids, depending on the ability of the patient to tolerate oral hydration. In the occasional sodium-overloaded patient, sodium excretion can be accelerated using loop diuretics or dialysis.

The management of hypernatremia secondary to diabetes insipidus varies according to whether the etiology is central or nephrogenic. As noted earlier, the two most suitable agents for correcting central diabetes insipidus (an ADH deficiency syndrome) are DDAVP and aqueous vasopressin. In nephrogenic diabetes insipidus, the renal collecting ducts are resistant to the action of ADH. Urinary water losses can be decreased by using salt and water restriction or thiazide diuretics to induce ECV contraction and enhance fluid reabsorption in the proximal tubules.

POTASSIUM

Potassium, the predominant intracellular cation, normally has a gradient of approximately 30 : 1 between the intracellular and extracellular spaces. Because of cell lysis during clotting, serum ($[K^+]$) is about 0.5 meq/liter higher than plasma $[K^+]$. Total body potassium in a 70-kg adult is approximately 4256 meq, of which 4200 meq is intracellular; of the 56 meq in the ECV, only 12 meq is located in the PV.

Total body potassium and potassium concentration are primarily regulated by three hormones: aldosterone, epinephrine, and insulin. Aldosterone increases renal reabsorption of sodium and excretion of potassium. Secretion of either epinephrine or insulin shifts potassium intracellularly and provides an important short-term response to hyperkalemia.

Potassium is also influenced independently by intrinsic renal mechanisms. Assuming a plasma $[K^+]$ of 4.0 meq/liter and a normal GFR of 180 1/day, 720 meq of potassium is filtered daily. Most is reabsorbed; usually, only the amount ingested (normally 40 to 120 meq/day) is lost. Dietary potassium intake, unless greater than normal, can be excreted as long as GFR exceeds 8.0 ml/min. Within the distal nephron, a magnesium-dependent sodium/potassium ATPase enzyme plays a critical role in potassium reabsorption.[175] Magnesium depletion impairs the activity of the enzyme, leading to renal potassium wasting.

Hypokalemia ($[K^+] < 3.0$ meq/liter) causes muscle weakness and, when severe, may even cause paralysis. The ratio of intracellular to extracellular potassium contributes to the resting potential difference across cell membranes and therefore to the integrity of cardiac and neuromuscular transmission. With chronic potassium loss, the ratio of intracellular to extracellular $[K^+]$ remains relatively stable; in contrast, acute redistribution of potassium from the extracellular to the intracellular space substantially changes resting membrane potentials.

Cardiac rhythm disturbances are among the most dangerous complications of potassium deficiency. Acute hypokalemia causes hyperpolarization of the cardiac cell and may lead to ventricular escape activity, reentrant phenomena, ectopic tachycardias, and delayed conduction. Despite the long-standing concern

of anesthesia personnel that preoperative chronic hypokalemia increases the incidence of intraoperative arrhythmias, a prospective study failed to confirm that suspicion.[176]

The plasma potassium concentration ($[K^+]$) poorly reflects total body potassium; hypokalemia may occur with normal, low, or high total body potassium stores. In uncomplicated hypokalemia, the potassium deficit exceeds 300 meq if plasma $[K^+]$ is less than 3.0 meq/liter and 700 meq if plasma $[K^+]$ is less than 2.0 meq/liter.

Hypokalemia may result from acute redistribution of potassium from the ECV to the ICV, in which case total body potassium will be normal, or from chronic depletion of total body potassium. Redistribution of potassium into cells occurs when the activity of the sodium-potassium ATPase pump is acutely increased by extracellular hyperkalemia or increased intracellular concentrations of sodium, as well as by insulin, carbohydrate loading (which stimulates release of endogenous insulin), β_2 agonists, and aldosterone. Both metabolic and respiratory alkalosis, as in acute therapeutic hyperventilation, lead to decreases in plasma $[K^+]$.[177] Metabolic acidosis and respiratory acidosis tend to cause an increase in plasma $[K^+]$. However, organic acidoses (i.e., lactic acidosis, ketoacidosis) have little effect on $[K^+]$, whereas mineral acids cause significant cellular shifts.

Causes of chronic hypokalemia include those associated with renal potassium conservation (extrarenal potassium losses; low urinary $[K^+]$) and those associated with renal potassium wasting. A low urinary $[K^+]$ suggests inadequate dietary intake or extrarenal depletion (in the absence of recent diuretic use). Diuretic-induced urinary potassium losses are frequently associated with hypokalemia, secondary to increased aldosterone secretion, alkalemia, and increased renal tubular flow. Aldosterone does not cause renal potassium wasting unless sodium ions are present; that is, aldosterone primarily controls sodium reabsorption, not potassium excretion. Renal tubular damage due to nephrotoxins such as aminoglycosides or amphotericin B may also cause renal potassium wasting.

Initial evaluation of hypokalemia includes a medical history (e.g., diuretic use), physical examination (e.g., cushingoid features, edema), measurement of serum electrolytes (e.g., magnesium), and arterial pH assessment. Measurement of 24-h urinary excretion of sodium and potassium may distinguish extrarenal from renal causes. Plasma renin and aldosterone levels may be helpful in the differential diagnosis.

The treatment of hypokalemia consists of potassium repletion, correction of alkalemia, and removal of offending drugs. Hypokalemia secondary only to acute redistribution may not require treatment. If total body potassium is decreased, oral potassium supplementation is preferable to intravenous replacement. Potassium is usually replaced as the chloride salt because coexisting chloride deficiency may limit the ability of the kidney to conserve potassium.

Potassium repletion must be performed cautiously, usually at a rate of 10 to 20 meq/h or less because the absolute deficit is unpredictable. The plasma [K$^+$] and the electrocardiogram (ECG) must be monitored during rapid repletion (>20 meq/h) to avoid hyperkalemic complications. Particular care should be taken in patients who have concurrent acidemia, type IV renal tubular acidosis, or diabetes mellitus, or in those patients receiving NSAIDs, angiotensin-converting enzyme (ACE) inhibitors, or β blockers, all of which delay movement of extracellular potassium into cells.

Hypokalemia associated with hyperaldosteronemia (e.g., primary aldosteronism, Cushing's syndrome) usually responds favorably to reduced sodium intake and increased potassium intake. Hypomagnesemia, if present, aggravates the effects of hypokalemia, impairs potassium conservation, and should be treated. In patients, such as those who have diabetic ketoacidosis, who are both acidemic and hypokalemic, potassium administration should precede correction of acidosis to avoid a precipitous decrease in plasma [K$^+$] as pH increases.

The most lethal manifestations of hyperkalemia ([K$^+$] > 5.0 meq/liter) involve the cardiac conducting system and include arrhythmias, conduction abnormalities, and cardiac arrest. In anesthesia practice, the classic example of hyperkalemic cardiac toxicity is associated with the administration of succinylcholine to paraplegic or quadriplegic patients.[178] If plasma [K$^+$] is less than 6.0 meq/liter, cardiac effects are negligible. As the concentration increases further, the ECG shows tall, peaked T waves, especially in the precordial leads. With further increases, the PR interval becomes prolonged, followed by a decrease in the amplitude of the P wave. Finally, the QRS complex widens into a pattern resembling a sine wave, as a prelude to cardiac standstill. Hyperkalemic cardiotoxicity is enhanced by hyponatremia, hypocalcemia, or acidosis. Because progression to fatal cardiotoxicity is unpredictable and often swift, the presence of hyperkalemic changes on the ECG mandates immediate therapy. The life-threatening cardiac effects usually require more urgent treatment than other manifestations of hyperkalemia. However, ascending muscle weakness appears when plasma [K$^+$] approaches 7.0 meq/liter, and may progress to flaccid paralysis, inability to phonate, and respiratory arrest.

Hyperkalemia may occur with normal, high, or low total-body potassium stores. Because the kidneys excrete potassium, severe renal insufficiency commonly causes hyperkalemia. Patients with chronic renal insufficiency can maintain normal plasma [K$^+$] despite markedly decreased GFR because urinary potassium excretion depends on tubular secretion rather than glomerular filtration if GFR exceeds 8 ml/min.

Drugs are now the most common cause of hyperkalemia.[179] Drugs that may limit potassium excretion include NSAIDs, ACE inhibitors, cyclosporin, and potassium-sparing diuretics such as triamterene. Drug effects most commonly occur in patients with other factors that predispose to hyperkalemia, such as diabetes mellitus, renal insufficiency, advanced age, or hyporeninemic hypoaldosteronism. ACE inhibitors are particularly likely to produce hyperkalemia in patients who have renal insufficiency[180] or severe congestive heart failure.[181]

In patients who have normal total body potassium, hyperkalemia may accompany a sudden shift of potassium from the ICV to the ECV because of acidemia, increased catabolism, or rhabdomyolysis. Pseudohyperkalemia, which occurs when potassium is released from cells in blood collection tubes, can be diagnosed by comparing serum and plasma K$^+$ levels from the same blood sample.

The treatment of hyperkalemia is aimed at eliminating the cause, reversing membrane hyperexcitability, and removing potassium from the body. Mineralocorticoid deficiency can be treated with 9-α-fludrocortisone (0.025 to 0.10 mg/day). Hyperkalemia secondary to digitalis intoxication may be resistant to therapy because attempts to shift potassium from the ECV to the ICV are often ineffective. In this situation, use of digoxin-specific antibodies has been successful.

Membrane hyperexcitability can be antagonized by translocating potassium from the ECV to the ICV, removing excess potassium, or (transiently) by infusing calcium chloride to depress the membrane threshold potential. Acute alkalinization using sodium bicarbonate (50 to 100 meq over 5 to 10 min in a 70-kg adult) transiently promotes movement of potassium from the ECV to the ICV. Bicarbonate can be administered even if pH exceeds 7.40; however, it should not be administered to patients with congestive cardiac failure or hypernatremia. Insulin, in a dose-dependent fashion, causes cellular uptake of potassium by increasing the activity of the sodium/potassium ATPase pump. Insulin increases cellular uptake of potassium *best* when high insulin levels are achieved by intravenous injection of 5 to 10 units regular insulin,[182] accompanied by 50 ml 50% glucose. β_2-Adrenergic drugs also increase potassium uptake by skeletal muscle and reduce plasma [K$^+$],[183] an action that may explain hypokalemia with severe, acute illness. The β_2 agonists have been used to treat hyperkalemia.[184]

Pending definitive treatment, rapid infusion of calcium chloride (1 ampule of $CaCl_2$ over 3 min, or 2 to 3 ampules of 10% calcium gluconate over 5 min) may stabilize cardiac rhythm. Calcium should be given cautiously if digitalis intoxication is likely. Potassium may be removed from the body by the renal or gastrointestinal routes. Furosemide promotes kaliuresis in a dose-dependent fashion. Sodium polystyrene sulfonate resin (Kayexalate), which exchanges sodium for potassium, can be given orally (30 g) or as a retention enema (50 g in 200 ml 20% sorbitol). However, sodium overload and hypervolemia are potential risks. Rarely, when temporizing measures are insufficient, emergency hemodialysis may remove 25 to 50 meq/h. Peritoneal dialysis is less efficient.

Summary

Appropriate fluid therapy for patients with neurologic disorders requires an understanding of the basic physical principles that govern the distribution of water between the intracellular and extracellular compartments. In the CNS, unlike peripheral tissues, osmolar gradients are the primary determinants of the movement of water. Changes in plasma oncotic pressure have negligible effects on brain water content. In contrast, administration of hypertonic solutions (e.g., 20% mannitol) results in a "dehydration" of normal brain tissue with a concomitant decrease in cerebral volume and ICP. Various monitoring modalities may help the clinician in the assessment of intravascular volume. Fluid administration should never be restricted to the point that cardiac output and blood pressure are compromised. Arterial hypotension after brain injury is an ominous sign that correlates with a marked increase in morbidity and mortality. In addition to management of intravascular volume, fluid therapy often must be modified to account for electrolyte disturbances. Of these, changes in $[Na^+]$ and $[K^+]$ are most important in patients with neurologic disease.

References

1. Bevan DR: Osmometry. 1. Terminology and principles of measurement. *Anaesthesia* 1978; 33:794.
2. Starling EH: On the absorption of fluids from the connective tissue spaces. *J Physiol* 1896; 19:312.
3. Peters RM, Hargens AR: Protein vs electrolytes and all of the Starling forces. *Arch Surg* 1981; 116:1293.
4. Fenstermacher JD, Johnson JA: Filtration and reflection coefficients of the rabbit blood-brain barrier. *Am J Physiol* 1966; 211:341.
5. Zornow MH, et al: The acute cerebral effects of changes in plasma osmolality and oncotic pressure. *Anesthesiology* 1987; 67:936.
6. Dodge PR, et al: Studies in experimental water intoxication. *Arch Neurol* 1960; 5:513.
7. Shenkin HA, et al: Restricted fluid intake: Rational management of the neurosurgical patient. *J Neurosurg* 1976; 45:432.
8. Warner DS, Boehland LA: Effects of iso-osmolal intravenous fluid therapy on post-ischemic brain water content in the rat. *Anesthesiology* 1988; 68:86.
9. Zornow MH, et al: Acute cerebral effects of isotonic crystalloid and colloid solutions following cryogenic brain injury in the rabbit. *Anesthesiology* 1988; 69:180.
10. Korosue K, et al: Comparison of crystalloids and colloids for hemodilution in a model of focal cerebral ischemia. *J Neurosurg* 1990; 73:576.
11. Little JR, et al: Treatment of acute focal cerebral ischemia with concentrated albumin. *Neurosurgery* 1981; 9:552.
12. Zornow MH, et al: Effect of a hypertonic lactated Ringer's solution on intracranial pressure and cerebral water content in a model of traumatic brain injury. *J Trauma* 1989; 29:484.
13. Badr KF, Ichikawa I: Prerenal failure: A deleterious shift from renal compensation to decompensation. *N Engl J Med* 1988; 319:623.
14. Henrich WL, et al: The role of renal nerves and prostaglandins in control of renal hemodynamics and plasma renin activity during hypotensive hemorrhage in the dog. *J Clin Invest* 1978; 61:744.
15. Henrich WL, et al: The influence of circulating catecholamines and prostaglandins on canine renal hemodynamics during hemorrhage. *Circ Res* 1981; 48:424.
16. Hall J, Robertson G: Diabetes insipidus. *Prob Crit Care* 1990; 4:342.
17. Needleman P, Greenwald JE: Atriopeptin: A cardiac hormone intimately involved in fluid, electrolyte, and blood-pressure homeostasis. *N Engl J Med* 1986; 314:828.
18. Cernacek P, et al: Renal dose response and pharmacokinetics of atrial natriuretic factor in dogs. *Am J Physiol* 1988; 255:R929.
19. Laragh JH: The endocrine control of blood volume, blood pressure and sodium balance: Atrial hormone and renin system interactions. *J Hypertens* 1986; 4(suppl 2):S143.
20. Murray MD, Brater DC: Adverse effect of nonsteroidal anti-inflammatory drugs on renal function. *Ann Intern Med* 1990; 112:559.
21. Arfors KE, Buckley PB: Role of artificial colloids in rational fluid therapy. In Tuma RF, et al (eds.): *The Role of Hemodilution in Optimal Patient Care.* München, W. Zuckschwerdt Verlag, 1989:100–123.
22. Stump DC, et al: Effects of hydroxyethyl starch on blood coagulation, particularly factor VIII. *Transfusion* 1985; 25:349.
23. Trumble ER, et al: Coagulopathy with the use of hetastarch in the treatment of vasospasm. *J. Neurosurg* 1995; 82:44.
24. Zikria BA, et al: Hydroxyethyl starch macromolecules reduce myocardial reperfusion injury. *Arch Surg* 1990; 125:930.
25. Zikria BA, et al: A biophysical approach to capillary permeability. *Surgery* 1989; 105:625.
26. Moorthy SS, et al: Increased cerebral and decreased femoral artery blood flow velocities during direct laryngoscopy and tracheal intubation. *Anesth Analg* 1994; 78:1144.
27. Brazeal BA, et al: Pentafraction for superior resuscitation of the ovine thermal burn. *Crit Care Med* 1995; 23:332.
28. Traber LD, et al: Pentafraction reduces the lung lymph response after endotoxin administration in the ovine model. *Circ Shock* 1992; 36:93.
29. Webb AR, et al: Advantages of a narrow-range, medium molecular weight hydroxethyl starch for volume maintenance in a porcine model of fecal peritonitis. *Crit Care Med* 1991; 19:409.
30. Dodd RY: The risk of transfusion-transmitted infection. *N Engl J Med* 1992; 327:419.
31. Rackow EC, et al: Fluid resuscitation in circulatory shock: A comparison of the cardiorespiratory effects of albumin, heta-

starch, and saline solutions in patients with hypovolemic and septic shock. *Crit Care Med* 1983; 11:839.

32. Weil MH, et al: Colloid oncotic pressure: Clinical significance. *Crit Care Med* 1979; 7:113.

33. Pearl RG, Halperin BD, Mihm FG, Rosenthal MH: Pulmonary effects of crystalloid and colloid resuscitation from hemorrhagic shock in the presence of oleic acid-induced pulmonary capillary injury in the dog. *Anesthesiology* 1988; 68:12.

34. Virgilio RW, et al: Crystalloid vs colloid resuscitation: Is one better? A randomized clinical study. *Surgery* 1979; 85:129.

35. Prough DS, Johnston WE: Fluid resuscitation in septic shock: No solution yet. *Anesth Analg* 1989; 69:699.

36. Baum TD, et al: Mesenteric oxygen metabolism, ileal mucosal hydrogen ion concentration, and tissue edema after crystalloid of colloid resuscitation in porcine endotoxic shock: Comparison of Ringer's lactate and 6% hetastarch. *Circ Shock* 1990; 30:385.

37. Linko K, Makelainen A: Cardiorespiratory function after replacement of blood loss with hydroxyethyl starch 120, dextran-70, and Ringer's acetate in pigs. *Crit Care Med* 1989; 17:1031.

38. Weed LH, McKibben PS: Experimental alteration of brain bulk. *Am J Physiol* 1919; 48:531.

39. Traverso LW, et al: Hypertonic sodium chloride solutions: Effect on hemodynamics and survival after hemorrhage in swine. *J Trauma* 1987; 27:32.

40. Velasco IT, et al: Hyperosmotic NaCl and severe hemorrhagic shock. *Am J Physiol* 1980; 239:H664.

41. Jelenko C III, et al: Studies in shock and resuscitation. I. Use of a hypertonic, albumin-containing fluid demand regimen (HALFD) in resuscitation. *Crit Care Med* 1979; 7:157.

42. Monafo WW, et al: Hypertonic sodium solutions in the treatment of burn shock. *Am J Surg* 1973; 126:778.

43. Shackford SR, et al: Hypertonic sodium lactate versus lactated Ringer's solution for intravenous fluid therapy in operations on the abdominal aorta. *Surgery* 1983; 94:41.

44. Gunn ML, et al: Prospective, randomized trial of hypertonic sodium lactate versus lactated Ringer's solution for burn shock resuscitation. *J Trauma* 1989; 29:1261.

45. Shackford SR, et al: Serum osmolar and electrolyte changes associated with large infusions of hypertonic sodium lactate for intravascular volume expansion of patients undergoing aortic reconstruction. *Surg Gynecol Obstet* 1987; 164:127.

46. Worthley LIG, et al: Treatment of resistant intracranial hypertension with hypertonic saline. Report of two cases. *J Neurosurg* 1988; 68:478.

47. Fisher B, et al: Hypertonic saline lowers raised intracranial pressure in children after head trauma. *J Neurosurg Anesth* 1992; 4:4.

48. Schertel ER, et al: Influence of 7% NaCl on the mechanical properties of the systemic circulation in the hypovolemic dog. *Circ Shock* 1990; 31:203.

49. Spital A, Sterns RD: The paradox of sodium's volume of distribution. Why an extracellular solute appears to distribute over total body water. *Arch Intern Med* 1989; 149:1255.

50. Badrick T, Hickman PE: The anion gap: A reappraisal. *Am J Clin Pathol* 1992; 98:249.

51. Mathieu D, et al: Effects of bicarbonate therapy on hemodynamics and tissue oxygenation in patients with lactic acidosis: A prospective, controlled clinical study. *Crit Care Med* 1991; 19:1352.

52. Mark NH, et al: Safety of low-dose intraoperative bicarbonate therapy: A prospective, double-blind, randomized study. *Crit Care Med* 1993; 21:659.

53. Leung JM, et al: Safety and efficacy of intravenous carbicarb in patients undergoing surgery: Comparison with sodium bi-

carbonate in the treatment of mild metabolic acidosis. *Crit Care Med* 1994; 22:1540.

54. Smith GJ, et al: A comparison of several hypertonic solutions for resuscitation of bled sheep. *J Surg Res* 1985; 39:517.

55. Mattox KL, et al: Prehospital hypertonic saline/dextran infusion for post-traumatic hypotension. The U.S.A. Multicenter Trial. *Ann Surg* 1991; 213:482.

56. Vassar MJ, et al: 7.5% sodium chloride/dextran for resuscitation of trauma patients undergoing helicopter transport. *Arch Surg* 1991; 126:1065.

57. Vassar MJ, et al: A multicenter trial for resuscitation of injured patients with 7.5% sodium chloride: The effect of added dextran 70. *Arch Surg* 1993; 128:1003.

58. Wisner DH, et al: Nuclear magnetic resonance as a measure of cerebral metabolism: Effects of hypertonic saline. *J Trauma* 1992; 32:351.

59. Waschke KF, et al: Coupling between local cerebral blood flow and metabolism after hypertonic/hyperoncotic fluid resuscitation from hemorrhage in conscious rats. *Anesth Analg* 1996; 82:52.

60. Norenberg MD, Papendick RE: Chronicity of hyponatremia as a factor in experimental myelinolysis. *Ann Neurol* 1984; 15:544.

61. Gross D, et al: Treatment of uncontrolled hemorrhagic shock with hypertonic saline solution. *Surg Gynecol Obstet* 1990; 170:106.

62. Bickell WH, et al: Immediate versus delayed fluid resuscitation for hypotensive patients with penetrating torso injuries. *N Engl J Med* 1994; 331:1105.

63. Natanson C, et al: Selected treatment strategies for septic shock based on proposed mechanisms of pathogenesis. *Ann Intern Med* 1994; 120:771.

64. Lanier WL, et al: The effects of dextrose infusion and head position on neurologic outcome after complete cerebral ischemia in primates: Examination of a model. *Anesthesiology* 1987; 66:39.

65. Longstreth WT Jr, et al: Neurologic outcome and blood glucose levels during out-of-hospital cardiopulmonary resuscitation. *Neurology* 1986; 36:1186.

66. Lam AM, et al: Hyperglycemia and neurological outcome in patients with head injury. *J Neurosurg* 1991; 75:545.

67. Sieber FE, et al: Glucose: A reevaluation of its intraoperative use. *Anesthesiology* 1987; 67:72.

68. Roberts JP, et al: Extracellular fluid deficit following operation and its correction with Ringer's lactate: A reassessment. *Ann Surg* 1985; 202:1.

69. Chiao JJC, et al: In vivo myocyte sodium activity and concentration during hemorrhagic shock. *Am J Physiol* 1990; 258:R684.

70. Shires GT, et al: Alterations in cellular membrane function during hemorrhagic shock in primates. *Ann Surg* 1972; 176:288.

71. Böck JC, et al: Post-traumatic changes in, and effect of colloid osmotic pressure on the distribution of body water. *Ann Surg* 1989; 210:395.

72. Zaloga GP, Hughes SS: Oliguria in patients with normal renal function. *Anesthesiology* 1990; 72:598.

73. Lipsitz LA: Orthostatic hypotension in the elderly. *N Engl J Med* 1989; 321:952.

74. Wong DH, et al: Changes in cardiac output after acute blood loss and position change in man. *Crit Care Med* 1989; 17:979.

75. Amoroso P, Greenwood RN: Posture and central venous pressure measurement in circulatory volume depletion. *Lancet* 1989; 2:258.

76. Riley LJ Jr, et al: Acute metabolic acid-base disorders. *Crit Care Clin* 1987; 5:699.

77. Goldring RM, et al: Respiratory adjustment to chronic metabolic alkalosis in man. *J Clin Invest* 1968; 47:188.

78. Ponce P, Santana A, Vinhas J: Treatment of severe metabolic alkalosis by "acid dialysis." *Crit Care Med* 1991; 19:583.

79. Douglas PS, et al: Unreliability of hemodynamic indexes of left ventricular size during cardiac surgery. *Ann Thorac Surg* 1987; 44:31.

80. Ellis RJ, Mangano DT, Van Dyke DC: Relationship of wedge pressure to end-diastolic volume in patients undergoing myocardial revascularization. *J Thorac Cardiovasc Surg* 1979; 78:605.

81. Hansen RM, et al: Poor correlation between pulmonary arterial wedge pressure and left ventricular end-diastolic volume after coronary artery bypass graft surgery. *Anesthesiology* 1986; 64:764.

82. Raper R, Sibbald WJ: Misled by the wedge? The Swan-Ganz catheter and LV preload. *Chest* 1986; 88:427.

83. Schiller NB, et al: Recommendations for quantitation of the left ventricle by two-dimensional echocardiography. *J Am Soc Echo* 1989; 2:358.

84. Thys DM, et al: A comparison of hemodynamic indices by invasive monitoring and two dimensional echocardiography. *Anesthesiology* 1987; 67:630.

85. Cheung AT, et al: Echocardiographic and hemodynamic indexes of left ventricular preload in patients with normal and abnormal ventricular function. *Anesthesiology* 1994; 81:376.

86. Reich DL, et al: Intraoperative transesophageal echocardiography for the detection of cardiac preload changes induced by transfusion and phlebotomy in pediatric patients. *Anesthesiology* 1993; 79:10.

87. Berk MR, et al: Reduction of left ventricular preload by lower body negative pressure alters Doppler transmitral filling patterns. *J Am Coll Cardiol* 1990; 16:1387.

88. Konstadt SN, et al: Validation of quantitative intraoperative transesophageal echocardiography. *Anesthesiology* 1986; 65:418.

89. Clements FM, et al: Simultaneous measurements of cardiac volumes, areas, and ejection fractions by transesophageal echocardiography and first-pass radionuclide angiography. *Anesthesiology* 1988; 69(3A):A4.

90. Urbanowicz JH, et al: Comparison of transesophageal echocardiographic and scintigraphic estimates of left ventricular end-diastolic volume index and ejection fraction in patients following coronary artery bypass grafting. *Anesthesiology* 1990; 72:607.

91. Leung JM, Levine EH: Left ventricular end-systolic cavity obliteration as an estimate of intraoperative hypovolemia. *Anesthesiology* 1994; 81:1102.

92. Stoddart MF, et al: Influence of alternation in preload on the pattern of left ventricular diastolic filling as assessed by Doppler echocardiography in humans. *Circulation* 1989; 79:1226.

93. Otto CM, Pearlman AS: Echocardiographic evaluation of ventricular diastolic filling and function. In *Textbook of Clinical Echocardiography*. Philadelphia, WB Saunders, 1995: 117–136.

94. Shoemaker WC, et al: Prospective trial of supranormal values of survivors as therapeutic goals in high-risk surgical patients. *Chest* 1988; 94:1176.

95. Tuchschmidt J, et al: Elevation of cardiac output and oxygen delivery improves outcome in septic shock. *Chest* 1992; 102:216.

96. Bishop MH, et al: Prospective, randomized trial of survivor values of cardiac index, oxygen delivery, and oxygen consumption as resuscitation endpoints in severe trauma. *J Trauma* 1995; 38:780.

97. Boyd O, et al: A randomized clinical trial of the effect of deliberate perioperative increase of oxygen delivery on mortality in high-risk surgical patients. *JAMA* 1993; 270:2699.

98. Hayes MA, et al: Elevation of systemic oxygen delivery in the treatment of critically ill patients. *N Engl J Med* 1994; 330:1717.

99. Gattinoni L, et al: A trial of goal-oriented hemodynamic therapy in critically ill patients. *N Engl J Med* 1995; 333:1025.

100. Cain SM: Oxygen delivery and uptake in dogs during anemic and hypoxic hypoxia. *J Appl Physiol* 1977; 42:228.

101. Shibutani K, et al: Critical level of oxygen delivery in anesthetized man. *Crit Care Med* 1983; 11:640.

102. Danek SJ, et al: The dependence of oxygen uptake on oxygen delivery in the adult respiratory distress syndrome. *Am Rev Respir Dis* 1980; 122:387.

103. Kaufman BS, et al: The relationship between oxygen delivery and consumption during fluid resuscitation of hypovolemic and septic shock. *Chest* 1984; 85:336.

104. Mohsenifar Z, et al: Relationship between O_2 delivery and O_2 consumption in the adult respiratory distress syndrome. *Chest* 1983; 84:267.

105. Clarke C, et al: Persistence of supply dependency of oxygen uptake at high levels of delivery in adult respiratory distress syndrome. *Crit Care Med* 1991; 19:497.

106. D'Orio V, et al: Lung fluid dynamics and supply dependency of oxygen uptake during experimental endotoxic shock and volume resuscitation. *Crit Care Med* 1991; 19:955.

107. Vermeij CG, et al: Independent oxygen uptake and oxygen delivery in septic and postoperative patients. *Chest* 1991; 99:1438.

108. Villar J, et al: Oxygen transport and oxygen consumption in critically ill patients. *Chest* 1990; 98:687.

109. Bhatt SB, et al: Effect of dobutamine on oxygen supply and uptake in healthy volunteers. *Br J Anaesth* 1992; 69:298.

110. Bakker J, Vincent J: Effects of norepinephrine and dobutamine on oxygen transport and consumption in a dog model of endotoxic shock. *Crit Care Med* 1993; 21:425.

111. Scalea TM, et al: Geriatric blunt multiple trauma: Improved survival with early invasive monitoring. *J Trauma* 1990; 30:129.

112. Fink MP: Gastrointestinal mucosal injury in experimental models of shock, trauma, and sepsis. *Crit Care Clin* 1991; 19:627.

113. Scalia S, et al: Persistent arteriolar constriction in microcirculation of the terminal ileum following moderate hemorrhagic hypovolemia and volume restoration. *J Trauma* 1990; 30:713.

114. Korein J, et al: Radioisotopic bolus technique as a test to detect circulatory deficit associated with cerebral death: 142 studies on 80 patients demonstrating the bedside use of an innocous IV procedure as a adjunct in the diagnosis of cerebral death. *Circulation* 1975; 51:924.

115. Jones TH, et al: Thresholds of focal cerebral ischemia in awake monkeys. *J Neurosurg* 1981; 54:773.

116. Symon L: Flow thresholds in brain ischaemia and the effects of drugs. *Br J Anaesth* 1985; 57:34.

117. Holbach KH, et al: Reversibility of the chronic post-stroke state. *Stroke* 1978; 7:296.

118. Hossmann KA, Olsson Y: Suppression and recovery of neuronal function in transient cerebral ischemia. *Brain Res* 1970; 22:313.

119. Sharbrough FW, et al: Correlation of continuous electroencephalograms with cerebral blood flow measurements during carotid endarterectomy. *Stroke* 1973; 4:674.

120. Kety SS, Schmidt CF: The determination of cerebral blood flow in man by the use of nitrous oxide in low concentrations. *Am J Physiol* 1945; 143:53.

121. Olesen J, et al: Regional cerebral blood flow in man determined by the initial slope of the clearance of intra-arterially injected ^{113}Xe. Theory of the method, normal values, error of measurement, correction for remaining radioactivity, relation to other flow parameters and response to $PaCO_2$ changes. *Stroke* 1971; 2:519.

122. Obrist WD, et al: Regional cerebral blood flow estimated by ^{133}Xenon inhalation. *Stroke* 1975; 6:245.

123. Bishop CCR, et al: Transcranial Doppler measurement of middle cerebral artery blood flow velocity: A validation study. *Stroke* 1986; 17:913.

124. Robertson CS, et al: Cerebral arteriovenous oxygen difference as an estimate of cerebral blood flow in comatose patients. *J Neurosurg* 1989, 70:222.

125. Gopinath SP, et al: Near-infrared spectroscopic localization of intracranial hematomas. *J. Neurosurg* 1993; 79:43.

126. Jobsis-Vandervliet FF, et al: Monitoring of cerebral oxygenation and cytochrome aa$_3$ redox state. In Tremper KK, Barker SJ (eds): *Advances in Oxygen Monitoring. International Anesthesiology Clinics.* Boston, Little, Brown, 1987:209–230.

127. Smith DS, et al: Reperfusion hyperoxia in brain after circulatory arrest in humans. *Anesthesiology* 1990; 73:12.

128. Delpy DT, et al: Quantitation of pathlength in optical spectroscopy. *Adv Exp Med Biol* 1989; 248:41.

129. Ferrari M, et al: Noninvasive determination of hemoglobin saturation in dogs by derivative near-infrared spectroscopy. *Am J Physiol* 1989; 256:H1493.

130. McCormick PW, et al: Clinical application of diffuse near-infrared spectroscopy to measure cerebral oxygen metabolism. *Hospimedica* 1990; 8:39.

131. Pollard V, et al: Validation in volunteers of a near-infrared spectroscope for monitoring brain oxygenation in vivo. *Anesth Analg* 1996; 82:269.

132. Pollard V, et al: The influence of carbon dioxide and body position on near-infrared spectroscopic assessment of cerebral hemoglobin oxygen saturation. *Anesth Analg* 1996; 82:278.

133. Whitley, JM, et al: Cerebral hemodynamic effects of fluid resuscitation in the presence of an experimental intracranial mass. *Surgery* 1991; 110:514.

134. Prough DS, et al: Hypertonic saline does not reduce intracranial pressure or improve cerebral blood flow after experimental head injury and hemorrhage in cats. *Crit Care Med* 1996; 24:109.

135. Robinson AG: DDAVP in the treatment of central diabetes insipidus. *N Engl J Med* 1976; 294:507.

136. Cobb WE, et al: Neurogenic diabetes insipidus: Management with dDAVP (1-desamino-8-D arginine vasopressin). *Ann Intern Med* 1978; 88:183.

137. Shucart WA, Jackson I: Management of diabetes insipidus in neurosurgical patients. *J Neurosurg* 1976; 44:65.

138. Chanson P, et al: Ultra low doses of vasopressin in the management of diabetes insipidus. *Crit Care Med* 1987; 15:44.

139. Wood JH, et al: Experimental hypervolemic hemodilution: Physiological correlations of cortical blood flow, cardiac output, and intracranial pressure with fresh blood viscosity and plasma volume. *Neurosurgery* 1984; 14:709.

140. Wood JH, et al: Hypervolemic hemodilution in experimental focal cerebral ischemia. Elevation of cardiac output, regional cortical blood flow, and ICP after intravascular volume expansion with low molecular weight dextran. *J Neurosurg* 1983; 59:500.

141. Wood JH, Snyder LL, Simeone FA: Failure of intravascular volume expansion without hemodilution to elevate cortical blood flow in region of experimental focal ischemia. *J Neurosurg* 1982; 56:80.

142. Wood JH, et al: Quantitative EEG alterations after isovolemic-hemodilutional augmentation of cerebral perfusion in stroke patients. *Neurology* 1984; 34:764.

143. Reasoner DK, et al: Marked hemodilution increases neurologic injury after focal cerebral ischemia in rabbits. *Anesth Analg* 1996; 82:61.

144. Scandinavian Stroke Study Group: Multicenter trial of hemodilution in acute ischemic stroke. I. Results in the total patient population. *Stroke* 1987; 18:691.

145. Italian Acute Stroke Study Group: Haemodilution in acute stroke: Results of the Italian Haemodilution Trial. *Lancet* 1988; 1:318.

146. The Hemodilution in Stroke Study Group: Hypervolemic hemodilution treatment of acute stroke. Results of a randomized multicenter trial using pentastarch. *Stroke* 1989; 20:317.

147. Hijdra A, et al: Prediction of delayed cerebral ischemia, rebleeding, and outcome after aneurysmal subarachnoid hemorrhage. *Stroke* 1988; 19:1250.

148. Voldby B, et al: Regional CBF, interventricular pressure, and cerebral metabolism in patients with ruptured intracranial aneurysms. *J Neurosurg* 1985; 62:48.

149. Klingelhöfer J, et al: Cerebral vasospasm evaluated by transcranial Doppler ultrasonography at different intracranial pressures. *J Neurosurg* 1991; 75:752.

150. Powers WJ, et al: Regional cerebral blood flow and metabolism in reversible ischemia due to vasospasm: Determination by positron emission tomography. *J Neurosurg* 1985; 62:539.

151. Nelson RJ, et al: Association of hypovolemia after subarachnoid hemorrhage with computed tomographic scan evidence of raised intracranial pressure. *Neurosurgery* 1991; 29:178.

152. Medlock MD, Dulebohn SC, Elwood PW: Prophylactic hypervolemia without calcium channel blockers in early aneurysm surgery. *Neurosurgery* 1992; 30:12.

153. Kirsch JR, et al: Cerebral aneurysms: Mechanisms of injury and critical care interventions. *Crit Care Clin* 1989; 5:755.

154. Zabramski JM, et al: Phase I trial of tissue plasminogen activator for the prevention of vasospasm in patients with aneurysmal subarachnoid hemorrhage. *J Neurosurg* 1991; 72:189.

155. Levy ML, Giannotta SL: Cardiac performance indices during hypervolemic therapy for cerebral vasospasm. *J Neurosurg* 1991; 75:27.

156. Berl T: Treating hyponatremia: Damned if we do and damned if we don't. *Kidney Int* 1990; 37:1006.

157. Lien YH, et al: Effects of hypernatremia on organic brain osmoles. *J Clin Invest* 1990; 85:1427.

158. Laureno R: Central pontine myelinolysis following rapid correction of hyponatremia. *Ann Neurol* 1983; 13:232.

159. Sterns RH, et al: Osmotic demyelination syndrome following correction of hyponatremia. *N Engl J Med* 1986; 314:1535.

160. Brunner JE, et al: Central pontine myelinolysis and pontine lesions after rapid correction of hyponatremia: A prospective magnetic resonance imaging study. *Ann Neurol* 1990; 27:61.

161. Verbalis JG, Drutarowsky MD: Adaptation to chronic hyposmolarity in rats. *Kidney Int* 1988; 34:351.

162. Ayus JC, et al: Rapid correction of severe hyponatremia in the rat: Histopathological changes in the brain. *Am J Physiol* 1985; 248:F711.

163. Karmel KS, Bear RA: Treatment of hyponatremia: A quantitative analysis. *Am J Kidney Dis* 1994; 21:439.

164. Sterns RH: Vignettes in clinical pathophysiology. Neurological deterioration following treatment for hyponatremia. *Am J Kidney Dis* 1989; XIII:434.

165. Ayus JC, Arieff AI: Symptomatic hyponatremia: Correcting sodium deficits safely. Extent of replacement may be more important than infusion rate. *J Crit Illness* 1990; 5:905.

166. Cluitmans FHM, Meinders AE: Management of severe hyponatremia: Rapid or slow correction? *Am J Med* 1990; 88:161.

167. Narins RG: Therapy of hyponatremia: Does haste make waste? *N Engl J Med* 1986; 314:1573.

168. Berl T: Treating hyponatremia: What is all the controversy about? *Ann Intern Med* 1990; 113:417.

169. Anderson RJ, et al: Hyponatremia: A prospective analysis of its epidemiology and the pathogenetic role of vasopressin. *Ann Intern Med* 1985; 102:164.

170. Ober KP: Endocrine crises: Diabetes insipidus. *Crit Care Clin* 1991; 7:109.

171. Seckl JR, et al: Neurohypophyseal peptide function during early postoperative diabetes insipidus. *Brain* 1987; 110:737.

172. Strange K: Regulation of solute and water balance and cell volume in the central nervous system. *J Am Soc Nephrol* 1992; 3:12.

173. Robertson GL: Differential diagnosis of polyuria. *Annu Rev Med* 1988; 39:425.

174. Griffin KA, Bidani AK: How to manage disorders of sodium and water balance. Five-step approach to evaluating appropriateness of renal response. *J Crit Illness* 1990; 5:1054.

175. Sweadner KJ, Goldin SM: Active transport of sodium and potassium ions. Mechanism, function, and regulation. *N Engl J Med* 1980; 302:777.

176. Vitez TS, et al: Chronic hypokalemia and intraoperative dysrhythmias. *Anesthesiology* 1985; 63:130.

177. Adrogué HJ, Madias NE: Changes in plasma potassium concentration during acute acid-base disturbances. *Am J Med* 1981; 71:456.

178. Tobey RE: Paraplegia, succinylcholine and cardiac arrest. *Anesthesiology* 1970; 32:359.

179. Rimmer JM, et al: Hyperkalemia as a complication of drug therapy. *Arch Intern Med* 1987; 147:867.

180. Textor SC, et al: Hyperkalemia in azotemic patients during angiotensin-converting enzyme inhibition and aldosterone reduction with captopril. *Am J Med* 1982; 73:719.

181. Maslowski AH, et al: Haemodynamic, hormonal, and electrolyte responses to captopril in resistant heart failure. *Lancet* 1981; 1:71.

182. DeFronzo RA, et al: Effect of graded doses of insulin on splanchnic and peripheral potassium metabolism in man. *Am J Physiol* 1980; 238:E421.

183. Vincent HH, et al: Effects of selective and nonselective β-agonists on plasma potassium and norepinephrine. *J Cardiovasc Pharmacol* 1984; 6:107.

184. Allon M, et al: Nebulized albuterol for acute hyperkalemia in patients on hemodialysis. *Ann Intern Med* 1989; 110:426.

185. Prough DS, et al: Effects of hypertonic saline versus lactated Ringer's solution on cerebral oxygen transport during resuscitation from hemorrhagic shock. *J Neurosurg* 1986; 64: 627.

186. Prough DS, et al: Effects on intracranial pressure of resuscitation from hemorrhagic shock with hypertonic saline versus lactated Ringer's solution. *Crit Care Med* 1985; 13:407.

187. Gunnar WP, et al: Resuscitation from hemorrhagic shock: Alterations of the intracranial pressure after normal saline, 3% saline and dextran-40. *Ann Surg* 1986; 204:686.

188. Schmoker JD, et al: Hypertonic fluid resuscitation improves cerebral oxygen delivery and reduces intracranial pressure after hemorrhagic shock. *J Trauma* 1991; 31:1607.

189. Prough DS, et al: Regional cerebral blood flow following resuscitation from hemorrhagic shock with hypertonic saline: Influence of a subdural mass. *Anesthesiology* 1991; 75:319.

190. Gunnar W, et al: Cerebral blood flow following hypertonic saline resuscitation in an experimental model of hemorrhagic shock and head injury. *Braz J Med Biol Res* 1989; 22:287.

191. Gunnar W, et al: Head injury and hemorrhagic shock: Studies of the blood brain barrier and intracranial pressure after resuscitation with normal saline solution, 3% saline solution, and dextran-40. *Surgery* 1988; 103:398.

192. Ducey JP, et al: A comparison of the cerebral and cardiovascular effects of complete resuscitation with isotonic and hypertonic saline, hetastarch, and whole blood following hemorrhage. *J Trauma* 1989; 29:1510.

193. Walsh JC, et al: A comparison of hypertonic to isotonic fluid in the resuscitation of brain injury and hemorrhagic shock. *J Surg Res* 1991; 50:284.

194. Battistella FD, Wisner DH: Combined hemorrhagic shock and head injury: Effects of hypertonic saline (7.5%) resuscitation. *J Trauma* 1991; 31:182.

195. Wisner DH, et al: Hypertonic saline resuscitation of head injury: Effects on cerebral water content. *J Trauma* 1990; 30:75.

Chapter 5

NEUROENDOCRINOLOGY

SATWANT K. TIWANA SAMRA

Neuroendocrinology is the study of the relationship between the nervous system and the endocrine system. The human endocrine system has two important functoins: to maintain internal homeostasis, that is, a balanced *milieu interieur*, and to facilitate reproduction. Both functions are accomplished by complex interactions of multiple hormones, the secretion of which is controlled by interactions and feedback loops between the central nervous system, the endocrine glands, and the target organs. Embryologic studies have shown that both the *endocrine* and *nervous* systems develop from the primitive ectoderm. Prohormones of several neuropeptides have been shown to be present in most animals, including single-celled organisms,[1,2] providing evidence that these two principal regulatory systems of the higher animals have evolved from primitive single-celled organisms. Evolution has resulted in an increase in the distance between the endocrine glands and the brain, and a hierarchy of neuroendocrine controls has thus developed. The hypothalamus serves as the highest signaling station, producing neurohormones which reach the pituitary gland via either a short portal circulation or along the axons of hypothalamic neurons. The pituitary gland in turn produces many hormones which affect the fluid and electrolyte balance as well as the metabolic and reproductive functions.

Despite the common embryologic origin of the nervous and endocrine systems, there are important differences in the functional organization of the two. The functional unit of the endocrine system is the secretory cell, which exercises its effects via the circulating blood, while the functional unit of the nervous system is the neuron, which participates in an organized network of point-to-point connections. Both the neuronal and endocrine tissues have secretory properties. Endocrine secretions (hormones) enter the bloodstream while neuronal secretions enter either the bloodstream (neurohormones) or the neuronal synapses (neurotransmitters, neuromodulators).

Neural control of glandular secretion is either *secretomotor* or *neurosecretory* in nature. *Secretomotor* control is mediated through nerves that have synapses directly on secretory cells. The regulation of secretion of saliva, sweat, gastric juice, renin, pancreatic hormones, and catecholamines exemplifies secretomotor control. The secretomotor nerves are part of the sympathetic and parasympathetic nervous system and, traditionally, secretomotor control has been attributed to the release of either norepinephrine (sympathetic) or acetylcholine (parasympathetic) at the nerve endings. More recent studies[3-8] have shown that both sympathetic and parasympathetic neurotransmitters may coexist at the same nerve terminals. Preganglionic sympathetic nerve fibers which were previously classified as cholinergic are now known to contain other biologically active peptides.[9] *Neurosecretory* control or *neurosecretion,* in a strict sense, is defined as the release of a *hormone* from a nerve terminal into the bloodstream. Until recently the classic example of the neurosecretory gland in mammals has been thought to be the pituitary gland, which releases several hormones into the bloodstream. Scharrer and coworkers[10] were the first to recognize that the appearance of certain hypothalamic neurons in mammals was modified by the state of hydration. These investigators, having shown the presence of bio-assayable antidiuretic hormone (ADH) in hypothalamic extracts, proposed that ADH and oxytocin, traditionally believed to be secretions of the posterior lobe of the pituitary, actually originated in the hypothalamus. These hormones are stored in the posterior lobe of the pituitary gland (neurohypophysis), from where they are released into the bloodstream. The term *neurosecretion* has therefore been broadened to include the release of any neuronal secretory product from a nerve ending. This secretion can be a *neurohormone* or a *neurotransmitter.* Neurosecretion is thus considered to be a fundamental property of all neurons. This chapter, however, will be confined to the discussion of secretion of *neurohormones* only. Neurohormone secretion in man is attributed predominantly to the hypothalamic-pituitary unit, although the presence of many of these peptides has been shown in other parts of the brain as well as in extracranial organs like gut and pancreas. It is important to emphasize that neurosecretory cells retain the functional structure and properties of neurons. They react to other neurons through synapses via neurotransmitters like acetylcholine. The hypothalamic neurons, which secrete hormones into the blood, thus are one of the major links by which the brain regulates metabolic and reproductive activities.

The close link between the nervous and endocrine systems is often not appropriately appreciated and in an atmosphere of specialized medicine most clinicians visualize these two functions as separate entities: one being in the field of endocrinology/gynecology and the other in neurology and neurosurgery. Most discussions of "neuroanesthesia" traditionally revolve around the intracranial hemodynamics and how these are affected by anesthetics. Very little space is devoted to the discussion of neuroendocrine mechanisms and dysfunction in textbooks of neuroanesthesia. One reason for a lack of appreciation of the neuroendocrine relationships is that the only endocrine abnormality that presents a clinical problem for anesthesiologists is the life-threatening hemodynamic instability in the perioperative period in patients with primary or secondary adrenal insufficiency. Since glucocorticoids are given to most neurosurgical patients during surgery, this complication seldom occurs.

Neuroendocrine dysfunction, however, plays a significant role in the management of neurosurgical patients in the perioperative period, particularly in the appropriate management of fluid and electrolyte balance. Moreover, patients with CNS pathology associated with neuroendocrine dysfunction may present for extracranial, nonneurosurgical procedures during which steroid supplementation may be overlooked. The purpose of this chapter is to review the anatomy and physiology of the neuroendocrine mechanisms and the pathophysiology of various disorders of the hypothalamic-pituitary control of the endocrine system. Discussion of the hypothalamic-pituitary-adrenal axis and of the hypothalamic-pituitary-thyroid axis will be included, while the hypothalamic-pituitary-gonadal axis will be omitted since it does not have a significant impact on perioperative management. In conclusion, pathologic lesions in the central nervous system commonly associated with neuroendocrine dysfunction, the neuroendocrine response to stress of surgery, and its modification by anesthetic techniques, will be summarized.

Anatomy and Physiology of Neuroendocrine Control

The gross anatomy of the interrelationships of the neuroendocrine system is diagramatically shown in Fig. 5-1. It can, theoretically, be divided into (a) the hypothalamic-pituitary control system and (b) the extrahypothalamic neurohormones, that is, somatostatin, peptide hormones of the gastrointestinal tract, and the atrial natriuretic factor. The anatomic relations and structural subdivisions of the hypothalamus and pituitary are shown in Fig. 5-2. The hypothalamus is a collection of specialized cells and nerve fiber tracts which regulates many of the body's autonomic functions, including temperature, blood pressure, hunger, thirst, blood volume, sleep, and sexual functions. The specialized nerve cells with secretory activities constitute the "endocrine hypothalamus" and are organized predominantly in the supraoptic and paraventricular regions of the hypothalamus. These cells contain neurosecretory material which consists of a complex of vasopressin and oxytocin and their specific proteins, called neurophysins. These hormones travel along the axons of the hypothalamic-neurohypophyseal tract to the posterior lobe of the pituitary gland (neurohypophysis) which is believed to be a downward growth of the hypothalamus. There these hormones are stored, awaiting release in response to appropriate stimuli (discussed later). Small nerve cells in the supraoptic part of the hypothalamus also produce anterior pituitary regulating hormones. Axons from these cells travel along the tuberohypophyseal tract (Fig. 5-3) to

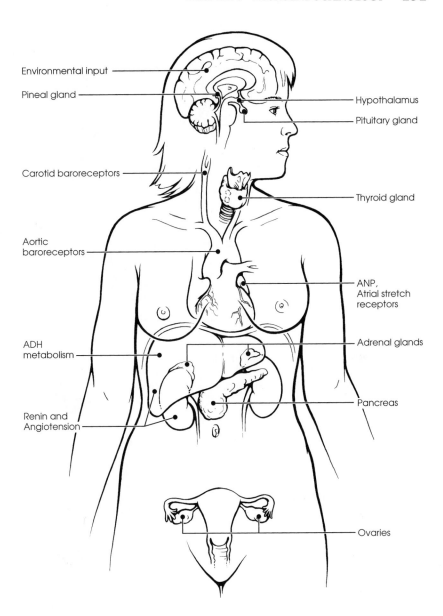

Figure 5-1   Gross anatomy of the human neuroendocrine system.

the anterior lobe of the pituitary (adenohypophysis). There, they connect with the capillary network of the pituitary portal system, which empties into the sinusoids of the anterior lobe of the pituitary gland. It is believed that sexual differences exist in the hypothalamus. During embryogenesis the gonads secrete steroid hormones that lead to the differentiation of neurons which regulate pituitary gonadotrophic hormones affecting male and female sexual behavior.

Hypothalamic-Pituitary Axis

The evidence for hypothalamic control of anterior pituitary hormone secretion is provided by several clinical and laboratory investigations. Early in the twentieth century,[11] hypopituitarism was reported to occur in patients with disease in the hypothalamic region. In a rodent model it was demonstrated that section of the hypophyseal stalk resulted in the loss of sexual function, which returned on regeneration of the hypothalamic-hypophyseal-portal circulation.[12] Extracranial transplantation or transplantation of the pituitary gland to the temporal lobe of the brain did not restore pituitary function, while transplantation to the hypothalamic region restored it.[13] These findings emphasize the role of the hypothalamic-hypophyseal portal circulation in the regulation of anterior pituitary hormone secretion.

HORMONES OF THE HYPOTHALAMUS AND THEIR RELEASE MECHANISMS

The hormones of the hypothalamus can be divided into (1) those stored in the posterior lobe of the pitu-

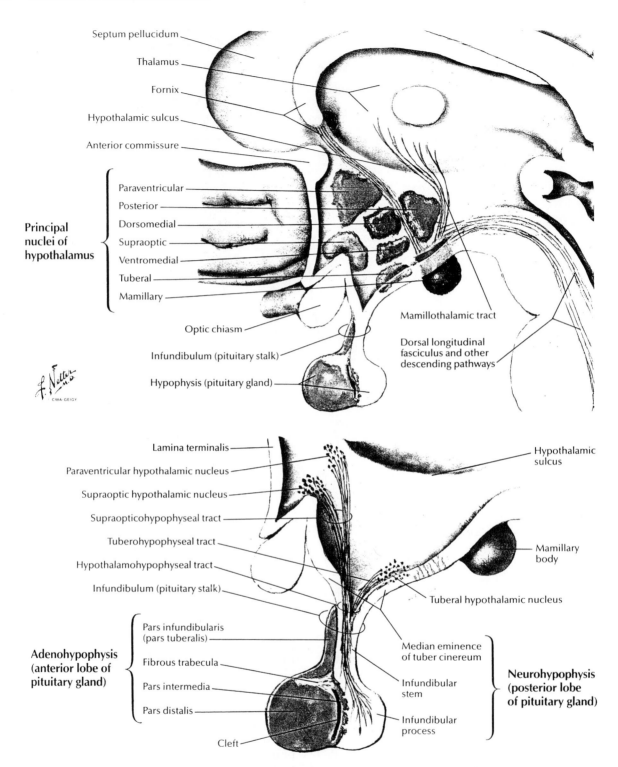

Figure 5-2   Hypothalamus and hypophysis. Modified from *The Atlas of Human Anatomy* by Frank H. Netter, MD, with permission.

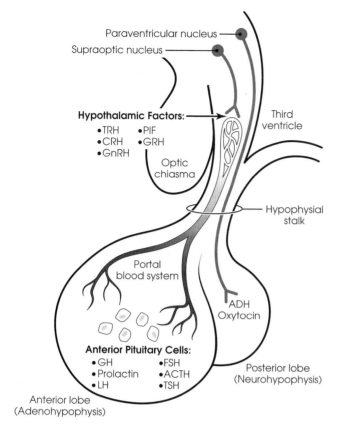

Figure 5-3   A schematic diagram of the functional anatomy of hypothalamic-pituitary axis of neurohormonal secretion.

ANTIDIURETIC HORMONE (ADH)   Also known as arginine vasopressin, antidiuretic hormone is a nonapeptide secreted by both the supraoptic and paraventricular hypothalamic nuclei. Its main physiologic effect is on the distal convoluted loop and on the collecting ducts of the nephrons in the kidney, where it promotes reabsorption of water. Without ADH the kidneys will excrete 20 to 30 liters of free water daily. The effective half life of ADH is 5 to 15 min, but the antidiuretic effect lasts 1.5 to 2 h. ADH is metabolized by both the liver and the kidney, and some of it is excreted unchanged by the kidney. In pharmacologic doses it has a pressor effect—hence the name vasopressin. Physiologically, the vasopressor effect is seen only in extreme hemorrhage. Vasopressin can modify the vascular effects of catecholamines at physiologic doses. In large doses it has some oxytocic and milk-ejecting activity and may stimulate bowel activity.

OXYTOCIN   The chemical structure of oxytocin is very similar to vasopressin, since both are nonapeptides. It differs from vasopressin in that leucine and isoleucine replace the amino acids arginine and phenylalanine in its molecule (Fig. 5-4). Its physiologic effect is to promote myometrial contractility (uterine contraction), and it plays a role in the onset of labor in pregnant women. Oxytocin also stimulates the myoepithelial cells of the acini of the breast and promotes lactation. The physiologic role of oxytocin in males is not clearly understood.

itary gland and (2) those controlling the secretion of hormones by the anterior lobe of the pituitary.

HORMONES STORED IN THE POSTERIOR PITUITARY
The chemical structure of the posterior pituitary hormones is shown in Fig. 5-4.

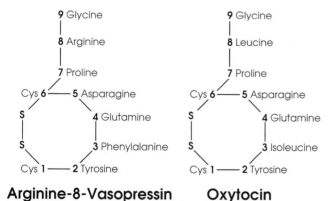

Arginine-8-Vasopressin   **Oxytocin**

Figure 5-4   Chemical structure of the hormones stored in the posterior lobe of the pituitary.

ANTERIOR PITUITARY REGULATING HORMONES
The evidence for hypothalamic control of hormone secretion by the anterior pituitary stems from two facts: (1) Crude extracts of hypothalamus, when injected into laboratory animals or added to pituitary tissue in vitro, release pituitary hormones. (2) Significant decrease in pituitary hormone levels occurs when the stalk of the pituitary is severed. The only exception is that prolactin secretion actually increases. It is therefore suggested that the hypothalamus provides hypophysiotropic hormones which include "releasing factors" for all anterior pituitary hormones and an "inhibiting factor" for prolactin. The chemical structures of the hypophysiotropic hormones have been identified predominantly by two groups of investigators,[14,15] who developed bioassays using extracts from the hypothalami of sheep and pigs. Several regulatory factors have thus been identified and chemically characterized. Some promote the secretion of anterior pituitary hormones and others inhibit it. These are diagrammatically summarized in Fig. 5-5 and discussed below.

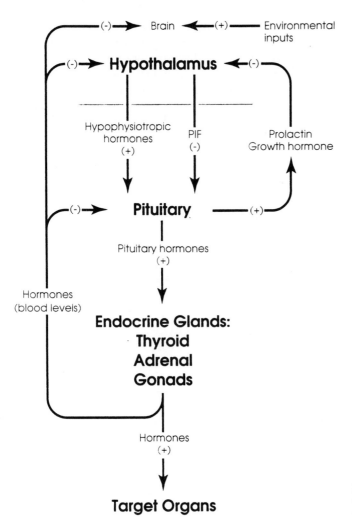

Figure 5-5 Hypothalamic hormones or releasing factors that control the secretion of hormones from the anterior lobe of pituitary. + = stimulates secretion; − = inhibits secretion.

THYROTROPIN-RELEASING HORMONE (TRH) This was the first hypophysiotropic hormone to be identified. It is a 3-amino acid cyclic peptide that stimulates the release of thyrotropin, a thyroid-stimulating hormone (TSH), from anterior pituitary cells. TRH undergoes a rapid enzymatic breakdown in tissues and body fluids. Over 70 percent of total brain TRH is found at extrahypothalamic sites, including motor nuclei of brainstem and anterior horn cells of the spinal cord. This bulbospinal distribution suggests that TRH may also function as a central regulator of the autonomic nervous system. TRH content is increased in the basal ganglia of patients with Huntington's disease. Substance P, a neurotransmitter, and TRH have been shown to coexist in certain cells along with serotonin.

Intravenous administration of TRH causes a rise in TSH level within 1 to 2 min, in contrast to the negative feedback effect of thyroxine, which takes 15 min to decrease TSH secretion. The site of action of TRH is at specific receptors on the cell membrane of the pituitary thyrotrophs. TRH also promotes prolactin secretion by the anterior pituitary. Additional physiologic and behavioral effects of TRH are not well understood. Early reports of beneficial effects, when used as a neuroleptic in patients suffering from chronic depression, have not been substantiated. Intrathecal injection of TRH is followed by a sensation of warmth in 100 percent, shivering in 75 percent, hypertension and tachycardia in 50 percent, diaphoresis in 30 percent, and nausea and vomiting in 15 percent of the patients. These actions suggest a role of TRH in centrally mediated autonomic stimulation. Intravenous administration of TRH is followed by genitourinary symptoms, which are not noted after intrathecal injections. It is possible that some of the above listed effects are due to TRH-breakdown products rather than TRH itself, but specific receptors for these breakdown products in humans have not yet been demonstrated.

CORTICOTROPIN-RELEASING HORMONE (CRH) It is a 41-amino acid peptide that promotes the secretion of adrenocorticotropic hormone (ACTH).

vided by Martin and Reichlin[20,21] and a
scope of this chapter. Suffice it to say th
of cell bodies that synthesize these neu
are located in the brainstem and midbra
ascend in the medial forebrain bundle
various forebrain structures including
mus, the limbic system (hippocampus, a
the cerebral cortex. These axons termin
the hypophysiotrophic neurons of the
An anatomic pathway is thus establis
adrenergic, noradrenergic, and cholin
can act directly to modulate secretion c
lamic hormones.

Various hypothalamic "releasing"
factors (listed earlier), secreted by the
are carried to the anterior lobe of th
capillaries that form the short hypothala
seal portal system. This portal system
with a capillary network that surrounds
anterior lobe. Reversal of blood flow r
occur, accounting for the presence of an
hormones in the hypothalamus. This r
in the portal system may be the basis f
back loop between the hypothalamus
The regulation of blood flow from th
pituitary and vice versa may be parti
upon the vasoactive substances secrete
rohypophysis. The major supply of bloc
hypophysis is via the hypothalamic-hy
tal circulation. The fact that the perfus
this vascular system is that of the venc
be one of the reasons why the enlarge
pregnant woman is highly susceptible t
to hemorrhagic shock, leading to the c
Sheehan's syndrome following postr
rhage.

DISORDERS OF THE HYPOTHALA

Pathologic lesions in the region of the
are predominantly of neoplastic origin.
tations are due either to anatomic effec
on the optic chiasm) or to abnormalit
production which present as pituita
(discussed later). Tumors in the region
amus may also produce disturbances i
sexual function, and sleep.

Gliomas occur most frequently in tl
optic chiasm and tuber cinereum. Invc
orly may produce optic atrophy or vist
while extension into the infundibular
cipitate diabetes insipidus. Other acc
tures may be failure of sexual maturity
temperature regulation, and obesity.
picture of a variable degree of anteric

GONADOTROPIN-RELEASING HORMONE (GnRH)   A
linear, 10-amino acid polypeptide which stimulates secretion of follicle-stimulating hormone (FSH) and luteinizing hormone (LH), it is sometimes also referred to
as luteinizing-hormone–releasing hormone (LHRH).

GROWTH-HORMONE–RELEASING   HORMONE   (GRH)
A 44-amino acid polypeptide, also known as *somatotropin*, it is responsible for the release of growth hormone (GH). It was first identified as an ectopic secretion by the pancreatic adenoma in patients with
acromegaly. An identical factor was subsequently
identified in the human hypothalamus.

SOMATOSTATIN   Also called somatotropin-release-
inhibiting factor (SRIF) or growth hormone inhibiting
factor (GIH), it has recently been isolated from the
hypothalamus. This 14-amino acid peptide is also
found in the pancreas, gastrointestinal tract and other
parts of the nervous system. Somatostatin blocks GH
release to all stimuli and lowers GH levels in acromegalic patients. Somatostatin is not clinically used in the
treatment of acromegaly because it has a short plasma
half life and needs to be administered as a continuous
infusion. In the pancreas, it inhibits the release of insulin and glucagon. In the nervous system it probably
serves as a neurotransmitter. It also inhibits the secretion of gastrin and vasoactive intestinal peptide in the
gastrointestinal tract.

In addition to these chemically isolated releasing
factors, there is presumptive evidence for the existence
of many other hypothalamic hormones, including a
prolactin releasing hormone (? vasoactive intestinal
peptide, VIP) and a prolactin release inhibiting hormone, PIH (? dopamine).

The actions of various hypothalamic hormones are
not absolutely clear. Various hypothalamic factors
have common properties: for example, somatostatin
not only blocks GH release but also inhibits TSH release by the pituitary in response to TRH without affecting TRH-induced prolactin secretion. Somatostatin
also has effects on the gut and pancreas. TRH stimulates prolactin release but does not promote secretion
of ACTH, LH, or FSH, the other hormones secreted by
the pituitary gland. Release of ACTH is controlled not
only by CRH but also by vasopressin and epinephrine,
and the two may be synergistic.

MECHANISMS OF RELEASE
OF THE HYPOTHALAMIC HORMONES

The difference in the hypothalamic regulation of anterior and posterior pituitary hormones is based on the
embryologic development of the two lobes of the pituitary gland. Developmentally, the posterior lobe of the

---

pituitary (neurohypophysis) is an extension of the
large neurons of the hypothalamus,[16] originating in the
supraoptic and paraventricular nuclei (Fig. 5-3), while
the anterior lobe of the pituitary (adenohypophysis)
consists of secretory cells. An important impact of this
developmental origin is that the neurohypophysis
merely acts as a storage site for hormones (oxytocin
and vasopressin) produced by the hypothalamus,
whereas the anterior pituitary hormones are synthesized by the secretory cells of the adenohypophysis
and their release is controlled by peptides produced
by the hypothalamus (listed earlier), grouped as hypophysiotropic hormones. The functions of the anterior
and posterior pituitary are thus regulated by the hypothalamus by different mechanisms, as discussed below.

POSTERIOR PITUITARY HORMONE
(VASOPRESSIN) REGULATION

Predominant control mechanisms involved in the release of vasopressin are

- Neural regulation
- Osmoregulation
- Volume regulation
- Other factors

NEURAL REGULATION   Many defined central and peripheral neural pathways influence the release of vasopressin.[16] One pathway travels through the midbrain
to the medial forebrain bundle, another through the
dorsal longitudinal fasciculus into the paraventricular
fibers. A third pathway involves the limbic system.
Stimulation of the midbrain reticular formation and of
the vagal nuclei increases vasopressin release. Centrally, α-adrenergic pathways stimulate vasopressin
release and β-adrenergic fibers inhibit it. Peripherally,
stimulation of the cut ends of the vagus and of the
ulnar nerve releases vasopressin.

OSMOREGULATION   The major physiologic function
of vasopressin is to regulate body fluid tonicity. Plasma
osmolality therefore is probably the most powerful
regulator of the vasopressin release. Changes in plasma
osmolality cause a change in the volume of the osmore-
ceptor cells in the hypothalamus and change the electrical activity of these cells, thus regulating vasopressin
release. Plasma osmolality is normally maintained
within a very narrow range. A 2 percent change in
osmolality initiates the response of either full diuresis
or full antidiuresis. The plasma osmolality at the initiation of antidiuresis is called the osmotic threshold for
vasopressin release. Normal value for the osmotic
threshold is 285 mosm. Plasma ADH level is approximately 2 pg/ml at this osmolality. ADH levels increase
abruptly with an increase in plasma osmolality above

285 mosm. Osmoregulation is me
hypothalamic cells, which act as
increased rate of electrical impulses
from these cells in response to intra
hypertonic saline.[17]

VOLUME REGULATION   Volume :
major factor that influences va:
Stretch receptors in the left atrium
in the carotid sinus and aortic ar
sponse via vagal stimulation. Left
by far the most sensitive. Atrial pi
up to 20 cm of water by balloon inf
to a 10 to 30 percent volume expar
vasopressin secretion by the pitu
creases in volume and atrial press
change or 6 percent volume expan
ported to be associated with dec
release.[18,19] Vasopressin release in
stimulation due to atrial stretch re
opposite to that noted after exper
of the cut end of the vagus nerve
increase in vasopressin secretion. T
be related to a difference in the nat
the stimuli. Redistribution of blood
system, without change in blood
left atrial pressure. Several peptic
activity (atrial natriuretic peptide, .
cently demonstrated. ANP may be
regulation of ADH secretion. On p
blood pools in the lower extrem
decrease in atrial pressure, and th
increase in ADH secretion after one
position. Atrial pressure changes
balloon inflation, volume expans
standing may occur during prolo
sure ventilation or in the Trendel
anesthetized patients, and may pla
cretion.
    Mediation of ADH response to
also occur through the carotid :
which send impulses along the
nerve. These baroreceptors respon
volume changes, as in acute hemo
ers believe that the baroreceptor:
and pulmonary veins also play a
vasopressin release.
    To summarize, left atrial barore
cipal mediators of small to mode
stimuli, whereas large volume chai
carotid and aortic baroreceptors.
levels do not correlate significantl
activity. Intraventricular injection
stimulate vasopressin release. Th
tionship between vasopressin an

CORTICOTROPHS   Make up about 15 percent of the adenohypophysis and are basophilic with conventional staining. These cells produce a large precursor molecule, proopiomelanocortin, with an approximate molecular weight of 31,000. It contains 240 amino acids and hence is classified as a glycoprotein. It breaks down into a 30-amino-acid-containing hormone (ACTH), also called corticotropin, and a β-lipotropic hormone. Biochemically active fragments of the β-lipotropic hormone are the endorphins and enkephalins, the opioid peptides that produce most of the actions of morphine. Endorphins may be secreted by corticotrophs under special circumstances.

GONADOTROPHS   Less than 10 percent of adenohypophyseal cells are gonadotrophs. These are medium-sized spherical or large oval cells which contain both follicle-stimulating and luteinizing hormones in the same cells.

THYROTROPHS   Least numerous of all cells. These are medium-sized angular cells, localized mainly in the anteromedial part of the gland, and take a basophilic stain.

PHYSIOLOGY AND RELEASE OF ANTERIOR PITUITARY HORMONES

The regulation of secretion of the pituitary hormones is the result of the integration of complex stimuli from higher centers in the brain and periphery. This concept is diagramatically shown in Figs. 5-1 and 5-3. An important factor in regulatoin of hormone secretion is the feedback mechanism between the target endocrine glands and the pituitary and between the pituitary and the hypothalamus (Fig. 5-6). A slight increase in plasma thyroxine level blocks the release of thyroid-stimulating hormone from the pituitary in response to thyrotropin-releasing hormone from the hypothalamus. Some hormones that do not act on target endocrine glands (e.g., growth hormone and prolactin) regulate their own secretion directly by acting on the hypothalamus. Anterior pituitary hormones are secreted in "pulses," the frequency and magnitude of which determine the peripheral blood levels. Increased secretion is noted during sleep but the reason for these nocturnal surges is not known. The physiologic actions of individual adenohypophyseal hormones are discussed below.

PROLACTIN

Prolactin is secreted by the lactotroph cells of the adenohypophysis. It has a molecular weight of 20,000. A precursor with a 40,000 molecular weight, probably a prohormone, constitutes a small portion of circulating prolactin in normal persons, but may be increased in

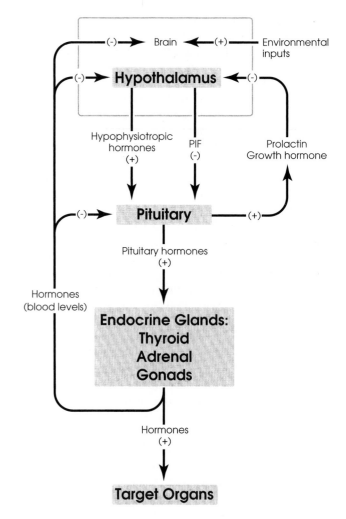

Figure 5-6   A schematic diagram of feedback mechanisms between hypothalamic-pituitary axis and extracranial components of neuroendocrine system.

patients with pituitary tumors. The only known physiologic function of prolactin in humans is to promote lactation in the female. It plays a minor role in the development of the breast in conjunction with estrogen and progesterone. Normal prolactin levels are 1 to 20 ng/ml in males and 1 to 25 ng/ml in females. During the third trimester of pregnancy, plasma prolactin levels increase but lactation is inhibited by high circulating levels of estrogen. After delivery, estrogen levels drop and lactation ensues. Suckling increases the circulating levels of prolactin, which promotes lactation and inhibits menstruation. Similarly, lactorrhea in patients with prolactin-secreting tumors of the pituitary may be accompanied by amenorrhea and anovulation (infertility). Possible mechanisms of anovulation associated with hyperprolactinemia include inhibition of GnRH by the hypothalamus, decreased responsiveness of pituitary gonadotrophs to GnRH, or decreased responsiveness of the ovaries to gonadotropins (FSH, LH) released by the pituitary.

Release of prolactin is episodic, and the nocturnal peak does not synchronize with the nocturnal peak of GH. Prolactin secretion is inhibited by the hypothalamus, but this "inhibiting factor" has not been precisely identified.[22] Dopamine causes a strong inhibition of prolactin release and may be the endogenous inhibiting factor. Prolactin secretion is also decreased by bromoergocryptine, which is clinically used to reduce the size of prolactin-producing pituitary tumors. Similarly, no definite "stimulating factor" has been identified, apart from a minor influence by TRH. Prolactin secretion is known to result from physical stimuli like suckling, stress, strenuous exercise, and sexual intercourse (in women). The physiologic function of prolactin in men is not known.

SOMATOTROPIN (GROWTH HORMONE)
It is a protein hormone with 191 amino acids. The biologic effect of somatotropin is to promote growth of skeleton, connective tissue, and viscera. Metabolic effects include stimulation of nucleic acid and protein synthesis, lipolysis, and decreased glucose utilization resulting in hyperglycemia, positive nitrogen balance, and decreased urea excretion. These effects are mediated via peptides called somatomedins, which are produced by the liver and transported in the blood by carrier proteins. Growth hormone exerts its effect via specific receptors on the cell membrane. Absence of these receptors results in dwarfism in the presence of normal blood levels of somatotropin. Although it is well accepted that growth hormone is required to obtain a normal body size during the first two decades of life, no sustained change in growth hormone secretion during childhood or adolescence is recorded.

Hypothalamic lesions, hypophyseal stalk resection, and pituitary transplantation away from hypothalamic regions result in decreased growth hormone secretion, suggesting that the hypothalamus promotes its secretion. Both somatostatin, which inhibits release of growth hormone, and somatotropin-releasing hormone (GRH), which promotes secretion of growth hormone, have been shown to be produced by the hypothalamus. Other factors that have been associated with increased levels of growth hormone include physical or emotional stress, hypoglycemia, sleep, estrogens, high doses of vasopressin, glucagon, L-dopa (after being converted to dopamine), and serotonin. The growth hormone rise during sleep is temporally different from the prolactin peak. Increase in growth hormone following stress is blunted by α-adrenergic blockade, suggesting an α-adrenergic mediation of this response. Growth hormone levels decrease with hyperglycemia, high doses of glucocorticoids and amino acids like arginine.

GONADOTROPINS
The pituitary produces two sex hormones, follicle-stimulating hormone (FSH) and luteinizing hormone (LH). In males, LH is also called interstitial-cell-stimulating hormone (ICSH). Both FSH and LH are glycoproteins, produced by common basophilic cells called gonadotrophs, although a few gonadotrophs with either only LH or only FSH are also present. The physiologic functions of the gonadotropins are different in men and women.

GONADOTROPINS AND OVARIAN FUNCTION FSH promotes growth of ovarian follicles to the point of rupture and promotes the secretion of estrogen by follicular cells. At midmenstrual cycle there is a surge of LH which facilitates ovulation, followed by secretion of progesterone from the corpus luteum. Ovarian steroid hormones (estrogen and progesterone) provide a negative feedback (for secretion of FSH and LH) to the pituitary. In the absence of ovarian hormones (during menopause, primary hypogonadism), serum FSH and LH levels rise to almost twice the normal concentration.

GONADOTROPINS AND TESTICULAR FUNCTION In males, FSH stimulates spermatogenesis and the production of an androgen-binding protein, inhibin, by the Sertoli cells. Inhibin is utilized in the transportation of testosterone. FSH is also essential for the development of LH receptors. LH promotes testosterone secretion by interstitial (Leydig) cells of the testes. The maturation of spermatozoa requires stimulation by both LH and FSH.[23] In therapeutic doses, testosterone administration inhibits only LH secretion. A combination of testosterone and "inhibin," a nonsteroidal peptide produced by the Sertoli cells of the testes, is required to suppress FSH secretion. Elevated LH levels are noted in aging males due to lack of testosterone secretion and hence to the absence of a negative feedback mechanism.

The gonadal hormones also provide feedback to the hypothalamus, which in turn controls the pituitary secretion of gonadotropins via GnRH. Puberty apparently occurs secondary to decreased sensitivity of the hypothalamus and pituitary to low levels of gonadal hormones, resulting in increased pulsatile secretion of LH during sleep.

THYROTROPIN (THYROID-STIMULATING HORMONE, TSH)
Thyrotropin is a glycoprotein, with molecular weight (30,000) similar to the gonadotropins. Its primary func-

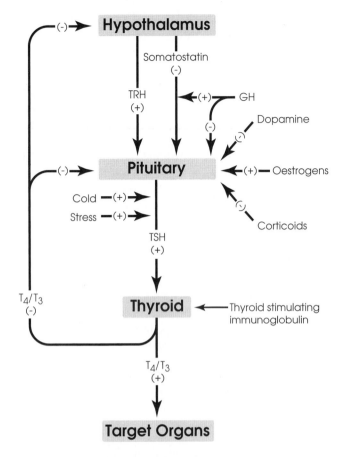

Figure 5-7 Hypothalamic-pituitary-thyroid axis showing feedback mechanisms involved in secretion of thyroid-stimulating hormone.

tion is to stimulate the synthesis of thyroxine in the thyroid gland. TSH secretion is regulated by TRH from the hypothalamus (positive feedback), on one side, and plasma triiodothyronine (T_3) and thyroxine (T_4) level, on the other (negative feedback), as shown in Fig. 5-7. This feedback mechanism is very sensitive, and a minimal decrease in blood thyroxine results in elevation of TSH levels, so that TSH levels can be used clinically as a useful tool for the early diagnosis of primary hypothyroidism and to evaluate the efficacy of thyroxine replacement therapy.[24] TSH levels are easily measured by radioimmunoassay at normal or high levels, but most assays are unable to distinguish between normal and low levels of TSH. Chronic treatment with excessive doses of thyroxine can result in low levels of TSH, which are reversible within 3 or 4 weeks of cessation of therapy.

CORTICOTROPIN (ADRENOCORTICOTROPIC HORMONE, ACTH)

Corticotropin is a 39-amino-acid polypeptide with a molecular weight of 4500. It is derived from a large

glycoprotein prohormone which is cleaved to give rise to ACTH and β-lipoprotein and its derivatives, as shown below.

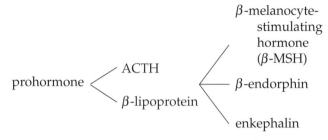

The major physiologic function of ACTH is the maintenance of adrenal function. Although ACTH controls the secretion of all three adrenal cortical steroid hormones—that is, glucocorticoids, mineralocorticoids, and androgens—its predominant effect is on glucocorticoid (cortisol) secretion. Mineralocorticoid (aldosterone) secretion is largely controlled by the renin-angiotensin system. Both ACTH and β-lipoprotein play a role in skin discoloration associated with adrenal insufficiency (Addison's disease).

The secretion of ACTH is controlled by at least three mechanisms:

1. Negative feedback: Cortisol inhibits the release of ACTH by the pituitary. After chronic administration of exogenous hydrocortisone, the hypothalamic-pituitary axis is suppressed and fails to provide a surge of endogenous glucocorticoids in response to stress. This suppression is noticed after approximately two weeks of exogenous steroid administration and persists for up to six months after cessation of therapy.
2. Diurnal variation: Like other pituitary hormones, ACTH secretion follows a diurnal rhythm. Adrenal activity is maximum in early morning, beginning around 4 A.M. There is a gradual fall in ACTH level and cortisol secretion, so that cortisol levels are lowest (about half) in the afternoon. This rhythm is abolished in central nervous system diseases and with sleep pattern alterations (e.g., in night-shift workers).
3. Stress response. Noxious stimuli (e.g., surgery and trauma) increase ACTH secretion in response to increased CRH secreted by the hypothalamus, which reaches the pituitary via the portal circulation. This mechanism overrides the other two, and the amount of ACTH increases proportionally with physical stress.

DISORDERS OF THE PITUITARY GLAND

Pituitary dysfunction can theoretically, for the sake of discussion, be divided into anterior pituitary gland dysfunction and posterior pituitary gland dysfunction.

In practice, however, patients may present with a combination of these disorders.

ANTERIOR PITUITARY GLAND DISORDERS

Clinical presentation of disorders of the pituitary gland can take any one of four forms: (1) enlargement of the sella turcica; (2) visual disturbances; (3) hypopituitarism; (4) hyperpituitarism. Patients may present with a single disturbance, or some or all of these may coexist. An acromegalic patient with a large tumor arising from the somatotrophs, leading to an enlargement of the sella turcica, may present with panhypopituitarism (due to destruction of other cells) and visual field defects (due to compression of the optic chiasm). Conversely, patients with pituitary tumors may be relatively free of any symptoms, often presenting to the gynecology clinic for investigation of infertility or amenorrhea, secondary to excessive prolactin secretion by a small prolactin-secreting pituitary tumor. The salient features of the four modes of presentation are discussed below.

Enlargement of Sella Turcica

This is frequently seen on x-ray images of the skull, done for a variety of indications; for example, following trauma, evaluation of the cervical spine, or investigation of headaches. The majority of these patients are obese, hypertensive, multiparous women. It is therefore suggested that enlargement of the pituitary during pregnancy with subsequent shrinkage after delivery may have something to do with this presentation. The differential diagnosis of an enlarged sella turcica, with or without evidence of erosion, is: primary pituitary tumor, the empty sella syndrome, and pituitary enlargement, secondary to primary hypothyroidism or primary hypogonadism. Disorders of primary hypothyroidism or hypogonadism are associated with lack of negative feedback and secondary hyperplasia of thyrotrophs or gonadotrophs, leading to enlargement of the pituitary and of the sella turcica. The empty sella syndrome is generally due to the presence of CSF in the sella. A small extension of a subarachnoid pouch below the diaphragma sellae, along the hypophyseal stalk where it passes through the diaphragm, is known to occur in 30 percent of the patients. If there is a rise in intracranial pressure or a vacuum in the sella (due to infarction of a pituitary tumor), the subarachnoid pouch fills with CSF—and further compresses the pituitary gland, and the sella appears empty. The majority of patients with empty sella have neither a pituitary tumor nor any endocrine disturbances indicating pituitary malfunction, and do not require surgery. Visual disturbances and endocrine abnormalities, if present, point to infarction of the pituitary tumor as the cause of the empty sella syndrome. Diagnosis can be confirmed by tomography.

Visual Disturbances

Close anatomic proximity of the optic chiasm to the pituitary gland makes it highly vulnerable to compression and displacement by an enlarged pituitary. Visual disturbances used to be the most common presenting feature in patients with large pituitary tumors. Recent advances in neuroimaging techniques can detect very small tumors, before they attain the size to cause chiasmal compression. Visual disturbances thus are no longer the leading presenting cause. When present, visual disturbances can be in the form of classic bilateral hemianopsia, when the pituitary tumor extends upward toward the roof of the sella, or there may be bilateral visual field defects, due to compression of the blood supply of the optic nerve and chiasm. Other tumors in this anatomic location (e.g., craniopharyngiomas) can also cause similar visual disturbances.

Hypopituitarism

A variety of endocrinopathies with varying clinical pictures can be the result of anterior pituitary malfunction. The fact that disorders of hypothalamic function or of the target endocrine glands can also result in a clinical picture similar to that of hypopituitarism has prompted the concept of primary, secondary, and tertiary endocrine deficiencies. Primary deficiencies occur due to absence of or diseases of target glands (i.e., gonads, thyroid, or adrenals); secondary deficiencies are due to defects of the pituitary, and tertiary disorders are due to diseases of the hypothalamus. Differentiation among these disorders can be made on the basis of endocrinologic evaluation. In primary deficiency the levels of target gland hormones (thyroxine, cortisol, estrogen, progesterone, testosterone) are low, with elevated hypophysiotropic hormones (GH, PRL, TSH, ACTH, FSH, and LH), due to the lack of negative feedback. In secondary deficiencies both target gland hormones and hypophysiotropic hormones are low, but the levels of the hypothalamic "releasing hormones" are elevated. Theoretically, decreased sensitivity of the hypothalamus to negative feedback can also result in endocrinopathies. It has been suggested that hyperadrenalism in Cushing's disease may be the result of a decreased sensitivity of the hypothalamus (higher setting for feedback) resulting in increased levels of CRH, leading to the development of pituitary corticotroph adenomas and ACTH elevation. Presence of diabetes insipidus generally suggests hypothalamic involvement, although massive enlargement of the anterior pituitary can also, over time, lead to destruction of the posterior pituitary lobe and to the development of diabetes insipidus.

The common cause of hypopituitarism is the destruction of normal pituitary tissue resulting from

Neoplasms: craniopharyngioma, adenomas, secondary metastases
Ischemia: infarction, necrosis, vasculitis
Infection: tuberculosis, sarcoidosis, meningitis
Physical injury: radiation, head trauma, surgery
Idiopathic: deficiency of one or more hormones.

The clinical picture in patients with hypopituitarism varies depending upon the number and extent of the hormones involved. Whether hypopituitarism develops before or after puberty, also affects the clinical presentation. The effects of individual hormone deficiencies are briefly listed below:

Prolactin deficiency. This defect results in failure to lactate. It is usually a result of pituitary necrosis secondary to postpartum hemorrhage.
Growth hormone deficiency. When present in childhood (prepuberty), it results in pituitary dwarfism. In adults it is a "silent" lesion. Failure to evoke a growth hormone response to provocative tests is a common finding in patients with hypothalamic-pituitary lesions. Growth hormone evaluation (discussed later) is thus an important diagnostic test for patients with suspected pituitary disease.
Gonadotropin deficiency. When present before puberty, it leads to lack of development of secondary sexual characteristics. In adult females it presents as primary or secondary amenorrhea or infertility. In adult males it is accompanied by testicular atrophy, loss of libido, and infertility.
Thyrotropin deficiency. Leads to hypothyroidism which is very similar to primary hypothyroidism, but less severe. Isolated TSH deficiency is rare. Accompanying features of growth hormone and/or gonadotropin deficiency and the presence of visual disturbances distinguish between primary and secondary hypothyroidism.
ACTH deficiency. This is the most serious, sometimes life-threatening, endocrine abnormality. It is discussed in detail later in this chapter.

Hyperpituitarism

Clinical syndromes of hyperpituitarism usually result from hypersecretion of prolactin, growth hormone, and ACTH. Hypersecretion of glycoprotein hormones of the pituitary (TSH, LH, and FSH) is rare, although ectopic secretion of these hormones is sometimes seen in patients with malignancy of the lungs. Development of hyperthyroidism and hypergonadism secondary to hyperpituitarism is therefore almost never seen in clini-

cal practice. Syndromes associated with the hypersecretion of PRL, GH and ACTH are discussed below.

HYPERPROLACTINEMIA Prolactinomas are the most commonly occurring pituitary tumors. Clinical presentation is a combination of either amenorrhea and galactorrhea in young women or visual disturbances with hypogonadism in males. Galactorrhea usually does not occur in males due to the lack of acinar tissue in the male breast. Rarely, however, galactorrhea may be present in male patients, and amenorrhea-galactorrhea may not occur in females. Other clinical features may be due to secondary hypofunction of other glands (hypothyroidism, adrenal insufficiency), which may result from compression of normal adenohypophyseal tissue by the growing prolactinoma.

Diagnosis is usually confirmed by high prolactin levels, that is, values above 100 to 150 ng/ml (normal range = 1 to 20 ng/ml in males and 1 to 25 ng/ml in females). In the absence of high resting levels of prolactin, provocative tests may be used. In normal subjects prolactin levels double in response to injecting TRH or chlorpromazine. In patients with a prolactinoma, this response is blunted. Rarely, however, the prolactin levels may rise even in the presence of a prolactinoma, suggesting storage of a prolactin precursor in the tumor.

The most effective (curative) treatment is surgical removal, which is usually accomplished by transsphenoidal hypophysectomy. Large size of the tumor may sometimes necessitate a frontal craniotomy. Treatment with radiation and/or bromocriptine (an ergot derivative) is reserved for patients who are poor candidates for surgery and anesthesia due to coexisting pulmonary or cardiovascular diseases. Preanesthesia evaluation should include clinical assessment for coexisting hypoadrenalism and hypothyroidism. Hypoadrenalism becomes less of a concern because these patients routinely receive glucocorticoids (dexamethasone) during surgery and in the immediate postoperative period, in anticipation of adrenal insufficiency which may develop after removal of ACTH-secreting pituitary tissue. Hypothyroidism is rare and when present it may be easily overlooked. Overall, in the absence of coexisting cardiovascular disease, these patients do not present an increased anesthetic risk. These tumors are not usually associated with increased vascularity or with a rise in intracranial pressure.

GROWTH HORMONE EXCESS Hypersecretion of GH can either be the result of a primary pituitary disorder that is, adenoma of GH-producing cells (somatotrophs) or be secondary to hypothalamic stimulation and increased production of GRH, leading to excess secretion of GH by the pituitary, without any evidence of pituitary microadenoma. When present, pituitary adenomas which produce GH are eosinophil tumors on light microscopy and show a presence of GH-granules on electron microscopy. Clinical presentation depends on the development of hypersecretion in relation to puberty, resulting in either gigantism (before puberty) or acromegaly (after puberty).

Gigantism is rarely seen in clinical practice. These patients are enormous due to delayed closure of the epiphyses of the long bones and hypertrophy of the soft tissues and viscera. Patients usually have a short life span. In younger age they are physically strong but later develop weakness due to myopathy and neuropathy. These patients rarely present for surgery. Anesthetic considerations are similar to those for acromegalic patients, discussed below.

Acromegaly develops due to excessive growth hormone secretion after fusion of long bone epiphyses (after puberty). Since growth of long bones is no longer possible, the predominant effect of excessive GH is seen on the bones of hands, feet, and face, and on soft tissues and viscera. Progress of the disease is slow and gradual; subtle changes in appearance are generally missed by the patient and by the family for a long time, until the tumor grows in size to cause visual disturbances or headaches.

Excessive growth hormone has both somatic and systemic effects. Generalized increase of soft tissue growth results in typical acromegalic facies with enlarged nose and mandible, thick lips, elevated nasolabial folds and prominent frontal sinuses. Early in the disease, joint spaces may be widened due to the enlargement of articular cartilages. Later on osteoarthritis may develop, resulting in joint pain and limitation of movement, including that of the temporomandibular joint. Osteoarthritis of the spine can lead to nerve root compression and paresthesias. Carpal tunnel syndrome is common due to rapid growth of soft tissue at the wrists. Systemic effects include increased basal metabolic rate and presence of hypertension in 95 percent of the patients. Visceral enlargement includes heart, kidneys, liver, adrenals and thyroid gland. Cardiac enlargement may be accompanied by congestive heart failure in the later stages. Renal enlargement is accompanied by increased glomerular filtration rate. Thyroid and adrenal function is generally normal. Glucose intolerance is seen in 50 percent of acromegalics, while 25 percent present with classical features of polyuria, polydipsia. Diabetes insipidus (discussed later) is rarely present. Other endocrine diseases may coexist with acromegaly. Multiple endocrine neoplasia (MEN, type I) with adenomas of the pituitary, pancreas, and parathyroid glands may present as acromegaly. A thorough examination of endocrine function, therefore, must be done in all acromegalics.

Diagnosis of acromegaly is made on the basis of classical physical appearance, enlarged sella on the CT scan, and elevated growth hormone secretion which is not suppressed after glucose ingestion or may even be paradoxically increased. The provocative test is to measure GH secretion after administration of TRH. In normal subjects TRH does not affect GH levels, while acromegalics may show an increase in GH levels.

Treatment is surgical removal either via the transsphenoidal approach (small tumors) or by an open craniotomy (large tumors). Radiation and medical therapy (with estrogens, progesterone, chlorpromazine, and bromocriptine) is reserved for patients in poor health and at increased anesthetic risk. Both surgery and irradiation may be required to control tumor growth in some patients.

Acromegaly is the only anterior pituitary disorder which has significant implications for anesthetic management. The large size of the patient may present difficulty in positioning on a narrow operating table. Thick skin is a minor inconvenience in vascular cannulation. The large size of the mandible and tongue, combined with the limitation of temporomandibular joint movement, may make endotracheal intubation difficult. At the conclusion of transsphenoidal surgery, presence of a nasal pack further adds to the difficulty in maintaining ventilation with bag and mask. Presence of blood in the oropharynx increases the risk of development of laryngospasm after tracheal extubation. Due caution, therefore, must be used in the extubation of the trachea in these patients. The systemic effects of acromegaly, that is, presence of hypertension and congestive failure, may necessitate appropriate invasive hemodynamic monitoring. The presence of multiple endocrine abnormalities must be kept in mind. Of greatest importance, however, is the presence of adrenal insufficiency. All patients scheduled for pituitary surgery, therefore, must be given intravenous glucocorticoids in anticipation of hypopituitarism in the perioperative period. Subclinical hypothyroidism with increased sensitivity to general anesthetics may be easily overlooked and must be borne in mind.

ACTH HYPERSECRETION (CUSHING'S DISEASE)   This results in the clinical picture of hypersecretion of adrenal glucocorticoids and must be differentiated from Cushing's syndrome, which is a nonspecific term referring to the hyperactivity of glucocorticoids due to any cause, including exogenous administration. Differentiation between Cushing's disease (a disorder of anterior pituitary functions) and Cushing's syndrome (hyperadrenalism) is made on the basis of loss of normal diurnal variations in ACTH and cortisol release in pituitary disorder. Other tests may include ACTH release in response to stress and the dexamethasone suppression test. ACTH release in response to stress, such as insulin-induced hypoglycemia, is impaired in Cushing's disease. The dexamethasone suppression test (discussed in detail later) helps to distinguish between Cushing's disease and Cushing's syndrome. After administratoin of a small dose of dexamethasone (0.5 mg every 6 h), the 24-h secretion of urinary 17-hydroxy steroids decreases to <3 mg/24 h in Cushing's disease but is >3 mg/24 h in Cushing's syndrome.

Most patients with Cushing's disease have identifiable pituitary adenomas, although enlargement of the sella turcica is seen in less than 10 percent of the cases. Selective removal of pituitary adenomas can generally be accomplished by microsurgery via the transsphenoidal approach and with good clinical results. The anesthetic considerations are the same as for obese, hypertensive patients.

EVALUATION OF ANTERIOR PITUITARY FUNCTION

Since the pituitary controls the hormone secretion of all endocrine glands, it is important to assess the effect of pituitary disease (usually a tumor) on the function of the target glands in all patients presenting for pituitary tumor resection. A thorough evaluation of the function of all endocrine glands is indeed costly. Fortunately, the hypofunction of only two endocrine glands, adrenals and thyroid, has clinically important, sometimes life-threatening consequences in the perioperative period. It is therefore a common practice to treat all patients with glucocorticoid supplementation during surgery and during the immediate postoperative period and to reserve the detailed endocrine function evaluation for postoperative follow-up. The effects of both the preexisting pituitary tumor and its surgical removal can thus be assessed at one time. A systematic approach to the evaluation of pituitary function is based on both clinical evaluation and laboratory investigations.

Clinical Evaluation

History and physical examination can provide valuable information about the cause and extent of pituitary hypofunction. A recent or remote history of postpartum hemorrhage, followed by failure to lactate, should alert clinicians to the presence of panhypopituitarism. Visual disturbances, when present, may point to chiasmal compression by a large pituitary tumor. Anosmia, especially when combined with congenital developmental defects like harelip and cleft palate, may suggest abnormality of hypothalamic function because of the developmental proximity of face and brain. Evidence of lactation (galactorrhea) may suggest either a lesion of the hypothalamus, hypophyseal stalk, or a prolactin-producing tumor of pituitary gland. Clinical

signs and symptoms of hypothyroidism are a rare presentation. The differential diagnosis between panhypopituitarism and anorexia nervosa in young women is important, since both can present with a clinical picture of malnutrition and menstrual disturbances (amenorrhea). Blood levels of glucose, thyroxine, and urinary steroids are low in both panhypopituitarism and anorexia. Normal plasma cortisol levels and growth hormone secretion in response to stress help to differentiate between the two conditions.

Endocrine Evaluation

The determination of random, resting blood or urinary levels of the anterior pituitary hormones has limited value because of the pulsatile (diurnal variation) nature of hypothalamic-pituitary hormone secretion. In the assessment of hypothalamic-pituitary function, greater reliance is therefore placed on the "provocative" tests for individual hormone secretion as discussed below.

PROLACTIN DEFICIENCY   The normal values of serum prolactin are 1 to 20 ng/ml in men and 1 to 25 ng/ml in women. These basal levels may be elevated in the presence of prolactin-producing pituitary adenomas. A positive provocative test produces a measurable increase in prolactin levels in response to TRH or chlorpromazine. In clinical practice testing for prolactin deficiency is rarely necessary.

GROWTH HORMONE RESERVE   Plasma GH levels are highly variable during the day and are closely related to blood glucose levels and to emotional and physical stress. Provocative tests, therefore, include response to exercise and to insulin or L-dopa administration. A value of GH greater than 6 ng/ml after moderate exercise (climbing stairs) is indicative of normal GH reserve. Alternatively if the patient is given an insulin injection (0.1 unit/kg), sufficient to decrease the plasma glucose level by 50 percent, and a value greater than 6 to 8 ng/ml of plasma GH is found in response to hypoglycemia, this indicates adequate response. In patients in whom induction of hypoglycemia may be risky (elderly, cerebrovascular or cardiovascular disease), L-dopa in a dose of 500 mg/70 kg is given orally. L-Dopa ingestion provokes GH release in 30 to 60 min, and a normal response is a GH level of 6 to 8 ng/ml. Induced hypoglycemia causes release of ACTH, cortisol, glucagon and epinephrine in addition to GH, and measurements of plasma levels of any of these hormones can also be used for pituitary function assessment. GH response to all stimuli is blunted in obese patients. The presence of hyperglycemia, corticosteroid and estrogen therapy also diminishes GH response.

ACTH DEFICIENCY   Hypoglycemia following insulin injection normally provokes ACTH release and a subsequent rise in the plasma ACTH and cortisol levels. A cortisol rise of 5 to 7 μg/100 ml or an absolute level of 15 μg/dl is considered a normal response. In patients clinically suspected of having pituitary-adrenal insufficiency, adequacy of adrenal function must be established by measuring either morning plasma cortisol levels or the 24-h urinary excretion of 17-hydroxyketosteroids, prior to doing provocative tests. If the patient has adrenal insufficiency, replacement therapy with synthetic glucocorticoids (dexamethasone 0.5 mg/day) should be started. This small dose of dexamethasone does not interfere with ACTH release in a provocative test. In patients in whom induction of hypoglycemia is contraindicated, metyrapone, a blocker of 11β-hydroxylase in the synthesis of cortisol, can be used. This block of the synthetic pathway causes an increase in ACTH by preventing the normal cortisol feedback inhibition of the hypothalamic-pituitary unit. A normal response is a rise in the urinary 17-hydroxyketosteroids due to the presence of 11β-deoxycortisol in response to increased ACTH. By itself 11β-deoxycortisol does not provide negative feedback for ACTH secretion.

THYROTROPIN DEFICIENCY The basal levels of TSH are useful in differentiating between primary and secondary hypothyroidism. In primary hypothyroidism, TSH levels are elevated while in secondary hypothyroidism they are low. Most clinically available radioimmunoassays, however, cannot differentiate between low and normal TSH levels. Provocative testing is done by giving intravenous TRH (400 to 500 μg). Normal response is a peak of TSH, approximately double the baseline value, 20 to 30 min after TRH injection. Some patients with normal response may be clinically mildly hypothyroid. Euthyroid and hyperthyroid patients do not respond to TRH provocation, thus limiting the clinical value of this provocative test.

GONADOTROPIN RESERVE Normal gonadal function (as evidenced by normal menstruation in women and normal sperm count in men) without hormone therapy is strong clinical evidence of the adequacy of hypothalamic-pituitary-gonadal function. Measurement of FSH and LH differentiates between primary and secondary hypogonadism. The levels of these hormones are elevated in primary and are decreased in secondary hypogonadism. The luteinizing-hormone–releasing hormone (LHRH), in a dose of 100 to 150 μg, is injected intravenously as a provocative test, and LH levels are measured at baseline and at 20-min and 30-min intervals. The peak of LH in response to LHRH injection correlates with baseline values. Therefore baseline LH values are often used clinically and provocative tests are rarely done.

ASSESSMENT AND TREATMENT OF PITUITARY HYPOFUNCTION AFTER PITUITARY SURGERY

It is well recognized that pituitary tumors may result in proliferation of one type of cells at the expense of others, resulting in hypersecretion of one pituitary hormone and insufficiency of others. Theoretically, therefore, every patient presenting for pituitary tumor resection must be thoroughly evaluated for the functional adequacy of all endocrine glands. Radioimmunoassay of all pituitary hormones is possible, but expensive. In surgical patients, the most critical problem is the presence of adrenal insufficiency, which, if overlooked, can be life-threatening. It is therefore customary to provide steroid supplementation to all patients and to postpone detailed endocrine evaluation till a later date when the effects of surgery on endocrine function can be assessed simultaneously. There are many regimens for steroid replacement in the perioperative period. A common practice is to administer 10 mg of dexamethasone at six-hour intervals on the day of surgery, with a rapid tapering of this dose in the postoperative period. At the time of discharge from the hospital (usually 4 to 6 days after surgery) the patients usually are to receive prednisone 5 mg in the morning and 2.5 mg in the afternoon. Return of normal ACTH secretion can be assessed approximately 1 month later, when the afternoon dose of prednisone can be omitted and the plasma cortisol level can be measured next morning. A value above 5 μg/dl indicates that a withdrawal of exogenous glucocorticoid will result in the assumption of normal ACTH secretion and in adequate endogenous adrenal response to stress.

A combined test for the assessment of pituitary reserve for all hormones has been used on an outpatient basis.[25] It involves the administration of TRH (200 μg), GnRH (100 μg), CRH (50 μg), and GRH (80 μg) intravenously in quick succession and the measurement of plasma levels of TSH, prolactin, ACTH, cortisol, FSH, LH, and GH, by radioimmunoassay, 20 min before and 120 min after the injection of the "releasing" hormones. Similar increases in all pituitary hormones have been reported after the administration of hypophysiotropic hormones in normal men and in posthypophysectomy patients, given either combined or separate injections.[25] While this test is expeditious and provides a thorough assessment of pituitary reserve, the cost involved in the estimation of all the hormones is not always justified. It is, therefore, common clinical practice to employ selective provocative tests for individual pituitary hormones, as suggested by the clinical manifestations in individual patients. Once an endocrine deficiency of "tropic" hormone(s)—for example, ACTH, TSH, FSH, LH—is established, return of function is unlikely and replacement with appropriate hormones is recommended. Mineralocorticoid replacement is not necessary in patients with normal adrenal glands because their secretion is controlled by the renin-angiotensin system and is not affected by the level of ACTH. Patients who develop persistent diabetes insipidus often require treatment with a vasopressin analogue, DDAVP.

POSTERIOR PITUITARY GLAND DISORDERS

The posterior pituitary gland is involved predominately in the storage and release of oxytocin and vasopressin (ADH), in response to stimuli from the hypothalamus which, in turn, receives stimuli from the higher brain centers (pain, emotion, stress) and from the periphery (atrial, aortic and carotid baroreceptors, plasma volume and osmolality). The physiologic functions of oxytocin pertain only to onset of labor and lactation. Therefore the common clinical disorders of the posterior pituitary are related mostly to disorders of ADH release. A decrease in ADH results in polyuria without glucosuria (hence named diabetes insipidus). An increase in ADH levels is seen in a syndrome of inappropriate antidiuretic hormone secretion (SIADH), thus named because the secretion of ADH is "inappropriate" in the presence of plasma hypoosmolality and hypervolemia. One of the features of SIADH is dilutional hyponatremia. A cerebral salt-wasting syndrome (CSWS), which produces hyponatremia due to a primary salt-wasting nephropathy of central origin, in patients with intracranial pathology, must therefore be considered in the differential diagnosis of SIADH. Similarly, the differential diagnosis of diabetes insipidus includes hysterical polydipsia or a psychiatric condition of compulsive water drinking (potomania). The clinical features, laboratory data, and appropriate therapy for these conditions are summarized in Table 5-1 and a brief discussion of each follows.

Diabetes Insipidus

This disorder of polyuria and polydipsia is associated either with the absence or the deficiency of endogenous ADH release in response to normal physiologic stimuli (neurogenic DI) or with failure of the kidney to respond to circulating ADH (nephrogenic DI).

ETIOLOGY   The causes of diabetes insipidus may be:

1. Hereditary: An autosomal dominant disorder.
2. Traumatic: Pituitary surgery, head injury.
3. Inflammatory: Meningitis, tuberculosis, sarcoidosis, histiocytosis, granulomatosis
4. Vascular: Sheehan's syndrome
5. Neoplastic: Lymphoma, leukemia, metastatic carcinoma of the lung, primary tumors in the vicinity of the hypothalamus or pituitary.
6. Idiopathic

CLINICAL PRESENTATION   This clinical syndrome is characterized by polyuria, that is, the passage of large quantities (2.5 to 24 liters/day) of dilute urine (sp gr < 1.004), with increased thirst and water intake. Onset is usually sudden, appearing from a few hours to 6 days after surgery in the pituitary region or after head trauma. Postoperative diabetes insipidus usually resolves in 2 to 3 days, but may reoccur after a normal interphase of 1 to 5 days and develop into a chronic syndrome. DI following head injury (with or without skull fracture) may last indefinitely, but usually resolves in a few days to few months, due to the regeneration of disrupted axons in the neurohypophyseal stalk. In patients with partial ADH insufficiency or during severe dehydration, urine specific gravity may be >1.004. The normal *interphase* is generally due to the release of ADH stored in the neurohypophysis prior to injury. If the normal function of the thirst center is preserved, patients ingest large quantities of fluid and dehydration seldom develops. If the underlying CNS pathology interferes with the function of the thirst center, or in postoperative patients, or in unconscious patients, fluid intake may be deficient and electrolyte disturbances, especially severe hypernatremia (170 to 180 meq/liter) may develop with further deterioration of CNS function.

DIAGNOSIS   DI is diagnosed by clinical history, by laboratory data (urine volume, specific gravity, ratio of serum/urine osmolality, serum electrolytes), and by the water deprivation test followed by administration of DDAVP. The clinical and laboratory parameters required to meet the criteria for the diagnosis of DI are listed in Table 5-1. The salient features of this disorder are low urine specific gravity and urine osmolality less than plasma osmolality. A cardinal feature of DI is the inability to concentrate urine in response to dehydration as tested by the water deprivation test. In this test, baseline determinations of plasma sodium, plasma osmolality, and urine osmolality are made, and the patient is deprived of fluids until the plasma sodium rises above 145 meq or the plasma osmolality rises above 295 mosm. The duration of fluid deprivation is variable, depending upon the severity of DI. Urine osmolality is measured at hourly intervals until it reaches a plateau, at which point a blood sample for the measurement of serum osmolality is drawn. The period of water deprivation may be continued until a decrease in body weight (due to loss of water) and no concentration of urine (as judged by repeated measurements of urine osmolality) is noted, provided the plasma sodium and osmolality do not reach too high a value. Then DDAVP, 1 μg, is injected subcutaneously and the measurements of urine and plasma osmolality are repeated. In normal subjects a rise in serum sodium

TABLE 5-1
Clinical and Laboratory Findings in Disorders of Posterior Pituitary (Neurohypophysis) Function

Parameter	Syndrome of Inappropriate ADH (SIADH)	Cerebral Salt Wasting Syndrome (CSWS)	Diabetes Insipidus (DI)
Blood pressure	Normal	Low or postural hypotension	Normal
Heart rate	Slow or normal	Resting or postural tachycardia	Normal or increased
Body weight	Normal or increased	Decreased	Normal or decreased
Glomerular filtration rate	Increased	Decreased	Increased
BUN, creatinine	Normal or low	Normal or high	Normal or high
Urine			
Volume	Normal or low	Normal or low	Increased
Specific gravity	High >1010	High >1010	Low <1004
Sodium	>25 meq	>25 meq	<25 meq
24-hour excretion of sodium	>30 meq	>30 meq	<30 meq
Osmolality	>Serum Osm	>Serum Osm	<Serum osm
Blood			
Volume	Increased	Decreased	Decreased
Hematocrit	Normal or low	Elevated	Elevated
Serum sodium	Low <135 meq	Low <135 meq	High
Osmolality	Low <280	Low	High
Treatment			
Salt (NaCl)	Supplement (±)	Supplement	Restriction
Water	Restrict	Supplement	Supplement
Timing after insult (rupture of aneurysm, trauma, surgery)	8th day (medium) (range 3–15 days)	4th–5th day (median) (range 2–10 days)	Few hours after insult, lasts 4–15 days followed by remission; rarely may progress to permanent stage
Plasma ADH level	High	Normal	Low

and serum osmolality, secondary to dehydration, causes the release of ADH, and urine osmolality reaches a value of 800 to 1500 mosm. In chronically debilitated or malnourished patients, urine osmolality may be 400 to 800 mosm, probably due to compromised renal function. The response to DDAVP injection helps to distinguish between patients with nephrogenic DI and those with DI due to hypothalamic-pituitary dysfunction. An increase in urine osmolality, after DDAVP, to 150 percent of pre-DDAVP value is suggestive of neurogenic DI, while a rise of 50 percent or less is indicative of nephrogenic DI. Distinction between hypothalamic and pituitary DI can be made by the fact that DI secondary to pituitary dysfunction is transient, since the vasopressin can be released from the stalk, while hypothalamic pathology results in permanent DI. Patients with psychogenic polydipsia may also show some increase in urine osmolality with water deprivation, which does not rise much more after DDAVP injection. Estimation of plasma ADH levels can provide definitive differentiation between neurogenic and nephrogenic DI. ADH levels are low (or absent) in the former and elevated in the latter disorder.

The integrity of osmoregulation of ADH release can be determined by a modification of the Hickey-Hare test, described by Moses and coworkers.[26] In this test the patient is given an oral water load of 20 ml/kg, over 15 to 20 min, and urine volume is measured every 15 min. Water load is maintained by intravenous fluids, replacing the fluid volume equal to the urine volume excreted every 15 min. When the urine volume is stable over three to six periods of 15 min each, a rapid salt load is administered by infusing 5% NaCl at the rate of 0.125 ml/kg per minute for 45 min. Urine collection is continued for three 15-min periods after infusion of hypertonic saline. From these samples free water clearance can be calculated according to the formula:

$$\text{Free water clearance} = \text{Urine volume (ml/min)} - \frac{\text{Urine vol} \times \text{Urine osmolality}}{\text{Serum osmolality}}$$

Measurements are made for each 15-min period. Free water clearance should fall to zero or to a negative value in normal individuals, due to ADH release in response to a rise in serum osmolality.

The osmotic threshold for ADH release is measured

by the infusion of 5% NaCl at a rate of 0.5 ml/kg per minute, after collecting of six to eight urine samples of equal volume over 15-min periods. During saline infusion, serum osmolality and urine volume are measured every 15 min. This procedure is continued either for 30 to 45 min after an abrupt cessation of urine output, or for a total of two hours of infusion time, or if a headache develops, whichever comes first. When an osmotic threshold is reached, ADH is released and there is an abrupt fall in free water clearance. Moses and Streeten[27] observed the osmotic threshold in normal subjects to be 285 to 292 mosm (mean = 288.5 ± SD 3.6). In patients with DI, osmotic threshold may be high or undetectable even after achieving a serum osmolality of 310 to 315 mosm or higher.

PATHOPHYSIOLOGY   The underlying cause of DI is either absent or decreased production or release of ADH (neurogenic DI) or the resistance of nephrons to circulating ADH (nephrogenic DI). Conceptually, four different pathophysiologic presentations of DI can be defined: (a) Minimal or no change in urine osmolality, with increasing serum osmolality after fluid deprivation. There is no evidence of ADH release in response to hypertonic saline infusion. These patients are not capable of producing any ADH. (b) Initially there is no change in urine osmolality, with rising serum osmolality, followed by an abrupt increase in urine osmolality as dehydration progresses. There is no evidence of an osmotic threshold during saline infusion. These patients have a defective osmoregulation and a higher threshold of the volume receptors that release ADH in response to hypovolemia. (c) Some rise in urine osmolality, with rising serum osmolality. There is an elevated osmotic threshold after saline infusion. These patients have a sluggish ADH release mechanism and are labeled as "high-set osmoreceptors." (d) Normal threshold of osmoreceptors and volume receptors, but a sluggish and subnormal ADH response.

TREATMENT   Prior to the availability of DDAVP, Pitressin nasal spray or Pitressin tannate in oil, given as an intramuscular injection, was the usual treatment. Pitressin nasal spray relieved polyuria for a few hours, while long-acting injections of 5 units of Pitressin tannate in oil were given three times a week. DDAVP nasal spray is effective for up to 12 h and, given twice a day, provides effective treatment.

A word of caution in planning treatment is to remember that DI is an essentially benign disorder and injudicious treatment can be harmful. Patients on oral intake seldom get dehydrated. Similarly, fluid and electrolyte balance can be easily maintained within normal limits in hospitalized patients. Fluid intake must be restricted for some time after DDAVP treatment to avoid a sudden fluid overload. An oversight, especially in postoperative patients receiving intravenous fluids, can lead to water intoxication with cerebral and pulmonary edema. It is therefore better to err on the side of undertreatment rather than overtreatment. Other drugs that have been tried in the treatment of DI are chlorpropamide (200 to 500 mg daily), clofibrate (500 mg every 6 h), and carbamazepine (400 to 600 mg daily). Thiazide diuretics sometimes act as antidiuretics in patients with nephrogenic DI.

Syndrome of Inappropriate Antidiuretic Hormone (SIADH)

The predominant feature of this disorder is dilutional hyponatremia due to excessive water retention (hypervolemia), secondary to continued ADH secretion in the presence of plasma hypoosmolality, hence the name, syndrome of "inappropriate" ADH (SIADH). It was first identified by Schwartz and Bartter[28] in 1957, in two patients with bronchogenic carcinoma, and is sometimes referred to as the Schwartz-Bartter syndrome.

ETIOLOGY   SIADH can result from a variety of clinical disorders listed below:

1. Central hypersecretion of ADH
   a. Hypothalamic disorders resulting from
      - Trauma
      - Surgery
      - Metabolic encephalopathy
      - Subarachnoid hemorrhage
      - Acute intermittent porphyria
      - Myxedema
      - Vascular Lesions
   b. Suprahypothalamic disorders
      - Cerebral infarction
      - Subdural hematoma
      - Infectious meningitis
2. Peripheral hypersecretion of ADH in response to
   - Pulmonary infections (tuberculosis)
   - Lung tumors (bronchogenic carcinoma)
   - Recumbent posture (coma)
3. Drugs
   - Vincristine
   - Chlorpropamide
   - Cyclophosphamide
   - Chlorothiazide
   - Carbamazepine
   - Chlorpromazine

As can be seen from the foregoing list, SIADH may be associated with a variety of intracranial and extracranial diseases. There is no specific anatomic site for lesions in the brain that is known to be associated with SIADH. It has been known to occur with acute subarachnoid hemorrhage, concussion, frontal lobotomy, craniotomy, subdural hematoma, brain tumor, cerebral infarction, brain abscess, meningitis, encephalitis, and diffuse microvascular disease. The lack of anatomic specificity of intracranial lesions resulting in SIADH has never been explained. It was proposed that the suprahypothalamic parts of the brain exerted an inhibitory influence on ADH secretion and that the above-named lesions lead to "denervation" of this inhibitory central mechanism, provoking ADH release. This hypothesis could not be proven in experimental studies. One common feature of the above-listed intracranial lesions is coma and recumbent position. It has been proposed that supine position, when prolonged, may lead to increased ADH secretion, due to malfunction of peripheral baroreceptors. Ectopic secretion of ADH is reported to occur most frequently in oat cell carcinoma of the lung, although it can also occur in carcinoma of the pancreas, duodenum, or bladder, lymphosarcoma, reticulum cell sarcoma, Ewing's sarcoma, Hodgkin's disease, and thymoma.

In addition to the drugs listed above, ADH secretion is known to increase in response to stress, as in the postoperative period, and in association with pain-relieving and tranquilizing drugs, especially in elderly patients.

PATHOPHYSIOLOGY   The classic features of SIADH include hyponatremia and plasma hypoosmolality. Urinary findings are natriuresis (loss of sodium in urine in the presence of hyponatremia) and high specific gravity. Urine osmolality is higher than plasma osmolality. ADH causes volume expansion, resulting in dilutional hyponatremia. Hyponatremia is exaggerated due to suppression of renin and aldosterone secretion, causing further natriuresis due to lack of sodium reabsorption by the proximal tubules of the nephrons. This mechanism explains why salt supplementation fails to correct hyponatremia unless it is supplemented by the normalization of plasma volume with fluid restriction. This fact also helps in the differential diagnosis of SIADH and other causes of hyponatremia. When a sodium load is administered, patients with SIADH promptly excrete sodium, while in those with hyponatremia due to volume depletion or edematous states (chronic congestive heart failure, liver failure) sodium is retained. Rare patients with SIADH may become volume-depleted (due to persistent vomiting) and may retain sodium after sodium loading. Similarly natriuresis may not be seen in SIADH patients with severe hyponatremia.

CLINICAL FEATURES   The symptoms of SIADH depend on both the degree of hyponatremia as well as the speed with which it develops. Levels of serum sodium up to 120 to 125 meq/liter are usually without any symptoms. When present, the early symptoms of SIADH are identical with those of water intoxication, presenting as anorexia, nausea, vomiting, lethargy, and irritability. There are subtle personality changes like inattentiveness, and forgetfulness, progressing to paranoia and delusions. With the fall of serum sodium to 110 meq/liter or below, neurological symptoms become more severe, progressing to lethargy, weakness, cramps, stupor, extrapyramidal signs, convulsions, and coma. Weight gain may be noted but peripheral edema is rare. The convulsions associated with SIADH do not respond to traditional anticonvulsant therapy. EEG abnormalities may be present, but are nonspecific. Symptoms usually disappear quickly after correction of the hyponatremia, but may persist in some cases for up to a week. Persistent mental changes are rare.

DIFFERENTIAL DIAGNOSIS   SIADH should be clearly differentiated from other causes of hyponatremia. Some of the salient features have been alluded to before and are outlined in Table 5-1. The distinguishing feature is that in SIADH there is hyponatremia without clinical evidence of hypovolemia or edema. Patients with SIADH have low BUN, creatinine, uric acid, and albumin. Urinary sodium concentration is greater than 25 meq/liter. Urine osmolality is greater than plasma osmolality.

The failure to excrete a water load normally is the diagnostic test of SIADH which differentiates it from other causes of hyponatremia. The water-loading test can be dangerous in the presence of congestive heart failure (CHF) and severe hyponatremia. It is therefore restricted to patients with serum sodium higher than 125 meq/liter and without clinical evidence of congestive heart failure. The test is performed by administering 20 ml/kg water orally over 15 to 20 min and collecting urine hourly for the next 4 h. A normal response is the excretion of 65 percent of the water in 4 h and the urine osmolality falling to less than 100 mosm during the test. In SIADH, the administration of NaCl corrects hyponatremia only transiently, since natriuresis sets in due to decreased renin and aldosterone secretion.

TREATMENT   The definitive treatment of SIADH in asymptomatic patients should be directed toward the treatment of the underlying cause. Patients with mild to moderate symptoms of water intoxication and hyponatremia should be treated with fluid restriction to 600 to 800 ml/day. Patients with severe symptoms or serum sodium levels below 120 meq/liter, especially if hyponatremia developed rapidly, may require NaCl supplementation to achieve serum sodium levels between 120 and 125 meq/liter. It is commonly accomplished by the intravenous administration of 200 to 400 ml of 3% to 5% NaCl slowly at a rate of 2 meq/h. Total fluid intake, both oral and intravenous must be restricted. Simultaneous administration of furosemide is recommended if hyponatremia is to be corrected expeditiously and hypervolemia is to be avoided. It may be important in the presence of CHF. When furosemide is given, a close watch for the development of hypokalemia must be kept, and treatment instituted when necessary. Treatment of hyponatremia must be initiated with caution. A rapid replacement of NaCl has been associated with central pontine myelinolysis and other brainstem, cerebellar, and cerebral disorders. Once normal levels of serum sodium are restored, fluid restriction must be maintained.

Other drugs have been tried in the treatment of SIADH. Lithium interferes with the effect of ADH on the kidney. The dose should be adjusted to achieve serum lithium levels of 0.3 to 0.6 meq/liter. Desmocycline, a tetracycline-like antibiotic, in doses of 600 to 1200 mg/day has been effective. Its use is restricted to situations where fluid restriction is difficult and treatment of the underlying cause of SIADH is impossible. When given desmocycline, the patient should be observed for renal toxicity and superimposed infections. Diphenylhydantoin also inhibits release of ADH from the pituitary. Narcotic antagonists have been reported to reduce ADH secretion in some cases.[29] Their role in the treatment of SIADH remains to be established.

Cerebral Salt-Wasting Syndrome (CSWS)

It has been long recognized that patients with intracranial pathology (variety of causes) develop hyponatremia with persistent urinary loss of sodium, even in the face of decreasing serum sodium levels. In the early 1950s this phenomenon was called the cerebral salt-wasting syndrome. The early investigators noted that CNS pathology somehow interfered with the kidney's ability to reabsorb sodium and treated these patients with salt supplementation. In 1957, Schwartz and Bartter[28] defined SIADH, changed the therapeutic approach to hyponatremia, and the traditional concept of the cerebral salt-wasting syndrome was abandoned. There is one major difference between these two syndromes. In SIADH water retention leads to an expanded blood volume and dilutional hyponatremia. In CSWS continued salt excretion by the kidneys results in secondary water loss and hence a decreased plasma volume. No blood volume studies had been done, either during the early observations on CSWS or by Schwartz and associates, who promoted the concept of SIADH and proposed the possibility that an unidentified natriuretic factor was produced by the brain.

Nelson and coworkers[30] in 1981 measured blood volumes in 12 neurosurgical patients who fulfilled the laboratory criteria of SIADH—that is, hyponatremia (<135 meq/liter), low serum osmolality (<280 mosm), and natriuresis (urine sodium > 25 meq/liter). Blood volumes were measured 24 to 48 hours after the laboratory investigations established the diagnosis of SIADH. The underlying CNS pathology in these patients was ruptured intracranial aneurysm (8), craniotomy for unruptured aneurysm (2), closed head injury (1), and traumatic carotid cavernous fistula (1). Fluids were not restricted and all patients had normal renal and adrenal function. Ten of the 12 patients had decreased intravascular volumes. These investigators therefore proposed that in these patients the primary defect might be the inability of the kidney to conserve sodium rather than hypervolemia and dilutional hyponatremia due to "inappropriate" secretion of ADH.

Nelson and coworkers, in a later study,[31] tested this hypothesis in a primate model of subarachnoid hemorrhage. Seven of the 9 monkeys became natriuretic and hyponatremic. Plasma ADH levels were elevated on the first postoperative day, but returned to the baseline values for the next 3 days. Plasma volume was slightly, but not significantly decreased. The ADH secretion response to both fluid and saline load was normal, suggesting that the primary defect was not an abnormal ADH response.

In a subsequent study of hyponatremia and cerebral infarction in 134 patients with subarachnoid hemorrhage, Wijdicks and associates[32] reported that hyponatremia developed in 44 (of 134) patients. Twenty-five of those who fulfilled the laboratory criteria of SIADH were treated with fluid restriction, and cerebral infarction developed in 21 of them. Six more of the 19 hyponatremia patients, not treated with fluid restrictions, also developed cerebral infarction, giving a total rate of cerebral infarction of 27/44 among the hyponatremic patients. By contrast only 19 out of 90 patients with normal serum sodium had cerebral infarction.

While it is not possible to draw firm conclusions about the cause and effect relationship between hyponatremia and its treatment and cerebral infarction, these data suggest that it is prudent to determine blood (plasma) volume in patients with subarachnoid hemorrhage who fulfill the criteria for SIADH, prior to the institution of treatment with fluid restriction.

Hypothalamic-Pituitary-Thyroid Axis

REGULATION OF TSH SECRETION

The pituitary-thyroid axis (Fig. 5-7) is the prime example of a feedback, self-regulation system in neuroendocrinology. Regulation of thyroid function is achieved by the interactions of hormones secreted by the hypothalamus, the pituitary, and the thyroid gland itself. The following hypothalamic hormones are involved: TRH, which stimulates secretion of TSH by the pituitary; somatostatin, which inhibits TSH secretion; and dopamine, which also has an inhibitory influence. TSH controls the synthesis and release of the thyroid hormones thyroxine (T_4) and triiodothyronine (T_3). Circulating blood levels of T_4 and T_3 provide a negative feedback to the pituitary gland. An additional factor that influences the secretion of TSH is the peripheral degradation of T_4, T_3, TSH, and TRH. Thyroid hormones bind to thyrotropes (pituitary cells) to suppress further TSH secretion. In experimental animals the negative feedback influence of T_3 is nearly 10 times stronger than that of T_4. Negative feedback of T_3 and T_4 for TRH secretion in man is questionable. Intrahypothalamic injections of T_4 and T_3 in experimental animals suppresses TSH secretion. Whether this effect is due to decrease in TRH, increase in somatostatin, or is a direct effect on the pituitary gland (via hypothalamic-hypophyseal portal circulation) is not clear. Anterior hypothalamic lesions in rats[33] decrease basal TRH secretion and modify, but do not totally prevent, TSH secretory response to blood levels of the thyroid hormones. Electrical stimulation of the anterior hypothalamic region also increases TRH secretion.

Somatostatin infusion suppresses TSH levels in hypothyroid patients[34] and blocks TRH-induced TSH secretion, suggesting an inhibitory influence of somatostatin on the pituitary. Similarly, dopamine infusion also lowers blood TSH levels in both normal and hypothyroid patients and decreases TSH secretion in response to TRH.[35] Dopaminergic agonists like bromocriptine inhibit, and dopamine antagonists like metoclopramide, stimulate TSH secretion.

Other hormones (e.g., glucocorticoids, estrogens, and growth hormones) regulate TSH secretion. Glucocorticoids have an inhibitory influence. Patients with Cushing's disease have a blunted TSH response to TRH even when T_4 levels are slightly lower than normal. This effect is apparently mediated via both hypothalamus and pituitary, resulting in reduced secretion of TRH and a reduced sensitivity of the pituitary gland to TRH. Estrogens increase the responsiveness of the pituitary to circulating TRH, resulting in higher secretion of TSH. This phenomenon may explain the higher prevalence of hyperthyroidism among women than among men. The basal levels of TRH in men, women, and prepubertal children are similar, but the TSH secretory response to exogenous TRH is higher in women, especially in the follicular phase of the menstrual cycle, when plasma estrogen levels are high. Estrogens probably have a direct effect on the thyrotropic cells of the pituitary. A reduction in the TRH-induced release of TSH by the pituitary is observed in acromegalic patients, suggesting that growth hormone modifies the secretion of TSH by the pituitary.

It has been postulated[36] that the functional GH state of patients with hypopituitarism determines the TSH response. Effect of GH may be mediated through the secretion of somatostatin, which reduces pituitary responsiveness to TRH.

Many drugs influence the pituitary-thyroid functional unit, by altering protein binding or the metabolism of T_3, T_4 hormones. Enzyme-inducing drugs like barbiturates, phenytoin, or chlorpromazine promote increased breakdown of T_4. Aspirin and phenytoin decrease protein binding of T_4, thus decreasing TSH secretion. Amiodarone, glucocorticoids, and propranolol inhibit T_4 to T_3 conversion, thus increasing TSH secretion in response to TRH.

Environmental factors also affect TSH secretion. Two important factors are the (a) exposure to cold and (b) physical or emotional stress. Exposure to cold in mammals has been known to increase plasma TSH and cause thyroid hypertrophy. Similar response is seen in the human newborn, but thyroid activation has not been demonstrated in adults. In experimental animals, stressful procedures like starvation, pain, restraint, and infection lead to the suppression of thyroid hormone secretion. In humans similar response may occur, but is much more difficult to demonstrate because simultaneous changes in the peripheral metabolism of the thyroid hormones occur. Patients with the *sick euthyroid syndrome*[37] show low T_3 levels early in the disease, and low T_3 and T_4 levels as the severity of the disease increases. The underlying cause is the failure of conversion of T_4 to T_3 in peripheral tissues, predominantly the liver. These changes are seen with starvation and are reversed with adequate nutrition. Severely starved patients may also have reduced TSH response to TRH.

Serum T_4 levels can be elevated in the absence of thyroid disease. Elevation of T_4 and T_3 is sometimes seen in depressed patients. This finding suggests a possible role of central neurotransmitter abnormalities in the pathogenesis of thyroid function abnormalities. In general, attempts to elucidate the role of neurotransmitters (GABA, acetylcholine, and neuropeptides) in the regulation of TSH secretion have given confusing and contradictory results,[38] in part due to a very heterogeneous neural input to the hypothalamus. The best-established neurotransmitter effect is that of norepinephrine, which stimulates TRH release in vitro. Many other peptides (e.g., neurotensin, VIP, cholecystokinin, bombesin, oxytocin, vasopressin, and substance P) influence TSH secretion in rats. Of these only bombesin has been studied in humans and has been shown to have no effect on pituitary-thyroid function. GABA administration inhibits TSH release in rat and human.

TSH SECRETION IN RESPONSE
TO EXOGENOUS TRH

TSH secretion in response to TRH varies in normal persons and in those with thyroid disease. Normally, the intravenous administration of TRH (10 to 500 μg) promotes rapid TSH secretion, with a peak response in 15 to 30 min, followed by a rise in T_3 and T_4 after 2 to 4 h. The degree of TSH increase varies depending upon the endogenous thyroid functional state. In primary hypothyroidism, an exaggerated TSH response is seen in 70 percent of the patients,[24,39] while in hyperthyroidism a markedly blunted response or no response is seen. This variation in response has popularized TRH testing in the diagnostic workup of mild thyrotoxicosis. Preservation of TSH responsiveness to TRH will exclude thyrotoxicosis in 95 percent of patients. TRH testing also helps to distinguish between disorders of the hypothalamus and the pituitary (secondary and tertiary hypothyroidism). Patients with TSH deficiency due to intrinsic pituitary disease (tumor, infarction) will not respond to TRH administration, while those with hypothalamic disorders will. Preservation of the TRH response, however, is not an absolute assurance of a normally functioning pituitary, nor is a sluggish response, as can be seen in elderly men, an absolute indication of pituitary disease. These findings, therefore, must be evaluated in conjunction with the entire clinical picture.

A few patients with hypothyroidism caused by pituitary or hypothalamic disease are known to have high TSH levels. The most likely explanation for this finding is the possibility of the secretion of a biologically inactive molecule with retained immunoreactivity so that it is considered as TSH during radioimmunoassays. Another explanation is the combination of subclinical intrinsic thyroid failure and pituitary disease.

DISORDERS OF THE HYPOTHALAMIC-PITUITARY-THYROID AXIS

The negative feedback loop of the pituitary-thyroid axis is so sensitive that a clinical picture of hyperthyroidism (persistent elevation of T_4 and T_3), secondary to either pituitary or hypothalamic disease, is rarely seen. In experimental circumstances, a mild elevation of T_3 and T_4 can be maintained with a continuous infusion of TRH. Clinical disorders of thyroid function, resulting from diseases of hypothalamic-pituitary-thyroid axis, therefore, almost always present as hypothyroidism which may be primary, secondary, or tertiary. The relative ease of assays for thyroid hormones (T_3, T_4) and TSH, combined with the availability of TRH, has now made it possible to differentiate between different levels of dysfunction within the hypothalamic-pituitary-thyroid axis, as shown in Table 5-2.

PRIMARY HYPOTHYROIDISM A long-standing thyroid hormone deficiency due to intrinsic diseases of the thyroid gland may lead to pituitary enlargement secondary to hypertrophy of the thyrotropes. This may appear clinically as visual disturbances and may be diagnosed as a pituitary tumor. Presence of high levels of TSH with low levels of T_4 and T_3 establishes the diagnosis of primary hypothyroidism rather than pituitary tumor, although very rarely the two can be concurrent.

SECONDARY HYPOTHYROIDISM Intrinsic pituitary disease leads to secondary hypothyroidism. These patients have low T_4 and T_3 values. TSH does not increase in response to TRH injection. Occasionally a patient with established pituitary disease may show an exaggerated TSH response to TRH. It is proposed that in those cases both the hypothalamus and the pituitary were diseased with sparing of a few thyrotropes, which respond to exogenous TRH. Rarely, isolated TSH deficiency unresponsive to TRH due to failure of development of the pituitary thyrotropes has been reported.

TERTIARY HYPOTHYROIDISM Availability of TRH for clinical use has made the diagnosis of hypothyroidism due to hypothalamic failure possible. Many of the cases previously diagnosed as idiopathic hypopituitarism are now known to be actually due to hypothalamic hypofunction. In tertiary hypothyroidism the patients have low TSH, low T_4, T_3 but a normal or exaggerated TSH response to TRH administration. Hypothalamic hypofunction may be secondary to tumor, trauma (surgery, section of pituitary stalk), or inflammation. Sheehan's syndrome sometimes develops secondary to infarction of the hypophyseal stalk.

HYPERTHYROIDISM As pointed out earlier, an overwhelming majority of the patients presenting with hyperthyroidism have intrinsic thyroid disease (Graves' disease, nodular goiter, thyroiditis). There have been, however, published cases of hyperthyroidism secondary to TSH-secreting pituitary tumors,[40] as well as due to a defect in the thyroid-pituitary negative feedback mechanism.[40,41] Diagnosis in these cases is based on high TSH levels with normal or high levels of T_3, T_4. In primary hyperthyroidism TSH levels are low, usually below 0.5 IU/ml. It should be emphasized that the commonly used radioimmunoassays for TSH are unable to detect low levels (<2.5 IU/ml), therefore many of these cases may be misdiagnosed. In secondary hyperthyroidism, the typical eye signs due to the orbital involvement seen in Graves' disease are missing. Patients with TSH-secreting pituitary adenomas have other concurrent endocrinopathies, like acromegaly. TSH secretion is not suppressed by exogenous thyrox-

TABLE 5-2
Differential Diagnosis of Hypothalamic-Pituitary-Thyroid Disorders

	T_4, T_3	TSH	TSH Response to TRH	Other Abnormalities
Primary hypothyroidism	Low	High	Exaggerated response	Increased prolactin secretion
Secondary hypothyroidism	Low	Low	No increase in TSH	
Tertiary hypothyroidism	Low	Low	Normal or exaggerated TSH secretion	
Primary hyperthyroidism	High	Low	Blunted or no response	
Secondary hyperthyroidism	High or normal	High	Normal	

ine administration but may be suppressed by glucocorticoids.

Thyrotoxicosis may develop due to a defect in the thyroid-pituitary negative feedback—that is, persistence of TSH secretion by the pituitary in the presence of elevated plasma T_3, T_4 levels. In this "secondary hyperthyroidism" the clinical picture is similar to that of Graves' disease, except that the typical signs of orbital infiltration are missing, and the patients are quite resistant to treatment with antithyroid drugs. This disorder is genetically transmitted as an autosomal dominant trait.

Hypothalamic-Pituitary-Adrenal Axis

The hypothalamic-pituitary-adrenal axis (Fig. 5-8) exemplifies the close interactions of the nervous system and the endocrine system in the maintenance of vital homeostatic functions, fluid and electrolyte balance, response to stress, and the circadian rhythm of endogenous hormone secretion. The adrenal gland in itself is a prime example of a neuroendocrine system. The adrenal medulla is a specialized part of the nervous system and in many ways can be considered the largest and an atypical sympathetic ganglion. Atypical, because it lacks the long postganglionic fibers typical of sympathetic ganglia. The adrenal medulla synthesizes epinephrine and norepinephrine while the adrenal cortex serves as an endocrine gland. The adrenal cortex synthesizes three groups of steroid hormones: glucocorticoids, mineralocorticoids, and sex hormones. Epinephrine and norepinephrine, in turn, control the secretion of adrenocortical steroids by affecting the secretion of corticotropin by the hypothalamus, thus completing the loop of neuroendocrine function. Adrenal hormones play a vital role in the maintenance of milieu interieur and survival.

It was more than a century ago, in 1855, that Thomas Addison first published his report on autopsy findings of the destruction of the adrenal glands in patients dying because of "pernicious anemia." This observation prompted the investigation of the effects of adrenalectomy in animal models and the observation that adrenalectomy was followed by death within a few days. The vital connection between adrenal hypofunction and mortality was thus identified. Effects of adrenal hyperfunction were described much later by Cushing in the 1920s, and the concept of central nervous control of adrenal function was developed in the 1940s.[42] Existence of corticotropin-releasing hormone, CRH (also called corticotropin-releasing factor, CRF), was proposed in the 1950s.[43,44]

The hypothalamic-pituitary-adrenal control axis is diagramatically illustrated in Fig. 5-8 and its components are discussed below.

CORTICOTROPIN-RELEASING HORMONE (CRH)

This hormone was first identified[43] by demonstrating the secretion of ACTH by pituitary slices, when incubated with hypothalmic slices in vitro and in extracts of posterior pituitary gland.[44] The chemical structure of CRH in humans is identical with that in rat and slightly different from that in sheep. Synthetic CRH, now commercially available, is a potent stimulator of ACTH in humans. It has a plasma half life of 11.6 min (α phase) and 73 min (β phase). After a bolus injection of CRH, elevation of ACTH is maintained for 2 to 3 h.[45] CRH also promotes the secretion of β-endorphin which is secreted from the same prohormone as ACTH. The normal level of CRF in human CSF is 8.6 $\pm$ 1.7 fmol/ml.

In addition to CRH, other neuropeptides are also involved in the control of ACTH secretion (Fig. 5-8) and have important interactions with CRH. Vasopressin has been known to be involved in the secretion of ACTH, and it has been debated[46] whether vasopressin and CRF are indeed the same substance, since both have been isolated from posterior pituitary extracts. The characterization and isolation of CRH in experi-

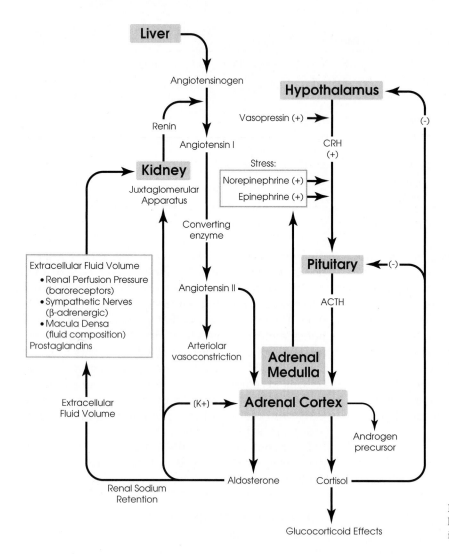

Figure 5-8 Schematic diagram of hypothalamic-pituitary-adrenal axis and its interaction with renin-angiotensin system.

mental animals has made the comparison of the potency of vasopressin and CRH possible, and it has been determined that CRH is about 1000 times more potent in releasing ACTH than vasopressin and that the effects of the two are synergistic.[47] Similarly, epinephrine and norepinephrine are also synergistic with CRH in enhancing ACTH secretion.[47,48]

NEGATIVE FEEDBACK REGULATION OF CRH
Hypothalamic CRH levels rise after adrenalectomy and decrease after glucocorticoid administration, suggesting a negative feedback effect of the circulating cortisol level. Mineralocorticoids do not have this negative feedback effect. Glucocorticoids given in the preoperative period do not suppress ACTH secretion because stress of surgery overrides the negative feedback effect of the exogenous glucocorticoids. Glucocorticoid receptors have been demonstrated in the brain.[49] Even very high doses of glucocorticoids cannot totally abolish the CRH secretion of hypothalamic neurons, and there is "breakthrough" secretion of some ACTH with

extreme stress in animals given high doses of corticoids.

The mechanism of action of CRH involves binding to pituitary membrane receptors. ACTH secretion is accompanied by a rapid increase in 3'5'-cyclic AMP which is blunted by corticoid administration. Normally, the CRH effect on the anterior pituitary is highly hormone-specific, but it may occasionally release GH in some patients with acromegaly.

ADRENOCORTICOTROPIC HORMONE (ACTH)

Human ACTH is a 39-amino-acid compound. Synthetic ACTH is available in a highly active form. ACTH and several other hormones synthesized by the anterior pituitary are derived from a common prohormone called proopiomelanocortin (POMC), the gene for which is localized on chromosome 2 in humans. The differences in hormones generated from POMC are due to the properties of distinct cell types in different parts of the brain and explain the close relationship of ACTH and α-melanocyte-stimulating hormone (α-MSH), a peptide similar in chemical structure to the ACTH amino-acid sequence of 1 to 13 amino acids. The POMC gene is widely distributed in the neurohypophyseal neurons, other parts of the brain, adrenal medulla, GI tract, pheochromocytoma, medullary thyroid carcinoma, and carcinoid, and may explain endocrine disorders in a wide variety of disease states. The rate of synthesis of POMC–messenger RNA is regulated by specific cell types. In the anterior pituitary gland, corticoids inhibit and CRH stimulates POMC-mRNA. In the intermediate lobe of lower animals (frogs and rats), glucocorticoids and CRH have no effect, while dopamine inhibits POMC-mRNA. In other parts of the brain, neither CRH nor glucocorticoids regulate POMC-mRNA synthesis. ACTH acts on the adrenal cortex through specific receptors on the cell membrane and promotes the synthesis of adrenal hormones.

NEURAL CONTROL OF ACTH SECRETION
Secretion of ACTH is regulated by both CRH and vasopressin in addition to other peptides (Fig. 5-8). The vasopressinergic system originates in the supraoptic and paraventricular nuclei. The principal projection of these neurons is to the neurohypophysis, but some neurons terminate near the hypophyseal capillary network. In addition, vasopressin secreted by the neurohypophysis may reach the adenohypophysis via retrograde blood flow. Specific CRH neurons are predominantly in the paraventricular nuclei. This neuron system contains a number of other peptides, including vasopressin, dynorphin, neurotensin, and vasogenic intestinal peptide (VIP). CRH is also contained in the oxytocinergic hypothalamic neurons that project onto the brainstem and spinal cord, and this pathway is thought to be involved in the autonomic regulation mentioned earlier. CRH neurons also receive extensive neural input from other parts of the brain, and thus bring ACTH secretion under the control of virtually all parts of the brain. Certain experimental stimuli (e.g., *E. coli* endotoxin, hemorrhage, surgery) promote ACTH secretion via the autonomic nervous system, virtually bypassing the hypothalamus. CRH neurons have also been identified extracranially in the adrenal medulla, lungs, liver, stomach, duodenum, and pancreas.

Intracerebroventricular administration of CRH in experimental animals causes remarkable sympathetic stimulation, evidenced by an increase of adrenal secretion of epinephrine and norepinephrine. The plasma levels of glucose and glucagon also rise. There is an elevation of BP and heart rate, locomotor activity, and emotionality in animals. It has been suggested that CRH may act both through the pituitary (ACTH secretion) and by alerting other parts of the brain for a "fight-or-flight" response.

NEGATIVE FEEDBACK OF ACTH SECRETION
ACTH secretion has a negative feedback mechanism similar to that described above for CRH. Adrenalectomy or primary disease of the adrenals (e.g., tuberculosis) leads to a high level of ACTH, while glucocorticoid administration suppresses ACTH levels. Glucocorticoids act both by suppressing mRNA coding of POMC (described above) and by reducing CRH receptors on the pituitary. Extrahypothalamic structures in the brain probably exert an inhibitory control on ACTH secretion, as evidenced by sustained high plasma cortisone levels in rats after isolation of the hypothalamus (by cutting the nerve fiber connections with the overlying brain).[50] Both activating and inhibitory functions of the midbrain and brainstem relative to ACTH secretion have been described in experimental animals. Responses probably depend upon the integrity of the afferents. Electrical stimulation of the limbic system (amygdala and lateral hypothalamus) also have been shown to increase ACTH levels in cats. ACTH secretion is also influenced by many other neurotransmitters. In humans, pituitary-adrenal response to insulin-induced hypoglycemia is blocked by propranolol and is suppressed by phentolamine, suggesting an adrenergic pathway. A serotonin-releasing agent (fenfluramine) stimulates ACTH release. ACTH secretion is also influenced by endogenous opioid neuropeptides.

ADRENAL HORMONES

As mentioned earlier, the adrenal glands are composed of cortex and medulla. Adrenal medullary hormones are the catecholamines: epinephrine and norepinephrine. The basic chemical structure of the hormones of the adrenal cortex is the steroid molecule (Fig. 5-9). Therefore, these are also called adrenal corticosteroids or corticoids for short. Based on their biologic effects, adrenal corticoids are divided into three categories (Fig. 5-9). A simplified interrelationship of the three categories is diagramatically shown in Fig. 5-10. The three categories of the adrenal cortical steroids are glucocorticoids, mineralocorticoids, and androcorticoids. The most important naturally occurring hormones in these three categories are cortisol, aldosterone, and androstenedione, respectively. The physiologic actions of the adrenal corticoids are described below.

GLUCOCORTICOIDS   Daily endogenous secretion of cortisol has been estimated to be approximately 20 mg. Normal resting plasma concentration is 10 to 20 μg/dl in the morning, and about half that in the afternoon.

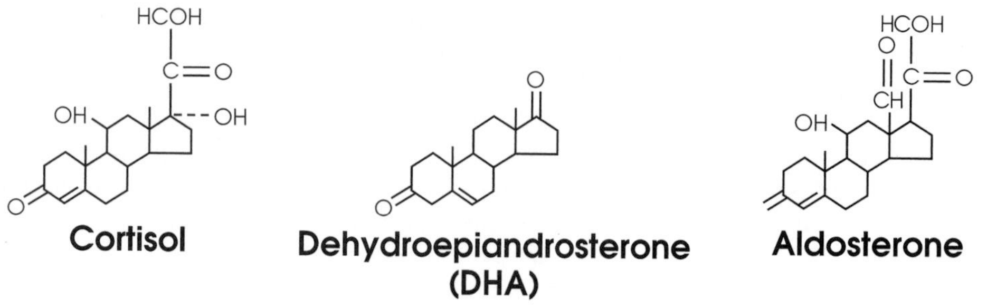

Cortisol   **Dehydroepiandrosterone (DHA)**   **Aldosterone**

Figure 5-9 Chemical structure of representatives of three classes of adrenal steroids: glucocorticoids (cortisol), mineralocorticoids (aldosterone), and androgens (dehydroepiandrosterone).

At midnight this level is 2 to 10 μg/dl. As the name implies, glucocorticoids are largely involved in the metabolism of carbohydrates, proteins, and fats. Cortisol promotes neoglucogenesis (conversion of amino acids and fats to glucose) and decreases glucose utilization by the cells. The net effect is an increase in the blood glucose level, a diabetogenic effect. In addition, cortisol also has a mild mineralocorticoid action, that is, it promotes the retention of sodium and the excretion of potassium. Cortisol also has weak androgenic effects. The anti-inflammatory effects of the glucocorticoids are the basis for their widespread use in clinical practice. The anti-inflammatory effect is secondary to the capability of glucocorticoids to (a) stabilize cell membranes, (b) reduce the permeability of the capillary membranes, and (c) inhibit the formation of bradykinin. Cortisol is the only hormone produced by the adrenal cortex that is essential for life. Cortisol also promotes the conversion of norepinephrine to epinephrine in the adrenal medulla and hence plays an important role in the maintenance of blood pressure and explains the life-threatening hemodynamic instability seen in patients with adrenal insufficiency under stressful situations, like the induction of anesthesia and surgery.

MINERALOCORTICOIDS   Aldosterone is the most important hormone of this group. Corticosterone and desoxycorticosterone also contribute to this action.

These hormones promote potassium excretion and sodium retention. The secretion and synthesis of mineralocorticoids are predominantly controlled by the renin-angiotensin system (Fig. 5-8), while ACTH plays a minor role. Aldosterone secretion is also stimulated by elevated serum potassium, while hypokalemia suppresses it.

SEX HORMONES   The principal androgen, dehydroepiandrosterone, is responsible for the masculinizing effects associated with adrenal hormone excess, since it is converted to testosterone and estradiol in the peripheral tissues. The release of androgens is controlled by ACTH. They are degraded in the liver and their metabolites are excreted as urinary 17-hydroxyketosteroids.

ACTH predominantly controls the release of corticosteroids and sex hormones. Although mineralocorticoid secretion is also initiated by ACTH, and a certain level of ACTH is necessary for continued secretion of aldosterone, the principal factor influencing aldosterone blood levels is the renin-angiotensin pathway rather than the adrenal-pituitary-hypothalamic axis. As a consequence, it is cortisol that provides the strongest negative feedback for ACTH and CRH secretion.

DYSFUNCTION OF THE ADRENAL GLAND

Clinically the disorders of the adrenal gland are associated with excessive secretion of adrenal medullary

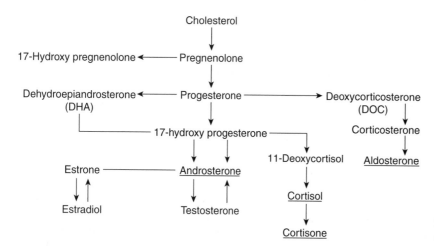

Figure 5-10 Major pathways of biosynthesis of adrenal cortical hormones.

neurotransmitters (pheochromocytoma), excessive secretion of adrenal corticoids, predominantly glucocorticoids due to primary adrenal hyperplasia (Cushing's syndrome), or secondary to hypothalamic-pituitary disease (Cushing's disease), or insufficient secretion of adrenal hormones (Addison's disease). As mentioned earlier, a discussion of neurotransmitters (and their disorders) is beyond the scope of this chapter; hence pheochromocytoma will not be discussed. A brief discussion of Cushing's syndrome/disease and Addison's disease is given below.

ADRENAL CORTICAL HYPERSECRETION

CUSHING'S SYNDROME AND CUSHING'S DISEASE. The term Cushing's syndrome is used to identify the clinical picture associated with the presence of excessive cortisol, which may be endogenous (disease of the adrenal gland) or exogenous (use of the synthetic glucocorticoids for therapeutic purposes). Cushing's disease, on the other hand, refers to increased cortisol secretion in response to increased blood levels of ACTH. Clinically Cushing's disease and Cushing's syndrome present an identical picture, and differentiation between the two can be made only on the basis of the laboratory investigations. The classical picture, as described by Cushing (hence the name), is that of a young female patient with truncal obesity, moon facies, short neck with a buffalo hump, plethoric skin with marked purplish striae, and easy bruisability. Hypertension, hirsutism, and osteoporosis are commonly present. Cushing's syndrome is nine times more frequent in women than in men.

The most common cause of Cushing's syndrome (in 75 percent of the cases) is bilateral benign hyperplasia of the adrenal cortex. Cushing's disease is secondary to excessive ACTH secretion, either due to a basophil adenoma of the pituitary gland or secondary to hypersecretion of CRH by the hypothalamus, as seen with hypothalamic gangliocytoma.[51] Other causes may be adrenal tumors (adenoma or carcinoma) or ectopic ACTH secretion by carcinoma of the lung or pancreas. Pituitary adenomas have been shown to exist in a majority (75 to 82 percent) of patients with Cushing's syndrome, and it is debatable whether adrenal hyperplasia is a primary or secondary phenomenon. In Cushing's disease, adrenal responses to stress and to suppressive doses of exogenous steroids are qualitatively normal but quantitatively abnormal. This suggests that the regulating mechanism is normal, but that a "high set point" for ACTH secretion exists. Further evidence for CNS pathology as the underlying cause of Cushing's syndrome is provided by the fact that the GH secretory rhythms are also abnormal in a large number of these patients.[52] Many patients with chronic depressive disorders have an abnormal exogenous ste-roid suppression test. Current clinical and experimental evidence suggests that most cases of Cushing's disease are due to intrinsic pituitary disease (microadenomas), but rarely secondary to excessive CRH production due to hypothalamic disease or ectopic ACTH secretion by extracranial malignancies (oat cell carcinoma of the lung, or carcinomas of the thymus, pancreas, thyroid, prostrate, and other organs), carcinoid, and neuroblastoma.

The clinical presentation of Cushing's disease secondary to extracranial malignancies is quite atypical. Explosive hyperadrenalism may develop early or late in the course of the disease with such rapidity that some of the typical features of Cushing's syndrome, like truncal obesity, may not have time to develop.[53] Electrolyte abnormalities, like hypokalemic alkalosis, are common, due to excess mineralocorticoids. Hypertension and diabetes mellitus are usually present. Another feature of Cushing's syndrome, secondary to ectopic ACTH, is the presence of abnormal skin pigmentation. Most often the presenting features of primary malignancy are helpful in the diagnosis although, rarely, these may not be prominent.

ADRENAL CORTICAL INSUFFICIENCY

ADDISON'S DISEASE. Acute or chronic adrenal corticoid deficiency is a life-threatening condition. The disease as first described by Addison, and which to date bears his name, was adrenal cortical insufficiency due to adrenal tuberculosis. These days, tuberculosis is a rare disease and most cases of adrenal hypofunction appear to be of unknown (idiopathic) origin, most probably an autoimmune disorder. The majority of cases show adrenal autoantibodies and polyglandular failure, most commonly thyroiditis (Hashimoto's disease) and diabetes mellitus. Adrenal insufficiency may occur secondary to pituitary disease (e.g., pituitary tumors) to infection, or to granulomas in the hypothalamic-pituitary region. If pituitary disease is the underlying cause, the resulting ACTH deficiency leads to a marked decrease of glucocorticoids (ACTH control). Mineralocorticoid levels (renin-angiotensin control) are relatively normal. Response to exogenous ACTH may be delayed due to secondary atrophy of the adrenal cortex. The clinical manifestations of secondary glucocorticoid deficiency are less severe than those of primary adrenal failure because some endogenous glucocorticoid secretion (due to ectopic ACTH) may continue in the presence of pituitary-hypothalamic disease. Clinically, hypoadrenalism may also be seen in patients following the prolonged use of exogenous glucocorticoids. In this situation, the glucocorticoids suppress endogenous ACTH secretion by negative feedback. A prolonged decrease in ACTH leads to aplasia (destruction) of the adrenal cortex which fails to provide a surge of corticosteroids in response to stress.

Primary adrenal insufficiency, due to adrenal disease, presents with muscle weakness, weight loss, and hypotension. Hyperpigmentation due to excessive melanotropin (melanocyte-stimulating hormone) production by the anterior pituitary is a common feature. Stress, trauma, and surgery can produce circulatory collapse with hypotension, hypovolemia, hyponatremia, and hyperkalemia. Prolonged volume depletion may result in diminished cardiac output and renal blood flow leading to an elevation of BUN. Hypovolemia is less likely in secondary adrenal insufficiency due to hypothalamic-pituitary disease.

ADRENOLEUKODYSTROPHY.   This is a sex-linked genetic disorder presenting as hypoadrenalism, affecting male patients exclusively.[54,55] In this disorder, adrenal insufficiency is assocaited with demyelination of the brain. Both adrenal failure and central demyelination are believed to be due to an enzymatic defect, but the precise abnormality has not yet been defined. The clinical features result from a combination of hypoadrenalism and CNS effects. The onset of the disease is in childhood between the ages of 4 and 16 years, presenting with personality change, dementia, vomiting, unsteady gate, ataxia, increasing pigmentation (especially on extensor surfaces and oral mucosa), cortical blindness, and quadriplegia, leading to death in 5 to 10 years.

LABORATORY DIAGNOSIS OF HYPOTHALAMIC-PITUITARY-ADRENAL AXIS DISORDERS

The disturbance of the diurnal rhythm of secretion of CRH, ACTH, and glucocorticoids is an early indication of the dysfunction of the hypothalamic-pituitary-adrenal axis. Most testing procedures are based on the measurement of glucocorticoids (cortisol) in blood or urine as indirect evidence of ACTH secretion, because these tests are easily available and less expensive. ACTH assays are available in specialized laboratories but are more expensive. Interlaboratory variations in the normal values of blood and urinary cortisol levels are overcome by resorting to "provocative tests" rather than relying on absolute values. The commonly used tests and their interpretations are discussed below

DIURNAL VARIATION OF CORTISOL SECRETION

Normal levels of plasma cortisol in the morning hours range between 10 and 25 μg/dl and fall to below 10 μg/100 ml in random samples drawn in the afternoon and evening (6 to 10 P.M.). Persistently low levels, below 6 μg/dl, suggest hypoadrenalism. Normal diurnal variation may be masked by episodic secretion of cortisol in stress-related situations—for example, in hospitalized patients undergoing invasive procedures. In this situation, diurnal variation should be seen on the following day. High normal values during both morning and afternoon, or high 24-h urinary excretion, will confirm the diagnosis of Cushing's syndrome. The normal values for urinary cortisol are 4 to 12 mg/24 h and are dependent upon total body muscle mass. As an alternative, urinary secretion of cortisol degradation products, that is, 17-hydroxyketosteroids, may be measured, but their level will be affected by the presence of liver disease.

ACTH STIMULATION TEST

Synthetic ACTH, 250 μg (25 units) in 500 ml normal saline, is given intravenously over 4 to 8 h, and plasma cortisol levels are measured before and after this injection. Twenty-four-hour urinary 17-hydroxyketosteroids are also measured before and after ACTH injection. In the normal population, plasma cortisol levels should rise to normal levels and urinary ketosteroid secretion should increase by 100 percent. For the sake of convenience, a one-hour Cortrosyn test has been widely used to screen for both ACTH deficiency and for primary adrenal failure. The normal response to a one-hour injection is a baseline value of plasma cortisol of 5 μg/dl, followed by an increase of 7 μg/dl and a maximum value of 18 μg/dl or greater. Lack of appropriate response in one hour can be due to a defect in either the pituitary or the adrenal glands. Prolonged ACTH deficiency, due to pituitary disease, can lead to adrenal atrophy and decreased adrenal sensitivity to ACTH. Repeated testing for three days may thus be necessary to differentiate between pituitary disease and adrenal disease as the underlying cause. Patients with pituitary disease will respond to ACTH stimulation, while those with primary adrenal disease will not respond.

METYRAPONE TEST FOR PITUITARY ACTH RESERVE

Metyrapone inhibits the biosynthesis of cortisol by blocking the enzyme 11β-hydroxylase. A decrease of plasma cortisol by metyrapone reduces negative feedback to the pituitary and should lead to a compensatory rise in plasma ACTH levels, followed by an increase in urinary 17-hydroxyketosteroids on the following day. This test is performed by giving metyrapone, 750 mg, every 4 h for six doses. A normal response is the doubling of urinary 17-hydroxyketosteroid excretion on the following day. In Cushing's disease, the response is supranormal. Either hypothalamic or pituitary disease can result in subnormal response because of the failure of the compensatory secretion of ACTH, which is normally present secondary to decreased plasma cortisol levels.

STRESS-INDUCED ACTH RESPONSE

Stress, induced by injection of insulin, pyrogens, and vasopressin, has been used to investigate pituitary reserve. Insulin-induced hypoglycemia is most commonly used, and helps to measure changes in GH and prolactin in addition to ACTH. Normally, a 50 percent reduction in blood glucose levels, induced by insulin injection, should increase the plasma cortisol level by 5 to 7 μg/dl, or an absolute plasma cortisol level of 15 μg/dl should be reached. All induced stress is unpleasant and may be dangerous in the presence of underlying CNS and cardiovascular disease. It is therefore a common practice to measure ACTH levels before and after a stressful situation (e.g., invasive diagnostic procedures), rather than to subject the patient to the additional induced stress of hypoglycemia. A lack of increased ACTH secretion, secondary to induced stress, does not differentiate between the hypothalamus or the pituitary as the underlying cause.

CRH SUPPRESSION TEST IN HYPOADRENALISM

It is at present not commonly available. Plasma ACTH and cortisol levels remain elevated for 2 to 3 h after a single injection of 1 μg/kg CRH in patients with normal pituitary-adrenal reserve. A normal response thus identifies underlying hypothalamic disease as the cause of hypoadrenalism.

DEXAMETHASONE SUPPRESSION TEST

Once the diagnosis of hyperadrenalism (Cushing's syndrome) has been made on the basis of (1) loss of diurnal variation in cortisol secretion; (2) persistent elevation of plasma cortisol levels > 25 μg/dl and (3) 24-h 17-hydroxyketosteroid > 18 mg/24 h, the dexamethasone suppression test can be used to identify the underlying cause, which may be primary adrenal disease (adenoma, carcinoma, hyperplasia), pituitary adenoma, or ectopic ACTH secretion by the other malignancies listed earlier.

This test is carried out by giving dexamethasone first at low doses (0.5 mg q.i.d.) and then high doses (2 mg q.i.d.) for 2 days. The suppression of cortisol secretion to <5 μg/dl at high doses, but not at low doses, points to a pituitary disease. Cortisol hypersecretion, due to primary adrenal disease or to ectopic ACTH secretion, is generally not affected by either dose regimen, although a few exceptions have been reported. Lack of dexamethasone suppression may be seen in obese patients, who may show suppression after a longer period.

CRH SUPPRESSION TEST IN HYPERADRENALISM

A normal or exaggerated increase in cortisol secretion is seen in response to CRH administration in patients with Cushing's disease of hypothalamic-pituitary origin. Patients with primary adrenal hyperplasia or ectopic ACTH secretion almost always show a suppressed response. A false-negative response to CRH is noted in 9 percent of the patients with Cushing's disease and compares favorably with 11 percent false-negative response to the dexamethasone suppression test[56] in this patient population. CRH administration also differentiates between Cushing's disease and the hyperadrenalism associated with psychiatric disorders, such as depression.[57] Response is normal in the former and is suppressed in depressed patients.

In addition to the endocrine evaluation tests listed above, radiologic investigations (i.e., CAT scan and MRI of the abdomen and skull) are useful in the diagnosis of hyperadrenalism associated with abnormalities of the hypothalamic-pituitary-adrenal axis.

Central Nervous System Pathology Associated with Neuroendocrine Problems

Early in this chapter we discussed neurotransmitter secretory and neurohormone secretory properties of the central nervous system. Although primarily only neurohormone secretion has been discussed in detail, it must be emphasized that in the intact organism both secretion and the physiologic effects of neurotransmitters and neurohormones are closely interrelated and essential for the proper functioning of the CNS. As an example, the hypothalamus, in addition to its role in regulating the secretion of hormones of the anterior and posterior pituitary, is also an important link in regulating many vital functions of the body—for example, water balance (through thirst and food intake), body temperature, consciousness, sleep, emotion, and behavior. The disorders of one function may thus have a close link with other body functions through neuroendocrine mechanisms that are not entirely clear-cut and well-understood. What complicates this understanding further is the fact that manifestations of underlying CNS pathology (e.g., hypothalamic disease) depend in part on the time course of the pathologic development. Relatively trivial acute trauma to the anterior part of the hypothalamus may result in fatal hyperthermia, while massive destruction of this region, if pathology has developed slowly (over years, as can occur with craniopharyngiomas and meningiomas), may be coexistent with near-normal hypothalamic function. The reason for such differences is not entirely clear, but it has been proposed that certain groups of hypothalamic neurons can regenerate after damage. Slow progress of the disease provides time for such regeneration, resulting in the maintenance of near-normal hypothalamic function. Diseases of the CNS in the region of the hypothalamus and the pituitary can thus have a wide variety of endocrine function involvement. Similarly, the etiology of the lesions of the hypothalamic-pituitary region is highly variable, and the preponderance of different diseases may depend on the age range of the patient population.

Various diseases associated with neuroendocrine abnormalities and their clinical manifestations are briefly summarized below. A detailed discussion of the individual pathologic conditions can be found in textbooks of neurology, neurosurgery and endocrinology.

DISEASES OF THE HYPOTHALAMUS

Table 5-3 summarizes the variety of pathologic lesions that have been known to develop in the hypothalamic region of the brain at different periods of life. As emphasized above, the functional impact of these lesions is highly variable. The common neurological manifestations of nonendocrine hypothalamic disorders are summarized in Table 5-4.

Based on a survey of 60 autopsy-proven cases of hypothalamic disease, Bauer[58] has reported the frequency of clinical signs and symptoms as summarized in Table 5-5. In addition, there is a high frequency of electrocardiographic changes and cardiac arrhythmias seen commonly in patients with subarachnoid hemorrhage and less commonly with cerebral ischemia, brain tumors and neurosurgical procedures. The cardiac arrhythmias include supraventricular and ventricular tachycardia and ventricular fibrillation. ECG abnormalities include prolonged QT interval, depressed or elevated ST segments, flat or inverted T waves, and the development of Q waves. These changes have been reported in the absence of coronary artery disease. The underlying cause of these cardiac abnormalities is intense central sympathetic stimulation, probably via β-adrenergic mechanisms, since treatment with propranolol (β-blocker) has ameliorated cardiac pathology. In experimental animals, electrical stimulation of the hypothalamus can induce similar arrhythmias, which can be prevented by vagotomy or with anticholinergic drugs, suggesting a vagal cholinergic mechanism.

DISEASES OF THE PITUITARY

A variety of pathologic lesions in the sella turcica and parasellar region, listed in Table 5-6, can compromise the function of the pituitary gland. The majority of pituitary tumors are first recognized by the clinical

TABLE 5-3
Etiology of Hypothalamic Disease by Age

1. *Premature infants and neonates*
   Intraventricular hemorrhage
   Meningitis: bacterial
   Tumors: glioma, hemangioma
   Trauma
   Hydrocephalus, kernicterus

2. *1 month to 2 years*
   Tumors: glioma, especially optic glioma
   Histocytosis X
   Hydrocephalus, meningitis
   "Familial" disorders: Laurence-Moon-Biedl, Prader-Labhart-Willi

3. *2 to 10 years*
   Tumors
      Craniopharyngioma
      Ganglioneuroma, ependymoma, medulloblastoma
   Meningitis
      Bacterial
      Tuberculous
   Encephalitis
      Viral and demyelinating
      Various viral encephalides and exanthematous demyelinating encephalides
   "Familial" disorders: diabetes insipidus, etc.

4. *10 to 25 years*
   Tumors
      Craniopharyngioma
      Glioma, hamartoma, dysgerminoma
      Histiocytosis X, leukemia
      Dermoid, lipoma, neuroblastoma
   Trauma
      Subarachnoid hemorrhage, vascular aneurysm, arteriovenous malformation
      Inflammatory diseases, meningitis, encephalitis, sarcoid, tuberculosis
      Associated with midline brain defects; agenesis of corpus callosum
      Chronic hydrocephalus or increased intracranial pressure

5. *25 to 50 years*
   Nutritional: Wernicke's disease
   Tumors
      Sarcoma, glioblastoma, lymphoma
      Meningioma, colloid cysts, ependymoma, pituitary tumors
   Vascular
      Infarct, subarachnoid hemorrhage
      Pituitary apoplexy
   Inflammation: encephalitis, sarcoid, meningitis

SOURCE: Adapted from Martin JB, Reichlin S: *Clinical Neuroendocrinology*, 2d ed. Philadelphia, FA Davis, 1987:410, with permission.

manifestations of hyperprolactinemia. Abnormalities of the individual pituitary hormones have been discussed before. Other clinical features that can be determined by taking a detailed history are headaches and disturbances of libido and of sleep.

Headaches are usually bitemporal or bifrontal and are the result of pressure in the diaphragma sellae. Suprasellar growth of the tumor may be accompanied by relief or absence of headache. Raised intracranial

TABLE 5-4
Neurologic Manifestations of Nonendocrine Hypothalamic Disease

Disorders of temperature regulation	Periodic Disease of hypothalamic origin
Hyperthermia	Diencephalic epilepsy
Hypothermia	Kleine-Levin syndrome
Poikilothermia	Periodic discharge syndrome of Wolff
Disorders of food intake	Narcolepsy
Hyperphagia (bulimia)	Disorders of the autonomic nervous system
Anorexia, aphagia	Pulmonary edema
Disorders of water intake	Cardiac arrhythmias
Compulsive water drinking	Sphincter disturbance
Adipsia or hypodipsia	Hereditary hypothalamic disease
Essential hypernatremia	Laurence-Moon-Biedl syndrome
Disorders of sleep and consciousness	de Morsier syndrome
Somnolence	Kallmann syndrome
Sleep-rhythm reversal	Miscellaneous
Akinetic mutism	Prader-Willi syndrome
Coma	Diencephalic syndrome of infancy
Disorders of psychic function	Cerebral gigantism
Rage behavior	
Hallucinations	

SOURCE: Adapted from Martin JB, Reichlin S: *Clinical Neuroendocrinology,* 2d ed. Philadelphia, FA Davis, 1987:380, with permission.

pressure, with nausea, vomiting, and papilledema, rarely develops. Visual disturbances and visual hallucinations are more common, but occur only when the tumor has attained a size large enough to cause chiasmal compression. A patient with a small pituitary tumor may have neither headaches nor visual disturbances.

Disturbances of libido usually result from gonadotropin deficiency. In men there may be accompanying impotence, which may be due either to the direct effect of increased prolactin levels or to decreased gonadotropin levels, secondary to negative feedback by prolactin.

TABLE 5-5
Symptoms and Signs of Hypothalamic Disease (From a Review of 60 Autopsy-Proven Cases)

Symptoms and Signs	Number of Cases
Sexual abnormalities (hypogonadism or precocious puberty)	43
Diabetes insipidus	21
Psychic disturbance	21
Obesity or hyperphagia	20
Somnolence	18
Emaciation, anorexia	15
Thermodysregulation	13
Sphincter disturbance	5

SOURCE: Adapted from Martin JB, Reichlin S: *Clinical Neuroendocrinology,* 2d ed. Philadelphia, FA Davis, 1987:380, with permission.

Treatment with bromocriptine (to shrink the pituitary tumor) results in the improvement of libido and impotence even though the testosterone levels are still lower than normal. Very rarely, hypersexuality with precocious puberty in boys is reported, secondary to hypothalamic disease (Klein-Levin syndrome).

Sleep disturbances may include insomnia, hypersomnia, or reversal of day/night rhythms. Details of the clinical presentations, pathophysiology, and treatment of individual lesions listed in Table 5-6 can be found in textbooks of neurology and neurosurgery.

NEUROENDOCRINE ROLE OF THE PINEAL GLAND AND PARAVENTRICULAR ORGANS

The pineal gland is a small gland (100 to 150 mg) attached to the roof of the third ventricle just under the corpus callosum. The functions of the pineal gland in humans are not clearly understood. Experimental work, however, suggests that it plays a role in the neuroendocrine control of the pituitary. In vertebrates, including humans, the embryologic origin of the pineal gland is from the ependymal cells of the epithalamic region of the third ventricle, where it is part of a family of secretory organs, including the subcommissural organ, area postrema, subfornical organ, median eminence, and neurohypophysis.[59,60] In lower animals (amphibians and fish), the pineal gland contains photoreceptors and serves as a "third eye," while in higher vertebrates it has glandular secretory features and sympathetic and parasympathetic nerve supply. Lack of a direct communicating channel between the pineal gland and the third ventricle suggests that pineal secretions that control hypothalamic-pituitary function reach there either via the bloodstream or through the CSF. The pineal gland has a rich blood supply (from the adjacent choroid plexus) and lacks a blood-brain barrier. The predominant cell type, pinealocyte, has secretory properties and a rich, postganglionic sympathetic nerve supply. A variety of neuropeptides, including vasopressin, renin-angiotensin, ACTH, and POMC-related peptides, are found in the pineal gland.[61] The best-known pineal secretions are serotonin, norepinephrine, and melatonin. The pineal gland also contains significant concentrations of hypothalamic hormones TRH, GnRH, and somatostatin. Impulses carried by sympathetic nerves to the pineal gland are modified by light and darkness. In both humans and experimental animals melatonin secretion is initiated minutes after the lights are turned off. It is suggested that the pineal gland, via melatonin, may be responsible for diurnal variations in hypothalamic-pituitary hormone secretion. This action is mediated through the sympathetic nerve supply (superior cervical ganglion), as suggested by the absence of circadian

TABLE 5-6
Tumors and Tumor-Like Conditions in the Sella Turcica and Parasellar Regions

Abscess	Glioma (optic nerve, infundibulum, posterior lobe hypothalamus)
Adenoma (pituitary)	
Aneurysm	Granular cell tumor (posterior lobe, stalk)
Angioma	Hamartoma (hypothalamus)
Carcinoma (pituitary)	Histiocytosis X
Carcinoma (sphenoid sinus, nasopharynx	Hypophysitis (chronic, lymphocytic)
	Leukemia
Chordoma	Lymphoma
Choristoma	Melanoma
Craniopharyngioma	Metastasis (carcinoma, sarcoma)
Cysts (various types)	Osteosarcoma
Fibroma	Paraganglioma
Fibrosarcoma	Plasmacytoma
Gangliocytoma	Sarcoidosis
Ganglioneuroma	Syphilis
Germinoma (ectopic pinealoma)	Teratoma
Giant cell granuloma	Tuberculosis

SOURCE: Adapted from Martin JB, Reichlin S: *Clinical Neuroendocrinology,* 2d ed. Philadelphia, FA Davis, 1987:440, with permission.

rhythm of melatonin secretion in quadriplegics. Immunohistology has localized melatonin at several other sites, including the outer nuclear layer of the retina, optic nerve, optic chiasma and gastrointestinal tract. The contribution of these extra-pineal sites to circulating melatonin is minimal, if any, since no circulating melatonin can be detected after pinealectomy. Radioactive melatonin is taken up by brain tissue, particularly the hypothalamus. The pharmacologic effects of melatonin include cessation of tremors and rigidity in Parkinson's disease, an increase in REM sleep and stages 3 and 4 of sleep. The potential significance of hypothalamic hormones, present in the pineal gland, is not known.

Physiologically, the best-known endocrine effects of the pineal gland are on gonadal development. In rats exposed to constant light (thus reducing melatonin secretion) development of the ovaries and testes is delayed. These effects are reversed by pinealectomy. Similarly, estrus can be induced in sheep by oral administration of melatonin.[62] In humans, an association between pinealomas and precocious puberty has been reported.[63] The effect of the pineal gland on other endocrine functions is less established.[64]

Clinically, the pineal gland has no specific, known function, but gains importance due to either calcification or tumor development. A calcified pineal gland is used by radiologists as a landmark to determine shifts in midline brain structures. Most often calcification occurs soon after puberty. It has therefore been hypothesized that the pineal gland may play a role in achieving puberty and having done that, it ceases to function and becomes calcified. On the other hand, normal weight and structure of pineal gland is maintained throughout life, in some species, suggesting that it may continue to play some role.

Tumors of the pineal gland are rare, accounting for less than 1 percent of the brain tumors. Pineal tumors are seen almost exclusively in young men and arise from a variety of cell components, as described by DeGirolami[65] and listed in Table 5-7. Many of these tumors arise in the pineal glands and infiltrate the third ventricle and hypothalamus or arise in the ventral hypothalamus. When pineal tumors extend to the hypothalamus, they produce the classical triad of diabetes insipidus, hypogonadism, and visual field defects. Although precocious puberty in children with pineal tumors has been reported, it is by no means a constant feature. In a large series of 177 cases of pineal tumors[66] with 56 cases under age 15, precocious puberty was reported in only one third of them. It is therefore believed that pineal tumors when associated with precocious puberty cause it the same way as other brain tumors—that is, by the destruction of the parts of the brain that normally inhibit gonadotropin secretion. An enlarging tumor in the pineal region invariably compresses the aqueduct of Sylvius, leading to development of hydrocephalus with characteristic headache, vomiting, and papilledema.

In addition to the pineal gland, other periventricular organs of ependymal origin (subcommissural organ, subfornical organ, organum vasculosum and the epen-

TABLE 5-7
Classification of the Tumors of the Pineal Region

A. Germ cell tumors
  1. Germinoma
     a. Posterior third ventricle and pineal
     b. Anterior third ventricle, suprasellar or intrasellar
     c. Combined lesions in anterior and posterior third ventricle, apparently noncontiguous, with or without foci of cystic or solid teratoma
  2. Teratoma
     a. Evidencing growth along two or three germ lines in varying degrees of differentiation
     b. Dermoid and epidermoid cysts with or without solid foci of teratoma
     c. Histologically malignant forms with or without differentiated foci of benign, solid, or cystic teratoma—teratocarcinoma, chorio-epithelioma, embryonal carcinoma (endodermal-sinus tumor of yolk-sac carcinoma), combinations of these with or without foci of germinoma, chemodectoma
B. Pineal parenchymal tumors
  1. Pinocytes
     a. Pineocytoma
     b. Pineoblastoma
     c. Ganglioglioma and chemodectoma
     d. Mixed forms exhibiting transitions between these
  2. Glia
     a. Astrocytoma
     b. Ependymoma
     c. Mixed forms and other less frequent gliomas (glioblastoma, oligodendroglioma, etc.)
C. Tumors of supporting or adjacent structures
  1. Meningioma
  2. Hemangiopericytoma
D. Nonneoplastic conditions of neurosurgical importance
  1. Degenerative cysts of pineal body lined by fibrillary astrocytes
  2. Arachnoid cysts
  3. Cavernous hemangioma

SOURCE: Adapted from Martin JB, Reichlin S: *Clinical Neuroendocrinology*, 2d ed. Philadelphia, FA Davis, 1987:363, with permission.

dymal lining of the third and fourth ventricles) share the neurosecretory properties of this gland. The precise functions of these organs are not clearly defined, and it is possible that secretion of yet unknown hormones and peptides into the CSF may exert yet unknown behavioral effects.

Neuroregulatory Peptides: A Link between Brain, Gut, and Pancreas

One of the most important advances in regulatory biology in the past two decades has been the discovery that identical peptides are present in the central and peripheral nervous systems and in the glandular cells of the gut and pancreas. This finding has led to a new understanding of the integration of the cellular function in both nervous system and endocrine system. It is likely that better understanding of molecular biology will shed further light in this area.

Several peptides, including opioid peptides, ACTH, growth hormone, TRH, cholecystokinin, substance P, neurotensin, vasoactive intestinal peptide (VIP), atrial natriuretic factor (ANF), and insulin, have been shown to be present both in the brain and in extracranial organs like gut, heart, and pancreas. Their presence in organs of such diverse function is intriguing and difficult to understand at first. This widespread distribution of the peptides, however, establishes the concept of a relationship between cells of the brain, an organ whose principal function is transmission of impulses, and the endocrine glands, which perform the same function mediated through hormones. This relationship is further substantiated by the embryologic origin of both (nervous system and endocrine system) from the primitive ectoderm. It is likely that during the course of evolution, the brain, an organ with the primary function of signal generation and transmission (to control other cellular functions), was compelled to develop alternate, nonaxonal mechanisms of signal transmission with the increasingly complex development of the organism (from single-cell organisms to higher animals). Nonaxonal, nonsynaptic routes of signal transmission through vascular and interstitial spaces thus developed and modified the endocrine cells which evolved in anatomically remote sites like the pancreas and the intestinal tract. Polypeptide signals released from these cells (endocrine glands) are still under the influence of the central nervous system (neuroendocrine control) and hormones released by endocrine glands exert an influence on the brain, thus establishing a two-way relationship between the nervous system and the endocrine system—and the relatively new discipline of neuroendocrinology.

Neuroendocrine Responses Related to Anesthesia and Surgery

Surgical trauma is accompanied by an alteration of the neuroendocrine system, involving changes in the secretion of pituitary, adrenal, thyroid, and pancreatic hormones, along with profound changes in autonomic nervous system activity. The overall stress response to surgery and anesthesia is therefore a result of the release of a combination of neuroendocrine hormones[67] and of the local release of cytokines.[68]

HORMONAL CHANGES

PITUITARY HORMONES

Secretion of most pituitary hormones, including ACTH, GH, prolactin, TSH, ADH, and beta-endorphins, is known to be increased during surgery and in the postoperative period.[69–74] The normal pulsatile, diurnal rhythm of anterior pituitary hormone secretion is also lost in the perioperative period,[75] and hormone secretion becomes a constant phenomenon. Elevation of different hormones begins with induction of anesthesia, reaches a peak level during surgery and gradually decreases in the postoperative period over the next 24 h (at which point measurements are stopped in most studies). TSH levels may be transiently elevated during surgery and return to a low-normal range in the postoperative period and remain at that level for the next 4 or 5 days. T_3, T_4 levels remain low during the postoperative period.

ADH levels remain elevated for up to 5 days after surgery,[73] even in the presence of increased plasma osmolality. A situation similar to SIADH thus exists and can theoretically contribute to the development of hyponatremia in the postoperative period. The development of hypervolemia secondary to ADH secretion has not been demonstrated in the postoperative period. The magnitude of ADH elevation has been shown to be proportional to the extent of surgical trauma.[73,76]

ADRENAL HORMONES

Elevation of both adrenal medullary catecholamines and adrenal corticoid hormones has been observed.[77–79] It is difficult to distinguish between the contributions of the adrenal medulla and of generalized sympathetic nervous system stimulation to the elevated levels of epinephrine and norepinephrine, which are discussed later. The elevation of cortisol[77] and aldosterone[79] levels is observed for several days after surgery. Increase in adrenal corticoids is probably due to increased secretion of ACTH, although it has been suggested that adrenal response to circulating ACTH may be exaggerated.[75] Increased blood levels of cortisol may be partly responsible for the development of hyperglycemia in the postoperative period.

PANCREATIC HORMONES

Plasma glucagon levels are increased[80] and insulin levels are low.[81] These hormonal changes, combined with elevated cortisol levels, account for the presence of hyperglycemia in postoperative patients. Endogenous insulin secretion, in response to infusion of glucose-containing solution, is also impaired.[81] It is possible that elevated levels of plasma catecholamines decrease insulin secretion.

AUTONOMIC NERVOUS SYSTEM ACTIVITY

Plasma catecholamine levels are shown to increase immediately after surgical incision and remain elevated for up to 5 days after surgery.[76,77] The nature of the surgical stimulus determines the magnitude and duration of the catecholamine elevation.[76] By using tracer techniques it has been shown[82] that elevation of norepinephrine in the postoperative period is due to increased production by the autonomic nervous system rather than to altered clearance. Although vagal stimuli, during surgery may lead to episodes of bradycardia and hypertension, postoperative patients almost always show an increase in heart rate for several days, suggesting that within the autonomic nervous system stimulation of the sympathetic nervous system predominates over its parasympathetic component in the postperative period.

RENIN-ANGIOTENSIN SYSTEM

Increase in plasma renin-angiotensin has been reported, but is thought to be dependent on the intravascular volume status rather than on surgical trauma.[83] Several investigators[83–85] have failed to show consistent elevation of plasma renin activity. Cardiopulmonary bypass, however, has been reported to be followed by elevated plasma renin levels.[86]

MECHANISMS AND PATHWAYS INVOLVED IN THE NEUROENDOCRINE RESPONSE TO SURGERY

Evidence for involvement of the sensory pathways from the site of surgical trauma in initiating neuroendocrine response has been provided by both experimental and clinical studies. In animals, hormonal alterations induced by thermal injury are prevented by denervation.[87] Similarly, the neurohormonal stress response to surgery is modified in paraplegic patients.[88] Several clinical studies (discussed later), however, have demonstrated that denervation produced by regional anesthesia, adequate to perform surgery, modifies but does not eliminate neuroendocrine response. These findings suggest that in addition to afferent neural signals some other mechanism, involving humoral mediators, also plays a part. It has been suggested that inflammatory mediators like the interleukins released by white blood cells at the surgical site may be involved.[89] Significant elevation of interleukins and of other tumor necrosis factors, after surgery, has not been consistently shown in clinical studies. It is possible that the levels of these factors are too low to be detected by currently available assays. Future studies with more refined techniques may shed more light on this mechanism.

CLINICAL IMPACT OF NEUROENDOCRINE ALTERATIONS ASSOCIATED WITH SURGERY

Neuroendocrine alterations, discussed above, lead to physiologic changes in cardiovascular parameters, metabolism, oxygen consumption, renal function, and electrolyte balance. Increased activity of the sympathetic nervous system (including adrenal medullary catecholamines) results in significant changes in heart rate (tachycardia), in hypertension, in increased cardiac output, and in dysrhythmias. In a patient with coronary artery disease these changes can precipitate myocardial ischemia or infarction due to increased myocardial oxygen consumption. Plasma catecholamine levels correlate with hypertension in the postoperative period.[77] Increased production of growth hormone, glucagon, cortisol, and epinephrine can produce hyperglycemia, commonly seen in the postoperative period in both diabetic and nondiabetic patients. Hyperglycemia can lead to osmotic diuresis, obtundation (hyperglycemic, hyperosmolar coma), impaired leukocyte function, and delayed wound healing. Hyperglycemia also relates to a poor outcome if ischemic neurological injury occurs in the perioperative period.[90] Other metabolic changes in the postoperative period include lipolysis and protein catabolism.[91,92]

Multiple factors, often working in opposite directions, influence fluid and electrolyte balance in the postoperative period. For example, increased ADH secretion causes fluid retention, while "third spacing" following surgical trauma causes fluid loss from the intravascular compartment. Similarly, increased plasma cortisol, aldosterone, and renin promote sodium reabsorption by the kidney, while increased

ADH, with an SIADH-like picture, can cause dilutional hyponatremia. Similarly, hypokalemia can occur due to increased excretion secondary to high aldosterone or to intracellular transmigration associated with increased catecholamine levels.[93] The total fluid-electrolyte picture resulting from a balance among all these opposing forces must be closely watched, and appropriate interventions must be made whenever necessary.

It can be seen from the foregoing account, that physiologic neuroendocrine changes, in response to surgery, have the potential to produce serious complications, especially in patients with preexisting cardiovascular and cerebrovascular disease. This knowledge has led to the concept of inhibiting or modifying the neuroendocrine response in the perioperative period.

NEUROENDOCRINE EFFECTS OF GENERAL ANESTHETICS

Endocrine and metabolic responses to anesthesia and surgery are significantly modified by the preoperative condition, including the nutritional status of the patients, and are therefore difficult to study. Further difficulty arises in separating the influence of anesthetics and of surgical trauma on the endocrine and metabolic responses. Limited information on this subject has therefore been collected by a small group of investigators. These studies have been conducted in a small number of relatively healthy (ASA I and II) patients scheduled for elective surgery, and the results may not be applicable to a large patient population undergoing a variety of surgical procedures under emergency situations. The study design in most investigations has involved obtaining blood levels of various hormones on the morning of the surgery (after premedication), at 15-min intervals for 45 min after induction of anesthesia but prior to surgical incision, and at 15, 30, 60, and 120 min after beginning of surgery. Not all hormones have been studied with all inhalation anesthetics. It should be emphasized that the effect of only a short duration of anesthesia (30 to 45 min) in the absence of surgical stimulus has been studied in humans. Even then it was noticeable that hormone levels 15 minutes after induction of anesthesia were similar to control value, and an increase was noticed after 30- and 45-min determinations. It is generally not feasible to make further observations without surgery. Influence of anesthesia alone is much less pronounced than the combined effect of anesthesia and surgery. Further difficulty in interpretation of data is presented by the fact that the nature of surgical procedures, and hence the extent of stress and injury posed by them, has varied with different anesthetics by different investigators.

TABLE 5-8
Effect of General Anesthetics on Neuroendocrine Function

Drugs	ACTH	Cortisol	Aldo-sterone	Renin	Hyper-glycemia	GH	Glucagen	THS	Thyroxine	T3	Testos-terone	LH (Males)	LH (Females)
						Hormones							
Diethyl ether	↑	↑↑	↑	→	↑↑	↑		→	↑	↓			
Cyclo-propane		↑			↑	→							
Methoxy-flurane		↗	↑			↑		→	→	↓		Plasma LH concentrations increase during surgery and decrease in postoperative period	No change during surgery or postoperative period is noted.
Halothane	↑	↑	↑	→↗	↑		↓	→	↑	↓	↓		
Enflurane	→	↘	↑	↑	↑	→				↓			
Isoflurane	↗	↗	↗	↗									
Sevoflurane	→	→	→										
Pentothal		↓				→		→	↓	↓	↓		
Ketamine		↑								↓			
Demerol		→								↓			
Demerol + Droperidol		↗								↓			
Droperidol + Penta-zocine	↑	↗				↑				↓	↓		
Droperidol + Fentanyl		→					↑	↓		↓			
Morphine	↓→	→				↑→				↓			

↑ = increase, ↓ = decrease, Ÿ = no change, ↗ = increase not statistically significant, ↘ = decrease not statistically significant. 60%–70% N₂O was used along with intravenous anesthetics and Seroflurane in most studies. N₂O was not used during studies with other inhalation anesthetics.
SOURCE: Data modified from Oyama.[94] Data for isoflurane and Sevoflurane is adapted from Matsuki, et al.[96] and Murakawa et al.[97]

The existing information has been reviewed by Oyama.[94] A summary of data derived from several investigations is presented in Table 5-8 and is discussed below.

ADRENOCORTICOTROPIN (ACTH)

ACTH levels rise intermittently in patients anesthetized with diethyl ether,[95] halothane, methoxyflurane, and neuroleptanesthesia with droperidol and pentazocine.[94] Several peaks of high levels of ACTH are identified in a single patient throughout the surgical procedure. This is accompanied by a steady rise in plasma cortisol level. Isoflurane anesthesia, 20 min after induction, produces a mild (1.7 times the control value) increase in plasma ACTH,[96] while sevoflurane, 20 min after induction, had no effect.[97] There is indirect evidence that high-dose morphine (4 mg/kg) also reduces ACTH secretion[98] in response to surgical stress. A smaller dose of morphine (1 to 2 mg/kg) does not affect ACTH secretion secondary to surgical stress.

ADRENAL HORMONES

Diethyl ether produces the strongest stimulation of adrenocortical activity.[95] Cyclopropane[99] and halothane[100] also produce marked elevation of cortisol, while methoxyflurane[101] and pentothal anesthesia do not alter it, or they produce a minimal decrease.[94] Balanced anesthesia with narcotics and neuroleptics does not have a significant effect on cortisol levels,[94] while high-dose morphine (4 mg/kg) has been shown to inhibit the rise of cortisol during surgery.[98] There was slight (not statistically significant) increase in plasma cortisol level after 30 min of isoflurane,[96] while sevoflurane had no effect[97] on plasma cortisol levels. In studies with halothane and methoxyflurane anesthesia, baseline values measured after premedication were below the normal range for that laboratory. Induction of anesthesia raised 17-OHCS levels to normal range. It was only after surgical incision that values above normal range were measured. In evaluating the effect of morphine,[98] it was noted that morphine response was dose-related. Cortisol elevation in response to surgical stress in patients anesthetized with 1 mg/kg morphine was similar to that during halothane anesthesia, while morphine 2 mg/kg blunted and 4 mg/kg abolished the cortisol rise. It was apparent that the effect of morphine was due to a decrease in ACTH secretion because administration of exogenous ACTH during surgery resulted in marked elevation of cortisol. Ketamine induction with 2 mg/kg followed by N₂O anesthesia resulted in signifciant increase in plasma cortisol 30 minutes after induction.[102]

ALDOSTERONE AND PLASMA RENIN ACTIVITY

Effect of several anesthetics on plasma aldosterone and renin activity was studied by Oyama[103] and coworkers. Aldosterone concentration increased 2.5 times the control values during 45 min of ether anesthesia, 2 times with enflurane-N_2O, 1.6 times with methoxyflurane-N_2O, and 1.5 times with halothane-N_2O anesthesia. There was further increase (to about 3 times) during surgery. Patients with spinal anesthesia did not show any change in aldosterone concentration with either anesthesia or surgery. Plasma renin activity was slightly increased with halothane and methoxyflurane-N_2O anesthesia and remained unchanged by ether. These data suggest that increased aldosterone secretion after induction of anesthesia (prior to beginning of surgery) is probably secondary to an increase in ACTH rather than activation of the renin-angiotensin system. Lack of increase in aldosterone in patients given spinal anesthesia was also accompanied by lack of alterations in ACTH and renin activity. These patients had relatively minor surgical procedures which presented less stress than those anesthesized with inhalation anesthetics. Plasma aldosterone and renin activity showed a slight but insignificant increase with halothane and isoflurane in another study,[96] while aldosterone remained unchanged with sevoflurane.[97]

INSULIN, GROWTH HORMONE, AND GLUCAGON

Carbohydrate metabolism is affected by multiple hormones; insulin, glucagon, cortisol, and catecholamines all affect serum glucose concentration. Blood glucose level, in turn, provides a feedback to secretion of growth hormone by the anterior pituitary. Growth hormone reduces peripheral utilization and uptake of glucose, increases retention of glycogen, and decreases glycolysis. Carbohydrate homeostasis therefore represents the net result of a complex interplay among pancreas, adrenal, and anterior pituitary glands.

It has long been appreciated that hyperglycemia developed during anesthesia with ether and cyclopropane and not during pentothal anesthesia.[94,104,105] Mechanisms responsible for development of hyperglycemia include hepatic glycogenolysis, decreased tissue glucose utilization, and decreased renal glucose clearance. An increase in sympathoadrenal activity is presumably largely responsible for these alterations. Plasma growth hormone levels increase during anesthesia with diethyl ether, methoxyflurane, and neuroleptics, while cyclopropane, enflurane, and thiopental[94,104,106] do not lead to an increase. Oyama has reported a 24 percent decrease in plasma glucagon levels following hal-

othane and neuroleptanesthesia (fentanyl, droperidol, N_2O) followed by a 33 percent increase above control values during surgery, reaching a peak level of a 60 percent increase above control values in the recovery room.[107]

THYROID HORMONES

Plasma TSH levels do not show an appreciable change during ether, halothane, methoxyflurane, or pentothal anesthesia.[94] Ether and halothane, however, lead to an increase in blood thyroxine levels, while methoxyflurane has no effect and pentothal decreases plasma thyroxine. All above anesthetics decreased plasma T_3 concentrations by 10 to 15 percent. A 50 percent decrease in T_3 was noticed on the first postoperative day, and it remained low (30 percent decrease) until the seventh postoperative day. Similar changes in T_3 have been reported with various intravenous drugs used to induce or supplement general anesthesia.[107]

SEX HORMONES

The alterations in plasma sex hormone levels differ between males and females. In men, venous plasma concentration of testosterone is decreased during anesthesia and surgery, and this decrease is noticed for up to 1 week in the postoperative period. The exact mechanism underlying this decreased testosterone level is not clearly understood but is most probably due to decreased testicular production of this hormone. It is unlikely that it is mediated via the anterior pituitary because the plasma levels of LH (anterior pituitary hormone) are actually increased during anesthesia and surgery and decrease in the postoperative period.[94]

In female patients, no specific changes in female hormones (compared with nonsurgical patients in the same phase of the menstrual cycle) could be attributed to anesthesia or surgery. Although females normally have very low levels of testosterone, a small decrease (25 percent compared with 50 to 80 percent decrease in males) in testosterone in the postoperative period is noticeable on the third postoperative day.[94]

ANTIDIURETIC HORMONE

It is common knowledge that ADH secretion increases in response to the stress of surgical procedures. Clinical studies documenting ADH secretion during surgery and separating the effect of surgery and anesthesia in humans are relatively few. Murakawa and coworkers[97] studied ADH secretion in 40 patients undergoing either abdominal or orthopedic surgery under sevoflurane anesthesia. Twenty minutes of sevoflurane anesthesia (prior to surgical incision) did not cause any change in plasma ADH levels. Patients undergoing orthopedic surgery showed a minimal (statistically insignificant) increase, while those having abdominal surgery showed a marked increase in ADH secretion. Stanley and colleagues[108] studied patients undergoing coronary artery bypass surgery with fentanyl-oxygen anesthesia. They noticed no change in ADH levels after anesthetic induction nor during intubation and the pre-bypass period. It was only after initiation of cardiopulmonary bypass that a marked elevation of ADH was noticed. In a subsequent publication[109] involving a similar patient population, it was documented that when either alfentanil-oxygen or sufentanil-oxygen anesthesia was used, the ADH increase even during extracorporeal circulation was abolished. The clinical significance of blocking this ADH response is yet to be determined.

MODIFICATION OF NEUROENDOCRINE RESPONSE BY ANESTHETIC TECHNIQUES

In the past two decades, a large number of clinical studies have evaluated the effect of the anesthetic technique on modification of the neuroendocrine response in the perioperative period. These studies have shown that neuroendocrine responses can be modified by (a) parenteral use of high-dose narcotics,[110,111] (b) neural blockade by local anesthetics (i.e., regional anesthesia),[112-114] (c) epidural or subarachnoid use of narcotics.[115]

PARENTERAL NARCOTICS

Opioids produce dose-related analgesia by modulating the nociceptive pathways within the central nervous system. High-doses narcotic techniques of anesthesia, commonly used in patients undergoing cardiac surgery, have been shown to decrease cortisol secretion when compared with patients anesthetized with an inhalation anesthetic.[110] High doses of potent narcotics have a similar effect in noncardiac surgery patients. The neuroendocrine effects of the narcotics may be due to blocking the pain stimuli or to other CNS effects, involving the mediation of stress response. Modifying neuroendocrine responses by high-dose narcotics is restricted to the patients requiring postoperative mechanical ventilation, because the ventilatory depression associated with high-dose narcotics is significant and large increases in stress hormones occur when the plasma narcotic levels fall.

REGIONAL ANESTHESIA

Intraoperative use of epidural anesthesia completely suppresses the neuroendocrine response to lower abdominal surgery,[113,114] provided that an extensive sympathetic block (T_4–S_5 level) is established, while in surgical procedures above the level of the umbilicus, the neuroendocrine response is modified but not com-

pletely suppressed.[116,117] The effect of neural blockade on modifying the neuroendocrine response is related to the intensity of the block. Epidural block, adequate for the surgical procedure, but with partial sympathetic blockade (levels below T_4), does not completely suppress the neuroendocrine response. Thus pain relief and stress response are not always coupled. These findings suggest not only that the neuroendocrine response is related to the nociceptive pathways, but that the nonnociceptive pathways (e.g., sympathetic nerve supply to adrenal glands) may be partly responsible for the neuroendocrine response to surgery. Similarly, use of intravenous patient controlled analgesia (PCA) postoperative analgesia relieves pain but the neuroendocrine response is unaltered.[118]

AXIAL NARCOTICS

The epidural or subarachnoid injection of small doses of narcotics provides intense analgesia without the ventilatory depression associated with high-dose narcotics used for general anesthesia. Either intra- or postoperative use of epidural narcotics has been reported to decrease postoperative plasma cortisol and urinary 17-ketosteroids in some studies[98,99] but not in others.[101,103] Differences in these observations may be attributed to the differences in types of surgical procedures and warrant further investigation. It should be emphasized that only the preincisional establishment of epidural anesthesia (with local anesthetics and narcotics) can prevent the stress response and that epidural anesthesia must be continued in the postoperative period to achieve the full benefit of abolishing the neuroendocrine response.[113]

In summary, epidural local anesthetics or narcotics effectively inhibit the neuroendocrine response to surgical procedures, especially after lower abdominal surgery, provided analgesia is established prior to the surgical incision and is maintained for several days postoperatively. Maximum effectiveness is achieved with local anesthetics used both intraoperatively and in the postoperative period. The results of some studies[120] involving a small number of patients suggest that utilizing prolonged postoperative epidural blockade may be associated with decreased cardiac morbidity in a selected patient population. More data need to be collected before a clear relationship between the reduction of neuroendocrine response and mortality related to elective surgery can be firmly established.

References

1. Roth J, et al: The evolutionary origins of hormones, neurotransmitters and other extracellular chemical messengers. *N Engl J Med* 1982; 306:523.

2. Roth J, et al: Intercellular communication: An attempt at unifying hypothesis. *Clin Res* 1983; 31:354.

3. Hokfelt T, et al: Coexistence of peptides and putative transmitters in neurons. *Adv Biochem Psychopharmacol* 1980; 22:1.

4. Lundberg JM, et al: Complementary role of vasoactive intestinal polypeptide and acetylcholine for cat submandibular blood flow and secretion. *Acta Physiol Scand* 1982; 3:329.

5. Lundberg, JM, et al: Vasoactive intestinal polypeptide in cholinergic neurons of exocrine glands: Functional significance of co-existing transmitters for vasodilation and secretion. *Proc Natl Acad Sci USA* 1980; 77:1651.

6. Lundberg, JM, et al: Organizational principles in the peripheral sympathetic system: Subdivision by co-existing peptides. *Proc Natl Acad Sci USA* 1982; 79:1303.

7. Schultzberg M, et al: Peptide neurons in the autonomic nervous system. *Adv Biochem Psychopharmacol* 1980; 25:341.

8. Schultzberg M, et al: Coexistence of classical transmitters and peptides in the central and peripheral nervous system. *Br Med Bull* 1982; 38:309.

9. Jan YN, et al: A peptide as possible transmitter in sympathetic ganglia of the frog. *Proc Natl Acad Sci USA* 1979; 76:1501.

10. Scharrer E, Scharrer B: *Neuroendocrinology*. New York, Columbia University, 1963.

11. Anderson E, Haymaker W: Breakthroughs in hypothalamic and pituitary research. In Swabb DF and Schade JP (eds): *Progress in Brain Research*. New York, W. Elsevier, 1974:1.

12. Harris GW, Jacobsohn D: Functional grafts of anterior pituitary gland. *Proc R Soc Ser B* 1952; 139:273.

13. Nisitovich-Winer M, Everett JW: Functional restitution of pituitary grafts retransplanted from kidney to median eminence. *Endocrinology* 1958; 63:916.

14. Guillemin R: Peptides in the brain: The new endocrinology of the neuron. *Science* 1978; 202:390.

15. Schally AV: Aspects of hypothalamic regulation of the pituitary gland: Its implications for the control of reproductive processes. *Science* 1978; 202:18.

16. Hayward JN: Neural control of the posterior pituitary. *Ann Rev Physiol* 1975; 37:191.

17. Schrier RW, et al: Osmotic and nonosmotic control of vasopressin release. *Am J Physiol* 1979; 236:F321.

18. Share L: Blood pressure, blood volume, and the release of vasopressin. In Knobil E, Sawyer W (eds): *Handbook of Physiology*. Washington DC, *American Physiological Society*, 1974:243–255.

19. Lester MC, Nelson PB: Neurological aspects of vasopressin release and syndrome of inappropriate secretion of antidiuretic hormone. *Neurosurgery* 1981; 8:735.

20. Martin JB, Reichlin S: Neuropharmacology of anterior pituitary regulation. In Martin JB, Reichlin S (eds): *Clinical Neuroendocrinology*, 2nd ed. Philadelphia, FA Davis, 1987:45–63.

21. Martin JB, Reichlin S: Neuroregulatory peptides. In Martin JB, Reichlin S (eds): *Clinical Neuroendocrinology*, 2nd ed. Philadelphia, FA Davis, 1987:559–574.

22. Neill JD: Neuroendocrine regulation of prolactin secretion. In Martin L, Gannong WF (eds): *Frontiers in Neuroendocrinology*, vol 6. New York, Raven Press, 1980:469–488.

23. Griffin JE, Wilson JD: Disorders of testes and male reproductive tract. In Wilson JD, Foster D (eds): *Textbook of Endocrinology*, 7th ed. Philadelphia, WB Saunders, 1985:259–311.

24. Snyder BJ, et al: Diagnostic value of thyrotropin releasing hormone in pituitary and hypothalamic disease. *Ann Intern Med* 1974; 81:751.

25. Cohen R, et al: Pituitary stimulation by combined administration of four hypothalamic releasing hormones in normal men and patients. *J Clin Endocrinol Metab* 1986; 62:892.

26. Moses A, Norman DD: Diabetes insipidus and syndrome of inappropriate antidiuretic hormone secretion (SIADH). *Adv Intern Med* 1982; 27:73.

27. Moses AM, Streeten DHP: Differentiation of polyuric states by measurement of responses to changes in plasma osmolality induced by hypertonic saline infusion. *Am J Med* 1967; 42:368.

28. Schwartz WB, et al: A syndrome of renal sodium loss and hyponatremia probably resulting from inappropriate secretion of antidiuretic hormone. *Am J Med* 1957; 23:529.

29. Hou S: Syndrome of inappropriate antidiuretic hormone secretion. In Reichlin S (ed): *The Neurohypophysis*. New York, Plenum, 1984:165–189.

30. Nelson PB, et al: Hyponatremia in intracranial disease—perhaps not the syndrome of inappropriate secretion of antidiuretic hormone (SIADH). *J Neurosurg* 1981; 55:38.

31. Nelson PB, et al: Hypernatremia and natriuresis in a monkey model. *J Neurosurg* 1984; 60:233.

32. Wijdicks EFM, et al: Hyponatremia and cerebral infarction in patients with ruptured intracranial aneurysms: Is fluid restriction harmful? *Ann Neurol* 1985; 17:137.

33. Martin JB, et al: Feedback regulation of TSH secretion in rats with hypothalamic lesions. *Endocrinology* 1970; 87:1032.

34. Lucke C, et al: The effect of somatostatin on TSH levels in patients with primary hypothyroidism. *J Clin Endocrinol Metab* 1975; 41:1082.

35. Scanlon MF, et al: The neuroregulation of human thyrotropin secretion. In Martin L, Gannong WF (eds): *Frontiers in Neuroendocrinology*, vol. 6. New York, Raven Press, 1980:333–380.

36. Cobb WE, et al: Growth hormone secretory status is a determinant of the thyrotropin response to thyrotropin releasing hormone in euthyroid patients with hypothalamic pituitary disease. *J Clin Endocrinol Metab* 1981; 52:324.

37. Engler D, Burger AG: The deiodination of iodothyronines and their derivatives in man. *Endocrine Rev* 1984; 5:151.

38. Krulich L: Neurotransmitter control of thyrotropin secretion. *Neuroendocrinol*, 1982; 35:139.

39. Vagenakis AG, et al: Hyper-response to thyrotropin releasing hormone accompanying small decreases in serum thyroid hormone concentrations. *J Clin Invest*, 1974; 54:913.

40. Ridgway EC: Glycoprotein hormone production by pituitary tumors. In Black P, et al (eds): Secretory Tumors of the Pituitary Glands, *Progress in Endocrine Research and Therapy*, vol 1. New York, Raven Press, 1984:343.

41. De Groot LJ, et al: *The Thyroid and Its Diseases*, 5th ed. New York, John Wiley and Sons, 1984.

42. Fortier C, Selye H: Adrenocorticotrophic effect of stress after severance of the hypothalamo-hypophyseal pathways. *Am J Physio* 1949; 159:433.

43. Guillemin R, Rosenberg B: Humoral hypothalamic control of anterior pituitary. A study with combined tissue cultures. *Endocrinology* 1955; 57:599.

44. Suffran M, Schally AV: Release of corticotropin by anterior pituitary tissue in vitro. *Can J Biochem* 1955; 33:408.

45. DeBold CR, et al: Effect of synthetic ovine corticotropin releasing factor: Prolonged duration of action and biphasic response of plasma adrenocorticotropin and cortisol. *J Clin Endocrinol Metab* 1983; 57:294.

46. Carlson DE, et al: Vasopressin-dependent and -independent control of the release of adrenocorticotropin. *Endocrinology* 1982; 110:680.

47. Lamberts SWJ, et al: Corticotropin releasing factor and vasopressin exert a synergetic effect on adrenocorticotropin release in man. *J. Clin Endocrinol Metab* 1984; 58:1087.

48. Gillies GE, et al: Corticotropin releasing activity of the new CRH is potentiated several times by vasopressin. *Nature* 1982; 299:355.

49. Fuxe K, et al: Mapping of glucocorticoid receptor immunoreac-

tive neurons in the rat telencephalon and diencephalon using a monoclonal antibody against rat liver glucocorticoid receptors. *Endocrinology* 1985; 117:1803.

50. Fortier C, Selye N: Adrenocorticotrophic effect of stress after severance of hypothalamo-hypophyseal pathways. *Am J Physiol* 1949; 159:433.

51. Asa SL, et al: Cushing's disease associated with an intraseller gangliocytoma producing corticotropin releasing factor. *Ann Intern Med* 1984; 101:789.

52. Gold PW, Chrousos GP: Clinical studies with corticotropin releasing factor. Implications for the diagnosis and pathophysiology of depression, Cushing's disease and adrenal insufficiency. *Psychoneuroendocrinology* 1985; 10:401.

53. Liddle GW, et al: The ectopic ACTH syndrome. *Cancer Res* 1965; 25:1057.

54. Moser HW, et al: Adrenoleukodystrophy: Survey of 303 cases—biochemistry, diagosis and therapy. *Ann Neurol* 1984; 16:628.

55. Schaumberg HH, et al: Adrenoleukodystrophy: Similar ultrastructural changes in adrenal cortical and Schwann cells. *Arch Neurol* 30:406, 19.

56. Hermus AR, et al: The corticotropin-releasing hormone test versus the high dose dexamethasone test in the differential diagnosis of Cushing's syndrome. *Lancet* 1986; 2:540.

57. Gold, WP, et al: Responses to corticotropin releasing hormone in the hypocorticalism of depression and Cushing's disease. *N Engl J Med* 1986; 314:1329.

58. Bauer HG: Endocrine and other clinical manifestations of hypothalamic disease: A survey of 60 cases with autopsies. *J Clin Endocrinol Metab* 1954; 14:13.

59. Kappers JA: The mammalian pineal organ. *J Neurovisceral Relations (Suppl)* 1969; 9:140.

60. Kappers JA: The pineal organ: An introduction. In Wholstenholme GEW, Knight J (eds): *The Pineal Gland.* (Ciba symposium). London, Churchill, 1971:3–33.

61. Vaughn MK: Pineal peptides, an overview. In Reilter R (ed): *The Pineal Gland.* New York, Raven Press, 1984:39–82.

62. Lincoln G: Melatonin as a seasonal time-cue—a commercial story. *Nature* 1983; 302:755.

63. Kitay JI: Pineal lesions and precocious puberty: A review. *J Clin Endocrinol Metab* 1954; 14:622.

64. Relkin R (ed): *The Pineal Gland.* New York, Elsevier Biomedical, 1983.

65. DeGirolami U, Schmidek HH: Clincopathological study of 53 tumors of pineal region. *J Neurosurg* 1973; 39:455.

66. Bing JF, et al: Pubertas precose: A survey of the reported anatomical findings. *J Mt Sinai Hosp* 1938; 4:935.

67. Smiley RM, et al: Alterations in β-adrenergic receptor system after thoracic and abdominal surgery. *Anesth. Analg* 1994; 79:821.

68. Weissman C: The metabolic response to stress, an overview and update. *Anesthesiology* 1990; 73:308.

69. Tsuji H, et al: Influences of splanchnic nerve blockade on endocrine metabolic responses to upper abdominal surgery. *Br J Surg* 1983; 70:437.

70. Newsome HH, Rose JC: The response of human adrenocorticotropic hormone and growth hormone to surgical stress. *J Clin Endocrinol* 1971; 33:481.

71. Arnetz BB, et al: Age related differences in the serum prolactin response during standardized surgery. *Life Sci* 1984; 35:2675.

72. Dubois M, et al: Surgical stress in humans is accompanied by an increase in plasma beta-endorphine immunoreactivity. *Life Sci* 1981; 29:1249.

73. Bormann BV, et al: Influence of epidural fentanyl on stress induced elevation of plasma vasopressin (ADH) after surgery. *Anesth Analg* 1983; 62:727.

74. Chen V, et al: Pituitary thyroid responses to surgical stress. *Acta Endocrinol* 1978; 88:490.

75. Udelsman R, et al: Responses of hypothalamic-pituitary-adrenal and renin-angiotensin axes and the sympathetic system during controlled surgical and anesthetic stress. *J Clin Endocrinol Metab* 1987; 64:986.

76. Chernow B: Hormonal responses to graded surgical stress. *Arch Intern Med* 1987; 147:1273.

77. Halter JB, et al: Mechanism of plasma catecholamine increases during surgical stress in man. *J Clin Endocrinol Metab* 1977; 45:936.

78. Sandberg AA, et al: The effects of surgery on the blood levels and metabolism of 17-hydroxy corticosteroids. *J Clin Invest* 1954; 33:1509.

79. Casey JH, et al: The pattern and significance of aldosterone secretion in postoperative patient. *Surg Gynecol Obstet* 1957; 105:179.

80. Goldberg NJ, et al: Insulin therapy in diabetic surgical patient: Metabolic response to low dose insulin infusion. *Diabetes Care* 1981; 4:279.

81. Halter JB, Pflug AE: Relationship of impaired insulin secretion during surgical stress to anesthesia and catecholamine release. *J Clin Endocrinol Metab* 1980; 51:1093.

82. Hilsted J, et al: Whole body clearance of norepinephrine. *J Clin Invest* 1983; 71:500.

83. Robertson D, Michelakis AM: Effect of anesthesia and surgery on plasma renin activity in man. *J Clin Endocrinol Metab* 1972; 34:831.

84. Hawkins, S, et al: Changes in pressor hormone concentrations in assocaition with coronary artery surgery. *Br J Anaesth* 1986; 58:1267.

85. Wallach R, et al: Pathogenesis of paroxysmal hypertension developing during and after coronary artery bypass surgery: A study of haemodynamic and humoral factors. *Am J Cardiol* 1980; 46:559.

86. Watkins L., et al: Angiotensin II levels during cardiopulmonary bypass: Comparison of pulsatile and nonpulsatile flow. *Surg Forum* 1979; 30:229.

87. Hume DM, Egdahl RH: The importance of the brain in the endocrine response to injury. *Ann Surg* 1959; 150:697.

88. Hume DM, et al: Direct measurement of adrenal secretion during operative trauma and convalescence. *Surgery* 1962; 52:174.

89. Rem J, et al: Postoperative changes in coagulation and fibrinolysis independent of neurogenic stimuli and adrenal hormones. *Br J Surg* 1981; 68:229.

90. Sieber FE, et al: Glucose: A re-evaluation of its intraoperative use. *Anesthesiology* 1987; 67:72.

91. Tsuji H, et al: Inhibition of metabolic responses to surgery with β-adrenergic blockade. *Br J Surg* 1980; 67:503.

92. Tsuji H, et al: Effects of epidural administration on postoperative nitrogen loss and catabolic hormones. *Br J Surg* 1987; 74:421.

93. Brown MJ, et al: Hypokalemia from beta$_2$-receptor stimulation by epinephrine. *N Engl J Med* 1983; 309:1414.

94. Oyama T: Endocrine response to general anesthesia and surgery. In Oyama T (ed): *Endocrinology and the Anesthetist.* New York, Elsevier Science Publishers, 1983:1–21.

95. Oyama T, et al: Plasma levels of ACTH and cortisol in man during diethyl ether anesthesia and surgery. *Anesthesiology* 1968; 29:559.

96. Matsuki A, et al: Pituitary adrenal functions during isoflurane anesthesia and surgery. In Matsuki A, et al (eds): *Endocrine Response to Anesthesia and Intensive Care.* Instructional Congress Series 893, New York, Elsevier Science Publishing Company Inc., 1989:111–118.

97. Murakawa T, et al: Effect of sevoflurane anesthesia and surgery on endocrine function in man. In Matsuki A, et al (eds): *Endocrine Response to Anesthesia and Intensive Care.* Instructional Congress Series 893, New York, Elsevier Science Publishing Company Inc., 1989:119–122.

98. Reiter CE, et al: Cortisol and growth hormone response to surgical stress during morphine anesthesia. *Anesth Analg* 1973; 52:1003.

99. Oyama T, Takazawa T: Effect of cyclopropane anesthesia and surgery on carbohydrate and fat metabolism in man. *Anesth Analg* 1972; 51:389.

100. Oyama T, et al: Effects of halothane anesthesia and surgery on adrenal cortical function in man. *Can J Anaesth* 1968; 15:258.

101. Oyama T, et al: Adrenocortical function related to methoxyflurane anesthesia and surgery in man. *Can J Anaesth* 1968; 15:362.

102. Oyama T, et al: Effects of ketamine on adrenocortical function in man. *Anesth Analg* 1970; 119:697.

103. Oyama T, et al: Effects of anesthesia and surgery on plasma aldosterone concentration and renin activity in man. *Br J Anaesth* 1973; 51:747.

104. Oyama T, Takazawa T: Effects of diethyl ether anesthesia and surgery on carbohydrate and fat metabolism in man. *Can J Anaesth* 1971; 18:298.

105. Bunker JP: Neuroendocrine and other effects on carbohydrate metabolism during anesthesia. *Anesthesiology* 1963; 24:515.

106. Oyama T, et al: Metabolic effects of anesthesia—effect of thiopental, nitrous oxide anesthesia on human growth hormone and insulin levels in plasma. *Can J Anaesth* 1971; 18:442.

107. Oyama T: Endocrine responses to anesthetic agents. *Br J Anaesth* 1973; 45:276.

108. Stanley TH, et al: Fentanyl-oxygen anesthesia for coronary artery surgery: Cardiovascular and antidiuretic hormone responses. *Can J Anaesth* 1979; 26:168.

109. DeLange S, et al: Antidiuretic and growth hormone responses during coronary artery surgery with Sufentanil-oxygen and alfentanil-oxygen anesthesia in man. *Anesth Analg* 1982; 61:434.

110. George JM, et al: Morphine anesthesia blocks cortisol, growth hormone response to surgical stress in humans. *J Clin Endocrinol Metab* 1974; 38:736.

111. Giesecke K, et al: High and low dose fentanyl anesthesia: Hormonal and metabolic responses during cholecystectomy. *Br J Anaesth* 1988; 61:575.

112. Breslow MJ, et al: Determinants of catecholamine and cortisol responses to lower extremity revascularization. *Anesthesiology* 1993; 79:1202.

113. Kehlet H: Modification of responses to surgery by neural blockage: Clinical implications. In Cousins MJ, Bridenbaugh PO (eds): *Neural Blockade in Clinical Anesthesia and Management of Pain.* Philadelphia, JB Lippincott, 1988:145–190.

114. Kehlet H: The stress response to surgery: Release mechanisms and the modifying effect of pain relief. *Acta Chir Scand* 1988; 550(suppl):22.

115. Rutberg H, et al: Effects of the extradural administration of morphine on bupivacaine on the endocrine response to upper abdominal surgery. *Br J Anasth* 1984; 56:233.

116. Tsuji H, et al: Attenuation of adrenocortical response to upper abdominal surgery with epidural blockade. *Br J Surg* 1983; 70:122.

117. Hjorts MC, et al: Effects of the extradural administration of local anesthetic agents and morphine on the urinary excretion of cortisol. Catecholamines and nitrogen following abdominal surgery. *Br J Anaesth* 1985; 57:400.

118. Moller IW, et al: Effect of patient controlled analgesia on plasma catecholamine, cortisol and glucose concentrations after cholecystectomy. *Br J Anaesth* 1988; 61:160.

119. Jorgensen BC, et al: Influence of epidural morphine on postoperative pain, endocrine, metabolic and renal responses to surgery—A controlled study. *Acta Anaesthesiol Scand,* 1982; 26:63.

120. Yeager MP, et al: Epidural anesthesia and analgesia in high risk surgical patients. *Anesthesiology* 1987; 66:729.

ELECTROENCEPH-ALOGRAM

IRA J. RAMPIL

The electroencephalogram (EEG) has challenged and fascinated investigators for more than a century. This apparently random variation of voltage detected on the scalp provides a portal into the otherwise covert activity of the central nervous system. A useful analogy exists between the electroencephalogram and the electrocardiogram as both provide a noninvasive indication of the changing membrane potential of millions of cells deep within the body. These distant echoes of ionic current can be interpreted to sense the vitality and function of their originating organs. The electrocardiogram consists of patterns that represent specific underlying physiologic events and sequences; unfortunately, the EEG does not permit us to link specific wave patterns with underlying function except in the special case of evoked potentials. The spontaneous EEG appears to be random tracings whose waves have no direct connection to known physiologic or behavioral activity. This does not imply that the brain's electrical function is random or chaotic, only that it is so complex that it appears so. Nonetheless, decades of empirical observation, coupled with clinical correlation, have allowed the evolution of the EEG into a diagnostic tool, a monitor of cerebral ischemia and "anesthetic depth," and a research tool for investigating the pharmacologic properties of psychoactive drugs despite the absence of understanding, until recently, of its neurophysiologic genesis.

History of the EEG

The discovery of a definitive role for electricity in the nervous system dates to 1791 and the work of Luigi Galvani, who described the effects of electricity on the peripheral nervous system.[1] Quantitative work involving biologic sources of electric currents began in earnest with the invention of the appropriate measuring instruments, particularly the string galvanometer. In 1875, Richard Caton reported his discovery of electric currents on the surface of the brains of rabbits and monkeys.[2,3] Caton even noted the change in epicortical currents with peripheral stimulation, thus providing the first description of evoked potentials. This work was published 28 years before the initial description of the electrocardiogram.[4]

The development of vacuum tube amplifiers in the first decades of the twentieth century permitted the detection of much smaller signals than the string galvanometer. This technology allowed Hans Berger to noninvasively detect and classify cortically derived electric currents on the human scalp.[5,6] His 1929 discovery and cataloguing of clinical correlations with the EEG earned Berger recognition as the "father" of electroencephalography. By 1932, Dietsch had performed laborious manual Fourier (harmonic) analysis on short segments of recorded EEG data[7] and noted differences in rhythmicity and harmonic content between normal and neuropathologic recordings. Adrian and Matthews[8] observed that anesthesia was associated with a slowing of the brain's electrical activity. In 1937, Gibbs, Gibbs, and Lennox of Boston reported the effects of ether, alcohol, barbiturates, and other drugs on human EEG recordings and suggested that EEG might be a useful intraoperative monitor.[9] This suggestion was not explored in earnest until the end of the following decade when a group at the Mayo Clinic led by Faulconer and Bickford began to report the results of their use of EEG. The Mayo group noted a consistent inverse relationship between barbiturate dose and overall EEG activity. This relationship stimulated their design of an automatic, EEG-servo-controlled barbiturate infusion or diethyl ether injection pump. In 1951, they reported a series of 50 operations in which an EEG-servo mechanism automatically controlled the delivery of anesthetic.[10] The concurrent development of cardiopulmonary bypass and concern about its potential negative impact on the brain provided additional motivation to examine intraoperative EEG phenomena. However, the overwhelming technical difficulty of EEG monitoring made intraoperative investigation difficult and routine use impractical. EEG equipment was cumbersome, unreliable, and expensive, and required a technician, and often a neurologist, to maintain it and interpret its recordings.

The need for expert professional interpretation was the technique's greatest failing, and several clever attempts were made to extract significant frequency and amplitude information from the EEG waveform using the analogue electronic technology of the day. Still cumbersome and expensive, these new devices were unpopular. The more capable Fourier analysis that Dietsch had used in the 1930s was too computationally intensive for the early minicomputers beginning to appear in laboratories by the mid-1960s. The development, in 1965, of the fast Fourier transform (FFT) algorithm by Cooley and Tukey of Bell Laboratories revolutionized the statistical analysis of EEG.[11] The FFT was a mathematical trick that allowed very rapid computer solutions to the problem of Fourier analysis, and its role in EEG analysis is described in detail below.

In 1971, Bickford described the advantages of displaying sequential frequency spectra in a trend-over-time plot he called a compressed spectra array (CSA).[12] For a time, the CSA also was impractical for intraoperative use because its computation required the presence of too large a computer, literally, a cabinet or desk-sized minicomputer[13] in the operating room. Maynard's introduction of the technologically and operationally simple cerebral function monitor (CFM), a device designed to detect brain death, appeared to solve both problems.[14] This compact, analogue-based device was briefly available commercially until its insensitivity to intraoperative EEG changes became apparent. Its failure decreased the interest of the anesthesia community in EEG monitoring for several years.

In the late 1970s, Nicolet made available a special-purpose signal-processing computer known as the Med-80. In addition to plotting EEG data in CSA format, this was the first device to give investigators the ability to quantify EEG in the form of band-power analysis. At about the same time, Fleming and Smith created a general-purpose digital microcomputer, the "BMC" (complete with analogue input and output), in a package less than a sixth of a cubic foot in volume and designed to fit as a standard module into a strip chart recorder system.[15] With software developed by Fleming, Quinn, Rampil, and Roxburgh, the BMC became the first practical real-time FFT-based EEG monitor for the operating room. Rampil and Sasse at the University of Wisconsin developed the spectral edge frequency (SEF) as a quantitative index of EEG activity and used it to determine the dynamic dose response of volatile anesthetics.[16,17] The SEF was the first quantitative EEG parameter successfully applied to the detection of cerebral ischemia[18] and to the study of pharmacodynamics.[17] In 1984, Moberg developed the first commercially successful computerized EEG monitor, the Neurotrac. Demetrescu developed a waveform analytic technique he called aperiodic analysis, which evolved into the Lifescan monitor.[19] Duffy and others pushed the computational frontiers with the development of brain mapping systems, which combined the simultaneous quantitative EEG data obtained from up to 32 electrodes to produce topographic maps of electrical activity and deviation from expected activity.[20] Higher-order spectral analysis, such as the bispectrum, was first reported by Dumermuth (Kleiner et al.[21]) and later refined by Chamoun into a clinical monitor.[22]

Physiology of the EEG

As noted above, there are some similarities between the electrocardiogram and the electroencephalogram. Significant differences exist, however, in their genesis and interpretation. While the ECG is created by a synchronous traveling wave of regenerative depolarization, the EEG is derived from subtle, subthreshold changes in neuronal membrane potentials. This chapter will provide only a brief overview of the relevant details of the genesis of the EEG; the interested reader is referred to more specialized texts.[23,24]

As in all living cells, the interior of a human neuron has a relative excess of negatively charged mobile ions creating a voltage difference across the cell membrane. The resting membrane potential of mammalian neurons is due predominantly to sodium (Na^+), potassium (K^+), and chloride (Cl^-). Each ion's contribution to the voltage across the membrane can be calculated by the Nernst equation (simplified for monovalent ions at 37°C):

$$V_{ion}(\text{millivolts}) = 61 \log \frac{\text{ion concentration}_{inside}}{\text{ion concentration}_{outside}}$$

This membrane potential is maintained relatively

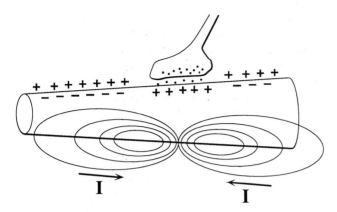

Figure 6-1 Local changes in membrane potential, like that which occurs in the postsynaptic membrane, lead to ionic current flow (I) in the extracellular space.

constant by sodium/potassium ion pumps, consuming a significant fraction of the cell's energy budget in the process. Due to the nontrivial impedance of axoplasm and extracellular fluid,[25] it is possible to charge a patch of cell membrane transiently to a transmembrane voltage different from that of neighboring regions of the same cell.[26] This focal perturbation in membrane potential occurs in postsynaptic membrane secondary to changes in receptor-mediated ion channel conductance. (For a review of ion channels, see Hille.[27]) As illustrated in Fig. 6-1, such regional differences in membrane potential lead to ionic current flow as the charges on each side of the membrane move along the electrochemical energy gradients. The membrane potential on a neuronal dendrite is most often the sum of focal postsynaptic potentials resulting from the activity of many thousands of synapses. If a region of membrane is depolarized to the opening threshold of the voltage-sensitive sodium channels, a regenerative action potential will form and propagate; otherwise, the membrane potential will tend to decay slowly to its stable baseline. Typically, there is a dynamic balance between depolarizing and hyperpolarizing (inhibitory) transmitters around the dendrite. Over time, the balance shifts from net inhibition to excitation and back, causing the postsynaptic membrane potential to oscillate with the current mixture of concentrations of neurotransmitters. These postsynaptic potentials are relatively long-lasting (tens to hundreds of milliseconds) compared with action potentials, but so small that the electric fields they generate usually cannot be detected at any distance from the cell. Larger currents will flow if, by chance, one part of the membrane is depolarized by an excitatory postsynaptic potential while a neighboring region is hyperpolarized by an inhibitory postsynaptic potential. Even these bipolar currents surrounding a single neuron within the brain are too small to be detected noninvasively with current technology.

However, the cytoarchitechure of the cerebral cortex has several features which combine to create currents large enough to be detected as the EEG. First, the cortex is densely populated with pyramidal cells notable for possessing single, large, relatively straight apical dendrites that are oriented perpendicular to the cortical surface.[28] Consequently, the dendrites of neighboring pyramidal cells are essentially parallel to one another. Second, afferent inputs to the pyramidal cells are relatively stratified and synchronous. That is, the neurons that provide incoming signals to pyramidal cells make synaptic connection to many neighboring pyramidal cells, and do so in approximately the same locations on each cell's dendrite.[26] The current loops that form around these cells tend to have similar instantaneous polarities and thus summate, greatly increasing the magnitude of the extracellular current flow, thereby permitting the detection of the mean currents on the scalp (Fig. 6-2).

Each pyramidal cell has thousands of afferent synapses, many of which derive from either neighboring cells, pyramidal cells in a homologous site in the contralateral cortex, or subcortical nuclei like the thalamus. Under some diverse circumstances, including deep sleep, certain drug intoxications (e.g., moderate doses of barbiturates or halothane, or high doses of opioid), calm relaxation, or some forms of head trauma, these afferents alter their firing patterns to increase the synchrony of pyramidal current loops, thus creating rela-

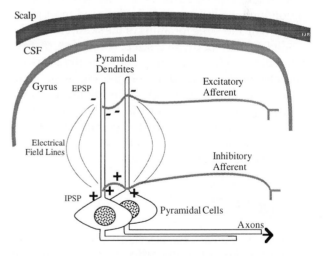

Figure 6-2 Cortical architecture provides the substrate from which the EEG is generated. Large pyramidal cells, particularly in layer 5, have long, straight dendrites which are oriented perpendicular to the cortical surface. Subthreshold, postsynaptic potentials of relatively long duration along the length of the dendrite create voltage differences and therefore current flow along the dendrite. Many thousands of neighboring pyramidal cells have similar postsynaptic potentials allowing the individual current flows to summate to the extent that they can be detected at the scalp.

tively high-voltage, rhythmic EEG patterns. Thalamo-cortical feedback loops[29,30] and thalamoreticular "pacemakers"[31] have been implicated in the genesis and control of these rhythms. The loss of synchroniza-tion is a natural consequence of alert consciousness and leads to a low-voltage, high-frequency jumble of wavelets.

The high degree of neuronal interconnection in the brain can produce interesting, but misleading EEG phenomena. For example, following a neuronal injury, there is often a reduction of neuronal activity in the corresponding area of the contralateral hemisphere. Known as diaschisis, this phenomenon probably is due to the extensive corticocortical pathways crossing the corpus callosum and may contribute to the inaccuracy sometimes apparent in the use of EEG to localize brain infarction.[32]

The clinician must remain cognizant that the EEG is predominantly a cortical phenomenon. Consequently, the bulk of the central nervous system is not directly involved in the production of the signals we observe of the scalp. For example, hemorrhage in the internal capsule, a common form of cerebrovascular accident leading to hemiplegia, seldom alters the EEG unless the hemorrhage is very large and induces coma. Likewise, EEG is an unreliable indicator of brain tumor.

Finally, from its site of origin in the cortex, the electric current associated with the EEG must traverse three "shells" of varying conductance, specifically the cerebrospinal fluid, the skull, and the scalp. Postsynaptic potential-derived currents are blended together in the conductive cerebrospinal fluid, forced through the many small and large foramina of the skull, and further blended in the conductive scalp. The effect of these intervening shells attenuates[33] and spatially blurs any focal electrical activity into neighboring areas of the scalp, significantly reducing the resolving power of noninvasive EEG measurements. If a very large number of electrode sites are used, it is possible to "deblur" the scalp signals mathematically using a technique known as the Laplacian operator.[34,35]

Normal EEG

Awake individuals vary widely in the characteristics of their baseline EEG. Interested readers are referred to any of the many excellent texts for details on the subject.[36,37] In general, EEG signals from awake adults contain a mixture of theta, alpha, and beta frequencies in varying combinations. Anxiety may cause a desyn-chronization and acceleration to primarily low-ampli-tude beta, while relaxation may result in prominent occipital alpha rhythms. True (nonartifactual) delta waves usually are a pathologic finding in awake, un-medicated adults, although normal in the deeper levels of natural sleep. The overall pattern of EEG changes in natural sleep is basically one of progressive slowing, except for the periods of REM sleep which are marked by fast, desynchronized activity.[38]

Intraoperatively, the activity of the central nervous system, and thus the EEG, is sensitive to change in many systemic parameters, including acid-base state, carbon dioxide concentration, and temperature that may alter oxygen delivery, metabolic requirements, or afferent cortical traffic. Additionally, the central nervous system will respond differently to different types of anesthetic or adjuvant agents and to different depths of anesthesia. Physiologic factors such as age, disease state, and electrolyte status will also have an effect. The panoply of confounding variables to consider when analyzing intraoperative EEG will be examined in more detail in the clinical sections that follow.

EEG Measurement Systems

ELECTRODES

To be useful to the clinician, the minute voltages traversing the scalp must be captured, enhanced, and displayed. The first step is transducing the scalp currents, converting them from ionic form into currents carried by electrons in metal, then via electronic circuitry into information. This sequence is implemented by placing pairs of electrodes according to a standardized system of sites that uses bony landmarks as reference points for placement (Fig. 6-3).[39] Electrodes are positioned at points 10 or 20 percent along inter-land-mark meridians, enabling the system (the "International 10-20") to provide intra- and interpatient repeatability of EEG recordings.

Because voltage is defined as difference in potential between two points, electrode sites must be considered in pairs. Groups of electrode pairs are called montages. The possible permutations of the 21 standard 10-20 electrode sites lead to thousands of possible montages. Multiple systems of defining and cataloguing montages of electrodes exist, many of which were defined without a theoretical (electronic) or logical basis. For example, the EEG literature distinguishes between "bipolar" and "unipolar," or "reference," montages when, by definition, any voltage measurement must be bipolar. These "bipolar" montages use two electrodes over cortical tissue, whereas "unipolar" montages place one over cortex, and one at a "quiet, distant" reference site. Unipolar montages are supposed to detect EEG preferentially from cortex directly under the scalp electrode, but actually do not, in part, because there is no true reference site. For a lucid discussion of the "fallacies" in the EEG literature, the reader is

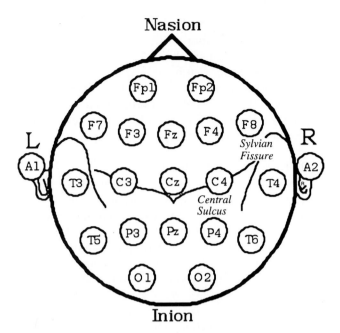

Nasion

Inion

Figure 6-3   The international 10-20 system for placement of EEG electrodes. This system employs symmetric bilateral placement to detect differences between the two sides of the cortex of any given patient. The essence of the system is that anteroposterior measurements are based on the distance between the nasion and the inion over the vertex in the midline; and five points—frontal pole (Fp), frontal (F), central (C), parietal (P), and occipital (O)—are marked along this line at certain percentages of the nasion-inion distance. This places a central line of electrodes one half the distance from the nasion to the inion. Lateral measurements are then based on the central coronal plane. Even numbers are used as subscripts for the points over the right heimsphere and odd numbers for those over the left hemisphere. Midline electrodes have the subscript Z.

of silver electrodes with silver chloride solution produces a very stable electrode potential and is the combination most often used. Many others (e.g., stainless steel and saline or extracellular fluid) generate unstable potentials, resulting in noise at the electrode interface that may be orders of magnitude larger than the EEG signal. Because the electrode potential also has capacitive effects, the fidelity of EEG signals through the electrode-electrolyte barrier also depends on the frequency content of the signals. Additionally, the electrode potential can be altered by motion of the electrode-electrolyte junction, which creates very large noise signals. A common motion-related artifact resembling a rhythmic oscillation occurs when an electrode is placed over the superficial temporal artery and "feels" the pulse. Accordingly, the characteristics of an ideal electrode include long-term electrical and mechanical stability, low frequency-related distortion, and low electrical contact impedance. However, the importance of the latter characteristic has declined over the past two decades, as will be discussed in the next section.

The electrodes most commonly used for diagnostic (nonsurgical) EEG monitoring are small ($\approx$1 cm) electrolyte-cream–filled metal cups which can be glued to either hairy or bare scalp using collodion-soaked cotton wads. These provide stable low-contact impedance for prolonged periods, but require a significant amount of time and skill to place correctly, making them less than ideal for use by anesthesia personnel in a busy operating room. A variant of the cream-filled cup electrodes is the Electro-Cap (Electrocap International, Dallas, TX), a nylon helmet with cup electrodes sewn into the appropriate "10-20" sites, thereby eliminating the need to place electrodes. Time still is required to abrade the skin below the electrodes with a blunt needle, inject the electrolyte cream, and test the electrode impedances. To keep the electrodes snug on the scalp, this device has a chin strap which would be in the surgical field during extracranial carotid surgery.

For use on hairy scalp, the primary alternatives to cup electrodes are subdermal needle electrodes, generally 30-gauge platinum or stainless steel wires with sharpened tips. The advantage of needle electrodes is that they are quickly and easily placed through any type of skin. Disadvantages include relatively high contact impedance (due to the small contact area), increased mechanical and boundary layer instability, high cost (unless resterilized and reused), and transient discomfort during placement. However, the discomfort is less than that of a lidocaine infiltration via a 25-gauge needle prior to venous cannulation. For use on nonhairy skin, the pre-gelled silver/silver chloride electrodes used in the operating room for electrocardiography are a good alternative. These electrodes are

referred to the landmark work of Nunez.[23] Katznelson has shown that the closer electrode pairs are, the more "focused" on local generators they become.[40] When multichannel EEG systems are used, a montage consisting of bilaterally symmetric sequential bipolar pairs of electrodes is frequently chosen (e.g., with reference to Fig. 6-3: Fp_1-F_3, F_3-C_3, C_3-P_3, P_3-O_1, and Fp_2-F_4, F_4-C_4, C_4-P_4, P_4-O_2).

The role of the electrode is to provide, as nearly as possible, an ideal electrical contact between the patient and the rest of the EEG system (e.g., amplifiers, filters, strip chart recorders, and/or computers). The biophysics of electrode interfaces is too complex for the scope of this chapter, and the interested reader is referred to Geddes's treatment of the subject.[41] Basically, the complex behavior of electrodes is secondary to the spontaneous development of a potential barrier at the surfaces of contact of metals with electrolyte solutions. The voltage characteristics of this barrier vary according to the specific combination of metals in the electrode and the electrolyte solution. The combination easily available, disposable and provide stable, low-impedance recordings if properly applied. The skin should be prepared by removing surface oils and some of the stratum corneum by abrasion, using either a dry gauze sponge or a small amount of Omni-Prep solution (a commercially available abrasive, conductive, adhesive liquid). Electrodes difficult to access intraoperatively may be additionally secured using tincture of benzoin, Mastisol, or adhesive tape.

The number and site of the electrodes used for a particular case should be determined by the motivation for monitoring (whether primarily for ischemia or drug effect) and relevant surgical factors such as the site of incision. Many neurologists and others trained in traditional, manually interpreted diagnostic EEG maintain that eight or more channels are mandatory for ischemia monitoring. Others, including this author, believe that one or two channels of EEG data are preferable to no data, that computer-assisted analysis likely is more sensitive to ischemia than is manual analysis on a per channel basis, and that oligo-channel systems are sensitive to even focal embolic events. The small body of literature addressing this issue is not decisive.[42,43] Because it is always prudent to place more than one pair of electrodes for intraoperative redundancy, the author suggests routine intraoperative use of two or four channels when EEG monitoring is indicated—the placement, testing, and maintenance of 10 or more electrodes is too time-consuming and distracting from other aspects of patient care for the anesthesiologist working alone.

AMPLIFIERS

The amplifiers used for EEG applications are quite similar to those used in electrocardiography; however, since the EEG is a smaller signal, the electrical specifications are more demanding. The most obvious specification is "gain," or the amount of amplification. Gain is specified in decibels, which is the log ratio of the output voltage over the input voltage:

$$dB \text{ (voltage)} = 20 \cdot \log_{10} \frac{\text{output}(\mu V)}{\text{input}(\mu V)} \text{ or } dB \text{ (power)}$$

$$= 10 \cdot \log_{10} \frac{\text{output}(\mu W)}{\text{input}(\mu W)}$$

EEG amplifiers usually have a gain of 100 to 120 dB (i.e., 10^5 to 10^6), while adequate gain for electrocardiographic amplifiers ranges from 60 to 80 dB.

The next important specification of an EEG amplifier is input impedance. Impedance is a measure of resistance to current flow which is appropriate to both alternating and direct current, essentially a measure of how much of the current flowing in the scalp is drained into the amplifier. The higher the input impedance, the less the perturbation of the biologic source. Early vacuum-tube–based amplifiers had input impedances in the range of $10^4 \Omega$ (ohms); current designs using insulated gate transistor op-amps have input impedances above $10^7 \Omega$. This thousandfold increase in input impedance decreases the dependence on carefully optimized electrode contact impedance (Fig. 6-4).

DIFFERENTIAL AMPLIFIERS

The most difficult problem in measuring EEG signals is "common-mode" noise—that is, an extraneous collection of undesirable voltages originating primarily outside the patient's body yet appearing uniformly at all electrode sites. The most frequent source of this type of noise is the AC power network running in the walls of the operating room. The 60 (or 50) Hz power lines radiate energy into their surroundings, and human bodies act as (capacitively coupled) antennae, resulting in 60-Hz skin voltage from power-line coupling to a patient that can be several orders of magnitude larger than the intrinsic EEG voltages. The best, but unfortunately an impractical way to eliminate power-line interference with EEG recordings, is to heavily shield the room where the patient is to be monitored. The next best technique, differential amplification, is the one actually used by essentially all bioelectric amplifiers. Differential amplification relies on the principle that power-line noise voltages are equal at all electrode sites on an individual and are thus "common-mode" signals, whereas EEG signal voltage differs at each electrode site. Differential amplifiers subtract the signal obtained at one electrode from that obtained at another. The common-mode signal should exactly cancel out, leaving only the EEG signal as the voltage difference between the two electrodes. The efficiency of this noise-canceling process is defined as the common-mode rejection ratio (CMRR) and is dependent on both the input impedance of the amplifier and on the electrode impedance.

CMRR's dual sensitivity is explained by the conservation of energy—that is, a current passing through a serial chain of resistors causes a voltage drop across each resistor that is proportional to the fraction of the chain's total resistance within the individual resistor (Fig. 6-4). In making contact with the patient, each lead has two impedances in series: the electrode impedance and the amplifier input impedance. In the older vacuum-tube-based amplifiers, the electrode impedance (e.g., 5 kiloΩ) was a large fraction of the amplifier input impedance (e.g., 10 kiloΩ), resulting in a relatively large decrease in the EEG voltage (in this case 33 percent) available to the amplifier, and a correspondingly high sensitivity of the CMRR to small differences in impedance between different pairs of electrodes. That

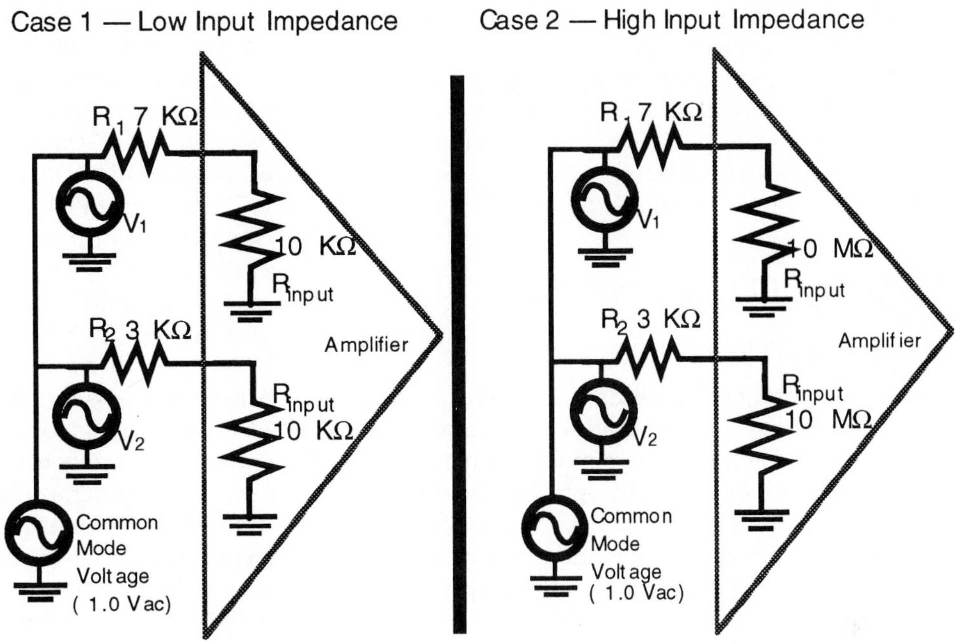

Case 1 — Low Input Impedance   Case 2 — High Input Impedance

Figure 6-4   Input resistor chain with CMRR example. When compared with older, low-input impedance amplifiers, integrated amplifiers with very-high-input impedance are insensitive to minor differences in patient contact impedance. For simplicity, the figure uses only ohmic resistance (R), not impedance (Z). In *case 1* with a mismatched pair of electrode resistances, a low-input resistance differential amplifier can produce only an 81.9 percent decrease in the common-mode voltage, whereas in *case 2* with the same mismatch, the high-input resistance amplifier produces a 99.96 percent decrease in common-mode voltage.

$$\text{Common Mode Voltage} = \left(\frac{R_1}{R_1 + R_{input}} - \frac{R_2}{R_2 + R_{input}} \right)$$

$$\text{Common Mode Noise Case 1} = \left(\frac{7}{17} - \frac{3}{13} \right) = 0.1809 \ \text{Volts}$$

$$\text{Common Mode Noise Case 2} = \left(\frac{7}{10007} - \frac{3}{10003} \right) = 0.0004 \ \text{Volts}$$

is, when the electrode impedance is a relatively large part of the total impedance, electrode voltage drops are relatively large. If the electrode resistances are not equal, by the time the signals get to the differential amplifier, the common-mode signal is no longer equal in each lead and does not completely cancel out. Because recent amplifier designs have input impedance in the range of 10 to 100 MΩ, the electrode impedance (e.g., 5 kΩ) is a much smaller fraction of the amplifier input impedance, resulting in a much smaller reduction in voltage (<0.05 percent) and a proportional decrease in the sensitivity of the CMRR electrode impedance and imbalance.

FILTERS

Another critical component of an EEG system is the filter in an electronic circuit or computer algorithm, which diminishes the contribution of specified frequencies while preserving others. The rational use of filters presumes that the information of interest in a complex signal lies in a different range of frequencies from that of the noise and artifact frequencies, as is often true of intraoperative EEG signals. Consequently, careful thought should be applied to the filter settings in an EEG system. Most systems have a bandpass type of filter which excludes frequencies outside a selectable passband. If the passband is set too narrowly, then relevant EEG information will be lost or distorted; if too wide, extraneous noise will contaminate the filter's output. In diagnostic EEG practice, a passband of 0.5 to 70 Hz is common.[44] However, the increased noise and artifact present in the operating room and intensive care unit, and the decreased high-frequency requirements for monitoring (in contrast to diagnosis), dictate a reduction in the filter pass range to perhaps 0.5 to 30 Hz to improve the signal-to-noise ratio.[45]

EEG data typically are recorded on a paper strip chart with 8 to 32 pressurized ink pen channels. The chart is a plot of voltage versus time. Most commonly, recording sensitivity is set so that 50 microvolts (μV) causes the recording pen to deflect 7 or 10 mm. The standard diagnostic horizontal axis speed is 30 mm per second or 108 meters of strip chart per hour; however, 15, even 5 mm/sec^{-1} has been advocated as adequate to demonstrate intraoperative changes relevant to the detection of ischemia, if not detailed patterns.[46]

Methods of EEG Interpretation

MANUAL INTERPRETATION

A trained observer of EEG examines several aspects of the signal tracings. A prime feature is wave amplitude. EEG waveform amplitude is measured from the peak of a wave to the following trough. The normal range of adult EEG amplitude is from 10 to 100 μV. Interpretation of absolute amplitude values must be tempered by recognition of many possible confounding variables such as electrode impedance, interelectrode distance, the type of electrode montage (discussed earlier), and the physiologic state of the patient.

Because the EEG voltage is a time-varying signal, the rate of voltage change can be evaluated most commonly, using frequency analysis. Conceptually, this is little more than classifying a segment of EEG as containing slow, medium, or fast waves, or some combination thereof. The first consistent rhythmic patterns detected in the apparent chaos were sinusoidal waves of 8 to 13 cycles/second (Hz) which Hans Berger named "alpha rhythms" in 1929.[6] Next, he discerned faster rhythms that he classified as "beta" (>13 Hz). Later authors defined "delta" (0 to 3 Hz), and "theta" (3 to 8 Hz) rhythms. To quantify frequency manually, the waves are measured either by measuring the distance between the zero voltage crossing points of an individual wavelet or by counting the wavelets over time. Since EEG is usually a complex mixture of different frequencies, manual quantitation can only approximate frequency content, but these visual ("eyeball") estimates by an educated observer are assumed to be sufficiently accurate in most cases of clinical diagnosis. Although many classic EEG studies are based on this simple four-frequency (alpha, beta, delta, theta) band analysis, there is no physiologic basis for rigidly defined band boundaries. During anesthesia, strict band descriptions lose their relevance because drugs cause smooth, continuous shifts in electrical activity patterns from beta range to delta and back in a reproducible manner. These drug-induced shifts are devoid of the prognostic significance they have in the nonanesthesia setting.

Waveshape is another characteristic examined in EEG tracings. It is generally difficult to ascribe meaning to particular waveshapes in the EEG recording, but there are exceptions. In routine neurologic diagnosis, the most important characteristic waveshapes are associated with epilepsy. These are spikelike shapes whose exact features depend to some extent on the underlying cause of the seizures. In fact, although the definition of a "spike" is a sharply pointed wave persisting 20 to 70 msec, the EEG diagnosis of epilepsy is far more complex, relying on recognition of such characteristics as the speed of onset of spiking, changes in spike frequency and amplitude during the ictal event, and postictal depression. Spike waves are common during enflurane anesthesia, but have no prognostic import (see below). Perhaps the best rationale for examining raw EEG waveforms along with computer-processed data in the operating room setting is the ability of the human operator to recognize the characteristic waveforms of different types of artifact.[47] The operating room is an electrically hostile environment for EEG signal gathering, combining hazards such as multiple patient-connected electronic devices (including monitors and electrosurgical units), the potential for motion artifact, or disruption of cables by personnel. Absolute vigilance is required to maintain the quality of incoming signals if EEG monitoring is to be accurate and useful during surgery. A short catalogue of artifact waveforms appears in Fig. 6-5. Additional discussion regarding the recognition and elimination of artifacts can be found below and in standard EEG texts.

Clinical (nonsurgical) electrodiagnosis uses eight or more electrodes distributed over the scalp in standardized montages to ascertain regional variations in EEG frequencies and amplitudes. For example, the well-known alpha rhythm is maximal over the occiput, which helps to distinguish it from the mu or motor rhythm that contains similar frequencies but is associated with different physiologic implications and is maximal over the precentral (motor) gyrus.

The EEG response to stimulation is the neurological equivalent of the cardiac stress test response. The central nervous system responds to stimuli such as pulsing light and sound; for example, stimuli normally block the relaxed-state alpha rhythm and cause subsequent desynchronization.

STATISTICAL BASIS OF AUTOMATED EEG PROCESSING

Historically, the interpretation of the EEG required heuristic and visual skills obtained only by years of training in electrophysiology. That brain waves could be assumed to be a (quasi-stationary) stochastic process was a major advance; that is, while samples of actual waves may appear random, taken in aggregate, their statistical measures are not random and vary only slowly over time when compared with the waves

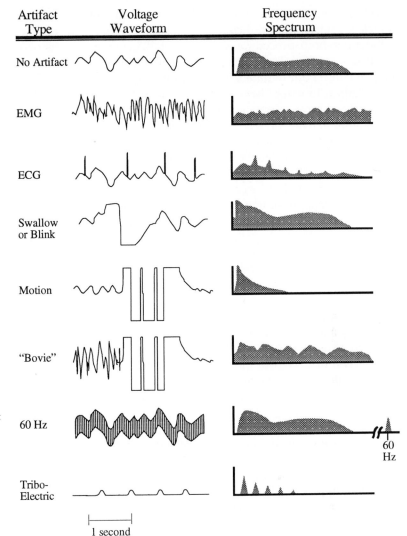

Artifact Type	Voltage Waveform	Frequency Spectrum

No Artifact

EMG

ECG

Swallow or Blink

Motion

"Bovie"

60 Hz

Tribo-Electric

60 Hz

1 second

Figure 6-5 Stylized artifacts are illustrated in both the time and frequency domains. Electromyographic artifact generally adds uniform, wideband (white) noise. Cardiac electrical activity adds a QRS pulse in the time domain, which translates to a series of blips in the frequency domain, spaced at intervals of the heart rate frequency. Swallows, blinks, and motion artifact are heavily weighted toward delta frequencies. Electrosurgical artifact ("Bovie") when present in small amount is white noise; if stronger, it saturates the EEG amplifier, producing flat-line EEG tracings. Power-line interference may significantly distort the time domain waveform, but generally leaves the spectral display unaltered, save a blip at 60 Hz. The triboelectric effect is created by mechanically deforming an insulator around a conductor—for example, a cardiac bypass roller pump creates the rhythmic pattern in the figure, which is then conducted by the blood in the body.

themselves. This assumption provided conceptual support for a mathematical analysis and, even, interpretation of EEG tracings without the continuous, single-minded effort of a trained electrophysiologist. The advent of integrated circuits then made it possible to introduce the compact, computer-based EEG analyzers which have renewed interest in perioperative EEG monitoring.

Computers can quantify various aspects of the EEG signal. The predominant advantages of this are two-fold: (1) Automated analysis compresses data and allows observation of long-term trends, and (2) these algorithms reduce the level of training and attention required for interpretation of intraoperative EEG. First, the computer translates the time-varying analogue signal into a form it can manipulate, a process known as digitizing that is performed by examining the signal at a rapid rate (e.g., 125 to 500 Hz) and determining the discrete digital number (composed of bits or bytes)

representing the voltage at each sampling time. Such a sample has a precision defined by the digitizing hardware and specified in bits: an 8-bit sample has a precision of 1 part in 256, a 12-bit sample resolves 1 part in 4096, and a 16-bit sample, 1 part in 65,536.

Shannon's sampling theorem dictates that the minimum acceptable sampling rate must be at least twice the highest frequency present in the recorded signal (not necessarily a frequency component generated by the brain), which is most often the 60-Hz power hum, but possibly a harmonic (multiple) of the hum. Therefore, the sampling rate must always be greater than 120 Hz, and 125 Hz (an 8.0-msec interval) often is chosen for convenience. Faster sampling rates provide more flexibility in signal processing but require faster (more costly) computer hardware. Failure to digitize at an adequate sampling rate produces a type of distortion known as aliasing, familiar to moviegoers as the phenomena leading to the appearance of vehicle wheels seeming to spin more slowly than the filmed vehicle's velocity would dictate.

For a one-hour procedure, digitizing at 125 Hz will result in 450,000 voltage measurements. Conventionally, an entire hour of data is not examined as a single unit. Rather, to assess EEG data in a timely fashion, the digitized array of data is divided into epochs with contiguous batches of ≈250 to 500 samples (2 to 4 s duration) each. An epoch, being a simple array of numbers, can be treated statistically; for example, a mean or variance can be calculated. The property of "stationarity" implies that, over time (from epoch to epoch), the statistics describing sequential epochs remain constant. Stationarity is an implicit assumption of many statistical tests. In fact, in biologic systems, true stationarity does not exist. However, when a subject maintains a constant neurobehavioral state, EEG output does appear to be quasi-stationary for up to 20 s at a time.[48,49] Stationarity usually is maintained over longer intervals during steady-state anesthesia. Some processing algorithms have been designed to sense and adapt to nonstationarity.[50,51] If quasi-stationarity was not present, many of our most valuable tools, such as trend-plotting, would be far less useful.

ARTIFACT DETECTION

EEG processing is truly a challenge of separating the wheat from the chaff. Before examining the problem of extraction of physiologically useful information from a random-appearing EEG signal, clinicians must be cognizant of inevitable contamination by extraneous "noise." In this context, noise or artifact is any undesirable signal—for example, the presence of electrocardiographic signal in the EEG leads would be considered noise because it would interfere with quantification and interpretation of the EEG. Most sources of such artifacts[47] can be controlled using simple preventive measures such as careful electrode application. Computerized EEG monitors are just as susceptible to the First Law of Computer Science as their general purpose brethren:

Garbage In, Garbage Out!

However, despite the best precautions—in electrode placement, and so on—artifact will still occur. The presence of artifact need not be considered entirely negative, because many artifacts actually contain potentially useful information, which may be extracted from the remaining EEG by sophisticated monitors. For example, a large electromyographic (EMG) signal from the frontalis muscle is common in frontal EEG leads during light anesthesia. Using bandpass filtering the Cerebrotrac monitor separates the EEG and EMG with (usually) minimal cross-interference and provides a separate indicator of EMG activity, which may have its own clinical uses. Several commercial monitors examine the amplitude of power-line frequencies and, if it exceeds a preset level, signal the operator to check for poorly connected electrodes. Many monitors contain other, limited forms of automatic artifact detection (such as looking for an amplitude exceeding some preset threshold) and flagging. For the present, the best detector remains a trained human observer, yet automated artifact detection schemes are essential in the processed EEG monitors used in the operating room and critical care settings. Once the raw data are transformed into the frequency domain for display (described later), it may be impossible to ascertain the presence of certain types of artifact (while enhancing the detection of other types) (Fig. 6-5). Additionally, the EEG waveform data must be audited to ensure that artifactual data are ignored if the EEG signal or its derivatives are being used to alter patient care. Ideally, a processed EEG monitor provides for simultaneous display of both raw (time-domain) EEG waves and the processed (usually frequency-domain) output in order to assure a degree of quality control.

QUANTITATIVE EEG (QEEG)

During the past 60 years, dozens of algorithms have been described to quantify and thereby refine or condense the information contained in the EEG. These may be divided taxonomically into at least three systems of classification:

| semantic versus statistical |
| time-domain versus frequency-domain |
| parametric versus nonparametric |

Semantic or syntactic analysis attempts to emulate directly the human observer in recognizing patterns of waveshapes. Statistical approaches use more numerically oriented algorithms. Frequency-domain analysis proceeds from the spectral content of an EEG epoch, while time-domain analysis uses the original voltage waveform. Parametric analysis makes a priori assumptions about the statistical nature of the "underlying generator" to build statistical models of the EEG. Parametric modeling is a statistical contrivance useful for predicting future activity and for producing sparse descriptions of the state of the EEG. In essence, parametric models are digital filters adjusted to take a truly random noise input and produce an output signal that has the same statistical descriptors (i.e., mean, variance, frequency content) as the currently observed EEG.

They are not models of the underlying physiology. The *parameters* of parametric models refer to the numerical coefficients of the filters, which match the model to the EEG. Parametric algorithms have been most often applied experimentally to diagnostic EEG[52] and have not been reported successful in real-time applications such as in the operating room and intensive care unit. Two factors discouraging their real-time use are the intensive computational load and their nonintuitive approach for clinicians without engineering backgrounds.

Nonparametric algorithms require only a degree of stationarity, but require no other a priori assumptions and do not use models. They are the most widely used in real-time analysis and are the only class of EEG analysis in common use in intraoperative monitoring, with frequency-domain algorithms currently more prevalent than devices using time-domain algorithms. The time- and frequency-domain-based nonparametric algorithms are discussed in more detail below.

TIME-DOMAIN ANALYSIS

One of the first[53] quantitative approaches to EEG analysis was the determination of average signal amplitude (a time-domain algorithm), usually implemented as the root-mean-square (RMS) or the mean of the absolute values of the EEG. This measurement is not influenced by the frequency content of the epoch from which it is calculated. In early clinical applications of EEG in the operating room, average amplitude parameters were considered adquate,[54,55] but EEG amplitude information is not normally distributed, suggesting that statistical comparisons of amplitude data may be inappropriate without first (log) transforming the data toward the normal distribution.[56,57] This statistical caveat applies to either the whole spectrum or band analysis.

Zero crossing frequency (ZXF) is also a time-domain algorithm[58,59] based on the assumption that most of the significant waves in the EEG waveform will cross the zero voltage axis and thus signify a boundary between waves. This algorithm measures the times between all the zero voltage crossings of an epoch of waveform, derives the mean interval and from it the "mean frequency." Although a crude estimator, because it tends to ignore the contributions of small-amplitude waves which might be superimposed on a larger wave (Fig. 6-6), variants of ZXF are simple to implement and seem to provide useful information.[60,61]

The "aperiodic" algorithm was first described by Demetrescu as a time-domain algorithm intended to address some of the shortcomings of the ZXF. Although related in concept to the ZXF, the aperiodic algorithm looks for "local" minima and maxima as the

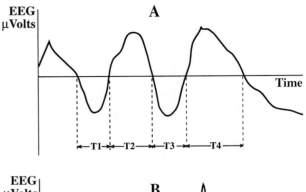

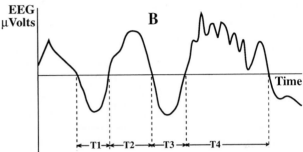

Figure 6-6 The original zero crossing display simply timed the intervals between sequential crossings of the zero voltage axis. This technique is simple to implement and is an accurate measure of mean frequency when the EEG signal consists of waves that are similar in frequency and amplitude, as in *A*. The zero crossing technique makes significant errors in estimating the mean frequency when the EEG consists of a mixture of wave amplitude and frequency. As illustrated in part *B*, small fast waves riding on a larger slow wave do not cross the zero axis and are therefore ignored.

boundaries of wavelets, not just zero crossing points. The peak-to-peak amplitude of each wave is retained, as well as the interval between adjacent minima (duration of the wavelet).[19] The resulting array of data for an epoch is plotted as a "telephone pole forest" as illustrated by Fig. 6-7.

Another example of a time-domain-based parameter is the burst suppression ratio (BSR).[62] This algorithm performs a type of morphologic assessment by evaluating the proportion of a given epoch in a state of electrical suppression (Fig. 6-8). The BSR can be a useful indicator of electric/metabolic depression due to the depressant effects of drugs such as thiopental, propofol, or isoflurane. Because of the morphologic recognition criteria, the time domain is the most successful arena for the automated detection of epileptiform activity as well as many forms of artifact.

The cerebral function monitor (CFM)[14] mentioned earlier was based on a time-domain approach/algorithm. This device displayed a single EEG parameter derived from a single channel of raw EEG via a complex sequence of filtering, logarithmic compression, and rectification. The predominant filter had a rising gain over the passband (2 to 12 Hz), thus emphasizing

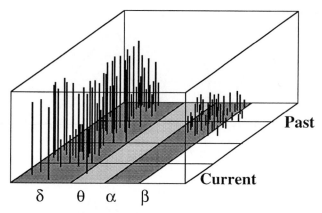

δ   θ   α   β

Figure 6-7   Aperiodic display as implemented on the Lifescan (Diatek, San Diego). This time-domain display depicts a four-minute trend where the newest information is drawn at the bottom of the "close" face of the "glass box." Wavelets are depicted as vertical bars whose height is proportional to the wavelet amplitude, and whose position on the bottom face of the cube is proportional to the frequency band, roughly $\log_{10}$ (frequency) horizontally, and recedes in depth with passing time. In this stylized cartoon there was activity in both the delta and alpha bands until two minutes prior to the current time, when the alpha activity ceased.

higher-frequency activity. Another way of explaining this filter is that it produced an output that was the product of the "average" frequency and amplitude within the passband. There have been anecdotal reports on the application of this device in anesthesia, intensive care, and neurology.[63] Unfortunately, the mapping from EEG input to CFM output was not unique—that is, many possible input waveforms with completely different characteristics could produce the same output. In particular, the CFM could not distinguish midfrequency, low-amplitude signals from low-frequency, high-amplitude signals. This characteristic rendered the CFM essentially useless for monitoring EEG for changes in anesthetic depth. For example, Sechzer and Ospina found no change in CFM output during 81 percent of anesthetic inductions with halothane and 91 percent of inductions with fentanyl. During induction with thiamylal, the CFM increased in 63 percent of patients, decreased in 10 percent, and was

unchanged in 27 percent.[64] Moreover, the device was insensitive to beta range frequencies, which are of considerable interest for intraoperative monitoring applications.[65]

FREQUENCY-DOMAIN ANALYSIS

Frequency-domain analysis first translates waveforms which are voltage magnitudes as a function of time into spectra which are magnitudes as a function of frequency. This process of conversion is akin to the action of a glass prism, which translates white light into a rainbow of the constituent frequencies. This type of conversion has its mathematical roots in the work of Baron Fourier, who was interested in the cyclic variations of tides. He discovered that any arbitrary waveform could be decomposed into a series of pure sine waves of differing frequencies, amplitudes, and phases. However, manual and even early computer solution of the Fourier transform for a particular set of data points was too time-consuming to be of practical use. Other approaches to frequency-domain analysis included the creation of large banks of analogues filters with narrow bandpasses, arrayed in parallel to emulate a true spectral analyzer.[66] It was not until Cooley and Tukey discovered a mathematical trick leading to the "fast Fourier transform" (FFT)[11] that frequency-domain analysis became practical for EEG processing.[67] The FFT algorithm results in a set of frequency bins, each containing the magnitude of the signal at that particular frequency. Although this algorithm still requires a great deal of numerical manipulation, current microprocessor chips can perform real-time EEG FFT analysis on four or more simultaneous channels. Special-purpose signal-processing chips can calculate FFTs with even greater speed.

SPECTRAL DISPLAYS

Once the spectrum has been calculated for a particular epoch, there are several popular approaches to displaying the data in a useful fashion. At present, the most commonly used is the compressed spectral array

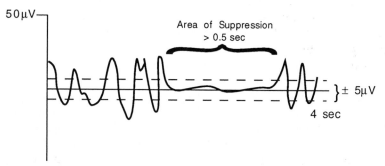

50μV

Area of Suppression > 0.5 sec

± 5μV

4 sec

Figure 6-8   The burst suppression ratio algorithm is a time-domain analysis technique which quantifies the degree of burst suppression.

CSA

DSA

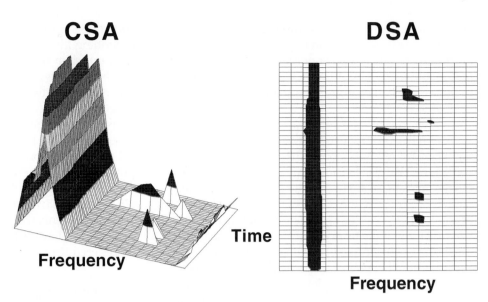

Figure 6-9   The creation of a spectral array display involves the transformation of a time-domain raw EEG signal into the frequency domain via the fast Fourier transform. This process is analogous to the creation of a light spectrum with a glass prism. A spectral histogram is calculated for short collections of sampled waveforms known as epochs. The resulting histograms are smoothed and plotted with hidden-line suppression for CSA displays or by converting each histogram value into a gray value for the creation of a DSA display.

(CSA) display technique which was popularized by Bickford.[12] The CSA is the now familiar "hill-and-valley" pseudo-three-dimensional plot of frequency versus power versus time. A second popular display technique is the density spectral array (DSA) introduced by Fleming and Smith.[68] The DSA uses gray-scale intensity or color changes to represent the EEG power at each frequency in each epoch. The CSA and DSA display essentially the same data, but there are some differences (Fig. 6-9). The DSA is more compact (i.e., more epochs can be comfortably viewed on a screen) and will not hide potentially important data as the CSA might "behind" earlier high peaks. On the other hand, the CSA provides superior dynamic range and resolution because it can display hundreds of digital steps in its graph, whereas the DSA usually is limited to 8 or 16 levels of intensity. Either of these display techniques achieves significant compression of EEG information, plotting up to an hour of data on a single screen or sheet of paper instead of the 308 feet of paper required by a traditional EEG recording. This compression may eliminate some of the nuances from the raw EEG signal, but the enhanced ability to detect trends is probably more valuable in operating room or critical care unit monitoring.

Interpretation of CSA/DSA plots still requires skill in pattern recognition. In an effort to simplify interpretation further, perhaps even to the point of automated diagnosis and alarms, many investigators have developed simple numerical parameters derived from the spectral histogram. One simple approach is to divide the spectrum into the classic neurological frequency bands (i.e., delta, theta, alpha, beta) and compute the total power for each band (by summing all the frequency bins contained in each band); the relative power then follows as the ratio of power in a band

divided by the total power in all four bands combined.[69] Multiple combinations and ratios of these band powers have been examined and reported. A recent example of this technology is the augmented delta ratio (ADR), defined as Power(8–20 Hz)/Power(1–4 Hz), and reported, in a single series, to be predictive of awakening and responsiveness following anesthesia.[70] The total power[71] or the delta band power[72] also has been reported as sensitive to cerebral ischemia during cardiopulmonary bypass surgery.

Another approach to condensing the information in the frequency spectrum is to treat the spectrum as a statistical distribution and use some measure of distributions. Three such descriptors have been cited in the anesthesia literature: the peak power frequency (PPF),[73] the median power frequency (MPF),[74] and the spectral edge frequency (SEF).[17] The PPF is the frequency in the spectrum that displays the highest power in a particular epoch—that is, the "mode" of the spectrum. The MPF is the frequency that bisects the power spectrum—that is, half the power is below and half above the MPF. In statistical terms, the SEF can be compared with the width of the distribution—that is, that frequency which is two standard deviations out from the mean. In practice, random variations in the spectrum require a pattern-matching algorithm rather than a strictly statistical approach to obtain a stable measure. The standard automated SEF algorithm is an attempt to emulate the visual recognition of a spectral edge. It searches from the high-frequency end of the spectrum downward, looking for the highest point in the spectrum that starts a contiguous frequency band of EEG activity at least 2 Hz wide, in which each frequency bin (each bin being 0.25 to 0.5 Hz wide) contains more power than some preset threshold. This approach disregards small random outliers in the higher frequencies. Some investigators have used simple percentile algorithms (e.g., 95th or 97th percentile power) in conjunction with other noise suppression techniques with reasonable success. Another view of the spectral distribution can be had by examining changes in its variance over time.[75]

Another recent approach to spectral analysis involves higher-order spectra. The bispectrum is the next higher-order analysis above the standard frequency spectrum. The bispectrum analyzes not only the frequency and phase angles of the components of a complex signal, but also the potential nonlinear interaction of some waves with others creating yet other waves.[76] Computation of the bispectrum starts with the Fourier transform of an epoch, but becomes far more intensive. For each possible pair of frequencies, f_1, f_2, the bispectrum $B(f_1, f_2)$ is the complex product of the Fourier transform at f_1, at f_2, and the complex conjugate of the Fourier transform at $f_1 + f_2$. Due to the stochastic nature of the EEG, the bispectrum of a single epoch is not a stable or reliable estimate of the true EEG state; therefore a moving average of the bispectrum of 10 to 20 epochs is used. The bispectrum calculation creates a two-dimensional array of results at each frequency pair; commercial implementations (e.g., Aspect Medical Systems, Natick, MA) use a proprietary algorithm to reduce this array to a single index value.[76]

Levy points out that the EEG usually is complex, may have a multimodal spectrum (i.e., more than one peak in the frequency spectrum), and therefore any single descriptor of spectral activity may not reflect the full range of EEG activity, particularly the appearance of additional modes, or peaks.[77] Whether this conclusion is actually germane to intraoperative monitoring with spectral parameters remains to be answered, because, to date, there are no clinical or physiologic correlations with the appearance of multimodal versus simpler EEG spectra. In the case of the SEF, the premise and the empiric observations that the highest frequencies are most sensitive to ischemia are not affected by the complexity or modality of the spectrum.

Physiologic Factors That Alter EEG

AGE

There are developmental changes in the EEG that progress from fetal patterns through senescence. Although specific changes with age are manifest in complex sets of patterns, the EEG generally progresses from predominantly slow frequencies in the neonate to higher frequencies through the end of the third decade. These changes appear to correlate with such maturational changes as increasing myelination. SEF has been used to demonstrate a quantitative measure of maturation of

cortical electrical activity in fetal lambs.[78] The literature describing EEG of anesthetized adults is growing rapidly, but data describing EEG effects in anesthetized children are few, despite a good foundation of information on EEG in awake children. In this author's experience, one may expect to see the same qualitative patterns in children undergoing anesthesia as those described below for adults.

From infancy onward, anesthetic agents increase in potency, and this effect is reflected in the EEG. At a fixed concentration of isoflurane (1.7%), older patients (78 ± 5 yr) had twice the degree of burst suppression as younger patients (28 ± 3 yr).[79] The differences between pediatric and adult EEG patterns should be carefully considered if intraoperative monitoring is necessary.

TEMPERATURE

Hypothermia causes progressive slowing and diminishes the amplitude of EEG activity.[80] During cooling, there is a strong correlation between tympanic membrane temperature and quantitative EEG analysis, such as SEF.[81] Depending on the type of concurrent anesthetic, the frequency-domain patterns will vary, as will the temperature at which electrical activity will cease. Patients undergoing cardiopulmonary bypass with moderate hypothermia (28° to 30°C) typically will have a sufficiently active EEG in which changes suggestive of cerebral ischemia can be detected, whereas cooler patients (<20°C) may have isoelectric EEG activity, rendering the modality useless for ischemic monitoring. Hypothermic depression or cessation of EEG activity is, on the other hand, believed to provide considerable protection to the transiently ischemic brain. EEG monitoring to determine the point at which electrocerebral silence occurs has been suggested as a more meaningful indicator of cerebral metabolic depression than core temperature monitoring in circulatory arrest surgery.[82] Hypothermia prolongs thiopental-induced suppression of cortical activity;[83] conversely thiopental often is necessary to induce complete electrical silence, even in deep hypothermia.[84] A recent report suggests that mild hyperthermia (2°C) during anesthesia does not grossly alter EEG characteristics.[85]

CARBON DIOXIDE

The EEG changes when arterial carbon dioxide tensions are outside the normal range. During extreme hypocapnia (P_{CO_2} < 20 to 25 mmHg), cerebral vasoconstriction may reduce cortical blood flow sufficiently to induce ischemia[86] and slowing of the EEG.[87,88] Although the intrinsic anesthetic effects of carbon dioxide (CO_2 narcosis) may initially accelerate EEG activity during mild hypercarbia, increasing P_{CO_2} leads to deeper anesthesia (MAC of carbon dioxide is 250 mmHg in dogs[89]) and slower EEG.[90,91] Rats exposed to supercarbia ($P_{CO_2} \approx 400$ mmHg) will have complete or near-complete depression of the EEG, and will seize briefly as P_{CO_2} is normalized before reverting to normal function and activity (Unpublished observation, Litt L, Rampil IJ, 1988). A recent study in humans receiving a nitrous oxide/narcotic anesthetic revealed EEG slowing with a decrease in the SEF and diffuse higher-frequency loss during mild hypercapnia ($Pa_{CO_2} = 50$ mmHg).[92] In the same study, moderate hypocapnia ($Pa_{CO_2} = 23$ mmHg) led to power increases in all bands, largest in the alpha range, and no change in the SEF. During stable desflurane anesthesia in man at 1.24 MAC, with or without nitrous oxide, changes in arterial carbon dioxide from 26 to 58 mmHg produced no change in EEG frequency content or in the degree of burst suppression.[93]

GLUCOSE

The brain requires a continuous supply of glucose to function normally. The minimum plasma glucose that provokes symptoms or alters the EEG varies widely.[94] Symptomatic hypoglycemia is associated with diminution of alpha rhythm, generalized slowing of the EEG, and may progress to grand mal seizures. Insulin-induced epileptiform seizures were, at one time, used in therapy of depression and schizophrenia. Hyperglycemia is associated with little change in EEG activity unless severe enough to cause obtundation and coma.

ELECTROLYTE BALANCE

Neuronal function is exquisitely sensitive to electrolyte imbalances that would interfere with synaptic function or impulse conduction. Hypocalcemia is epileptogenic and results in slow background EEG activity with bursts of spikes[95]; frank seizures may occur at calcium levels below 6.0 mg/dl.[96] Hypercalcemia is associated with EEG slowing when calcium levels exceed 13 mg/dl.[97] Hyponatremia also is associated with EEG slowing.

ENDOCRINE AND METABOLIC DISORDERS

EEG activity appears to be sensitive to circulating thyroid hormone.[98] Hyperthyroidism is associated with acceleration of normal alpha rhythms, even into the beta range, while hypothyroidism is associated with slowing and low-voltage tracings.

The EEG of patients with hepatic encephalopathy or renal failure usually slows, usually in proportion to the serum ammonia[99] or urea nitrogen[100] levels, respectively.

EEG Patterns in Anesthesia

ISCHEMIA

The metabolic and functional consequences of oxygen deprivation depend on the circumstances of the episode. Hypoxia is physiologically different from ischemia, and ischemia should be further classified by whether it is focal or global. Under normal conditions in adults, the brain receives a global average of 50 cc/100 g per min of blood flow and consumes, on average, 3.5 cc/100 g per min of oxygen. When blood flow decreases below 40 percent (about 20 cc/100 g per min) of normal or arterial hemoglobin saturation falls below 60 percent, the neuronal electrical activity becomes depressed.[101] When cerebral blood flow falls below 25 to 30 percent of normal (about 12 to 15 cc/100 g per min), electrical activity ceases, although the cells remain metabolically viable, at least for some period of time. At cerebral blood flow values below 20 percent of normal, cellular damage occurs quickly—that is, in 4 to 5 min at normothermia—unless cerebroprotective agents are used. If sudden ischemia occurs, for example, as may happen during a cardiac arrest or carotid artery clamping, EEG activity will begin to change within 15 to 30 s.

The pattern of EEG change with hypoxia or ischemia may vary according to the type and severity of insult, but typically the pattern progresses from an initial loss of high-frequency activity to an increase in relatively synchronized delta activity, and finally a decrease in the amplitude of all activity. Prompt restoration of blood flow and substrate supply generally will restore EEG activity to normal. A typical ischemic pattern is shown in Fig. 6-10. Clute and Levy examined the EEG during 93 episodes of brief, intentional cardiac arrest in 10 patients anesthetized with volatile anesthesia,[102] and found that the EEG detectably changed in only 88 percent of asystolic episodes; of those, 93 percent had "classic" changes involving acute slowing (to delta or theta). Remaining episodes were characterized by an isolated loss of delta activity with preservation of higher frequencies. A comparable study by Konstadt and associates in 15 patients anesthetized with high-dose opioids revealed that only 60 percent produced spectral EEG changes that could be identified as ischemic[103] during brief asystole.

Restoration of oxygen transport after the onset of neuronal damage can produce a wide variety of EEG patterns, ranging from slight, diffuse slowing of normal activity, frontal intermittent rhythmic delta activity (FIRDA pattern), epileptiform activity, monotonic, nonblockable alpha rhythm (alpha coma), to electrocerebral silence.

Ischemia of white matter (i.e., internal capsular stroke) may not produce significant EEG changes. The

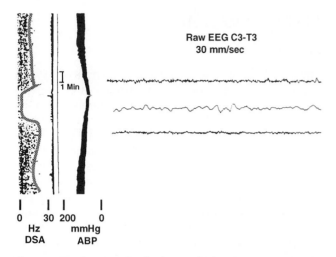

Figure 6-10 An example of ischemic changes as portrayed by a density spectral array display. In this case, the recording begins at the bottom of the figure and ends at the top, a total of just over 17 minutes. The raw EEG tracings on the right side of the figure correspond to the activity present at the time in the DSA tracing at the same vertical level of the graph. The initial spectral edge frequency (drawn in gray) is in the range 20 to 24 Hz, compatible with the moderately light halothane-fentanyl anesthetic. The arterial pressure decreases slowly until the systolic pressure is 80 mmHg. At this point, the EEG changes with a complete loss of alpha, theta, and beta activity and retains only intermittent delta. The spectral edge falls from 20 to less than 5 Hz in less than one minute. When, after three minutes of ischemia, the blood pressure rises above 80 mmHg, the EEG activity promptly returns to its baseline pattern. It is noteworthy that the raw EEG tracings are separated by 11 pages of strip chart, whereas the corresponding tracing of the DSA required three inches of paper for the same period of time.

territorial boundaries between the major arterial supplies to the brain are known as watershed areas, and the cerebral cortex in these areas is thought to be particularly sensitive to ischemia resulting from reduced cerebral perfusion pressure. Despite the anatomic localization of these watersheds, the EEG findings following acute watershed ischemia frequently reveal ipsilateral hemisphere-wide slowing, often accompanied by spike waves.[104] The concept of using EEG to monitor for excessive hypotension developed with Beecher, who, early in the development of the EEG, noted that feline EEG activity changed with hypotension.[105] EEG may therefore be useful in monitoring the adequacy of cerebral perfusion during surgery benefiting from induced hypotension, such a total hip arthroplasty in elderly patients with impaired cerebral autoregulation, or in younger patients at risk due to management with combined hypotension and hemodilution.

Systemic hypoxemia progressively, reversibly slows EEG activity. The EEG appears to change sooner than brainstem auditory evoked potentials in rabbits subjected to hypoxic hypoxia.[106] Persistent hypoxemia results in EEG silence followed by neuronal necrosis.

The EEG, however, is not an effective substitute for pulse oximetry because significant EEG changes do not occur until the arterial hemoglobin saturation falls below 60 percent[107] in awake subjects. With gradual onset of hypoxemia, EEG activity may accelerate transiently prior to slowing. This excitation is thought to be secondary to increased afferent traffic from peripheral chemoreceptors.[108]

ANESTHETIC DRUG EFFECTS ON THE EEG

Anesthetic drugs are administered to alter CNS function. Therefore, it is not surprising that they alter the EEG. The EEG effects of these drugs can be classified into one of three categories (Fig. 6-11). True general anesthetics create a dose-dependent biphasic EEG response, first described by Martin, Faulconer, and Bickford in 1959 with reference to ether.[109] These observations remain relevant as a similar response can be observed with halothane, isoflurane, desflurane, thiopental, and propofol, among others. During light anesthesia, the EEG desynchronizes and accelerates, corresponding to the phase of excitement or disinhibition. Increasing the dose leads to progressive synchronization, slowing and depression of the EEG, corresponding typically to anesthesia adequate for surgery. Increasing doses beyond that adequate for surgical anesthesia can produce burst suppression and even electrocortical silence. Administration of opioids produces a different dose response in EEG, that is, a mono-

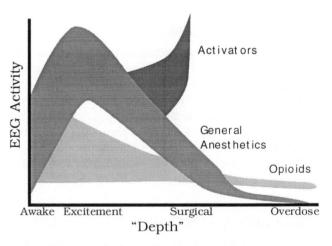

Figure 6-11 General template of anesthetic effect on EEG. The original template of Martin, Bickford, and Faulconer showed a biphasic change in EEG power with a decreasing population variance as depth increased. This pattern remains valid with current anesthetics and frequency-domain quantitation of EEG. Activators of EEG, such as ketamine and enflurane, may cause seizures at a depth beyond the excitement phase. Narcotics have a sigmoidal effect where very small doses cause no change and very large doses plateau in their response, which is short of complete EEG suppression.

tonic slowing of EEG, without an excitement phase. The EEG depression ends at a plateau of delta range activity and does not progress to cortical inactivity even at very high doses. The third pattern resembles the first, except that certain drugs (such as enflurane, ketamine, etomidate) can induce, at what would nominally be considered adequate anesthetic doses, a secondary increase in EEG activity progressing up to and including epileptiform activity.

VOLATILE ANESTHETICS

Induction and halothane,[110-112] enflurane,[113] isoflurane,[114,115] sevoflurane,[116,117] or desflurane[93] is associated with the loss of occipital alpha rhythms and the genesis of frontally maximal, relatively well-synchronized alpha to beta range activity. This activity may resemble sleep spindles or a fast version of alpha rhythm. In a spectral display, it will create an alpha-beta band of activity, usually separated from the delta activity by the theta region of the spectrum containing relatively little activity. Once this anesthetic-induced fast activity appears, its dominant frequency changes inversely with anesthetic concentration, and the distribution of its energy over the scalp changes. With induction of anesthesia, the occipital dominance of this alpha-beta range activity shifts to the frontal region.[118] The topographic distribution of delta-range activity also changes during anesthesia and stimulation,[119] and the loss of anesthetic-induced localization may be a marker of arousal.[120] Desflurane anesthesia does not appear to produce significant regional differences in EEG with changing doses, just a slight blunting of the difference (frontal versus occipital) in median frequency that existed in awake subjects.[93]

The prototypical drug-induced fast activity observed with anesthesia invites comparison but should not be confused with alpha pattern coma, a postischemic or trauma pattern signifying a very poor prognosis. At surgical levels of anesthesia (>1.0 MAC), the volatile agents begin to differ in their EEG effects. Isoflurane and desflurane induce burst suppression at a concentration above 1.2 MAC without further slowing of the EEG activity within the remaining bursts.[62,93] In dogs, the profound EEG suppression occurring early in exposure to desflurane may decrease, suggesting acute tolerance to the drug.[121] This effect has been sought but not detected in swine[62] and in humans.[122] Enflurane is associated with epileptiform activity,[113] particularly "spike-and-wave" complexes or even frank seizures at concentrations above 1.5 MAC. Hypocapnia accentuates this apparent increase in excitability. Halothane causes a reasonably linear slowing in the "fast" activity.[112,123] Burst suppression does not occur at clinically relevant concentrations of halothane. Intense noxious (tetanic) stimulation of the sciatic nerve in dogs receiving less than one MAC of halothane activates EEG (with desynchronization) and increases cerebral oxygen consumption, but provokes little change in dogs receiving more than one MAC.[124] Similar changes have been reported in adult humans following skin incision, whereas stimulation in children anesthetized with halothane tended to produce high-voltage slow waves.[110]

NITROUS OXIDE

The effects of nitrous oxide on the EEG depend on the conditions of its administration. Given alone, in subanesthetic concentrations (30 to 70 percent), nitrous oxide induces a frontally dominant, fast rhythmic activity having an average peak frequency of 34 Hz[125] and persisting for up to 50 min following exposure. When combined with other volatile anesthetics, nitrous oxide decreases the amplitude and increases the frequency of the anesthetic-induced fast activity in dogs[126] and rabbits.[127] If sufficient isoflurane is given to cause burst suppression, the addition of nitrous oxide will diminish the fraction of time in the suppression phase in animals[127,128] and humans.[129] The aforementioned findings suggest nitrous oxide antagonizes general anesthesia. However, when nitrous oxide is added to halothane or isoflurane anesthesia at concentrations that do not elicit burst suppression, delta activity may increase and alpha/beta activity may decrease,[129-131] suggesting nitrous oxide increases anesthetic effect. Avramov has reported that administration of nitrous oxide to humans receiving a steady-state concentration of halothane changed the sequence of EEG patterns over the course of approximately one hour—changed in manner suggesting the development of tolerance to nitrous oxide.[131]

PARENTERAL ANESTHETICS

Barbiturates follow the standard general anesthetic dose-response: small doses cause drug-induced fast activity, while higher doses increase EEG depression, culminating in burst suppression, then electrocerebral silence, if the dose is high enough.[132,133] The topographic sequence of EEG changes (Fig. 6-12) appears to be similar to those seen with volatile anesthetics. The appearance of fast activity corresponds with clinically apparent excitement phenomena and substantial delta activity with insensibility present.[133] This consistent pattern of EEG response during barbiturate anesthesia was used by Bickford and colleagues[54] in the late 1940s to automatically control thiopental anesthesia in surgical patients, and later by Cosgrove and Smolen[74] in rabbits. Schwilden and colleagues have reported using median power frequency to control methohexital sedation in volunteers. In their study it was possible to maintain a steady median power frequency of 2 to 3

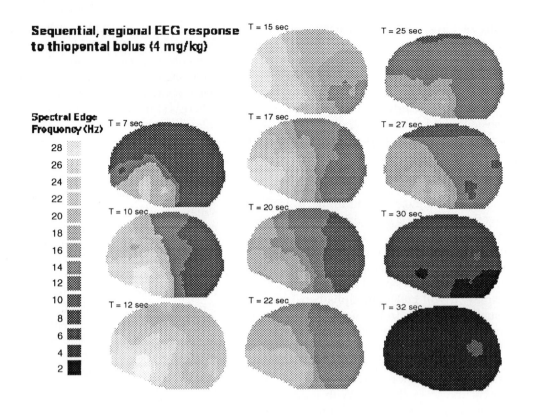

Figure 6-12 A sequence of "snapshots" at 2.5-s intervals displaying the changing distribution of EEG frequency content (in this case, spectral edge frequency) over the scalp following a bolus injection of 4.0 mg/kg thiopental. In frames T = 7 through T = 17, there is a prominent focus of frontotemporal fast activity which spreads posteriorly during this interval. Starting about T = 15, extreme slowing and suppression begin occipitally and spread anteriorly, enveloping the entire cortex by T = 30.

Hz, but this EEG pattern was not clearly correlated with an acceptable anesthetic state.[134]

Methohexital (0.5 mg/kg) appears to enhance interictal epileptiform activity in predisposed patients while seeming to diminish seizure propagation, whereas thiopental does not,[135] although both are used to localize seizure foci during epilepsy surgery.[136,137]

ETOMIDATE AND PROPOFOL

Propofol[138,139] and etomidate[140,141] are nonbarbiturate hypnotics that produce EEG changes similar to those induced by barbiturates (Fig. 6-11). Induction of anesthesia with these agents often is associated with myoclonic activity.[142] During such episodes the EEG is free of epileptiform activity, suggesting these movements are mediated at subcortical or spinal sites.[140,143] Like methohexital, etomidate in small doses (0.1 mg/kg) enhances interictal activity of epileptic foci[144] and may produce a generalized seizure in patients with epilepsy. At higher doses, etomidate causes burst suppression and a reduction in $CMRO_2$ similar to that observed with thiopental.[145] Propofol may enhance[146] or reduce[147] interictal spike activity in patients with complex partial epilepsy. The cerebral metabolic depression and relatively preserved hemodynamic stability associated with etomidate may confer cerebral protection during temporary occlusion for aneurysm surgery.[148] Etomidate also increases the amplitude of somatosensory evoked potentials.[149]

KETAMINE

Ketamine is a dissociative agent that produces a different EEG pattern than general anesthetic agents. The onset of sedation results in a high-amplitude, rhythmic theta activity, often accompanied by a significant increase in beta range activity.[150] Ketamine can provoke frank seizure activity in patients with epilepsy, but only rarely in normal subjects.[151]

BENZODIAZEPINES

When used in small doses as premedicants or as adjuvants to induction of anesthesia, benzodiazepines induce significant, predominantly frontal beta range activity[152] and decrease alpha activity.[153] Increased beta activity or beta/alpha band power ratio may be associated with the onset of amnesia.[154] Increasing benzodiazepine dosage is associated with generalized slowing to the theta/delta range, apparently without burst suppression.[155] Flumazenil promptly restores EEG activity to a pre-benzodiazepine state.[155] Aside from their salutary effects on patients, premedication with a benzodiazepine frequently simplifies EEG interpretation during induction and maintenance of anesthesia because additional anesthetics cause only a decrease in EEG frequency rather than the biphasic response. The relatively high-frequency EEG produced by benzodiazepines may possibly increase the sensitivity of ischemia detection schemes that quantify the alpha and beta range of the spectrum (i.e., SEF). Diazepam is widely used as an anticonvulsant, but it also induces fast activity and possibly even spikelike activity in patients with epilepsy.

OPIOIDS

The EEG effects of opioids differ from those of the general anesthetics, as illustrated in Fig. 6-11. Generally, there is little or no excitement phase when mu-subtype agonists (morphine, fentanyl, sufentanil, alfentanil) are administered, but, instead, a steady decline in frequency content until only delta activity remains.[156–158] There is no further change in the EEG with increasing dose. Burst suppression does not occur with narcotics. Peripheral muscle rigidity is not associated with cortical seizure activity,[159] but rather appears to be a direct effect of narcotics on specific areas of the brainstem, particularly nucleus raphe pontis and dorsal periaqueductal gray.[160] Seizures do not occur during clinical administration of opioids, but have been noted in dogs given extremely high doses (i.e., fentanyl 4 mg/kg intravenously)[161] and in the presence of normeperidine, a metabolite of meperidine.

ALPHA₂-ADRENERGIC AGENTS

The administration of α_2-adrenergic agonists appears to increase the potency of commonly used general anesthetics. This anesthetic-like effect is associated with EEG slowing and a reduction in anesthetic requirement. For example, the addition of clonidine to isoflurane/nitrous oxide anesthesia in patients slows the EEG while simultaneously allowing reduction in the inspired concentration of isoflurane.[162] Similarly, dexmedetomidine reduces the dose of thiopental required to produce burst suppression in volunteers, an effect that may be explained pharmacokinetically rather than pharmacodynamically.[163]

MUSCLE RELAXANTS

Nicotinic antagonists administered for neuromuscular blockade generally are considered to be highly polar molecules that transfer minimally through the blood-brain barrier and thus are likely to have little effect on the EEG. However, a number of exceptions have been identified. For example, although succinylcholine is not thought to enter the cerebrospinal fluid or directly affect the central nervous system, intravenous bolus administration appears to cause an increase in EEG activity and cerebral blood flow that resembles arousal and persists far longer (5 min) than might be expected from electromyographic fasciculation artifact.[164] This effect may be due to increased afferent neural traffic from intrafusal fibers in fasciculating muscle. Pancuronium, on the other hand, appears to prolong the isoelectric phase of burst suppression that occurs with isoflurane anesthesia in dogs.[165]

Atracurium is metabolized to a large extent by nonenzymatic Hofmann elimination. One of the metabolites of this process is laudanosine, a compound long known to be a convulsant and cerebral stimulant.[166] While it is unlikely that a patient will receive a sufficient dose of atracurium intraoperatively for laudanosine to cause convulsions, administered doses may be sufficient to increase EEG activity and perhaps alter the depth of anesthesia.[167] Small doses of atracurium or pancuronium adminstered directly into the intrathecal space cause grand mal seizures and rapid demise of rats.[168]

Clinical Indications and Practice

CAROTID SURGERY

The most important indication for EEG monitoring presently is risk for focal ischemia. As indicated earlier, the EEG provides a convenient indicator of failing cerebral activity that can permit timely therapeutic intervention which may prevent or minimize neurological damage. The best-documented demonstration of this principle is the use of selective shunting during carotid endarterectomy.[169–171] Sundt and his colleagues compared regional cerebral blood flow (intracarotid ^{133}Xe injection with a single detector over the ipsilateral sensorimotor cortex) and continuous surveillance of 16 raw EEG tracings by a neurologist with patient outcome in a large clinical series.[172] They found that all major, new postoperative deficits were preceded by intraoperative EEG change, and that the EEG changes correlated with regional cerebral blood flow measurements. In 1979, Chiappa[173] compared an 8-channel EEG strip recording with a 4-channel computerized compressed spectral array display and concluded that the CSA *"proved to be of greater utility than did routine EEG methods."* In 1983, Rampil and colleagues defined specific, quantitative criteria with which to diagnose the occurrence of significant ischemia [rapid (<1 min) decrease in SEF to ≤50 percent of prior baseline, persisting 10 minutes or longer] and found these criteria to be accurate in predicting new postoperative neurological deficits in preoperatively intact patients undergoing carotid endarterectomy with general anesthesia.[18] Russ[174] and Baker,[175] using similar spectral edge criteria, obtained similar results. However, abnormalities present in the EEG of patients with preoperative stroke rendered the SEF criteria less useful in those patients.[18] Another report noted that during carotid surgery with cervical plexus regional block, computerized EEG monitoring using criteria developed for general anesthesia may not be accurate.[176] Given the high variability of EEG in awake patients, this result is not surprising. Further, in light of the previously described anatomic and physiologic limitations, EEG monitoring can never be expected to have 100 percent sensitivity and specificity, as the occasional case report will attest.[177] Ischemia of many, perhaps most, subcortical areas would produce no detectable change in EEG; it is fortuitous that EEG monitoring during anesthesia is as sensitive as it appears to be.

Despite its putative accuracy, the utility of EEG monitoring during carotid surgery remains a matter of debate.[178,179] EEG should only be considered useful in patient care if it can be used to initiate and guide therapeutic maneuvers for the treatment of ischemia. Three such maneuvers have been proposed (although they lack outcome data): selective intraluminal shunting, induced arterial hypertension, and barbiturate protection. Arterial shunting provides some degree of continued perfusion during carotid artery clamping at the risk of increased embolization. It would therefore be prudent (in theory) to place a shunt only in patients whose brain indicates a need for additional perfusion following carotid clamping. The efficacy of computerized EEG-based selective shunting was examined by Tempelhoff,[180] who used as a diagnostic criterion either a decrease in SEF of ≥50 percent[18] or a decrease in total EEG spectral power >30 percent. When selective shunting was used, EEG remained a useful predictor of postoperative outcome, yet the question of whether EEG-based selective shunting improves patient outcome remains unanswered. For example, a shunt placed during persistent EEG changes indicative of ischemia does not assure resolution of the ischemia.[181] Moreover, the alternative therapy, routinely elevating arterial blood pressure with phenylephrine during this operation, is a maneuver that ap-

pears to triple the risk of myocardial ischemia.[182] EEG may therefore be useful to "titrate" the demands of the brain against the workload of the heart, although at present there are no data to support this patient management technique. Finally, EEG evidence of cerebral ischemia may suggest administration of thiopental,[183] which has been shown to be relatively safe,[184] but again data from controlled clinical trials are lacking.

There is no consensus among clinicians who use computerized EEG monitoring on the best methodology for carotid surgery. Experience in interpretation is probably a more significant factor in the successful use of this technology than the number of simultaneous channels monitored or any other factor. If the clinician believes the EEG to be useful for detecting ischemia during carotid surgery, then certain limitations must be placed on the anesthetic technique to preserve adequate cortical activity for diagnosis. For example, large doses of opioids or barbiturates, or high concentrations of isoflurane or desflurane, will render the EEG very slow or even isoelectric and therefore an insensitive background for ischemic changes. A mixture of low-dose isoflurane, fentanyl, and benzodiazepines often works well, maintaining an SEF in the 15 to 20 Hz range. Some clinicians use the EEG to titrate the anesthetic dosing to achieve stable barbiturate coma for prospective brain protection, rendering the prior point moot. The author prefers a two- or four-channel CSA/DSA system with bilaterally symmetric bipolar leads over the cortical convexity (i.e., F_3-C_3/F_4-C_4 and C_3-P_3/C_4-P_4). These lead pairs cross watershed regions of the middle cerebral arteries and should detect ischemia due to inadequate collateralization during carotid cross-clamping. Focal ischemia due to emboli is probably very common during carotid surgery.[185] Emboli may occur anywhere in the hemispheres and therefore one cannot anticipate the best electrode sites a priori. Most quantitative EEG monitors allow the clinician to adjust the analysis update rate within a range of 2 s to several minutes per update. In the context of ischemia monitoring, the fastest update rate is most desirable. The analysis algorithm chosen should be sensitive to both loss of alpha/beta power and changes in delta power. The author finds the simultaneous display of the raw EEG, a CSA or DSA display, and current SEF value for each channel to be most convenient.

CARDIAC SURGERY

The advent of cardiopulmonary bypass and interest in what that particular physiologic trespass did to the brain was an early motivating factor in the development of intraoperative EEG monitoring. As neuropsychiatric testing has become more sophisticated and widespread, it is clear that there is a high risk (up to 60 percent) of damage following cardiopulmonary bypass. In a prospective study of 65 patients, Soltaniemi found that 37 percent of these patients developed new (mostly transient) neurological deficits within 10 days of surgery and an additional 21 percent who were neurologically asymptomatic had pathologic EEG changes.[186]

In 1981, the National Center for Health Care Technology (Office of Health Technology Assessment) of the Department of Health and Human Services formally assessed the literature and solicited comments[187] from device manufacturers, physicians, and other interested parties regarding the value of intraoperative EEG monitoring during cardiac surgery. The resulting report[188] concludes:

> There is little published data based on well-designed studies regarding the clinical effectiveness of brain wave monitoring during open-heart surgery. . . . It appears that there is no clear role for routine EEG monitoring during open-heart surgery and in the immediate postoperative period for patient management.

Since this 1981 report, there has been some progress toward collecting data that objectively support the use of intraoperative EEG monitoring for cardiac surgery. First, the direct intraoperative utility of EEG monitoring has been supported by case reports citing timely detection of cerebral ischemia which might have otherwise gone undetected—one involving an aortic cannula dissection,[189] another involving a pump malfunction,[190] and yet another, vertebrobasilar arterial kinking.[191] Second, Nussmeier and coworkers demonstrated that the use of EEG to titrate sufficient doses of thiopental during normothermic cardiopulmonary bypass reduced postoperative neuropsychiatric deficits.[192] Zaidan[193] also used EEG burst suppression to titrate thiopental during hypothermic cardiopulmonary bypass but found no benefit to thiopental administration. Finally there have been two reports of improved patient outcome using EEG monitoring. Arom and colleagues reported a reduction of postoperative neuropsychiatric deficits from 44 percent to 5 percent with the use of total EEG power in a 16-lead montage to diagnose and actively treat presumptive cerebral ischemia during cardiac surgery.[71] Other investigators indicated that adjustment of perfusion pressure based on changes in delta range power reduced postoperative disorientation.[72] Independent verification of the beneficial results of these reports is eagerly awaited by clinicians hoping to use EEG monitoring to improve patient care. However, delta power changes may not always provide reliable ischemia monitoring, as documented in a recent study where as many computer-tagged "ischemic" events occurred in the control group as in the patients with verifiable ischemia.[194]

ELECTROCORTICOGRAPHY

Occasionally, the need to localize eloquent or epileptogenic regions of cortex requires direct recording from the cortex. In these cases, a neurosurgeon will place an array of sterile, ball-shaped ($\approx$2 mm diameter) metal electrodes on the pial surface using a positioning frame which is bolted to the skull. Electrocorticographic (ECog) signals are usually interpreted by a neurologist using a multichannel strip-chart recorder. The anesthesiologist also plays an important role in these cases, in light of the frequent requirement for a complete paradigm shift from the usual goals of anesthetic management. Specifically, the anesthetic state usually is created to maximally depress and disrupt the normal function of the CNS, whereas the goal during ECog for seizure focus localization must be to preserve, as much as possible, the usual state of CNS and neuronal function. Many anesthetic agents obviously alter neuronal function which may mask or otherwise alter the sought-after EEG patterns. The specific anesthetic plan should therefore be determined in consultation with the neurologist and surgeon and will depend on the relative weight of intraoperative ECog data in guiding the extent of the surgical resection.

It is becoming common in otherwise routine neurosurgical cases to use ECog to help localize eloquent cortex and avoid incidental resection of these areas in the approach to a lesion. For example, prior to resecting a deep, posterior frontal lobe tumor, a surgeon may wish to know accurately the extent of the primary motor cortex. At present, the most effective localization is performed by the surgeon who directly stimulates the cortex with 2 to 20 volts AC using a small, hand-held probe, and looks for peripheral motor activity in the unparalyzed patient. The ECog recording electrodes are used to detect and minimize stimulation-induced seizures. In the future, localization may be accomplished preoperatively using PET (positron emission tomography) or functional MR (magnetic resonance) imaging.

BRAIN PROTECTION

Thiopental and similar agents frequently are used to reduce cerebral metabolic demand and to provide a measure of brain protection in procedures where transient ischemia may occur.[183,184,195–197] One posited mechanism for the efficacy of these agents is the reduction in electrical/synaptic activity. Because these agents have a relatively wide range of pharmacokinetic and pharmacodynamic parameters in any given population, the most efficacious means of administration uses the occurrence of EEG burst suppression as a nearly direct indicator of the desired metabolic effect.[183,192,198,199] This type of EEG monitoring can be done with just a few channels, since burst suppression is a rather global phenomena. In monitoring for this purpose, examination of the raw waveforms for suppression is far more useful and accurate than looking for slowing in a computerized spectral array.

DEPTH OF ANESTHESIA OR SEDATION

Much investigation has focused on the use of EEG as a means to quantify the clinical anesthetic effect in individual patients. The generic dose-response of the EEG is well known, but it is not directly clinically useful. Unfortunately, much of the existing literature has focused on dose-response curves rather than specific correlates of individual patient responsiveness or level of consciousness. It has proven difficult to formulate a quantitative EEG factor that will correlate reliably with patient responsiveness independent of the mixture of anesthetic agents. The first demonstration that this might be possible showed that the SEF immediately prior to laryngoscopy predicted the magnitude of the blood pressure response that followed.[200] That is, patients with adequate anesthesia—slow EEG (SEF < 14 Hz)—had small increases in blood pressure, whereas patients with light anesthesia (SEF ≥ 14 Hz) experienced large increases. This SEF criterion, however, was proven sensitive to changes in induction drugs. In the former study, anesthesia was induced with thiopental, yet a later study using predominantly fentanyl found that the SEF was a good predictor of hemodynamic response only once the discriminant frequency was altered to 10 Hz.[201] In another study, SEF failed to correlate with hemodynamic response to surgical incision.[202]

Several investigators attempted to correlate EEG with the probability of patient movement in response to surgical incision or other noxious stimulation. To date, all of these results have been less than successful in producing an EEG parameter that can accurately predict movement in individuals.[203–205] Even the presence of burst suppression in the EEG did not guarantee immobility.[203,204] In a prospective, multicenter trial, a bispectrum-derived index did vary with probability of patient movement, but the predictive value was low (the slope of the response curve was shallow) and accuracy was further diminished in the presence of opioids.[206] These rather disappointing findings may be understood in light of recent findings that neither the cerebral cortex (and the intrinsic EEG generators)[207] nor the brainstem[208] is necessary to mediate anesthetic-induced immobility.

While the spinal cord may mediate immobility, it is rather likely that the cortex is a site at which anesthetics act to cause unconsciousness and amnesia. It would seem reasonable to seek EEG correlation with clinical phenomena such as amnesia, inability to follow verbal commands, or emergence. Here, too, the use of frequency spectrum–derived indices like spectral edge or median power frequency has met with limited success.[154,205,209–211] It is possible that higher-order brain functions, such as consciousness and memory, may be reflected in more subtle EEG markers than gross frequency changes. A new bispectrum-derived index (BIS3, Aspect Medical Systems), which is tuned to detect interfrequency dependencies, may provide a useful tool for this type of monitoring. Preliminary tests of BIS3 to assess level of sedation and amnesia are very encouraging.[212,213]

References

1. Brazier MAB: *A History of Neurophysiology in the 17th and 18th Centuries: From Concept to Experiment.* New York, Raven, 1984, pp 205–217.
2. Caton R: The electric currents of the brain. *Br Med J* 1875; 2:278 Aug 28.
3. Brazier MAB: *A History of Neurophysiology in the 19th Century.* New York, Raven, 1988, pp 185–194.
4. Einthoven W: Die galvanometrische registrirung des menschlichen capillar-elektrometers in der physiologie. *Pfluegers Arch Ges Physiol* 1903; 99:472.
5. Berger H: Über das elektroenkephalogramm des menchen. *Arch Psychiatr Nervenkr* 1929; 87:527.
6. Gloor P: *Hans Berger on the Electroencephalogram of Man.* Amsterdam, Elsevier, 1969.
7. Dietsch G: Fourier-analyse von elecktrenenkephalogrammen des menschen. *Plfuegers Arch Ges Physiol* 1932; 230:106.
8. Adrian ED, Matthews BHC: The interpretation of potential waves in the cortex. *J Physiol* 1934; 81:440.
9. Gibbs FA, et al: Effect on the electroencephalogram of certain drugs which influence nervous activity. *Arch Intern Med* 1937; 60:154.
10. Soltero DE, et al: The clinical application of automatic anesthesia. *Anesthesiology* 1951; 12:574.
11. Cooley JW, Tukey JW: An algorithm for the machine calculation of complex Fourier series. *Math Comp* 1965; 19:297.
12. Bickford RG, et al: The compressed spectral array (CSA). A pictorial EEG. *Proc San Diego Biomed Symp* 1972; 11:365.
13. Myers RR, et al: The use of on-line telephonic computer analysis of the EEG in anesthesia. *Br J Anaesth* 1973; 45:664.
14. Maynard D, et al: A continuous monitoring device for cerebral activity. *Electroencephalogr Clin Neurophysiol* 1969; 27:672.
15. Fleming RA, et al: An inexpensive general purpose biomedical computer system. *Proc San Diego Biomed Symp* 1976; 15:79.
16. Smith NT, et al: Does thiopental or N_2O disrupt the EEG during enflurane? *Anesthesiology* 1979; 51:S4.
17. Rampil IJ, et al: Spectral edge frequency—A new correlate of anesthetic depth. *Anesthesiology* 1980; 53:S4.
18. Rampil IJ, et al: Prognostic value of computerized EEG analysis during carotid endarterectomy. *Anesth Analg* 1983; 62:186.
19. Gregory TK, Pettus DC: An electroencephalographic processing algorithm specifically intended for analysis of cerebral electrical activity. *J Clin Monit* 1986; 2:190.
20. Duffy FH, et al: Brain electrical activity mapping (BEAM): A method for extending the clinical utility of EEG and evoked potential data. *Ann Neurol* 1979; 5:309.

21. Kleiner B, et al: Analysis of the interrelations between frequency bands of the EEG by means of the bispectrum. *Electroencephalogr Clin Neurophysiol* 1969; 27:693.

22. Kearse LAJ, et al: Bispectral analysis of the electroencephalogram during induction of anesthesia may predict hemodynamic responses to laryngoscopy and intubation. *Electroencephalogr Clin Neurophysiol* 1994; 90:194.

23. Nunez PL: *Electric Fields of the Brain: The Neurophysics of EEG.* New York, Oxford, 1981.

24. Speckmann EJ, Elger CE: Introduction to the neurophysiological basis of the EEG and DC potentials. In Niedermeyer E, Lopes da Silva F (eds): *Electroencephalography: Basic Principles, Clinical Applications, and Related Fields,* 3d ed. Baltimore, Williams & Wilkins, 1993, pp 15–26.

25. Kuffler SW, et al: *From Neuron to Brain: A Cellular Approach to the Function of the Nervous System.* Sunderland, MA, Sinauer Associates, 1984. p 100.

26. Elul R: The genesis of the EEG. *Int Rev Neurobiol* 1972; 15:227.

27. Hille B: *Ionic Channels of Excitable Membranes.* Sunderland, MA, Sinauer Associates, 1992.

28. White EL: *Cortical Circuits. Synaptic Organization of the Cerebral Cortex: Structure, Function, and Theory.* Boston, Birkhäuser, 1989, pp 19–29.

29. Andersen P, Anderson SA: Thalmic origin of cortical rhythmic activity. In Creutzfeldt O (eds): *Handbook of Electroencephalography and Clinical Neurophysiology,* Vol 2C. Amsterdam, Elsevier, 1974, pp 90–118.

30. Steriade M: Cellular substrates of brain rhythms. In Niedermeyer E, Lopes da Silva F (eds): *Electroencephalography: Basic Principles, Clinical Applications, and Related Fields,* 3d ed. Baltimore, Williams & Wilkins, 1993, pp 27–62.

31. McCormick DA, Pape HC: Properties of a hyperpolarization-activated cation current and its role in rhymic oscillation in thalamic relay neurons. *J Physiol (Lond.)* 1990; 431:291.

32. Jonkman EJ, et al: The use of neurometrics in the study of patients with cerebral ischaemia. *Electroencephalogr Clin Neurophysiol* 1985; 61:333.

33. Cooper R, et al: Comparison of subcortical, cortical, and scalp activity using chronically indwelling electrodes in man. *Electroencephalogr Clin Neurophysiol* 1965; 18:217.

34. Hjorth B: An on-line transformation of EEG scalp potentials into orthogonal source derivations. *Electroencephalogr Clin Neurophysiol* 1975; 39:526.

35. Koles ZJ, et al: Computed radial-current topography of the brain: patterns associated with the normal and abnormal EEG. *Electroencephalogr Clin Neurophysiol* 1989; 72:41.

36. Chatrian GE, Lairy GC: The EEG of the waking adult. In Remond AJG (ed): *Handbook of Electroencephalography and Clinical Neurophysiology, vol 6a,* Amsterdam, Elsevier, 1976.

37. Kiloh LG: *Clinical Electroencephalography,* 4th ed. London, Butterworth, 1981.

38. Erwin CW, et al: A review of electroencephalographic features of normal sleep. *J Clin Neurophysiol* 1984; 1:253.

39. Jasper H: Report of committee on methods of clinical exam in EEG. *Electroencephalogr Clin Neurophysiol* 1958; 10:370.

40. Katznelson RD: EEG recording, electrode placement, and aspects of generator localization. In Nunez P (eds): *Electric Fields of the Brain: The Neurophysics of EEG.* New York, Oxford, 1981, pp 176–213.

41. Geddes LA, Baker LE: *Principles of Applied Biomedical Instrumentation.* New York, Wiley-Interscience, 1989, pp 315–452.

42. Spackman TN, et al: A comparison of aperiodic analysis of the EEG with standard EEG and cerebral blood flow for detection of ischemia. *Anesthesiology* 1987; 66:229.

43. Kearse LAJ, et al: Computer-derived density spectral array in detection of mild analog electroencephalographic ischemic

44. International Federation of the Societies of Electroencephalography and Clinical Neurophysiology: *Recommendations for the Practice of Clinical Neurophysiology.* Amsterdam, Elsevier, 1983, p 49.

45. International Federation of the Societies of Electroencephalography and Clinical Neurophysiology: *Recommendations for the Practice of Clinical Neurophysiology.* Amsterdam, Elsevier, 1983, p 64.

46. Blume WT, Sharbrough FW: EEG monitoring during carotid endarterectomy and open heart surgery. In Niedermeyer E, Lopes da Silva F (eds): *Electroencephalography: Basic Principles, Clinical Applications, and Related Fields.* Baltimore, Williams & Wilkins, 1993, pp 747–756.

47. Rampil IJ: Intelligent detection of artifact in the EEG. In Gravenstein JS, et al (eds): *The Automated Anesthesia Record and Alarm Systems.* Boston, Butterworths, 1987, pp 175–190.

48. Isaksson A, Wennberg A: Spectral properties of nonstationary EEG signals, evaluated by means of Kalman filtering: Application examples from a vigilance test. In Kellaway P, Petersén I (eds): *Quantitative Analytic Studies in Epilepsy.* New York, Raven, 1976, pp 389–402.

49. Levy WJ: Effect of epoch length on power spectrum analysis of the EEG. *Anesthesiology* 1987; 66:489.

50. Bodenstein G, Praetorius HM: Feature extraction from the encephalogram by adaptive segmentation. *Proc IEEE* 1977; 65:642.

51. Barlow JS: Methods of analysis of nonstationary EEGs, with emphasis on segmentation techniques: a comparative review. *J Clin Neurophysiol* 1985; 2:267.

52. Lopes da Silva F: EEG Analysis: Theory and Practice. In Niedermeyer E, Lopes da Silva F (eds): *Electroencephalography: Basic Principles, Clinical Applications, and Related Fields,* 3d ed. Baltimore, Williams & Wilkins, 1993, pp 1097–1123.

53. Loomis AL et al: Electrical potentials of the human brain. *J Exp Psychol* 1936; 19:249.

54. Bickford RG: Automatic electroencephalographic control of general anesthesia. *Electroencephalogr Clin Neurophysiol* 1950; 2:93.

55. Brazier MAB: Some actions of anesthetics on the nervous system. *Fed Proc* 1960; 19:626.

56. John ER, et al: Developmental equations for the electroencephalogram. *Science* 1980; 210:1255.

57. Gasser T, et al: Transformation towards the normal distribution of broad band spectral parameters of the EEG. *Electroencephalogr Clin Neurophysiol* 1982; 53:119.

58. Burch NR: Period analysis of the EEG on a general-purpose digital computer. *Ann NY Acad Sci* 1964; 115:827.

59. Klein FF: A waveform analyzer applied to the human EEG. *IEEE Trans Biomed Eng* 1976; 23:246.

60. Pronk RAF, Simons AJR: Automatic recognition of abnormal EEG activity during open heart and carotid surgery. *Electroncephalogr Clin Neurophysiol (EEG Suppl)* 1982; 36:590.

61. Rampil IJ, Smith NT: Comparison of EEG induces during halothane anesthesia. *J Clin Monit* 1985; 1(Abs):89.

62. Rampil IJ, et al: I653 and isoflurane produce similar dose-related changes in the electroencephalogram of pigs. *Anesthesiology* 1988; 69:298.

63. Prior P: *Monitoring Cerebral Function.* Amsterdam, Elsevier/North Holland, 1979.

64. Sechzer PH, Ospina J: Cerebral function monitor: Evaluation in anesthesia/critical care. *Curr Therap Res* 1977; 22:335.

65. Cucchiara RF, et al: An electroencephalographic filter-processor as an indicator of cerebral ischemia during carotid endarterectomy. *Anesthesiology* 1979; 51:77.

pattern changes during carotid endarterectomy. *J Neurosurg* 1993; 78:884.

66. Matousek M, et al: Automatic assessment of randomly selected routine EEG records. In Dolce G KH (ed): *CEAN—Computerized EEG Analysis.* Stuttgart, Fisher, 1975, pp 421–428.

67. Dumermuth G: Fundamentals of spectral analysis in electroencephalography. In Remond A (ed): *EEG Informantics: A Didactic Review of Methods and Applications of EEG Data Processing.* Amsterdam, Elsevier, 1977, pp 83–105.

68. Fleming RA, Smith NT: Density modulation: A technique for the display of three variable data in patient monitoring. *Anesthesiology* 1979; 50:543.

69. Matousek M, Petersén I: Frequency analysis of the EEG in normal children and in normal adolescents. In Kellaway P, Petersén I (eds): *Automation of Clinical Electroencephalography.* New York, Raven, 1973, pp 75–102.

70. Long CW, et al: A comparison of EEG determinants of near-awakening from isoflurane and fentanyl anesthesia. Spectral edge, median power frequency, and delta ratio. *Anesth Analg* 1989; 69:169.

71. Arom KV, et al: Effect of intraoperative intervention on neurologic outcome based on electroencephalographic monitoring during cardiopulmonary bypass. *Ann Thorac Surg* 1989; 48:476.

72. Edmonds HLJ, et al: Quantitative electroencephalographic monitoring during myocardial revascularization predicts postoperative disorientation and improves outcome. *J Thorac Cardiovasc Surg* 1992; 103:555.

73. Stockard JJ, Bickford RG: The neurophysiology of anaesthesia. In Gordon E (ed): *A Basis and Practice of Neuroanaesthesia.* Amsterdam, Elsevier, 1975.

74. Cosgrove RJ, Smolen VF: Systems for automatic feedback-controlled administration of drugs: Analog and digital optimal-adaptive control of thiopental anesthesia. *Proc San Diego Biomed Symp* 1978; 17:261.

75. Young WL, et al: Electroencephalographic monitoring for ischemia during carotid endarterectomy. *J Clin Monit* 1988; 4:78.

76. Sigl JC, Chamoun NG: An introduction to bispectral analysis for the electroencephalogram. *J Clin Monit* 1994; 10:392.

77. Levy WJ: Electroencephalography. In Lake CL (ed): *Clinical Monitoring.* Philadelpha, Saunders, 1990, p 705.

78. Szeto HH: Spectral edge frequency as a simple quantitative measure of the maturation of electrocortical activity. *Pediatr Res* 1990; 27:289.

79. Schwartz AE, et al: Electroencephalographic burst suppression in elderly and young patients anesthetized with isoflurane. *Anesth Analg* 1989; 68:9.

80. Brechner VL: *Practical Electroencephalography for the Anesthesiologist.* Springfield, IL, Charles Thomas, 1962, pp 80–90.

81. Russ W, et al: Spectral analysis of the EEG during hypothermic cardiopulmonary bypass. *Acta Anaesthesiol Scand* 1987; 31:111.

82. Mizrahi EM, et al: Hypothermic-induced electrocerebral silence, prolonged circulatory arrest, and cerebral protection during cardiovascular surgery. *Electroencephalogr Clin Neurophysiol* 1989; 72:81.

83. Quasha AL, et al: Hypothermia plus thiopental: Prolonged electroencephalograph suppression. *Anesthesiology* 1981; 55:636.

84. Rung GW, et al: Thiopental as an adjunct to hypothermia for EEG suppression in infants prior to circulatory arrest. *J Cardiothor Vasc Anesth* 1991; 5:337.

85. Lopez M, et al: Mild core hyperthermia does not alter electroencephalographic responses during epidural-enflurane anesthesia in humans. *J Clin Anesth* 1993; 5:425.

86. Alexander SC, et al: Cerebral carbohydrate metabolism of man during respiratory and metabolic alkalosis. *J Appl Physiol* 1968; 24:66.

87. Yamatani M, et al: Hyperventilation activation on EEG recording in childhood. *Epilepsia* 1994; 35:1199.

88. Achenbach-Ng J, et al: Effects of routine hyperventilation on PCO_2 and PO_2 in normal subjects: Implications for EEG interpretations. *J Clin Neurophysiol* 1994; 11:220.

89. Eisele JH, et al: Narcotic properties of carbon dioxide in the dog. *Anesthesiology* 1967; 28:856.

90. Litt L, et al: Cerebral intracellular ADP concentration during hypercarbia: An *in vivo* ^{31}P nuclear magnetic resonance study in rats. *J Cereb Blood Flow Metab* 1986; 6:389.

91. Smith LJ, et al: Effects of altered arterial carbon dioxide tension on quantitative electroencephalography in halothane-anesthetized dogs. *Am J Vet Res* 1994; 55:467.

92. Kalkman CJ, et al: Influence of changes in arterial carbon dioxide tension on the electroencephalogram and posterior tibial nerve somatosensory cortical evoked potentials during alfentanil/nitrous oxide anesthesia. *Anesthesiology* 1991; 75:68.

93. Rampil IJ, et al: The electroencephalographic effects of desflurane in humans. *Anesthesiology* 1991; 74:434.

94. Ziegler DK, Presthus J: Normal electroencephalogram at deep levels of hypoglycemia. *Electroencephalogr Clin Neurophysiol* 1957; 9:523.

95. Kurtz D: The EEG in parathyroid dysfunction. In Remond A (ed): *Handbook of Electroencephalography and Clinical Neurophysiology,* vol 15C. Amsterdam, Elsevier, 1976, pp 77–87.

96. Corriol J, et al: Electroclinical correlations established during tetanic manifestations induced by parathyroid removal in the dog. In Gastaut H, et al (eds): *The Physiopathogenesis of the Epilepsies.* Springfield, IL, Charles Thomas, 1969, pp 128–140.

97. Spatz R, et al: Zur bedeutung elektroenzephalograpischer veränderungen beim hyperkalzämie-syndrom. *ZEEG-EMG* 1977; 6:14.

98. Pohunkova D, et al: Influence of thyroid hormone supply on EEG frequency spectrum. *Endocrinol Exp* 1989; 23:251.

99. Cohn R, Castell DO: The effect of acute hyperammoniemia on the electroencephalogram. *J Lab Clin Med* 1966; 68:195.

100. Hughes JR: Correlations between EEG and chemical changes in uremia. *Electroencephalogr Clin Neurophysiol* 1980; 48:583.

101. Jones TH, et al: Thresholds of ischemia in awake monkeys. *J Neurosurg* 1981; 54:773.

102. Clute HL, Levy WJ: Electroencephalographic changes during brief cardiac arrest in humans. *Anesthesiology* 1990; 73:821.

103. Konstadt SN, et al: The effects of global normothermic hypoperfusion on the processed electroencephalogram in patients. *J Cardiothorac Vasc Anesth* 1991; 5:214.

104. Niedermeyer E: Cerebrovascular disorders and EEG. In Niedermeyer E, Lopes da Silva F (eds): *Electroencephalography: Basic Principles, Clinical Applications, and Related Fields,* 3d ed. Baltimore, Williams & Wilkins, 1993, pp 311.

105. Beecher HK, et al: Effects of blood pressure changes on cortical potentials during anesthesia. *J Neurophysiol* 1938; 1:324.

106. Pierelli F, et al: Early auditory evoked potential changes during hypoxic hypoxia in the rabbit. *Exp Neurol* 1986; 94:479.

107. Cohen PJ, et al: Effects of hypoxia and normocarbia on cerebral blood flow and metabolism in conscious man. *J Appl Physiol* 1967; 23:183.

108. Hugelin A, et al: Activation réticulaire et corticule d'origine chémoceptive au cours de l'hyoxie. *Electroencephalogr Clin Neurophysiol* 1959; 11:325.

109. Martin JT, et al: Electroencephalography in anesthesiology. *Anesthesiology* 1959; 20:359.

110. Oshima E, et al: EEG activity during halothane anaesthesia in man. *Br J Anaesth* 1981; 53:65.

111. Pichlmayr I, Lips U: Halothane-effekte im elektroencephalogram. *Anaesthesist* 1980; 29:530.

112. Yli-Hankala A, et al: EEG spectral power during halothane

anaesthesia. A comparison of spectral bands in the monitoring of anaesthesia level. *Acta Anaesthesiol Scand* 1989; 33:304.

113. Neigh JL, et al: The electroencephalographic pattern during anesthesia with Ethrane: Effects of depth of anesthesia, P_aCO_2, and nitrous oxide. *Anesthesiology* 1971; 35:482.

114. Clark DL, et al: Neural effects of isoflurane (forane) in man. *Anesthesiology* 1973; 39:261.

115. Eger EI II, et al: The electroencephalogram in man anesthesized with forane. *Anesthesiology* 1971; 35:504.

116. Scheller MS, et al: The effects of sevoflurane on cerebral blood flow, cerebral metabolic rate for oxygen, intracranial pressure, and the electroencephalogram are similar to those of isoflurane in the rabbit. *Anesthesiology* 1988; 68:548.

117. Koitabashi T, et al: Quantitative analysis of electroencephalographic (EEG) activity during sevoflurane anesthesia. *Masui(Jpn J Anesthesiol)* 1992; 41:1946.

118. Tinker JH, et al: Anterior shift of the dominant EEG rhythm during anesthesia in the Java monkey: Correlation with anesthetic potency. *Anesthesiology* 1977; 46:252.

119. Kochs E, et al: Surgical stimulation induces changes in brain electrical activity during isoflurane/nitrous oxide anesthesia. A topographic electroencephalographic analysis. *Anesthesiology* 1994; 80:1026.

120. Scherer GB, et al: Differences in the topographical distribution of EEG activity during surgical anaesthesia and on emergence from volatile anesthetics. *Int J Clin Monit Comput* 1994; 11:179.

121. Lutz LJ, et al: The cerebral functional, metabolic, and hemodynamic effects of desflurane in dogs. *Anesthesiology* 1990; 73:125.

122. Rampil IJ, et al: No EEG evidence of acute tolerance to desflurane in swine. *Anesthesiology* 1991; 74:889.

123. Sugiyama K, et al: Relationship between changes in power spectra of electroencephalograms and arterial halothane concentration in infants. *Acta Anaesthesiol Scand* 1989; 33:670.

124. Kuramoto T, et al: Modification of the relationship between cerebral metabolism, blood flow, and electroencephalogram by stimulation during anesthesia in the dog. *Anesthesiology* 1979; 51:211.

125. Yamamura T, et al: Fast oscillatory EEG activity induced by analgesic concentrations of nitrous oxide in man. *Anesth Analg* 1981; 60:283.

126. Smith NT, et al: Does thiopental or N_2O disrupt the EEG during enflurane? *Anesthesiology* 1979; 51:S4(abstr).

127. Kaieda R, et al: The effects of anesthetics and $PaCO_2$ on the cerebrovascular, metabolic, and electroencephalographic responses to nitrous oxide in the rabbit. *Anesth Analg* 1989; 68:135.

128. Drummond JC, et al: The effect of nitrous oxide on cortical cerebral blood flow during anesthesia with halothane and isoflurane, with and without morphine, in the rabbit. *Anesth Analg* 1987; 66:1083.

129. Yli-Hankala A, et al: Nitrous oxide-mediated activation of the EEG during isoflurane anaesthesia in patients. *Br J Anaesth* 1993; 70:54.

130. Yli-Hankala A: The effect of nitrous oxide on EEG spectral power during halothane and isoflurane anaesthesia. *Acta Anaesthesiol Scand* 1990; 34:579.

131. Avramov MN, et al: Progressive changes in electroencephalographic responses to nitrous oxide in humans: A possible acute drug tolerance. *Anesth Analg* 1990; 70:369.

132. Kiersey DK, et al: Electro-encephalographic patterns produced by thiopental sodium during surgical operations: descriptions and classification. *Br J Anaesth* 1951; 23:141.

133. Clark DL, Rosner BS: Neurophysiologic effects of general anesthetics. I. The electroencephalogram and sensory evoked responses in man. *Anesthesiology* 1973; 38:564.

134. Schwilden H, et al: Closed-loop feedback control of methohexital anesthesia by quantitative EEG analysis in humans. *Anesthesiology* 1987; 67:341.

135. Paul R, Harris R: A comparison of methohexitone and thiopentone in electrocorticography. *J Neurol Neurosurg Psychiatry* 1970; 33:100.

136. Ford EW, et al: Methohexital anesthesia in the surgical treatment of uncontrollable epilepsy. *Anesth Analg* 1982; 61:997.

137. Wyler AR, et al: Methohexital activation of epileptogenic foci during acute electrocorticography. *Epilepsia* 1987; 28:490.

138. Hazeaux C, et al: Electroencephalographic impact of propofol anesthesia. *Ann Fr Anesth Reanim* 1987; 6:261.

139. Seifert HA, et al: Sedative doses of propofol increase beta activity of the processed electroencephalogram. *Anesth Analg* 1993; 76:976.

140. Ghoneim MM, Yamada T: Etomidate: A clinical and electroencephalographic comparison with thiopental. *Anesth Analg* 1977; 56:479.

141. Doneicke A, et al: Plasma concentration and EEG after various regimens of etomidate. *Br J Anaesth* 1982; 54:393.

142. Reddy RV, et al: Excitatory effects and electroencephalographic correlation of etomidate, thiopental, methohexital, and propofol. *Anesth Analg* 1993; 77:1008.

143. Borgeat A, et al: Propofol and spontaneous movements: An EEG study. *Anesthesiology* 1991; 74:24.

144. Ebrahim ZY, et al: Effect of etomidate on the electroencephalogram of patients with epilepsy. *Anesth Analg* 1986; 65:1004.

145. Milde LN, et al: Cerebral functional, metabolic and hemodynamic effects of etomidate in dogs. *Anesthesiology* 1985; 63:371.

146. Samra SK, et al: Effects of propofol sedation on seizures and intracranially recorded epileptiform activity in patients with partial epilepsy. *Anesthesiology* 1995; 82:843.

147. Rampil IJ, et al: Propofol sedation may disrupt interictal epileptiform activity from a seizure focus. *Anesth Analg* 1993; 77:1071.

148. Batjer HH, et al: Use of etomidate, temporary arterial occlusion, and intraoperative angiography in surgical treatment of large and giant cerebral aneurysms. *J Neurosurg* 1988; 68:234.

149. McPherson RW, et al: Effects of thiopental, fentanyl, and etomidate on upper extremity somatosensory evoked potentials in humans. *Anesthesiology* 1986; 65:584.

150. Schultz A, et al: Ketamine effects in electroencephalograms: Typical patterns and spectralanalytic profiles. *Anaesthesist* 1990; 39:222.

151. Modica PA, et al: Pro- and anticonvulsant effects of anesthetics (Part II). *Anesth Analg* 1990; 80:433.

152. Greenblatt DJ, et al: Pharmacokinetic and elecroencephalographic study of intravenous diazepam, midazolam, and placebo. *Clin Pharmacol Ther* 1989; 45:356.

153. Fink M, et al: Blood levels and electroencephalographic effects of diazepam and bromazepam. *Clin Pharmacol Ther* 1976; 20:184.

154. Veselis RA, et al: The EEG as a monitor of midazolam amnesia: Changes in power and topography as a function of amnesic state. *Anesthesiology* 1991; 74:866.

155. Fleischer JE, et al: Cerebral effects of high-dose midazolam and subsequent reversal with RO 15-1788 in dogs. *Anesthesiology* 1988; 68:234.

156. Chi OZ, et al: Power spectral analysis of EEG during sufentanil infusion in humans. *Can J Anaesth* 1991; 38:275.

157. Sebel PS, et al: Effects of high-dose fentanyl anesthesia on the electroencephalogram. *Anesthesiology* 1981; 55:203.

158. Wauquier A, et al: Electroencephalographic effects of fentanyl sufentanil and alfentanil anaesthesia in man. *Neuropsychobiology* 1984; 11:203.

159. Benthuysen JL, et al: Physiology of alfentanil-induced rigidity. *Anesthesiology* 1986; 64:440.

160. Weinger MB, et al: Brain sites mediating opiate-induced mus-

cle rigidity in the rat: Methylnaloxonium mapping study. *Brain Res* 1991; 544:181.

161. de Castro J, et al: Comparative study of cardiovascular, neurological and metabolic side effects of 8 narcotics in dogs. Pethidine, piritramide, morphine, phenoperidine, fentanyl, R 39 209, sufentanil, R 34 995. II. Comparative study on the epileptoid activity of the narcotics used in high and massive doses in curarised and mechanically ventilated dogs. *Acta Anaesthesiol Belg* 1979; 30:55.

162. Gabriel A, et al: Clonidine: An adjunct in isoflurane N_2O/O_2 relaxant anaesthesia. Effects on EEG power spectra, somatosensory and auditory evoked potentials. *Anaesthesia* 1995; 50:290.

163. Buhrer M, et al: Dexmedetomidine decreases thiopental dose requirement and alters distribution pharmacokinetics. *Anesthesiology* 1994; 80:1216.

164. Lanier WL, et al: Cerebral stimulation following succinylcholine in dogs. *Anesthesiology* 1986; 64:551.

165. Schwartz AE, et al: Pancuronium increases the duration of electroencephalographic burst suppression in dogs anesthetized with isoflurane. *Anesthesiology* 1992; 77:686.

166. Chapple DJ, et al: Cardiovascular and neurological effects of laudanosine: Studies in mice and rats, and in conscious and anaesthetized dogs. *Br J Anaesth* 1987; 59:218.

167. Shi W, et al: Laudanosine (a metabolite of atracurium) increases the minimum alveolar concentration of halothane in rabbits. *Anesthesiology* 1985; 63:584.

168. Szenohradszky J, et al: Central nervous system effects of intrathecal muscle relaxants in rats. *Anesth Analg* 1993; 76:1304.

169. Baker JD, et al: An evaluation of electroencephalographic monitoring for carotid surgery. *Surgery* 1975; 78:787.

170. Blackshear WM, et al: Advantages of continuous electroencephalographic monitoring during carotid surgery. *J Cardiovasc Surg* 1986; 27:146.

171. Cho I, et al: The value of intraoperative EEG monitoring during carotid endarterectomy. *Ann Neurol* 1986; 20:508.

172. Sundt TM, et al: Correlation of cerebral blood flow and electroencephalographic changes during carotid endarterectomy with results of surgery and hemodynamics of cerebral ischemia. *Mayo Clin Proc* 1981; 56:533.

173. Chiappa KH, et al: Results of electroencephalographic monitoring during 376 endarterectomies: Use of a dedicated minicomputer. *Stroke* 1979; 10:381.

174. Russ W, et al: Experience with a new spectral analysing system (CSA) during carotid surgery. *Anaesthesist* 1985; 34:85.

175. Baker AB, Roxburgh AJ: Computerised EEG monitoring for carotid endarterectomy. *Anaesth Intensive Care* 1986; 14:32.

176. Silbert BS, et al: The processed electroencephalogram may not detect neurologic ischemia during carotid endarterectomy. *Anesthesiology* 1989; 70:356.

177. Bowdle TA, et al: Intraoperative stroke during carotid endarterectomy without a change in spectral edge frequency of the compressed spectral array. *J Cardiothorac Anesth* 1988; 2:204.

178. Sundt TM: The ischemic tolerance of neural tissue and the need for monitoring and selective shunting during carotid endarterectomy. *Stroke* 1983; 14:93.

179. Ferguson GG: Intraoperative monitoring and internal shunts: Are they necessary in carotid endarterectomy? *Stroke* 1982; 13:287.

180. Tempelhoff R, et al: Selective shunting during carotid endarterectomy based on two-channel computerized electroencephalographic/compressed spectral array analysis. *Neurosurgery* 1989; 24:339.

181. Rampil IJ, et al: Computerized EEG monitoring and carotid artery shunting. *Neurosurgery* 1983; 13:276.

182. Smith JS, et al: Does anesthetic technique make a difference?

Augmentation of systolic blood pressure during carotid endarterectomy: Effects of phenylephrine versus light anesthesia and of isoflurane versus halothane on the incidence of myocardial ischemia. *Anesthesiology* 1988; 69:846.

183. Hicks RG, et al: Thiopentone cerebral protection under EEG control during carotid endarterectomy. *Anaesth Intensive Care* 1986; 14:22.

184. Frawley JE, et al: Thiopental sodium cerebral protection during carotid endarterectomy: Perioperative disease and death. *J Vasc Surg* 1994; 19:732.

185. Jansen C, et al: Impact of microembolism and hemodynamic changes in the brain during carotid endarterectomy. *Stroke* 1994; 25:992.

186. Soltaniemi KA: Cerebral outcome after extracorporeal circulation. *Arch Neurol* 1983; 40:75.

187. Scientific Evaluation of Medical Technology. *Federal Register,* March 3, 1981, p 14972.

188. National Center of Health Services Research: *Public Health Service Assessment of EEG Monitoring During Open Heart Surgery,* V3(1). Department of Health and Human Services, Rockville, MD, 1983.

189. Michaels I, Sheehan J: EEG changes due to unsuspected aortic dissection during cardiopulmonary bypass. *Anesth Analg* 1984; 63:946.

190. el-Fiki M, Fish KJ: Is the EEG a useful monitor during cardiac surgery? A case report. *Anesthesiology* 1987; 67:757.

191. Steele ER, et al: Compressed spectral array EEG monitoring during coronary bypass surgery in a patient with vertebrobasilar artery insufficiency. *Anesth Analg* 1987; 66:271.

192. Nussmeier NA, et al: Neuropsychiatric complications after cardiopulmonary bypass: Cerebral protection by a barbiturate. *Anesthesiology* 1986; 64:165.

193. Zaidan JR, et al: Effect of thiopental on neurologic outcome following coronary artery bypass grafting. *Anesthesiology* 1991; 74:406.

194. Adams DC, et al: The reliability of quantitative electroencephalography as an indicator of cerebral ischemia. *Anesth Analg* 1995; 81:80.

195. Todd MM, et al: The neurologic effects of thiopental therapy following experimental cardiac arrest in cats. *Anesthesiology* 1982; 57:76.

196. Pappas TN, Mironovich RO: Barbiturate-induced coma to protect against cerebral ischemia and increased intracranial pressure. *Am J Hosp Pharm* 1981; 38:494.

197. Smith DS, et al: Barbiturates as protective agents in brain ischemia and as free radical scavengers in vitro. *Acta Physiol Scand Suppl* 1980; 492:129.

198. Sano T, et al: A comparison of the cerebral protective effects of etomidate, thiopental, and isoflurane in a model of forebrain ischemia in the rat. *Anesth Analg* 1993; 76:990.

199. Metz S, Slogoff S: Thiopental sodium by single bolus dose compared to infusion for cerebral protection during cardiopulmonary bypass. *J Clin Anesth* 1990; 2:226.

200. Rampil IJ, Matteo RS: Changes in EEG spectral edge frequency correlates with the hemodynamic response to laryngoscopy and intubation. *Anesthesiology* 1987; 67:139.

201. Sidi A, et al: Estimating anesthetic depth by electroencephalography during anesthetic induction and intubation in patients undergoing cardiac surgery. *J Clin Anesth* 1990; 2:101.

202. Ghouri AF, et al: Electroencephalogram spectral edge frequency, lower esophageal contractility, and autonomic responsiveness during general anesthesia. *J Clin Monit* 1993; 9:176.

203. Rampil IJ, Laster MJ: No correlation between quantitative electroencephalographic measurements and movement response

to noxious stimuli during isoflurane anesthesia in rats. *Anesthesiology* 1992; 77:920.

204. Hung OR, et al: Thiopental pharmacodynamics. II. Quantitation of clinical and electroencephalographic depth of anesthesia. *Anesthesiology* 1992; 77:237.

205. Dwyer RC, et al: The electroencephalogram does not predict depth of isoflurane anesthesia. *Anesthesiology* 1994; 81:403.

206. Sebel PS, et al: Bispectral analysis for monitoring anesthesia—a multicenter study. *Anesthesiology* 1993; 79:A178(abstr).

207. Rampil IJ, et al: Anesthetic potency (MAC) is independent of forebrain structures in the rat. *Anesthesiology* 1993; 78:707.

208. Rampil IJ: Anesthetic potency is not altered after hypothermic spinal cord transection in rats. *Anesthesiology* 1994; 80:606.

209. Drummond JC, et al: A comparison of median frequency, spectral edge frequency, a frequency band power ratio, total power, and dominance shift in the determination of depth of anesthesia. *Acta Anaesthesiol Scand* 1991; 35:693.

210. Levy WJ: Power spectrum correlates of changes in consciousness during anesthetic induction with enflurane. *Anesthesiology* 1986; 64:688.

211. Withington PS, et al: Assessment of power spectral edge for monitoring depth of anaesthesia using low methohexitone infusion. *Int J Clin Monit Comput* 1986; 3:117.

212. Kearse L, et al: The bispectral index correlates with sedation/hypnosis and recall: Comparison using multiple agents. *Anesthesiology* 1995; 83:A507.

213. Flaishon R, et al: Detection of consciousness following thiopental: Isolated forearm and bispectral EEG (BIS). *Anesthesiology* 1995;83:A515.

Chapter 7

EVOKED POTENTIALS

TOD B. SLOAN

Basic Evoked Potential Technology

Although the technology used is relatively sophisticated, evoked potentials are rather simple in concept, and several excellent books have been written on their use.[1-4] Whereas the electroencephalogram (EEG) is the measurement of the spontaneous electrical activity of the brain (cerebral cortex), evoked potentials are a measurement of the electrical potentials produced in response to a stimulus ("evoked"). They allow assessment of defined neural tracts, including peripheral and subcortical regions. They have gained popularity because they can be measured without patient cooperation. Thus they are useful for diagnosis of patients during altered states of consciousness (e.g., head trauma), during anesthesia (e.g., intraoperative monitoring), and during sedative therapy (e.g., barbiturate coma).

The most commonly utilized evoked potentials are those produced by stimulation of the sensory system, the sensory evoked potentials (SEPs). The three commonly used types include somatosensory evoked potential (SSEP), in which peripheral nerves are stimulated using electric pulses sufficient to depolarize the nerve; brainstem auditory evoked response (BAER), produced by stimulation in the ear with brief sound bursts; and visual evoked potentials (VEP), produced by stimulation of the eye by light.

Since these evoked electrical potentials are very small (less than 10 μV), signal averaging is used to resolve them from the much larger EEG and electrocardiogram (ECG) activity. This method involves stimulating the nervous system and measuring the response for a set window of time (the time to see the activity of interest). A second stimulation follows and the electrical activity at each time point following stimulation is averaged. This is repeated for several hundred or thousand times, and the evoked response becomes apparent. This occurs because the unwanted background activity (noise) averages to zero, since it is unrelated to the stimulus. However, since the desired signal always follows the stimulation by a set time (it is related to the stimulus), it consistently builds while the noise is diminished. Technically, the ratio of the signal to noise builds by the square root of the number of averages. Because of this need for signal averaging, evoked potentials did not become widely available until the development of inexpensive digital computer averagers (Fig. 7-1).

A typical evoked response consists of a plot of voltage versus time (Fig. 7-2). The voltage is measured using three electrodes. A differential amplifier compares the activity of an active electrode (placed near the neural structure producing the desired electrical activity) with the activity at a reference electrode somewhere else. This difference is compared with a ground electrode and presented to the averager after filtering and converting to digital information. This use of a differential amplifier allows removal of a large amount of noise which is common to all of the electrodes. This plot of voltage versus time typically has an artifact of stimulation at time zero (coincident with the stimulation) and then a subsequent series of peaks and valleys at later times. Peaks may be positive or negative (with respect to the active electrode) and may be plotted upward or downward depending on the convention of the technique and individual. Peaks are often labeled by the polarity [positive (P) or negative (N)] followed by the time in milliseconds from stimulation. Hence the cortical N_{20} of the median nerve SSEP is a negative peak occurring about 20 ms after stimulation. Some responses have peaks defined by convention using roman numerals (brainstem auditory evoked response)

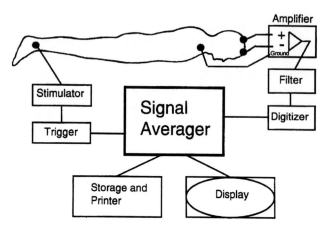

Figure 7-1 Block diagram of evoked potential machine. An evoked potential machine consists of stimulating and recording components that are synchronized by a trigger. At the same time the trigger activates the stimulation to the nervous system, it begins the signal acquisition process. The evoked response is recorded via three patient electrodes. The active (+) and reference (−) electrodes are amplified by a differential amplifier and compared to a ground electrode. The resulting signal is filtered to remove extraneous noise and converted to digital information for processing by the averager. After a sufficient number of responses are averaged, the response can be stored, printed, and displayed. For some responses (particularly muscle responses), the output can also be played through a loudspeaker for audible feedback.

or letters (cortical auditory response, electroretinogram).

The peaks (and valleys) are thought to arise from specific neural generators (often more than one neural structure) and therefore can be used to follow the response at various points along the stimulated tract. The information recorded is usually the amplitude (peak to adjacent trough) and the time from the stimulation to the peak (called latency). In addition, the time between peaks (interwave latency or conduction time) is occasionally measured.

SOMATOSENSORY EVOKED RESPONSES

The electrophysiologic technique with the greatest degree of potential use is the somatosensory evoked po-

tential (SSEP). In this technique a peripheral nerve is stimulated and the neural response is measured. Stimulation produces both dromic (propagating in the normal direction) and antidromic (propagating opposite to normal) neural transmission in both the sensory and motor pathways. The dromic motor stimulation elicits a muscle response and the dromic sensory response initiates the SSEP. Nerves stimulated tend to be large mixed motor and sensory nerves (e.g., posterior tibial, common peroneal, ulnar, and median), although pure sensory nerves can also be used. Mixed nerves have an advantage over pure sensory nerves in that stimulation of the nerve can be verified by motor activity in peripheral muscles. Recordings can be made over the peripheral structures (e.g., peripheral nerves, brachial plexus) during muscle relaxation to confirm stimulation (Fig. 7-3).[2]

The length of the neural tract involved makes the SSEP potentially one of the most widely usable monitors because of the many neural structures that can be assessed (peripheral nerves, plexus components, spinal cord tracts, brainstem structures, and sensory cortex). The interwave latency between the response recorded over the cervical spine (thought to be a response of brainstem structures) and the response recorded over the sensory cortex has been of particular interest and is termed *central conduction time* (CCT).

It is currently thought that the incoming volley of neural activity from the upper extremity represents primarily the activity in the pathway of proprioception and vibration. Stimulation of the peripheral nerve causes a response that ascends the ipsilateral dorsal column, synapses near the nucleus cuneatus, decussates near the cervicomedullary junction, ascends via the contralateral medial lemniscus, synapses in the ventroposterolateral nucleus of the thalamus, and finally projects to the contralateral parietal sensory cortex (Fig. 7-3).[5] The response from the lower extremity is anatomically similar to that of the upper extremity except that a portion of the response appears to travel via anterolateral spinal pathways (see below).

An occasional patient who exhibits a motor deficit when the SSEP is unaltered highlights the anatomy

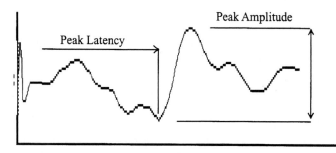

Time after Stimulation (milliseconds)

Figure 7-2 Typical evoked potential response. A typical evoked response consists of a plot of average voltage (vertical) versus time after stimulation (horizontal). Normally seen is a voltage deflection at the time of stimulation due to the electrical effect of the stimulator (artifact of stimulation). The peak of interest (corresponding to the neural generators desired for assessment) is measured by the time from stimulation ("latency") and amplitude (measured peak to adjacent peak of opposite polarity).

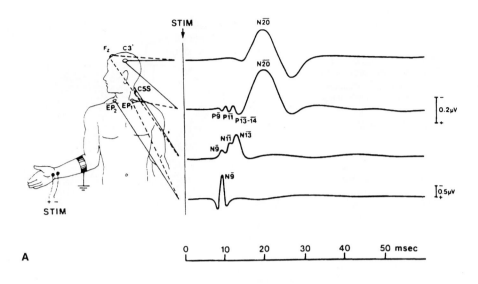

A

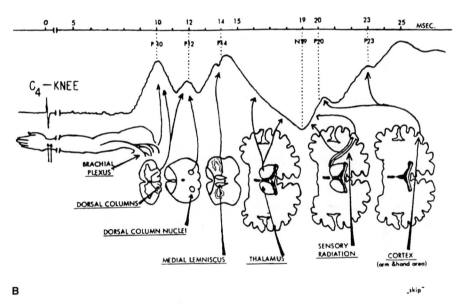

Figure 7-3 Example of the somatosensory evoked potential. The upper extremity (median n.) SSEP can be recorded at several locations (*A*) including the antecubital fossa (not shown), Erb's point (EP2—over the brachial plexus), cervical spine (C5S), and with various electrode combinations over the sensory cortex. (Reproduced with permission from Spehlmann R.[2]) Shown in *B* is the corresponding anatomy of the peaks of the median nerve SSEP. [Reproduced with permission from Weiderholt WC, et al: Stimulating and recording methods used in obtaining short-latency somatosensory evoked potentials (SSEPs) in patients with central and peripheral neurologic disorders. *Ann NY Acad Sci* 388:349, 1982.]

B

involved in the SSEP. The intensity used for SSEP stimulation evokes a response in the motor axons (resulting in peripheral muscle activity), but this response fails to ascend the spinal cord, due to interruption of the motor pathway in the anterior horn cell. Larger sensory axons are also stimulated and pass to the central nervous system. Ventrolateral pain pathways are not stimulated.[6] The responses recorded from stimulation of the upper extremity are thought to be primarily those traveling in the dorsal column–medial lemniscal pathways associated with proprioception and vibration. Recordings following stimulation of the lower extremity appear to include additional components that pass in the spinocerebellar pathways.[6,7] The contribution of the spinocerebellar pathways located more anteriorly in the spinal cord may explain why the SSEP is altered

in anterior cord ischemia and correlates with motor function[8] (Fig. 7-4).

DERMATOMAL EVOKED POTENTIALS

Several variations of SSEP have been developed in order to overcome some of the anatomic limitations of the evoked response. One problem of the traditional SSEP is that the response travels into the cord via several nerve roots. Hence the SSEP may not reflect pathology in only one component root. Dermatomal evoked potentials (DEPs) were developed to overcome this problem (Fig. 7-5).[9–12] The DEP is produced by stimulation of specified cutaneous dermatomal regions. The specific anatomic paths stimulated by the DEP are unknown, but the amplitude of the cortically

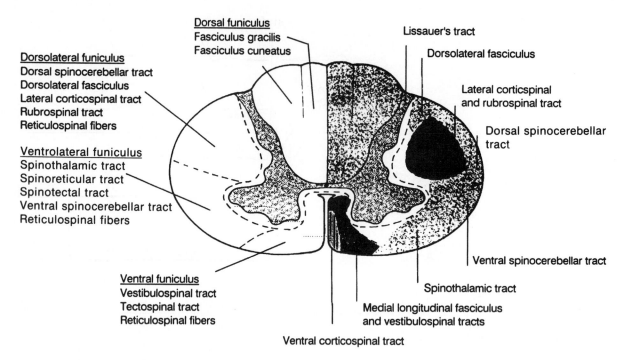

Figure 7-4 Cross section of spinal cord indicating the location of various neural pathways. (Reproduced with permission from Hickey et al.[8])

recorded response appears to be related to the somatotopic representation of the dermatome. Using this method individual nerve roots can be tested. This also allows testing of spinal function in regions without mixed nerves such as the thoracic region. Unfortunately, controversy surrounds the exact dermatome distribution in some regions (e.g., L_5), and poor amplitude of responses in areas of regions with small cerebral representation (such as the thoracic region) limit this technique to some extent.

BRAINSTEM AUDITORY EVOKED RESPONSES

A second widely used evoked response is the brainstem auditory evoked response (BAER) (Fig. 7-6). The BAER is produced when sound activates the cochlea following transmission through the external and middle ear. Vibrations activate the hair cells in the cochlea which results in a nerve impulse that travels to the brainstem via the eighth cranial nerve. The nerve impulse travels via the brainstem acoustic relay nuclei and lemniscal pathways until the cortical auditory cortex is activated. Numerous reviews have been published concerning assessment of the hearing system with BAER.[13-22]

In the first 10 ms after stimulation, three major peaks are usually seen: wave I is generated by the extracranial portion of cranial nerve VIII; wave III from the auditory pathway nuclei in the pons; and wave V from high pons or midbrain (lateral lemniscus and inferior colliculus).[17,22] Occasionally a wave II is seen, and wave IV may be resolvable from V (IV and V often blend together).

The neural pathway of the BAER appears to follow the normal hearing pathways (Fig. 7-6). Responses to auditory stimulation can also be recorded over the auditory cortex (cortical AEP) (Fig. 7-7) or cortical association areas (response about 300 ms after auditory stimulation, P300). These responses appear to be related to the auditory sensory cortex and cerebral cognitive function areas, respectively.

BAER testing is frequently conducted outside of the operating room using stimulation with "clicks" delivered by headphones. These clicks have a broad spectrum of frequency content, with significant stimulation in the 1000 to 4000 hertz (Hz) range. Clicks are classified as "condensing" if the initial sound wave is moving toward the tympanic membrane and "rarefaction" if the sound wave is initially moving away. These two stimuli produce slightly different responses. Often, stimulation that alternates between the two will be used ("alternating"), so that the electrical artifact of stimulation is canceled. Other types of sound have also been used for stimulation, including tone "pips," which have a more defined frequency content.

Usually only one ear is stimulated at a time, in order to focus on the neural pathway from that ear. Since the stimulation sound is conducted through the bone, it may also stimulate the contralateral cochlea. In order to further reduce this contribution from the nonstimu-

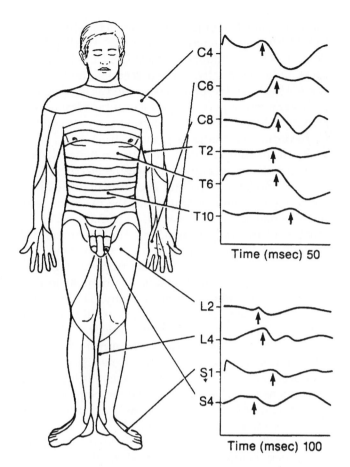

Figure 7-5   Dermatomal evoked potentials can be recorded over the sensory cortex following cutaneous stimulation at several dermatome levels. (Reproduced with permission from Sloan et al.[12])

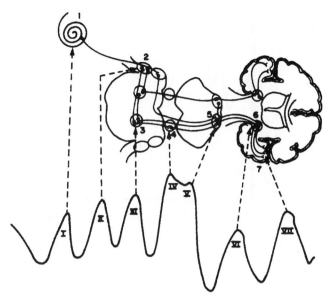

Figure 7-6   Normal BAER tracing and its generators. Peaks I through VII of the BAER are produced by neural generators near (1) organ of Corti and extracranial c.n. VIII; (2) cochlear nucleus; (3) superior olivary complex; (4) lateral lemniscus; (5) inferior colliculus; (6) medial geniculate body; (7) auditory radiation. (Reproduced with permission from Aravabhumi et al.[22])

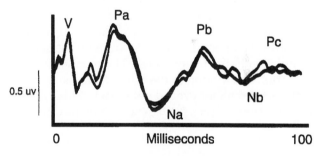

Figure 7-7   Example of cortical AEP recorded over the parietal cortex. Wave V of the BAER can be seen in the first 10 ms, followed by the cortical peaks (Pa, Na, Pb, Nb, and Pc).

lated ear, "white" noise may be delivered to that ear to mask the bone conducted click.

VISUAL EVOKED RESPONSES

Visual evoked potentials (VEPs) are produced by light stimulation of the eyes (Fig. 7-8). The most effective stimulation appears to be one with very high contrast, such as a checkerboard on which squares alternate between white and black. This requires that the patient focus on the stimulation pattern but allows stimulation of select portions of the visual field (e.g., hemifields, quadrants). For patients unable to focus or cooperate, VEPs also can be produced by light flash stimulation, including through the closed eyes. The VEP response appears different for these two types of stimulation and may not measure the same physiologic response. The traditional VEPs are recorded by electrodes over the occipital cortex and appear to be generated by the visual cortex.[1]

The neural response to visual stimulation can be recorded by electrodes placed near the eye. These re-

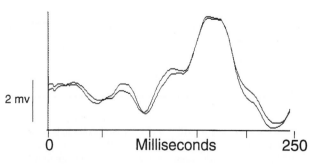

Figure 7-8   Typical VEP to light emitting diode stimulation recorded over the occipital cortex.

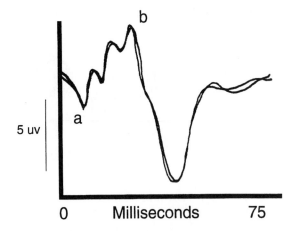

Figure 7-9 Typical electroretinogram (ERG) to flash stimulation recorded from electrodes placed near the eye.

sponses are of the retina and are termed the electroretinogram (ERG) (Fig. 7-9). By manipulating the color and intensity of the stimulus, the responses of the rods and cones can be separated.

MOTOR EVOKED RESPONSES

Because motor function is often considered more important clinically than sensory function, efforts have focused on the development of evoked responses from the motor system. The earliest attempts to produce motor evoked potentials (MEPs) were by transcranial stimulation of the motor cortex. The pioneering work of Merton and Morton in 1980[23] has led to the transcranial electrical motor evoked potential (tcEMEP) monitoring system[24-30] (Fig. 7-10). A second method utilized

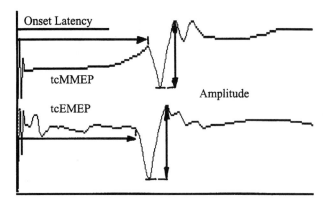

Figure 7-10 Examples of transcranial magnetic (*top*, tcMMEP) and electrical (*bottom*, tcEMEP) motor evoked potentials recorded in the hand. Measurements of the recorded compound muscle action potential include onset latency (time to the beginning of the complex) and amplitude (measured from most negative to most positive peak of the complex).

for transcranial stimulation is magnetic stimulation (tcMMEP), as pioneered by Barker[23,28,29,31-33] (Fig. 7-10). Both of these techniques produce sufficient intracortical stimulation to activate the descending motor pathways. The evoked response is recorded as the resultant peripheral motor nerve response or peripheral muscle activity, CMAP (compound muscle action potential), by recording electrodes near these structures.

The major clinical difference between these two cortical stimulation techniques is that the electrical technique is moderately painful because cutaneous pain receptors are stimulated, whereas the magnetic technique is painless (as long as direct stimulation of the muscles of the scalp is avoided). For this reason the magnetic technique is favored in awake patients.

These techniques also differ electrophysiologically. Transcranial electrical stimulation is thought to activate the corticospinal neurons directly. The resulting descending volley of activity in the spinal tracts consists of a "D" wave followed by a series of "I" waves produced by additional cortical activation from cortical internuncial activity. In contrast, magnetic stimulation produces only the "I" waves,[28,29] except at high magnetic intensities where a "D" wave can be produced.[34] The presence of a D wave explains the shorter onset-latency of the electrical technique and the differences in susceptibility of the two techniques to anesthetic drugs (see below). These cortical stimulation techniques both produce pure motor tract stimulation that passes down the lateral corticospinal and ventral corticospinal tracts.[35] Synaptic blocking of transmission in sensory pathways prevents antidromic sensory pathway activation.

Transcranial stimulation of the cerebellum has also been studied.[25] This appears to produce a response in the vestibulospinal, rubrospinal, fastigiospinal, and reticulospinal pathways. Although these latter pathways may be more important for ambulation, the transcranial techniques remain the focus of most transcranial monitoring techniques.

The descending D and I waves travel to the anterior horn cells in the spinal cord. When sufficient D and I waves have activated the anterior horn cell, a descending wave travels out along the motor components of the peripheral nerve, and a muscle response is elicited. Recording methodology is similar for MEP and SEP, except that under most circumstances the MEP response is much larger, requiring fewer signal averages to resolve the signal. In the case of recording MEP by the muscle response, the compound muscle action potential (CMAP) response (recorded by electrodes placed near the muscle belly) is often sufficiently large that only a single stimulation is utilized, and averaging is not required. This single response capability is fortunate for tcMMEP, because stimulation rates are slow due to the time needed to recharge the magnetic impulse device and allow the heat produced in the stimulation probe to be dissipated.[36]

The MEP response generated in the underlying motor nerve or the muscle near the recording electrode is measured similar to the SEP (Fig. 7-10). Latency of onset is measured as the time from stimulation to the beginning of the peak. Amplitude is measured as the peak to peak voltage of the response. As with the SEP, the latency of onset is a measure of average conduction velocity, and amplitude is a measure of the response strength. In addition to latency and amplitude, some researchers refer to threshold. The threshold is the lowest amount of magnetic or electrical energy that still elicits an MEP response. This is presumably a measure of the ease of motor cortex stimulation. By varying the stimulator location on the scalp, a wide variety of motor nerves and muscle groups can be tested.

It should be noted that the safety of the MEP technique has not been resolved entirely. It is possible that delivering energy to the cerebral cortex by either electrical or magnetic means may produce a cerebral injury resulting in a seizure focus (kindling). A variety of theoretical and practical considerations suggest that injury is unlikely with the current methodology.[37] Further, many individuals have been studied, suggesting that if injury does occur it is rare. Activation of a latent seizure focus may occur in an individual with epilepsy. Attempts to activate seizure foci in known well-controlled epileptics using magnetic stimulation have failed to produce seizures. However, a magnetic stimulator was able to activate the seizure focus in 12 of 13 patients with medically intractable complex partial seizures.[38] Because the magnetic stimulus did not produce seizure foci outside of the known epileptic focus, the magnetic technique was suggested as a method of activating and identifying seizure foci prior to surgical ablation.[38] Hence, the unmasking of a latent epileptic is possible.

MULTIMODALITY EP

Multimodality evoked potentials are testing schemes that use some combination of these evoked responses (most commonly including SSEP and BAER). Such testing appears to have a greater degree of usefulness than individual studies, since the combination allows assessment of different areas of the CNS.

Diagnostic Uses of Evoked Potentials

Evoked responses have a variety of uses for assessment of the nervous system. As diagnostic tools, they can be used for objective, quantifiable measurements of neural function. For example, they have been utilized in the diagnosis of acoustic neuroma (BAER) and multiple sclerosis (VEP). Perhaps the most important usage has been to assess neural tracts when a clinical examination is not feasible. Assessments of patients with head injury, with spinal cord injury, and during surgical procedures conducted with general anesthesia are important applications.

ELECTROPHYSIOLOGIC ASSESSMENT IN HEAD INJURY

Electrophysiologic evaluation of head-injured patients using sensory evoked potentials has been utilized in many centers. The neurologic assessment of the head-injured patient using a clinical examination may be limited by sedative drugs, neuromuscular blocking agents, or deep coma. Electrophysiologic testing using the EEG or sensory evoked potentials (SEPs) has been suggested as an adjunct to the clinical exam or as a replacement when the latter cannot be performed.

In contrast to studies such as computed tomography or magnetic resonance imaging, which assess structure, the electrophysiologic studies evaluate the functioning of the central nervous system (CNS) structures being tested. This utility in functional assessment has led to the use of electrophysiologic studies for diagnosis, guidance of management, observation of the effects of therapeutic maneuvers, monitoring of viability, and estimation of prognosis for recovery. Review of the literature suggests that these monitoring modalities can be integrated effectively into care of the head-injury patient.

The utility of SEPs during head-injury management includes assessment of neurologic function in specific neural pathways, as well as detection of further CNS insults that occur from secondary processes. SEPs have been shown to be responsive to conditions such as hypoxia, hypotension, elevated intracranial pressure (ICP), cerebral edema, and the formation of delayed mass lesions that can serve as secondary injury forces.[39] Suggestions for the use of SEPs in the ICU include (1) as an adjunct to the clinical neurologic examination; (2) as a diagnostic tool to localize neurologic injury; (3) to monitor the clinical condition for deterioration, or to assess the effectiveness of therapy; (4) to assess the adequacy for the CNS of routinely measured physiologic variables; (5) to assist in determining the prognosis for outcome; and (6) to assist in the determination of brain death.

SEPs have been advocated because they are much less affected by analgesic and sedative drugs than the EEG. Even during barbiturate coma, when the EEG is near isoelectric, the SSEP and BAER can still be recorded. The responses are not, however, without technical problems. For example, with SSEP, edema and swelling may make peripheral nerve stimulation difficult, and spinal cord or peripheral nerve injury may preclude SSEP recording despite normal brainstem and cortical function. Similarly, head trauma frequently has associated injury to the external hearing apparatus (external or middle ear, cochlea, or cranial nerve VIII),[40-44] and preexisting hearing abnormalities may also make recording or interpretation of BAER difficult. Further, since evoked responses are small, electrical noise in the intensive care unit (ICU) may make their measurement a challenge.

Despite these limitations, a variety of studies with SSEP suggest that it can play a role in the diagnosis of cerebral dysfunction from ischemia and from elevated ICP.[45] The CCT has been used as an index of some of these generalized variables. As opposed to the BAER, the CCT and cortical components of the SSEP can be used to assess neurological function at a higher CNS level.

Studies in ICU patients have identified several situations in which neurologic assessment by BAER has been useful.[40] BAERs have been correlated with the level of structural coma and the site of lesions in the brainstem, and have been proposed as a quantitative means of grading neurologic status.[40] Other uses include assistance in evaluating patients during chemical sedation or paralysis, when the clinical examination is rendered useless. It has also been found useful with deep coma and after hypoxic episodes. When intracranial pressure is elevated, BAER can be used to identify uncal herniation.[40] In one study, the BAER was able to warn of impending disaster by changing before pupillary signs occurred.[39]

BAER has also been advocated when contemplating the diagnosis of brain death (e.g., the presence of peripheral nerve VIII activity with no peaks present from the brainstem).[46] Although most criteria for brain death utilize the clinical examination and EEG, the BAER can potentially assist in diagnosis during periods when a question arises about the EEG because of the effect of residual sedative drugs. Advocates suggest that the BAER may allow a more prompt diagnosis that then facilitates expeditious and proper patient management.

In general the VEP has not been reported to be of as much usefulness as BAER or SSEP. York has described the use of an early peak as a noninvasive measure of elevated ICP.[47] This has prompted its use for ICU monitoring and for risk assessment for elevated ICP in head injury, where clinical evaluation might otherwise suggest the patient does not have elevated ICP. Perhaps the most favorable reports of the usefulness of the VEP have been where the response of the retina (electroretinogram) and VEP were simultaneously recorded.[48] These studies suggested that this combination could detect optic nerve injury and other organic visual system defects.

ASSESSMENT OF OUTCOME IN HEAD INJURY

The enthusiasm for the use of SEP for prognostic information gained momentum in the 1970s when several investigators integrated these studies into ICU care. In general, the predictive value of the SEP may be superior to the EEG, because many of the extraneous factors that influence the EEG (e.g., sedative medications) have a markedly reduced effect on the SSEP.

Of the SEP types, the SSEP has enjoyed the most favorable results for outcome prediction. Several studies have suggested that the SSEP from median nerve stimulation is capable of predicting both favorable and unfavorable outcomes with a high degree of accuracy.[47-71] Grading schemes for classifying SSEP responses include the presence or absence of responses usually seen in normal individuals, the time between stimulation and the peaks, or the time between peaks (conduction time). Of particular interest with the SSEP is the CCT, which provides an index of cortical abnormality that is independent of peripheral dysfunction.

Many studies have shown that the absence of the cortical SSEP responses or severely abnormal cortical responses correlate with poor outcome, whereas normal responses correlate with good outcome. However, the association with outcome is not perfect. For example, two children have recovered after having absent SSEPs.[57] In numerous other studies, patients have had poor outcome after normal SSEPs. Many of these relate to secondary deterioration processes or death from nonneurological causes.

In studies in which they have been compared, the SSEP has been shown to be superior to the BAER.[49,50,54,56,57,62,70,72] A possible explanation for this is that the SSEP has measurement components of both the brainstem and the cortex, while the BAER is solely brainstem in origin. A patient may have severe cortical damage despite normal BAERs. Not surprisingly, the literature is occasionally conflicting regarding the predictive power of the BAER. For example, BAER has been shown to correlate with prognosis in some studies,[39,44,52-54,64-66,68,70,73-87] and shown not to correlate with outcome in other studies.[42,56,62,80,88] In some of these studies, the predictive nature was dependent on when the recordings were done and on the clinical setting. In some studies the cortical AEP was more predictive than the short latency BAER,[63,89] consistent with the finding that the cortical responses of the SSEP appear to be more useful for prediction than the subcortical BAER.

In studies in which the VEP has been compared with the SSEP and BAER, the VEP has consistently been shown to be less predictive of outcome.[54,57,62,70,74] However, several studies have shown that abnormalities in the VEP are related to outcome,[43,57–59,62,66,70,75] perhaps because of its cortical nature. Several other studies have shown that the VEP provides little information about outcome.[52,54,56,67]

The inconsistency of findings with individual modalities suggests that lesions or injury in several locations may be fatal, but that they may be detected in different neural pathways tested by different SEP modalities. Hence, the most effective approach may be the combination of several modalities to increase the predictive power by testing the widest area of neural tissue.

Greenberg and colleagues popularized the use of all three SEP modalities (SSEP, VEP, BAER) in what was termed *multimodality evoked potentials*.[58,59,75] Using a grading system of waveform abnormalities, the responses were scaled I to IV and compared with outcome. If any of the three responses was absent or severely abnormal, this correlated with persistent neurologic dysfunction in that neural pathway.[58] If only mild to moderate abnormalities were seen, eventual recovery was predicted. Further, the degree of abnormality of the cortically recorded components of the responses correlated with the duration of coma. During the first three days after injury, the SEP could be used to predict outcome. Insufficient studies with motor evoked potentials to date limit comment on its usefulness.

Differences between studies may also explain the varying ability of the SEPs to predict outcome after head injury. Several common findings are suggested by these studies. First, the most predictive situation is when the degree of neural injury is such that the SEPs are absent or seriously abnormal. In this case the possibility for meaningful survival is very poor. On the other extreme, if the degree of neural injury is so minimal that the SEPs are normal or minimally altered, then the possibility of a good recovery is excellent. Intermediate degrees of abnormality are not as predictive. The reasons for this lack of correlation may also explain why the extremes are not entirely predictable. These reasons include drugs or intervening conditions that impair the testing but are not related to neurologic outcome.

Examples of nonneural causes for poor responses include drug-induced coma depressing the EEG, and auditory pathology interfering with the BAER. Reasons for poor outcome despite normal responses after injury include death by nonneural processes or secondary injury processes that may cause deteriorations. Finally, treatment protocols may salvage marginally functioning tissues and improve outcome. It is perhaps the ability to detect neural deterioration that makes SEPs a monitoring tool more valuable than a simple predictor of outcome.[39]

The value of SEPs in predicting outcome is similar to their value in operative monitoring in that they are tools that should be integrated into the other methods of evaluation to guide therapy and evaluate the effectiveness of management and treatment modalities. The numerous studies cited here suggest that the multimodality approach is most effective to assist in patient management.

EVOKED POTENTIALS IN SPINAL CORD INJURY

Evoked potentials have found utility in the diagnosis and management of spinal trauma. In spinal cord injury, evoked potentials have been used for diagnosis of residual function and to assess improvement by repeated measurement during rehabilitation. Evoked potentials have also been utilized as a tool to monitor spinal cord function during surgery and during studies of spinal cord injury.

The use of evoked responses in human spinal cord injury was prompted by findings in experimental spinal cord injury and by their success in diagnosis of other human spinal abnormalities. Evoked responses have been used extensively in animal experimentation.[12,90] In general, mild trauma is associated with transient loss of sensory responses, followed by return; this pattern appears to mimic clinical function in the animals studied. Moderate trauma is associated with loss of evoked responses, which return if there is ultimate clinical recovery, or deteriorate if there is not, mimicking the clinical picture. In these animals, the deterioration appears to occur only where complete paraplegia results.[91] Finally, very severe experimental trauma causes a loss of evoked responses that mimics the complete loss of clinical function observed.[12,90] The apparent close correlation of the sensory evoked response with the degree of trauma and eventual function has made it a valuable tool for experimental studies, since it offers an assessment of spinal cord function without complete clinical evaluation.

Numerous studies have been conducted with the SSEP in human spinal cord injury.[52,91–98] In general, the SSEP appears to match the clinical examination. In the acute phase (1 week postinjury), amplitude changes predominate, with latency shifts occurring in the later phase (over 6 weeks).[91] Transient abnormalities have been seen commonly between the third and sixth days, consistent with cord edema. As would be expected because of the different tracts involved in the SSEP, some patients with no motor function but with sensory function had an intact SSEP. In addition, in some cases of complete clinical loss of all function, the SSEP was present, indicating residual neural function (or at least that some sensory pathways were anatomically intact but not clinically functional). SSEP improvement or deterioration in patients appeared to follow changes in the clinical exam. The SSEP also responded appropriately to maneuvers such as surgery that were associated with improved clinical function.[96,99,100]

In order to evaluate spinal cord injury more thoroughly, dermatomal evoked responses (DEPs) have been utilized.[101–103] In general these allow a more thorough evaluation of function at spinal levels, since they are able to detect sensory function in anatomic regions not tested by the major nerves. They also test the component roots of major nerves where several roots contribute to the SSEP response. Of interest is one case report in which sacral dermatomal responses were present in a patient with no recordable lower extremity SSEP who had eventual functional recovery.[104] As suggested by this report, dermatomal responses may be more sensitive than SSEP or clinical exam for residual neural function,[102] although their prognostic value remains in question.[101]

Motor evoked potentials have also been studied following acute human spinal cord injury.[105–108] The evoked response generally mimicked the clinical examination. In some patients an MEP was present with some clinical motor function but the SSEP was absent (pointing out the topographically different neural pathways being tested).[108] In some other patients, an MEP was present in the absence of clinical function (probably indicating that the axonal pathways were intact but not clinically functional).[107]

Although the clinical exam remains the most powerful examination in the spinally injured patient, it has been suggested that evoked responses be used in acute human spinal injury to objectively evaluate spinal function when the clinical examination is difficult (e.g., head injury, coma, anesthesia, or chemical muscle paralysis). The routine monitoring of somatosensory evoked responses in spinal-cord-injured patients with residual function is supported by outcome studies in these patients[109] and several other types of spinal surgeries.

Evoked responses may also be helpful in the differentiation of a complete lesion (no function below the level of injury) from an incomplete lesion (residual function present), in which more aggressive therapy is often employed because of greater potential for recovery. Further, since the clinical exam can be subjective, or differ between observers, evoked responses may objectively measure improvement with therapy. Evidence suggests that evoked responses may be more sensitive to residual function than the clinical exam,[12] and SSEP changes often precede clinical improvement.[95]

PREDICTION OF OUTCOME WITH SPINAL CORD INJURY

Numerous studies have attempted to utilize evoked responses to provide prognostic information, allowing selective application of medical and surgical treatment. Most studies have shown that the complete absence of SSEP in a clinically complete patient is reliably followed by no recovery of function. A few authors have suggested that the evoked response acquired within four hours of injury is predictive, but that the prognostic value diminishes as the time of recording increases post injury.[99,110] Measurements in chronic spinal cord injury bear no correlation with useful function. Some authors have been unable to elicit useful prognostic information from any measurements. Therefore, except for evoked response recordings acquired shortly after injury, the evoked responses may not provide more information than that which is discernible by a thorough clinical exam and may not provide any extra prognostic information.

Intraoperative Evoked Potential Monitoring

Just as evoked responses are useful adjuncts to the clinical exam in the ICU, they may also be utilized during surgical procedures with anesthesia and muscle relaxants. Selective application to surgical procedures where neural injury is a well-recognized complication appears to improve (but not eliminate) the risk of these complications. As discussed below, intraoperative monitoring has been successfully utilized in numerous surgical procedures.

Currently, it is considered by some to be a standard of care in surgical correction of scoliosis since the Scoliosis Research Society published its position statement acknowledging its value (see below). The NIH has published the results of a consensus conference for surgery of acoustic neuromas (vestibular schwannoma) and indicated monitoring should be used (see below). The standard of electrophysiologic monitoring of procedures is further confused by the legal ruling of Judge Learned Hand (*U.S. vs Carroll Towing 159 Fed 169*). Ruling on a different kind of monitoring, he stated that the failure to utilize monitoring may be malpractice if the cost of monitoring a large number of patients is less than the cost of a single bad outcome prevented by that monitoring. Since bad neurologic outcome is usually quite expensive (particularly when involving young individuals or litigation), monitoring can be useful even if all injury cannot be prevented, and even if the expense is not negligible.

This financial balance can be calculated for scoliosis. The American Society of Neurophysiologic Monitoring (ASNM) conducted a survey in 1993 to determine the costs of monitoring spinal surgery. This survey revealed that the actual cost (not billing) of monitoring is $609.00 for an average scoliosis procedure in 1993. In this surgery, the risk of neurologic injury and paralysis (in healthy patients and simple corrections) is about 1 percent. If paralysis occurs, the cost "to society" for a surviving paraplegic is very conservatively $1,000,000.00. At $609.00 per case, 1642 patients could be monitored for the cost of one complication. Since 16 of these patients are predicted to become paralyzed (1 percent of 1642), if monitoring could prevent more than one such outcome, it would be cost-effective, and the ruling of Judge Learned Hand would suggest that the failure to monitor is negligent.

This latter analysis has resulted in a general "rule of thumb" that procedures with neurologic risk of severe injury above 1 percent will likely be cost-effectively monitored if it can be incorporated into the surgery. It is important to recognize that several caveats apply to this situation. First, monitoring must be available to assess a neural pathway that has a direct correlation with the injured neural pathway. Second, the surgical procedure must have identifiable components that could be reversible or accomplished in different ways if monitoring indicates that neural compromise is occurring.

Several books and articles have been written to discuss the methods and applications of intraoperative electrophysiologic monitoring[17,18,111–119] as well as monitoring in the neurosurgical intensive care unit.[120–125] Guidelines have been published by the American Electroencephalographic Society.[126,127] The American Academy of Neurology published an assessment of intraoperative monitoring, concluding that "considerable evidence favors the use of monitoring as a safe and efficacious tool in clinical situations where there is significant nervous system risk, provided its limitations are appreciated."[128]

Examples of some of the types of procedures in which intraoperative monitoring has been utilized are shown in Table 7-1. In general, the somatosensory evoked response and the brainstem auditory evoked response have been used most extensively. This monitoring has been used for a wide variety of surgical procedures, most notably those on the spinal cord and on the brainstem.

PERIPHERAL NERVE SURGERY

The SSEP technique has been considered "indispensable" for intraoperative evaluation and monitoring during surgical procedures of peripheral nerves and plexus regions.[120,129,130] For example, stimulation of nerves allows identification of intact nerves or nerve trunks in injury areas when peripheral function has been lost. The identity of residual function in damaged nerves ("neuroma in continuity") and identification of a preganglionic or postganglionic injury of a plexus allows selective and focused repair. The SSEP technique has the capacity to detect neural continuity in some situations in which the clinical exam is not possible, or in which function may be insufficient to allow an accurate clinical exam.[120,131] Similarly, evoked responses have been used to reduce sciatic nerve injury with hip procedures.[132–134]

SPINAL SURGERY

Intraoperative monitoring has been widely applied in surgical procedures on the spine. Corrective procedures for the abnormality resulting from scoliosis have been of particular interest.

WAKE-UP TEST
Early studies with Harrington rod placement indicated that paralysis resulting from overcorrection of a deformity could be identified with the "wake-up" test.[135] In this test, the Harrington rods were placed and the curvature was corrected; the patient was then awakened to verify motor function. This procedure worked poorly with patients who were not amenable to such tests (e.g., retarded individuals). In addition, there were occasional injuries that occurred during the wake-up.[35] Further, advances in corrective methods (notably hardware techniques) changed the period of risk from one identifiable event (spine straightening with Harrington rod distraction) to multiple potentially deleterious events (sublaminar wires, multiple hooks, pedicle screws, etc.). Therefore, a more continuous method of assessment, preferably one independent of patient cooperation, was desirable.

There is still controversy regarding the question of whether the wake-up test should be performed if sensory or motor evoked response monitoring is also performed.[136] One author suggests that in children "electrophysiologic monitoring has now superseded the wake-up test as an index of spinal cord function."[137] In several studies, the wake-up test usually correlates with the SSEP.[35] In one study of 1168 cases, the two always correlated, and the authors concluded, "there is probably no need to use wake-up testing."[138] However, other authors point out the occasional false-negative case and continue to recommend wake-up testing.[35,139,140]

SOMATOSENSORY EVOKED RESPONSES
The use of the SSEP in the operating room and intensive care unit has been discussed in several reviews.[7,17,18,34,35,124,131,141–150]

Several basic studies in animals have set the scientific

TABLE 7-1
Examples of Procedures Monitored with Evoked Potentials

Spine Procedures	**Posterior Fossa Surgery**
Scoliosis	Acoustic neuroma
Stabilization and correction of fractures	Cerebellopontine angle tumors
Decompression	Retromastoid craniectomy
Tumors	Space-occupying infarcts
AVMs (resection and embolization)	Microvascular decompression
Syringomyelia	Relief of hemifacial spasm
Vascular Surgery	**Sella or Parasellar Procedures**
Carotid endarterectomy	Transsphenoidal pituitary procedures
Aortic aneurysm	Supratentorial frontal procedures
Bronchial artery embolization	Repair of basilar skull fracture
Spinal angiography and transvascular embolization	**Skull Base Surgery**
Joint Surgery	Tumors
Hip or knee replacement	Cavernous sinus
Shoulder arthroscopy	**Stereoencephalotomy**
	Parkinson's disease
	Other movement disorders
	Intractable pain

basis of monitoring by examining both motor and sensory function. Croft and associates[151] examined monitoring in cats during injury with graded weights applied directly on the spinal cord. Sensory function was assessed by recording cortically generated SSEPs, and motor function was assessed by cortical stimulation and recording from the sciatic nerve. Each monitoring technique was altered in parallel with injury, and both appeared to correlate with postoperative motor function. Kojima and coworkers[152] used an epidural screw to produce spinal canal narrowing anteriorly at C_5. The SSEP was monitored at C_I after sciatic nerve stimulation. Motor recovery and histologic changes in the cord correlated with the SSEPs. When slight SSEP latency changes occurred (but with normal amplitude), some animals had mild motor deficits (50 to 60 percent canal compression). However, at greater degrees of compression, when the SSEP amplitude was lost, postoperative paralysis occurred. These findings continued to support the relationship of sensory monitoring (SSEP) and motor function.

Of greater interest are two studies where monitoring of motor tracts and sensory tracts was conducted during the spinal trauma. The first study involved epidural spinal compression by a balloon in cats.[153] The SSEP was monitored at the scalp and spine using sciatic nerve stimulation. Motor tract monitoring was done using stimulation of the cerebral pedicle and sciatic nerve recording. These two monitoring modalities had parallel changes in their values during compression. In the second study,[154] cats were anesthetized and SSEP monitoring established using sciatic nerve stimulation and recording from Kirschner wires placed in vertebral bodies and surface electrodes or needle electrodes placed in paraspinous muscles. For study, a distraction apparatus was placed and L_1–L_2 distracted in 4-mm increments for 10 min and released. During the release period the SSEPs were recorded and a wake-up test conducted to assess sensory and motor function in the legs. For analysis of the SSEP, the amplitude of the waves produced was measured. Studies with animals indicate that the cortical amplitude of the somatosensory evoked response from hind limb stimulation correlated with loss of motor function when spine distraction was excessive (Fig. 7-11).[154,155] These have led to the wide application of the SSEP in scoliosis surgery as a supplement to the wake-up test. As experience has increased, it has become clear that the use of the SSEP is associated with reduction in rates of neural injury during corrective procedures for scoliosis. These animal studies confirm that mechanical cord changes from surgical manipulation cause simultaneous changes in sensory and motor pathways. This close correlation may not apply for neurovascular insults.

Intraoperative SSEP monitoring is usually accomplished by placing stimulating and recording electrodes prior to induction of anesthesia or as shortly thereafter as possible. Recording is begun as quickly as possible in order to begin establishing an operative baseline under anesthesia. This early baseline serves two important purposes. First, it allows determination of whether the anesthetic technique is favorable for monitoring. If not, then there is time to adjust the type and amounts of anesthesia agents to find a suitable anesthetic technique prior to the period of neural vulnerability from the procedure.

Second, the early acquisition of responses allows monitoring during the period of patient positioning and may therefore warn of potential hazards to the neural system not related to spine manipulation. One

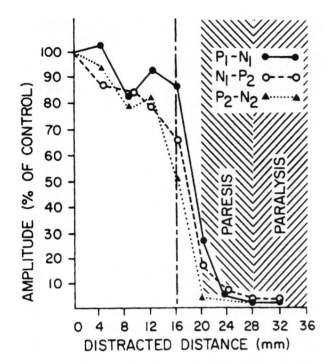

Figure 7-11 Correspondence between loss of evoked potential amplitude (three peaks shown vertically as percentage of predistraction value) and clinical motor dysfunction during experimental spinal cord distraction (distance shown on horizontal axis). (Reproduced with permission from Nordwall et al.[154])

report detected loss of posterior tibial SSEP and motor responses (stimulation of the motor cortex and recording in the soleus muscle) during dissection of the spine, prior to distraction or instrumentation.[156] No further surgery was conducted and the patient awakened with a motor deficit, suggesting monitoring may be important for other periods than those expected to cause injury. Other authors have studied the use of the SSEP to evaluate viability of the spinal cord during deliberate hypotension or deliberate hemodilution.[117] These SSEP changes indicated the viability of the spinal cord may have been threatened by anesthetic maneuvers otherwise thought to be innocuous.

Throughout the surgical procedure monitoring is conducted as often as possible. Like other types of monitoring (e.g., blood pressure), it needs to be conducted as rapidly as possible to be sensitive to intraoperative events. When the monitored response changes, a determination must be made rapidly whether this indicates that potential neural compromise could be causing the evoked response change. A variety of criteria have been offered by numerous authors as to what constitutes a "significant change" in the evoked response. Generally a sudden increase in latency of 10 percent or decrease in amplitude of 50 percent, or both, is considered significant. However, other criteria have

been utilized and the issue of which baseline to use is not resolved. Certainly abrupt changes are easy to recognize, but more subtle changes may be more difficult to recognize. An alternate approach is to utilize statistics to determine when the recorded response deviates from the expected response.

When it is determined that the response has changed, the monitoring team must rapidly attempt to ascertain the cause. Generally speaking, the causative event is likely technical, physiologic, anesthetic, or patient-related. Usually the monitoring team will repeat the response or seek confirmation of the change by recording other, related responses (e.g., the left-leg SSEP when the right SSEP changes). During this time technical factors need to be reassessed to ensure that the monitoring equipment is functioning properly and not the cause of the change. Here, recording from multiple locations can verify that the stimulus is adequate and that a single recording electrode is not the source of the problem. Furthermore, multiple locations can help anatomically locate the region of neural tissue affected (e.g., cortical versus subcortical).

If the problem is not technical, the possible contributions of altered physiology (e.g., hypotension) or sudden change in anesthetic depth need to be evaluated. These can often be assessed by reviewing the physiologic monitoring and anesthetic delivery with the anesthesiologist. These factors are discussed near the end of this chapter.

The surgeon needs to be aware of the changes in monitoring if a patient compromise could be causing the evoked response change. Notification of the surgical team needs to be done as close to the event as possible so they can assess if some surgical or positioning step can be reversed or changed so as to improve neural viability. Certainly, information 10 to 15 min old will be unlikely to be helpful. The surgeon also needs to be notified if the monitoring is of poor quality. In this situation the surgeon needs to know that the monitoring is unlikely to be of value because responses are poor.

Clearly, when a monitored change occurs, the response of the monitoring team must be rapid and encompass all possible explanations, if timely feedback is to be given to the surgeon. At the time of writing, monitoring remains an "art" that is best done by an individual who can integrate all of the technical, physiologic, anesthetic, and patient factors. As yet, no machine has surfaced to replace the human element.

The value of the SSEP in experimental procedures has been matched by several studies in human surgery indicating that monitoring is predictive of neural outcome.[35,109,138,142,157–160] Evaluating 295 patients undergoing stabilization for spinal instability (trauma), the neurologic injury rate decreased from 6.9 to 0.7 percent with

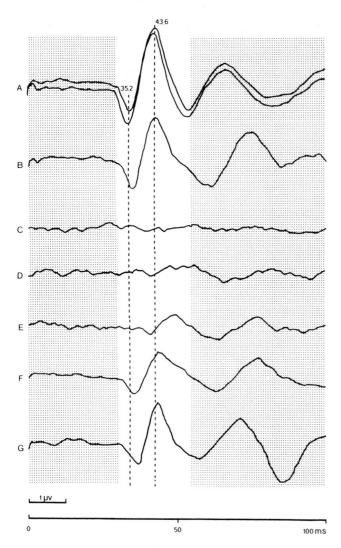

Figure 7-12 Example of an SSEP monitoring case. (*A*) Normal baseline recordings the afternoon prior to operation; (*B*) after induction of anesthesia; (*C*) responses were abolished after passing through the wires around the laminae; (*D*) wake-up test was positive; (*E*) after 15 min poorly defined potentials reappeared; (*F*) after closure of wound evoked potentials showed a little increased latency P_{40} and N_{50} measuring 4.1 and 2.0 ms, respectively, with normal overall waveform (*G*). (Reproduced with permission from Mostegl et al.[162])

SSEP monitoring.[109] Evaluating 100 procedures on the cervical spine, one series noted a reduction of paraplegia from 3.7 percent to none, coincident with the use of SSEP monitoring.[161] Although studies such as these, which are based on historical controls, need to be evaluated with caution, the implication is clear. An example of SSEP monitoring is seen in Fig. 7-12.[162]

The Scoliosis Research Society and the European Spinal Deformities Society reviewed over 51,000 surgical cases.[136,163] In this study, the occurrence of a neurologic deficit without SSEP warning ("false-negative") was 0.63 percent; SSEP changes were seen in the remainder

of the patients experiencing a deficit. The report indicated that surgical teams with the most experience in monitoring had a neurologic complication rate less than half of the rate of less experienced teams. The author concluded that "these results confirm the clinical efficacy of experienced SSEP spinal cord monitoring."[163]

Perhaps the most compelling testament of the efficacy of SSEP in spinal surgery has been prepared by the Scoliosis Research Society.[164] Their position statement reviews the evidence of efficacy and concludes that "neurophysiological monitoring can assist in the early detection of complications and possibly prevent postoperative morbidity in patients undergoing operations on the spine." This has made monitoring during scoliosis correction a virtual standard of care.

As with the wake-up test, the correlation of SSEP monitoring and neural injury is not exact, since cases of neural injury without intraoperative warning have occurred (although rare events). The dissociation of monitoring and outcome may be due to several factors:

1. The primary pathways of the SSEP are thought to be posterior column proprioception and vibration pathways that are vascularly and topographically distinct from the motor pathways.
2. In some cases the monitoring was not properly conducted (i.e., monitoring bilateral pathways or monitoring the wrong pathway).
3. Structures were injured which were not amenable to monitoring (e.g., injury to nerve roots by pedicle screws).
4. The injurious event may have occurred postoperatively or at a time other than during the monitored part of the case (e.g., formation of a compressing hematoma during patient awakening at the conclusion of the procedure).

Concern about an occasional patient (usually less than 1 percent of injuries) who experiences a motor deficit when the SSEP fails to provide a warning reinforces that the SSEP does not monitor the motor pathways directly. Certainly, mechanical effects on the cord may involve both the anterior (motor) and posterior elements, thus altering the SSEP. The contribution of the more anteriorly located spinocerebellar pathways activated in the lower extremity SSEP may explain the response of the SSEP to anterior cord ischemia[165] and the close correlation with motor function that would otherwise not be expected for the dorsal columns during some types of cord vascular compromise (such as anterior spinal artery ischemia).

An important consideration during monitoring is the specific roots carrying the SSEP signal. Obviously, the use of the median or ulnar nerve SSEP would not be predicted to be useful for spinal procedures in the lower thorax or lumbar regions. In one report, the use of the femoral nerve SSEP was advocated to improve the monitoring of thoracolumbar fracture stabilization.[166] The authors noted changes in the femoral nerve SSEP not reflected in posterior tibial or common peroneal SSEP responses and concluded that the femoral nerve SSEP improves monitoring of the L_2–L_4 roots.

The SSEP has been successfully used to monitor procedures to relieve herniated nucleus pulposus.[167] The experience of many authors has varied with this report, generally concluding that chronic nerve irritation recovers slowly with few SSEP changes, whereas relief of acute nerve compression may be reflected in the SSEP. Unfortunately, since the SSEP monitors multiple nerve roots, it is possible that monitoring may not reflect nerve dysfunction, because the other component nerves can form a normal SSEP.[168] Thus some authors have not found the SSEP useful for isolated lumbar root lesions. For more specific monitoring, dermatomal evoked responses have been developed, in which the dermatome of the nerve of interest is stimulated and the cortical response is recorded. Dermatomal responses have also been advocated to monitor nerve roots during release of lumbar spinal stenosis to determine the success of nerve decompression.[169,170]

Another variation of the SSEP has been to stimulate the cauda equina via percutaneously placed electrodes because the amplitude of the response is at least twice the traditional SSEP of peripheral nerve stimulation. This has been advocated in patients for whom peripheral SSEP is not recordable.[171] Similarly, epidural stimulated evoked responses may be useful in other spinal regions where conventional SSEP is absent. One example is that of a cervicomedullary ependymoma that was monitored by cortical potentials from epidural stimulation (the SSEP was absent).[172]

In order to improve the monitoring of the SSEP, many variations of the technique have been developed. Because anesthesia can influence the monitoring of cortical responses (see below), recording locations near the spinal cord have been developed, since they are less affected by anesthesia. Placement of needle electrodes in the spine bony elements,[173] intraspinous ligament,[174] or subdural or epidural space[160] has been advocated as a simple and stable technique. One study evaluated different spinal recording locations[165] and concluded that the epidural recording location was superior. Problems with perispinal recording locations included marked variability due to motion and dislodgment by the surgeon. When recording from the epidural space, several peaks can be discerned (Fig. 7-13).[144] These peaks may represent responses in different neural pathways, and several authors suggest that the response in the spinocerebellar tract may be differ-

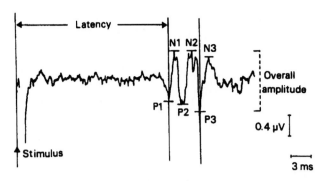

Figure 7-13 Typical somatosensory evoked potential (SSEP) recorded in the extradural space. Seen are three positive peaks (P_1, P_2, P_3) and three negative peaks (N_1, N_2, N_3). (Reproduced with permission from Loughnan and Hall.[144])

entiated from the dorsal columns.[175–178] Studies have also explored the placement of the stimulating epidural electrode to specifically monitor motor tracts.[179,180]

Epidural electrodes, placed percutaneously or directly by the surgeon, have become popular. They can be used for recording responses from peripheral (SSEP) or cortical (transcranial motor cortex) stimulation. They can be used for stimulation with recording of cortical responses or peripheral neural or muscle (CMAP) responses, or recording at both locations simultaneously.[181] They have become commonplace in Japan and Europe, and despite its invasive nature, this technique appears remarkably safe.[35,149] Some authors consider epidural recording and stimulation to be superior to the SSEP[177,181] and the recording locations near the cord to provide "the most important information obtained in the intraoperative period."[119] Although the specific anatomy of the epidurally monitored neural tracts is largely unknown, they appear useful for monitoring.[119] One study with 60 patients suggested that scalp recorded responses from epidural electrodes were superior to peripheral nerve stimulation because of the ability to record well-defined responses.[177] Another study compared epidural and peripheral nerve stimulation for responses recorded epidurally.[182] The authors concluded that epidural stimulation produced larger amplitude (allowing faster updates and recording time) and was more sensitive to spinal cord insults.

MOTOR EVOKED POTENTIALS IN SPINAL SURGERY

Monitoring of spinal surgery using motor tract techniques has been of great interest, since motor function is usually considered more important clinically than sensory function. As such, several motor tract methods have been employed.

Monitoring using transcranial MEPs has also been

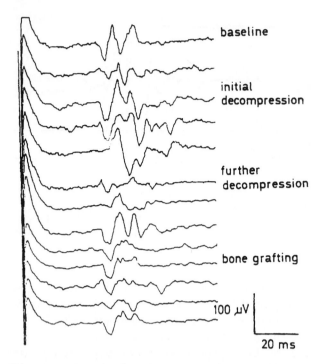

baseline

initial
decompression

further
decompression

bone grafting

100 μV

20 ms

Figure 7-14 Example of tcEMEP monitoring: Intraoperative tcEMEP recordings from the leg during surgery on an old T_{10} compression fracture. The amplitude did not change significantly in the initial stage of decompression, but decreased suddenly on dural retraction and recovered gradually after waiting. On further decompression and bone grafting, persistent amplitude reduction of more than 50 percent of baseline was noted despite stable latency. Postoperatively, this patient suffered from increased spasticity of the lower extremities. (Reproduced with permission from Yang et al.[183])

successful (Fig. 7-14).[183] Jones studied 34 patients undergoing spinal surgery with tcEMEP.[155] The technique was sensitive to intraoperative spinal manipulation and loss of motor conduction correlated with neurologic injury. Another study in 8 patients demonstrated stable recordings with good correlation to outcome using tcMMEP.[184] The authors concluded that the magnetic technique may be more sensitive than the electrical technique for stimulation.

Responses to transcranial stimulation can also be recorded in the epidural space, over peripheral nerves, and from muscle activity. The epidural recordings are preferred by some because of the problems with anesthetic effects at the anterior horn cell or neuromuscular junction.[143] The disadvantage of epidural recordings is that they likely represent activation of bilateral pathways, whereas recordings from muscles can differentiate unilateral changes.[143]

A second method of monitoring the motor tracts is stimulation of the spinal cord. Stimulation methods include epidural electrodes and electrodes placed near or in the vertebral bodies. After stimulation, recording can be accomplished in muscles, nerves, and from the

epidural space. Clearly, recording a muscle response is an indication of motor function. However, monitoring along the peripheral nerve or near the spinal cord may record responses from dromic passages along descending motor pathways as well as antidromic responses traveling downward in sensory tracts.[185] The mixed nature of these latter responses makes it difficult to determine which tract is being monitored, but does not reduce the value of these responses. However, epidurally recorded responses may not correlate as well with outcome in terms of muscle function as a muscle response.

One popular spinal cord stimulation technique was pioneered by Owen and is termed the neurogenic motor evoked potential (NMEP)[150,186] (Fig. 7-15). In this technique, stimulating electrodes are placed percutaneously near the vertebral bodies at adjacent levels cephalad to the level of surgery. Recording electrodes are placed near a peripheral nerve, such as the sciatic nerve. Studies with spinal cord lesioning suggest that the response recorded in the sciatic nerve is due to pure motor tract transmission, while the response in the spinal cord is mixed dromic and antidromic tract transmission.[187] This interpretation has been challenged, since during isoflurane anesthesia, the motor component is preferentially blocked,[143] and recordings in sensory nerves show responses that cannot be motor in origin.

Studies suggest that NMEP responses are less variable, less subject to anesthesia and a more valid monitor of motor function than lower extremity SSEP.[186,188] One case report of the NMEP detecting a change that was not reflected in the SSEP has been published,[189] similar to reports with transcranial magnetic MEP.[190]

Spinal-to-spinal evoked responses using epidural electrodes have become common in Japan. An excellent example of the application of this technique is the segmental recording of ascending and descending responses during surgery for relief of myelopathy.[191] Recording at various levels allowed identification of the regions of the cord that were neurologically involved, as well as prediction of the degree of improvement from the surgery.

Motor evoked potentials have been used to monitor areas such as the cauda equina where traditional SSEP responses cannot be used.[192–194] Stimulation techniques include epidural electrodes cephalad to the surgical site and recording of spontaneous muscle activity. For operations such as tethered cord, specific tissue in the operative field can be stimulated in an attempt to determine which tissue should be resected or left.

An important variation has been to monitor individual nerve roots during the placement of pedicle screws for fixation of metal support structures to the vertebra. If these screws are not placed fully in the body and

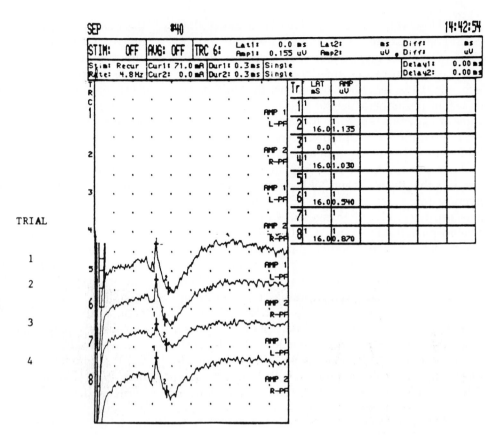

Figure 7-15 Example of NMEP recording from electrodes near the sciatic nerve, with stimulation cephalad to the spinal operative site. (Reproduced with permission from Owen et al.[186])

pedicles of the vertebra, they may impinge on the nerve roots in the vicinity. Dermatomal evoked responses have been used in this setting; however, difficulties with anesthesia and time needed for response acquisition have made dermatomal responses less useful than mechanically or electrically elicited muscle recordings in the distribution of the nerve root.[195–201] Techniques using passive muscle recordings can continually monitor nerve root integrity, with neurotonic discharges providing early warning of potential nerve compromise. They can also be used specifically to test screw placement. These studies suggest that improper screw placement may be as high as 19 percent.[202]

The MEP for monitoring the spinal cord has achieved substantial popularity despite the long track record of the SSEP. This is likely because most insults are probably mechanical in nature and effect the SSEP as well as the MEP. However, vascular insults may produce a potential disparity between these two techniques, making their difference an important issue. Such a disparity might be important in aortic vascular procedures where anterior artery ischemia is possible and prevention of paralysis is based on detection of ischemia, particularly in the thoracic region of the spinal cord. Since the SSEP is thought to be conducted primarily in the posterior columns, the SSEP will likely reflect primarily posterior spinal artery perfusion. Since the

motor tracts are located in the anterior cord, they may be more responsive to anterior spinal artery perfusion.

The thoracic spinal cord is particularly vulnerable to ischemia, since it is not well vascularly collateralized and may have only one anterior feeding vessel between T_4 and L_4.[148] A single anterior spinal artery runs from the vertebral arterial supply down the ventromedial sulcus. The vascular supply is rather variable, and may have several radicular branches including the thyrocervical trunk and artery of Adamkiewicz (AA), arising from the aorta at T_9–L_2. During thoracic aorta surgery, blood flow to the AA may be compromised, leading to anterior spinal ischemia. Even if distal aorta perfusion is provided (supplying the AA), critical radicular branches may be lost during thoracic graft placement, leading to spinal infarction. Monitoring with the SSEP or motor evoked responses has been advocated to identify adequate distal perfusion of the AA or to identify critical radicular arteries so as to prompt reanastomosis.[203,204]

There are examples of patients in whom anterior artery ischemia or infarcts have had unchanged intraoperative SSEP but who awaken with absent motor function.[205] This difference of vascularity between the anterior and posterior spinal cord has led to conclusions that dorsal column SSEP would be of poor value for monitoring during aortic cross-clamping procedures. However, studies of spinal cord blood flow (SCBF) demonstrate a correlation of the SSEP and the SCBF in white or gray matter[206] and demonstrate that aortic occlusion causes anterior as well as posterior ischemia. Thus, regardless of whether the SSEP is mediated in posterior or lateral tracts, it is affected by anterior ischemia. Studies in the lamb suggest that the SSEP (epidural stimulation) and cortically generated MEP behaved similarly with aortic cross-clamping.[207]

Observation of the SSEP in human aortic occlusion suggests that the SSEP and MEP can be utilized effectively during vascular surgery.[206,208–212] The monitoring may also detect adverse changes in SCBF, such as when cerebrospinal fluid pressure (CSFP) is elevated, reducing the net spinal cord perfusion pressure (SCPP).[213,214] Thus the SSEP may be able to monitor spinal cord perfusion abnormalities due to both reduced blood supply and increased CSFP. Studies using epidural stimulated and recorded responses during aortic cross-clamping suggest that the portion of the response thought to be mediated via gray matter is more sensitive to ischemia than the long tracts in the dorsal column.[178] Experience using motor evoked potentials resulting from transcranial magnetic stimulation is promising. One study noted successful monitoring in 10 of 13 patients using recordings from the cauda equina or leg muscles.[215] In this study, the prediction of short-term motor outcome was exact, without false-positive or false-negative occurrences.

MONITORING WITH MULTIPLE TECHNIQUES

Because of the various tracts involved in a surgical region, some authors have advocated the use of several modalities during one monitoring session.[131,182,216–219] One study used motor evoked potentials from transcranial electrical stimulation simultaneously with lower extremity elicited SSEP, with responses recorded from epidural electrodes caudal and cephalad to the spinal surgical site.[131,149,218,219] The authors indicated that these responses are stable during a variety of anesthetic techniques (including complete neuromuscular blockade) and resistant to a variety of artifacts. Using simultaneous monitoring, the authors noted that although both pathways often responded during presumed spinal insults, the effect appeared first in the motor tracts. This observation matches the experimental observation that mechanical compression affects the motor tracts before the sensory tracts.[34]

Another case report supporting multimodality monitoring demonstrated loss of SSEP with preserved MEP.[220] Despite intact motor function, the loss of sensory function as predicted by the monitoring made ambulation very difficult. Based on experiences of this kind, some authors have indicated that monitoring of motor responses as a sole technique may be less advan-

tageous than a combined technique.[176] Another study utilized long latency reflex activity in the leg muscles after common peroneal stimulation.[216] The authors conclude that this reflex activity is more sensitive to spinal cord compromise than long tract monitoring.

Simultaneous monitoring has been advocated for surgery on the cauda equina.[200,201] Conventional SSEP recording is useful during this procedure, but only for the regions of the nervous system traversed by SSEP pathways from the lower extremity. Hence, sacral function may be missed, and muscle recordings can be used to record lower nerve motor function. In a report of median nerve SSEP during syringoendoscopy, the authors noted a postoperative motor deficit without SSEP changes[221] but sensory changes correlated with the SSEP. The authors concluded that both motor and sensory pathways should be monitored. Such multimodality monitoring is similarly suggested in some patient subsets where SSEP is more difficult to record, such as neuromuscular scoliosis.[219,222,223]

For procedures in the very high cervical spine (C_1/C_2), multimodality monitoring including the BAER has been suggested and has been utilized to detect cord and vertebral artery compromise at the cervicomedullary junction.[34,116] One example has been the detection of inadequate positioning in the lateral position for retromastoid craniectomy.[224]

SELECTIVE DORSAL RHIZOTOMY

Selective dorsal rhizotomy (SDR) has been advocated to relieve leg spasticity and thereby improve gait in cerebral palsy.[131] In this surgical procedure, a laminectomy is used to expose the $L_2–S_2$ ventral and dorsal nerve roots. Recording electrodes are placed in numerous leg muscles to observe evoked compound muscle action potentials. The ventral root can be differentiated from the dorsal root by its lower threshold for stimulation, with response in the innervated muscles. The dorsal root is teased into 3 to 7 rootlets and stimulated at 50 Hz. If an excessive muscle response is generated, the rootlet is marked for sectioning (at least one rootlet is spared at each spinal level). Other rootlets innervating muscles which are known to be particularly troublesome may also be sectioned. If excessive lesioning is done, morbidity is high. Electrophysiologic monitoring has been used to selectively limit lesioning and improve the outcome. These procedures, guided by the intraoperative electrophysiology, appear to improve the spasticity.

DREZ LESIONS

SSEPs have been used during dorsal root entry zone lesionings.[120] During these procedures, the SSEP can be used to identify the location of the desired lesion by noting a nerve action potential at the desired root. Continued SSEP response during lesioning suggests preservation of sensory activity, thereby helping to avoid one of the most common complications of a DREZ lesion.

POSTERIOR FOSSA PROCEDURES

Intraoperative monitoring is frequently utilized during surgery on the posterior fossa. A variety of monitoring methods have been used, including SSEP, BAER, and monitoring of several cranial nerves. Cranial nerve monitoring is usable when the specific site of surgery is in the vicinity of the cranial nerve. BAER can be used to monitor the integrity of the auditory apparatus (cochlea) and neural pathways between the lower pons to the level of the inferior colliculus in the midbrain.

In addition to BAER, the SSEP can monitor the specific pathways of proprioception and vibration as they traverse the entire brainstem. One study of over 200 patients undergoing operations for skull base tumors demonstrated the general use of BAER and SSEP for monitoring of the brain.[225] In this series, one patient who lost the BAER awoke with no hearing, and marked persistent changes in the BAER and SSEP have correlated with postoperative brainstem dysfunction.

The most common monitoring applications in the posterior fossa are to preserve facial nerve function and hearing. Many of the procedures in the posterior fossa are for benign tumors, which may grow to a large size (4 cm). Surgical removal is complicated by the delicate process of avoiding cranial nerves that may be obscured or intertwined with the tumor. Since cranial nerve involvement is common with tumors over 2 cm,[226] monitoring of cranial nerve function is a useful adjunct to the surgical procedure. Although the most commonly involved nerves are VIII (hearing) and VII (facial), several other cranial nerves can be monitored when appropriate.

BRAINSTEM AUDITORY EVOKED RESPONSES
Headphone stimulators may be unacceptable in the operating room due to their size. Hence most monitoring paradigms utilize small earphone stimulators similar to those used with personal stereo sets. Some investigators prefer to use a short plastic tubing between the earphone and the ear, so that the electrical artifact of stimulation is physically removed from the recording electrodes and contributes less to the recording.

The most important recording electrode for the BAER is placed near (mastoid), on, or in the ear. The reference electrode is usually placed at the top of the head (Cz, vertex), and a ground electrode is placed elsewhere on the head (often Fz, forehead). Two means

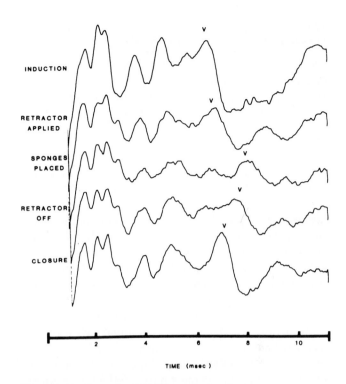

Figure 7-16 Example of BAER monitoring during a microvascular decompression procedure in the posterior fossa. Typical latency increases in wave V (marked) are seen associated with retractor placement. (Reproduced with permission from Friedman et al.[16])

of presenting the tracings are used based on individual preferences for whether the peaks (I–V) should be presented upward or downward.

Since several generators are seen with the BAER, it can be used to find the anatomic location of the neural insult and assist the surgeon. Shifts in latency that delay wave I without changes in interwave latencies may reflect reduction in hearing from external or middle ear changes, such as fluid in the middle ear. Examination of effects on waves I, III, and V may allow identification of brainstem injury. It is important to note that below the obex of the brainstem, the structures producing the BAER are ipsilateral to the ear stimulated, whereas above the obex the structures are primarily contralateral. An example of BAER monitoring is shown in Fig. 7-16.[16]

In general, anesthetic effects on the BAER are not dramatic. Slow shifts may be seen as the concentration of inhalational agents changes (halothane, enflurane, isoflurane). Nitrous oxide is generally benign unless it causes changes in middle ear pressure. Some changes can be seen with shifts in body temperature and will be most dramatic if cold irrigation fluids are applied into the surgical fields.

The cochlear nerve, which is responsible for hearing and has been termed one of the most fragile cranial

TABLE 7-2
Procedures Where BAER Has Been Suggested

Acoustic neuromas	Large tumors in the posterior fossa
Cerebellopontine angle tumors	
Microvascular decompression of c.n. V, VII, and VIII	Trigeminal neuralgia
	Hemifacial spasm
Brainstem hematoma removal	Glossopharyngeal neuralgia
Posterior circulation surgery	Disabling vertigo
	Cochlear implant surgery

nerves,[13] is frequently involved in tumors of the posterior fossa. Hearing is often impaired, and hearing preservation in tumor removal has been studied extensively (notably with acoustic neuromas). It has been suggested that BAER monitoring be utilized for several surgical procedures (Table 7-2).

Many studies have shown an improvement in hearing outcome using BAER in vestibular schwannoma (acoustic neuroma).[14,15,227-230] However, with large tumors, or some other tumor types or locations, the involvement of the cochlear nerve in the tumor makes hearing preservation more difficult.[13] The assessment of improvement in hearing is also confounded between studies using varying definitions of hearing, failing to differentiate among surgical procedures and preoperative pathology, and failing to correlate intraoperative events with postoperative results.[13,231]

Several studies show that hearing outcome is related to preoperative hearing impairment and to tumor size.[228,232,233] One study nicely demonstrated how outcome is related to tumor size. With tumors less than 5 mm in diameter, anatomic preservation (AP) was 100 percent and normal hearing (NH) at 1 year postoperatively was 100 percent.[228] For tumors 6 to 15 mm, AP was 100 percent and NH was 92 percent. For tumors 16 to 25 mm, AP was 90 percent and NH 83 percent. Finally, for tumors >25 mm, AP was 88 percent and NH 75 percent. In this study, the most important variable correlating with outcome was the normalcy of wave V at the end of the case. Another study suggested that intraoperative BAER amplitude changes were more important than latency changes[234] as a predictor of outcome.

Perhaps the most common changes seen intraoperatively with BAER recording are increases in V latency and I–V interwave latency with retractor placement. Many of these changes, if mild, are reversible and have been considered part of a routine procedure.[16,235] However, more significant changes have prompted attempts to reposition the retractor to reduce direct injury to the cochlear nerve.[13] The viability of the cochlea is thought to be threatened frequently by vascular obstruction or vasospasm[13]; therefore identification of

wave I is extremely important, and transient changes may be indicative of injury processes. Often an abrupt and complete loss of wave I is due to loss of cochlear blood supply with resultant loss of useful hearing. Changes in wave V are less clearly correlated with outcome; wave V can be lost due to desynchronization in the pathways, and hearing may be retained even with its loss.[13,236] The latter situation probably happens less than 5 percent of the time. In general, if waves I and V are preserved, hearing is usually preserved, but if they are both lost, there is little chance of preservation of hearing postoperatively.

Since the BAER is of small amplitude, thousands of responses must be recorded to acquire an adequate average. Frequently the responses are abnormal and/or smaller than normal due to the effects of the tumor. The time interval (one to several minutes) required to acquire sufficient responses for averaging may reduce the sensitivity of this technique to neural injury during tumor removal. Thus many monitoring teams utilize the BAER with cochlear microphonics and cochlear nerve action potentials to provide additional evaluation of the auditory system.

Cochlear microphonics are recordings directly from an electrode placed in the inner ear near the cochlear capsule (promontorium).[237-242] The larger amplitude of this signal, due to the close proximity of the electrode to the cochlea, allows much faster recording (Fig. 7-17).[243] Although these signals monitor the viability of the cochlea (integrity of the blood supply), they will not monitor the intracranial portion of the nerve.

Recordings from the exposed intracranial portion of the eighth cranial nerve (cochlear nerve action potentials) have also been used, and similarly improve the time to a usable response because of the large signal amplitude.[13,244-248] However, this location may place the recording electrode in the immediate operative field, making the dissection difficult or causing the electrode to be moved (particularly with large tumors). The nerve action potential can also be utilized to locate the cochlear nerve by using an exploring recording electrode.[19,249] Studies suggest that the recording of cochlear microphonics or cochlear nerve action potentials may be superior for monitoring and predicting useful postoperative hearing.[240,242,246,248,250,251]

Another alternative to the BAER is to place the recording electrode in the lateral recess of the fourth ventricle and allow recording from the cochlear nucleus.[252] This allows recording updates in 15 to 20 s. Monitoring of the auditory pathway has also been accomplished by electrical stimulation of the promontory in deaf individuals. This procedure has been useful in monitoring cochlear implant surgery[19] and is important for determination of the suitability of the patient to receive an implant. Monitoring has also been accom-

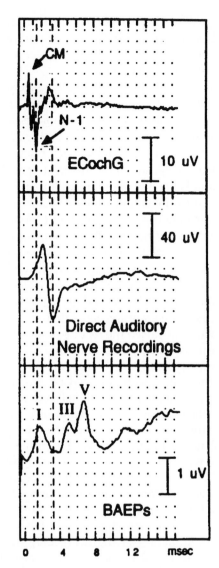

Figure 7-17 Recordings of the electrochochleogram (*top*, EcochG), direct auditory nerve recordings (*middle*), and BAER (*bottom*). (Reproduced with permission from Levine.[243])

plished by stimulation of the cochlear nucleus via the implant in a patient with an implant in place at the time of surgery to remove a tumor.[253]

Monitoring in the posterior fossa is not confined to procedures for tumor removal. Any procedure that may place adjacent, monitorable structures at risk may be appropriate for monitoring. In addition, these techniques may be useful during any procedure in which general brainstem manipulation or compression puts the brainstem at risk of injury from positioning or changes in vascular supply.[14,17]

The BAER is often used during procedures for microvascular decompression for relief of hemifacial spasm, trigeminal neuralgia, or glossopharyngeal neuralgia. It is also used in conjunction with procedures to relieve tinnitus and disabling positional vertigo,[113,254] during decompression of space-occupying defects in the cerebellum,[255] and for removal of cerebellar vascular malformations.[256]

FACIAL NERVE MONITORING

Because of the importance of facial nerve function to the patient, extensive experience is available with facial nerve monitoring, particularly in the posterior fossa where many of the tumors are slow-growing and commonly involve cranial nerves. The frequent involvement of the facial nerve with tumors in the cerebellopontine angle and acoustic neuromas (currently known as vestibular schwannomas) has led to the application of facial nerve monitoring during these surgeries in an attempt to salvage function. Despite the fact that most patients have intact nerves, facial nerve weakness is usual with tumors over 4 cm (100 percent) and common (85 percent) with smaller tumors. Since recovery often occurs (two-thirds of patients) if the nerve is left intact, monitoring to retain structural integrity can be highly useful and important to patient outcome.[13,226]

Initial efforts at monitoring involved visible identification of activity of the facial muscles after stimulation of the nerve in the operative field. Improvement in this technique involved the use of mechanical detectors on the face to detect muscle activity.[13,257] Although insensitive to the artifacts of electrocautery, the mechanical response was also insensitive to small changes and was not specific to facial nerve irritation; mechanical monitoring would unfortunately detect the response to stimulation of the muscles of mastication innervated by the trigeminal nerve.

Current methods use muscle recordings in the specific muscles of the facial nerve, with display on an oscilloscope and audible confirmation of muscle EMG activity after stimulation. These techniques have superior outcome to the mechanical methods,[258] with preservation of the nerve being directly related to the initial size of the tumor. Preservation of both anatomic and physiologic function has been reported in over 86 percent of patients[226,257]; anatomic preservation rates as high as 99.2 percent have been reported.[13]

Facial nerve monitoring is usually accomplished by placing closely spaced bipolar recording electrodes in the orbicularis oris and orbicularis oculi (with an indifferent or ground electrode elsewhere on the face). The EMG recordings are presented on an oscilloscope screen as well as played through a loudspeaker system (with suppression during cautery). Additional recording sets may be placed in other muscles (of other cranial nerves) to monitor other nerves of interest as well as to identify artifact.

This monitoring system will detect several types of

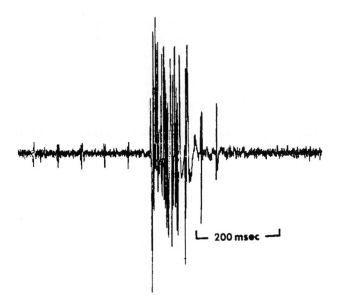

Figure 7-18 Example of burst activity from facial nerve monitoring during mechanical stimulation. (Reproduced with permission from Prass and Luders.[259])

physiologic activity in the muscle.[113,122] Two basic types of spontaneous activity have been identified.[13,259,260] First are phasic "bursts" of activity (Figs. 7-18 and 7-19). These neurotonic discharges are brief (less than 1 s), relatively synchronous motor unit discharges that result from single discharges of multiple facial nerve axons. These are usually caused by mechanical stimulation of the nerve (nearby dissection, ultrasonic aspiration or drilling, retraction), but can also be caused by thermal (irrigation, lasers, drilling, electrocautery) and chemical/metabolic insults. They serve to indicate to the surgeon that the nerve is in the immediate vicinity

of the surgical field. These short bursts of activity are not usually associated with injurious stimuli, and often indicate that the nerve remains intact and is in the vicinity of the operative field.[260]

More injurious stimuli can cause the second type of response. Tonic or "train" activity is an episode of continuous, synchronous motor unit discharges in trains of neurotonic activity lasting up to several minutes. This is usually associated with traction on the nerve (particularly lateral to medial traction[260]). The audible sounds have a more musical quality and have been likened to the sound of an outboard motorboat engine, swarming bees, popping corn ("popcorn"), or an aircraft engine ("bomber"). The bomber pattern of 50 to 100 Hz activity has been called the sound ("swan song") of dying neurons.[13] These trains are often associated with nerve compression, traction, or ischemia and are thought to be an indication of nerve injury. The proposed mechanism of the repetition of discharge is that the insult has raised the resting membrane potential to, near, or above threshold and represents an evolving injury pattern.[259]

Monitoring can also be utilized by the surgeon to locate the facial nerve by intentional electrical stimulation. Here, the surgeon can use a hand-held stimulating probe to stimulate the nerve at rates of 1 to 5 Hz. The facial nerve monitor shows repetitive bursts in synchrony with the stimulation (sounding like a machine gun). This allows the nerve to be localized, confirming identification or integrity, and identifying structures for sections that are not the nerve (i.e., strands of tissue in the dissection). It is likely that functional stimulation of the nerve may be possible with as few as 1 to 2 percent of the nerve fibers remaining intact.[261] By stimulating at several locations

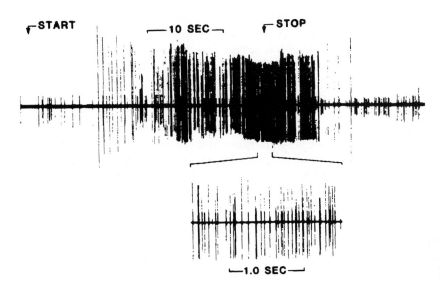

Figure 7-19 Example of sustained neurotonic discharge from facial nerve monitoring during potential injury to the nerve. (Reproduced with permission from Prass and Luders.[259])

along the nerve, the surgeon can identify the site of a conduction block. Since some investigators believe that sharp dissection may injure or sever the nerve without warning, they advocate the use of surgical instruments that are constantly providing a stimulus, so that when the nerve is approached, the stimulation will act as an early warning.[262]

By recording the response in several muscles on an oscilloscope (where the individual waveforms can be seen), different cranial nerves can be differentiated and located. This differentiation may be particularly important when the trigeminal nerve is stimulated. This is because the trigeminal nerve innervates the masseter and temporalis muscles, which, because of their larger size and proximity to the facial nerve recording locations, may produce artifact in the facial nerve monitoring that is confused for an intact facial nerve. Here, the response distribution (in the muscles) and latency (time from stimulation to response) can be used to differentiate the nerves (e.g., the latency for true facial nerve response is 6 to 8 ms whereas the latency for trigeminal response is 3 to 4 ms).

Spatial mapping of the nerve is dependent on the type and size of stimulus (for which controversy surrounds the best technique). This mapping is complicated by the fact that most facial nerves are anterior to acoustic neuromas, while most approaches are from the posterior.[13] Small stimuli are used to specifically identify the nerve, and larger stimuli are used to assure that the nerve is not in the immediate vicinity. Spatial mapping also can be used to locate the facial colliculus on the floor of the fourth ventricle when nearby brainstem lesions are being resected.[263]

The value of identifying nerve integrity is that over 60 percent of patients with intact nerves will regain at least partial function several months postoperatively, whereas loss of response is associated with a poor outcome.[122] One author reported that a direct correlation exists between the amplitude of the facial muscle CMAP and the degree of postoperative weakness.[264] Another study revealed that if the stimulation threshold of the nerve is increased, there is a suggestion that the nerve may be injured.[122] Finally, there is good correlation between the final stimulation threshold and clinical outcome.[13] A very high threshold or no response carries a 50 percent chance of a significant, long-term palsy.[13]

Several studies have demonstrated an improvement in outcome in posterior fossa surgery with monitoring.[122,265] The case is sufficiently strong for maintenance of facial nerve integrity that an NIH consensus panel has concluded, "The benefits of routine intraoperative monitoring of the facial nerve have been clearly established. This technique should be included in surgical therapy. . . . Routine monitoring of other cranial nerves should be considered."[266] This has established facial nerve monitoring as a routine part of acoustic neuroma surgery in cases where monitoring can be accomplished.

Usually muscle relaxant medications are avoided in the portion of surgery during which facial nerve monitoring is utilized.[13,112,113,267] However, controlled infusions of muscle relaxants have been used[122] since neurotonic discharges are often present when a 50 percent neuromuscular block has been achieved. However, some authors have indicated that spontaneous activity from nerve irritation is difficult to detect during controlled relaxation, particularly small amplitude responses of injured or poorly functioning nerves.[13,113,122] In addition, muscle relaxants decrease the CMAP amplitude, and amplitude is normally proportional to the number of axons able to conduct a response. Thus, when quantitative measurement of the CMAP is used as a measurement of the functional integrity of the nerve, muscle relaxants are clearly controversial.

Alternative methods of recording the facial nerve has been proposed. One technique involves stimulation of the nerve at the stylomastoid foramen; the antidromic response is recorded in the operative field by a hand-held electrode.[267] This is awkward because of the need for a hand-held stimulator in the operative field, and remains less useful than the continuous recording of muscle activity. The nerve action potential can also be recorded at the stylomastoid foramen, instead of muscle activity. Both of these methods allow complete neuromuscular relaxation, but they have been criticized because there is lack of audible feedback to the surgeon, and because it is not known if these methods are as sensitive to injury from manipulation of the nerve.[13]

A less commonly used method to continuously assess the facial nerve is termed *BFER* (*brainstem facial evoked response*).[13] This method is based on the crossed auricular response to sound that controls ear movement in animals. This technique uses the recording of the facial nerve response at the mastoid after stimulation of the contralateral ear by sound. Wide applicability of this technique is limited by lack of availability of the digital computer filtering needed for monitoring.

OTHER CRANIAL NERVES

Monitoring of the motor component of other cranial nerves has been used extensively in surgery on the base of the skull[17,18,112,131,267–270] and cavernous sinus,[267] as well as with surgery in the posterior fossa. Many other cranial nerves can be monitored by recording the muscle activity of innervated muscle in response to intentional stimulation of the nerves (Table 7-3). Methods have been described for monitoring cranial nerves III–

TABLE 7-3
Recording Locations for Motor Cranial Nerve Monitoring

I	Olfactory	(Not measured)
II	Optic	VEP
III	Oculomotor	Inferior rectus
IV	Trochlear	Superior oblique
V	Trigeminal	Masseter, temporalis
VI	Abducens	Lateral rectus
VII	Facial	Orbicularis oculi, orbicularis oris
VIII	Auditory	BAER
IX	Glossopharyngeal	Posterior soft palate (stylopharyngeus)
X	Vagus	Vocal folds, special endotracheal tubes, cricothyroid muscle
XI	Spinal accessory	Sternocleidomastoid, trapezius
XII	Hypoglossal	Tongue, genioglossus

VII and IX–XIII, usually by techniques similar to those for the facial nerve discussed above. Since cardiovascular changes are possible with stimulation of c.n. IX and X, and potentially harmful muscle activity possible with stimulation of c.n. XI, caution has been suggested in repeated stimulation of these nerves.[113]

Trigeminal Evoked Responses
Trigeminal evoked responses can be monitored by electrodes on the scalp,[113,271] with electrical stimulation of the nerve (face, gums, tooth pulp). This method has been used to test the integrity of the sensory component of c.n. V during procedures to correct trigeminal neuralgia.[118,272] However, it has not come into wide use for monitoring nerve integrity. Another method proposed for monitoring of the extraaxial nerve is stimulation of the face using electrodes inside the supraorbital, infraorbital, or mental foramina and recording from the trigeminal root entry zone.[267] This monitoring has been advocated in skull base surgery such as during tumors involving Meckel's cave, the medial middle fossa floor, or the cavernous sinus.

Vagal Innervation of the Larynx
Of recent interest has been monitoring of the vagal innervation of the larynx. This can be done using electrodes placed in the false vocal cords via direct laryngoscopy,[273] surface electrodes placed in the larynx,[274] or a specially designed endotracheal tube with electrode contacts on each lateral surface. This monitoring has been advocated in resection of tumors of the lower brainstem, thyroidectomy, and parathyroidectomy.[273,274]

Lower Cranial Nerves
Monitoring of the lower cranial nerves (c.n. IX, X, XI, and XII) is important during resection of large low

brainstem lesions because injury may cause airway collapse and inadequate protection from aspiration of gastric contents. In addition, these nerves are commonly involved in tumors in the pediatric surgical population (e.g., glioma and astrocytoma).

MONITORING THE CEREBRAL CORTEX
Extensive experience has been gained in monitoring during supratentorial neurosurgery. In general, monitoring is most effective when used for localization of the sensory-motor strip and for assessment of the viability of specific neural pathways (particularly identification of ischemia). Evoked potentials, a general monitor of cerebral well-being, are probably less useful than the EEG, since the EEG can assess a much larger scope of cortex (admittedly only the surface) than the specific pathways of evoked potentials.

Evoked potentials have been used as a general monitor of cerebral well-being to minimize cortical injury from retractor pressure[275,276] (Fig. 7-20). Such injuries are estimated to occur in 5 percent of intracranial aneurysm procedures and 10 percent of cranial base proce-

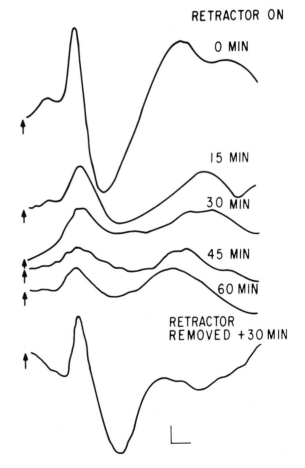

Figure 7-20 Alterations in SSEP due to cortical brain retraction. (Reproduced with permission from Bennett et al.[276])

dures, and evoked potentials have been advocated to allow identification of unfavorable perfusion in cortical tissue under retractors. One advantage of evoked responses is that viability can be monitored, and the surgeon can be warned when normally innocuous retractor pressures become significant, causing relative hypotension or selective vessel occlusion with inadequate collateral flow.

CORTICAL LOCALIZATION

Evoked potentials have also been termed *indispensable* for localization of the sensory-motor strip in the exposed cortex.[120,277] The localization is accomplished by recording the cortical component (N_{20}) of the median nerve SSEP using bipolar recording strips placed on the cortex (Fig. 7-21).[130,131] The gyrus separating the motor and sensory strip (rolandic fissure) is identified by a phase reversal of the response. This effect is thought to be due to a horizontal dipole generator that is located in the gyrus wall below the surface.[120,121] Procedures involving removal of cortical tissue, particularly structures deep to the surface, have been facilitated by identification of the sensory cortex using direct cortical recordings from SSEP stimulation. Location of the sensorimotor strip can be used to guide surgery for removal of deeper tumors.[277]

Recordings from deep structures can be utilized to identify the location of depth probes in preparation for lesioning. For example, placement of thalamotomy lesions for Parkinson's disease and other movement disorders can be assisted by recordings from the tip of the lesion probe.[133,226,278,279] Similarly depth recordings have been used during lesioning for pain syndromes.[280]

VASCULAR PROCEDURES

Monitoring has also been applied to procedures on the supratentorial structures. A large body of research demonstrates the effect of cerebral ischemia on the cortical responses of the SSEP. This monitoring has been utilized to detect cerebral ischemia perioperatively in subarachnoid hemorrhage associated with intracranial aneurysm rupture and during intraoperative procedures in which cerebral ischemia may occur.

Since the cortical response of the upper extremity SSEP is generated by cortex supplied by the middle cerebral artery, the SSEP has been utilized during carotid endarterectomy or procedures on aneurysms of the middle cerebral artery. Numerous studies have shown that the amplitude of the cortical response to SSEP stimulation is markedly diminished by reductions in cerebral blood flow. Therefore the SSEP can be used to detect cerebral ischemia, signaling the need for changes in operative management, including shunt placement.[281]

The relationship of SSEP changes to outcome in ca-

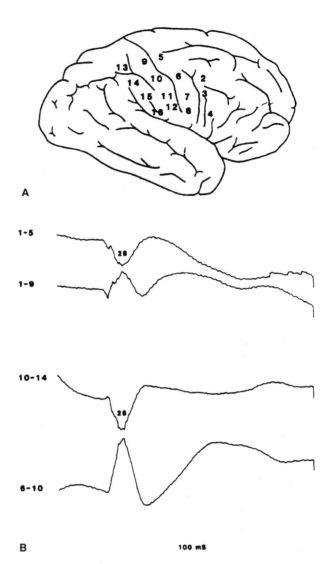

Figure 7-21. Cortical localization using SSEP. (*A*) Schematic diagram of exposed hemisphere during an epilepsy operation. The sites where recording electrodes have been placed are numbered. The site of electrode 1 (temporalis muscle) is not shown. (*B*) The contralateral median nerve is stimulated, and the cortical somatosensory evoked potential is recorded directly from the surface of the brain. A phase reversal is observed as the recording montage is shifted from electrode 5 to electrode 9, identifying the intervening fissure as the central sulcus. Likewise, bipolar recordings reveal a phase reversal centered on electrode 10, identifying this brain area as the site of generation of the potential (hand somatosensory cortex). (Reproduced with permission from Friedman and Grundy.[130])

rotid endarterectomy has been demonstrated,[282] and analysis of over 3000 patients in several studies suggests that the SSEP can be more specific than the EEG, although less sensitive to ischemia[111] and anesthesia.[283] An example of cortical SSEP loss with carotid occlusion is shown in Fig. 7-22.[284]

Although EEG is often employed during vascular procedures (notably carotid endarterectomy), advo-

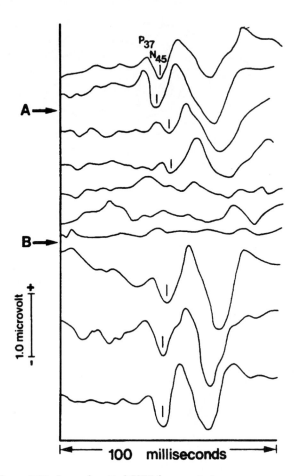

Figure 7-22 Loss of cortical SSEP from posterior nerve stimulation during carotid artery occlusion. Selected serial SSEP tracings taken from beginning of surgery (*top*) through surgical closure (*bottom*). Complete loss of recognizable cortical evoked responses is seen after placement of anterior neck retractor and occlusion of carotid artery flow (*A*). These responses return following replacement of the retractor (*B*). (Reproduced with permission from Sloan et al.[284])

cates of the SSEP indicate that it has the ability to detect injuries in structures deep to the cortical surface. In addition, one author suggests that the SSEP can be used to identify the need for shunt placement.[285] They shunted only when EEG and SSEP were both altered and noted that this reduced the shunt rate and attendant risks of shunting. Drawbacks of the SSEP include limitation of the scope of neural monitoring when compared with the EEG which can monitor a larger area of the cortex. Strokes have been observed in patients undergoing carotid endarterectomy despite absence of SSEP recording changes.[286] Comparison studies of the EEG and SSEP in carotid endarterectomy suggest they are of similar sensitivity in detection of ischemia, but neither is clearly superior for monitoring.[287]

Cortical responses from lower extremity SSEP are from cortex supplied by the anterior cerebral artery; therefore monitoring can be utilized during surgical

treatment of aneurysms of anterior vascular structures. Several studies have evaluated changes with temporary clipping to determine the integrity of collateral flow and the tolerance to use of a temporary clip. In one study[288] the SSEP was lost between 1 and 30 min after temporary clip placement; only the patient in whom the loss occurred within 1 min had a poor outcome. A similar study of temporary clipping of the middle cerebral artery or internal carotid artery showed 10 min as a permissible occlusion time.[289] Its ability to detect ischemia has also allowed monitoring to be of use during arteriovenous malformation management.[120]

Correlation between outcome and findings on monitoring in anterior circulation aneurysms has been observed,[121,123,290-295] confirming the usefulness of this modality in aneurysm surgery. Studies suggest that the amplitude of the cortical SSEP response is the most sensitive indicator of ischemia. The CCT has also been found useful as an index of ischemia.[295,296]

In addition, a very quick loss of cortical SSEP response (loss occuring in less than 1 min) after clipping is highly associated with development of neurological deficit. However, a slow loss with prompt recovery after release of the clip appears associated with the presence of collateral circulation, with a markedly reduced neural morbidity rate. One author suggests that when the N_{20} of the median nerve SSEP disappears slowly (over 4 min), 10 additional min of occlusion can be tolerated safely.[297] Examining experience with 228 aneurysms, Schramm[292] comments that the SSEP is particularly useful with multilobed and giant aneurysms, trapping procedures, and temporary occlusion.

In addition to its obvious use intraoperatively to determine tolerance of cortical tissue to deliberate hypotension, temporary clipping,[289] or the identification of inadvertent occlusion of a vessel by a clip,[293] monitoring can be used to identify ischemia from vasospasm. SSEP can also be used to detect interactions of dual events (e.g., retractor pressure[275] and hypotension, retractor pressure and temporary clipping, deliberate hypotension and hyperventilation) to identify ischemia that might otherwise not be predicted. For the detection of ischemia, monitoring of central conduction time has been advocated.[114,298] Evoked responses have been used during neuroradiologic procedures such as occlusion of vessels (e.g., AVM) or during streptokinase dissolution of occluding blood clots.[299]

Monitoring during vascular procedures on the posterior circulation has been more problematic than with the anterior circulation.[114,300] Some authors have found cranial nerve monitoring useful.[112] One author suggests that monitoring with BAER may be less useful in vascular procedures, since the known tolerance of the

BAER to ischemia may limit changes seen in response to levels of ischemia that directly threaten viability (perhaps as low as a cerebral perfusion pressure of 7 mmHg[114]). Another author suggests that the regions of brainstem ischemia produced during these procedures may be too small to be detected by SSEP or BAER.[301] This differs from anterior circulation monitoring, in which an "early warning" is seen in cortical SSEP at ischemia levels well above the level of blood flow associated with injury (cerebral blood flows below 15 cc/min per 100 g).[114] Because of these limitations, one author proposes that BAER and SSEP monitoring should be used simultaneously in posterior circulation surgery.[302]

VISUAL EVOKED POTENTIALS

Monitoring of visual evoked potentials appears to have limited application in the operating room. Perhaps the classical application is in procedures near the anterior visual pathways (such as pituitary gland), in which monitoring may allow identification of encroachment on the optic chiasm. Use of VEP monitoring during these procedures has been recommended, particularly when tumor location may obscure differentiation of the tumor tissue from normal optic nerve tissue.[303] VEP has also been used for monitoring during craniofacial procedures such as those on the orbit.[304]

Technical problems have limited the application of large, bulky, light-emitting diode "goggles," but smaller stimulators made with contact lenses or scleral caps are more useful. Studies during operative monitoring of VEP have demonstrated that manipulation of the optic pathways leads to response changes; however, response variations do not always correlate with manipulation.[305,306] In many series, monitoring does not consistently correlate with visual outcome. Therefore, one group has concluded that this lack of consistency makes the VEP a less effective monitor than other modalities. At least one author believes VEP can be of value, particularly with skull base surgery.[267] Perhaps a better stimulator than the traditional LED flash stimulation is needed to improve predictive value; the LED or flash VEP does not seem to be as specific for alteration in the visual pathways during surgery as the traditional pattern reversal techniques usable in an awake patient. It may not be a coincidence that favorable reports have been with more innovative types of stimulation (scleral cap or contact lense stimulators[267]) as these methods may monitor different neural tracts.

Alterations in Evoked Responses

PHYSIOLOGIC EFFECTS

The SEP and MEP are measures of neural function and are responsive to a variety of factors independent of

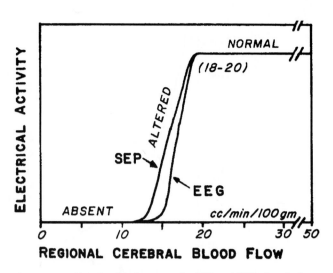

Figure 7-23 Relationship between the SEP and EEG electrical response and regional cerebral blood flow. (Reproduced with permission from Sloan.[323])

surgical insults. Therefore, intraoperative monitoring must distinguish changes associated with physiologic alterations and anesthesia, in order to improve the sensitivity of monitoring to surgical factors and ensure optimal neural environment monitoring.

Evoked responses have been used to assess cortical viability during procedures unassociated with surgical intervention on brain structures. For example, cortical AEP has been advocated during open heart surgery to monitor for cortical ischemia,[307] and during extracranial procedures to detect changes associated with local retractor pressure.[275] Evoked potentials have been utilized during interventional neuroradiologic procedures in which patient consciousness may be altered by anesthetic drugs.[299] Evoked responses have also been noted to be of value in surgery to detect improper patient positioning.[14,224,308–310]

BLOOD FLOW

Numerous studies[295,311–315] have demonstrated a threshold relationship between regional cerebral blood flow and cortical evoked responses. Although clinical function becomes abnormal at about 25 cc/min per 100 g (about one half of the normal 50 cc/min per 100 g), the SSEP remains normal until blood flow is reduced to about 20 cc/min per 100 g (Fig. 7-23).[323] At blood flows between 13 and 18 cc/min per 100 g the SSEP is altered and lost.[316–322] Experimental models have included middle cerebral artery occlusion, systemic hypotension (with and without carotid artery occlusion), and cerebral missile injury. Global hypotension is associated with SSEP cortical loss at higher rates of cerebral blood flow than with middle cerebral artery occlusion, suggesting that subcortical flow reduction contributes to the loss in hypotension.[317,318]

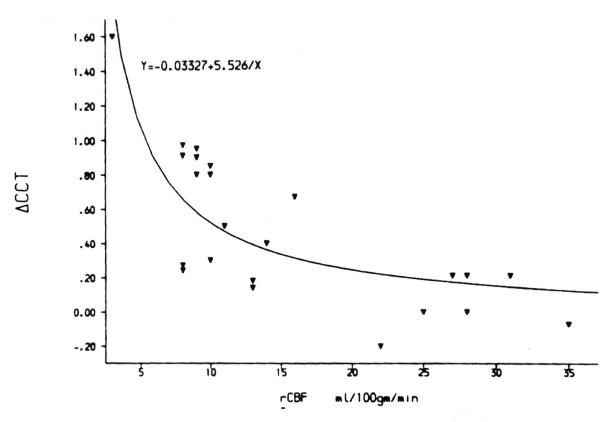

$$Y=-0.03327+5.526/X$$

Figure 7-24 The relationship between absolute regional cerebral blood flow (rCBF) levels and changes in the CCT in the postocclusive phase. (Reproduced with permission from Hargadine and Snyder.[116])

In some patients neural dysfunction occurs at higher blood pressure than expected. During spinal surgery, the effects of hypotension may be aggravated by spinal distraction, such that an acceptable limit of systemic hypotension cannot be determined without monitoring.[324-326] The relation of SSEP to ischemia is obviously the key to monitoring in cerebral vascular surgery. The CCT bears a parametric relationship to cerebral blood flow[16,316] during ischemia, again indicating that the cortex is more sensitive to blood flow reductions than subcortical structures (Fig. 7-24).

In addition to systemic hypotension, regional hypoperfusion can also be detected by the evoked response if it involves the neural structures generating the response. Examples include peripheral nerve ischemia from positioning, tourniquets or vascular interruption,[327-329] spinal cord ischemia from aortic interruption or mechanical distortion, carotid artery interruption,[283] vertebrobasilar insufficiency aggravated by head extension, cerebral artery constriction by vasospasm, and cerebral ischemia due to retractor pressure.[311]

INTRACRANIAL PRESSURE

Another physiologic variable affecting the evoked responses that can have adverse consequences on neu-

ronal survival is raised intracranial pressure. Several studies have shown that reductions in amplitude and increase in latency of cortically generated visual, somatosensory, and auditory evoked responses occur with increasing intracranial pressure (Fig. 7-25). BAER

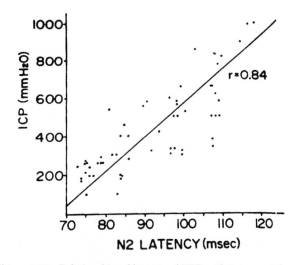

Figure 7-25 Relationship of latency of VEP with intracranial pressure. (Reproduced with permission from York et al.[47])

responses are altered as uncal herniation occurs.[330] These changes with intracranial pressure can occur after induction and during closure of intracranial surgeries. As anesthetic management may contribute to the cause as well as treatment of raised intracranial pressure, the anesthesiologist should be aware of these changes. As with raised intracranial pressure, raised cerebrospinal fluid pressure can reduce spinal cord perfusion pressure in procedures in which aortic mean arterial pressure is reduced. SSEP has been used to guide CSF pressure management during thoracic aorta procedures to reduce the risk to the spinal cord.[213,214,331] The relationship of the VEP to ICP has suggested the VEP as a means of noninvasive ICP testing.[47]

HYPOXEMIA

Hypoxemia can also cause evoked potential deterioration. This has been recorded in one case when the Pa_{O_2} reached 41 mmHg[332] before other clinical parameters had changed. Fortunately, a variety of other monitors currently make unexpected systemic hypoxemia unlikely.

BLOOD RHEOLOGY

Since changes in hematocrit can alter both oxygen-carrying capacity and blood viscosity, the maximum oxygen delivery is often thought to occur in a midrange hematocrit (30 to 32 percent). Evoked response changes with hematocrit are consistent with this optimum range. In a study of VEPs and upper extremity SSEP in the baboon, Nagao[333] observed an increase in amplitude with mild anemia, an increase in latency at hematocrits of 10 to 15 percent, and further latency changes and amplitude reductions at hematocrits below 10 percent. These changes were partially restored by an increase in the hematocrit. It is unlikely, however, that evoked response alterations due to isolated hematocrit changes will be seen, since a hematocrit change will probably occur slowly and other events (such as changes in blood pressure, blood volume, body temperature, or electrolyte concentrations) may occur coincident with the hematocrit change.

VENTILATION

One physiologic variable that may be associated with evoked response changes but may not signal adverse neural changes is ventilation. Mild hypocapnia has been associated with minimal change in the SSEP response[334]; however, alterations in cortically generated latency and amplitude have been observed as ventilation is altered beyond the extremes of arterial or end-tidal carbon dioxide concentrations routinely employed during anesthesia and surgery.[311] The most significant changes occur when the carbon dioxide is extremely low and may indicate cerebral ischemia from

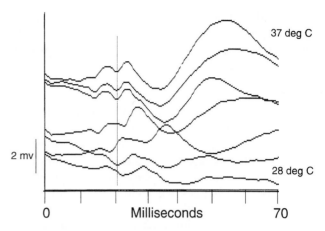

Figure 7-26   Changes in the cortical SSEP (median nerve) with whole body hypothermia as esophageal temperature is lowered from 37° to 28° centigrade (98.6° to 82.4° F).

vasoconstriction associated with excessive hyperventilation (carbon dioxide tensions below 20 mmHg). It is not clear whether the evoked response changes are due to changes in cerebral blood flow or cerebrospinal fluid pH, or other cerebral changes altered by ventilation. However, hypocapnia may aggravate hypotension due to arterial vasoconstriction. This effect has been suggested to contribute to alterations in SSEP during spinal surgery.[14]

TEMPERATURE

Hypothermia can also alter evoked responses by changing nerve depolarization (increased action potential duration,[335] reduced conduction velocity,[336,337] and decreased synaptic function[338]), resulting in increases in latency and decreases in amplitude of evoked responses.[339] These changes have been observed in visual,[340,341] brainstem auditory,[342–344] cortical auditory,[307] and somatosensory evoked potentials.[339,345,346] Hypothermia appears to affect synaptic function more than conduction,[346] probably primarily by interference in the postsynaptic membrane.[338] Thus changes are more prominent at the cephalic end of long neural tracts (such as the SSEP) or in components of responses associated with multiple synaptic elements (Fig. 7-26). Hence, responses recorded from peripheral nerves are minimally affected, while those produced by cortical structures are markedly affected.[339,345]

Whole body hypothermia, either inadvertent or intentional, is the most obvious temperature change that occurs during surgery. Although changes in whole body (or central core) temperature may occur gradually, some acute changes in regional temperature can occur and result in evoked response alterations. For example, cold irrigation solutions applied to the spinal cord,[347] brainstem, or cortex routinely cause evoked response changes. These cold irrigation solutions may also irritate the nerve, causing increased muscular activity if the nerve has motor components.[17] Similarly, extremity cooling (as from cold intravenous solutions) can alter the SSEP.

OTHER

Changes in a variety of other physiologic variables may produce alterations in the evoked responses during surgical monitoring. Significant reduction in blood volume can alter evoked responses due to changes in blood flow distribution, despite absence of significant blood pressure changes (e.g., extremity ischemia altering the SSEP as blood flow to central organs is spared). An increase in superior vena caval pressure during cardiopulmonary bypass has been associated with SSEP changes.[348]

Other physiologic events may occur too slowly to be noted as changes in the evoked response. For example, changes in glucose,[349] sodium, potassium, and other electrolytes important in the neurochemical environment and affecting neural depolarization and conduction are likely to result in evoked response changes.

MOTOR RESPONSES AND PHYSIOLOGY

Because MEP is a relatively new monitoring modality, studies of the impact of physiologic variables and anesthesia are sparse. However, since the responses are initiated by a cortical activation, it is not surprising that physiologic and pharmacologic factors affecting cortical SEP responses have parallel effects on initiation of the MEP response. However, once the MEP is initiated, the response is propagated and produced by the peripheral motor systems, potentially making it somewhat resistant to physiologic and pharmacologic effects.

For example, while cortical SEP responses can be altered by the extremes of ventilation (Pa_{CO_2}) tcMMEP upper extremity responses are not altered between an end-tidal CO_2 of 20 to 60 mmHg. However, the strength of the magnetic field needed to initiate a response (threshold) was increased at the extremes of ventilation.[350] This is consistent with initiation being a cortical event, but propagation and final response being subcortical or peripheral.

As with the SSEP, MEP is sensitive to spinal cord ischemia associated with thoracic aortic clamping,[207,351,352] and a decrease in response has been shown to correlate with reduced spinal cord blood flow.[207,353] MEP studies using cortically generated MEPs and recorded epidurally are sensitive to ischemia but not anterior horn cell injury. This is postulated to be due to persistent conduction in the corticorporeal tracts.[353] This is in contrast to recording of peripheral nerve or muscle response with MEPs, in which anterior horn cell injury can destroy the anterior horn cell function

that is required to translate the descending neural signal into a peripheral nerve response.[351]

MEPs and SEPs are both sensitive to spinal cord events produced by vascular ischemia (aortic cross-clamping) or mechanical compression (epidural balloon). However, because these tracts are topographically removed from one another, MEP and SSEP may be different in their sensitivity to ischemia.[207]

With hypothermia, the tcMMEP demonstrated a gradual increase in onset as temperature decreased from 38° to 32° C (100.4° to 89.6° F) esophageal. An increase in stimulation threshold was also observed at lower temperatures. This is consistent with both cortical initiation and peripheral conduction being affected by the drop in temperature.[354]

Increased intracranial pressure, probably by virtue of its affect on cortical structures, produces a gradual increase in onset of the tcMMEP until a response can no longer be initiated (i.e., threshold exceeded the capacity of the stimulator). The increase in latency suggests that the central component of the motor pathway is altered in its conduction velocity.[355]

CONCLUSIONS—PHYSIOLOGY

Several basic concepts have been demonstrated by analysis of the effects of physiologic changes on evoked responses. These include (1) the need to monitor continually so as to detect an evolving baseline, (2) the need to interpret evoked response changes in the context of the whole surgical environment (e.g., methodology, physiology, anesthetic as well as surgical procedure), (3) deviations from normal physiologic environments are not always deleterious to the neural system but may cause evoked response changes, and (4) in general, physiologic disturbances tend to affect the cortically generated peaks more than they affect the responses recorded from brainstem and more peripheral neural structures.

Clearly the most "monitoring favorable" environment would be for the anesthesiologist to maintain normal physiologic parameters (i.e., normothermia, normocarbia, and normotension), as these are optimally supportive of neural function and evoked response amplitude and latency. However, since reasonable deviations from normal are often innocuous or even desirable (such as hyperventilation with intracranial procedures) and can be protective (such as hypothermia), physiologic changes routinely used for procedures should be followed when they offer benefit to the patient. However, physiologic parameters should be held as constant as possible during periods where monitoring for neural compromise is needed (i.e., during portions of the surgical procedure when the nervous system is most at risk). If evoked response deteriorations occur without obvious relation to other causes (i.e., methodologic, pharmacologic, or surgical), the anesthesiologist must determine if a deleterious physiologic disturbance (such as relative hypotension) may be contributing to neural compromise. Correcting the disturbance, if possible, may improve monitoring as well as neural safety.

ANESTHESIA

An understanding of the alterations in evoked responses with anesthesia is necessary for provision of monitoring in the operating room and proper interpretation of intraoperative changes. There are several important generalizations that apply to the pharmacologic effects of anesthetic agents on evoked responses. These include: (1) Most anesthetics decrease the amplitude and increase the latency of evoked responses. (2) Anesthetic effects, like physiologic effects, are generally more pronounced in the cortically generated peaks. Thus, responses of the brainstem are usually little affected, and those of the spinal cord and peripheral nerve virtually unaffected. (3) Anesthetic effects appear to be dose-related. (4) Patients appear to differ in the degree to which they are affected by anesthesia (i.e., a dose that will produce adequate anesthesia and monitoring in one patient may be inadequate for either in another patient). (5) During periods of acute neural risk, a steady state of anesthesia is important.

During surgical monitoring, SEP responses will inevitably be altered when compared with preoperative recordings (usually amplitude decreased and latency increased). The anesthesiologist needs to strive to choose anesthetic drugs that leave sufficient response to allow monitoring, if consistent with a safe and adequate anesthetic. Fortunately this is usually possible by judicious choice and adjustment of anesthetic drugs (see below).

PREOPERATIVE MEDICATIONS

Preoperative medications can alter the amplitude and latency of the SSEP. This has been shown for meperidine (increased amplitude of median nerve SSEP[356]), droperidol,[357] and diazepam (decreased amplitude and increased latency of visual evoked responses[358]). Even the anticholinergics (atropine, scopolamine, and L-hyoscyamine[359]) can cause changes in the cortical evoked responses that appear coincident with sedation.[359,360]

ANESTHETIC AGENTS—OVERVIEW

Himwich proposed a concept of CNS stratification with respect to anesthesia effects.[361] He proposed that as anesthetic depth is increased, the cerebral cortex is depressed by the anesthetic before the subcortical diencephalon. At deeper levels the mesencephalon and pons are gradually affected until the vital centers of the

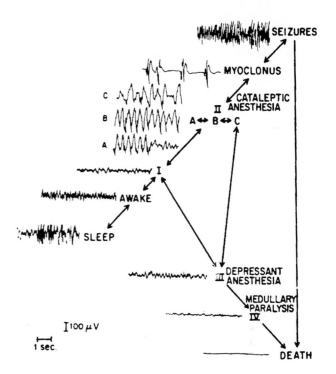

Figure 7-27 Cortical EEG stages typical of anesthesia. (Reproduced with permission from Winters.[363])

medulla are depressed at the deepest levels. Evoked responses appear to follow this pattern, with cortical responses being affected more than subcortical responses at any given level of anesthesia.

Since the most prominent anesthetic effects are on the cortically generated responses, it is not surprising that anesthetic effects on evoked responses are similar to anesthetic effects on the EEG (which is also cortically derived). In 1967 Winters[362] proposed a schema for anesthesia effects on cortical SEP that mimics a similar schema for anesthetic effects on the EEG (Figs. 7-27 and 7-28).[363] This has been observed in the VEP, where agents will decrease or increase cortical SEP in parallel to their effects on the EEG.[359] Unfortunately, most drugs in common use today produce a dose-related depression of the EEG, so that they decrease the evoked response (decrease in amplitude and increase in latency), making the choice of anesthetic medications challenging during intraoperative monitoring of cortical SEP.

Because of the correlation of cortical evoked responses and the EEG, there has been interest in using SEP for quantifying the depth of anesthesia.[364–367] The modality receiving the most attention has been the cortical AEP. Unfortunately, no drug-independent measure of depth of anesthesia has evolved.

The effects of anesthetic depression have been shown in an extensive study by Angel and Gratton,[368] in which numerous anesthetic agents were examined

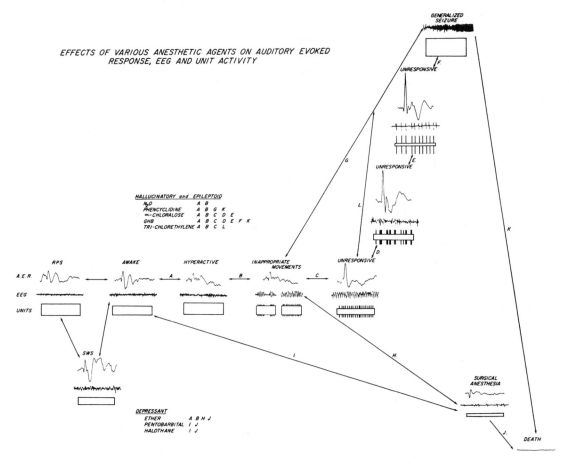

Figure 7-28 Cortical SSEP stages typical of anesthesia. (Reproduced with permission from Winters et al.[362])

using the cortical SSEP from forepaw stimulation in the rat. All of the agents used (ethyl carbonate, pentobarbital, thiopental, Althesin, ketamine, trichloroethylene, halothane, methoxyflurane, dimethyl ether, ethylvinyl ether, cyclopropane, enflurane, and chloroform) produced a dose-dependent decrease in amplitude and increase in latency. An ED$_{50}$ was calculated for 50 percent depression of amplitude, which correlated with the lipid solubility of the agents. Since lipid solubility is known to correlate with anesthetic potency (Meyer-Overton theory), this suggested that the cortical evoked potential changes paralleled anesthetic depth. Of interest are other studies that suggest evoked potential depression is pressure-reversible, similar to anesthesia effects.[368,369]

Although changes in evoked potentials parallel the depth of anesthesia, the degree of evoked potential depression between agents differs when compared using the known MAC values of the agents in the rat. This suggests that agents may differ in degree of cortical depression at equivalent levels of surgical anesthesia. This phenomenon is well known for the EEG (i.e.,

isoflurane is more depressant than halothane, and enflurane may be excitatory).

Although the evoked potential effects of anesthetics appear to parallel their anesthetic potency, specific anesthetic agents may differ depending on the specific loci of neural structures that may be excited or depressed. This was nicely demonstrated by Rosner, who reviewed the dose-related effects of several anesthetics on different neural areas (notably the mesencephalic reticular formation, thalamus, and cerebral cortex).[370] In an extensive discussion of barbiturates and inhalational agents, Rosner demonstrated that differences in neural depression and excitation correlated with differences in EEG patterns with increasing doses of these agents. Rosner ordered anesthetic agents based on ability to depress cortical evoked responses (nitrous oxide > ether > chloroform > halothane, methoxyflurane, and trichloroethylene).

Thus, at equivalent depths of anesthesia, some agents (nitrous oxide) may produce a greater degree of cortical evoked potential depression than other agents. Rosner did not systematically evaluate comparative

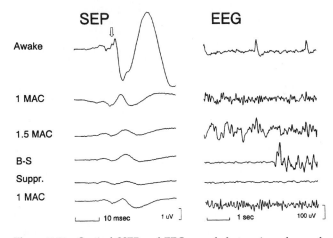

Figure 7-29 Cortical SSEP and EEG recorded at various doses of isoflurane. (Reproduced with permission from Porkkala et al.[385])

anesthetic effects on different modalities (e.g., VEP, SSEP, BAER), but evidence was presented that agents may affect modalities differently because of specific effects at various neural loci. For example, barbiturates and nitrous oxide depress the anterolateral spinal cord pathways more than the dorsal column pathways. This suggests that the detection of anterior spinal artery ischemia using lower extremity SSEPs will be hampered at large doses of these agents.

VOLATILE INHALATIONAL AGENTS
SSEP

Many studies have been conducted evaluating responses with inhalational anesthetic agents. The SSEP has been studied with halothane,[371–378] enflurane,[193,372,373,379–381] isoflurane,[373,376,377,379–390] and nitrous oxide.[373,376,381,386,389–391]

In general, all inhalational agents produce a dose-related increase in latency and reduction in amplitude of the cortically recorded SSEP responses (Fig. 7-29). Smaller effects are seen on the response recorded over the cervical spine, and minimal effects are seen in epidural or peripherally recorded responses. This suggests the prominent effects are at the cortical level with a uniform change in all the generator sites.[380] Several studies support the potency of the agents (when compared on a MAC basis) in the order nitrous oxide (most potent) > isoflurane > enflurance > halothane.[373,381,389,390] Studies of nitrous oxide in a hyperbaric chamber confirm the depressant nature of its effect at higher doses (Fig. 7-30).[391] At the time of writing, desflurane appears similar in potency and effects to isoflurane. Sevoflurane is similarly depressant, but ranking is not possible at this writing.

Although the most prominent effect is cortical, effects in the subcortical area occur. Studies of recordings at Erb's point (brachial plexus from upper extremity

stimulation) and over the cervical spine show minimal changes (0 to 9 percent), and they are not dose-related.[372,374,383] Changes in the H reflex[193] suggests an additional effect at the spinal level as well. Depth electrode studies in the spinal cord suggest that halothane and nitrous oxide may have effects in laminae I–VI and thereby account for the changes seen in epidural recordings and cervical spinal recordings from posterior tibial nerve stimulation. Although the effects of inhalational agents appear to be dose-related, changes in some studies appear to plateau at low concentrations. For example, the major latency increase often occurs at 0.5 to 1 percent inspired concentration with minimal effects at higher concentrations.[392] This nonlinear effect suggests that the drugs may have their greatest effect at low concentrations.[383] The more prominent effect at

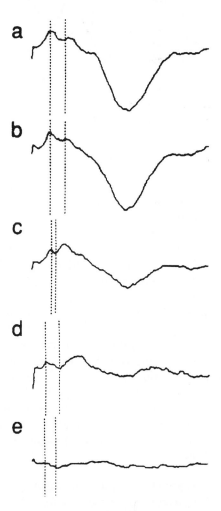

Figure 7-30 Somatosensory evoked potentials were cortically recorded after hindlimb stimulation in rats during anesthesia with N_2O and O_2 at hyperbaric pressures of 2.25 ATA (atmospheres absolute pressure). The end-tidal N_2O concentrations at which the evoked potentials were recorded were (a) 0%; (b) 31% (0.31 ATA); (c) 68% (0.68 ATA); (d) 118% (1.18 ATA); (e) 164% (1.64 ATA). (Reproduced with permission from Russell and Graybeal.[391])

EFFECT OF ISOFLURANE ON BAEP

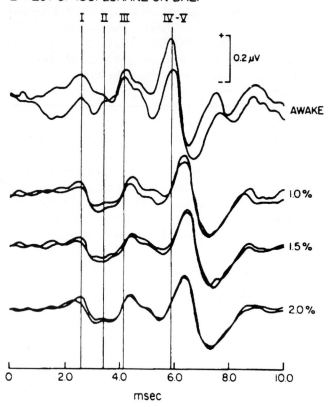

Figure 7-31 Influence of isoflurane alone on BAER. Latency of peaks III and IV–V increased at 1.0 percent but plateaued with increasing anesthetic depth. (Reproduced with permission from Manninen et al.[392])

higher cortical structures is consistent with a synaptic location of effect similar to hypothermia.[393,394]

Several investigators have successfully monitored SSEP cortical responses during 1.0 to 1.5 percent inspired halothane[371] and to a lesser extent with isoflurane and enflurane.[395] This has led some investigators to the erroneous conclusion that cortical SSEP responses can always be recorded with these agents. Several studies have demonstrated that successful monitoring can be conducted during inhalational anesthesia when low concentrations are used or when subcortical peaks are followed.[376,383] When nitrous oxide is combined with isoflurane, the effect is not predictable, suggesting that a drug interaction occurs.[390] Because of this unpredictability, and the more potent depressant effect of the combination (based on MAC equivalents), many investigators prefer to avoid nitrous oxide during recording.

Auditory Responses (BAER, Cortical AEP)
BAER has been studied with halothane,[377,396–398] enflurane,[386,399,400] isoflurane,[377,384,389,391,398,401,402] and nitrous oxide.[389,405] Cortical AEP has been studied with halothane,[396,397,404] enflurane,[396,400] isoflurane,[389,402,405] and nitrous oxide.[389,405]

As a subcortical response, the BAER is much less affected by inhalational agents (Fig. 7-31). The more prominent latency changes occur in wave V, with wave III having less and wave I being little affected (amplitude changes are minimal). Nitrous oxide can increase middle ear pressure[406] and hearing threshold,[407] thereby presenting the possibility for disproportionate effects on BAER and cortical AEP responses when eustachian tube dysfunction occurs.

As with the SSEP, all agents produce a dose-related increase in latency and decrease in amplitude of the cortical AEP (Fig. 7-32). The rank order of the effect of anesthetic agents on the auditory system is similar to the effects on the SSEP.[405] Since the changes appear to be related to depth of anesthesia, the cortical AEP has been investigated as a measure of anesthetic depth. Cognitive studies reveal that the alterations seen during nitrous oxide correlate with decreased hearing threshold,[407] level of sedation,[408] and decreased reaction time with a task.[409] Of interest is the change in response when stimulation due to intubation occurs at a stable anesthetic concentration.[405] This change mimicks a lower concentration of agent. This suggests the degree of evoked response change may reflect the level of stimulation as well as the amount of anesthetic present.

VEP
VEP has been studied with halothane,[372,410,411] enflurane,[412,413] isoflurane,[384] and nitrous oxide.[411] The electro-

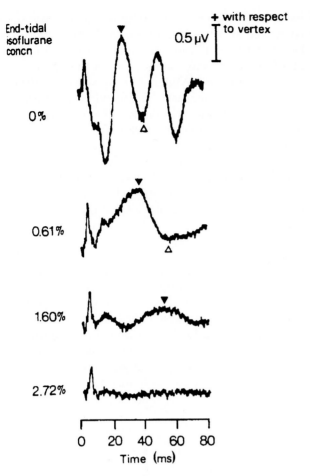

Figure 7-32   Effect of increasing end-tidal isoflurane on the early cortical components of the cortical AEP. The latencies of Pa (▼) and Nb (△) increase, and the amplitudes decrease, with increasing isoflurane concentration. (Reproduced with permission from Heneghan et al.[302])

retinogram (ERG) has been studied with halothane,[411] enflurane,[413] and nitrous oxide.[411] These studies suggest that both the ERG and cortically derived VEP are affected, with increases in latency and decreases in amplitude (Fig. 7-33).

Motor Evoked Responses

The tcMMEP has been studied with halothane,[414] enflurane,[415] isoflurane,[416] and nitrous oxide.[414] The tcEMEP has been studied with halothane,[417–419] enflurane,[417,418] isoflurane,[416–418,420–423] and nitrous oxide.[424]

The transcranial motor responses appear to be the most easily abolished by inhalational agents (Figs. 7-34, 7-35). As with sensory responses, these changes increase with increasing anesthetic concentration. However, the major effect may occur at low concentrations (e.g., less than 0.2 to 0.5 percent isoflurane[418,422]). Hence, even at low concentrations, it may not be possible to use these agents if single pulse transcranial motor responses are to be monitored.[415,420]

Studies comparing tcMMEP and tcEMEP suggest that the magnetic technique is more sensitive to the inhalational agents.[416] Since the number of I waves is known to be reduced with inhalational anesthesia,[421] this differential effect between types of stimulation suggests that the tcMMEP is more sensitive because it relies totally on I wave production. High magnetic strength tcMMEP (which produces D waves) appears to overcome this cortical effect. Since tcEMEP is easily recorded in the epidural space at concentrations of anesthetic agent that abolish a peripheral response, it appears that the most prominent anesthetic effect on tcEMEP is at the anterior horn cell level.[417,419] One novel approach to overcoming the anesthetic depression of tcEMEP and tcMMEP has been to use repetitive stimulation with closely spaced stimuli (2 to 5 ms).[149,425]

Studies on NMEP or epidurally stimulated responses show minimal effects of anesthesia. However, the above-described effects at the anterior horn cell suggest that anterior horn cell depression may change the mixture of dromic motor and antidromic sensory contributions to the recorded responses in mixed peripheral nerves.

Comparison of Modalities

When comparing a large number of studies, patterns emerge regarding the relative sensitivity of evoked responses and the relative effects of the inhalational agents. The anesthetic effect appears to mimic the more prominent effects of physiology on cortical structures (i.e., cortical structures are more affected than subcortical and peripheral structures). This differential effect probably results from a pre- or postsynaptic effect on

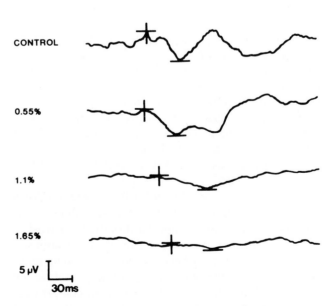

Figure 7-33   Visual evoked potentials during isoflurane anesthesia. (Reproduced with permission from Sebel et al.[384])

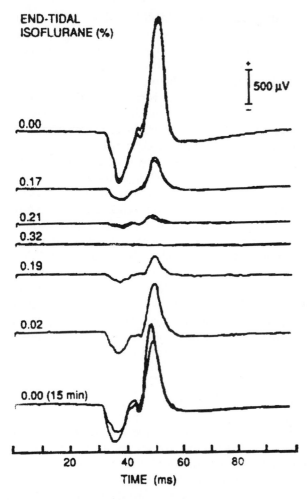

END-TIDAL ISOFLURANE (%)

500 μV

0.00

0.17

0.21

0.32

0.19

0.02

0.00 (15 min)

TIME (ms)

Figure 7-34 Motor evoked responses to transcranial electrical stimulation during nitrous oxide/sufentanil anesthesia before, during, and after administration of isoflurane (0.3% end-tidal). (Reproduced with permission from Kalkman et al.[420])

the transmission of sensory signals. This synaptic effect has been demonstrated for a variety of agents,[426–428] and many agents are known to have their primary effect at the synapse. The relative susceptibility of the various monitoring modalities to isoflurane for latency change is: SSEP (Erb's), SSEP (spinal cord), BAER I < BAER II < BAER V < SSEP (cortex) < VEP (cortex) < cortical AEP < tcMMEP,tcEMEP. Based on susceptibility to amplitude changes: SSEP (Erb's), SSEP (spinal), BAER I < BAER III < BAER V < cortical AEP < SSEP (cortex) < VEP (cortex) < tcMMEP,tcEMEP. This order follows the general pattern of increasing susceptibility with increasing cephalad location (and perhaps increasing synaptic contribution to the pathways and response), as well as cortical motor evoked potentials being more sensitive than sensory evoked potentials. Among the currently available volatile agents (halothane, enflurane, isoflurane), a consistent pattern of degree of evoked depression emerges. Halothane appears to

have the least effects and isoflurane the greatest when compared at equi-MAC levels. Desflurane appears to be similar to isoflurane, and insufficient studies with sevoflurane prevent comment about this agent.

Consistent with Winters'[362] proposal and effect on the EEG, enflurane has the capability of causing an increase in cortical excitability, which appears to enhance cortical evoked potentials. This is similar to the production of cortical irritability and seizure activity. This effect has been observed in the rat VEP and BAER using depth electrodes[429] at concentrations over 1.5 percent (MAC = 2.21 percent[418]). It is unknown if this tendency contributes to the altered order of SSEP depression.

NITROUS OXIDE
Studies with nitrous oxide are not always consistent, particularly when studies are compared in which nitrous oxide has been used alone (in awake patients), added to a patient anesthetized with volatile inhalational agents, or added to anesthesia with intravenous agents such as fentanyl. When used alone, nitrous oxide tends to produce graded amplitude and latency changes in a dose-dependent manner,[407,430–434] with mi-

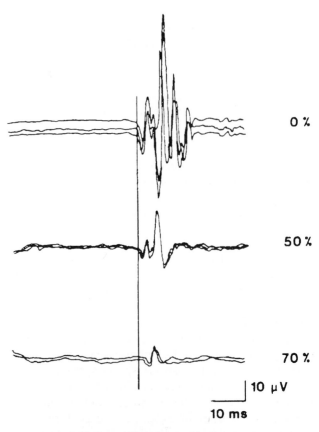

0 %

50 %

70 %

10 μV

10 ms

Figure 7-35 Successive tcEMEP responses recorded from the foot at concentrations of inhaled N_2O of 0, 50, and 70% in the same subject. (Reproduced with permission from Jellinek et al.[424])

nor or no changes in subcortical responses.[374,401] When added to inhalational anesthetics, nitrous oxide may cause additional changes in latency and amplitude[374] or have no apparent additive effect.[392,435] In cases in which nitrous oxide is added to intravenous agents, amplitude changes predominate, without latency change.[381,436-438] Hence nitrous oxide may be more "context-sensitive" in its effects (i.e., the actual effect may vary with the other anesthetics already present).

Nitrous oxide has generally been assumed to have a mild effect on monitoring, probably because its anesthetic potency is minimal. However, several studies document marked depressant effects when combined with inhalational agents[374,384] or with opioid agents[381,437,438] and when used or studied alone.[381,407-409,430-434] In contrast, occasional studies suggest no additional effect of nitrous oxide when added to volatile agents.[435]

CONCLUSION—INHALATIONAL ANESTHESIA

Inhalational agents have occasionally been referred to as the "horrible halogenated hydrocarbons" because of their ability to reduce amplitude with cortical evoked responses and effectively prevent intraoperative recording. As above, this effect is dose-dependent, patient-dependent, and monitoring-modality-dependent. Among the SSEP responses, lower extremity responses appear to be more sensitive than upper extremity responses,[439] perhaps due to the anatomic location of the sensory cortex[18] or differences in the somatotopic organization of the sensory cortex. However, inhalational agents (including nitrous oxide) may be very acceptable anesthetic choices when peripheral and subcortical responses are monitored.

INTRAVENOUS ANALGESIC AGENTS

Because the inhalational anesthetic agents have marked depressant effects on cortical evoked potentials and motor evoked potentials, anesthesiologists frequently choose intravenous analgesics (opioids or ketamine) supplemented with intravenous sedative agents (barbiturates, benzodiazepines, etomidate, propofol, or droperidol) when monitoring is required.

Opioid Agents

The effects of the opioid analgesics on evoked responses are generally mild; effects are maximal when the drug effect is peaking and then remain rather stable. Studies have been conducted with fentanyl, alfentanil, sufentanil, morphine, and meperidine.

Results are somewhat similar for most evoked sensory modalities, including the SSEP,[339,356,440-448,455] SSEP (spinal recordings),[448,449,455] BAER,[441,450,451] cortical AEP,[443,452,453] and VEP.[441,454]

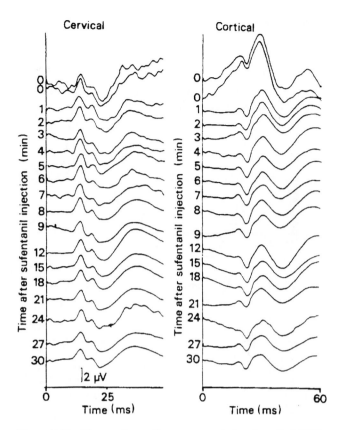

Figure 7-36 Changes in median nerve cervical and cortical SSEP recording with time in one patient after sufentanil 5 mcg kg^{-1}. Two baseline recordings at time zero are shown. (Reproduced with permission from Kimovec et al.[455])

Generally little effect is seen with systemic opioids when given alone (Figs. 7-36, 7-37).[345] One study of meperidine used as a premedicant demonstrated enhanced SSEP amplitude.[356] Opioid effects are minimal on spinal or subcortical recordings, with depression of amplitude and increases of latency in cortical responses and occasional loss of late cortical peaks (over 100 ms), particularly with doses producing sedation. The effects are reversed with naloxone,[443,448,454] suggesting that the effect is a mu receptor effect.

As a consequence of this minimal effect, total intravenous anesthesia with opioids and sedative drugs is often used when recording of responses is not possible in the presence of inhalational agents. One study using constant infusion of fentanyl suggests that the change in evoked responses may be reduced by this infusion method when compared with intermittent bolus dosing.[447] This also potentially avoids transient bolus effects seen when drugs are injected. Studies with transcranial motor evoked responses using electrical[456] and magnetic[457,458] methods also show mild amplitude decreases and latency increases which permit continuation of recording.

The spinal application of morphine[459] or fentanyl[460]

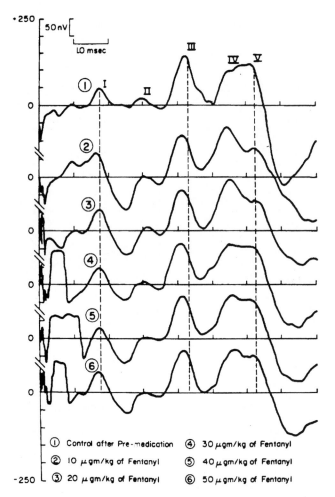

Figure 7-37 Composite tracings of 10 patients showing effect of incremental doses of fentanyl on morphology and latencies of brainstem auditory evoked potentials. (Reproduced with permission from Samra et al.[450])

produces minimal changes in the SSEP. A similar lack of effect was observed in a study using dermatomal evoked responses.[461] Consistent with lack of spinal effect, spinally applied fentanyl failed to alter the H reflex.[460]

Ketamine
An alternative analgesic to opioids and the inhalational agents is ketamine. Ketamine provides excellent analgesia and hypnosis, but hallucinatory activity and increases in intracranial pressure in patients with cortical abnormalities limit its usefulness.

Ketamine has been studied with BAER,[462–464] SSEP,[465] cortial AEP,[466,467] VEP,[468] and tcMMEP.[469,470] Minimal effects were observed. Studies in the SSEP have shown an increase in cortical amplitude, suggesting an enhancing effect (Fig. 7-38).[471] Muscle responses and spinal recorded responses to spinal stimulation are also enhanced at doses that do not produce spike and wave

activity in the EEG.[472] Cortical excitement may also be responsible for the appearance of additional peaks in the rat VEP with ketamine.[468]

These studies suggest that ketamine is a desirable agent for use when monitoring evoked responses which are usually susceptible to anesthetic effects (notably dermatomal evoked responses and transcranially elicited motor evoked responses) (Fig. 7-39). Some investigators prefer to supplement the ketamine with midazolam to reduce the likelihood of hallucinations.

SEDATIVE-HYPNOTIC DRUGS
In some patients, excellent anesthesia for cortical evoked response recording can be provided with analgesia from opioids or ketamine, supplemented with nitrous oxide or low-dose inhalational agents. However, in some patients the depressant characteristics of these supplemental agents reduce the size of the evoked response below that acceptable for monitoring (i.e., the desired response cannot be reliably distinguished from background noise). In these circumstances, the anesthesiologist may choose to supplement with intravenous sedative agents rather than the inhaled agents (e.g., opioids or ketamine for analgesia and ketamine or sedative-hypnotics for sedation). Numerous studies have been conducted to evaluate agents including thiopental, midazolam, propofol, etomidate, and droperidol as supplements to opioid analgesia.

Barbiturates
Thiopental has been used by infusion to provide supplemental sedation during intravenous anesthesia. Because of a prolonged pharmacologic half-life due to slow metabolism, infusion rates must be kept low (1 to 3 mg/kg per h) to allow awakening shortly after the conclusion of surgery. Although this produces excellent sedation during intracranial procedures, an unacceptably high incidence of awareness during spine procedures has been observed. This problem has prompted a change to other agents with shorter pharmacologic half-lives or superior amnesia.

Thiopental, however, remains a frequent drug for induction (Fig. 7-40). Studies on evoked responses with anesthesia induction with thiopental,[440,458,473–482] pentobarbital,[483,484] or methohexital[474] have been conducted. Modalities studied have included SSEP, cortical AEP, BAER, and tcMMEP.

These studies demonstrate decreases in amplitude and increases in latency of cortical sensory responses with increasing effects on longer latency waves and minimal effects on the brainstem responses. The pattern of SSEP change with thiopental was consistent with redistribution of the drug.[473] This suggests that marked changes should be expected shortly following

Within the figure:
+250
50 nV
LO msec
III
I   II   IV   V
① Control after Pre-medication   ④ 30 μgm/kg of Fentanyl
② 10 μgm/kg of Fentanyl   ⑤ 40 μgm/kg of Fentanyl
③ 20 μgm/kg of Fentanyl   ⑥ 50 μgm/kg of Fentanyl
-250

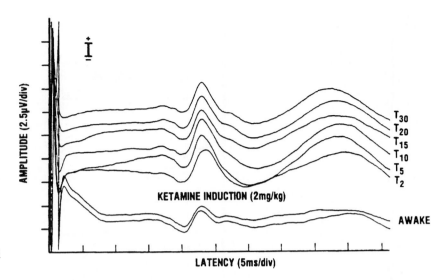

Figure 7-38 Example of SCEP waveforms before and after induction with ketamine at times 2, 5, 10, 15, 20, and 30 min. (Reproduced with permission from Schubert et al.[471])

induction (with resolution in 15 to 20 min) or shortly following bolus delivery during a monitoring session.

Studies with thiopental demonstrate that the effect is minimal on subcortically recorded responses, with progressive effects on later responses, most notably late responses. For example, BAER is virtually unaffected at doses of pentobarbital that produce coma.[463,477,485] Changes in the BAER are not seen until dosages are sufficient to produce cardiovascular collapse.[486] The SSEP can be recorded with thiopental sufficient to produce a silent EEG.[485,487]

The tcMMEP, however, was more sensitive to barbiturates, with amplitude depression at doses below that affecting the SSEP and lasting for a longer period of time after induction. In one study, induction eliminated the tcMMEP response for a period of 45 min,[458]

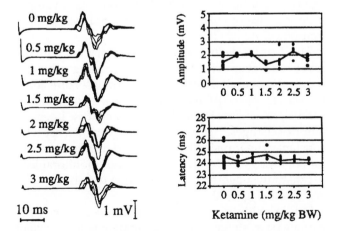

Figure 7-39 Transcranial magnetic motor evoked potentials and ketamine. Four single recordings at each step of 0 mg/kg body weight (BW) to 3 mg/kg BW are superimposed. Tables show mean values of amplitude and latency with 12 recordings at baseline and 4 recordings at each dosage step. (Reproduced with permission from Kothbauer et al.[470])

suggesting that it may be a poor induction drug for monitoring of this modality. These studies suggest a drug effect in the cortex.

Benzodiazepines

Midazolam, in doses consistent with induction of anesthesia and in the absence of other agents, produces a mild depression of cortical SSEP.[482,488] An initial increase in latency and decrease in amplitude gradually resolve (Fig. 7-41). Because of midazolam's excellent amnestic qualities, an infusion of midazolam is chosen by some anesthesiologists to maintain a steady level of supplemental hypnosis during opioid analgesia. Similarly, midazolam is an excellent supplemental hypnotic when used with ketamine.

Evoked responses have been studied following diazepam 10 to 20 mg or 0.1 mg/kg.[441,489] The median nerve SSEP demonstrated mild decreases in amplitude for early peaks (N_{18}, P_{22}), moderate decreases in amplitude for late peaks (N_{60}), and loss of very late peaks (200 to 400 msec). Curiously, middle latency peaks (N_{35} to N_{60}) usually increased in amplitude. Diazepam at 0.2 mg/kg[490] resulted in 10 to 20 percent decreases in very early epidural responses, whereas the subsequent, later peaks increased 10 to 20 percent. There was no change in BAER.[278] Studies on the cortical AEP and VEP showed similar small amplitude decreases and latency increases. Therefore, a benzodiazepine-opioid combination has been advocated for SEP recording.[441,491,492]

In addition to possible cortical locations for the benzodiazepine effect, an effect at the spinal cord has been suggested by a study of posterior tibial stimulation.[490] Diazepam produced a marked decrease in the amplitude of the H reflex with no effect on the M reflex. Since the first peak of the electrospinogram was decreased, this is consistent with drug effect at the dorsal root.

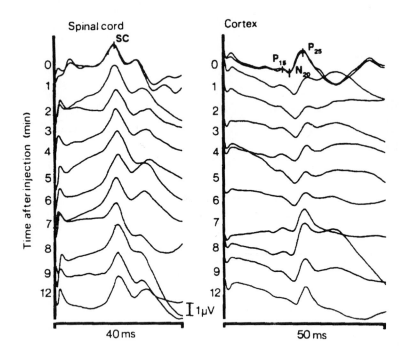

Figure 7-40 SSEP responses recorded from the cervical and cortical electrodes before (0) and at several times up to 12 min following the injection of thiopentone (4 mg/kg). (Reproduced with permission from Sloan et al.[473])

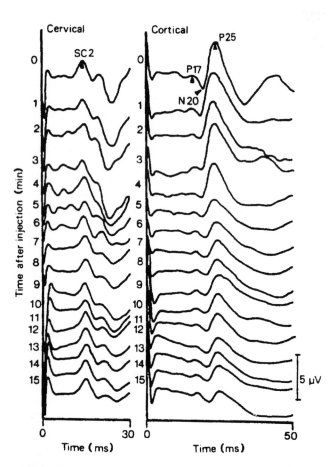

Figure 7-41 SSEP responses recorded from the cervical and cortical electrodes are shown before and at 1-min intervals after the injection of midazolam (0.2 mg/kg). (Reproduced with permission from Sloan et al.[488])

As with thiopental, midazolam produced prolonged marked depression of tcMMEP, suggesting it also may be a poor induction agent for recording.[456,493,494] This has been interpreted as inhibition of cortical pyramidal cell neurons.

Etomidate

Etomidate has also been studied with sensory and motor evoked responses. Studies with the BAER,[495] cortical AEP,[495] and VEP[496] suggest that doses used for induction of anesthesia produce little effect. However, when the same dose was given during a fentanyl-nitrous oxide anesthetic, a VEP amplitude depression was observed.[496] Studies with the SSEP demonstrate an amplitude increase of cortical components following injection (Fig. 7-42).[440,478,482,497]

This amplitude increase appears coincident with the myoclonus seen with the drug, suggesting a heightened cortical excitability (no evidence of seizure activity was seen).[488] The increase has raised concern that a transient increase in amplitude may confuse interpretation of changes.[440] However, a sustained increase with constant drug infusion has been used to enhance cortical recordings that were otherwise not monitorable.[492] A cat study suggests that the location of enhancement is cortical (Fig. 7-43).[498]

Studies with transcranial elicited motor evoked potentials have suggested that etomidate is an excellent agent for induction and monitoring of these modalities.[183,456,458,474,499,500] Of several intravenous agents studied, etomidate had the least degree of amplitude depression after induction doses or continual intravenous infusion. Latency (onset) changes were not observed

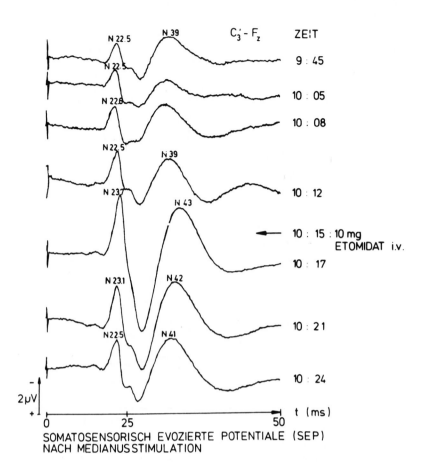

Figure 7-42 Cortical SSEP from median nerve stimulation before and following 10 mg etomidate. (Reproduced with permission from Russ et al.[478])

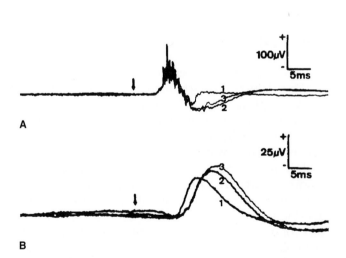

Figure 7-43 Effect of etomidate on the amplitude and latency of thalamic (*A*) and cortical (*B*) evoked potentials in an animal. Trace 1 in both *A* and *B* is control response; traces 2 and 3 were recorded 5 and 10 min, respectively, after injection of 3 mg/kg etomidate. Note difference in *A* and *B* in scales of amplitude. Different amplifier gain settings were used to facilitate simultaneous viewing of thalamic and cortical potentials on the oscilloscope. (Reproduced with permission from Samra and Sorkin.[498])

and amplitude enhancement of muscle responses was not observed except at very small dosages with depression at high dosages.[500]

Unlike thiopental, etomidate also offers a relatively fast clearance rate, making it an excellent supplemental hypnotic agent. Despite the known effect of depression of cortisol production, short-term administration appears safe. This may not be an issue with many surgeries in which steroid agents are given routinely. However, when not given as a part of the surgery, it is unclear if supplemental steroids should be given when etomidate is used.[492]

Ketamine and etomidate are therefore unique agents in the intravenous armamentarium, as they have the ability to enhance cortical evoked responses while contributing to anesthesia. It is unknown if this increase in cortical excitability increases risk to these neural structures during surgery. It is similarly unknown if monitoring by any active, stimulatory technique (i.e., evoked potentials) increases the risk to the structures tested (even using a depressant anesthetic technique).

Propofol

Since intravenous anesthetic agents have been recommended to reduce the amount of inhalational agents,

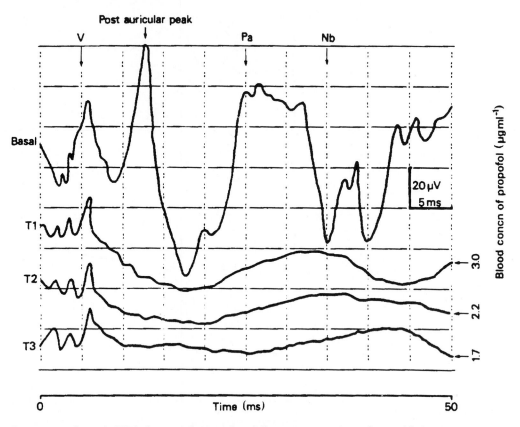

Figure 7-44 Cortical AEP before anesthesia and at different concentrations of propofol. Arrows indicate the position of waves V, Pa, and Nb. (Reproduced with permission from Chassard et al.[501])

propofol has been studied. Propofol's fast clearance makes it an excellent sedative drug provided by infusion. Propofol induction doses produce amplitude depression in cortical AEP[501,502] and cortical SSEP[503–505] with rapid recovery after cessation of infusion. One report of propofol used without other major anesthetic agents demonstrated a 15 percent increase in cortical SSEP amplitude.[506] The latencies of the BAER were increased without significant amplitude decreases (Fig. 7-44).[501,507]

When the SSEP is recorded in the epidural space, propofol had no significant effect. This is consistent with the postulated site of anesthetic action of propofol on the cerebral cortex.[508] Studies with transcranial electrical or magnetic motor evoked potentials have demonstrated a depressant effect on response amplitude, also consistent with a cortical effect.[456,474,509] Propofol has been used in tcEMEP when the recordings are epidural.[419]

Droperidol

Droperidol also appears to be an acceptable anesthetic agent during monitoring. It appears to have minimal effects when combined with an opioid on SSEP,[510] VEP,[511] and tcMMEP.[457,483] The use of a droperidol-opioid ("neurolept") technique has the additional advan-

tage of not depressing cortical seizure activity (thus making it useful for seizure focus identification and ablation) and provides excellent anesthesia for awake intubation and positioning when required (such as with spinal surgery).

REGIONAL ANESTHESIA

Major conduction anesthesia (i.e., epidural or spinal) does not appear to be an acceptable alternative to general anesthesia for spinal procedures, since the evoked responses are eliminated by dosages of local anesthetic agents which provide anesthesia. This has been seen with intravenous regional block[512] and specific nerve blocks.[513] Certainly local anesthesia placed away from the evoked response neural pathway (such as scalp anesthesia for awake craniotomy) would be satisfactory for monitoring unless systemic absorption is substantial.

In addition to the specific effects of local anesthetics on regional nerve function, systemically infused agents can cause an effect probably due to influence on sodium ion channels. In a cat study, Javel saw a dose-related increase in latency of auditory evoked response peaks with systemic infusions of lidocaine.[514] In this study, brain stem-generated peaks "split" at higher lidocaine concentrations (>1 mg/min), suggesting

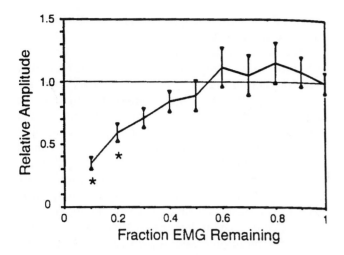

Figure 7-45 Plot of tcMMEP amplitude as recorded from thenar muscles (plotted versus the fraction of a single twitch remaining following median nerve stimulation). (Reproduced with permission from Sloan and Erian.[522])

components from several generators that blend normally to form each peak might be affected differently. However, at lower doses systemic lidocaine produces only minor changes.[515]

MUSCLE RELAXANTS

Muscle relaxants are generally thought to have no effect on the sensory evoked responses.[516–518] In fact, SEPs may actually improve with muscle relaxation because EMG interference is reduced in electrodes near muscle groups such as over the cervical spine. This effect may be responsible for the enhancement seen with low doses of propofol[506] and demerol.[356] When excessive EMG activity appears in these electrodes, the monitorist may be able to indicate the need for additional relaxant (should moderate neuromuscular block be desired). Partial neuromuscular blockade also has the advantage of reducing body motion during stimulation that can be disturbing in the operative field.

As discussed previously, the use of muscle relaxants with facial nerve monitoring is controversial. However, several reports of successful recording of MEP muscle response have appeared.[37,215,519–521] In these studies, a single twitch response is maintained at 10 to 20 percent of baseline using a constant infusion of muscle relaxant. This is consistent with animal studies showing a nonlinear effect of atracurium[522] and vecuronium[523] on tcMMEP responses (Fig. 7-45). Many authors use closed-loop control systems to monitor the twitch and control the infusion. Because of varying muscle sensitivity to muscle relaxants, the neuromuscular blockade may need to be monitored in the muscle groups being used for CMAP monitoring.

CHOICE OF ANESTHESIA FOR EVOKED RESPONSE MONITORING

OVERVIEW

As with any surgical anesthetic, a variety of factors determine the choice of agent. These include (1) the patient (i.e., interaction of anesthetic agents with the patient's pathophysiology), (2) the surgical requirements (i.e., unusual requirements such as awake positioning, wake-up test), and (3) the specific modalities of sensory evoked responses to be utilized for monitoring.

With respect to the monitored evoked responses, the surgeon must evaluate, in conjunction with the monitorist, the neural structures that will be at risk to determine which evoked response peaks of the various stimulation techniques are most appropriate.

SUBCORTICAL RESPONSES

If the monitored peaks are entirely from peripheral nerves (e.g., during evaluation of neuroma in situ), spinal cord (e.g., invasive spinal cord electrodes), or brainstem (e.g., BAER), then any anesthetic technique (except regional) will usually be acceptable. Under these circumstances, the anesthetic should be chosen based on considerations of the patient and surgical procedure. If a muscle response is to be monitored, then avoidance of muscle relaxants should be considered. As noted above, controversy surrounds the effects of partial neuromuscular block. If inhalational agents can be used without problems, then simply avoiding muscle relaxants during periods of monitoring is an obvious consideration.

Many individuals prefer to monitor cortical responses during subcortical surgery (notably spinal surgery), since these may allow detection of events that may injure cortical structures (e.g., carotid occlusion during anterior neck surgery[284]). If no recordable cortical evoked response can be identified, the surgeon and anesthesiologist may be able to assist the monitorist in the placement of invasive recording electrodes that will allow the detection of responses not recordable by surface electrodes. For subcortical surgery, recording electrodes placed along the spinal cord or near the brain stem may allow recording due to the lesser degree of anesthetic effect on these structures. Unfortunately, subcortical responses are often of lower amplitude, thus making them more susceptible to artifact or noise. This problem is usually reduced when an invasive electrode is placed near the generator tissue.[17] One recent report indicated successful intraoperative spinal cord monitoring of a group of patients with a variety of neuromuscular disorders by recording the response to lower extremity stimulation at the cervical spine.[376] Because of the reduced effects of anesthesia, the authors were able to monitor despite halothane or isoflurane anesthesia (up to 0.6%) with opioids and nitrous oxide in this traditionally difficult to monitor group of patients.

CORTICAL RESPONSES

When cortically generated evoked responses are desired for monitoring, certain agents that would otherwise be acceptable for the patient and surgery may prove unfavorable for monitoring. Often, the inhalational agents will be acceptable in low concentrations, but usually not in concentrations sufficient to provide anesthesia without supplementation with intravenous agents (e.g., opioids and sedative agents).

Hence, most techniques utilize low-dose inhalational agents (0.25 to 0.5 MAC) or nitrous oxide with opioid supplementation. However, if the monitorist is unable to obtain adequate, repeatable, reliable responses, these agents may need to be reduced or replaced with intravenous agents. There is often time between the induction of the anesthetic and the time of greatest surgical risk for the necessary anesthetic adjustment. Occasionally, a total intravenous anesthetic will be required; the anesthetic is usually initiated with an opioid analgesic (or ketamine if appropriate), and supplemental agents are added as appropriate to provide sedation and hypnosis.

Just as patients appear to vary in the effect of anesthetic agents on cardiovascular and autonomic tone, individual patients appear to respond with different degrees of change of the evoked responses to anesthetic agents. Hence patients need to be evaluated individually as to the effect of anesthesia on the evoked responses, and what may be an acceptable anesthetic with one patient may not be acceptable with the next.

A knowledge of the preoperative evoked responses (if tested) can be useful. If the preoperative responses are of large amplitude and well defined, then the patient may tolerate a moderate amount of anesthetic depression and still be monitored. Alternatively if the preoperative responses are poorly defined and of low amplitude, then a depressant anesthetic will probably be unacceptable, since the decrease in amplitude due to anesthesia will render them unrecordable. If preoperative responses are not available, older patients and those with existing neurologic impairment are at greater risk for significant anesthetic depression. In general,[524] older patients and patients with marked neurologic abnormalities in the pathway to be monitored have smaller, poorly defined evoked responses under anesthesia and are therefore more sensitive to depressant agents such as the inhalational agents. One explanation for this effect is that injured spinal neurons become demyelinated, causing an increased sensitivity to anesthesia and environmental changes.[525]

If poor preoperative responses are due to EMG inter-ference, the operative responses may actually improve with anesthesia due to a reduction in the EMG by anesthesia and muscle relaxants. Also, if the recording technique used preoperatively is different than that used for monitoring (e.g., the methodology used for diagnostic purposes is often different than that for monitoring), the preoperative study may not predict the intraoperative recording. It should be noted that the maximal stimulation rate during anesthesia is slower than that during preoperative testing.[311] Anesthesia appears to make the nervous system more prone to fatigue. Hence the monitoring response may often be improved during anesthesia by slowing the stimulation rate. If the patient has preexisting neurologic disease in the monitored neural pathway, or if consultation with the monitorist reveals poor preoperative responses, the anesthesiologist may wish to simply begin the anesthetic using opioids with supplementation with an intravenous hypnotic agent.

If the monitored response remains unacceptably small with opioid-sedative anesthetic, then the use of enhancing agents such as etomidate or ketamine may be useful. Despite these efforts, in a few patients (fewer than 1 percent in the author's experience) an anesthetic approach will not be found that will allow monitoring to be conducted while conditions remain surgically and anesthetically adequate.

CRANIOTOMY

If the required response is cortical and a craniotomy has been conducted, the anesthetic problem may be aggravated by the inability to place recording electrodes near the generator sources. Since amplitude falls off by the square of the distance, this distance may compound anesthetic depression. This problem may be partially solved by placing sterile recording electrodes along the craniotomy flap or in the surgical area. Scalp, dura, or cortical strip electrodes may allow larger responses due to closer proximity to the cortical generator (the scalp response is about one-twentieth the size of the signal recorded on the cortical surface).

MOTOR EVOKED RESPONSES

Because the anesthetic effect on the spinal column is less than on the cortex, anesthetic choice for spinal responses after epidural or spinal column stimulation (NMEP) appears to be rather broad except for muscle relaxant considerations (above). However, providing surgical anesthesia for monitoring of transcranial stimulated MEP may be more challenging than anesthesia for surgery with cortical SEP monitoring. First, volatile agents are poorly tolerated.[33] Thus, reliance on opioids or ketamine is frequently employed. Second, muscle relaxants, if used, must be carefully controlled (such as with a relaxant infusion) so as not to obliterate EMG responses (if needed for monitoring).[33] This sensitivity to volatile agents and obliteration by neuromuscular blocking agents is a challenging combination for providing anesthesia. Hence a light stage of anesthesia is needed, probably by intravenous agents. Fentanyl has been suggested to be useful in reducing background spontaneous muscle contractions and associated motor unit potentials in addition to providing surgical analgesia.[524] Additional studies and experience will be needed to provide a more thorough guide to anesthesia when transcranially stimulated MEP recording is desired.

OVERALL ANESTHESIA GOAL

Regardless of the anesthetic agents chosen, the anesthetic goal should be to provide a constant level of anesthetic during the critical surgical periods. A bolus drug injection or a change in inhaled concentration might produce a sudden change in the evoked response that could simulate, obscure, or eliminate an indication in the evoked response that neuronal injury is occurring. For example, a bolus of sodium thiopental, by reducing amplitude and increasing latency, can mimic injury. Likewise, the elimination of nitrous oxide at a critical time might allow an increase in amplitude that offsets a simultaneous decrease that would usually be indicative of neural injury.

Thus, during the procedure, the maintenance anesthetic should be adjusted prior to the critical surgical periods and then held constant. If further adjustments are necessary, their timing should be considered in the surgical and monitoring context so as to minimize confusion with neural injury. Because of the lesser degree of depression with the intravenous agents, and because of the ability to provide a constant effect by infusion techniques, several excellent total anesthetic approaches have been developed for use during cortical evoked response recording.

Fortunately, most anesthetic regimes that are acceptable for monitoring during spinal procedures are also compatible with the conduct of a wake-up test. For this reason, some investigators have popularized the use of intravenous infusions so as to allow predictable wake-up tests.[442]

Conclusion

Evoked responses have become a valuable adjunct to the clinical neurologic examination, especially in circumstances in which the clinical examination is hampered by injury or medications that interfere with patient participation. They have become important additions for functional assessment to complement the many studies available for structured assessment of the nervous system. The recent implementation of evoked responses from the motor pathways has nicely complemented sensory pathway responses in patient assessment and monitoring.

References

1. Chiappa KH: *Evoked Potentials in Clinical Medicine.* New York, Raven Press, 1990.
2. Spehlmann R: *Evoked Potential Primer.* Boston, Butterworth Publishers, 1985.
3. Luders H: *Advanced Evoked Potentials.* Boston, Kluwer Academia Publishers, 1989.
4. Morocutti C, Rizzo PA (eds): *Evoked Potentials, Neurophysiological and Clinical Aspects.* New York, Elsevier, 1985.
5. Perot PL, Vera CL: Scalp-recorded somatosensory evoked potentials to stimulation of nerves in the lower extremities and evaluation of patients with spinal cord trauma. *Ann NY Acad Sci* 1982; 388:359.
6. York DH, et al: Utilization of somatosensory evoked cortical potentials in spinal cord injury: Prognostic limitations. *Spine* 1983; 8:832.
7. Gugino V, Chabot RJ: Somatosensory evoked potentials. *Int Anesthesiol Clin* 1990; 28(3):154.
8. Hickey R, et al: Functional organization and physiology of the spinal cord. In Porter SS (ed): *Anesthesia for Surgery of the Spine.* New York, McGraw-Hill, 1995:15.
9. Scarff TB, et al: Dermatomal somatosensory evoked potentials in children with myelomeningocele. *Z Kinderchir Grenzgeb* 1979; 28(4):384.
10. Eisen A, et al: Evaluation of radiculopathies by segmental stimulation and somatosensory evoked potentials. *Can J Neurol Sci* 1983; 10:178.
11. Green J, et al: Dermatomally stimulated somatosensory cerebral evoked potentials in the clinical diagnosis of lumbar disc disease. *Clin Electroencephalogr* 1983; 14:152.
12. Sloan TB, et al: Evaluation of spinal cord function by means of evoked potentials. In Meyer P (ed): *Surgery of Spine Trauma.* New York, Churchill-Livingstone, 1989;121–136.
13. Yingling CD: Intraoperative monitoring of cranial nerves in skull base surgery. In Jackler RK, Brackmann DE (eds): *Neurotology.* St. Louis, Mosby, 1994:967–1002.
14. Grundy BL, et al: Intraoperative monitoring of brain-stem auditory evoked potentials. *J Neurosurg* 1982; 57:674.
15. Abramson M, et al: Intraoperative BAER monitoring and hearing preservation in the treatment of acoustic neuromas. *Laryngoscope* 1985; 95:1318.
16. Friedman WA, et al: Intraoperative brain-stem auditory evoked potentials during posterior fossa microvascular decompression. *J Neurosurg* 1985; 62:552.
17. Moller AR: *Evoked Potentials in Intraoperative Monitoring.* Baltimore, Williams & Wilkins, 1988.
18. Nuwer MR: *Evoked Potential Monitoring in the Operating Room.* New York, Raven Press, 1986.
19. Kileny PR, et al: Neurophysiologic intraoperative monitoring; I. Auditory function. *Am J Otol* 1988; 9 (Suppl):17.
20. Daspit CP, et al: Monitoring of intraoperative auditory brain stem responses. *Otolaryngol Head Neck Surg* 1982; 90:108.
21. Luders H: Surgical monitoring with auditory evoked potentials. *J Clin Neurophysiol* 1988; 5:261.
22. Aravabhumi S, et al: Brainstem auditory evoked potentials: Intraoperative monitoring technique in surgery of posterior fossa tumors. *Arch Phys Med Rehabil* 1987; 68:142.

23. Merton PA, Morton HB: Stimulation of the cerebral cortex in the intact human subject. *Nature* 1980; 285:227.

24. Levy WJ, et al: Motor evoked potentials from transcranial stimulation of the motor cortex in humans. *Neurosurgery* 1984; 15:214.

25. Levy WJ Jr: Clinical experience with motor and cerebellar evoked potential monitoring. *Neurosurgery* 1987; 20:169.

26. Amassian VE, Cracco RQ: Human cerebral cortical responses to contralateral transcranial stimulation. *Neurosurgery* 1987; 20:148.

27. Rothwell JC, et al: Motor cortical stimulation in intact man: Physiological mechanisms and application in intraoperative monitoring. In Desmedt, JE (ed): *Neuromonitoring in Surgery.* Amsterdam, Elsevier, 1989:71–98.

28. Day BL, et al: Electric and magnetic stimulation of human motor cortex: Surface MEG and single motor unit responses. *J Physiol* 1989; 412:449.

29. Day BL, et al: Different sites of action of electrical and magnetic stimulation of the human brain. *Neurosci Lett* 1987; 75:101.

30. Rothwell JC, et al: Motor cortex stimulation in intact man. *Brain* 1987; 110:1173.

31. Barker AT, et al: Noninvasive magnetic stimulation of the human cortex. *Lancet* 1985; 1:1106.

32. Edmonds H Jr, et al: Transcranial magnetic motor evoked potentials (tcMMEP) for functional monitoring of motor pathways during scoliosis surgery. *Spine* 1989; 14:683.

33. Shields CB, et al: Intraoperative use of transcranial magnetic motor evoked potentials. In Chokroverty S (ed): *Magnetic Stimulation in Clinical Neurophysiology.* London, Butterworths, 1990:173–184.

34. Sood S, et al: Somatosensory and brainstem auditory evoked potential in congenital craniovertebral anomaly: Effect of surgical management. *J Neurol Neurosurg Psychiatry* 1992; 55:609.

35. Ben-David B: Spinal cord monitoring. *Orthop Clin North Am* 1988; 19:427.

36. Cracco RQ, et al: Transcranial stimulation: Technique and interpretation of the effects of stimulating motor and non-motor cortical regions in man. In Desmedt JE (ed): *Neuromonitoring for Surgery.* Amsterdam, Elsevier, 1989:61–70.

37. Lee WY, et al: Intraoperative monitoring of motor function by magnetic motor evoked potentials. *Neurosurgery* 1995; 36:493.

38. Hufnagel A, et al: Activation of the epileptic focus by transcranial magnetic stimulation of the human brain. *Ann Neurol* 1990; 27:49.

39. Mackey-Hargadine JR, Hall JW III: Sensory evoked responses in head injury. *Central Nervous System Trauma* 1985; 2:187.

40. Hall JW III, Mackey-Hargadine J: Auditory evoked responses in severe head injury. *Seminars in Hearing* 1984; 5:313.

41. Keith RW, et al: Auditory brainstem response testing in the surgical intensive care unit. *Seminars in Hearing* 1983; 4:385.

42. Alster J, et al: Density spectral array, evoked potentials, and temperature rhythms in the evaluation and prognosis of the comatose patient. *Brain Injury* 1993; 7:191.

43. Newton PG, et al: The dynamics of neuronal dysfunction and recovery following severe head injury assessed with serial multimodality evoked potentials. *J Neurosurg* 1982; 57:168.

44. Seales D, et al: Brainstem auditory evoked responses in patients comatose as a result of blunt head trauma. *Trauma* 1979; 19:347.

45. Hall JW III, Tucker DA: Sensory evoked responses in the intensive care unit. *Ear Hear* 1986; 7:220.

46. Hall JW III, et al: Auditory brain-stem response in determination of brain death. *Arch Otolaryngol* 1985; 111:613.

47. York PH, et al: Relationship between visual evoked potentials and intracranial pressure. *J Neurosurg* 1981; 55:916.

48. Greenberg RP, Ducker TB: Evoked potentials in the clinical neurosciences. *J Neurosurg* 1982; 56:1.

49. Hutchinson DO, et al: A comparison between electroencephalography and somatosensory evoked potentials for outcome prediction following severe head injury. *Electroencephalogr Clin Neurophysiol* 1991; 78:228.

50. Walser H, Sutter M: *Koma.* New York, Thieme, Stuttgart, 1986.

51. Ganes T, Lundar T: EEG and evoked potentials in comatose patients with severe brain damage. *Electroencephalogr Clin Neurophysiol* 1988; 69:6.

52. Anderson DS, et al: Multimodality evoked potentials in closed head trauma. *Arch Neurol* 1984; 41:369.

53. Cant BR, et al: The assessment of severe head injury by short-latency somatosensory and brain-stem auditory evoked potentials. *Electroencephalogr Clin Neurophysiol* 1986; 65:188.

54. Dauch WA: Prediction of secondary deterioration in comatose neurosurgical patients by serial recording of multimodality evoked potentials. *Acta Neurochir (Wein)* 1991; 111:84.

55. de la Torre JC, et al: Somatosensory evoked potentials for the prognosis of coma in humans. *Exp Neurol* 1978; 60:304.

56. Duric S, Klopcic-Spevak M: Multimodal evoked potentials and the blink reflex in patients with primary brainstem lesions. *Med Pregl* 1992; 45:432.

57. Firsching R, Frowein RA: Multimodality evoked potentials and early prognosis in comatose patients. *Neurosurg Rev* 1990; 13:141.

58. Greenberg RP, et al: Evaluation of brain function in severe human head trauma with multimodality evoked potentials. Part 2: Localization of brain dysfunction and correlation with post-traumatic neurological conditions. *J Neurosurg* 1977; 47:163.

59. Greenberg RP, et al: Evaluation of brain function in severe human head trauma with multimodality evoked potentials. Part I: Evoked brain-injury potentials, methods, and analysis. *J Neurosurg* 1977; 47:150.

60. Gutling E, et al: Dissociation of frontal and parietal components of somatosensory evoked potentials in severe head injury. *Electroencephalogr Clin Neurophysiol* 1993; 88:369.

61. Hume AL, et al: Central somatosensory conduction time in comatose patients. *Ann Neurol* 1979; 5:379.

62. Lindsay K, et al: Evoked potentials in severe head injury—analysis and relation to outcome. *J Neurol Neurosurg Psychiatry* 1981; 44:796.

63. Lutschg J, et al: Brain-stem auditory evoked potentials and early somatosensory evoked potentials in neurointensively treated comatose children. *Am J Dis Child* 1983; 137:421.

64. Mahapatra AK: Evoked potentials in severe head injuries: A prospective study of 40 cases. *J Indian Med Assoc* 1990; 88:217.

65. Mauguiere F, et al: Aspects des potentiels evoques auditifs it somesthesiques precoces dans les comas neurologiques et la mort cerebrale. *Rev EEG Neurophysiol* 1982; 12:280.

66. Narayan RK, et al: Improved confidence of outcome prediction in severe head injury: A comparative analysis of the clinical examination, multimodality evoked potentials, CT and ICP. *J Neurosurg* 1981; 54:751.

67. Pfurtscheller G, et al: Clinical relevance of long-latency SEPs and VEPs during coma and emergence of coma. *Electroencephalogr Clin Neurophysiol* 1985; 62:88.

68. Riffel B, et al: Early prognostic assessment using evoked potentials in severe craniocerebral trauma. *Eed EMG Z Elektroenzephalogr Elektromyogr Verwandte Geb* 1987; 18:192.

69. Rumpl E, et al: Central somatosensory conduction time and short latency somatosensory evoked potentials in post-traumatic coma. *Electroencephalogr Clin Neurophysiol* 1983; 56:583.

70. Vilalta J, et al: Evaluation of post-traumatic coma using evoked potentials. *Rev Esp Anestesiol Reanim* 1989; 36:255.

71. Zentner J, Ebner A: Somatosensory and motor evoked potentials in the prognostic assessment of traumatic and non-traumatic comatose patients. *Eed EMG Z Elektorenzephalogr Elecktromyogr Verwandte Geb* 1988; 19:267.

72. Synek VM: Revised EEG coma scale in diffuse acute head injuries in adults. *Clin Exp Neurol* 1990; 27:99.

73. Serafini G, et al: The use and the potential of auditory electrophysiology in patients in posttraumatic coma. *Acta Otorhinolaringol Esp* 1993; 44:291.

74. Facco E, et al: Is the auditory brain-stem response (ABR) effective in the assessment of post-traumatic coma? *Electroencephalogr Clin Neurophysiol* 1985; 62:332.

75. Greenberg RP, et al: Prognostic implications of early multimodality evoked potentials in severely head-injured patients. *J Neurosurg* 1981; 55:227.

76. Hall J, et al: Auditory brainstem abnormalities in experimental and clinical acute severe head injury. *Trans Pa Acad Ophthalmol Otolaryngol* 1983; 36:83.

77. Hall JW, et al: Auditory function in acute severe head injury. *Laryngoscope* 1982; 95:321.

78. Kaga D, et al: Auditory short, middle and long latency responses in acutely comatose patients. *Laryngoscope* 1985; 95:321.

79. Karnaze D, et al: Auditory evoked potentials in coma after closed head injury: A clinical-neurophysiologic coma scale for predicting outcome. *Neurology* 1985; 35:1122.

80. Rosenberg M, et al: Auditory brain-steam and middle- and long-latency evoked potentials in coma. *Arch Neurol* 1984; 41:835.

81. Mjoen S, et al: Auditory evoked brainstem responses (ABR) in coma due to severe head trauma. *Acta Otolaryngol* 1983; 95:131.

82. Ottaviani F, et al: Auditory brain-stem (ABRs) and middle latency auditory responses (MLRs) in the prognosis of severely head-injured patients. *Electroencephalogr Clin Neurophysiol* 1986; 65:196.

83. Rosenblum WI, et al: Midbrain lesions: Frequent and significant prognostic feature in closed head injury. *Neurosurgery* 1981; 9:613.

84. Tsubokawa T, et al: Assessment of brainstem damage by the auditory brainstem response in acute severe head injury. *J Neurol Neurosurg Psychiatry* 1980; 43:1005.

85. Daly DM, et al: Early evoked potentials in patients with acoustic neuroma. *Electroencephalogr Clin Neurophysiol* 1977; 43:151.

86. Uziel A, Benezsch J: Auditory brainstem responses in comatose patients: Relationship with brainstem reflexes and levels of coma. *Electroencephalogr Clin Neurophysiol* 1978; 45:515.

87. Zuccarello M, et al: Importance of auditory brainstem responses in the CT diagnosis of traumatic brainstem lesions. *AJNR* 1983; 4:481.

88. Becker DP, et al: Prognosis after head injury. In Youmans JR (ed): *Neurological Surgery*, 3d ed. Philadelphia, WB Saunders, 1990:2194–2229.

89. Rappaport M, et al: Evoked brain potentials and disability in brain-damaged patients. *Arch Phys Med Rehabil* 1977; 85:333.

90. Hirschfeld A, Young W: Trends in spinal cord injury research. In Alderson JD, Frost EM (eds): *Spinal Cord Injuries: Anesthetic and Associated Care*. Boston, Butterworths, 1990:199–232.

91. Young W: Correlation of somatosensory evoked potentials and neurological findings to spinal cord injury. In Tator CH (ed): *Early Management of Acute Spinal Cord Injury*. New York, Raven Press, 1982:153–165.

92. Perot PL: The clinical use of somatosensory evoked potentials in spinal cord injury. *Clin Neurosurg* 1973; 20:367.

93. Perot PL: Somatosensory evoked potentials in the evaluation of patients with spinal cord injury. In Marley TP (ed): *Current Controversies in Neurosurgery*. Philadelphia, WB Saunders, 1976:160–167.

94. Sedgwick EM, et al: Spinal cord potentials in traumatic paraplegia and quadriplegia. *J Neurol Neurosurg Psychiatry* 1980; 48:823.

95. Rowed DW, et al: Somatosensory evoked potentials in acute spinal cord injury: Prognostic value. *Surg Neurol* 1978; 9:203.

96. Spielholz NI, et al: Somatosensory evoked potentials and clinical outcome in spinal cord injury. In Popp AJ (ed): *Neural Trauma*. New York, Raven Press, 1979:217–222.

97. Cracco RQ: Spinal evoked responses: Peripheral nerve stimulation in man. *Electroencephalogr Clin Neurophysiol* 1973; 35:379.

98. Dorfman LJ, et al: Use of cerebral evoked potentials to evaluate spinal somatosensory function in patients with traumatic and surgical myelopathies. *J Neurosurg* 1980; 52:654.

99. Nash CL, et al: The unstable thoracic compression fracture. Its problems and the use of spinal cord monitoring in the evaluation of treatment. *Spine* 1977; 2:261.

100. Larson SJ, et al: Lateral extracavitary approach to traumatic lesions of the thoracic and lumbar spine. *J Neurosurg* 1976; 45(6):628.

101. Katz RT, et al: Somatosensory evoked and dermatomal-evoked potentials are not clinically useful in the prognostication of acute spinal cord injury. *Spine* 1991; 16:730.

102. Date ES, et al: Somatosensory evoked responses to dermatomal stimulation in cervical spinal cord injured and normal subjects. *Clin Electroencephalogr* 1988; 19:144.

103. Jorg J, et al: Diagnostic value of somatosensory evoked potentials in cases with chronic progressive para- and tetraspastic syndromes. In Courjon J, et al. (eds): *Clinical Applications of Evoked Potentials in Neurology*. New York, Raven Press, 1982:347–358.

104. Schrader SC, et al: Detection of sacral sparing in acute spinal cord injury. *Spine* 1987; 12:533.

105. Thompson PD, et al: Examination of motor function in lesions of the spinal cord by stimulation of the motor cortex. *Ann Neurol* 1987; 21:389.

106. Caramia MD, et al: Neurophysiologic evaluation of the central nervous impulse propagation in patients with sensorimotor disturbances. *Electroencephalogr Clin Neurophysiol* 1988; 70:16.

107. Gianutsos J, et al: A noninvasive technique to assess completeness of spinal cord lesions in humans. *Exp Neurol* 1987; 98:34.

108. Dimitrijevic MR, et al: Assessment of corticospinal tract integrity in human chronic spinal cord injury. In Rossini PM, Marsden CD (eds): *Non-Invasive Stimulation of the Brain and Spinal Cord: Fundamentals and Clinical Applications*. New York, Alan Liss, Inc, 1988:243–253.

109. Meyer PR, et al: Operative complications resulting from thoracic and lumbar spine internal fixation. *J Clin Orthop* 1988; 237:125.

110. Rohdewald P, et al: Changes in cortical evoked potential as correlates of the efficacy of weak analgesics. *Pain* 1982; 12:329.

111. Fisher RS, et al: Efficacy of intraoperative neurophysiological monitoring. *J Clin Neurophysiol* 1995; 12:97.

112. Kawaguchi M, et al: Introperative electrophysiologic monitoring of cranial motor nerves in skull base surgery. *Surg Neurol* 1995; 43:177.

113. Moller AR: Neurophysiological monitoring in cranial nerve surgery. *Neurosurgery Quarterly* 1994; 5:55.

114. Jacobson GP, Tew JM Jr: Intraoperative evoked potential monitoring. *J Clin Neurophysiol* 1987; 4:145.

115. Symon L, et al: Evoked potential monitoring in neurosurgical practice. In Symon L (ed): *Advances in Technical Standards in Neurosurgery*. Wien, Springer-Verlag, 1986; 14:25–71.

116. Hargadine JR, Snyder E: Brainstem and somatosensory evoked

potentials: Application in the operating room and intensive care unit. *Bull Los Angeles Neurol Soc* 1982; 47:62.

117. Grundy BL: Intraoperative monitoring of sensory-evoked potentials. *Anesthesiology* 1983; 58:72.

118. Grundy BL: Monitoring of sensory evoked potentials during neurosurgical operations: Methods and applications. *Neurosurgery* 1982; 11(4):556.

119. Erwin CW, Erwin AC: Up and down the spinal cord: Intraoperative monitoring of sensory and motor spinal cord pathways. *J Clin Neurophysiol* 1993; 10:425.

120. Friedman WA: Somatosensory evoked potentials in neurosurgery. *Clin Neurosurg* 1988; 34:187.

121. Emerson RG, Turner CA: Monitoring during supratentorial surgery. *J Clin Neurophysiol* 1993; 10:404.

122. Cheek JC: Posterior fossa intraoperative monitoring. *J Clin Neurophysiol* 1993; 10:412.

123. Djuric S, et al: Somatosensory evoked potential monitoring during intracranial surgery. *Acta Neurochir (Wien)* 1992; 119:85.

124. Nuwer MR: Electroencephalograms and evoked potentials. *Neurosurg Clin North Am* 1994; 5:647.

125. Jordan KG: Continuous EEG and evoked potential monitoring in the neuroscience intensive care unit. *J Clin Neurophysiol* 1993; 10:445.

126. Anonymous: American Electroencephalographic Society guidelines for intraoperative monitoring of sensory evoked potentials. *J Clin Neurophysiol* 1987; 4:397.

127. Anonymous: Guideline eleven: Guidelines for intraoperative monitoring of sensory evoked potentials. American Electroencephalographic Society. *J Clin Neurophysiol* 1994; 11:77.

128. Anonymous: Assessment: Intraoperative neurophysiology. Report of the Therapeutics and Technology Assessment Subcommittee of the American Academy of Neurology. *Neurology* 1990; 40:1644.

129. Kaplan BJ, et al: Intraoperative electrophysiology in treatment of peripheral nerve injuries. *J Fla Med Assoc* 1984; 71:400.

130. Friedman WA, Grundy BL: Monitoring of sensory evoked potentials is highly reliable and helpful in the operating room. *J Clin Monit* 1987; 3:38.

131. Harper CM, Nelson KR: Intraoperative electrophysiological monitoring in children. *J Clin Neurophysiol* 1992; 9:342.

132. Porter SS, et al: Intraoperative cortical somatosensory evoked potentials for detection of sciatic neuropathy during total hip arthroplasty. *J Clin Anesth* 1989; 1:170.

133. Vrahas M, et al: Intraoperative somatosensory evoked potential monitoring of pelvic and acetabular fractures. *J Orthop Trauma* 1992; 6:50.

134. Stone RG, et al: Evaluation of sciatic nerve compromise during total hip arthroplasty. *Clin Orthop* 1985; 201:26.

135. Vauzelle C, et al: Functional monitoring of spinal cord activity during spinal surgery. *Clin Orthop* 1973; 93:173.

136. Dawson EG, et al: Spinal cord monitoring. Results of the Scoliosis Research Society and the European Spinal Deformity Society survey. *Spine* 1991; 16(8 Suppl):S361.

137. Whittle IR, et al: Intra-operative spinal cord monitoring during surgery for scoliosis using somatosensory evoked potentials. *Aust N Z J Surg* 1984; 54:553.

138. Forbes HJ, et al: Spinal cord monitoring in scoliosis surgery. Experience with 1168 cases. *J Bone Joint Surg Br* 1991; 73:487.

139. Ben-David B, et al: Anterior spinal fusion complicated by paraplegia. A case report of a false-negative somatosensory-evoked potential. *Spine* 1987; 12:536.

140. Ben-David B, et al: Posterior spinal fusion complicated by posterior column injury. A case report of a false-negative wake-up test. *Spine* 1987; 12:540.

141. Nash CL, Brown RH: Current concepts review. Spinal cord monitoring. *J Bone Joint Surg* 1989; 71:627.

142. Brown RH, et al: Cortical evoked potential monitoring. A system for intraoperative monitoring of spinal cord function. *Spine* 1984; 9:256.

143. Deletis V: Intraoperative monitoring of the functional integrity of the motor pathways. *Adv Neurol* 1993; 63:201.

144. Loughnan BA, Hall GM: Spinal cord monitoring 1989. *Br J Anaesth* 1989; 63:587.

145. Whittle IR, et al: Intra-operative recording of cortical somatosensory evoked potentials as a method of spinal cord monitoring during spinal surgery. *Aust N Z J Surg* 1986; 56:309.

146. Nuwer MR, Dawson EC: Intraoperative evoked potential monitoring of the spinal cord. A restricted filter, scalp method during Harrington instrumentation for scoliosis. *Clin Orthop* 1984; 183:42.

147. Lesser RP, et al: Early somatosensory potentials evoked by median nerve stimulation: Intraoperative monitoring. *Neurology* 1981; 31:1519.

148. Lebwohl NH, Calancie B: Perioperative neurologic deficit: Surgical practices and intraoperative monitoring. *Spine: State of the Art Reviews* 1992; 6:403.

149. Loughnan BA, Fennelly ME: Spinal cord monitoring. *Anaesthesia* 1995; 50:101.

150. Owen JH: Intraoperative stimulation of the spinal cord for prevention of spinal cord injury. *Adv Neurol* 1993; 63:271.

151. Croft TJ, et al: Reversible spinal cord trauma: A model for electrical monitoring of spinal cord function. *J Neurosurg* 1972; 35:402.

152. Kojima Y, et al: Evoked spinal potentials as a monitor of spinal viability. *Spine* 1979; 4:471.

153. Bennett MH: Effects of compression and ischemia on spinal cord evoked potentials. *Exp Neurol* 1983; 80:508.

154. Nordwall A, et al: Spinal cord monitoring using evoked potentials recorded from feline bone. *Spine* 1979; 4:486.

155. Jones SJ, et al: A system for the electrophysiological monitoring of the spinal cord during operations for scoliosis. *J Bone Joint Surg Br* 1983; 65:134.

156. Noel P, et al: Neurophysiologic detection of a unilateral motor deficit occurring during the noncritical phase of scoliosis surgery. *Spine* 1994; 19:2399.

157. Mostegl A, Bauer R: The application of somatosensory-evoked potentials in orthopedic spine surgery. *Arch Orthop Trauma Surg* 1984; 103:179.

158. Wilber RG, et al: Postoperative neurological deficits in segmental spinal instrumentation. A study using spinal cord monitoring. *J Bone Joint Surg Am* 1984; 66:1178.

159. Dinner DS, et al: Intraoperative spinal somatosensory evoked potential monitoring. *J Neurosurg* 1986; 65:807.

160. Whittle IR, et al: Recording of spinal somatosensory evoked potentials for intraoperative spinal cord monitoring. *J Neurosurg* 1986; 64:601.

161. Epstein NE, et al: Evaluation of intraoperative somatosensory-evoked potential monitoring during 100 cervical operations. *Spine* 1993; 18:737.

162. Mostegl A, et al: Intraoperative somatosensory potential monitoring. A clinical analysis of 127 surgical procedures. *Spine* 1988; 13:396.

163. Nuwer MR, et al: Somatosensory evoked potential spinal cord monitoring reduces neurologic deficits after scoliosis surgery: Results of a large multicenter survey. *Electroencephalogr Clin Neurophysiol* 1995; 96:6.

164. Scoliosis Research Society: Position Statement on Somatosensory Evoked Potential Monitoring of Neurologic Spinal Cord Function During Surgery, Park Ridge, Illinois, September 1992.

165. Apel DM, et al: Avoiding paraplegia during anterior spinal surgery. The role of somatosensory evoked potential monitor-

ing with temporary occlusion of segmental spinal arteries. *Spine* 1991; 16(8 Suppl):S365.

166. Robinson LR, et al: The efficacy of femoral nerve intraoperative somatosensory evoked potentials during surgical treatment of thoracolumbar fractures. *Spine* 1993; 18:1793.

167. Gepstein R, Brown MD: Somatosensory-evoked potentials in lumbar nerve root decompression. *Clin Orthop* 1989; 245:69.

168. Harper CM Jr, et al: Lumbar radiculopathy after spinal fusion for scoliosis. *Muscle Nerve* 1988; 11:386.

169. Herron LD, et al: Intraoperative use of dermatomal somatosensory-evoked potentials in lumbar stenosis surgery. *Spine* 1987; 12:379.

170. Keim HA, et al: Somatosensory evoked potentials as an aid in the diagnosis and intraoperative management of spinal stenosis. *Spine* 1985; 10:338.

171. Lueders H, et al: Surgical monitoring of spinal cord function: Cauda equina stimulation technique. *Neurosurgery* 1982; 11:482.

172. Morioka T, et al: Usefulness of epidurally evoked cortical potential monitoring during cervicomedullary glioma surgery. *J Clin Monit* 1991; 7:30.

173. Maccabee PJ, et al: Evoked potentials recorded from scalp and spinous processes during spinal column surgery. *Electroencephalogr Clin Neurophysiol* 1983; 56:569.

174. Hahn JF, et al: Simple technique for monitoring intraoperative spinal cord function. *Neurosurgery* 1981; 9:692.

175. Vanderstraeten G, et al: Spinal cord monitoring. State of the art. Results in Harrington and C.D. instrumentation for scoliosis. *Acta Orthop Belg* 1992; 58(Suppl 1):99.

176. Koyanagi I, et al: Spinal cord evoked potential monitoring after spinal cord stimulation during surgery of spinal cord tumors. *Neurosurgery* 1993; 33:451.

177. Machida M, et al: Spinal cord monitoring. Electrophysiological measures of sensory and motor function during spinal surgery. *Spine* 1985; 10:407.

178. Okamoto Y, et al: Intraoperative spinal cord monitoring during surgery for aortic aneurysm: Application of spinal cord evoked potential. *Electroencephalogr Clin Neurophysiol* 1992; 84:315.

179. Satomi K, Nishimoto GI: Comparison of evoked spinal potentials by stimulation of the sciatic nerve and the spinal cord. *Spine* 1985; 10:884.

180. Levy WJ: Spinal evoked potentials from the motor tracts. *J Neurosurg* 1983; 58:38.

181. Burke D, Hicks R: Intraoperative monitoring of corticospinal function. *Electroencephalogr Clin Neurophysiol* 1995; 94:89.

182. Morioka T, et al: Direct spinal versus peripheral nerve stimulation as monitoring techniques in epidurally recorded spinal cord potentials. *Acta Neurochir (Wien)* 1991; 108:122.

183. Yang LH, et al: Intraoperative transcranial electrical motor evoked potential monitoring during spinal surgery under intravenous ketamine or etomidate anaesthesia. *Acta Neurochir (Wien)* 1994; 127:191.

184. Jellinek D, et al: Noninvasive intraoperative monitoring of motor evoked potentials under propofol anesthesia: Effects of spinal surgery on the amplitude and latency of motor evoked potentials. *Neurosurgery* 1991; 29:551.

185. Pereon Y, et al: Could neurogenic motor evoked potentials be used to monitor motor and somatosensory pathways during scoliosis surgery? *Muscle Nerve* 1995; 18:1215.

186. Owen JH, et al: The clinical application of neurogenic motor evoked potentials to monitor spinal cord function during surgery. *Spine* 1991; 16(suppl):S385.

187. Laschinger JC, et al: Direct noninvasive monitoring of spinal cord motor function during thoracic aortic occlusion. (Reply.) *J Vasc Surg* 1988; 7:177.

188. Phillips LH 2nd, et al: Direct spinal stimulation for intraopera-

tive monitoring during scoliosis surgery. *Muscle Nerve* 1995; 18:319.

189. Mustain WD, Kendig RJ: Dissociation of neurogenic motor and somatosensory evoked potentials. A case report. *Spine* 1991; 16:851.

190. Rosenberg JN: Somatosensory and magnetic evoked potentials in a postoperative paraparetic patient: *Case report. Arch Phys Med Rehabil* 1991; 72:154.

191. Baba H, et al: Spinal cord evoked potentials in cervical and thoracic myelopathy. *Int Orthop* 1993; 17:82.

192. Legatt AD, et al: Electrical stimulation and multichannel EMG recording for identification of functional neural tissue during cauda equina surgery. *Childs Nerv Syst* 1992; 8:185.

193. Mavroudakis N, et al: Spinal and brain-stem SEPs and H reflex during enflurane anesthesia. *Electroencephalogr Clin Neurophysiol* 1994; 92:82.

194. Shinomiya K, et al: Intraoperative monitoring for tethered spinal cord syndrome. *Spine* 1991; 16:1290.

195. Calancie B, et al: Intraoperative evoked EMG monitoring in an animal model. A new technique for evaluating pedicle screw placement. *Spine* 1992; 17:1229.

196. Cass JR, Ducker TB: Two thoracolumbar spinal tumors causing pain and gait problems. *J Spinal Disord* 1994; 7:270.

197. Toleikis JR, et al: The use of dermatomal evoked responses during surgical procedures that use intrapedicular fixation of the lumbosacral spine. *Spine* 1993; 18:2401.

198. Owen JH, et al: The use of mechanically elicited electromyograms to protect nerve roots during surgery for spinal degeneration. *Spine* 1994; 19:1704.

199. Hormes JT, Chappuis JL: Monitoring of lumbosacral nerve roots during spinal instrumentation. *Spine* 1993; 18:2059.

200. Kothbauer K, et al: Intraoperative motor and sensory monitoring of the cauda equina. *Neurosurgery* 1994; 34:702.

201. Phillips LH 2d, Park TS: Electrophysiological monitoring during lipomyelomeningocele resection. *Muscle Nerve* 1990; 13:127.

202. Calancie B, et al: Stimulus-evoked EMG monitoring during transpedicular lumbosacral spine instrumentation. Initial clinical results. *Spine* 1994; 19:2780.

203. Laschinger JC, et al: Definition of the safe lower limits of aortic resection during surgical procedures on the thoracoabdominal aorta: Use of somatosensory evoked potentials. *JACC* 1983; 2:959.

204. Lam AM, Teturswamy G: Monitoring of evoked responses during carotid endarterectomy and extracranial-intracranial anastomosis. *Int Anesthesiol Clin* 1984; 22:107.

205. Zornow MH, et al: Preservation of evoked potentials in a case of anterior spinal artery syndrome. *Electroencephalogr Clini Neurophysiol* 1990; 77:137.

206. Kaplan BJ, et al: Effects of aortic occlusion on regional spinal cord blood flow and somatosensory evoked potentials in sheep. *Neurosurgery* 1987; 21:668.

207. Hitchon PW, et al: Response of spinal cord blood flow and motor and sensory evoked potentials to aortic ligation. *Surg Neurol* 1990; 34:279.

208. Zornow MH, Drummond JC: Intraoperative somatosensory evoked responses recorded during onset of the anterior spinal artery syndrome. *J Clin Monit* 1989; 5:243.

209. Grabitz K, et al: Spinal evoked potential in patients undergoing thoracoabdominal aortic reconstruction: A prognostic indicator of postoperative motor deficit. *J Clin Monit* 1993; 9:186.

210. Stuhmeier KD, et al: Use of the electrospinogram for predicting harmful spinal cord ischemia during repair of thoracic or thoracoabdominal aortic aneurysms. *Anesthesiology* 1993; 79:1170.

211. de Mol BA, et al: Experimental and clinical use of somatosen-

sory evoked potentials in surgery of aneurysms of the descending thoracic aorta. *Thorac Cardiovasc Surg* 1990; 38:146.

212. Fava E, et al: Evaluation of spinal cord function by means of lower limb somatosensory evoked potentials in reparative aortic surgery. *J Cardiovasc Surg (Torino)* 1988; 29:421.

213. Grubbs PE, et al: Somatosensory evoked potentials and spinal cord perfusion pressure are significant predictors of postoperative neurologic dysfunction. *Surgery* 1988; 104:216.

214. Maeda S, et al: Prevention of spinal cord ischemia by monitoring spinal cord perfusion pressure and somatosensory evoked potentials. *J Cardiovasc Surg (Torino)* 1989; 30:565.

215. Herdmann J, et al: Magnetic stimulation for monitoring of motor pathways in spinal procedures. *Spine* 1993; 18:551.

216. Leppanen R, et al: Intraoperative lower extremity reflex muscle activity as an adjunct to conventional somatosensory-evoked potentials and descending neurogenic monitoring in idiopathic scoliosis. *Spine* 1995; 20:1872.

217. Glassman SD, et al: Correlation of motor-evoked potentials, somatosensory-evoked potentials, and the wake-up test in a case of kyphoscoliosis. *J Spinal Disorders* 1993; 6:1948.

218. Burke D, et al: Assessment of corticospinal and somatosensory conduction simultaneously during scoliosis surgery. *Electroencephalogr Clin Neurophysiol* 1992; 85:388.

219. Hicks RG, et al: Monitoring spinal cord function during scoliosis surgery with Cotrel-Dubousset instrumentation. *Med J Aust* 1991; 154:82.

220. Kalkman CJ, et al: Severe sensory deficits with preserved motor function after removal of a spinal arteriovenous malformation: Correlation with simultaneously recorded somatosensory and motor evoked potentials. *Anesth Analg* 1994; 78:165.

221. Wagner W, et al: Intra-operative monitoring during syringo-endoscopy: Results of median nerve stimulated somatosensory evoked potentials in nine patients. *Acta Neurochir (Wien)* 1993; 123:187.

222. Ashkenaze D, et al: Efficacy of spinal cord monitoring in neuromuscular scoliosis. *Spine* 1993; 18:1627.

223. Williamson JB, Galasko CS: Spinal cord monitoring during operative correction of neuromuscular scoliosis. *J Bone Joint Surg Br* 1992; 74:870.

224. Grundy BL, et al: Evoked potential changes produced by positioning for retromastoid craniectomy. *Neurosurgery* 1982; 10:766.

225. Gentili F, et al: Monitoring of sensory evoked potentials during surgery of skull base tumours. *Can J Neurol Sci* 1985; 12:336.

226. Daube JR: Recent applications of electrophysiologic monitoring during surgery. *Electroencephalogr Clin Neurophysiol Suppl* 1987; 39:231.

227. Harper CM, et al: Effect of BAEP monitoring on hearing preservation during acoustic neuroma resection. *Neurology* 1992; 42: 1551.

228. Nadol JB Jr, et al: Preservation of hearing and facial nerve function in resection of acoustic neuroma. *Laryngoscope* 1992; 102:1153.

229. Fischer G, et al: Hearing preservation in acoustic neurinoma surgery. *J Neurosurg* 1992; 76:910.

230. Sindou M, et al: Lessons from brainstem auditory evoked potential monitoring during microvascular decompression for trigeminal neuralgia and hemifacial spasm. In Schramm J, Moller AR (eds): *Intraoperative Neurophysiological Monitoring.* Berlin, Springer-Verlag, 1991:293–300.

231. Jannetta PJ, et al: Technique of hearing preservation in small acoustic neuromas. *Ann Surg* 1984; 200:513.

232. Nadol JB Jr, et al: Preservation of hearing in surgical removal of acoustic neuromas of the internal auditory canal and cerebellar pontine angle. *Laryngoscope* 1987; 97:1287.

233. Slavit DH, et al: Auditory monitoring during acoustic neuroma removal. *Arch Otolaryngol Head Neck Surg* 1991; 117:1153.

234. Schramm J, et al: Detailed analysis of intraoperative changes in monitoring brain stem acoustic evoked potentials. *Neurosurgery* 1988; 22:694.

235. Grundy BL, et al: Reversible evoked potential changes with retraction of the eighth cranial nerve. *Anesth Analg* 1981; 60:835.

236. Mustain WD, et al: Inconsistencies in the correlation between loss of brain stem auditory evoked response waves and postoperative deafness. *J Clin Monit* 1992; 8:231.

237. Sabin HI, et al: Intraoperative electrochochleography to monitor cochlear potentials during acoustic neuroma surgery. *Acta Neuchir (Wien)* 1978; 85:110.

238. Ojemann RG, et al: Use of intraoperative auditory evoked potentials to preserve hearing in unilateral acoustic neuroma removal. *J Neurosurg* 1984; 61:938.

239. Levine, RA: Monitoring auditory evoked potentials during cerebellopontine angle tumor surgery: Relative value of electrocochleography, brainstem auditory evoked potentials, and cerebellopontine angle recordings. In Schramm J, Moller AR (eds): *Intraoperative Neurophysiological Monitoring.* Berlin, Springer-Verlag, 1991:193–204.

240. Symon L, Jellinek DA: Monitoring of auditory function in acoustic neuroma surgery. In Schramm J, Moller AR (eds): *Intraoperative Neurophysiological Monitoring.* Berlin, Springer-Verlag, 1991:205–213.

241. Lambert PR, Ruth RA: Simultaneous recording of noninvasive ECoG and ABR for use in intraoperative monitoring. *Otolaryngol Head Neck Surg* 1988; 98:575.

242. Lenarz T, Ernst A: Intraoperative monitoring by transtympanic electrocochleography and brainstem electrical response audiometry in acoustic neuroma surgery. *Eur Arch Otorhinolaryngol* 1992; 249:257.

243. Levine RA. Short-latency auditory evoked potentials: Intraoperative applications. *Int Anesthesiol Clin* 1990; 28:147–153.

244. Hashimoto I, et al: Brainstem auditory evoked potentials recorded directly from human brain-stem and thalamus. *Brain* 1981; 104:841.

245. McDaniel AB, et al: Retrolabyrinthine vesticular neurectomy with and without monitoring of eighth nerve potentials. *Am J Otol* 1985; Suppl:23.

246. Silverstein H, et al: Hearing preservation after acoustic neuroma surgery using intraoperative direct eighth cranial nerve monitoring. *Am J Otol* 1985; Suppl:99.

247. Nedzelski JM, et al: Hearing preservation in acoustic neuroma surgery: Value of monitoring cochlear nerve action potentials. *Otolaryngol Head Neck Surg* 1994; 111:703.

248. Silverstein H, et al: Hearing preservation after acoustic neuroma surgery with intraoperative direct eighth cranial nerve monitoring: Part II. A classification of results. *Otolaryngol Head Neck Surg* 1986; 95:285.

249. Colletti V, Fiorino FG: Electrophysiologic identification of the cochlear nerve fibers during cerebello-pontine angle surgery. *Acta Otolaryngol (Stockh)* 1993; 113:746.

250. Rowed DW, et al: Intraoperative monitoring of cochlear and auditory nerve potentials in operations in the cerebellopontine angle: An aid to hearing preservation. In Schramm J, Moller AR (eds): *Intraoperative Neurophysiological Monitoring.* Berlin, Springer-Verlag, 1991:214–223.

251. Kveton JF: The efficacy of brainstem auditory evoked potentials in acoustic tumor surgery. *Laryngoscope* 1990; 100:1171.

252. Moller AR, et al: Preservation of hearing in operations on acoustic tumors: An alternative to recording brain stem auditory evoked potentials. *Neurosurgery* 1994; 34:688.

253. Waring MD: Electrically evoked auditory brainstem response

monitoring of auditory brainstem implant integrity during facial nerve tumor surgery. *Laryngoscope* 1992; 102:1293.

254. Kalmanchey R, et al: The use of brainstem auditory evoked potentials during posterior fossa surgery as a monitor of brainstem function. *Acta Neurochir (Wien)* 1986; 82:128.

255. Krieger D, et al: Monitoring therapeutic efficacy of decompressive craniotomy in space occupying cerebellar infarcts using brain-stem auditory evoked potentials. *Electroencephalogr Clin Neurophysiol* 1993; 88:261.

256. Schwartz DM, et al: Intraoperative monitoring of brainstem auditory evoked potentials following emergency evacuation of a cerebellar vascular malformation. *J Clin Monit* 1989; 5:116.

257. Dickens JRE, Graham SS: A comparison of facial nerve monitoring systems in cerebellopontine angle surgery. *Am J Otol* 1991; 12:1.

258. Jako GJ: Facial nerve monitor. *Trans Am Acad Ophthalmol Otolaryngol* 1965; 69:340.

259. Prass RL, Luders H: Acoustic (loudspeaker) facial electromyographic monitoring: Part 1. Evoked electromyographic activity during acoustic neuroma resection. *Neurosurgery* 1986; 19:392.

260. Prass RL, et al: Acoustic (loudspeaker) facial EMG monitoring: II. Use of evoked EMG activity during acoustic neuroma resection. *Otolaryngol Head Neck Surg* 1987; 97:541.

261. Gantz BJ: Intraoperative facial nerve monitoring. *Am J Otol* 1985; Suppl:58.

262. Kartush JM: Electroneurography and intraoperative facial monitoring in contemporary neurotology. *Otolaryngol Head Neck Surg* 1989; 101:496.

263. Katsuta T, et al: Physiological localization of the facial colliculus during direct surgery on an intrinsic brainstem lesion. *Neurosurgery* 1993; 32:861.

264. Harner SG: Intraoperative monitoring of the facial nerve. *Laryngoscope* 1988; 98:209.

265. Synopsis of a panel held at the annual meeting of the American Otological Society: Indications for cranial nerve monitoring during otologic and neurotologic surgery. *Am J Otol* 1994; 15:611.

266. National Institutes of Health (NIH) Consensus Development Conference (held December 11–13, 1991). Consensus Statement 9, 1991.

267. Stechison MT: Neurophysiologic monitoring during cranial base surgery. *J Neurooncol* 1994; 20:313.

268. Albin MS: Anesthetic management of posterior fossa surgery in the sitting position. *Acta Anaesthesiol Scand* 1976; 20:117.

269. Kartush J, Bouchard K (eds): *Neuromonitoring in Otology and Head and Neck Surgery.* New York, Raven Press, 1992.

270. Tos M, Thomsen J (eds): *Acoustic Neuroma.* Amsterdam, Kugler, 1992.

271. Soustiel JF, et al: Monitoring of brain-stem trigeminal evoked potentials. Clinical applications in posterior fossa surgery. *Electroencephalogr Clin Neurophysiol* 1993; 88:255.

272. Sweet WH, et al: Treatment of trigeminal neuralgia and other facial pains by retrogasserian injection of glycerol. *Neurosurgery* 1981; 9:647.

273. Lipton RJ, et al: Intraoperative electrophysiologic monitoring of laryngeal muscle during thyroid surgery. *Laryngoscope* 1988; 98:1292.

274. Rea JL, Khan A: Recurrent laryngeal nerve location in thyroidectomy and parathyroidectomy: Use of an indwelling laryngeal surface electrode with evoked electromyography. *Operative Techniques in Otolaryngology—Head and Neck Surgery* 1994; 5:91.

275. Andrews RJ, Bringas JR: A review of brain retraction and recommendations for minimizing intraoperative brain injury. *Neurosurgery* 1993; 33:1052.

276. Bennett M, et al: Evoked potential changes during brain retraction in dogs. *Stroke* 1977; 8:487.

277. Firsching R, et al: Lesions of the sensorimotor region: Somatosensory evoked potentials and ultrasound guided surgery. *Acta Neurochir (Wien)* 1992; 118:87.

278. Birk P, et al: Somatosensory evoked potentials in the ventrolateral thalamus. *Appl Neurophysiol* 1986; 49:327.

279. Pratt H: Evoked potentials in the operating room: Three examples using three sensory modalities. *Isr J Med Sci* 1981; 17:460.

280. Greenberg RP, Fleischer AS: Intraoperative monitoring of brain function with evoked potentials during neurosurgical procedures. *Ariz Med* 1983; 40:389.

281. Markand ON, et al: Monitoring of somatosensory evoked responses during carotid endarterectomy. *Arch Neurol* 1984; 41:375.

282. Russ W, et al: Intraoperative somatosensory evoked potentials as a prognostic factor of neurologic state after carotid endarterectomy. *Thorac Cardiovasc Surg* 1985; 33:392.

283. Russ W, Fraedrich G: Intraoperative detection of cerebral ischemia with somatosensory cortical evoked potentials during carotid endarterectomy—presentation of a new method. *Thorac Cardiovasc Surg* 1984; 32:124.

284. Sloan TB, et al: Reversible loss of somatosensory evoked potentials during anterior cervical spine fusion. *Anesth Analg* 1986; 65:96.

285. Fava E, et al: Role of SEP in identifying patients requiring temporary shunt during carotid endarterectomy. *Electroencephalogr Clin Neurophysiol* 1992; 84:426.

286. Horsch S, et al: Intraoperative assessment of cerebral ischemia during carotid surgery. *J Cardiovasc Surg (Torino)* 1990; 31:599.

287. Lam AM, et al: Monitoring electrophysiologic function during carotid endarterectomy: A comparison of somatosensory evoked potentials and conventional electroencephalogram. *Anesthesiology* 1991; 75:15.

288. Mizoi K, Yoshimoto T: Intraoperative monitoring of the somatosensory evoked potentials and cerebral blood flow during aneurysm surgery: Safety evaluation for temporary vascular surgery. *Neurol Med Chir (Tokyo)* 1991; 31:318.

289. Mizoi K, Yoshimoto T: Permissible temporary occlusion time in aneurysm surgery as evaluated by evoked potential monitoring. *Neurosurgery* 1993; 33:434.

290. Friedman WA, et al: Evoked potential monitoring during aneurysm operation: Observations after fifty cases. *Neurosurgery* 1987; 20:678.

291. Schramm J, et al: Surgical and electrophysiological observations during clipping of 134 aneurysms with evoked potential monitoring. *Neurosurgery* 1990; 26:61.

292. Hyman SA, et al: Median nerve somatosensory evoked potentials as an indicator of ischemia in a case involving an aneurysm of the internal carotid artery. *Neurosurgery* 1987; 21:391.

293. Schramm J, et al: Intraoperative SEP monitoring in aneurysm surgery. *Neurol Res* 1994; 16:20.

294. Bojanowski WM, et al: Reconstruction of the MCA bifurcation after excision of a giant aneurysm. *J Neurosurg* 1988; 68:974.

295. Symon L, et al: Perioperative use of somatosensory evoked responses in aneurysm surgery. *J Neurosurg* 1984; 60:269.

296. Carter LP, et al: Somatosensory evoked potentials and cortical blood flow during craniotomy for vascular disease. *Neurosurgery* 1984; 15:22.

297. Symon L, et al: Assessment of reversible cerebral ischaemia in man: Intraoperative monitoring of somatosensory evoked response. *Acta Neurochir (Wien)* 1988; Suppl 42:3.

298. Symon L, et al: Central conduction time as an index of ischaemia in subarachnoid haemorrhage. *J Neurol Sci* 1979; 44:95.

299. Hacke W, et al: Monitoring of hemispheric or brainstem func-

tions with neurophysiologic methods during interventional neuroradiology. *AJNR* 1983; 4:382.

300. Little JR, et al: Brain stem auditory evoked potentials in posterior circulation surgery. *Neurosurgery* 1983; 12:496.

301. Little JR, et al: Electrophysiological monitoring during basilar aneurysm operation. *Neurosurgery* 1987; 20:421.

302. Manninen PH, et al: Evoked potential monitoring during posterior fossa aneurysm surgery: A comparison of two modalities. *Can J Anaesth* 1984; 41:92.

303. Costa e Silva I, et al: The application of flash visual evoked potentials during operations on the anterior visual pathways. *Neurol Res* 1985; 7:11.

304. Handel N, et al: Monitoring visual evoked response during craniofacial surgery. *Ann Plast Surg* 1979; 2:257.

305. Cedzich C, Schramm J: Monitoring of flash visual evoked potentials during neurosurgical operations. *Int Anesthesiol Clin* 1990; 28:165.

306. Raudzens PA: Intraoperative monitoring of evoked potentials. *Ann NY Acad Sci* 1982; 388:308.

307. Kileny P, et al: Middle-latency auditory evoked responses during open-heart surgery with hypothermia. *Electroencephalogr Clin Neurophysiol* 1983; 55:268.

308. McPherson RW, et al: Somatosensory evoked potential changes in position-related brain stem ischemia. *Anesthesiology* 1984; 61:88.

309. Mahla ME, et al: Detection of brachial plexus dysfunction by somatosensory evoked potential monitoring. A report of two cases. *Anesthesiology* 1984; 60:248.

310. Witzmann A, Reisecker F: Somatosensory and auditory evoked potential monitoring in tumor removal and brainstem surgery. In Desmedt JE (ed): *Neuromonitoring for Surgery*. Amsterdam, Elsevier, 1989:219–241.

311. Symon L, Murota T: Intraoperative monitoring of somatosensory evoked potentials during intracranial vascular surgery. In Desmedt JE (ed): *Neuromonitoring for Surgery*. Amsterdam, Elsevier, 1989:263–302.

312. Branston NM, et al: Relationship between the cortical evoked potential and local cortical blood flow following acute middle cerebral artery occlusion in the baboon. *Exp Neurol* 1974; 45:195.

313. Branston NM, et al: Recovery of the cortical evoked response following temporary middle cerebral artery occlusion in baboons: Relation to local blood flow and P_{O_2}. *Stroke* 1976; 7:151.

314. Astrup J, et al: Cortical evoked potentials and extracellular K^+ and H^+ at critical levels of brain ischemia. *Stroke* 1977; 8:51.

315. Brierley JN, Symon L: The extent of infarcts in baboon brains 3 years after division of the middle cerebral artery. *J Neuropathol Appl Neurobiol* 1979; 3:271.

316. Hargadine JR, et al: Central conduction time in primate brain ischemia—a study in baboons. *Stroke* 1980; 11:637.

317. Gregory PC, et al: Effects of hemorrhagic hypotension on the cerebral circulation. II. Electrocortical function. *Stroke* 1979; 10:719.

318. Lesnick JE, et al: Alteration of somatosensory evoked potentials in response to global ischemia. *J Neurosurg* 1984; 50:490.

319. Crockard HA, et al: Somatosensory evoked potentials, cerebral blood flow and metabolism following cerebral missile trauma in monkeys. *Surg Neurol* 1977; 7:281.

320. Branston NM, et al: Comparison of the effects of ischaemia on early components of the somatosensory evoked potential in brainstem, thalamus, and cerebral cortex. *J Cereb Blood Flow Metab* 1984; 4:68.

321. Branston NM, et al: Somatosensory evoked potentials in experimental brain ischemia. In Pfurtscheller G, et al (eds): *Brain Ischemia: Quantitative EEG and Imaging Techniques. Progress in Brain Research*, Vol 62. Amsterdam, Elsevier, pp 185–199.

322. Kobrine AI, et al: Relative vulnerability of the brain and spinal cord to ischemia. *J Neurol Sci* 1980; 45:65.

323. Sloan T: American Society of Anesthesiology: *Refresher Courses*, October 1985, Lecture 211.

324. Brodkey JS, et al: Reversible spinal cord trauma in cats: Additive effects of direct pressure and ischemia. *J Neurosurg* 1972; 37:591.

325. Dolan EJ, et al: The effect of spinal distraction on regional blood flow in cats. *J Neurosurg* 1980; 53:756.

326. Griffiths IR, et al: Spinal cord blood flow and conduction during experimental cord compression in normotensive and hypotensive dogs. *J Neurosurg* 1979; 50:353.

327. Yamada T, et al: Tourniquet-induced ischemia and somatosensory evoked potentials. *Neurology* 1981; 31:1524.

328. Fava E, et al: Evaluation of spinal cord function by means of lower limb somatosensory evoked potentials in reparative aortic surgery. *J Cardiovasc Surg* 1988; 29:421.

329. North RB, et al: Monitoring of spinal cord stimulation evoked potentials during thoracoabdominal aneurysm surgery. *Neurosurgery* 1991; 28:325.

330. Nagao S, et al: Acute intracranial hypertension and auditory brainstem responses. Part 1. Changes in the auditory brainstem and somatosensory evoked responses in intracranial hypertension in cats. *J Neurosurg* 1979; 51:669.

331. Oka Y, Miyamoto T: Prevention of spinal cord injury after cross-clamping of the thoracic aorta. *J Cardiovasc Surg* 1987; 28:398.

332. Grundy BL, et al: Intraoperative hypoxia detected by evoked potential monitoring. *Anesth Analg* 1981; 60:437.

333. Nagao S, et al: The effects of isovolemic hemodilution and reinfusion of packed erythrocytes on somatosensory and visual evoked potentials. *J Surg Res* 1978; 25:530.

334. Shubert A, et al: Loss of cortical evoked responses due to intracranial gas during posterior fossa craniectomy in the seated position. *Anesth Analg* 1986; 65:203.

335. Klee MR, et al: Temperature effects on resting potential and spike parameters of cat motoneurons. *Exp Brain Res* 1974; 19:789.

336. Kraft H: Effects of temperature and age on nerve conduction velocity in the guinea pig. *Arch Phys Med Rehabil* 1972; 53:328.

337. Desmedt JE: Somatosensory evoked potentials in neuromonitoring. In Desmedt JE (ed): *Neuromonitoring for Surgery*. Amsterdam, Elsevier, 1989:1–22.

338. Weight FF, Erulkar SD: Synaptic transmission and effects of temperature at the squid giant synapse. *Nature* 1976; 261:720.

339. Dolman J, et al: The effect of temperature, mean arterial pressure, and cardiopulmonary bypass flows on somatosensory evoked potential latency in man. *Thorac Cardiovasc Surg* 1986; 34:217.

340. Reilly EL, et al: Visual evoked potentials during hypothermia and prolonged circulatory arrest. *Electroencephalogr Clin Neurophysiol* 1978; 45:100.

341. Wolin LR, et al: Electroretinogram and cortical evoked potentials under hypothermia. *Arch Ophthalmol* 1964; 72:521.

342. Doyle WJ, Fria TJ: The effects of hypothermia on the latencies of the auditory brainstem response (ABR) in the rhesus monkey. *Electroencephalogr Clin Neurophysiol* 1985; 60:258.

343. Stockard JJ, et al: Effects of hypothermia on the human brainstem auditory response. *Ann Neurol* 1978; 3:368.

344. Kaga K, et al: Effects of deep hypothermia and circulatory arrest on the auditory brain stem responses. *Arch Otorhinolaryngol* 1979; 225:199.

345. Hume AL, Durkin MA: Central and spinal somatosensory conduction times during hypothermic cardiopulmonary bypass and some observations on the effects of fentanyl and

isoflurane anesthesia. *Electroencephalogr Clin Neurophysiol* 1986; 65:46.

346. Budnick B, et al: Hypothermia-induced changes in rat short latency somatosensory evoked potentials. *Electroencephalogr Clin Neurophysiol* 1981; 51:19.

347. Coles JG, et al: Intraoperative management of thoracic aortic aneurysm. *J Thorac Cardiovasc Surg* 1983; 85:292.

348. Hill R, et al: Alterations in somatosensory evoked potentials associated with inadequate venous return during cardiopulmonary bypass. *J Cardiothorac Anesth* 1987; 1:48.

349. Deutsch E, et al: Auditory nerve brainstem evoked potentials and EEG during severe hypoglycemia. *Electroencephalogr Clin Neurophysiol* 1983; 55:714.

350. Sloan TB: Alteration in ventilation does not alter the onset of cortical magnetic motor evoked potentials. *Anesth Analg* 1991; 72:S261.

351. Svensson LG, et al: Influence of preservation or perfusion of intraoperatively identified spinal cord blood supply on spinal motor evoked potentials and paraplegia after aortic surgery. *J Vasc Surg* 1991; 13:355.

352. Laschinger JC, et al: Direct noninvasive monitoring of spinal cord motor function during thoracic aortic occlusion: Use of motor evoked potentials. *J Vasc Surg* 1988; 7:161.

353. Elmore JR, et al: Failure of motor evoked potentials to predict neurologic outcome in experimental thoracic aortic occlusion. *J Vasc Surg* 1991; 14:131.

354. Sloan TB: Mild hypothermia alters cortical magnetic evoked potentials. *Anesth Analg* 1991; 72:S260.

355. Sloan TB, Levin D: Raised intracranial pressure alters magnetic cortical evoked potentials. *J Neurosurg Anesth* 1991; 3:242.

356. Anonymous: Society proceedings: 32nd Annual Meeting of the Southern Electroencephalographic Society. *Electroencephalogr Clin Neurophysiol* 1980; 50:177P.

357. Kalkman CJ, et al: Intraoperative monitoring of spinal cord function. A review. *Acta Orthop Scand* 1993; 64:114.

358. Boker T, Heinze HJ: Influence of diazepam on visual pattern-evoked potentials with due regard to nonstationary effects. *Neuropsychobiology* 1984; 11:207.

359. Domino EF, et al: Effects of various general anesthetics on the visually evoked response in man. *Anesth Analg* 1963; 42:735.

360. Herz A, et al: Pharmacologically induced alterations of cortical and subcortical evoked potentials compared with physiological changes during the awake-sleep cycle in cats. *Electroencephalogr Clin Neurophysiol* 1967; 26:164.

361. Himwich HE: *Brain Metabolism and Cerebral Disorders.* Baltimore, Williams & Wilkins, 1951.

362. Winters WD, et al: The neurophysiology of anesthesia. *Anesthesiology* 1967; 28:65.

363. Winters WD: Effects of drugs on the electrical activity of the brain: Anesthetics. *Annu Rev Pharmacol Toxicol* 1976; 16:413.

364. Plourde G, Picton TW: Long-latency auditory evoked potentials during general anesthesia: N1 and P3 components. *Anesth Analg* 1991; 72:342.

365. Thornton C: Evoked potentials in anaesthesia. *Eur J Anaesthesiol* 1991; 8:89.

366. Stark JA, et al: Electroencephalogram and evoked potential analysis: A model-based approach. *Int Anesthesiol Clin* 1993; 31:121.

367. Schwender D, et al: Motor signs of wakefulness during general anaesthesia with propofol, isoflurane and flunitrazepam/fentanyl and midlatency auditory evoked potentials. *Anaesthesia* 1994; 49:476.

368. Angel A, Gratton DA: The effect of anaesthetic agents on cerebral cortical responses in the rat. *Br J Pharmacol* 1982; 76:541.

369. Angel A, et al: Pressure reversal of the effect of urethane on the evoked somatosensory cortical response in the rat. *Br J Pharmacol* 1980; 70:241.

370. Rosner BS, Clark DL: Neurophysiologic effects of general anesthetics: II. Sequential regional actions in the brain. *Anesthesiology* 1973; 39:59.

371. Wang AD, et al: The effects of halothane on somatosensory and flash visual evoked potentials during operations. *Neurol Res* 1985; 7:58.

372. Sebel PS, et al: Effects of halothane and enflurane on far and near field somatosensory evoked potentials. *Br J Anaesth* 1987; 59:1492.

373. Salzman SK, et al: Effects of halothane on intraoperative scalp-recorded somatosensory evoked potentials to posterior tibial nerve stimulation in man. *Electroencephalogr Clin Neurophysiol* 1986; 65:36.

374. Peterson DO, et al: Effects of halothane, enflurane, isoflurane, and nitrous oxide on somatosensory evoked potentials in humans. *Anesthesiology* 1986; 65:35.

375. Baines DB, et al: Effect of halothane on spinal somatosensory evoked potentials in sheep. *Br J Anaesth* 1985; 57:896.

376. Abel MF, et al: Brainstem evoked potentials for scoliosis surgery: A reliable method allowing use of halogenated anesthetic agents. *J Pediatr Orthop* 1990; 10:208.

377. Bimar-Blanc MC, et al: Effets de l'isoflrane et de l'holothane sur les potentiels evoques auditifs et somesthsiques. *Ann Fr Anesth Reanim* 1988; 7:279.

378. Loughnan BA, et al: Effects of halothane on somatosensory evoked potentials recorded in the extradural space. *Br J Anaesth* 1989; 62:297.

379. Stone JL, et al: A comparative analysis of enflurane anesthesia on primate motor and somatosensory evoked potentials. *Electroencephalogr Clin Neurophysiol* 1992; 84:180.

380. Shimoji K, et al: The effects of anesthetics on somatosensory evoked potentials from the brain and spinal cord in man. In Gomez QJ, et al (eds): *Anaesthesia—Safety for All.* Amsterdam, Elsevier, 1984:159–164.

381. McPherson RW, et al: Effects of enflurane, isoflurane, and nitrous oxide on somatosensory evoked potentials during fentanyl anesthesia. *Anesthesiology* 1985; 62:626.

382. Vandesteene A, et al: Topographic analysis of the effects of isoflurane anesthesia on SEP. *Electroencephalogr Clin Neurophysiol* 1993; 88:77.

383. Samra Satwant K, et al: Differential effects of isoflurane on human median nerve somatosensory evoked potentials. *Anesthesiology* 1987; 66:29.

384. Sebel PS, et al: Evoked potentials during isoflurane anaesthesia. *Br J Anaesth* 1986; 58:580.

385. Porkkala T, et al: Somatosensory evoked potentials during isoflurane anaesthesia. *Acta Anaesthesiol Scand* 1994; 38:206.

386. Perlik SJ, et al: Somatosensory evoked potential surgical monitoring. Observations during combined isoflurane-nitrous oxide anesthesia. *Spine* 1992; 17:273.

387. Mason DG, et al: Sequential measurement of the median nerve somatosensory evoked potential during isoflurane anaesthesia in children. *Br J Anaesth* 1992; 69:567.

388. Mason DG, et al: Effects of isoflurane anaesthesia on the median nerve somatosensory evoked potential in children. *Br J Anaesth* 1992; 69:562.

389. Thornton C, et al: Somatosensory and auditory evoked responses recorded simultaneously: Differential effects of nitrous oxide and isoflurane. *Br J Anaesth* 1992; 68:508.

390. Lam AM, et al: Isoflurane compared with nitrous oxide anaesthesia for intraoperative monitoring of somatosensory-evoked potentials. *Can J Anaesth* 1994; 41:295.

391. Russell GB, Graybeal JM: Direct measurement of nitrous oxide

MAC and neurologic monitoring in rats during anesthesia under hyperbaric conditions. *Anesth Analg* 1992; 75:995.

392. Manninen PH, et al: The effects of isoflurane and isoflurane-nitrous oxide anesthesia on brainstem auditory evoked potentials in humans. *Anesth Analg* 1985; 64:43.

393. Hosick EC, et al: Neurophysiological effects of different anesthetics in conscious man. *J Appl Physiol* 1971; 31:892.

394. Griffiths R, Norman RI: Effects of anaesthetics on uptake, synthesis and release of transmitters. *Br J Anaesth* 1993; 71:96.

395. Fujioka J, et al: The effects of enflurane on somatosensory evoked responses simultaneously recorded from brain, spinal cord and peripheral nerve in man. *Masui* 1984; 33:698.

396. Thornton C, et al: Effects of halothane or enflurane with controlled ventilation on auditory evoked potentials. *Br J Anaesth* 1984; 56:315.

397. Sainz M, et al: Brainstem and middle latency auditory evoked responses in rabbits with halothane anaesthesia. *Acta Otolaryngol (Stockh)* 1987; 103:613.

398. Lloyd-Thomas AR, et al: Quantitative EEG and brainstem auditory evoked potentials: Comparison of isoflurane with halothane using the cerebral function analysing monitor. *Br J Anaesth* 1990; 65:306.

399. Dubois MY, et al: Effects of enflurane on brainstem auditory evoked responses in humans. *Anesth Analg* 1982; 61:898.

400. Thornton C, et al: Enflurane anaesthesia causes graded changes in the brainstem and early cortical auditory evoked response in man. *Br J Anaesth* 1983; 55:479.

401. Schmidt JF, Chremmer-Jorgensen B: Auditory evoked potentials during isoflurane anaesthesia. *Acta Anaesthesiol Scand* 1986; 30:378.

402. Heneghan CPH, et al: Effect of isoflurane on the auditory evoked response in man. *Br J Anaesth* 1987; 59:277.

403. Duncan PG, et al: Preservation of auditory-evoked brainstem responses in anaesthetized children. *Can Anaesth Soc J* 1979; 26:492.

404. James MFM, et al: Halothane anaesthesia changes the early components of the auditory evoked response in man. *Br J Anaesth* 1982; 54:787P.

405. Newton DEF, et al: Early cortical auditory evoked response in anaesthesia: Comparison of the effects of nitrous oxide and isoflurane. *Br J Anaesth* 1989; 62:61.

406. Rosenblum SM, et al: Brainstem auditory evoked potentials during enflurane and nitrous oxide anesthesia in man. *Anesthesiology* 1982; 57:A159.

407. Houston HG, et al: Effects of nitrous oxide on auditory cortical evoked potentials and subjective thresholds. *Br J Anaesth* 1988; 61:606.

408. Lader M, Norris H: The effects of nitrous oxide on the human auditory evoked response. *Psychopharmacologia* 1969; 16:115.

409. Jarvis MJ, Lader MH: The effects of nitrous oxide on the auditory evoked response in a reaction time task. *Psychopharmacologia* 1971; 20:201.

410. Uhl RR, et al: Effect of halothane anesthesia on the human cortical visual evoked response. *Anesthesiology* 1980; 53:273.

411. Raitta C, et al: Changes in the electroretinogram and visual evoked potentials during general anesthesia. *Graefes Arch Clin Exp Ophthanol* 1979; 211:139.

412. Chi OZ, Field C: Effects of enflurane on visual evoked potentials in humans. *Br J Anaesth* 1990; 64:163.

413. Raitta C, et al: Changes in the electroretinogram and visual evoked potentials during general anaesthesia using enflurane. *Graefes Arch Clin Exp Ophthalmol* 1982; 218:294.

414. Firsching R: Effects of halothane and nitrous oxide on transcranial magnetic evoked potentials. *Anasthesiol Intensivmed Notfallmed Schmerzther* 1991; 26:381.

415. Stone JL, et al: A comparative analysis of enflurane anesthesia on primate motor and somatosensory evoked potentials. *Electroencephalogr Clin Neurophysiol* 1992; 84:180.

416. Sloan T, Angell D: Differential effect of isoflurane on motor evoked potentials elicited by transcortical electric or magnetic stimulation. In Jones SS, et al (eds): *Handbook of Spinal Cord Monitoring*. Hingham, MA, Kluwer Academic Publishers, 1993:362–367.

417. Zentner J, et al: Influence of halothane, enflurane, and isoflurane on motor evoked potentials. *Neurosurgery* 1992; 32:298.

418. Haghighi SS, et al: Suppression of motor evoked potentials by inhalation anesthetics. *J Neurosurg Anesth* 1990; 2:73.

419. Loughnan BA, et al: Effects of halothane on motor evoked potentials recorded in the extradural space. *Br J Anaesth* 1989; 63:561.

420. Kalkman CJ, et al: Low concentrations of isoflurane abolish motor evoked responses to transcranial electrical stimulation during nitrous oxide/opioid anesthesia in humans. *Anesth Analg* 1991; 73:410.

421. Hicks RG, et al: Some effects of isoflurane on I waves of the motor evoked potential. *Br J Anaesth* 1992; 69:130.

422. Haghighi SS, et al: Depressive effect of isoflurane anesthesia on motor evoked potentials. *Neurosurgery* 1990; 26:993.

423. Calancie B, et al: Isoflurane-induced attenuation of motor evoked potentials caused by electrical motor cortex stimulation during surgery. *J Neurosurg* 1991; 74:897.

424. Jellinek D, et al: Effects of nitrous oxide on motor evoked potentials recorded from skeletal muscle in patients under total anesthesia with intravenously administered propofol. *Neurosurgery* 1991; 29:558.

425. Taniguchi M, et al: Modification of cortical stimulation for motor evoked potentials under general anesthesia: Technical description. *Neurosurgery* 1993; 32:219.

426. Somjen G: Effects of anesthetic on spinal cord of mammals. *Anesthesiology* 1967; 28:135.

427. Judge SE: Effect of general anaesthetics on synaptic ion channels. *Br J Anaesth* 1983; 55:191.

428. Richards CD: Actions of general anaesthetics on synaptic transmission in the CNS. *Br J Anaesth* 1983; 55:201.

429. Yeoman RR, et al: Enflurane effects on acoustic and photic evoked responses. *Neuropharmacology* 1980; 19:481.

430. Benedetti C, et al: Effect of nitrous oxide concentration on event-related potentials during painful tooth stimulation. *Anesthesiology* 1982; 56:360.

431. Harkins SW, et al: Effects of nitrous oxide inhalation on brain potentials evoked by auditory and noxious dental stimulation. *Prog Neuropsychopharmacol Biol Psychiatry* 1982; 6:167.

432. Chapman CR, et al: Event-related potential correlates of analgesia: Comparison of fentanyl acupuncture and nitrous oxide. *Pain* 1982; 14:327.

433. Fenwick P, et al: Contingent negative variation and evoked potential amplitude as a function of inspired nitrous oxide concentration. *Electroencephalogr Clin Neurophysiol* 1979; 47:473.

434. Zenter J, Ebner A: Nitrous oxide suppresses the electromyographic response evoked by electrical stimulation of the motor cortex. *Neurosurgery* 1989; 24:60.

435. Chi OZ, Field C: Effects of isoflurane on visual evoked potentials in humans. *Anesthesiology* 1986; 65:328.

436. Schubert A, et al: The effect of ketamine on human somatosensory evoked potentials and its modification by nitrous oxide. *Anesthesiology* 1990; 72:33.

437. Sloan TB, Koht A: Depression of cortical somatosensory evoked potentials by nitrous oxide. *Br J Anaesth* 1985; 57:849.

438. Zentner J, et al: Influence of anesthetics—nitrous oxide in particular—on electromyographic response evoked by transcranial electrical stimulation of the cortex. *Neurosurgery* 1989; 24:253.

439. Nuwer MR, Dawson E: Intraoperative evoked potential monitoring of the spinal cord: Enhanced stability of cortical recordings. *Electroencephalogr Clin Neurophysiol* 1984; 59:318.

440. McPherson RW, et al: Effects of thiopental, fentanyl, and etomidate on upper extremity somatosensory evoked potentials in humans. *Anesthesiology* 1986; 65:584.

441. Loughnan BL, et al: Evoked potentials following diazepam or fentanyl. *Anaesthesia* 1987; 42:195.

442. Taniguchi M, et al: Total intravenous anesthesia for improvement of intraoperative monitoring of somatosensory evoked potentials during aneurysm surgery. *Neurosurgery* 1992; 31:891.

443. Velasco M, et al: Effect of fentanyl and naloxone on human somatic and auditory-evoked potential components. *Neuropharmacology* 1984; 23:359.

444. Van Beem, H, et al: Spinal monitoring during vertebral column surgery under continuous alfentanil infusion. *Eur J Anaesthesiol* 1992; 9:287.

445. Schubert A, et al: The effect of high-dose fentanyl on human median nerve somatosensory-evoked responses. *Can J Anaesth* 1987; 34:35.

446. Pathak KS, et al: Effects of fentanyl and morphine on intraoperative somatosensory cortical-evoked potentials. *Anesth Analg* 1984; 63:833.

447. Pathak KS, et al: Continuous opioid infusion for scoliosis fusion surgery. *Anesth Analg* 1983; 62:841.

448. Lee VC: Spinal and cortical evoked potential studies in the ketamine-anesthetized rabbit: Fentanyl exerts component-specific, naloxone-reversible changes dependent on stimulus intensity. *Anesth Analg* 1994; 78:280.

449. Mongan PD, Peterson RE: Intravenous anesthetic alterations on the spinal-sciatic evoked response in swine. *Anesth Analg* 1993; 77:149.

450. Samra SK, et al: Fentanyl anesthesia and human brain-stem auditory evoked potentials. *Anesthesiology* 1984; 61:261.

451. Samra SK, et al: Scopolamine, morphine, and brain-stem auditory evoked potentials in awake monkeys. *Anesthesiology* 1985; 62:437.

452. Plourde G, Boylan JF: The long-latency auditory evoked potential as a measure of the level of consciousness during sufentanil anesthesia. *J Cardiothorac Vasc Anesth* 1991; 5:577.

453. Schwender D, et al: Anesthesia with increasing doses of sufentanil and midlatency auditory evoked potentials in humans. *Anesth Analg* 1995; 80:499.

454. Chi OZ, et al: Effects of fentanyl anesthesia on visual evoked potentials in humans. *Anesthesiology* 1987; 67:827.

455. Kimovec MA, et al: Effects of sufentanil on median nerve somatosensory evoked potentials. *Br J Anaesth* 1990; 65:169.

456. Kalkman CJ, et al: Effects of propofol, etomidate, midazolam, and fentanyl on motor evoked responses to transcranial electrical or magnetic stimulation in humans. *Anesthesiology* 1992; 76:502.

457. Ghaly RF, et al: The effect of neuroleptanalgesia (droperidol-fentanyl) on motor potentials evoked by transcranial magnetic stimulation in the monkey. *J Neurosurg Anesth* 1991; 3:117.

458. Glassman SD, et al: Anesthetic effects on motor evoked potentials in dogs. *Spine* 1993; 18:1083.

459. Schubert A, et al: The effect of intrathecal morphine on somatosensory evoked potentials in awake humans. *Anesthesiology* 1991; 75:401.

460. Chabel C, et al: Effects of intrathecal fentanyl and lidocaine on somatosensory-evoked potentials, the H-reflex, and clinical responses. *Anesth Analg* 1988; 67:509.

461. Lund C: Effect of extradural morphine on somatosensory evoked potentials to dermatomal stimulation. *Br J Anaesth* 1987; 59:1408.

462. Cohen MS, Britt RH: Effects of sodium pentobarbital, ketamine, halothane, and chloralose on brainstem auditory evoked responses. *Anesth Analg* 1982; 61:338.

463. Bobbin RP, et al: Effects of pentobarbital and ketamine on brain stem auditory potentials. *Arch Otolaryngol* 1979; 105:467.

464. Church MW, Gritzke R: Effects of ketamine anesthesia on the rat brain-stem auditory evoked potential as a function of dose and stimulus intensity. *Electroencephalogr Clin Neurophysiol* 1987; 67:570.

465. Schubert A, et al: The effect of ketamine on human somatosensory evoked potentials and its modification by nitrous oxide. *Anesthesiology* 1990; 72:33.

466. Schwender D, et al: Mid-latency auditory evoked potentials in humans during anesthesia with S(+) ketamine—a double-blind, randomized comparison with racemic ketamine. *Anesth Analg* 1994; 78:267.

467. Schwender D, et al: Mid-latency auditory evoked potentials during ketamine anesthesia in humans. *Br J Anaesth* 1993; 71:629.

468. Hetzler BE, Berger LK: Ketamine-induced modification of photic evoked potentials in the superior colliculus of hooded rats. *Neuropharmacol* 1984; 23:473.

469. Ghaly RF, et al: Effects of incremental ketamine hydrochloride doses on motor evoked potentials (MEPs) following transcranial magnetic stimulation: A primate study. *J Neurosurg Anesth* 1990; 2:79.

470. Kothbauer K, et al: The effect of ketamine anesthetic induction on muscle responses to transcranial magnetic cortex stimulation studied in man. *Neurosci Lett* 1993; 154:105.

471. Schubert A, et al: The effect of ketamine on human somatosensory evoked potentials and its modification by nitrous oxide. *Anesthesiology* 1990; 72:33.

472. Kano T, Shimoji K: The effects of ketamine and neuroleptanalgesia on the evoked electrospinogram and electromyogram in man. *Anesthesiology* 1974; 40:241.

473. Sloan TB, et al: Effects of thiopentone on median nerve somatosensory evoked potentials. *Br J Anaesth* 1989; 63:51.

474. Taniguchi M, et al: Effects of four intravenous anesthetic agents on motor evoked potentials elicited by magnetic transcranial stimulation. *Neurosurgery* 1993; 33:407.

475. Schwender D, et al: Effects of thiopentone on mid-latency auditory evoked potentials and their frequency analysis. *Anasth Intensivmed Notfallmed Schmerzther* 1991; 26:375.

476. Schwender D, et al: Midlatency auditory evoked potentials and purposeful movements after thiopentone bolus injection. *Anaesthesia* 1994; 49:99.

477. Cohen MS, Britt RH: Effects of sodium pentobarbital, ketamine, halothane, and chloralose on brainstem auditory evoked responses. *Anesth Analg* 1982; 61:338.

478. Russ W, et al: Somatosensorisch evozierte Potentiale unter thiopental und etomidate. *Anaesthesist* 1986; 35:679.

479. Stockard JJ, et al: Effects of centrally acting drugs on brainstem auditory responses. *Electroencephalogr Clin Neurophysiol* 1977; 43:550.

480. Allison T, et al: The effects of barbiturate anesthesia upon human somatosensory evoked responses. *Electroencephalogr Clin Neurophysiol* 1963; 24:68.

481. Abrahamian HA, et al: Effects of thiopental on human cerebral somatic evoked response. *Anesthesiology* 1963; 24:650.

482. Koht A, et al: Effects of etomidate, midazolam, and thiopental on median nerve somatosensory evoked potentials and the additive effects of fentanyl and nitrous oxide. *Anesth Analg* 1988; 67:435.

483. Kalkman CJ, et al: Effects of droperidol, pentobarbital, and ketamine on myogenic transcranial magnetic motor-evoked responses in humans. *Neurosurgery* 1994; 35:1066.

484. Smith DI, Kraus N: Effects of chloral hydrate, pentobarbital, ketamine, and curare on the auditory middle latency response. *Am J Otolaryngol* 1987; 8:241.

485. Newlon PG, et al: Effects of therapeutic pentobarbital coma on multimodality evoked potentials recorded from severely head-injured patients. *Neurosurgery* 1983; 12:613.

486. Marsh RR, et al: Resistance of the auditory brain stem response to high barbiturate levels. *Otolaryngol Head Neck Surg* 1984; 92:685.

487. Drummond JC, et al: The effects of high dose sodium thiopental on brainstem auditory and median nerve somatosensory evoked responses in humans. *Anesthesiology* 1985; 63:249.

488. Sloan TB, et al: Effects of midazolam on median nerve somatosensory evoked potentials. *Br J Anaesth* 1990; 64:590.

489. Prevec TS: Effect of valium on the somatosensory evoked potentials. In Desmedt JE (ed): *Clinical Uses of Cerebral Brainstem and Spinal Somatosensory Evoked Potentials*. Basel, Karger, 1980:311–318.

490. Kaieda R, et al: Effects of diazepam on evoked electrospinogram and evoked electromyogram in man. *Anesth Analg* 1981; 60:197.

491. Schwender D, et al: Mid-latency auditory evoked potentials and intraoperative wakefulness during general anesthesia with propofol, isoflurane, and flunitrazepam/fentanyl. *Anaesthesist* 1991; 40:214.

492. Sloan TB, et al: Improvement of intraoperative somatosensory evoked potentials by etomidate. *Anesth Analg* 1988; 67:582.

493. Ghaly RF, et al: The effect of an anesthetic induction dose of midazolam on motor potentials evoked by transcranial magnetic stimulation in the monkey. *J Neurosurg Anesth* 1991; 3:20.

494. Schonle PW, et al: Changes of transcranially evoked motor responses in man by midazolam, a short acting benzodiazepine. *Neurosci Lett* 1989; 101:321.

495. Thornton C, et al: Effect of etomidate on the auditory evoked response in man. *Br J Anaesth* 1985; 57:554.

496. Chi OZ, et al: Visual evoked potentials during etomidate administration in humans. *Can J Anaesth* 1990; 37:452.

497. Kochs E, et al: Increase of somato-sensorically evoked potentials during induction of anaesthesia with etomidate. *Anaesthetist* 1986; 35:359.

498. Samra SK, Sorkin LS: Enhancement of somatosensory evoked potentials by etomidate in cats: An investigation of its site of action. *Anesthesiology* 1991; 74:499.

499. Lumenta CB: Effect of etomidate on motor evoked potentials in monkeys. *Neurosurgery* 1991; 29:480.

500. Sloan, T, Levin D: Etomidate amplifies and depresses transcranial motor evoked potentials in the monkey. *J Neurosurg Anesth* 1993; 5:299.

501. Chassard D, et al: Auditory evoked potentials during propofol anaesthesia in man. *Br J Anaesth* 1989; 62:522.

502. Savoia G, et al: Propofol infusion and auditory evoked potentials. *Anaesthesia* 1988; 43(suppl):46.

503. Maurette P, et al: Propofol anaesthesia alters somatosensory evoked cortical potentials. *Anaesthesia* 1988; 43(suppl):44.

504. Freye E, et al: Somatosensory-evoked potentials during block of surgical stimulation with propofol. *Br J Anaesth* 1989; 63:357.

505. Scheepstra GL, et al: Median nerve evoked potentials during propofol anaesthesia. *Br J Anaesth* 1989; 62:92.

506. Zentner J, et al: Propofol increases amplitudes of SEP. *Funct Neurol* 1991; 6:411.

507. Purdue JAM, Cullen PM: Brainstem auditory evoked response during propofol anaesthesia in children. *Anaesthesia* 1993; 48:192.

508. Angel A, LeBeau F: A comparison of the effects of propofol with other anaesthetic agents on the centripetal transmission of sensory information. *Gen Pharmacol* 1992; 23:945.

509. Keller BP, et al: The effects of propofol anesthesia on transcortical electric evoked potentials in the rat. *Neurosurgery* 1992; 30:557.

510. Bertens APMG: Effects of an analgesic, fentanyl, and of a sedative, droperidol, on the somatosensory evoked potentials in dogs. *Electromyogr Clin Neurophysiol* 1988; 28:433.

511. Russ W, et al: Influence of neuroleptanalgesia on human visual evoked potentials. *Anaesthesist* 1982; 31:575.

512. Lang E, et al: Median nerve blockage during diagnostic intravenous regional anesthesia as measured by somatosensory evoked potentials. *Anesth Analg* 1993; 76:118.

513. Benzon HT, et al: Somatosensory evoked potential quantification of ulnar nerve blockade. *Anesth Analg* 1986; 65:843.

514. Javel E, et al: Auditory brainstem responses during systemic infusion of lidocaine. *Arch Otolaryngol* 1982; 108:71.

515. Schubert A, et al: Systemic lidocaine and human somatosensory-evoked potentials during sufentanil-isoflurane anaesthesia. *Can J Anaesth* 1992; 39:569.

516. Domino EF, Corssen G: Visually evoked response in anesthetized man with and without induced muscle paralysis. *Ann NY Acad Sci* 1964; 112:226.

517. Harker LA, et al: Influence of succinylcholine on middle component auditory evoked potentials. *Arch Otolaryngol* 1977; 103:133.

518. Sloan TB: Nondepolarizing neuromuscular blockade does not alter sensory evoked potentials. *J Clin Monit* 1994; 10:40.

519. Stinson LW, et al: A computer-controlled, closed-loop infusion system for infusing muscle relaxants: Its use during motor-evoked potential monitoring. *J Cardiothorac Vasc Anesth* 1994; 8:40.

520. Kalkman CJ, et al: Intraoperative monitoring of tibialis anterior muscle motor evoked responses to transcranial electrical stimulation during partial neuromuscular blockade. *Anesth Analg* 1992; 75:584.

521. Tabaraud F, et al: Monitoring of the motor pathway during spinal surgery. *Spine* 1993; 18:546.

522. Sloan TB, Erian R: Effect of atracurium induced neuromuscular blockade on cortical motor evoked potentials. *Anesth Analg* 1993; 76:979.

523. Sloan TB, Erian R: Effect of vecuronium induced neuromuscular blockade on cortical motor evoked potentials. *Anesthesiology* 1993; 78:966.

524. Daube JR, Harper CM: Surgical monitoring of cranial and peripheral nerves. In Desmedt JE (ed): *Neuromonitoring for Surgery*. Amsterdam, Elsevier, 1989:115–138.

525. Nuwer M: Monitoring spinal cord injury with cortical somatosensory evoked potentials. In Desmedt JE (ed): *Neuromonitoring for Surgery*. Amsterdam, Elsevier, 1989:151–162.

Chapter 8

MONITORING TECHNOLOGY
Capnography, Intracranial Pressure, Precordial Doppler, and Transcranial Doppler

LEONID BUNEGIN

ON THE ORIGINS OF INTRAOPERATIVE MONITORING

The successful demonstration of ether anesthesia in 1846 by Morton at the Massachusetts General Hospital was the first and perhaps the most significant step toward the institution of regular patient monitoring during surgery. Prior to this event, the overriding concern of most surgeons was to get in and out as quickly as possible, recognizing the excruciating pain associated with surgery on conscious patients. A primary concern was to insure a minimum of movement by the patient during the procedure; thus, surgical assistants had the task of holding the patient still until either the procedure was complete or the mercy of unconsciousness drew a curtain on the patient's pain. In either case, monitoring the patient's physiologic state had little priority (Fig. 8-1).[1]

Three months after the introduction of ether anesthesia in England, Francis Plomley of Maidstone characterized three states of consciousness, or lack thereof, following inhalation of ether. He himself inhaled the vapors; he also observed the reactions of others who breathed ether.[2]

Upon learning of the successful demonstration of ether anesthesia in October of 1846 by Morton in Boston, (Fig. 8-2) John Snow, an English physician who ultimately devoted his practice to anesthesia, published a volume in 1847 describing a series of 80 anesthetic procedures in patients ranging in age from children to octogenarians. Most significant to patient monitoring was that Snow, recognizing Plomley's three stages of anesthesia, utilized the most commonly available monitoring devices of the era—namely, his senses—to "monitor" the physical conditions of his patients during induction of unconsciousness by the inhalation of sulfuric ether. In doing so, Snow was able to define two additional levels or stages through which the individual passed during the establishment of ether anesthesia.[3] In addition, he demonstrated that by paying careful attention to a patient's physical signs, anesthesia of sufficient depth to render optimal indifference to pain could be consistently and safely produced.

Shortly thereafter, chloroform was recognized to have anesthetic properties. In Edinburgh, James Young Simpson began inducing anesthesia with it in his obstetric practice (Fig. 8-3).[4] Chloroform was cheaper, more potent, and more pleasant than ether, but it could cause sudden death if used inappropriately. In 1855, the eminent surgeon James Syme (also of Edinburgh) (Fig. 8-4) lectured that if the patient's respiration were "monitored" during chloroform anesthesia, the sudden death sometimes associated with this anesthetic could be avoided.[5] Simpson also believed that by monitoring the breathing and pulse, chloroform anesthesia could be administered safely.[4] The extraordinary anesthetic safety record compiled by John Snow using both ether and chloroform was attributed in no small way to his vigilant patient monitoring practices.[6]

With two potent anesthetics available for eradicating pain during surgery, the need to choose not only which to use, but the depth to which anesthesia was to be taken, ushered in the practice of patient monitoring. Surgical procedures no longer needed to be races to the finish line. Longer and more complex operations could be attempted requiring extended and better-controlled anesthesia, which in turn necessitated more consistent monitoring practices.

The earliest reports in the literature on the use of anesthetics for cranial surgery were in 1881 by Macewen,[7] Durante in 1884,[8] and Bennett and Godlee in

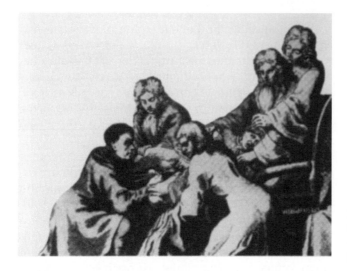

Figure 8-1 Surgical assistants hold patient still while lithotomist removes a stone via the perineum. (From Bettman OL: *A Pictorial History of Medicine.* Charles C. Thomas, 1956. Reprinted by permission.)

1885.[9] From the onset, controversy arose over which of the two agents was better. Chloroform produced quieter anesthesia and tended not to "congest" the brain, but depression of blood pressure and respiration were complications. The safer ether inductions were slower and associated with coughing and straining reactions attributed to the irritant properties of the drug. Subsequent rises in arterial pressure, dilation of the vessels of the brain, and increases of cranial tension caused the pioneering neurosurgeon Victor Horsley to recommend against its use.[10]

Early surgical anesthesia emphasized primarily the

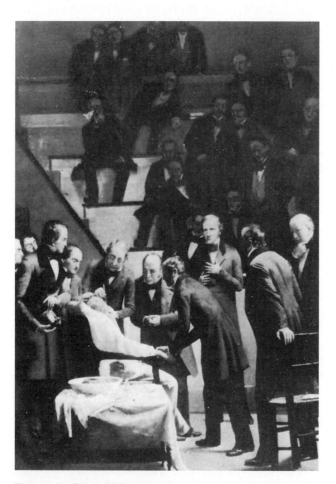

Figure 8-2 Original Ether Day, Boston, October 16, 1846. Dr. Morton (*left*) holds inhaler while Dr. J. C. Warren excises tumor on the jaw of Gilbert Abbott. (From Bettman OL: *A Pictorial History of Medicine.* Charles C. Thomas, 1956. Reprinted by permission.)

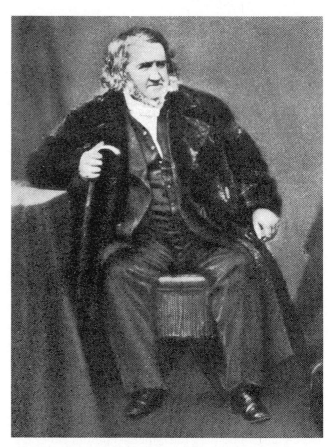

Figure 8-3 James Young Simpson of Edinburgh, introduced chloroform anesthesia. (From Bettman OL: *A Pictorial History of Medicine.* Charles C. Thomas, 1956. Reprinted by permission.)

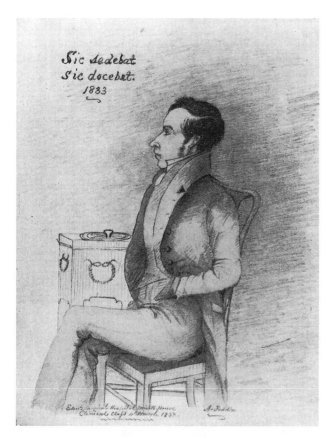

Figure 8-4   Sketch by Alexander Peddie, a student, of James Syme lecturing on surgery. (From Guthrie D: *A History of Medicine.* JB Lippincott, 1946. Reprinted by permission.)

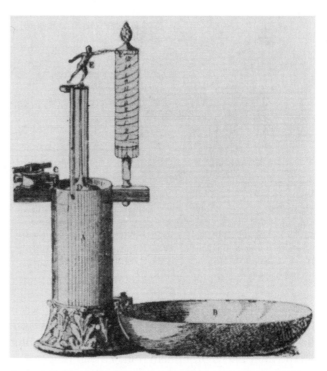

Figure 8-6   Water clock developed by Herophilus for measuring patient's pulse rate. (From Bettman OL: *A Pictorial History of Medicine.* Charles C. Thomas, 1956. Reprinted by permission.)

production of narcosis for pain relief, evaluating depth in terms of respiration, pulse, and other observable physical signs available to the five senses.[6,11] The next evolutionary step in patient monitoring took the form of a recommendation by F. B. Harrington to keep formal records during surgical procedures that utilized anesthesia. In 1894, Harvey Cushing and E. A. Codman

were the first to record times of administration and quantity of anesthetic, drugs, pulse, and respiration (Fig. 8-5).[12]

Even before physicians began expanding the notion of intraoperative monitoring of patients, technology was developing the tools that would significantly impact the ability to assess a patient's physiologic state.

About 300 B.C., Herophilus described the use of a water clock to measure the pulse rate (Fig. 8-6). He associated this measure with the state of his patients' health.[13] Steven Hales demonstrated a method in which

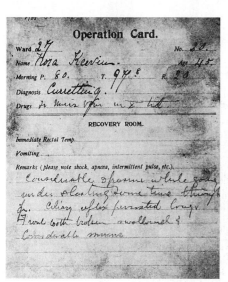

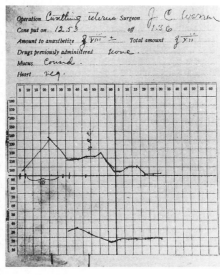

Figure 8-5   Anesthesia chart designed and used by E. A. Codman and Harvey Cushing during an operation on November 30, 1894. (From Beecher.[12] Reprinted by permission.)

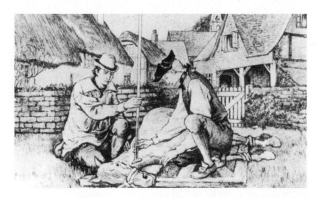

Figure 8-7 Hales measures blood pressure of a mare tied to an old field door. Glass pipe inserted into the jugular vein showed a column of blood 12 inches in height when animal was still, and 64 inches when animal was excited. (From Bettman OL: *A Pictorial History of Medicine.* Charles C. Thomas, 1956. Reprinted by permission.)

direct cannulation of an artery provided a measurement of arterial pressure in 1733 (Fig. 8-7).[14] In 1816, Laennec introduced the stethoscope, a device that would later play a prominent role in the intraoperative measurement of arterial pressure (Fig. 8-8).[15] Poiseuille's contribution to blood pressure measurement came in 1828, when he suggested that the long vertical glass tube that was connected to the artery in Hales' method could be replaced with a U tube in which mercury was used to counterbalance intravascular pressure.[16] On a more theoretical level, Christian Doppler presented a paper to the Royal Bohemian Society of Sciences in Prague in 1842 describing how the perception of frequency changes relative to the motion of the source or observer (Fig. 8-9).[17] This principle, now known as the Doppler effect, is the basis of precordial venous air embolism detection, echocardiography, and more recently transcranial sonography. In 1863, Marey described a sphygmograph, which recorded radial artery pulse oscillations on a smoked glass plate (Fig. 8-10).[18] Interestingly, a device of this design is believed to have recorded radial artery pulse waves during anesthesia using both ether and chloroform. These recordings appeared in *Principles and Practice of Surgery* by D. H. Agnew, published in 1881.[19]

Invention of the thermometer is credited to Sanctorious, some time between 1561 and 1636. These early instruments, however, were unscaled, influenced by atmospheric conditions, and gave only relative indications of temperature change. In 1714, Fahrenheit introduced the first scaled thermometer; this was followed in 1742 by Celsius' scaling approach based on the freezing and boiling points of water (Fig. 8-11).[20] Carl Wunderlich's publication of *The Temperature in Diseases* in 1868 spurred a great deal of interest in clinical temperature monitoring. While the importance of temperature was apparent, the thermometer did not come into regu-

lar use until after 1870, when Albutt introduced a design that is essentially the present-day clinical thermometer.[20] Almost simultaneously (1870), Fick was working out the principles governing the measurement of cardiac output.[21] Fick's principles provided the foundation for the subsequent development of dye dilution and thermodilution methods for measuring cardiac output.

In 1881, Basch demonstrated improvements to Marey's sphygmograph designs (Fig. 8-12).[22] While this device and that of Marey were probably not used routinely for intraoperative monitoring, they did represent the first experimental responses to the growing perception that monitoring the arterial pulse could significantly improve the safety of anesthetic administration. Not until 1896, when Riva-Rocci described *A New Sphygmomanometer* that could rapidly and repeatably measure radial artery pressure noninvasively, was the

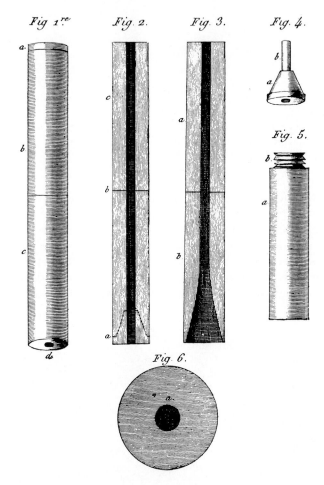

Figure 8-8 Laennec's wooden stethoscope. The cylinder (*Fig. 1*) was made of two pieces, screwed together (*Fig. 5*), with a detachable funnel fitted into one end (*Fig. 4*). *Figures 2* and *3* show sections of the instrument with and without the funnel, while the end view (*Fig. 6*, natural size) illustrates the relative size of the bore. (From Guthrie D: *A History of Medicine.* JB Lippincott, 1946. Reprinted by permission.)

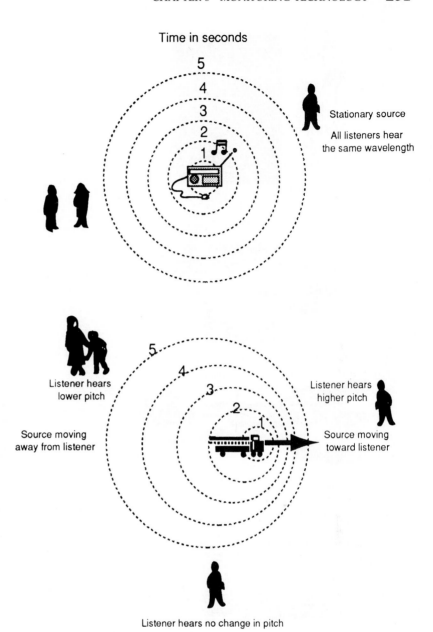

Time in seconds

Figure 8-9 The Doppler effect occurs when a source of waves is moving relative to the observer of the waves. The result is a change in the apparent frequency of the waves. Sound waves will seem to change in pitch. (From Trefil J, and Hazen RM: *The Sciences: An Integrated Approach.* John Wiley, 1994. Reprinted by permission.)

way cleared for routine intraoperative pressure monitoring (Fig. 8-13).[23] Cushing, upon learning of Riva-Rocci's blood pressure armlet, was able to secure a model in 1901 from Dr. Orlandi in Pavia, bringing it back to Johns Hopkins Hospital for regular use during neurosurgical operations.[12] By incorporating systolic blood pressure with measurements of pulse rate, respiration, and etherization on his anesthetic record, Cushing was the first to attempt a comprehensive intraoperative monitoring program. While it may be a stretch to consider Cushing as the progenitor of neurologic monitoring, it was in the neurosurgical patient that the first comprehensive monitoring was attempted. Thus, Cushing could well be considered to have stood at the

doorway of modern neurologic monitoring practice. By 1903, Cushing and others were reporting systolic arterial pressures in relation to various anesthetics and surgical procedures.[24,25] By this time, Cushing had also described the relationship of intracranial pressure to systemic pressure regulation.[26]

In 1903, Einthoven demonstrated for the first time the measurement of bioelectric potentials using a galvanometer to monitor the electrocardiogram.[27] While Caton recognized the presence of cerebral bioelectric potentials in 1875, 50 years would pass before Berger in 1925 recorded these potentials from the human scalp.[28] Within a short time, Berger and others recognized that anesthetics profoundly affected the electroencephalo-

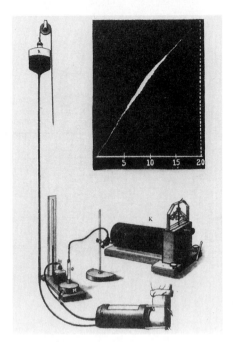

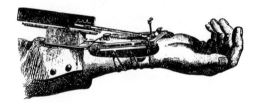

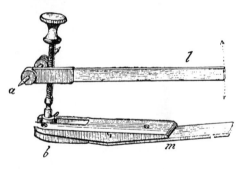

Figure 8-10   Marey's pulse recorder (*A*) showing adjustable lever in contact with the radial artery, and (*B*) an arm-occluding method of blood pressure measurement. (From Geddes LA: *Handbook of Blood Pressure Measurement.* Humana Press, 1991. Reprinted by permission.)

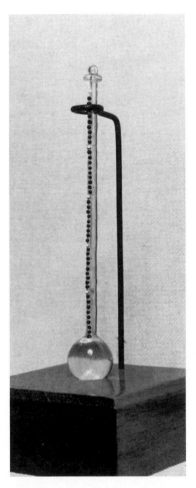

Figure 8-11   Thermometer constructed in 1657 at the Accademia del Cimento in Florence. (From Margotta R: *The Story of Medicine.* Golden Press, 1968. Reprinted by permission.)

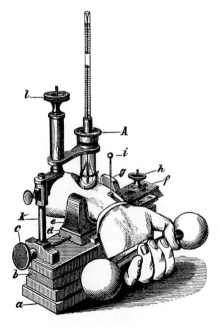

Figure 8-12   Von Basch's sphygmomanometer. (From Crile.[25] Reprinted by permission.)

gram, and they proposed the use of EEG to monitor depth of anesthesia (Fig. 8-14).[29] The first attempts to monitor the brain related exclusively to the need to control anesthetic depth, and it would take several decades of technological advances in the areas of electronics, engineering, materials, and manufacturing before these newly developed monitoring devices could be used to expand understanding in physiology and pharmacology sufficient to make clear the need to monitor the brain in terms of its own unique physiology.

The measurement of heart rate, blood pressure (ei-

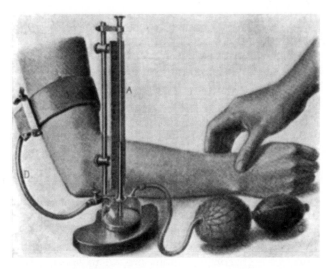

Figure 8-13   Riva-Rocci's sphygmomanometer. (From Janeway TC: *The Clinical Study of Blood Pressure, a Guide to the Sphygmomanometer.* D Appleton and Co, 1910. Reprinted by permission.)

ther by direct arterial cannulation or by sphygmanometric techniques), temperature, cardiac output, as well as listening to the sound of the beating heart, have all become routine monitoring practices, not only in general surgical procedures, but also in those involving the central nervous system. Theoretical concepts such as the Doppler principle, and even the somewhat esoteric quantum atomic theories have spawned the development of instruments like the precordial and transcranial Doppler and infrared absorption carbon dioxide analyzers. Early instruments designed to measure the brain's biopotentials have evolved into sophisticated monitors capable of examining the action potential of specific cell groups in the brain following stimulus, or of evaluating both motor and sensory pathways of the CNS. Devices that can perform spectral analysis of the brain's biopotentials have provided the opportunity for immediate and continuous asssessment of brain status during prolonged periods of anesthesia. In the absence of direct access to the patient's control centers, reliance falls on externally applied monitoring equipment for physiologic management.

Capnometery—Capnography

The measurement of inspired and expired carbon dioxide (CO_2) during the ventilatory cycle is termed capnometery or capnography. The term capnometery arises from the Greek *capnos,* meaning smoke, and the suffix *meter,* a means for measurement. Additionally, capnograph and capnogram come about from adding the Greek words *graphein,* to write, or *gramma,* that which is written, as a suffix to capnos. A capnograph or capnogram is therefore a graphic representation of inhaled and exhaled CO_2 concentrations in the ventilatory gas delivered to a patient during ventilatory support. As one might suspect, a capnogram or capnograph is generated by a capnometer; however, not all capnometers produce capnograms or capnographs. Modern devices often deliver data in the form of a digital readout of the peak expired end tidal CO_2 in terms of either a percentage or partial pressure of the ventilatory gas mixture.

PHYSICAL AND CHEMICAL PROPERTIES OF CO_2

Carbon dioxide is formed by the oxidation of free or bound carbon with excess oxygen, producing a molecule containing a single carbon atom covalently bonded to two oxygen atoms (Fig. 8-15). Its density is approximately 1.5 times that of air, and it can be poured from one container to another. CO_2 is a tasteless, odorless, and colorless gas at room temperature. The mole-

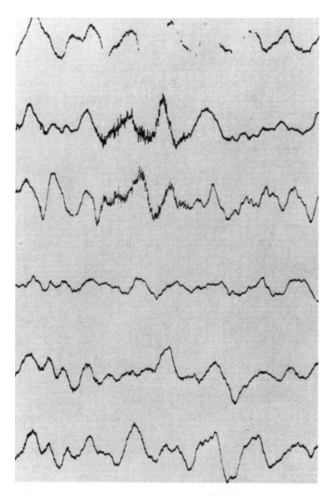

Figure 8-14   Portion of an electroencephalograph tracing made by Berger in 1929. (From Margotta R: *The Story of Medicine.* Golden Press, 1968. Reprinted by permission.)

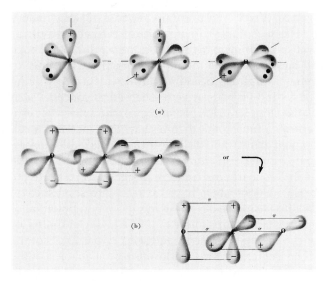

Figure 8-15 Orbital representation of a molecule of CO_2. (From Brescia F, et al: *Fundamentals of Modern Chemistry: A Modern Introduction.* Academic, 1966. Reprinted by permission.)

cule itself has an atomic mass of 44, is highly soluble in polar solvents, and can easily be ionized to form charged fragments. Structurally, CO_2 is a linear molecule, with each oxygen double-bonded to a central carbon at 180°, with both symmetric and asymmetric vibrational modes. CO_2 is also stable and relatively inactive and does not burn or support combustion. It readily dissolves in water, forming carbonic acid, which is weak and unstable. A 2 to 3 percent mixture in air can be breathed with no apparent ill effects. Above 5 percent, however, panting is produced, and at 50 percent CO_2 can be tolerated for only a short time. Atmospheric concentrations are approximately 3 parts in 10,000 in rural areas, and can be as high as 1 part in 100 in a crowded, poorly ventilated room.

MEASURING CO_2 IN VENTILATORY GASES

The measurement of carbon dioxide during ventilation requires methodology capable of continuous sampling, with a fast response time, and one that can distinguish CO_2 from other gases, notably nitrous oxide (N_2O). The instrumentation currently in use is based on both the physical and chemical properties of CO_2 and utilizes infrared (IR) spectroscopy, (IR absorption and IR scattering), mass spectrometry, and colorimetric endpoint technologies.

For a capnometer to be clinically useful, a capacity to detect CO_2 in the range of 0 to about 10 percent with an accuracy no less than 10 percent of the actual value is required. In addition, the precision of the measurement, that is the ability to replicate measurements con-

sistently, should be within 1 mmHg when using a calibration gas source.

In order to insure accurate measurements, it is essential that detailed two-point calibration procedures be carried out periodically. This enables an assessment of long-term stability and helps to establish the frequency of such a calibration. From a practical standpoint, a one-point calibration prior to each monitoring period insures that the capnometer is producing accurate measurements.

There are several approaches for calibrating a capnometer. The oldest and most reliable method utilizes compressed gas cylinders of precision mixtures of CO_2 in air, spanning the range of the capnometer. Gas is introduced directly into the sampling port, and the low and high concentrations are set to specific CO_2 values by adjusting the zero and gain controls. Another approach utilizes calibration cuvettes that contain the appropriate calibration gas mixtures. This method is particularly useful in mainstream capnometers based on IR technologies. The cuvettes replace the airway adapter during calibration; as before, zero and gain are adjusted to reflect the specific concentrations of CO_2 in the cuvette.

Another factor that can potentially influence the accuracy of the capnometric measurement is interference. In the IR and mass analysis methods, other substances such as nitrous oxide can have IR absorption bands and mass peaks close enough to the absorption bands and mass peaks of CO_2, so that the output measurement reflects a combination of both the CO_2 and interfering substance concentrations. Corrections for this interference have been implemented in most modern capnometers and include output offsets based on empiric determinations of the interfering gas's effect on the CO_2, or measurement of the interfering gas and correcting for it directly.

The response time of an instrument is another important consideration in capnography. Response time reflects the ability of an instrument to track a continuously changing condition, ultimately affecting the accuracy of the measurement (Fig. 18-16). Too slow a response may result in low end-tidal values and spuriously high inspiratory values. In addition, a low frequency response will significantly affect the shape of the wave form, providing more an estimate of the mean over a given time period while obscuring the instantaneous variations that occur during a ventilatory cycle.

Essentially, two factors affect the frequency response of an instrument. The first is the time it takes for a representative sample to reach the instrument detector and is referred to as *delay time*. In general, detectors that are located directly in the mainstream of the ventilatory gas flow (mainstream capnometers) have very low delay times, the frequency response being depen-

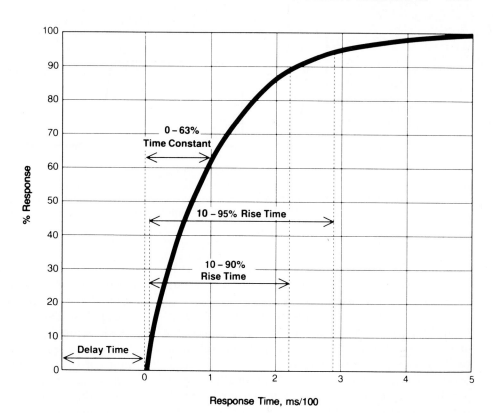

Figure 8-16 Schematic representing various aspects of a signal response. (From Gravenstein JS, et al: *Capnography in Clinical Practice.* Butterworths, 1989. Reprinted by permission.)

dent mostly on the frequency response of the detector and supporting electronics. In devices that draw a sample from the ventilatory gas flow and carry out the analysis on the periphery (sidestream capnometers), flow rate and sampling tube diameter and length are the principal factors in determining the delay time. A second factor affecting instrument response time is the response time of the detectors and supporting electronics. Also known as the rise time, this is the time needed for the instrument to reflect the true concentration of CO_2 following detector contact with the sample. Thus, the response time of a capnometer must be fast enough to insure that the readout is at least 95 percent of the true value at any given point in the ventilatory cycle, and must provide sufficient fidelity so as not to obscure fine detail in the wave form (Fig. 8-17).

Several additional factors having potentially significant effects in CO_2 measurements include choice of the sampling catheter material, gas diffusion effects, temperature, and pressure induced spectral absorption band broadening.

In sidestream capnometers, the material from which the sampling catheter is made also affects both the accuracy and frequency response of the instrument. Materials that have a high coefficient of permeability to CO_2 (Teflon, high- and low-density polyethylene) will permit CO_2 to diffuse out of the sample volume radially, rendering the measured value lower than the true value, as well as significantly reducing waveform fidelity. This effect is directly proportional to the catheter surface area and wall thickness. Thus, long, thin-walled catheters will have the greatest effect on CO_2 measurement.

The CO_2 waveform can also be distorted by axial diffusion out of the sample volume into adjacent space ahead and behind the sample (Fig. 8-18). In narrow catheters, the radial component can be minimized, assuming a low permeability catheter is used, leaving only the axial component to be considered. Axial diffusion tends to smear the waveform, causing successive cycles to blend together, thus reducing resolution. Small sample volumes and long delay times will affect the output to a greater extent than will larger sample volumes having short delay times.

Pressure or collision broadening occurs when molecules of CO_2 collide with other molecules in the gas such as N_2O, causing the spectral absorption band to widen. As pressure in the system increases during the ventilatory cycle the probability of molecular collision also increases, affecting the absorption of infrared energy by CO_2.[30,31] Corrections for these errors have been calculated empirically, tested experimentally, and implemented in instrument designs.[32,33]

Because the temperature range of the patient's expired gas will be within a narrow range, the effect of temperature on the CO_2 measurement will be slight.

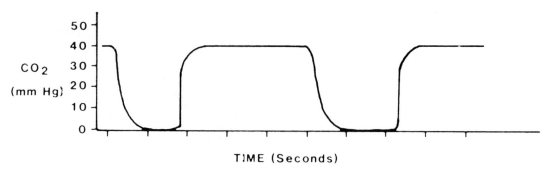

Figure 8-17 A normal capnogram. The ordinate represents CO_2 concentration and can be expressed in mmHg or kPa partial pressure or volume percent. The abscissa presents time in seconds.

Correction for temperature effects, however, must be taken into consideration when attempting to correlate end-tidal CO_2 with arterial p_{CO_2}.

Two approaches to capnometry are currently practiced clinically. The mainstream capnometer places the analysis cell directly in the ventilation circuit, optimally as close to the patient's mouth as possible (Fig. 8-19). This approach produces high quality capnographs having excellent fidelity with an imperceptible delay time. However, the weight of the analysis cell places additional stress on the ventilation tubing and patient airway. Cells are easily damaged and subject to errors stemming from the accumulation of water vapor or other secretions on the cell windows. While the typical cell is small, it does increase mechanical dead space.

In sidestream capnometers, gas samples are aspirated from the airway into an analysis cell within the body of the instrument (Fig. 8-20). While many of the problems associated with mainstream capnometers are eliminated, sidestream capnometry introduces its own unique complications.[34-39] Most notably, sample tube obstruction resulting from water vapor condensation or entrainment of airway secretions is a common occurrence. Aspirated gas must be dried or otherwise filtered in order to prevent complications. In addition, the analysis delay time depends not only on the length of the sampling tube, increasing as the length of the tube increases, but also on aspiration flow. Aspiration flows of 150 ml/min are normally used when analyzing gas in adult circuits. Flow that is too low tends to smear the capnogram, reducing fidelity, whereas too rapid an aspiration flow may actually steal gas from the ventilatory cycle, producing underventilation, particularly in the smaller patient.[34] Sampling port location also requires careful consideration to minimize contamination by ambient air.[35] Finally, exhaust gas from the sidestream capnometer must be scavenged in order to eliminate the possibility of contaminating the operating room with anesthetic gases.[40,41]

SPECTRAL BASED CAPNOMETERY

INFRARED ABSORPTION
Carbon dioxide has four fundamental vibrational modes, two of which are infrared-active (Fig. 8-21). An

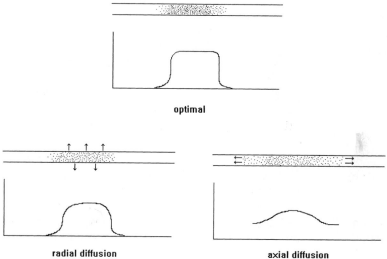

Figure 8-18 The effect of radial and axial diffusion in the sampling catheter on the capnograph waveform.

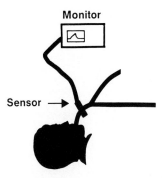

Figure 8-19   In the mainstream capnograph the sample cell is located within the ventilation tubing as close to the mouth as possible. (From Hess D: Capnometry and capnography: Technical aspects, physiologic aspects, and clinical application. *Resp Care* 1990; 35:6, 557. Reprinted by permission.)

asymmetric stretch vibration absorbs IR radiation at a wavelength of 4.26 μm, and a bending vibration absorbs at 14.99 μm.[42] Most absorption instruments utilize the 4.26 μm wavelength for analysis, as it falls in between two intense water vapor absorption bands with the N_2O and CO bands, offering minimal interference when appropriate band pass filtering is employed (Fig. 8-22).

All capnometers utilizing IR absorption technology have similar configurations: an infrared radiation source; analysis cell through which gas samples pass; a detector or transducer that converts the intensity of the analysis light beam to an electrical signal proportional to concentration; and a means for displaying the signal. This configuration is often employed in single-beam mainstream instruments (Fig. 8-23). A collimated infrared beam passes through a sample cell, typically positioned at the end of the endotracheal tube, onto a detector. Interposed between the sample cell and the detector is a chopper wheel on which are positioned two additional cells, one containing CO_2, the other N_2. As the wheel rotates past the sample cell, the infrared

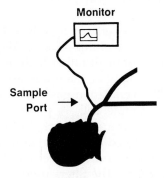

Figure 8-20   The sidestream capnograph continuously draws ventilatory gases through a catheter into the sample cell located within the instrument. (From Hess D: Capnometry and capnography: Technical aspects, physiologic aspects, and clinical application. *Resp Care* 1990; 35:6, 557. Reprinted by permission.)

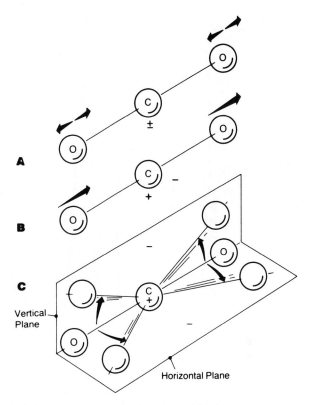

Figure 8-21   Vibrational modes for CO_2. (*A*) Non-infrared active symmetric vibration with no net displacement of charge. (*B*) Infrared active (4.26 μm) asymmetric vibration resulting in a net charge displacement. (*C*) Infrared active (15 μm) bending vibration resulting in a net charge displacement. (From Gravenstein JS, et al: *Capnography in Clinical Practice.* Butterworths, 1989. Reprinted by permission.)

analysis beam passes alternately through each of the additional cells. An alternating electric potential (voltage) is developed by the detector that is proportional to the sample cell concentration of CO_2. When the solid portion of the chopper passes in front of the detector, dark current (or small residual electrical output present when no radiant energy is impinging on the detector) can be measured and utilized to correct baseline drift.

To improve stability and specificity, the infrared analysis beam can be split in two, one beam passing through a reference cell and the other through a sample cell (Fig. 8-24). The intensity differential between the two beams results in a signal that is proportional to the concentration of CO_2 in the sample cell. Interference from N_2O and other interfering gases is minimized through the use of appropriate band pass filters. This design lends itself particularly well to sidestream capnometers. Both the single and double beam configurations are specified as the nondispersive type (NDIR). The incident infrared analysis beam is of a fairly narrow bandwidth that cannot be dispersed into its component wavelengths. Dispersive type analyzers are not commonly used in monitoring CO_2 in the clinical arena. In these instruments, a broad band infrared beam is

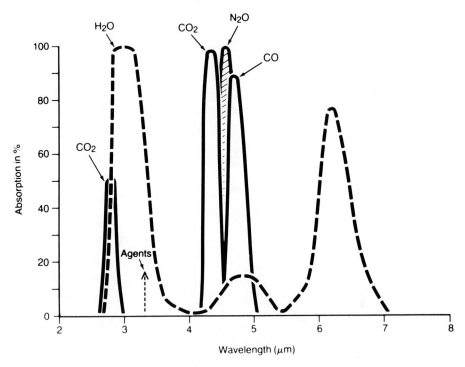

Figure 8-22 Infrared absorption spectra for CO_2 and potentially interfering gases. (From Gravenstein JS, et al: *Capnography in Clinical Practice*. Butterworths, 1989. Reprinted by permission.)

split into its component wavelengths and absorption by a sample volume is measured at specified frequencies.

RAMAN SCATTERING

In infrared absorptive spectroscopy, light energy induces a leap from one allowed vibrational state to a higher allowed vibrational state only if the energy of the incident light is equal to the difference between the allowed states. It is possible, however, for light of higher frequencies, namely those in the visible and ultraviolet ranges, to be partially absorbed, increasing the amplitude of molecular vibration only very slightly.[43] The remaining unabsorbed light is re-emitted at a lower frequency (Fig. 8-25). This, in principle, is Raman scattering. Because the probability of this type of interaction is small, the intensity of the reemitted or scattered light is very low. The intensity of the scattered radiation is, however, proportional to the concentra-

tion of the scattering species, and can therefore be utilized for quantification. Since the portion of the incident light absorbed by a molecule is dependent on its rotational and vibrational states, the frequency shift in the reemitted light is unique for each molecular species and can be used as an identifying signature. Unlike infrared absorption that occurs only when the molecular vibrational mode is asymmetric, Raman scattering requires that a vibrational state exist, either symmetric or asymmetric. Monoatomic species with no vibrational states about a bond will not be Raman active. Thus, most if not all physiologic and anesthetic gases can be measured by Raman scattering.[44] In addition to the Raman scattering, another form of scattering occurs in which the incident radiation is reemitted without alteration or shift in frequency. This is known as Rayleigh scattering, and is a potential source of interference.

Since the Raman scattered light is of low intensity, practical applications of this principle require that the incident light beam be of rather high intensity. Typically, argon laser light at 488 nm is used to irradiate a portion of the ventilation gas that is continuously drawn into a sample cell. A photomultiplier tube (PMT) positioned at a right angle to the sample cell measures the scattered radiation after it is conditioned by passing through a collection lens, battery of filters, and a focusing lens. The filters used in conditioning the scattered light remove Rayleigh interference, and provide a narrow band-pass at 523.4 nm for CO_2 Raman scattered light to reach the PMT.[44] Interference

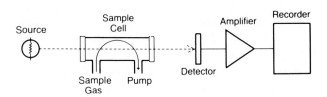

Figure 8-23 Schematic of a single beam nondispersive capnometer. This is a nonselective broad-band design that functions accurately only when CO_2 is the only absorbing species in the sample gas. (From Gravenstein JS, et al: *Capnography in Clinical Practice*. Butterworths, 1989. Reprinted by permission.)

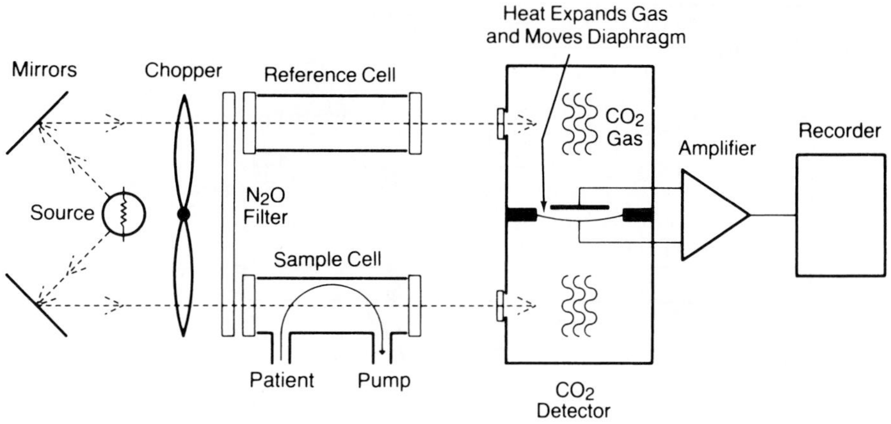

Figure 8-24 Schematic of a double-beam nondispersive capnometer. A reference cell and selective detector monitors the infrared light source and provides selectivity and sensitivity to CO_2. Interference from N_2O is removed by blocking radiation in the N_2O absorption band. (From Gravenstein JS, et al: *Capnography in Clinical Practice.* Butterworths, 1989. Reprinted by permission.)

from Raman scattered radiation by other gases is minimized by careful selection of band-pass filters. By adding an additional PMT, and a filter wheel that intermittently imposes narrow band-pass filters specific for other respiratory and anesthetic gases between the sample cell and the PMT, intermittent estimates of their concentrations can be made simultaneously along with CO_2 (Fig. 8-26).

MASS SPECTROMETRY

In mass spectrometry, sample gas is aspirated into a vacuum chamber where molecules in the gas are positively ionized by bombardment with a stream of highly energized electrons. During this process, the parent molecule is also fragmented into ions of smaller mass. Separation of the ion mixture occurs during acceleration through a magnetic field. As the ions move through the magnetic field, they travel in a curved path with a radius that is dependent on their velocity,

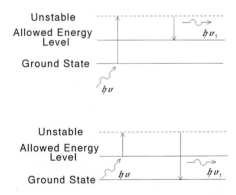

Figure 8-25 Energy level diagram describing Raman scattering. Upper diagram shows a Stokes' emission: instantaneous re-emission of a photon with longer wavelength than the incident light. Lower diagram shows anti-Stokes emission: instantaneous emission of a photon with a shorter wavelength than the incident light.

charge/mass ratio, and the strength of the magnetic field through which they pass. Particles of a specific charge/mass ratio can be focused to impact onto a detector by varying either the velocity of the ion or the strength of the magnetic field through which it passes. In order to maintain the integrity of the focused ion beams, the system operates under a high vacuum so as to reduce the probability of collision with ambient particles. A detector current that arises from the impacting ions becomes a function of the sample concentration. The mass spectrum is also exceedingly useful for molecular species identification, because bombardment of a given molecular species by high energy electrons produces a family of positively charged fragments with a mass distribution dependent on the parent species.

Two types of mass spectrometers are currently in clinical use. One relies on a fixed acceleration potential and magnetic field strength to separate the ionic fragments according to their mass (Fig. 8-27). In general, the ionic fragments produced from physiologic gases and inhalational anesthetics will bear only a single charge. Thus, the radius of their travel will be a function of mass and velocity if the acceleration potential and magnetic field strength are held constant. Heavier particles will have a large radius of travel while lighter fragments will move in a tight radius. Detectors can then be precisely positioned in a dispersion chamber along the focal plane of the ionic beams so that ions of a specific mass will fall upon that detector. In this type of configuration, not only can CO_2 be measured continuously, O_2, N_2O, N_2, and various anesthetic agents can also be monitored simultaneously.[45–52]

The second type of mass spectrometer functions much like a mass filter (Fig. 8-28). Following ionization, ions are accelerated into a chamber in which four parallel rods are oriented in a square pattern. Opposing rods are energized by both a DC potential and a radio frequency. The fields are tuned so that the trajectory

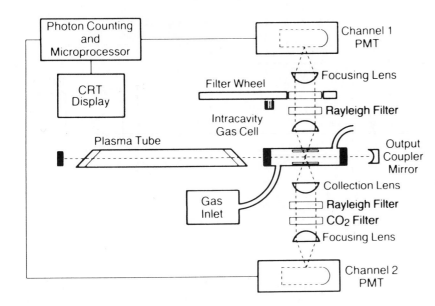

Figure 8-26 Schematic representation of a Raman spectrometer for CO_2 measurement. The gas sample aspirated through the sample cell is irradiated by monochromatic light from an argon laser. Rayleigh scatter is blocked by filters that absorb the incident frequency. In a dual channel instrument, CO_2 is monitored continuously by one channel, while the other provides discontinuous monitoring of other relevant gases by intermittent imposition of narrow band-pass filters specific to those gases. (From Gravenstein JS, et al: *Capnography in Clinical Practice.* Butterworths, 1989. Reprinted by permission.)

of a specific mass ion follows the longitudinal axis, utlimately colliding with a detector. The trajectories of the other ionic fragments follow paths that lead to collisions with one of the four rods. Altering the field characteristics in a controlled fashion permits scanning several mass levels, allowing for analysis of several gases. The detector current, as in the fixed magnetic field/detector configuration, is also proportional to the concentration of the sample.

Because of size, bedside use of mass spectrometers is not practical. Sidestream sampling is essentially the only alternative for ventilatory gas analysis. In addition to size considerations, the expense of mass spectrometry systems is prohibitive for dedicated single-patient use. Rotary values connected to the sample port permit multiplexing or sharing the system between several operating rooms, providing discontinuous sequential monitoring. In order to admit a gas sample into the ionization chamber without compromising the high vacuum, a molecular leak into the ionization chamber is established. A separate vacuum pump draws the patient gas sample through a long capillary tube past the sample port at the mass spectrometer. The high vacuum (10^{-6} mmhg) in the ionization chamber draws the gas past a needle valve adjusted to permit a leak of 10^{-4} ml/sec.

As with infrared capnometry, capnometry using mass spectroscopy is plagued by interference from

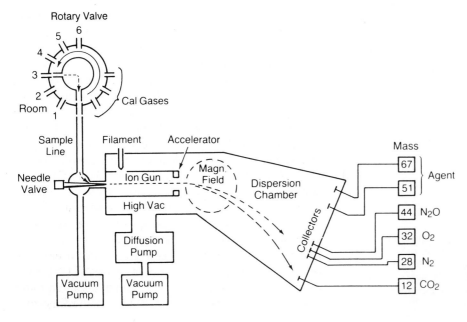

Figure 8-27 A fixed detector mass spectrometer configured for multiple site sampling. Calibration and patient gases are sequentially sampled through a rotary valve and are admitted into the ionization chamber through a low flow molecular leak. Following ionization and fragmentation, particles are accelerated and move through a fixed magnetic field for dispersal. Discrete detectors located in the focal plane collect the charged particles outputting an electrical current proportional to their concentration. (From Gravenstein JS, et al: *Capnography in Clinical Practice.* Butterworths, 1989. Reprinted by permission.)

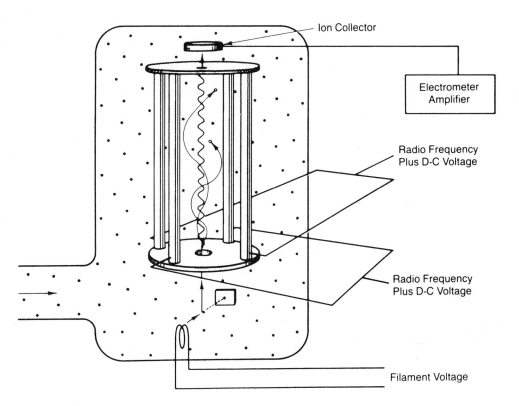

Figure 8-28   In a quadropole mass spectrometer, charged particles are accelerated through a tuned radio frequency and DC electric field. Particles of a specific mass are focused on the detector while all others collide with one of the four poles thus preventing them from being detected. Scanning a mass range is achieved by continuously retuning the radio and electric fields so that the charged particles of the specific mass range are focused onto the detector sequentially. (From Gravenstein JS, et al: *Capnography in Clinical Practice.* Butterworths, 1989. Reprinted by permission.)

N_2O. Both CO_2 and N_2O have nearly identical molecular weights, and thus the spectral peak for both gases occurs at the same mass band. During the ionization process not only is the parent molecule ionized but additional ion fragments of the parent molecule are formed. Fortunately, any of these fragments can be used for quantification. As long as the ionization conditions are consistent, the parent molecule will fractionate in a fixed relationship into ion fragments (Fig. 8-29). In order to resolve N_2O and CO_2, the spectral bands for N_2O^+ parent, and C^+ fragment are monitored. Anesthetic agents are handled somewhat differently. Halothane (mol wt 197.4), isoflurane (mol wt 184.5), and enflurane (mol wt 184.5) all fracture into ionic fragments having molecular masses of 67 and 51. The ratio of these fragments for each anesthetic, however, is different and can be used for identification and quantification.

COLORIMETRIC CAPNOMETERY

Since colorimetric CO_2 monitors rely on chemical indicators, they require no electrical power and need no calibration or maintenance.[53] Carbon dioxide in exhaled gas is exposed to a hygroscopic material containing a pH indicator. Hydration of the CO_2 results in the formation of carbonic acid, which dissociates to produce hydrogen ions causing a color change in the indicator (Fig. 8-30). Careful selection of the indicator allows a reasonably accurate estimation of CO_2 over a fairly broad range of concentrations (less than 2.3 mmHg to greater than 15.2 mmHg). Design considerations include the use of stable reagents and assurance that no toxic compounds or vapors form during hydration reactions and that the indicator color change does not occur in the red-green spectrum.[53] Metacresol purple fulfills these criteria. It is stable and nontoxic. When CO_2 is at or below 2.3 mmHg the indicator is purple. A CO_2 range between 3.8 and 7.6 mmHg produces a purple-yellow color; yellow appears when CO_2 is greater than 15.2 mmHg.[53] Colorimetric CO_2 monitoring is particularly useful for verifying endotracheal tube position. Additionally, in situations where capnometers are unavailable, colorimetric methods may be an expedient, temporary substitute.

Colorimetric methods have the significant drawback in that breath-to-breath analysis is not possible. Additionally, when pulmonary blood flow is reduced, a low end-tidal CO_2 may be measured, typically between 3.8 and 15.2 mmHg. When attempting to verify intubation, this condition may cause some confusion. Colorimetric instrumentation still lacks the ability to measure in the hypercapnic range, limiting its usefulness in monitoring intraoperative and postoperative respiratory depression.[53]

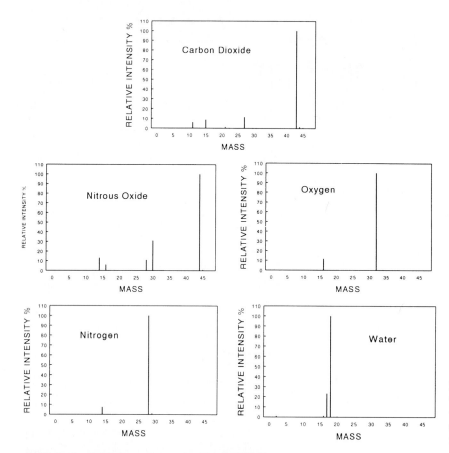

Figure 8-29 The fragmentation pattern for various components normally found in ventilatory gas samples. Peak intensity is calculated as a percentage of the largest fragment population.

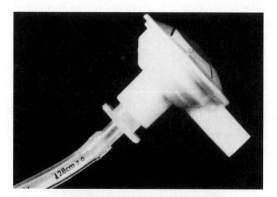

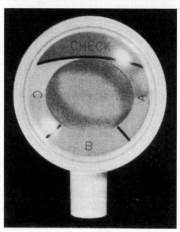

Figure 8-30 Side and top views of a colorometric end-tidal CO_2 detector. The device is normally interposed between the endotracheal tube and ventilatory tubing. CO_2 in the expired gas is hydrated increasing acidity in proportion to its concentration. A chemical indicator impregnated in the matrix of the unit changes color in response to the pH change. (From Goldberg et al.[53] Reprinted by permission.)

Intracranial Pressure Monitoring

CRANIAL CONTENTS

The cranial chamber is a rigid container approximately 1900 ml in volume. The contents of the cranium can be divided into three separate compartments. The brain or tissue compartment (including extracellular water), encompasses 80 percent of the cranial vault. Cerebrospinal fluid makes up 10 percent, and blood occupies the remaining 10 percent.[54] Partial compartmentalization of the brain results from the various attachments of the dura. The right and left hemispheres are incompletely separated by the falx cerebri; the supratentorial cerebral hemispheres are partially separated from the infratentorial cerebellum, brain stem, pons, and medulla by the tentorium cerebelli.[54] CSF circulates freely between these tentorial divisions through the communicating subarachnoid space, which also connects six large reservoirs or cisterns containing CSF at the base of the brain. Within the substance of the brain are located four additional irregular cavities called ventricles. Two lateral ventricles communicate via intraventricular foramen with a single medial cavity, the third ventricle. The aqueduct of Sylvius provides the primary CSF communication path between the third and fourth ventricles. The spinal cord with its associated cerebrospinal fluid and dural sac form an additional compartment. CSF moves freely through the subarachnoid space between the various compartments of the craniospinal axis.[55] Under normal circumstances, pressure is transmitted uniformly throughout the CSF channels.[55]

The brain is composed of two types of tissue with significantly different viscoelastic properties. The white matter is composed primarily of axons and myelinated fibers supported within a matrix of astroglial cells. The gray matter surrounds the white matter, forming the outer layer of the brain. It contains dense populations of cells and dendrites with connecting axons and synapses.[56] Throughout both gray and white matter, arteries and veins course vertically, spawning capillary beds at right angles. Pressures within these vessels range from 120 mmHg to less than 5 mmHg, their distribution having a significant effect on the brain's responses to deforming stresses.

ELEVATED INTRACRANIAL PRESSURE

Intracranial pressure (ICP) less than 15 mmHg are typically normal. Increasing the volume in one of the compartments establishes an initial pressure differential between the other compartments. If the CSF pathways remain open, the pressure gradient can quickly equilibrate by shifting CSF, extravascular water, or blood volume to the other compartments. If the initial increase in volume is not too large, ICP can remain within normal ranges. The ability to compensate for changes in compartmental volume by shifting the excess to other compartments, is termed *intracranial compliance* (Fig. 8-31). The compliance mechanism prevents sustained elevations in pressure as long as there is CSF or blood that can be displaced. When the intruding volume approaches the compensation limit, ICP rises abruptly with only small additional increases in intracranial volume. When an elevation in intracranial pressure in excess of 20 mmHg is sustained, ICP is considered to be abnormally high.

At extremely high intracranial pressures, gradients may develop between compartments, resulting in displacement or herniation of brain tissue. Portions of the brain can become compressed against bony ridges of the skull, resulting in ischemia and necrosis. The most commonly identified herniation associated with elevated ICP, transtentorial or uncal, occurs when a mass lesion in the supratentorial space displaces brain tissue through the tentorial hiatus.[57-59] Displacement of tissue from one supratentorial compartment to an adjacent compartment across the falx cerebri is called *cingulate* or *subfalcial herniation. Rostrocaudal herniation* also occurs when ICP pressure gradients force the cerebellum and brain stem through the foramen magnum. Following head injury, the development of edema often results in brain herniation through the skull fracture.

To maintain normal function, the brain requires uninterrupted delivery of oxygen and nutrients by the blood. From a hydrodynamic perspective, in order for flow to occur, a pressure gradient must exist between

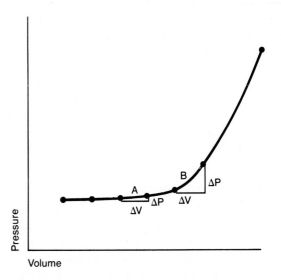

Figure 8-31   In an idealized intracranial pressure-volume relationship, the change in volume *V* at (*A*) results in a small change in pressure *P*, *P/V* or elastance is small. When elastance is high (*B*), the same *V* results in a substantially greater *P*. (From Bruce.[61] Reprinted by permission.)

the inlet and outlet points of a conduit system. In general, the gradient between the systemic arterial and central venous pressures induces blood flow through organs. In the brain, however, the arterial pressure at which blood flow begins must be greater than the pressure within the closed cranium. This pressure gradient, the perfusion pressure, is a function of the intracranial pressure rather than the central venous pressure as it is in other organ systems. Thus, significant elevations in ICP can influence the delivery of blood to the brain.[60–62]

REFLEX RESPONSES TO INTRACRANIAL HYPERTENSION

The brain can make adjustments in response to elevated ICP. Reflex cerebral vasodilation decreases cerebrovascular resistance, resulting in acute increases in cerebral blood flow and volume. Plateau waves, which are acute and sustained increases in ICP, are believed to be a consequence of this reflex mechanism. Systemic hypertension and baroreceptor-mediated bradycardia first described by Cushing and known as "Cushing's reflex" occur when the intracranial pressure approaches or equals the systemic arterial pressure.[26,63,64]

While the purpose of these compensatory mechanisms is to increase perfusion of the brain, they ultimately may aggravate intracranial hypertension. The eventual consequence of reducing cerebrovascular resistance or elevating arterial pressure is the expansion of cerebral blood volume. Under conditions of autoregulatory impairment that may be found following traumatic brain injury, tumors, or large doses of direct cerebrovasodilators, cerebral blood flow becomes a direct function of cerebral perfusion pressure. Any increase in systemic pressure is mirrored by an increase in blood flow and volume—hence, elevation of ICP. Increased systemic pressure also elevates the hydrostatic pressure gradient between the tissue and blood compartments. Water can then move into the extravascular space, further aggravating the situation, particularly when blood-brain barrier function is impaired.

COMPARTMENT CHANGES AND INTRACRANIAL HYPERTENSION

Intracranial hypertension can be caused by changes in the volume of any one or combination of intracranial compartments. Factors predominantly affecting the brain tissue and interstitial volumes are tumors, vasogenic and cytotoxic edema, and interstitial edema. Head trauma may also contribute to the formation of both cellular edema and vascular hemorrhage, or hyperemia. Elevation of intracranial tension can result

from obstruction of CSF pathways and alteration of CSF production or absorption.

Intracranial hypertension rarely results from changes in only the cerebrovascular compartment. Exceptions include hematomas secondary to vascular compartment rupture and arteriovenous malformations. However, when the intracranial compliance is already compromised, even small changes in the volume of the vascular compartment can become profound. Since normal cerebrovasculature is sensitive to CO_2 levels, hypocapnia can be used to induce vasoconstriction, which effectively reduces cerebral blood volume. A 4 percent change in cerebral blood flow is realized for every mmHg change in Pa_{CO_2}, resulting in approximately a 2 ml/100 g per min change in CBF or a 0.04 ml/100 g change in cerebral blood volume.

Anesthetics and other pharmacologic agents with potent vasodilating properties may also affect ICP, particularly when the brain's compensatory mechanisms are impaired. Inhalational agents such as halothane and isoflurane, as well as vasodilators such as nitroglycerin, nitroprusside, hydralazine, and calcium antagonists all have been reported to exacerbate ICP increases. On the other hand, beta- and alpha-adrenergic blocking agents such as esmolol, propranolol, and labetalol have not been associated with increased ICP.

INTRACRANIAL PRESSURE MONITORING

Since clinical deterioration may follow intracranial hypertension, the goal of monitoring intracranial pressure is to permit early and rapid intervention so as to minimize cranial compartment shifts, as well as the preservation of cerebral perfusion pressure.[62,65–69] Because elevated ICP does not always produce symptoms, ICP evaluation based on clinical signs may be unreliable, nonspecific, and not quantitative. Under some conditions such as posterior fossa and temporal lobe pathology, ICP measurements may be within normal ranges.[61,62]

INDICATIONS

The need to monitor ICP intraoperatively can be based on three factors. The first is the preoperative neurologic status; the second, the nature of the intracranial pathology; and the third is the duration of the proposed surgical procedure.[70] Patients with head trauma or subarachnoid hemorrhage having a 5 or less on the Glasgow coma scale will have increased intracranial pressure and may need to be monitored.[70] In patients with known intracranial pathology, monitoring ICP can be effective for initial preoperative stabilization and control during surgery.[71] Computed axial tomographic studies suggest that compressed ventricles and/or basal cisterns, the extent of midline shift, and the pres-

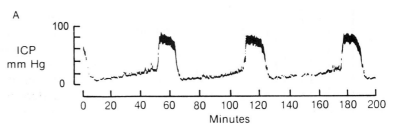

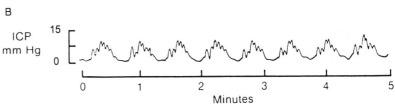

Figure 8-32 *A.* Plateau waves most often associated with poor neurologic outcome. *B.* Normal ICP trace showing respiratory fluctuations. [From Sokoll MD: Monitoring intracranial pressure. In Blitt CD (ed): *Anesthesia Monitoring in and Critical Care Medicine.* Churchill Livingstone, 1985. Reprinted by permission.]

ence of subarachnoid blood are strong indicators of elevated ICP, and can be used as an aid in making decisions about the need for monitoring.[72,73]

In disease states such as Reye's syndrome, or in massive strokes where the development of edema can be a possibility, outcome may be favorably influenced by monitoring and controlling ICP.[74,75] During therapy for elevated ICP, direct monitoring can be of assistance, especially in establishing the dosage regimen of osmotic agents.[76] Postoperatively, ICP monitoring should be considered when the possibility of an increased ICP would have serious consequences. This may occur when autoregulation impairment is suspected (as in large AVMs), or when brain swelling becomes a problem intraoperatively.

MEASUREMENT OF INTRACRANIAL PRESSURE
Normal ICP is in the range of 10 to 15 mmHg. When a sustained increase in ICP exceeds 20 mmHg, an abnormal condition is believed to exist (Fig. 8-32). Normal ICP traces depict respiratory and cardiac oscillations and never show sustained rises. ICP measurements are relative and most commonly reference to the external ear canal.

The intraventricular, subarachnoid, and epidural spaces are the principal sites for monitoring ICP. The subarachnoid and epidural spaces are less invasive, but are subject to waveform dampening, do not allow removal of CSF, and may not accurately reflect global pressure. Infectious complications are common to all methods of monitoring.

Intraventricular, subarachnoid, and epidural ICP measurements can be expected to yield the same estimates of global intracranial pressure only when there is free communication of the CSF between the various compartments of the intracranial space. In instances where space-occupying lesions are found intracranially, lumbar pressure is often significantly lower than intracranial pressure.[77] Occlusion of the tentorial inci-

sura or the foramen magnum can result when herniating brain tissue blocks communication between the intracranial and spinal compartments.[78,79] In contrast, when intracranial pressure is elevated subsequent to increases in the volume of cerebrospinal fluid, communication throughout the craniospinal axis is maintained, with both lumbar and intracranial pressures reflecting comparable values.[80]

There are essentially two main classes of ICP monitoring devices, those in which ICP is coupled to an extracranial transducer by a fluid column and those in which small transducers are inserted intracranially. Five methods are generally available for ICP monitoring; these include ventriculostomy, subarachnoid bolt, subdural transducers, epidural transducers, and fiberoptic catheters.[70]

Many of the pressure transducers used in association with ventriculostomy, subarachnoid bolts, and catheters rely on strain gauge technology. The basis of this technology relates a mechanical deformation in a conducting element to a change in the ability of that element to carry electrical current. Stretching or straining a wire increases its length and decreases its diameter. Associated with this deformation is a proportional increase in electrical resistance. Compression strain has the reverse effect. Shortening and thickening the wire proportionally reduces its electrical resistance.[81] This principle led the way to the development of the strain gauge, a very fine wire arranged in a reciprocating pattern bonded to a backing (Fig. 8-33).[82] For pressure measurement, the strain gauge is bonded to a diaphragm that has one side open to the atmosphere, while the other side is exposed to the pressure source. Changes in pressure deform the diaphragm, similarly deforming the strain gauge and resulting in a proportional change in electrical resistance. To detect the small change in resistance, the strain gauge output is directed into a Wheatstone bridge circuit, in which the resistance causes a current imbalance (Fig. 8-34). The

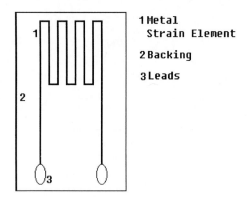

Figure 8-33 Schematic diagram of a metal foil strain gauge. Maximum sensitivity to strain is achieved when the reciprocating pattern of the metal foil is parallel to the strain.

magnitude of the imbalance is proportional to the resistance change, which is in turn proportional to the applied pressure.

The newer disposable pressure transducers are solid-state piezoelectric devices. Piezoelectric crystals, when mechanically strained, produce an electrical potential proportional to the strain. When bonded to a diaphragm in a manner similar to strain gauges, they produce an output voltage proportional to the applied pressure.

LUMBAR PRESSURE

Shortly after the practice of measuring cerebrospinal fluid pressure via lumbar puncture was introduced by Quincke, the significance of this measure was demonstrated in relation to a variety of pathologic conditions, including intracranial tumors.[83-85] While there exists a general consensus that lumbar pressure in excess of

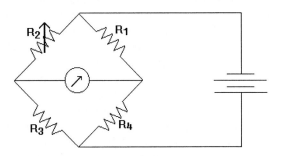

Figure 8-34 A Wheatstone bridge showing the strain sensing element R2 (strain gauge) as a variable resistor. Because resistances R3 and R4 are equal, current entering the bridge will be equally divided between them. Balancing the transducer such that the resistances R2 and R4 are also equal results in equivalent amounts of current flowing through both resistors. Since current flow on both sides of the bridge are equal, there is no deflection of the meter. Application of pressure to the transducer, alters the resistance in R2 unbalancing the current in the bridge and causing the meter to deflect in proportion to the imbalance.

200 mmH$_2$O constitutes an abnormal condition, significant disagreements have developed with regard to the indications for lumbar puncture, its reliability, and its accuracy.[80] There are two primary objections to the diagnostic use of lumbar puncture in intracranial hypertension. The first is the potential for causing brain stem compression at either the tentorial incisura or the foramen magnum when CSF pressure in the spinal compartment is either purposely or inadvertently reduced.[86-89] The second is that CSF pressure at the lumbar level is not an accurate reflection of intracranial pressure under all conditions of cranial pathology.[67,77,79,90-92] In spite of these risks, long-term monitoring of cerebrospinal fluid via lateral cannulation of the C1-C2 subarachnoid space has been suggested as a viable alternative to ventricular cannulation in patients with small or compressed lateral ventricles.[93]

VENTRICULOSTOMY

Ventriculostomy or cannulation of the lateral cerebral ventricle represents the gold standard for intracranial pressure measurement, in that this method provides simultaneous diagnostic and therapeutic access.[94] While it is the most invasive of all the ICP monitoring methods, it is also the most accurate and versatile, permitting the recording of pressure waves with excellent fidelity, allowing the drainage of CSF for treatment of intracranial hypertension and assessment of intracranial compliance. Ventricular cannulation, however, is not without risk. Besides the potential for hemorrhage on insertion, an infection rate as high as 21 percent and a 2 to 5 percent failure rate have been reported.[70] If the cannula is not precisely positioned within the fluid reservoir, accidental aspiration of brain tissue can occur. While placement of ventricular catheters is straightforward in patients with normal-sized ventricles, ventriculostomy is contraindicated in those with severe compression or distortion of the ventricular system or coagulopathy.[70]

When using this approach to monitor ICP, the ventricular catheter is connected to a drainage bag by fluid tubing. The drainage bag is positioned at a fixed level above the head in order to maintain a set pressure and provide additional space into which CSF can be displaced. A pressure transducer can be connected to a side port located between the catheter and drainage bag. However, before an accurate measure of ICP can be made, the channel to the drainage bag must be closed; otherwise, the fluid column established by the height of the drainage bag will be the pressure that is measured. Care must be taken to avoid precipitous drainage or the unintended injection of fluid. Inadvertently dropping the drainage bag would create a sudden negative pressure within the ventricles, resulting

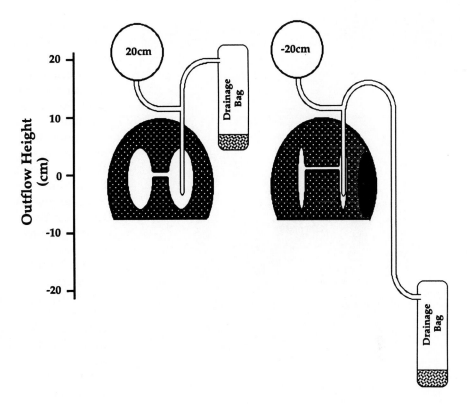

Figure 8-35 Schematic showing proper drainage bag position relative to patient. Elevating the bag 20 cm above the interauricular line elevates the ICP to 20 cmH₂O (*left*). Bag positions lower than the head induce siphoning of CSF into the bag leading to negative ICP and ventricular collapse (*right*). Complications on the order of tissue aspiration and or subdural hematoma formation subsequent to bridging vessel rupture are possible. (From Todd.[70] Reprinted by permission.)

in their collapse and possible hemorrhage from torn bridging veins (Fig. 8-35).[70] The system should never be connected to a pressurized bag commonly used for arterial line infusion, nor should a CVP, PA, or arterial pressure transducer be shared in order to measure ventricular pressure. Maintenance of sterility of the system is of paramount importance.

SUBARACHNOID BOLT

Substantially less invasive and somewhat more easily placed than a ventricular catheter, the subarachnoid bolt is screwed into a burr hole drilled into the skull. An incision in the underlying dura establishes communication with subarachnoid CSF and fluid-filled tubing conveys pressure fluctuations to an externally located transducer, typically referenced to the ear canal. To ensure that there is sufficient fluid for pressure transmission, and to maintain the opening of the bolt clear of obstruction, periodic flushing with small volumes of fluid are necessary.[80] The subarachnoid bolt is particularly useful in patients who demonstrate distorted lateral ventricles or the presence of coagulopathy (Fig. 8-36).[70] The risks of causing hemorrhage during insertion or of developing an infection during monitoring are significantly less than for ventriculostomy.[95,96]

The subarachnoid bolt is not without disadvantages. CSF cannot be drawn through the bolt; thus, the main therapeutic advantage to communication with the CSF

compartment is lost. In addition, compliance measurements also cannot be made. Highly edematous brain or tissue displaced in the direction of the bolt's position by a mass lesion increases the potential for tissue herniation into the opening of the bolt. This condition causes almost 20 percent of bolt placements to ultimately fail because pressure fluctuations are seriously damped by the occluding herniation.[95] In an acute focal lesion, the accuracy of subarachnoid bolt measurements may be questionable. Pressure differences as high as 40 mmHg between right- and left-side bolts have been reported.[97] When compared to ventriculostomy measurements, subarachnoid bolt estimates have been shown to be approximately 15 mmHg lower.[98]

SUBDURAL CATHETERS

Essentially a variant of the subarachnoid bolt technique, subdural catheters were introduced in order to improve on the failure rate of subarachnoid bolts. The device is nothing more than a fluid-filled catheter that is threaded into the subdural or subarachnoid space (Fig. 8-37).[95,99–101] Clinical data seem to indicate that while the failure rate is somewhat improved, and the infection rate is comparable to that of the subarachnoid bolt, pressure measurements are typically lower than ventricular pressures.[101] Insertion requires a comparatively large cranial opening, thus precluding bedside application. This technique may be most useful for

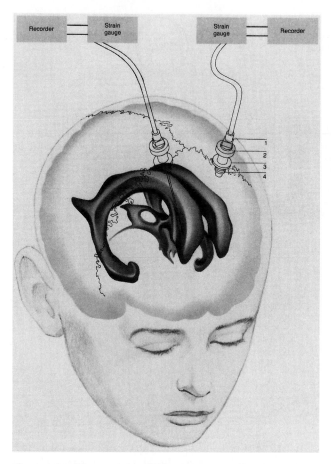

Figure 8-36 Measurement of ICP using ventriculostomy, and subarachnoid bolt. 1. Intravenous tubing connector. 2. Flange fits into handle for screwing bolt into twist drill hole. 3. Seal 4. Threaded end is screwed into twist drill hole. (From Bruce.[61] Reprinted by permission.)

postoperative monitoring in craniotomy patients, where the advantages of placement outweigh the limitations.[102,103]

EPIDURAL TRANSDUCERS

A great many epidural devices for measuring intracranial pressure have been introduced since the mid-1960s. While epidural transducers seem to offer a reduced risk for brain infection and trauma, accuracy of the measurement, and the ability to zero and calibrate in situ have become major concerns.[104-114] Nevertheless, epidural monitoring has been shown to be clinically useful in patient care.[104,105,115-119] Of the myriad of devices described in the literature, few have enjoyed any commercial success.

Ladd Fiberoptic Transducer

The Ladd fiberoptic sensor is based on a pressure switch concept (Fig. 8-38). The active elements are housed within a hollow cylindrical silicone shroud 10 mm in diameter and 1 mm high. Centrally posi-

tioned on one of the internal cylindrical surfaces is a pillar to which a mirror is attached (sensing surface). Entering the shroud from one side parallel to the plane of the sensing surface is a pneumatic tube within which is a bundle of three parallel optical fibers. The optical fiber bundle is aligned with the mirror so that light emanating from the central fiber is reflected onto the two outer fibers, illuminating each one equally. The application of pressure to the sensing surface alters the alignment of the mirror relative to the fiberoptic bundle, unbalancing the amount of light that the outer fibers receive. A photodetector continuously compares the intensity of the light returning from each fiber. When an intensity imbalance is detected, a small air compressor is activated that pressurizes the cylindrical shroud, returning the mirror alignment to where the outer optical fibers are once again illuminated equally. This balance pressure is equal to the epidural pressure. The continuous balancing cycle follows pressure changes, providing what appears to be continuous epidural ICP monitoring. In reality this sensor produces discrete pressure readings over a given time interval. If the balancing interval is kept short, reasonable fidelity can be achieved. Superimposed over the basal ICP are respiratory waves caused by the slight restriction of venous return following elevation of intrathoracic pressure during inspiration. In addition a reflection of systemic pressure fluctuation is also seen over the top of the respiratory waves. In order to resolve the latter frequency components, the balancing frequency of the ICP monitor must at a minimum be twice that of the frequency being measured (Nyquist theorem). Other-

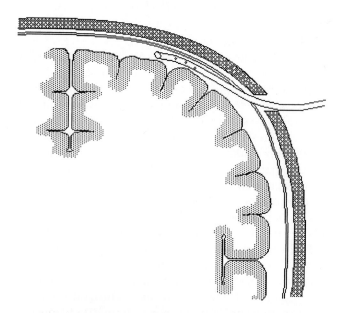

Figure 8-37 Position of a subarachnoid catheter for measuring ICP. Catheter is connected to a strain gauge transducer and output can be recorded and or displayed visually on a CRT.

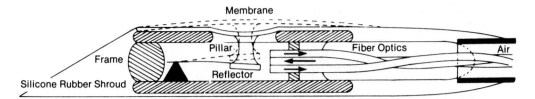

Figure 8-38 The Ladd epidural transducer in cross-section. [From Sokoll MD: Monitoring intracranial pressure. In Blitt CD (ed): *Monitoring in Anesthesia and Critical Care Medicine.* Churchill Livingstone, 1985. Reprinted by permission.]

wise, the frequency components that are observed will be aliased or will appear lower than the actual frequency.

Experimentally, and in limited clinical experience, the Ladd sensor used epidurally has shown reasonably good correlation to ventricular and cisternal pressure.[111,112] Few infections have also been reported, and, after an initial learning curve with respect to handling the unit, failure from breakage is low.

While the Ladd unit has good sensitivity and fidelity, and has been demonstrated to be stable over long periods, the major drawback to its use is its inability to rezero once it has been inserted subdurally. Since the transducer that measures the balancing pressure is external to the sensor, its calibration and zeroing are straightforward. However, to zero the sensor, that is, to verify that the fiberoptic bundle and mirror are correctly aligned, stress applied to the sensing surface must be relieved. After placement subdurally, this is not possible without removing the sensor. No facility is available for removing CSF; thus, compliance testing is precluded. Placement of the sensor requires a large opening in the skull if used for epidural insertion. As a final consideration, the sensors are expensive, of single use, and require proprietary electronics for interfacing with the outside world.

CAMINO FIBEROPTIC TRANSDUCER

Another approach to fiberoptic implementation for ICP measurement is embodied by the Camino transducer (Fig. 8-39). Two parallel optical fibers, transmitting/receiving, are positioned within a 4F hollow flexible catheter aligned opposite a diaphragm that seals the catheter tip. Internally, the diaphragm is reflective. Externally, applied pressure deforms the diaphragm. Light from the transmitting fiber is reflected onto the receiving fiber. The amount of reflected light is proportional to the extent of deformation, which is in turn proportional to the applied pressure. The returning light is converted to an electrical signal, amplified, and displayed as a continuous pressure waveform.[113] Since the Camino device does not rely on counterbalancing pressure, frequency response is quite good.

The Camino device can be placed via a small burr hole that can be inserted at the bedside. The fiberoptic catheter can be positioned within the ventricles, subdurally, or within the cortical parenchyma. Parenchymal insertion directly measures tissue pressure. Because there is no need for fluid coupling to an external transducer, pressure wave damping, and catheter occlusion are avoided. Placement through a hollow catheter allows ICP measurement as well as CSF drainage. Excellent correlations between ventricular pressures using standard ventriculostomies and the Camino fiberoptic transducer have been reported.[120–122] While some evaluations have shown good agreement with subdural and intraparenchymal measurements, others have demonstrated somewhat less encouraging correlations.[123–127]

Calibration verification prior to insertion requires pressurization of the catheter tip by a means that maintains the unit's sterility. Immersion in a sterile fluid column or insertion into a pressurization chamber are among the few options available for external calibration. These options, unfortunately, carry the potential for contamination. Additionally, the fiberoptic transducer cannot be rezeroed after insertion, although zero drift has not proved to be a significant problem (0.75 mmHg/8 h).[124]

GAELTEC TRANSDUCER TIPPED CATHETER

The Gaeltec transducer, based on thin film strain gauge technology, houses a strain gauge in the tip of a flexible 5F double lumen tube (Fig. 8-40). The end of the tube is sealed and a diaphragm to which a strain gauge is bonded seals the side hole of one of the lumina. An elastic shroud encases the catheter tip so as to include the diaphragm and the side hole opening of the second lumen. In use, external pressure causes deformation of the diaphragm, which in turn deforms the strain gauge, resulting in an electrical resistance change proportional to the applied pressure. For all practical purposes, the Gaeltec transducer functions identically to the standard strain gauge transducer previously described. A unique innovation in this device, however, allows in-situ zeroing and calibration. Because the two lumina within the catheter can be made to communicate at the opposite end, inflation with a small volume

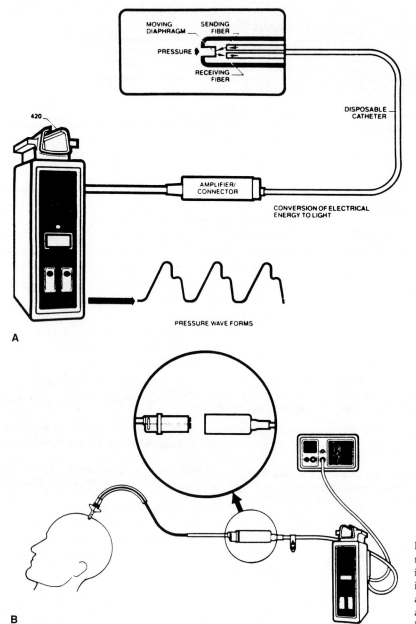

Figure 8-39 (*A*) The Camino fiberoptic ICP monitoring system. The catheter tip which is implanted intracranially is shown in detail in the inset. (*B*) Schematic describing the general application and configuration of the transducer and intervening electronics. (From Yablon et al.[124] Reprinted by permission.)

of air expands the encasing shroud, simultaneously applying pressure to both sides of the diaphragm. This results in no net deformation of the diaphragm or strain gauge, a condition equivalent to no external application of pressure. The electronic circuitry can then be zeroed, and monitoring continued following release of the inflating air. Calibration is similarly straightforward. When air is instilled into only the lumen communicating with the shroud, it expands and applies pressure to only one side of the diaphragm, resulting in a deformation proportional to the specifically applied pressure. Gain can then be adjusted to reflect the calibration pressure. Using this approach, calibration can

be achieved both prior to insertion or in situ without compromising sterility.

The transducer has a flat frequency response to 4 kHz and a linear pressure range from 0 to 150 mmHg, and can be coupled electronically to most standard monitoring systems.[114] While the stability of strain gauge devices is always a concern, the Gaeltec device exhibits minimal baseline drift.[114]

In experimental and clinical evaluations as both an epidural and subdural pressure sensor, the Gaeltec device displayed positive correlation to conventional methods of measurement. Both epidural and subdural pressures also have been correlated well against direct

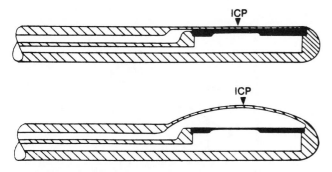

Figure 8-40   Cross-sectional diagram of the Gaeltec transducer. The upper diagram depicts the normal operating configuration. The lower panel shows the transducer in zero check mode. The membrane deflection is exaggerated for clarity. (From Roberts et al.[114] Reprinted by permission.)

ventricular pressure assessments.[101,114,128-130] Intraventricular or intraparenchymal insertion is not approved in the United States. Inflation of the zeroing/calibration shroud, particularly intraparenchymally, could result in serious injury to brain tissue. Rupture of the shroud could also introduce biologic contaminants directly into the substance of the brain.

While the Gaeltec transducer has many significant advantages over other approaches for monitoring intracranial pressure, the unit does have a high cost. Because of design limitations, the Gaeltec transducer cannot measure negative pressures, and exhibits difficulties in reproducing ICP waveforms when pressure is below 5 mmHg. As with fiberoptic devices, it is relatively delicate, and is prone to breakage during sterilization, insertion, zeroing, calibration, removing, and cleaning.[114] Radio wave frequencies from beeper systems have, in at least one instance, been shown to produce artifact significant enough to affect waveform interpretation.[131]

NONINVASIVE MEASUREMENT
Intracranial Pressure from the Anterior Fontanelle
In recent years, considerable attention has been paid to the development of a noninvasive approach for evaluating intracranial pressure in newborns and infants. Instrumentation for estimating neonatal ICP has generally been designed to take advantage of the anterior fontanelle window of the newborn cranium. These devices have met with little acceptance because of a lack of consistent correlation to ICP, high sensitivity of transducer output to patient position and motion, lack of continuous monitoring capability in some designs, inability to correct for zero drift and to calibrate in situ, and poor reproducibility after successive reapplications of the sensor to a given fontanelle. The failure of previous anterior fontanelle transducer designs seems to be the result of inconsistent application of the

principles governing measurement, pressure/volume relationships, and material properties of skin.

In general, ICP in the neonate can be perceived as the result of the cranial contents exerting a force onto the inner table of the skull. Nonrigid areas such as the anterior fontanelle in the cranial vault will therefore be visibly deformed in proportion to the force applied to this area (Fig. 8-41). With respect to atmospheric pressure, a positive ICP will cause a fontanelle bulge, whereas a negative ICP will cause a fontanelle concavity. Zero ICP with respect to the atmosphere results in the anterior fontanelle membrane lying flat within the plane of the scalp. Anterior fontanelle membrane deformation in response to pressure is likely to be nonlinear because of the nonuniform nature of skin elasticity. Transducer designs utilizing fontanelle deformation or fontanelle tension as a basis for estimating ICP may be subject to considerable error resulting from inconsistent membrane elasticity due to varying levels of hydration, nutrition, and temperature.

Accurate estimates of ICP can be made, however, if transcutaneous compression of the fontanelle membrane can be assumed to be small and the cranial bones forming the fontanelle are relatively firmly attached to one another. Then the pressure applied to the intracranial side of the anterior fontanelle membrane would be transmitted extracranially by the membrane with little attenuation. A pressure-sensing device firmly attached to the scalp overlying the cranial bone margin

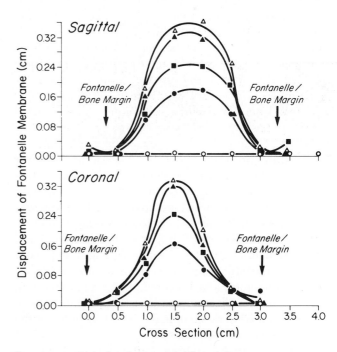

Figure 8-41   Sagittal and coronal profiles of the anterior fontanelle membrane in a neonatal cranial model at various ICPs. ○–0 mmHg, ●–10 mmHg, ■–20 mmHg, ▲–30 mmHg, △–40 mmHg. (From Bunegin et al.[142] Reprinted by permission.)

of the anterior fontanelle would therefore have the same pressure exerted onto its diaphragm as that being exerted onto the inner table by the intracranial contents. In essence, the scalp overlying the cranial bone margin of the anterior fontanelle acts as a stable reference point from which reliable estimates of ICP can be made.

Accurate estimates of ICP from the anterior fontanelle also depend on other variables, which include transducer cross-sectional diameter, position on the anterior fontanelle, transducer application pressure, and attachment technique.

It is essential that the transducer base have sufficient diameter so that its outer edges will rest on the area beyond the anterior fontanelle membrane-cranial bone interface. This produces a consistent and stable reference from which measurements can be made. It is also important that the transducer be positioned directly over the apex of the anterior fontanelle. Transducer positions that are skewed may result in inconsistent referencing and transmission of pressure to the transducer diaphragm.

After positioning, sufficient pressure must be applied to the transducer to ensure firm contact with the reference points. With insufficient transducer application pressure, the anterior bulge prevents transducer contact with the reference points and lower estimates of ICP can occur. Excessive application pressure does not significantly affect ICP estimates in the infant cranial model when transducer cross-section diameter is sufficiently large to contact the scalp adjacent to the bony margin of the fontanelle. However, in humans damage to tissue at the contact sites may result from decreased tissue perfusion. Application pressures slightly higher than the actual ICP are necessary for accurate estimations of ICP from the fontanelle.

Transducer application techniques have varied widely, most often involving the use of adhesive media.[132–139] These techniques seem to be useful only for short-duration applications because significant drift occurs in the transducer output with their use. Adhesives will tend to slip over time, and, in combination with gradual tape stretching, invariably lead to lower estimates of ICP. The use of elastic bandages may reduce the component of output drift due to material relaxation; however, the adhesive slippage component may stil introduce significant error into the ICP estimate. Transducer attachments utilizing a harness with elastic straps will provide adequate application pressure over a wide range of ICPs so that accuracy of the estimates can be maintained.

Properly affixed anterior fontanelle monitors can have a better frequency response than ventricular catheters. Catheter damping, the result of catheter tip obstruction or accidental introduction of air into the pres-

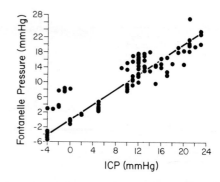

Figure 8-42 A least squares fit of all AFP vs. ventricular ICP measurements obtained from three ICU neonates previously instrumented with a ventriculostomy and anterior fontanelle transducer. The correlation between AFP and ICP is significant to a 95 percent confidence interval. (From Bunegin et al.[142] Reprinted by permission.)

sure lines, would be avoided. It can also be used together with or after removal of the ventricular cannula and can be maintained indefinitely without risk of infection. Also, patient movement and positional changes should not substantially affect AFM output.

In most published reports dealing with the measurement of anterior fontanelle pressure, the two devices that have been predominantly used are the applanation transducer and the Ladd fiberoptic sensor.[132,135,138,140,141] For applanation devices, difficulty in correlating AFP and ICP occurred when the base place of the transducer was not circumferentially in contact with the bony margins of the fontanelle.[135,137,138] Accurate estimates of ICP from the fontanelle could be made only when there was firm contact between the base plate of the transducer and the bony margin of the fontanelle (Fig. 8-42).[135,137,138] The bony margin of the fontanelle seems to offer a stable reference from which ICP estimates can be made accurately. Unfortunately, the applanation devices require minimal patient positional changes and are prone to motion artifact. Also, these devices have no means for in-situ calibration or baseline correction.

Studies in which AFP was monitored using fiberoptic systems have been contradictory in terms of the effect of application pressure on sensor output.[133,137,140] Some investigators report that AFP correlates very well with ICP and is not affected by application pressure; others have demonstrated quite convincingly that the application pressure on a fiberoptic sensor does affect sensor output.[137,140] In those studies, a 12-*g* force applied to the fiberoptic sensor seemed to provide the best correlation between fontanelle pressure and ICP. Greater pressure resulted in higher than actual estimates of the ICP from the fontanelle. Application pressure does affect AFP, but only when the transducer base plate is not in contact with the scalp adjacent to the bony margins of the fontanelle. Transducers with smaller cross-sectional diameters than the smallest dimension of the anterior fontanelle tend to "float" on the fontanelle, and their output (AFP) then depends on the extent to which the application device presses them into the fontanelle window.[142]

Doppler Technology

The Doppler principle was formulated by an Austrian physicist Christian Doppler in 1842 in an attempt to explain observed positional aberrations of stars that were greater than could be ascribed to parallax alone.[17] This wave theory describes the relationship between the observed frequency of radiation emanating from an object and the velocity of that object. Doppler described the effect in terms of a ship sailing directly into oncoming waves. The ship would encounter wave fronts more frequently and of greater amplitude than a ship at rest. Sailing directly away from oncoming waves, reduces the frequency of encounters as well as the amplitudes of the waves. This frequency shift, known as Doppler shift, is proportional to the difference in velocity between the observer and the source of the waves. Thus, a stationary observer could in principle measure the velocity of moving objects by measuring the frequency change or shift in the radiation reflected from that object. The first application of this principle for medical uses was in 1960 by Satamura and Kaneko, who developed an instrument for measuring blood circulation.[197] Subsequent to this work, a profusion of instrumentation evolved for noninvasive monitoring of the various aspects of circulation, from the precordial Doppler for detecting air embolism to the sophistication of imaging the working cardiac muscle and the fetus in utero.

THE DOPPLER PRINCIPLE

The Doppler effect occurs during relative motion between an observer and a radiation source. This radiation can of course span acoustical and electromagnetic spectra. Whenever movement of the source and observer are toward one another, the observer perceives a frequency greater than that actually emanating from the source. In the reverse, when the observer and source are moving apart, the frequency perceived by the observer is less than the actual frequency emanating from the source. In medical instrumentation, the observer, that is, the transducer, is stationary and serves a dual purpose. As the observer, it detects wave fronts coming from the moving source. Since the objects that are being observed do not radiate frequencies that are easily detected, the transducer additionally broadcasts acoustical radiation, typically in the 1 to 20 mHz range. The transducer can then observe the reflected radiation from the objects of interest, comparing the transmitted and the received frequencies.

In a situation where the source, (e.g., a red blood cell) is stationary relative to the transducer, the frequency of the reflected acoustic energy will be identical to that originally transmitted. If the blood cells were moving toward the transducer with a velocity v_b, then during one cycle or period T of the incident wave, the blood cell would traverse a distance that is the product of its velocity and the duration of the wave period, that is $v_b T$. Since the period T of a wave is equal to the reciprocal of its frequency $1/f$, then the distance traveled by the blood cell becomes v_b/f. This is the amount by which the incident wavelength λ is shortened. So the wavelength λ_r of the reflected acoustic energy observed by the transducer can be given by:

$$\lambda_r = \lambda - \left(\frac{v_b}{f}\right) \tag{1}$$

Since $\lambda = v/f$, the wavelength received by the transducer is:

$$\lambda_r = \frac{v}{f} - \frac{v_b}{f} = \frac{v - v_b}{f} \tag{2}$$

Recasting this equation in terms of the reflected frequency by substituting λ_r with v_r/f_r results in:

$$\frac{v_r}{f_r} = \frac{v - v_b}{f} \tag{3}$$

Taking the reciprocal of both sides and rearranging gives:

$$f_r = f\left(\frac{v_r}{v - v_b}\right) \tag{4}$$

Since the velocity of the reflected wave v_r is the sum of the transmitted wave velocity v and the velocity of the blood cell v_b, then:

$$f_r = f\left(\frac{v + v_b}{v - v_b}\right) \tag{5}$$

By dividing the numerator and denominators by v and simplifying, an exact expression for the reflected frequency is developed:

$$f_r = f\left(\frac{1 + \dfrac{v_b}{v}}{1 - \dfrac{v_b}{v}}\right) \tag{6}$$

Additional algebraic manipulation is necessary to recast this expression into a more useful form, and is presented without comment:

$$f_r = \frac{\left(1 + \dfrac{v_b}{v}\right)}{\left(1 - \dfrac{v_b}{v}\right)} \times \frac{\left(1 + \dfrac{v_b}{v}\right)}{\left(1 + \dfrac{v_b}{v}\right)} = \left(\frac{1 + 2\dfrac{v_b}{v} + \left(\dfrac{v_b}{v}\right)^2}{1 - \left(\dfrac{v_b}{v}\right)^2}\right) \quad (7)$$

Since the velocity of the blood cell v_b (<6 m/s) will be substantially less than the velocity of the transmitted wave v(1540 m/s, velocity of sound in blood) $(v_b/v)^2$ will be negligibly small, further simplifying the expression for the frequency of the reflected wave to:

$$f_r = \left(1 + 2\frac{v_b}{v}\right) = f + 2f\frac{v_b}{v} \quad (8)$$

The Doppler shift is defined as the difference between the incident and reflected frequencies and is expressed as:

$$f_{ds} = f - f_r \quad (9)$$

Substituting Equation 8 for the reflected frequency f_r:

$$f_{ds} = f - f + 2f\frac{v_b}{v} = 2f\frac{v_b}{v} \quad (10)$$

In early Doppler instruments this frequency was directed to amplifiers for output to speakers and to recorders for velocity analysis.

PRECORDIAL DOPPLER

Venous air embolism has come to be recognized as a significant complication affecting diagnostic, therapeutic, and surgical interventions.[143] The notion that venous air embolism is restricted to neurosurgical procedures is a common misconception. Ample numbers of clinical reports of its incidence during surgical procedures of the head, neck, chest, as well as in obstetric procedures were published during the nineteenth century.[144-151] In this century, incidents of venous air embolism have been reported during abdominal, gynecologic, neurosurgical, orthopedic, plastic, and vascular surgery.[152-174] No reliable hard data are available on the overall occurrence of VAE. Periodic aspiration of previously positioned right atrial catheters in neurosurgical sitting position cases, or detection via an esophageal stethoscope roughly approximated an incidence of 6 percent.[175,176] Since the introduction of the precordial Doppler, the incidence of VAE detection has been estimated to range between 10 and 33 percent in neurosurgical cases in the sitting position.[177-181] En-

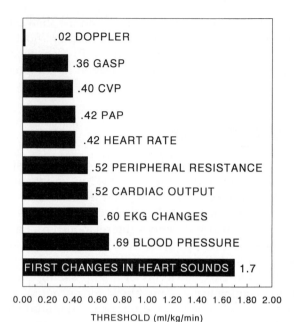

Figure 8-43 Synopsis of various methods used for the detection of venous air embolism and their relative sensitivity. (From Gildenberg et al.[185] Reprinted by permission.)

trance of air into the venous circulation can occur whenever a gradient exists between the right atrium and an open vein. A gradient as small as a 5 cm is sufficient to permit venous entrainment of air.[182] A lethal volume of air, 100 ml, can be entrained through a 14-gauge needle within a second at a gradient of 5 cm H_2O.[173,183] The volume of air that ultimately enters the venous circulation is a function of the body position, depth of anesthesia, intrathoracic, and central venous pressures. Death results primarily from acute obstruction of blood flow to the right heart and pulmonary outflow tract, leading to a reduced cardiac output and subsequent cardiac standstill.[184]

Several approaches have been attempted for detecting VAE sufficiently early to institute effective therapy (Fig. 8-43).[185] Of these, precordial Doppler is by far the most effective and sensitive method. Volumes as small as 0.1 ml can easily be detected.[154,175,184,186-190] The performance, however, is a function of the position of the transducer, with optimal results occurring when the transducer is transmitting its ultrasonic beam directly at the superior vena cava and right atrium. In this position, air will be detected before it enters the pulmonary circulation. In most people it will be located over the third to sixth intercostal space to the right of the sternum.[191] Confirmation of the correct position can easily be carried out by the injection of a small volume of saline thought the right atrial catheter. A distinct transient "whoosh" is heard as the saline passes through the Doppler ultrasonic field. Alternatively,

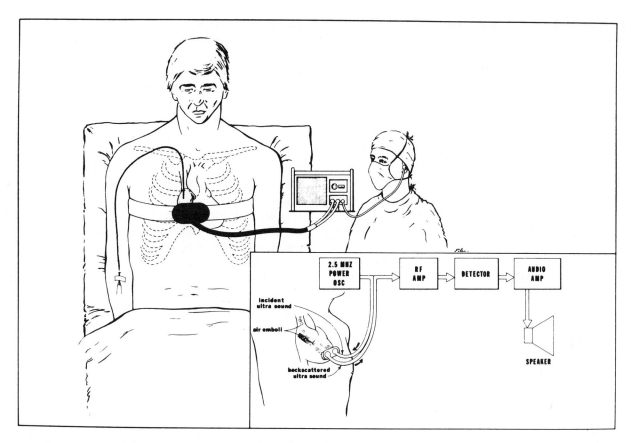

Figure 8-44 A precordial Doppler transducer properly positioned over the right atrium and secured with a circumferential strap. The inset shows a simplified schematic of Doppler cardiac auscultation. (From Maroon and Albin.[191] Reprinted by permission.)

0.25 to 0.5 ml of carbon dioxide or air can be injected while one listens for the characteristic "chirp" (Fig. 8-44).[191]

The precordial Doppler is not specifically designed for measuring blood velocity in the SVC or right atrium. The Doppler shift arising from moving blood is a characteristic swishing sound synchronous with the venous flow velocity. The ability to detect air stems from the extremely high acoustical reflectivity of air emboli relative to blood components. The result is a "high-pitched scratching noise similar to that produced when a phonograph needle slides across a moving record."[186] Others have described the audio signature of air emboli as a "hollow metallic chirp, scratchy, chirping, or roaring noise."[53]

While Doppler technology has been used to advantage in detecting air emboli, additional information is encoded in the reflected ultrasonic beam. In addition to frequency shifts, which are indicative of velocity of a reflector, the amplitude of the reflected signal, can provide a notion about the nature of the reflector. The amplitude of an echo indicates not only what percentage of the originally transmitted beam was reflected,

but also can provide information about the medium through which it has passed. The mechanism by which reflection occurs requires the recognition that the speed with which sound waves travel varies as a function of the medium through which they move. A medium, therefore, can be viewed as offering resistance to transmission of sound waves. This resistance is termed impedance (Z) and is defined as the product of the density of the medium and the velocity of sound in that medium. Thus, high-density material, such as liquid, will support high sound velocities, resulting in high acoustical impedance; low density media, such as air, will have low acoustic impedance. In a medium of uniform acoustic impedance, sound waves will be transmitted uniformly with little reflection. if, on the other hand, a medium contains elements that have different acoustic impedances, the boundary between the two impedances offers a surface from which the sound wave can be reflected. The fraction of the incident beam that is reflected depends on the impedance difference of the two media. Greater differences result in larger reflections. A reflectance coefficient (α_R) can therefore be defined as the square of the ratio of the difference and sum of the two impedances.[192] Expressed mathematically:

$$\alpha_R = \left(\frac{Z_2 - A_1}{Z_2 + Z_1}\right)^2 \qquad (11)$$

where Z_1 = acoustic impedance of medium 1; Z_2 = acoustic impedance of medium 2. Because there is a large impedance difference between blood ($Z_b = 1.6 \times 10^{-6}$ kg/m² per s) and air ($Z_a = 0.0004 \times 10^{-6}$ kg/m² per s), as much as 99.9 percent of the incident ultrasound beam can be reflected back, accounting for its unusual sensitivity and the distinctive "roar" that is heard when air passes the precordial Doppler transducer.

After initial reflection, there arises a suspicion that the precordial Doppler may further yield information regarding the volume of air entering the right atrium. After all, more air increases the area of acoustically reflecting surface, permitting a greater fraction of the incident ultrasonic beam to be reflected back for detection. While this logic is in principle correct, other factors such as body position and atrial geometry complicate its application. As an example, in patients undergoing neurosurgical procedures in the sitting position, air emboli entering the superior vena cava are buoyed up by a force equal to the weight of the volume of blood that they displace. This buoyancy is opposed by a force exerted on them by the flowing blood and is proportional to the surface area of the emboli, density, and square of the velocity of the blood. The emboli will pass through the Doppler field to the pulmonary circulation if this force is greater than the buoyant force acting on them. Otherwise, they will float upward. In view of the pulsatory flow pattern within the cava and right atrium, an air-blood vortex is formed where entering air is churned, subsequently fractionating into microemboli that are passed into the pulmonary circulation. The portion of this vortex lying within the Doppler field would continuously reflect back incident radiation, resulting in an output proportional not only to the volume of the emboli but also to the time the emboli spends in the Doppler field.

Most precordial Doppler devices operate in the ultrasonic frequency range, emitting an acoustic frequency between 1 and 3 MHz. At these frequencies, the energy is not damaging to tissue, easily generated, and capable of moving through tissue without overwhelming attenuation. To produce and detect these frequencies, Doppler transducers rely on another physical phenomenon called the *piezoelectric effect*. Discovered by Pierre and Jacques Curie in 1880, it is a property of some crystalline substances that an electrical potential develops across the crystal in response to mechanical deformation. The phenomenon also operates in reverse, in that placing the crystal into an electric field causes it to deform. In general, precordial Doppler transducers have at least two piezoelectric crystals. An oscillating electrical potential with a frequency in the desired range (2.5 MHz) is continuously applied across one of the crystals, causing it to vibrate at the same frequency and broadcasting or transmitting sound waves outward. A second crystal positioned adjacent to the transmitter is deformed by the reflected or returning acoustic energy, generating an oscillating electrical potential identical to the frequency and proportional to the amplitude of the returning wave. The frequencies of the transmitted and reflected waves are compared, and the difference is directed to an audio output device following suitable amplification.

A disconcerting feature of early Doppler units was radio frequency interference emanating from electrocautery usage. The ultrasonic transducer readily picks up the signal, which completely obliterates the cardiac signals. This difficulty, however, has been overcome by instituting better electromagnetic shielding, and including cut-off circuitry as a part of the audio portion of the instrument. Deactivation of the Doppler occurs within 10 ms when radio frequency interference from cautery is detected (3 to 300 kHz). This band range is well below the acoustic frequency used by the instrument (2.5 MHz). The unit reactivates after a 200-msec delay. Because the period of deactivation is very brief, the probability of missing significant air embolization is small.

Various treatments of venous air embolism have been proposed during the past several decades. Durant and coworkers introduced the left decubitus position with the head lowered (Duran's maneuver) which keeps air in the apex of the right ventricle, maintaining the patency of the pulmonary outflow tract.[193] Stallworth and associates suggested transthoracic aspiration of air in the heart, a procedure that never gained popularity because of its invasive nature.[194] Ericsson and coworkers developed closed chest cardiac massage for treatment of venous air embolism, showing it to be a simple, noninvasive, and effective technique.[195] Michenfelder and associates introduced the use of the right atrial catheter for aspirating air from the heart. The latter method has proved to be the most effective approach for dealing with venous air embolism.[175] Subsequent clinical findings suggested that despite aspiration of large volumes of air during air embolism episodes, reasonably large amounts of air were still entering the pulmonary circulation.[182] This study led to the discovery that in neurosurgical procedures utilizing the sitting position, entering venous air emboli accumulated in the superior vena cava just outside the right atrium.[196] In order to maximize the amount of aspirated air, the position of the right atrial catheter

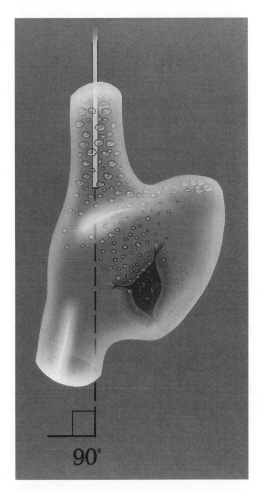

90°

Figure 8-45 Orientation of a catheter within an air-blood vortex in the superior vena cava at the confluence of the right atrium for optimal embolus aspiration.

tip had to be within the air-blood vortex churning just outside the right atrium in the vena cava. With the addition of side holes to form multi-orificed aspiration catheters, further improvements in clearing venous air embolism were realized (Fig. 8-45).[196]

While the combination of multi-orificed aspiration catheter design and improved catheter positioning dramatically increases the probability of clearing lethal venous air embolism, this method of treatment is only as effective as the method used for detecting the emboli. The precordial Doppler together with echocardiography are currently the only methods that have sufficient sensitivity and reliability to detect venous air emboli before they enter the pulmonary circulation.

TRANSCRANIAL DOPPLER

While significant technological development for noninvasive assessment of extracranial blood flow, air bub-

ble detection, and structural imaging continues at a rapid pace, little effort has been directed until recently toward similar analysis for the intracranial environment. The overriding obstacle was a belief that the skull could not be penetrated by ultrasonic energy, thus rendering the intracranial environment inaccessible. This assumption was subsequently shown to be incorrect, and the ability to measure blood flow velocity in cerebral vessels in a noninvasive manner was demonstrated.[198] Since this demonstration, the field of transcranial Doppler sonography, as has become known, has ballooned with new knowledge of the physiologic and anatomic aspects of the cerebral circulation and new technological developments in instrumentation.

All transcranial Doppler (TCD) instruments have several components and features in common. Because bone and soft tissue offer significant attenuation to higher ultrasonic frequencies between 3 and 10 MHz, TCD instruments operate at the much lower frequency of 2 MHz. In comparison to continuous wave Doppler transducers like those found in precordial devices, TCD transducers emit ultrasonic pulses at regular intervals. Pulsed transducers utilize a single piezoelectric crystal for both transmission of the ultrasonic pulse and detection of the reflected signal. This design allows for depth discrimination and the ability to evaluate blood flow velocity within vessels located at various distances from the brain surface. The ultrasonic beam diameter is converged by refraction through plastic lenses to encompass the cross-section of the cerebral vessels and ranges from 3×3 mm to 6×6 mm, depending on the instrument and the desired settings. Combined with depth discrimination (range gating), the ultrasonic beam samples a specific volume called the sample volume that is defined by the product of the cross-sectional area of the incident ultrasonic beam and the distance the beam travels during a pulse interval. The echo contains information about the distribution of blood flow velocities in the flow lamina within the vessel as well as artifact caused by cardiac wall-thumping and transducer movement. From here, the signal is high-pass filtered to remove high frequency artifact, then subjected to fast Fourier transform analysis, generating a frequency spectrum characteristic of the velocity profile within the sample volume. The spectrum for that time interval is displayed by plotting on the ordinate axis and assigning the amplitude of each frequency a proportional gray scale intensity. Repetition of this process for subsequent echoes results in an accumulation of discrete slices in time displaying the blood velocity profile within the segment of vessel on which the sample volume is focused. TCD devices can also discriminate directionality by comparing the frequency shift of the echo to the parent pulse. A higher frequency indicates advancing movement; a lower frequency indicates receding movement.

Since the introduction of the first TCD, new systems have evolved rapidly and can now generate 3D representations of the vascular segment under evaluation. Ultrasonic systems utilizing color-coded B-mode technology for direct vessel segment visualization have also been developed.[199-201] These instruments can produce an impression of dimensionality by rapidly scanning the region of interest with an ultrasonic beam through a range of depths, creating a series of 2D images that are then melded together.[202] Improvements in transducer sensitivity have allowed intracranial components of the venous circulation to also be insonated.[198] Methods for microemboli detection, blood-brain barrier disruption, and improved sampling through the temporal window are currently under development.[203-209]

The primary obstacle to transcranial Doppler examination of blood flow velocity in cerebral vessels has been the skull. The acoustic properties of the bone are such that only low ultrasonic frequencies can penetrate. A cancellous layer called the diploe is sandwiched between inner and outer layers of dense ivory bone. Thickness of the layers varies, with the inner layer somewhat convoluted to conform to the surface contour of the brain.[210] The porous nature of the diploe favors the absorption and scattering of high frequency energy and can reduce the power of the transmitted ultrasonic beam by as much as 80 percent. The convolutions of the inner table also act as acoustic lenses, refracting the incident ultrasonic beams in an unpredictable fashion.[211] The thinnest part of the skull and the most ultrasonically conductive is found in the temporal area. In this region, the diploe is at its minimum, and the minute bony spicules responsible for scattering the ultrasonic energy are absent.[211]

Ultrasonic examination of the brain is facilitated through the ultrasonically conductive portions of the skull. Several windows for peering into the intracranial environment are available (Fig. 8-46). In addition to the temporal area or window, the orbital window and the foramen magnum window are commonly used for examinations. The transorbital approach provides access to the ophthamic artery and the carotid siphon (Fig. 8-47).[212,213] In addition, portions of the anterior and the middle cerebral artery can be insonated.[213,214] Transorbital insonation, however, should never be attempted at transducer output energies above 25 percent of maximum. While the energy levels known to cause tissue injury far exceed those available in clinical instrumentation, minimizing ultrasonic exposure to the eye is prudent.[213,215,216] The temporal window provides access to the anterior, middle, and posterior cerebral arteries, as well as the termination of the internal

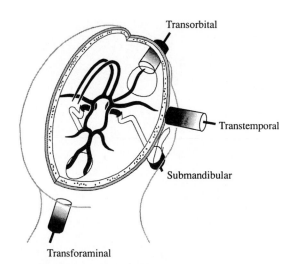

Figure 8-46 Various natural acoustical windows through which ultrasonic beam penetration into the calvarium can occur with minimal beam attenuation. (From Fujioka KA, and Douville CM: Anatomy and freehand examination techniques. In Newell DW, and Aaslid R (eds): *Transcranial Doppler.* Raven, New York, 1992. Reprinted by permission.)

carotid artery (Fig. 8-48).[24] The foramen magnum window allows insonation of the vertebral and basilar arteries (Fig. 8-49).[213,215,217,218]

The transducer or probe is essentially a cylindrical housing with a piezoelectric crystal located at the tip. The plane of the crystal is oriented parallel to the end of the housing, so that when in use the plane of the crystal will be parallel to the surface to which it is applied. A curved plastic acoustic lens focuses the ultrasonic beam to a distance of 40 to 60 mm from the end of the probe. In order to facilitate transmission of the ultrasonic beam, a small amount of transmission gel is used at the interface between transducer and skin surface. A brief oscillating electrical potential is applied across the crystal surfaces, inducing it to vibrate at a frequency and with an amplitude close to the applied voltage (usually 2 MHz). The efficiency of conversion from electrical to mechanical energy is quite high. As much as 90 percent of the energy in the electrical pulse is converted to mechanical energy (crystal oscillation), which in turn generates the ultrasonic burst.[199] The burst is actually a longitudinal ultrasonic wave that is propagated outward along an axis perpendicular to the plane of the crystal. In a longitudinal wave, the particles of the medium are displaced in the direction of the wave travel, with regions of compression preceded and followed by a regions of rarification. The wavelength is defined as the distance between the centers of alternate compression or rarefied regions (Fig. 8-50).

The transducer emits ultrasonic pulses at regular intervals called the *pulse repetition frequency (PRF)*

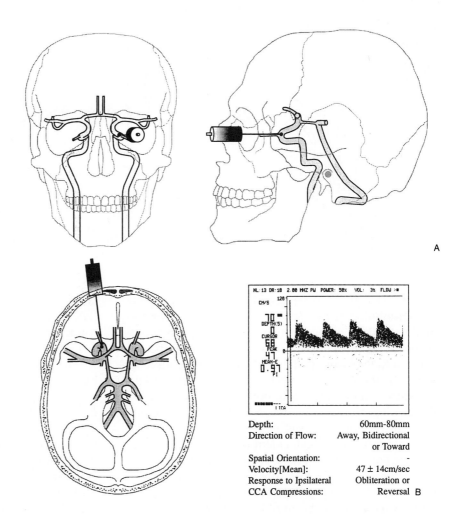

Figure 8-47 Transorbital insonation of the carotid siphon. (*A*) Placement of the transducer. (*B*) Doppler waveforms and vessel identification criteria. Spectrum describes flow velocity in the parasellar portion with blood flow in the direction of the transducer. (From Fujioka KA, and Douville CM: Anatomy and freehand examination techniques. In Newell DW, and Aaslid R (eds): *Transcranial Doppler.* Raven, New York, 1992. Reprinted by permission.)

Depth:	60mm-80mm
Direction of Flow:	Away, Bidirectional
	or Toward
Spatial Orientation:	-
Velocity[Mean]:	47 ± 14cm/sec
Response to Ipsilateral	Obliteration or
CCA Compressions:	Reversal B

(Fig. 8-51). The wave pulse travels through the medium at a velocity *v* for a distance *L*, where a reflecting structure such as a blood cell is encountered. A portion of the pulse wave is reflected back toward the transducer, returning over the distance L. The time needed for the transmission to travel to the reflector and return is therefore $T = 2L/v$. *Range-gating* is the process by which the transducer detection circuitry is activated for a brief period around the time T. Echoes returning from reflectors at different distances will have traveled for different periods, subsequently returning to the transducer during times when the detection circuitry is deactivated. Echoes returning at around time T induce the crystal to vibrate, producing an oscillating electrical voltage equivalent to the frequency of the returning echo. The ability to activate the detection circuitry at a desired time allows information from a specified depth to be returned, as L or the depth of the reflector is vT/2.

Resolution refers to the ability to distinguish between

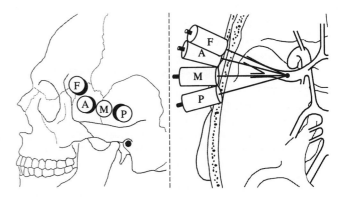

Figure 8-48 The profile in the left panel shows four possible probe locations in the transtemporal window; frontal, anterior, middle, and posterior. The right panel depicts probe angulation relative to the probe location for appropriate insonation of the middle cerebral artery. (From Fujioka KA, and Douville CM: Anatomy and freehand examination techniques. In Newell DW, and Aaslid R (eds): *Transcranial Doppler.* Raven, New York, 1992. Reprinted by permission.)

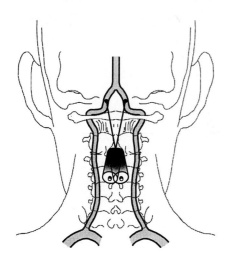

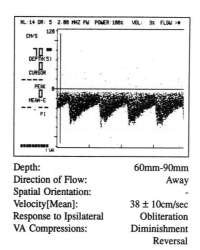

Depth:	60mm-90mm
Direction of Flow:	Away
Spatial Orientation:	-
Velocity[Mean]:	38 ± 10cm/sec
Response to Ipsilateral	Obliteration
VA Compressions:	Diminishment
	Reversal

Figure 8-49 Insonation of the intracranial portions of the vertebral arteries through the transforaminal window is achieved by slight angulation of the transducer from the midline. The Doppler waveform and vessel identification criteria are shown in the panel to the right. Basilar artery insonation is also possible and is accomplished by a direct midline approach. (From Fujioka KA, and Douville CM: Anatomy and freehand examination techniques. In Newell DW, and Aaslid R (eds): *Transcranial Doppler.* Raven, New York, 1992. Reprinted by permission.)

adjacent structures. Transcranial Doppler devices provide resolution at two levels. *Lateral resolution,* or the ability to discriminate between structures within a plane perpendicular to the axis of the ultrasonic beam, is equal to the beam diameter. Reflectors separated by less than the beam diameter will appear as a single structure. The ability to differentiate particles along the axis of the ultrasonic beam is *axial resolution* and depends on the number of cycles in the pulse as well as the frequency of the incident beam.[219]

Since the sample volume is relatively large, between 9 and 12 mm^3, it will encompass the entire cross-section of the vessel segment of interest. The echo's frequency will be the sum of the multitude of Doppler shifts, corresponding not only to the range of blood cell velocities found in the flow lamina of the vessel, but also high-frequency noise and artifact. After filtration to remove the noise and artifact, the echo signal is digi-

tally processed, using a fast Fourier transformation (FFT) algorithm converting the original signal to a distribution of its component frequencies. Digitally, the echo can be represented as a series of discrete points within a temporal domain. The number varies with instrument design and can range from 32 to 8129 points. In general, a 64-point FFT provides better than 2 percent full scale resolution, and allows sufficient accuracy for most Doppler applications. Spectral resolution can be increased by augmenting the number of points representing the returning echo; however, the associated increase in processing time causes the display to lag relative to "real time."[199] Each frequency in the spectrum is assigned a gray-scale intensity or color for display. The frequencies for a sample are displayed vertically on a time scale. Subsequent samples are plotted chronologically, resulting in a frequency profile representative of the blood flow velocity within the

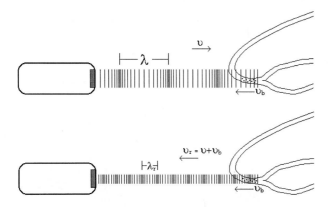

Figure 8-50 The upper panel shows the incident Doppler pulse. λ represents the wavelength, and v the velocity of the incident beam. v_b is the velocity of the blood with the arrows indicating direction. In the lower panel, the reflected ultrasonic beam has a velocity that is the sum of the incident velocity v and the velocity of the blood v_b. The increased velocity of the reflected beam results in a proportional shortening of its wavelength λ_r.

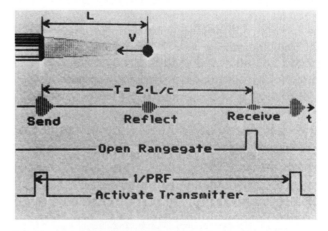

Figure 8-51 Ultrasonic bursts are directed towards a reflector at distance L and velocity v with a predetermined pulse repetition frequency (PFR). The returning echoes are detected at time T which corresponds to the depth setting of the instrument. (From Aaslid.[199] Reprinted by permission.)

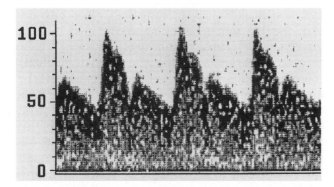

Figure 8-52   A typical middle cerebral artery Doppler spectral display when the sample volume is centered on the straight segment of the vessel. (From Aaslid.[220] Reprinted by permission.)

insonated vessel, assuming the pulse repetition rate is at least twice the cardiac rate (in reality it is substantially greater) (Fig. 8-52).

In precordial Doppler technology, the primary concern is the detection of air bubbles, and the Doppler beam tends to be broad, covering a large portion of the right side of the heart. The beam is also oriented at a large angle relative to the direction of the flow axis. While the rhymic "swishing" of the flowing blood is discernible, it is the sharp "hollow metallic chirp" arising from the distinct acoustic boundary formed by air and blood that is of interest. Neither flow direction nor velocity estimates need to be made. In TCD sonography, both direction and flow velocity are the primary focus. The direction parameter is easily determined, in that reflectors moving away from the transducer produce a Doppler shifted echo with a longer wavelength than the parent beam, while those moving toward the transducer produce an echo with a shorter wavelength. Determining the true velocity, however, requires that the angle Θ between the axis of flow and the axis of the incident ultrasonic beam be known. When both are superimposed, that is, Θ is zero, the apparent velocity will be identical to the true velocity. At angles other than zero, the apparent velocity will be lower and is related to the true velocity by the expression $v_a = |v_t| \times \cos \Theta$. In practice, the flow axis of interest is rarely known. Thus, there is a high probability that the measured velocity is an underestimation of the actual. The error can be minimized if Θ can be kept small (Fig. 8-53). For insonation angles of less than 30° the error in the velocity estimate will be less than 13.5 percent. Further increases in the angle rapidly increases the error, exceeding 50 percent at insonation angles greater than 60°.[220] If the angle is known, this effect can be corrected by the application of the formula[220]:

$$V = \frac{v}{2 \times \cos \Theta} \times \frac{f_{ds}}{f} \qquad (12)$$

In addition to errors that can result from insonation angle deviations, anatomic variations in cerebral vessel location and orientation, temporal window thickness and area, inappropriate sample volume, and improper adjustment of gain and dynamic response can further exacerbate difficulties in interpreting Doppler velocity profiles.

While ultrasound examination has been accepted as essentially harmless at the power densities of commercial TCD instruments, two conditions arise that inevitably present a possibility of injury. Ultrasound-induced cavitation, a nonthermal effect, generates microbubbles in the fluid encompassed by the sample volume. When the cavitation is stable, no clinical risk has been associated with this phenomenon.[219] In transient cavitation, the sudden collapse of the bubbles can cause a shockwave with enough energy to disrupt tissue integrity.[221] In vitro studies have also demonstrated the formation of free radicals, and sonotoxins that can have potentially mutagenic effects on tissue.[222-224] As yet none of these conditions have been identified during in vivo use. Power densities in excess of 3300 W/cm² are believed to be required for cavitation in soft tissue.[211] Commercially available instruments operate at power densities well below 1000 W/cm².

Conversion of some of the ultrasonic energy in the insonation beam to heat is unavoidable. Since attenuation in the bone is greater than in soft tissues, heating in bone can be as much as 50 times greater than in soft

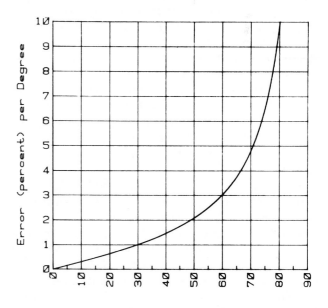

Figure 8-53   The relationship between the angle of insonation and error in velocity measurement. Small angles of insonation produce small errors. Errors, however, increase extremely rapidly at angles in excess of 60 degrees. (From Aaslid.[199] Reprinted by permission.)

tissue. Nonetheless, temperature rises of more than 1°C have not been reported, and are considered inconsequential.[225] With the introduction of high-power Doppler for simultaneous bilateral monitoring, the potential for significant heating of brain tissue in the beam overlap region was recognized. Bench simulations of continuous bilateral insonation at 530 mW/cm² for 8 h showed that the net temperature rise in the fluid of the simulation amounted to 0.75×10^{-2}°C/h in the overlap region. In acute animal studies where insonation was through temporal window craniotomies (the attenuating effect of the bone was eliminated) brain tissue temperature was elevated by no more than 0.4°C after 8 h of continuous insonation at a power density of 530 mW/cm² for each transducer. This study further demonstrated no neurologic or histopathologic sequelae.[226,227]

Adverse effects on the eye as a result of insonation through the transorbital window should always be a concern. Formation of cataracts has been described, but this requires several times more power than available in current diagnostic equipment.[216] Limiting both the power output of the transducer to 10 to 25 percent of maximum and the duration of insonation can significantly reduce the risk of injury.[213,215,216]

Wave form analysis resulting from a single cardiac cycle has evolved as a common clinical and scientific tool for evaluating intracranial hemodynamics. Indices of pulsatility have grown in popularity in part from their insensitivity to the angle of insonation, thus relying on relative changes in the wave form as opposed to absolute values. The most commonly used indices are the *Pulsatility Index* ($PI = (v_s - v_d)/v_m$), *Index of Resistance* ($IR = (v_s - v_d)/v_s$, and *AB Ratio* ($AB = v_s/v_d$); where v_s is the systolic velocity, v_d is the diastolic velocity, and the v_m is the mean velocity.[228-230] Other approaches, in particular fast Fourier transformation analysis of the velocity wave form, produce a component distribution of sine or cosine waves which can then be correlated to physiologic conditions or responses.

Since the introduction of these indices a significant body of information has been developed correlating each index to various cerebrohemodynamic parameters, including cerebral blood flow (CBF), intracranial pressure (ICP), cerebrovascular resistance (CVR), and cerebral compliance (C_c).[230-246] Additionally, the effects of pharmacologic agents, ventilation, and surgical manipulations on PI have been studied.[240,241,247-258] While the focus of this work has been the correlative nature between basal cerebral vessel indices and cerebrovascular hemodynamics, little attention has been given to the systemic hemodynamic influences on indices of pulsatility as well as the indirect effects by those factors which affect systemic function. A variety of systemic factors such as Pa_{O_2}, Pa_{CO_2}, heart rate, blood pressure, and vascular compliance all appear to affect these ratios.[242-249,255,259,260] Thus, the absolute value of an index may not always reliably characterize the intracranial conditions unless information about the systemic hemodynamic profile is available.[244,246-258,260,261] In order to develop a better appreciation for the indices of pulsatility, it may perhaps be useful to examine these indices from a more theoretical perspective. These are mathematical expressions, but interesting physiologic implications can come to light upon inspection of the expressions as the variables approach the limits of their ranges. Additionally, reassessment of the indices in terms of system hemodynamic parameters may provide useful insight into those factors that have an influence on their values.

The Pulsatility Index as defined by Gosling is:

$$PI = \frac{V_{sys} - V_{dia}}{V_{mean}} \quad (13)$$

where V_{sys}, V_{dia}, and V_{mean} are systolic, end-diastolic, and mean blood flow velocities. If the V_{mean} term in the denominator is redefined using the classic hemodynamic approximation[262]:

$$mean = \frac{1}{3}(systolic - diastolic) + diastolic \quad (14)$$

then the PI expression becomes:

$$PI = \frac{V_{sys} - V_{dia}}{\frac{1}{3}(V_{sys} - V_{dia}) + V_{dia}} \quad (15)$$

As the blood flow velocity pulse amplitude becomes smaller, that is, $V_{sys} - V_{dia}$ approaches zero, the value of the PI expression also approaches zero, consistent with the idea of increasing compliance.

If increases in intracranial compliance are attributed to decreases in the volume of the extravascular compartment, the accompanying reduction in transmural pressure on the cerebral vascular walls reduces the rigidity of the conduit, permitting expansion into the newly available space during systole. The resulting increase in cross-sectional area during systole would result in a reduction in blood flow velocity pulse amplitude ($V_{sys} - V_{dia}$). When the $V_{sys} - V_{dia} = 0$, then $PI = 0$, suggesting cessation of pulsatility as a result of either infinite compliance or termination of cardiac function. On the other hand, as the blood flow velocity pulse amplitude increases, as might be expected with decreasing intracranial compliance, intuitively PI would be expected to increase proportionately. However, as the $V_{sys} - V_{dia}$ term continues to increase, the

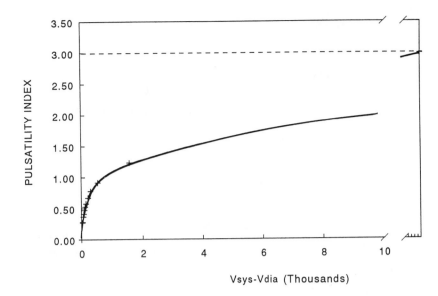

Figure 8-54 As the systolic-diastolic velocity difference increases, the pulsatility index tends, asymptotically, toward a value of 3. The *PI* function is not linear but rater exponential in nature.

V_{dia} term in the denominator becomes increasingly smaller with respect to $V_{sys} - V_{dia}$ and eventually becomes insignificant. At this point, the ratio $(V_{sys} - V_{dia}):[(V_{sys} - V_{dia}) + V_{dia}]$ in the *PI* expression approaches 1; thus, *PI* must asymptotically approach 1 over 1/3, or 3. What this means is that *PI* is not linearly related to compliance. Uniform increases in pulse velocity differences result in a progressively smaller affect on the *PI* (Fig. 8-54). It seems then if *PI* is to be a useful index of any condition such as CO_2 reactivity, ICP, CVR, CBF, or C_c, then the boundaries at which *PI* becomes an unreliable representation must be established. Figure 8-55 represents the results of varying intracranial compliance on pulsatility index in a computer simulation of an intracranial system based on the pressure, volume relationships as derived by Marmarou and coworkers.[264] The simulation also includes mathematical expressions relating patient age and vascular elasticity, which were delineated by the work of Hallock and associates.[263] Simulations were run for both young (29 to 31 years) and old (71 to 78 years) patients for comparison. While this simulation may not define the curves location in the graphical quadrant precisely relative to clinical reality, it is, however, sufficient to point out that, under similar physiologic conditions, PI may vary substantially as a function of vascular elasticity. It needs to be remembered, that PI not only reflects changes in intracranial compartment volumes and pressures, but is significantly influenced by systemic dynamics. Measures such as CO_2 relativity, ICP, and CBF are themselves highly influenced by systemic dynamics as well as reflecting the intracranial compliance conditions. Similar arguments can be made for the other pulsatility indices that rely only on the systolic and diastolic velocity measures within the cerebral vessels. Other factors which influ-

ence the value of these ratios should also be considered when interpreting the indices of pulsatility relative to cerebrohemodynamic events.

It is clear that blood flow in cerebral vessels—hence, blood flow velocity—is a function of the ability of the heart to generate an output. The proportion of the cardiac output that reaches the cerebral circulation is also significantly influenced by the systemic compliance and cerebrovascular and systemic vascular resistances. These measures are themselves subject to influence by pharmacologic agents, respiratory state, and metabolic considerations. Correlation of cerebrodynamics with what is essentially an arbitrary ratio runs the risk of generating relationships without the benefit of a theoretical basis, and may have no meaning outside the specific conditions that existed during the reported observations.

Shortly after its introduction, the innate ability of transcranial Doppler to detect emboli, particularly gaseous microbubbles, was recognized. As in precordial Doppler, the large difference in acoustic impedance between blood and microbubbles in the cerebral vessels results in an interface that is highly reflective to ultrasound and can be used as the basis for embolus detection paradigms. Neuropsychologic and neurologic sequelae following cardiopulmonary bypass have been the subject of recent clinical interest. Post-coronary bypass cognitive and neurologic deficits have been related to several intraoperative conditions, among which are age, duration of bypass, and inadequate cerebral perfusion.[265–275] Advances in Doppler sonography have enabled clinical studies to monitor not only intracerebral hemodynamics during coronary bypass, but also to generate evidence that implicates embolic phenomena in the development of postoperative neuropsychologic deficits.[204,276–280,281,282] Much of the

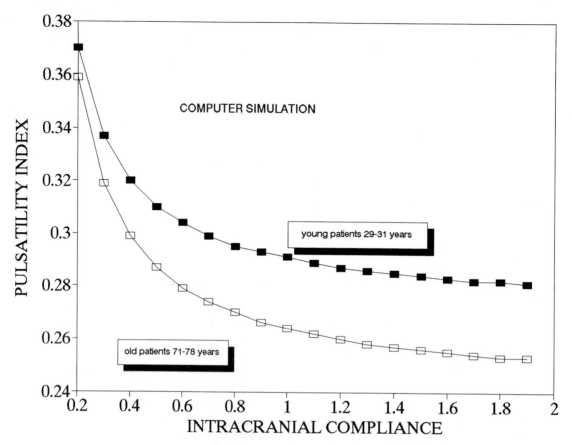

Figure 8-55 A computer simulation of the effect of intracranial compliance on pulsatility index in young and old patients. The simulation is based on intracranial pressure-volume relationships derived by Marmarou et al.[264] and includes mathematical expressions relating vascular elasticity and age.[263]

work correlating embolic incidents and psychological deficits relates patient neuropsychologic status to total number of emboli detected in the MCA without consideration for type and volume. Discrimination between gaseous and particulate emboli, however, has been less concrete. Albin and coworkers reported successful discrimination between gaseous and particulate emboli in a primate animal model based on peak Doppler shifts and maximal amplitude of the reflected signal. Qualitative differences in the geometric shape and gray scale intensity (signal amplitude) in the video image of the Doppler shift were identified. Distinct qualitative differences in the audio output that resulted from gaseous and particulate emboli were also described.[205] Spencer and associates, on the other hand, concluded that the TCD spectrograms recorded during their study did not exhibit sufficient differences between air bubbles and formed-element emboli to warrant a claim of embolic differentiation.[204] More recently, Russell and coworkers and Markus and Brown demonstrated a limited ability to differentiate between the various types of emboli based on the intensity of the reflected

signal. They were also able to quantify embolic volumes based on amplitude and signal duration measures.[206,207] Unfortunately, the particulate types they studied all gave similar signal amplitude and duration profiles such that mixtures of the embolic types could not be resolved.

Using the criterion described by Albin and coworkers for detection and identification of air emboli, Mitzel and associates reported that alterations in the six-week postoperative neuropsychologic status of CABG patients could not be statistically correlated to incidences of air embolism.[283] This may, in part, be due to a threshold relationship between these two measures, in that the brain may be able to tolerate small amounts of air, declining in function only after the entrainment of a threshold volume.[284] Thus, an estimation of embolic volume may be more useful than incidence data in developing a cause and effect relationship between neuropsychologic deficits and cerebral air embolism.

Based on the hypotheses that: (1) the distinctive audible qualities that are heard when gaseous emboli pass through insonated cerebral vessels can be used to identify air emboli; and (2) that the total power of those frequencies is proportional to the volume of the microbubbles, Bunegin and coworkers examined the characteristics of the TCD audio output during air embolic episodes and demonstrated an analytic approach that could permit the isolation and volume estimation of embolic air.

The extremely high ultrasonic reflectivity of gaseous microbubbles renders detection of gaseous emboli within the cerebral circulation using pulsed TCD a relatively simple process. Hills and Grulke demonstrated that single bubbles as small as 0.03 μl could be detected with Doppler ultrasound; they also described the effect of bubble velocity on the detection limit.[286] In an in vitro model, Sellman and coworkers described the detection of microbubbles on the order of 0.5 nl.[287] The smallest microbubble (0.5 μl) detected by Albin and coworkers produced a very high amplitude spike, having a peak Doppler shift of at least 3000 Hz, while particulates (latex microspheres) produced spikes of significantly smaller amplitude, having Doppler shifts that did not exceed 2400 Hz (Fig. 8-56).[205]

FFT analysis of the TCD audio segments obtained from the in vivo primate model indicated that the principal frequencies that appeared consistently in the spectrum when air emboli were present in the MCA are between 250 and 500 Hz (Fig. 8-57). These findings were somewhat surprising in that the identifying Doppler shifts for air were expected to be in excess of 2500 Hz. While these frequencies were present and measurable, the amplitude of the lower harmonics (250 to 500 Hz) were several orders of magnitude greater and more consistent than the parent frequencies.

The quantitation of microbubble volumes, however, is somewhat more complex than simple detection, and requires that the gaseous microemboli pass through the insonated portion of the cerebral vessel one time without entrapment in turbulent flow patterns or vortices. Otherwise, the resultant Doppler signal will arise from more than a single interaction with the same microbubble, producing an overestimation of the volume measurement. Flow through the MCA is laminar (Reynolds number less than 100) for all but the most extraordinary conditions. The microemboli are also small enough to offer little resistance, and thus are swept through the MCA at velocities comparable to that of the blood.

The first hypothesis imposes the constraint that the Doppler beam reflected from gaseous microemboli contains frequencies that can be used to unambiguously identify air emboli. The dominant frequencies specific to artifact generated by sensor movement and electrocautery appear to be lower and their power attenuated by an order of magnitude over the frequencies associated with gaseous microbubbles (Fig. 8-57).

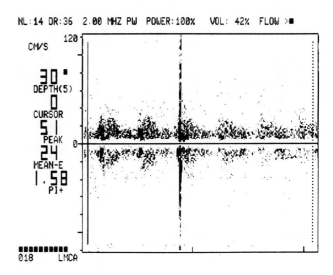

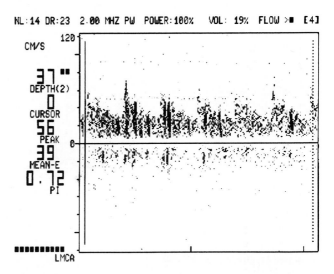

Figure 8-56 Doppler spectral display of 0.5 μl of air in the middle cerebral artery of a rhesus monkey. Doppler spectral display of 50 μm diameter latex microspheres used to simulate solid particulate emboli. The acoustical impedance is close to that of solid particulate.

While Albin and coworkers[205] were able to recognize qualitative differences in both the video and audio Doppler signals between gaseous and particulate emboli in an in vivo primate model, Spencer and associates[204] were unable to distinguish between the two in the clinical setting. This confusion is not surprising in that the resolution of the various commercially available TCD monitors may vary substantially and may not be any greater than that needed to provide a visual description of the blood flow velocity envelope in as close to real time as possible. To achieve this, data acquisition, frequency analysis, assignment of gray scale intensities to the frequencies, and finally modulation to video output signals must all occur in an extremely short time in order to achieve "real time" dis-

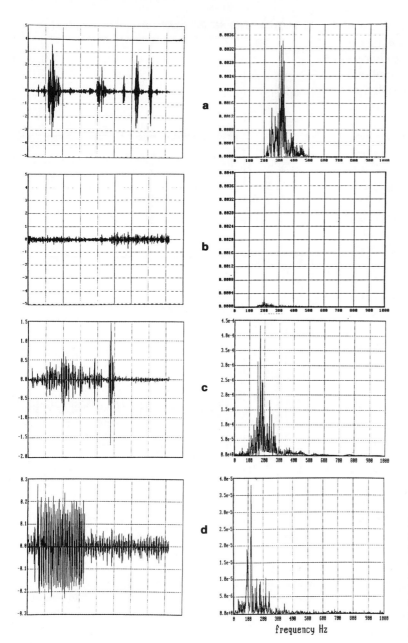

Figure 8-57 Transcranial Doppler audio signals and respective frequency domain spectra obtained from the middle cerebral artery of a primate during; (*a*) air embolism, (*b*) background, (*c*) transducer movement (artifact), and (*d*) electrocautery (artifact). The Doppler shifts in the left panels represent a 4-s observation window. The ordinates of all graphs represent volts. (From Bunegin et al.[203] Reprinted by permission.)

play. Rates and duration of data acquisition must therefore be kept to a minimum, followed by an FFT spectral analysis using as few points as necessary for blood flow velocity envelope resolution (typically 32 to 64 point FFT).[199] Sampling windows of 10 ms are typical in pulsed Doppler equipment and can only provide a maximal resolution of 100 Hz, which may not be sufficient resolution for discrimination between air and particulates.[288] Additionally, Spencer and associates' observations were made in a clinical setting where absolute conformation of the nature of the detected emboli was not possible. The identification of those TCD images could, at best, be educated estimates. Since the audio signal represents the raw Doppler shift, it may contain the information necessary for discrimination between air and particulate emboli. Extracting that information, however, appears to require more robust signal analysis than can be managed on line by currently used TCD equipment.

The characteristic "hollow metallic auditory chirp" that has become accepted by many TCD users as the definitive signature of air emboli appears to be the product of component frequencies that lie between 250 and 500 Hz. Latex microspheres between 1 and 25 μm in diameter produced a sound similar to a "crackle" during experiments in a primate model.[205] Since the acoustic impedance and density of latex is similar to formed elements of blood components, it is likely that

Doppler signals both in terms of frequency shift and amplitude will be comparable to those of particulate emboli.[288] Both background and artifact also produce dominant harmonics (125 and 300 Hz, respectively) that appear only minimally to overlap those of gaseous microbubbles and that are substantially lower in amplitude.

The second hypothesis that the intensity or amplitude of the Doppler signal reflecting from gaseous microbubbles is proportional to the microbubble size also appears to be confirmed. Several studies have described the relationship between reflected ultrasonic energy and bubble size.[289-292] Sellman and coworkers demonstrated a positive exponential association between bubble diameter and Doppler amplitude between 10 and 160 μm.[287] Two recently published reports confirm a similar correlation for thrombus, platelet, atheroma, and fat emboli.[206,207] J. R. Klepper and M. A. Moehring point out, however, that the ultrasonic beam returning from the highly reflective air blood interface can quickly saturate the video amplifiers of the TCD monitor, resulting in a maximum intensity rail-to-rail spike for all but the smallest gas bubbles.[293] The audio amplifiers in the TCD equipment used in this study do not appear to be limited to the same extent as the video amplifier circuits. While the video image of a 0.75 μl bubble produces a full scale deflection of high intensity, the total power for audio frequencies between 307 and 450 Hz appears to increase linearly up to approximately 40 μl bubble volumes in in vivo experiments and 20 to 40 μl in the bench experiments. Bubble volumes greater than 50 μl could not be differentiated based on the total power of the signature frequencies between 307 and 450 Hz. This suggests that the audio amplifiers are being saturated by the signal arising from the larger bubbles (Fig. 8-58).

Doppler velocity envelopes observed in the in vitro and in vivo experiments were similar in shape and frequency composition. The thin-walled silicone for MCA simulation combined with a flow capacitor provided the facility for fine-tuning the flow patterns in the in vitro model. Additionally, the simulated blood solution used in the bench evaluation appeared to reflect incident ultrasonic frequencies similarly to blood. In a previous study, Spencer and coworkers demonstrated that there were no differences between a suspension of Sephadex microspheres and sheep's blood when evaluating Doppler waveforms in vitro.[285] Miles and associates and Spencer and coworkers also showed that flow and Doppler measures of pulsatility index and resistance index in their in vitro models correlated well with in vivo measurements.[285,294]

Even though these results appear encouraging, it should be remembered that they were obtained under

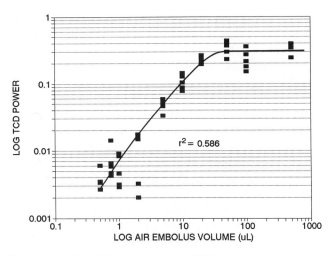

Figure 8-58 Graph shows an exponential least-squares regression analysis correlating spectral power in the 307 to 450 frequency band and gaseous microbubble volume in an in-vitro middle cerebral artery model. (From Bunegin et al.[203] Reprinted by permission.)

highly controlled conditions. Great care was taken to ensure that all aspects of the audio signal manipulation, that is, volume settings on the TCD, record and playback amplification, and acquisition parameters were consistent throughout the volume range studied. However, the effects of small changes in sensor position relative to the insonated vessel that could occur during the course of monitoring on the linearity and slope of the correlation have not been evaluated. Other potential sources of error have been identified by Butler.[295] Detection errors from encapsulated or coalesced bubbles would tend to reduce the reflected signal. An encapsulating layer around the air bubble would absorb a portion of the signal energy, resulting in underestimation.[295] Coalesced bubbles, accumulating as foam, will present a non-uniform surface scattering the incident sound energy and possibly reflecting signals containing complex waveforms that could be difficult to interpret.[295] It is certainly possible that some combination of these factors may have played a role in the tenfold difference in slope between the in vivo and in vitro calibration curves. Additionally, accurate focusing of the Doppler beam may have been hampered by the small dimension of the primate cranium. If the MCA was in reality closer to the probe than the minimum possible beam focal length (2.5 cm), less energy would be reflected, resulting in lower total power values for the emboli. Other detection difficulties that Butler identified as significant using continuous wave insonation could possibly be avoided with pulsed wave equipment. The ability to set the focal depth permits adjustment for optimal response. Insonation at an angle of 0 to 20° from the vessel axis usually will result in the Doppler field encompassing the entire vessel cross-section, allowing detection of larger more buoyant bubbles. Axial insonation with pulsed wave equipment may also minimize the effect of overlying bubbles.

A significant amount of work is still needed to further delineate this approach. Important evaluations include: the effect of bubble velocity, in terms of their location in the cardiac cycle, on the accuracy of the volume estimate; recalibration using calibrated microbubbles such as those described by Hills and Butler[296]; and evaluating the various detection errors described by Butler on the calibration accuracy. While still in the preliminary stages of development, this technique may provide a promising starting point for development of algorithms that would be suitable for automated embolic air detection and volume estimation.

References

1. Siegrist HE: Surgery before anesthesia. *Bull School Med U Maryland* 1944; 31:116.
2. Plomley F: Operations upon the eye. *Lancet* 1847; 1:134.
3. Snow J: *On the Inhalation of the Vapor of Ether*. London, John Churchill, 1847.
4. Simpson WG (ed): *Works of Sir JY Simpson*. New York, Appleton, 1872.
5. Sykes WS: *Essays on the First Hundred Years of Anesthesia: The Scottish Chloroform Legend—Syme and Simpson as Practical Anaesthetist*. Huntington, NY Robert Krieger, 1972.
6. Snow J: *On Chloroform and Other Anaesthetic: Their Action and Administration*. London, John Churchill, 1858.
7. Macewan W: Intracranial lesions—illustrating some points in connexion with the localization of cerebral affections and the advantages of aseptic trephining. *Lancet* 1881; 2:541.
8. Durante F: A contribution to endocranial surgery. *Lancet* 1884; 2:654.
9. Bennett AH, Godlee RJ: A case of cerebral tumor. *Med Chir Trans* 1885; 68:243.
10. Horsley V: On the technique of operations on the central nervous system. *BMJ* 1906; 2:411.
11. Guedel AE: Third stage of anesthesia: A subclassification regarding the significance of the position and movement of the eyeball. *Am J Q Suppl Anesth Analg* 1920; 34:53.
12. Beecher HK: The first anesthesia records (Codman, Cushing). *Surg Gynecol Obstet* 1940; 71:689.
13. Hamburger WW: Development of knowledge concerning the measure and rhythm of the pulse. *J Mt Sinai Hosp* 1941; 8:585.
14. Hales S: *Statistical essays: Containing haemastaticks, 1733*. Republished, vol 22, New York Academy of Medicine. New York, Hafner Publishing, 1964.
15. White PD: The evolution of our knowledge about the heart and its diseases since 1628. *Circulation* 1957; 15:915.
16. Klopp EH: Poiseuille's contributions to medical science. *Surg Gynecol Obstet* 1974; 139:95.
17. Doppler C: Uber das farbige Licht der Dopplesterne und einiger anderer Gistirne des Himmels 1843; *Abhandl Konigl Bohm Ges*, 2:465.
18. Marey EJ: *Physiologie Médicale de la Circulation du Sang. Basée sur l'Étude graphique des Mouvements du Coeur et du Pouls Arteriel avec Application aux maladies de l'Appareil Circulatorie*. Paris, Adrien Delahaye, 1863.
19. Agnew DH: *Principles and Practice of Surgery*. Philadelphia, Lippincott, 1881.
20. McGrew RE: *Encyclopedia of Medical History*. New York, McGraw-Hill, 1985.
21. Fick A: Uber den Messung de blut quantum inden Herzentrikeln. *Arch Med Gez Wurzburg* 1870; 16:1872.
22. von Basch S: Ein Verbesserter Sphygmo-und Cardiograph. *Z Kn Med* 1881; 2:654.
23. Riva-Rocci S: Un novo sfigmomanometro. *Gazz Med Torino* 1896; 47:981.
24. Cushing H: On routine determinations of arterial tension in operating room and clinic. *Boston Med Surg J* 1903; 148:250.
25. Crile GW: Blood pressure. In *Surgery, an Experimental and Clinical Approach*. Philadelphia, Lippincott, 1903.
26. Cushing H: Concerning a definite regulatory mechanism of the vaso-motor center which controls blood pressure during cerebral compression. *Johns Hopkins Hosp Bull* 1901; 12:290.
27. Einthoven W: Die galvanometrische Registrirung des menschlichen Capillarelektrometers in der Physiologie. *Arch Ges Physiol* 1903; 99:472.
28. Martins JT, et al: Electroencephalography in anesthesiology. *Anesthesiology* 1959; 20:359.
29. Gibbs FA, et al: Effect on electro-encephalogram of certain drugs which influence nervous activity. *Arch Int Med* 1937; 60:154.
30. Sveringhaus JW, et al: Correction factors for infrared carbon dioxide pressure broadening by nitrogen, nitrous oxide, and cyclopropane. *Anesthesiology* 1961; 22:429.
31. Ammann ECB, Galvin RD: Problems associated with the determination of carbon dioxide by infrared absorption. *J Appl Physiol* 1968; 25:333.
32. Cormack RS, Powell JN: Improving the performance of infrared carbon dioxide meter. *Br J Anaesth* 1972; 44:131.
33. Kennell EM, et al: Correction factors for nitrous oxide in the infrared analysis of carbon dioxide. *Anesthesiology* 1973; 39:441.
34. Schena J, et al: Mechanical influences on the capnogram. *Crit Care Med* 1984; 12:672.
35. Gravenstein N, et al: Factors influencing capnography in the Bain circuit. *J Clin Monit* 1985; 1:6.
36. Epstein RA, et al: Determinants of distortion in CO_2 catheter sampling systems: A mathematical model. *Resp Physiol* 1980; 41:127.
37. From RP, Scamman FL: Ventilatory frequency influences accuracy of end-tidal CO_2 measurements. Analysis of seven capnometers. *Anesth Analg* 1988; 67:884.
38. van Genderingen HR, Gravenstein N: Capnogram artifact during high airway pressures caused by a water trap. *Anesth Analg* 1987; 66:185.
39. Lerou JGC, et al: The influence of tube geometry on performance of long sampling tubes in respiratory mass spectrometry. *Clin Phys Physiol Meas* 1986; 7:125.
40. Lawson D, Jelenich S: Capnographs: A new operating room pollution hazard. *Anesth Analg* 1985; 64:377.
41. Cozanitis DA, Paloheimo MPJ: Operating room pollution from capnographs. *Anesth Analg* 1986; 65:990.
42. Carver CD: A special collection of infrared spectra from the Coblentz Society Inc, Kirkwood, MO, 1980.
43. Bauman RP: *Absorption Spectroscopy*. New York, Wiley, 1962.
44. VanWagenen RA, et al: Dedicated monitoring of anesthetic and respiratory gases by Raman scattering. *J Clin Monit* 1986; 2:215.
45. Fowler KT, Hugh-Jones P: Mass spectrometry applied to clinical practice and research. *BMJ* 1957; 1:205.

46. McAslan TC: Automated respiratory gas monitoring of critically injured patients. *Crit Care Med* 1976; 4:255.

47. Ayres SM: Use of mass spectrometry for evaluation of respiratory function in the critically ill patient. *Crit Care Med* 1976; 4:219.

48. Riker JB, Haberman B: Expired gas monitoring by mass spectrometry in a respiratory intensive care unit. *Crit Care Med* 1976; 4:223.

49. Yakulis R, et al: Mass spectrometry monitoring of respiratory variables in an intensive care unit. *Resp Care* 1978; 23:671.

50. Ozanne GM et al: Multipatient anesthetic mass spectrometry: Rapid analysis of data stored in long catheters. *Anesthesiology* 1981; 55:62.

51. Grevisse P, et al: Turning the mass spectrometer into an easy to handle clinical instrument for routine multipatient surveillance of respiratory and anesthetic gases during anesthesia. *Acta Anaesthesiol Belg* 1987; 38:37.

52. Banks ST, et al: Anesthesia gas monitoring: Central system or stand-alone? *Med Instrum* 1988; 22:160.

53. Goldberg JS, et al: Colorimetric end-tidal carbon dioxide monitoring for tracheal intubation. *Anesth Analg* 1990; 70:191.

54. Kuhl DE, et al: Local cerebral blood volume determined by three-dimensional reconstruction of radionuclide scan data. *Circ Res* 1975; 36:610.

55. Pollock LJ, Boshes B: Cerebrospinal fluid pressure. *Arch Neurol Psychiatry* 1936; 36:931.

56. Schmitt FO, et al: Brain cell microenvironment. *Neurosci Res Prog Bull* 1969; 7(4):277.

57. Jefferson G: The tentorial pressure cone. *Arch Neurol Psychiatry* 1938; 40:857.

58. Jennett WB, Stern WE: Tentorial herniation, the midbrain and pupil. Experimental studies in brain compression. *J Neurosurg* 1960; 17:598.

59. Southerland S: The tentorial notch and complications produced by herniations of the brain through the aperture. *Br J Surg* 1958; 17:422.

60. Bruce DA, et al: Regional cerebral blood flow, intracranial pressure and brain metabolism in comatose patients. *J Neurosurg* 1973; 38:131.

61. Bruce DA: *The Pathophysiology of Increased Intracranial Pressure.* Kalamazoo MI, The Upjohn Company, 1978.

62. Overgaard J, Tweed WA: Cerebral circulation after head injury. Part 1: Cerebral blood flow and its regulation after closed head injury, with emphasis on clinical correlations. *J Neurosurg* 1976; 41:531.

63. Cushing H: Some experimental and clinical observations concerning states of increased intracranial tension. *Am J Med Sci* 1902; 124:375.

64. Cushing H: The blood pressure reaction of acute cerebral compression, illustrated by cases of intracranial hemorrhage. *Am J Med Sci* 1903; 125:1017.

65. Browder J, Meyers R: Observation on the behavior of the systemic blood pressure following craniocerebral injury. *Am J Surg* 1936; 31:402.

66. Marshall LF, Bowers SA: Medical management of head injury. *Clin Neurosurg* 1982; 29:312.

67. Marshall LF, et al: Outcome with aggressive treatment in head injuries. Part I: The significance of intracranial pressure monitoring. *J Neurosurg* 1979; 50:20.

68. Ropper AH, et al: Head position, intracranial pressure and compliance. *Neurology* 1981; 13:184.

69. Wilkinson HA: Intracranial pressure monitoring: Techniques and pitfalls. In: Copper PR (ed): *Head Injury.* Baltimore, Williams & Wilkins, 1982.

70. Todd MM: Monitoring in Neuroanesthesia. In: Saidman LJ,

Smith NT (eds): *Monitoring in Anesthesia.* London, Butterworth-Heinemann, 1993.

71. Marshall LF, et al: The National Coma Data Bank. Part 2: Patients who talk and deteriorate. *J Neurosurg* 1983; 59:285.

72. Hassler O: Arterial pattern of human brainstem. Normal appearance and deformation in expanding supratentorial conditions. *Neurology* 1967; 17:368.

73. Hayashi M, et al: Ventricular size and isotope cisternography in patients with acute transient rises of intracranial pressure (plateau waves). *J Neurosurg* 1982; 57:797.

74. Bruce DA, et al: Cerebrospinal fluid pressure monitoring in children: Physiology, pathology, and clinical usefulness. *Adv Pediatr* 1977; 24:233.

75. James HE, et al: Methodology for intraventricular and subarachnoid continuous recording of intracranial pressure in clinical practice. *Acta Neurochir(Wien)* 1976; 33:45.

76. Marshall LF, et al: Mannitol dose requirements in brain-injured patients. *J Neurosurg* 1978; 48:169.

77. Smyth GE, Henderson WR: Observations of the cerebrospinal fluid pressure on simultaneous ventricular and lumbar punctures. *J Neurol Physiol* 1938; 1:226.

78. Finney LA, Walker AE: *Transtentorial Herniation.* Springfield, IL, Charles C Thomas, 1962.

79. Kaumann GE, Clark WK: Transmission of increased intracranial pressure across the tentorium in man. *Surg Forum* 1969; 20:437.

80. Wilkinson HA: Intracranial pressure. In: Youmans JR (ed): *Neurological Surgery.* Philadelphia, WB Saunders, 1990.

81. Tomlinson H: On the increase in resistance to the passage of electric current produced on stretching. *Proc R Soc* (Lond) 1876; 25:451.

82. Simmonds EE: U.S. Patent 2,292,549, 1942.

83. Quincke H: Uber Meningitisserosa und Verwandte Zustande. *Dtsch Z Nervenheilk* 1897; 9:149.

84. Ayer JB: Analysis of lumbar cerebrospinal fluid in sixty-seven cases of tumors and cysts of the brain. *Res Publ Ass Nerv Ment Dis* 1927; 8:189.

85. Jackson JH: The management of acute cranial injuries by the early exact determination of intracranial pressure, and its relief by lumbar drainage. *Surg Gynecol Obstet* 1992; 34:494.

86. Hirschberg R: Traitment de la meningite tuberculeuse. *Bull Gen Therap Med Chir Obstet Pharmaceut,* Paris, 1984.

87. Duffy GP: Lumbar puncture in the presence of intracranial pressure. *BMJ* 1969; 1:407.

88. Hollis PH, et al: Neurological deterioration after lumbar puncture below complete spinal subarachnoid block. *J Neurosurg* 1986; 64:253.

89. Ingvar S: On the danger of leakage of the cerebrospinal fluid after lumbar puncture. *Acta Med Scand* 1923; 58:67.

90. Hodgson JS: The relation between increased intracranial pressure and intraspinal pressure. Changes in the cerebrospinal fluid in increased intracranial pressure. *Res Publ Assoc Res Nerv Ment Dis* 1927; 8:182.

91. Kahn AJ: Effects of variation in intracranial pressure. *Arch Neurol Psychiatr* 1944; 51:508.

92. Langfitt TW et al: Transmission of increased intracranial pressure I. Within the craniospinal axis. *J Neurosurg* 1964; 21:989.

93. Papo I, et al: Traumatic cerebral mass lesions: Correlations between clinical, intracranial pressure and computed tomographic data. *Neurosurgery* 1980; 7:337.

94. Lundberg N: Continuous recording and control of ventricular fluid pressure in neurosurgical practice. *Acta Psychiatr Neurol Scand* 1960; 149(Suppl):1.

95. North B, Reilly P: Comparison among three methods of intracranial pressure recording. *Neurosurgery* 1986; 18:730.

96. Aucoin PJ, et al: Intracranial pressure monitors. Epidemiologic study of risk factors and infections. *Am J Med* 1986; 80:369.

97. Weaver DD, et al: Differential intracranial pressure in patients with unilateral mass lesions. *J Neurosurg* 1982; 56:660.

98. Mendelow AD, et al: A clinical comparison of subdural screw pressure measurements with ventricular pressure. *J Neurosurg* 1983; 58:45.

99. Yano M, et al: Intracranial pressure in head injured patients with various intracranial lesions is identical throughout the supratentorial intracranial compartment. *Neurosurgery* 1987; 21:688.

100. Sugiura K, et al: Intracranial pressure monitoring by subdurally placed silicone catheter: Technical note. *Neurosurgery* 1985; 16:241.

101. Barlow P, et al: Clinical evaluation of two methods of subdural pressure monitoring. *J Neurosurg* 1985; 63:578.

102. Constantini S, et al: Intracranial pressure monitoring after elective intracranial surgery. A retrospective study of 514 consecutive patients. *J Neurosurg* 1988; 69:540.

103. Rossenwasser RH, et al: Intracranial pressure monitoring in the posterior fossa: A preliminary report. *J Neurosurg* 1989; 71:503.

104. Coronoeos NJ, et al: Measurement of extradural pressure and its relationship to other intracranial pressures. *J Neurol Neurosurg Psychiatry* 1973; 36:514.

105. Coronoeos NJ, et al: Comparison of extradural with intraventricular pressure in patients after head injury. In: Brock M, Dietz H (eds): *Intracranial Pressure.* Berlin, Springer-Verlag, 1972.

106. Fasol P, et al: Intracranial pressure monitoring by fiberoptic technique. In: Ishii S et al (eds): *Intracranial Pressure V.* Berlin, Springer-Verlag, 1983.

107. Gobit W, et al: Experience with an intracranial pressure transducer readjustable in vivo. Technical note. *J Neurosurg* 1974; 39:272.

108. Gosch HH, Kindt GW: Subdural monitoring of acute increased intracranial pressure. *Surg Forum* 1972; 23:405.

109. Nornes H, Serck-Hanssen F: Miniature transducer for intracranial pressure monitoring in man. *Acta Neurol Scand* 1970; 46:203.

110. Ream AK, et al: Epidural measurement of intracranial pressure. *Neurosurgery* 1979; 5:36.

111. Ivan LP, et al: Intracranial monitoring with the fiberoptic transducer in children. *Childs Brain* 1980; 7:303.

112. Ivan LP, Choo SH: A comparative study of epidural and cisternal pressure in dogs. *J Neurosurg* 1982; 57(4):511.

113. Shellok FG: A fiberoptic transducer-tipped pressure catheter. *Med Elec* 1985; 16:103.

114. Roberts PA, et al: Experimental and clinical experience with a new solid state intracranial pressure monitor with in vivo zero capability. In: Nagai IH, Brock M (eds): *Intracranial Pressure V.* Berlin, Springer-Verlag, 1983:104.

115. Cheek WR, et al: Device for extradural monitoring of intracranial pressure: Technical note. *Neurosurgery* 1979; 5:692.

116. Gobeit W: The influences of dexamethasone on intracranial pressure in patients with severe head injury. In: Pappius HM, Feindel W (eds): *Dynamics of Brain Edema.* New York, Springer-Verlag, 1976.

117. Rylander HE, III, et al: Chronic measurement of epidural pressure with an induction-powered oscillator transducer. *J Neurosurg* 1976; 44:465.

118. Schettini A, et al: Experimental approach for monitoring surface brain pressure. *J Neurosurg* 1971; 34:38.

119. Turner JM, et al: Further experience with extradural pressure monitoring. In: Lunberg N, et al (eds): *Intracranial Pressure II.* Berlin, Springer-Verlag, 1974.

120. Ostrup RC, et al: Continuous monitoring of intracranial pressure with a miniaturized fiberoptic device. *J Neurosurg* 1987; 67:206.

121. Chambers IR, et al: A clinical evaluation of the Camino subdural screw and ventricular monitoring kits. *Neurosurgery* 1990; 26:421.

122. Crutchfield JS, et al: Evaluation of a fiberoptic intracranial pressure monitor. *J Neurosurg* 1990; 72:482.

123. Schicner DJ, Young RF: Intracranial pressure monitoring: Fiberoptic monitor compared with the ventricular catheter. *Surg Neurol* 1992; 37(4):251.

124. Yablon JS, et al: Clinical experience with a fiberoptic intracranial pressure monitor. *J Clin Monit* 1993; 9(3):171.

125. Artru F, et al: Monitoring intracranial pressure with intraparenchymal fiberoptic transducer. Technical aspects and clinical reliability. *Ann Fr Anesth Reanim* 1992; 11(4):424.

126. Gambardella G, et al: Intracranial pressure monitoring in children: comparison of external ventricular device with the fiberoptic system. *Childs Nerv Syst* 1993; 9(8):470.

127. Tasker RC, Matthew DJ: Cerebral intraparenchymal pressure monitoring in non-traumatic coma: Clinical evaluation of a new fiberoptic device. *Neuropediatrics* 1991; 22(1):47.

128. Lebkowsli WJ: The control of intracranial pressure using computerized data system—our observations. *Ann Med Univ Bialystok Poland* 1993; 38(1):93.

129. Weinstabl C, et al: Comparative analysis between epidural (Gaeltec) and subdural (Camino) intracranial pressure probes. *J Clin Monit* 1992; 8(2):116.

130. Lebkowski W, et al: Intracranial epidural implantation of a Gaeltec ITC/b sensor in the light of our experience. *Neurol Neurochir Polska* 1988; 22(5):476.

131. Betsch, Aschoff A: Measurement artifacts in Gaeltec intracranial pressure monitors due to radio waves from personal beeper systems. *Anesth Intens Notfall Schmerz* 1992; 27(1):51.

132. Hill A, Volpe JJ: Measurement of intracranial pressure using the Ladd intracranial pressure monitor. *J Pediatr* 1981; 98:974.

133. Hobar JD, et al: Effect of application force on non-invasive method for measurement of intracranial pressure. *J Pediatr* 1980; 66:455.

134. Menke JA, et al: The fontanelle tonometer: A non-invasive method for measuring intracranial pressure. *J Pediatr* 1982; 100:960.

135. Robinson RO, et al: Non-invasive method for measuring intracranial pressure in newborn infants. *Dev Med Child Neurol* 1977; 19:305.

136. Salmon JH, et al: The fontogram: A non-invasive intracranial pressure monitor. *Pediatrics* 1977; 60:721.

137. Walsh P, Logan WJ: Continuous and intermittent measurement of intracranial pressure by the Ladd Monitor. *J Pediatr* 1983; 102:439.

138. Wealthall SR, Smallwood R: Methods of measuring intracranial pressure via the fontanelle without puncture. *J Neurol Neurosurg Psychiatry* 1974; 37:88.

139. Kaiser AM, Whitelaw AG: Non-invasive monitoring of intracranial pressure—fact or fancy? *Dev Med Child Neurol* 1987; 29(3):320.

140. Myberg DZ, et al: Comparison of non-invasive and direct measurements of intracranial pressure. *Pediatrics* 1980; 65:473.

141. Vidyasagar D, Raju TNK: A simple non-invasive technique of measuring intracranial pressure in the newborn. *Pediatrics* 1977; 59:951.

142. Bunegin L, et al: Intracranial measurement from the anterior fontanelle utilizing a pneumoelectronic switch. *Neurosurgery* 1987; 20(5):726.

143. Bailey H: Air embolism. *J Int Coll Surg* 1956; 25:675.

144. Amussat JZ: *Recherches sur l'introduction accidentelle de l'air dans les Veins.* Paris, Germer Baillier, 1839.

145. Barlow M: An attempt to remove a tumor on the neck: Entrance of air in vein. Sudden death. *Med Chir Trans* 1830; 16:28.

146. Cormack JR: *Presence of Air in Organs of Circulation* (thesis). Edinburgh, John Carfrae, 1837:56.

147. Erichsen JE: On the proximate cause of death after spontaneous introduction of air into the veins, with some remarks on the treatment of the accident. *Edinburgh Med Surg J* 1844; 61:1.

148. Legailois E: Des maladies occasionees par la résorbtion de pus. *J Hebdomadaire Med* 1829; 3:166.

149. Senn N: An experimental and clinical study of air embolism. *Surg Ann* 1885; 2:197.

150. Warren JC: Two cases of accidents from admission of air into veins during surgical operations. *J Med Sci* 1832; 20:545.

151. Cormack JR: The entrance of air by the open mouths of uterine veins, considered as a cause of danger and death after parturition. *London Med J* 1850; 2:928.

152. Adams VI, Hirch CS: Venous air embolism from head and neck wounds. *Arch Pathol Lab Med* 1989; 113:498.

153. Ahmat KP, et al: Fatal air embolism following anesthesia for insertions of peritoneovenous shunt. *Anesthesiology* 1989; 70:702.

154. Albin MS, et al: Anesthetic management of posterior fossa surgery in the sitting position. *Acta Anaesth Scand* 1976; 20:117.

155. Albin MS, et al: Venous air embolism during lumbar laminectomy in the prone position: Report of three cases. *Anesth Analg* 1991; 73:346.

156. Albin MS, et al: Venous air embolism during radical retropubic prostatectomy. *Anesth Analg* 1992; 74:151.

157. Baggish MS, Daniell JF: Death caused by air embolism associated with neodymium:yttrium-aluminum-garnet laser surgery and artificial sapphire tips. *Am J Obstet Gynecol* 1989; 161:877.

158. Bohrer H, Luz M: Bypass associated air embolism during liver transplantation. *Anaesth Intensive Care* 1990; 18:265.

159. Buckland RW, Manners JM: Venous air embolism during neurosurgery. *Anaesthesia* 1976; 31:633.

160. Fatteh A, et al: Fatal air embolism in pregnancy resulting from orogenital sex play. *Forensic Sci* 1973; 2:247.

161. Hybels RL: Venous air embolism in head and neck surgery. *Laryngoscope* 1980; 90:946.

162. Kuhn M, et al: Acute pulmonary edema caused by venous air embolism after removal of a subclavian catheter. *Chest* 1987; 92:364.

163. Lang SA, et al: Fatal air embolism in an adolescent with Duchenne muscular dystrophy during Harrington instrumentation. *Anesth Analg* 1989; 69:132.

164. Lee SK, Tanswell AK: Pulmonary vascular air embolism in the newborn. *Arch Dis Child* 1989; 64:507.

165. Lowdon JD, Tidmore TJ Jr: Fatal air embolism after gastrointestinal endoscopy. *Anesthesiology* 1988; 69:622.

166. Naulty SJ, et al: Air embolism during radical hysterectomy. *Anesthesiology* 1982; 57:420.

167. Nagi SH, Stinchfield EE: Air embolism during hip arthroplasties. *BMJ* 1974; 3:460.

168. Perchau RA, et al: Pulmonary interstitial edema after multiple venous air emboli. *Anesthesiology* 1983; 45:364.

169. Phillips RIL, Mulliken JB: Venous air embolism during a craniofacial procedure. *Plast Reconstr Surg* 1988; 82:155.

170. Rich RE: Fatal pulmonary air embolism following lysis of adhesions. *Surgery* 1952; 32:126.

171. Stoney WS, et al: Air embolism and other accidents using pump oxygenators. *Ann Thorac Surg* 1980; 29:336.

172. Wadhwa RK, et al: Gas embolism during laparoscopy. *Anesthesiology* 1978; 48:74.

173. Yeakel AE: Lethal air ebolism from plastic blood storage container. *JAMA* 1968; 204:267.

174. Younker D, et al: Massive air embolism during cesarian section. *Anesthesiology* 1986; 65:77.

175. Michenfelder JD, et al: Air embolism during neurosurgery—a new method of treatment. *Anesth Analg* 1966; 45:390.

176. Smith C: An endo-oesophageal stethoscope. *Anesthesiology* 1954; 15:566.

177. Standefer M, Bay JW, Trusso R: The sitting position in neurosurgery: A retrospective analysis of 488 cases. *Neurosurgery* 1984; 14:649.

178. Matjasko J, et al: Anesthesia and surgery in the seated position: Analysis of 554 cases. *Neurosurgery* 1985; 17:695.

179. Munson ES, et al: Early detection of venous air embolism using a Swan-Ganz catheter. *Anesthesiology* 1975; 42:223.

180. Standefer M, et al: The sitting position in neurosurgery: A retrospective analysis of 488 cases. *Neurosurgery* 1984; 14:649.

181. Young ML, et al: Comparison of surgical and anesthetic complications in neurosurgical patients experiencing venous air embolism in the sitting position. *Neurosurgery* 1986; 18:157.

182. Albin MS, et al: Clinical considerations concerning detection of venous air embolism. *Neurosurgery* 1978; 3:380.

183. Flanagan JP, et al: Air embolism: A lethal complication of subclavian puncture. *N Engl J Med* 1969; 281(9):488.

184. Chang JL, et al: Analysis and comparison of venous air embolism detection methods. *Neurosurgery* 1980; 7(2):135.

185. Gildenberg PL, et al: The efficacy of Doppler monitoring for the detection of venous air embolism. *J Neurosurgery* 1981; 54:75.

186. Maroon JC, et al: Detection of minute venous air emboli with ultrasound. *Surg Gynecol Obstet* 1968; 127:1236.

187. Brechner VL, Bethune RWM: Recent advances in monitoring pulmonary air embolism. *Anesth Analg* 1971; 50:255.

188. Edmonds-Seal J, Prys-Roberts C, Adams AP: Air embolism: A comparison of various methods of detection. *Anaesthesia* 1971; 26:202–208.

189. English JB, et al: Comparison of venous air embolism monitoring methods in supine dogs. *Anesthesiology* 1978; 48:425.

190. Gildenberg PL, et al: The efficacy of Doppler monitoring for detection of venous air embolism. *J Neurosurg* 1981; 54:74.

191. Maroon JC, Albin MSA: Air embolism diagnosed by Doppler ultrasound. *Anesth Analy* 1974; 53(3):399.

192. Russell D: The detection of cerebral emboli using Doppler ultrasound. In: Newell DW, Aaslid R (eds): *Transcranial Doppler.* New York, Raven Press, 1992.

193. Durant TM, et al: Pulmonary (venous) air embolism. *Am Heart J* 1947; 33:269.

194. Stallworth JM, et al: Aspiration of the heart in air embolism. *JAMA* 1950; 143:1250.

195. Ericsson JA, et al: Closed chest cardiac message for the treatment of venous air embolism. *N Engl J Med* 1964; 270:1353.

196. Bunegin L, et al: Positioning the right atrial catheter. *Anesthesiology* 1981; 55(4):343.

197. Satamura S, Kaneko Z: Ultrasonic blood rheograph. *Proc 3d Int Conf Med Electr* 1960:254.

198. Aaslid R, et al: Noninvasive transcranial Doppler ultrasound recording of flow velocity in basal cerebral arteries. *J Neurosurg* 1982; 57:769.

199. Aaslid R: The Doppler principle applied to measurement of blood flow velocity in cerebral arteries. In: Aaslid R (ed): *Transcranial Sonography.* Wien/New York, Springer-Verlag, 1986.

200. Niederkorn K, et al: Three-dimensional transcranial Doppler blood flow mapping in patients with cerebrovascular disorders. *Stroke* 1988; 19:1335.

201. Bogdahn U, et al: Transcranial color-coded real-time sonography in adults. *Stroke* 1990; 21:1680.

202. Jeschke B: Transcranial Doppler sonography. *Psych Neurol Med Psychiatry* 1989; 41(6):321.

203. Bunegin L, et al: Detection and volume estimation of embolic air in the middle cerebral artery using transcranial Doppler sonography. *Stroke* 1994; 25(3):593.

204. Spencer MP, et al: Detection of middle cerebral artery emboli during carotid endarterectomy using transcranial Doppler ultrasonography. *Stroke* 1990; 21:415.

205. Albin MS, et al: The transcranial Doppler can image microaggregates of air and particulate matter. *J Neurosurg Anesthesiol* 1989; 1:134.

206. Markus HS, Brown MM: Differentiation between different pathological cerebral embolic materials using transcranial Doppler in an in vitro model. *Stroke* 1993; 24:1.

207. Russell D, et al: Detection of arterial emboli using Doppler ultrasound in rabbits. *Stroke* 1991; 22:253.

208. D'Arrigo JS, et al: Lipid coated uniform microbubbles for earlier sonographic detection of brain tumors. *J Neuroimaging* 1991; 1:134.

209. Fies F: Air microbubbles as a contrast medium in transcranial Doppler sonography. *J Neuroimaging* 1991; 1:173.

210. White DN, et al: The acoustic characteristics of the skull. *Ultrasound Med Biol* 1978; 4:225.

211. Grolimund P: Transmission of ultrasound through temporal bone. In: Aaslid R (ed): *Transcranial Doppler Sonography.* Vienna, Springer-Verlag, 1986.

212. Spencer MP: Intracranial carotid artery diagnosis with transorbital pulsed wave (PW) and continuous wave (CW) Doppler ultrasound. *J Ultrasound Med* 1983; 2:(suppl)61.

213. Aaslid R: Transcranial Doppler examination techniques. In: Aaslid R (ed): *Transcranial Doppler Sonography.* New York, Springer-Verlag, 1986.

214. Gomez CR: *Transcranial Doppler.* In: American Society for Neuroimaging Neurosonology course, Orlando, FL, 1991.

215. Saver JL, Feldmann E: Basic transcranial Doppler examination: Technique and anatomy. In: Babikian VL, Wechsler LR (eds): *Transcranial Doppler Ultrasonography.* St. Louis, CV Mosby, 1993.

216. Sokollu A: Destructive effect of ultrasound on ocular tissue. In: Reid JM, Sikov MR (eds): *Interaction of Ultrasound and Biological Tissues.* US Department of Health Publication 73, 1972.

217. Budingen DHJ, et al: Subclavian steal: Transcranial Doppler sonography of the basilar artery. *Ultraschall Med* 1987; 8:218.

218. Ringelstein EB, et al: Non-invasive diagnosis of intracranial lesions in the vertebrobasilar system. A comparison of Doppler sonographic and angiographic findings. *Stroke* 1985; 16(5):848.

219. Tegeler CH, Eicke M: Physics and principles of transcranial Doppler ultrasonography. In: Babikian VL, Wechsler LR (eds): *Transcranial Doppler Ultrasonography.* St. Louis, CV Mosby, 1993.

220. Aaslid R: Developments and principles of transcranial Doppler. In Newell DW, Aaslid R (eds): *Transcranial Doppler.* New York, Raven Press, 1992.

221. Kremkau FW: Biologic effects and safety. In: Rumack CM, et al (eds): *Diagnostic Ultrasound, Vol. 1.* St Louis, Mosby-Year Book, 1991.

222. Christman CL, et al: Evidence for free radical production in aqueous solutions by diagnostic ultrasound. *Ultrasonics* 1987; 25(1):31.

223. Atchley AA, et al: Acoustic cavitation and bubble dynamics. In: Suslick KS (ed): *Ultrasound: Its Chemical, Physical and Biological Effects.* New York, VCH Publishers, 1988.

224. Doida Y, et al: Conformation of an ultrasound-induced mutation in two in-vitro mammalian cell lines. *Ultrasound Med Biol* 1990; 16:699.

225. American Institute of Ultrasound in Medicine, Bioeffects Committee: Bioeffects considerations for the safety of diagnostic ultrasound. *J Ultrasound Med Biol* 1988; 7(suppl):S1–S38.

226. Bunegin L, et al: Bench simulation of brain fluid heating during bilateral high power insonation. *Anesthesiology* 1995; 38(3A):A511.

227. Bunegin L, et al: The effect of bilateral high power ultrasonic beams on cerebral tissue temperature. *Anesthesiology* 1995; 38(3A):A512.

228. Gosling RG, King DH: Arterial assessment by Doppler shift ultrasound. *Proc R Soc Med* 1974; 67:447.

229. Planiol T, et al: La circulation carotidenne et cérébrale. Progres réalisés dans l'étude par les méthodes physiques externes. *Nouv Presse Med* 1973; 37:2451.

230. Stuart B, et al: Fetal blood velocity wave forms in normal pregnancy. *Br J Obstet Gynaecol* 1980; 87:780.

231. McCallum WD, et al: Fetal blood velocity waveforms. *Am J Obstet Gynecol* 1978; 132:425.

232. Marshall K, et al: Myocardial contractility and ultrasonically measured blood velocity in fetal lamb. In: Gill RW, Dadd MJ (eds): *World Federation for Ultrasound in Medicine and Biology,* 85. Sydney, Australia, Pergamon Press, 1985:256.

233. Gosling RG, et al: The quantitative analysis of occlusive peripheral arterial diseases by a non-intrusive ultrasonic technique. *Angiology* 1971; 22:52.

234. Seiler RW, Nirkko AC: Effect of Nimodipine on cerebrovascular response to CO_2 in asymptomatic individuals and patients with subarachnoid hemorrhage: A transcranial Doppler ultrasound study. *Neurosurgery* 1990; 27(2):247.

235. Hassler W, et al: Transcranial Doppler ultrasonography in raised intracranial pressure and in intracranial circulatory arrest. *J Neurosurg* 1988; 68:745.

236. Klingelholfer J, et al: Evaluation of intracranial pressure from transcranial Doppler studies in cerebral disease. *J Neurol* 1988; 235:159.

237. Klingelholfer J, et al: Intracranial flow patterns at increasing intracranial pressure. *Klin Wochenschr* 1987; 65:542.

238. Fischer A, Livingstone J: Transcranial Doppler and real time cranial sonography in neonatal hydrocephalus. *J Child Neurol* 1989; 4:64.

239. Lindegaard K-F, et al: Assessment of intracranial hemodynamics in carotid artery disease by transcranial Doppler ultrasound. *J Neurosurg* 1985; 63:890.

240. Markwalder TM, et al: Dependency of blood flow velocity in the middle cerebral artery on end tidal carbon dioxide partial pressure—a transcranial ultrasound Doppler study. *J Cereb Blood Flow Metab* 1984; 4(3):368.

241. Hauge A, et al: Changes in cerebral blood flow during hyperventilation and CO_2-breathing measured transcutaneously in humans by a bidirectional, pulsed, ultrasound Doppler blood velocitymeter. *Acta Physiol Scand* 1980; 110(2):167.

242. Downing GJ, et al: Comparison of the pulsatility index and input impedance parameters in a model of altered hemodynamics. *J Ultrasound* 1991; 10:317:21.

243. Thompson RS, Trudinger BJ: Doppler waveform pulsatility index and resistance, pressure and flow in the umbilical placental circulation: An investigation using a mathematical model. *Ultrasound Med Biol* 1990; 16(5)449.

244. Legarth J, Thorup E: Characteristics of Doppler blood-velocity waveforms in a cardiovascular in-vitro model. II. The influence of peripheral resistance, perfusion pressure, and blood flow. *Scand J Clin Lab Invest* 1989; 49:459.

245. Legarth J, Nolsoe C: Doppler blood velocity waveforms and

the relation to peripheral resistance in the brachial artery. *J Ultrasound Med* 1990; 9:449.

246. Guilioni M, et al: Correlations among intracranial pulsatility, intracranial hemodynamics, and transcranial Doppler waveform. *Neurosurgery* 1988; 22:807.

247. Beasley MG, et al: Changes in internal carotid artery flow velocities with cerebral vasodilation and constriction. *Stroke* 1979; 10(3):331.

248. Dahl A, et al: A comparison of transcranial Doppler and cerebral blood flow studies to assess cerebral vasoreactivity. *Stroke* 1992; 23(1):15.

249. Provinciali L, et al: Investigation of cerebrovascular reactivity using transcranial Doppler sonography. Evaluation and comparison of different methods. *Funct Neurol* 1990; 5(1):33.

250. Schregel W, et al: Transcranial Doppler sonography: Halothane increases average blood flow velocity in the middle cerebral artery. *Anaesthesist* 1988; 37(5):305.

251. Werner C, et al: Effects of sufentanil on cerebral blood flow, cerebral blood flow velocity, and metabolism in dogs. *Anesth Analg* 1991; 72(2):177.

252. Werner C, et al: The effects of propofol on cerebral blood flow in correlation to cerebral blood flow velocity in dogs. *J Neurosurg Anesth* 1992; 4(1):41.

253. Werner C, et al: Cerebral blood flow in correlation to cerebral blood flow velocity during isoflurane anesthesia. *J Neurosurg Anesth* 1991; 3(3):236.

254. Raju TN, Kim SY: The effect of hematocrit alterations on cerebral vascular CO_2 reactivity in newborn baboons. *Pediatr Res* 1991; 29:385, 1991.

255. Brouwers PJ, et al: Transcranial pulsed Doppler measurements of blood flow velocity in the middle cerebral artery: Reference values at rest and during hyperventilation in healthy children and adolescents in relation to age and sex. *Ultrasound Med Biol* 1990; 16(1):1.

256. Halsey JH, et al: Blood velocity in the middle cerebral artery and regional cerebral blood flow during carotid endarterectomy. *Stroke* 1989; 20(1):53.

257. Harders A, Gilsbach J: Transcranial Doppler sonography and its application in extracranial-intracranial bypass surgery. *Neuro Res* 1985; 7:129.

258. Taylor RH, et al: Cerebral haemodynamics in infants during cardiopulmonary bypass. *Can J Anaesth* 1990; 37:S153.

259. Legarth J, Thorup E: Characteristics of Doppler blood-velocity waveforms in a cardiovascular in-vitro model. I. The model and the influence of heart rate. *Scand J Clin Lab Invest* 1989; 49:451.

260. Mari G, et al: Fetal heart rate influence of the pulsatility index in the middle cerebral artery. *J Clin Ultrasound* 1991; 19:149.

261. Gnudi G, et al: A simulation study of the hemodynamic factors influencing the carotid pulsatility index. Atti dell'Accademia della Scienze dell'Istituto di Bologna Serie XIV, Tomo I, 1983–84:115.

262. Berne RM, Levy MN: The arterial system. In: *Cardiovascular Physiology*, 3d ed. St Louis, CV Mosby, 1992:103.

263. Marmarou A, et al: A non-linear analysis of the cerebrospinal fluid system and intracranial pressure dynamics. *J Neurosurg* 1975; 48:523.

264. Hallock P, Benson IC: Studies on elastic properties of isolated human aorta. *J Clin Invest* 1937; 16:595.

265. Rodewald G, et al: Central nervous system risk factors in heart surgery. *Z Kardiol* 1990; 79(suppl):13.

266. Tilsner V, et al: Noncardiac risk factors in heart surgery—the blood coagulation system. *Kardiol* 1990; 79(suppl):63.

267. Blumenthal JA, et al: A preliminary study of the effects of cardiac procedures on cognitive performance. *Int J Psychosom* 1991; 38(1–4):13.

268. Shaw P, et al: Early neurological complications of coronary bypass. *BMJ* 1985; 291:1384.

269. Newman SP, et al: Acute neuropsychological consequences of coronary artery bypass surgery. *Curr Psychol Res Rev* 1987; 6:115.

270. Stump DA, et al: Cardiopulmonary bypass time and neuropsychological deficits after cardiac surgery. *2nd International Conference, The Brain and Cardiac Surgery, Proceedings Abstracts* 1993:3.

271. Delphin E, et al: Cerebral dysfunction after cardiac surgery in elderly patients. *2nd International Conference, The Brain and Cardiac Surgery, Proceedings Abstracts.* 1993:4.

272. Roach GW, et al: Risk factors for adverse CNS outcome in patients following coronary bypass surgery (CABG) preliminary results of the multicenter study of perioperative ischemia. *2nd International Conference, The Brain and Cardiac Surgery, Proceedings Abstracts* 1993:13.

273. Newman MF, et al: Cerebral blood flow regulation during cardiopulmonary bypass: Correlation with postoperative neurologic and neuropsychologic deficits. In: Willner AE, Rodewald G (eds): *Impact of Cardiac Surgery on the Quality of Life.* New York, Plenum Press, 1990:137.

274. Stump DA, et al: Cerebral blood flow declines independently of metabolism during hypothermic cardiopulmonary bypass. In: Willner AE, Rodewald G (eds): *Impact of Cardiac Surgery on the Quality of Life.* New York, Plenum Press, 1990:265.

275. Pokar H, et al: The role of prolonged cardiopulmonary bypass time for cognitive dysfunctions after coronary artery bypass surgery. *2nd International Conference, The Brain and Cardiac Surgery, Proceedings Abstracts* 1993:19.

276. Spencer MP, et al: The use of ultrasonics in the determination of arterial aeroembolism during open heart surgery. *Ann Thorac Surg* 1969; 8:489.

277. Ries F, et al: Clinical applications and perspectives of TCD-signal enhancement with standardized air microbubbles. *J Cardiovasc Technol* 1989; 8:177.

278. Clayton RH, et al: Clinical comparison of two devices for detection of microemboli during cardiopulmonary bypass. *Clin Phys Physiol Meas* 1990; 11(4):327.

279. van der Linden J, Casimir-Ahn H: When do cerebral emboli appear during open heart operations? A transcranial Doppler study. *Ann Thorac Surg* 1991; 51(2):237.

280. Pugsley WB, et al: Relationship between microembolic event counting and neuropsychological deficit in patients undergoing coronary artery bypass. *2nd International Conference, The Brain and Cardiac Surgery, Proceedings Abstracts.* 1993:9.

281. Strottmann JM, et al: Ultrasonic emboli detection during routine cerebral angiography. *2nd International Conference, The Brain and Cardiac Surgery, Proceedings Abstracts.* 1993:28.

282. Padayachee TS, et al: The detection of microemboli in the middle cerebral artery during cardiopulmonary bypass: A transcranial Doppler ultrasound investigation using membrane and bubble oxygenators. *Ann Thorac Surg* 1981; 44:298.

283. Mitzel H, et al: Neuropsychological change and statistical artifact. *J Neurosurg Anesth* 1991; 3(3):241.

284. Fries CC, et al: Experimental cerebral gas embolism. *Ann Surg* 1957; 145(4):461.

285. Spencer JAD, et al: Validation of Doppler indices using blood and water. *Ultrasound Med* 1991; 10:305.

286. Hills BA, Grulke DC: Evaluation of ultrasonic bubble detectors in-vitro using calibrated microbubbles at selected velocities. *Ultrasonics* 1975; 13(4):181.

287. Sellman M, et al: Doppler ultrasound estimation of microbubbles in the arterial line during extracorporeal circulation. *Perfusion* 1990; 5:23.

288. Evans DH, et al: Origin of the Doppler power spectrum. *Dopp-*

ler Ultrasound: Physics, Instrumentation and Clinical Applications. Chichester, John Wiley, 1989:115.

289. Semb BKH et al: Doppler ultrasound estimation of bubble removal by various arterial line filters during extracorporeal circulation. *Scand J Thorac Cardiovasc Surg* 1982; 16:55.

290. Hatteland K, et al: Comparison of bubble release from various types of oxygenators. *Scand J Thorac Cardiovasc Surg* 1985; 19:125.

291. Hatteland K, Semb BKH: Gas bubble detection in fluid lines by means of pulsed Doppler ultrasound. *Scand J Thorac Cardiovasc Surg* 1985; 19:119.

292. Lubbers J, van den Berg JW: An ultrasonic detector for micro gas emboli in a blood flow line. *Ultrasound Med Biol* 1976; 2:301.

293. Klepper JR, Moehring MA: Personal communication, 1992.

294. Miles RD, et al: Relationships of five Doppler measurements with flow in an in-vitro model and clinical findings in newborn infants. *J Ultrasound Med* 1987; 6:597.

295. Butler B: Biophysical aspects of gas bubbles in blood. *Med Instr* 1985; 12(2)59.

296. Hills BA, Butler BD: A method of producing calibrated micro-bubbles for air embolism studies. *J Appl Physiol: Respirat Environ Exerc Physiol* 1981; 51(2):524.

Chapter 9
NEUROBEHAVIORAL EVALUATION

RAYMOND M. COSTELLO

HOWARD C. MITZEL

SANDRA L. SCHNEIDER

Tradition of Scientific Psychology

The history of psychology reflects a concern with the mind-body connection, a dilemma with philosophical roots going back to Descartes in the seventeenth century. Springing from roots in philosophy, psychology has focused on the "immaterial" aspects of brain function, measuring immanent aspects of brain observable in the realm of mind or consciousness.[1] In this immaterialist tradition, William James's seminal text, *The Principles of Psychology*,[2] considered topics of both mind and body, still of central concern to psychology more than a century later. James included chapters on the sensory and nervous systems, judgment, attention, memory, emotion, and consciousness. For James and his followers, consciousness, although a topic of mind, was not distinct from body, because it exists within human experience. The mode of investigation for the study of consciousness was phenomenologic, with a typical "experiment" involving the introduction of a stimulus followed by a verbal description of its sentient experience.

At about the same time in Europe, the mind-body problem was under investigation from a very different, but powerful, experimentalist perspective, by physiologists and early psychologists like Weber, Fechner, von Helmholtz, and Wundt. A typical experiment involved the presentation of a stimulus with a known physical property, such as the brightness of a light or the loudness of a tone, followed by a judgment of the magnitude of the stimulus by a human subject. This line of inquiry became known as "psychophysics" and early on developed investigatory techniques which included multiple trials from a single subject, multiple subjects, and strictly controlled experimental protocols. By knowing the physical characteristics of the inputs to the sensory system, these early psychologists developed psychophysical "laws," which mathematically related physical events (e.g., spectrum values of sound or light) to human behavior (e.g., judgments of loudness or brightness). These relationships are still in use today, particularly in applied areas of investigation such as the development of new fragrances and foods.

The success of the early psychophysicists profoundly influenced American psychology, and from the 1920s through the 1950s the "behaviorist" tradition associated with John B. Watson dominated scientific psychology. During this period, investigation into things of mind retrenched. The mind-body problem became focused on the study of only those variables with highly observable, quantifiable attributes. Behavioral psychology researchers thought of stimuli as inputs and behavior as outputs. Their research objective was to quantify the relationship between inputs and outputs with no regard to mental "processing" in between. Animal conditioning and learning studies, involving endless combinations of stimuli in the form of reinforcement schedules, were a primary preoccupation associated with this tradition. Although this tradition of inquiry is now regarded as substantively impoverished,[3] great methodologic strides continued to be made in the development of the experimental design. Sir Ronald Fisher's *The Design of Experiments*[4] appeared during this period, introducing the analysis of variance to the scientific community. This seminal introduction married experimental design to statistics for the first time. This in turn led to the development of increasingly complex and elegant experimental designs, which have become the hallmark of the practice of scientific psychology today.

In the late 1950s British and American psychologists, in defiance of the behaviorist tradition, began to study aspects of cognitive process and triggered the "cognitive revolution"[5] in psychology. This revolution resulted in the revival of many of the "mentalistic" topics defined as the purview of psychology by James[2] but pursued under rigorous scientific practice gained from a century of experimental psychology. British psychologist Donald Broadbent[6] began the study of attention, which pertains to the ability to prepare, direct, and control one's mental resources, as required, for example, to drive a car in heavy traffic, to write a note while simultaneously conducting a telephone conservation, or to distinguish and follow one conversation from among many in a crowded room. The assessment of attentional resources is now an important aspect of neurobehavioral evaluation and is an explicit component task in nearly all neuropsychological test batteries.

Similarly, American psychologist George Miller[7] began the study of "immediate," or short-term, memory in the early 1960s, experimentally distinguishing this aspect of memory from long-term memory, based on its limited capacity. Miller's careful laboratory experiments demonstrated that most people can only remember between five and nine single digits. These experiments are now embodied in the "digit span test," a component task in a number of the most commonly administered neuropsychological batteries. In turn, long-term memory research has undergone a great deal of theoretical development through laboratory study and clinical observation. For example, retrograde amnesiacs' loss of memory for personal detail, but retention of semantic information, combined with confirming laboratory results, have resulted in the theoretical distinction of separate autobiographical and semantic long-term memory systems.[8] This distinction has become important in the evaluation and distinction between cortical and subcortical dementias. Butters and associates,[9] for example, found that Huntington disorder patients (presumably with a "subcortical" dementia) are severely impaired in general retrieval of information, whether or not the task is "semantic" in nature. Letter retrieval tasks require words to be retrieved which begin with a particular letter, allowing phonemic cues to be effective aids in the retrieval process. Category recall tasks require recall of members of categories (e.g., animals or fruits) and require an intact semantic memory capacity. Whereas Huntington patients do poorly on both types of task, patients with senile dementia of the Alzheimer's type do much more poorly on category retrieval tasks than on letter recall tasks. Many neuropsychological tests in use today have this scientific laboratory pedigree, which provides testing and assessment with a unique grounding in a theoretical basis of psychology.

Tradition of Individual Psychological Assessment

In the public perception, clinical, educational, and industrial psychology have long been associated with objective tests to measure psychopathology and intellectual ability, to aid in employment screening and placement, and in more recent decades, to assess neuropsychopathology. Supported by a century of development in the mathematically based theory of measurement, educational, intellectual, personality, and aptitude testing now represents a multibillion-dollar industry in the United States. This tradition of individual assessment originates with Darwinian concepts of adaptation and change, which so revolutionized the life sciences in the nineteenth century. American psychologist James M. Cattell, who trained with the European psychophysicist Wundt, became interested in the source of individual differences among experimental subjects. Collaborating with Sir Francis Galton, Cattell began the development of tests of reaction time and sensory discrimination as objective indicators of mental and intellectual functioning.[10] At about the same time, the French government commissioned physician Alfred Binet to develop tests to identify intellectually subnormal children for school placement. The result, just after the turn of the century, was a 30-item test which became known as the Binet-Simon Scale. American revisions, which are still in use today, came to be known as the Stanford-Binet, yielding the now familiar intelligence quotient (IQ), defined as the ratio of "mental" age to chronological age. During World War I, the U.S. Army commissioned the development of aptitude tests to classify recruits, which spurred later use in industrial settings for personnel selection and classification. Following World War II, intelligence testing became common in U.S. public schools to assist in tracking children, and achievement tests came into widespread use for educational assessment and college admissions decisions.

This assessment history is important in modern neurobehavioral testing for reasons beyond its methodologic contributions to measurement theory. Many of the early aptitude screening batteries included tasks of motor fluency and reaction time, which have been adapted in modern neuropsychological test batteries. More important, intellectual ability, often as indicated by years of formal education, is closely associated with performance on most neuropsychological tasks. For that matter, performance on virtually all psychological tasks is correlated to some degree, including motor, reaction time, scholastic achievement, and tests of specific abilities like memory and reasoning. Inconsistencies in this expected pattern of correlated relationships, or differential changes across testing domains in individual performance, provide important information to clinicians in making diagnostic and treatment decisions. This pattern of general correlation of performance has been known to psychologists throughout this century, and explains Cattell's early use of simple motor and choice reaction time tasks to measure general mental functioning.

This result, combined with the availability of large samples of uniformly administered tests, has played an important part in the development of theories of intelligence. Using newly available correlational methods just after the turn of the century, Charles Spearman proposed a general or *g* factor of intelligence, implying that intellectual functioning is a stable trait. Although he later modified this theory to a multifactor model for intelligence,[10] the concept of intelligence as a unitary concept persists in the everyday discourse of our culture, encouraged by the assignment of a sole IQ score. Multifactor theories of intelligence continue to predominate in modern educational psychology, in part due to the considerable descriptive and predictive successes of the multivariate statistical methods employed to reduce test items to factored scales. A great deal of measurement theory has grown up around these techniques, in which mental abilities (e.g., verbal or numerical fluency) are conceptualized as latent traits, i.e., stable quantifiable properties of an individual's mental functioning.

With methodologic roots in experimental design, modern cognitive theorists provide a somewhat different, more fluid and process-oriented account of human intellectual ability. Basic processes like memory storage, retrieval, and search, combined with attention and short-term memory, become enhanced and supplemented through developmentally learned strategies. The broad latent constructs and factors originated by Spearman and his collaborators to explain intellectual ability are viewed by modern cognitive theorists as statistical artifacts of the complex web of interacting processes studied by cognitive scientists. Sternberg's work[11] is exemplary of this process approach to intellectual ability. Interestingly, the more "molecular" level accounts of cognitive process have close analogues with theories of neural function at the level of the brain. Early network-like theories of "spreading activation"[12-13] in verbal processing have rapidly evolved into elegant computational theories of neural network architecture.[14-15] The advent of nuclear imaging techniques such as PET have recently begun to demonstrate physiologic evidence for network-based cognitive theories of verbal processes, the latter pieced together by years of laboratory experimentation on the part of scientific psychologists. In the decade of the brain, what has traditionally been a problem of mind for cognitive science is now becoming a question of body for the newly evolving neurosciences. In the years to come, cognitive theory will continue to inform and influence neuroscience and neurobehavioral evaluation.

The symbiotic model of scientific laboratory and clinical practice we have described here for neuropsychology is familiar to physicians. Medical clinical practice is informed by centuries of work in anatomy and decades of results from physiology, pharmacology, microbiology, and other disciplines. Likewise, clinical practice and research have informed all of these sciences to one degree or another. In more recent years, clinicians are becoming increasingly concerned with practices that may affect human cognitive functioning, juxtaposing traditional concerns with healing of the body and concerns of mind. Neurobehavioral evaluation is squarely situated on the crux of the mind-body problem, a dilemma that psychology has grappled with for more than a century in both clinical and scientific modes. Modern neuropsychological evaluation is informed by both a scientific tradition emphasizing the testing and development of theory and by a clinical tradition in which objective assessment of individuals occurs in the context of psychological theory.

Neurobehavioral Testing in a Clinical Research Setting

In the previous section, we sketched the history of the two traditions in psychology: scientific inference and individual assessment. Although these traditions share a theoretical base and many identical statistical methods, their aims are quite different. Scientific psychology is concerned with the testing and advancement of psychological theory. Experimental design is the engine for scientific studies, where characteristically the objective is to draw an inference from some (usually) small sample to a population, thereby permitting the generalization of some principle or result. In the classical design situation, the sample is partitioned, preferably by random assignment, into an "experimental" condition which receives a stimulus or "treatment" of some sort, and a "control" condition which does not. Often the stimuli and the measures used to assess experimental outcomes are developed exclusively for the experiment at hand. This can raise issues as to the validity and reliability of measures. It is often misunderstood, even by some experimentalists, that a primary purpose of the control is to represent a (no-treatment) condition in which the outcome confirms some known or prior expectation. In this way, control conditions serve to bolster the credibility of the effect, if any, of the treatment and the measurement of its outcome. Classical experimentation represents a problem of generalizability. The credibility of this inference rests strongly on conditions that are *internal* to the design of the experiment.

Assessment represents a different problem, one that is essentially inductive in nature. When objective tests are employed for assessment purposes, the aim is usually to make a decision about a particular individual or sometimes a group of individuals, as in the case of some educational testing applications. In clinical situations, test results are usually employed as only one of several informational inputs to the decision maker. Interviews or histories are also relevant informational inputs in what is a process of judgment. The role of the objective test is to place the individual, quantitatively, in the context of a population. The specific aim of developers of objective tests is to order the population with respect to some attribute(s) (e.g., short-term memory ability), and then to permit the clinician to estimate the place of the individual in that ordering. In a sense, this is the scientific inference problem turned on its head. The reliability and validity of the assessment instrument must be known in advance and standardized or "normed" on populations to which the tests belongs. This procedure functions logically as the control group in scientific inference problems. Modern commercial test developers can spend years and much money completing this process before a test is released for general use.

Clinical research often requires the incorporation of both scientific and individual assessment objectives. A clinician may want to know if a practice or treatment has an outcome for a particular group (a question of generalizability), but may also wish to know if an outcome was realized for specific individuals (a question of assessment). Unfortunately for the clinical researcher, objectives pertaining to both generalizability and assessment are often not compatible within the same study. For example, random assignment is often not a viable procedure, forcing designs to "weaker" inference situations. Standardized instruments may take too long to administer, exceed available financial constraints, or be inapplicable in a specific research design calling for repeated administrations to assess change. The remainder of this chapter considers these difficult issues that confront clinical researchers.

Neurobehavioral Psychology (Neuropsychology) and Psychometrics

Neurology and psychology are both devoted to the study of brain-behavior relationships. With roots in natural science, neurology has focused on the "material" aspects of brain and brain function, measuring size and structural properties of brain itself, and electrophysiologic or other "molecular" events reflecting certain behavioral properties of brain as a functioning biological system.[16] The historical aim of clinical and scientific neurologic investigations of brain has been to understand various disease processes affecting physical properties of brain thought to correlate with clinical or symptomatic deterioration of biologic functioning.

Somewhere between the disciplines of neurology and psychology, intermediate disciplines have developed, with measurement tools and clinical and scientific aims reflecting theoretical goals and investigative strategies of either the natural sciences or philosophy. Behavioral neurology is an extension beyond the traditional concerns of neurology into the traditional realm of psychology. The scientific constructs and clinical measuring instruments of behavioral neurology go beyond the typical preoccupation with signs such as the "reflex" or subjective measures of "motor strength" into the area of "mental status."[16] Neuropsychology is an applied specialty area within psychology with scientific constructs and clinical measuring instruments extending beyond the traditional concerns of philosophical and laboratory psychology into the traditional realm of neurology. Purely sensory or motor phenomena are of as much interest to the neuropsychologist as are more "complicated" mental functions characterizing memory, learning, and reasoning.[17] Neurobehavioral evaluation is a generic term used by some behavioral neurologists and some neuropsychologists to refer to the instrumentation used by either as they attempt to map brain-behavior relationships. Only some of the instruments of neurobehavioral evaluation are common to neurologists and neuropsychologists, while most are discipline-specific.

The measurement tradition within psychology is characterized by the apt label of psychometrics. Psychometrics is concerned primarily with psychological "test" construction. Psychological tests are systematic procedures to confirm or document the amount to which some human, or psychological, attribute, ability, or property of "mind" exists. Although an "impressionistic" tradition of psychological testing is a valued measurement enterprise for many psychologists working in clinical areas, primarily in psychiatric settings, the psychometric tradition emphasizes the systematic, objective aspects of measurement for comparing the behavior of persons to each other or to themselves at different times. Impressionists often work with instruments such as Rorschach's test[18] or other "projective" techniques where "quality" or "kind" or "subjectivity" of performance is the valued output. Psychometricians typically work with instruments such as Wechsler's Scales of Intelligence[19] or other "objective" techniques where "quantity" of performance is the valued output. The neurobehavioral tests of many neurology clinicians can be characterized as impressionistic, as the scales used to rate behaviors typically are subjective, with little attention paid to concepts such as the distributional properties of the test. The neurobehavioral tests of typical neuropsychologists or psychometricians are rigorously objective, with in-depth studies of distributional properties. Yet even among neuropsychologists, differences in emphasis with regard to "product" versus "process" are also obvious. Collections of clinical tests used to map brain functions range from the battery proposed by Ralph Reitan known as the Halstead-Reitan Neuropsychology Test Battery (HRNTB), emphasizing a fixed, standardized battery of tests to be employed in each and every case and concerned with quantitative output,[20] to Christensen's Luria Neuropsychological Investigation,[21] which is more concerned with techniques particularized to the apparent clinical needs of the individual case, to the "process" approach of Edith Kaplan, concerned with the quality, or the how and why, of performance, irrespective of the test battery used.[22]

Just as psychometricians are preoccupied with the statistical aspects of tests and test construction, psychologists of all specialty areas are preoccupied with sample statistics, statistical inference, and accurate generalizations to populations. The experimental laboratory psychologist typically works with animal or human subjects in highly controlled conditions which facilitate refined measurements with normal distributions and small error terms, isolated from the confounding influence of extraneous information or nuisance variables. The psychometrician, clinical psychologist, neuropsychologist, or neurobehavioral evaluator seldom is afforded the luxury of this sort of measurement paradigm. Clinical situations with information on single cases, with much missing data, and with no applicable normative data are commonplace and render inferential statistics impossible. Statistics in the clinical case often are merely descriptive, with little value beyond the individual case, and serve a primary purpose to document clinical status at different time points. In intermediate, "experimental-clinical" situations where tests can be administered to a number of persons, inferences about general principles of theoretical concern and generalizations to large populations of persons become matters of some interest and require essential knowledge about psychometrics and about statistics.

A central concern in psychometrics is to produce tests with known statistical properties. The essential statistical properties of tests reflect the central tendency (average score, modal score, or median score) and variability of scores (different sorts of ranges and measures of deviation about the average score) and the shape of the distribution of scores obtained either from an individual person tested many times or from various persons from populations of interest to whom comparisons are to be made. These statistical properties become the "normative" data used to describe the relative standing at any given time of any given person over

time or relative to a population with matching demographic characteristics, usually chronologic age, gender, and educational attainment.

It is often desirable for distributions of test scores to be shaped as though they reflect "normal" curves with known statistical properties.[23] Raw scores on tests can be subjected to various normalizing "transformations" to facilitate comparisons within or across persons. By definition, scores on tests distributed normally will vary, whether the variation is within or across persons. Sixty-eight percent of all scores will vary within two standard deviation raw score units, 34 percent or one standard deviation on either side of the average score. Thirty-two percent of all scores will vary by more than one standard deviation, 16 percent on either side of the average score.

Scores vary even in the "normal" case, sometimes considerably, depending on the "reliability" of the test, from the score that best reflects the central tendency of the person tested over time or of the sample of persons representing a given population. Any individual will produce a range of scores on any given test, the central tendency of which is thought to reflect the "true" score, and deviations from which are thought to reflect varying degrees of "error" of measurement. Samples of people from the same population will also distribute themselves within a range from high to low on any given test. This fact of measurement variability complicates the interpretation of any given score on any particular test. No psychological test score has any meaning except with reference to some standard of comparison. Consistency, in measurement parlance, reflects the degree of reliability of the measuring device. The measure of central tendency is often thought to reflect the "true" score of the individual tested repeatedly, or of the normative population matching the person's demographic characteristics. In the "normal" case, deviations from this central tendency are thought to reflect inconsistencies of measurement and suggest measurement unrealiability. Psychometricians go to great lengths to minimize "error variance," or unreliability of their tests, to facilitate interpretation or understanding of any particular test score. Highly reliable tests will have small standard errors of measurement (i.e., small standard deviations of scores when applied to the individual case tested an infinite number of times). If this were not so, any particular score for an individual would be of little usefulness, as the psychometrician or neurobehavioral evaluator would not know where, in her own range of scores, the examinee happens to be scoring at any particular time. Once a standard error of measurement is known for a test, the psychometrician can state with a confidence of 2 : 1 that any obtained score of an individual lies within a band +1 to −1 standard deviation units, as about 67 percent

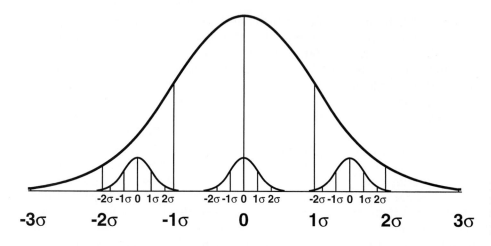

Figure 9-1 Distribution of scores for all persons on a particular ability measure and three hypothetical persons on many trials.

of an individual's scores will fall within this range. Small standard errors of measurement suggest that any person can be compared with a reference group with some confidence that the comparison is meaningful and reflects a "true" placement of the person within the range of the population characteristic and not one likely to be accounted for by chance. The distribution of test scores for any particular individual can match closely the distribution of test scores for a population reference group, or can be very different (Fig. 9-1), reflecting a performance in a tail of the reference distribution.

Neurobehavioral Evaluation and Experimental Design

As early as the 1920s it was obvious to psychological investigators, then working primarily in educational settings, that the development of "statistics" as strategies for organizing data was far beyond that of the "design" of experiments to collect adequate and valid data upon which to use statistics.[24] The experimental laboratory psychologist could, then and today, design experiments with rigorous control over "environmental" variables so that the yield of experimental data was rich in terms of "internal" validity and "external" validity, or generalizability; most investigators working in natural settings could not. Internal validity is a basic requirement that, when met, permits the experimenter to draw conclusions with confidence about the effect of an experimental variable. Without the assurance of internal validity, no amount of statistical manipulation or analysis of data is helpful in permitting unequivocal conclusions of "causal" relationships between experimental, or independent, variables and criterion, or dependent, variables. Yet, then and even somewhat now, statistics textbooks simply assumed that data warranted analysis, with little consideration

of how the data were acquired and how meaningful any statistical manipulation might be. As limitations of poorly collected data were recognized in educational settings, more and more attention was devoted to the design of research, especially those designs termed *quasi-experimental*, a term intended to reflect situations in which only limited control of environmental conditions was permitted because of ethical or situational circumstances. The same limitations are obvious in many clinical research situations. Consequently, clinical investigators are now as concerned about questions of design as they are about questions of statistics.[25]

In the "natural" setting, e.g., the classroom, clinic, or surgical suite, the conditions of experimental observation are not optimal relative to the "laboratory" setting of the neurobiologist or experimental psychologist. Often, the true designs of the experiment are not permissible or are impossible in the natural setting, and data are collected with "preexperimental" or various "quasi-experimental" procedures that reflect the inherent liabilities of doing scientific work in these contexts. The neurobehavioral evaluator and her clinical research team must be informed about quasi-experimental procedures and the threats to internal and external validity inherent in their use, whether designing studies of their own or reviewing studies of others. Campbell and Stanley[24] list *three* preexperimental designs: (1) one-shot case study, (2) one-group pretest-posttest design, (3) static-group comparison; *ten* quasi-experimental designs: (1) time series, (2) equivalent time samples design, (3) equivalent materials samples design, (4) nonequivalent control group design, (5) counterbalanced designs, (6) separate-sample pretest-posttest designs, (7) separate-sample pretest-posttest control group designs, (8) multiple time series, (9) institutional cycle design, (10) regression discontinuity; and *eight* threats to internal validity: (1) history, (2) maturation, (3) testing, (4) instrumentation, (5) regression, (6) selection, (7) mortality, (8) interactions of previous sources of invalidity. A brief review of their text, with reference to a few designs encountered commonly in clinical research circumstances, outlines common issues for the neurobehavioral evaluator working in clinical contexts familiar to neuroanesthesiology.

PREEXPERIMENTAL DESIGNS

Whether applied to an individual clinical case or to a group of cases, the preexperimental one-shot case study is encountered commonly in clinical situations. Often, because of the unique circumstances surrounding the clinical presentation of an interesting individual case, the clinical researcher has no alternative but to study a particular individual, with no possibility for "control" of extraneous variables which might influence the clinical phenomenon of concern. Although the case study might be quite informative for the clinician, Campbell and Stanley[24] declare that the design has almost no scientific value, and include the design as a minimum reference point from which to understand other designs. Examples of the one-shot case study would be clinical situations for which data collection is possible only after exposure to a purported experimental variable (e.g., an individual is encountered after a stroke in an area of the brain of particular interest to the investigator). Data are collected on any of various psychometric instruments and analyzed in relationship to what might have been expected if the experimental clinical variable had not been present. Sometimes, comparisons of results on standardized tests to norms underlying the standardization are made, but such "implicit" comparisons contribute only equivocally to scientific wisdom, even if they play an important role in the development of clinical lore.

In the one-group pretest-posttest preexperimental design, a pretest is obtained from an individual case or from a group of individuals similar to each other on some interesting characteristic. Exposure to an experimental condition then occurs and is followed by posttesting on the same or parallel measures as used in the pretest. Although very common in clinical situations, this design is described as a "bad example" of quasi-scientific research and is most useful as a point of reference for instruction about threats to internal validity by the confounding of extraneous variables with the experimental condition of interest. Significant threats to internal validity are inherent in this and any setup in which randomization to groups, experimental isolation of cases, or experimental control of extraneous influences cannot be achieved to rule out possible rival competing hypotheses.

History, maturation, testing, instrumentation, statistical regression, and their interactions are possible sources of internal invalidity. History, as an uncon-

trolled rival hypothesis, suggests that many "extraorganismic" or environmental events, besides the experimental condition, might occur between pretest and posttest, any of which might pose an alternative explanation for research findings. The longer the duration between pretest and posttest, the more plausible does history become as a rival hypothesis. *Maturation* is a term used to include all of the "intraorganismic" changes that might occur between pretest and posttest, any of which might be construed as a rival hypothesis for explanation of presumed relationships. Pretesting itself can also have an effect that rivals that of the experimental condition. Practice effects are ubiquitous, noteworthy examples of how performances can be influenced simply as a result of an initial exposure to a criterion variable. In some circumstances, "reactive" arrangements also provide a rival hypothesis for explanation of research results. When test-takers know what is being measured and why, at least sometimes they modify their responses either to comply with experimenter expectations or to defy them. Use of nonreactive measuring instruments is nearly always recommended, but in the clinical case this recommendation is often ignored. To the clinician measuring "depressed mood," for example, a face-valid measure of depression, like the Beck Depression Inventory,[26] seems an obvious choice. To the scientist knowledgeable about threats to internal and external validity, however, choice of a reactive instrument is seldom preferred, so as to avoid the problem of the act of measuring changing that which is being measured. Instrumentation characteristics such as "drift" or "decay" can be extremely important sources of variation in criterion measures. An example of instrumentation decay is an unpredictable change in a criterion score, caused by occasional drifting of attention, or fatigue of an external rater observing a clinical research subject performing a task purportedly influenced by the experimental condition. Another threat to internal validity is statistical regression. Statistical regression is considered a "tautologic" result of an imperfect correlation between pretest and posttest. The less reliable is the pretest-posttest correlation, the greater is the likelihood of statistical regression. The more extreme is the pretest score, the more likely it is to contain a larger amount of measurement error, and the more likely it is to regress to the grand mean on retest. Finally, if contrast groups are selected because of their extremity on a pretest measure, statistical regression is very likely to pose an alternative explanation for retest findings.

Another preexperimental design often encountered in clinical situations is the static-group comparison. In this situation, an individual or group of individuals has been exposed to an experimental condition, and the researcher attempts to assess the significance of the condition by developing a comparison group of persons not exposed. The researcher may attempt to control for effects of extraneous variables through matching or statistical covariance techniques, but the design is still very problematic. The essential problem for the design is that randomization to groups has not assured that groups are similar on the criterion variable of interest at pretest. Usually the experimental group is a convenience group, not selected scientifically from a larger population, and not assigned at random to the experimental condition. Self-selection artifact and differential experimental "mortality," or differential loss of subjects from groups, pose the most likely threats to internal validity. Matching is seldom adequate to control for sources of extraneous variance, as the researcher seldom is in a position to know what matching variables are crucial influences on the criterion variable. Also, matching on some variables, even if important influences on criterion variables, often systematically unmatches on other measured variables which might be equally crucial with regard to their effect on dependent measures.

QUASI-EXPERIMENTAL DESIGNS

Only a few of the ten quasi-experimental designs of Campbell and Stanley[24] are encountered frequently enough to warrant attention here. Quasi-experimental designs are not recommended if true experimental designs can be used. It is only when true experimental designs cannot be implemented that quasi-experimental designs become interesting mechanisms to help in the scientific process of phenomenologic or morphologic description, or ruling out of plausible, rival, competing explanations of purportedly causal relationships.

The single-case or single-group time series experiment is common in psychological studies and in some neurological studies as well. Basic to the time series study is a number of observations made on a variable or on multiple variables considered crucial to the process being investigated. These observations are interrupted by the imposition of an experimental variable and then repeated. Designs typically are variations of an "Off-On-Off" model, where the "Off" and "On" refer to the absence or presence of the experimental condition. History and instrumentation are considered threats to internal validity for this design, while interaction of pretesting, and/or selection, and the experimental variable, and reactive arrangements are considered threats to external validity.

Possible outcomes in a time series experiment are displayed in Fig. 9-2. An effect attributable to the experimental condition might be warranted in outcomes A, E, and F. In outcome A, it is apparent that the dependent variable is highly reliable and changes systematically after introduction of the experimental variable. In outcome E, a learning curve or practice effect is obvious in the dependent variable, which is reversed after exposure to the experimental condition. In outcome F, the preexposure learning curve is reversed after exposure to the experimental condition, and the effect is observed to be short-lived when the learning curve is resumed after washing out the effect of the experimental condition. In outcome D, no effect whatever is observed over time, as the dependent criterion never varies slope, prior to or after exposure to the experimental condition. Outcomes B and C are the interesting outcomes, as they reflect interpretive dilemmas investigators face when they do not have access to the history of the responding subject beyond a single or very few pretests. If only the O_4–O_5 lag is compared between outcomes A, B, and C, no differences would be apparent, and the investigator would be likely to conclude that the experimental condition is effective in producing a change in the dependent criterion. The

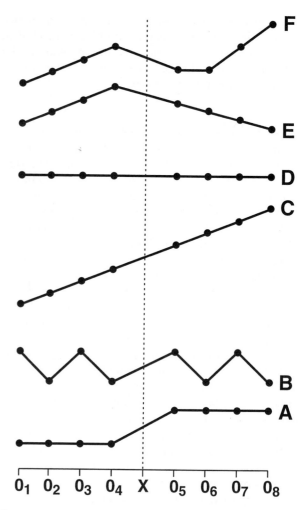

Figure 9-2 Possible outcomes in a time series experiment.

time series experiment captures the history of the respondent for some period of time prior to exposure, however, and outcomes B and C reveal obvious alternative, rival hypotheses. Criterion unreliability is exposed in outcome B and a learning curve is exposed in outcome C.

These few outcome possibilities do not exhaust all outcome possibilities. Time lags before effects are obvious are possible, as are shifts in slopes of criterion measures. It is important, in use of time series paradigms, that investigators declare, a priori, expected relationships with regard to time and effect and with regard to shape or slope of effect. The more closely expected relationships match observed ones, the more likely the experimenter understands causal relationships, and the less necessary does "statistical" testing of relationships become. When statistical testing is necessary because the empirical relationships have not been predicted beforehand, then problems of autocorrelation—that is, correlation between adjacent observations in the time series which exceeds correlation between nonadjacent lags—become prominent concerns. Tests of intercepts and slopes then become important statistical observations. Assumptions about linearity of relationships also can become problematic, especially if the natural time course of the dependent phenomenon is nonlinear, or if the effect of the experimental condition is gradual and confounded with history.

A very common design in clinical situations is the nonequivalent control group design. In this design, two groups, an experimental and control group, are studied, each having been given the pretest. This design is differentiated from a true experimental pretest-posttest control group design by the lack of random assignment of the experimental condition to the group that is to experience it. In the clinical research context, the experimental group is ordinarily a convenience group of individuals required by their physical or psychological condition to undergo the experimental condition (e.g., individuals needing a coronary bypass grafting procedure). The control group is ordinarily a convenience group of persons with a different physical status, undergoing a different procedure (e.g., individuals needing a total knee replacement), for whom the researcher is unable to demonstrate similarity on the independent variables known or suspected to influence the dependent criteria. In some cases, the investigator attempts to simulate preexperimental sampling equivalence through *post hoc* matching of experimental subjects with control subjects similar on variables thought to be important extraexperimental influences. In other cases, the investigator attempts to simulate preexperimental sampling equivalence through statistical covariance techniques, sometimes applied even

after subject matching. All the sources of threats to internal validity operate in this design, irrespective of the investigator's usually futile attempts to rule out rival hypotheses. Analysis of covariance with unreliable covariates is a very common problem, as the assumption of homogeneity of regression can almost never be accepted. In situations where the covariate is differentially correlated with the criterion (i.e., the correlation between covariate and criterion is different for the experimental group and for the control group), the covariance analysis will systematically overcorrect one group and undercorrect the other. Although use of regressed change scores, as opposed to simple gain scores, sometimes helps in controlling variation from extraneous sources, this seldom yields unequivocal findings. Matching also seldom controls for the practically ubiquitous problem of statistical regression, especially when groups are selected to be extreme at pretest on variables important to the pretest-posttest change, or when respondents are self-selected to the experimental condition. "Undermatching" and "matching-regression" effects are notorious problems rendering any conclusion of experimental effect subject to question as a pseudoeffect.

Primary Mental Abilities and the Structure of Intellect

Tests of cognitive functions that might be helpful in reflecting the kinds of change in mental functions of interest to neuroanesthesiologists are numerous. The rich measurement tradition in psychology is characterized by comprehensive assessment of various human abilities, with many purported tests of mental functions. It is also characterized by a statistical tradition which distills correlational relationships among tests into root abilities through the statistical procedure of factor analysis. L. L. Thurstone and J. P. Guilford, pioneers in the development of factor analysis, discovered purported "primary" mental abilities (PMAs), thought to explain distinctive patterns of intertest correlations.[27] In the factor analytic tradition, the "meaning" of any test is defined by its pattern of concordant and discordant correlations with others comprising the full data base of an investigation.

Thurstone suggested that tests of mental abilities could be distilled into six fundamental dimensions or PMAs.[27] He labeled these basic cognitive operations *verbal* (vocabulary or word meaning), *number* (arithmetic), *spatial* (pattern recognition and geometric figure copying), *word fluency* (rapid word recall), *memory* (rote learning of words, designs, or numbers), and *reasoning* (rule induction from particular instances). Some tests of complex intellectual performance may require combinations of PMAs. Thurstone's tests can be grouped by content (i.e., words versus numbers versus shapes) and by mental "process" (i.e., memory, fluency, and reasoning).

Guilford extended Thurstone's work and developed a "structure of intellect" (SOI) model composed of five types of mental "operation" (memory, cognition, convergent thinking, divergent thinking, and evaluation), three types of "content" (figural, symbolic, and behavioral), and six kinds of "product" (units of information, classes of units, relations between units, systems of information, transformations, and implications). His three-dimensional ($5 \times 3 \times 6$) SOI model permits classification of a test into one of 120 types.[27] Each type represents a distinctly different cognitive ability.

K. W. Schaie[28] has devoted his lifetime to Thurstone's model and has tracked more than 5000 persons in six study waves to map the longitudinal course of intellectual development. He developed tests used as markers for Thurstone's PMAs and has given comprehensive sets of these tests to a broad population, considered representative of the top 75 percent of the socioeconomic spectrum, in six waves from 1956 to 1991. He demonstrated that PMAs generally tend to increase until about age 40 to 45, stabilize until about age 50 to 55, and then begin a gradual decline until death. Thurstone's verbal PMA, which Schaie labels "verbal meaning," measured by various tests of vocabulary, is the most robust ability, continuing to develop well into the age 50s and resisting significant decline until sometime in the 60s. In contrast, "word fluency," measured as the ability to learn new associations between words, related semantically or not, and the ability for rapid recall of words belonging to a certain category, tends to peak earlier, perhaps in the early 40s, and decline earlier and more rapidly. Gender effects are obvious in the longitudinal data, favoring women on verbal meaning and inductive reasoning tasks, and men on spatial orientation and number tasks. This work is important in that neurobehavioral evaluators, working in neuroanesthesiology contexts where patient cohorts may vary widely in terms of chronologic age or in terms of gender ratios, may have to consider these dimensions as confounding variables when analyzing data.

Neuropsychological Tests and Primary Mental Abilities

The neuropsychological battery of tests used in ordinary clinical contexts which require comprehensive evaluation of memory, motor, sensory, perceptual, and reasoning abilities are extensive, time-consuming, and labor-intensive. It is not uncommon for the HRNTB to require 6 to 8 h to administer and score. This time frame might be much longer and extended over a period of days when the examinee is sufficiently impaired so as to tolerate only brief testing periods at any one sitting. The time taken to understand the output protocol and to write a comprehensive report summarizing findings in a format understandable to persons who might have limited knowledge of neuropsychological constructs results sometimes in an investment of 10 to 12 h until the report is logged into the medical record.

Few tests of the HRNTB match the PMA prototypes. Rather, many of the HRNTB tests developed out of a neurological tradition and measure pure motor fluency (index finger tapping), pure motor strength (grip strength measured with a dynamometer), pure sensory-perceptual acuity (finger recognition), sensory-perceptual acuity with a cognitive component in which a verbal label must be selected to match haptic or acoustic input (fingertip number writing, tactile form recognition, speech sounds perception), spatial pattern recognition in which the input is either haptic (Tactual Form Recognition Test) or visual (Trail Making Test) and the output is motor, cognitive reasoning (Category Test), and aphasia (Reitan-Indiana Aphasia Screening Test).

The Luria-Nebraska Neuropsychological Battery (LNNB) is another test that has evolved out of the neurological tradition.[29] The LNNB is composed of 269 specific tests, grouped into purported ability scales. The Motor Scale comprises items of motor coordination and speed, but also items requiring praxis to verbal command or visual model. The Tactile Scale requires tactile category discriminations and pure sensory acuity. The Visual Scale requires tests of gnosis, but also circular clock-reading and directional tasks. Receptive Speech items test phoneme recognition and language comprehension. Expressive Speech items test word articulation and language fluency. Writing items test the motor aspects of written language. Reading items require letter recognition and reading comprehension. Arithmetic items test the recognition of mathematical signs and basic arithmetic skills. Memory items measure immediate and short-term memory for verbal and nonverbal input. Intellectual Processes items measure concept formation. Scale scores are combined to yield an overall measure of brain dysfunction labeled the Pathognomonic Scale. A Left Hemisphere Scale and a Right Hemisphere Scale are derived from tests of purported sensory-motor strip functioning.

Neuroanesthesiology research projects that require an assessment of some PMAs seldom provide a clinical context for a comprehensive neuropsychological study. In these instances, specific tests are chosen from the various test batteries in common use or from an array of other tests derived from the psychometric tradition. Many of Thurstone's original 56 tests provide prototype tests of mental functions of particular interest to neurobehavioral evaluators in neuroanesthesiology settings. Although there is no consensus about which tests best canvas the PMAs in neuroanesthesiology practice where only limited evaluation times are common, some tests are used frequently.

Verbal meaning is considered an important ability, as the vocabulary tests used as markers reflect educational attainment and experience in a social world where language facility is an important adaptation tool. Vocabulary attainment is also usually insensitive to the effect of brain injury and under many circumstances can be used as an index of premorbid intellectual-cognitive status. Parallel forms, equal in level of difficulty, are simple to construct using the vocabulary subtest of the WAIS-R, which lists words in increasing order of difficulty. Using the 40 words from the WAIS-R, four parallel 10-word tests of equal difficulty can be constructed with no overlapping words. Scoring of answers is usually straightforward, with high levels of inter-rater reliability. Test-retest reliability estimates are usually very high, even over extended periods between testing occasions. In a review of 11 studies, Matarazzo and coworkers[30] report a median test-retest reliability, over retest intervals of 1 to 416 weeks, of .85 for vocabulary. Wechsler[19] reports a vocabulary reliability of .94 for 18- to 19-year-olds, .95 for 25- to 34-year-olds, and .96 for 45- to 54-year-olds. A multiple-choice version, as found in the Wechsler Adult Intelligence Scale–Revised, Neuropsychological Instrument (WAIS-RNI), can be substituted when an oral model of response is not possible, or if the respondent suffers from a word-finding deficit as opposed to a word-meaning deficit. As vocabulary tests are robust, they might be insensitive to subtle effects of brain impairment and might underestimate the degree of disability acquired as a result of surgery, anesthetic, or some other condition of interest in neuroanesthesiology. When vocabulary ability is impaired and not an artifact of anomia, word-finding deficit, or some other condition masquerading as a vocabulary deficit, the clinical condition of the respondent is likely to be very impaired and other, "neighborhood" signs of impairment are often obvious.

Word fluency measures are also common in neuroanesthesiology applications. Tests of word fluency are related to tests of verbal ability like vocabulary, but are much more sensitive to the effects of aging, transient impairment of attention, concentration, memory, or other factors that result in more chronic language dysfunction. As fluency of oral speech is an important adaptation tool, tests of word fluency of varius sorts are often included even in short neurobehavioral batteries. The Controlled Oral Word Fluency Test[31] requires the respondent to recall as many words as possible, each within a 1-min time span, for the letters F, A, and S. Parallel forms are possible using nearly any letter of the alphabet. As some letters consistently result in more word retrievals than others, care must be taken to assure equality of difficulty across forms. Scoring is simple, requiring only tabulation of words that "count," that is, words that begin with the designated letter, are not plurals (if the singular form has been given) or proper names, or words beginning with the same prefix. Rules can be relaxed or tightened to fit particular requirements of the testing circumstances. Inter-rater reliability is quite high. Test-retest reliability, under the same or similar testing circumstances, is also high, but can vary considerably depending upon intervening historical or maturational variables. Olin and Zelinski[32] report a 12-month test-retest reliability of .89 for 60 normal elderly persons with an average age of 71. The F-A-S test is much more sensitive to disruptive effects on brain function than are tests of verbal ability like the vocabulary test. The F-A-S test is also quite sensitive to attention problems and disruptive mood states, sometimes making it difficult to determine what factors influence performance downward. Other tests of verbal fluency include word finding to specified categories—for example, animals in a zoo, articles of clothing, things in a grocery store, synonyms, or antonyms. Speed of response is crucial in word fluency tests, whether they are oral, written, or recognition tests. Any factor that can disrupt speed of responding can disrupt language fluency tests.

Pure motor skills, although not "mental" abilities, per se, are often included in neurobehavioral batteries. Tests of finger dexterity, for example, are easy to administer and are very sensitive to any condition that impairs the sensorium. They are reasonable surrogate measures of general alertness, sometimes preferred to clinical estimates of intactness of sensorium, because they can be precisely quantified. They can also be used as covariates for other more complicated tests involving a combination of mental abilities when the investigator wants to partial out variance possibly attributable to motor speed. The Finger Oscillation Test (FOT), a simple test of index finger-tapping speed, is commonly used to map, bilaterally, fine motor dexterity. Typically, a number of trials, two or more, of 10 seconds each are allowed for the index finger of each hand on a standardized finger-tapping apparatus. Reitan's criterion for stability of measurement is the average of five consecutive trials that differ by no more than five taps. Other investigators simply average tapping speed over two or more trials for each hand. Inter-rater reliability estimates are typically quite high, as the instrumentation for measurement is highly standardized and permits little variation across examiners. With minimum historical or maturational events intervening between retests, test-retest reliability can be expected to be reasonable, although the test is sensitive to many nonspecific effects and wide performance variation is possible. Cronbach[27] reports test-retest reliability correlation over one to four years from .59 to .72. When a simple "cognitive" dimension is added to a motor speed task, such as in letter cancellation tests (e.g., the respondent is confronted with a paper upon which letters are scattered about and is instructed to use a pencil to strike through as many of a certain letter as can be found in a certain time frame), the test is considered to be one of "attention," "vigilance," or "perceptual speed," thought also to be surrogate measures of intactness of sensorium.[33] When comprehensive neuropsychological evaluation is required, if the respondent does sufficiently poorly on tasks such as letter cancellation, often more detailed evaluation is delayed until clinical status improves. Individuals who perform poorly on simple tests purportedly of sustained attention tend generally to do poorly across the board, and the informational yield of extensive testing is nullified.

Numeric ability is important, as keeping track of the quantity of things is obviously an important adaptation requirement. A test of arithmetic competency is standard in intellectual evaluations and is highly determined by academic classroom experience. Inter-rater reliability estimates of most arithmetic tests are very high, as tests are highly standardized. Parallel forms are simple to devise. Test-retest reliability estimates are also high, as the test is saturated with educational attainment and general intelligence variance. Wechsler[19] reports arithmetic test-retest reliability of .79 for 18- to 19-year-olds, .81 for 25- to 34-year-olds, and .86 for 45- to 54-year-olds. Matarazzo and associates[30] report a median test-retest reliability of .74 when retest intervals vary from 1 to 416 weeks. Test-retest reliability estimated on young persons still learning arithmetic skills will reflect continuing learning and be lower than estimates drawn on persons no longer in learning environments. Digit recall, forward and backward, is a test of number facility which merges into a memory test. Test-retest reliability tends to vary widely, as tests of digit span are highly sensitive to any distractor that influences sustained attention and to any factor that influences memory abilities, per se. Matarazzo and associates[30] report a median test-retest reliability estimate of .79, and Youngjohn and coworkers' estimate[34] is .73 over a 13- to 41-day interval for 115 normal, highly educated volunteers ranging in age from 17 to 82. Wechsler[19] reports a coefficient of .71 for 18- to 19-year-olds and .66 for 25- to 54-year-olds.

Memory tasks are considered essential in most neuropsychological applications. Without an intact memory ability, individuals are locked into an experiential world without object constancy or a sense of history. The influence of a poor memory upon the conduct of lives is immeasurable, so great attention is paid by test constructors and investigators to include at least one, but preferably many, measures of memory in test batteries. Memory tests vary widely in terms of content domain and in retrieval process parameters. Verbal, visual, symbolic, and tactual content are highly variable, with process requirements varied between recognition and recall, and time spans from immediate to delayed, over various intervals. Word fluency tasks such as the F-A-S have memory components, as do vocabulary and arithmetic tasks, as memory is an ubiquitous requirement for nearly all perceptual and cognitive tasks. Memory tasks can also consume considerable testing time; tests of delayed recall are very sensitive to conditions that compromise brain function, whereas tests of immediate memory may not be as sensitive. Encoding and retrieval are different aspects of memory function and are considered by some to be best measured with different tasks. To test delayed recall, at a minimum, requires 30-min intervals between memory trials. When multiple content domains are surveyed, testing time can be extensive. Youngjohn and associates[34] studied various memory tests, from novel computerized tests to standard, manual tests used commonly in clinical situations. A number of their novel computerized tests are very interesting. As an example, a test of memory of oral prose listened to while engaging in a distracting motor task (i.e., listening to a weathercast while engaging in a simulated automobile driving task) produced a test-retest reliability coefficient of .72. This test is purported to correlate with other tests of verbal memory. A test of "misplaced objects," which requires respondents to "hide" objects in different rooms of a house and then locate them again after a delay of about 40 min, yielded a test-retest correlation of .78. This test is purported to correlate with others that measure a "verbal-visual associative memory" ability. A novel test of facial memory, purportedly a test of visual memory, produced a test-retest correlation of .60 for immediate memory and .18 for memory delayed for 40 min. A traditional measure of memory of oral prose, the ability to remember stories involving some action scene (e.g., a women robbed of money who reports it to police; an ocean liner which sinks during a storm), produced a test-retest reliability coefficient of .55. Another traditional test of verbal associative memory, which requires the respondent to learn associations between words, some of which are related semantically (e.g., east-west) and some of which are not (e.g., gold-walk), produced a test-retest correlation of .72. Benson's Visual Retention Test,[35] a traditional test of visual memory, produced a test-retest reliability coefficient of .57 for number correct.

Chelune and coworkers[36] examined the Wechsler Memory Scale–Revised, a standard clinical measure, with 136 epilepsy patients, some of whom underwent temporal lobectomies, over about a 10-month retest interval. Test-retest correlations were consistent for general memory (.84), verbal memory (.83), visual memory (.81), and delayed recall (.81). Clearly, some memory tests are preferable to others as stability over test occasions is important. Low test-retest reliability coefficients, especially if historical and maturational variables are minimal, suggest that the test is especially prone to statistical regression artifact. This is a prime concern of Olin and Zelinski[32] in their assessment of Folstein's Mini-Mental Status Examination (MMSE), a test in common use in psychiatric settings.

Thurstone's spatial factor is tapped by many different tests of visual-perceptual or tactual content. Knowing where one is in space or how to analyze a spatial configuration for purposes of identification is an important perceptual ability with considerable adaptation significance. Some tests require a simple "choice" to be made as an output parameter (e.g., recognizing letters in inverted position or degraded in some way; counting the number of sides a geometric solid might have when some sides are hidden from view). Many other tests of spatial-perceptual ability require a speeded motor output and are referred to as visuomotor tests. The WAIS has a number of tests of spatial ability. The Block Design Test requires the respondent to construct geometric patterns from blocks, which are variously colored, to match a two-dimensional picture. Matarazzo and associates[30] report a median test-retest reliability coefficient of .76 for Block Design. Wechsler[19] reports coefficients of .86, .83, and .82 for his three age groups, 18 to 19, 25 to 34, and 45 to 54, respectively. The Object Assembly Test is a simple picture puzzle type test which requires the respondent to recognize a familiar pattern (e.g., a manikin, a face, a hand, and an elephant) when presented in disassembled form, and then to reassemble the pattern. Some respondents assemble the pattern without ever recognizing it in terms of being able to give it a verbal label, yet others recognize the pattern, but cannot assemble it. Matarazzo and associates[30] report a median test-retest reliability of .73 for Object Assembly. Wechsler[19] reports coefficients of .65, .68, and .71 for groups with increasing ages. The Digit Symbol Test (DST) is complicated in that a combination of PMAs is required for fluent completion. The test requires the respondent to learn associations between numbers from 1 to 9 and symbols like a hyphen, circle, or X. Working from a model, the respondent fills in boxes with the symbol that corresponds to each number in an associated box. Spatial patterns must be differentiated, numbers must be distinguished, associations must be learned, calligraphy must be sufficient to render drawings recognizable,

and perceptual-motor speed is necessary to complete the task quickly. Matarazzo and associates[30] report a median test-retest correlation of .80 for DST. Youngjohn and associates[34] criticize the DST as a test with little "face" or "ecologic" validity, but credit it as a test with considerable test-retest reliability (.88). Wechsler[19] reports a reliability coefficient of .92 for 18- to 19-year-old subjects.

Reasoning tests vary in difficulty from simple to very complex across instruments, and even on items within the same instrument. Reasoning tests are the most "face-valid" tests of "general" intelligence as they require mental operations consistent with common ideas as to what constitutes "intelligent" behavior. Raven's Progressive Matrices Test (RPMT) is a reasoning test developed more than 50 years ago, yet it is still very popular.[27] The RPMT requires the respondent to see relationships among two-dimensional analogy problems. A pattern design with a missing detail is presented, with multiple options permitted as selections to complete the pattern. Specific conceptual principles define options across items. The principles vary systematically in difficulty, as the respondent progresses through the test. Parallel forms are simple to construct. The RPMT is an excellent component in a neurobehavioral test battery, as it is highly correlated with measures of general intelligence, even in samples of persons varying widely in terms of primary language use, reading ability, or educational level. The Wisconsin Card Sorting Test (WCST) is of more recent development and requires the respondent to induce principles permitting correct sorts of stimulus cards with targets that vary, singly or in various combinations, on three dimensions, color, form, and number.[37] The examiner rewards matches on a particular dimension up to a certain number, and then repeatedly shifts to another principle which is to be discovered as the "correct" principle. Respondents who perform poorly on the test "perseverate" a sorting principle long after it has been declared inapplicable by the examiner, or "fail to maintain" a cognitive set defining a correct sorting principle throughout the full series where it could apply correctly. Respondents who do well maintain and shift cognitive sets in response to feedback from the examiner as to the appropriateness of their choices. Numerous "scores" can be computed from the WCST, any of which might be a sensitive measure for neurobehavioral evaluation purposes.

Common Issues in Neurobehavioral Evaluation in Neuroanesthesiology

Although tests used by neurobehavioral evaluators working in clinical practice settings might be quite different from those used in clinical research settings, neurobehavioral evaluators in either setting work similarly. The primary diagnostic function of neurobehavioral evaluation is the precise measurement of motor, sensory, or cognitive phenomena considered important in the fine-grained, clinical diagnostic articulation of neurological disease or disorder. In the clinical practice setting, labor-intensive, comprehensive measurement of many brain-behavior relationships permits the assessment of the strengths and weaknesses of the individual case to be compared with normative standards of persons of similar gender, age, and education. Deviations from normative expectations permit diagnostic speculation of brain dysfunction lateralized or localized to specific brain areas probabilistically associated with similar patterns of deficit. Patterns of neurobehavioral deficit, recognizable to the trained clinician as coherent or internally consistent patterns, provide the basis for treatment planning to remediate deficits or to educate family members of affected persons about reasonable expectations for recovery or sustained difficulties to which they may have to adapt along with their affected family member. In the clinical research setting, precise measurement is no less important, but may be limited to specific brain-behavior functions thought to be crucial to the clinical process under investigation. Diagnostic ramifications may be less important in the research setting, giving way to concerns about accurate measurement of immediate effect or longer-term change. In the clinical practice setting, knowledge of experimental design and statistics may be relatively unimportant, whereas in the clinical research setting, knowledge of the scientific basis of practice may be crucial in guiding conclusions about safety and risk of experimental procedures.

CLINICAL CASE EXAMPLE

In the clinical setting, the neurobehavioral evaluator may be asked to determine if a patient's presenting complaints can be documented with standardized tests when they might not be obvious in an ordinary clinical workup. Results from such an evaluation might have considerable consequence with regard to vocational rehabilitation planning or disability determination. Such was the case when a young man presented to his family practice doctor with a complaint of headache and a concern about arithmetic and concentration errors he was making on his job. Neither the headache, nor the errors were typical for him. He became frightened that something was seriously wrong, and he was beginning to lose confidence in himself and his ability to succeed in his job. Neurological examination was essentially within normal limits, but his complaints about new onset headache were persistent and he was referred to neuroradiology for computerized tomogra-

phy scanning of his head. A large pituitary tumor was revealed, radiation and surgical treatment were recommended, and he was referred for a comprehensive neuropsychological assessment to establish a pretreatment baseline.

The neurobehavioral assessment battery used in this case included the WAIS-R to document general intellectual ability. The WAIS-R includes 11 subtests, 6 mediated by language used to compute a "Verbal Intelligence Quotient" (VIQ), and 5 visuomotor tests used to compute a "Performance Intelligence Quotient" (PIQ). All 11 subtests contribute to an overall "Full Scale Intelligence Quotient" (FSIQ). Various of the subtests are also used as markers of PMAs. The Information, Vocabulary, and Comprehension subtests assess verbal meaning; DST, Arithmetic, and Digit Span assess numerical ability; Block Design, Object Assembly, and Picture Arrangement assess spatial ability or perceptual scanning ability. The WCST was used to assess reasoning, and the Trail Making Test (TMT) to assess spatial ability and perceptual-motor speed. In the TMT-A, the patient scans an array of scattered numbers and connects them in consecutive order. In TMT-B, the patient scans an array of scattered numbers and letters and connects them in a consecutive alphanumeric sequence, 1-A-2-B-3-C, and so on. The FOT was used as a measure of motor fluency. The F-A-S was used to assess verbal fluency. The WMS was used to assess memory functions. The Clinical Analysis Questionnaire (CAQ) was used to document personality characteristics.[38] The same battery (i.e., the tests described in Table 9-1 and others not listed as they do not contribute new information to the discussion) was used to document neurobehavioral status at one year and three years after surgery and radiation treatment.

The value of a comprehensive neurobehavioral evaluation is demonstrated by this case. On the "intelligence" measures, a clear trend in an improved ability to think and problem-solve is indicated. Although changes may not be significant in a statistical sense, this trend is reflected in the PMAs of verbal meaning and verbal fluency, number, and reasoning. The reasoning test is especially impressive. Spatial and motor tests suggest performance stability in these areas. Memory tests, however, tell a different story. Immediate memory scores reflect attention and concentration and are essentially unimpaired. Delayed memory scores, however, are truer tests of ability to store information to provide a sense of familiarity and history. Prior to surgery and radiation treatment, delayed memory scores are within normal limits, with very little erosion noted over an approximate 30-min delay. After treatment, however, nearly 100 percent erosion is noted for both oral prose and figural memory (savings scores nearly 0 percent). The implications of this find-

TABLE 9-1
Neurobehavioral Psychometric Tests That Documented Clinical Status before Surgical Resection and Radiation Treatment of a Large Pituitary Tumor and at One and Three Years after Treatment

Primary Mental Ability	Marker Test	Pretreatment Scores	One Year Posttreatment	Three Years Posttreatment
Verbal				
Meaning	Vocabulary	9	10	10
	Comprehension	10	11	10
	Information	9	8	9
Fluency	F-A-S	34	32	39
Number	Arithmetic	7	6	10
	Digit Span	9	10	12
	Digit Symbol	11	10	10
Motor	Finger-Tapping	51	48	48
Spatial	Block Design	11	12	11
	Object Assembly	12	12	10
	Picture Arrangement	11	13	15
	Trails-A	23	30	32
	Trails-B	59	62	59
Reasoning	WCST			
	Conceptual Level %	52	66	86
	Perseverative Responses	25	25	5
	Trials to Completion	128	128	86
Memory	Oral Prose (OP)	19	11	13
	Word Associates (WA)	10	7	7
	Figures* (F)	14	14	38
	Delayed OP	14	0	1
	Delayed WA	10	8	7
	Delayed F*	11	0	0
Intelligence	VIQ	91	93	100
	PIQ	108	110	114
	FSIQ	97	99	106
Personality	Social Interest	4.25	5.00	4.25
	Emotionality	7.25	5.25	2.50
	Experimenting	4.00	3.50	4.00
	Trusting	5.00	4.67	4.67
	Depression	8.00	4.50	4.00
	Irrationality	7.25	5.00	5.25

* Same figural memory test used for pretreatment and one-year posttreatment. Different test used for three-year posttreatment.

ing for this young man are substantial. Although he was remarkable in his adaptation to his memory deficit, noted here as positive changes in Emotionality, Depression, and Irrationality on his personality test, he is essentially totally disabled in his ability to return to his former employment capacity or to learn any new vocation that requires memory of cognitive information, verbal or figural. He had attempted to remediate his cognitive skills by auditing classes in a local university. Although immediate learning was unimpaired and he could not be distinguished from other students on casual observation by his teachers, he performed very poorly on academic examinations which required delayed recall of information. Thus, both aspects of real life performance, retained ability to learn and lost ability to remember, are reflected in this comprehensive neurobehavioral evaluation.

RESEARCH EXAMPLE

In the research setting, precise measurement of targeted neurobehavioral abilities and knowledge of research design and data analysis are essential.[39] "Mental status" is an important consideration whenever risk and outcome from surgical procedures that employ anesthetics are assessed. Mental status, however, is usually defined poorly in ordinary clinical situations. A popular scale measuring degree of "alertness," from "comatose" to "fully alert and oriented," is often the only measure of mental status recorded for medico-

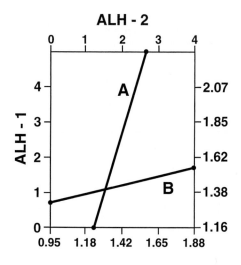

A = Regression line showing
best prediction from
pre-test to post-test
.227 ALH-1 + 1.164 = ALH-2

B = Regression line showing
best prediction from
post-test to pre-test
.234 ALH-2 + 0.948 = ALH-1

A

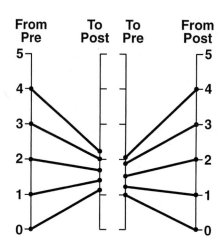

$r_{(ALH\text{-}1 \text{ and } ALH\text{-}2)} = .230$

ALH = Associate Learning-
Hard Word Pairs

B

Figure 9-3   Forward (pretest to posttest) and backward (posttest to pretest) prediction demonstrates statistical regression artifact from unreliable tests with poor test-retest correlation coefficients.

legal documenting purposes. Scales like Folstein's MMSE are both simple and multidimensional, so that many abilities are measured poorly, and no ability is measured well. If changes occur on such multidimensional tests of mental status, it is impossible to determine what PMA has been affected, positively or negatively, and to differentiate "real" change from artifactual change induced by measurement unreliability. Experience from our laboratory in measuring effects on "mental status" of surgical procedures requiring coronary artery bypass grafting (CABG) is illustrative.

In a series of 38, male, cardiovascular, surgical cases requiring CABG, eight tests were used to document mental status (Folstein's MMSE, Trails A and B, FOT, Associate Learning [of words not related semantically], DST, Vocabulary, and F-A-S). Each person was assessed immediately presurgery, approximately one week postsurgery, and approximately 6 weeks postsurgery.[40] Seven-day, test-retest correlations ranged from .23 for the semantically-unrelated word pairs of the Associate Learning task to .92 for the DST.

Forward (pretest or posttest) and backward (posttest to pretest) prediction demonstrates that tests with poor test-retest reliability produce change scores that are unreliable because of the confounding effect of statistical regression.[24] Using data from the unrelated word pairs of the Associate Learning task, Fig. 9-3A demon-

strates the classical configuration of forward and backward regression lines that obtains when an unreliable test is used. The two regression lines are very dissimilar in terms of slope. The statistical regression for categories of pre and post scores is demonstrated in Fig. 9-3B, where a classical "fanlike" configuration (i.e., the "smart" get "duller" and the "dull" get "smarter") obtains with unreliable tests. Youngjohn and associates[34] report a test-retest correlation of .72 for an Associate Learning test similar to that reported here, where a correlation of .23 was found. The Youngjohn test differs in an important respect, however, in that "easy" words (i.e., words related semantically) were used as well as words not semantically related. Only "hard" word pairs were reported by Mitzel and coworkers,[40] because the "easy" word pairs seldom were missed by any respondent. When all words are used, inflated test-retest correlations can be found. Although more "reliable" in that respondents maintain their approximate rank orders across testing trials, less pre-post change is observed, and effects of independent variables are very likely to be underestimated.

Using data from the DST, Fig. 9-4A reflects the similarity between forward and backward regression lines that obtains when reliable tests are used. The lines are very similar in slope and nearly overlapping. As test-retest correlations diverge, so too do the regression lines diverge from each other. Figure 9-4B demon-

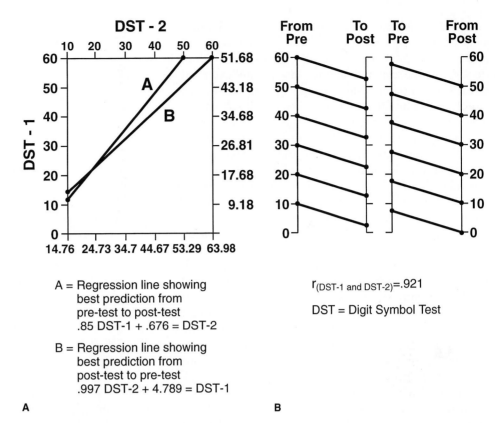

Figure 9-4 Forward (pretest to posttest) and backward (posttest to pretest) prediction demonstrates that reliable tests with good test-retest correlation coefficients produce change scores free of statistical regression artifact.

A = Regression line showing best prediction from pre-test to post-test
.85 DST-1 + .676 = DST-2

B = Regression line showing best prediction from post-test to pre-test
.997 DST-2 + 4.789 = DST-1

$r_{(DST\text{-}1 \text{ and } DST\text{-}2)}=.921$

DST = Digit Symbol Test

strates the classical, parallel shape of regression lines from categorical scores when going in either a forward or a backward prediction direction. Slopes are negative when scores decrease, on average, from pretest to posttest. Thus, Matarazzo and associates,[30] Youngjohn and coworkers,[34] Wechsler,[19] and Mitzel and others[40] all produced findings with the DST that suggest good psychometric properties, recommending its use in clinical research settings where brief, targeted, "cognitive" measures are needed. The DST is complicated in that it is not a "pure" test of a single PMA. This is the basis of Youngjohn's criticism that the DST lacks "ecologic" validity. As a general measure of "mental status," however, with implications for prediction of performance on other lengthier tests or on comprehensive batteries, the DST is likely to perform excellently, as regression artifact should not be a consideration.

Clinical research investigators seldom choose tests specifically because they are purported to measure particular PMAs. In many cases, change scores across various dimensions vary widely. When this happens, the investigator is hard pressed to determine which test to "believe" in terms of representing the effect of the independent variable or experimental condition under investigation. Factor analysis can sometimes be helpful in defining root abilities that link performance on various of the tests used in any study. Assuming the conditions for a proper factor analysis have been met, scores

on various tests can be summed to reflect the root ability. Psychometric properties of the derived test scores should be improved, as increased test "length" or increased number of observations of an ability usually improves reliability of measurement. The Mitzel and associates data[40] are illustrative.

Principal components analysis is one method of determining the root factors that explain variance in a correlation matrix that summarizes the interrelationships among various tests.[41] Prior to factor analysis, transformation of the raw scores to stanine scores permits easy summing of scores to derive root measures. Transforming of scores also eliminates influence of "metric" and normalizes distributions so that artifactual factors will not be "discovered."[42] Characteristically, only root dimensions that reach a certain size as indicated by their "eigen" values are considered. When Mitzel and associates' seven baseline measures[40] are analyzed, two factors, rotated to orthogonal simple structure, are suggested. All tests but FOT "load" the first factor and only FOT loads the second. The first root dimension can be labeled a "general cognitive" factor, while the second can be labeled a "motor fluency" factor.

A common factor labeled "g" is consistently derived from factor analyses of batteries of cognitive tests.[27] The attribute of persons that purportedly contributes to the generation of "g" is commonly referred to as "general intelligence." "g" theorists propose that persons who do well on one kind of cognitive task will also do well on others. Conversely, people who do not do well on one kind of cognitive task are not expected to do well on others. Measures of "g" can be derived simply as arithmetic sums of scores on all subtests of a battery after transforming scores to a common metric and demonstrating through a factor analytic process that a common factor is derivable. Individuals can then be studied on a longitudinal basis to determine if their "mental capacity" has changed as a result of experimental circumstances. The Mitzel and coworkers[40] study is illustrative of this process.

A common factor "general cognition" is derivable by adding scores on six subtests used by Mitzel (Associate Learning is dropped because of poor test-retest reliability; MMSE is dropped because its distribution could not be normalized) after transforming scores to stanines, subtest by subtest. Raw scores on each subtest are pooled for all three test occasions and each score in the aggregate pool is transformed on a common stanine metric. Mean scores on the three test occasions (pre-CABG, immediately post-CABG, and six-week follow-up CABG) are determined. Baseline mean is 5.224 for the 38 subjects. Postsurgical mean is 4.719, and follow-up mean is 5.404. The postsurgical mean is significantly lower than either the baseline mean (t = 4.668) or the follow-up mean (t = 7.015). The baseline mean does not differ significantly from the follow-up mean (t = 1.727). The test-retest correlation between baseline and postsurgery is .91; between baseline and follow-up is .927; and between postsurgery and follow-up is .906. A conclusion drawn from analysis of mean differences attributable to time of testing is that surgery appears to depress cognitive functioning in the week immediately following the surgery, but the effect is eliminated by six weeks, as the group returns to baseline. A conclusion drawn from analysis of test-retest correlations is that the rank order of individuals appears to be essentially unaffected by the surgery or follow-up period. The "smarter" subjects at baseline tend to remain so throughout the longitudinal series and the "duller" subjects retain their relative rank throughout the follow-up period.

Figure 9-5 is a graphic depiction of how the 38 men undergoing the CABG procedure fare from baseline to six-week follow-up. This graph depicts what is considered to be a "stable" phenomenon reflecting group "change" and somewhat less stable, but still reliable, indicators of individual fluctuations (i.e., intraindividual variability rather than intraindividual change) about the group trend line. The slope of the regression line suggests that a stable group trend has occurred, with modest intraindividual fluctuations on a highly reliable test. The intraindividual fluctuations are

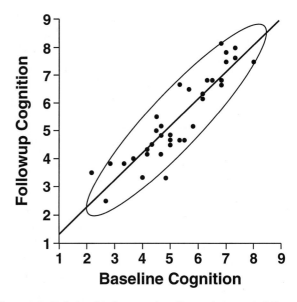

Figure 9-5 Relationship between baseline and six-week follow-up scores on a reliable measure of general cognitive ability for 38 men undergoing coronary artery bypass grafting.

densely packed about the group trend line with only two outliers obvious, as the pretest score is highly predictive of the follow-up score. One of the outliers is in the left tail of the graph suggesting that a "dull" person, although still dull at follow-up, became somewhat less dull than was predicted for him. The second outlier is at the sample mean at pretest and appears to have declined after the surgery, as he does not return to the baseline predicted for him. The first case "changes" less than one standard deviation of what is predicted for him, but the second case "changes" slightly more than one standard deviation. In this research situation, the two outliers are simply considered examples of intraindividual variability somewhat more extreme than is characteristic of the majority of cases studied. If this was a clinical situation, however, the second case would be under consideration as having suffered somehow from the surgical procedure. Although many cases do not perform as well at follow-up as they did at baseline, changes are small and within expectations given ordinary intraindividual fluctuations. The rather large fluctuation or "change" for the single negative outlier might require the clinician to examine this case further for possible neuropsychological compromise. Without the rather sophisticated analysis of change scores from a scientific research perspective, however, it would be impossible for the clinician to have identified this single individual as a person who may be at risk for neurobehavioral deficit. Thus, the concept of "intraindividual variability" would adequately explain results of this study for the neurobehavioral scientist. But the neurobehavioral clinician would be interested in the concept of "intraindividual change" as a risk management consideration. Resolution of the two perspectives in a single study such as this one is difficult.

Summary

Neurology and psychology approach the mind-body problem from different theoretical perspectives, with different practical implications for the problem of scientific measurement and clinical application. Neurology has focused on the material aspects of brain and brain function, measuring size, gross anatomy, and electrophysiologic properties of brain as a functioning biologic system, with a historical scientific aim to understand basic biologic function and a historical clinical aim to understand disease process. Psychology has focused on the immaterial aspects of brain, measuring immanent aspects of brain function observable in the realm of mind or consciousness, with a historical scientific aim of discovering how sensory information is transformed into "knowledge" and a historical clinical aim to understand psychopathology or distorted knowledge. Behavioral neurology and neuropsychology are intermediate disciplines shared by neurologists and psychologists interested in scientific and clinical neuroscience. Neurobehavioral evaluation is a generic term to characterize the measurement strategies common to scientists and clinicians working in these intermediate disciplines.

Psychophysics was perhaps the earliest neurobehavioral discipline. Biologically oriented psychologists with strong backgrounds in experimental, laboratory psychology set the tone for the importance of a scientific background necessary to plan, conduct, and interpret sound studies emphasizing controlled, precise measurement strategies. Behavioral psychology was also scientistic in its orientation and emphasized the importance of operational definition of constructs as manifest behavior, and eschewed hypothetical, "mentalistic" notions. Although impressionistic psychologists interested in nonobservable, mentalistic notions never conceded to the behaviorists, the recent emergence of "cognitive" psychology represents a kind of revival of a mentalist tradition, more or less acceptable to the behaviorist camp. This is partly because the development of statistics, the wedding of statistical concepts to the experimental laboratory, and the application of laboratory approaches to clinical problems altered the earliest mentalist approaches, establishing the scientific method as a preferred means of neurobehavioral investigation.

The tradition of individual psychological assessment, or individual differences, has a long history,

the modern features of which include measurement of aptitudes and skills (such as might be useful in occupational endeavors) and of intelligence (useful in predicting success in academic pursuits). Such assessment originates with Darwinian concepts of adaptation and change and is obviously important in predicting "survival" in various social and clinical settings. Its scientific emphasis is perhaps less than that of other psychological specialties and its practical or clinical applications perhaps more than that of other psychological specialties. Although obvious in other psychology traditions, it is within the tradition of individual psychological assessment that the symbiotic model, of the scientific laboratory interfacing with clinical practice, is most apparent.

The essential aim of scientific psychology is the advancement of psychological theory. Scientific inferences are drawn from generally small samples and generalized to larger populations, resulting in theoretical "laws" once sufficient replications of the inference accumulate. The credibility of the inference rests on conditions internal to the design of experiments used to produce it. The essential aim of individual assessment psychology, however, is inductive in nature. Observations are made on single individuals with an intention to place the individual in the context of a population ordered with respect to some attribute of interest. The reliability and validity of the assessment instruments must be known in advance and standardized or normed on populations to which the individual belongs. The normative data function as the control group in the scientific tradition.

Scientific research in the clinical situation requires the incorporation of scientific and individual assessment objectives and methodologies. A research clinician may want to know if a treatment has an outcome for a particular group (a question of generalizability) and also may want to know if the outcome was realized for specific individuals (a question of assessment). These questions are often difficult to answer within any particular study, whether the study is of a single individual or of groups of individuals. It is the complexity of this sometimes incompatibility that the bulk of this chapter addresses.

No particular approach dominates the neurobehavioral landscape. Clinical neurobehavioral measurement approaches vary from fixed, standardized batteries emphasizing patterns of numerical output as preferred bases for induction, to fluid, ad hoc batteries designed to mirror the theoretical expectations of each individual examinee and emphasizing the process by which problems are solved as the preferred unit of observation. The statistical procedure of factor analysis proposes cognitive abilities as latent traits which can be measured in the individual assessment tradition.

Most neuropsychology test batteries will canvas at least six purported primary mental abilities derived as a result of factor analysis: verbal meaning, word fluency, number, spatial, memory, and reasoning. One structure of intellect model characterizes intelligence as five types of mental operation, three types of mental content, and six kinds of mental product, yielding a scheme capable of classifying tests into 120 different types. Few neuropsychology tasks are pure measures of a single primary mental ability and most are measures of various combinations of primary mental abilities. Profiles of primary mental abilities vary among individuals, with age, gender, and educational backgrounds important causal or confounding influences. Often, in the individual case, primary mental abilities must be broadly and redundantly canvased to permit valid clinical conclusions to be drawn about pathologic brain function. A clinical case example is provided, demonstrating that the structure of a young man's intellect remained essentially intact after a neurosurgical procedure, except for the primary mental ability of memory, which was devastated in his case, with grave prognostic implications for his subsequent adaptational capability. Many intelligence theorists emphasize "g" or a broad, general attribute by which persons can be ordered. Factor analysis can be used to produce "g" factors which can be highly statistically reliable and, therefore, excellent probes for neurobehavioral research. A research example is provided to demonstrate how a broad general cognitive measure was used to track the cognitive behavioral outcomes of men who underwent coronary artery bypass grafting.

Neurobehaviorists working in neuroanesthesiology settings may have many research and clinical objectives. The essential objective, however, is to produce and apply rigorously reliable and valid psychometric tests in individual clinical or clinical research settings to help neuroanesthesiologists to make the kinds of decisions necessary to, and to understand the effects of, the treatments they apply in research or clinical contexts. The evaluation of pharmacologic anesthetic agents and adjuvants, and of immediate, transitory, or residual effects of medical procedures such as neurosurgery are examples. The information generated by neurobehaviorists may help to characterize the behavioral implications of neurological diagnoses, to monitor the trajectory of cognitive recovery after injury or treatment, and to educate patients, family, or professionals about treatment needs or adaptational limitations of affected individuals.

Neurobehavioral evaluation is both a scientific and clinical skill. Rigorous training in neuroscience and supervised experience in clinical applications are essential prerequisites to success in neurobehavioral projects.

References

1. Watson RI: *The Great Psychologists: From Aristotle to Freud.* Philadelphia, JB Lippincott, 1968.
2. James W: *The Principles of Psychology.* Cambridge MA, Harvard University Press, 1983.
3. Lachman R, et al: *Cognitive Psychology and Information Processing.* Hillsdale, NJ, LEA, 1979.
4. Fisher R: *The Design of Experiments,* 8th ed. Edinburgh, Oliver & Boyd, 1966.
5. Baars BJ: *The Cognitive Revolution in Psychology.* New York, Guilford, 1986.
6. Broadbent DE: *Perception and Communication.* New York, Pergamon, 1958.
7. Miller GA: The magical number seven, plus or minus two: Some limits on our capacity for processing information. *Psychol Rev* 1966; 63:81.
8. Tulving E: Episodic and semantic memory. In Tulving E, Donaldson W (eds): *Organization and Memory.* New York, Academic, Chap 10, 1972:382.
9. Butters N, et al: Episodic and semantic memory: A comparison of amnesic and demented patients. *J Clin Exp Neuropsychol* 1987; 9:470.
10. Anastasi A: *Psychological Testing,* 5th ed. New York, Macmillan, 1982.
11. Sternberg RJ: *Beyond IQ: A Triarchic Theory of Human Intelligence.* New York, Cambridge University Press, 1985.
12. Craik FIM, Lockhart RS: Levels of processing: A framework for memory research. *J Verbal Learn Verbal Behav* 11:671, 1972.
13. Anderson JR, Bower GH: *Human Associative Memory.* Washington, DC, Winston and Sons, 1973.
14. Anderson JR: *The Architecture of Cognition.* Cambridge, MA, Harvard University Press, 1983.
15. McClelland JL, Rumelhart DE: *Parallel Distributed Processing,* vols I and II. Cambridge, MA, The MIT Press, 1986.
16. Reeves AG: *Disorders of the Nervous System.* Chicago, Year Book Medical, 1981.
17. Joseph R: *Neuropsychology, Neuropsychiatry, and Behavioral Neurology.* New York, Plenum, 1990.
18. Rorschach H: *Psychodiagnostics: A Diagnostic Test Based on Perception.* Berne, Switzerland, Hans Huber, 1969.
19. Wechsler D: *The Measurement and Appraisal of Adult Intelligence.* Baltimore, Williams & Wilkins, 1958.
20. Wedding D, et al (eds): *The Neuropsychology Handbook.* New York, Springer, 1986.
21. Christensen AL: *Luria's Neuropsychological Investigation.* New York, Spectrum, 1975.
22. Boll T, Bryant BK: *Clinical Neurospsychology and Brain Function: Research, Measurement, and Practice.* Washington, DC, American Psychological Association, 1988.
23. Cohen RJ: *Sixty-Five Exercises in Psychological Testing and Assessment.* Mountain View, CA, Mayfield, 1992.
24. Campbell DT, Stanley JC: *Experimental and Quasi-Experimental Designs for Research.* Chicago, Rand McNally, 1966.
25. Chassan JB: *Research Design in Clinical Psychology and Psychiatry.* New York, Irvington Publishers, 1979.
26. Beck AT, et al: The measurement of pessimism: The hopelessness scale. *J Consult Clin Psychol* 1974; 42:861.
27. Cronbach LJ: *Essentials of Psychological Testing.* New York, Harper & Row, 1960.
28. Schaie KW: The course of adult intellectual development. *Am Psychol* 1994; 49(4):304.
29. Wedding D, et al (eds): *The Neuropsychology Handbook: Behavioral and Clinical Perspectives.* New York, Springer, 1986.
30. Matarazzo JD, et al: Test-retest reliability and stability of the

WAIS: A literature review with implications for clinical practice. *J Clin Neuropsychol* 1980; 2(2):89.

31. Benton AL, Hamsher K deS: *Multilingual Aphasia Examination: Manual of Instruction.* Iowa City, AJA Associates, 1983.

32. Olin JT, Zelinski EM: The 12-month reliability of the Mini-Mental State Examination. *Psychol Assess* 1991; 3(3):427.

33. Mesulam M (ed): *Principles of Behavioral Neurology.* Philadelphia, FA Davis, 1985.

34. Youngjohn JR, et al: Test-retest reliability of computerized, everyday memory measures and traditional memory tests. *Clin Neuropsychol* 1992; 6(3):276.

35. Benton AL: *The Revised Visual Retention Test*, 4th ed. New York, Psychological Corporation, 1974.

36. Chelune GJ, et al: Individual change after epilepsy surgery: Practice effects and base-rate information. *Neuropsychology* 1993; 7(1):41.

37. Heaton SK: *Wisconsin Card Sorting Test Manual.* Odessa, Florida, Psychological Assessment Resources, 1981.

38. Krug, SE: *Clinical Analysis Questionnaire Manual.* Champaign, IL, Institute for Personality and Ability Testing, 1980.

39. Brown DL: *Risk and Outcome in Anesthesia.* Philadelphia, JB Lippincott, 1988.

40. Mitzel HC, et al: Neuropsychological change and statistical artifact. *J Neurosurg Anesthesiol* 1991; 3(3):241.

41. Wilkinson L, et al: *Systat Statistics.* Evanston, IL, Systat Inc., 1992.

42. Gorsuch RL: *Factor Analysis.* Philadelphia, WB Saunders, 1974.

Chapter 10

CARDIOVASCULAR MANAGEMENT IN THE PATIENT WITH NEUROLOGIC DYSFUNCTION

MARK F. NEWMAN

Cardiovascular disease remains the most significant cause of mortality in the United States today. More than 25 percent of the population has cardiovascular disease, with one out of every two deaths attributable to this disease.[1] In addition, one-third of the entire health care resources of the United States are appropriated to the diagnosis and treatment of cardiovascular disease.[1] Not only is coronary disease prominent in the population as a whole, but greater than one-third of the 25 million patients who undergo noncardiac

surgery have coronary artery disease, risk factors for coronary artery disease, or are over the age of 65 years.[1,2] Four percent of this entire population, or approximately one million patients, suffer cardiovascular morbidity during the perioperative period, resulting in an overall in-hospital and long-term cost exceeding $22 billion annually in the United States.[1] Cardiovascular complications remain the primary source of morbidity and mortality in most major surgical procedures, and although we have reduced the cardiovascular disease death rate by 20 to 30 percent, the predominant influence of aging will offset this decreased mortality by increasing the incidence of coronary artery disease.[3-6] This trend is illustrated in Table 10-1.

Preoperative cardiac assessment of any patient undergoing noncardiac surgery relies primarily on a well-conducted history and understanding the defined likelihood of coexisting coronary disease in patients with vascular disease. Determination of the need for further evaluation or treatment can be directed by logical algorithms and clinical judgment of whether the knowledge gained will alter the perioperative management without adding significant risk. This type of assessment strategy utilizes resources appropriately and minimizes the likelihood of false-negative or false-positive testing that can result from using inappropriate testing in low- or high-risk populations.

The preoperative cardiac assessment of the patient with neurological disease is complicated in some cases (subarachnoid hemorrhage, acute head injury, and others) by centrally mediated ECG changes, arrhythmias, and myocardial damage that may necessitate far greater care and monitoring than would normally be predicted by other risk factors. This chapter attempts to describe the preoperative cardiac assessment of patients with neurological disease in generic terms related to the likelihood of coronary artery disease, valvular disease, congestive heart failure, dysrhythmias, and congenital heart disease. This is followed by sections describing the particular cardiovascular complications and considerations in patients with cerebrovascular occlusive disease, subarachnoid hemorrhage, severe head injury, and spinal cord injury.

Cardiovascular Risk Evaluation

CORONARY ARTERY DISEASE

The evaluation of a patient's coronary artery disease or risk of coronary artery disease relies primarily on history. Several factors including previous myocardial infarction, smoking, strong family history of atherosclerotic coronary disease, male sex, age, and diabetes remain the primary predictors of significant coronary

TABLE 10-1
Coronary Artery Disease: Incidence, Prevalence, Mortality, and Cost Projections

Year	Incidence	Prevalence	Mortality	Cost*
1980	692,117	5,977,405	432,613	31.9
1985	729,235	6,700,639	486,428	35.3
1990	759,583	7,230,904	540,557	37.8
1995	792,006	7,625,001	567,798	39.9
2000	834,522	7,973,869	596,777	42.0
2005	888,438	8,385,046	608,434	44.4
2010	953,750	8,939,816	637,304	47.4

*In billions of 1980 dollars.

SOURCE: From Frye et al.[3] with permission.

artery disease. The incremental value of further preoperative evaluation such as noninvasive stress testing in patients at risk for coronary artery disease relates obviously and directly to the prevalence of coronary artery disease in the population being tested. Diamond and colleagues appropriately noted that it seemed less reasonable to assess the value of history given the test results, than to assess what is the value of the test results given the history.[7] Consequently the recommendations to perform a test should be predicted on evidence that the evaluation will add to that which is already known, thereby reducing our uncertainty. Several studies[8-10] found that multiple historical predictors of coronary artery disease were highly predictive in delineating the significance of coronary artery disease in an individual patient. From Bayes' theorem, it is clear that the incremental value of exercise testing with cardiac imaging as a screen for severe disease will be minimal for high- and low-risk groups based on their pretest likelihood (see Fig. 10-1). The remaining approximately 50 percent of the population who are at intermediate risk of severe coronary artery disease represent the group in which noninvasive testing would have the greatest impact. In this manner such tests could be used cost effectively.

Hubbard and coworkers showed that by utilizing history components including age, angina, presence of diabetes, male gender, and prior evidence of myocardial infarction, they could classify patients into low, intermediate and high risk groups for severe coronary artery disease (left-main or three-vessel disease) (see Fig. 10-2 and Table 10-2).[10] Those patients predicted to be at high risk, approximately 39 percent of the total group, had a prevalence of severe coronary disease of nearly 50 percent (see Table 10-2), whereas those predicted to be at low risk (14 percent of the population) had a prevalence of only 9 percent of three-vessel or left-main disease.[10] The remaining 47 percent of patients were at intermediate risk and had 25 percent prevalence of severe disease. It is clear that the incremental value of exercise testing with cardiac imaging is greatest in those patients at intermediate risk. Patients at high risk would benefit most from coronary arteriography (since negative noninvasive studies add little information), whereas in patients at low risk for severe disease, the predictive probability of noninvasive testing is marginal and further evaluation prior to surgery will provide little additional assistance to the anesthesia team.

Which noninvasive testing to use for the diagnosis of coronary artery disease in the intermediate-risk population remains somewhat controversial. Stress exercise testing with the addition of thallium-201 or other modalities appears to have the greatest predictive power.[11,12] However, other modalities such as exercise or dobutamine stress echocardiography have produced similar excellent results in recent studies.[13] The combination of excellent history with the appropriate use of noninvasive testing tended to yield the best overall results.[14] Reports from the Massachusetts General Hospital and the University of Virginia demonstrated a clear statistical incremental value of the combination of clinical and exercise variables over clinical variables alone, and the highest statistical power was achieved when thallium-201 variables were combined with clinical and exercise variables[14] (Fig. 10-3).

PREVIOUS MYOCARDIAL INFARCTION

In addition to its obvious predictive value in identifying patients with coronary artery disease, prior myocardial infarction (MI) has been associated with increased perioperative cardiac complications in many epidemiologic studies.[15-19] The impact of prior myocardial infarction on the likelihood of perioperative cardiac morbidity and mortality relates to the timing of the infarction in relation to the planned surgery (Table 10-3). The highest risk of reinfarction appears to be in those patients who undergo surgery less than three months after their myocardial infarction. After six months the perioperative reinfarction rate seems to stabilize at between 2 to 6 percent (see Table 10-3). The most encompassing studies on the impact of previous infarction on reinfarction rate and mortality all show relatively similar results.[15,16,20-25,18,19,26-39]

There exists a significant amount of confusion on the study conducted by Rao showing a vast decrease in perioperative reinfarction rate attributable to the use of monitoring techniques as well as prolonged ICU stay of 72 h.[15] The overall perioperative reinfarction rate was decreased from 7.7 to 1.9 percent for all time periods combined and from 36 to 5.8 percent when surgery occurs within three months of a previous myo-

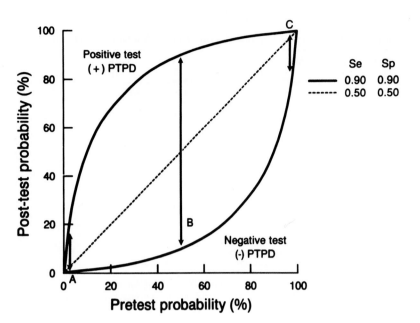

Figure 10-1 Posttest probability plotted as a function of pretest probability of coronary artery disease (Bayes' theorem). The dashed line represents a test of no incremental value because the posttest probability equals pretest probability of disease. A positive result for a test with 90 percent sensitivity is represented by the upper curve and a negative test with a specificity of 90 percent is represented by the lower curve. Note that patients with a very high or very low pretest probability derive a modest incremental change in posttest probability (patients A and C), whereas patients at intermediate pretest likelihood (patient B) derive the greatest increase in posttest probability. (From Christian TF: The incremental value of noninvasive stress testing for the diagnosis of coronary artery disease. *ACC Curr J Rev* 3:60–64, 1994, with permission.)

cardial infarction.[15] The aid of invasive monitoring in allowing rapid treatment of cardiovascular variables when these values deviate from the normal was used to explain the difference in outcome between the two groups. The increased monitoring applied to two periods, both the intraoperative period and the first 72 h postoperatively. Monitoring for 72 h may have been critical since the majority of reinfarction tends to occur between 24 and 96 h after surgery[15,16,18,19,25,31–45] (Table 10-4). Reduction in perioperative morbidity was also noted in vascular surgery patients in whom normalization of hemodynamics assessed with a pulmonary artery catheter was undertaken for three days in an ICU

postoperatively.[45] While both Rao's and Berlauk's studies have potential flaws, they demonstrate the advantages of close hemodynamic control in the perioperative period in reducing perioperative morbidity and mortality, especially in those patients who are less than six months after a myocardial infarction. Regardless of the potential deficiencies associated with lack of randomization or historical controls, these studies confirm that the perioperative reinfarction rate is higher in the first six months after a previous MI. Therefore in situations of truly elective surgery, postponement of surgery in those patients who have had an MI less than six months earlier should reduce the morbidity and mortality associated with anesthesia. Potentially, the less severe the coronary disease the more likely the patient's anticipated survival curve will mimic that of patients who do not have coronary disease and are probably at less risk for perioperative events.[45–49]

The decision tree in Fig. 10-4 from the work of Mantha and colleagues describes a preoperative evaluation

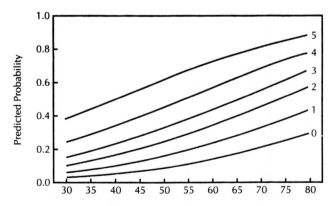

Figure 10-2 Composite graph estimating the probability of severe coronary artery disease based on a 5-point risk score that awards one point for each of the following variables: male gender, typical angina, history and electrocardiographic evidence of myocardial infarction, diabetes, and use of insulin. Each curve shows the probability of severe coronary artery disease as a function of age for a given risk score. (From Hubbard et al.,[10] with permission.)

TABLE 10-2

Separation of Patients Based on Clinical Predictors According to the Probability of Having Left-Main or Three-Vessel Coronary Artery Disease (CAD)

Group	Total No. of Patients	Patients with Left-Main or Three-Vessel CAD, No. (%)
Low probability, <15%	96	9(9)
Intermediate probability, 15 to 35%	322	79(25)
High probability, <35%	262	127(48)
Total	680	215(32)

TABLE 10-3
Incidence of Perioperative Myocardial Infarction or Mortality in Patients with Previous Myocardial Infarction

Time from MI Operation (mo)	Arkins et al. 1963 Mort	Topkins and Artusio 1959–1964 Reinf	Mort	Fraser et al. 1960–1964 (Mort)	Tarhan et al. 1975–1976 Reinf	Mort	Sapala et al. 1970–1974 Reinf	Mort	Steen et al. 1980 Reinf	Mort	Von Knorring 1981 Reinf	Mort
0–3	11/27(40)	12/22(54.5)	•	19/38(38)	3/8(37)	•	6/7(86)	6/7(86)	2/18(27)	•	4/16(25)	•
4–6	•	•	•	•	3/19(16)	•			2/18(11)			
7–12	•	9/36(25.0)	•	•	2/42(5)	•					2/11(18)	•
13–18	•	11/49(22.4)	•	•	1/27(4)	•						
19–24	•		•	•	1/21(4)	•	9/159(5.7)	3/159(1.9)			10/89(11)	•
25–36	•	3/51(5.9)	•	•	11/232(5)	•			30/544(5.4)			
>36	•	5/493(1.0)	•	•		•						
Unknown	•	3/7(42.8)	•	•	7/73(5.6)	•					9/41(22)	•
Total patients with MI		43/658(6.5)	31/658(4.7)		28/422(6.6)	15/422(3)	15/166(9)	9/166(5.4)	36/587(6.1)	25/587(4.2)	25/157(15.9)	7/157(4)

NOTE: Mort, mortality; Reinf, reinfarction. Number in parentheses denotes percentage.
SOURCE: From Roizen MF: Preoperative evaluation. In Miller RD (ed): *Anesthesia*, New York, Churchill-Livingstone, 1994, with permission.

to assess whether vascular surgery patients have *significant* ischemic heart disease.[50] The utilization of history is followed by the extensive utilization of noninvasive and invasive cardiac evaluations. The premise is based on the logical but unproven theory that PTCA or CABG prior to vascular surgery reduces the combined risk of perioperative morbidity and mortality. When the morbidity and mortality of PTCA and CABG are combined with that of the eventual procedure it becomes less logical or clear that myocardial revascularization reduces overall risk.

The type of surgery must be delineated and the urgency of that procedure stratified to best utilize our limited preoperative evaluation resources. An additional nomogram utilizing different stratification criteria and an alternative decision tree is shown in Fig. 10-5. Differing recommendations based on surgery type for patients having less-invasive surgery are cov-

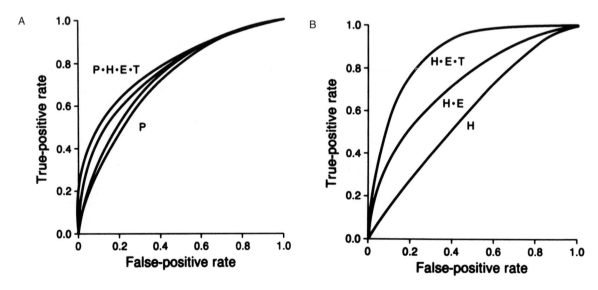

Figure 10-3 *A.* Receiver-operating characteristics curves demonstrating the incremental value of pretest probability (P), probability and history (second curve from bottom), probability and history and exercise ECG (E) (third curve from the bottom), and probability and history and exercise and thallium variables (T) in patients with normal rest electrocardiograms. *B.* The same analysis in patients with abnormal rest ECGs. (From Ladenheim et al. *Am J Cardiol* 59:270, 1987, with permission.)

Time from MI Operation (mo)	Goldman et al 1975–1976		Eerola et al 1970–1974		Schoeppel et al 1980		Reo et al. 1973–1976		Rao et al. 1976–1982		Shah et al. 1983–1986	
	Reinf	Mort	Reinf	Mort	Reinf	Mort	Reinf	Mort	Reinf	Mort	Reinf	Mort
0–3	1/22(4.5)	5/22(23)	1/12(8)	1/12(8)	0/1(0)	0/1(0)	4/11(30)	•	3.52(5.8)	•	1/23(4.3)	
4–6		1/17(5.9)	0/1(0)	0/8(0)	0/8(0)	0/8(0)	8/31(26)	•	2/36(2.3)	•	0/18(0)	
7–12	0/13(0)						6/127(5)	•	1/104(1.0)	•		
13–18		1/13(8)					6/114(5)	•	4/258(1.6)	•	10/74(5.7)	
19–24					0/10(0)	0/10(0)						
25–36			4/82(4.9)	1/82(12)			4/81(5)	•	4/235(1.7)	•		
>36	2/66(3.3)	2/66(3.3)			0/26(0)	0/26(0)						
Unknown												
Total patients with MI		9/109(8.9)			3/53(5.7)	2/53(3.8)	28/364(7.7)	15/364(4.1)	14/733(1.9)	5/733(0.7)	13/275(4.7)	3.275(1.1)

ered by a separate nomogram (Fig. 10-6). A nomogram individualized for patients undergoing carotid endarterectomy is included in the section on cerebrovascular occlusive disease.

VALVULAR DISEASE

History along with the basic physical examination remains the primary mechanism for evaluating patients with valvular disease. Patients with asymptomatic murmurs do not represent significant incremental risk in overall outcome. However, patients with a history of poor exercise tolerance in connection with a new murmur deserve further evaluation, such as echocardiography.

Determination of the type of valvular heart disease is imperative in patients undergoing noncardiac surgical procedures because of the markedly different hemodynamic strategies involved in the management of ste-

notic and regurgitant lesions. Each valvular lesion has unique characteristics and differing management goals that can significantly impact overall outcome.[51–53] Therefore, the type of lesions that exist in a particular patient should be determined preoperatively, not necessarily to allow further preoperative intervention, but to more appropriately decide monitoring strategies, hemodynamic goals, and potential need for antibiotic endocarditis prophylaxis.

While the long-term prognosis and potentially the perioperative risk in patients with valvular heart disease depend on the extent of the disease,[54,55] aortic disease, particularly aortic stenosis, has been consistently identified as a factor increasing perioperative risk.[56] Important once again is that the preoperative history and physical examination appear to be sensitive and specific indicators of disease and disease stage[57] (Table 10-5).

TABLE 10-4
When Do Myocardial Infarctions Occur after Vascular Surgery?

Investigators	Year Published	Examined Prospectively	POSTOPERATIVE				
			Day 0	Day 1	Day 2	Day 3	Day 4
Plumlee and Boettner	1972	No	11/24	3/24	1/24	2/24	
Tarhan et al.	1972	No		14/71	8/71	22/71	13/71
Rao et al.	1983	No		8/28	7/28	10/28	3/27
		No		3/14	4/14	7/14	
Becker and Underwood	1987	?	11/28	6/28	9/28	0/28	1/28
Total (4 studies)			22	34	29	41	17

SOURCE: From Roizen MF: Preoperative evaluation. In Miller RD (ed): *Anesthesia.* New York, Churchill-Livingstone, 1994, with permission.

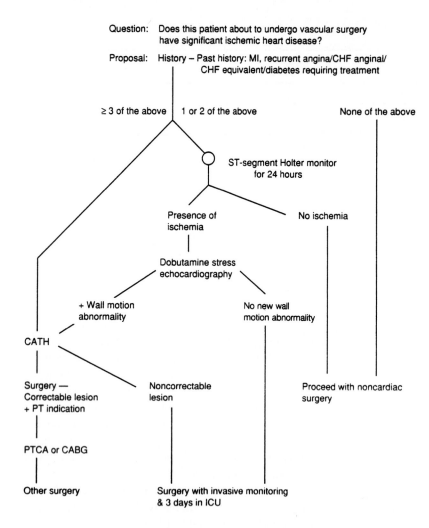

Question: Does this patient about to undergo vascular surgery
            have significant ischemic heart disease?

Proposal: History – Past history: MI, recurrent angina/CHF anginal/
            CHF equivalent/diabetes requiring treatment

Figure 10-4   Assessment of cardiac risk in patients undergoing vascular surgery. Twenty-four-hour ST Holter is utilized as a screening tool in low and intermediate risk patients. This decision tree should be contrasted with those in Figs. 10-5 and 10-6, which represent alternative plans from other authors for patients undergoing less-invasive procedures. (From Mantha et al,[50] with permission.)

Management of Patients with Valvular Lesions

STENOTIC LESIONS

AORTIC STENOSIS

Aortic stenosis is typically classified as being valvular, subvalvular, or supravalvular. Pure valvular aortic stenosis is the most common, accounting for more than three-quarters of the obstructive lesions. The primary cause of aortic stenosis has changed in recent years from a rheumatic origin to calcific degeneration of congenital bicuspid or tricuspid aortic valves. Senile degeneration of normal aortic valves occurs in approximately 30 percent of patients over the age of 65 years.

Mild forms of aortic stenosis may be asymptomatic for many years in patients or be first recognized by the typical systolic crescendo-decrescendo murmur. With increasing age, calcification of the valve often occurs, resulting in the development of symptoms. Any of the triad of symptoms including angina, syncope, or congestive heart failure heralds a life expectancy of less than five years without intervention.

Obviously the degree of aortic stenosis is of concern when the patient presents for neurologic surgery. In a patient with a previously unrecognized murmur and evidence of symptoms, further cardiologic evaluation is necessary to determine the extent of valvular disease, which can usually be done with a simple echocardiogram. Patients with severe to critical aortic stenosis have markedly increased perioperative morbidity and thus should receive correction of their lesion prior to all but urgent or emergent surgery. Patients with mild to moderate aortic stenosis with varying symptom levels can be managed if the anesthesiologist understands the hemodynamic goals and the anesthetic implications of the lesion.

Hemodynamic goals for aortic stenosis include maintenance of preload, contractility, and systemic vascular resistance (SVR). Heart rate should be controlled at baseline or lower to minimize increases in oxygen consumption and allow adequate time for ejec-

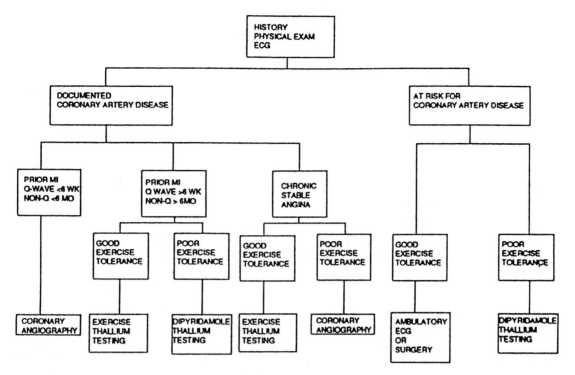

Figure 10-5   Proposed algorithm for patients undergoing surgical procedures associated with *high risk* of perioperative myocardial ischemia (e.g., abdominal aortic aneurysm resection). In these patients, further cardiovascular evaluation to delineate the extent of coronary artery disease is warranted if the information obtained influences clinical care. (From Fleisher LA, Barash PG: *Anesth Analg* 74:586–98, 1992, with permission.)

tion. The obvious conclusion is to maintain predetermined, well-tolerated hemodynamic values in the patient with aortic stenosis (see Table 10-6). Marked reductions in systemic vascular resistance that can occur with regional anesthesia or high-dose inhalation anesthetics should be avoided to reduce the likelihood of developing decreased coronary perfusion and ongoing myocardial ischemia of the hypertrophied myocardium. Understanding the hemodynamic goals allows the anesthesiologist to most appropriately manage the patient with little morbidity and mortality in the intraoperative or postoperative period.

MITRAL STENOSIS

The primary cause of mitral stenosis remains rheumatic heart disease which leads to scarring of the mitral valve leaflets. Fusion of the commissures is often seen, leading to the development of a funnel-shaped mitral apparatus that becomes secondarily calcified. Similar to patients with aortic stenosis, the patients with mitral stenosis may remain asymptomatic for many years. However, as increasing stenosis and calcification occur, symptoms begin to appear most often associated with exercise or high-cardiac-output states. The mortality of symptomatic mitral stenosis is high, with 20 percent of patients dying within one year of diagnosis. Again

the severity of the mitral stenosis determines the necessity for further evaluation and intervention prior to neurological surgery. The progression of mitral stenosis is slow and insidious, and therefore only critical mitral stenosis typically requires intervention prior to planned procedures. Hemodynamic goals in patients with mitral stenosis are very similar to those states for aortic stenosis (see Table 10-6). Goals should be to maintain left ventricular preload and contractility while maintaining or controlling heart rate to allow adequate time for emptying. Maintenance of systemic vascular resistance as with aortic stenosis is also a key part of the plan. If the patient is in sinus rhythm, all attempts should be made to maintain rhythm and maintain rate control if at all possible. Right ventricular failure can occasionally occur with increasing pulmonary vascular resistance such that all attempts should be made to maintain overall cardiac contractility and reduce pulmonary vascular resistance to reduce potential postoperative problems of right-sided congestive failure.

REGURGITANT LESIONS

AORTIC REGURGITATION

Aortic regurgitation is a significantly different lesion from aortic stenosis, representing a volume rather than

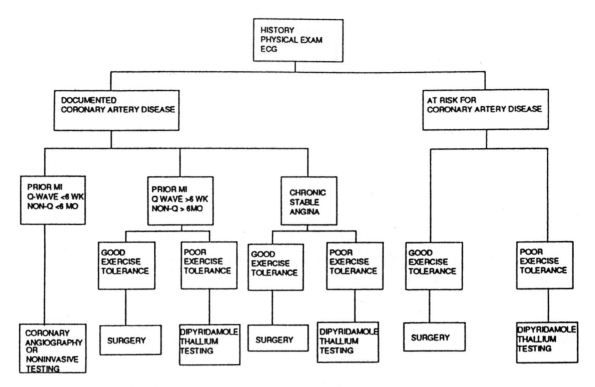

Figure 10-6 Proposed algorithm for patients undergoing surgical procedures at low to moderate risk of perioperative myocardial ischemia (e.g., peripheral procedures). Further evaluation is not warranted in those with good exercise tolerance. (From Fleisher LA, Barash PG: *Anesth Analg* 74:586–98, 1992, with permission.)

TABLE 10-5
Bedside Diagnosis of Systolic Murmurs: Sensitivity, Specificity, and Predictive Value of Diagnostic Maneuvers

					PREDICTIVE VALUE	
Maneuver	Response	Murmur	Sensitivity (%)	Specificity (%)	Positive (%)	Negative (%)
Inspiration	Increase	Right-sided	100	88	67	100
Expiration	Decrease	Right-sided	100	88	67	100
Muller maneuver	Increase	Right-sided	15	92	33	81
Valsalva maneuver	Increase	Hypertrophic cardiomyopathy	65	96	81	92
Squatting to standing	Increase	Hypertrophic cardiomyopathy	95	84	59	98
Standing to squatting	Decrease	Hypertrophic cardiomyopathy	85	85	61	99
Leg elevation	Decrease	Hypertrophic cardiomyopathy	85	91	71	96
Handgrip	Decrease	Hypertrophic cardiomyopathy	85	75	46	95
Handgrip	Increase	Mitral regurgitation and ventricular septal defect	68	92	84	81
Transient arterial occlusion	Increase	Mitral regurgitation and ventricular septal defect	78	100	100	87
Amyl nitrite inhalation	Decrease	Mitral regurgitation and ventricular septal defect	80	90	84	87

SOURCE: From Lembo[57] and Roizen MF: Preoperative evaluation. In Miller RD (ed): *Anesthesia*. New York, Churchill-Livingstone, 1994, with permission.

TABLE 10-6
Management of Valvular Heart Lesions

	LV Preload	Heart Rate	Contractile State	SVR	PVR
Aortic stenosis	↑	↓ →	→	↑	→
Mitral stenosis	↑	↓	→	↑	↓
Aortic regurgitation	↑	↓	→	↑	→
Mitral regurgitation	↑ →	↓	→	↑	↓

pressure overload of the left ventricle. With chronic aortic regurgitation, changes in volume occur slowly, such that by the time there are symptoms, left ventricular dysfunction secondary to left ventricular damage may be partially irreversible. Hemodynamic management for patients with aortic regurgitation is markedly different from that for aortic stenosis (see Table 10-6). In aortic regurgitation maintenance of heart rate, contractility, and left ventricular preload are the preeminent features. Systemic vascular resistance should be decreased in order to decrease the regurgitant fraction and improve forward flow. Obviously this has to be balanced against coronary perfusion but typically is the overall goal in the management of patients with aortic regurgitation. The anesthetic management should be designed along these goals as well as maintaining normal contractility in a depressed heart.

MITRAL REGURGITATION

Mitral regurgitation may be either *chronic* due to valvular degeneration or more rarely rheumatic heart disease, or *acute* often associated with papillary muscle dysfunction or rupture with myocardial ischemia or poor coaptation due to bacterial endocarditis. The hemodynamic consequences of chronic and acute mitral regurgitation differ markedly. Chronic mitral regurgitation is typically minimally symptomatic for many years, but the onset of more severe symptoms typically heralds a rapid downhill course unless surgical intervention occurs. Approximately three-quarters of these patients develop atrial fibrillation, which obviously decreases their overall cardiac output.

Mitral regurgitation patients are similar in many ways to patients with aortic regurgitation. Systemic vascular resistance should again be decreased to improve forward flow. The indication to increase preload in these patients is not universal as some patients may show mitral valve annular dilatation with increasing volume resulting in an increasing regurgitant fraction. Adequate monitoring to assess different interventions in these patients is thus needed often either with pulmonary artery catheterization or with transesophageal echocardiography.

In the anesthetic management of these patients, care

should be taken to minimize heavy premedication leading to hypercarbia and potentially significant increases in pulmonary vascular resistance. As previously noted, pulmonary artery catheters or transesophageal echocardiography may be helpful in judging the impact of anesthetic or other surgical interventions.

Of additional prime importance in patients with valvular heart disease is maintenance of the patient's normal rhythm. Patients with a decreased ejection fraction or significant mitral or aortic stenosis deteriorate rapidly with the onset of atrial fibrillation or flutter, as the atrial component of left ventricular filling can be critical in maintaining cardiac output. Maintenance of preoperative antiarrhythmic therapy and careful consideration to maintain normal sinus rhythm or to maintain adequate rate control in those patients already in atrial fibrillation are essential to maintaining adequate cardiac output perioperatively.

Mitral valve prolapse is an interesting entity unto itself occurring in approximately 5 to 17 percent of otherwise healthy people. Mitral valve prolapse can be associated with von Willebrand syndrome and polycystic kidney disease, and the presence of one condition requires a search for potential existence of another, at least by history and physical exam. Mitral valve prolapse is occasionally asymptomatic but also results in potential palpitations, atypical chest pain, dizziness, and on rare occasions sudden death. Supraventricular arrhythmias occur in more than half of the patients with mitral valve prolapse, with ventricular arrhythmias occurring perioperatively in a significant percentage as well.[58-60] The occurrence of occasional cerebral ischemia has resulted in the chronic use of aspirin or other anticoagulants in patients with mitral valve prolapse, and the potential for endocarditis has led to a recommendation for prophylaxis with antibiotics prior to known bacteremic events.[58-60,61]

Patients who have any form of known valvular heart disease as well as those with intracardiac or intravascular shunts should be protected against endocarditis when they will undergo a known bacteremic procedure. Endocarditis has occurred in a sufficiently significant number of patients with hypertrophic cardiomyopathy and mitral valve prolapse to warrant their inclusion in this prophylactic regimen as well. The degree of bacteremia varies with different surgical procedures, with the greatest degree occurring with dental extraction 30 to 80 percent, down to the lowest percentage occurring with nasotracheal intubation (16 percent) or oral-tracheal intubation (0 percent).[62,63] Thus, since oral-tracheal intubation is associated with little bacteremia, the decision for antibiotic prophylactics is based on the patient's procedure, typically being instituted prior to instrumentation of the GI tract, gallbladder, pharynx, or genitourinary tract. The choice of prophylactic antibiotics should be aimed at the most commonly occurring pathogens[64] (Table 10-7). The guidelines of the American Heart Association state that all antimicrobial prophylaxis should be started 30 min to an hour rather than 24 h before known bacteremic events in order to reach therapeutic levels without superinfecting the patients with unusual pathogens.[64,65]

Cardiac valve prostheses represent an interesting further challenge in managing chronic anticoagulation perioperatively. Recommendations vary by author, but typically in those patients with aortic valve prostheses, anticoagulation can be suspended for several days without significant risk. However, due to the increased risk of thromboembolic events with mitral valve prostheses, approximately 5 percent, patients with these prostheses should have their period of anticoagulation curtailed through the utilization of preoperative vitamin K or fresh frozen plasma.[66] Typically the reinstitution of anticoagulation within 12 h postoperatively is indicated, with heparin therapy followed by reintroduction of oral agents.[67,68]

Left Ventricular Dysfunction (Congestive Heart Failure and Cardiomyopathy)

Congestive heart failure has been recognized as a potential risk factor in patients undergoing surgical procedures since the work of Skinner and Pearce in 1964.[56] They found a significant correlation between the patient's preoperative functional capacity and postoperative cardiac morbidity and mortality especially in patients undergoing significant intrathoracic or intraabdominal procedures. The significance of congestive heart failure was further emphasized by Goldman and associates[69] in 1977 and indicated by a number of other researchers.[15,20,22,34,36,42–46,48,54,70–80]

O'Keefe and coworkers demonstrated that 95 percent of patients with a normal electrocardiogram had a normal left ventricular ejection fraction.[135] Such patients with normal left ventricular ejection fraction have an excellent prognosis, and it is difficult to justify the routine use of cardiac imaging as a means to assess left ventricular function in these patients. However, in patients with signs and symptoms of CHF or with an abnormal ECG, functional evaluation by the use of echocardiography or MUGA may yield valuable information.

Physical signs of congestive heart failure correlate to a greater degree than history in predicting risk, indicating that preoperative therapy to reduce the degree of congestive failure may improve outcome. This is further delineated by the work of Skinner and Pearce

in which the New York Heart Association classification was predictive of the overall cardiac morbidity and mortality associated with surgical procedures.[56] Therefore, in patients in whom evidence of clinical CHF exists, data support delaying surgery until optimization of functional status can be accomplished.

Dysrhythmias

Prior to the routine use of electrocardiograms, Ernstene in the 1950s noted two intraoperative cardiac dysrhythmias that he described as "heart standstill" and "ventricular fibrillation."[81] Ernstene noted at that time that detection of these dysrhythmias was of such fundamental importance that the time may have come for an inexpensive oscilloscope to be part of every anesthetist's armamentarium.[81] While Ernstene's remarks may seem modest in relation to our current monitoring practices, several studies have delineated preoperative and perioperative dysrhythmias as potential predictors of adverse cardiac outcomes.[36,43,69] In the most careful and extensive evaluation of the significance of preoperative arrhythmias in cardiac outcome, Mangano and colleagues[70] utilized two-channel Holter ECG monitoring for up to 2 days preoperatively, during operation, and for up to 2 days postoperatively in 474 men undergoing elective noncardiac surgery. Three types of adverse cardiac outcomes were assessed including ischemic events, congestive heart failure, and ventricular tachycardia. History of arrhythmia correlated with an increased risk of postoperative congestive heart failure but not with ischemic events or ventricular tachycardia.

Dysrhythmias, particularly bradyarrhythmias, often are an indication for the use of pacemakers. The type of pacemaker placed and indication for such have markedly changed since the early 1980s. Typically the majority of pacemakers were placed for bradyarrhythmias after tachycardia, bradytachy syndrome, sick sinus syndrome, or AV conduction disorders. Insertion of pacemakers typically allows an increase in heart rate to provide augmentation of cardiac output and, with dual-chamber pacing or demand pacing, the ability to retain atrioventricular synchrony. More complex pacemakers are now being employed to provide better cardiac output in stressful situations and to decrease myocardial wall stress or to treat ventricular tachyarrhythmias.

In the preoperative evaluation of the patient with pacemakers, the anesthesiologist must understand a significant portion of the pacemaker's programming in order to know how it would respond to electrocautery or other electrical interference or patient factors in the perioperative period. From Shapiro[82] we see the

TABLE 10-7
Endocarditis Prophylaxis: Recommended Antibiotic Regimens[a]

	Dosage for Adults	Dosage for Children (In No Case to Exceed Adult Dose)
Dental and upper respiratory procedures tonsilloadenoidectomy, nasal intubation, nasogastric tube placement, (e.g., bronchoscopy) likely to produce bacteremia		
Oral		
Amoxicillin	3 g 1 h before procedure and 1.5 g 6 h later	50 mg/kg
Amoxicillin (penicillin) allergy: use		
erythromycin ethylsuccinate or	800 mg	20 mg/kg 1 h before procedure and 10 mg/kg 6 hr later
erythromycin stearate or	1 g PO 2 h before procedure and half the initial dose 6 h later	
clindamycin	300 mg orally 1 h before procedure and 150 mg 6 h after initial dose	10 mg/kg and 5 mg/kg 6 h later
Parenteral		
Ampicillin	2 g IM or IV 30 min before procedure	50 mg/kg IM or IV 30 min before procedure
Penicillin allergy: use clinda-mycin	300 mg IV 30 min before procedure	10 mg/kg IV 30 min before procedure
Gastrointestinal and genitourinary procedures (i.e., GI or GU surgery, or instrumentation or surgery involving a tissue possibly contaminated with GI or GU organisms		
Parenteral		
Ampicillin	2 g IM or IV 30 min before procedure	50 mg/kg IM or IV 30 min before procedure
plus gentamicin	1.5 mg/kg (not to exceed 80 mg) IM or IV 30 min before procedure	2.0 mg/kg IM or IV 30 min before procedure
plus amoxicillin	1.5 g PO 6 h after ampicillin and gentamicin or 50 mg/kg repeat ampicillin and gentamicin after initial dose	50 mg/kg
Penicillin		
Amoxicillin allergy: use vanco-mycin	1 g IV infused slowly over 1 h beginning 1 hr before procedure	20 mg/kg IV infused slowly over 1 h beginning 1 h before procedure
plus gentamicin	1.5 mg/kg (not to exceed 80 mg) IM or IV 30 min before procedure	2.0 mg/kg IM or IV 30 min before procedure
Oral		
Amoxicillin	3 g 1 hr before procedure and 1.5 g 6 h after initial dose	50 mg/kg 1 h before procedure and 25 mg/kg 6 h after initial dose

[a] The frequently used cephalosporins are not recommended. A single dose of the parenteral drugs is probably adequate, because bacteremias after most oral cavity and diagnostic procedures are of short duration. However, one or two follow-up doses may be given at 8- to 12-hour intervals in selected patients, such as hospitalized patients judged to be at higher risk.
SOURCE: From Dajani et al.,[64] with permission.

following areas that an anesthesiologist should determine prior to taking a patient with a pacemaker to the operating room: (1) The indication for placement of the pacemaker; (2) the default rhythm; (3) the type of pacemaker. Pacemakers have traditionally been given a five-letter code (see Table 10-8); however, the majority of a pacemaker's actions can be delineated by the first three letters indicating chamber paced, chamber sensed, and the sensing pattern. An example of this would be a DDD pacemaker, in which the initial D represents dual or double pacing of the atrium and ventricle. The second D indicates the chamber sensed, and again relates to double or dual sensing. The third D indicates demand mode relating the complete capability to have atrioventricular synchrony through atrial

demand for ventricular output or complete AV pacing; (4) how to detect deterioration of battery function increased (or decreased) rate; (5) how to change the mode or the part of the pacemaker that is of a radio frequency type. While the anesthesiologist may not have performed these changes, the magnet and program device should be available near the operating room at the time of surgery; (6) current rate in sensitivity settings of the pacemaker; (7) whether the pacemaker is currently functioning as well as the underlying rhythm.[82]

Due to potential complications of setting the patients in demand or inhibitory mode, including sensing of electrocautery which can inhibit pacemaker function, most pacemakers can be converted to a fixed rate, and the anesthesiologist should understand how this can

TABLE 10-8
Traditional Five-Letter Code for Pacemaker Systems

1st Letter Chamber Paced	2nd Letter Chamber Sensed	3rd Letter Mode of Response	4th Letter (If Used) Programmable Features	5th Letter (If Used) Arrhythmia Treatment
A = atrium	A = atrium	T = triggered	P = programmable	B = burst
V = ventricle	V = ventricle	I = inhibited	M = multiprogrammable	N = normal
D = double	D = double	D = double	O = not programmable	S = scanning
	O = non	O = not applicable	R = rate modulated	E = external

be accomplished as well as having the necessary equipment to accomplish this immediately available. Obviously the ground plate for the electrocautery should be as far from the pulse generator as possible. Although not typically utilized, a bipolar form of electrocautery is preferable to minimize the flow of current through the pacemaker.

The proper perioperative utilization of pacemakers depends on the anesthesiologist's understanding of the pacemaker function, underlying disease, ongoing treatment, and what implications these have in relation to the patient's overall outcome.

Congenital Heart Disease

Successful treatment of many congenital heart lesions has resulted in a significant increase in the number of adult patients presenting for surgical procedures with either corrected or partially corrected congenital heart defects. Adequate history taking as well as understanding of the congenital defect, or residual defect, is essential for the anesthesiologist to appropriately manage the patient. The following section divides congenital lesions into four major categories. The management for the different lesions in a particular category is fairly similar. The basic understanding of these defects will assist the anesthesiologist in management of either adult or pediatric patients with CHD undergoing neurological procedures (Table 10-9).

SHUNT LESIONS

Shunt lesions are intracardiac connections between chambers or extracardiac connections from the pulmonary artery to the aorta where the shunt flow depends on the relative resistance on either side of the shunt, either pulmonary vascular resistance (PVR) or systemic vascular resistance (SVR).[83] Blood flows via the pathway of least resistance, making vascular resistance a major determinant of shunt flow. Typically, if no obstruction of flow occurs in the right ventricle (RV), systemic pressure and SVR exceed right ventricular

pressure, pulmonary artery pressure and PVR, so left-to-right shunting occurs. This shunt results in increased pulmonary blood flow with these primary results: (1) Volume overload of the pulmonary circulation; (2) excessive pulmonary blood flow, resulting in progressive elevation of pulmonary vascular resistance; and (3) increased cardiac work for the left ventricle (LV).[84] A prolonged increase in pulmonary blood flow can result in fixed pulmonary arterial changes especially without early correction. The increased demand for cardiac output on a noncompliant LV of a newborn usually results in increased heart rate and eventually left ventricular congestive heart failure if the LV is unable to sustain adequate systemic perfusion.

Right-to-left shunts occur when appropriate connection exists and pulmonary vascular resistance or pulmonary outflow tract obstruction causes PVR to exceed SVR, thus reversing the normal shunt. These patients are cyanotic and hypoxemic, with pressure overloaded right ventricles. Representative defects include tetralogy of Fallot, pulmonary atresia with VSD, and Eisenmenger's complex. The resultant problems are a combination of reduced pulmonary flow, cyanosis and hypoxia, and right ventricular outflow obstruction with pressure overload and possible right ventricular failure.

MIXING LESIONS

Mixing lesions make up the largest group of cyanotic congenital heart lesions. These lesions have large communications between the pulmonary and systemic circulations. Because the communication is so large and has nearly complete mixing the pulmonary to systemic flow ratio (Qp/Qs ratio) is not dependent on the shunt but is totally dependent on vascular resistance or outflow obstruction. Common mixing lesions are listed in Table 10-9.

OBSTRUCTIVE LESIONS

Obstructive lesions involving the aorta, pulmonary outflow track, or mitral valve often leave newborns

TABLE 10-9
Classification and Manifestations of Congenital Heart Disease

Physiologic Classification	Manifestations
Shunts	
Left to right	
VSD	Volume-overloaded ventricle
ASD	Develop CHF
PDA	
AV Canal	
Right to left	Pressure-overloaded ventricle
Tetralogy of Fallot	Cyanotic
Pulmonary atresia/VSD	Hypoxemic
Eisenmenger's complex	
Mixing lesions	
Transposition/VSD	Variable: pressure v volume overload
Tricuspid atresia	Usually cyanotic
Anomalous venous return	
Univentricular heart	
Obstructive lesions	
Interrupted aortic arch	Ventricular dysfunction
Critical aortic stenosis	Pressure-overloaded ventricle
Critical pulmonic stenosis	Ductal dependence
Hypoplastic left heart syndrome	
Coarctation of the aorta	
Mitral stenosis	
Regurgitant lesions	
Ebstein's anomaly	Volume overloaded
Other secondary causes	

with pressure overloaded small dysfunctional ventricles proximal to the lesions. The aortic lesions including critical aortic stenosis, coarctation of the aorta, hypoplastic left heart syndrome, or interrupted aortic arch leave systemic perfusion dependent on PDA flow. The right ventricular obstructive lesions cause dependency on the PDA for pulmonary blood flow. The left ventricular obstructive lesions are associated with (1) profound left ventricular failure; (2) impaired coronary perfusion with increased ectopy; (3) systemic hypotension; and (4) PDA-dependent systemic circulation.[84] Right ventricular obstructive lesions lead to a right ventricular failure and decreased pulmonary blood flow. Mild to moderate forms of these diseases may remain asymptomatic for years. The neonatal forms of left ventricular obstruction other than coarctation carry high morbidity and mortality. Morbidity is associated with the severity of the disease pathophysiology.

REGURGITANT LESIONS

Ebstein's malformation of the tricuspid valve, a spiraling displacement of the annulus and leaflets of the tricuspid valve into the right ventricle with associated tricuspid regurgitation, is the only true regurgitant lesion. Regurgitant lesions associated with other anomalies are similar to regurgitant lesions in adults. Volume overload and ventricular failure occur without adequate treatment.

PREOPERATIVE EVALUATION OF CONGENITAL HEART DISEASE

The adequate preoperative evaluation of the child or adult with congenital heart disease most importantly includes a good history and physical examination. It is also important to note that approximately 25 percent of the patients with congenital heart disease have associated noncardiac anomalies.[85] Airway abnormalities are of particular significance, including the cervical spine instability and enlarged tongue associated with trisomy 21, micrognathia, microstomia, or cleft palate. Changes in pulmonary vascular resistance from hypoxia exaggerate difficulties during induction and necessitate adequate evaluation of the patient's airway. Preoperative evaluation should include hematocrit, electrolyte count, and potentially arterial blood gas if indicated. Many severe congenital heart lesions will have undergone full or partial correction prior to neurosurgical procedures; however, traumatic injuries preclude further correction and place the anesthesiologist in an important role in understanding the necessary management of lesions.

Preoperative preparation and planning are essential to the appropriate care of the child or adult with congenital heart disease. Coordination of NPO status, premedication, as well as cardiac medications is imperative to the successful anesthetic and procedure. Time and care must be taken to explain procedures and orient patients and parents to dispel misinformation or misgivings; of particular importance in the pediatric cases may be allowing the parents to arrive in the operating room with the child to minimize crying and other problems that may be of particular importance in cyanotic congenital heart disease and neurosurgical procedures.

Typically neonates or infants are given clear liquids until 2 to 3 h prior to the procedure. In older children solid foods usually are withheld after midnight and clear liquids given until 3 to 4 h before the procedure begins. It is therefore very important to correlate scheduling for the operating room in these patients, who are so prone to becoming dehydrated and potentially hypotensive and acidotic.

Obviously, overall anesthetic management of these patients depends on the lesion present and the extent of the neurosurgical procedure undertaken. Basic understanding of the impact of anesthetic agents as well

TABLE 10-10
Medical Characteristics of NASCET-Eligible Patients

Medical Condition (Based on History)	Symptomatic Patients (%) ($n = 2256$)
Angina	24
Previous myocardial infarction	20
Hypertension	60
Claudication	15
Smoking: current	37
previous	40
Diabetes	19

as different adrenergic agents available is essential to the anesthesiologist's successful care of the patient with congenital heart disease.

Differential Risk and Cardiovascular Management in Patients with Neurologic Disease

OCCLUSIVE CEREBROVASCULAR DISEASE

Occlusive disease of the carotid or cerebral vessels secondary to atherosclerosis or atherosclerotic plaques represents a situation in which the majority of patients are also at significant risk for moderate to severe coronary artery disease. In fact, the development of atherosclerosis in peripheral or central vessels obviously indicates a high probability of coronary atherosclerosis, and the risk factors for both disease processes overlap markedly (Table 10-10). Cardiac complications have been reported to be the primary source of mortality associated with carotid endarterectomy (CEA).[86-88] Therefore, in this group, the evaluation process is similar to that described in the initial section on coronary artery disease.

If a patient has a stable angina pattern without evidence of previous MI or diabetes or is otherwise at low risk, then the patient should in all cases be assumed to have coronary artery disease but proceed without further evaluation. Patients who have unstable angina including a progressive component, pain at rest, or no improvement with medical treatment should be considered for further evaluation. In this high-risk population that evaluation most likely represents coronary arteriography. As was previously mentioned in the section on coronary artery disease, in this high-risk group the patients have coronary artery disease and thus noninvasive testing offers very little to our perioperative management. In diabetic patients or patients in whom the history predicts intermediate risk of severe

coronary artery disease, noninvasive exercise stress testing with or without thallium may be of significant benefit in further decision making. In patients who cannot exercise, dobutamine stress echocardiography is most likely of greater incremental value than dipyridamole thallium.[13]

Additional perioperative testing in patients with suspected coronary artery disease is only beneficial if it is likely to alter the perioperative plan. This could potentially be in patients with three-vessel disease or left main disease in whom the symptomatology or severity of the coronary artery disease would indicate the necessity for coronary artery bypass surgery prior to or simultaneous with carotid endarterectomy. The literature is confusing in relation to the best management in patients of this variety, with individual surgeon or institutional preference determining the typical progression of intervention.[87,89-91] Many institutions will do coronary artery bypass grafting followed at a later date by carotid endarterectomy unless the patient is having active TIAs or ongoing symptoms with their cerebrovascular disease.[89,90] In those cases some institutions will select the carotid endarterectomy first versus other institutions combining the carotid endarterectomy with the CABG.[87,89-91] There is little consensus among the many small studies evaluating the efficacy and safety of the many different processes.[87,89-97] It is impossible to make a simple recommendation based on the current literature, and each case must be judged on its own merit.[89] From the standpoint of risk reduction and overall mortality, it has been shown that patients who undergo carotid endarterectomy after coronary artery bypass are at lower risk of myocardial injury during endarterectomy. However, this doesn't take into account the approximately 7 percent or greater myocardial infarction rate or the 2 percent mortality rate also associated with CABG. It is difficult to show a significant improvement in overall cardiac morbidity and mortality if CABG precedes correction of the cerebrovascular disease, even though CABG in this population significantly reduces symptoms and prolongs life.[98] While the percutaneous coronary angioplasty (PTCA) carries less acute risk of morbid or mortal events than CABG, there are no data showing that it significantly reduces perioperative morbidity, and due to the prothrombotic effects of surgical stress, a significant delay between PTCA and surgery would seem warranted.

The decision tree shown in Fig. 10-7 represents a blueprint for cardiac evaluation in patients undergoing CEA based on the work of Hubbard and others using history to predict *severe* (three-vessel or left main) coronary artery disease. Branches are placed in this decision tree to allow readers to insert their institutional bias in relation to delaying surgery or considering combined

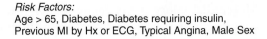

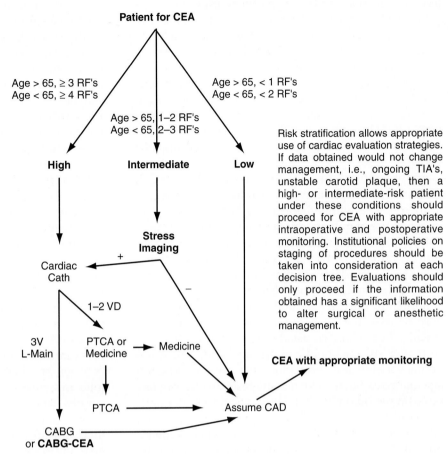

Figure 10-7 Preoperative cardiac (coronary artery disease) assessment algorithm for patients undergoing CEA. Decisions should be based on the likelihood that the information gained will alter the anesthetic or surgical management of the patient. Based on institutional practice related to the timing of CABG and CEA a logical evaluation scheme can be adopted. CEA = carotid endarterectomy, RF's = risk factors, VD = vessel disease, PTCA = percutaneous transluminal angioplasty, CABG = coronary artery bypass grafting, Hx = history, MI = myocardial infarction, CAD = coronary artery disease, L-Main = left main coronary disease.)

CABG/CEA procedures. The likelihood of acting on the information to change surgical or anesthesia planning should determine whether noninvasive or invasive cardiac testing is utilized. Patients should receive CABG surgery or PTCA based most importantly on its ability to improve long-term symptoms and survival, which is significant in left main and three-vessel disease.[98] Patients in whom survivability is not improved with CABG or PTCA should begin medical therapy as indicated and proceed for their CEA with understanding of their risk.

Regardless of the results of perioperative testing the anesthesiologist should assume the patient has significant coronary artery disease. Mangano showed that with dipyridamole thallium imaging, ischemia occurred similarly in those with positive and negative preoperative exams.[134] Perioperative monitoring and postoperative care should be based on the extent of predicted risk and early perioperative observations. In the current climate of cost containment, 72 h of ICU care with extensive hemodynamic monitoring is not warranted with CEA without data similar to that from

Rao[15] in major vascular surgery showing an outcome benefit.

SUBARACHNOID HEMORRHAGE

Subarachnoid hemorrhage (SAH), like other acute neurological injuries, may result in cardiac ischemic changes or cardiac injury in patients who otherwise, according to history, are at low risk for significant coronary artery disease. After subarachnoid hemorrhage, injury to the posterior hypothalamus may stimulate the release of norepinephrine from the adrenal medulla and sympathetic cardiac efferents.[99] Norepinephrine, either through direct toxicity or via significant elevation of myocardial afterload, produces ischemic changes in the subendocardium.[100] Pathologic examination of the myocardium after SAH reveals microscopic subendocardial hemorrhages and myocytolysis.[101] Based on history or other evaluations, the ischemic ECG changes and myocardial damage of subarachnoid hemorrhage cannot be satisfactorily explained by coronary atherosclerosis or thrombosis.

Myocardial injury is frequently scattered rather than confined to a particular coronary distribution.[102] Although elevation of plasma creatinine phosphokinase (CPK) and its cardiac specific isoenzyme (CPK-MB) occurs in 50 percent of patients with subarachnoid hemorrhage,[103] the total CPK and ratio of CPK-MB to total CPK is rarely consistent with a transmural infarction. Ventricular wall dysfunction is seen in one-fourth to one-third of the patients with subarachnoid hemorrhage.[104,105] Patients with poor ventricular function suffered greater morbidity, including pulmonary edema, intramural thrombus formation, and embolic stroke.

Abnormalities in electrocardiographic (ECG) rhythm and morphology are seen in 50 to 80 percent of the patients with subarachnoid hemorrhage[106] and therefore are of only marginal value in assessing these patients. A variety of changes have been reported including prolongation of Q-T interval, p wave changes, u waves, and dysrhythmias including ventricular tachycardia and fibrillation. The most common ECG abnormalities involve ST and T wave changes which may or may not be associated with myocardial ischemia. ECG changes usually occur during the first 48 h after subarachnoid hemorrhage, and their duration is variable and correlation with myocardial damage marginal. Some evidence suggests that prophylactic administration of beta blockers and autonomic antagonists can improve the outcome in patients with subarachnoid hemorrhage,[107–109] while other evidence does not.[110,111] Even though the evidence supporting their use is not unanimous, beta blockers can hopefully reduce ischemia and potentially dysrhythmia thresholds associated with higher levels of catecholamines.

Cardiac dysrhythmias occur in up to 90 percent of the patients with subarachnoid hemorrhage and vary from occasional PVCs to any form of ventricular or supraventricular rhythm abnormalities, including ventricular tachycardia and fibrillation.[110] Life-threatening dysrhythmias may occur in patients during the first 48 h after subarachnoid hemorrhage, but the development of ventricular fibrillation is frequently preceded by torsades des pointes.[112] In those cases where torsades was followed by life-threatening ventricular dysrhythmias the QT interval was significantly prolonged.[112]

While most ECG abnormalities following subarachnoid hemorrhage appear to be neurogenic rather than cardiogenic in nature, patients do sustain myocardial infarction, and the previously noted lack of correlation between ECG abnormalities and myocardial ischemia predicts a difficult management dilemma.[113] The clinical debate is whether cardiac injury warrants delay of surgery and further cardiac evaluation.[113,114] Cardiac enzymes in assessment of ventricular function may be helpful in suspicious cases. However, even if myocardial ischemia is present, it may have minimal impact on overall mortality.[115] Consequently the decision to postpone surgery must be balanced against the course of the disease, especially with respect to the risk of vasospasm. Significant cardiopulmonary edema or malignant dysrhythmias may warrant the postponement of surgery until adequate medical management can be obtained. Clinical or diagnostic evidence of myocardial dysfunction may be helpful in assessing the need for pulmonary artery catheter monitoring, transesophageal echocardiography, or other additional cardiac monitoring in the perioperative period.

Regardless of the extent of myocardial involvement associated with subarachnoid hemorrhage the hemodynamic goals of anesthetic management of subarachnoid hemorrhage or coronary artery disease remain extremely similar. Maintaining hemodynamic stability in response to varying levels of stimulation is obviously important to prevent ischemia and also to reduce risk of aneurysm rupture. Anticipating particularly painful stimuli should allow the additional use of rapid-acting anesthesia or sympathetic blockers, to minimize hemodynamic swings. Obviously blood pressure after aneurysm clipping must be balanced between providing adequate flow through higher systolic pressures and maintaining reasonable oxygen supply-demand ratios. In cases where myocardial ischemia or potentially infarction and related dysrhythmias are suspected pulmonary artery catheters can give additional evidence of the impact this hypertensive therapy has in relation to myocardial performance and diastolic function.

SEVERE HEAD INJURY

Severe head injury represents an interesting cardiopulmonary evaluation for the anesthesiologist. This injury is associated with a massive alpha-adrenergic discharge resulting in significant systemic and pulmonary vasoconstriction which can lead to neurogenic pulmonary edema (Fig. 10-8). Therefore in the evaluation of the patient with severe head injury, hypotension not associated with significant bradycardia should direct the anesthesiologist to look for other potential sources of hypovolemia or bleeding that may explain these unusual changes. Severe head injury or blunt trauma to the chest should also make one alert to potential lung injuries, including pulmonary contusion, or cardiac contusion that could lead to other significant complications in addition to neurogenic pulmonary edema.[116]

As previously noted for subarachnoid hemorrhage, electrocardiographic changes occurring with acute CNS injury have been described by many clinical in-

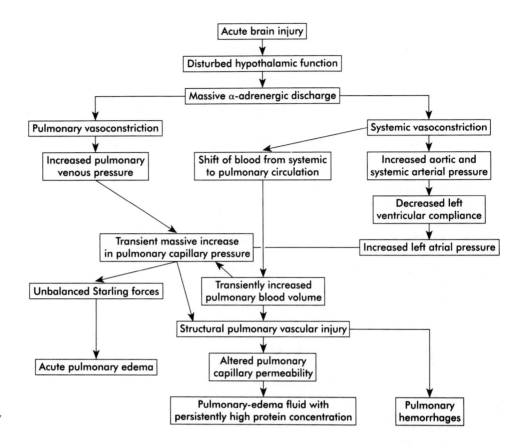

Figure 10-8   Hypothesized mechanism of neurogenic pulmonary edema. [From Matjasko MJ: Multisystem sequelae of severe head injury. In Cottrell JE, Smith DS (eds): *Anesthesia and Neurosurgery*, 3d ed. Chicago, Mosby Year Book, 1994, with permission.]

vestigators.[117–121] The pathogenesis of the varied electrocardiographic abnormalities after head injury or other CNS abnormalities, including CVA, is less than well delineated. While central autonomic stimulation occurring in addition to the massive alpha-adrenergic discharge with cortical hypothalamic or brainstem levels may account for these observations,[122,123] the correlation between the levels of ECG abnormalities and intracranial hypertension or electrolyte imbalance is not well defined. Some authors report a correlation,[105] and others show no indication of an association among intracranial hypertension, electrolyte imbalance, and ECG changes.[122]

Due to these ECG changes, as well as occasional isolated serum CPK and CPK-MB levels in patients with severe head injury, full evaluation of the heart through either cardiac catheterization or echocardiography is necessary prior to utilization of a patient's heart as a donor for cardiac transplantation.[105,109,124]

Preoperative assessment of the patient's hemodynamic status must take into account that the patient is typically hypertensive for a reason. Therefore, great caution should be exercised in attempts to reduce systemic pressure to decrease myocardial oxygen consumption, as this may lead to the possible negative effects on cerebral perfusion in patients with increased intracranial pressure. The physician must balance the

potential positive and negative effects on the brain and the cardiac system before developing an interventional plan for controlling hypertension or minimizing changes in intracranial pressure.

SPINAL CORD INJURY

Typically preoperative assessment of the patient with an acute spinal cord injury would demonstrate spinal shock—that is, hypotension, bradycardia, and increased venous capacitance, the degree of which would depend on the level of the spinal cord injury. This typical spinal shock picture occurs after a transient period of hypertension. Experimental animal models of acute transection of the spinal cord have additionally shown acute increases in pulmonary capillary wedge pressure, extravascular lung water, and intracranial pressure with increased brain water, blood-brain barrier permeability, and a decrease in cerebral blood flow.[125] While pretreatment with phentolamine prior to the spinal cord transection prevented the increase in mean arterial pressure it did nothing to change the cerebral response.[126] As seen with acute head injury, occasionally spinal cord injuries are associated with neurogenic pulmonary edema, originally named by Sarnoff and Sarnoff.[127] Neurogenic pulmonary edema appears to be characterized by a number of components including (1) the absence of cardiopulmonary pathology to act as the primary process; (2) an extraordinarily rapid onset; (3) the inhibition of the pulmonary edema by an alpha-adrenergic blocker anesthetic for central nervous system depression; (4) similarity to fulminant onset of pulmonary edema found with epinephrine infusion at high doses; (5) high protein content of pulmonary edema exudate, and (6) the initial transitory increase in pulmonary and systemic vascular resistance.[128]

The acuteness of the secondary brain and pulmonary consequences of spinal cord injury serves to emphasize the vulnerability of these patients with acute transection and the necessity for their transport to adequate centers within the first few hours. In the 1960s Albin and associates[129,130] and White and associates[131] emphasized the rapidity of the intrinsic physiopathologic response to transection and the need for rapid movement to a center where evaluation and therapy could be initiated. With both the brain and the lungs at risk, the potential of associated head injury, hypoxia, hypercarbia, and hypovolemia could have, and probably does have, devastating effects. While this section describes the cardiopulmonary sequelae of SCI, it is obvious that adequate stabilization of the spine must occur to prevent further injury.

In addition to these cerebral and pulmonary complications, suspicion should exist for associated cardiovascular disturbances. Several studies have found that persistent bradycardia, heart rates of less than 60 beats per min for one day, occurred in 100 percent of the patients with severe cervical spinal cord injury.[132] This finding was less common in those with milder cervical injury or thoracolumbar injury, 35 and 13 percent respectively. Hypotension on at least two consecutive measurements or primary cardiac arrest occurred mainly in the severe cervical injury group, with frequencies of 68 and 16 percent respectively.[132] Supraventricular arrhythmias occurred in severe cervical and milder cervical injury groups at rates of 19 and 6 percent.

Consideration of the patient's hemodynamic status prior to anesthesia induction is extremely important. Further myocardial depression with reduction of cardiac output and mean arterial pressure due to anesthetic or narcotic analgesia must be avoided. Respiratory alkalosis produced by hyperventilation should be avoided, because it may further depress the myocardium. As with severe injuries, one must be vigilant of the potential that hypotension may be due to other associated injuries or hemorrhagic shock. During spinal shock marked blood loss and hypovolemia are poorly tolerated since there is no normal sympathetic response. Cure must be taken in spinal cord injury as with closed head injury to maintain spinal cord

perfusion pressure, as hypotension may drop perfusion pressure below the autoregulatory limit described by Hickey and colleagues.[133] Systemic perfusion should be gauged from urine output or other clinical and laboratory factors, including lactic acid production. If questions exist as to the adequacy of perfusion, additional monitoring of CVP or PA catheter should be instituted. Fluid therapy should first be instituted with inotropes if necessary. Care should be used in supporting pressure with an alpha agonist as this may worsen rather than improve perfusion.

References

1. National Center for Health Statistics: *Health, 1989.* United States 1099, DHHS Publication Report Number 89-1232.
2. Mangano DT: Perioperative cardiac morbidity. *Anesthesiology* 1990; 72:153.
3. Frye RL, et al: Task Force III: Major demographic and epidemiologic trends affecting adult cardiology. *J Am Coll Cardiol* 1988; 12:840.
4. Weinstein MC, et al: Forecasting coronary heart disease incidence, mortality, and cost: The coronary heart disease policy model. *Am J Public Health* 1987; 77:1417–1426.
5. National Center for Health Statistics: *Vital Statistics of the United States 1980, 1985.* DHHS Publication Report Number 85-1101.
6. Thom TJ, et al: Factors in the decline of coronary heart disease mortality. In Conner WE (ed): *Coronary Heart Disease.* JB Lippincott, Philadelphia, 1985:5–18.
7. Diamond GA: Penny wise. *Am J Cardiol* 1988; 62:806.
8. Pryor DB, et al: Value of the history and physical in identifying patients at increased risk for coronary artery disease. *Ann Intern Med* 1993; 118:81.
9. Pryor DB, et al: Estimating the likelihood of severe coronary artery disease. *Am J Med* 1991; 90:553.
10. Hubbard BL, et al: Identification of severe coronary artery disease using simple clinical parameters. *Arch Intern Med* 1992; 152:309.
11. Christian TF, et al: Noninvasive identification of severe coronary artery disease using exercise tomographic thallium-201 imaging. *Am J Cardiol* 1992; 70:14.
12. Christian TF, et al: The incremental value of thallium-201 imaging for the detection of three vessel coronary disease in patients with normal rest electrocardiograms. *Circulation* 1992; 86:1865.
13. Dagianti A, et al: Stress echocardiography: Comparison of exercise, dipyridamole and dobutamine in detecting and predicting the extent of coronary artery disease. *J Am Coll Cardiol* 1995; 26(1):18.
14. Pollock SG, et al: Independent and incremental prognostic value of tests performed in hierarchical order to evaluate patients with suspected coronary artery disease: Validation of models based on these tests. *Circulation* 1992; 85:237.
15. Rao TLK, et al: Reinfarction following anesthesia in patients with myocardial infarction. *Anesthesiology* 1983; 59:499.
16. Mauney FM, et al: Postoperative myocardial infarction: A study of predisposing factors, diagnosis and mortality in a high risk group of surgical patients. *Ann Surg* 1970; 172:497.
17. Okuda S, et al: Effect of acute reduction in blood pressure on renal function of rats with diseased kidneys. *Nephron* 1987; 45:311.

18. Arkins R, et al: Mortality and morbidity in surgical patients with coronary artery disease. *JAMA* 1964; 190:485.

19. von Knorring J: Postoperative myocardial infarction: A prospective study in a risk group of surgical patients. *Surgery* 1981; 90:55.

20. Charlson ME, et al: Postoperative renal dysfunction can be predicted. *Surg Gynecol Obstet* 1989; 169:303.

21. Charlson ME, et al: Preoperative characteristics predicting intraoperative hypotension and hypertension among hypertensives and diabetics undergoing noncardiac surgery. *Ann Surg* 1990; 212:66.

22. Charlson ME, et al: Risk for postoperative congestive heart failure. *Surg Gynecol Obstet* 1991; 172:95.

23. Schneider AJL, et al: Morbidity prediction using pre- and intraoperative data. *Anesthesiology* 1979; 51:4.

24. Eerola M, et al: Risk factors in surgical patients with verified preoperative myocardial infarction. *Acta Anaesthesiol Scand* 1980; 24:219.

25. Garraway WM, Whisnant JP: The changing pattern of hypertension and the declining incidence of stroke. *JAMA* 1987; 258:214.

26. Apfelbaum J, et al: An automated method to validate preoperative test selection: First results of a multicenter study, abstracted. *Anesthesiology* 1989; 71:A928.

27. Borer JS, et al: Limitations of the electrocardiographic response to exercise in predicting coronary artery disease. *N Engl J Med* 1975; 293:367.

28. Proudfit WL, et al: Selective cine coronary angiography: Correlation with clinical finding in 1000 patients. *Circulation* 1966; 33:901.

29. Goldschlager N: Use of a treadmill test in the diagnosis of coronary artery disease in patients with chest pain. *Ann Intern Med* 1982; 97:383.

30. Weiner DA, et al: Exercise stress testing. Correlations among history of angina, ST-segment response and prevalence of coronary artery disease in the Coronary Artery Surgery Study (CASS). *N Engl J Med* 1979; 301:230.

31. Topkins MJ, Artusio JF: Myocardial infarction and surgery: A five year study. *Anesth Analg* 1964; 43:715.

32. Fraser JG, et al: Anesthesia and recent myocardial infarction. *JAMA* 1972; 199:318.

33. Tarhan S, et al: Myocardial infarction after general anesthesia. *JAMA* 1972; 199:318.

34. Sapala JA, et al: Operative and nonoperative risks in the cardiac patient. *J Am Geriatr Soc* 1975; 23:529.

35. Steen PA, et al: Myocardial reinfarction after anesthesia and surgery. *JAMA* 1976; 239:2566.

36. Goldman L, et al: Cardiac risk factors and complications in noncardiac surgery. *Medicine (Baltimore)* 1978; 57:357.

37. Schoeppel SL, et al: Effects of myocardial infarction on perioperative cardiac complications. *Anesth Analg* 1983; 62:493.

38. Knapp RB, et al: The cerebrovascular accident and coronary occlusion in anesthesia. *JAMA* 1962; 182:332.

39. Shah KB, et al: Reevaluation of perioperative myocardial infarction in patients with prior myocardial infarction undergoing noncardiac operations. *Anesth Analg* 1990; 71:231.

40. Plumlee JE, Boettner RB: Myocardial infarction during and following anesthesia and operation. *South Med J* 1972; 65:886.

41. Becker RC, Underwood DA: Myocardial infarction in patients undergoing noncardiac surgery. *Cleve Clin J Med* 1987; 54:25.

42. Eagle KA, Boucher CA: Cardiac risk of noncardiac surgery. *N Engl J Med* 1989; 321:1330.

43. Detsky AS, et al: Predicting cardiac complications in patients undergoing non-cardiac surgery. *J Gen Intern Med* 1986; 1:211.

44. Gerson MC, et al: Cardiac prognosis in noncardiac surgery. *Ann Intern Med* 1985; 103:832.

45. Berlauk JF, et al: Preoperative optimization of cardiovascular hemodynamics improves outcome in peripheral vascular surgery: A prospective, randomized clinical trial. *Ann Surg* 1991; 214:289.

46. Lowenstein E, et al: Perioperative myocardial reinfarction: A glimmer of hope—a note of caution, editorial. *Anesthesiology* 1983; 59:493.

47. Mahar LJ, et al: Perioperative myocardial infarction in patients with coronary artery disease with and without aorta-coronary bypass grafts. *J Thorac Cardiovasc Surg* 1978; 76:533.

48. Kennedy JW, et al: Clinical and angiographic predictors of operative mortality from the Collaborative Study in Coronary Artery Surgery (CASS). *Circulation* 1981; 63:793.

49. Bruschke AVG, et al: Progress study of 590 consecutive nonsurgical cases of coronary disease followed 5–9 years. *Circulation* 1973; 47:1147.

50. Mantha S, et al: Relative effectiveness of four preoperative tests for predicting adverse cardiac outcomes after vascular surgery; a meta-analysis. *Anesth Analg* 1994; 79(3):422.

51. Thompson RC, et al: Perioperative anesthetic risk of noncardiac surgery in hypertrophic obstructive cardiomyopathy. *JAMA* 1985; 254:2419.

52. Selzer A: Changing aspects of the natural history of valvular aortic stenosis. *N Engl J Med* 1987; 317:91.

53. Kirklin JW, Pacifico AD: Surgery for acquired valvular heart disease (2nd of 2 parts). *N Engl J Med* 1973; 288:194.

54. Higgins TL, et al: Stratification of morbidity and mortality outcome by preoperative risk factors in coronary artery bypass patients. *JAMA* 1992; 267:2344.

55. O'Keefe JH, et al: Risk of noncardiac surgical procedures in patients with aortic stenosis. *Mayo Clin Proc* 1989; 64:400.

56. Skinner JF, Pearce ML: Surgical risk in the cardiac patient. *J Chronic Dis* 1964; 17:57.

57. Lembo NJ, et al: Bedside diagnosis of systolic murmurs. *N Engl J Med* 1988; 318:1572.

58. Nishimura RA, et al: Echocardiographically documented mitral-valve prolapse: Long term follow-up of 237 patients. *N Engl J Med* 1985; 313:1305.

59. Bor DH, Himmelstein DU: Endocarditis prophylaxis for patients with mitral valve prolapse: A quantitative analysis. *Am J Med* 1984; 76:711.

60. Swartz MH, et al: Mitral valve prolapse: A review of associated arrhythmias. *Am J Med* 1977; 62:377.

61. Clemens JD, et al: A controlled evaluation of the risk of bacterial endocarditis in persons with mitral-valve prolapse. *N Engl J Med* 1982; 307:776.

62. Berry FA, et al: A comparison of bacteremia occurring with nasotracheal and orotracheal intubation. *Anesth Analg* 1973; 52:873.

63. Shull HJ, et al: Bacteremia with upper gastrointestinal endoscopy. *Ann Intern Med* 1975; 83:212.

64. Dajani AS, et al: Prevention of bacterial endocarditis. Recommendations by the American Heart Association. *JAMA* 1990; 264:2919.

65. Antimicrobial prophylaxis in surgery. *Med Lett Drugs Ther* 1992; 34:5.

66. Tinker JH, Tarhan S: Discontinuing anticoagulant therapy in surgical patients with cardiac valve prostheses: Observations in 180 operations. *JAMA* 1978; 239:738.

67. Cade JF, et al: Guidelines for the management of oral anticoagulant therapy in patients undergoing surgery. *Med J Aust* 1979; 2:292.

68. Katholi RE, et al: The management of anticoagulant during noncardiac operations in patients with prosthetic heart valves: A prospective study. *Am Heart J* 1978; 96:163.

69. Goldman L, et al: Multifactorial index of cardiac risk in noncardiac surgical procedures. *N Engl J Med* 1977; 297:845.

70. Mangano DT, et al: Association of perioperative myocardial ischemia with cardiac morbidity and mortality in men undergoing noncardiac surgery. *N Engl J Med* 1990; 323:1781.

71. American Society of Anesthesiologists Task Force on Pulmonary Artery Catheterization: Practice guidelines for pulmonary catheterization. *Anesthesiology* 1993; 78:380.

72. Backer CL, et al: Myocardial reinfarction following local anesthesia for ophthalmic surgery. *Anesth Analg* 1980; 59:257.

73. Wolf GL, et al: Intra-ocular surgery with general anesthesia. *Arch Ophthalmol* 1975; 93:323.

74. Naylor CD, et al: Pulmonary artery catheterization: Can there be an integrated strategy for guideline development and research promotion? *JAMA* 1993; 269:2407.

75. Roizen MF: Anesthesia goals for surgery to relieve or prevent visceral ischemia. In Roizen MF (ed): *Anesthesia for Vascular Surgery.* New York, Churchill-Livingstone, 1990:171.

76. Eagle KA, et al: Combining clinical and thallium data optimizes preoperative assessment of cardiac risk before major vascular surgery. *Ann Intern Med* 1989; 110:859.

77. Boucher CA, et al: Determination of cardiac risk by dipyridamole-thallium imaging before peripheral vascular surgery. *N Engl J Med* 1985; 312:389.

78. Raby KE, et al: Correlation between preoperative ischemia and major cardiac events after peripheral vascular surgery. *N Engl J Med* 1989; 321:1296.

79. Lette J, et al: Usefulness of the severity and extent of reversible perfusion defects during thallium-dipyridamole imaging for cardiac risk assessment before noncardiac surgery. *Am J Cardiol* 1989; 64:276.

80. Hultgren HN, et al: Unstable angina, comparison of medical and surgical management. *Am J Cardiol* 1977; 39:734.

81. Ernstene AC: The management of cardiac patients in relation to surgery. *Circulation* 1951; 4:430.

82. Shapiro WA, et al: Intraoperative pacemaker complications. *Anesthesiology* 1985; 63:319.

83. Berman WJ: The hemodynamics of shunts in congenital heart disease. In Johansen Burggren KM (ed): *Cardiovascular Shunts: Phylogenetic, Ontogenetic, and Clinical Aspects.* New York, Raven Press, 1985:399.

84. Greeley WJ, Kern FH: Anesthesia for pediatric cardiac surgery. In Miller RD (ed): *Anesthesia.* New York, Churchill-Livingstone, 1990:1653.

85. Rashkind WJ: Historical aspects of surgery for congenital heart disease. *J Thorac Cardiovasc Surg* 1982; 84:619.

86. Hertzer NR, Lees CD: Fatal myocardial infarction following carotid endarterectomy. *Ann Surg* 1981; 194:212.

87. O'Donnell TF, et al: The impact of coronary artery disease on carotid endarterectomy. *Ann Surg* 1983; 198:705.

88. Towne JB, et al: First phase report of cooperative Veterans Administration asymptomatic carotid stenosis study—operative morbidity and mortality. *J Vasc Surg* 1990; 11:252.

89. Dunn EJ: Concomitant cerebral and myocardial revascularization. *Surg Clin North Am* 1986; 66:385.

90. Fode NC, et al: Multicenter retrospective review of results and complications of carotid endarterectomy in 1981. *Stroke* 1986; 17:370.

91. Kaul TK, et al: Surgical management in patients with coexistent coronary and cerebrovascular disease. Long-term results. *Chest* 1994; 106(5):1349.

92. Thompson J, et al: Concomitant carotid and coronary artery reconstruction. *Am Surg* 1982; 195:712.

93. Ennix CL, et al: Improved results of carotid endarterectomy in patients with symptomatic coronary disease: An analysis of 11,546 consecutive carotid operations. *Stroke* 1979; 10:122.

94. Bernhard VM, et al: Carotid artery stenosis: Association with surgery for coronary artery disease. *Arch Surg* 1972; 105:837.

95. Emery RW, et al: Coexistent carotid and coronary artery disease. *Arch Surg* 1983; 118:1035.

96. Urschel HC, et al: Management of concomitant occlusive disease of the carotid and coronary arteries. *J Thorac Cardiovasc Surg* 1976; 72:829.

97. Turnipseed WD, et al: Postoperative stroke in cardiac and peripheral vascular disease. *Ann Surg* 1980; 192:365.

98. Jones RH, et al: Long-term survival benefit of CABG and PTCA in patients with coronary artery disease. *J Thorac Cardiovasc Surg* 1996; 111(5):1013.

99. Cruickshank JM, et al: Possible role of catecholamines, corticosteroids, and potassium in production of electrocardiographic abnormalities associated with subarachnoid haemorrhage. *Br Heart J* 1974; 36:697.

100. Botterell EH, et al: Hypothermia and interruption of the carotid or carotid and vertebral circulation in the surgical management in intracranial aneurysms. *J Neurosurg* 1956; 13:1.

101. Doshi R, Neil-Dwyer G: A clinicopathologic study of patients following a subarachnoid hemorrhage. *J Neurosurg* 1980; 52:295.

102. Geenhoot JH, Reichenbach DD: Cardiac injury and subarachnoid hemorrhage. *J Neurosurg* 1969; 30:521.

103. Kaste M, et al: Heart type creatinine kinase isoenzyme (CKMB) in acute cerebral disorders. *Br Heart* 1978; 40:802.

104. Davies KR, et al: Cardiac function in aneurysmal subarachnoid hemorrhage: A study of electrographic and echocardiographic abnormalities. *Br J Anaesth* 1991; 67:58.

105. Pollick C, et al: Left ventricular wall motion abnormalities in subarachnoid hemorrhage. An echocardiographic study. *J Am Coll Cardiol* 1988; 12:600.

106. Marion DW, et al: Subarachnoid hemorrhage and the heart. *Neurosurgery* 1986; 18:101.

107. Cruickshank JM, et al: Reduction of stress catecholamine-induced cardiac necrosis by beta-selective blockade. *Lancet* 1987; 2:585.

108. Neil-Dwyer G, et al: Beta-blockage benefits patients following a subarachnoid hemorrhage. *Eur J Clin Pharmacol Suppl* 1984; 28:25.

109. Neil-Dwyer G, et al: Beta-blockers, plasma total creatinine kinase and creatinine kinase myocardial isoenzymes and prognosis in subarachnoid hemorrhage. *Surg Neurol* 1986; 25:163.

110. Dipasquale G, et al: Holter detection of cardiac arrhythmias in intracranial subarachnoid hemorrhage. *Am J Cardiol* 1987; 59:596.

111. Grad A, et al: Effect of elevated plasma norepinephrine on electrocardiographic changes in subarachnoid hemorrhage. *Stroke* 1991; 22:746.

112. Andreoli A, et al: Subarachnoid hemorrhage: Frequency and severity of cardiac arrhythmias. A survey of 70 cases studied in the acute phase. *Stroke* 1987; 18:558.

113. Koselko P, et al: Subendocardial hemorrhage and ECG changes in intracranial bleeding. *Br Med J* 1964; 1:1479.

114. Rudehill A, et al: A study of ECG abnormalities and myocardial specific enzymes in patients with subarachnoid hemorrhage. *Acta Anaesthiol Scand* 1982; 26:344.

115. Van Gijn J, Van Dongen KJ: The time course of aneurysmal haemorrhage on computed tomograms. *Neuroradiology* 1982; 23:153.

116. Thomas DGT, et al: Serum myelin-basic-protein assay in diagnosis and prognosis of patients with head injury. *Lancet* 1978; 1:113.

117. Byer E, et al: Electrocardiogram with large, upright T waves and long QT intervals. *Am Heart J* 1947; 33:796.

118. Jacobson SA, Danufsky P: Marked electrocardiographic

changes produced by experimental head trauma. *J Neuropathol Exp Neurol* 1954; 13:462.

119. Marks J: Central nervous system influence in the genesis of atrial fibrillation. *Ohio State Med J* 1956; 52:1054.

120. Hersch C: Electrocardiographic changes in head injuries. *Circulation* 1961; 23:853.

121. Rotem M, et al: Life-threatening torsades des pointes arrhythmias associated with head injury. *Neurosurgery* 1988; 23:89.

122. Hersch C: Electrocardiographic changes in subarachnoid hemorrhage, meningitis, and intracranial space-occupying lesions. *Br Heart J* 1964; 26:785.

123. Weinberg SJ, Fuster JM: Electrocardiographic changes produced by localized hypothalamic stimulations. *Ann Intern Med* 1960; 53:332.

124. Kaste M, et al: Creatinine kinase isoenzymes in acute brain injury. *J Neurosurg* 1981; 55:511.

125. Albin MS, et al: Brain and lungs at risk after cervical cord transection: Intracranial pressure, brain water, blood-brain barrier permeability, cerebral blood flow and extravascular lung water changes. *Surg Neurol* 1985; 24:191.

126. Albin MS: Epidemiology, physiopathology and experimental therapeutics of acute spinal cord injury. *Crit Care Clin* 1987; 3:441.

127. Sarnoff SJ, Sarnoff LC: Neurohemodynamics of pulmonary edema. The role of sympathetic pathways in the elevation of pulmonary and systemic vascular pressure following the intracranial injection of fibrin. *Circulation* 1952; 6:51.

128. Theodore J, Robin ED: Speculations in neurogenic pulmonary edema (NPE). *Am Rev Respir Dis* 1976; 113:405.

129. Albin MS, et al: Study of functional recovery produced by delayed localized cooling after spinal injury in primates. *J Neurosurg* 1968; 29:113.

130. Albin MS, et al: Effect of localized cooling in spinal cord trauma. *J Trauma* 1969; 9:1000.

131. White RJ: Current status of spinal cord cooling. *Clin Neurosurg* 1973; 20:400.

132. Lehman KG, et al: Cardiovascular abnormalities accompanying acute spinal cord injury in humans: Incidence, time course and severity. *J Am Coll Cardiol* 1987; 10:46.

133. Hickey R, et al: Autoregulation of spinal cord and cerebral blood flow: Is the cord a microcosm of the brain? *Stroke* 1987; 17:1183.

134. Mangano DT, et al: Dipyridamole thallium-201 scintigraphy as a preoperative screening test. A reexamination of its predictive potential. Study of Perioperative Ischemia Research Group. *Circulation* 1991; 84:493.

135. O'Keefe JH Jr, et al: Value of normal electrocardiographic findings in predicting resting left ventricular function in patients with chest pain and suspected coronary artery disease. *Am J Med* 1989; 86:658.

136. American Society of Anesthesiologists Task Force on Pulmonary Artery Catheterization: Practice guidelines for pulmonary catheterization. *Anesthesiology* 1993; 78:380.

Chapter 11 _____

CONSCIOUSNESS, DELIRIUM, AND COMA

CLAUDIO BASSETTI

MICHAEL S. ALDRICH

Consciousness [from the Latin *cum* (with) and *scire* (to know)] is the prerequisite for higher mental activities and corresponds to the subjective experience that arises from the interaction of the self with the inner and outer world. Because of its mainly subjective quality, and because of the numerous psychological, physiologic, and philosophical contexts in which this term is applied, it is difficult to formulate a universally satisfactory definition of consciousness.[1-3] From a pragmatic viewpoint, consciousness can be defined as a state of awareness of environment and self that is produced by a central nervous system (CNS) process that gives significance to stimuli from the external and internal environments and allows appropriate behavior to occur. It can be viewed as having two dimensions: wakefulness (arousal, alertness, or vigilance) and awareness (the sum of cognitive and emotional functions). These two dimensions reflect the two critical CNS components required to maintain consciousness: the brainstem ascending reticular activating system (ARAS) with the medial diencephalic structures to which it projects, and the cerebral cortex with its associated white matter tracts, subcortical nuclei, and descending corticofugal systems.

Wakefulness corresponds to the cortical "tone" necessary to run the cognitive apparatus and depends on the integration of the ARAS with the descending (corticoreticular) pathways that modulate its function. The ARAS, first described by Moruzzi and Magoun[4] almost 50 years ago, is viewed today as a functional system composed of different subunits. Anatomically, one can differentiate two major projection routes: the dorsal or "thalamic route," and the ventral or "extrathalamic route" (Fig. 11-1).[5] Physiologically, different components of the ARAS are responsible for the activation of mental, EEG, motor, and vegetative functions. As a consequence, the three basic states of being—wakefulness, rapid eye movement (REM) sleep, and non-REM (NREM) sleep—and their disturbances can be expressed in terms of the specific profile of activation or impairment of these components. Pharmacologically, noradrenergic, dopaminergic, serotoninergic, and cholinergic pathways constitute the best characterized but not the only transmitter systems involved in the different functions of the ARAS.

Awareness is the result of arousal, attention, and higher cognitive functions. Directing and maintaining attention to a specific task depends upon the function of the prefrontal cortex of the right hemisphere and its descending connection to the thalamus.[6,7] These pathways allow selective gating of external inputs and consequently the choice between environmentally driven and internally driven behavior.[8,9] The "aroused and attentive" brain is finally enabled by multiple partially segregated corticosubcortical circuits to perform such higher cognitive functions as memory, thinking, and language.[10] Awareness has been suggested to "arise" from the simultaneous activation of these brain areas over a few milliseconds, a synchronization which

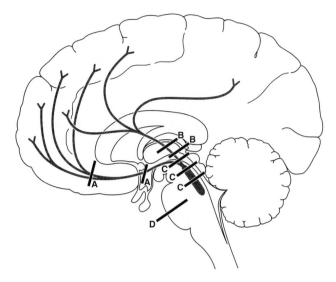

Figure 11-1 Schematic representation of the *ascending reticular activating system* (ARAS), with ventral pathway projecting from the pons and mesencephalon to the subthalamus-hypothalamus and frontal forebrain and dorsal pathway to the paramedian thalamus and cortex. Effects of focal lesions are depicted: a = akinetic mutism, b = hypersomnia, c = coma, d = locked-in syndrome.

in turn may depend on intrinsic oscillatory properties of thalamocortical projections.[11]

From a clinical and pathophysiologic viewpoint, disturbances of consciousness traditionally have been divided into disorders of wakefulness, due to impaired arousal, and disorders of awareness with preserved wakefulness, due to primary cerebral dysfunction. *Disorders of wakefulness* are expressions of direct or indirect dysfunction of the ARAS and always impair awareness. The spectrum of *disorders of awareness* is wide and includes relatively isolated dysfunction of such specific functions as memory or language, or a more diffuse disturbance of mental activities as occurs with dementia or the vegetative state.

In clinical practice arousal and awareness are often affected together, but the profile of involvement of arousal and of cognitive, motor, and vegetative functions may differ depending on the topography, nature, and time-course of the underlying lesion.[12] Examples include the so-called dissociated states, such as alert with insufficient motor arousal (akinetic mutism), coma with near-normal EEG (alpha coma), and dreaming in the awake state (peduncular hallucinosis).[13–17] Disturbances of consciousness, therefore, should be defined by the specific profile of dysfunction as assessed by clinical examination and paraclinical tests.

Disorders of Wakefulness (Impaired Arousal)

Depending on the type—auditory, tactile, or noxious—and the intensity of stimulation needed to arouse the patient, several levels of disturbed wakefulness can be differentiated: (1) hypervigilance (hyperalertness), (2) somnolence, (3) stupor, and (4) coma.

HYPERVIGILANCE

Although decreased arousal is most often encountered in organic brain disorders, the opposite occasionally is observed. Hypervigilance may be caused by an increase in activity of systems maintaining wakefulness, as can be seen in delirium following benzodiazepine or alcohol withdrawal, or by impairment of sleep-promoting mechanisms as can occur with encephalitic or neoplastic lesions of the anterior hypothalamus, after thalamotomy, or in the course of fatal familial insomnia.[18,19]

SOMNOLENCE AND OBTUNDATION

These descriptors, along with drowsiness, pathologic sleepiness, and hypersomnia, refer to states in which patients are drowsy or appear asleep and show little interest in the environment. Although verbal stimuli are usually sufficient to elicit speech and appropriate motor behavior, responses are slow and patients fall asleep easily when not stimulated.

STUPOR

With stupor, a more advanced stage of impaired arousal, patients usually appear to be asleep and awaken only when stimulated with a loud voice or vigorous shaking. They may be agitated or combative at such times but they do not communicate in a meaningful way apart from monosyllabic sounds, groans, and simple behaviors. They return to a sleeplike state as soon as stimulation ceases.

COMA

Coma (from the Greek *coma* = sleep) refers to a sleeplike state of unarousability in which consciousness is completely absent. Comatose patients keep their eyes closed even after painful stimuli, are not capable of any comprehensible verbal response, do not obey commands, and do not localize painful stimuli, although they may make posturing and reflexive responses. Coma is rarely a permanent state, probably because of redundancy of activating systems, and most patients either die or regain identifiable sleep-wake cycles after a few days or weeks.[20,21] Prolonged coma and *brain death* are discussed in Chap 38.

Disorders of Awareness

DELIRIUM

Delirium is the most common disturbance of consciousness encountered in clinical practice and may

TABLE 11-1
Diagnostic Criteria for Delirium

A. Reduced attention

B. Disorganized thinking

C. At least two of the following:
   Reduced level of consciousness
   Perceptual disturbances (illusions, hallucinations)
   Disturbed sleep-wake cycle
   Increased or decreased psychomotor activity
   Disorientation
   Amnesia

D. Development over hours to days, often with a fluctuating course

affect 5 to 10 percent of hospitalized patients. Despite the many possible causes, the clinical picture is relatively constant, with reduced ability to maintain attention, disturbance of immediate memory, and disorganized, slowed, and impoverished thinking (Table 11-1). Disorientation, altered short-term and long-term memory, and illusions and hallucinations are frequently but not invariably present.[22,23] Although delirium usually is accompanied by decreased arousal and psychomotor slowing, occasionally—for example, in the course of alcohol and benzodiazepine withdrawal—it is characterized by hypervigilance and enhanced psychomotor activity.[22] Occasionally, there is a "dreamy" or "twilight" state associated with partial loss of contact with the outer world. The severity of delirium typically waxes and wanes, occasionally from minute to minute, and may be interrupted by relatively lucid moments. Exacerbation of delirium in the night hours is typical and is called "sundowning." Associated nighttime insomnia and daytime hypersomnia are common.

Delirium may result from an underlying dementing illness and can be caused by any cerebral or extracerebral disorder that can lead to coma. Toxic-metabolic encephalopathies and drug and alcohol withdrawal states are the most common extracerebral causes.[22] Ictal and postictal states, focal brain lesions more commonly of the right hemisphere, and meningoencephalitic disorders are typical primary cerebral causes.[24-27] In elderly subjects, particularly those with dementia or other brain damage, delirium may be precipitated by dehydration, pulmonary or urinary infection, hypoxia, cardiac failure, urinary retention, and a variety of drugs.[23,28]

Delirium must be differentiated from isolated memory impairment as occurs in the syndrome of *transient global amnesia* (TGA). Although such patients may be anxious and disoriented, they have normal arousal, attention, and concentration.[29,30]

PERSISTENT VEGETATIVE STATE

Although some comatose patients regain full consciousness, others "awaken" into a persistent vegeta-

tive state (PVS) characterized by preserved autonomic and vegetative functions despite severe mental impairment.[31] Although spontaneous eye opening, yawns, chewing, grimacing, and other reflex motor actions occur along with spontaneous respiration and physiologic features of sleep and wakefulness, the lack of awareness and cognition is apparent in the inability of such patients to respond in a learned manner to external stimuli and the absence of sustained, reproducible, purposeful, or voluntary responses to stimulation.[32,33] The term PVS is preferable to apallic syndrome, coma vigile, or neocortical death syndrome because it does not imply a specific pathoanatomic substrate.

The PVS may follow coma from head injury or anoxia and may also occur as the terminal stage of dementing illnesses. The reduction in cognitive and metabolic activity is usually associated with extensive damage to cortex and subcortical structures, with relative sparing of brainstem structures; preserved brainstem function accounts for the persistence of autonomic functions and sleep-wake cycle.[34] Less commonly PVS can follow more or less selective damage of paramedian thalamic structures, emphasizing the key role of these structures in cognitive processes.[11,35] The PVS is discussed in more detail in Chap. 38.

Coma-like Conditions

Several conditions, including PVS, can be mistaken for coma (Table 11-2). Differentiation is important because of the differences in the level of awareness, degree of suffering, etiology, and prognosis.

AKINETIC MUTISM

This term describes a state of silent immobility associated with an alert appearance as indicated by optic fixation and following eye movements.[36] Despite the wakeful appearance, these patients almost always have markedly impaired cognitive functions. The immobility is usually not associated with significant spasticity or rigidity and is best interpreted as an extreme form of lack of spontaneous and evoked behavior (*abulia*) caused by disruption of reticulothalamofrontal and extrathalamic activating reticulofrontal afferents. These patients are mute but not speechless and akinetic but not paralyzed: repetitive stimuli can bring them to say a few understandable words and to move purposefully.

Akinetic mutism most often follows large bilateral basal-medial lesions of the frontal lobes involving orbital and septal cortex, cingulate gyrus, and the limbic system, due to bilateral cerebral artery occlusion, vasospasm following subarachnoid hemorrhage, or decom-

TABLE 11-2
Coma and Coma-like Conditions

	Coma	Akinetic Mutism	Locked-in Syndrome	Vegetative State
Self-awareness	Absent	Present	Present	Absent
Motor function	Not purposeful	Paucity of movements Purposeful possible	Absent	Not purposeful
Suffering	No	Yes	Yes	No
Respiration	Disturbed	Normal	Normal or disturbed	Normal
Sleep-wake cycles	Mostly absent	Present Often hypersomnia	Present	Present
EEG	Theta-delta or alpha coma	Slowing or normal	Normal or near normal	Variable[a]
Lesion site	Bihemispheric or brainstem	Frontodiencephalic or midbrain	Pontine base	Bihemispheric or bithalamic

[a] From almost normal tracing to theta-delta or almost isoelectric EEG.
SOURCE: From Multi-Society Task Force,[33] with permission.

pensating communicating hydrocephalus[37–39] (Fig. 11-1). Patients usually exhibit other "frontodiencephalic signs" such as urinary incontinence and forced grasping as well as frontally dominant slowing on EEG. Less commonly, akinetic mutism occurs in patients with bilateral lesions of basal ganglia or thalamus, or with incomplete lesions of the midbrain reticular formation[40–44] (Fig. 11-1). In these patients, hypersomnia and such disturbances of eye movements as vertical gaze palsy, third nerve palsy, and skew deviation are usually present while the EEG may show a near-normal pattern.

CATATONIA

This syndrome, first described by Kahlbaum over 100 years ago, is characterized by staring; a perplexed appearance with mutism and lack of reaction to surroundings; motor signs including increased tone, unusual posturing, catalepsy (an immobile position that is constantly maintained), and waxy rigidity (flexibilitas cerea); and such bizarre repetitive behaviors as verbigerations, grimacing, echolalia, and echopraxia.[45] The presence of motor signs and repetitive behaviors differentiates catatonia from akinetic mutism.

Although schizophrenia and depression are the most common causes, organic conditions including drug intoxication and withdrawal, metabolic encephalopathies, and focal brain damage to frontal lobes, basal ganglia, and diencephalon must be considered in the differential diagnosis.[45–47]

LOCKED-IN SYNDROME

This term was introduced in 1966 by Plum and Posner[20] to denote a condition described by Alexander Dumas in *Le compte de Monte-Cristo* and by Emil Zola in *Thérèse*

Raquin. In this deefferented state, there is paralysis of the extremities, the lower cranial nerves, and horizontal gaze while vertical eye movements and blinking are preserved. The locked-in syndrome (LiS) differs from akinetic mutism in that awareness of self and environment is preserved so that the patient is conscious, at least to some degree, and is able to communicate by means of eye movements and blinking. Decerebrate posturing, ocular bobbing, skew deviation, respiratory difficulties, and involuntary crying, grimacing, yawning, or groaning may accompany LiS.[48,49] The EEG is usually normal or only mildly abnormal.[50,51]

Ventral pontine lesions (Figs. 11-1 and 11-2) are the usual cause of LiS, although midbrain stroke, diffuse cerebral hypoxia after cardiac arrest, encephalitis, severe polyradiculoneuropathy, tumor, abscess, trauma, and pontine myelinolysis have been reported.[51–55] Bilateral deep hemispheric strokes, usually involving the capsula interna, can cause a bilateral disruption of corticospinal and corticobulbar pathways (*anarthric tetraparesis*) with preservation of consciousness.[56–59] Preserved horizontal eye movements differentiate this syndrome from the LiS.

SLEEP AND HYPERSOMNIA

Even though comatose patients usually maintain a sleeplike appearance, there are important differences between sleep and coma. Sleep is a natural, periodic, reversible, and active process requiring appropriate interactions of a number of brainstem and diencephalic structures, whereas stupor and coma are associated with metabolic depression of the brainstem and cerebral hemispheres. Stimulation of some of the structures that compose the sleep system induces sleep, whereas lesions of these areas may induce disordered sleep-wake regulation. Although the specific functions of

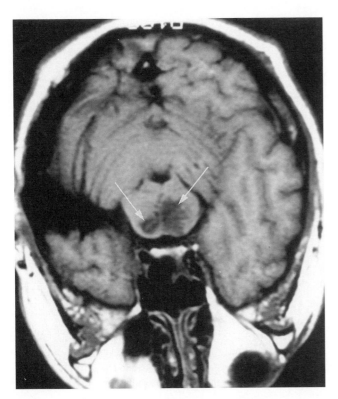

Figure 11-2 *Locked-in syndrome.* Brain CT of a 36-year-old man with bilateral pontine infarction due to basilar artery thrombosis. (*Arrows*, pontine infarctions.) (Courtesy of D. Quint, Neuroradiology Department, University of Michigan Hospitals, Ann Arbor, Michigan.)

sleep are not well defined, the restoration of alertness and vigor brought about by sleep is one of its most important characteristics; coma, whether induced by diseases or by general anesthesia, lacks this general restorative quality.

Although sleep and disturbances of arousal are produced by physiologically distinct processes, pathologic sleepiness related to brain disorders can closely resemble physiologic sleepiness caused by sleep deprivation, particularly when somnolence is caused by lesions of the paramedian thalamic and thalamohypothalamic areas (Fig. 11-3).[60,61] Hypersomnia in such cases is frequently accompanied by physiologic sleep postures, quiet breathing, and yawning.[62–65] With more caudal lesions of the mesencephalic and pontine tegmentum, decreased arousal is associated with nonphysiologic decorticate or decerebrate postures with pyramidal signs.[60]

Pathophysiology of Altered States of Consciousness

Two principal groups of pathologic processes impair consciousness. One group consists of diffuse toxic-met-abolic encephalopathies that decrease the function of both cerebral hemispheres. The second group consists of focal lesions that impair, directly or indirectly by mass effect, the critical areas of the brainstem and diencephalon that are involved in the maintenance of consciousness. In clinical practice, it is useful to divide the latter group into two types: (1) supratentorial lesions and (2) subtentorial lesions. Subtentorial lesions account for about 15 percent of cases of coma in patients admitted to hospital without traumatic or other readily apparent causes and supratentorial structural lesions for about 20 percent. Toxic-metabolic disorders are responsible for the remaining two thirds.[20]

TOXIC-METABOLIC ENCEPHALOPATHIES

These disorders disrupt brain function and lead to coma by preventing substrate utilization, by the effects of exogenous or endogenous toxins, or by the effects of temperature, electrolyte, or hormone imbalance. The brain relies entirely on glucose to supply its energy needs via the oxygen-requiring citric acid cycle and to a much lesser degree via anaerobic glycolysis. About 3.3 ml oxygen/min and 5.5 mg glucose/min are re-

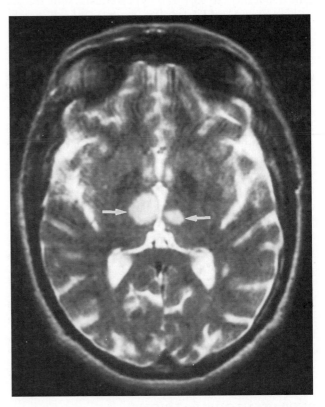

Figure 11-3 *Bilateral paramedian thalamic stroke.* Brain MRI of a 51-year-old patient who presented with initial coma and subsequently severe hypersomnia with up to 17 h of sleep behavior per day. (*Arrows*, thalamic infarcts.) (Courtesy of Prof. G. Schroth, Neuroradiology Department, University of Bern Hospital, Bern, Switzerland.)

quired for each 100 g brain tissue along with certain cofactors, such as thiamine. Since the brain has virtually no energy reserve, deprivation for even a short time of one or more of these substrates at normothermia produces encephalopathy and altered consciousness. While metabolic encephalopathies impair consciousness more or less in proportion to their severity, the type of metabolic disturbance is also important in determining the degree of impairment. In addition to global disturbances, metabolic disorders may produce such focal disturbances as aphasia or hemiparesis, particularly among the elderly.[20]

Since the primary site of dysfunction is the cerebral cortex, the EEG and cortical evoked potentials—which primarily reflect the activity of thalamocortical neurons—can be helpful, together with the clinical examination, in assessing the severity and the course of metabolic encephalopathies, but they are usually not useful for determining etiology.[66–68]

Initial stages of diffuse encephalopathy are characterized by delirium that at first may be subtle or transient and manifest only as irritability, restlessness, and mild attentional deficits. Later, hallucinatory elements and such neurological signs as appendicular ataxia, gait instability, dysarthria, hyperreflexia, and tremor may appear. The EEG is usually only mildly abnormal, with generalized slowing or frontal intermittent rhythmic delta activity (FIRDA). More advanced stages are accompanied by severe delirium and stupor along with grasping and other frontal release signs, flapping tremor (also called asterixis or negative myoclonus), multifocal myoclonus, focal or generalized seizures, hyperreflexia, and pyramidal signs including bilateral Babinski signs. Mild focal deficits and nuchal rigidity with hyperproteinorrhachia and mild pleocytosis occasionally occur in the absence of focal brain damage or CNS infection.[69] The EEG usually demonstrates generalized slowing, often accompanied by epileptiform activity and triphasic waves.[67] With severe encephalopathy, patients become comatose and a variety of "pseudostructural" eye movement disturbances can appear, including downbeat nystagmus, ocular bobbing, skew deviation, horizontal or vertical gaze deviations, and opsoclonus.[70] The EEG demonstrates severe slowing and amplitude reduction and eventually only an intermittent burst-suppression pattern.[67] Finally, more robust electrophysiologic parameters such as the cortical short-latency SEP also are abolished.

SUPRATENTORIAL LESIONS

Although a few studies have suggested a left-hemispheric dominance for wakefulness and a right-hemispheric dominance for attention, higher cognitive functions and awareness appear to decline in cortical

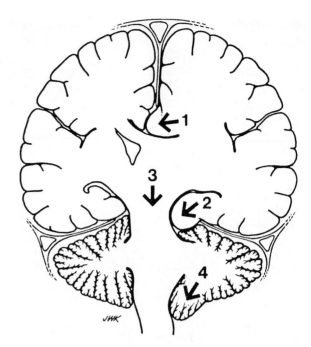

Figure 11-4   The *herniation syndromes*. (From Wilkins RH, Rengachary SS: *Neurosurgery*. New York, McGraw-Hill Book Company, 1985, by permission of the publisher.)

lesions roughly in proportion to the amount of cortex that is damaged or destroyed rather than in relation to any particular area.[7,26,71–74]

In patients with expanding intracerebral processes, pressure gradients between different intracranial compartments can lead to several types of herniation (Fig. 11-4). Disturbances of consciousness in such patients traditionally have been attributed to brainstem distortion and secondary ischemia occurring with two herniation syndromes: the *uncal syndrome* and the *central syndrome*.[20,75] While the two patterns show distinct differences during their early phases, the differences disappear as the level of dysfunction progresses to the midbrain and below. Furthermore, recent studies suggest that disturbances of consciousness in supratentorial lesions may be the expression of lateral displacement of deep brain structures rather than downward herniation.

Complications of both herniation processes include hydrocephalus and secondary vascular lesions. Compression of the posterior cerebral artery at the tentorium can cause occipital infarction. Brainstem hemorrhages (of *Duret*) can occur as a consequence of acute brainstem compression in the presence of rapidly expanding, large supratentorial lesions and can lead to deep coma and death. Intraventricular bleeding or lumbar puncture in the presence of an expanding mass can cause sudden downward herniation of the cerebellar tonsils in the foramen magnum with cardiopulmonary failure.

In general, the acute effects of cortical and subcortical lesions on consciousness are more severe than the chronic effects, and impaired alertness can occur with acute lesions in the absence of other signs of mass effect. The sudden loss of consciousness that may occur at the onset of acute hemispheric strokes and the usually short-lasting stupor or coma sometimes observed in isolated, focal hemispheric strokes without significant perifocal edema are usually explained by a transitory functional depression of the contralateral hemisphere referred to as *diaschisis*.[74,76]

Uncal Syndrome

The uncal syndrome, which usually occurs with laterally placed lesions of the temporal lobe, refers to herniation of the medial temporal lobe into the space between the edge of the tentorium and the midbrain (Fig. 11-5). Its most striking clinical feature is the *dilated pupil* on the side of the expanding mass. Although compression of the third nerve by the herniating uncus against the petroclinoid ligament, the free edge of the tentorium, or the posterior cerebral artery is the traditional explanation for pupillary dilatation, other mechanisms are often responsible.[77,78] For example, stretching and distortion of the nerve in its subarachnoid course can cause pupillodilation before actual herniation of the temporal lobe through the tentorial notch and may explain the rapid pupillary contraction that can occur with antiedematous treatment.[79] Pupillodilation also can occur from an intraparenchymatous fascicular or nuclear third nerve lesion secondary to mechanical distortion of the midbrain.[80] Decreased alertness correlates better with the degree of lateral displacement and distortion of the upper brainstem, associated with lateral shift of the supratentorial mass, than it does with the degree of downward transtentorial herniation; in fact, third nerve palsy can occur in patients with temporal herniation but without alteration of consciousness.[81] Hence, transtentorial herniation may not be the crucial event in the appearance of stupor and coma in patients with the uncal syndrome.[82-85]

Cheyne-Stokes respirations (see "Respiration" below) may be seen in the early stages of the uncal syndrome, occasionally accompanied by sighs and yawns, and although they are not specific their occurrence in the setting of a mass lesion should alert the clinician to the potential for further neurological deterioration.[86] The absence of the Cheyne-Stokes pattern, however, does not provide assurance that the patient is stable, since the uncal syndrome may develop even when respiration is entirely normal.

Once pupillodilation has appeared, herniation and death can occur within a few hours, even in patients with brain tumors who have been stable for weeks. As the uncal syndrome progresses to involve the midbrain, coma and ophthalmoplegia occur, with fixed pupils of 5 to 8 mm diameter. Compression of the contralateral cerebral peduncle against the tentorium can produce hypertonus, hemiparesis, and pyramidal signs that are *ipsilateral* to the mass.[87] Further progression leads to changes identical to those that occur with the central syndrome.

Central Syndrome

The central syndrome, which refers to the downward displacement of the upper brainstem through the tentorium (Fig. 11-4), typically occurs with medially situated frontal, parietal, or occipital lesions and with rapidly advancing compression (<24 h). It begins with the diencephalic stage, characterized by a reduction in alertness. Agitation, confusion, drowsiness, or stupor may be apparent along with conjugate or roving and slightly divergent eye movements and small pupils that are attributed to injury to pupillodilatory fibers in the hypothalamus.[75] Progressive brainstem dysfunction is indicated clinically by coma, decerebrate or decorticate rigidity, and fixed midposition pupils of moderate size. As the level of brainstem dysfunction reaches the lower pons, eye movements cease, even with caloric stimulation, and the patient becomes flaccid. Tidal volume decreases, while more or less regular patterns of respiration may continue. Once the level of dysfunction reaches the upper medulla, respirations become ataxic due to disruption of pathways connecting pontomedullary respiratory centers. With continued caudal progression, the respiratory rate slows and long periods of apnea occur before breathing finally stops.

SUBTENTORIAL LESIONS

Stupor and coma with subtentorial lesions occur by direct or indirect disruption of the reticular activating system and its projection pathways. Disturbances of consciousness may develop rapidly and without the initial lateralized motor signs characteristic of supratentorial lesions. Intrinsic brainstem processes that cause direct ARAS injury are almost invariably accompanied by disturbances of eye movements due to dysfunction of the extensive oculomotor pathways that accompany the ARAS. Indirect injury of the ARAS occurs by compression and can be associated with upward herniation of the midbrain through the tentorium cerebelli or with downward herniation of the medulla through the foramen magnum.

Unlike diffuse encephalopathic and supratentorial lesions, the EEG correlates poorly with the degree of impairment of arousal in subtentorial lesions.[88] Occa-

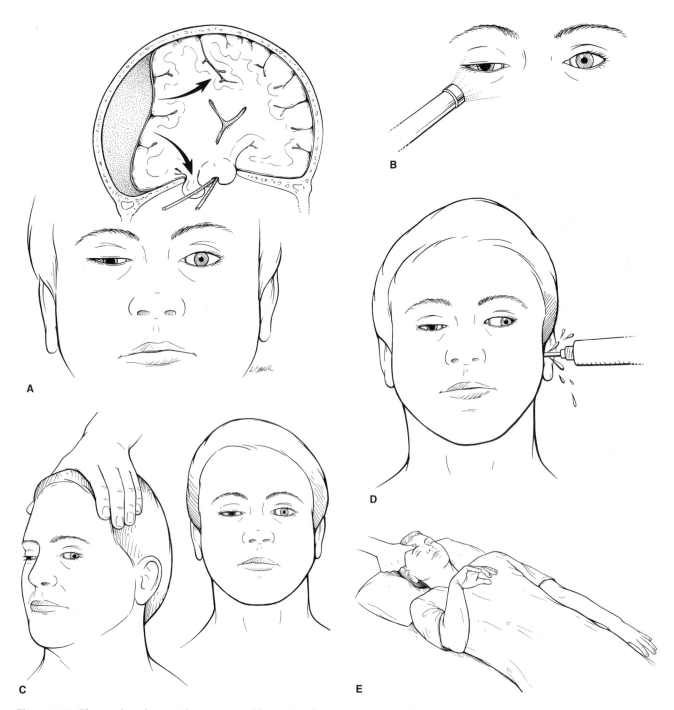

Figure 11-5 The *uncal syndrome* with transtentorial herniation due to a supratentorial mass (*A*). Clinical findings include unilateral nonreactive mydriasis (*B*), absent adduction of the homolateral eye on oculocephalic (*C*) and ventibuloocular (*D*) reflex testing, and pain response diminished contralaterally (*E*).

sionally, a dissociation between clinical state and EEG may be observed, such as in cases with only a mildly reduced level of consciousness but with severe EEG slowing, or of coma with unreactive alpha EEG activity.[13,15] On the other hand, significant disturbances of sleep architecture and abnormalities of somatosensory

evoked potentials and auditory evoked potentials are more commonly seen with infratentorial than with supratentorial lesions. Reduced numbers of sleep spindles and decreased amounts of non-rapid-eye-movement (NREM) sleep can be seen in thalamohypothalamic lesions, whereas a decrease of both rapid-eye-movement (REM) and NREM sleep usually occurs with mesencephalopontine lesions.[62,89–93]

Intrinsic Lesions

With intrinsic lesions, the severity of altered consciousness is roughly proportional to the extent of tissue destruction of the ARAS.[20] In *thalamohypothalamic lesions* (Fig. 11-3), coma is often only transient even with bilateral lesions, probably because thalamic and extrathalamic projections of the ARAS are already separated and cannot both be affected by a single lesion. Initial coma or stupor evolves frequently to a somnolent state with apathy and akinetic mutism, often accompanied by amnesia and vertical gaze deficits. Persistent stupor and coma are more frequent in mesencephalopontine lesions because a single bilateral lesion can disrupt most of the ARAS. *Midbrain lesions* usually cause coma with fixed moderately dilated pupils and asymmetric motor findings with decorticate or decerebrate posturing. Cranial nerve III palsy and other eye movement and pupillary abnormalities can be observed (see "Neurological Examination," later). *Rostral pontine lesions* may cause coma or hypersomnia associated with bilateral sensorimotor signs, pseudobulbar palsy, pinpoint pupils, cranial nerves IV and V palsies, internuclear ophthalmoplegia (INO), or ocular bobbing. *Caudal pontine lesions* usually do not cause severe disturbances of consciousness but produce ataxic or apneustic respirations, horizontal gaze palsy due to destruction of the pontine center for lateral gaze, and palsies of cranial nerves VI to VIII. *Medullary* and *high spinal cord lesions* typically do not affect the level of arousal,[20,60,64] whereas deficits of cranial nerves IX through XII, respiratory disturbances, and downbeat nystagmus are common clinical findings.

Extrinsic Lesions

Upward herniation is most commonly due to cerebellar lesions; other causes include subdural or epidural hematomas and acoustic neuromas. The clinical picture is related to midbrain dysfunction and is indicated by downward gaze deviation with upward gaze paresis, decerebrate posturing, and fixed, moderately dilated pupils.[94] Occasionally, the combination of absent oculocephalic response and normal pupillary reflex can be seen in early upward herniation.

Downward herniation (Fig. 11-4) through the foramen magnum, which can occur with any enlarging subtentorial or supratentorial lesion, leads not only to coma but also to rapid circulatory and respiratory failure due to compression of neurons of the floor of the IVth ventricle that are involved in blood pressure and ventilatory control. Homolateral hemiparesis may occur as an early sign of downward herniation, related to compression against the clivus of the pyramid contralateral to the mass.[95]

Clinical Signs of Disturbances of Consciousness

GENERAL EXAMINATION

Temperature, Heart Rate, and Blood Pressure

As fever *per se* is not a cause of stupor or coma, *hyperthermia* in patients with disturbances of consciousness should always suggest infection. Other causes are thyrotoxicosis, heatstroke, and anticholinergic overdose. *Hypothermia* can cause stupor or coma (see "Disordered Temperature Regulation," later). Wernicke's encephalopathy may be associated with hypothalamic damage and hypothermia that is typically not accompanied by shivering.[79]

Hypertension—common after subarachnoid hemorrhage, stroke, head trauma, and other conditions associated with increased intracranial pressure—also occurs following withdrawal from antihypertensive treatment and with aortic dissection, thermal burns, and acute renal disease. The *Kocher-Cushing reflex*, which refers to hypertension associated with bradycardia and irregular breathing, is a late sign of increased intracranial pressure due to lower brainstem distortion that is seen most often in comatose children with posterior fossa lesions.[96] *Hypotension* can occur with blood and volume loss, sepsis, cardiac disease, barbiturate and other intoxications, Wernicke's encephalopathy, and Addison's crisis.

Neurogenic heart disease refers to arrhythmias, repolarization abnormalities that may suggest acute myocardial infarction, creatine kinase elevations, and structural cardiac changes that can accompany status epilepticus, subarachnoid hemorrhage, and stroke and may explain the occurrence of sudden death in patients with these conditions.[97–99] Potentially lethal cardiovascular abnormalities may occur with both left-sided and right-sided hemispheric lesions, particularly with large lesions that involve the insular cortex, and are the basis for the practice of continuous ECG monitoring during the first 1 to 3 days after large strokes or hemorrhages.[99–102] The pathogenesis appears to be related to increased sympathetic activity.[103,104]

Repetitive episodes of autonomic dysfunction with profuse sweating, tachycardia, transient fever, facial flushing, hyperventilation, and spontaneous motor activities (opisthotonus and decorticate or decerebrate postures) have been referred to as "*diencephalic seizures*" and can be seen in patients who are in coma or in a vegetative state.

TABLE 11-3
Disturbances of Breathing in Brain Lesions

Findings in patients with breathing disturbances and acute brain damage. Three fourths of the patients had decreased level of consciousness.

a) *Frequency* of different breathing patterns (130 patients)
   Periodic: 29 patients
   Irregular: 38 patients
   Tachypnea (>25/min): 31 patients
   Combination of 2 or 3: 32 patients

b) *Sites of damage* different breathing patterns (200 patients)
   Periodic: unilateral hemispheric ($n = 30$), bilateral hemispheric ($n = 17$), brainstem ($n = 15$)
   Irregular: unilateral hemispheric ($n = 21$), bilateral hemispheric ($n = 21$), brainstem ($n = 30$)
   Tachypnea: unilateral hemispheric ($n = 27$), bilateral hemispheric ($n = 20$), brainstem ($n = 19$)

SOURCE: From North and Jennett,[106] with permission.

Respiration

Several types of breathing disturbance may occur with stupor and coma. Although recognition of these types can help to determine the affected area of the nervous system, the contribution for anatomic diagnosis has probably been overestimated. In fact, the most common causes of changes in respiration in these patients are aspiration, sedation, metabolic acidosis or alkalosis, hyperthermia or hypothermia, and infections. Furthermore, the three breathing patterns often associated with CNS injury—periodic breathing, irregular breathing, and tachypnea—all may occur with supratentorial or infratentorial processes (Table 11-3).[105,106]

Cheyne-Stokes respiration (CSR, Fig. 11-6) refers to periodic waxing and waning of respiratory amplitude and rate, with apnea at the nadir of the cycle. It is more common in light NREM sleep than in deep NREM sleep or REM sleep.[107,108] The cycle duration may be 20 to 90 s with apneas lasting up to 30 s, and the level of arousal in somatic and autonomic functions is higher in the waxing phase as indicated by phasic motor activities, pupillodilation, arousals, and increase in heart rate and intracranial blood flow velocity.[79,109] The aberrant ventilatory control responsible for this pattern is complex and includes circulatory and neurogenic factors.[108] Delayed peripheral feedback can be caused by, for example, congestive heart failure with prolonged circulation time, whereas hemispheric dysfunction can change the setpoint of central chemoreceptors leading to abnormally increased ventilatory response to hypercapnia and an abnormally decreased or absent ventilatory response to hypocapnia. While CSR is often seen early in metabolic encephalopathy or as an early sign of impending transtentorial herniation, it is not specific for these conditions, can occur with a wide variety of neurological conditions, and does not imply a poor

prognosis.[86,106] In stroke patients, for example, CSR may occur in as many as 59 percent of patients with supratentorial lesions and 40 percent of those with infratentorial lesions.[110] *Posthyperventilation apnea* probably reflects mechanisms similar to those involved in CSR.

Causes of coma associated with *hyperventilation* and metabolic acidosis (*Kussmaul respiration*) include diabetic ketoacidosis, uremia, hyperosmolar states, and lactic acidosis. Hyperventilation with respiratory alkalosis can be caused by hepatic encephalopathy, salicylate intoxication, sepsis, or psychogenic factors. Less commonly, hyperventilation is related to increased intracranial presure or to focal hemispheric or brainstem damage. In these cases of *"central neurogenic" hyperventilation* (metronomic breathing), the arterial oxygen pressure is above 70 to 80 mmHg, and it is the increased regularity rather than the increased rate of breathing (up to 30 to 40/min) that is characteristic.[111] This pattern of breathing is nonspecific and can also occur as a result of coexisting cardiopulmonary disorders that affect stretch receptors in the lungs.[106,111]

Infarctions affecting the pneumotaxic center in the dorsolateral pons rostral to the motor trigeminal nerve nucleus can lead to an unusual respiratory pattern called *apneustic breathing*.[112] This breathing pattern—characterized by a pause at full inspiration, abnormally prolonged expiration, and a 2- or 3-s pause at the end of expiration—can also occur with anoxic brain injury, meningitis, and hypoglycemic coma.

"Ataxic breathing" (Biot's respiration) refers to an irregular respiratory pattern of variable rate and ampli-

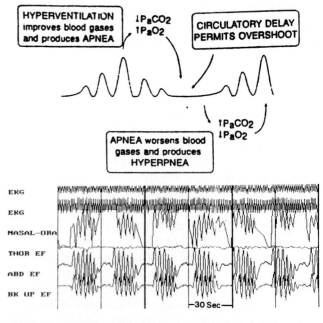

Figure 11-6 *Cheyne-Stokes respiration.* Schematic description of pathogenesis (*above*) and a recording (*below*). (From Yamashiro and Kryger[108] with permission.)

tude that may be seen in association with medullary infarction or pontomedullary compression from cerebellar hemorrhage or infarction. Acute demyelination caused by poliovirus or other viral infections that affect the brainstem is another cause of ataxic breathing. Since ataxic breathing may proceed quickly to *respiratory failure* and is especially susceptible to the respiratory depressant effects of sedatives, assisted ventilation is required as soon as the pattern is evident. Although respiratory failure usually indicates bilateral medullary damage, unilateral strokes involving the nucleus tractus solitarius, nucleus ambiguus, and the medullary reticular formation occasionally may cause respiratory failure involving both automatic and voluntary control.[113,114]

Neurogenic lung edema refers to alveolar noncardiac pulmonary edema that may develop following head trauma, status epilepticus, subarachnoid hemorrhage, and medullary lesions.[103,115] The pathogenesis is complex and probably relates to increased central sympathetic activity leading to left atrial hypertension, systemic hypertension, pulmonary venoconstriction, and reduction in pulmonary vascular compliance.[103]

Persistent *hiccup*, more common in men that in women and thought to represent a disinhibited gastrorespiratory reflex, usually occurs with thoracoabdominal diseases and as a drug side effect but can occur also after tegmental brainstem injury, and rarely after focal supratentorial damage.[20,116,117]

Others

Skin changes such as needle marks (opiate intoxication), increased pigmentation (Addison's crisis, porphyria), cherry-red discoloration (CO poisoning), icterus (hepatic failure), gynecomastia and spider nevi (alcoholism), petechiae (diffuse intravascular coagulation), ecchymosis (trauma), linear hemorrhages under the nails (endocarditis and sepsis), "blue toes" (cholesterol emboli), "raccoon" eyes (orbital ecchymosis of anterior base skull fracture), hematoma over the mastoid (Battle sign of basilar skull fracture), petechial rash (meningoccocemia), and vesicular or maculopapular rash (drug reactions) may reveal the etiology of delirium, stupor, and coma.

Meningismus may occur with meningitis, subarachnoid hemorrhage, tonsillar herniation, spinal trauma, and rarely with metabolic encephalopathy and can be absent in the first hours after subarachnoid hemorrhage.[118] Nuchal rigidity can be disclosed by a positive *Kernig's sign* (flex thigh to 90 degrees with knee bent, when knee is straightened pain is reported in the hamstrings) or a positive *Brudzinski's sign* (flexion of patient's neck elicits involuntary hip flexion).

Fundus examination can reveal papilledema from increased intracranial pressure; retinal, subhyaloid, or

TABLE 11-4
Neurologic Examination of the Patient in Coma

Date: including time after onset of coma

Medications: particularly sedatives, analgesics, and muscle relaxants

Vital signs: temperature, blood pressure, pulse, breathing

Observation: spontaneous activities (eye opening, posture, seizures, and myoclonus)

Level of arousal: Glasgow coma scale, mental status

Brainstem functions: spontaneous eye movements, corneal reflex, pupillary reflex, oculocephalic and vestibuloocular reflex

Lateralizing signs: muscle tone, reflexes, pyramidal signs

Meningeal signs

vitreous hemorrhage from subarachnoid hemorrhage; retinal hemorrhages from embolism (*Roth's spots*); and cholesterol emboli (*Hollenhorst's plaques*). Venous pulsations usually disappear when intracranial pressure (ICP) is elevated, but papilledema may not always be present.

Ear examination may reveal hemotympanum, tympanic perforation, or otorrhea from skull base fracture.

NEUROLOGIC EXAMINATION

The neurologic examination is essential to determine level of consciousness, brainstem function, and the presence or absence of lateralizing signs (Table 11-4). This assessment usually allows the differentiation between coma due to a structural lesion and that due to toxic-metabolic dysfunction, which is of paramount importance in directing management. The time of the examination and the patient's medications should be noted.

Although it is often possible to determine the topography of the underlying lesions from the neurologic examination, the examiner must be aware of *false localizing* symptoms or signs, often caused by transtentorial or foraminal herniation and increased intracranial pressure.[119] The most common false localizing signs are homolateral hemiparesis due to compression of the midbrain peduncle against the contralateral tentorium edge in supratentorial masses and unilateral or bilateral abducens palsy with increased intracranial pressure. Less common are focal epileptic seizures in hydrocephalus, anisocoria following seizures, ipsilateral gaze deviation in supratentorial lesions, cerebellar signs in supratentorial masses, and upward gaze palsy in patients with somnolence or frontal lobe disorders.

Mental Status

The bedside examination of mental status assesses level of arousal, orientation, attention, memory, and

TABLE 11-5
Mental Status Assessment in Patients With Disturbances of Consciousness

1. *Level of arousal*: hypervigilant, normal, somnolent, stuporous, comatose

2. *Attention*: digit span (normal ≥5), serial sevens or backward spelling of words

3. *Orientation*: time (year, month, date, day, season), space (state, town, county, hospital, floor, room), situation, person

4. *Memory*: recall of 4 phonemically and semantically unrelated words after 10 min (normal ≥2), and after 30 min (after repetition at 5 to 10 min, normal ≥3)

5. *Language*: spontaneous speech fluency; naming animals (normal ≥15 in 1 min); naming of colors, body parts, room objects, parts of objects; repetition of words and sentences; comprehension; writing; reading

6. *Right-hemispheric functions*: visual or sensory neglect (simultaneous application of stimuli); visuoconstructive abilities (copy a cube or star, or draw a clock)

7. *Writing sample*: name, date, simple sentence, and drawing of spiral to detect tremor

selective left and right hemisphere functions (Table 11-5).[26,120] *Language* is a left hemispheric function in 99 percent of right-handed subjects and 75 percent of left-handed subjects. The writing sample allows objective documentation and can be used for subsequential comparison, for example, in metabolic encephalopathy. A rapid global neuropsychological assessment of the awake patient can be obtained with the Folstein Mini-Mental State test.[120]

Eyes

PUPILS. Pupillary size and reactions are under the control of the parasympathetic and sympathetic systems (Fig. 11-7). The "horizontal" parasympathetic pathway runs from the midbrain tectum with the oculomotor nerve to the eye. The "vertical" sympathetic pathway runs from the hypothalamus homolaterally down the dorsal brainstem to the intermediolateral columns of the upper cervical cord, ascends via peripheral fibers to the superior cervical ganglion (preganglionic fibers), and then travels together with the carotid and ophthalmic artery to the eye (postganglionic fibers).

Bilateral pupillary reactivity is preserved in most comatose patients with metabolic-toxic encephalopathy. Thus, the light reflex is the single most helpful sign in distinguishing metabolic from structural causes of coma (Fig. 11-8). Although in metabolic encephalopathy the pupils may be small and poorly reactive, sufficiently bright light will generally produce some reaction. Exceptions to this rule occur with overdoses of barbiturates, glutethimide, and drugs with anticholinergic properties such as tricyclic antidepressants,

which produce widely dilated and fixed pupils. Hypothermia can be accompanied by small and unreactive pupils.[121] Opiate overdose and organophosphate intoxication can cause small pupils in which the light reaction may be visible only with a magnifying glass. Pontine lesions characteristically produce *pinpoint pupils* due to interruption of descending sympathetic pathways and perhaps also to irritation of parasympathetic fibers. Insufficient illumination, the effects of systemic or local drugs, and ocular diseases are common confounders of pupillary examination.

Bilateral unreactive pupils in a comatose patient may occur with midbrain disease, bilateral third nerve palsy, or intoxication. Tectal and pretectal midbrain lesions often lead to large pupils that are unreactive to light although they may respond in the noncomatose patient to accommodation, a phenomenon referred to as near-light dissociation. Dorsal tegmental midbrain lesions produce fixed irregular pupils of normal size. Central midbrain lesions may cause a nuclear syndrome of the third nerve that is characterized by unreactive pupils of 4 to 5 mm in diameter and, even in unilateral lesions, by bilateral ptosis.[122] Ventral midbrain lesions can affect the intraaxial portion of the third nerve and cause an oculomotor palsy usually, but not invariably, accompanied by pupillary dilation.[123] Severe diffuse brain anoxia can lead to dilated and unreactive pupils; the pupils usually normalize within the first postresuscitation hour in patients with good outcome.[124,125]

Asymmetry of pupils (*anisocoria*), even of minor degree (2 mm), suggests unilateral dilation (mydriasis), as in oculomotor palsy, or contraction (miosis), as in Horner's syndrome. A *unilateral dilated and unreactive pupil*, usually associated with other oculomotor findings, suggests a third nerve lesion that can occur with midbrain lesions, but most commonly is due to extraaxial oculomotor compression from transtentorial herniation or posterior communicating artery aneurysm. Somnolence and anisocoria, the homolateral pupil being wider and unreactive, are the first signs of transtentorial herniation, and usually precede extraocular motor abnormalities.[86] Once the homolateral pupil is dilated, further evolution can be monitored with the opposite pupil, which first exhibits a diminished light reaction, then a decrease in size, and finally a reenlargement.[126] Although a unilateral dilated pupil without other third nerve findings is often due to topical application of pupillodilators or local eye trauma, it can be the first sign of an expanding aneurysm. *Oval pupils* are related to a nonuniform paresis of the sphincter pupillae and can be seen as a transitional form of third nerve compression or in the course of midbrain processes.[127-129] *Horner's syndrome* refers to homolateral miosis and ptosis with preserved light reflex. Hypohidro-

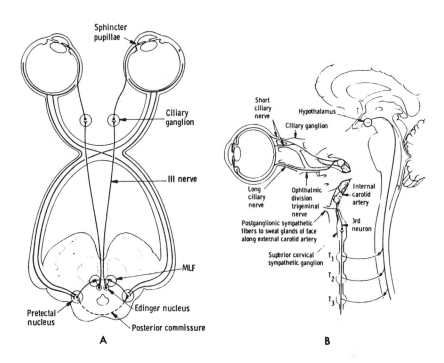

Figure 11-7 *Pupillary control. A.* The parasympathetic pupilloconstrictor pathway. *B.* The sympathetic pupillodilator pathway. (From Plum and Posner,[20] with permission.)

sis of the face and hemibody may also occur. A central Horner's syndrome can occur with pontine and medullary lesions but rarely with supratentorial lesions.[20,130,131] In thalamic or hypothalamic lesions both pupils are usually small and reactive (diencephalic pupils), but a homo- or contralateral Horner's syndrome has also been described.[20,132–134] Dissection or occlusion of the carotid artery can cause a homolateral peripheral Horner's syndrome.

Occasionally, one or both pupils show spontaneous constriction and dilation. This phenomenon, called *hippus*, can be seen with meningitis and with barbiturate or paraldehyde poisoning.[79]

The *ciliospinal reflex* refers to bilateral pupillodilation following painful stimuli and is thought to represent a spinal cord reflex with sensory afferents and sympathetic efferents. Its diagnostic and prognostic value in comatose patients is limited.

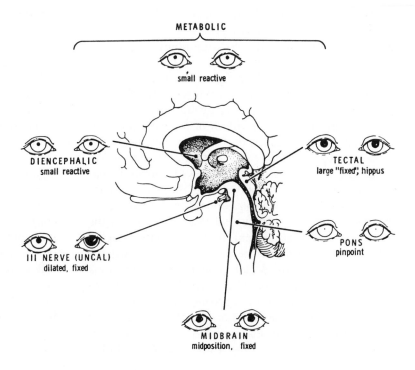

Figure 11-8 *Pupils in the unresponsive patient.* (From Plum and Posner,[20] with permission.)

EYELID AND EYE MOVEMENTS. Voluntary eye movements are difficult or impossible to test in patients with disturbances of consciousness, and the examiner must limit the examination to spontaneous and reflex eye movements. The presence of spontaneous and conjugate eye movements in the vertical and horizontal planes implies integrity of the oculomotor nuclei and the pathways connecting them bilaterally, including the medial longitudinal fasciculus (MLF), and therefore indicates the absence of significant damage between the midbrain and the lower pons.

In most patients with acute coma, the eyes are closed due to tonic contraction of the orbicularis oculi and there is no spontaneous blinking. If the eyes are opened passively and released, they close briskly in light coma and more smoothly and gradually in deeper coma. Patients with psychogenic unresponsiveness may resist eye opening and are unstable voluntarily to mimic the passive eye closure of coma. On rare occasions—for example, in some patients with hepatic coma, hyponatremia, or cerebellar hemorrhage—attempts to open the eye passively elicit a *reflex blepharospasm* that is similar to the resistance to eye opening that typifies psychogenic unresponsiveness.[79] Spontaneous or light-evoked *blinking* is also typical of psychogenic unresponsiveness but can be observed in coma.[79,135,136] *Spontaneous eye opening* usually indicates improvement in arousal levels but in the absence of improvement of other functions it may represent the first sign of transition into a vegetative state. *Rhythmic eye opening* associated with vertical eye movements or divergent-convergent eye movements occasionally may represent the only clinical manifestation of seizure activity in coma or after intraventricular hemorrhage.[137-139] Tonic lid retraction and *widely fixed eye opening* are rare findings in patients with coma due to large pontine lesions.[140] Occasionally, ipsi-, contra, or bilateral *ptosis* without pupillary changes may accompany extensive frontal lobe injury or diffuse cortical damage, presumably due to dysfunction of supranuclear eyelid opening.[141]

Although the resting position of the eyes can help to localize the topography of the lesion causing altered consciousness, almost any neuroophthalmological syndrome may occur on occasion with metabolic encephalopathies or drug intoxications. Slight divergence of the eyes can be seen in sleep and in light stages of metabolic coma. Supratentorial lesions involving the frontal eye fields reduce tonic output from the affected side and lead to *horizontal gaze deviation* toward the affected hemisphere so that patients appear to "look to" the side of the lesion. In most such cases, the eyes will cross the midline with vigorous oculocephalic maneuvers. Irritative lesions of the frontal eye fields, such as epileptic foci, have the opposite effect, so that patients "look away" from the lesion. Rarely, this phenomenon can occur with thalamic hemorrhage or with other hemispheric diseases (*"wrong-way eyes"*).[79,142,143] Pontine lesions that affect the paramedian pontine center for lateral gaze and midbrain lesions that affect the descending pathways responsible for its cortical control can produce an ipsilateral gaze palsy in which the eyes do not move across the midline during oculocephalic testing.[144] The combined involvement of the pontine center for lateral gaze and the homolateral MLF leads to the *one and a half syndrome*, in which the only preserved horizontal eye movement is abduction of the contralateral eye. Occasionally the side of gaze deviation alternates (*Ping-Pong gaze*), and the eyes can remain for up to 1 to 2 min in the lateral position.[145-146] Ping-Pong gaze may occur in comatose patients with bihemispheric and brainstem stroke, hepatic encephalopathy, hydrocephalus, and carbon monoxide intoxication. *Downgaze palsy* indicates a bilateral midbrain lesion, whereas *upgaze palsy* can be due to a unilateral or bilateral lesion of the dorsal mesencephalic tegmentum.[122] *Downward gaze deviation*, which usually occurs with posterior diencephalic and rostral midbrain dysfunction, for example, with compression by pinealoma, can also be seen in hydrocephalus, in hepatic coma, after caloric stimulation in patients with coma due to sedative drugs, and in psychogenic disturbances.[147-149] Forced downward-inward gaze with miosis (*tip of nose syndrome*) is typical for thalamic hemorrhage.[79,150] *Upward gaze deviation*, which usually occurs with a midbrain lesion, is a poor prognostic sign when it occurs in diffuse hypoxic encephalopathy.[151] *Skew deviation*—a divergence of the vertical axes of the eyes not due to oculomotor palsy or restrictive ophthalmopathy—is common in structural brainstem lesions and rare in metabolic encephalopathies and drug intoxications.[152,153] *Monocular eye deviation* usually indicates an oculomotor, trochlear, or abducens palsy.

Nystagmus is rare in coma since the fast component usually corresponds to a cortical corrective movement that disappears with decreasing arousal. A variety of other spontaneous eye movements may be seen in comatose patients, including *slow roving eye movements*—slow, random, mainly horizontal conjugate or dysconjugate movements—which occur in light sleep and in coma with intact brainstem function. As they cannot be mimicked voluntarily, their presence excludes psychogenic states. *Ocular bobbing*, a rapid downward movement of the eyes, usually with an excursion of one-fourth or one-third of the normal voluntary range, followed by a slow return to midposition, usually occurs with horizontal gaze palsy in patients with pontine and cerebellar lesions and occurs occasionally with hydrocephalus, anoxia, hepatic encephalopathy, and hypoglycemia.[154,155] Variations of ocular bobbing include *reverse ocular bobbing*, a rapid upward movement with slow return to midposition that can occur with metabolic encephalopathy or with anoxia, and *ocular dipping*, a slow downward movement of full range with rapid return to midposition that may accompany anoxic encephalopathy.[156] *Vertical ocular myoclonus* refers to spontaneous, vertical, pendular, full-range 1 or 2 Hz movements of the eyes that may occur in patients who are either locked-in or comatose following pontine stroke.[157] *Seesaw nystagmus*, disconjugate rotatory nystagmus in which the eyes alternately move up and down, is most often due to mesodiencephalic lesions but can also occur with pontomedullary tegmental damage.[158]

Convergence nystagmus is an "intermittent, quick, jerking movement of convergence in which the eyeballs rhythmically move toward each other and then slowly return to the midposition before the next movement" that usually but not invariably indicates a bilateral lesion of the midbrain tegmentum.[159,160] Convergence nystagmus in association with abnormal pupils and vertical gaze palsy is called *Parinaud's syndrome.* Downward gaze preference (setting-sun sign), skew deviation, lid retraction (*Collier's sign*), and ptosis may also be present.[161] Less commonly, dorsal midbrain lesions can give rise to convergence spasm or convergence paralysis. *Convergence spasm*, also called "pseudo-sixth palsy" because it can be mistaken for bilateral abducens palsy, usually involves both eyes, although one eye can be involved preferentially or in isolation.[162,163] *Retractory nystagmus*, defined as an irregular jerking of the eyes backward into the orbit, is another sign of midbrain involvement that is probably caused by simultaneous activation of all six extraocular muscles. *Opsoclonus*—saccadic oscillations that are multidirectional without a consistent intersaccadic interval—can be observed as a paraneoplastic syndrome with neuroblastoma as well as in patients with toxic-metabolic encephalopathies, meningoencephalitis, and head trauma.[70]

CORNEAL REFLEXES.   Corneal reflexes are mediated by afferents of the fifth nerve and efferents of the third and seventh nerves. Bilaterally intact responses—eye closure and upward movement of the eyes following corneal stimulation—imply intact brainstem tegmental pathways from the third nerve nucleus in the midbrain to the seventh nerve nucleus in the pons. The corneal reflex is usually retained until deep coma, and the most common cause for an absent response is insufficient corneal stimulation. On occasion, corneal stimulation evokes contralateral jaw deviation (*corneomandibular reflex*), a reflex that has no localizing or prognostic value and can be seen on occasion also in elderly awake subjects. A rapid test of corneal reflex can be made by touching the eyelashes.

OCULOCEPHALIC AND VESTIBULOOCULAR REFLEXES (Fig. 11-9).   These reflexes are useful tests of pontomesencephalic function. The *oculocephalic reflex*, which should be tested only after exclusion of cervical spine injury, is elicited by passive rapid rotation of the head to either left or right; upward and downward head movements can also be performed. In the normal awake individual, the response consists of an initial slow phase in the opposite direction to the head rotation followed by a resetting quick phase that returns the eye to midposition. The presence of the quick phase implies an intact pontomesencephalic reticular formation and, at most, mild depression of level of consciousness. Absent quick phases with preservation or enhancement of slow phases, often referred to as "*positive doll's eye phenomenon*" or "positive doll's head maneuver," are typical of patients with depressed sensorium and an intact brainstem, as occurs in the early stages of metabolic encephalopathies.[164] Unilateral absence of the quick phase suggests a unilateral brainstem lesion, although this finding can be seen occasionally with acute unilateral hemispheric lesions.

The *vestibuloocular reflex* (*VOR*), tested with caloric stimulation of the external ear canal, is preserved in up to one third of patients in whom oculocephalic responses are absent.[165] The reflex should be tested after inspection of the ear to rule out tympanic rupture. With the head elevated to 30 degrees, cold stimuli (100 to 150 ml of ice water given in 30 to 60 s) evoke downward currents of the endolymph in the lateral semicircular canal and tonic firing of the vestibular nerve. The result is excitation of the ipsilateral lateral rectus and the contralateral medial rectus, producing ipsilateral deviation of the eyes within 15 to 60 s. Warm stimuli have the opposite effect and should be tested 3 to 5 min later. With either cold or warm stimuli, awake persons develop nystagmus as the tonic deviation is interrupted by quick phases in the opposite direction. The mnemonic "COWS" (cold opposite, warm same) describes the expected direction of the quick phase. Patients who are comatose from bihemispheric dysfunction and have intact oculomotor pathways develop sustained eye deviation with unilateral caloric stimulation and downward movement of both eyes with bilateral simultaneous ice-water irrigation. With metabolic coma, caloric responses are initially brisk but become sluggish or disappear entirely as coma deepens. With lesions of the MLF, ipsilateral responses are preserved while contralateral responses are absent due to interruption of pathways to the contralateral oculomotor nuclei (*internuclear ophthalmoplegia*, INO). Although intact caloric responses are a useful sign of preserved brainstem function in comatose patients, the absence of responses or the presence of INO does not necessarily indicate brainstem injury.

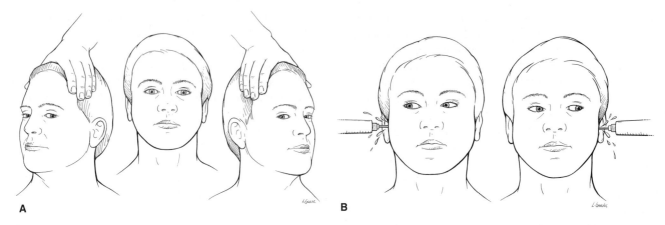

Figure 11-9 *Normal oculocephalic* (doll's eye maneuver, *A*) and *vestibuloocular reflexes* (ice calorics, *B*).

Vestibular disorders, drugs such as phenytoin, phenothiazines, lithium, beta blockers, and barbiturates, and less commonly metabolic diseases can eliminate oculovestibular responses or depress them asymmetrically causing INO.[70] On the other hand, the presence of both the slow and quick phase of the response rules out a significant organic disturbance of consciousness and may be useful in identification of psychogenic unresponsiveness.

Motor Functions

The degree of impairment of motor functions usually parallels the severity of disturbance of consciousness. Because of the anatomic segregation of the two systems, however, a dissociation between the two functional systems can occur, as in patients with locked-in syndrome or in those with decerebrate posturing but without loss of consciousness.[64]

POSTURE AND SPONTANEOUS MOTOR ACTIVITIES. Organic disturbances of consciousness are accompanied by unnatural body positions. An exception is represented by coma and hypersomnia following paramedian thalamic stroke in which patients can present sleeplike postures.[65]

Spontaneous motor activities are frequently seen in comatose patients, and asymmetry in movements of the face or extremities may help to identify a focal cause of coma. *Yawning*, *sneezing*, and *blinking* may occur with light coma, whereas *hiccup*, *cough*, and spontaneous *swallowing* can be observed also in deep coma. *Orofacial dyskinesias*, including protrusion of the tongue, puffing of the cheeks, chewing, and protrusion of the lips, *bruxism*, and *trismus*, can be seen in all stages of coma.[79,166,167] *Crying* and other involuntary motor patterns can occur in patients with locked-in syndrome or persistent vegetative state, and *laughing* can herald pontine infarction or pontine myelinolysis.[49,168]

Focal *seizures* usually point to a supratentorial lesion but can also be seen with hypoglycemia and other metabolic encephalopathies. Generalized seizures and multifocal *myoclonus* are frequent with postanoxic coma and with uremic or hyponatremic encephalopathy.[66,169–173] Occasionally myoclonus can be elicited only by acoustic or tactile stimuli or is limited to the periocular muscles. *Shivering* or tonic-clonic spasms of one extremity can be seen in subtentorial lesions and probably indicate a partial dysfunction of corticospinal pathways.[79,174,175] Multifocal shivering can be seen in metabolic encephalopathies or can follow withdrawal from muscle relaxants.[170] *Asterixis* refers to lapses of posture in tonically active muscles ("negative myoclonus" or flapping tremor) which can best be observed while the patient is holding out the arms with dorsiflexed hands, protruding the tongue, or abducting and flexing the hips. Asterixis is often preceded by *tremor* and both are most often seen in metabolic encephalopathies, but they can be accentuated unilaterally in the presence of concomitant or preexisting focal brain damage. Unilateral asterixis suggests focal brain damage.[176] *Automatic stepping* can be seen in the pontomedullary stage of central herniation and probably represents an automatism generated within the spinal locomotion center.[177] In patients with brain death, neck flexion can be followed by arm and hip flexion; apnea testing can be accompanied by automatic shoulder adduction and internal rotation with elbow flexion and arching of the back (*Lazarus sign*); and undulating plantar flexion of the toes can be elicited by plantar stimulation.[83]

MOTOR RESPONSES TO STIMULI. Motor responses should be assessed after verbal stimuli, followed if necessary by noxious stimulation with sternal rub or a pinch at the base of the nails. A voluntary response with localization of the pain stimulus and *nonreflex withdrawal* of the limb must be differentiated from stereotyped reactions. The distinction can be made by stimulating the inner part of arms or legs: only abduction is then a nonstereotyped withdrawal response.

Four principal patterns of stimulation-induced stereotyped motor activity have been differentiated but in clinical practice a combination of the four patterns is often seen.[178] The first pattern, *decorticate rigidity* with triple flexion of the upper extremities and extension and adduction of the lower extremities, usually occurs with the lightest forms of coma, associated with dysfunction at the diencephalomesencephalic level. *Decerebrate rigidity*, the second pattern, presents with extensor posturing of all extremities, opisthotonus and jaw clenching, and usually occurs in deeper coma, with dysfunction at the mesencephalopontine level. The third pattern, extensor movements of the arms and weak flexor movements of the legs, and the fourth, flaccidity of all extremities, usually occur with deep coma accompanied by dysfunction at the pontomedullary level. These general associations of specific brainstem levels with specific motor responses do not apply for all patients; for example, decorticate or decerebrate rigidity or both can occur with diffuse metabolic encephalopathies, with sedative drug-induced coma, and with bihemispheric lesions without midbrain compression.[79,179–181] Furthermore, as decerebrate posturing may occur in patients with preserved consciousness and in the absence of other brainstem signs, its presence does not indicate *per se* an anatomically defined brainstem lesion but probably indicates dysfunction of specific reticulospinal or vestibulospinal descending motor pathways.[178,180,182]

Bilateral *Babinski signs* can be observed in delirium and coma of various causes and do not imply a structural lesion.[183] An asymmetric plantar response is diagnostically more useful as it suggests focal brain disease. *Frontal release signs* such as grasp, self-grasp, suck, and snout can be observed in patients with confusional states and somnolence but they disappear in coma. Their presence usually rules out a psychogenic disturbance of consciousness. Asymmetry of these signs may help with diagnosis of focal brain damage in patients with delirium.[184]

COMA AND DELIRIUM SCALES

The need for standardized assessments of disturbances of consciousness for inter- and intraindividual comparisons prompted the creation of clinical scales. The *Glasgow coma scale* (GCS, Table 11-6), the most widely adopted coma scale, is useful in both traumatic and nontraumatic coma and defines responsiveness with three scales—arousal (eye opening), activity (motor response), and awareness (speech)—that correspond to the components of conscious activity and that have

TABLE 11-6
Glasgow Coma Scale

Response	Reaction	Score
Best motor response	Obeys	6
	Localizes	5
	Withdraws	4
	Abnormal flexion	3
	Extensor response	2
	Nil	1
Verbal response	Orientated	5
	Confused conversation	4
	Inappropriate words	3
	Incomprehensible sounds	2
	Nil	1
Eye opening	Spontaneous	4
	To speech	3
	To pain	2
	Nil	1
		Score 3–15

a low rate of observer variability.[185–191] Disadvantages of the GCS are its poor discrimination of mild disturbances of consciousness (GCS >13) and the lack of assessment of brainstem reflexes and functions. Alternative scales such as the Glasgow-Pittsburgh coma scale[192] and the Innsbruck coma scale, which include brainstem functions, have been proposed but have not found wide acceptance. "Observer's assessment of alertness/sedation scale,"[193] the "delirium scale,"[120] and the Mini-Mental State scale assess mild alterations of consciousness and confusional states.

Etiology of Delirium and Coma

The differential diagnosis of delirium and coma is extensive (Table 11-7). In 500 patients who presented with coma of unknown cause, 326 had diffuse toxic-metabolic encephalopathies, half of them related to exogenous toxins; 101 had supratentorial focal lesions; 65 had subtentorial focal lesions; and 8 had psychogenic unresponsiveness.[20]

DIFFUSE TOXIC-METABOLIC AND MULTIFOCAL ENCEPHALOPATHIES

Lack of Oxygen or Unavailability of Essential Substrates

ISCHEMIA AND ANOXIA. Cerebral blood flow of <20 ml/100 g per min or a partial pressure of oxygen of <40 mmHg in arterial blood leads to reduced consciousness.[77,194] Brief periods of ischemia from decreased cardiac output or from decreased vascular resistance cause syncope. Failure to restore blood flow and oxygenation leads to irreversible damage, first to mitochondria and subsequently to neuronal cell bodies. The interval between the onset of hypoxia and the occurrence of irreversible damage varies depending on the severity of hypoxia and ischemia and may be as short as 4 min in complete anoxia. While depletion of adenosine triphosphate (ATP) is a critical factor in the development of irreversible damage associated with hypoxia, at least four other types of events have been identified that may also contribute to neuronal injury.[20,195] The first is delayed hypoperfusion, or the "no-reflow phenomenon," a period of reduced cerebral blood flow associated with a marked increase in cerebral vascular resistance that occurs 15 to 20 min following resuscitation from anoxic-ischemic events. The second is the production of cytotoxic metabolites

TABLE 11-7
Etiology of Delirium and Coma

1. *Diffuse toxic-metabolic encephalopathies*
   Lack of oxygen or unavailability of essential substrates
      Ischemia-anoxia (including cardiac arrest, hypertensive encephalopathy, subarachnoid hemorrhage)
      Hypoglycemia
      Thiamine deficiency (Wernicke's encephalopathy)
   Endogenous toxins
      Hepatic failure
      Renal failure
      Pancreatic failure
      Idiopathic recurrent stupor
      Acute intermittent porphyria
   Electrolyte-osmolality disorders
      Hyper- and hypoosmolality
      Hyper- and hyponatremia
      Others (hyper- and hypomagnesemia, hypophosphatemia)
   Endocrine disorders
      Hyper- and hypothyroidism, Hashimoto's encephalopathy
      Adrenal insufficiency
      Hyper- and hypocalcemia
   Epileptic states
      Postictal state
      Partial-complex status epilepticus
      Absence status epilepticus
   Infectious and inflammatory CNS disorders
      Meningitis, encephalitis
      Vasculitis
      Septic encephalopathy
   Disordered temperature regulation
      Hypothermia
      Heat stroke
   Drug intoxication-withdrawal, poisoning

2. *Supratentorial processes*
      Stroke
      Head trauma
      Neoplasms
      Abscess

3. *Subtentorial processes*
      Stroke
      Pontine myelinolysis
      Migraine

4. *Psychogenic disturbances*

of arachidonic acid, the third is the production of oxygen free-radicals, and the fourth is neuronal influx of calcium ions.[196] Pathologic changes are characterized by cortical laminar necrosis, watershed infarcts, and rarely, white matter lesions.

Common causes of anoxic and ischemic encephalopathies include cardiac arrest, respiratory arrest associated with drowning or suffocation, carbon monoxide poisoning, prolonged hypotension, and vasospasm. Hypoxic-ischemic injury also occurs with conditions associated with increased vascular resistance such as subarachnoid hemorrhage, hypertensive encephalopathy, disseminated intravascular coagulation, bacterial meningitis, and cerebral edema.

The clinical features of *global cerebral ischemia* reflect the selective vulnerability of specific brain areas such as the hippocampus, cerebellar and cerebral cortex, and basal ganglia. The most common sequela is an amnesic syndrome from hippocampal damage. In these patients, unlike amnesics with alcoholic Korsakoff's syndrome, orientation is preserved and confabulations are usually absent.[197] More extensive cerebral damage can lead to cortical blindness, dementia, or vegetative state. Cerebellar damage may cause spontaneous or action myoclonus and ataxia, and basal ganglia lesions may lead to a parkinsonian syndrome. Flaccid brachial biparesis ("*man-in-the-barrel syndrome*") or tetraparesis probably reflects cervical spinal cord ischemia.[198,199]

The recovery of clinical and electrophysiologic function after diffuse cerebral hypoxia follows a characteristic caudorostral pattern that can help in predicting outcome.[124,125] Most patients with good outcome awaken from coma within the first three days.[200,201] Rarely, clinical deterioration follows a few days or weeks after initial improvement. This *delayed postanoxic encephalopathy* corresponds to diffuse demyelination or focal cavitating lesions of the basal ganglia and can be seen after carbon monoxide poisoning, strangling, cardiac arrest, and cardiac surgery.[202,203]

Multifocal small cortical strokes, often due to cardioembolism, can present with a clinical picture similar to metabolic-toxic encephalopathy consisting of headache, delirium, stupor and coma, seizures, and fluctuating neurologic signs. Another cause is *diffuse intravascular coagulation*, which can also lead to intracerebral hemorrhages and sinus venous thrombosis. In *thrombotic thrombocytopenic purpura*, neurologic symptoms appear in association with systemic bleeding, fever, renal insufficiency, hemolytic anemia, and thrombocytopenia.[204] *Cholesterol embolization* may occur after arterial trauma during catheter placement in elderly patients and may present with multiple strokes and mental changes that are typically accompanied by retinal emboli (Hollenhorst plaques), skin lesions (livedo reticularis), and kidney and neuromuscular involvement.[205] A similar multisystem "pseudoencephalopathic" picture can be seen in the hereditary or acquired *antiphospholipid syndrome.*[206,207] Intracerebral hemorrhages complicating *thrombolysis* and *anticoagulation* are more frequent in patients above 70 years of age, are often large, and may be fatal.[208–210]

Hypertensive encephalopathy is now a relatively rare condition that usually follows withdrawal of hypertensive treatment, acute renal disease, or trauma.[69] Markedly elevated blood pressure with diastolic BP usually >120 to 130 mmHg is accompanied by headaches, visual blurring, generalized seizures, papilledema, fluctuating neurologic signs, delirium, stupor, and coma.[210] Involvement of the kidney, heart, and retina is frequent and brain CT or MRI typically shows white matter changes that are diffuse or more prominent in parietooccipital areas.[211] The fibrinoid necrosis of arterioles found in hypertensive encephalopathy may result from endothelial damage with local thrombosis.

Subarachnoid hemorrhage (SAH) caused by intracranial aneurysms, arteriovenous malformations, or vasculitis can lead to disturbances of consciousness due to increased intracranial pressure; vasospasm, which often occurs 1 to 2 weeks after the bleeding; or hydrocephalus due to blockage by blood of spinal fluid resorption.[20] Clinical presentations include "sentinel" headaches, which can precede the major bleed by days or weeks, acute severe headache, meningeal signs, ocular hemorrhages, delirium, and coma.[212] Hyperthermia and the syndrome of inappropriate antidiuretic hormone (SIADH) can occur as a consequence of hypothalamic damage.

Pulmonary diseases can be complicated by an encephalopathy associated with hypoxia and CO_2 retention (*CO_2 narcosis*). Altered consciousness usually appears when arterial P_{CO_2} rises acutely above 75 mmHg and probably relates to CSF acidosis.[213] Patients present with headache, delirium, tremor and asterixis, myoclonus, and occasionally papilledema.[20] Although acute CO_2 retention with acidosis may lead to encephalopathy, most persons with chronically elevated P_{CO_2}, somnolence, and neurophysical deficits probably have unrecognized obstructive sleep apnea along with chronic hypoventilation due to obesity or other causes.

HYPOGLYCEMIA. Lethargy, confusion, agitation, or coma may occur with hypoglycemia, occasionally complicated by seizures, focal neurological signs, and hypothermia, but clinical signs do not correlate strongly with levels of blood glucose. For example, coma can occur with levels as high as 28 mg/dl while stupor and confusion without coma can occur at levels as low as 8 mg/dl.[214] The highly variable clinical responses to low blood glucose suggest that metabolic insufficiency from depletion of substrate is not the only effect of hypoglycemia. Rapidity of onset of hypoglycemia is one determinant of the severity of encephalopathy, and increases in ammonia and alterations of amino acid concentrations in the brain may also contribute.[20] Insulin is the most common cause of hypoglycemia, particularly when taken in combination with inhibitors of angiotensin converting enzyme or beta blockers that blunt the typical adrenergically mediated warning symptoms of hypoglycemia.[215] Hypoglycemia also can occur with sepsis, alcoholism, hepatic failure, alimentary disturbances, retroperitoneal sarcoma, or insulinoma.[216] Hypoglycemic episodes exceeding one hour in duration may lead to an amnesic state resembling Korsakoff's syndrome or to other permanent neurologic sequelae.

WERNICKE'S ENCEPHALOPATHY. Thiamine is an essential cofactor for decarboxylation of pyruvate to form acetate and for the action of thiamine transketolase in the hexose monophosphate shunt. *Thiamine deficiency* is the cause of Wernicke's encephalopathy, a triad of confusional states with severely disturbed memory and confabulations, ataxia, and ocular abnormalities including gaze-evoked nystagmus, abducens palsy, INO, vertical nystagmus, paralysis of conjugate vertical or horizontal gaze, and impaired vestibular responses.[70] The complete syndrome may be present in only a minority of cases, and thiamine deficiency should always be considered when encephalopathy occurs in the setting of alcoholism, malnutrition, bariatric surgery, dialysis, or hyperemesis gravidarum.[217,218] Pathologically, there is hemorrhagic neuronal damage involving the periaqueductal areas and the regions surrounding the IIId and IVth ventricles, which occasionally can be visualized on brain MRI.

OTHERS. *Vitamin B_{12} deficiency* almost never causes stupor or coma although it can cause dementia or delirium, sometimes accompanied by visual disturbances, anemia, and signs of spinal cord degeneration. *Vitamin B_1 deficiency* (beriberi) and *nicotinic acid deficiency* (pellagra) are rare causes of amnesic syndromes or delirious states but they do not cause coma.

Endogenous Toxins

HEPATIC ENCEPHALOPATHY. Hepatic encephalopathy is the second most frequently encountered metabolic brain dysfunction after ischemic-hypoxic encephalopathy. Although the mechanisms responsible for hepatic encephalopathy are not entirely known, increased levels of gamma-aminobutyric acid (GABA) in an animal model of hepatic encephalopathy and of endogenous benzodiazepines in body fluids of patients with hepatic encephalopathy, as well as the clinical and EEG improvement produced by benzodiazepine antagonists, suggest that increased GABA-ergic tone plays a role in its development.[219–222] Although high levels of ammonia, the clearance of which is reduced in hepatic encephalopathy, may affect cerebral blood flow and regulation of GABA, serum ammonia concentrations do not always correlate well with the degree of encephalopathy.[223] A manganese neurotoxicity has been suggested to play a role in the pathogenesis of chronic hepatic encephalopathy and could be responsible for the symmetric hypersignals of the basal ganglia that can be found in the T1-weighted brain MRI of these patients.[224] The severity of encephalopathy correlates well with EEG findings, although triphasic EEG waves, thought originally to be specific for hepatic encephalopathy, can occur with other diffuse encephalopathies[67] (see "Paraclinical Studies," later in this chapter).

Features of hepatic encephalopathy include abrupt or insidious onset of altered consciousness, asterixis, hyperventilation with respiratory alkalosis, multifocal myoclonus, seizures, increased muscle tone with hyperreflexia, pyramidal signs, and decorticate or decerebrate posturing, even in the absence of superimposed structural brainstem lesions.[179] Oculomotor abnormalities in obtunded or comatose patients with hepatic failure may include ocular bobbing, skew deviation, tonic downward gaze deviation, dysconjugate eye movements, and nystagmus. The stupor and coma associated with fulminant hepatic failure and with Reye's syndrome are due to hepatic encephalopathy as well as to increased intracranial pressure and brain edema.[225]

UREMIC ENCEPHALOPATHY. Uremic encephalopathy usually occurs when the glomerular filtration rate falls below about 10 percent of normal, but the correlation between the degree of uremia and the severity of encephalopathy varies.[226] As with hepatic encephalopathy, the severity of mental changes correlates well with EEG changes.[67] Brain metabolism and oxygen consumption are reduced, and electrolyte imbalances, endogenous toxins, metabolic alkalosis, and drug toxicity contribute to the encephalopathy.[69,227] Accumulation of conjugated metabolites of midazolam may cause coma in patients with renal failure who receive conventional dosages of this short-acting benzodiazepine.[228]

As with hepatic failure, clinical features of uremic encephalopathy are nonspecific and may include delirium, stupor, tremor, asterixis, seizures, multifocal myoclonus, and coma.[181,229] Tetanus is frequent and nuchal rigidity and mild CSF pleocytosis can be observed, but focal signs are rare.[69,118] Headaches, sudden cortical blindness, and papilledema may occur in the *dysequilibrium syndrome* of hemodialysis.[69]

OTHERS. The existence of *pancreatic encephalopathy* in patients with acute pancreatic disease remains controversial, and most disturbances of consciousness can be attributed to such complications of the abdominal process as hypoglycemia, sepsis, renal failure, fat embolism, and electrolyte changes.[230]

Idiopathic recurrent stupor, a recently described syndrome that usually affects middle-aged persons, is characterized by recurrent episodes of stupor that can persist for hours to days without abnormal vital signs. The EEG displays nonreactive diffuse 13 to 16 Hz beta activity. The syndrome is related to an increase in endogenous benzodiazepine-like activity identified as endozepine-4, a probable modulator of the GABA receptor, and clinical symptoms and EEG changes can be reversed by flumazenil, a benzodiazepine antagonist.[231,232]

Acute intermittent porphyria is an autosomal dominant disorder of pyrrole metabolism. Symptoms can be precipitated by a variety of medications including antiepileptics, barbiturates, sulfonamides, and analgesics. The clinical picture may include delirium, seizures, ascending paralysis, vomiting, and abdominal pain.

Electrolyte and Osmolality Abnormalities

Hyponatremia, which occurs in 2.5 percent of hospitalized patients, can occur with euvolemia, hypovolemia, or hypervolemia.[233] In euvolemic states, SIADH is a common cause and may result from brain tumors, brain trauma, subarachnoid hemorrhage, stroke, and meningoencephalitis. SIADH may also occur with certain drugs including carbamazepine, thiazides, and tricyclic antidepressants; with pulmonary diseases; and rarely as a postoperative complication in otherwise healthy women.[234] The rate of change in sodium concentration is probably a more significant contributor than the serum level to brain swelling, the major factor in the pathogenesis of mental status changes.

The clinical picture is characterized by anorexia, headaches, cramps, decreased level of consciousness (usually when sodium level <115 to 120 mmol/liter), generalized tonic-clonic and nonconvulsive seizures, multifocal myoclonus, asterixis, and occasionally focal signs.[20] Rapid correction of hyponatremia can cause central pontine myelinolysis, which can lead to a secondary deterioration of the level of consciousness (see later in this chapter). Hyponatremia is not a benign condition: Chronic neurologic sequelae may occur in 6 to 60 percent of patients, depending on the population considered.[233]

Fluid shift into the brain and encephalopathy with cerebral edema also occur in the *dysequilibrium syndrome* and following correction of *diabetic ketoacidosis*.

Hyperosmolar states, usually due to *hypernatremia* or

hyperglycemia, or both, can lead to a diffuse encephalopathy. The usual causes of hypernatremia are dehydration, fever, burns, diabetes insipidus, and defective thirst mechanism.[69] Nonketotic hyperglycemic hyperosmolality with glucose levels as high as 1200 mg/dl can occur in older patients with type II diabetes mellitus. Hyperosmolality leads to brain dehydration and shrinking and can cause tearing of small blood vessels with intradural, subarachnoid, or intracerebral hemorrhage.

Clinically, patients present with signs of systemic dehydration and altered consciousness, occasionally accompanied by seizures, eye movement disturbances including opsoclonus, and focal signs.[20] Seizures occasionally appear during rehydration.[235] Mortality may be as high as 20 percent but clinically significant sequelae are present in only a minority of survivors.[235]

Patients with *hypomagnesemia* can occasionally present with delirium, nystagmus, and seizures, but tremor, myoclonus, and muscular weakness with respiratory failure are more common. *Hypophosphatemia* with levels below 1 mg/dl may occur with intravenous hyperalimentation, vomiting or gastric suction, sepsis, burns, treatment of ketoacidosis, and hepatic failure. Mental changes including stupor and coma are frequent and can mimic Wernicke's encephalopathy.[69] Acute flaccid areflexic paralysis may also occur. *Hypokalemia*, *hyperkalemia*, and *hypermagnesemia* can lead to progressive muscle weakness with tetraparesis, speech difficulties, and oculomotor disturbances that resemble the locked-in syndrome.

Endocrine Disorders

Hypothyroidism may cause delirium and coma (myxedema coma) that can be triggered by bacterial infections, trauma, stroke, and anesthesia, particularly in elderly women and in winter.[69,236] Patients may present with typical skin changes, myotonic reactions, bradycardia, ataxia, altered consciousness, and six "hypo's" (hypotension, hypoventilation, hypothermia, hyporeflexia, hypoglycemia and hyponatremia).[237] A recent phosphorus magnetic-resonance spectroscopy study demonstrated that hypothyroidism is accompanied by decreased brain metabolism that is proportional to the increase in thyroid-stimulating hormone and can be reversed by treatment.[238] With appropriate treatment the mortality of myxedema coma has dropped from 60 to 70 percent to 15 to 20 percent.[236] *Hyperthyroidism* can present with hyperthermia, tachycardia, delirium, tremor, but only rarely with coma accompanied by prominent and reversible pyramidal signs.[239] *Hashimoto's encephalitis* is a rare steroid-responsive condition that is associated with high titers of antithyroid antibodies and presents clinically with altered consciousness, seizures, myoclonus, strokelike episodes, elevation of CSF protein, and diffuse EEG abnormalities.[240]

Adrenal insufficiency (Addison's crisis) is a rare cause of seizures, papilledema, delirium, and coma in patients who usually first present with weight loss, hyperpigmentation, hypotension, generalized weakness, hyporeflexia, and electrolyte changes.[241] *Cushing's syndrome* and iatrogenic steroid excess can be accompanied by depression or delirium with insomnia, agitation, and hallucinations.

Hypercalcemia is most commonly observed in patients with cancer or primary hyperthyroidism. Thirst, polyuria, headache, nausea, vomiting, and muscle weakness often precede nonspecific encephalopathic signs, delirium, and coma.[242] *Hypocalcemia*—a poor prognostic sign in critically ill patients that occurs in hypoalbuminemia, sepsis, acute pancreatitis, and severe crush injury—presents with tetany, cramps, paresthesias, and seizures, but coma and other disturbances of consciousness are rare.[20,69] Hypocalcemia due to hypoparathyroidism can be complicated by brain edema, papilledema, and delirium.[243] For *pituitary apoplexy*, see under "Neoplasms," later.

Epileptic States

Significant impairment or loss of consciousness secondary to epileptic activities most commonly but not invariably implies involvement of both hemispheres.[3] Prolonged *generalized tonic-clonic seizures*—which produce metabolic derangements and neuronal damage independent of the effects of hypotension, acidosis, and hypoxia—can lead to *postictal stupor* and obtundation that usually resolve within a few hours but occasionally can last longer than one day.[244]

Two other epileptic syndromes can be associated with prolonged periods of altered consciousness. *Partial complex status epilepticus* (PCS), which usually arises from the frontal lobe or the temporal lobe, is characterized by repetitive episodes of psychomotor, psychosensory, or psychoaffective symptoms with automatisms that are separated by more or less lucid intervals and that are accompanied by focal EEG changes.[245,246] Less commonly there is a prolonged stuporous or delirious state. *Absence status epilepticus* (ASE) is associated with disorientation, perseverations, delusions, hallucinations, and a lack of spontaneous activity.[247] ASE can occur spontaneously; following benzodiazepine withdrawal, metrizamide myelography or contrast arteriography; in association with a variety of metabolic encephalopathies; or rarely after focal brain damage.[248–251]

Patients with ASE or PCS usually but not always have a history of seizures.[252–255] When PCS or ASE occur in middle-aged or elderly patients without a prior history of epilepsy, they may be mistaken for psychogenic disorders or metabolic encephalopathies.[251,256] Electroencephalography is usually diagnostic.[257,258]

Infectious and Inflammatory Diseases of the CNS

Bacterial meningitis causes disturbances of consciousness through a variety of effects on the CNS. Cerebral edema and obstructive hydrocephalus can lead to herniation while vasculitis, cerebral vein thrombosis, and diffuse intravascular coagulation can lead to diffuse or multifocal hypoxic-ischemic injury. Transient stenoses of intracranial vessels are present in up to 50 percent of patients and are associated with focal brain damage and a poor outcome.[259] Seizures, hyponatremia, and sepsis may contribute to metabolic disturbances.[260] Clinical presentation includes headache, fever, meningismus, and somnolence. In fulminant courses of bacterial meningitis and in immunocompromised patients, the initial CSF may not show a pleocytosis and meningeal signs may be lacking.

Recurrent meningitis is a rare condition that presents with episodes of delirium or stupor associated with fever and headaches that can recur over years. This syndrome can be caused by herpes simplex type II infection (Mollaret's meningitis), or it may occur secondary to an intracranial epidermoid cyst.[261]

Herpes *encephalitis* is the most common form of sporadic encephalitis and typically presents with fever, headaches, and behavioral and neuropsychological disturbances that evolve rapidly into delirium and stupor. Associated findings include periodic sharp waves over the temporal lobes on EEG, lymphocytic hemorrhagic pleocytosis on CSF examination, and temporal lobe abnormalities on brain MRI.[262] Once coma supervenes, prognosis is almost invariably poor.[263] A variety of other viruses may cause encephalitis, sometimes associated with intractable seizures, severe neurological damage, death, or all three. Among nonviral infectious disorders, Lyme disease, legionnaires disease, *Mycoplasma pneumoniae*, and rickettsial disorders can induce encephalitis.

In patients with *HIV infection* a meningoencephalitic picture can be caused by HIV meningitis, toxoplasmosis, cryptococcosis, tuberculosis, syphilis, cytomegalovirus, and neoplastic infiltration.[264] The additional presence of focal signs suggests toxoplasmosis or infection with JC virus (progressive multifocal encephalopathy). An encephalopathy with myoclonus, periodic epileptiform discharges, and rapid reversal under zidovudine treatment can be the first manifestation of the AIDS-dementia complex.[265]

Postviral encephalomyelitis is a disorder that resembles acute encephalitis and occurs mainly in children after infections with measles, varicella-zoster, Epstein-Barr, or other viruses. Manifestations may include seizures, altered consciousness, ataxia, multifocal neurologic signs, and MRI evidence of acute demyelination.[266]

Delirium, stupor, and coma are not infrequent in the course of sepsis but a clear cause is often missing. The term *septic encephalopathy* has been used for this condition which is typically accompanied by tachycardia, hypotension, and respiratory insufficiency. Cerebral microabscesses and diffuse hypoxic-ischemic damage are the presumed causes.[69,267] In a prospective study of neurologic complications of critical medical illnesses, a metabolic encephalopathy was the most frequently encountered complication, and a septic encephalopathy was found to be the second most common form.[268]

Vasculitis of the CNS can present with protean symptomatology that includes headaches, focal symptoms and signs related to ischemic stroke or intracerebral hemorrhage, seizures, cranial neuropathies, visual disturbances, movement disorders, delirium, stupor and coma. Diagnosis is sometimes difficult, as CSF examination, erythrocyte sedimentation rate, and cerebral angiography may be normal in some cases. The differential diagnosis includes an idiopathic systemic vasculitis (e.g., polyarteritis nodosa, Wegener's granulomatosis, Sjögren syndrome); a systemic neoplastic, paraneoplastic, infectious, or drug-induced vasculitis; and an isolated vasculitis of the central nervous system.[269] In patients with known systemic vasculitis, the distinction between primary vasculitic CNS involvement, side effects of medication, encephalopathy secondary to systemic organ involvement, and opportunistic infection may be problematic.[270]

Disordered Temperature Regulation

Depression of consciousness with *hypothermia* is proportional to reductions in cerebral blood flow and oxygen consumption and can occur in hypoglycemia, hypothyroidism, barbiturate intoxication, alcoholism, Wernicke's encephalopathy, poisoning, sepsis, and exposure.[20] Temperatures of 32 to 35°C (89.6 to 95°F) are associated with confusion and lethargy; as the temperature falls to 27 to 32°C (80.6 to 89.6°F), verbal responses are usually still present, although the pupils react sluggishly. At temperatures of 20 to 24°C (68 to 75.2°F), patients are stuporous with no verbal responses and sluggish or unreactive small pupils, although they may still respond purposefully to pain.[121] At temperatures below 20°C (68°F) the EEG becomes isoelectric.

Neurogenic hyperthermia is rare and can occur with pontine lesions and with hypothalamic damage from subarachnoid hemorrhage, often in association with SIADH. Increased *sweating* without hyperthermia can occur with supratentorial and infratentorial damage, usually contralaterally to the lesion, presumably due to involvement of a pathway that runs with corticospinal fibers and inhibits contralateral sweating.[133,271–275] Hyperthermia without sweating and with dilated pupils is characteristic of intoxication with atropine or other anticholinergics.

Stupor or coma with intact pupils and extraocular movements, sometimes accompanied by delirium or convulsions, characterizes *"heat stroke,"* which usually occurs with body temperatures above 42°C (107.6°F). Sweating is often absent and the condition may be complicated by cardiovascular collapse, bleeding disorders, and hepatic or renal failure. Decreased cerebral metabolism accompanies severe hyperthermia.[276] Rare sequelae of hyperthermia include cerebellar ataxia, neuropsychological deficits, and polyneuropathy.[277]

Exogenous Toxins and Their Withdrawal

Deliberate or unintentional drug intoxications and poisonings—many of which are overdoses of sedatives, hypnotics, tricyclic antidepressants, opiates, ethanol, cocaine, or other psychoactive drugs—account for 25 to 30 percent of all cases of nontraumatic coma.

Sedative drugs, especially *barbiturates*, tend to depress vestibular function. As a result, nystagmus is usually a feature of mild intoxication, and oculocephalic responses are usually reduced or absent in the comatose patient. Reactive pupils, hypothermia, and respiratory depression often accompany the altered consciousness. Muscle tone is usually decreased but decerebrate posturing following painful stimuli is occasionally present and does not rule out a good outcome.[180] The association of normally reactive pupils with impaired oculocephalic/oculovestibular reflexes distinguishes barbiturate coma from coma due to a structural brainstem lesion. *Benzodiazepine overdose*—generally less dangerous than barbiturate overdose—is characterized by a decreased level of consciousness with relatively preserved cardiovascular and respiratory functions. Withdrawal from benzodiazepines resembles withdrawal from ethanol, but seizures and delirium are rare and usually occur only after abrupt discontinuation of high doses of short-acting benzodiazepines.[278]

Tricyclic antidepressant overdose may cause hyperthermia and cardiac conduction defects in addition to seizures and coma. Cardiac arrhythmias may persist for several days after overdose because of the long half-lives of some tricyclic and tetracyclic antidepressants. *Lithium* intoxication is characterized by nystagmus and other eye movement disorders, including INO and opsoclonus; by ataxia, myoclonus, and tremor; by cardiac arrhythmias; by delirium and rarely coma.[70,279] Hyperosmolar coma due to diabetes insipidus induced by lithium has been reported.[280] Occasionally, neurological deficits can persist after acute intoxication.[281]

The *neuroleptic malignant syndrome*—stupor, catatonic rigidity, hyperthermia, hyperhidrosis, cardiovascular instability, and elevation of serum creatine kinase—occurs in 0.07 to 0.15 percent of persons treated with neuroleptics and is attributed to a profound reduction in central dopaminergic function.[282] Rarely, it can also occur during withdrawal from dopamine or from *dopamine agonists* and be complicated by delirium and respiratory depression.[283] *Serotonin syndrome* is a potentially lethal condition of increased serotonin action caused by various combinations of serotomimetic drugs, with or without MAO inhibitors. Clinical features include mental status changes, shivering, tremor, myoclonus, rigidity, seizures, hyperreflexia, autonomic instability, hyperthermia, diarrhea, and flushing.[284,295] *Malignant hyperthermia*, clinically similar to the neuroleptic malignant syndrome, is related to administration of halogenated inhalation anesthetics or depolarizing muscle relaxants and is due to a disorder of calcium regulation in skeletal muscles.

Opioid overdoses produce sedation, nausea, delirium, very small reactive pupils, bradycardia, and respiratory depression. Inhalation of *heroin pyrolysate* ("brown sugar" or "Chinese heroin") has been linked to an acute and frequently lethal demyelinating and spongiform disease of the CNS that resembles other toxic leukoencephalopathies and presents clinically with delirium, catatonia, cerebellar signs,[286] and occasionally rhabdomyolysis (personal observation).

Hypothermia, eye movement paralysis, respiratory depression, and reactive pupils are characteristic of deep coma from *ethanol* overdose. Symptoms of ethanol withdrawal are usually most pronounced at 24 to 36 h and include nervousness, insomnia, agitation, generalized tumor, nausea, and autonomic hyperactivity. Repeated generalized seizures related to withdrawal typically appear within 7 to 30 h of abstinence and usually precede delirium tremens. Prolonged postictal confusion, repeated seizures, and focal seizures suggest the possibility of focal brain damage.[217] *Delirium tremens*, the most severe form of withdrawal from ethanol, usually occurs within 3 to 5 days of cessation of drinking, can persist for several days, and is fatal in 5 to 10 percent of cases. Patients present with a hypervigilant confusional state with hallucinations and autonomic dysfunction including tachycardia, sweating, and hyperthermia.[217]

Amphetamine and *cocaine* intoxication may present with delirium, tremor, hyperthermia, hyperhidrosis, mydriasis, tachycardia, cardiac arrhythmias, and hypertension. Neurologic complications include seizures, movement disorders (tic, chorea, or dystonia), transient monocular blindness, cerebral vasculitis, ischemic strokes, intracerebral hemorrhage, and subarachnoid hemorrhage.[287–291] *Phencyclidine* ("angel dust"), lysergic acid diethylamide (*LSD*), and less commonly *marijuana* can be the cause of hypervigilant delirium with complex hallucinations usually associated with tremor, ataxia, seizures, and such signs of autonomic hyperactivity as tachycardia and hyperhidrosis. *Inhalants* such as gasoline, rubber cement, and spray paints containing toluene, benzene, hydrocarbons, and other ingredients can cause nausea, nystagmus, hyporeflexia, involuntary movements, delirium, and in higher doses, stupor and coma. A toxic leukoencephalopathy can lead to permanent brain damage.[292]

Poisoning with *arsenic, manganese, mercury*, and less commonly *lead* may be accompanied by delirium. Intoxications with *methanol, paraldehyde*, and *ethylene glycol* cause metabolic acidosis, abdominal pain, seizures, stupor, and coma. Neurologic sequelae such as blindness do not correlate with the degree of acidosis. *Pesticides* that inhibit cholinesterase cause accumulation of acetycholine and produce salivation, miosis, abdominal cramps, muscle weakness, insomnia, seizures, delirium, stupor, and coma. *Carbon monoxide* intoxication presents first with nonspecific symptoms such as headache, vomiting, and chest pain; focal brain neurological deficits, seizures, cardiac complications, and coma occur when carboxyhemoglobin concentrations exceed 40 to 50 percent. Long-term sequelae include parkinsonism and a sometimes fatal delayed postanoxic encephalopathy (discussed earlier in this section).

The list of nonpsychotropic drugs that can cause altered consciousness is almost endless and includes cardiovascular compounds, anticholinergic agents, nonsteroidal anti-inflammatory agents, antihistaminics, antibiotics, and bronchodilators.[293] *Salicylate* poisoning leads to encephalopathy, neurogenic hyperventilation, and respiratory alkalosis with increased organic acid production and aciduria. In late stages metabolic acidosis can be seen as well. Several *antineoplastic drugs*, including FK 506, OKT3, ifosfamide, L-asparaginase, and procarbazine, are potential causes of encephalopathies. *Cyclosporin* neurotoxicity presents clinically with headache and tremor, and in more severe cases with delirium, cortical blindness, tetraspasticity with hyperreflexia, seizures, and coma.[294] Radiologic studies may show a diffuse leukoencephalopathy as well as brain edema that occasionally causes brainstem compression.[294,295]

SUPRATENTORIAL LESIONS

In 67 patients described by Plum and Posner,[20] focal supratentorial causes of altered consciousness were stroke (*n* = 12), hemorrhage (*n* = 20), neoplasm (*n* = 11), head trauma (*n* = 21) and abscess (*n* = 3).

Stroke

Brief and transient loss of consciousness (syncope) occurs in 6 percent of patients with hemispheric stroke and is less common in patients with TIA and lacunar stroke.[296] Coma develops in 5 to 18 percent of those with ischemic stroke and 31 to 55 percent of those with

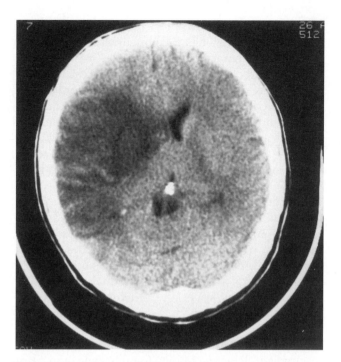

Figure 11-10 *Ischemic stroke.* Brain CT of a patient with right middle cerebral artery infarction with mass effect. (Courtesy of D. Quint, Neuroradiology Department, University of Michigan Hospitals, Ann Arbor, Michigan.)

intracerebral hemorrhage.[76,297] Age, stroke size, and occipital or right temporoparietal location are risk factors for delirium in stroke patients.[27,71,298–300] Partial-complex seizures and secondary toxic-metabolic disturbances may also affect consciousness in patients with stroke.[301]

In hemispheric ischemic stroke, *coma* usually appears after 2 to 5 days of progressive decrease in level of arousal, and usually due to bilateral infarcts or to edema with mass effect leading to the uncal or less commonly the central syndrome (Fig. 11-10). Early signs of brain edema include headache, somnolence, and pupillary abnormalities and may be followed by Cheyne-Stokes respiration and Babinski's sign on the side opposite of the hemiparesis.[80,86] On occasion, prolonged disturbances of consciousness and bilateral motor signs can be seen in patients with unilateral stroke without mass effect. In these cases a remote neural or vascular dysfunction (Monakow's diaschisis) may be responsible.

Initial coma or delirium is particularly common in unilateral or bilateral *paramedian thalamic and thalamomesencephalic infarcts* (Fig. 11-3), due most commonly to embolic occlusion of small often unpaired thalamic-subthalamic perforating arteries arising from the rostral basilar artery.[42,62,303] Because of the absence of lateralizing signs, coma may be initially assumed to be of toxic-metabolic origin. A triad of hypersomnia, vertical eye movement deficits, and amnesia that fol-

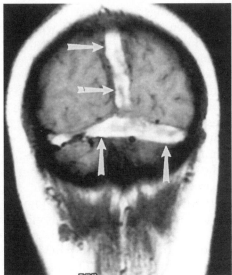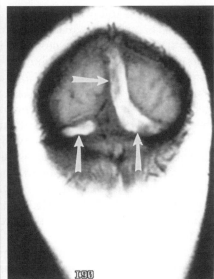

Figure 11-11 *Sinus venous thrombosis.* Coronal, noncontrast-enhanced, T1-weighted brain MRI of an 18-year-old patient who presented following otitis media with neck and head pain but no neurologic deficits. (*Arrows*—thrombus in superior sagittal and transverse dural venous sinuses.) (Courtesy of D. Quint, Neuroradiology Department, University of Michigan Hospitals, Ann Arbor, Michigan.)

lows awakening of the patient is characteristic (the paramedian diencephalic syndrome).[304] Hypersomnia may be severe with more than 20 h of sleep per day. Altered sleep architecture, amnesia, abulia, and depression may persist for months or years.[38,62,305,306]

Intracerebral hemorrhage (ICH) typically presents with sudden headache and vomiting during activity, followed over minutes to hours in more than 50 percent of cases by altered consciousness and progressive motor deficits. Level of consciousness and prognosis are functions of the size of the hemorrhage, with coma typical when the clot exceeds 2 to 3 cm in diameter.[76,307] The clinical syndrome is determined by the site of the bleed, the most common being the basal ganglia (50 percent), the cerebral white matter (15 to 20 percent), the thalamus (15 percent), the cerebellum (10 to 15 percent), and the pons (5 percent).[308] Coma at the onset is more common with basal ganglia or pontine hemorrhage than with lobar hemorrhages. Although preceding TIA, occurrence in sleep, and regression of deficits in the first 6 h suggest ischemic stroke, the differentiation of ischemic stroke from small ICH is not always possible on clinical grounds alone.[309] Hypertension, arteriovenous malformations, and bleeding into brain tumors are common causes of ICH; other causes include intoxication with cocaine, amphetamine, phenylpropanolamine, or alcohol; carotid endarterectomy or cardiac surgery; anticoagulation and thrombolytic treatments; exposure to cold; and vasculopathies due to amyloidosis or vasculitis.[208,209,310,311]

Sinus venous thrombosis, a disorder that often proved fatal in the pre-CT/MRI era due to delayed diagnosis, is characterized by headaches with bilateral and fluctuating sensorimotor deficits, seizures, blurred vision with papilledema, and decreased level of conscious-

ness (Fig. 11-11). It can present also with a more subtle clinical picture of isolated intracranial hypertension with headaches and papilledema or with isolated abducens palsy. Altered consciousness and seizures occur in only a minority of patients, and the outcome is usually favorable.[312] Causes include intracranial infections, vascular or neoplastic processes, and such systemic disorders as cancer, infection, coagulopathy, pregnancy and puerperium, polycythemia, and heart failure. The cause remains undetermined in up to one third of cases.

Head Trauma

Brain damage after head trauma can be classified by its location (diffuse, local, or multifocal), its time course (immediate or delayed), and its severity, which can be estimated from the duration of initial loss of consciousness, from the severity of subsequent amnesia, and from the initial Glasgow coma scale (GCS).[184] A minor head injury, defined by a GCS score of 15 and posttraumatic amnesia of less than 24 h (most commonly <1 h), accounts for 95 percent of all head traumas and is associated with fracture in less than 10 percent. A GCS score of 9 to 14 occurs in 4 percent of cases and defines a mild-moderate head injury with skull fracture in about a third of cases and a mortality of 3 to 9 percent. A GCS score <8 is found in 1 percent of cases and corresponds to a severe head injury with skull fracture in more than 50 percent and a mortality rate of 35 to 40 percent.[313] Loss of consciousness for more than 1 h and posttraumatic amnesia for more than 24 h also indicate significant head trauma.[189]

Cerebral concussion (commotio cerebri) refers to an acute and transient loss of consciousness following closed head trauma that can last for seconds, minutes, or hours and is followed by a more or less prolonged *posttraumatic amnesia* (which can be present even without initial loss of consciousness). Although loss of consciousness formerly was attributed to temporary dysfunction of the ARAS,[314] *acute diffuse axonal injury* with damage of axons and small vessels by shearing forces generated by sudden deceleration is probably the principal cause of disturbance of consciousness and neuropsychological sequelae. Along with diffuse axonal damage, focal lesions in the corpus callosum and upper brainstem occur and may extend from the subcortical white matter to the centrum semiovale, internal capsule, and brainstem.[315] Brain MRI is more sensitive than brain CT in the detection of these focal and multifocal lesions.[316]

Occasionally, most commonly in children, trivial trauma without initial loss of consciousness can be followed after a lucid interval by prolonged stupor, focal convulsions, and cortical blindness.[20] The outcome is usually benign and the relationship to migraine coma (discussed later in this chapter) and the sometimes fatal syndrome of *delayed encephalopathy following mild head trauma* in adults is unclear. Diffuse brain edema appears to be the cause.[317,318]

Focal brain injury (contusio cerebri) most commonly occurs in the frontotemporal areas due to direct or indirect (contrecoup) trauma, and can be complicated by *acute subdural hematoma* due to injury to veins or sinuses with rapid clinical deterioration.

The classical clinical presentation of *epidural hematoma* from temporal bone fracture with tearing of the middle meningeal artery consists of brief posttraumatic loss of consciousness, a lucid interval of a few hours, and then stupor with ipsilateral pupillary dilation and contralateral hemiparesis (uncal syndrome).[20,319] This presentation occurs in only a minority of cases: Loss of consciousness may not occur initially or may be prolonged without a lucid interval; pupillary dilatation may be absent or contralateral; hemiparesis may be ipsilateral (*Kernohan's phenomenon*); and secondary deterioration may occur over longer intervals of up to several days. Also, the *lucid interval* has little diagnostic value: It occurs with epidural, intracerebral, and subdural hematoma as well as in patients with no focal mass lesions.[318] *Chronic subdural hematoma*, which can run an indolent course, occurs with trauma, alcoholism, coagulopathies, and after shunting for normal-pressure hydrocephalus. The most common symptoms are headaches, delirium, and transient focal deficits; less commonly patients present with seizures or prolonged focal neurological deficits.[320,321] A frequent misdiagnosis is diffuse metabolic-toxic encephalopathy, particularly in the 25 percent of patients with bilateral hematomas. In *traumatic subdural hygroma* there is an accumulation of cerebrospinal fluid in the subdural space without associated cerebral contusion. Patients present with a decreased level of consciousness and seizures, usually without focal neurological signs.[322]

Neoplasms

Neoplasms present with focal neurologic deficits, seizures, headache, altered consciousness, and such pseudolocalizing signs as abducens palsy. Disturbances of consciousness may result from shifts of structures caused by gradients of increased intracranial pressures in different intracerebral compartments, from seizures and postictal states, from bleeding into the neoplasm (most commonly in glioblastoma, lymphoma, melanoma, choriocarcinoma, renal cell carcinoma, and bronchial carcinoma), from obstruction of CSF circulation (typical in cysts of the third ventricle), from infiltration of the ARAS, from accompanying metabolic disturbances such as SIADH, or from side effects of drugs such as steroids used to control vasogenic edema.[323]

Pituitary apoplexy refers to sudden bleeding or necrosis within a pituitary macroadenoma, and presents with headache, meningeal signs, visual loss, unilateral or bilateral ophthalmoplegia, stupor and occasionally coma caused by direct compression of the upper brainstem or by sudden increase in intracranial pressure related to bleeding.[20]

SUBTENTORIAL LESIONS

The most common causes of intrinsic lesions of the brainstem are vascular disease and demyelinating processes.

Stroke

Brainstem stroke, such as basilar artery thrombosis, thrombosis or embolism of perforating branches of the basilar artery, and pontine hemorrhages, may produce abrupt loss of consciousness.

Basilar artery thrombosis is caused by atheromatous disease, dissecton, or embolism. The clinical picture includes preceding vertebrobasilar TIA, early disturbances of consciousness, headache, vertigo, eye movement disorders (internuclear ophthalmoplegia, conjugate gaze palsy, ocular bobbing, nystagmus, skew deviation), pseudobulbar signs, ataxia, disturbed breathing, and bilateral motor deficits.[324–326] The course is usually unfavorable although spontaneous recovery has been reported and early thrombolysis may alter the course.[327]

The *top of the basilar syndrome* is caused by occlusive lesions of the rostral tip of the basilar artery and its branches.[152] The clinical picture is heterogeneous and reflects the involvement of occipitotemporal cortices, paramedian thalamus, midbrain, and superior cerebellum. Patients may present with cortical blindness, amnesia, and pupillary and eye movement disturbances including the pretectal syndrome. Disturbances of consciousness are frequent and include peduncular hallucinosis, delirium, stupor, and coma.[328,329]

Peduncular hallucinosis (PH) refers to a hallucinatory syndrome first observed in mesencephalic and upper pontine strokes that can also follow thalamic lesions.[330-335] Vivid visual hallucinations, which typically appear in the predormitum, are commonly accompanied by nighttime insomnia and daytime hypersomnia. The syndrome appears to represent the intrusion of REM sleep processes into wakefulness.[16]

Pontine hemorrhage presents with headache and vomiting, sudden coma, pinpoint pupils, tetraplegia, absent oculovestibular reflexes, disturbed breathing, and hyperthermia.[308] The usual cause is hypertension and the course is often fatal. Rarely, pontine hemorrhage is limited to the tegmentum and patients survive; in these cases an arteriovenous malformation should be suspected.[336,337]

Initial symptoms of *cerebellar infarcts* and *hemorrhages* typically include headache, nausea, vomiting, and vertigo. The most common signs are gait disturbance, dysarthria, nystagmus, and somnolence. Altered consciousness is common with hemorrhages over 1.5 cm in diameter. Particularly insidious are infarcts in the territory of the anterior inferor cerebellar artery (AICA), which can present initially with headache, vertigo, and nystagmus alone and can be mistaken for peripheral vestibular disease. As the brainstem is compressed laterally, coma and symptoms similar to those of intrinsic brainstem disease appear. In cerebellar infarct the course is often protracted and coma can occur up to 10 days after onset of symptoms due to compression of the brainstem from ischemia or obstructive hydrocephalus, from upward herniation, or from downward herniation.[338]

The clinical presentation of *subarachnoid hemorrhage* in the posterior circulation is similar to that of the anterior circulation.

Others

Brainstem demyelination associated with *multiple sclerosis* usually has a gradual onset with consciousness more often impaired than completely lost.

Central pontine myelinolysis (CPM, Fig. 11-12) refers to an acute syndrome of osmotic demyelination, first described in alcoholism and malnutrition,[339] that is linked to rapid correction of hyponatremia. The syndrome can be prevented in most cases of hyponatremia by gradual correction of sodium concentration, although the ideal rate of correction remains controversial, and water restriction alone may be safer than the use of hypertonic saline solutions.[340] Patients usually

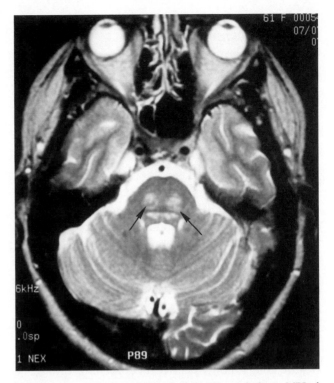

Figure 11-12 *Central pontine myelinolysis.* T2-weight brain MRI of 49-year-old man with alcoholic cirrhosis two weeks after liver transplantation, complicated by multifactorial encephalopathy (hepatorenal insufficiency, sepsis, cyclosporin toxicity). (*Arrows*—increased signal from midpons.) (Courtesy of D. Quint, Neuroradiology Department, University of Michigan Hospitals, Ann Arbor, Michigan.)

present 3 to 5 days after correction of hyponatremia with pseudobulbar palsy, tetraparesis, ophthalmoparesis, and coma. Delirium, locked-in syndrome, and seizures can also be observed. Although the outcome may be fatal, patients with less dramatic presentations have a good outcome. In 10 percent of cases of CPM, there is also myelinolysis of supratentorial white matter.[341]

Basilar migraine can be familial, typically affects young females, and presents with recurrent episodes of headache with nausea and vomiting, vertigo, tinnitus and hearing loss, diplopia and eye movement disorders, visual fields deficits, ataxia, bilateral sensorimotor deficits, and disturbances of consciousness that range from syncope to delirium and coma.[342-344] Rarely, altered consciousness may persist for hours to days.[345]

Migraine coma (also called *meningitic migraine*) is a rare familial condition that shares some features of basilar migraine and presents with recurrent episodes of migrainous headaches, often triggered by trivial head trauma, and complicated by hemiparesis, ataxia, delirium and psychosis, coma, fever, CSF pleocytosis, and brain edema.[346] Its relationship to autosomal dominant *hemiplegic migraine* and autosomal dominant cerebral arteriopathy with subcortical infarcts is unclear.[347-350]

Brainstem encephalitis can be seen in infections with Lyme disease, syphilis, listeriosis, herpes simplex, and as a paraneoplastic syndrome.

Stupor and coma are late manifestations of *brainstem tumors*. "*Cerebellar fits*"—brief attacks of loss of consciousness with headache, opisthotonus, and extensor posturing—can be observed in cerebellar tumors and indicate herniation of the tonsils through the foramen magnum.[64]

PSYCHOGENIC STATES

Psychiatric causes of altered responsiveness include conversion disorder, catatonia, psychotic depression, fugue states, and malingering. Although several signs help to distinguish psychogenic from organic causes of unresponsiveness, no one feature is completely reliable.[351] Furthermore, organic signs do not exclude a psychogenic cause since organic disorders may predispose patients to conversion symptoms. Nonetheless, findings on eye and motor examination are often helpful. Slow roving eye movements and the gradual eye closure that follows passive eye opening cannot be duplicated voluntarily; hence their presence helps to confirm neurologic dysfunction. Most patients with psychogenic coma will either resist passive eye opening or will close their eyes briskly following passive eye opening. However, reflex blepharospasm accompanying metabolic or structural brain disease can lead to similar findings. Furthermore, rhythmic eye opening, orofacial dyskinesias, alternating extreme gaze (Ping-Pong gaze), and forced downward gaze can be seen also in organic coma.[166] Normal vestibuloocular (caloric) reflexes, normal EEG with reactive occipital alpha activity, and normal motor evoked potentials in paralyzed limbs support a diagnosis of psychogenic unresponsiveness.

Initial Assessment of Delirium and Coma

CLINICAL APPROACH TO THE DIFFERENTIAL DIAGNOSIS OF DELIRIUM AND COMA

The management of a comatose patient should be directed initially at stabilizing the cardiopulmonary status. Airway patency should be assessed, and if obstruction is apparent, an oral airway, nasal trumpet, or endotracheal tube should be inserted. If respiratory efforts are slow, shallow, or absent, mechanical ventilation should be instituted after the rate and rhythm of spontaneous respiratory efforts have been noted. Blood pressure, oxygen saturation (pulse oximeter), and carotid pulse should be assessed and, if necessary, measures to correct arrhythmias and increase cardiac output and cerebral perfusion should be instituted. Blood should be obtained for laboratory tests, and simultaneously an intravenous line should be inserted and at least 25 ml of 50% glucose should be injected. In the absence of proven hypoglycemia, greater amounts of glucose should be avoided, since hyperglycemia may aggravate ischemic brain damage.[352] Thiamine, 100 to 300 mg, should be infused with glucose to prevent Wernicke's encephalopathy.

The next step should be a rapid and complete neurological assessment (Table 11-4). The combination of mode of onset of coma, motor signs, and pupillary reactions often allows one to determine the most probable pathophysiology (Table 11-8) and to initiate rational diagnostic and therapeutic interventions.

Delirium or Coma With Focal Signs

If the examination shows focal signs and suggests the presence of the uncal or central syndrome or brainstem compression from a posterior fossa mass, measures should be instituted to reduce intracranial pressure and a computed tomography (CT) brain scan should be obtained promptly. Focal signs can be observed also in a variety of metabolic-toxic encephalopathies as described above.

Delirium or Coma With Meningeal Signs and Without Focal Signs

If meningitis or subarachnoid hemorrhage is suspected and no focal findings or papilledema is apparent, a lumbar puncture should be performed immediately without waiting for a CT scan. The mortality associated with delayed antibiotic treatment is much higher than the risk associated with lumbar puncture.[353] A normal brain CT scan within the first 12 h does not rule out subarachnoid hemorrhage, and spectrophotometric analysis of CSF should be performed.[354] Metabolic encephalopathies, stroke, migraine, and seizures occasionally can be accompanied by slight pleocytosis (10 to 20 cells/mm³) and mild meningeal signs.

Delirium or Coma Without Focal or Meningeal Signs

Such patients are likely to have a toxic-metabolic encephalopathy, particularly if consciousness fluctuates and pupillary reflexes are preserved. Structural lesions that can mimic a toxic-metabolic encephalopathy include paramedian thalamic strokes, sinus venous thrombosis, bilateral subdural hematomas, and meningitis. Coma with absent oculocephalic/vestibuloocular reflexes and normal pupillary responses is typical of drug intoxication. A narcotic antagonist, such as naloxone, and a benzodiazepine antagonist, flumazenil, should be injected if there is the slightest suspicion of narcotic overdose or benzodiazepine intoxication. Flumazenil can induce clinical improvement also in hepatic and uremic encephalopathy and in the syndrome of idiopathic recurrent stupor.

TABLE 11-8
General Rules for Pathophysiologic Differential Diagnosis of Coma

	Onset of Coma	Motor Signs	Pupils	OCR/VOR[a]
Supratentorial lesion	Gradual	Unilateral or bilateral Asymmetric	Reactive or unilateral areactive	Preserved
Subtentorial lesion	Often sudden	Bilateral Asymmetric	Unreactive or reactive	Absent
Metabolic-toxic encephalopathy	Often gradual (initial delirium)	Bilateral Symmetric	Reactive	Preserved (=endogenous) Absent (=exogenous)

[a] Oculocephalic reflexes and vestibuloocular reflexes.

Assessment to this point will indicate whether additional emergency treatment is necessary. The physician can now proceed to obtain a complete history from relatives, friends, or others with pertinent information and to perform a complete physical examination and paraclinical tests.

PARACLINICAL STUDIES

Laboratory Studies

Laboratory testing should include electrolytes, glucose, renal and liver function tests, a complete blood count with differential, prothrombin time, arterial blood gases, creatine phosphokinase, thyroid function tests, urinalysis, serum osmolality, plasma cortisol level, and serum vitamin levels; tests for porphyria should be performed if indicated. If drug overdose is suspected, blood and urine should be obtained for drug analysis, and after appropriate protection of the airway, the gastric contents should be aspirated for drug removal and analysis and to look for pill fragments. The prognostic value of CSF creatine phosphokinase, CSF lactate, and serum neuronal specific enolase remains to be confirmed.[355–359]

Neuroradiologic Imaging

Brain CT gives reliable information about the presence of brain hemorrhage, supratentorial lesions, midline shift, ventricular size, and status of basal cisterns. In acute mass lesions, midline shift at the pineal level of 3 to 4 mm is usually associated with somnolence, 5 to 9 mm with stupor, and above 9 mm with coma.[78] CT is more sensitive than MRI in detection of intraventricular blood, subarachnoid blood, and foreign bodies.

Brain MRI is superior for examination of the posterior fossa, for diagnosis of sinus venous thrombosis and arterial dissections, and for detection of diffuse axonal injuries. It is also more sensitive in the diagnosis of brain infarction, leukoencephalopathy, focal or diffuse brain edema, CT-isodense subdural hematoma, herpes encephalitis, and myelinolysis.

The clinical relevance of *MRI-spectroscopy* and other functional studies in diagnosis and prognosis of delirious and comatose states remains to be established.[238,355,360]

Electroencephalography (EEG)

The EEG remains the most useful clinical electrophysiologic test in patients with altered consciousness. The EEG can be helpful in (1) separating psychogenic from organic unresponsiveness; (2) detecting the presence of status epilepticus; (3) assessing the severity of a toxic-metabolic encephalopathy; (4) determining the presence of lateralized or focal processes; and (5) detecting the persistence of a physiologic arousal cycle.[67,361,362] The major limitations of the EEG are related to the subjective nature of its interpretation and to the alteration or suppression of EEG activity by sedatives and anesthetics.

In the locked-in syndrome and in psychogenic unresponsiveness, the presence of normally distributed and *reactive alpha activity* document the preserved state of consciousness.

The clinical differentiation between toxic-metabolic encephalopathy and nonconvulsive *status epilepticus* can be difficult and may be possible only with EEG evaluation. Also, the EEG may be the only way to recognize seizures in patients in coma, especially if muscle relaxants are used.[172,363] In postanoxic and other metabolic encephalopathies, serial EEG studies with assessment of the severity of slowing of the background activity, the degree of reactivity to external stimuli, and the presence of specific EEG patterns may be helpful in monitoring the evolution and determining the prognosis.[66,67,364–366]

A graded EEG scale for prognostication in nontraumatic coma has been suggested. An EEG grade I (normal or near-normal tracing), with spontaneous variations and normal reactivity to external stimuli, carries a good prognosis.[366,367] In the presence of an EEG grade II or III (theta-delta dominance), prognosis is uncertain. EEG grade IV or V, with *generalized periodic activities*, *burst suppression*, or an *isoelectric* pattern, almost invariably predicts a poor outcome.[368]

A few EEG features are relatively specific for delirium or coma. *Focal periodic epileptiform activities* (also

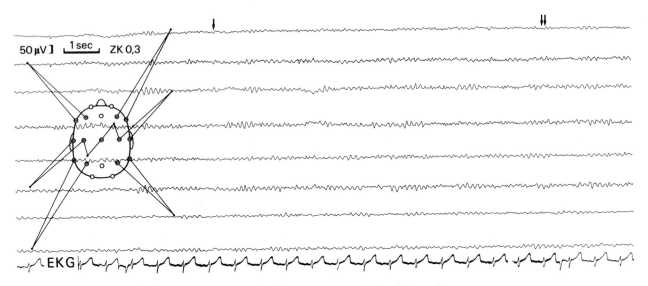

Figure 11-13 *Alpha coma.* Diffuse nonreactive alpha EEG activity to external stimuli (*arrow*) in a 47-year-old patient comatose 34 h after cardiac arrest and resuscitation.

called periodic lateralized epileptiform discharges or *PLEDs*) are characteristic for herpes encephalitis but can also be seen over one or both hemispheres (*BIPLEDs*) after stroke, with subacute sclerosing pan-encephalitis, or with Jakob-Creutzfeldt disease.[369] *Triphasic waves*—typical of hepatic coma—can be observed also in patients with focal or diffuse encephalopathies from a variety of causes and have little prognostic significance.[66,67,370–373]

In comatose patients, nonreactive 10- to 12-Hz alpha activity (*alpha coma*, Fig. 11-13) or slower 5- to 7-Hz theta activity (*theta coma*) on EEG usually, but not invariably, heralds a poor outcome, with the exception of coma due to drug intoxication.[17,66,374–378] The recording of spindles in comatose patients (*"spindle coma"*) has been associated with a poor outcome in nontraumatic states, but with a good outcome after head trauma.[67,362,379–382] The prognostic utility of the EEG is limited to the acute phase of disturbances of consciousness. Later on, EEG and clinical recovery may dissociate. For example, in the vegetative state the EEG may be almost isoelectric or it may show only mildly slowed occipital alpha activities.

Evoked Potentials

Sensory evoked potentials test somatosensory (medial lemniscus) and auditory (lateral lemniscus) pathways in the brainstem, and can localize conduction defects within a few centimeters. Furthermore, the analysis of cortical evoked responses allows the assessment of thalamocortical volleys. Motor evoked potentials (MEPs) provide information about the functional integrity of motor pathways.

With the exception of MEPs, evoked potentials are not appreciably affected by therapeutic doses of central depressant and muscle relaxant drugs. However, evoked potentials test only specific pathways and small portions of the cerebral cortex and tend to be more resistant than the EEG to partial damage. Their preservation does not imply complete structural integrity of the system tested and does not guarantee a full clinical recovery. Preservation of middle-latency somatosensory evoked potentials has been associated with good clinical outcome in postanoxic coma, whereas the absence of early somatosensory evoked potentials in nontraumatic and traumatic coma following median nerve stimulation predicts a poor outcome.[52,359,367,383–389] The usefulness of brainstem auditory evoked potentials in comatose patients is limited by their anatomic specificity for auditory pathways and the topography of the generators. Mechanical distortion of the brainstem is usually accompanied by alterations or loss of waves III through V and preservation of wave I, whereas lesions above the lower midbrain and lesions below the midbrain but not reaching the lateral tegmentum may be accompanied by normal responses. However, BAEP can help in monitoring the effect of intracranial pressure treatment in patients with coma due to an acute supratentorial mass.[390]

In the locked-in syndrome and stroke, motor evoked potentials may predict the degree of recovery of motor functions.[52,391,392]

Intracranial Pressure Monitoring

Intracranial pressure (ICP) at midhead level in the supine position normally is less than 10 mmHg and varies with arterial pressure and breathing. Elevation of ICP is dangerous because it contributes to pressure gradients and herniations and because it may decrease cerebral blood flow. Significant elevations of ICP can occur

TABLE 11-9
Early Prognostic Criteria in Nontraumatic Coma

	GCS at 48–72 h BR at 6–124 h	EEG-Grade (at 12–72 h)	SEP (at 12–72 h)
favorable	≥8 normal BR	I	normal
uncertain	5–7 normal BR	II, III, IV*	abnormal cortical resp.
unfavorable	<5 >1 BR absent	IV, V	absent cortical resp.

NOTE: CGS = Glasgow coma score; BR = brainstem reflexes (corneal, pupillary, oculocephalic); EEG Grade: see text; SEP = median nerve somatosensory evoked potentials; IV* = "alpha-theta coma."[366]

without clinical signs, and conversely herniation symptoms can appear before the mean ICP is increased.[393] The indications for ICP monitoring remain controversial, and proof that ICP monitoring improves outcome is lacking for both traumatic and nontraumatic coma.[96] Increased ICP occurs in 50 percent of adults in coma after head trauma, and the persistence of a pressure >20 mmHg usually heralds a poor outcome.[96] Increased ICP is often seen also after ischemic stroke and intracranial hemorrhage, after cardiac arrest due to respiratory arrest,[385] and less commonly in meningoencephalitis, intracranial tumors, and metabolic encephalopathies.

PROGNOSIS OF ALTERED STATES OF CONSCIOUSNESS

Prognosis of altered consciousness depends upon duration, severity, and underlying etiology. Prediction of individual outcome—a difficult task with important medical, ethical, and socioeconomic implications—is important for counseling of families, for triage decisions, for decisions concerning resuscitation, and for future clinical investigations of brain-resuscitative measures.[394,395] Because of inherent theoretical limitations in the early prediction of outcome and the tendency for poor prognoses to be self-fulfilling, prognostication should be cautious and made in the context of a particular patient's age, comorbidity, and psychosocial status.[395] Overly optimistic predictions are preferable to overly pessimistic ones that may lead to withdrawal of care from a patient with potential for recovery.

Despite these limitations, a reasonable prognosis can be formulated in most cases within a few days of brain injury based on repeated clinical examinations, EEG, and evoked potentials (Table 11-9). The Glasgow outcome scale—analogous to the Glasgow coma scale—defines five outcome categories: (1) good recovery with resumption of normal occupational and social activities, (2) moderate disability with independence in ac-

tivities of daily living, (3) severe disability with essentially complete dependency, (4) persistent vegetative state, and (5) death.[396]

Nontraumatic Coma

A good outcome in these patients—defined as full recovery or only moderate disability—occurs in only 12 percent of those in coma for >6 h, and 3 percent of those in coma for >1 week.[397] The absence of more than one of the corneal, pupillary, and vestibuloocular brainstem reflexes at 24 h is followed by a poor outcome in >95 percent of patients.[397] A GCS <6 in the first 72 h is associated with a risk of death or vegetative state at 2 weeks of 85 percent, compared with 47 percent for a GCS of 6 to 8.[188] On day 3 of coma, abnormal brainstem responses, absent verbal response, absent withdrawal response to pain, creatine levels above 1.5 mg%, and age of 70 years or older are independently associated with 2-month mortality. When four or five of these risk factors are present the 2-month mortality is 97 percent.[398] For patients with a similar depth of coma, prognosis is better with drug-induced and toxic-metabolic encephalopathies than with stroke or cardiac arrest. For patients in nontraumatic coma for >6 h, the likelihood of a good outcome is <10 percent following stroke or cardiac arrest and >20 percent with hepatic coma.[397] Patients with drug-induced coma have an eightfold greater likelihood of awakening within 2 weeks than patients with other causes of nontraumatic coma and similar GCS.[188]

Only 10 to 20 percent of patients in coma with *postanoxic encephalopathy* make a good recovery, and most of these awaken within the first 3 days.[192,200,201,399-401] Unlike coma after head trauma, age does not seem to affect prognosis.[402] The presence of decorticate or decerebrate posturing does not rule out good recovery.[20,179] Because of the greater vulnerability of the cerebral cortex to hypoxia as compared with the brainstem, recovery usually occurs in a caudorostral pattern, and the maximal recovery time that can still be followed by good outcome depends on the function considered.[124,125] Although the absence of brainstem reflexes for more than 6 to 24 h, a GCS <5 for more than 2 or 3 days, generalized myoclonus for more than 30 min, and coma for more than 1 week all herald a poor outcome, accurate clinical prognosis within the first 2 or 3 days is often not possible, as these predictors do not apply to the majority of patients.[124,125,169,172,187,192,401,403,404] In these situations electrophysiologic studies can be of assistance. The presence of an EEG grade IV or V and the absence of early cortical SEP are reliable predictors of a poor outcome unless the recording took place within the first 2 to 8 h after resuscitation.[66,124,125,364-366,383,389,405,406] In a prospective study of 60 patients, the combination of GCS at 48 h, SEP, and EEG allowed a correct prediction

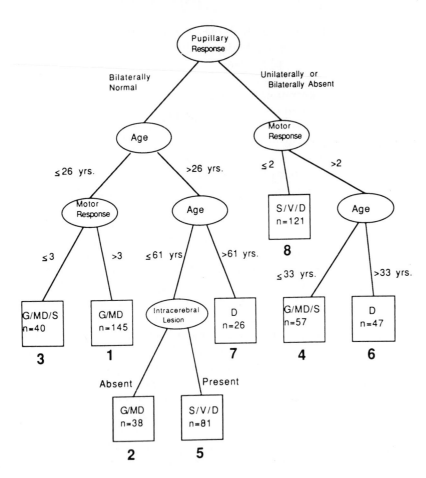

Figure 11-14 *Prediction tree based on 555 severely head-injured patients.* The predicted 12-month outcomes (defined by the Glasgow outcome scale) are: GO = good recovery; MD = moderately disabled; S = severely disabled; V = vegetative; D = dead. Squares denote five prognostic subgroups. The number below the squares represents the prognostic rank of each subgroup based on the proportion of good (G/MD) outcomes. (From Choi et al,[415] with permission.)

in 77 percent of patients with no falsely pessimistic predictions.[406]

The level of consciousness is one of the best predictors of outcome in ischemic and hemorrhagic *stroke*.[76,307,407] The short-term fatality rate is 80 percent in comatose patients, 60 percent in stuporous patients, and 40 percent in somnolent patients after stroke.[408] Less than 10 percent of ischemic stroke patients who require intubation, and less than 5 percent of those in coma from stroke have a satisfactory outcome.[397,409] Early detection and surgical treatment of patients with decreasing level of consciousness due to cerebellar stroke can improve prognosis.[410]

Prognosis in *cerebral hemorrhage* is poor when the patient is over age 70, when the hemorrhage is >60 ml in volume, and when there is intraventricular extension.[69] For patients with intracerebral hemorrhage and a GCS <8 on the day of admission, the 30-day mortality is 78 percent.[307] Whether hemorrhagic stroke has a worse outcome than ischemic stroke remains controversial, and a recent study of 1000 patients suggests that initial stroke severity may be more relevant for stroke prognosis.[411]

Prognosis in *hepatic coma* depends on the underlying hepatic disease, its course (fulminant or long-standing), and the cause that precipitates hepatic encepha-

lopathy.[69] Overall, 20 to 30 percent of patients eventually have a good outcome.[397] However, loss of pupillary, corneal, or vestibuloocular reflexes heralds a poor outcome in >95 percent of cases. In other toxic-metabolic encephalopathies and in status epilepticus, prognosis depends on the underlying disease and associated conditions and is generally better than in coma due to structural brain disorders. In deep coma, however, the same clinical and electrophysiologic prognostic criteria discussed for postanoxic encephalopathy can be applied.[66,67,397]

Traumatic Coma

In 1107 cases of traumatic coma for >6 h, only 26 percent had a good outcome at 3 months.[412] The absence of pupillary reflexes and spontaneous or reflex eye movements at 24 h is followed by a poor outcome in 95 percent of patients.[185] At 6 h after head trauma a GCS <6 carries a risk of death or vegetative state of 65 percent compared with 20 percent for those with a GCS of 6 to 8.[412] Age seems to affect prognosis more in coma after traumatic brain injury than after nontraumatic brain damage.[402,413] Decerebrate rigidity in the early phase of acute head injury does not rule out a good outcome.[78]

In addition to clinical status, the type of lesion that

causes coma affects prognosis. In patients with similar GCSs, acute subdural hematoma is associated with a worse prognosis than epidural hematoma.[412] Independent of clinical status, a midline shift of the pineal gland >15 mm, the obliteration of basal cisterns, the presence of subarachnoid blood on brain CT, and persistent ICP >20 mmHg usually predict a poor outcome.[96,414] The combination of age, pupillary reflexes, motor responses, and CT findings allowed the accurate prediction of the Glasgow outcome score at 12 months in 78 percent of 555 severely head-injured patients (Fig. 11-14).[415]

The early reappearance on the EEG of sleeplike activities, spindles, and normal reactivity are favorable prognostic signs in posttraumatic coma, whereas the bilateral absence of early cortical SEP is a poor prognostic sign.[362,367,379,381,382,384–388,392] As with postanoxic coma, a prognostic approach based on clinical examination and electrophysiologic tests is superior to purely clinical prognostication.[384,388]

Persistent Vegetative State

Persistent vegetative state (PVS) develops in 1 to 14 percent of patients with prolonged traumatic coma and 12 percent of those with prolonged nontraumatic coma.[33] Among patients in a vegetative state 1 month after brain injury, 24 percent of 434 posttraumatic cases, and 4 percent of 169 nontraumatic cases had a good recovery or a moderate disability at a follow-up 12 months after brain injury. Provided that the diagnosis is accurate, prognosis worsens with longer duration of PVS: Among patients in a vegetative state 6 months after brain injury, only 4 percent of 123 posttraumatic cases and none of 50 nontraumatic cases had good recovery of moderate disability at follow-up 12 months after brain injury.[33,416] Thus the PVS appears to be essentially permanent 3 months after nontraumatic and 12 months after traumatic brain injury, although there are single case reports of recovery with moderate disability after nontraumatic PVS lasting 18 months and traumatic PVS lasting for 36 months.[417,418]

Locked-in Syndrome

The mortality of the locked-in syndrome (LiS) is 41 percent of those with nonvascular causes and 67 percent of those with vascular etiology. Functional recovery, which usually takes place in the first 3 months, is more rapid and complete in nonvascular than in vascular cases.[51,419] A good outcome with motor recovery and independent life is possible, although rare.[48,63,419–421] Early recovery or preservation of horizontal eye movements and motor evoked potentials represents a good prognostic sign in vascular LiS.[63,421,422]

References

1. Baumgartner G: Gehirn und Bewusstsein. *Schweiz Med Wochenschr* 1992; 122:4.
2. Fredericks JAM: Consciousness. In *Handbook of Clinical Neurology,* vol 3. Amsterdam, North-Holland Publishing Company, 1974:48–61.
3. Gloor P: Consciousness as a neurological concept in epileptology: A critical review. *Epilepsia* 1986; 27(Suppl 2):S14.
4. Moruzzi G, Magoun HW: Brainstem reticular formation and activation of the EEG. *Electroencephalogr Clin Neurophysiol* 1949; 1:455.
5. Jones BE: Basic mechanisms of sleep-wake states. In Kryger MH, et al (eds): *Principles and Practice of Sleep Medicine,* 2d ed. Philadelphia, WB Saunders Co, 1994:145–162.
6. Jonides J, et al: Spatial working memory in humans as revealed by PET. *Nature* 1993; 363:623.
7. Knight RT: Decreased response to novel stimuli after prefrontal lesions in man. *Electroencephalogr Clin Neurophysiol* 1984; 59:9.
8. Lhermitte F, et al: Human autonomy and the frontal lobes. Part I: Imitation and utilization behaviour: A neuropsychological study of 75 patients. *Ann Neurol* 1986; 19:326.
9. Lhermitte F: Human autonomy and the frontal lobes. Part II: Patient behaviour in complex and social situations: The environmental syndrome. *Ann Neurol* 1986; 19:335.
10. Damasio AR: Category-related recognition defects as a clue to the neural substrates of knowledge. *Trends in Neurosci* 1990; 13:95.
11. Llinas RR, Paré D: Of dreaming and wakefulness. *Neuroscience* 1991; 44:521.
12. Koella WP: A partial theory of sleep. *Eur Neurol* 1986; 25:9.
13. Cravioto H, et al: A clinical and pathologic study of akinetic mutism. *Neurology* 1960; 10:10.
14. Feldman SM, Waller HJ: Dissociation of electrocortical activation and behavioural arousal. *Nature* 1962; 4861:1320.
15. Loeb C, Poggio G: Electroencephalogram in a case with pontomesencephalic haemorrhage. *Electroencephalogr Clin Neurophysiol* 1953; 5:295.
16. Mahowald MW, Schenck CH: Dissociated states of wakefulness and sleep. *Neurology* 1992; 42:44.
17. Westmoreland BF, et al: Alpha-Coma. *Arch Neurol* 1975; 32:713.
18. Bricolo A: Insomnia after bilateral stereotactic thalamotomy in man. *J Neurol Neurosurg Psychiatry* 1967; 30:154.
19. Lugaresi E, et al: Fatal familial insomnia and dysautonomia with selective degeneration of thalamic nuclei. *N Engl J Med* 1986; 315:997.
20. Plum F, Posner JB: *The Diagnosis of Stupor and Coma.* Philadelphia, FA Davis, 1980.
21. Villablanca J: Electroencephalogram in the permanently isolated forebrain of the cat. *Science* 1962; 138:44.
22. Lipowski ZJ: *Delirium: Acute Confusional State.* New York, Oxford University Press, 1990.
23. Taylor D, Lewis S: Delirium. *J Neurol Neurosurg Psychiatry* 1993; 56:742.
24. Bassetti C, Regli F: Les états confusionnels aigus. Analse de 64 cas observés en milieu neurologique. *Schweiz Rundsch Med Prax* 1994; 8:226.
25. Dunne JW, Edis RH: Inobvious stroke: A cause of delirium and dementia. *Aust N Z J M* 1986; 16:771.
26. Mesulam M: Attention, confusional states, and neglect. In Mesulam M (ed): *Principles of Behavioural Neurology.* Philadelphia, FA Davis, 1985:125–168.
27. Mori E, Yamadori A: Acute confusional state and acute agitated delirium. *Arch Neurol* 1987; 44:1139.
28. Lipowski ZJ: Delirium in the elderly patient. *N Engl J Med* 1989; 320:578.
29. Fisher DM, Adams RD: Transient global amnesia. *Acta Neurol Scand* 1964; 40:1.
30. Hodges JR, Warlow CP: The aetiology of transient global amnesia. A case control study of 114 cases with prospective follow-up. *Brain* 1990; 113:639.

31. ANAC: Persistent vegetative state: Report of the American Neurological Association committee on ethical affairs. *Ann Neurol* 1993; 33:386.

32. Jennett B, Plum F: Persistent vegetative state after brain damage. *Lancet* 1972; 1:734.

33. Multi-Society Task Force: Medical aspects of the persistent vegetative state (first of two parts). *N Engl J Med* 1994; 330:1499.

34. Kinney HC, Samuels MA: Neuropathology of the persistent vegetative state. A review. *J Neuropathol Exp Neurol* 1994; 53:548.

35. Kinney HC, et al: Neuropathological findings in the brain of Karen Ann Quinlan. The role of the thalamus in the persistent vegetative state. *N Engl J Med* 1994; 330:1469.

36. Cairns H, et al: Akinetic mutism with an epidermoid cyst of the 3rd ventricle. *Brain* 1941; 64:273.

37. Barris RW, Schuman HR: Bilateral anterior cingulate gyrus lesions. Syndrome of the anterior cingulate gyri. *Neurology* 1953; 3:44.

38. Bassetti C, et al: Spontaneous intracranial dissection in the anterior circulation. *Cerebrovasc Dis* 1994; 4:170.

39. Buge A, et al: "Mutisme akinétique" et ramollissement bicingulaire. *Rev Neurol* 1975; 131:121.

40. Bogousslavsky J, et al: Loss of psychic self-activation with bithalamic infarction. *Acta Neurol Scand* 1991; 83:309.

41. Brage D, et al: Syndrome nécrotique tegmento-thalamique avec mutisme akinétique. *Rev Neurol* 1961; 104:126.

42. Castaigne P, et al: Paramedian thalamic and midbrain infarcts: Clinical and neuropathological study. *Ann Neurol* 1981; 10:127.

43. Lhermitte F, et al: Troubles de la conscience et mutisme akinétique. *Rev Neurol* 1963; 109:115.

44. Segarra J: Cerebral vascular disease and behaviour. I. The syndrome of the mesencephalic artery. *Arch Neurol* 1970; 22:408.

45. Gelenberg AJ: The catatonic syndrome. *Lancet* 1976; 1:1339.

46. Fisher CM: Catatonia due to disulfiram toxicity. *Arch Neurol* 1989; 46:798.

47. Hauser P, et al: Benzodiazepine withdrawal delirium with catatonic features. *Arch Neurol* 1989; 46:696.

48. Bauer G, et al: Varieties of the locked-in syndrome. *J Neurol* 1979; 221:77.

49. Bauer G, et al: Involuntary motor phenomena in the locked-in syndrome. *J Neurol* 1980; 223:191.

50. Hawkes CH, Bryan-Smith L: The electroencephalogram in the locked-in syndrome. *Neurology* 1974; 24:1015.

51. Patterson JR, Grabois M: Locked-in syndrome: A review of 139 cases. *Stroke* 1986; 17:758.

52. Bassetti C, et al: Multimodal electrophysiological studies including motor evoked potentials in patients with locked-in syndrome: Report of six patients. *J Neurol Neurosurg Psychiatry* 1994; 57:1403.

53. Drury I, et al: Fulminating demyelinating polyradiculoneuropathy resembling brain death. *J Neurol Neurosurg Psychiatry* 1987; 50:42.

54. Karp JS, Hurtig H: Locked-in state with bilateral midbrain infarcts. *Arch Neurol* 1974; 30:176.

55. Thadani VM, et al: Locked-in syndrome for 27 years following a viral illness: Clinical and pathologic findings. *Neurology* 1991; 41:498.

56. Chia LG: Locked-in state with bilateral internal capsule infarcts. *Neurology* 1984; 34:1365.

57. DeSmet Y, et al: Infarctus putamino-capsulo-caudés bilatéraux symétriques et simultanés. *Rev Neurol* 1990; 146:415.

58. Ferbert A, Thron A: Bilateral anterior cerebral artery territory infarction in the differential diagnosis of basilar artery occlusion. *J Neurol* 1992; 239:162.

59. Nicolai A, Lazzarino LG: Transient locked-in state in a patient with bilateral simultaneous infarctions of the internal capsule. *Cerebrovasc Dis* 1993; 3:383.

60. Castaigne P, Escourolle R: Etude topographique des lésions anatomiques dans les hypersomnies. *Rev Neurol* 1967; 116:547.

61. Davison C, Demuth EL: Disturbances in sleep mechanism: A clinicopathologic study. V. Anatomic and neurophysiologic considerations. *Arch Neurol Psychiatry* 1946; 55:364.

62. Bassetti C, et al: Hypersomnia following paramedian thalamic stroke. *Ann Neurol* 1996; 39:471.

63. Façon E, et al: Hypersomnie prolongée engendrée par des lésions bilatérale du système activateur médial. Le syndrome thrombotique de la bifuraction du tronc basilaire. *Rev Neurol* 1958; 98:117.

64. Cairns H: Disturbances of consciousness with lesions of the brainstem and diencephalon. *Brain* 1952; 75:109.

65. Catsman-Berrevoets CE, Harskamp F: Compulsive pre-sleep behaviour and apathy due to bilateral thalamic stroke. *Neurology* 1988; 38:647.

66. Bassetti C, Karbowski K: Prognostischer Wert der Elektroenzephalographie bei nicht-traumatischen Komata. *Schweiz Med Wochenschr* 1990; 120:1425.

67. Markand ON: Electroencephalography in diffuse encephalopathies. *J Clin Neurophysiol* 1984; 1:357.

68. Obrecht R, et al: Value of EEG in acute confusional states. *J Neurol Neurosurg Psychiatry* 1979; 42:75.

69. Wijdicks EFM: *Neurology of Critical Illness.* Philadelphia, FA Davis, 1995.

70. Leigh RJ, Zee DS: *The Neurology of Eye Movements.* Philadelphia, FA Davis, 1991.

71. Albert ML, et al: Cerebral dominance for consciousness. *Arch Neurol* 1976; 33:453.

72. Chapman LF, Wolff HJ: The cerebral hemispheres and the highest integrative functions of man. *Arch Neurol* 1959; 1:357.

73. Dougherty JH et al: Hypoxic-ischemic brain injury and the vegetative state. Clinical and neuro-pathologic correlation. *Neurology* 1981; 31:991.

74. Slater R, et al: Diaschisis with cerebral infarction. *Stroke* 1977; 8:684.

75. McNealy DE, Plum F: Brainstem dysfunction with supratentorial mass lesions. *Arch Neurol* 1962; 7:10.

76. Melo TP, et al: An emergency room-based study of stroke coma. *Cerebrovasc Dis* 1992; 2:93.

77. Ropper A: Evoked potentials in cerebral ischemia. *Stroke* 1986; 17:3.

78. Ropper AH: Acute increased intracranial pressure. In Asbury AK, et al (eds): *Diseases of the Nervous System.* Philadelphia, WB Saunders, 1986:1064–1073.

79. Fisher CM: The neurological examination of the comatose patient. *Acta Neurol Scand* 1969; 45:1.

80. Ropper AH, Shafran B: Brain edema after stroke. Clinical syndrome and intracranial pressure. *Arch Neurol* 1984; 41:26.

81. Feldman E, et al: MRI demonstrates descending transtentorial herniation. *Neurology* 1988; 38:384.

82. Inao S, et al: Magnetic resonance imaging assessment of brainstem distortion associated with a supratentorial mass. *J Neurol Neurosurg Psychiatry* 1993; 56:280.

83. Ropper AH: Unusual spontaneous movements in brain-dead patients. *Neurology* 1984; 34:1089.

84. Ropper A: Lateral displacement of the brain and level of consciousness in patients with an acute hemispheral mass. *N Engl J Med* 1986; 314:953.

85. Ropper AH: A preliminary MRI study of the geometry of brain displacement and level of consciousness with acute intracranial masses. *Neurology* 1989; 39:622.

86. Ropper AH, Shafran B: Brain edema after stroke. Clinical features and ICP. *Arch Neurol* 1984; 41:725.

87. Wolf RFE, et al: Kernohan's notch and misdiagnosis. *Lancet* 1995; 345:259.

88. Chase TN, et al: Clinical and electroencephalographic manifestations of vascular lesions of the pons. *Neurology* 1968; 18:357.

89. Autret A, et al: A syndrome of REM and non-REM sleep reduction and lateral gaze paresis after medial tegmental pontine stroke. *Arch Neurol* 1988; 45:1236.

90. Guilleminault C, et al: Pseudo-hypersomnia and pre-sleep behaviour with bilateral paramedian thalamic lesions. *Brain* 1993; 116:1549.

91. Kushida CA, et al: Cortical asymmetry of REM sleep EEG following unilateral pontine hemorrhage. *Neurology* 1991; 41:598.

92. Markand ON, Dyken ML: Sleep abnormalities in patients with brainstem lesions. *Neurology* 1976; 26:769.

93. Valldeoriola F, et al: Absence of REM sleep, altered NREM sleep and supranuclear horizontal gaze palsy caused by a lesion of the pontine tegmentum. *Sleep* 1993; 16:184.

94. Cuneo RA, et al: Upward transtentorial herniation. Seven cases and a literature review. *Arch Neurol* 1979; 36:618.

95. Kanis KB, Ropper AH: Homolateral hemiparesis as an early sign of cerebellar mass effect. *Neurology* 1994; 44:A226.

96. Ropper AH, Rockoff MA: Physiology and clinical aspects of raised intracranial pressure. In Ropper AH (ed): *Neurological and Neurosurgical Intensive Care Medicine*, 3d ed. New York, Raven Press, 193:11–27.

97. Beard EF, et al: Spontaneous subarachnoid hemorrhage simulating myocardial infarction. *Am Heart J* 1959; 58:755.

98. Dimant J, Grob D: Electrocardiographic changes and myocardial damage in patients with acute cerebrovascular accidents. *Stroke* 1977; 8:448.

99. Lavy S, et al: The effect of acute stroke on cardiac functions as observed in an intensive stroke care unit. *Stroke* 1974; 5:775.

100. McDermott MM, et al: ST segment depression detected by continuous electrocardiography in patients with acute ischemic stroke or transient ischemic attack. *Stroke* 1994; 25:1820.

101. Oppenheimer S: The anatomy and physiology of cortical mechanisms of cardiac control. *Stroke* 1993; 24(Suppl I):I6.

102. Sander D, Klingelhöfer J: Changes of circadian blood pressure patterns and cardiovascular parameters indicate lateralization of sympathetic activation following hemispheric brain infarction. *J Neurol* 1995; 242:313.

103. Samuels M: Cardiopulmonary aspects of neurologic diseases. In Ropper AH (ed): *Neurological and Neurosurgical Intensive Care Medicine*, 3rd ed. New York, Raven Press, 1993:103–119.

104. Yuki K, et al: Coronary vasospasm following subarachnoid hemorrhage as a cause of stunned myocardium. *J Neurosurg* 1991; 75:308.

105. Lee MC, et al: Respiratory rate and pattern disturbances in acute brainstem infarction. *Stroke* 1976; 7:382.

106. North JB, Jennett S: Abnormal breathing patterns associated with acute brain damage. *Arch Neurol* 1974; 31:338.

107. Power WR, et al: Sleep-stage dependent Cheyne-Stokes respiration after cerebral infarct: A case study. *Neurology* 1982; 32:763.

108. Yamashiro Y, Kryger MH: Review: Sleep in heart failure. *Sleep* 1993; 16:513.

109. Wardlaw JM: Cheyne-Stokes respiration in patients with acute ischaemic stroke: Observations on middle cerebral artery blood velocity changes using transcranial Doppler ultrasound. *Cerebrovasc Dis* 1993; 3:377.

110. Nactmann A, et al: Cheyne-Stokes respiration in ischemic stroke. *Neurology* 1995; 45:820.

111. Leigh RJ, Shaw DA: Rapid regular respiration in unconscious patients. *Arch Neurol* 1976; 33:356.

112. Plum F, Alvord EC: Apneustic breathing in man. *Arch Neurol* 1964; 10:101.

113. Bogousslavsky J, et al: Respiratory failure and unilateral caudal brainstem infarction. *Ann Neurol* 1990; 28:668.

114. Devereuaux MW, et al: Automatic respiratory failure associated with infarction of the medulla. *Arch Neurol* 1973; 29:46.

115. Simon RP, et al: Medullary lesion inducing pulmonary edema: A magnetic resonance imaging study. *Am Neurol* 1991; 30:727.

116. Al Deeb SM, et al: Intractable hiccup induced by brainstem lesion. *J Neurol Sci* 1991; 103:144.

117. Askenazy JJM: About the mechanism of hiccup. *Eur Neurol* 1992; 32:159.

118. Madonikc MJ, et al: Pleocytosis and meningeal signs in uremia: Report on sixty-two cases. *Arch Neurol Psychiatry* 1950; 64:431.

119. Gassel MM: False localizing signs. *Arch Neurol* 1961; 4:526.

120. Strub RL, Black FW: *The Mental Status Examination in Neurology*. Philadelphia, FA Davis, 1993.

121. Fischbeck SH, Simon RP: Neurological manifestations of accidental hypothermia. *Ann Neurol* 1981; 10:384.

122. Bogousslavsky J, Meienberg O: Eye-movement disorders in brainstem and cerebellular stroke. *Arch Neurol* 1987; 44:141.

123. Kumar P, Ahmed I: Pupil-sparing oculomotor palsy due to midbrain infarct (letter). *Arch Neurol* 1992; 49:348.

124. Jörgensen EO, Malchow-Möller A: Natural history of global and critical brain ischaemia. *Resuscitation* 1981; 9:217.

125. Jörgensen EO, Malchow-Möller A: Natural history of global and critical brain ischaemia. *Resuscitation* 1981; 9:131.

126. Ropper AH: The opposite pupil in herniation. *Neurology* 1990; 40:1707.

127. Fisher CM: Oval pupils. *Arch Neurol* 1980; 37:502.

128. Selhorst JB, et al: Midbrain corectopia. *Arch Neurol* 1976; 33:193.

129. Wilson SA: Ectopia pupillae in certain mesencephalic lesions. *Brain* 1906; 29:524.

130. Appenzeller O: *The Autonomic Nervous System*. New York, Elsevier Biomedical, 1982.

131. Keane JR: Oculosympathetic paresis. Analysis of 100 hospitalized patients. *Arch Neurol* 1979; 36:13.

132. Austin CP, Lessel S: Horner's syndrome from hypothalamic infarction. *Arch Neurol* 1991; 48:332.

133. Bassetti C, Staikov I: Hemiplegia vegetativa alterna. *Stroke* 1995; 26:702.

134. Garcin R, Kipfer M: Syndrome de Claude Bernard-Horner et troubles oculo-sympathiques dans les lésions du thalamus optique. *Rev Neurol* 1939; 71:121.

135. Brierly JB, et al: Neocortical death after cardiac arrest. *Lancet* 1971; 2:560.

136. Tavy DL, et al: Persistence of the blink reflex to sudden illumination in a comatose patient. *Arch Neurol* 1984; 41:323.

137. McCarty GE, Marshall DW: Transient eyelid opening associated with postanoxic EEG suppression-burst suppression. *Arch Neurol* 1981; 38:754.

138. Mori E, et al: Transient eye opening with EEG suppression-burst pattern in postanoxic encephalopathy (letter). *Arch Neurol* 1983; 40:189.

139. Nelson KR, et al: Divergent-convergent eye movements and transient eyelid opening associated with an EEG burst-suppression pattern. *J Clin Neuro Ophthalmol* 1986; 6:43.

140. Keane JR: Spastic eyelids. Failure of levator inhibition in unconscious states. *Arch Neurol* 1975; 32:695.

141. Caplan LR: Ptosis. *J Neurol Neurosurg Psychiatry* 1974; 37:1.

142. Pessin MS, et al: "Wrong-way eyes" in supratentorial hemorrhage. *Ann Neurol* 1981; 9:79.

143. Tijssen CC: Contralateral conjugate eye deviation in acute supratentorial lesions. *Stroke* 1994; 25:1516.

144. Zackon DH, Sharpe JA: Midbrain paresis of horizontal gaze. *Ann Neurol* 1984; 16:495.

145. Averbuch-Heller L, Meiner Z: Reversible periodic alternating gaze deviation in hepatic encephalopathy. *Neurology* 1995; 45:191.

146. Ishikawa H, et al: Short-cycle periodic alternating (Ping-Pong) gaze. *Neurology* 1993; 43:1067.

147. Keane JR, Rawlison DG: Sustained downward deviation. Two cases without structural pretectal lesions. *Neurology* 1976; 26:594.

148. Rosenberg ML: The eyes in hysterical states of unconsciousness. *J Clin Neuro Ophthalmol* 1982; 2:259.

149. Simon RP: Forced downward ocular deviation. Occurrence during oculovestibular testing in sedative drug-induced coma. *Arch Neurol* 1978; 35:456.

150. Kumral E, et al: Thalamic hemorrhage: A prospective study of 100 patients. *Stroke* 1995; 26:964.

151. Keane JR: Sustained upgaze in coma. *Ann Neurol* 1981; 9:409.

152. Caplan LR, Goodwin JA: Dysconjugate gaze in hepatic coma. *Ann Neurol* 1980; 8:328.

153. Keane JR: Ocular skew deviation. Analysis of 100 cases. *Arch Neurol* 1975; 32:185.

154. Drake JME, et al: Ocular bobbing in metabolic encephalopathy. *Neurology* 1982; 32:1029.

155. Fisher CM: Ocular bobbing. *Arch Neurol* 1964; 11:543.

156. Ropper AH: Ocular dipping in anoxic coma. *Arch Neurol* 1981; 38:297.

157. Keane JR: Acute vertical ocular myoclonus. *Neurology* 1986; 36:86.

158. Keane JR: Intermittent see-saw eye movements. *Arch Neurol* 1978; 35:173.

159. Schnyder H, Bassetti C: Bilateral convergence nystagmus in unilateral dorsal midbrain stroke due to occlusion of the superior cerebellar artery. *Neuro Ophthalmol* 1996; 16:59.

160. Segarra JM, Ojeman RJ: Convergence nystagmus. *Neurology* 1961; 11:883.

161. Keane JR: The pretectal syndrome: 206 patients. *Neurology* 1990; 40:684.

162. Caplan LR: "Top of the basilar" syndrome. *Neurology* 1980; 30:72.

163. Gomez CR, et al: Acute thalamic esotropia. *Neurology* 1988; 38:1759.

164. Buettner UW, Zee DS: Vestibular testing in comatose patients. *Arch Neurol* 1989; 46:561.

165. Mueller-Jensen A, et al: Outcome prediction in comatose patients: Significance of reflex eye movement analysis. *J Neurol Neurosurg Psychiatry* 1987; 50:389.

166. Noda S, et al: Orofacial dyskinesia in stupor and coma. *Neurology* 1988; 38:1331.

167. Pratap-Chand R, Gourie-Devie M: Bruxism: Its significance in coma. *Clin Neurol Neurosurg* 1985; 87:113.

168. Wali GM: "Fou rire prodromique" heralding a brainstem stroke. *J Neurol Neurosurg Psychiatry* 1993; 56:209.

169. Krumholz A, et al: Outcome from coma after CPR: Relation to seizures and myoclonus. *Neurology* 1988; 38:401.

170. Snyder BD, et al: Neurologic prognosis after cardiopulmonary arrest: III. Seizure activity. *Neurology* 1980; 30:1292.

171. Stark RJ: Reversible myoclonus with uremia. *Br Med J* 1981; 282:119.

172. Wijdicks EFM, et al: Prognostic value of myoclonus status in comatose survivors of cardiac arrest. *Ann Neurol* 1994; 35:239.

173. Wijdicks EFM, Sharbrough FW: New-onset seizures in critically ill patients. *Neurology* 1993; 43:1042.

174. Bassetti C, et al: Isolated infarcts of the pons. *Neurology* 1996; 46:165.

175. Kaufmann DK, et al: Involuntary tonic spasms of a limb due to a brainstem lacunar infarction. *Stroke* 1994; 25:217.

176. Feldmeyer JJ, et al: Asterixis uni- or bilatéral en cas de lésion thalamique ou pariétale: un trouble moteur afférentiel? *Schweiz Med Wochenschr* 1984; 114:167.

177. Hanna JP, Frank JI: Automatic stepping in pontomedullary stage of central herniation. *Neurology* 1995; 45:985.

178. Bricolo A, et al: Decerebrate rigidity in acute head injury. *J Neurosurg* 1977; 47:680.

179. Conomy J, Swash M: Reversible decerebrate and decorticate postures in hepatic coma. *N Engl J Med* 1968; 278:876.

180. Greenberg DA, Simon RP: Flexor and extensor postures in sedative drug-induced coma. *Neurology* 1982; 32:448.

181. Tyler HR: Neurologic disorders in renal failure. *Am J Med* 1968; 44:734.

182. Halsey JH, Downie AW: Decerebrate rigidity with preservation of consciousness. *J Neurol Neurosurg Psychiatry* 1966; 29:350.

183. Babinski J: Du phénomène des orteils et de sa valeur sémiologique. *Semi Méd* 1898; 18:321.

184. Ropper AH: Self-grasping: A focal neurological sign. *Ann Neurol* 1982; 12:575.

185. Jennett B, Teasdale G: Predicting outcome in individual patients after severe head injury. *Lancet* 1976; 1:1031.

186. Jennett B, et al: Prognosis of patients with severe head injury. *Neurosurgery* 1979; 4:283.

187. Mullie A, et al: Predictive value of Glasgow coma score for awakening after out-of-hospital cardiac arrest. *Lancet* 1988; 1:137.

188. Sacco RL, et al: Non traumatic coma. Glasgow coma score and coma etiology as predictors of 2-week outcome. *Arch Neurol* 1990; 47:1181.

189. Teasdale GM: Head injury. *J Neurol Neurosurg Psychiatry* 1995; 58:526.

190. Teasdale G, Jennett B: Assessment of coma and impaired consciousness. A practical scale. *Lancet* 1974; 2:81.

191. Teasdale G, et al: Observer variability in assessing impaired consciousness and coma. *J Neurol Neurosurg Psychiatry* 1978; 41:603.

192. Edgren E, et al: Prediction of outcome after cardiac arrest. *Crit Care Med* 1987; 15:820.

193. Chernik D, et al: Validity and reliability of the observer's assessment of alertness/sedation scale. Study with intravenous midazolam. *J Clin Psychopharmacol* 1990; 10:2244.

194. Sundt TM, et al: Cerebral flow measurements and electroencephalograms during carotid endarterectomy. *J Neurosurg* 1974; 41:310.

195. White R, et al: Brain ischemic anoxia. Mechanisms of injury. *JAMA* 1984; 251:1586.

196. Siesjö BK: Pathophysiology and treatment of focal cerebral ischemia. Part I: Pathophysiology. *J Neurosurg* 1992; 77:169.

197. Volpe BT, Hirst W: The characterization of an amnesic syndrome following hypoxic ischemic injury. *Arch Neurol* 1983; 40:436.

198. Caronna JJ, Finklestein S: Neurological syndromes after cardiac arrest. *Stroke* 1978; 9:517.

199. Sage JI, vanUitert RL: Man-in-the-barrel syndrome. *Neurology* 1986; 36:1102.

200. Longstreth WT, et al: Prediction of awakening after out-of-hospital cardiac arrest. *N Engl J Med* 1983; 308:1378.

201. Longstreth WT, et al: Neurologic recovery after out-of-hospital cardiac arrest. *Ann Intern Med* 1983; 98:588.

202. Dooling EC, Richardson EP: Delayed encephalopathy after strangling. *Arch Neurol* 1976; 33:196.

203. Plum F, et al: Delayed neurological deterioration after anoxia. *Arch Intern Med* 1962; 110:18.

204. Rock GA, et al: Comparison of plasma exchange with plasma infusion in the treatment of thrombotic thrombocytopenic purpura. *N Engl J Med* 1991; 325:392.

205. Gress DR: Case records of the Massachussetts General Hospital. *N Engl J Med* 1991; 324:113.
206. Briley DP, et al: Neurologic disease associated with antiphospholipid antibodies. *Ann Neurol* 1989; 25:221.
207. Coull BM, et al: Multiple cerebral infarctions and dementia associated with anticardiolipin antibodies. *Stroke* 1987; 18:1107.
208. Aldrich MS: Cerebrovascular complications of streptokinase infusion. *JAMA* 1985; 253:1777.
209. Maggioni AP, et al: The risk of stroke in patients with acute myocardial infarction after thrombolytic and antithrombotic treatment. *N Engl J Med* 1992; 327:1.
210. Jellinek EH, et al: Hypertensive encephalopathy with cortical disorders of vision. *Quart J Med* 1964; 33:239.
211. Weingarten L, et al: Acute hypertensive encephalopathy: Findings on spin-echo and gradient-echo MR imaging. *Am J Radiol* 1994; 162:665.
212. Linn FHH, et al: Prospective study of sentinel headache in aneurysmal subarachnoid haemorrhage. *Lancet* 1994; 344:590.
213. Posner JB, Plum F: Spinal fluid pH and neurologic symptoms in systemic acidosis. *N Engl J Med* 1967; 277:605.
214. Malouf R, Brust JCM: Hypoglycemia: Causes, neurological manifestations, and outcome. *Ann Neurol* 1985; 17:421.
215. Herings RMC, et al: Hypoglycemia associated with use of inhibitors of angiotensin converting enzyme. *Lancet* 1995; 345:1195.
216. Service FJ: Hypoglycemic disorders. *N Engl J Med* 1995; 332:1144.
217. Charness ME, et al: Ethanol and the nervous system. *N Engl J Med* 1989; 321:442.
218. Harper C: The incidence of Wernicke's encephalopathy in Australia. A neuropathologic study of 131 cases. *J Neurol Neurosurg Psychiatry* 1983; 46:593.
219. Banksy G, et al: Reversal of hepatic coma by benzodiazepine antagonist (Ro 15-1788). *Lancet* 1985; 1:1324.
220. Basile AS, et al: Differential responsiveness of cerebellar Pukinje neurons to GABA and benzodiazepine ligands in an animal model of hepatic encephalopathy. *J Neurosci* 1988; 8:2414.
221. Mullen KD, et al: "Endogenous" benzodiazepine activity in body fluids of patients with hepatic encephalopathy. *Lancet* 1990; 336:81.
222. Pomier-Layrargues G, et al: Flumazenil in cirrhotic patients in hepatic coma: A randomized double-blind placebo-controlled crossover trial. *Hepatology* 1994; 19:32.
223. Bleck TP: Neurologic consequences of fulminant hepatic failure. *Mayo Clin Proc* 1995; 70:195.
224. Krieger D, et al: Manganese and chronic hepatic encephalopathy. *Lancet* 1995; 346:270.
225. Wijdicks EFM, et al: Clinical and radiologic features of cerebral edema in fulminant hepatic failure. *Mayo Clin Proc* 1995; 70:119.
226. Hughes JR: Correlation between EEG and clinical changes in uremia. *Electroencephalogr Clin Neurophysiol* 1980; 48:583.
227. Mahoney CA, Arieff AI: Uremic encephalopathies: Clinical, biochemical and experimental features. *Am J Kidney Dis* 1982; 2:324.
228. Bauer TM, et al: Prolonged sedation due to accumulation of conjugated metabolites of midazolam. *Lancet* 1995; 346:145.
229. Lockwood AH: Neurologic complications of renal disease. *Neurol Clin* 1989; 7:617.
230. Pallis CA, Lewis PD: *The Neurology of Gastrointestinal Disease.* London, Saunders, 1974.
231. Tinuper P, et al: Idiopathic recurring stupor: A case with possible involvement of the gamma-aminobutyric acid (GABA)eric system. *Ann Neurol* 1992; 31:503.
232. Tinuper P, et al: Idiopathic recurrent stupor. *Neurology* 1994; 44:621.
233. Mulloy AL, Caruana RJ: Hyponatremic emergencies. *Med Clin North Am* 1995; 79:155.
234. Arieff AI: Hyponatremia, convulsions, respiratory arrest and permanent brain damage after elective surgery in healthy women. *N Engl J Med* 1986; 314:1529.
235. Morris-Jones PH, et al: Prognosis of the neurological complications of acute hypernatremia. *Lancet* 1967; 2:1385.
236. Jordan RM: Myxedema coma. Pathophysiology, therapy, and factors affecting prognosis. *Med Clin North Am* 1995; 79:185.
237. Newmark SR, et al: Myxedema coma. *JAMA* 1974; 230:884.
238. Smith CD, Ain KB: Brain metabolism in hypothyroidism studied with 31P magnetic-resonance spectroscopy. *Lancet* 1995; 345:619.
239. Newcomer J, et al: Coma and thyrotoxicosis. *Ann Neurol* 1983; 14:689.
240. Shaw PJ, et al: Hashimoto's encephalopathy: A steroid-responsive disorder associated with high anti-thyroid antibody titers—report of 5 cases. *Neurology* 1991; 41:228.
241. Jefferson A: A clinical correlation between encephalopathy and papilledema in Addison's disease. *J Neurol Neurosurg Psychiatry* 1956; 19:21.
242. Lemann J, Donatelli AA: Calcium intoxication due to primary hyperparathyroidism. *Ann Intern Med* 1964; 60:447.
243. Grant DK: Papilledema and fits in hypoparathyroidism. *Quart J Med* 1953; 86:243.
244. Delgado-Escueta AV, Bajorek JG: Status epilepticus: Mechanisms of brain damage and rational management. *Epilepsia* 1982; 23:S29.
245. Ballenger CE, et al: Partial complex status epilepticus. *Neurology* 1983; 33:1542.
246. Williamson PD, et al: Complex partial status epilepticus: A depth-electrode study. *Ann Neurol* 1985; 18:647.
247. Guberman A, et al: Nonconvulsive generalized status epilepticus: Clinical features, neuropsychological testing, and long-term follow-up. *Neurology* 1986; 36:1284.
248. Hess R, et al: Borderline cases of petit mal status. *Eur Neurol* 1971; 5:137.
249. Niedermeyer E, et al: Absence status (petit mal status) with focal characteristics. *Arch Neurol* 1979; 36:417.
250. Thomas P, et al: De novo absence status epilepticus as a benzodiazepine withdrawal syndrome. *Epilepsia* 1993; 34:355.
251. Wullimann R, et al: Confusional state due to nonconvulsive generalized status epilepticus (abstract). *Electroencephalogr Clin Neurophysiol* 1995; 95:5P.
252. Dunne JW, et al: Non-convulsive status epilepticus: A prospective study in an adult general hospital. *Quart J Med* 1987; 238:117.
253. Thomas P, et al: "De novo" absence status of late onset: Report of 11 cases. *Neurology* 1992; 42:104.
254. Tomson T, et al: Nonconvulsive status epilepticus: High incidence of complex partial status. *Epilepsia* 1986; 27:276.
255. Walsh GO, Delgado-Escueta AV: Status epilepticus. *Neurol Clin* 1993; 4:835.
256. Lee SI: Nonconvulsive status epilepticus. *Arch Neurol* 1985; 42:778.
257. Rohr-Lefloch J, et al: Etats confusionnels d'origine épileptique intérêt de l'EEG fait en urgence. *Rev Neurol* 1988; 144:425.
258. Treiman DM: Electroclinical features of status epilepticus. *J Clin Neurophysiol* 1995; 12:342.
259. Müller M, et al: Clinical relevance and frequency of transient stenoses of the middle and anterior cerebral arteries in bacterial meningitis. *Stroke* 1995; 26:1399.
260. Pfister HW, et al: Spectrum of complications during bacterial meningitis. Results of a prospective clinical study. *Arch Neurol* 1993; 50:575.
261. Ruben S: Mollaret's Meningitis. *West J Med* 1994; 160:459.

262. Smith RR, Arvin MC: Neuroradiology of intracranial infection. *Semin Neurol* 1992; 12:248.

263. Whitley RJ: Viral encephalitis. *N Engl J Med* 1990; 323:242.

264. Berger JR, Levy RM: The neurologic complications of human immunodeficiency virus infection. *Med Clin North Am* 1993; 77:1.

265. Thomas P, Borg M: Reversible myoclonic-encephalopathy revealing the AIDS-dementia complex. *Electroencephalogr Clin Neurophysiol* 1994; 90:166.

266. Paskavitz JF, et al: Acute arcuate fiber demyelinating encephalopathy following Epstein-Barr virus infection. *Ann Neurol* 1995; 38:127.

267. Jackson AC, et al: The encephalopathy of sepsis. *Can J Neurol Sci* 1985; 12:303.

268. Bleck TP, et al: Neurologic complications of critical medical illnesses. *Crit Care Med* 1993; 21:98.

269. Moore PM: Vasculitis of the central nervous system. *Semin Neurol* 1994; 14:307.

270. Futrell N, et al: Central nervous system disease in patients with systemic lupus erythematosus. *Neurology* 1992; 42:1649.

271. Awada A, et al: Excessive sweating: An uncommon sign of basilar artery occlusion. *J Neurol Neurosurg Psychiatry* 1991; 54:277.

272. Kim BS, et al: Contralateral hyperhidrosis after cerebral infarction. *Clinicoanatomic correlations in five cases. Stroke* 1995; 26:896.

273. Korpelainen JT, et al: Hyperhidrosis as a reflection of autonomic failure in patients with acute hemispheral brain infarction. *Stroke* 1992; 23:1271.

274. Labar DR, et al: Unilateral hyperhydrosis after cerebral infarction. *Neurology* 1988; 38:1679.

275. List CF, Peet MM: Sweat secretion in man. Disturbances of sweat secretion with lesions of the pons, medulla and cervical portion of the cord. *Arch Neurol Psychiatry* 1939; 42:1098.

276. Meyer JS, Handa J: Cerebral blood flow and metabolism during experimental hyperthermia (fever). *Minn Med* 1967; 50:37.

277. Mehta AC, Baker RT: Persistent neurological deficits in heat stroke. *Neurology* 1970; 20:336.

278. Busto U, et al: Withdrawal reaction after long-term therapeutic use of benzodiazepines. *N Engl J Med* 1986; 315:854.

279. Corbett JJ, et al: Downbeating nystagmus and other ocular motor defects caused by lithium toxicity. *Neurology* 1989; 39:481.

280. MacGregor DA, et al: Hyperosmolar coma due to lithium-induced diabetes insipidus. *Lancet* 1995; 346:413.

281. Apte SN, Langston JW: Permanent neurological deficits due to lithium toxicity. *Ann Neurol* 1983; 13:453.

282. Buckley PF, Hutchinson M: Neuroleptic malignant syndrome. *J Neurol Neurosurg Psychiatry* 1995; 58:271.

283. Riley DE, et al: Acute respiratory failure from dopamine agonist withdrawal. *Neurology* 1992; 42:1843.

284. Bodner RA, et al: Serotonin syndrome. *Neurology* 1995; 45:219.

285. Kline SS, et al: Serotonin syndrome versus neuroleptic malignant syndrome as a cause of death. *Clin Pharm* 1989; 8:510.

286. Wolters EC, et al: Leucoencephalopathy after inhaling "heroin" pyrolysate. *Lancet* 1982; 2:1233.

287. Cardoso F, Jankovic J: Movement disorders. In Brust JCM (ed): *Neurologic Complications of Drug and Alcohol Abuse,* Philadelphia, WB Saunders, 1993:625–638.

288. Choy-Kwong M, Lipton RB: Seizures in hospitalized cocaine users. *Neurology* 1989; 39:425.

289. Libman RB, et al: Transient monocular blindness associated with cocaine abuse. *Neurology* 1993; 43:228.

290. Mody CK, *et al.* Neurologic complications of cocaine abuse. *Neurology* 1988; 38:1189.

291. Tapia JF, Golden JA: Case record of the MGH. *N Engl J Med* 1993; 329:117.

292. Rosenberg NL, et al: Toluene abuse causes diffuse central nervous system white matter changes. *Ann Neurol* 1988; 23:611.

293. Abramowicz M: Drugs that cause psychiatric symptoms. *Med Letter* 1989; 31:113.

294. deGroen PC, et al: Central nervous toxicity after liver transplantation. *N Engl J Med* 1987; 317:861.

295. Nussbaum ES, et al: Cyclosporine A toxicity presenting with acute cerebellar edema and brainstem compression. *J Neurosurg* 1995; 82:1068.

296. Bousser MG, et al: Pertes de connaissance brèves au cours des accidents ischémiques cérébraux. *Ann Med Interne (Paris)* 1981; 132:300.

297. Gustafson Y, et al: Acute confusional state (delirium) in stroke patients. *Cerebrovasc Dis* 1991; 1:257.

298. Devinski O, et al: Confusional states following posterior cerebral artery infarction. *Arch Neurol* 1988; 45:160.

299. Gustafson Y, et al: Acute confusional state (delirium) soon after stroke is associated with hypercortisolism. *Cerebrovasc Dis* 1993; 3:33.

300. Mesulam M, et al: Acute confusional states with right middle cerebral infarction. *J Neurol Neurosurg Psychiatry* 1976; 39:84.

301. Boller F, et al: Paroxysmal "nightmares." *Neurology* 1975; 25:1026.

302. Bogousslavsky J, et al: Manic delirium and frontal-lobe syndrome with paramedian infarction of the right thalamus. *J Neurol Neurosurg Psychiatry* 1988; 51:116.

303. Gentilini M, et al: Bilateral paramedian thalamic artery infarcts. *J Neurol Neurosurg Psychiatry* 1987; 50:900.

304. Meissner I, et al: The paramedian diencephalic syndrome: A dynamic phenomenon. *Stroke* 1987; 18:380.

305. Castaigne P, et al: Ramollissement pédonculaire médian, tegmentothalamique avec ophtalmoplégie et hypersommie. *Rev Neurol* 1962; 106:357.

306. Katz DI, et al: Dementia following strokes in the mesencephalon and diencephalon. *Arch Neurol* 1987; 44:1127.

307. Tuhrim S, et al: Prediction of intracerebral hemorrhage survival. *Ann Neurol* 1988; 24:258.

308. Kase CS, et al: Intracerebral hemorrhage, in Barnett HJM, et al (eds): *Stroke. Pathophysiology, Diagnosis, and Management* 2d ed. New York, Churchill Livingstone, 1992:561–616.

309. Weir CJ, et al: Poor accuracy of stroke scoring systems for differential clinical diagnosis of intracranial hemorrhage and infarction. *Lancet* 1994; 344:999.

310. Caplan LR: Intracerebral hemorrhage revisited. *Neurology* 1988; 38:624.

311. Hart RG, et al: Oral anticoagulants and intracranial hemorrhage. Facts and hypotheses. *Stroke* 1995; 26:1471.

312. Ameri A, Bousser MG: Cerebral venous thrombosis. In Barnett HJM, Hachinski VC (eds): *Cerebral Ischemia: Treatment and Prevention,* Philadelphia, WB Saunders, 1992:87–111.

313. Miller JD: Head injury. *J Neurol Neurosurg Psychiatry* 1993; 56:440.

314. Foltz EL, Schmidt RP: The role of the reticular formation in the coma of head injury. *J Neurosurg* 1956; 13:145.

315. Adams JH, et al: Diffuse axonal injury due to nonmissile head injury in humans: An analysis of 45 cases. *Ann Neurol* 1982; 12:557.

316. Mittl RL, et al: Prevalence of MR evidence of diffuse axonal injury in patients with mild head injury and normal head CT findings. *Am J Neurorad* 1994; 15:1583.

317. Bruce DA, et al: Diffuse cerebral swelling following head injuries in children: The syndrome of "malignant brain edema." *J Neurosurg* 1981; 54:170.

318. Lobato RD, et al: Head-injured patients who talk and deteriorate into coma. *J Neurosurg* 1991; 75:256.

319. McKissock W, et al: Extradural hematoma: Observations on 125 cases. *Lancet* 1960; 2:167.

320. Black DW: Mental changes resulting from subdural hematoma. *Br J Psychol* 1984; 145:1139.

321. Robinson RG: Subdural hematoma: Surgical management in 133 patients. *J Neurosurg* 1984; 61:263.

322. Greenberg MS: *Handbook of Neurosurgery.* Lakeland, Florida, Greenberg Graphics, 1994.

323. Weaver DD, et al: Differential intracranial pressure in patients with unilateral mass lesions. *J Neurosurg* 1982; 56:660.

324. Ferbert A. et al: Clinical features of proven basilar artery occlusion. *Stroke* 1990; 21:1135.

325. Kubick CS, Adams RD: Occlusion of the basilar artery: A clinical and pathological study. *Brain* 1946; 69:73.

326. Loeb C, Meyer JS: *Strokes Due to Vertebrobasilar Disease.* Springfield, Charles C Thomas, 1965.

327. Hacke W, et al: Intra-arterial thrombolytic therapy improves outcome in patients with acute vertebrobasilar occlusive disease. *Stroke* 1988; 19:1216.

328. Mehler MF: The neuro-ophthalmologic spectrum of the rostral basilar artery syndrome. *Arch Neurol* 1988; 45:966.

329. Mehler MF: The rostral basilar artery syndrome. *Neurology* 1989; 39:9.

330. Catafau JS, et al: Peduncular hallucinosis associated with posterior thalamic infarction. *J Neurol* 1992; 239:89.

331. Feinberg WF, Rapcsack SZ: Peduncular hallucinosis following paramedian thalamic infarction. *Neurology* 1989; 39:1535.

332. Geller TJ, Bellur SN: Peduncular hallucinosis: Magnetic resonance imaging confirmation of mesencephalic infarction during life. *Ann Neurol* 1987; 21:602.

333. Lhermitte J: L'hallucinose pédonculaire. *Encephale* 1932; 27:422.

334. Lhermitte MJ: Syndrome de la calotte du pédoncule cérébral. Les troubles psychosensoriels dans les lésions mésocéphaliques. *Rev Neurol* 1922; 29:1359.

335. VanBogaert L: L'hallucinose pédonculaire. *Rev Neurol* 1927; 43:608.

336. Caplan LR, Goodwin JA: Lateral tegmental brainstem hemorrhages. *Neurology* 1982; 32:252.

337. Kilpatrick TJ, et al: Lateral tegmental pontine hemorrhage due to vacular malformation. *Cerebrovasc Dis* 1991; 1:108.

338. Amarenco P: L'infarctus du cervelet: un modèle pour l'étude des mécanismes de l'ischémie vertébrobasilaire. *Sang Thrombose Vaisseux* 1992; 4:583.

339. Adams RD, et al: Central pontine myelinolysis: A hitherto undescribed disease occuring in alcoholic and malnourished patients. *Arch Neurol* 1959; 81:154.

340. Harris CP, et al: Symptomatic hyponatremia: Can myelinolysis be prevented by treatment. *J Neurol Neurosurg Psychiatry* 1993; 56:626.

341. Laureno R, Karp BI: Pontine and extrapontine myelinolysis following rapid correction of hyponatremia. *Lancet* 1988; 2:439.

342. Bickerstaff ER: Basilar artery migraine. *Lancet* 1961; 1:15.

343. Frequin SFFM, et al: Recurrent prolonged coma due to basilar artery migraine. A case report. *Headache* 1991; 31:75.

344. Sturzenegger M, Meienberg O: Basilar artery migraine: A follow-up study of 82 cases. *Headache* 1985; 25:408.

345. Lee CH, Lance JW: Migraine stupor. *Headache* 1977; 17:32.

346. Fitzsimons RB, Wolfenden WH: Migraine coma. Meningitic migraine with cerebral oedema associated with a new form of autosomal dominant cerebellar ataxia. *Brain* 1985; 108:555.

347. Baudrimont M, et al: Autosomal dominant leukoencephalopathy and subcortical ischemic stroke. A clinico-pathological study. *Stroke* 1993; 24:122.

348. Feely MP, et al: Episodes of confusion or psychosis in familial hemiplegic migraine. *Acta Neurol Scand* 1982; 65:369.

349. Joutel A, et al: A gene for familial hemiplegic migraine maps to chromosome 19. *Nature Genetics* 1993; 5:40.

350. Jung H, et al: Cerebral autosomal dominant arteriopathy with subcortical infarcts and leucoencephalopathy: A clinico-pathological and genetic study of a Swiss family. *J Neurol Neurosurg Psychiatry* 1995; 59:138.

351. Hopkins A: Pretending to be unconscious. *Lancet* 1973; 1:312.

352. Kushner M, et al: Relation of hyperglycemia early in ischemic brain infarction to cerebral anatomy, metabolism, and clinical outcome. *Ann Neurol* 1990; 28:129.

353. Archer BD: Computed tomography before lumbar puncture in acute meningitis: A review of the risks and benefits. *Can Med Assoc J* 1993; 148:961.

354. van derWee N, et al: Detection of subarachnoid haemorrhage on early CT: Is lumbar puncture still needed after a negative scan. *J Neurol Neurosurg Psychiatry* 1995; 58:357.

355. Berek K, et al: Early determination of neurologic outcome after prehospital cardiopulmonary resuscitation. *Stroke* 1995; 26:543.

356. DeGiorgio CM, et al: Serum neuron-specific enolase in human status epilepticus. *Neurology* 1995; 45:1134.

357. Longstreth WT, et al: Cerebrospinal fluid and serum creatine kinase BB activity after out-of-hospital cardiac arrest. *Neurology* 1981; 31:455.

358. Roine RO, et al: Neurological outcome after out of hospital cardiac arrest: Prediction by cerebrospinal fluid enzyme analysis. *Arch Neurol* 1989; 46:753.

359. Rothstein TL, et al: Predicting outcome in hypoxic-ischemic coma. A prospective clinical and electrophysiological study. *Electroencephalogr Clin Neurophysiol* 1991; 79:101.

360. Bowler JV, et al: Contribution of diaschisis to the clinical deficit in human cerebral infarction. *Stroke* 1995; 26:100.

361. Evans BM: Patterns of arousal in comatose patients. *J Neurol Neurosurg Psychiatry* 1976; 39:392.

362. Evans BM, Bartlett JR: Prediction of outcome in severe head injury based on recognition of sleep related activity in the polygraphic electroencephalogram. *J Neurol Neurosurg Psychiatry* 1995; 59:17.

363. Simon RP, Aminoff MJ: Electrographic status epilepticus in fatal anoxic coma. *Ann Neurol* 1986; 20:351.

364. Hockaday JM, et al: Electoencephalographic changes in acute cerebral anoxia from cardiac or respiratory arrest. *Electroencephalogr Clin Neurophysiol* 1965; 18:575.

365. Prior PF: *The EEG in Acute Cerebral Anoxia.* Amsterdam, Excerpta Medica, 1973.

366. Synek VM: Value of revised EEG coma scale for prognosis after cerebral anoxia and diffuse head injury. *Clin Electroencephalogr* 1990; 21:25.

367. Gütling E, et al: EEG reactivity in the prognosis of severe head injury. *Neurology* 1995; 45:915.

368. Kuroiwa Y, Celesia GC: Clinical significance of periodic EEG patterns. *Arch Neurol* 1980; 37:15.

369. de la Paz D, Brenner RP: Bilateral independent periodic lateralized epileptiform discharges. Clinical significance. *Arch Neurol* 1981; 38:713.

370. Bahamon JE, et al: Prognostic significance of EEG triphasic waves in patients with altered state of consciousness. *J Clin Neurophysiol* 1989; 6:313.

371. Fisch BJ, Klass DW: The diagnostic specificity of triphasic waves patterns. *Electroencephalog Clin Neurophysiol* 1988; 70:1.

372. Karnaze DS, Bickford RG: Triphasic waves: A reassessment of their significance. *Electroencephalogr Clin Neurophysiol* 1984; 57:193.

373. Townsend JB, Drury I: Triphasic waves in coma from brainstem infarction. *Eur Neurol* 1991; 31:47.

374. Austin E, et al: Etiology and prognosis of alpha coma. *Neurology* 1988; 33:773.

375. Carroll WM, Mastaglia FL: Alpha and beta coma in drug intoxication uncomplicated by cerebral hypoxia. *Electroencephalogr Clin Neurophysiol* 1979; 46:95.

376. Grindal AB, et al: Alpha-pattern coma: 24 cases with 9 survivors. *Ann Neurol* 1977; 1:371.

377. Soerensen K, et al: Prognostic significance of alpha frequency EEG rhythm in coma after cardiac arrest. *J Neurol Neurosurg Psychiatry* 1978; 41:840.

378. Wilkus RJ, et al: Electroencephalogram and sensory evoked potentials. Findings in an unresponsive patient with pontine infarct. *Arch Neurol* 1971; 24:538.

379. Bergamasco B, et al: EEG sleep patterns as a prognostic criterion in post-traumatic coma. *Electroencephalogr Clin Neurophysiol* 1968; 24:374.

380. Britt CW: Nontraumatic "spindle coma": Clinical, EEG, and prognostic features. *Neurology* 1981; 31:393.

381. Chatrian GE, et al: Electroencephalographic patterns resembling those of sleep in certain comatose states after injuries to the head. *Electroencephalogr Clin Neurophysiol* 1963; 15:272.

382. Rumpl E, et al: Incidence and prognostic value of spindles in posttraumatic coma. *Electroencephalogr Clin Neurophysiol* 1983; 56:420.

383. Brunko E, Zegers deBeyl D: Prognostic value of early cortical somatosensory evoked potentials after resuscitation from cardiac arrest. *Electroencephalogr Clin Neurophysiol* 1987; 66:15.

384. Greenberg R, et al: Evaluation of brain function in severe human head trauma with multimodality evoked potentials. *J Neurosurg* 1977; 47:188.

385. Judson J, et al: Early prediction of outcome from cerebral trauma by somatosensory evoked potentials. *Crit Care Med* 1990; 18:363.

386. Lindsay K, et al: Somatosensory and auditory brainstem conduction after head injury: A comparison with clinical features in prediction of outcome. *Neurosurgery* 1990; 26:278.

387. Madl C, et al: Early prediction of individual outcome after cardiopulmonary resuscitation. *Lancet* 1993; 341:855.

388. Narayan RK, et al: Improved confidence of outcome prediction in severe head injury. A comparative analysis of the clinical examination, multimodality evoked potentials, CT scanning, and intracranial pressure. *J Neurosurg* 1981; 54:751.

389. Walser H, et al: Early cortical median nerve somatosensory evoked potentials. Prognostic value in anoxic coma. *Arch Neurol* 1986; 42:32.

390. Krieger D, et al: Serial somatosensory and brainstem auditory evoked potentials in monitoring of acute supratentorial lesions. *Crit Care Med* 1995; 23:1123.

391. Ferbert A, et al: Transcranial magnetic stimulation in pontine infarction: Correlation to degree of paresis. *J Neurol Neurosurg Psychiatry* 1992; 55:294.

392. Ying Z, et al: Motor and somatosensory evoked potentials in coma: Analysis and relation to clinical status and outcome. *J Neurol Neurosurg Psychiatry* 1992; 55:470.

393. Frank JI: Large hemispheric infarction, deterioration, and intracranial pressure. *Neurology* 1995; 45:1286.

394. Gray WA, et al: Unsuccessful emergency medical resuscitation. Are continued efforts in the emergency department justified? *N Engl J Med* 1991; 325:1393.

395. Shewmon DA, DeGiorgio CM: Early prognosis in anoxic coma. *Neurol Clin* 1989; 7:823.

396. Jennett B, Bond M: Assessment of outcome after severe brain damage. A practical scale. *Lancet* 1975; 1:480.

397. Levy DE, et al: Prognosis in nontraumatic coma. *Ann Intern Med* 1981; 94:293.

398. Hammel MB, et al: Identification of comatose patients at high risk for death or severe disability. *JAMA* 1995; 273:1842.

399. Abramson NS, et al: Randomized clinical study of a calcium-entry blocker (Lidoflaxine) in the treatment of comatose survivors of cardiac arrest. *N Engl J Med* 1991; 324:1225.

400. Bedell SE, et al: Survival after cardiopulmonary resuscitation in the hospital. *N Engl J Med* 1983; 309:569.

401. Levy DE, et al: Predicting the outcome from hypoxic-ischemic coma. *JAMA* 1985; 254:1171.

402. Rogove HJ, et al: Brain resuscitation Clinical Trial and 11 study groups. Old age does not negate good cerebral outcome after cardiopulmonary resuscitation: Analysis from the brain resuscitation clinical trials. *Crit Care Med* 1995; 23:18.

403. Earnest MP, et al: Quality of survival after out-of-hospital cardiac arrest: Predictive value of early neurologic evaluation. *Neurology* 1979; 29:56.

404. Edgren E, et al: Assessment of neurological prognosis in comatose survivors of cardiac arrest. *Lancet* 1994; 343:1055.

405. Scollo-Lavizzari G, Bassetti C: Prognostic value of EEG in post-anoxic coma after cardiac arrest. *Eur Neurol* 1987; 26:161.

406. Bassetti C, et al: Prognosis of coma after cardiac arrest: A prospective study of 60 patients. *Neurology* 1994; 44:A345.

407. Hénon H, et al: Early predictors of death and disability after acute cerebral ischemic event. *Stroke* 1995; 26:392.

408. Asplund K, Britton M: Ethics of life support in patients with severe stroke. *Stroke* 1989; 20:1107.

409. Grotta J, et al: Elective intubation for neurologic deterioration after stroke. *Neurology* 1995; 45:640.

410. Shenkin HA, Zavala M: Cerebellar strokes: Mortality, surgical indications and results of ventricular drainage. *Lancet* 1982; 2:429.

411. Jörgensen HS, et al: Intracerebral hemorrhage versus infarction: Stroke severity, risk factors, and prognosis. *Ann Neurol* 1995; 38:45.

412. Gennarelli TA, et al: Influence of the type of intracranial lesion on outcome from severe head injury. *J Neurosurg* 1982; 56:26.

413. Datz DI: Traumatic brian injury: Predicting course of recovery and outcome of patients admitted to rehabilitation. *Arch Neurol* 1994; 51:661.

414. Eisenberg HM, et al: Initial CT findings in 753 with severe head injury. *J Neurosurg* 1990; 73:688.

415. Choi SC, et al: Prediction tree for severely head-injured patients. *J Neurosurg* 1991; 75:251.

416. Childs L, et al: Accuracy of diagnosis of persistent vegetative state. *Neurology* 1993; 43:1465.

417. Higashi K, et al: Five-year follow-up study of patients with persistent vegetative state. *J Neurol Neurosurg Psychiatry* 1981; 44:552.

418. Rosenberg GA, et al: Recovery of cognition after prolonged vegetative state. *Ann Neurol* 1977; 2:167.

419. McCusker EA, et al: Recovery from the locked-in syndrome. *Arch Neurol* 1982; 39:145.

420. Rae-Grant AD, et al: Posttraumatic extracranial vertebral artery dissection with locked-in syndrome: A case with MRI documentation and unusually favorable outcome. *J Neurol Neurosurg Psychiatry* 1989; 52:1191.

421. Yang CC, et al: Early smooth horizontal eye movements: A favourable prognostic sign in patients with locked-in syndrome. *Arch Phys Med Rehabil* 1989; 70:230.

422. Towle VL, et al: Electrophysiologic studies on locked-in patients: Heterogeneity of findings. *Electroencephalogr Clin Neurophysiol* 1989; 73:419.

NEUROLOGIC SYNDROMES AND DISORDERS WITH THEIR ANESTHETIC IMPLICATIONS

DIANE SOLOMON

DALE SOLOMON

MAURICE ALBIN

Patients with congenital or acquired neurologic syndromes or disorders will sometimes require surgical intervention to correct associated disease or for unrelated surgical problems. While the prevalence of these syndromes ranges from common to very rare, proper perioperative management requires specific knowledge of the pathophysiology, optimal medical treat-

ment, and proper anesthetic interventions. In this chapter, we will review a number of these neurologic conditions and discuss what is known about their anesthetic and perioperative management.

Movement Disorders

PARKINSON'S DISEASE (PARALYSIS AGITANS)

Reported since antiquity, this condition was often called the "shaking palsy" and was described in a 66-page fascicle by James Parkinson in 1817.[1] In the opening chapter of his book, Parkinson mentions that the disease is characterized by "Involuntary tremulous motion, with lessened muscular power, in parts not in action and even when supported; with a propensity to bend the trunk forwards, and to pass from a walking to a running pace: the senses and intellects being uninjured." The problem of rigidity ("cogwheel"), dementia, or slow movement was not touched on in the essay. Paralysis agitans can produce symptoms of involuntary dysesthesia, masklike facies, alternating tremor, stooped posture, gait abnormalities, cogwheel rigidity, slowness of movements, autonomic system dysfunction, decrease of associated movements, disturbances of postural control, and decreased olfactory function. It is important to realize that the classical disease state described by Parkinson is a distinct clinical, idiopathic entity. This is opposed to states with symptoms similar to Parkinson's Disease (PD), yet having a more rapid evolution with recognition of the etiologic factors which have been labeled as Parkinson's Syndrome (PS). PS can be suspected after CNS trauma, encephalitis, carbon monoxide, manganese and other metallic intoxications, encephalitis, brain tumors (rare), and drugs such as phenothiazines, butyrophenones, reserpine, and phenylbutylpiperidines.

Essentially, PD is one of aging, beginning between the fourth and seventh decades of life, the peak occurring in the sixth decade. The incidence of onset in the seventh decade is about 3.0 percent.[2] In the United States alone there are approximately 500,000 patients with PD[3] and about 40,000 new cases develop each year.[4]

The pathophysiology of PD is important and is characterized by the loss of pigmented cells in the brain stem, principally in the substantia nigra and locus ceruleus. This cellular depletion gives rise to gliosis and eosinophilic intracytoplasmic inclusions named Lewy bodies, and they are seen in most cases of PD and occasionally in postencephalitic PS. The biochemistry of PD involves the decrease of dopamine in the caudate and putamen. Interestingly, tyrosine beta-hydroxylase, the rate limiting enzyme for dopamine, is decreased with age. Thus, it appears that PD mainly affects the nigrostriatal dopaminergic system. The synthetic neurotoxin 1-methyl-4-phenyl-1,2,3,6-tetra-hydropyridine (MPTP) selectively destroys dopaminergic neurons in the substantia nigra with similar clinical responses. However, no neuronal loss in the locus ceruleus nor Lewy bodies can be seen after MPTP injection.[5] Albin and coworkers[6] believe that striatal neuronal projection to the medial globus pallidus and substantia nigra pars reticulata have decreased activity, while projection to the lateral globus pallidus has a higher order of activity. This results in a disinhibition of the major output centers of the basal ganglia and increased inhibition of ventral-anterior and ventral-lateral thalamic, mediodorsal thalamic, and the centromedian-parafascicular neurons. This suggests that in PD there is an increase in basal ganglion output.

Medical treatment depends largely on the seriousness of symptoms and stage of the disease. Hoehn and Yahr have developed a universally recognized scale[7] consisting of 5 stages:

Stage I: Unilateral involvement

Stage II: Bilateral involvement but no postural abnormalities

Stage III: Bilateral involvement with mild postural imbalance; the patient leads an independent life

Stage IV: Bilateral involvement with postural instability; the patient requires substantial help

Stage V: Severe, fully developed disease; the patient is restricted to bed and chair

In general, patients in Stage I or II may require no medication, or only an anticholinergic (benztropine, biperiden, procyclidine) or a dopamine agonist such as amantadine, or a combination of both. These anticholinergics may relieve the slow frequency, pill rolling rest tremor typical of PD. The major standby in the treatment of PD is L-dihydroxyphenylalanine (L-dopa or levodopa) in stages III, IV, and V. L-Dopa is used as a replacement for the lost striatal dopamine and is combined with a decarboxylase inhibitor (carbidopa) to prevent its rapid metabolic turnover in blood. Levodopa has been shown to improve the akinesia, postural disorder, and at times the rest tremors.[8–10] The side effects of levodopa can be nausea; hypotension; depression with delusions; development of involuntary movements such as choreoathetosis, dystonia of limbs, neck, and trunk, restlessness, head wagging, grimacing, and dyskinesia of tongue and lips.[11] A long-acting form of carbidopa/levodopa is available and is helpful for patients with end of dose motor fluctuations or those requiring frequent dosing. Bromocriptine or pergolide are employed because of their stimulating effects on dopamine receptors and are used in patients not responding well to levodopa. Deprenyl (selegiline hydrochloride) is a monoamine oxidase (MAO)B inhibitor and thought to have a role in inhibiting dopamine metabolism and thus reducing oxidative stress. Deprenyl is itself metabolized to amphetamine derivatives which may exert a weak antiparkinsonism response.[3,10] Propranolol can suppress the fast-frequency action tremor which sometimes occurs in PD patients in addition to the typical pill rolling tremor. Metoprolol is also used and may be a safer beta-blocker in patients with asthma. Since many of the drugs used in PD and PS therapy have marked systemic effects, drug interaction responses are important.[11] These interaction responses are very important in the preoperative evaluation, intraoperative management, and postoperative anesthesia care, and are noted in Table 12-1.[12–42]

In the patients with PD who become resistant to medical therapy, three other approaches are available including stereotactic surgery, tissue transplants, and electroconvulsive therapy. There are a growing group of clinicians who feel that neuroablative procedures may be useful not only in those PD patients who are resistant to drug therapy, but also can be employed to treat tremor and rigidity in the younger age group.[43,44] It appears that patients with a thalamotomy prior to medical treatment suffer fewer side effects when on levodopa treatment.[43,44] These results are due in large part to major improvements in stereotactic techniques. Dyskinesias due to levodopa therapy have been treated by lesions in the ventralis intermedius nucleus (VIM) of the thalamus as well as in the ventralis oralis posterior (VOP). The study of Kelly and Gillingham regarding lesioning the thalamic ventralis oralis anterior (VOA) in 58 patients showed that 88 percent had no signs of rigidity 2 years after the thalamotomy.[43,45] Recently, lesions of the internal and/or external segments of globus pallidus (pallidotomy) have been used for resolution of PD symptoms that are resistant to medical treatment.[46]

ANESTHESIA FOR THE PATIENT WITH PARKINSON'S DISEASE

Management of anesthesia is based on knowledge of the disease process and potential adverse drug effects. Phenothiazines, butyrophenones, and metoclopramide are avoided because of their ability to antagonize the effects of dopamine in the basal ganglia. Anesthetic agents that sensitize the heart to arrhythmias, such as halothane, are excluded because of the concern that halothane could precipitate cardiac arrhythmias in patients receiving levodopa, although this has not been documented. There has been one case report of a hyperkalemic response after succinylcholine administra-

TABLE 12-1
Drug Interactions to Levodopa

Drug	Response
Tricyclic antidepressants[12–14]	Slow gastric emptying, enhances degradation of levodopa to inactive form in GI tract.
Benzodiazepines[15–17]	Mechanisms not clear, with 5 cases reported in deterioration of PD after diazepam and chlordiazepoxide.
Beta blockers (Propranolol)[18–24]	May antagonize beta-adrenergic effects of dopamine due to levodopa intake. May enhance levodopa responses in patients with PD and tremor. May increase levodopa stimulation of growth hormone secretion.
Clonidine[25,26]	Inhibits levodopa responses by stimulating central alpha-adrenergic receptors. Seven patients had exacerbation of PD.
Guanethidine[27]	Hypotensive effect of guanethidine increased with levopoda in 2 patients.
Methyldopa[28–30]	Inhibits response to levodopa and may cause an additive hypotensive response.
MAO inhibitors[31–35]	The degradation of dopamine involves MAO; hence MAO inhibitors ↓ dopamine breakdown and levodopa increases dopamine concentration—this will ↑ norepinephrine formation. Hypertensive responses have been reported with nialamide and phenelzine. The use of MAO inhibitors in patients on levodopa can result in worsening of akinesia and tremor. A favorable clinical response was noted with levadopa and the MAO inhibitor L-deprenil.
Papaverine[35,36]	PD worsened following papaverine possibly due to dopamine receptors blockade.
Phenylephrine[37]	Suggested that levodopa or its metabolites may involve competitive inhibition on alpha receptors since levodopa produces mydriasis following topical phenylephrine.
Pyridoxine[38–40]	Increases metabolism of levodopa, decreasing availability in brain. Pyridoxine reverses improvement with levodopa in PD.
Phenothiazines and butyrophenones	Phenothiazines may block dopamine receptors in the CNS. Extrapyramidal symptoms are well-known side effects of the phenothiazines. Haloperidol may have the same effect.
Phenytoin[41]	Phenytoin controlled levodopa dyskinesias but also suppressed therapeutic effect in controlling PD. If phenytoin is to be used, the dose of levodopa should be increased.[108]
Reserpine[42]	Implicated as a causal agent in PD by depleting brain of dopamine.[36,7]

tion in a patient with Parkinson's disease, but this report was clouded by the complex nature of the case.[47] A subsequent series of seven patients with severe Parkinson's disease who received succinylcholine during surgery for adrenal medullary to caudate transplantation did not develop hyperkalemia after the succinylcholine.[48] There has also been one case report of an acute dystonic reaction after alfentanil in a patient with untreated Parkinson's disease.[49] The MAO inhibitor selegiline, has been used to prevent degradation of dopamine in the brain of patients with Parkinson's disease. It is an MAO type B inhibitor (intestinal MAO is type A, while most of that in brain is type B). Although drug interactions may be less common with this drug than with nonselective MAO inhibitors, there has been one case report of a severe adverse reaction (agitation, stupor, muscle rigidity, hyperthermia) between selegiline and the narcotic meperidine (pethidine).[50]

Autonomic dysfunction may be seen in patients with Parkinson's disease. Gastrointestinal dysfunction may be manifested by difficulties in swallowing saliva and in more advanced cases, solid foods. The most common cardiovascular symptom is orthostatic hypotension, which may be exacerbated by antiparkinsonian drugs (levodopa, bromocriptine). Postoperatively, patients with Parkinson's disease have been shown to be more susceptible to developing confusion and hallucinations.[51] Drug therapy is resumed as soon as possible in the postoperative period to avoid recurrent extrapyramidal symptoms.

Stereotactic and ablative procedures are almost always carried out under local anesthesia. The use of intravenous low-dose narcotics for pain and glycopyrrolate to prevent bradycardia are part of the anesthetic conduct as well as patient monitoring for blood pressure, heart rate, EKG, and pulse oximetry. These anesthetic techniques are addressed in depth in Chaps. 21 and 22. Adrenal medullary transplants have not been successful for the most part, but fetal tissue transplants which include substantia nigra neurons are probably more effective. The use of electroconvulsive shock therapy in patients with depression and PD have, at times, showed evidence of symptom attenuation (see Chap. 23).

HUNTINGTON'S DISEASE

Huntington's disease is a neurodegenerative disorder of the central nervous system which causes dementia, psychiatric illness, and movement disorders. Because the disease consists of both neurologic and psychiatric abnormalities, the term Huntington's disease is now favored over Huntington's chorea. It is a disease which has probably existed for many centuries, but was not fully described until 1872 when George Huntington reported on families from Long Island, New York, who were treated by himself, his father, and his grandfather. Because he had knowledge of several generations of families with the disease, Huntington was able to describe not only the signs and symptoms of the disease, but also the hereditary nature of its transmission.[52,53]

Huntington's disease occurs in 3 to 10 persons per 10,000 population. Male/female frequency is the same. The prevalence throughout Europe is nearly uniform (except for Finland), and while the disease has a very low prevalence in Asians and other peoples without European ancestry, it does occur in all populations.[54,55]

Huntington's disease is inherited in an autosomal dominant fashion with 100 percent penetrance; the phenotypic appearance is identical in homo- or heterozygotes. There is a very low spontaneous mutation rate. The genetic abnormality in HD has been found to reside in the terminal end of the short arm of chromosome 4, at 4p16.3. There resides a novel gene encoding a protein product (huntingtin) with a predicted molecular weight of 348 kDa and containing a polymorphic stretch of CAG repeats (coding for glutamine) near the amino terminus of the protein. Transcripts from this gene are expressed widely in nonneuronal tissue and within virtually all neurons, arguing against the hypothesis that HD is caused by selective regional expression of the gene product in affected areas of brain.[56]

How the protein product of this genetic sequence, or the expanded CAG sequence (translated as polyglutamine) acts within neurons to cause the neuropathy of HD is currently unknown. The polyglutamine and/ or huntingtin may cause neuronal death by slow deposition of abnormal proteins in nerve cells or by interference with normal genetic transcription because of the presence of the abnormal proteins or the excessive CAG sequence.[57] Excitotoxicity mediated through NMDA receptors has also been strongly implicated in the pathogenesis of HD.[56]

Whatever the biochemical cause, HD results in progressive atrophy and gliosis of the striatum, particularly the caudate nucleus. There is early cell loss in the putamen, and later in the globus pallidus, pre-frontal cortex, and elsewhere in the brain.[58] MR, CT, and PET scanning can detect and verify the lesions associated with HD. The chorea is explained on the basis of loss of GABA-ergic neurons in the striatum (caudate plus putamen) which provide inhibitory striatopallidal projections. Dopaminergic pathways seem to be at least relatively preserved.[53,59]

The average age of onset is in the late 30s or early 40s, but the disease can be detected at an early age by genetic testing. The age of onset of the disease is partially genetically determined, and is to a certain degree explained by the repeat length of the CAG sequence; greater repeat lengths tend to cause earlier onset of the disease.

The majority of the time, HD presents with chorea and athetosis. Chorea presents as involuntary, random, jerking movements of the extremities, torso, face, and truncal muscles, and athetosis as sinuous writhing movements which are slower and more distal. At first these movements may be mistaken for tics or mannerisms. There may be head-bobbing and rolling, a dancing gait, and uncontrolled hand and finger movements described as "piano-playing." The eye muscles are affected early, with delayed saccades, fixation instability, abnormal smooth pursuit, and loss of opticokinetic nystagmus. Dysarthria can progress to unintelligible speech. Late in the course, dystonia and bradykinesia/ akinesias often replace choreoathetosis.[60]

A large subset of patients with HD develop severe disabling psychiatric and behavioral disturbances prior to the onset of chorea.[61] Early in the proces there is impaired cognition and inability to pay attention or concentrate. Dementia often supervenes. Personality disorders are common: anxiety, irritability, explosiveness, and sexual deviation are often reported. Major depression is common; a high suicide rate is part of the disease, as noted by Huntington in his original report. Many patients will be nutritionally depleted, either as a consequence of difficulty chewing and swallowing food, or because hypermetabolism outweighs adequate caloric intake.[53]

There is no specific treatment to block the progression of the disease. Neuroleptic agents (phenothiazines, butyrophenones, thioxanthenes, and other heterocyclic antipsychotic drugs), because of their dopamine blocking properties, are useful in ameliorating psychiatric symptoms and suppressing abnormal movements. Haloperidol has the longest record of use, but comparative trials are lacking.

Many patients will be prescribed anti-depressant medications, particularly the selective serotonin reuptake inhibitors (e.g., sertraline, fluoxetine).

The course of the disease will last 1 to 2 decades. Death often comes as the result of pneumonia, choking, malnutrition, and suicide or other self-destructive behavior.

ANESTHESIA FOR THE PATIENT WITH HUNTINGTON'S DISEASE

The published anesthetic experience with HD consists primarily of case reports and small series of a few patients. Nevertheless, because of the relatively high prevalence of the disease, and the predilection of patients with HD for traumatic injury, including dental trauma due to involuntary movements, anesthesiologists would be expected to encounter such patients with some regularity.

Involvement of the oral, pharyngeal, and laryngeal muscles may place these patients at risk for aspiration of gastric contents during induction of anesthesia. Attempts to preoperatively decrease the volume or acidity of gastric fluid are warranted (e.g., H2 blockers), and prokinetic agents are probably safe although metoclopramide has been reported to cause choreiform movements.[62]

Several agents have been used for induction of anesthesia in patients with Huntington's disease. Thiopental has been reported to have an exaggerated and prolonged effect,[63] and an animal model of HD shows altered sensitivity to thiopental.[64] Nevertheless, normal or reduced doses of thiopental[65–70] have been used successfully for induction of anesthesia as have midazolam[71] and propofol.[72,73]

Succinylcholine has been reported to have a prolonged effect[68] perhaps because of an increaed incidence of pseudocholinesterase deficiency,[74] but this has not been verified and succinylcholine is probably safe when its use is warranted.[65] The response to nondepolarizing muscle relaxants is normal.

The volatile anesthetic agents appear to be safe, although postanesthetic shivering has been reported to cause toxic spasms.[66] Centrally acting anticholinergic drugs should be avoided as they may exacerbate the movement disorder.[70]

DYSTONIAS

Dystonias are sustained contractions of muscles which result in abnormal twisting or postures. They may be sustained or intermittent and focal or generalized. Dystonias are classified by the patient's age of onset, the distribution of the muscles affected, and the etiology. Most adult-onset dystonias are idiopathic, or primary, excluding drug reactions. Secondary dystonias involve other areas of the central nervous system in addition to the basal ganglia, so that the clinical manifestations are not limited to a disorder of movement. There are several hereditary neurometabolic and degenerative neurologic disorders that may cause dystonia secondarily. Most are rare, but younger patients and those with progressive or generalized dystonia should always be screened for Wilson's disease because it is more common and treatable. Wilson's disease is an autosomal recessive disorder with progressive lenticular degeneration and liver cirrhosis which is associated with prominent dystonic posturing. It is caused by a defect of copper metabolism and decreased ceruloplasm synthesis (the serum enzyme that binds cop-

per). The improvement after treatment with penicillamine is sometimes dramatic.[75] Dystonia may also result from anoxic brain injury, heavy metal toxicity, encephalitis, and focal cerebral disease, including stroke, head trauma, multiple sclerosis, and brain tumors.[76]

Autosomal dominant classical childhood-onset dystonia or dystonia musculorum deformans has been linked to chromosome 9q and a gene designated DYT1.[77,78] Although there is incomplete penetrance and clinical heterogeneity in carriers of this gene, included are the patients with generalized, disfiguring dystonia. These children, failing medication, have much to gain by sterotactic thalamotomy. Unfortunately, the progression of disease is not halted and serious risks include dysarthria (following bilateral thalamotomy) and hemiparesis.[79]

The focal dystonias common in adulthood include blepharospasm (forced, involuntary eye closure), oromandibular dystonia (face, jaw, or tongue), cervical dystonia or torticollis (neck), writer's cramp (action-induced dystonic contraction of hand muscles), and spasmodic dysphonia. Blepharospasm begins with increased blinking and often progresses to a debilitating disorder of functional blindness. The onset is in the fifth to sixth decades. A patient who presents with dystonia in one area may develop dystonia in other cranial-cervical areas over time.[80] When blepharospasm is associated with spasms in the face, jaw, or neck, it is called Meige's syndrome. There is electrophysiologic evidence of hyperexcitability of the facial nucleus that in most patients has no demonstrable underlying cause. However, there have been reports of abnormal brain stem auditory evoked potentials at the pons in patients with Meige's syndrome or blepharospasm.[81]

Torticollis or cervical dystonia is the most common form of focal dystonia presented for treatment. The scalene, sternocleidomastoid, and trapezius muscles are most often affected. These patients may have neck rotation, flexion, extension, head tilt, lateral shift, or a combination of these.[82,83] Patients with a twisted neck should be evaluated for secondary, structural abnormalities. If there are any findings on history or examination suggestive of an orthopedic cause (atlantoaxial dislocation, cervical fracture, degenerative disc disease, osteomyelitis, or Klippel-Feil syndrome), magnetic resonance imaging of the cervical spine should be performed.[84]

Treatment is individualized and, for the most part, based on empiric trials rather than systematic drug trials. Physical therapy has limited benefit in mildly affected patients. Pharmacotherapeutic agents that may be useful in small doses early in therapy include anticholinergics, baclofen, and benzodiazepines.[85] Of children with dystonia, 5 to 10 percent have a form associated with diurnal variation which responds to low dose carbidopa/levodopa (½ to 1 carbidopa 25 mg/levodopa 100 mg TID).[86] Most patients with focal dystonia are now treated with local injections of botulinum toxin. Seventy to ninety-two percent obtain relief of abnormal postures with injections repeated every 3 to 6 months. Side effects may include excessive weakness in the injected or adjacent muscles, but this can usually be avoided with proper selection of muscles for injection and by reducing the dose. Resistance develops in some patients and appears to be linked to the development of antibodies.[87–90]

In medically intractable cases of dystonia, surgical procedures may be beneficial. For torticollis, denervation of the anterior roots of the upper cervical nerves and sometimes the spinal accessory nerve can provide relief.[91] Similarly, blepharospasm is sometimes treated with orbital myectomy when botulinum therapy has been unsuccessful. Fixed lesions, such as infarction of the basal ganglia or post-traumatic lesions are associated with hemidystonia and have the best surgical response to thalamotomy.[92] Thalamotomy is performed using local anesthesia so that the patient can give feedback in assessing the effect of electrical stimulation and lesion placement on the dystonia.

ANESTHESIA FOR THE PATIENT WITH DYSTONIA

Very few published accounts exist of anesthetic management of patients with dystonia or torticollis. Surgical release or application of halo devices may be undertaken in patients with torticollis.[93] Airway considerations are paramount, as prolonged contraction will cause facial asymmetry and fixation of the head, jaw, and cervical spine even in the presence of complete pharmacologic neuromuscular blockade. Based on clinical judgment, many patients will require awake tracheal intubation prior to induction of general anesthesia. Alternatively, maintenance of spontaneous ventilation during induction of anesthesia, or placement of a laryngeal mask airway, would seem appropriate. When kyphoscoliosis is present, the patient should be evaluated for restrictive lung disease, and appropriate precautions taken to assure adequate pulmonary function in the postoperative period. There appears to be no contraindication to succinylcholine, since the muscle is normal and in fact overstimulation of neuromuscular receptors is occurring.[94,95]

For lower extremity surgery, spinal or epidural anesthesia would seem ideal except that positioning may be a problem in the patient with extreme dysmorphism.

Anesthetic considerations for patients undergoing awake craniotomy for thalamotomy are reviewed in Chap. 22.

Finally, it should be noted that severe dystonic reactions and opisthotonos can occur during and after the administration of general anesthesia, usually but not always after antidopaminergic drugs have been given.[96,97]

HEMIFACIAL SPASM

Hemifacial spasm (HS) involves irregular contractions usually beginning in the orbicularis occuli and then spreading to the other muscles on one side of the face, demonstrating motor hyperactivity of the facial nerve (FN). The pathophysiology is distinct from blepharospasm and the dystonias and is believed to be compression of the FN by a vessel near the root exit zone. Brain tumors, such as gliomas of the cerebellopontine angle may cause HS. Magnetic resonance imaging should be done unless the symptoms are longstanding and typical. Atypical features include facial sensory changes, deafness, sustained chronic contractions, or younger patients in the first two decades of life.[98] Traditional medical therapy (anticonvulsants, benzodiazepines, and weak anticholinergics) are not usually effective for HS, but botulinum toxin has given good results in some patients.[99] Good surgical candidates, especially those who do not respond to botulinum therapy, should be referred for surgery. The surgical procedure to treat this condition is exactly the same as for trigeminal neuralgia (Jannetta procedure) and similarly a plastic sponge is interposed between the nerve and the artery.[100] The anesthetic considerations are similarly covered in Chap. 29 on posterior fossa surgery.

Neurocutaneous Diseases

NEUROFIBROMATOSIS TYPE I

There are two types of neurofibromatosis. Type I (NF1) was first discribed by von Recklinghausen in 1882.[101] It is a relatively common autosomal dominant disorder and has a widespread, but widely variable effect on the tissues of mesodermal and ectodermal origin. Type II (NF2), or bilateral acoustic neurofibromatosis, is distinct from Type I both clinically and genetically. The diagnostic criteria for the two disorders are listed in Table 12-2.[102]

NF1 is a progressive systemic disease with an incidence of 1 in 3000.[103] Pathologically, there is an abnormality of neural crest cell development which adversely affects migration and localization of neural crest cells and secondarily affects the supporting mesenchymal elements. Not all the protean disease manifestations are explained by this pathologic model, however, and the search for a more complete understanding is currently focused on molecular genetics.

The NF1 gene has been mapped to 17q11.2 and codes

TABLE 12-2
Criteria for Diagnosis of the Neurofibromatoses

Neurofibromatosis 1

NF1 may be diagnosed when two or more of the following are present:
* Six or more café au lait macules whose greatest diameter is more than 5 mm in prepubertal patients and more than 15 mm in postpubertal patients.
* Two or more neurofibromas of any type, or one plexiform neurofibroma.
* Freckling in the axillary or inguinal region.
* Optic glioma
* Two or more Lisch nodules (iris hamartomas).
* A distinctive osseous lesion such as sphenoid dysplasia or thinning of long-bone cortex, with or without pseudarthrosis.
* A parent, sibling, or child with neurofibromatosis 1 according to the above criteria.

Neurofibromatosis 2

NF2 may be diagnosed when one of the following is present:
* Bilateral eighth-nerve masses seen with appropriate imaging techniques (computed tomography or magnetic resonance imaging).
* A parent, sibling, or child with neurofibromatosis 2 and either unilateral eighth-nerve mass or any two of the following: neurofibroma, meningioma, glioma, schwannoma, or juvenile posterior subcapsular lenticular opacity.

SOURCE: Adapted from Conference Statement, National Institutes of Health Concensus Development Conference: Neurofibromatosis. *Arch Neurol* 1988; 45:575; with permission.

for a tumor suppressor protein named neurofibromin. Its inactivation by a mutation results in activity of the *ras* oncogene.[104] It may also have a regulatory role in the growth and development of connective tissues through an effect on microtubular function.[105] The molecular diagnosis involves identification of mutations which may include deletions, translocations, and point mutations.[106] Because of the large size of the gene and the wide range of mutations described, standard DNA diagnostic analysis is, so far, not routinely practical.[107] There is tremendous variability of the manifestations of NF1 even within affected members of a family who have the same germline mutation. Affected individuals have one nonfunctional NF1 gene in every cell in the body as a result of their inherited or germline mutation. The clinical features of NF1 are believed to arise when a somatic mutation also occurs in a given cell. The variability of somatic mutations in terms of timing, number, and location leads to the clinical variability of the disease and makes it impossible to predict the course in a given individual.[107] There may also be other modifying genes involved.[108]

As Table 12-2 shows,[102] the consistent features of NF1 are café-au-lait spots, freckling in the axilla and other intertriginous areas, lisch nodules (pigmented iris hamartomas), multiple neurofibromas, and bony lesions. Neurofibromas are benign except when compressing structures or causing disfigurement, but up to 7 percent undergo malignant transformation to become neurofibrosarcomas and malignant schwannomas. The neurofibromas increase more rapidly at puberty and during pregnancy[109,110] and sometimes form after blunt trauma.[103] Hyperpigmented lesions overlying midline plexiform neurofibromas often indicate spinal cord involvement.[111] Bony abnormalities include pseudo-arthrosis, usually of the tibia or radius, sphenoid dysplasia which results in an abnormal orbit and leads to exophthalmos, scalloping of the vertebra, and kyphoscoliosis, not infrequently requiring surgical intervention.

Other characteristics which are common with NF1 include postnatal macrocephaly independent of brain tumors or hydrocephalus, although cases of aqueductal stenosis with secondary hydrocephalus were reported in 29 patients in a review by Senveli and coworkers.[112] Optic nerve gliomas occur in 15 to 20 percent, but are less likely to invade the optic nerve than in non-NF patients.[113] Patients complain of impaired vision and may present with proptosis and nystagmus. Hypertension in a NF1 patient should prompt a search for renal artery stenosis on the basis of an extramural or intramural neurofibroma and pheochromocytoma. Pheochromocytoma probably occurs in less than 1 percent of patients and does not present in childhood, but screening adults with urine catecholamines is recommended. Hypertension may be idiopathic and have its onset in childhood. All NF1 patients should have their blood pressure monitored.[103]

Because learning difficulties occur in approximately 40 percent of NF1 patients, they should undergo neuropsychiatric evaluation. The learning disabilities have been attributed by some to small neuronal hamartomas or deep heterotopias.[114,115] As many as 60 percent of children with NF1 have high signal focal areas on magnetic resonance imaging (prolonged T2), primarily in the globus pallidus, brain stem, and cerebellum which Duffner and colleagues[116] postulated were developmental abnormalities such as glial nodules or hamartomas, but these were not found to be predictive of learning problems in their study of 47 children. Mental retardation and seizures occur in 5 percent. Mental retardation dates from birth and is nonprogressive. If mental status changes occur later in life, hydrocephalus or an intracranial tumor should be ruled out. An increased incidence of seizure disorder in NF1 patients is independent of brain tumors and mental retardation,[115] but a search for intracranial tumors should always take place following new onset seizures. Headaches, a frequent complaint, are worrisome as a sign of intracranial tumor, hydrocephalus, or pheochromocytoma, but most are benign tension-type or migrainous.

Malignant tumors that are more common in neurofibromatosis than in the population at large include sarcomas, malignant schwannomas, leukemia, Wilms' tumor, rhabodomyosarcomas, and medullary thyroid carcinomas.[103] Spinal tumors are frequently meningiomas. Precocious puberty due to hypothalamic gliomas or hamartomas may occur.[117,118]

Other endocrine anomalies reported in different age groups include obesity, hypoglycemia, diabetes insipidus, parathyroid adenomas and hyperparathyroidism, goiter, myxedema, and gigantism or acromegaly.[118] Endocrine dysfunction is not a common feature of NF1, but there may be overlap with the multiple-endocrine-neoplasia syndromes in selected patients accounting for some of the reports of endocrine problems.[103,119] Congenital heart defects, particularly pulmonic stenosis may be relatively frequent in NF1.[120] There are also reports of idiopathic hypertrophic cardiomyopathy,[121] but it is unclear whether these occurred in association with NF1 by chance. Intracranial occlusive arterial disease is the most common neurovascular manifestation of neurofibromatosis and is often associated with a moya-moya pattern of collateral circulation. Cervical arteriovenous fistulae and aneurysms are the most common nonocclusive neurovascular anomalies. Intracranial saccular aneurysms also occur, usually in association with occlusive intracranial disease.[122,123]

Patients with NF1 are usually followed by a multidisciplinary team consisting of a coordinating neurologist, dermatologist, ophthalmologist, and orthopedist. Other specialists are consulted as the need arises. Patients with neurologic symptoms should receive magnetic resonance imaging (MRI) of the brain and/or spinal cord. Macrocephaly should prompt screening imaging to rule out hydrocephalus and brain tumors. Patients with seizure disorders are imaged, an electroencephalogram is obtained and anticonvulsants are given. Nonprogressive optic gliomas may be followed closely with ophthalmologic examinations and MRIs. Other neural tumors should be treated as in the general population. If there is increased intracranial pressure or compression of other structures, resection is indicated. If the tumor has characteristics of malignancy,

a biopsy followed by decompression, chemotherapy, or XRT is done, depending on tumor type. Kyphoscoliosis may require bracing or spinal fusion. Pseudoarthrosis is recently being treated with wide resection and free vascularized bone grafts.[124] Soft tissue disfigurements are difficult to repair and recur, although exophthalmos due to sphenoid dysplasias may be surgically corrected. Patients with NF1 and hypertension should be evaluated for pheochromocytoma, including 24-h VMA and metanephrines and serum catecholamines. Renal artery stenosis should be evaluated with DSA or angioplasty. Abnormal blood indices should prompt a search for leukemia, especially in children. Neuropsychological testing to screen for learning disabilities is indicated due to the high association. Importantly, genetic and supportive counseling should be provided.

NEUROFIBROMATOSIS TYPE II

The gene for NF2 has been mapped to 22q12. The gene codes for a protein called by the acronym *merlin*, which stands for moesin-ezrin-radixin-like protein, another tumor suppresser protein.[104] The autosomal dominant penetrance is greater than 95 percent so that all offspring have a 50 percent chance of developing bilateral acoustic neuromas.[125] Individuals with NF2 may have café-au-lait lesions and/or one or more small neurofibromas, but they do not have Lisch nodules or axillary freckling (See Table 12-2).[102] Conversely, patients with NF1 may suffer an acoustic neuroma, but do not develop bilateral acoustic neuromas. The age of onset of NF2 is typically during the teens, but ranges from the first to seventh decades.[126] Loss of hearing in one ear is usually the earliest symptom of NF2. It is often accompanied by intermittent ringing or roaring in the ear. Imbalance and loss of sense of direction may occur and facial weakness, sensory changes, and headache sometimes develop, depending on the size and location of the tumor. Presenile subcapsular cataracts occur in up to 50 percent of those affected with NF2.[127]

As with NF1, pregnancy in patients with NF2 is associated with an exacerbation of symptoms and growth of tumors.[128]

MRIs, audiograms, and brain stem auditory evoked responses assist in identifying and managing the acoustic neuromas.[129,130] Management requires balancing the risk of deafness with tumor removal against the risk of continued tumor growth, but modern surgical techniques have vastly improved the surgical risks. Subtotal tumor resection is sometimes advocated to delay progression of hearing loss.[131] Thorough skin examinations with a Wood's light and ophthalmologic evaluations are also indicated.

Central nervous system tumors are common in NF2.

Schwann cell tumors are the most common and meningiomas and gliomas are next. Spinal tumors occur frequently and are largest in the cervical region, warranting routine studies.[126] Although most are benign glial hamartomas or low-grade gliomas and remain unchanged over time, it cannot be predicted which will have neoplastic growth and these should be followed closely by MRI. Stereotactic biopsy can be done if accessible.

ANESTHESIA FOR THE PATIENT WITH NEUROFIBROMATOSIS

Patients with NF1 may undego surgery to excise tumors that compromise vital structures, to relieve renal artery stenosis, to repair aneurysms, for ventriculoperitoneal shunting, and a variety of other reasons. Preoperative evaluation of patients with NF1 requires identification of concomitant disease and verification of optimized medical management of these diseases. Perhaps most important to identify are: (1) pheochromocytoma, (2) intracranial mass lesions and intracranial hypertension, (3) endocrinopathies, (4) congenital heart disease, (5) presence of tumors impinging on the airway, including laryngeal involvement, (6) restrictive lung disease, (7) pulmonary interstitial fibrosis and pulmonary hypertension, and (8) cervical spine instability.[132–135] The tongue may be large and gross facial asymmetry may be present. In addition, a tumor involving the cranial nerves which control the pharynx and larynx may make patients more susceptible to regurgitation and aspiration of gastric contents during induction of anesthesia.

No anesthetic agent has been shown to cause adverse effects in NF1. Case reports describe an exaggerated response to nondepolarizing muscle relaxants[136–139] and to succinylcholine,[139] but others report resistance or a normal response to succinylcholine.[137,138]

Spinal or epidural anesthesia carries the risk that unrecognized lumbar tumors may not become clinically evident until after performance of the procedure, thereby implicating the procedure as the cause of the neurologic problem. However, when airway or other considerations warrant its use, neuraxial blockade may be chosen. Ideally, neuroimaging studies should rule out spinal tumors which are in the path of the needle or intracranial tumors which are blocking CSF pathways, causing herniation should the dura be punctured.[140] Epidural analgesia for labor and vaginal delivery has been reported,[140] but because tumors increase in size and number during pregnancy, a careful neurologic exam should be done prior to epidural analgesia and consideration given to performing MR imaging of the spine and brain.

Patients with NF2 will undergo anesthesia for excision of acoustic neuromas or other CNS tumors. The anesthetic management of the patient with acoustic neuroma is discussed in Chap. 29.

TUBEROUS SCLEROSIS

Tuberous sclerosis (TS) is an autosomal dominant disorder characterized by involvement of nearly all organ systems and tissues with hamartomas. Because the clinical expression of TS is so variable, the incidence of the disease is unknown, but is believed to be present in 1 in 6000 to 10,000 individuals.[141,142] Depending on the family, TS has been linked to genes on chromosomes 9 or 16, which at least in the latter represents a tumor suppressor gene.[142] Over half of cases are new mutations.

The diagnostic criteria for TS put forth by the National Tuberous Sclerosis Association are listed in Table 12-3.[143] Seizures beginning at an early age are the most common presenting symptom, occurring in more than 90 percent of patients. Mental retardation, learning difficulties, and abnormal behavior are also very common, but at least half of patients have normal intellect. CNS tumors include subependymal nodules, cortical hamartomas (tubers), areas of focal cortical hypoplasia, heterotopic gray matter, and giant cell astrocytomas. Tumors may enlarge to the point of causing new focal deficits, obstructing CSF pathways, or causing intracranial hypertension. Hemorrhage within a large tumor or hydrocephalus may require urgent neurosurgical intervention.

As many as two-thirds of patients with TS will develop cardiac rhabdomyomas. Presenting symptoms and signs are due to obstruction of right or left ventricular outflow, cardiac arrhythmias including heart block and ventricular dysfunction due to replacement of contractile muscle by tumor.[144,145]

The respiratory system is rarely affected, but cystic lung disease with an obstructive pattern and progressive hypoxemia are reported. Lymphangiomyomatosis may result in pulmonary fibrosis and progressive dyspnea. Smooth muscle proliferation in the pulmonary arterial vasculature may lead to pulmonary hypertension and right heart failure.[144]

Renal angiomyolipoma may manifest as hematuria, progressive renal failure, or hypertension. The tumors are benign and are removed only for recurrent gross hematuria or when there is renal artery compression. Renal cysts occur frequently and may progress to cause renal failure due to parenchymal compression or collective system compression. Renal cell carcinoma is rare.[146] Renal failure is the most common cause of death.

ANESTHESIA FOR THE PATIENT WITH TUBEROUS SCLEROSIS

Patients with tuberous sclerosis may require craniotomy for tumor excision or cortical resection for intrac-

TABLE 12-3
Diagnostic Criteria for Tuberous Sclerosis Complex

Primary Features

Facial angiofibromas[a]
Multiple ungual fibromas[a]
Cortical tuber (histologically confirmed)
Subependymal nodule or giant cell astrocytoma (histologically confirmed)
Multiple calcified subependymal nodules protruding into the ventricle (radiographic evidence)
Multiple retinal astrocytomas[a]

Secondary Features

Affected first-degree relative
Cardiac rhabdomyoma (histologic or radiographic confirmation)
Other retinal hamartoma or achromic patch[a]
Cerebral tubers (radiographic confirmation)
Noncalcified subependymal nodules (radiographic confirmation)
Shagreen patch[a]
Forehead plaque[a]
Pulmonary lymphangiomyomatosis (histologic confirmation)
Renal angiomyolipoma (radiographic or histologic confirmation)
Renal cysts (histologic confirmation)

Tertiary Features

Hypomelanotic macules[a]
"Confetti" skin lesions[a]
Renal cysts (radiographic evidence)
Randomly distributed enamel pits in deciduous and/or permanent teeth
Hamartomatous rectal polyps (histologic confirmation)
Bone cysts (radiographic evidence)
Pulmonary lymphangiomyomatosis (radiographic evidence)
Cerebral white-matter "migration tracts" or heterotopies (radiographic evidence)
Gingival fibromas[a]
Hamartoma of other organs (histologic confirmation)
Infantile spasms

Definite TSC:

Either one primary feature, two secondary features, or one secondary plus two tertiary features.

Probable TSC:

Either one secondary plus one tertiary feature, or three tertiary features.

Suspect TSC:

Either one secondary feature of two tertiary features.

---

[a] Histologic confirmation is not required if the lesion is clinically obvious; TSC = tuberous sclerosis complex.
SOURCE: Reprinted from Roach ES, et al: Diagnostic criteria: Tuberous sclerosis complex. Report of the Diagnostic Criteria Committee of the National Tuberous Sclerosis Association. *J Ch Neurol* 1992; 7(2):221, with permission.

table seizures, laser treatment of angiofibromas, cardiac surgery for rhabdomyomas, kidney surgery for renal angiomyolipomas or renal cyst excision, or orthopedic surgery.[147]

Most patients will have an associated seizure disorder, and routine perioperative management of patients with seizures should be carried out. A variety of cardiac arrhythmias may be present, including Wolf-Parkinson-White syndrome,[144] and a preoperative ECG should be obtained. Preoperative Holter monitoring may be required in symptomatic patients. Echocardiography and MRI are useful in detecting the presence and functional significance of cardiac tumors. Patients with pulmonary symptoms should undergo further evaluation with PFTs, chest x-ray, and arterial blood gas analysis.

Renal failure due to cyst formation or as a result of renal angiomyolipomas can be detected by routine blood chemistry, and the etiology confirmed by ultrasonography or CT scanning of the kidneys.

Rarely, endocrine glands can be affected by tumor growth, and signs and symptoms of endocrine dysfunction should be sought.

Finally, tumors of the tongue, palate, pharynx, and larynx may interfere with airway management. A thorough preanesthetic evaluation of the airway is advocated.

Again, there is no support in the literature for the

TABLE 12-4
Diagnostic Criteria for Von Hippel-Lindau Disease

Column A	Column B
Retinal angiomatosis	Pheochromocytoma
Cerebellar hemangioma	Pancreatic cysts
Spinal hemangioma	Epididymal cysts
	Renal cysts
	Renal cell cancer

NOTE: Diagnosis depends on the presence of one finding from column A plus one from column B or two symptoms from column A or one symptom from either column in a patient with a positive family history.
SOURCE: From Lesho EP: Recognition and management of von Hippel-Lindau disease. *Am Fam Physician* 1994; 50:1269, with permission.

use of one anesthetic agent over another, but avoidance of agents which are epileptogenic is advocated. Because of the possibility that CNS tumors may be present in the lumbar spine, spinal or epidural anesthesia is avoided unless CNS imaging has ruled out the presence of a potentially harmful tumor.

VON HIPPEL-LINDAU DISEASE

Von Hippel-Lindau (VHL) disease is a rare single gene disorder characterized by (1) retinal and cerebellar hemangioblastomas, (2) cysts of the kidney, pancreas, and epididymis, and (3) renal carcinoma. There may also be hemangioblastomas of the medulla and spinal cord, cysts and hemangiomas of the other visceral organs, and in some families, phenochromocytoma.[148]

VHL is considered to be a rare disease with a prevalence of 1 in 40,000 to 100,000.[149,150] Inheritance is in an autosomal dominant fashion with a variable but usually high degree of penetrance. The VHL gene was identified in 1993 to chromosome 3p,[151] which most likely represents a tumor suppressor gene. Genetic testing now allows the presymptomatic diagnosis of the disease in most susceptible families.

The diagnostic criteria for VHL disease are listed in Table 12-4. The incidence of major organ involvement is listed in Table 12-5. Most patients will present by the third decade of life, often much earlier, usually with retinal angiomas or signs of a cerebellar tumor.[152] Presenting complaints are related to disturbances in vision, symptoms of posterior fossa tumor, and in patients with pheochromocytoma, palpitations, or sequelae of hypertension. About 10 percent of all patients with VHL disease will develop a pheochromocytoma but in some families the prevalence is much higher.[148]

The central nervous system is affected by hemangioblastomas. They are found most frequently in the cerebellum, with a prevalence of 66 percent in autopsy studies.[148]

Cerebellar hemangioblastoma may present as a slow-growing tumor with gradual onset of cerebellar symptoms and signs, including those related to intracranial hypertension. Alternatively, bleeding into the tumor or subarachnoid hemorrhage may cause the sudden onset of symptoms and a rapid increase in intracranial pressure.

Hemangioblastomas may also be found in the medulla oblongata and spinal cord. While between 10 and 30 percent of patients with VHL disease have spinal cord tumors, most are asymptomatic. Most spinal tumors are located in the cervical and thoracic spinal cord, but they may be located anywhere along the spine. Supratentorial hemangioblastomas are rare. At least 50 percent of deaths in VHL disease are related to the presence of CNS tumors.

The kidneys may be affected by cysts, hemangiomas, benign adenomas, and malignant hypernephromas which can metastasize. Renal disease may manifest as hematuria or elevated creatinine.

Frequently, patients with VHL disease are polycythemic, probably because of increased erythropoietin activity.

Patients with VHL disease should have an annual physical and ophthalmologic examination, peripheral blood cell count, urinalysis, and CT of the abdomen. Annual evaluation of urinary catecholamines is carried out, and biannual MRI of the posterior fossas has been advised.

Prognosis and outcome in VHL disease depends entirely on the incidence of malignant renal tumors, the natural history of cerebellar hemangioblastomas, and

TABLE 12-5
Major Organ Involvement in von Hippel-Lindau Disease

Organ	Lesion	Patients Affected (%)
Eye	Hemangioblastoma; retina, optic disc	24–73
Central nervous system	Hemangioblastoma; cerebellum, medulla oblongata, cord	22–66
Kidney	Cysts, cancer, hemangioma, adenomas	56–83
Pancreas	Cysts, cancer, hemangioblastomas, hemangiomas	9–72
Adrenal	Pheochromocytoma, adenomas, cysts, cortical	7–17
Epididymis	Cysts, hemangiomas, adenomas	7–27
Liver	Cysts, adenomas, hemangiomas	17

SOURCE: From Michels VV: Von Hippel-Lindau disease. In Gomez M (ed): *Neurocutaneous Diseases.* Butterworths, Boston, 1987:53–66, with permission.

complications related to the occurrence of pheochromocytoma.

ANESTHESIA FOR THE PATIENT WITH VON HIPPEL-LINDAU DISEASE

Patients with VHL disease will present for posterior fossa tumor excision, removal of adrenal tumors, nephrectomy, and eye surgery. During the preanesthetic evaluation, a search must be carried out for clinical manifestations of the disease which might cause perioperative morbidity. Of greatest concern are ruling out the presence of: (1) pheochromocytoma, (2) intracranial tumors causing hydrocephalus and/or increased intracranial pressure, (3) renal dysfunction due to cysts or renal cell carcinoma, and (4) increased intraocular pressure due to retinal lesions. Cerebellar hemangioblastomata are at risk of spontaneous hemorrhage due to hypertensive episodes.

Only a few case reports concerning anesthetic management exist in the medical literature. Epidural anesthesia for management of cesarean delivery has been reported,[153,154] but others argue against its use because of the possibility of the subclinical presence of tumors in the lumbar area of the spinal cord, cauda equina, meninges, nerve roots, and vertebrae.[155]

STURGE-WEBER SYNDROME

Sturge-Weber syndrome is a congenital malformation characterized by: (1) angiomatous malformations of the skin, most often on the face in a unilateral distribution of the trigeminal nerve, (2) telangiectatic venous angiomatosis of the ipsilateral leptomeninges and brain, and (3) choroidal angioma with or without buphthalmos or glaucoma.[156] Patients with Sturge-Weber syndrome may have either one or varying combinations of these manifestations. Angiomata may be present on the skin of both sides of the face, the torso, and extremities, and may involve the mucous membranes of the nose, oropharynx, tongue, larynx, and trachea. In addition, vascular malformations may be found in the pituitary, thymus, lung, spleen, and lymph nodes.[157] Cerebral atrophy due either to parenchymal calcium deposition or vascular ischemia may result in spastic hemiparesis, hemianopsia, or cortical hemisensory deficit contralateral to the cerebral deficit. There is a high incidence of mental retardation. Up to 90 percent of patients have seizures, often appearing in the first months of life.

Despite the presence of angiomas, intracranial hemorrhage is rare. However, heart failure due to a large shunt has been reported.[158] In addition, there is an association with a variety of congenital heart defects including septal defects, valvular stenosis, and transportation of the great vessels.

TABLE 12-6
Organs Affected by Hemangiomas in Sturge-Weber

Airway and Respiratory System	Endocrine System	Central Nervous System
Lip	Pituitary	Brain
Oropharynx	Thyroid	Spinal cord
Tongue	Testes	Dura
Larynx		
Trachea		
Lungs		

About 30 percent of patients will develop glaucoma associated with a choroidal angioma.

ANESTHESIA FOR THE PATIENT WITH STURGE-WEBER SYNDROME

Patients with Sturge-Weber syndrome will require surgery for eye disease, repair of congenital malformations, intraabdominal catastrophes secondary to vascular abnormalities, and intracranial procedures. Many patients will be young because of ocular problems which manifest at a young age. A careful evaluation of organs which may be affected with angiomas should be carried out (Table 12-6). Many patients will have a seizure disorder, and therapeutic drug concentrations of anticonvulsants should be verified in the preoperative period.

Angiomata of the lip, oral cavity, tongue, larynx, and trachea should be identified when possible as they may impinge on the airway or may hemorrhage due to the trauma of laryngoscopy, intubation, or tracheal suctioning.[159] Use of soft, well-lubricated endotracheal tubes and gentle tracheal suctioning has been advised.[160]

Patients with a large intracranial angioma may suffer from high-output cardiac failure and signs and symptoms should be elicited during the preanesthetic evaluation. In addition, the high prevalence of congenital cardiac malformations makes the cardiac evaluation even more important.

When glaucoma is present, careful attention should be paid to an anesthetic technique which avoids increases in intraocular pressure, including avoidance of straining, coughing, and valsalva maneuver. In addition, large elevations in arterial or venous pressure may cause bleeding of intracranial hemangiomas.[157]

There is no literature to support the use of one anesthetic agent over another, except avoidance of agents which may promote seizure activity in susceptible patients. Spinal or epidural anesthesia are avoided because of the possibility of hemangiomas in the path of the needle.

Finally, patients should be monitored in the intra- and postoperative period for the onset of DIC with

TABLE 12-7
Clinically Definite MS—Schumacher Criteria

1. Neurologic examination reveals objective abnormalities of CNS function.
2. Examination or history indicates involvement of two or more parts of CNS.
3. CNS disease predominantly reflects white matter involvement.
4. Involvement of CNS follows one of two patterns:
   a. Two or more episodes, each lasting at least 24 hrs. and a month or more apart.
   b. Slow or stepwise progression of signs and symptoms over at least 6 months.
5. Patient 10 to 50 years old at onset.
6. Signs and symptoms cannot better be explained by other disease process.

SOURCE: From Schumacher GA, et al: Problems of experimental trials of therapy in multiple sclerosis: Report by the panel on evaluation of experimental trials of therapy in multiple sclerosis. *Ann NY Acad Sci* 1965; 122:552, with permission.

attendant bleeding diathesis, organ dysfunction, and thrombocytopenia.[161]

Multiple Sclerosis and Devic's Neuromyelitis Optica

Multiple sclerosis (MS) is a demyelinating disease of the central nervous system. Its prevalence in the United States and Europe ranges from 15 to 145 per 100,000.[162] Immunologic abnormalities are believed to be at the core of the pathogenesis of MS, but disease susceptibility is also influenced by genetics and environmental factors. Distance of residence from the equator increases the risk of MS and a viral precipitant is suspected by many.[163,164] Recent preliminary work has implicated herpes simplex virus.[165,166] Patients with MS develop a spectrum of neurologic symptoms including difficulties with vision, impaired coordination, numbness and tingling, weakness, gait problems, fatigue, decreased respiratory function, bladder dysfunction, paroxysmal disorders, pain, spasticity, and behavioral disorders. Optic neuritis is frequently the first manifestation of MS,[167] but the clinical course is highly variable and unpredictable. The diagnosis of MS relies mainly on clinical criteria.

The Schumacher criteria have been widely used for many years to define MS (Table 12-7).[168] These criteria are often synopsized into the statement, "multiple abnormalities of central nervous system function disseminated over time and space"; that is, lesions occurring a month or more apart and in different areas of the white matter of the CNS. The clinical criteria were expanded by Rose and coworkers to include guidelines for probable MS and possible MS, with fulfillment of

the Schumacher criteria designated as clinically definite MS (Table 12-8).[169] Laboratory tests and imaging studies are helpful in supporting the clinical diagnosis of MS and eliminating alternative diagnoses. Abnormal evoked responses, cerebrospinal fluid abnormalities of IgG synthesis and oligoclonal bands, and MRI white matter lesions on T2-weighted images are supportive in the appropriate clinical context,[170] but none of these tests are specific for multiple sclerosis. The diagnostic criteria currently being used in research protocols includes laboratory-supported categories to help delineate the role that ancillary tests may play in making the diagnosis (Table 12-9).[170]

The sensitivity of MRI in detecting demyelinating lesions has been particularly helpful in confirming the clinical diagnosis of MS.[171] Over 95 percent of patients with clinically proven MS have periventricular white matter lesions on MRI[172,173] and MRI is more likely than CT, evoked responses, or CSF examinations to demonstrate abnormalities in patients with MS.[174] The importance of considering age and the clinical context when interpreting MRI lesions cannot be overly emphasized.[175] Twenty to 30 percent of the elderly have periventricular white matter lesions not attributable to MS.[176,177] Patchy white matter lesions may also be seen in small vessel ischemia, neurosarcoidosis, Sjogren's syndrome, vitamin B_{12} deficiency, complicated migraine, Lyme disease, and several vasculitides. These include some of the neurologic diseases which should be considered in the differential diagnosis of MS.[178]

The course of MS is classified as relapsing-remitting, in which subacute exacerbations resolve in weeks to months; relapsing-progressive, in which exacerbations leave significant residual disability[179]; or chronic-progressive, in which there is a persistent deteriorating course. There is evidence that the chronic-progressive

TABLE 12-8
Clinical Diagnosis of Multiple Sclerosis

Clinically Definite MS
Fulfilling Schumacher criteria

Probable Multiple Sclerosis

1. Relapsing/remitting symptoms with only one neurologic sign commonly associated with MS; or
2. Documented single episode with signs of multifocal white matter disease with complete or partial recovery.
3. No better explanation.

Possible Multiple Sclerosis

1. Relapsing/remitting symptoms without documented signs; or
2. Objective signs insufficient to establish more than one site of CNS involvement.
3. No better explanation.

SOURCE: From Rose AS, et al: Criteria for the clinical diagnosis of multiple sclerosis. *Neurology* 1976; 26:20, with permission.

TABLE 12-9
Washington (Poser) Criteria for the Diagnosis of Multiple Sclerosis

Category	Attacks	Clinical		Paraclinical	CSF OB/IgG
Clinically Definite					
CD-MS A1	2	2			
CD-MS A2	2	1	and	1	
Laboratory-Supported Definite					
LSD-MS B1	2	1	or	1	+
LSD-MS B2	1	2			+
LSD-MS B3	1	1	and	1	+
Clinically Probable					
CP-MS C1	2	1			
CP-MS C2	1	2			
CP-MS C3	1	1	and	1	
Laboratory-Supported Probable					
LSP-MS D1	2				+

NOTE: CD = clinically definite; LSD = laboratory-supported definite; CP = clinically probable; LSP = laboratory-supported probable; CSF = cerebrospinal fluid; OB = oligoclonal bands.
SOURCE: From Poser CM, et al: New diagnostic criteria for multiple sclerosis: Guidelines for research protocols. *Ann Neurol* 1983; 13:227, with permission.

form has a different pathogenesis from relapsing-remitting[180] so that these patients are studied separately in clinical trials. Many patients with relapsing-remitting MS, however, develop the chronic-progressive form over time, designated as secondary-progressive. Illustrating the variability of this disease, about one-third of patients have a benign form and remain unimpaired after many years, but a small percentage (3 to 12 percent) of patients develop severe disability within months to a few years.[181] During pregnancy, MS usually becomes relatively quiescent, but an increase in postdelivery exacerbations has been documented.[182]

The hallmark of MS is the white-matter plaque which can occur throughout the CNS, but particularly vulnerable sites include the optic nerve, brain stem, spinal cord, and periventricular regions. An inflammatory response characterizes the acute lesions, but the pathogenesis of MS is not known. The model widely held is that T-cell receptors respond to antigens presented by MHC class II molecules on macrophages and astrocytes. Proliferation and stimulation of helper T cells and cytokine secretion follows, resulting in a breakdown of the blood-brain barrier, widespread oligodendrocyte death, and demyelination.[183] Specific MHC class II alleles (DRw15 and DQw6) are associated with an increased risk of MS.[184] Candidate antigens are myelin basic protein[185] and myelin oligodendrocyte glycoprotein (MOG).[186] Quantitative study of antigen-specific T cells has proved that the number of T cells directed against myelin proteins is increased in MS spinal fluid and peripheral blood.[187] An endothelial cell

abnormality may be instrumental in allowing the entry of T cells reactive to myelin antigens into the CNS.[183] Abnormalities of cell adhesion molecules which allow lymphocyte migration across endothelial cells have been implicated.[188]

The evidence is strong for MS being an autoimmune disease, but it remains circumstantial. It is uncertain whether the T-cell response is primary or secondary, and the candidate antigens are not specific for MS.[189,190] Nevertheless, the current understanding of the pathogenesis of MS has directed attempts to control the disease through treatment and in clinical trials by altering the immunologic processes believed to lead to demyelination.

Treatment of MS is directed toward the resolution of acute attacks, prevention of attacks, and slowing of progression. Acute attacks of sufficient severity to warrant treatment are those which cause significant discomfort and disability. Milder attacks will usually subside in 1 to 2 weeks without treatment,[191] although reduced activity appears to be helpful toward promoting the resolution of exacerbations. For disabling acute attacks, high-dose methylprednisolone (6 to 15 mg/kg per day) given as daily intravenous pulses for 3 to 10 days, and usually followed by an oral prednisone taper from 60 mg for 10 to 21 days, has largely replaced the use of corticotropin (ACTH).[192–194] Eighty-five percent of patients with relapsing-remitting MS will show significant objective neurologic improvement as early as 3 to 5 days into the treatment course. The treatment benefit is not sustained and is not as good for progressive MS, benefitting approximately 50 percent of these patients, primarily by reducing spasticity. High-dose IV methylprednisolone therapy reduces intrathecal immunoglobulin production,[195-199] plaque edema, and gadolinium enhancement evidenced by serial CT and MR scans.[171,200,201]

Oral prednisone alone for treatment of acute exacerbations is no longer recommended due to the results of the Optic Neuritis Treatment Trial which showed an increased relapse rate in those patients treated only with oral prednisone. However, patients with optic neuritis treated with high-dose IV methylprednisolone followed by an oral steroid taper had a reduced risk of developing clinical evidence of MS for 2 years.[202] This therapy is usually well tolerated. Side effects include insomnia, restlessness, euphoria, and weight gain. Rarely, aseptic necrosis of the femoral or humoral head occurs.

Interferons (IFNs) have been studied for the treatment of MS due to their antiviral and immunomodulatory activities.[203] Copolymer-1 (Cop1, Copaxone) is a synthetic polymer composed of four amino acids that resembles myelin basic protein and may induce myelin basic protein-specific suppressor cells.[204] Two class I interferons and copolymer-1 have recently been evaluated in well-designed clinical trials. The trials enrolled similar patients (young and ambulatory with active, relapsing-remitting, clinically definite disease) and found a similar effect on reduction of the attack rate, although differences in design and primary outcome measures make direct comparisons difficult.

IFNβ-1b (Betaseron) is the only interferon currently approved for the treatment of relapsing-remitting MS patients. It was expeditiously approved in the United States in 1993, based on the results of the University of British Columia IFNβ Multiple Sclerosis Study Group trial and is now in wide use. In this trial, IFNβ-1b was randomized to 372 patients and, when given at a high dose of 80 mU alternate day subcutaneous injections, was shown to reduce clinical attacks by about one-third compared to placebo.[205] After a median follow-up of about 4 years, this reduction was sustained for most patients, but neutralizing antibody to IFNβ had developed in 38 percent and there was a decreased effect over time in those patients.[206] Most interesting, there was a decrease in the progression of lesion burden on annual quantitative MRI in the treated patients.[207] The study was not powered to determine an effect on the progression of disability and further study is required to address this important question. Systemic "flu-like" side effects were common during the first 1 to 3 months of therapy (occurring in 52 percent), but could be decreased by cautious concomitant use of ibuprofen or other non-steroidal anti-inflammatory drugs. A small percentage of patients (3 to 8 percent)

were unable to tolerate the drug due to persistence of the flu-like symptoms. An increase in depressive symptoms associated with IFNβ treatment has been documented with suicide attempts occurring in 2 percent. Injection site reactions occurred in 80 percent, but treatment discontinuation due to skin reactions occurred in only 1 to 3 percent. Liver enzyme elevations and mild leukopenia were common in the early weeks of therapy, but were not associated with clinical liver disease or opportunistic infections in the trial, and usually returned to normal in 3 to 4 months.[206]

Cop1 is not yet available for use, but it is currently being reviewed by the FDA and approval is expected. It is given as a daily subcutaneous injection and has been shown to reduce the mean number of relapses by 29 percent.[204] In the placebo-controled trial, there was a trend toward a more profound effect on relapses for patients with the least clinical disability.[208] Systemic postinjection reactions and skin reactions occur with Cop1.[204]

The third product recently studied is IFNβ-1a (Avonex), an interferon produced in mammalian cells which is native sequence and normally glycosylated (IFNβ-1b is nonglycosylated and mutated to improve stability).[203] IFNβ-1a is given intramuscularly on a weekly schedule. Publication of the detailed results of the phase III study of IFNβ-1a is pending, but because preliminary data suggest the effect of IFNβ-1a is similar to IFNβ-1b and Cop1 (and they will likely be comparably high-priced), factors dictating the choice of therapy may be route of administration, frequency of dosing, and individual response to side-effect profiles. The mechanism of action of the interferons differs from the mechanism of Cop1, so that one possibility of the future may be using a combination of these drugs.

The results of trials using immunosuppressant therapies in MS have been variable. This, in addition to their unfavorable side-effect profiles, limit the enthusiasm for their use. Probably best tolerated is azathioprine, a purine analogue which exerts its maximal immunosuppressive effect after 3 to 6 months of daily use. Metaanalysis of seven controlled trials, studying either exacerbating or chronic progressive MS,[209-214] showed a small but significant benefit.[215] The number of patients remaining relapse-free after 3 years was similar to that achieved with IFNβ-1b.[215] There was only a small and unsustained reduction in progressive disability. Azathioprine therapy is associated with an increase in malignancies, especially non-Hodgkin's lymphoma.[216] Other complications include leukopenia, thrombocytopenia, macrocytic anemia, hypersensitivity pancreatitis, and toxic hepatitis.[193] About 10 percent of patients discontinue therapy due to side effects—most commonly, drug-related fever, rash, and gastrointestinal intolerance.[214,216]

The use of cyclophosphamide, an alkylating agent with both cytotoxic and immunosuppressive mechanisms, in the treatment of chronic progressive MS is controversial. Initial optimism waned when later trials did not substantiate a benefit and the potential toxicity was experienced in clinical practice. Even in one of the early positive studies, a significant reduction in progression after 12 months was not sustained at 2 years.[217] Bimonthly booster injections did not prolong the benefit in one study,[218] and extended the benefit in only 14 percent of patients in another.[219] The Northeast Cooperative Sclerosis Treatment Group[220] has suggested that cyclophosphamide be given only to patients younger than 40 years and that those with a secondary progressive course rather than primary progressive will more likely benefit. Others point out that the most positive studies showed stabilization for not more than 12 to 18 months so that cyclophosphamide should be reserved for those patients likely to significantly progress during that time period.[193] The side effects of cyclophosphamide therapy include scalp alopecia, hemorrhagic cystitis, nausea and vomiting, leukopenia with complicating infections, myocarditis, gonadal suppression and amenorrhea, interstitial pulmonary fibrosis, and increased malignancies.[193]

Until more effective therapy becomes available, much of the management of patients with MS must focus on symptomatic treatment. Spasticity is treated with baclofen, sometimes with the addition of valium in refractory cases. High doses of baclofen (>80 mg/day) are sometimes used and there is usually a tradeoff, with increased weakness a result of improved spasticity. Sudden withdrawal of baclofen has been associated with seizures and confusion.[221] Fatigue is a frequent complaint of MS patients, affecting 76 to 92 percent.[222-225] It is improved with amantadine, 100 mg twice daily.[226] The mechanism is unknown, but higher levels of β-endorphin and β-lipotropin, and lower levels of lactate have been measured in patients responding to amantadine.[227] Pemoline is sometimes used to treat fatigue, but a recent study did not show any benefit compared to placebo.[226] Heat has been recognized to exacerbate fatigue and other MS symptoms in many patients, so that cool temperatures will sometimes lessen fatigue. Two potassium channel blockers are being studied in the control of heat sensitivity, but seizures and other complications may limit their use.[228-230]

Other symptomatic treatment for MS is directed toward depression[231] and emotional lability. The former responds to the usual antidepressant therapies and the latter is often improved with low doses of amitriptyline or imipramine. Patients with MS may also have a neurobehavioral disorder of "la belle indifference" or inappropriate euphoria. There is a cheerful optimism despite severe disability which requires no treatment, but is sometimes quite striking.[231]

Paroxysmal pain syndromes, especially tic douloureux (trigeminal neuralgia) and dystonias are common in MS and are usually treated with carbamazepine. If unsuccessful, a trial of phenytoin is given, but rhizotomy is sometimes required for tic douloureux. Unfortunately, it often recurs on the other side at a later date.[232]

Neurogenic bladder is common in MS and may be spastic, with irritative symptoms, or flaccid, with obstructive symptoms. Anticholinergic medications, such as propantheline bromide or oxybutynin are used for a small, spastic bladder and care must be given to avoid excessive cholinergic blockade when tricyclic antidepressants are used concurrently. Confusion and short-term memory loss may also occur with anticholinergic therapy, especially if there is baseline impairment. A flaccid bladder is usually controlled with intermittent catheterization, but occasionally a cholinergic antagonist and α-adrenergic blocker such as phenoxybenzamine or antispasmodic like diazepam, baclofen, tizanidine, or chlorpromazine is used.[233]

Devic's neuromyelitis optica (DNO) is a rare disorder which is considered by some to be a subtype of multiple sclerosis. Others, based on pathologic data, argue that it is a distinct neurological syndrome. DNO is characterized by the acute or subacute onset of myelopathy preceded or followed within days or weeks by blindness in one or both eyes due to optic neuritis.[234] The myelopathy usually affects the cervical and/or thoracic spinal cord and is often associated with a clinical syndrome of complete spinal cord section, that is, paralysis, bowel and bladder dysfunction, and, depending on the level of the lesion, respiratory compromise. The course may be progressive, relapsing or, rarely, remitting.[235] Patients with progressive disease may die within 2 to 4 years. Those who survive tend to have lasting neurologic deficits.

Magnetic resonance imaging of the spinal cord shows swelling and cavitation.[236] Pathologically, the spinal cord lesions are marked by necrosis of both the gray and white matter. In a recent series of eight patients,[235] five with pathologic data showed no inflammatory cell infiltrates and enlarged, hyalinized vessels. The optic nerves and chiasm were demyelinated, some with cavitation. In contrast to the multiple demyelinated lesions typically seen in MS, no other demyelinated or necrotic lesions were detected in the brain, brain stem, or cerebellum. Neither were white matter lesions seen on MRI during life, and oligoclonal bands were identified in the CSF of only one patient. This information gives support to the argument that DNO is pathophysiologically distinct from MS. Until the etiology of MS is better understood, it will be difficult to resolve this issue.

Treatments used for MS have been used for DNO with variable results. Steroids, corticotropin, cyclophosphamide, plasmapheresis, and lymphocytoplasmapheresis have been used.[235-237] There have been several reports of patients becoming steroid-dependent with relapses occurring when attempts to reduce steroid doses have been attempted.

ANESTHESIA FOR THE PATIENT WITH MULTIPLE SCLEROSIS

Scattered demyelination in the brain and spinal cord of patients with MS may affect sensory, motor, autonomic, optic, and integrative pathways of neurologic function. Respiratory function may be affected by lesions in the cervical or thoracic spinal cord or in the respiratory control centers in the medulla oblongata, even in the absence of bulbar or limb paralysis.[238] Pulmonary function studies and arterial blood gases should be obtained preoperatively to assess the pulmonary reserve, especially when kyphoscoliosis is present. In patients with moderately severe MS, maximal inspiratory and expiratory pressure generation is about half-normal, and the ventilatory response to elevations of arterial P_{CO_2} is significantly impaired.[239] Total lung capacity, residual volume, and vital capacity may be close to normal, but maximal voluntary ventilation and maximal inspiratory and expiratory pressure generation can be significantly decreased.[240] Pharyngeal and laryngeal motor involvement will place some patients at risk for aspiration of gastric contents during induction of anesthesia, especially when gastric emptying is delayed. Patients with high thoracic or spinal cord lesions are at risk for autonomic hyperflexia, and symptoms of this process should be elicited during the preanesthetic interview. Symptoms of syncope, vasomotor instability, or orthostatic hypotension may indicate involvement of autonomic vascular control pathways, and be a harbinger of hemodynamic instability in the perioperative period.

A few of the medications used to treat the side effects of MS have known anesthetic implications. Baclofen and dantrolene, sometimes used to treat spasticity, can potentiate the effect of nondepolarizing muscle relaxants. Patients taking carbamazepine may be resistant to nondepolarizing muscle relaxants. Diazepam may potentiate the sedative effects of anesthetic drugs. A history of recent (within 1 year) steroid use should be elicited, and perioperative stress steroid coverage should be provided when adrenal suppression cannot be excluded. Cyclophosphamide may result in pancytopenia, pulmonary fibrosis, and myocarditis.

Preoperative counseling should include informing the patient that anesthesia and / or perioperative stress may exacerbate the disease.[241-243] For example, in the first three months after delivery, postpartum patients have a relapse rate up to three times that of the nonpregnant population, even in the absence of regional or general anesthesia.[244] Fever or hyperthermia can exacerbate the disease process by slowing conduction in demyelinated nerve fibers.[245] Because fever is a common sequelae of most surgery, many cases of worsening of the disease may be linked to hyperpyrexia.

Most clinicians favor the choice of general over spinal or epidural anesthesia for patients with MS, because the normally unpredictable waxing and waning of the disease may be unfairly linked to neuraxial anesthesia in the postoperative period. Certainly, spinal anesthesia has been implicated in postoperative exacerbations of the disease, which may be related to enhanced susceptibility of demyelinated neurons to the neurotoxic effects of local anesthetics.[246] Nevertheless, MS should be considered a *relative* contraindication to spinal surgery and successful outcomes where spinal anesthesia was judged preferable have been reported.[247]

Epidural anesthesia is probably safer than spinal anesthesia in patients with MS because of the lower local anesthetic concentrations found in the central and peripheral spinal cord after epidural anesthesia.[248] The relapse rate of women who received epidural analgesia for vaginal delivery did not exceed that of women who received local infiltration.[249] Of those women who had received epidural analgesia and suffered a relapse, however, all had been given bupivacaine of a concentration greater than 0.25%. Thus, caution is urged when performing epidural anesthesia using higher concentrations and larger doses of local anesthetics.

The volatile anesthetics have not been shown to exacerbate the disease.[250,251] Avoidance of the use of enflurane in patients with associated seizures is advocated. There is no substantiation supporting or denigrating the use of a particular intravenous or inhaled anesthetic over another.

The use of muscle relaxants can be problematic. As in other cases of upper motor neuron disease, the use of succinylcholine is associated with massive release of intracellular potassium from muscle tissue, which may result in cardiac arrest.[252] Because MS is often a cyclic or progressive disease, succinylcholine is not safe even in patients with longstanding disease. Nondepolarizing muscle relaxants will have a variable pharmacodynamic effect in patients with MS. On the one hand, as in other diseases which cause denervation of skeletal muscle, an increase in skeletal muscle acetylcholine receptors and a clinical resistance to nondepolarizing muscle relaxants has been reported.[253] In addition, patients taking antiseizure medications such as phenytoin and carbamazepine would be expected to be resistant to muscle paralysis by nondepolarizing relaxants. On the other hand, patients who have borderline respiratory muscle strength and decreased muscle mass preoperatively would be expected to be more susceptible to the effects of nondepolarizing relaxants. Also, a myasthenic-like syndrome has been associated with MS, which again would potentiate the effects of this class of muscle relaxants.[254] Finally, as mentioned previously, baclofen and dantrolene may potentiate muscle relaxation. Close monitoring and titration of muscle relaxants and use of the minimally necessary dose is advocated. Because of the risk of hemodynamic instability due to autonomic insufficiency, verification of adequate intravascular volume replacement and minute-to-minute observation of blood pressure are advised. Episodes of hypertension should be avoided, as increased vascular hydrostatic pressures in the presence of a deficient blood-brain barrier may lead to focal vasogenic cerebral edema. Because of alterations in the blood-brain barrier, the CNS may be more susceptible to the ability of local anesthetics to produce seizures. This may be especially true in patients with a preexisting seizure disorder. For these reasons, a diminution in maximum dose of local anesthetics given to patients with MS has been proposed.[250]

In the postoperative period, elevated temperatures should be treated very aggressively to prevent hyperthermia-associated exacerbations of the disease. Postoperative neurologic evaluation may detect worsening of the disease and the need for more aggressive medical therapy.

Trigeminal Neuralgia (Tic Doloreux)
(See also Chap. 22)

An estimated 5000 to 10,000 new cases of trigeminal neuralgia (TN) occur annually in the United States,[255] with a higher incidence in women than in men. The absolute etiology and pathophysiology are not clear and the literature has indicated the role of trauma, dental problems and infections, viral disease, tumors, vascular compression, demyelination, skull base distortions, and brain stem pathway pathology as being causative factors. One finding brought to our attention by the pioneering work of Jannetta,[256] involved the high incidence of vascular channels impinging on the root entrance zone of the trigeminal nerve (CN V). Patients with TN experience brief repetitive paroxysmal spasms of unilateral lancinating pain involving one or more division(s) of the CN V. This pain is often described as similar to a "bolt of lightning" or "electric shock-like." Usually the pain is triggered by nonpainful tactile stimuli such as a light touch on the face, a breeze, talking, chewing, or eating. Interestingly, 1 to 2 percent of patients with multiple sclerosis (MS) will be found to have associated TN.[257] Histologically, a demyelinating plaque is seen at the root entry zone of CN V. The diagnosis is made by history and neurologic examination. An MRI will help to rule out MS and might demonstrate flow voids of vascular loops adjacent to the root entry zone, with CN V distortion. This type of scanning will also rule out AVM, aneurysms, and aberrant vessels. Neurophysiologic testing may indicate abnormal responses in evoked potentials and electromyography in the affected side when compared to the normal contralateral side.

Medical treatment of TN employs two mainstay drugs, phenytoin and carbamazepine. The side effects of carbamazepine include sedation, obtundation in coordination, disequilibrium, decrease in cognition, liver toxicity, and abnormal hematological responses. With phenytoin, the side effects can include a cutaneous rash, disequilibrium, liver toxicity, cardiac irregularities, and sedation. Secondary drugs that may help these patients include baclofen and chlorphenesin carbamate.

The surgical approach is considered when medical treatment has failed and two types of procedures have been developed. The first, partial percutaneous neurolysis of CN V, can be carried out with radiofrequency lesioning,[258] percutaneous chemoneurolysis with glycerol,[259] or percutaneous compression of the gasserian ganglion with a balloon catheter.[260] The procedures noted above are performed in either the operating room or in the radiology suite. Many anesthetic techniques are available and we have carried out these procedures using neurolept analgesia with droperidol and fentanyl as well as midazolam. The needle is inserted into the cheek, lateral to the corner of the mouth, and into the foramen ovale. The stylet is then withdrawn, an electrode is inserted into the needle, and stimulation is carried out until complete localization takes place. At this point, a radiofrequency lesion, glycerol, or insertion of a balloon catheter takes place. On occasion, brief anesthesia can be instituted with methohexital or propofol during the more painful part of the procedure.

The second type of procedure is the vascular decompression of the CN V (Jannetta procedure),[261] which is carried out under general anesthesia. Entering the posterior fossa, the root entry zone is approached and CN V and the vessel impinging on it are separated and a piece of plastic material interposed between these structures. The anesthetic aspect is similar to any posterior fossa surgery and is covered in Chap. 29.

Dementia

Dementia is an acquired syndrome of intellectual impairment which interferes with social and vocational function. It is a disease process and not a normal part of aging, but its incidence increases dramatically over the age of 65, affecting 15 to 20 percent of individuals.[262] The intellectual impairment of dementia is associated with deficits in language, memory, visuospatial skills, and cognition. Memory loss and personality changes are often the earliest signs, heralding the onset of disease. Dementia must be differentiated from delirium, a condition which impairs consciousness and can often be reversed when the underlying metabolic or other causes are treated.

Cognitive impairment without functional decline has been termed "age-associated memory impairment" and is considered by some to be a normal part of aging. Neuropsychological testing has identified problems with timed tasks, episodic memory, and incidental learning in these individuals. In contrast to patients with dementia, verbal intellect, immediate memory, long-term memory, retrieval of over-learned material, and semantic memory remain intact. Many of these people will develop progressive dementia if followed over time, however, so that the distinction between very early Alzheimer disease and normal aging can be difficult.[263]

Alzheimer disease (AD) is the most common type of dementia, affecting up to 75 percent of demented patients.[264,265] It is estimated that there will be at least 7 million AD patients in the United States by the early twenty-first century.[266,267] AD is classified as a cortical dementia in which the memory impairment occurs early, followed temporally by anomia and then more widespread cognitive impairment and behavioral alterations. At present, no laboratory test short of a brain biopsy or autopsy study confirms the diagnosis of AD. The diagnosis is made based on sets of criteria and tests of exclusion. The diagnostic criteria most widely used are the NINCDS-ADRDA task force criteria developed in 1984 and the DSM-IV guidelines.[268,269]

The evaluation of the demented patient begins with a skillful history. Even in the early stages, it is important to interview a family member in addition to the patient, as the patient will often deny or be unaware of behavioral changes or many of the other observations a family member will contribute. The time course of the illness is an important focus. An insidious course will differentiate AD from acute causes of dementia such as stroke or infection and subacute etiologies such as hydrocephalus and Creutzfeldt-Jakob disease. Questions about job performance and activities of daily living are specifically addressed to establish whether a decreased level of functioning is present. It is also useful to question the patient regarding a depressed mood and to obtain any family history of AD or other dementia.

Mental status evaluation must first confirm that there is no impairment of consciousness (except in the very late stages of dementia). Waxing and waning of alertness is the hallmark of delirium and warrants a different evaluation. Attention, sensorium, recent and remote memory, language, praxis, visuospatial skills, calculations, and judgment must be tested. Folstein's Mini-Mental Status Examination is a screening instrument often used at the bedside to assist with documentation of deficits (Table 12-10).[270] Its strengths are brevity and convenience. Any mental status evaluation must take into account the patient's baseline cognitive abilities, education, primary language, and age. Age specific norms have been developed for the Mini-Mental Status Examination.[271] Bedside screening tools are not comprehensive or diagnostic and are usually followed by more in-depth neuropsychological testing when dementia is suggested.

The neurologic examination is often normal early in AD. Primitive reflexes, such as the snout, glabellar, or grasp, and impairment of graphesthesia may be early findings.[272] Although difficulties with gait, myoclonus, and extrapyramidal signs may be seen in late AD, the presence of these disturbances early on should alert the clinician to other etiologies of dementia. Extrapyramidal signs are prominent in the subcortical dementias associated with the degenerative neurologic diseases of Parkinson, Huntington, and progressive supranuclear palsy. Myoclonus is seen early in Jakob-Cruetzfeld disease and gait difficulties may be a presenting finding in normal pressure hydrocephalus and stroke-related dementia. Early focal abnormalities also signal neurologic pathology other than AD.

The laboratory evaluation of a patient being evaluated for dementia should include routine screening for metabolic, toxic, infectious, and other treatable conditions. The Centers for Disease Control recommends that a CBC, sedimentation rate, electrolytes, BUN/creatinine, liver function tests, calcium, thyroid function tests, serum B_{12} level, syphilis serology, and HIV antibody testing be performed. Drug levels should be checked for any potentially toxic medications. In a review of 11 studies by Clarfield, 13.2 percent of 2889 subjects were found to have potentially reversible causes of dementia. Of these, metabolic abnormalities accounted for 16 percent of the cases and drugs for 28 percent. Depression was identified as etiologic in 26 percent (Table 12-11).[264]

An imaging study of the brain should be performed to rule out structural lesions and to assist with differ-

TABLE 12-10
Folstein's MINI MENTAL STATUS EXAMINATION[a]

Test	Score
What is the year, season, date, day, month?	5
Where are you: state, county, town, place, floor?	5
Name three objects: State slowly and have patient repeat (repeat until patient learns all three).	3
Do reverse serial 7s (five steps) or spell "WORLD" backwards.	5
Ask for three unrelated objects above.	3
Name from inspection a pencil, a watch.	2
Have patient repeat, "No if's, and's, or but's."	1
Follow a three-stage command (1 point each). (Take a paper in your hand, fold it, and put it on the floor)	3
Read and obey, "Close your eyes."	1
Write a simple sentence.	1
Copy intersecting pentagons.	1

[a] Out of a possible total score of 30, most patients with true dementia score below 15, whereas those with uncomplicated depression score above 25. Mixed or transient cognitive impairments produce scores in between normal persons and those with irreversible dementia.

SOURCE: From Folstein MF, Folstein SE, McHugh PR: Mini-Mental State: a practical method for grading the cognitive state of patients for the clinician. *J Psychiatr Res* 1975; 12:189, with permission.

entiating AD from multi-infarct dementia. While some have advocated only imaging those patients in high risk groups.[273,274] most clinicians agree that identifying a potentially treatable lesion even in a relatively few patients (Larson estimates 4 percent) is worthwhile, especially considering that the test is readily available and noninvasive.[275,276] CT and MRI are nonspecific in AD. Cerebral atrophy may be seen, but brain atrophy on imaging studies does not necessarily correlate with brain function. Normal individuals may have marked

TABLE 12-11
Summary of 103 Cases Reported with Partially and Completely Reversed Dementia

Condition	Reversed Dementia Partly *n*	Reversed Dementia Completely *n*	Total[a] *n* (%)	Cumulative % *n* (%)
Drugs	17[b]	12	29 (28.2)	28.2
Depression	18	9	27 (26.2)	54.4
Metabolic	10	6	16 (15.5)	69.9
Thyroid	6	1	7 (6.8)	—
B_{12}	—	1	1 (1.0)	—
Calcium	2	—	2 (1.9)	—
Hepatic	2	—	2 (1.9)	—
Other	—	4	4 (3.9)	—
Normal pressure hydrocephalus	8	3	11 (10.7)	80.6
Subdural hematoma	5	1	6 (5.8)	86.4
Neoplasm	4	—	4 (4.0)	90.4
Other	9	1	10 (9.7)	100.0
TOTAL[c]	71 (68.9)	32 (31.1)	103 (100)	—

[a] Total includes all cases of partially and completely reversed dementia.
[b] Includes four cases of alcohol abuse.
[c] Figures are *n*(%).

SOURCE: From Clarfield AM: The reversible dementias: Do they reverse? *Ann Intern Med* 1988; 109:476, with permission.

atrophy and those with early AD may not.[277] Progressive cortical atrophy on serial imaging, prominent in the temporoparietal lobes, is supportive of AD. Single-photon emission computed tomography (SPECT) has shown decreased regional blood flow in the temporal and parietal lobes in studies of AD patients. If this pattern is seen, it may be helpful in identifying probable AD.[278,279]

Lumbar punctures are not helpful and therefore not recommended in the evaluation of a patient with typical AD.[280,281] If the patient has any of the following characteristics and there are no contraindications, CSF studies should be done: The patient is under age 55; has rapidly progressive or unusual dementia; is immunosuppressed; or there is suspicion of CNS vasculitis (particularly in patients with collagen vascular diseases), cancer, suspicion of CNS infection, reactive serum antitreponemal syphilis serology, or hydrocephalus.[276] EEGs are also not helpful in routine cases of AD. EEG tracings will be normal early and show nonspecific slowing later in the disease. EEG should be obtained when Creutzfeldt-Jakob disease, seizures, or encephalitis are possibilities.

The histopathology of AD is characterized by generalized cortical neuronal dropout with more severe neuronal loss in the nucleus basalis of Meynert, an area high in acetylcholine production. There is neuronal granulovacuolar degeneration, most extensive in Somner's sector of the hippocampus. Neurofibrillary tangles and neuritic plaques must be seen in sufficient numbers on microscopic examination to meet pathologic criteria for a definite diagnosis of AD.[282] The neuritic plaques contain a core of amyloid. Amyloid is also found in the walls of small blood vessels near the plaques.[283,284] The role of amyloid and its precursor peptide, beta amyloid precursor protein, have been the focus of recent genetic research and searches for biological markers.[285]

The neurochemical defect of AD is decreased acetylcholine and choline acetyl transferase activity, the enzyme involved in the synthesis of acetycholine.[286] It is unclear whether the reduction in the acetylcholine neurotransmitter is primary, or is a secondary effect resulting from neuronal loss in areas high in acetylcholine production (the nucleus basalis of Meynert).[287] The concentration of amino acid transmitters, particularly glutamate, is also reduced in cortical and subcortical areas.[288]

There is also evidence of a complement mediated inflammatory response in AD. Reactive microglia have been found embedded in the amyloid of neuritic plaques, as well as antigens of major histocompatibility complex glycoproteins.[289] Increased cytokines and proteins associated with complement activation (the acute phase protein alpha-1-antichymotrypsin) have also

been identified.[290] Several epidemiologic and case-control studies have shown a sparing effect on AD by taking NSAIDs, sparking further interest in a potential inflammatory role in AD.[291-296]

At least four chromosomes have been implicated in the development of AD. Chromosome 21 codes for the β-amyloid precursor protein gene and is linked to some cases of familial AD.[297,298] Chromosome 14 is a potential locus of early-onset familial AD[299,300] and chromosome 1 carries a gene, STM-2, which has recently been linked to some early onset familial AD.[301] Chromsome 19 is a potential locus of late-onset AD, both sporadic and familial.[302] Chromsome 19 carries the apolipoprotein E (ApoE) allele which is one of several risk factors for AD.[303-306]

ApoE is found in plaques, neurofibrillary tangles, and vascular amyloid.[307] A commercial test for the ApoE genotype is available to physicians. It has been estimated that the ApoE allele increases the risk of AD twofold.[308] However, there are many other variables which affect this risk, including age, female gender, history of head trauma, myocardial infarction, and other genetic influences.[276] The ApoE gene is neither necessary nor sufficient for development of AD and, although it is a significant risk factor for AD, ApoE typing will rarely provide clinically useful information.[308]

Tetrahydroaminoacridine (THA) was the first drug to be approved by the Food and Drug Administration for the treatment of mild to moderate dementia of the Alzeheimer's type. Its primary mechanism of action is as a competitive, reversible acetylcholinesterase inhibitor. It may also increase the synthesis, turnover, and release of serotonin, norepinephrine, and dopamine.[309] Three large clinical trials have shown a significant improvement or slowing of decline in some cognitive test scores in AD patients.[310-312] The response is dose-related, but many patients are unable to tolerate higher doses due to the side-effects of nausea, vomiting, diarrhea, and anorexia. Elevated liver enzymes occur in one-third of patients, requiring SGPT monitoring every 2 weeks for 18 weeks, then every 3 months at stable doses.

In those patients for whom THA is not an option, medical management is primarily directed toward addressing problem behaviors and preventing unnecessary or premature functional decline. Depression may be seen early in AD and is often treated with one of the serotonin receptor inhibitors due to their favorable side-effect profile. Agitation and delusions may improve in the setting of a structured, simple, and familiar environment with frequent orientation, but very low doses of an antipsychotic are sometimes required. Providing support and respite for the caregiver may help to maintain the patient at home. Being attentive to

TABLE 12-12
Differential Diagnosis of the Dementias

Alzheimer disease

Lewy Body disease

Vascular dementia

Extrapyramidal syndromes with dementia
  Parkinson's disease
  Huntington's disease
  Wilson's disease
  Progressive supranuclear palsy
  Spinocerebellar degenerations
  Miscellaneous extrapyramidal syndromes

Slow viral dementias
  Creuzfeld-Jakob disease
  Gerstmann-Straussler

Chronic meningitis
  Neurosyphilis
  Granulomatous and fungal infections

Toxic and metabolic dementias

Hydrocephalic dementias

Nonprogressive dementias
  Traumatic
  Postanoxic

Neoplastic dementias

Myelin diseases with dementia

Dementias associated with psychiatric disorders

Cognitive impairment without functional decline

intercurrent illnesses and anticipating end-of-life decisions are also important management issues.

Areas of investigation in AD treatment include antioxidant therapy with selegiline and others.[313–316] Retrospective and epidemiologic data suggest the NSAIDs may be associated with a less rapid decline in some areas of cognition.[291,295,296,317] Trophic factors, including nerve growth factor, compounds affecting amyloidogenesis, and lipoprotein-lowering agents are also being studied.[318]

The differential diagnosis of dementia is extensive (Table 12-12). As many as 20 percent of patients with dementia are estimated by some investigators to have Lewy body disease which is underrecognized and not clearly delineated in terms of diagnostic criteria.[319] It is characterized by cognitive deficits similar to those of AD, prominent psychiatric problems, and extrapyramidal signs (often lacking a resting tremor).[319,320] Pathologically, there are many plaques and diffuse cortical and brainstem Lewy bodies, but few neurofibrillary tangles.[321]

Differentiating vascular dementia from AD and other forms of dementia is important because of the possibility of halting the process by means of pharmacologic intervention. Advances in imaging techniques have dramatically increased the identification of ischemic white matter lesions and lacunar strokes and

their relationship to dementia. A history of strokes and/or transient ischemic events and other risk factors for stroke such as hypertension, diabetes mellitus, smoking, hyperlipidemia, family history, age, and male gender predispose to vascular dementia. Stepwise episodes of sudden-onset deterioration are consistent, but vascular dementia may occur without these defining events. Vascular dementia is unlikely if there is an early, severe, and progressive memory deficit, language problems, apraxia or agnosia not explained by focal vascular lesions, or no focal neurologic signs.[322,323] Approximately 10 percent of demented patients have mixed dementia, with features of both AD and vascular disease. It is often clinically difficult to decide whether one entity or both contributes to the dementia.[276,324]

An uncommon type of cortical dementia, Pick disease, affects the frontal and/or anterior lobes. These patients have extravagant personality changes and stereotyped language output, but appear clinically similar to AD in the late stages. Subcortical dementias are clinically differentiated by early psychomotor retardation and forgetfulness, or difficulty with retrieval of information, rather than an inability to make new memories.[325] Parkinson disease, Huntington disease, progressive supranuclear palsy, Wilson disease, and early AIDS dementia are associated with subcortical dementia. Jacob-Creutzfeldt disease is a rare, rapidly progressive dementia associated with seizures and early myoclonus. Neurosyphilis may cause dementia or "general paresis" and is routinely screened for using the VDRL. The clinical triad of ataxia, incontinence, and dementia can be associated with normal pressure hydrocephalus. Unfortunately, it is difficult to identify those patients who may improve with a shunt and there is high morbidity associated with shunting.[326] The elderly and alcoholics are at increased risk for subdural hematomas. Chronic subdurals cause dementia, but often symptoms are fluctuating and occur in tandem with headaches and focal signs. Toxic and metabolic abnormalities are often associated with delirium, but can present in a more chronic way and should always be considered. Drug intoxication, thyroid disease, B_{12} deficiency, and hyponatremia are examples.[327]

Many patients with primary dementia develop a secondary depression and benefit from treatment of their depression. A dementia syndrome which reverses with antidepressant therapy has been termed "pseudodementia" and occurs in up to 10 percent of the depressed elderly.[328] Recent studies have shown, however, that many of these people will later develop irreversible dementia, suggesting that the depression may unmask an underlying early dementia. Regardless, there is a potential substantial benefit from treating the depression. Depression decreases concentration, response time, and motivation, and may be difficult to differentiate from dementia, especially in the elderly.[329] A more acute onset and rapid progression, and a positive history of depression in the patient or the family, will assist in recognizing depression. Also, depressed persons tend to give "don't know" answers whereas demented persons usually attempt incorrect answers on tasks. The absence of dyspraxia, agnosia, and language problems may be helpful in identifying depression.[330,331]

ANESTHESIA FOR THE PATIENT WITH DEMENTIA

Perioperative management of the patient with dementia requires a thorough preoperative medical and neurologic assessment, meticulous intraoperative care, and special postoperative management. Preoperative evaluation should ascertain that those illnesses which can cause or exacerbate cognitive dysfunction are identified, and that medical treatment has been optimized. Most patients with dementia should have had a complete neurologic evaluation prior to elective surgery. Scrutiny of patients' medication lists should identify drugs which may predispose to cognitive dysfunction in the post-operative period. For example, high dose steroids, antiemetic drugs, opioids, anticholinergics, and many other pharmacologic agents have been implicated in causing CNS dysfunction. The need for these drugs must be reevaluated prior to surgery to eliminate them as a possible cause of postoperative neurologic dysfunction. Drugs with well-known CNS side effects and a narrow therapeutic index should have their serum concentration verified prior to anesthesia and surgery. If such tests have not been performed recently, patients taking tacrine should have liver function tests surveyed.

The baseline neurologic function should be documented prior to administration of anesthesia. This allows identification of worsening function in the postoperative period and intervention as needed. No anesthetic technique has been shown to result in superior outcome in the patient with dementia. In normal elderly patients, general anesthesia does not pose a greater risk than regional anesthesia for postoperative cognitive impairment.[332,333] Whether this is true in patients with dementia has not been formally studied. Compared to normal patients, patients with impaired preoperative cognitive function may have delayed recovery to baseline function after general anesthesia[334] and local anesthesia with sedation.[335] Volatile anesthetics can disturb sleep-wake cycles, cognition, and behavior for up to several days after general anesthesia, presumably because of their long half-life in brain tissue. It seems reasonable to assume therefore that regional anesthesia with light sedation would most quickly return patients to their baseline level of function.

Anticholinergic drugs, when used for that purpose or as a side effect of their primary action, have a well-known detrimental effect on cognitive function.[336] When anticholinergic drugs are needed, compounds with quaternary ammonium moieties, such as glycopyrrolate, cause less cognitive dysfunction because of their inability to cross the blood-brain barrier.

THA, through its anticholinesterase effects, can exaggerate the action of succinylcholine.[337] In addition, THA may increase the incidence of salivation, nausea, and bradycardia in surgical patients.[338] Ergoloid mesylates, a commonly used pharmacologic agent for the treatment of dementia, may cause platelet dysfunction.[339,340]

Because many patients have dementia as the result of extracranial or intracranial cerebrovascular disease, close attention should be paid to maintaining baseline cerebral perfusion pressure[341] and preventing hyperventilation-induced cerebral vasoconstriction. In addition, careful titration of anesthetic agents is mandatory in elderly patients and those with low levels of arousal.

Postoperatively, it is very important to maintain a normal *milieu intérieur*. Small perturbations in physiological parameters may have profound effects of an abnormal brain. Medications with CNS side effects are avoided as much as possible. Discomfort and pain may result in restlessness, agitation, and confusion. Besides surgical pain, occult causes of discomfort may include tight surgical dressings, bladder or gastric distention, IV infiltration, and nausea. Because natural sleep patterns may be disturbed for several days after surgery, it is important to allow patients to remain aware of the light-dark cycle, and to keep patients oriented to time of day.

Patients with preoperative dementia and cognitive dysfunction are at increased risk for surgical complications after general,[342] orthopedic,[343,344] and cardiac[345] surgical procedures. This knowledge must be conveyed to patients and their families during preoperative counseling.

Idiopathic Intracranial Hypertension

Idiopathic intracranial hypertension (IIH), also known as pseudotumor cerebri or benign intracranial hypertension, is a syndrome which results in elevated intracranial pressure without an intracranial mass lesion. Because the disease often results in visual loss, the term *benign* intracranial hypertension is no longer favored.

Of patients with IIH, more than 90 percent are women and more than 90 percent are obese.[346] Patients with systemic arterial hypertension also have a higher incidence of the disease.[347] The diagnosis may be made from childhood all through the adult years, with most patients being diagnosed in the fourth decade of life.

The cause of IIH remains unknown. The most likely etiology is a disturbance of CSF reabsorption by the arachnoid granulations. Reduced conductance to CSF outflow would require that intracranial pressure rises until CSF resorption equals production. Brain parenchyma demonstrates increases in interstitial fluid content and intracellular water content, a factor which would cause reductions in brain elastance and prevent ventricular dilation. In fact, hydrocephalus is not an accompaniment of IIH.

Medical disorders which may secondarily cause intracranial hyptertension must be ruled out before making the diagnosis of IIH. These disorders can be grouped into: (1) disease of the arachnoid granulations secondary to inflammatory scarring (meningitis, subarachnoid hemorrhage), (2) obstruction to venous drainage (venous sinus thrombosis, bilateral neck dissection, superior vena cava syndrome, elevated right heart pressure), (3) endocrine disorders (Addison's disease, hypoparathyroidism, steroid withdrawal), (4) AV malformations, and (5) other, including hypervitaminosis A and drug reaction, especially to tetracycline.[346]

The diagnosis of IIH is based on clinical examination with confirmatory imaging and lab studies. Headache is nearly ubiquitous and is the most common presenting symptom, often being described as nonlocalized, pulsatile, worse in the morning, and exacerbated by Valsalva maneuver and movement. Nausea frequently occurs. Over half of patients report visual obscurations and pulsatile intracranial noise, and about one-third complain of diplopia or visual loss. Several other complaints are common, indicating retrobulbar pain, shoulder/arm pain, motor incoordination, and weakness and numbness.

On examination, papilledema is the most common physical finding, but its absence does not rule out the diagnosis of IIH, especially in children.[348] Visual field defects and loss of visual acuity are due to optic nerve compression and neuronal death as a consequence of increased intracranial pressure. About one-fourth of patients have demonstrable VI nerve palsy, a false localizing sign caused by increased intracranial pressure. Consciousness and mentation are normal and despite the plethora of complaints, the remaining neurologic exam is usually normal.

Prior to lumbar puncture (LP), the presence of a CSF pathway obstruction or mass lesion causing papilledema is ruled out by CT or MR head scan. When brain stem findings are present, special effort must be made to image the posterior fossa. In patients with IIH, the brain is normal in appearance by CT or MRI, with normal or small ventricles. Specific MRI windows may demonstrate increased brain water.

The LP should demonstrate an opening pressure >200 mmH$_2$O in the non-obese and >250 mmH$_2$O in the obese patient. The CSF should otherwise be normal.

The goal of treatment is to relieve symptoms and to prevent permanent loss of vision. Treatment of blood pressure and weight reduction are effective in some patients. Failing that, corticosteroids and diuretics are the most commonly used medications to treat IIH. Steroids are effective but require a fairly long therapeutic duration and taper. Acetazolamide, a carbonic anhydrase inhibitor, decreases CSF production and reduces papilledema at doses of 1 to 4 g/day. Furosemide may also be effective therapy, but thiazide and other diuretics are less helpful.

Surgical intervention (optic nerve sheath fenestration or lumbar subarachnoid-peritoneal shunt) are reserved for those patients with intractable headache or progressive visual loss despite medical therapy.

ANESTHESIA FOR THE PATIENT WITH IDIOPATHIC INTRACRANIAL HYPERTENSION

Careful preoperative documentation of the current visual abnormalities is important to adequately assess postoperative dysfunction. A thorough medication history is taken to discover recent (within 1 year) use of steroids and to document current diuretic usage. Patients who may be adrenally suppressed due to recent steroid ingestion should have perioperative stress steroid coverage.

For patients taking acetazolamide, a metabolic acidosis may develop which would make these patients more susceptible to hypoventilation-induced respiratory acidosis. For patients taking other diuretics, hypokalemia may develop. In either case, blood chemistry should be analyzed prior to surgery.

Patients with the diagnosis of IIH will have had CT or MRI of the head during their diagnostic work-up. If these patients have remained stable, then spinal or epidural anesthesia is safe, since lumbar CSF drainage is in fact therapeutic.[349,350] For patients whose signs and symptoms of the process have worsened since last being imaged, an enhanced CT or MRI should be repeated preoperatively to rule out development of a mass lesion or obstructive hydrocephalus as the primary cause of intracranial hypertension. Dural puncture in this case could result in tonsillar herniation of the brain. In patients with a lumbar shunt, it is probably best to avoid spinal or epidural anesthesia unless it can be ascertained that the path of the needle will not impinge on the catheter.

General anesthesia can be safely performed in IIH if drugs and techniques are used that prevent increases in intracranial pressure. It would seem prudent to use inhaled and intravenous drugs which do not increase the rate of CSF formation or the resistance to absorption. These drugs include isoflurane, N_2O, etomidate, pentothal, propofol, and the opioids (alfentanil, fentanyl, and sufentanil).[351]

Subacute Combined Degeneration

Subacute combined degeneration (SCD) is a myeloneuropathy affecting the spinal cord, brain, optic nerves, and peripheral nerves. Vitamin B_{12} (cobalamin) deficiency is the most common cause, but folate deficiency has also been reported to cause SCD.[352] In 1978, Layzer[353] reported on 15 patients who developed clinical signs and symptoms of SCD after abuse of or occupational exposure to N_2O. It is now well established that N_2O, which inactivates cobalamin by irreversibly oxidizing the cobalt core from the active reduced Co (I) state to the inactive Co (III) state,[354] can, in some patients, cause a functional B_{12} deficiency which results in a neurologic disease indistinguishable from SCD. Methylcobalamine is an essential cofactor in the enzymatic conversion of homocysteine and methyltetrahydrofolate to methionine and tetrahydrofolate by methionine synthase. Methionine is the precursor for S-adenosylmethionine (SAM) which is required for methylation reactions during myelin synthesis. While SAM does not appear to be depleted in neural tissue of animals with experimentally induced cobalamin deficiency, methionine is protective against the onset of SCD. Still, the exact mechanism by which cobalamin deficiency and methionine synthase dysfunction cause SCD remains uncertain.[355-357]

The neuropathy of SCD takes the form of demyelination and axonal loss primarily in the posterior and lateral columns of the spinal cord. The process usually begins in the upper or midthoracic region, spreading both longitudinally along the spinal cord and anteriorly to involve the anterior columns. The brain and peripheral nerves are affected more rarely.

Symptoms of the disease are related to dysfunction of the posterior columns, corticospinal tract, spinothalamic tracts, and peripheral nerves. Parasthesias of the hands and feet, numbness, unsteady gait, muscle stiffness and weakness, and eventually paraplegia are the usual presentation.

On examination, loss of vibration sense is the most consistent finding, along with loss of proprioception. Motor signs may include muscle weakness, spasticity, and clonus. The patient may exhibit Lhermitte's sign (sudden electric-like shocks extending down the spine on flexing the head). The patellar and Achilles reflexes are variable, depending on whether peripheral, sensory, or motor tracts are most affected. The gait is ataxic, progressing to weakness, spasticity, and eventually to paraplegia. Mental signs are frequent, including confusion, depression, personality changes, and dementia. The majority of affected patients will exhibit the megaloblastic anemia characteristic of vitamin B_{12} deficiency. However, a large subset of patients with SCD can have a normal hematocrit and normal mean cell volume.[358] When cobalamin deficiency is suspected, serum B_{12} deficiency is verified by serum assay. MRI can reveal the spinal cord abnormalities.[259] Treatment of SCD is with intramuscular B_{12} (and folate in confirmed cases of folate deficiency). The response to treatment depends primarily on the duration of the illness: Full recovery can be expected if therapy is instituted within a few weeks of onset of symptoms, but in longstanding disease only a halting of the progression of the disease can be expected.[360]

N_2O-INDUCED NEUROPATHY

In vitro, N_2O has been shown to oxidize the cobalt ion in cobalamin, therby rendering cobalamin inactive.[354] N_2O may also inactivate methionine synthase through the action of hydroxy free radicals formed by the interaction of N_2O with the cobalamin.[356] At a 50% concentration in humans, N_2O inhibits the activity of hepatic methionine synthase by about 50 percent after 2 h, with activity declining almost linearly with longer exposure.[361,362] The duration of methionine synthase inhibition after exposure to N_2O is uncertain but appears to be several days.[363]

Most reports of N_2O-induced neuropathy, proposed recently to be termed "anesthesia paresthetica,"[364] have occurred in patients who received prolonged or repeated exposure to N_2O, or who had overt, borderline, or subclinical cobalamin deficiency.[353,359,364,365-369]

Several agents may be protective against or reverse the adverse effects of N_2O. Methionine, a product of the enzyme inhibited by N_2O, may counteract the effects of N_2O both at a biochemical level and after clinical signs have appeared.[363,367] Folinic acid (formyltetrahydrofolic acid, leucovorin) appears to be protective against measurable biochemical abnormalities of DNA synthesis caused by N_2O.[356] The hydroxy-radical scavenger dimethylthiourea has been shown to diminish N_2O-induced inactivation of methionine synthase, lending credence to the hypothesis that N_2O inactivates the enzyme through formation of free radicals.[370] Finally, administration of B_{12} prior to N_2O exposure does *not* appear to be protective against N_2O-induced neuropathy, against substantiating the theory of cobalamin-N_2O interactions being causative.

Thus, in susceptible patients, N_2O can cause the neurologic syndrome of SCD. Patients at risk include those with known vitamin B_{12} deficiency, laboratory evidence of megaloblastic anemia, and those with low cobalamin stores due to pernicious anemia, HIV infection, B_{12} deficient vegetarian diets, gastric resection, and old age.[356] The use of N_2O in these groups of patients should be avoided.

Abnormal Central Nervous System Drug Responses

ANTIPSYCHOTIC DRUGS AND OTHER DOPAMINE AGONISTS

DRUG-INDUCED DYSTONIAS

Acute dystonic reactions may occur secondary to neuroleptics and other dopamine antagonists, especially in young males. Symptoms include involuntary movements of limbs, facial grimacing, torticollis, oculogyric crisis, tongue protrusion, trismus, opisthotonus, and, rarely, laryngospasm. Metoclopramide and promethazine (both dopamine antagonists) may rarely be associated with these reactions in cumulative preoperative and postoperative doses.[371] Treatment begins with abrupt withdrawal of the etiologic medication and giving parenteral diphenhydramine hydrochloride (50 mg) or benztropine mesylate (1 to 2 mg). An oral anticholinergic should be continued every 4 to 6 h over the next 24 to 48 h, especially if the inciting agent was given as a depot injection.

TARDIVE DYSKINESIAS

Tardive dyskinesia (TD) consists of hyperkinetic stereotyped movements, typically of the face, tongue, neck, and limbs.[372] The pathophysiology is believed to involve supersensitivity of the dopamine receptors of the striatonigral pathway secondary to chronic dopamine blockade. Antipsychotic medications are most often causative, but TD may also occur following treatment with the antiemetics promethazine, prochlorperazine, and metaclopramide. Approximately 20 percent of patients develop TD after long-term neuroleptic use.[373] Up to 80 percent of patients treated with levodopa for Parkinson disease develop dyskinesias late in the disease and course of therapy.[374]

Neuroleptic-induced TD usually occurs after at least 3 months of therapy.[375] Advanced age is a risk factor for acquiring TD, as probably are both length of drug exposure and cumulative drug dose. Female sex, organic mental disorder, and maximum drug dosage have also been reported as risk factors.[373,376,377]

Neuroleptic-induced TD is frequently irreversible. Withdrawal of medication is desirable if possible. This should be done slowly to decrease the potential of a psychotic relapse and possible worsening of the dyskinesia. When the neuroleptic is stopped, the sensitized

dopamine receptors are unblocked and a worsening of movement may occur. In patients who tolerate a gradual neuroleptic taper there may be some improvement, but rarely is there complete resolution of symptoms. Treatment with reserpine is sometimes helpful, but its anticholinergic side effects and association with depression limit its use. Recent reports suggest that benzodiazepines may help alleviate movements by suppressing the GABA receptors of the striatonigral pathway.[378,379] Calcium channel blockers,[380–383] vitamin E,[384,385] propranolol,[386–388] clonidine,[389–391] and bromocriptine[392] have also been found effective in small studies. Increasing the neuroleptic will often suppress the abnormal movements for a while, but the underlying pathologic process is worsened with a poorer prognosis in the long term.

Levodopa dyskinesias resolve when the levodopa dose is decreased.[374] Unfortunately, the alternative to dyskinesias in Parkinson disease is often profound bradykinesia or akinesia and many patients prefer dramatic dyskinesias to complete loss of function. Pallidotomy may be an option for some patients who have progressed beyond the benefit of medical management (see "Parkinson's Disease," above).[393]

Respiratory dyskinesia is of special interest to anesthesiologists. Usually seen in the context of typical TD, it may occur in isolation. It is defined as an irregular, tachypneic pattern of breathing due to respiratory muscle involvement of TD.[394] Affected patients complain of shortness of breath and have uncompensated respiratory alkalosis. It has been theorized that the respiratory alkalosis is uncompensated due to its intermittency, since TD resolves with sleep.[395] Pharyngeal dyskinesia associated with dysphagia and laryngeal dyskinesia associated with grunts, gasps, and interrupted speech often accompany the respiratory problem. Complications reported in addition to the uncompensated respiratory alkalosis include respiratory compromise and aspiration pneumona.[396–398] Similar to other forms of TD, respiratory dyskinesia may occur as a result of neuroleptic, antiemetic, or levodopa use and, more rarely, idiopathically.

NEUROLEPTIC MALIGNANT SYNDROME

Neuroleptic malignant syndrome (NMS) is an idiosyncratic reaction that occurs in one of two pharmacologic settings:

1. After withdrawal of dopaminergic agonists used for treatment of Parkinsonism
2. After administration of drugs that cause central dopaminergic blockade of the striatum. These drugs would include many drugs used in the perioperative period (chlorpromazine droperidol, metoclopramide, compazine), neuroleptics used primarily in

TABLE 12-13
Neuroleptic Malignant Syndrome Etiologic Agents

Neuroleptic Drugs

Phenothiazines
Butyrophenones
Thioxanthenes
Other Dopamine antagonists
  Metoclopramide (Reglan)
  Sulpride
  Sultopride
  Zuclopenthixol
  Tetrabenazine

Nonneuroleptic Agents

Tricyclic antidepressants
  Desipramine (Norpramin, Pertofrane)
  Amoxapine (Asendin)
  Maptrotiline (Ludiomil)
  Trimipramine
  Dothiepin
  Amitriptyline (Elavil)
  Fluoxetine (Prozac)

Monoamine oxidase inhibitors
  Phenelzine (Nardil)

Benzodiazepines
  Diazepam (Valium)
  Lorazepam (Ativan)

Anticonvulsants
  Carbamazepine (Tegretol)
  Phenytoin (Dilantin)

Withdrawal parkinsonian medication
  Ethopropazine (Parsidol)
  Levodopa/Carbidopa (Sinemet)
  Amantadine
  Bromocriptine (Parlodel)

Lithium
  With Clozapine
  With Carbamazapine
  With Phenelzine
  With Chlorpromazine
  With antiparkinsonian agents
  With Doxepin

Estrogen
  Possible trigger in patients on neuroleptics

SOURCE: From Lev R, Clark RF: Neuroleptic malignant syndrome presenting without fever: Case report and review of the literature. *J Emerg Med* 1994; 12:49, with permission.

psychiatry (butyrophenones, phenothiazines, and thioxanthenes), and many other drugs (Table 12-13). NMS most often occurs when these drugs are administered at dosages within the therapeutic range.[399] NMS occurs in about 1 in 100 to 1 in 1000 patients treated with neuroleptic medications.[400] Since other drugs besides neuroleptics can cause the illness, the name "drug-induced central hyperthermic syndrome" has been proposed, a term which identifies the pathophysiology and distinguishes the disease from malignant hyperthermia.[401]

Because dopamine is an integral neurotransmitter both in thermoregulatory neural pathways of the hypothalamus and in striatal motor projections, interference with dopaminergic activity can lead to impairment of temperature regulation and drug-induced parkinsonism. Fever results from altered thermoregulation in the face of increased thermogenesis due to exaggerated muscle activity, such as tremor and/or rigidity. Thus NMS should be suspected in the proper pharmacologic setting when parkinsonism or other movement disorders, such as dystonia, are associated with fever. Autonomic instability, altered mental status, and elevation in creatine kinase may be present.[400] Criteria for diagnosing NMS are listed in Table 12-14.[402] Metabolic changes in peripheral skeletal muscle have also been implicated in the pathogenesis of the disease.[403]

The onset of NMS can occur hours to days after administration of neuroleptic drugs or withdrawal of antiparkinson drugs. While NMS has been reported to present without fever, hyperthermia and increased muscle tone occur in close to 100 percent of patients with NMS.[399] Temperatures as high as 41°C have been reported.

The rigidity of NMS is commonly the lead-pipe type, but akinesia, dyskinesia, waxy flexibility, and cogwheeling have been reported. Involvement of the chest wall may impair ventilation. Dysautonomia may present as pallor, diaphoresis, tachycardia, cardiac arrhythmias, and blood pressure swings. Nearly all patients will have mental status changes including confusion, delirium, agitation, or frank coma. No laboratory studies are diagnostic. The CPK is usually elevated because of unrelenting muscle contraction. There may be lactic acidosis superimposed on respiratory acidosis. Death is usually due to respiratory insufficiency of aspiration pneumonia.[404]

Fever and movement disorder may also be seen in a variety of other clinical situations (Table 12-15). Encephalitis and meningitis may have a similar presentation, as may idiopathic or drug-induced parkinsonism with ongoing infection, heat stroke, malignant hyperthermia, and alcohol or benzodiazepine withdrawal.

TABLE 12-14
Criteria for the Diagnosis of NMS

Major Criteria	Minor Criteria
Fever	Tachycardia
Rigidity	Abnormal blood pressure
Elevated serum CPK	Tachypnea
	Altered level of consciousness
	Diaphoresis
	Leukocytosis

SOURCE: From Levenson JL: Neuroleptic malignant syndrome. *Am J Psychiat* 1985; 142:1137, with permission.

TABLE 12-15
Differential Diagnosis of Neuroleptic Malignant Syndrome

Primary Central Nervous System Disorders

Infections (viral encephalitis, human immunodeficiency virus, postinfectious encephalomyelitis)

Tumors

Cerebrovascular accidents

Seizures

Major psychoses (lethal catatonia)

Systemic Disorders

Infections

Metabolic conditions

Endocrinopathies (thyroid storm, pheochromocytoma)

Autoimmune disease (systemic lupus erythematosus)

Heatstroke

Toxins (salicylates, dopamine inhibitors and antagonists, stimulants, psychedelics, monoamine oxidase-inhibitors, anesthetics, anticholinergics, alcohol or sedative withdrawal)

SOURCE: From Caroff SN, Mann SC: Neuroleptic malignant syndrome. *Med Clin North Am* 1993; 77:185, with permission.

Lethal catatonia, a psychiatric disorder resulting in continuous uncontrollable motor activity and hyperthermia, is often included in the differential diagnosis. Central anticholinergic syndrome may cause fever and abnormal motor responses and physostigmine should be therapeutic in this condition. Monoamine oxidase inhibitors taken in conjunction with meperidine or tricyclic antidepressants or selective serotonin reuptake inhibitors can cause a NMS-like syndrome termed "serotonin syndrome."[405]

The initial treatment of NMS is supportive. Neuroleptic medication is stopped. Adequate oxygenation and ventilation are assured if necessary, with tracheal intubation, mechanical ventilation, and muscle paralysis. Nondepolarizing muscle relaxants will provide paralysis in NMS. Hyperpyrexia is treated with cooling blankets, cool water baths, and antipyretics. Cardiovascular stability is achieved with fluid and vasopressors in the hypotensive patient, and with vasodilators or β-blockers when severe hypertension is present. Dantrolene can improve the muscle rigidity and aid in lowering fever, but an improvement in mortality has not been consistently demonstrated with the use of dantrolene.[406] The dopamine agonists, levodopa-carbidopa (Sinemet), amantadine, and bromocriptine can shorten the duration of the illness and probably lessen mortality.[399] A stepped approach to drug therapy based on the degree of temperature elevation has been proposed.[406] When myoglobinuria is present, vigorous fluid therapy and alkalization of the urine are necessary to prevent renal failure.

Since 1980 the overall mortality of NMS has declined from 30 to 10 percent or less.[399,407] Excess mortality occurs when NMS is associated with myoglobinemia and renal failure.

Patients with a history of NMS may present for surgery. It is probably safe to rechallenge patients with antidopaminergic drugs if their use is felt necessary, but a period of at least 2 weeks should have passed since recovery from the acute episode.[399,408]

Succinylcholine has been used many times in patients with NMS, although a case of succinylcholine-induced hyperkalemia has been reported.[409] Nondepolarizing muscle relaxants are safe to use. Patients with a history of NMS have been repeatedly anesthetized with volatile anesthetics, emphasizing the basic difference in pathophysiology between NMS and malignant hyperthermia.

LITHIUM

Abnormal neurologic response to lithium may include choreoathetotic, dystonic movements of the trunk and limb, diffuse myoclonus, and perioral tremor, all probably due to hypersensitivity of dopamine receptors in the basal ganglia because of receptor blockade with antipsychotic medication.[410,411]

Therapeutic levels of lithium range from 0.5 to 1.5 meq/liter. Even with therapeutic levels, ECG changes can occur with QRS widening and atrioventricular heart block, as well as hypotension. Besides the dyskinetic symptoms seen at or above 1.5 meq/liter, dizziness, nystagmus, stuttering, nausea, diarrhea, fatigue, polydipsia, and polyuria may occur. At levels of 3.5 meq/liter, the symptoms may resemble those of Creutzfeldt-Jakob disease.

There are a number of important drug interactions seen with lithium. The loss of sodium due to diuretics may increase the serum lithium concentration and bring about the symptoms of lithium toxicity. The duration of action of succinylcholine and pancuronium may be prolonged with lithium.[412,413]

It has been shown that acetazolamide may impair the proximal tubular reabsorption of lithium ions, increasing lithium excretion.[414] Haloperidol and lithium combine to have an inhibitory effect on striatal adenylate cyclase which may result in extrapyramidal symptoms.[415] It has also been noted that indomethacin (and possibly ibuprofen) reduces renal lithium clearance and increases the lithium levels. This may be due to indomethacin-induced prostaglandin inhibition.[416] Lithium toxicity was also noted in patients given methyldopa after being on stabilized lithium therapy.[417,418]

The information on lithium described above indicates the need for vigilance in the anesthetic evaluation of a large segment of our psychiatric population with bipolar disorder who have been treated with lithium.

ALCOHOL

In this section we will briefly review some of the effects of alcohol on the CNS and drug interactions, and relate the anesthetic implication concerning the use and abuse of this drug. It has been noted by Courville that ". . . alcohol is the most common form of poisoning."[419] In 1985, an estimated 10.6 million Americans were dependent on alcohol with another 7.3 million being involved in some variant of abuse with this substance. About 10 percent of occupational injuries and nearly 50 percent of marital violence can be attributed to alcohol, with 40 percent of the traffic deaths also being related to ethanol. Alcoholism is indeed a protean disease affecting many corporeal systems, especially the CNS.[420]

Ethanol has a depressive effect on the CNS. It is metabolized in the liver and several enzyme systems are utilized. Ethanol, with its principal metabolite acetaldehyde and its intermediaries, many of which are free radicals, has the potential to trigger diverse reactions including CNS cell aggregates.[421] Its global effects include altering platelet metabolism[422]; increasing the risk for hemorrhagic stroke,[423] reducing blood linoleic acid levels and inducing or exaggerating essential fatty acid (EFA) deficiency states; and blocking metabolism of linoleic acid to EFA metabolites which are important in brain structure, and enhancing conversion of the linoleic acid metabolite dihomo-betalinoleic acid to prostaglandin E_1. These effects noted above may explain the euphoria seen with ethanol, the fatty liver, and the alcohol withdrawal syndrome[424]; the production spasms of cerebral blood vessels[425] as an important cause of "essential" hypertension[426] and the fetal alcohol syndrome since it crosses the placenta; involving the endorphin system and subsequent psychogenics of drug-seeking behavior[427]; and altering the function of the NMDA system in the brain.[428] Ethanol can also be found to increase factor VIII coagulant activity, VIII-related antigen, and VIII ristocetin cofactor, providing an explanation as to why intoxication with ethanol increases susceptibility to cerebral thrombosis,[429] producing an increase in bilateral CBF[430] with intoxication. Ethanol can develop a very toxic addictive homologue called cocaethylene (COCE) when mixed with cocaine. COCE has a half-life more than three times that of cocaine and may explain the cocaine-related heart attacks or stroke when cocaine levels are low.[431]

Ethanol is an analgesic equivalent to intravenous morphine and superior to saline.[432] It has also been evaluated as an agent for induction of anesthesia by

Dundee and Isaac.[433] They noted that the dose required for sleep showed a wide variation and methohexital was often needed to complete the induction. The incidence of emergence delirium was high and recovery delayed when supplemental methohexital was used.

We will touch upon some of the important clinical CNS responses including the abstinence syndrome, Wernicke-Korsakoff Syndrome, polyneuropathy, and the fetal alcohol syndrome.

The abstinence (or withdrawal) syndrome has both a *minor* and a *major* form. The minor or early syndrome can demonstrate nausea and vomiting, flushed facies, insomnia, diaphoresis, convulsions, and visual and auditory hallucinations. Usually these symptoms begin within 7 to 8 h after drinking is halted, peak within 24 h, and subside over several days. In a few patients, these early symptoms of alcohol withdrawal may herald delirium tremens (DTs). The major withdrawal form, called the DTs, manifests as confusion; tremor and jactitations; delusions and hallucinations; and autonomic hyperactivity such as fever and diaphoresis, tachycardia, and dilated pupils. Unlike the early form, the DTs begin 48 to 96 h after drinking has stopped, with peak onset about 72 h. Although the major is less frequent than the minor, it is generally more serious, with a 5 to 10 percent mortality.

Treatment of the minor withdrawal and the major DT symptoms should be oriented to correct any fluid and electrolyte imbalance that may exist; hence the need for a blood chemistry profile with electrolytes, liver, renal, and glucose profiles. An ECG and chest and skull films, as well as a CT scan of the brain, should be carried out to rule out cardiac, pulmonary, and intracranial pathology, since associated injuries are not uncommon. Appropriate fluids should be given to correct any electrolyte and hypovolemia problems. Glucose solutions should be used sparingly since these patients are probably thiamine and B vitamin deficient and may be propelled into Wernicke's syndrome by using up the remaining stores of B_1. In the minor withdrawal syndrome, the therapeutic goal is to put the patient at rest and enhance sleep. Numerous drugs have been used to control withdrawal symptoms, ranging from the phenothiazines to the benzodiazepines, yet the superiority of these drugs over oral paraldehyde has not been proven in a randomized controlled study.[434,435] Medications such as diazepam (10 mg), or midazolam (2 mg), can be given parenterally, and repeated at 30-min intervals until the patient is calm, yet awake. In the case of withdrawal seizures, anticonvulsants are generally not needed since these seizures begin very early during the withdrawal and probably have stopped by the time medical treatment is available. On the other hand, status epilepticus secondary to ethanol withdrawal should be treated as status due to any other etiology. In general, Wernicke's disease is a reversible entity.

The Wernicke-Korsakoff syndrome[436,437] (WKS) is usually applied to the alcoholic with a background of nutritional deficiency (especially the B vitamin group), who has impaired retentive memory combined with ophthalmoplegia, ataxia, and problems in mentation. It must be pointed out that Wernicke's disease may be seen in patients who are not alcoholics. The Korsakoff psychosis (usually severe and irreversible), where the patient may be alert and responsive yet have a severe impairment of retentive memory, can also be observed in other neurologic conditions (such as in temporal lobe infarctions, 3d ventricular tumors, or after herpes simplex encephalitis). The mortality rate from acute Wernicke's disease is about 17 percent and those who respond to treatment with thiamine start to improve within hours or days—with alleviation of the ocular symptoms being extraordinarily dramatic. About 40 percent of these patients recover completely from their ataxia within 3 to 4 weeks after commencement of treatment. While many of the mental symptoms clear quickly after thiamine administration, the amnestic symptoms may recover incompletely. Treatment of WKS involves use of B complex vitamins with large doses of B_1 in the acute stage (50 to 100 mg IV and IM) and balanced diet. Care should be taken about the use of glucose during the acute phase since it may deplete the already low stores of B_1 and further exacerbate the WKS. All patients with a history of WKS or severe alcoholics who are having surgery should be given B complex vitamins, added to the intravenous solutions the night before and prior to entering the surgical suite.

It is thought that the polyneuropathy found associated with alcoholics[438] involves depletion of nutritional components, particularly the B vitamin complex. Symptomatic patients demonstrate weakness, paresthesias, and pain—often referred to the distal portion of the limbs which can progress proximally if no treatment is initiated. The lower extremities appear to be affected before the upper ones. The paresthesias include constant aches in the legs, sharp pains, cramping and tightness in muscles of feet and calves, burning feelings in soles, sweating of soles and hands and fingers, and postural hypotension. Again, treatment consists of adequate nutrition including the B vitamin complex. It would be wise to avoid conduction anesthesia in these patients.

The fetal alcohol syndrome (FAS) is important because of the significant number of congenital anomalies that arise from this condition. It has been reported that the FAS may be the major cause of mental retardation in the West with a worldwide incidence of 1.9 per 1000 live births.[439,440] Most of the cases reported have been in infants born to severely alcoholic mothers who imbibed during their pregnancy. Many of these newborns are hyperactive and irritable, resembling those with alcohol withdrawal. Pathologically, cerebellar malformations, schizencephaly, agenesis of the corpus callosum, and arrhinencephaly have been reported.[441]

Disulfiram[442] (DS) has had a renaissance in the past decade as a means of sensitizing the alcoholic to ethanol in a supervised program. It is thought that DS markedly accelerates the metabolism of ethanol into acetaldehyde causing nausea, vomiting, flushing, tachycardia, dypsnea, and blurred vision vertigo. There is also an increased serum phenytoin[443] level within 4 h of administration of the first dose of DS. In patients on DS, the dose of phenytoin should be reduced. Along the same lines, DS increases the hypothrombonemic effect and plasma levels of warfarin.[444] Similarly, the dose of oral anticoagulant should be decreased or if possible, stopped. Because of the potentially hazardous side effects, all medication should be checked for alcohol content prior to oral intake. Patients with pulmonary and cardiac problems should be cautioned about the side effects of DS.

Summary

Patients with a variety of neurologic syndromes and disorders, both rare and common, will periodically need surgical interventions. Knowledge of the overt and occult disease processes associated with the illness will allow physicians to provide optimal perioperative care. An index of rare neurologic syndromes not otherwise addressed in this textbook is provided in Table 12-16.

TABLE 12-16
Index of Neurologic Syndromes and Their Anesthetic Implications

Name	Description	Anesthetic Implications
Albright's osteodystrophy (pseudohypoparathyroidism)	Ectopic bone formation. Mental retardation. Rare familial disease.	Hypocalcemia—Possible ECG conduction defects, neuromuscular problems. Convulsions.
Alport syndrome	Nephritis and nerve deafness. Renal pathology variable.	Renal failure in 2d–3d decade. Care with drugs excreted via kidneys.
Alström syndrome	Obesity, blindness by seven years. Hearing loss. Diabetes after puberty—glomerulosclerosis.	Renal impairment. Management of diabetes and obesity.
Ataxia-telangiectasia	Cerebellar ataxia. Skin and conjunctival telangiectasia. Decreased serum IgA & IgE. 10% development reticuloendothelial malignancy. Diabetes.	Defective immunity—recurrent pulmonary and sinus infections. Bronchiectasis.
Central core disease	Congenital myopathy. Hypotonia and proximal weakness.	Risk for malignant hyperthermia. Sensitive to thiopental. Care with muscle relaxants.
Charcot-Marie-Tooth[445,446] (peroneal muscular atrophy)	Peripheral neuropathy affecting muscles of feet and legs, then hands and arms and muscles of respiration, cardiac arrhythmias.	Respiratory muscle involvement. Normal response to succinylcholine and nondepolarizing relaxants in chronic disease. Avoid succinylcholine in acute disease.
Cockayne syndrome[447]	Mental retardation, premature aging, microcephaly, hypertension, renal insufficiency, diabetes, emphysema, asthma, blindness, multiple organ involvement.	Difficult intubation, asthma, hypothermia, fragile skin.
Conradi's syndrome (Condrodystrophia calcificans congenita)	Chondrodystrophy with contractures, saddle nose, mental retardation. Associated congenital heart disease and renal anomalies.	Problems are those of associated renal and cardiac disease.
Craniosynostoses		
Apert's syndrome	Acrocephalosyndactyly. Relative prognathism. Mental retardation.	Difficult intubation. Possibly raised intracranial pressure, associated congenital heart disease.
Carpenter's syndrome	Acrocephalosyndactyly. Associated congenital heart disease.	Hypoplastic mandible. Possibly difficult intubation.
Chotzen syndrome	Acrocephalosyndactyly. Beaked nose with deviated nasal septum, prognathism.	May be difficult intubation. Associated renal anomalies and possible impaired renal excretion of drugs.
Noack's syndrome	Craniosynostosis and digital anomalies. Obesity.	May be difficult to intubate because of skull deformity.
Cretinism (congenital hypothyroidism)	Absent thyroid tissue or defective synthesis thyroxine and goiter.	Airway problems—large tongue, goiter. Respiratory center very sensitive to depression. CO_2 retention common. Hypoglycemia, hyponatremia, hypotension. Low cardiac output. Transfusion poorly tolerated.
Cri-du-Chat syndrome	Chromosome 5-P abnormal. Abnormal cry, microcephaly micrognathia. Congenital heart disease.	Airway problems—stridor, laryngomalacia. Possibly difficult intubation.
Familial periodic paralysis	Episodic weakness associated with hypokalemia. Also hyperkalemic and normokalemic forms. Overlap with hyperthyroidism and paramyotonia congenita.	Monitor serum K+. Limit use of dextrose. Monitor ECG. Avoid relaxants.
Farber's disease (lipogranulomatosis)	Sphingomyelin deposition. Widespread visceral lipogranulomas especially in the central nervous system.	Deposits in larynx—careful intubation. Generalized systemic involvement leading to cardiac, renal failure.
Friedreich's ataxia[448]	Ataxia, dysarthria, cardiomyopathy, diabetes, scoliosis, restrictive lung disease, upper and lower motor neuron disease.	Preoperative cardiac evaluation, risk of cardiac failure, abnormal response to muscle relaxants, probable hyperkalemic response to succinylcholine.
Glycogen Storage Diseases		
Von Gierke's disease Type I	Hepatomegaly, enlarged kidneys, severe attacks of hypoglycemia.	Monitor blood sugar and acid-base balance (IV glucose infusion). Diazoxide for hypoglycemia.
Pompe's disease Type II	Muscle deposits—severe hypotonicity. Massive cardiomegaly. Death before 2 years of age.	Extreme care, avoidance respiratory depressants, muscle relaxants, cardiac depressants. Large tongue may cause airway problem.

TABLE 12-16
Index of Neurologic Syndromes and Their Anesthetic Implications (*Continued*)

Name	Description	Anesthetic Implications
Glycogen Storage Diseases (*Continued*)		
Forke's disease Type III	Hepatomegaly, hypoglycemia, growth retardation, proximal and distal myopathy in some patients.	
Anderson's disease Type IV	Debrancher enzyme deficiency.	Possibility of hypoglycemia under anesthesia.
McArdle's disease Type V	Cramping and weakness of muscles with exercise.	Muscles affected including cardiac muscle; care with cardiac depressant drugs.
Hallervorden-Spatz disease[449]	Iron deposits in globus pallidus, substantia nigra, and red nucleus. Dementia, dystonia, scoliosis, facial spasm.	Airway fixation, possible hyperkalemic response to succinylcholine. Limited pulmonary reserve.
Histiocytosis X (Hand-Schuller-Christian and Letterer-Siwe Disease)	Histiocytic granulomata in viscera and bones, lungs, larynx, teeth loss.	Laryngeal fibrosis, pulmonary infiltration, respiratory failure, cor pulmonale, DI with sella turcica involvement, steroid history, pancytopenia.
Holoprosencephaly[450]	Facial abnormalities, mental retardation, temperature instability, seizures, apnea, cardiac defects (dextrocardia, septal defects).	Difficult airway, temperature swings, apnea, limited cardiac reserve, hypoglycemia.
Klinefelter syndrome (gonosomal aneuploidy)	Tall stature, reduced intelligence. Vertebral collapse due to osteoporosis. High incidence of psychosis, asthma, diabetes, and mediastinal tumors.	No described anesthetic problem. Care in positioning.
Klippel-Feil syndrome	Congenital fusion two or more cervical vertebrae leading to neck rigidity.	Difficult airway and intubation.
Klippel-Trenaunay-Weber syndrome (angio-osteohypertrophy)	Vascular malformation of the spinal cord with vascular cutaneous nevi, hypertrophy of extremity, and thrombocytopenia.	Arteriovenous fistulae and anemia lead to high cardiac output state. Thrombocytopenia in visceral hemangiomata.
Laurence-Moon-Biedl syndrome	Obesity, retinitis pigmentosa. Polydactyly. Mental retardation.	May be associated with cardiac defects, renal disease and occasionally diabetes insipidus.
Lesch-Nyhan syndrome	Hyperuricemia and mental retardation. Renal failure by age ten years.	High serum uric acid leads to red cell damage and renal stones. Care with renally excreted drugs.
Leukodystrophy[451]	Inherited defect in formation of myelin; spasticity, arrested development, motor dysfunction, scoliosis, poor upper airway control, seizures, movement disorder.	Risk of aspiration, seizures, temperature fluctuations, ? succinylcholine-induced hyperkalemia, increased respiratory depression.
Adrenoleukodystrophy	Hypoadrenalism.	
Alexander disease	Onset <1 year of age.	
Canavan disease	Macrocephaly, increased water content of brain, increased cell membrane permeability.	
Krabbe disease	Onset at 4–6 months.	
Metachromatic leukodystrophy	Fever, abdominal pain, gallbladder disease.	
Pelizaeus-Merybacker	Progressive CNS deterioration.	
Lipid Storage diseases		
Fabry disease	Ceramide deposits in cells of blood vessels, renal tubules, and nerve cells. Lancinating neuropathic pain.	Cerebrovascular symptoms—hypertension, myocardial ischemia (before 3d or 4th decade). Renal failure. Care with renally excreted drugs. Brain infarctions.
Gaucher disease	Cerebroside accumulation in CNS, liver, spleen, etc.	Pulmonary disease from aspiration (pseudobulbar palsy). Hepatosplenomegaly, hypersplenism may cause platelet deficiency.
Neimann-Pick disease	Sphingomyelin and cholesterol accumulation in CNS, marrow, liver, and spleen. Diffuse infiltration of lungs. Epilepsy, ataxia, and mental retardation.	Anemia and thrombocytopenia due to marrow and spleen involvement. Pulmonary insufficiency, pneumonia.
Tay Sach disease	Gangliosidosis. Blindness an progressive dementia and degeneration of CNS.	No described anesthetic hazard. Progressive neurologic loss leads to respiratory complications. Supportive measures only treatment.

TABLE 12-16
Index of Neurologic Syndromes and Their Anesthetic Implications (*Continued*)

Name	Description	Anesthetic Implications
Lowe syndrome (oculocerebrorenal syndrome)	Male only. Cataract, glaucoma. Mental retardation. Hypotonia. Renal acidosis, proteinuria, osteoporosis, and rickets.	Check electrolyte and acid-base balance. Check serum Ca^{2+} (treated with Vitamin D and Ca^{2+}). Care with drugs excreted via kidneys.
Maple-syrup urine disease (branched chain ketonuria)	Amino acid disturbance treated by diet only. Severe neurologic damage and respiratory disturbances.	General supportive measures.
Meckel's syndrome	Microcephaly, micrognathia, and cleft epiglottis. Congenital heart disease. Renal dysplasia.	Intubation may be difficult. Cardiac problems. Renal failure in infancy—care with renally excreted drugs.
Mucopolysaccharidoses[452]		
Hurler syndrome Type I	Mental retardation, macroglossia, valvular heart disease, cardiac failure, short neck, thoraco-lumbar kyphosis.	Difficult airway. Frequent upper respiratory infection. Abnormal tracheobronchial cartilages. Severe coronary artery disease at early age, valvular, and myocardial involvement.
Hunter syndrome Type II	Stiff joints, dwarfing, hepatosplenomegaly. Pectus excavatum and kyphoscoliosis. Valvular and coronary heart disease. Mental retardation.	Difficult airway. Upper airway obstruction due to infiltration of lymphoid tissue and larynx. Pneumonias. Possible hypersplenism. Cardiac failure.
San-Filippo syndrome Type III	CNS malfunction in childhood progresses to mental retardation and dementia. No hepatosplenomegaly or cardiac problems.	Difficult airway.
Morquio-Ullrich syndrome Type IV	Severe dwarfing. Aortic incompetence. Thoracic deformities. Unstable atlantoaxial joint.	Cardiorespiratory symptoms by 2d decade. Severe kyphoscoliosis with poor lung function. All develop spinal cord damage from atlanto-occipital subluxation.
Scheie syndrome Type V	Corneal clouding, hernias. Joint stiffness, especially in hands and feet. Aortic valve invovement. Same as Hurler's (Type I) except normal intelligence and height.	Aortic incompetence by 3d decade. Joint stiffness—care in positioning. May be difficult intubation.
Maroteaux-Lamy syndrome Type VI	Myocardial involvement. Kyphoscoliosis and chest infection. Hepatosplenomegaly. Macroglossia.	Difficult airway. Heart failure by age 20. Care with cardiac depressant drugs. Chronic respiratory infection with poor lung reserve. Hypersplenism, anemia, thrombocytopenia.
Myotonic dystrophy	Weakness and myotonia. Ptosis, cataracts, partial baldness, and gonadal atrophy. Cardiac conduction defects and arrhythmias. Impaired ventilation. Delayed gastric emptying. Diabetes.	Avoid succinylcholine which causes myotonia in 50%. Nondepolarizing drugs do not relax myotonia. Neostigmine induces myotonia. Monitor ECG. Limited pulmonary reserve. Extremely sensitive to respiratory depressants, use regional or inhalational agents, IPPV post-op if necessary. Halothane may cause post-op shivering and myotonia. Pulmonary complications due to poor cough.
Olivopontocerebellar atrophy[453,454]	Gait or limb ataxia, tremor, parkinsonism, spasticity, dystonia, dementia, anterior column, and corticospinal tract degeneration leading to atrophy or fasciculations.	Presumed hyperkalemic response to succinylcholine. Upper airway obstruction.
Osler-Weber-Rendu syndrome (hemorrhagic telangiectasia)	No coagulation abnormalities. Associated pulmonary A-V fistula. Angiomas may form in spinal cord or column.	Blood loss may be impossible to control. IV may be difficult to maintain due to poor tissues. More than 90% have recurrent chest infection, dyspnea, cyanosis, clubbing by age 60.
Patau syndrome (trisomy 13)	Mental retardation in 100%. Microcephaly, micrognathia, and/or dextrocardia. Cleft lip or palate. Congenital heart disease. Usually fatal by three years.	Difficult intubation. Usually VSD.
Phenylketonuria	Phenylalanine hydroxylase deficiency. Vomiting, irritability, mental retardation, hypertonia, convulsions. Very sensitive to narcotics and other CNS depressants.	Inhalation induction and maintenance. Continue antiepileptic drugs. Tendency to hypoglycemia—dextrose infusion.

TABLE 12-16
Index of Neurologic Syndromes and Their Anesthetic Implications (*Continued*)

Name	Description	Anesthetic Implications
Porphyria	Paralysis, psychiatric disorder. Autonomic imbalance—hypertension, tachycardia. Abdominal pain precipitated by drugs, infections, etc.	Many drugs will induce porphyria including barbiturates, etomidate, benzodiazepines, and some local anesthetics. Generally regarded as safe: Propofol, droperidol, opiates, N_2O, muscle relaxants, neostigmine, atropine. *Controversial:* ketamine, volatile anesthetics.
Prader-Willi syndrome	*Neonate*—Hypotonia, poor feeding, absent reflexes. *Second phase*—Hyperactive, uncontrollable polyphagia, mental retardation.	Obesity of extreme proportions leading to cardiopulmonary failure.
Progeria (Hutchinson-Gilford syndrome)	Premature aging starts 6 months–3 yr. Cardiac disease—ischemia, hypertension, cardiomegaly.	Anesthesia as for adults with myocardial ischemia.
Rett syndrome (first reported in 1967 by Rett)	Only in females, 1 in 10,000 to 12,000 live births; leading cause of prolonged mental retardation in females due to failure of brain maturation. Characterized by autistic behaviors; spasticity, abnormal breathing patterns; seizures; scoliosis; lack of use of hands which they wring or suck; many deaths due to cardiac arrhythmias.	No case reports in the literature implicating anesthesia. Perioperative care relates to presenting problems.
Rieger syndrome	Myotonic dystrophy and other myopathies. Hypoplasia or maxilla, abnormal teeth, mental retardation. Occasional imperforate anus.	Anesthetic requirements dictated by associated muscle disease—see amyotonia congenita, myotonic dystrophy.
Riley-Day syndrome (familial dysautonomia)	Deficiency of dopamine hydroxylase. Hyper- and hypotensive attacks, absent lacrimation, abnormal sweating. Insensitive to pain. Poor suckling and swallowing.	Emotional lability. Recurrent aspiration, pneumonia and chronic lung disease. Labile blood pressure—care with volatile anesthetics. Sensitive to adrenergic and cholinergic drugs. Respiratory center insensitive to CO_2—need IPPV. Avoid respiratory depressants.
Rubinstein syndrome	Mental retardation, microcephaly. Frequent chest infections. Swallowing abnormality. Congenital heart and kidney disease.	Repeated aspiration leads to pneumonia and chronic lung disease.
Sebaceous linear nevi	Linear nevi from forehead to nose. Hydrocephalus, mental retardation, associated with coarctation and hypoplasia of aorta. Congenital neurocutaneous disorder.	Cardiovascular complications.
Shy-Drager syndrome	Orthostatic hypotension. Diffuse degeneration of CNS and autonomic nervous system. Decreased sweating. Hypersensitive to angiotensin and epinephrine.	Labile pulse and blood pressure possibly due to defective baroreceptor response. Titrate anesthesia carefully. Treat hypotension with infusion phenylephrine.
Smith-Lemli-Opitz syndrome	Mental retardation. Genital and skeletal anomalies—micrognathia. Thymic hypoplasia. 3q or 2p gene duplication.	Airway and intubation problems. Pneumonia, possible increased susceptibility to infection.
Sotos syndrome (cerebral gigantism)	Acromegalic features without a known neuroendocrine defect. Dilated ventricles but normal intracranial pressure.	All features non-progressive. Possible airway problems due to acromegalic skull. No other described problems.
Spinal muscular atrophy		
Progressive infantile spinal muscular atrophy (Amyotonia congenita)	Anterior horn cell degeneration	Sensitive to thiopental (reduced muscle mass) and respiratory depressants. Care with muscle relaxants.
Werdnig-Hoffman disease (early onset spinal muscular atrophy)	Earlier onset and more severe muscular dystrophy than in Kugelberg-Welander. Feeding difficulties, aspiration, usually death before puberty.	Chronic respiratory problems. Minimal anesthesia required. Avoid muscle relaxants and respiratory depressant drugs. Ventilatory support may be required and weaning may be difficult.
Kugelberg-Welander disease (late onset juvenile spinal muscular atrophy)	Initial involvement peripheral muscles. Prognosis good for life, poor for ambulation.	May require spinal fusion. Extreme care with thiopentone, muscle relaxants. Avoid respiratory depressant drugs.

TABLE 12-16
Index of Neurologic Syndromes and Their Anesthetic Implications (*Continued*)

Name	Description	Anesthetic Implications
Supravalvular aortic stenosis syndrome (idiopathic infantile hypercalcemia—William syndrome)	Hypercalcemia and mental retardation. Abnormal facies. Cardiac dyspnea, angina. Therapy—low calcium diet, steroids. Cardiac surgery.	Fixed cardiac output and ischemia. History of steroids. Monitor serum Ca^{2+}.
Tangier disease	High triglycerides with low HDL and low serum cholesterol. Orange tonsils and rectal mucosa. Splenomegaly. 50% neurologic abnormality. Asymmetric sensorimotor neuropathy. Premature coronary disease.	Anemia and thrombocytopenia due to hypersplenism. Abnormal EMG—care with muscle relaxants. Beware premature ischemic heart disease.
Thomsen disease	See myotonia congenita	
Tourette syndrome[455]	Tics, echolalia, coprolalia, ballistic movements.	QT interval prolongation secondary to medications; worsening of condition due to anxiety.
Werner syndrome	Premature aging, diabetes. Early cataracts. Bony lesions like osteomyelitis. Cardiac infarction and failure. Increased tumors.	Anesthesia as for adult with myocardial ischemia.
Zellweger syndrome (cerebro-hepatorenal syndrome)	Hepatomegaly and neonatal jaundice. Polycystic kidneys. Associated congenital heart disease. Muscular hypotonia. Dysmorphia of skull and face. Seizures.	Hypoprothrombinemia. Care with renally excreted drugs and muscle relaxants.

SOURCE: Adapted from Jones AEP, Pelton DA. An index of syndromes and their anaesthetic implications. *Can Anaesth Soc J* 1976; 23, with permission.

References

1. Parkinson J: *An Essay on the Shaking Palsy.* London, Sherwood, Neely and Jones, 1817.
2. Broe GA: The neuroepidemiology of old age. In Tallis R (ed): *The Clinical Neurology of Old Age.* Chichester, Wiley, 1989: 61–65.
3. Adams RD, Victor M: *Principles of Neurology,* 5th ed. New York, McGraw-Hill, 1993.
4. Rajut AH, et al: Epidemiology of parkinsonism: Incidence classification and mortality. *Ann Neurol* 1984; 16:278.
5. Snyder SH, D'Amato RJ: MPTP: A neurotoxin relevant to the pathophysiology of Parkinson's disease. *Neurology* 1986; 36:250.
6. Albin RL, et al: The functional anatomy of the basal ganglia disorders. *Trends Neurosci* 1989; 12:366.
7. Hoehn MM, Yahr MD: Parkinsonism: Onset progression and mortality. *Neurology* 1967; 17:427.
8. Young RR: The differential diagnosis of Parkinson's disease. *Int J Neurol* 1977; 12:210.
9. Fahn S, et al (eds): *Recent Advances in Parkinson's Disease.* New York, Raven, 1986.
10. Growdon JH: Medical treatment of extrapyramidal disease. In KJ Isselbacher, et al (eds): *Update III: Harrison's Principles of Internal Medicine.* New York, McGraw-Hill, 1982.
11. Hawsten PD: *Drug Interactions.* Philadelphia, Lea and Fibiger, 1985.
12. Jefferson JW: A review of the cardiovascular effects and toxicity of tricyclic antidepressants. *Psychosom Med* 1975; 37:160.
13. Morgan JP, et al: Imipramine-mediated interference with levodopa absorption from the gastrointestinal tract. *Neurology* 1975; 25:1029.
14. Rampton DS: Hypertensive crisis in a patient given sinemet, metoclopramide and amitriptyline. *Br Med J* 1977; 3:607.
15. Wodak J, et al: Review of 12 months' treatment with L-DOPA in Parkinson's disease, with remark on unusual side effects. *Med J Aust* 1972; 2:1277.
16. Hunter KR, et al: Use of levodopa with other drugs. *Lancet* 1970; 2:1283.
17. Yosselson-Superstine S, Lipman AG: Chlordiazepoxide interaction with levodopa. *Ann Intern Med* 1982; 96:259.
18. Kissel P, et al: Levodopa-Propranolol therapy in parkinsonian tremor. *Lancet* 1974; 1:403.
19. Camanni F, Massara: Enhancement of levodopa-induced growth-hormone stimulation by propranolol. *Lancet* 1974; 1:942.
20. Whitsett TL: Propranolol blockade of positive inotropic effects of L-dopa in dog and man. *Pharmacologist* 1970; 12:213.
21. Duvoisin RC: Hypotension caused by L-dopa. *Br Med* 1970; 3:47.
22. Collu R, et al: Re-evaluation of levodopa-propranolol as a test of growth hormone reserve in children. *Pediatrics* 1978; 61:242.
23. Lotti G, et al: Enhancement of levodopa-induced growth hormone stimulation by practolol. *Lancet* 1974; 2:1329.
24. Sandler M, et al: Oxpernolol and levodopa in parksinsonian patients. *Lancet* 1975; 1:168.
25. Shoulson I, Chase TN: Clonidine and the anti-parkinsonian response to L-dopa or piribedil. *Neuropharm* 1976; 15:25.
26. Tarsy D, et al: Clonidine in Parkinson's disease. *Arch Neurol* 1975; 32:134.
27. Morgan JP, Bianchine JR: The clinical pharmacology of levodopa. *Rational Drug Ther* 1971; 5:1.
28. Gibberd FB, Small E: Interaction between levodopa and methyldopa. *Br Med* 1973; 2:90.
29. Cotzias GC, et al: L-Dopa in Parkinson's syndrome. *N Engl J Med* 1969; 281:272.
30. Kofman O: Treatment of Parkinson's disease with L-Dopa: A current appraisal. *Can Med Assoc J* 1971; 104:483.
31. Friend DG, et al: The action of L-dihydroxyphenylalanine in patients receiving nialamide. *Clin Pharmacl Ther* 1965; 6:362.

32. Hunter KR et al: Monoamine oxidase inhibitors and L-DOPA. *Br Med* 1970; 3:388.

33. Kott E, et al: Excretion of dopa metabolites. *N Engl J Med* 1971; 284:395.

34. Birkmayer W, et al: Implications of combined treatment with madopar and L-deprenil in Parkinson's disease. *Lancet* 1977; 1:439.

35. Duvoisin RC: Antagonism of levodopa by papaverine. *JAMA* 1975; 231:845.

36. Posner DM: Antagonism of levodopa by papaverine. *JAMA* 1975; 233:7658.

37. Godwin-Austen RB, et al: Mydriatic response to sympathomimetic amines in patients treated with L-DOPA. *Lancet* 1969; 2:1043.

38. Bianchine JR, Sunyapridakul L: Interactions between levodopa and other drugs: Significance in the treatment of Parkinson's disease. *Drugs* 1973; 6:364.

39. Carter AB: Pyridoxine and parkinsonism. *Br Med J* 1973; 4:236.

40. Mars H: Levodopa, carbidopa and pyridoxine in Parkinson's disease. Metabolic interactions. *Arch Neurol* 1974; 30:444.

41. Mendez JS, et al: Diphenylhydantoin blocking of levodopa effects. *Arch Neurol* 1975; 32:44.

42. Bianchine JR, Sunyapridakul L: Interactions between levodopa and other drugs: Significance in the treatment of Parkinson's disease. *Drugs* 1973; 6:364.

43. Kelly PJ, Gillingham FJ: The long term results of stereotactic surgery and L-dopa in patients with Parkinson's disease. A 10 year follow-up study. *J Neurosurg* 1980; 53:332.

44. Ojemann GA, Ward AA Jr: Abnormal movement disorders. In Youmans JR (ed): *Neurological Surgery: A Comprehensive Reference Guide to the Diagnosis and Management of Neurological Problems,* 3d ed. Philadelphia, WB Saunders, 1990:4227–4262.

45. Cardoso F, et al: Outcome after stereotactic thalamotomy for dystonia and hemiballismus. *Neurosurgery* 1995; 36:501.

46. Lozano AM, et al: Effect of Gpi pallidotomy on motor function in Parkinson's Disease. *Lancet* 1995; 346(8987):1383.

47. Grovlee GP: Succinylcholine-induced hyperkalemia in a patient with Parkinson's disease. *Anesth Analg* 1980; 59:444.

48. Nuizzi DA, et al: The lack of effect of succinylcholine on serum potassium in patients with Parkinson's disease. *Anesthesiology* 1989; 71:322.

49. Nietz B: Acute dystonia after alfentanil in untreated Parkinson's disease. *Anesth Analg* 1991; 72:557.

50. Zornberg GL, et al: Severe adverse reaction between pethidine and selegiline. *Lancet* 1991; 337:246.

51. Golden WE, et al: Acute post-operative confusion and hallucinations in Parkinson's disease. *Ann Intern Med* 1989; 111:218.

52. Folstein S: *Huntington's Disease.* Johns Hopkins University Press, Baltimore, 1989.

53. Furtado S, Suchowersky O: Huntington's disease: Recent advances in diagnosis and management. *Ann NY Acad Sci* 1992; 648:6.

54. Harper PS: The epidemiology of Huntington's disease. *Human Genetics* 1992; 89:365.

55. Leung CM, et al: Huntington's disease in Chinese: A hypothesis of its origin. *J Neurol Neurosurg Psychiat* 1992: 55:681.

56. Albin RL, Tagle DA: Genetics and molecular biology of Huntington's disease. *Trends Neurosci* 1995; 18:11.

57. La Spada AR, et al: Trinucleotide repeat expansion in Neurological disease. *Ann Neurol* 1994; 36:814.

58. Forno LS: Neuropathologic features of Parkinson's, Huntington's, and Alzheimer's diseases. *Ann NY Acad Sci* 1992; 648:6.

59. Gusella JF, MacDonald ME: Huntington's disease. *Semin Cell Biol* 1995; 6:21.

60. Purdon SE, et al: Huntington's disease: Pathogenesis, diagnosis and treatment. *J Psychiat Neurosci* 1994; 19:359.

61. Mendez MF: Huntington's disease: Update and review of neuropsychiatric aspects. *Int J Psychiatry Med* 1994; 24:189.

62. Patterson J: Choreiform movement associated with metoclopramide. *Southern Med J* 1986; 79:1465.

63. Davies DD: Abnormal response to anaesthesia in a case of Huntington's chorea. *Br J Anaesth* 1966; 38:490.

64. Sandberg PR, et al: Pentobarbitone anaesthesia in an animal model of Huntington's disease. *Br J Anaesth* 1981; 53:442.

65. Costarino A, Gross JB: Patients with Huntington's chorea may respond normally to succinylcholine. *Anesthesiology* 1985; 63:570.

66. Harris MN: Anaesthesia, atracurium and Huntington's chorea. *Anaesthesia* 1984; 39:66.

67. Blanloeil Y, et al: Anaesthesia in Huntington's chorea. *Anaesthesia* 1982; 37:695.

68. Farina J, Rauscher LA: Anaesthesia and Huntington's chorea. A report of two cases. *Br J Anaesth* 1977; 49:1167.

69. Browne MG: Anaesthesia in Huntington's chorea. *Anaesthesia* 1983; 38:65.

70. Gaubatz CL, Wehner RJ: Anesthetic considerations for the patient with Huntington's disease. *AANA J* 1992; 60:41.

71. Rodrigo MR: Huntington's chorea: Midazolam, a suitable induction agent? *Br J Anaesth* 1987; 59:388.

72. Soar J, Matheson KH: A safe anaesthetic in Huntington's disease. *Anaesthesia* 1993; 48:743.

73. Kaufman MA, Erb T: Propofol for patients with Huntington's chorea? *Anaesthesia* 1990; 45:889.

74. Whittaker M: Plasma cholinesterase variants and the anaesthetist. *Anaesthesia* 1980; 35:174.

75. Starosta-Rubinstein S, et al: Clinical assessment of 31 patients with Wilson's disease. *Arch Neurol* 1987; 44:365.

76. Marsden DC: Investigation of dystonia. *Adv Neurol* 1988; 50:35.

77. Ozelius L, et al: Human gene for torsion dystonia located on chromosome 9q32-q34. *Neuron* 1989; 2:1427.

78. Ozelius LJ, et al: Strong allelic association between the torsion dystonia gene (DYT1) and loci on chromosome 9q34 in Ashkenazi Jews. *Am J Hum Genet* 1992; 50:619.

79. Cardoso F, et al: Outcome after stereotactic thalamotomy for dystonia and hemiballismus. *Neurosurgery* 1995; 36:501.

80. Patrinely JP, Anerson RL: Essential blepharospasm: A review. *Geriatr Ophthalmol* 1986; 2:27.

81. Holds JB, et al: Brainstem auditory evoked potentials in essential blepharospasm. *Invest Ophthalmol Vis Sci* 1989; 30(Suppl): 411.

82. Chan J, et al: Idiopathic cervical dystonia: Clinical characteristics. *Mov Disord* 1991; 6:119.

83. Jankovic J, et al: Cervical dystonia: Clinical findings and associated movement disorders. *Neurology* 1991; 41:1088.

84. Brin MF: Torticollis (Cervical Dystonia). In Johnson RT, Griffin JW (eds): *Current Therapy in Neurologic Disease,* 4th ed. St. Louis, MO, Mosby-Year Book, 1993:266–270.

85. Greene P, et al: Analysis of open-label trials in torsion dystonia using high dosages of anticholinergics and other drugs. *Mov Disord* 1988; 3:46.

86. Fink JK, et al: Clinical and genetic analysis of progressive dystonia with diurnal variation. *Arch Neurol* 1991; 48:908.

87. National Institutes of Health Consensus Development Conference Statement: Clinical use of botulinum toxin. *Arch Neurol* 1991; 48:1294.

88. Greene P, et al: Double-blind, placebo-controlled trial of botulinum toxin injections for the treatment of spasmodic torticollis. *Neurology* 1990; 40:1213.

89. Taylor DJN, et al: Treatment of blepharospasm and hemifacial spasm with botulinum A toxin: A Canadian multicentre study. *Can J Ophthalmol* 1991; 26:133.

90. Jankovic J, Brin M: Therapeutic uses of botulinum toxin. *N Engl J Med* 1991; 324:1186.

91. Bertrand C, et al: Technical aspects of selective denervation for spasmodic torticollis. *Appl Neurophysiol* 1982; 45:326.

92. Andrew J, et al: Stereotaxic thalamotomy in 55 cases of dystonia. *Brain* 1983; 106:981.

93. Oh I, Nowacek CJ: Surgical release of congenital torticollis in adults. *Clin Orthop* 1978; 131:141.

94. Walajahi FH, Karasic LH: Anesthetic management of a patient with dystonia musculorum deformans. *Anesth Analg* 1984; 63:616.

95. Davis NL, David R: Anesthetic management of a patient with dystonia musculorum deformans. *Anesthesiology* 1975; 42:630.

96. Dehring DJ, et al: Postoperative opisthotonus and torticollis after fentanyl, enflurane, and nitrous oxide. *Can J Anaesth* 1991; 38:919.

97. Stemp LI, Taswell C: Spastic torticollis during general anesthesia: Case report and review of receptor mechanisms. *Anesthesiology* 1991; 75:365.

98. Digre K, Corbvett JJ: Hemifacial spasm: Differential diagnosis, mechanism and treatment. *Adv Neurol* 1988; 49:151.

99. Taylor DJN, et al: Treatment of blepharospasm and hemifacial spasm with botulinum A toxin: A Canadian multicentre study. *Can J Ophthalmol* 1991; 26:133.

100. Janetta PS, et al: Etiology and definitive microsurgical treatment of hemifacial spasm: Operative techniques and results in forty-seven people. *J Neurosurg* 1977; 47:321.

101. Crump T: Translation of case reports in (Ueber die multiplen Fibrome der Haut und ihre Beziehung zu den multiplen Neuromon by F. V. Recklinghausen). *Adv Neurol* 1981; 29:259.

102. Conference Statement, National Institutes of Health Consensus Development Conference: Neurofibromatosis. *Arch Neurol* 1988; 45:575.

103. Riccardi VM: Von Recklinghausen neurofibromatosis. *N Engl J Med* 1981; 305:1617.

104. Rosenberg RN, Iannaccone ST: The prevention of neurogenetic disease. *Arch Neurol* 1995; 52:356.

105. Gutmann DH, Collins FS: The neurofibromatosis type 1 gene and its protein product, neurofibromin. *Neuron* 1993; 10:335.

106. Gutmann DH, Collins FS: Recent progress toward understanding the molecular biology of von Recklinghausen neurofibromatosis. *Ann Neurol* 1992; 31:555.

107. Gutmann DH, Collins FS: Neurofibromatosis type 1: Beyond positional cloning. *Arch Neurol* 1993; 50:1185.

108. Easton DF, et al: Analysis of variation in expression of neurofibromatosis (NF1): Evidence for modifying genes. *Am J Hum Genet* 1993; 53:305.

109. Jarvis GJ, Crompton AC: Neurofibromatosis and pregnancy. *Br J Obstet Gynaecol* 1978; 85:844.

110. Weissman A, et al: Neurofibromatosis and pregnancy. An update. *J Reprod Med* 1993; 38:890.

111. Riccardi VM: Pathophysiology of neurofibromatosis. IV. Dermatologic insights into heterogeneity and pathogenesis. *J Am Acad Dermatol* 1980; 3:157.

112. Senveli E, et al: Association of von Recklinghausen's neurofibromatosis and aqueduct stenosis. *Neurosurgery* 1989; 24:99.

113. Rubenstein AE, et al: Neurologic aspects of neurofibromatosis. *Adv Neurol* 1981; 29:11.

114. Lott IT, Richardson EP: Neuropathological findings and the biology of neurofibromatosis. *Adv Neurol* 1981; 29:23.

115. Rosman NP, Pearce J: The brain in multiple neurofibromatosis (von Recklinghausen's disease): A suggested neuropathological basis for the associated mental defect. *Brain* 1967; 90:829.

116. Duffner PK, et al: The significance of MRI abnormalities in children in neurofibromatosis. *Neurology* 1989; 39:373.

117. Laue L, et al: Precocious puberty associated with neurofibromatosis and cystic gliomas. Treatment with luteinizing hormone releasing hormone analogue. *AJDC* 1985; 130:1097.

118. Saxena KM: Endocrine manifestations of neurofibromatosis in children. *Am J Dis Child* 1970; 120:265.

119. Knudson AG: A geneticist's view of neurofibromatosis. *Adv Neurol* 1981; 29:237.

120. Neiman HL, et al: Neurofibromatosis and congenital heart disease. *Am J Roentgenol Radium Ther Nucl Med* 1974; 122:146.

121. Fitzpatrick AP, Emanuel RW: Familial neurofibromatosis and hypertrophic cardiomyopathy. *Br Heart J* 1988; 60:247.

122. Schievink WI, et al: Neurovascular manifestations of heritable connective tissue disorders. A review. *Stroke* 1994; 25:889.

123. Sobata E, et al: Cerebrovascular disorders associated with von Recklinghausen's neurofibromatosis. A case report. *Neurosurgery* 1988; 22:544.

124. Mathoul C, et al: Congenital pseudoarthrosis of the forearm: Treatment of six cases with vascularized fibular graft and a review of the literature. *Microsurgery* 1993; 14:252.

125. Eldridge R: Central neurofibromatosis with bilateral acoustic neuroma. *Adv Neurol* 1981; 29:57.

126. Martuza RL, Eldridge R: Neurofibromatosis 2 (Bilateral acoustic neurofibromatosis). *N Engl J Med* 1988; 328:684.

127. Pearson-Webb MA, et al: Eye findings in bilateral acoustic (central) neurofibromatosis: Association with presenile lens opacities and cataracts but absence of Lisch nodules. *N Engl J Med* 1986; 315:1553.

128. Allen J, et al: Acoustic neuroma in the last months of pregnancy. *Am J Obstet Gynecol* 1974; 119:516.

129. Truhan AP, Filipek PA: Magnetic resonance imaging. Its role in the neuroradiologic evaluation of neurofibromatosis, tuberous sclerosis, and Sturge-Weber syndrome. *Arch Dermatol* 1993; 129:219.

130. Ojemann RG, et al: Use of intraoperative auditory evoked potentials to preserve hearing in unilateral acoustic neuroma removal. *J Neurosurg* 1984; 61:938.

131. Miyamoto RT, et al: Contemporary management of neurofibromatosis. *Ann Otol Rhinol & Laryngol* 1991; 100:38.

132. Lovell AT, et al: Silent, unstable cervical spine injury in multiple neurofibromatosis. *Anaesthesia* 1994; 49:453.

133. Crozier WC: Upper airway obstruction in neurofibromatosis. *Anaesthesia* 1987; 42:1209.

134. Chang-Lo M: Laryngeal involvement in von Recklinghausen's Disease: A case report and review of the literature. *Laryngoscope* 1977; 87:435.

135. Abel M: Emergency medicine and anesthesiology aspects of neurofibromatosis in childhood. *Anasthesie Intensivtherapie Notfallmedizin* 1985; 20:76.

136. Manser J: Abnormal responses in von Recklinghausen's Disease. *Br J Anaesth* 1970; 42:183.

137. Baraka A: Myasthenic response to muscle relaxants in von Recklinghausen's disease. *Br J Anaesth* 1974; 46:701.

138. Naguib M, et al: The response of a patient with von Recklinghausen's disease to succinylcholine and atracurium. *Middle East J Anesthesiol* 1988; 9:429.

139. Magbagbeola J: Abnormal responses to muscle relaxants in a patient with von Recklinghausen's disease (Multiple Neurofibromatosis). *Br J Anaesth* 1974; 46:701.

140. Dounas M, Mercier FJ, Lhuissier C, Benhaumou D: Epidural analgesia for labour in a parturient with neurofibromatosis. *Can J Anaesth* 1995; 42:420.

141. Kwiatkowski DJ, Short MP: Tuberous sclerosis. *Arch Dermatol* 1994; 130:348.

142. Webb DW, Osborne JP: Tuberous sclerosis. *Arch Dis Child* 1995; 72:471.

143. Roach ES, et al: Diagnostic criteria: Tuberous sclerosis complex. Report of the Diagnostic Criteria Committee of the Na-

tional Tuberous Sclerosis Association. *J Child Neurol* 1992; 7:221.

144. Lie JT: Cardiac, pulmonary and vascular involvements in tuberous sclerosis. *Ann NY Acad Sci* 1991; 615;58.

145. Gomez MR: Tuberous slcerosis. In Gomez MR (ed): *Neurocutaneous Diseases: A Practical Approach.* Butterworths, Boston, 1987:30–52.

146. Bernstein J, Robbins T: Renal involvement in tuberous sclerosis. *Ann NY Acad Sci* 1991; 615:36.

147. Lee JJ, et al: Anaesthesia and tuberous sclerosis. *Br J Anaesth* 1994; 73:421.

148. Michels VV: Von Hippel-Lindau disease. In Gomez M (ed): *Neurocutaneous Diseases.* Butterworths, Boston, 1987:53–66.

149. Lesho EP: Recognition and management of von Hippel-Lindau disease. *American Family Physician* 1994; 50:1269.

150. Maher ER: Von Hippel-Lindau disease. *Eur J Cancer* 1994; 30A:1987.

151. Latif F, et al: Identification of the von Hippel-Lindau disease tumor suppressor gene. *Science* 1993; 260:1317.

152. Maher ER, Moore AT: Von Hippel-Lindau disease. *Br J Opthalmol* 1992; 76:743.

153. Matthews AJ, Halshaw J: Epidural anaesthesia in von Hippel-Lindau disease. Management of childbirth and anaesthesia for caesarean section. *Anaesthesia* 1986; 41:853.

154. Ogasawara KK, et al: Pregnancy complicated by von Hippel-Lindau disease. *Obstet Gynecol* 1994; 85:829.

155. Joffe D, et al: Caesarean section and phaeochromocytoma resection in a patient with Von Hippel-Lindau disease. *Can J Anaesth* 1993; 40:870.

156. Gomez M, Bebin EM: Sturge-Weber syndrome. In Gomez M (ed) *Neurocutaneous Diseases.* Butterworth, Boston, 1987:356–357.

157. Batra RK, et al: Anaesthesia and the Sterge-Weber syndrome. *Can J Anaesth* 1994; 41:133.

158. Anderson FH, Duncan GW: Sturge-Weber disease with subarachnoid hemorrhage. *Stroke* 1974; 5:509.

159. Reich DS, Wiatrak BJ: Upper airway obstruction in Sturge-Weber and Klippel-Trenaunay-Weber syndromes. *Ann Otol Rhinol Laryngol* 1995; 104:364.

160. de Leon-Casasola OA, Lema MJ: Anaesthesia for patients with Sturge-Weber disease and Klippel-Trenaunay syndrome. *J Clin Anesth* 1991; 3:409.

161. Garcia JC, et al: Recurrent thrombotic deterioration in Sturge-Weber Syndrome. *Child's Brain* 1981; 8:427.

162. Goodkin DE: Interferon beta-1b. *Lancet* 1994;344:1057.

163. Ellison GW: Multiple sclerosis: A fever blister on the brain. *Lancet* 1974; 2:664.

164. Nelson DA: Dorsal root ganglia may be reservoirs of viral infection in multiple sclerosis. *Med Hypotheses* 1993; 40:278.

165. Sander VJ, et al: Herpes simplex virus in postmortem multiple sclerosis brain tissue. *Arch Neurol* 1996; 53:125.

166. Challoner PB, et al: Plaque-associated expression of human herpes virus 6 in multiple sclerosis. *Proc Natl Acad Sci USA* 1995; 92:7440.

167. Ebers GC: Optic neuritis and multiple sclerosis. *Arch Neurol* 1985; 42:702.

168. Schumacher GA, et al: Problems of experimental trials of therapy in multiple sclerosis: Report by the panel on evaluation of experimental trials of therapy in multiple sclerosis. *Ann NY Acad Sci USA* 1965; 122:552.

169. Rose AS, et al: Criteria for the clinical diagnosis of multiple sclerosis. *Neurology* 1976; 26:20.

170. Poser CM, et al: New diagnostic criteria for multiple sclerosis: Guidelines for research protocols. *Ann Neurol* 1983; 13:227.

171. Goodkin DE, et al: The use of brain magnetic resonance imaging in multiple sclerosis. *Arch Neurol* 1994; 51:505.

172. Ormerod IEC, et al: The role of NMR imaging in the assessment of multiple sclerosis and isolated neurological lesions. *Brain* 1987; 110:1579.

173. Paty DW, et al: MRI in the diagnosis of MS. *Neurology* 1988; 38:180.

174. Gebarski SS, et al: The initial diagnosis of multiple sclerosis: Clinical impact of magnetic resonance imaging. *Ann Neurol* 1985; 17:469.

175. National Multiple Sclerosis Society Working Group on Neuroimaging for the Medical Advisory Board: Use of magnetic resonance imaging in the diagnosis of multiple sclerosis: Policy statement. *Neurology* 1986; 36:1575.

176. Bradley WG Jr, et al: Patchy, periventricular white matter lesions in the elderly. *Noninvasive Med Imaging* 1984; 1:35.

177. Awad IA, et al: Incidental subcortical lesions identified on magnetic resonance imaging in the elderly. *Stroke* 1986; 17:1085.

178. Rudick RA, et al: Multiple sclerosis: The problem of misdiagnosis. *Arch Neurol* 1986; 43:578.

179. Weinshenker BG, et al: The natural history of multiple sclerosis: A geographically based study. Predictive value of the early clinical course. *Brain* 1989; 112:1419.

180. Revez T, et al: A comparison of the pathology of primary and secondary progressive multiple sclerosis. *Brain* 1994; 117:759.

181. Matthews WB, et al: *McAlpine's Multiple Sclerosis,* 2d ed. New York, Churchill Livingstone, 1991.

182. Birk, K, et al: Clinical course of multiple sclerosis during pregnancy and the puerperium. *Arch Neurol* 1990; 47:738.

183. ffrench-Constant C: Pathogenesis of multiple sclerosis. *Lancet* 1994; 343:271.

184. Olerup O, Hillert J: HLA class-II associated genetic susceptibility in multiple sclerosis: A critical evaluation. *Tissue Antigens* 1990; 38:1.

185. Allegretta M, et al: T cells responsive to myelin basic protein in patients with multiple sclerosis. *Science* 1990; 247:718.

186. Linington C, et al: T cells specific for the myelin oligodendrocyte glycoprotein mediate an unusual autoimmune inflammatory response in the central nervous system. *Eur J Immunol* 1993; 23:1364.

187. Olsson T: Immunology of multiple sclerosis. *Curr Opin Neurol Neurosurg* 1992; 5:195.

188. Cannella B, et al: Relapsing autoimmune demyelination: A role for vascular addressins. *J Neuroimmunol* 1991; 35:295.

189. Ebers GC: Treatment of multiple sclerosis. *Lancet* 1994; 343:275.

190. Wang WZ, et al: Myelin antigen reactive T cells in cerebrovascular disease. *Clin Exp Immunol* 1992; 88:157.

191. Herndon RM: Multiple sclerosis. In Rakel RE (ed): *Conn's Current Therapy.* Philadelphia, WB Saunders, 1995:848–855.

192. Barnes MP, et al: Intravenous methylprednisolone for multiple sclerosis in relapse. *J Neurol Neurosurg Psychiatry* 1985; 48:157.

193. Mitchell G: Update on multiple sclerosis therapy. *Med Clin N Am* 1993; 77:231.

194. Goodkin DE: Role of steroids and immunosuppression and effects of interferon beta-1b in multiple sclerosis. *West J Med* 1994; 161:292.

195. Dureili L, et al: High-dose intravenous methylprednisolone in the treatment of multiple sclerosis: Clinical-immunologic correlations. *Neurology* 1986; 36:238.

196. Huston DB, et al: Immune suppression for multiple sclerosis. *N Engl J Med* 1983; 309:240.

197. Tourtellotte WW, et al: Multiple sclerosis de novo CNS IgG synthesis: Effect of ACTH and corticosteroids. *Neurology* 1980; 30:1155.

198. Warren KG, et al: Effect of methylprednisolone on CSF IgG parameters, myelin basic protein and anti-myelin basic protein in multiple sclerosis exacerbations. *Can J Neurol Sci* 1986; 13:25.

199. Trotter JL, Garvey WF: Prolonged effects of large-dose methylprednisolone infusion in multiple sclerosis. *Neurology* 1980; 30:702.

200. Barkhof F, et al: Quantitative MRI changes in gadolinium-DTPA enhancement after high-dose intravenous methylprednisolone in multiple sclerosis. *Neurology* 1991; 41:1219.

201. Burnham JA, et al: The effect of high-dose steroids on MRI gadolinium enhancement in acute demyelinating lesions. *Neurology* 1991; 41:1349.

202. Beck RW, et al: The effect of corticosteroids for acute optic neuritis on the subsequent development of multiple sclerosis. *N Engl J Med* 1993; 329:1764.

203. Jacobs L, et al: Results of a phase III trial of intramuscular recombinant interferon as treatment for multiple sclerosis. *Ann Neurol* 1994; 36:259.

204. Johnson KP, et al: Copolymer 1 reduces relapse rate and improves disability in relapsing-remitting multiple sclerosis: Results of a phase III multicenter, double-blind, placebo-controlled trial. *Neurology* 1995; 45:1268.

205. IFNB Multiple Sclerosis Study Group: Interferon beta-1b is effective in relapsing-remitting multiple sclerosis. I. Clinical results of a multicenter, randomized, double-blind, placebo-controlled trial. *Neurology* 1993; 43:655.

206. IFNB Multiple Sclerosis Study Group, Univ Brit Columbia MSMRI Analysis Group: Interferon beta-1b in the treatment of multiple sclerosis: Final outcome of the randomized controlled trial. *Neurology* 1995; 45:1277.

207. Filippi M, Paty DW, Kappos L, et al: Correlations between changes in disability and T_2-weighted brain MRI activity in multiple sclerosis: A follow-up study. *Neurology* 1995; 45:255.

208. Wolinsky JS: Copolymer 1: A most reasonable alternative therapy for early relapsing-remitting multiple sclerosis with mild disability. *Neurology* 1995; 45:1245.

209. Swinburn WR, Liversedge LA: Long-term treatment of multiple sclerosis with azathioprine. *J Neurol Neurosurg Psychiatry* 1973; 36:124.

210. Mertin J, et al: Double-blind controlled trial of immunosuppression in the treatment of multiple sclerosis: Final report. *Lancet* 1982; 2:351.

211. Goodkin DE, et al: The efficacy of azathioprine in relapsing-remitting multiple sclerosis. *Neurology* 1991; 41:20.

212. Ellison GW, et al: A placebo-controlled, randomized, double-masked, variable dosage, clinical trial of azathioprine with and without methylprednisolone in multiple sclerosis. *Neurology* 1989; 39:1018.

213. Milanese C, et al: Double blind controlled randomized study on azathioprine efficacy in multiple sclerosis—Preliminary results. *Ital J Neurol Sci* 1988; 9:53.

214. British and Dutch Multiple Sclerosis Azathioprine Trial Group: Double-masked trial of azathioprine in multiple sclerosis. *Lancet* 1988; 2:179.

215. Yudkin PL, et al: Overview of azathioprine treatment in multiple sclerosis. *Lancet* 1991; 338:1051.

216. Kinlen LJ: Incidence of cancer in rheumatoid arthritis and other disorders after immunosuppressive treatment. *Am J Med* 1985; 78(suppl A):44.

217. Hauser SL, et al: Intensive immunosuppression in progressive multiple sclerosis: A randomized, three-arm study of high-dose intravenous cyclophosphamide, plasma exchange, and ACTH. *N Engl J Med* 1983; 308:173.

218. Goodkin DE, et al: Cyclophosphamide in chronic progressive multiple sclerosis: Maintenance vs. nonmaintenance therapy. *Arch Neurol* 1987; 44:823.

219. Weiner HL, et al: Intermittent cyclosphosphamide pulse therapy in progressive multiple sclerosis: Final report of the Northeast Cooperative Multiple Sclerosis Treatment Group. *Neurology* 1993; 43:910.

220. Canadian Coop MSS: The Canadian cooperative trial of cyclophosphamide and plasma exchange in progressive multiple sclerosis. *Lancet* 1991; 337:441.

221. Terrence CF, Fromm GHY: Complications of baclofen withdrawal. *Arch Neurol* 1981; 38:588.

222. Krupp LB, et al: Fatigue in multiple sclerosis. *Arch Neurol* 1988; 45:435.

223. Fisk JD, et al: The impact of fatigue on patients with multiple sclerosis. *Can J Neurol Sci* 1994; 21:9.

224. Freal JE, et al: Symptomatic fatigue in multiple sclerosis. *Arch Phys Med Rehabil* 1984; 65:135.

225. Murray TJ: Amantadine therapy for fatigue in multiple sclerosis. *Can J Neurol Sci* 1985; 12:251.

226. Krupp LB, et al: Fatigue therapy in multiple sclerosis: Results of a double-blind, randomized, parallel trial of amantadine, pemoline, and placebo. *Neurology* 1995; 45:1956.

227. Rosenberg GA, Appenzeller O: Amantadine, fatigue and multiple sclerosis. *Arch Neurol* 1988; 45:1104.

228. Stefoski D, et al: 4-Aminopyridine in multiple sclerosis: Prolonged administration. *Neurology* 1991; 41:1344.

229. Davis FA, et al: Orally administered 4-aminopyridine improves clinical signs in multiple sclerosis. *Ann Neurol* 1990; 27:186.

230. Bever CT Jr, et al: Preliminary trial of 3,4-diaminopyridine in patients with multiple sclerosis. *Ann Neurol* 1990; 27:421.

231. Minden SL, Schiffer RB: Affective disorders in multiple sclerosis: Review and recommendations for clinical research. *Arch Neurol* 1990; 47:98.

232. Jensen TS, et al: Association of trigeminal neuralgia with multiple sclerosis: Clinical and pathological features. *Acta Neurol Scand* 1982; 65:182.

233. Noseworthy JH: Therapeutics of multiple sclerosis. *Clin Neuropharmacol* 1991; 14:49.

234. Shibasaki H, et al: Clinical studies of multiple sclerosis in Japan: Classical multiple sclerosis and Devic's disease. *J Neurol Sci* 1974; 23:215.

235. Mandler RN, et al: Devic's neuromyelitis optica: A clinicopathological study of 8 patients. *Ann Neurol* 1993; 34:162.

236. Aguilera AJ, et al: Lymphocytoplasmaphoresis in Devic's syndrome. *Transfusion* 1985; 25:54.

237. Piccolo G, et al: Devic's neuromyelitis optica: Long-term follow-up and serial CSF findings in two cases. *J Neurol* 1990; 237:262.

238. Aisen M, et al: Diaphragmatic paralysis without bulbar or limb paralysis in multiple sclerosis. *Chest* 1990; 98:499.

239. Tantucci C, et al: Control of breathing and respiratory muscle strength in patients with multiple sclerosis. *Chest* 1994; 105:1163.

240. Smeltzer SC, et al: Respiratory function in multiple sclerosis. Utility of clinical assessment of respiratory muscle function. *Chest* 1992; 101:479.

241. Siemkowic E: Multiple sclerosis and surgery. *Anaesthesia* 1976; 31:1211.

242. Baskett P, Armstrong R: Anaesthetic problems in multiple sclerosis. *Anaesthesia* 1970; 25:39.

243. Bamford C, et al: Anesthesia in multiple sclerosis. *Can J Neurol Sciences* 1978; 5:41.

244. Korn-Lubetski I, et al: Activity of multiple sclerosis during pregnancy and periperium. *Ann Neurol* 1984; 16:229.

245. Guthrie TC, Nelson DA: Influence of temperature changes on multiple sclerosis: Critical review of mechanisms and research potential. *J Neurol Sci* 1995; 129:1.

246. Alderson JD: Intrathecal diamorphine and multiple sclerosis. *Anaesthesia* 1990; 45:1084.

247. Leigh J, et al: Intrathecal diamorphine during laparotomy in a patient with advanced multiple sclerosis. *Anaesthesia* 1990; 45:640.

248. Bromage P: Mechanism of action of extradural analgesia. *Br J Anaesth* 1975; 47:199.

249. Bader AM, et al: Anesthesia for the obstetric patient with multiple sclerosis. *J Clin Anesth* 1988; 1:21.

250. Jones RM, Healy T: Anaesthesia and demyelinating disease. *Anaesthesia* 1980; 35:879.

251. Kohno K, et al: Sevoflurane anesthesia in a patient with multiple sclerosis. *Masui* 1994; 43:1229.

252. Cooperman LH: Succinylcholine-induced hyperkalemia in neuromuscular disease. *JAMA* 1970; 213:1867.

253. Brett RS, et al: Measurements of acetylcholine receptor concentration in skeletal muscle from a patient with multiple sclerosis and resistance to atracurium. *Anesthesiology* 1987; 66:837.

254. Cendrowski W: Multiple sclerosis associated with defective neuromuscular transmission. *J Neurol* 1975; 209:297.

255. Yoshimasee F, et al: Tic douloureux in Rochester, Minnesota, 1945–1968. *Neurology* 1972; 22:952.

256. Jannetta PS: Arterial compression of the trigeminal nerve at the pons in patients with trigeminal neuralgia. *J Neurosurg* 1967; 26:159.

257. Rushton JF, Olofson RA: Trigeminal neuralgia associated with multiple sclerosis: Report of 35 cases. *Arch Neurol* 1965; 13:383.

258. Nugent GR: Techniques and results of 800 percutaneous radiofrequency thermocoagulations for trigeminal neuralgia. *Appl Neuro Physiol* 1982; 45:504.

259. Hakanson S: Trigeminal neuralgia treated by the injection of glycerol into the trigeminal astern. *Neurosurgery* 1981; 9:638.

260. Mullan S, Lichtor T: Percutaneous microcompression of the trigeminal ganglion for trigeminal neuralgia. *J Neurosurg* 1954; 11:299.

261. Jannetta PS: Microsurgical approach to the trigeminal nerve for tic douloureux. In Krayenbuhl H, et al (eds): *Progress in Neurological Surgery*, vol 7. Basel, S. Karger, 1976:180–200.

262. Small GW, et al: Diagnosis and treatment of dementia in the aged. *West J Med* 1981; 135:469.

263. Morris JC, et al: Very mild Alzheimer's disease: Informant-based clinical, psychometric, and pathologic distinction from normal aging. *Neurology* 1991; 41:469.

264. Clarfield AM: The reversible dementias: Do they reverse? *Ann Intern Med* 1988; 109:476.

265. Evans DA, et al: Prevalence of Alzheimer's disease in a community population of older persons. *JAMA* 1989; 262:2551.

266. United States Congress, Office of Technology Assessment: Losing a million minds: Confronting the tragedy of Alzheimer's disease and other dementias. Washington, DC, 1987.

267. Evans DA, et al: Estimated prevalence of Alzheimer's disease in the United States. *Milbank Q* 1990; 68:267.

268. McKhann G, et al: Clinical diagnosis of Alzheimer's disease: Report of the NINCDS-ADRDA Work Group under the auspices of the Department of Health and Human Services Task Force on Alzheimer's Disease. *Neurology* 1984; 34:939.

269. American Psychiatric Association: *Diagnostic and Statistical Manual of Mental Disorders*, 4th ed. Washington DC, American Psychiatric Press, 1995.

270. Folstein MF, et al: Mini-Mental State: A practical method for grading the cognitive state of patients for the clinician. *J Psychiatr Res* 1975; 12:189.

271. Bleecker ML, et al: Age-specific norms for the Mini-Mental State Exam. *Neurology* 1988; 38:1565.

272. Koller WC, et al: Primitive reflexes and cognitive function in the elderly. *Ann Neurol* 1982; 12:302.

273. Larson EB, et al: Diagnostic tests in the evaluation of dementia: A prospective study of 200 elderly outpatients. *Arch Intern Med* 1986; 146:1917.

274. Siu AL: Screening for dementia and investigating its causes. *Ann Intern Med* 1991; 115:122.

275. Katzman R: Should a major imaging procedure (CT or MRI) be required in the workup of dementia: An affirmative view. *J Fam Pract* 1990; 31:401.

276. Corey-Bloom J, et al: Diagnosis and evaluation of dementia. *Neurology* 1995; 45:211.

277. Erkinjuntti T, et al: Temporal lobe atrophy on magnetic resonance imaging in the diagnosis of early Alzheimer's disease. *Arch Neurol* 1993; 50:305.

278. Jagust WJ, et al: Alzheimer's disease: Age at onset and single-photon emission computed tomographic patterns of regional cerebral blood flow. *Arch Neurol* 1990; 47:628.

279. Johnson KA, et al: Lofetamine I^{123} single photon emission computed tomography is accurate in the diagnosis of Alzheimer's disease. *Arch Intern Med* 1990; 150:752.

280. Becker PM, et al: The role of lumbar puncture in the evaluation of dementia: The Durham Veterans Administration/Duke University study. *J Am Geriatr Soc* 1985; 33:397.

281. Hammerstrom DC, Zimmer B: The role of lumbar puncture in the evaluation of dementia: The University of Pittsburgh study. *J Am Geriatr Soc* 1985; 33:397.

282. Henderson JM, Hubbard BM: Definition of Alzheimer disease. *Lancet* 1985; 1:408.

283. Clinton J, et al: Amyloid plaque: Morphology, evolution, and etiology. *Mod Pathol* 1992; 5:439.

284. McKee AC, et al: Neuritic pathology and dementia in Alzheimer's disease. *Ann Neurol* 1991; 30:156.

285. Selkoe DJ: The molecular pathology of Alzheimer's disease. *Lancet* 1991; 1:1342.

286. Bowen DM, et al: Neurotransmitter-related enzymes and indices of hypoxia in senile dementia and other abiotrophies. *Brain* 1976; 99:459.

287. Whitehouse PJ, et al: Basal forebrain neurons in the dementia of Parkinson's disease. *Ann Neurol* 1983; 13:243.

288. Sasaki H, et al: Regional distribution of amino acid transmitters in postmortem brains of presenile and senile dementia of Alzheimer type. *Ann Neurol* 1986; 19:263.

289. McGeer PL, Rogers J: Anti-inflammatory agents as a therapeutic approach to Alzheimer's disease. *Neurology* 1992; 42:447.

290. McGeer PL, et al: Activation of the classical complement pathway in brain tissue of Alzheimer patients. *Neurosci Lett* 1989; 107:341.

291. Broe GA, et al: A case-control study of Alzheimer's disease in Australia. *Neurology* 1990; 40:1698.

292. Jenkinson ML, et al: Rheumatoid arthritis and senile dementia of the Alzheimer's type. *Br J Rheumatol* 1988; 28:86.

293. McGeer PL, et al: Anti-inflammatory drugs and Alzheimer's disease. *Lancet* 1990; 335:1037.

294. Henderson AS, et al: Environmental risk factors for Alzheimer's disease: Their relationship to age of onset and to familial or sporadic types. *Psychol Med* 1992; 22:429.

295. Breitner JCS, et al: Inverse association of anti-inflammatory treatments and Alzheimer's disease: Initial results of a co-twin control study. *Neurology* 1994; 44:227.

296. Rich JB, et al: Nonsteroidal anti-inflammatory drugs in Alzheimer's disease. *Neurology* 1995; 45:51.

297. Murrell J, et al: A mutation in the amyloid precursor protein associated with hereditary Alzheimer's disease. *Science* 1991; 254:97.

298. Salbaum JM, et al: The promoter of Alzheimer's disease amyloid A4 precursor gene. *EMBO J* 1988; 7:2807.

299. Schellenberg GD, et al: Genetic linkage evidence for a familial

Alzheimer's disease locus on chromosome 14. *Science* 1992; 258:668.

300. Pericak-Vance M, et al: Genetic evidence for a novel familial Alzheimer's locus on chromosome 14. *Nature Genet* 1992; 2:330.

301. Levy-Lahad E, et al: A familial Alzheimer's disease locus on chromosome 1. *Science* 1995; 269:970.

302. Pericak-Vance M, et al: Linkage studies in familial Alzheimer disease: Evidence for Chromosome 19 linkage. *Am J Hum Genet* 1991; 48:1034.

303. Saunders AM, et al: Association of allele E 4 with late-onset familial and sporadic Alzheimer's disease. *Neurology* 1993; 43:1467.

304. Corder EH, et al: Gene dose of apolipoprotein E type 4 allele and the risk of Alzheimer's disease in late onset families. *Science* 1993; 261:921.

305. Brousseau T, et al: Confirmation of the E4 allele of the apolipoprotein E gene as a risk factor for late-onset Alzheimer's disease. *Neurology* 1994; 44:342.

306. Peacock ML, Fink JK: ApoE allelic association with Alzheimer's disease. *Neurology* 1994; 44:339.

307. Strittmatter WJ, et al: Apolipoprotein E: High avidity binding to BA amyloid and increased frequency of type 4 allele in late-onset familial Alzheimer's. *Proc Natl Acad Sci USA* 1993; 90:1977.

308. Seshadri S, Drachman DA, Lippa CF: Apolipoprotein E E4 allele and the lifetime risk of Alzheimer's disease. *Arch Neurol* 1995; 52:1074.

309. Crismon ML: Tacrine: First drug approved for Alzheimer's disease. *Ann Pharmacother* 1994; 28:744.

310. Davis KL, et al: A double-blind placebo controlled multicenter study of tacrine for Alzheimer's. *N Engl J Med* 1992; 327:1253.

311. Farlow M, et al: A controlled trial of tacrine in Alzheimer's disease. *JAMA* 1992; 268:2523.

312. Knapp MJ, et al: A 30-week randomized controlled trial of high-dose tacrine in patients with Alzheimer's disease. *JAMA* 1993; 271:985.

313. Schneider LS, et al: A pilot study of low-dose L-deprenyl in Alzheimer's disease. *J Geriatr Psy & Neur* 1991; 4:1143.

314. Schneider LS, et al: A double-blind crossover pilot study of e-deprenyl combined with cholinesterase inhibitors in Alzheimer's disease. *Am J Psychiatry* 1993; 150:321.

315. Claus JJ, et al: Nootropic drugs in Alzheimer's disease: Symptomatic treatment with primeracetam. *Neurology* 1991; 41:570.

316. Spagnoli A, et al: Long-term acetyl-e-carnitine treatment in Alzheimer's disease. *Neurology* 1991; 41:1726.

317. Rogers J, et al: Clinical trial of indomethacin in Alzheimer's disease. *Neurology* 1993; 43:1609.

318. Davis KL, Haroutunian V: Strategies for the treatment of Alzheimer's disease. *Neurology* 1993; 43(suppl 4):552.

319. Olichney JM, et al: The spectrum of disease with diffuse Lewy Bodies. *Adv Neurol* 1995; 65:159.

320. Lennox G: Lewy body dementia. *Baillieres Clin Neurol* 1992; 1:653.

321. Pollanen MS, et al: Pathology and biology of the Lewy body. *J Neuropathol Exp Neurol* 1993; 52:183.

322. Roman GC, et al: Vascular dementia: Diagnostic criteria for research studies. Report of the NINDS-AIREN International Workshop. *Neurology* 1993; 43:250.

323. Roman GC: Senile dementia of the Binswanger type. A vascular form of dementia in the elderly. *JAMA* 1987; 258:1782.

324. Fischer P, et al: Prospective neuropathological validation of Hachinski's Ischemic Score in dementias. *J Neurol Neurosurg Psychiatry* 1991; 54:580.

325. Cummings JL, Benson DF: Subcortical dementia review of an emerging concept. *Arch Neurol* 1984; 41:874.

326. Friedland RP: "Normal" pressure hydrocephalus and the saga of the treatable dementias. *JAMA* 1989; 262:2577.

327. Friedland RP: Alzheimer's disease: Clinical features and differential diagnosis. *Neurology* 1993; 43(suppl 4):S45.

328. Weytingh MD, et al: Reversible dementia: More than 10% or less than 1%? A quantitative review. *J Neurol* 1995; 242:466.

329. Johnson J, et al: Differential diagnosis of dementia, delirium and depression. Implications for drug therapy. *Drugs & Aging* 1994; 5:431.

330. Caine ED: Pseudodementia. Current concepts and future directions. *Arch Gen Psychiat* 1981; 38:1359.

331. Yesavage J: Differential diagnosis between depression and dementia. *Am J Med* 1993; 34:23S.

332. Nielson WR, et al: Long-term cognitive and social sequelae of general versus regional anesthesia during arthroplasty in the elderly. *Anesthesiology* 1990; 73:1103.

333. Ghoneim MM, et al: Comparison of psychologic and cognitive functions after general or regional anesthesia. *Anesthesiology* 1988; 69:507.

334. Chung F, et al: Age-related cognitive recovery after general anesthesia. *Anesth Analg* 1990; 71:217.

335. Chung F, et al: Cognitive impairment after neuroleptanalgesia in cataract surgery. *Anesth Analg* 1989; 68:614.

336. Simpson KH, et al: Comparison of the effects of atropine and glycopyrrolate on cognitive function following general anaesthesia. *Br J Anaesth* 1987; 59:966.

337. Davies-Lepie SR: Tacrine may prolong the effect of succinylcholine. *Anesthesiology* 1994; 81:524.

338. Hartvig P, et al: Pharmacokinetics and effects of 9-amino-1,2,3,4-tetrahydroacridine in the immediate postoperative period in neurosurgical patients. *J Clin Anesth* 1991; 3:137.

339. Sinzinger H: Double blind study of the influence of co-degocrine on platelet parameters in healthy volunteers. *Eur J Clin Pharmacol* 1985; 28:713.

340. Fouque F, Vargaftig BB: Adrenaline/PAF acether synergism on human platelets: Involvement of hydergine. *J Pharmacol* 1985; 16(Suppl 3):129.

341. Gustafson Y, et al: Acute confusional states in elderly patients treated for femoral neck fracture. *J Am Geriatr Soc* 1988; 36:525.

342. Hirashima T, et al: Prognostic analysis for postoperative complications of abdominal surgery in the elderly. *Nippon Ronen Igakkai Zasshi* 1992; 29:635.

343. Wood DJ, et al: The ASNIS guided system for fixation of subcapital femoral fractures. *Injury* 1991; 22:190.

344. Davis FM, et al: Prospective, multi-centre trial of mortality following general or spinal anaesthesia for hip fracture surgery in the elderly. *Br J Anaesth* 1987; 59:1080.

345. Nussmeier NA: Neuropsychiatric complications of cardiac surgery. *J Cardiothorac Vasc Anesth* 1994; 8:13.

346. Wall M: Idiopathic intracranial hypertension. *Neurologic Clinics* 1991; 9:73.

347. Wall M, et al: Symptoms and disease associations in pseudotumor cerebri: A case-control study. *Neurology* 1989; 39:210.

348. Amacher A, Spence J: Spectrum of benign intracranial hypertension in children and adolescents. *Childs Nerv Syst* 1985; 1:81.

349. Aboulesh E, et al: Benign intracranial hypertension and anesthesia for cesarean section. *Anesthesiology* 1985; 63:705.

350. Palop R, et al: Epidural anesthesia for delivery complicated by benign intracranial hypertension. *Anesthesiology* 1979; 50:159.

351. Artru A: Cerebrospinal fluid. In Cottrell J, Smith D (eds): *Anesthesia and Neurosurgery.* Mosby, St. Louis, 1994:93.

352. Ravakhah K, West BC: Case report: Subacute combined degeneration of the spinal cord from folate deficiency. *Am J Med Sci* 1995; 310:214.

353. Layzer RB: Myeloneuropathy after prolonged exposure to nitrous oxide. *Lancet* 1978; 2:1227.

354. Banks R, et al: Reactions of gases in solution III. Some reactions of nitrous oxide with transition metal complexes. *J Chem Soc* 1968; 3:2886.

355. Metz J: Cobalamin deficiency and the pathogenesis of nervous system disease. *Ann Rev Nutr* 1992; 12:59.

356. Louis-Ferdinand RT: Myelotoxic, neurotoxic and reproductive adverse effects of nitrous oxide. *Adverse Drug React Toxicol Rev* 1994; 13:193.

357. Surtees R: Biochemical pathogenesis of subacute combined degeneration of the spinal cord and brain. *J Inherit Metab Dis* 1993; 16:762.

358. Lindenbaum J, et al: Neuropsychiatric disorders caused by cobalamin deficiency in the absence of anemia or macrocytosis. *N Engl J Med* 1988; 318:1720.

359. Timms SR, et al: Subacute combined degeneration of the spinal cord: MR findings. *Am J Neuroradiol* 1993; 14:1224.

360. Adams R, Victor M: Principles of Neurology, 4th ed. McGraw-Hill, New York, 1989:833.

361. Koblin DD, et al: Nitrous oxide inactivates methionine synthetase in human liver. *Anesth Analg* 1982; 61:75.

362. Royston BD, et al: Rate of inactivation of human and rodent hepatic methionine synthase by nitrous oxide. *Anesthesiology* 1988; 68:213.

363. Christensen B, et al: Preoperative methionine loading enhances restoration of the cobalamin-dependent enzyme methionine synthase after nitrous oxide anesthesia. *Anesthesiology* 1994; 80:1046.

364. Kinsella LJ, Green R: Anesthesia paresthetica: Nitrous oxide-induced cobalamin deficiency. *Neurology* 1995; 45:1608.

365. Holloway KL, Alberico AM: Postoperative myeloneuropathy: A preventable complication in patients with B$_{12}$ deficiency. *J Neurosurg* 1990; 72:732.

366. Schilling RF: Is nitrous oxide a dangerous anesthetic for vitamin B$_{12}$-deficient subjects? *JAMA* 1986; 255:1605.

367. Stacy CB, et al: Methionine in the treatment of nitrous-oxide-induced neuropathy and myeloneuropathy. *J Neurol* 1992; 239:401.

368. Flippo TS, Holder WD Jr: Neurologic degeneration associated with nitrous oxide anesthesia in patients with vitamin B$_{12}$ deficiency. *Arch Surg* 1993; 128:1391.

369. Blanco G, Peters H: Myeloneuropathy and macrocytosis associated with nitrous oxide abuse. *Arch Neurol* 1983; 40:416.

370. Koblin D, Tomerson B: Dimethylthiourea, a hydroxy radical scavenger, impedes the inactivation of methionine synthase by N$_2$O in mice. *Br J Anaesth* 1990; 64:214.

371. Bateman DN, et al: Extrapyramidal reactions to metoclopramide and prochlorperazine. *Q J Med* 1989; 71:307.

372. Stacy M, et al: Tardive stereotypy and other movement disorders in tardive dyskinesias. *Neurology* 1993; 43:937.

373. Kane JM, Smith JM: Tardive dyskinesia: prevalence and risk factors. *Arch Gen Psychiatry* 1982; 39:473.

374. Nutt JG: Levodopa-induced dyskinesia: review, observations, and speculations. *Neurology* 1990; 40:340.

375. Schooler NR, Kane JM: Research diagnosis for tardive dyskinesia. *Arch Gen Psychiatry* 1982; 39:486.

376. Mukherjee S, Rosen AM, Cardena C, et al. Tardive dyskinesia in psychiatric outpatients: A study of prevalence and association with demographic, clinical, and drug history variables. *Arch Gen Psychiatry* 1982; 39:466.

377. Smith JM, Baldessarini RJ: Changes in prevalence, severity, and recovery in tardive dyskinesia with age. *Arch Gen Psychiatry* 1980; 37:1368.

378. Thaker GK, et al: Clonazepam treatment of tardive dyskinesia: A practical GABA mimetic strategy. *Am J Psychiatry* 1990; 147:445.

379. Thaker GK, et al: Brain gamma-aminobutyric acid abnormality in tardive dyskinesia. *Arch Gen Psychiatry* 1987; 44:522.

380. Falk WE, et al: Diltiazem for tardive dyskinesia and tardive dystonia. *Lancet* 1988; 8589:824.

381. Kushnir SL, Ratner JT: Calcium channel blockers for tardive dyskinesia in geriatric psychiatric patients. *Am J Psychiatry* 1989; 146:1218.

382. Leys D, et al: Diltiazem for tardive dyskinesia. *Lancet* 1988; 8579:250.

383. Ross JL, et al: Diltiazem for tardive dyskinesia. *Lancet* 1987; 8527:268.

384. Elkashef AM, et al: Vitamin E in the treatment of tardive dyskinesia. *Am J Psychiatry* 1990; 147:505.

385. Lohr JB, et al: Alphatocopherol in tardive dyskinesia. *Lancet* 1987; 8538:913.

386. Chaudhry R, et al: Efficacy of propranolol in a patient with tardive dyskinesia and extrapyramidal syndrome. *Am J Psychiatry* 1982; 139:674.

387. Kulik FA, Wilbur R: Propranolol for tardive dyskinesia and extrapyramidal side effects (pseudoparkinsonism) from neuroleptics. *Psychopharmacol Bull* 1980; 16:18.

388. Schrodt GR Jr, et al: Treatment of tardive dyskinesia with propranolol. *J Clin Psychiatry* 1982; 43:328.

389. Freedman R, et al: Clonidine therapy for coexisting psychosis and tardive dyskinesia. *Am J Psychiatry* 1980; 137:629.

390. Freedman R, et al: Clonidine treatment of schizophrenia: Double-blind comparison to placebo and neuroleptic drugs. *Acta Psychiatr Scand* 1982; 65:35.

391. Lechin F, Van Der Dijs B: Clonidine therapy for psychosis and tardive dyskinesia. *Am J Psychiatry* 1981; 138:390.

392. Lieberman JA, et al: Treatment of tardive dyskinesia with bromocriptine: A test of the receptor modification strategy. *Arch Gen Psychiatry* 1989; 46:908.

393. Laitinen LV, et al: Leksell's posteroventral pallidotomy in the treatment of Parkinson's disease. *J Neurosurg* 1992; 76:53.

394. Rich MW, Radwang SM: Respiratory dyskinesia: An under-recognized phenomenon. *Chest* 1994; 105:1826.

395. Weiner WJ, et al: Respiratory dyskinesia: Extrapyramidal dysfunction and dyspnea. *Ann Intern Med* 1978; 88:327.

396. Goswami U, Channabasavanna SM: On the lethality of the acute respiratory component of tardive dyskinesia. *Clin Neurol Neurosurg* 1985; 87:99.

397. Sakamoto J, Hayasaka K: A case of respiratory dyskinesia. *Clin Psychiatr* 1987; 29:433.

398. Yassa R, Lal S: Respiratory irregularity and tardive dyskinesia: A prevalance study. *Acta Psychiatr Scand* 1986; 73:506.

399. Caroff SN, Mann SC: Neuroleptic malignant syndrome. *Med Clin North Am* 1993; 77:185.

400. Heiman-Patterson TD: Neuroleptic malignant syndrome and malignant hyperthermia. Important issues for the medical consultant. *Med Clin North Am* 1993; 77:477.

401. Heyland D, Sauve M: Neuroleptic malignant syndrome without the use of neuroleptics. *Can Med Assoc J* 1991; 145:817.

402. Levenson JL: Neuroleptic malignant syndrome. *Am J Psychiat* 1985; 142:1137.

403. Dickey S: The neuroleptic malignant syndrome. *Prog Neurobiol* 1991; 36:425.

404. Schneider SM: Neuroleptic malignant syndrome: Controversies in treatment. *Am J Emerg Med* 1991; 9:360.

405. Keltner N, Harris CP: Serotonin syndrome: A case of fatal SSRI/MAOI Interaction. *Perspect Psychiatr Care* 1995; 33:33.

406. Gratz SS, et al: The treatment and management of neuroleptic malignant syndrome. *Prog Neuropsychopharmacol Biol Psychiatry* 1992; 16:425.

407. Lev R, Clark RF: Neuroleptic malignant syndrome presenting

without fever: Case report and review of the literature. *J Emerg Med* 1994; 12:49.

408. Granner MA, Wooten GF: Neuroleptic malignant syndrome or parkinsonism hyperpyrexia syndrome. *Semin Neurol* 1991; 11:228.

409. George AL, Wood CA: Succinylcholine-induced hyperkalemia complicating the neuroleptic malignant syndrome. *Ann Intern Med* 1987; 106:172.

410. Synder SH: Receptors, neurotransmitters and drug responses. *N Engl J Med* 1979; 300:465.

411. Baldressarini RJ: Drugs and treatment of psychiatric disorders. In Gilman AG, Rail TW, Nies AS, Taylor P (eds). *The Pharmacological Basis of Therapeutics*, 8th ed. New York, McGraw-Hill, 1990:383–435.

412. Hill GE, et al: Lithium carbonate and neuromuscular blocking agents. *Anesthesiology* 1977; 46:122.

413. Martin BA, Kramer PM: Clinical significance of the interaction between lithium and a neuromuscular blocker. *Am J Psychiat* 1982; 139:1326.

414. Thomsen K, Schou M: Renal lithium excretion in man. *Am J Physiol* 1968; 215:823.

415. Louden JB, Waring H: Toxic reactions to lithium and haloperidol. *Lancet* 1976; 2:1088.

416. Ragheb M, et al: Interaction of indomethacin and ibuprofen with lithium in manic patients under a steady lithium level. *J Clin Psychiatry* 1980; 41:397.

417. O'Regan JB: Adverse interaction of lithium carbonate and methyldopa. *Can Med Assoc J* 1976; 115:385.

418. Byrd GJ: Methyldopa and lithium carbonate: Suspected interaction. *JAMA* 1975; 223:320.

419. Courville CB: *Effects of Alcohol on the Nervous System of Man.* Los Angeles, San Lucas Press, 1955.

420. Toward a National Plan to Combat Alcohol Abuse and Alcoholism: Administrative Document, draft report to the National Institute on Alcohol Abuse and Alcoholism. Research Triangle Park, NC, Research Triangle Institute, 1985.

421. Albin MS, Bunegin L: An experimental study of craniocerebral trauma during alcohol intoxication. *Crit Care Med* 1986; 14:841.

422. Haut MJ, Cowan DH: The effect of ethanol on hemostatic properties of human blood platelets. *Am J Med* 1974; 56:22.

423. Donahue RP, et al: Alcohol and hemorrhagic stroke: The Honolulu heart program. *JAMA* 1986; 255:2311.

424. Horrobin DF: Essential fatty acids, prostaglandins, and alcohol: An overview. *Alcohol Clin Exp Res* 1987; 11:2.

425. Alburo BM, et al: Alcohol-induced spasms of cerebral blood vessels: Relation to cerebrovascular accident and sudden death. *Science* 1983; 20:331.

426. Glieberman L, Hartung E: Alcohol usage and blood pressure: A review. *Human Biol* 1986; 58:1.

427. Blum K, Topel H: Opioid peptides and alcoholism: Genetic deficiency and chemical management. *Funct Neurol* 1986; I:71.

428. Adahma Bulletin. *JAMA* 1989; 261:2604.

429. Hillbom M, et al: Can ethanol intoxication affect hemocoagulation to increase the risk of brain infarction in young adults. *Neurology* 1983; 33:381.

430. Mathew RJ, Wilson WH: Regional cerebral blood flow changes associated with ethanol intoxication. *Stroke* 1986; 17:1156.

431. Medical News and Perspectives. *JAMA* 1992; 267:1043.

432. Janies MFM, et al: Analgesic effect of ethyl alcohol. *Br J Anaesth* 1978; 50:139.

433. Dundee JW, Isaac M: Clinical studies of induction agents. XXIX: Ethanol. *Br J Anaesth* 1969; 41:1063.

434. Gessner PK: Drug therapy of the alcohol withdrawal syndrome. In Majchrowicz E, Moble EP (eds): *Biochemistry and Pharmacology of Ethanol,* vol II. New York, Plenum Press, 1979:375–435.

435. Bacon MK: Cross-cultural studies in drinking. In Bourne PG, Fox R (eds): *Alcoholism: Progress in Research and Treatment.* New York, Academic Press, 1973:171–174.

436. Victor M, et al: *The Wernicke-Korsakoff Syndrome and Related Neurologic Disorders Due to Alcoholism and Malnutrition,* 2d ed. Philadelphia, Davis, 1989.

437. Adams RD, Victor M: *Principles of Neurology,* 5th ed. New York, McGraw-Hill, 1993.

438. Behse F, Buchtal F: Alcoholic neuropathy: Clinical, electrophysiological, and biopsy findings. *Ann Neurol* 1977; 2:95.

439. Abel E, Sokol RJ: Incidence of fetal alcohol syndrome and economic of FAS-related anomalies. *Drug Alcohol Depend* 1987; 19:51.

440. Schenker S, et al: Fetal alcohol syndrome: Current status of pathogenesis. *Alcohol Clin Exp Res* 1990; 14:635.

441. Peiffer J, et al: Alcohol embryo- and fetopathy: Neuropathology of 3 children and 3 fetuses. *J Neurol Sci* 1979; 41:125.

442. Kitson TM: The disulfiram-ethanol reaction: A review. *J Stud Alcohol* 1977; 38:96.

443. Olesen OV: Disulfiram (Antabuse) as inhibitor of phenytoin metabolism. *Acta Pharmacol Toxicol* 1966; 24:317.

444. O'Reilly RA: Interaction of sodium warfarin and disulfiram in man. *Ann Intern Med* 1973; 78:73.

445. Greenberg RS, Parker SD: Anesthetic management for the child with Charcot-Marie-Tooth disease. *Anesth Analg* 1992; 74:305.

446. Antognini JF: Anaesthesia for Charcot-Marie-Tooth disease: A review of 86 cases. *Can J Anaesth* 1992; 39:398.

447. O'Brien FC, Ginsberg B: Cockayne syndrome: A case report. *AANA* 1994; 62:346.

448. Kubal K, et al: Spinal anesthesia in a patient with Friedreich's ataxia. *Anesth Analg* 1991; 72:257.

449. Roy RC, et al: Anesthetic management of a patient with Hallervorden-Spatz disease. *Anesthesiology* 1983; 58:382.

450. Katende RS, Herlich A: Anesthetic considerations in holoprosencephaly. *Anesth Analg* 1987; 66:908.

451. Tobias JD: Anaesthetic considerations for the child with leukodystrophy. *Can J Anaesth* 1992; 39:394.

452. Kempthorne PM, Brown TCK: Anaesthesia and the mucopolysaccharidoses: A survey of techniques and problems. *Anaesth Intensive Care* 1983; 11:203.

453. Schiffman FL, Golbe LI: Upper airway dysfunction in olivopontocerebellar atrophy. *Chest* 1992; 102:291.

454. Harasawa I, et al: Anesthesia for a patient with olivopontocerebellar atrophy. *Masui* 1994; 43:1066.

455. Morrison JE Jr, Lockhart CH: Tourette syndrome: Anesthetic implications. *Anesth Analg* 1986; 65:200.

Chapter 13 ────────────────────

NEUROANESTHESIA AND NEUROMUSCULAR DISEASES

JAMES W. ALBERS

JOHN J. WALD

The relationship between anesthesia and neuromuscular disease involves two separate but closely associated problems. First are the patients who require special consideration when administered anesthesia because they have a neuromuscular disease that influences their response to anesthetic agents. Alternatively, they may require medications that have a potential influence upon anesthesia. The second relates to anesthetic complications that produce neuromuscular impairments, independent of any underlying neurologic disease.

An example of a specific neuromuscular disease that poses anesthetic problems is myasthenia gravis. Thymectomy frequently is recommended for myasthenic patients, and important perioperative considerations include identification of medications used to treat myasthenia gravis that may influence anesthesia (e.g., corticosteroid or anticholinesterase agents), choice of anesthetic agents, and postanesthesia decisions including the timing of extubation. Other examples of procedures in patients with neuromuscular disorders requiring special anesthetic consideration

include diagnostic biopsy in Lambert-Eaton myasthenic syndrome, tracheotomy in Guillain-Barré syndrome or motor neuron disease, or any procedure requiring anesthesia in a patient with polyneuropathy who may have unusual susceptibility to nerve injury. Issues related to specific effects of anesthesia upon the peripheral nervous system are also important, including the potential problem of anesthesia-related worsening or exacerbation of a neuromuscular disorder such as inflammatory polyneuropathy or polymyositis.

Several neuromuscular disorders are associated with anesthesia. The best known associations are anesthetic-induced malignant hyperthermia and postanesthetic mononeuropathy or plexopathy. There also are patients who develop critical illness neuropathy or myopathy after prolonged paralysis after receiving neuromuscular blocking agents. Further, some patients with neuromuscular disorders, including those with cervical spondylosis, are susceptible to postanesthetic impairments attributed to spinal cord or anterior horn cell ischemia. While controversial, these problems frequently are attributed to tissue compression or intraoperative hypotension. In some, the mechanisms of injury are well understood, whereas in others the associations are speculative. Of equal importance are a group of neuromuscular disorders that mimic anesthesia complications, including idiopathic brachial plexopathy, postoperative Guillain-Barré syndrome, and development of an isolated mononeuropathy during the postoperative recovery phase. Recognition of these disorders has important medicolegal implications.

Role of the Neuromuscular Specialist

The most important role of the neuromuscular specialist in relationship to the anesthesiologist involves anticipation of potential anesthesia-related problems in patients with known or suspected neuromuscular disease. This commonly relates to the neurologist's familiarity in evaluating and treating specific diseases such as myasthenia gravis or polyneuropathy. As such, the neurologist participates in decisions involving preanesthetic medical management, selection of anesthetic agents, and timing of elective operations and postanesthetic extubation. The neurologist occasionally identifies patients with neuromuscular diseases potentially associated with malignant hyperthermia or other anesthetic-related complications.

The second role of the neuromuscular specialist relates to identifying peripheral nervous system impairments developing during or after anesthesia. In addition to the clinical history and neurologic examination, the neurologist frequently uses specialized evaluations including nerve conduction studies and

453

needle electromyography to localize a peripheral impairment, estimate the time of onset, and establish etiology. Occasionally other aspects of nerve conduction studies such as repetitive motor nerve stimulation identify neuromuscular junction impairments in patients with prolonged paralysis after receiving neuromuscular blocking agents.[1-4] These studies are important in evaluating peripheral neuromuscular disorders, and their application will be reviewed for specific disorders, with special attention to use of these techniques in establishing the causation and prognosis of any new peripheral nervous system impairment.

Role of the Anesthesiologist

The role of the anesthesiologist parallels that of the neuromuscular specialist. Both are expected to anticipate potential anesthetic problems posed by the presence of an underlying neuromuscular disorder, and both are involved in identifying anesthetic-related complications involving the peripheral nervous system. The anesthesiologist also has an important role in the intensive care of patients, many of whom have or acquire neuromuscular problems. The unique experience of the anesthesiologist frequently is required during the treatment of patients with respiratory failure or dysphagia related to a primary neuromuscular disease.

Acute respiratory failure and dysphagia leading to aspiration are among the most important emergencies caused by neuromuscular diseases, and their evaluation and treatment typically involve the combined efforts of the anesthesiologist and neuromuscular specialist. A unique feature of respiratory failure in patients with neuromuscular disorders is the rapid transition from unlabored breathing to decompensation and hypoventilation. Intubation should not be delayed until the usual signs of tachypnea, reduced vital capacity, and hypercarbic blood gases are apparent, because decompensation occurs abruptly with muscular fatigue. This is especially true in conditions such as myasthenia gravis, where reliance on resting respiratory rate or blood gases may provide false reassurance of stability. One of the earliest signs of impending respiratory fatigue is nonspecific anxiety or agitation. Simply asking patients whether they are tiring provides useful information, and noting their ability to produce a forceful, explosive cough indicates good respiratory muscle reserve.[5] An intact cough also indicates the airway can be protected from aspiration. Quantitative measures of pulmonary function include vital capacity and maximal inspiratory force. Threshold values for intubation are a vital capacity less than 15 ml/kg and inspiratory force less than 15 mmHg.[6-8] However, the rate of decline in the vital capacity is as important as the absolute value. Early intubation is important in neuromuscular disorders, when conditions are stable and proper preparations can be made for a safe elective procedure.

A second consideration regarding timing of intubation relates to protecting the airway from aspiration in the presence of dysphagia.[9] Intubation should be considered even when respiratory function is adequate, because aspiration occurs in the setting of adequate respiratory function in disorders such as myasthenia gravis and Guillain-Barré syndrome. Nasal regurgitation of liquids and frequent coughing while eating or drinking can be confirmed by observing the patient drinking water. Formal assessment can be made by viewing the mechanics of swallowing liquid barium or barium-coated cookies under fluoroscopy.[10] A nasogastric feeding tube should be placed at the time of intubation.[9] Insertion of a nasal gastric tube without intubation may improve intake, but does not protect the airway and may stimulate secretions and increase the relative risk of aspiration.

Anesthesia in Neuromuscular Disorders

The anesthesiologist frequently participates in the treatment of patients with neuromuscular diseases. This participation includes involvement as an expert in respiratory support of patients with respiratory failure, as well as in administration of anesthesia to patients having surgery unrelated (or remotely related) to their underlying neuromuscular disorder. Of importance are complications of anesthetic agents affecting the neuromuscular system. Because patients with underlying neuromuscular disorders present special problems, selected peripheral disease will be described, including a review of special anesthesia considerations.

COMPLICATIONS OF ANESTHESIA AFFECTING NEUROMUSCULAR DISEASES

EFFECT OF ANESTHESIA UPON THE NEUROMUSCULAR SYSTEM

Anesthesia, of course, affects the peripheral nervous system. Many of these effects are desired, for example, muscle relaxation and anesthesia. However, in patients with underlying neuromuscular disorders these effects can be exaggerated. Specific examples of underlying conditions with altered responsiveness follow.

Neuromuscular Blockers in Neuromuscular Junction Disease

Neuromuscular transmission begins with presynaptic nerve depolarization causing entry of calcium ions through voltage-gated calcium channels. This leads to fusion of the acetylcholine (ACh) containing vesicles with the axonal membrane, diffusion of the ACh across the synaptic cleft, and activation of the postsynaptic ACh receptor (AChR). This activation opens sodium channels, leading to depolarization of the muscle membrane, release of calcium from the sarcoplasmic reticulum, and the development of muscle contraction.[11] Typically, the amount of ACh released is greater than required to activate all AChRs in the junction, a concept described as the "margin of safety" in neuromuscular junction transmission. Reduction in this safety margin is the basis for electrophysiologic testing of neuromuscular junction transmission and determining the level of neuromuscular blockade during anesthesia. Anesthetic muscle relaxants exploit these interactions to produce desired effects; however, these interactions also account for exaggerated responses.

Competitive neuromuscular blockers such as curare bind to the AChR without causing channel opening. Depolarizing blocking agents lead to channel opening with binding to the AChR. Other agents block the response to ACh without binding directly to the AChR.[11] Patients with neuromuscular junction disease (e.g., myasthenia gravis) have a reduced safety margin, as the ACh released with motor nerve depolarization may not cause activation of all AChRs present. As such, these patients are extremely sensitive to nondepolarizing agents. They also respond abnormally to depolarizing agents, demonstrating resistance. Anticholinesterase medications, used to treat disorders of neuromuscular junction transmission and capable of reversing nondepolarizing agents, inhibit plasma cholinesterase, causing increased intensity and duration of response to succinylcholine.[12] Myasthenic patients are sensitive to other medications not typically considered neuromuscular junction blockers, including analgesics, antiarrhythmics, and antibiotics.[13] These effects again relate to the diminished safety margin of transmission. While they are most important in patients with marginal function (e.g., those with borderline ventilation), these effects further illustrate the caution required when using medication in patients with neuromuscular junction transmission defects.

Motor neuron disorders with rapid denervation and reinnervation (such as in ALS) can produce a similar alteration in the neuromuscular junction safety margin. This leads to similar responses to nondepolarizing agents.[14] Succinylcholine has caused hyperkalemia, contracture, and cardiac arrest in these patients and should be avoided if significant motor nerve disease (motor neuron disease or sensorimotor polyneuropathy) is identified.[15]

Depolarizing Agents in Muscle Disease

Patients with underlying muscle disease respond variably to succinylcholine. In patients with myotonic disorders, particularly myotonic dystrophy, the response to succinylcholine may be normal, myotonia may disappear, or excessive myotonia may develop with contracture.[14] Similar unpredictable response is reported in the muscular dystrophies.[14,16]

Abnormal Cardiovascular Responses in Neuropathy with Autonomic Involvement

Dysautonomia may be *primary* (due to central nervous system involvement such as Parkinson's disease, multiple system atrophy, or Shy-Drager syndrome or due to peripheral nervous system involvement such as hereditary sensory autonomic neuropathy or autonomic degeneration) or *secondary* to medications or a disorder such as diabetic polyneuropathy, amyloidosis, or Guillain-Barré syndrome. Symptoms and signs include dizziness or light-headedness associated with postural blood pressure change, decreased or absent heart rate variability during normal respiration or Valsalva maneuver, altered temperature regulation with decreased sweating, and impotence. Cardiovascular compensatory mechanisms may fail, leading to severe hypotension after postural change, blood loss, or increased intrathoracic pressure. Dysautonomia may cause supersensitivity to sympathomimetic medications, presumably due to increased numbers of receptors.[17]

NEUROMUSCULAR COMPLICATIONS THAT RESULT FROM ANESTHESIA

Several neuromuscular problems appear only after anesthesia or prolonged assisted ventilation. Although some problems such as malignant hyperthermia have an underlying genetic predisposition, they develop unexpectedly unless a similar problem has occurred in another family member.

Malignant Hyperthermia

Malignant hyperthermia associated with anesthesia is an autosomal dominant disorder having an incidence of about 1 in 50,000 persons exposed to inhalation anesthesia.[18,19] In susceptible patients, exposure to the neuromuscular blocker succinylcholine or halogenated anesthetic agents produces a hypermetabolic state of skeletal muscle, presumably related to increased concentration of calcium from defective membrane regulation. Malignant hyperthermia is categorized as a membranopathy because of the identified abnormality of the calcium release channel of the lateral cisterns in the sarcoplasmic reticulum involving the ryanodine receptor.[20,21] The resultant abnormality produces muscle rigidity, hyperpyrexia, tachycardia and other dysrhythmia, and dramatically increased oxygen consumption.[22] During an attack, serum creatine kinase and myoglobin become elevated. Without prompt reversal of triggering mechanisms, malignant hyperpyrexia and cardiac dysrhythmia occur, as does rhabdomyolysis, depending upon the variable degree of muscle rigidity and resultant muscle fiber necrosis.[22]

Identification of susceptible individuals is imprecise. A positive family history of anesthetic difficulty or death, or a history of unexplained tachycardia or hyperpyrexia with previous procedures is important, although as many as 50 percent of patients with documented malignant hyperthermia had prior anesthesia without recognized difficulty.[23] The association of a hyperpyrexic state with cardiac arrest, elevated serum creatine kinase, and myoglobinuria in a patient with known muscular dystrophy suggests a special susceptibility.[16] Similarly, patients with idiopathic elevation of serum creatine kinase, presumably related to an underlying metabolic myopathy, should be considered at risk for developing malignant hyperthermia. Development of in vitro muscle contracture to caffeine or halothane suggests increased susceptibility to malignant hyperthermia.[24]

Treatment consists of discontinuation of the anesthetic agent and administration of intravenous dantrolene sodium, an inhibitor of calcium ion release.[25] Agents such as pancuronium cause flaccid muscle paralysis but have no effect upon malignant hyperthermia. However, dantrolene is associated with recognized side effects including muscle weakness and fatigue when administered to patients thought to be susceptible to malignant hyperthermia.[26] These side effects do not obviate the usefulness of dantrolene in treating patients with malignant hyperthermia, but should be a consideration when deciding when the prophylactic use is indicated in potentially susceptible patients.[26]

Prolonged Assisted Ventilation

The anesthesiologist frequently contributes to the management of patients undergoing prolonged assisted ventilation in the critical care unit. These patients typically have multiple medical complications, making them vulnerable to a variety of neuromuscular problems. Because the individual problems are addressed in subsequent sections, they will be mentioned here as an introduction. The most common problem relates to disuse atrophy and weakness, a normal physiologic consequence of prolonged inactivity. In some patients, this decompensation makes it difficult to wean them from the respirator or to resume previous activities. For patients with preexisting neuromuscular impairments this poses special difficulty and may represent the difference between independent existence and the need for complete assistance in activities of daily living. A severe axonal sensorimotor polyneuropathy (critical illness polyneuropathy) and an acute quadriplegic myopathy are two clinically similar disorders that may develop.[27,28] Critical illness polyneuropathy, however,

TABLE 13-1
Myopathies with Cardiac Involvement

Carnitine deficiency: Cardiomyopathy

Polymyositis/dermatomyositis: Cardiomegaly, congestive heart failure, conduction abnormality

Mitochondrial myopathy, Kearns-Sayre syndrome: Cardiac conduction block

Duchenne, Becker muscular dystrophy: Sinus arrhythmias, cardiomyopathy

Debranching enzyme deficiency: Cardiomyopathy

Emery-Dreifuss: Arrhythmias, heart block

Myotonic dystrophy: Complete heart block, arrhythmias

includes sensory loss and develops in association with sepsis and multiorgan failure, whereas acute quadriplegic myopathy usually is associated with administration of neuromuscular blocking and corticosteroid medications. Prolonged effects of neuromuscular blocking drugs like vecuronium in patients with renal insufficiency may mimic myopathy.[29]

SPECIFIC NEUROMUSCULAR DISEASES
MYOPATHY

There are several types of myopathy, ranging from acquired inflammatory myositis associated with other medical conditions to congenital myopathy present at birth. The anesthesiologist will likely encounter these patients, as they frequently require surgical procedures, including diagnostic muscle biopsy and feeding tube placement. Furthermore, in patients with underlying muscle disease or elevated creatine kinase (CK), malignant hyperthermia is of concern (see above). Besides limb-muscle weakness, a number of other conditions will be of concern to the anesthesiologist, including cardiac (Table 13-1) and diaphragmatic involvement (Table 13-2).

TABLE 13-2
Myopathies with Diaphragmatic Involvement

Dystrophies: Duchenne, myotonic,[a] facioscapulohumeral, limb-girdle, oculopharyngeal

Congenital myopathies: Nemaline rod,[a] centronuclear.[a]

Metabolic myopathies: Acid maltase deficiency[a]

Mitochondrial myopathies

Inflammatory myopathies: Polymyositis, dermatomyositis

Endocrine myopathies: Hypo- or hyperthyroidism, hyperadrenocorticosteroidism

Myosin-deficient myopathies: Use of corticosteroids, neuromuscular blocking agents

Acute steroid myopathies

[a] Present with ventilatory failure.

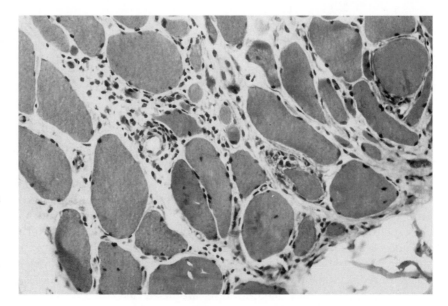

Figure 13-1 Muscle biopsy from patient with polymyositis, demonstrating inflammatory infiltrate involving vessels, interstitium, and muscle, with muscle fibers undergoing degeneration and regeneration. (Original magnification ×200. Courtesy of Mila Blaivas, University of Michigan Medical Center, Department of Pathology.)

Inflammatory Myopathy

The term *inflammatory myopathy* typically denotes three diseases—polymyositis (PM), dermatomyositis (DM), and inclusion-body myositis (IBM). These disorders involve primarily but not exclusively skeletal muscle with invasion by inflammatory cells (Fig. 13-1). DM is a form of ischemic-inflammatory myopathy involving a humoral autoimmune attack directed primarily against muscle blood vessels.[30] PM involves a cell-mediated autoimmunity directed primarily against muscle fibers.[31,32] In contrast, IBM is a distinct form of inflammatory myopathy in which the role of autoimmunity is unknown, but inclusions are apparent on muscle biopsy (Fig. 13-2).[33,34] The major symptom in inflammatory myopathy is proximal weakness, though distal weakness (in IBM) or skin changes (in DM) are important in clinical classification. Dysphagia, esophageal dysmotility, and slowed gastric emptying occur, though ventilatory muscle weakness or ventilatory failure is rare, occurring most often in PM.[35] Cardiac muscle also may become inflamed, leading to cardiomegaly, congestive heart failure, or conduction abnormality including atrioventricular block, supraventricular tachycardia, and ventricular tachycardia.[36,37] Pulmonary involvement ranges from aspiration pneumonia, related to pharyngeal weakness, to interstitial lung disease, which can affect up to 10 percent of patients.[38] Patients over 50 years of age with inflammatory myopathy, DM in particular, are felt to be at increased risk of malignancy.[39] The malignancy may be apparent before the muscle disease is discovered.

Evaluation of patients with suspected inflammatory

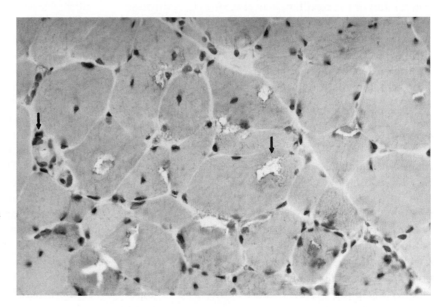

Figure 13-2 Muscle biopsy from patient with inclusion-body myositis. Note the dark rimmed vacuoles (*arrow*) and inflammation (*arrow*). (Original magnification ×400. Courtesy of Mila Blaivas, University of Michigan Medical Center, Department of Pathology.)

myopathy includes physical examination for proximal weakness, search for other associated disorders, electromyography, and possible muscle biopsy. Serum CK is elevated in up to 90 percent of patients, and other cellular enzymes (e.g., lactate dehydrogenase, LDH) are also often elevated without underlying hepatic disease. Elevated erythrocyte sedimentation rate (ESR) and the presence of autoantibodies may lead to the diagnosis of an associated collagen vascular disorder. The Jo-1 autoantibody is present in patients with associated intrinsic lung disease,[40] while SS-A (Ro) suggests underlying Sjögren syndrome and may be associated with cardiac damage.[41]

Corticosteroids are used almost uniformly to treat PM and DM.[42] If patients cannot tolerate corticosteroid side effects, or unusually high doses of corticosteroids are required, cytotoxic agents such as azathioprine, cyclophosphamide, and methotrexate are used as "steroid-sparing agents." Intravenous immune globulin may also be effective.[43] IBM usually does not respond to any treatment, though treatment with immunosuppressant medications is often attempted, particularly if there is biopsy evidence of prominent inflammation. The lack of response to immunosuppression may be helpful in differentiating IBM from PM.

Metabolic Myopathy
The term *metabolic myopathy* implies defective glycogen, lipid, or purine metabolism. Patients typically complain of exercise-induced muscle pain, exercise intolerance, and may experience myoglobinuria or progressive muscle weakness related to underlying metabolic defects. The major source of adenosine triphosphate (ATP), required for muscle contraction, is oxidative phosphorylation of glycogen, followed by conversion of the resultant acetyl-CoA to CO_2 through the tricarboxylic acid cycle. During intense activity anaerobic metabolism of glycogen produces lactate through glycolysis. Lipid also may be metabolized through intermitochondrial processes to produce ATP. Thus, any metabolic defect causing impairment of substrate availability (glycogen, lipid) or ATP extraction from substrate can lead to underlying muscle pathology. Furthermore, with accumulation of substrate, progressive muscle weakness may become superimposed or intermittent or exercise-induced weakness and fatigue. Diagnosis depends upon the clinical presentation and usually requires biopsy for histologic and biochemical evaluation.

Myopathies due to defective glycogen metabolism are rare. Myophosphorylase deficiency (McArdle's disease) is one of the most common of many potential enzyme deficiencies (e.g., phosphofructokinase deficiency, phosphoglycerate mutase deficiency). Myoglo-

binuria with renal failure is common.[16,44] These disorders are characterized by intolerance of high-intensity exercise (e.g., sprinting) with attacks of muscle cramping, stiffness, and weakness. Many patients note improvement in function after a brief rest ("second-wind phenomenon").[45] The diagnosis can be suspected when there is a failure of lactate production during the ischemic forearm exercise test, and can be confirmed by very low or absent levels of phosphorylase activity on muscle biopsy. Serum CK is often elevated between attacks, and there is the potential association with malignant hyperthermia. Acid maltase deficiency is important to the anesthesiologist, as this condition may present during infancy or later in life with respiratory failure and resultant pulmonary hypertension due to diaphragm involvement.[46] Glycogen debranching enzyme deficiency may cause cardiomyopathy.[47]

Lipid metabolism occurs within the mitochondria. This requires carnitine and carnitine palmitoyl transferase (CPT) to carry the long-chain fatty acids across the mitochondrial membranes. Deficiency of carnitine may be inherited or secondary to a number of underlying conditions, including organic acidurias with renal loss of acid-bound carnitine, inability to produce carnitine due to liver failure, medications causing depletion (e.g., valproic acid), or pregnancy. Carnitine deficiency may cause a progressive weakness similar to other myopathies, or produce intermittent "Reye syndrome-like" attacks including hypoglycemia and liver dysfunction. CPT deficiency is recessively inherited, variably expressed, and frequently causes myoglobinuria, particularly after stressors such as infection, hypoglycemia, general anesthesia, or exercise.[48,49] Strength, CK, and EMG are usually normal between attacks. Recognition of this disorder is important, as glucose is required during general anesthesia.[50] Provocative factors promoting crises in patients with carnitine deficiency include fasting, fever, and overexertion; treatment of an acute attack requires correction of the resultant acidosis.[51]

Mitochondrial Myopathy
Mitochondrial myopathy is a specific form of metabolic myopathy, as the mitochondria are the site of the electron transport chain, generating the majority of ATP required for muscle function through oxidative phosphorylation. The disorder may be inherited, acquired with exposure to mitochondrial toxins, or develop as part of normal aging. A number of proteins required for mitochondrial function are encoded by mitochondrial DNA present within the mitochondria in multiple copies, while others are encoded by nuclear DNA. As the mitochondrial DNA is that present in the ovum (with very little contribution from the sperm) at conception, nearly all mitochondrial genes are inherited

maternally. However, as nuclear DNA is required for mitochondrial function, dominant, recessive, or X-linked inheritance of mitochondrial disorders is possible. The multiple copies of mitochondrial DNA are randomly distributed between dividing cells, leading to unequal proportions of mutated mitochondrial DNA in cells destined to become certain tissues or organs.

Organs with the greatest energy requirements (nervous system, muscle, gastrointestinal system) most commonly exhibit dysfunction related to impaired energy production with mitochondrial disease. The specific organ affected, however, is also determined by the *mitotic segregation* of mitochondria during development and by *heteroplasmy*, the presence of variable proportions of normal and abnormal mitochondrial DNA in a given cell (as there are multiple copies of mitochondrial DNA present in each mitochondrion, and many mitochondria present in each cell).[44]

Progressive external ophthalmoplegia (PEO) is a common finding in patients with mitochondrial muscle disease, and is associated with ptosis, limb weakness, and other systemic features suggesting a particular syndrome. Lactate and pyruvate are often elevated. Confirmation of the diagnosis can be obtained through muscle biopsy if abnormal accumulations of mitochondria are discovered. When stained with modified trichrome, these accumulations appear red, thus the term *ragged red fiber* (Fig. 13-3). Sampling error can lead to false-negative muscle biopsy. When examined electron-microscopically, the mitochondria often contain nonspecific inclusions. The genetic defects responsible for a number of the mitochondrial disorders are now known, and confirmation can be obtained commercially.[52,53]

Attempts at defining specific syndromes have been confounded by significant overlap; however, there are certain features of these syndromes of importance to the anesthesiologist. The Kearns-Sayre syndrome includes PEO, mitochondrial myopathy, retinal pigmentary degeneration, and cardiac conduction block.[44] There may be associated ventilatory dysfunction.[54] These patients frequently require pacemaker placement. Another mitochondrial defect that is associated with limb weakness, seizures, and myoclonus has been called <u>my</u>oclonic <u>e</u>pilepsy with <u>r</u>agged <u>red f</u>ibers (MERRF). A similar syndrome, with "strokelike episodes" rather than seizures, has been termed mitochondrial <u>my</u>opathy, <u>e</u>ncephalopathy, <u>l</u>actic <u>a</u>cidosis, and <u>s</u>trokelike episodes (MELAS). Treatment for these disorders with mitochondrial cofactors such as coenzyme Q is suggested but only occasionally effective.[55,56] Supportive care, appropriate anticonvulsants when required, and treatment of associated conditions are necessary.

Muscular Dystrophy

Muscular dystrophies are inherited, progressive disorders causing muscle weakness but also involving other organs. The best understood and recognized dystrophy is Duchenne muscular dystrophy (DMD), an X-linked disorder of boys and adolescent males causing progressive weakness. The findings of elevated CK, proximal weakness (leading to the classical "Gowers' sign," pushing the thorax upward with the hands against the thighs to compensate for proximal extensor weakness when arising), and calf pseudohypertrophy (replacement of muscle by fat and connective tissue) suggest the diagnosis. The diagnosis can be confirmed by analysis for dystrophin, a cytoskeletal protein that is absent in this disorder.[57-59] Joint contractures and scoliosis develop early in the course of the disease. Most boys with DMD have ECG abnormalities, sinus arrhythmias being most common, though symptoms are rare. Gastric hypomotility may occur.[60] Intellectual impairment is common, though the causation of this is unknown. Another X-linked form of muscular dystrophy causing less rapidly progressive weakness is Becker muscular dystrophy. This is due to decreased or abnormal dystrophin. Similar, though less severe changes are seen in organs other than muscle.

Treatment of DMD includes physiotherapy, bracing, surgical release of contracture, and spinal stabilization. Patients with DMD react adversely to halogenated anesthetics and neuromuscular depolarizing agents, developing a syndrome similar to malignant hyperthermia, and thus these agents should be used with caution, if at all.[16,61] Prednisone treatment has recently been shown to temporarily improve strength and function.[62] In a retrospective report of 54 patients with DMD, respiratory support was required in the later stages when the respiratory vital capacity approached 10 percent of the predicted value.[63]

There are a number of other muscular dystrophies with important implications regarding anesthesia. Myotonic muscular dystrophy, a multisystem, dominantly inherited disorder presenting with limb weakness, is the most common adult muscular dystrophy. Patients with myotonic muscular dystrophy have facial muscle wasting and weakness with frontal baldness producing a well-recognized "hatchet face." Myotonia, sustained contraction related to repetitive muscle membrane depolarization, is present clinically (percussion myotonia) and during EMG testing, though it rarely causes symptoms. Most patients with myotonic muscular dystrophy will have some type of cardiac conduction abnormality, including complete heart block, as well as arrhythmias.[64] Treatment of the arrhythmias, or use of antiarrhythmics to treat myotonia, can be confounded by the cardiac conduction abnormalities.[65] Congestive heart failure, cardiac valvular

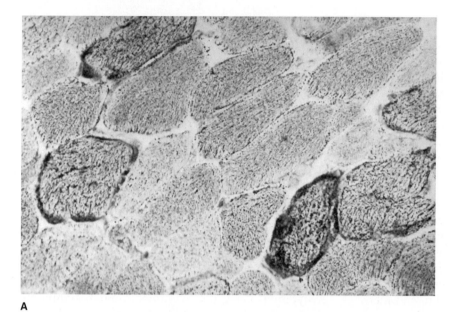

A

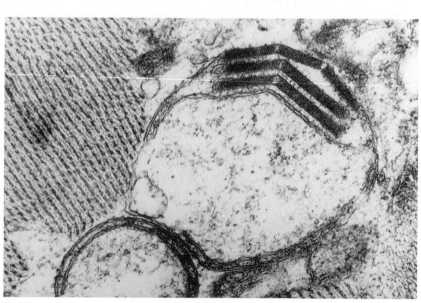

B

Figure 13-3 Muscle biopsy from patient with mitochondrial myopathy, demonstrating "ragged red fibers." *A.* Note dark-staining abnormal mitochondrial grouping. (Original magnification ×400.) *B.* Enlarged mitochondria with classic "parking lot" inclusions. (Original electron microscopy magnification ×200,000. Courtesy of Mila Blaivas, University of Michigan Medical Center, Department of Pathology.)

disease, impaired GI motility,[66] ventilatory muscle involvement, decreased responsiveness to hypoxia and hypercapnia,[67] prolonged contraction after administration of succinylcholine,[68] and hypersensitivity to medications can complicate anesthesia.[69,70] Emery-Dreifuss dystrophy is another X-linked dystrophy that may be associated with early cardiac involvement, primarily arrhythmias and heart block.[71] It is most often recognized by the prominent upper extremity contractures that develop.

Congenital Myopathy

Abnormalities attributed to congenital myopathy usually are present at birth, and congenital myopathy is associated with nonprogressive weakness in the majority of patients. These patients are of most interest to the anesthesiologist due to an increased risk of malignant hyperthermia associated with these disorders. Furthermore, these patients may develop respiratory compromise, and they occasionally present with respiratory involvement in adulthood. Diagnosis is based on evidence of weakness, myopathic EMG abnormalities, an elevated CK, and charcteristic morphologic changes on muscle biopsy.

Family History of Myopathy

Asymptomatic family members of patients known to have myopathy may be important to identify. Female carriers of Duchenne dystrophy may be identified by elevated CK levels (elevated CK is present in up to 70 percent, but this decreases with increasing age) or genetic analysis.[72] Up to 8 percent of female carriers may develop mild myopathic weakness.[73] Similarly, asymptomatic patients with myotonic muscular dystrophy may be identified during EMG testing when characteristic myotonic discharges are found, during physical examination if percussion myotonia or typical facies are identified, or by examination for excessive repeats on DNA testing, which is very sensitive and specific if an affected family member has an increased number of repeats.[74–76]

NEUROMUSCULAR JUNCTION DISEASES

Myasthenia Gravis

Myasthenia gravis is a disease of the neuromuscular junction that is characterized by weakness and rapid fatiguability of voluntary muscles. Because it is so frequently encountered by the anesthesiologist compared with other neuromuscular disorders, it will be discussed in greater detail. Myasthenic gravis is an immunologic disorder manifested by serum antibodies against acetylcholine receptors (AChRs) with possible cell-mediated immune abnormalities, as well.[77,78] The origin of the abnormal immune response is unclear, but the thymus gland has been implicated in the process, perhaps as the source of acetylcholine receptor-like autoantigen or as a reservoir of B cells secreting acetylcholine receptor antibodies (AChR Abs).[79] The resultant pathophysiology is a decreased number of AChRs at the postsynaptic neuromuscular junction, producing impaired neuromuscular transmission.[80]

CLINICAL FEATURES   The incidence of idiopathic myasthenia gravis is about 50 per 100,000 population, with a prevalence of 50 to 125 per 1,000,000 population.[81] Overall, there is a slight female to male predilection. The onset age in women is usually in the third decade, compared with the fifth and sixth decades for men. There is an occasional familial occurrence, but myasthenia is not considered a hereditary disorder. Transient neonatal myasthenia gravis affects infants of myasthenic mothers.[82] Involvement is temporary, and relates to transplacental transmission of AChR Abs. Involvement usually manifests itself within 1 week of delivery and resolves within 3 to 4 months. There are a variety of congenital myasthenic syndromes that are hereditary, many of which clinically resemble myasthenia gravis, in spite of differing pathophysiologies.

Characteristic symptoms include weakness and fatigibility of skeletal muscles. The distribution of weakness includes ocular, bulbar, and symmetric proximal limb involvement. Most patients have extraocular muscle involvement (ptosis and diplopia) at some time during the course of their illness, and about one-third of patients develop dysarthria or dysphagia. Isolated respiratory distress is an uncommon presenting feature. Occasional patients are identified with postoperative respiratory depression related to drug-induced

neuromuscular blockade.[83] Myasthenic weakness varies in severity hour-to-hour and day-to-day, increasing with repetitive activity and improving with rest.

Myasthenia gravis is characterized by unsustained remissions and exacerbations. Permanent remission without treatment is considered rare. Patients who demonstrate a fluctuating course typically stabilize after 5 to 7 years when the risk of severe progression diminishes. The onset, exacerbation, or resistance to treatment is associated with infection, surgery, emotional upset, immunization, or change in thyroid function, among other factors. Patients typically are aware of temperature sensitivity, worsening with increased temperature and improving when cooled. This temperature difference may, in fact, account for much of the hour-to-hour variation in weakness. Pregnancy has an unpredictable effect upon myasthenia, but the postpartum period is not associated with worsening.[84] Nevertheless, labor, lack of sleep, and exhaustion frequently precipitate weakness. Neurologic signs are limited to weakness of skeletal muscles without abnormality of reflexes, coordination, or sensation.

Myasthenic crisis is defined as acute weakness of bulbar and respiratory muscles that requires respiratory support.[79,85] Crisis commonly is associated with infection, perhaps because of attendant fever, and also is reported after immunization, surgery, pregnancy, stress, or no apparent antecedent event. The term *myasthenic crisis* is reserved for patients with impending respiratory failure, whether it be from poor diaphragm contractility or frequent aspiration because of bulbar dysfunction. Patients demonstrate poor response to anticholinesterase medications. Signs of impending deterioration include restlessness, difficulty sleeping, tachycardia, and nonspecific anxiousness. The signs occur in the absence of evidence suggesting cholinergic overdose. Cholinergic crisis is uncommon and is characterized by increased weakness after receiving cholinergic medications. Associated nicotinic side effects include muscle cramping and fasciculations. Muscarinic side effects include abdominal cramps, diarrhea, palpitations, sweating, increased secretions, salivation, tearing, bradycardia, and increased urinary frequency.

DIAGNOSTIC TESTING   The diagnosis of myasthenia gravis is established using a combination of clinical, pharmacologic, immunologic, and electrodiagnostic evaluations.

Pharmacologic. Edrophonium (Tensilon) is a short-acting anticholinesterase used to identify reversible weakness associated with myasthenia.[86] The inhibition of cholinesterase prolongs ACh availability, increasing the probability of depolarizing the muscle fiber. Clinically weak muscles that can be easily observed or tested (e.g., levator palpebrae, orbicularis oculi, extraocular muscles, diaphragm, specific limb muscles) are identified. Evaluation of a few moderately involved muscles is preferable to examination of multiple muscles, and observing a clinically weak muscle is preferable to evaluating for abnormal fatigue in a strong muscle. The cholinergic effects of edrophonium are sufficient to preclude masking in most situations. Many physicians mask the patient to the active drug by beginning with a placebo injection. A test dose of 2 mg of edrophonium is given IV, and if no adverse reaction results within 2 min, an additional 3 mg and 5 mg are given at 2-min intervals. Edrophonium is effective within 20 to 60 s, and has a duration of 2 to 10 min. Over 80 percent of patients with moderately severe generalized myasthenia gravis have a positive response. However, specificity for myasthenia gravis is poor because any weakness associated with partial denervation and reinnervation may be reversed. The usefulness in evaluating effective treatment by anticholinesterase medications is also limited because individual muscles may be undertreated, overtreated, or adequately treated. Edrophonium is relatively contraindicated in the evaluation of cholinergic crises because the additional anticholinesterase may precipitate respiratory failure. If use is deemed necessary, the dose is limited to 1 or 2 mg.

Laboratory. AChR Abs that interfere with the nicotonic AChR are found in the serum of almost 90 percent of patients with myasthenia gravis.[87-90] Antibodies react with a variety of determinants on the AChR and are involved in antigenic modulation and complement-mediated AChRs. AChR binding Abs react with epitopes other than ACh binding sites and are the primary immunologic diagnostic test for myasthenia gravis. Other antibodies exist, including blocking Abs that react with the AChR binding site in approximately 50 percent of myasthenia gravis patients, and AChR modulating Abs that bind to AChR sites on the surface of muscle cells.[79,91] The major Ab-mediated effect is AChR loss due to accelerated degradation.[79] False-positive results are rare (some patients with LEMS, motor neuron disease, and D-penicillamine-associated myasthenia). Antistriatal muscle (striational) Abs are found in a high percentage of patients with thymoma (about 80 percent), and less commonly in myasthenia gravis patients without thymoma (about 30 percent). Antibody-negative patients who have otherwise typical myasthenia gravis have circulating AChR Abs that are not detected by radioimmunoassay, and passive transfer produces loss of functional AChRs in experimental animals.[79,92,93] There is a limited correlation of titer with clinical involvement for groups of patients but better correlation with clinical status in the individual patient. Because of an associated increase of other immune-mediated disorders in patients with myasthenia gravis, the laboratory evaluation includes a search for these other problems, including hypo- or hyperthyroidism.[94,95]

Imaging. Abnormalities of the thymus gland are frequently identified on conventional chest x-rays as an abnormal mediastinal mass. Computed tomography and MRI are the most sensitive methods for identifying a mediastinal mass.

Electrophysiologic. The electrophysiologic defect in myasthenia gravis is impaired neuromuscular transmission. This impairment is demonstrated as a decremental motor evoked response to repetitive motor nerve stimulation at low rates (3 Hz).[96,97] The decrement reflects the reduced safety factor from depletion of immediately available ACh quanta prior to mobilization, reducing the probability of a suprathreshold endplate potential, thereby reducing the probability of muscle fiber depolarization. The decrement is increased 2 to 4 min after 1 min of volitional exercise (Fig. 13-4). This postexercise exhaustion is related to depletion of the immediately available acetylcholine quanta. Single-fiber electromyography (SFEMG) is an extremely sensitive test of neuromuscular transmission commonly used in establishing the diagnosis of myasthenia gravis.[97,98] Nevertheless, an abnormal SFEMG is not specific for myasthenia gravis, and false-positive studies occur in a variety of disorders associated with partial denervation and reinnervation (e.g., motor neuron disease, polymyositis, chronic neuropathy).

TREATMENT   The treatment of myasthenia gravis has changed substantially during the past 25 years, in part due to advances in assisted ventilation in intensive care units with respiratory support.[99,100] In addition to symptomatic treatment, a variety of additional treatments exist including those directed toward elimination of the causative antigen and others related to suppression of the immune response.[101,102]

Symptomatic. The traditional treatment involves administration of anticholinesterase medications such as pyridostigmine (Mestinon). Mestinon is well tolerated by most patients and has a relatively predictable response. Onset is within 30 min of ingestion with a peak effect at 90 to 120 min. The effect terminates by 4 h. The starting dosage for most patients is 60 mg every 3 to 4 h while awake. This can be increased by 30-mg increments to a maximum of 180 mg every 4 h, although higher doses may produce weakness. Dosage is individualized throughout the day. Muscarinic side effects, particularly abdominal cramping and diarrhea, can be limited by Robinul (glycopyrrolate), 1 mg given one to three times per day. Intravenous mestinon (approximately one-thirtieth the oral dosage) is available for hospitalized patients unable to take oral medications. A variety of adjunctive medications such as ephedrine are thought to facilitate acetylcholine release and are used to supplement anticholinesterase agents.

Thymectomy. The thymus gland plays an important

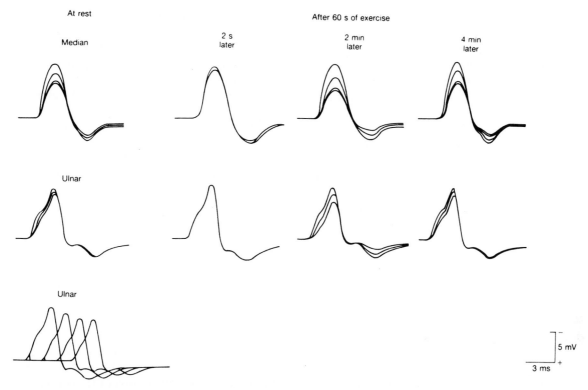

Figure 13-4   Motor responses following 3-Hz repetitive stimulation of the median and ulnar nerves, recording from thenar and hypothenar muscles, respectively, in a patient with myasthenia gravis. Four superimposed responses are shown at rest and after 60 s of exercise (recording 2 s, 2 min, and 4 min later). The repair of the decrement immediately after exercise reflects postactivation facilitation. The increased decrement 2 min later reflects postactivation exhaustion. Calibration: 3 ms and 5 mV. (Reprinted with permission from Albers JW, Sanders DB. *Repetitive Stimulation.* American Academy of Neurology Annual Course No. 350. Minneapolis, American Academy of Neurology, 1989:13–29.)

but poorly understood role in myasthenia gravis. Thymoma is present in 10 to 20 percent of myasthenic patients, usually presenting after the third decade. Of patients undergoing therapeutic thymectomy, 60 percent demonstrate thymic hyperplasia. Of patients with thymoma, 25 percent are malignant. The distinction of benign vs. malignant thymoma is best made by the surgeon (not the pathologist) based upon adherence or infiltration of adjacent structures. Interestingly, most patients without myasthenia who undergo thymectomy for thymoma eventually develop myasthenia gravis. Thymectomy is a conventional but previously controversial treatment of myasthenia gravis. Nevertheless, there is a general consensus that patients with generalized myasthenia should have thymectomy.[103,104] Uncontrolled studies report improvement following thymectomy in 50 to 80 percent of patients.[79,105] Thymectomy is unquestionably indicated in all patients with thymoma to prevent local spread to adjacent tissues. Some physicians reserve thymectomy for myasthenia gravis patients without thymoma for only those who do not respond to medical treatment including corticosteroids, whereas others recommend thy-

mectomy in any myasthenic patient (usually excluding purely ocular myasthenia gravis), independent of severity. Because of management problems characteristic to myasthenia gravis postoperatively, there is broad consensus that thymectomy should be restricted to centers with facilities and experience for such care.[79]

Therapeutic plasma exchange (TPE). TPE is used commonly to treat myasthenic crisis or to stabilize patients with moderately severe involvement before thymectomy.[106] In many ways, myasthenia gravis is the model disease to demonstrate the efficacy of TPE: A specific antibody associated with the illness is known, TPE effectively removes that antibody from the circulation, and objective measures are available to quantify immunologic and neurologic responses.[107] In general, improvement occurs days to weeks after initiating a series of five single-volume exchanges performed over 10 to 14 days. The improvement follows the reduction in Ab levels. Occasional patients demonstrate improvement almost immediately after the first exchange, although this may relate to cooling rather than removal of some neuromuscular blocking agent. Unfortunately, the effects of TPE are short-lived, and patients almost always demonstrate eventual return to baseline, usually within weeks to months. Presumably, the time between TPE-related improvement and subsequent relapse relates to the rate at which AchR Abs are produced. Because of this, almost all patients undergoing TPE are started on some other form of treatment, usually corticosteroids.[108]

While there are risks to TPE, in general, they are not substantial. These include difficulty with venous access and risks associated with change in plasma volume or change of serum constituents, including normal clotting mechanisms. Its major application in myasthenia gravis involves patients who would benefit from rapid improvement in strength, particularly those requiring respiratory support.

Immunosuppression. Beginning in the mid-1970s, a variety of immunotherapies became available for patients poorly controlled by anticholinesterase medications. Numerous treatment protocols exist for chronic immunosuppression, with the most commonly used medications being corticosteroids, azathioprine, and cyclosporin.[79,109,110] The best-studied treatments involve long-term administration of corticosteroids, and improvement is reported in over 80 percent of patients.[101,106,111] Because of the well-established early deterioration (over weeks) after administration of high-dose oral corticosteroids, many physicians prefer to begin with a low (20 mg/day) dose and gradually increase over weeks to approximately 1 mg/kg per day in a single morning dose.[109,111–113] This is maintained for 4 to 12 weeks, unless there are complications, at which time the medication is tapered eventually to an alternate-day low-dose schedule. Alternatively, others begin with a full-dose alternate-day schedule (2 mg/kg per day) in an effort to minimize corticosteroid-induced side effects. Regardless of the schedule, the majority of patients require a maintenance schedule indefinitely, typically in the range of 5 to 20 mg on alternate days. High-dose intravenous pulse therapy using methylprednisolone has been recommended for any patient with incapacitating or life-threatening exacerbation of generalized myasthenia gravis.[114] In limited trials, response has been reported within several days. The advantages to this form of therapy are rapid improvement with fewer side effects compared with high-dose daily corticosteroids. This can be used in conjunction with daily corticosteroids, anticholinesterase inhibitors, and therapeutic plasma exchange. A recommended schedule includes 2 g of methylprednisolone administered IV over 12 h, repeated at 5-day intervals for a total of two to three courses depending upon the degree of response.[114]

It is not known whether cytotoxic agents such azathioprine or cyclophosphamide offer any clinical or immunologic advantage over corticosteroids.[106] Azathioprine is often recommended as a corticosteroid-sparing agent.[115] It is cytotoxic primarily to T cells and the mechanism of action in myasthenia gravis may relate to reduced products of T-cell-dependent AChR Abs. When used in isolation, improvement usually is delayed for 4 to 6 months. The most impressive evidence of its efficacy is the striking remission rate after it has been discontinued in seemingly stable myasthenia gravis patients. Azathioprine is typically started at 50 mg/day and increased by a similar amount every 1 to 2 weeks to a total dose of a 2 to 3 mg/kg per day. Complete blood count and liver function studies are monitored weekly for the first 4 to 6 weeks and then monthly for the next 6 months because of the common occurrence of a drug-related hepatitis and neutropenia.

Cyclosporin has recently been evaluated because of its inhibition of interleukin-2, resulting in impairment of T-lymphocyte-dependent immune response mechanisms.[116] It is most commonly used to prevent organ rejection after transplantation, but trials involving myasthenia gravis have demonstrated efficacy. Cyclosporin is administered in divided doses of approximately 5 mg/kg per day. Effectiveness is apparent within several months, slower than corticosteroids but faster than azathioprine. Unfortunately, renal toxicity and hypertension limit general application.

GENERAL ANESTHESIA CONSIDERATIONS The expertise of the anesthesiologist is required at several points during the clinical course of a typical myasthenic patient. The anesthesiologist may be involved unwittingly in the treatment of a patient with latent or undiagnosed myasthenia who is undergoing surgery for an unrelated reason. Conversely, the anesthesiologist may be involved during the early portion of myasthenic crisis in an established myasthenic patient who requires respiratory support. Most commonly, the anesthesiologist becomes involved prior to elective thymectomy, when there are multiple considerations related to administration of general anesthesia.

The first decision involves timing of the thymectomy. Thymectomy almost always is an elective procedure, and most neurologists agree that the optimal time to perform the operation is after the patient has been medically stabilized. This sometimes requires treatment with TPE or treatment with corticosteroids.[117,118] Most surgeons prefer that the operation be performed prior to the use of corticosteroids, but the overall control of the myasthenia dictates this decision. The most important neuromuscular preoperative considerations relate to pulmonary and swallowing functions. The best indicator of respiratory function is repeated measurements of the forced vital capacity. Patients with a vital capacity less than 1.5 liters are poor surgical candidates because any deterioration in function likely results in prolonged intubation. Similarly, patients with satisfactory respiratory function but prominent dysphagia are at risk for recurrent aspiration. Either problem is a strong indication to postpone surgery.

Additional preoperative decisions relate to medications used to treat myasthenia gravis. Any patient who has received preoperative corticosteroids will require a preoperative steroid supplementation.[119] Anticholinesterase medications frequently are withheld at least 6 h prior to surgery because they increase secretions. Only rarely are anticholinesterase medications required to maintain respiratory or bulbar function, and these patients are poor candidates for elective thymectomy until stabilized. Atropine frequently is used to reduce tracheal secretions, independent of whether anticholinesterase medications are administered. Glycopyrrolate also can be used to limit secretions in situations where the side effect of atropine (such as tachycardia) are undesirable.[120]

Most general anesthetic agents, including Fluothane, nitrous oxide, and cyclopropane, are appropriate for myasthenic patients.[120] Ether and chloroform are contraindicated because of their known adverse effects upon neuromuscular transmission.[120] Additional anesthetic considerations include intraoperative use of neuromuscular blockade in patients with myasthenia. Because of the decreased number of AChRs, sensitivity to nondepolarizing neuromuscular blocking drugs that compete with ACh such as tubocurarine, pancuronium, atracurium, and vecuronium is greatly increased, producing prolonged flaccid paralysis.[2,3] Because of this increased sensitivity to neuromuscular blocking agents, their use should be avoided or minimized whenever possible, although atracurium or vecuronium can be given in small doses, with recovery induced by an anticholinesterase drug.[3,121,122] It should be anticipated that a prolonged neuromuscular blockade may occur. Myasthenic patients may show resistance to succinylcholine, a depolarizing neuromuscular blocking drug that acts like ACh but is not broken down by acetylcholinesterase.[2,3] However, once neuromuscular blockade is achieved, the resultant paralysis is prolonged, and several short-acting anesthetic drugs including ketamine and propanidid potentiate the action of succinylcholine.[83]

The presence of myasthenia gravis always influences postoperative extubation decisions.[117] It is common practice to evaluate the patient's level of consciousness and extremity strength prior to extubation. In patients with myasthenia, results of extremity strength testing may be misleading, because extremity strength may be normal but respiratory function markedly impaired, making it necessary to delay extubation. Patients with a forced vital capacity of less than about 1 liter are unable to protect their airway, because of inadequate cough. These patients also may have bulbar weakness with dysphagia and recurrent aspiration, making it important that a strong cough be present prior to extubation. Physicians experienced in the care of myasthenic patients recognize that extubation under these circumstances almost always results in emergent reintubation, usually within minutes to hours of extubation. Postoperative fatigue, fever, and a variety of other factors contribute to the importance of careful observation of the myasthenia patient. In a prospective evaluation of 53 myasthenic patients undergoing thymectomy, 41 had removal of the endotracheal tube in the recovery room, whereas 12 had delayed extubation.[117] The only factor predicting prolonged mechanical ventilation was the degree of bulbar involvement.

Anticholinesterase medications can be restarted after extubation, if required. If they cannot be given orally, intravenous administration is possible but rarely required. Many commonly administered postoperative medications, including several antibiotics and antiarrhythmics, have neuromuscular blocking properties, and the anesthesiologist should be aware of their presence.[83] In general, their use is not absolutely contraindicated in any myasthenic patient whose general medical condition requires use of such drugs, but they should be administered under close observation, with special attention to respiratory depression.

Lambert-Eaton Myasthenic Syndrome

Several disorders other than myasthenia gravis demonstrate impaired neuromuscular transmission. The most important of these neuromuscular junction disorders is the Lambert-Eaton myasthenic syndrome (LEMS). Like myasthenia gravis, LEMS also is an immunologic-mediated disease, but unlike myasthenia gravis, the immune response is directed toward the presynaptic voltage-gated calcium channel as opposed to the postsynaptic AChR.[123] IgG has been shown to react with calcium channels on the presynaptic junction, and this interaction presumably results in damage to calcium channels, decreased calcium entry during depolarization, and decreased ACh release.

CLINICAL FEATURES   LEMS is characterized by progressive weakness of proximal more than distal muscles, diminished reflexes, and autonomic features including dry mouth and impotence.[124] The distribution of weakness includes symmetric proximal more than distal muscles. Bulbar muscles are usually spared, but occasional patients have extraocular involvement with ptosis, and respiratory weakness may be a presenting complaint or occur as a prolonged consequence after administration of neuromuscular blocking drugs.[125,126] The weakness on clinical examination often is less than expected given the patient's functional disability. This finding probably reflects the facilitation of strength that occurs on repeated trials on examination of single muscles but which interferes with normal activities. The most characteristic feature of LEMS is the association with certain malignancies or connective tissue diseases. LEMS is typically one component of a paraneoplastic syndrome associated with small cell carcinoma of the lung or other malignancy.[124,127] In young-onset LEMS, malignancy is uncommon but presentation in association with systemic lupus erythematosus or other autoimmune disorder is common.[128]

DIAGNOSTIC TESTING *Immunologic.* Antineuronal calcium channel antibodies are frequently identified by radioimmunoassay in LEMS patients. Approximately 50 percent of LEMS patients have Abs that bind to calcium channels extracted from small cell lung carcinoma.[123,129] This occurs in about 75 percent of LEMS patients with malignancy and about 30 percent of LEMS patients without malignancy. The same Abs are found in patients with small cell carcinoma who do not have LEMS.[123] Non-organ-specific antinuclear antibodies are found in approximately one-third of patients with LEMS and malignancy.

Electrodiagnosis. Electrodiagnostic abnormalities include low-amplitude motor responses with markedly abnormal facilitation immediately after brief voluntary exercise. Facilitation is defined as the difference between the response amplitude before and after facilitation divided by the initial amplitude, expressed as percentage. The amount of facilitation usually exceeds 100 percent in LEMS, and values greater than 500 percent are common (Fig. 13-5). There also is markedly abnormal facilitation to 50-Hz stimulation. Because 50-Hz stimulation is painful, it usually is unnecessary except for occasional use in patients unable to perform voluntary exercise. Unlike myasthenia gravis, identified abnormalities are relatively uniform in all muscles of individual patients with LEMS.

TREATMENT Attention to any identified underlying disorder such as a small cell carcinoma or a systemic connective tissue disease is the primary treatment.[130] Originally, guanidine was used to facilitate release of ACh, but its undesirable side effects, including bone marrow suppression, limit its application.[127,131] Symptomatic treatment of the motor impairment sometimes results from administration of anticholinesterase medications, although the effectiveness in LEMS is limited compared with the marked response in myasthenia.[132] Immunosuppressive protocols including use of TPE, corticosteroids, cyclosporin, cyclophosphamide, and azathioprine are of proven efficacy, limited primarily by the long duration from treatment initiation to onset

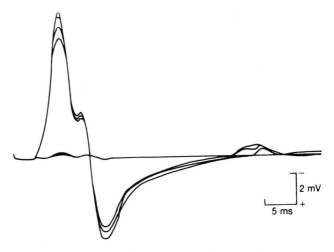

Figure 13-5 Motor responses following 3-Hz repetitive supramaximal ulnar motor nerve stimulation, recorded from hypothenar muscle in a patient with Lambert-Eaton myasthenic syndrome. Lower tracing represents the markedly reduced amplitude with a small decrement in rested muscle. Upper tracing recorded immediately after 10 s of maximal voluntary contraction, representing marked postexercise facilitation. Calibration: 5 ms and 2 mV. (Reprinted with permission from Albers JW, Sanders DB. *Repetitive Stimulation.* American Academy of Neurology Annual Course No. 350. Minneapolis, American Academy of Neurology, 1989:13–29.)

of neurologic improvement.[102,133–136] More recently, 3,4-diaminopyridine and human intravenous immune globulin (IVIG) have been proven effective in reversing the presynaptic blockage of ACh release.[132,137–139]

GENERAL ANESTHESIA CONSIDERATIONS The anesthesiologist may be involved with patients with LEMS during diagnostic bronchoscopy or during surgical procedures related to an underlying malignancy, and involvement may occur in the treatment of a patient with undiagnosed LEMS undergoing surgery for malignancy. Ventilatory failure unrelated to surgery is uncommon but does occur.[125,126] Because respiratory involvement is uncommon, timing of required surgical procedures is rarely dictated by the patient's neurological status. Nevertheless, assessment of preanesthesia respiratory function is always appropriate, and some patients may require treatment before proceeding with surgery.[125] Like patients with myasthenia gravis, patients with LEMS often are taking medications such as corticosteroids, anticholinesterases, or 3,4-diaminopyridine that require special attention. All medications having a direct effect on the neuromuscular junction can be withheld at least 6 h prior to surgery and resumed postoperatively. Additional considerations include intraoperative use of neuromuscular blocking medications. Because of the sensitivity of LEMS patients to these nondepolarizing neuromuscular blocking agents, they should be avoided or minimized if possible.[3,125] If used, prolonged neuromuscular blockade should be anticipated, and postoperative extubation delayed until respiratory function has been carefully assessed.

The dysautonomia of LEMS poses potential consideration, but rarely has a direct effect upon anesthetic considerations. Unlike the profound dysautonomia sometimes associated with Guillain-Barré syndrome, dysautonomia in LEMS is typically mild. Impaired temperature regulation because of impaired sweating is a feasible consideration, as is instability of blood pressure. The potential association of pseudoobstruction is another postoperative consideration.[140]

POLYNEUROPATHY

Polyneuropathy is common in the general population, and the anesthesiologist encounters patients with peripheral nerve disorders on a daily basis. A few forms of polyneuropathy have rapid onset with progression to respiratory and autonomic insufficiency. For these patients, the anesthesiologist has an important support role. Other patients have polyneuropathy as an incidental or secondary finding, usually unrelated to the reason they require the anesthesiologist's services. Because these patients may be at increased susceptibility for compressive neuropathy or plexopathy, recognition is important.

Inflammatory Neuropathy

The most common acquired polyneuropathies associated with rapid deterioration leading to respiratory arrest are the inflammatory demyelinating polyneuropathies. These neuropathies are acquired disorders of unknown but presumed immunologic cause. There are acute and chronic forms with many clinical similarities, differing primarily in their onset and relapse rates. The neuropathy is characterized as idiopathic in most patients. However, the association with a systemic disorder such as plasma cell dyscrasia influences the clinical evaluation of these patients. Familiarity with the inflammatory neuropathies is important to the anesthesiologist because of the frequent development of respiratory failure requiring prolonged respiratory support, often in association with clinically significant dysautonomia.

CLINICAL FEATURES Guillain-Barré syndrome is the acute form of inflammatory polyneuropathy, and is also known as inflammatory polyneuritis, postinfectious polyneuritis, or acute inflammatory demyelinating polyneuropathy (AIDP).[141-144] Although the specific immune trigger is unknown, antecedent events temporally related to onset are identified in over 75 percent of patients. Reported antecedent events occurring within the month prior to the onset of polyneuropathy include respiratory and gastrointestinal tract infections, other viral and bacterial infections, immunization, and surgery.[142,145,146] For most patients, the first neurologic symptoms include nonspecific paresthesias or distal weakness, often in association with back and muscle pain. Lower extremity weakness is a common initial complaint, and most patients recognize progression over days in a distal to proximal fashion. Cranial nerves are commonly involved, typically producing facial weakness, difficulty chewing, and dysphagia.[147-149] Bladder or bowel dysfunction is unusual.[150] Early after onset, weakness is most prominent in distal compared with proximal muscles, although proximal weakness may be severe early in the clinical course. Facial weakness occurs frequently, most easily identified by incomplete eyelid closure. Extraocular muscles are rarely involved, and pupillary muscles are spared. Objective sensory loss usually consists of mild distal vibratory loss. Muscle stretch reflexes are absent or markedly reduced.[150]

Chronic inflammatory demyelinating polyneuropathy (CIDP) is a progressive or relapsing polyneuropathy that resembles Guillain-Barré syndrome, except for its temporal profile, its likelihood of relapse, and its association with a systemic illness.[142,151-154] CIDP is characterized by symmetric weakness with or without cranial nerve involvement, areflexia, and elevated cerebrospinal fluid protein.[143,153] Sensory loss in distal extremities often is striking, and occasional patients demonstrate sensory ataxia or postural tremor. The course of CIDP is prolonged compared with Guillain-Barré syndrome, with the interval from onset to peak impairment typically exceeding three months. Unlike the Guillain-Barré syndrome, the course in CIDP is highly variable with approximately 50 percent of patients having a progressive course, one-third a relapsing course, and one-sixth a monophasic course.[153] Rare patients with CIDP demonstrate rapid deterioration indistinguishable from Guillain-Barré syndrome patients.

DIAGNOSTIC TESTING *Laboratory.* Laboratory findings in inflammatory neuropathy include cerebrospinal fluid albuminocytologic dissociation by the second or third week of illness.[142] There may be a mild cerebrospinal fluid pleocytosis, but white blood cell counts above 40 cells per mm^3 suggest alternative diagnoses.[150] Because CIDP is frequently associated with a systemic illness such as plasma cell dyscrasia, multiple myeloma, systemic lupus erythematosus, HIV-1 infection, or lymphoma, the laboratory evaluation of these patients reflects a search for suspected systemic disorders.[142]

Electrodiagnostic. As in other peripheral nervous system disorders, the electrodiagnostic examination is the

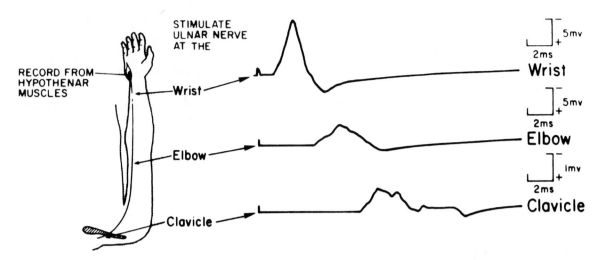

Figure 13-6 Motor responses recorded from hypothenar muscles following stimulation of ulnar nerve at distal and proximal sites. Abnormal responses obtained from patient with inflammatory polyneuropathy demonstrating abnormal temporal dispersion with partial conduction block, increased duration with proximal stimulation, and decreased conduction velocity. (Modified with permission from Albers JW: Clinical neurophysiology of generalized polyneuropathy. *J Clin Neurophysiol* 1993; 10:149.)

primary method of establishing a diagnosis. Hallmarks of acquired demyelinating polyneuropathy include evidence of substantial slowing of conduction velocity and prolongation of distal latencies (greater than can be explained by axonal loss lesion alone), partial conduction block and abnormal temporal dispersion of motor responses, and absent or prolonged F wave latencies.[142,155,156] Representative motor conduction studies are shown in Fig. 13-6 for a patient with an inflammatory polyneuropathy.

TREATMENT   General principles of supportive care and monitoring for autonomic dysfunction are important for patients with inflammatory polyneuropathy. The advent of respiratory intensive care units dramatically reduced mortality to its current rate of approximately 2 to 5 percent.[157] In addition, TPE and IVIG are of demonstrated efficacy in Guillain-Barré syndrome,[157–160] and corticosteroids and other forms of immunosuppression are indicated for patients with CIDP.[161–165]

Ventilatory support. Ventilatory support is required in about one-third of Guillain-Barré syndrome patients, usually during the second or third week after onset.[149] Because most deaths in Guillain-Barré syndrome are associated with respiratory complications, the most important evaluation relates to respiratory function. All Guillain-Barré syndrome patients should be monitored for respiratory deterioration and respiratory failure managed.[5,6] Respiratory failure requiring ventilator assistance is less common in CIDP than in Guillain-Barré syndrome,[142] but occasional patients require respira-

tory support during a severe exacerbation or during the terminal phase of their illness.

Admission of patients with inflammatory neuropathy to the intensive care unit for monitoring of respiratory and autonomic functions depends upon the severity of involvement, rate of progression, and accompanying findings. The anesthesiologist frequently is involved in decisions regarding intubation and respiratory support. In general, the urgency of the need for intubation is measured by the rate of deterioration or the level of respiratory impairment.[5] Respiratory failure rarely occurs abruptly in patients with good respiratory function unless the immediate course is complicated by aspiration, cardiac dysrhythmia, or pulmonary embolism. The ability to cough is a good screening indicator of sufficient respiratory function, and the forced vital capacity should be monitored if the patient is stable. False-low recordings may be obtained if mouth closure on the spirometer is poor. The decision and timing of elective intubation depend upon several factors, including the extent and rate of respiratory deterioration. Intubation should be accomplished if the forced vital capacity is equal to or less than 15 ml/kg, or if there is a rapid decline in function, clinical evidence of hypoxia, known or suspected aspiration with poor tracheopulmonary toilet, or signs of respiratory fatigue.[142] Arterial blood gases represent a poor measure of respiratory function in acute Guillain-Barré syndrome, and hypercapnia is a late finding that is a poor threshold criterion for intubation. Low P_{O_2} combined with a low or normal P_{CO_2} indicates shunting from early atelectasis and may precede respiratory failure.[142] Hypercapnia generally precedes hypoxia, but is a relatively late finding of respiratory failure and a dangerous criterion for elective intubation.

Dysautonomia occurs commonly in Guillain-Barré syndrome and occasionally in CIDP patients. It usually consists of constipation, urinary hesitancy, and impaired thermoregulation. Most deaths relate to medical complications of respiratory paralysis, but about 50 percent are sudden and presumably related to dysautonomia.[143,157,166] The most threatening consequences of autonomic dysfunction include cardiac dysrhythmia (usually bradycardia), labile pulse rate, and labile blood pressure resulting in fluctuating hypotension and hypertension.[143] In general, dysautonomia poses the greatest problem during prolonged ventilation. It is not directly related to the extent of weakness, although catastrophic cardiac dysrhythmia and blood pressure lability are unusual in patients with mild functional impairment. Autonomic dysfunction and significant arrhythmia occurred in 11 of 100 patients reported by Winer and Hughes.[166] All of those who developed serious cardiac dysrhythmia were receiving mechanical ventilation and 7 died; arrhythmias were often preceded by wide fluctuations of pulse or blood pressure and transient asystole following tracheal suction.[166]

Any suspicion of autonomic instability requires monitoring in an intensive care setting. Autonomic instability resulting in hypotension or new hypertension occurs in 10 to 15 percent of AIDP patients. Hypotension should be managed with administration of fluids, and sympathomimetics should be avoided.[142] Hypertension should be treated using short-acting medications such as nitroprusside or propranolol. Minor cardiac dysrhythmias occur in about 20 percent of hospitalized patients, but arrhythmias sufficiently severe to affect blood pressure or require medication occur in about 5% of patients.[142] Dysrhythmias commonly involve second- or third-degree AV block. Effective treatment results from temporary pacemaker insertion.[142] The syndrome of inappropriate antidiuretic hormone secretion (SIADH) is associated with Guillain-Barré syndrome, and there may be a resultant hyponatremia.[167] Nonambulatory patients require antiembolic protection, including support stockings and low-dose heparin.

Therapeutic plasma exchange and IVIG. TPE and IVIG are of proven efficacy in the treatment of Guillain-Barré syndrome if initiated within the first 3 to 4 weeks.[157,168] If treatment is completed within the first 4 weeks of illness, there is an increased frequency of limited relapse requiring additional TPE.[169] Patients with CIDP also respond to TPE and IVIG, although, unlike Guillain-Barré syndrome patients, the response is usually short-lived.[170] Most patients with CIDP require prolonged treatment, usually with immunomodulating agents.

Corticosteroids and other forms of chronic immunosuppression are of proven efficacy in CIDP, but have no apparent role in the treatment of Guillain-Barré syndrome.[153,162] Patients with CIDP and immune system disorders often experience remission of their polyneuropathy with treatment of the underlying systemic illness. IVIG is of proven efficacy in Guillain-Barré syndrome and CIDP, although treatment-associated relapse has been a concern.[171,172]

Immunosuppression. Corticosteroids are of unproved efficacy in Guillain-Barré syndrome, and were thought to have a detrimental effect in the initial controlled studies.[128,173] A single recent study has suggested efficacy of methylprednisolone when combined with IVIG.[174] However, corticosteroids are of demonstrated efficacy in controlled clinical trials in CIDP.[162] Schedules similar to those described for the treatment of myasthenia gravis patients are used.[170]

GENERAL ANESTHESIA CONSIDERATIONS Patients with inflammatory neuropathy who require anesthesia pose special problems because of potential autonomic instability, particularly in those with Guillain-Barré syndrome. Special considerations related to autonomic dysfunction are identical with those described above regarding treatment of Guillain-Barré syndrome. These patients requiring anesthesia also are at risk for SIADH and may develop hyponatremia.[167] Patients receiving short-term anticoagulation should have heparin discontinued during any operative procedure.

Porphyric Neuropathy

The hepatic porphyrias are disorders of heme synthesis associated with overproduction of porphyrins or precursors, delta-aminolevulinic acid (ALA) and porphobilinogen (PBG). They include acute intermittent porphyria (AIP), hereditary coproporphyria, and variegate porphyria; all have been associated with acute deterioration resembling the Guillain-Barré syndrome, although central nervous abnormalities are frequently present.[175-178]

CLINICAL FEATURES During an acute attack, unexplained abdominal pain likely related to dysautonomia may be associated with constipation, nausea, and vomiting, sometimes leading to surgical exploration. Gastrointestinal complaints may coexist with or precede mental status changes ranging from mild confusion to psychosis. Initial manifestations of neuropathy consist of weakness, with or without sensory loss, sometimes progressing to quadriplegia requiring respiratory support. Reflexes usually disappear. Dysautonomia is characterized by unstable blood pressure and cardiac dysrhythmia. Cutaneous manifestations consist of photosensitivity in hereditary coproporphyria and var-

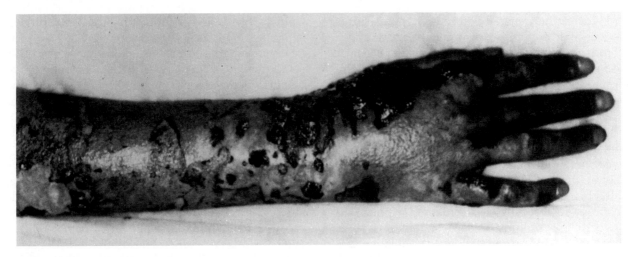

Figure 13-7 Skin lesions in a photodistribution in patients with biochemical evidence of coproporphyria taken during an acute attack consisting of quadriparesis and respiratory failure. The skin lesions were characterized by mechanical fragility, multiple blisters and bullae, and rupture of bullae into open sores.

iegate porphyria but not in acute intermittent porphyria (Fig. 13-7). A variety of precipitating events exist, including many medications, as well as stress, pregnancy, fasting, and infection.[175] The diagnosis should be considered in any patient with suspected Guillain-Barré syndrome.

DIAGNOSTIC TESTING Biochemical classification of the porphyrias involves identification of abnormal excretion of heme precursors. This requires analysis of urine for ALA, PBG, and uroporphyrin; stool for protoporphyrin and coproporphyrin; and blood cells for the specific enzyme deficiency. Identification is not always straightforward, and the distinction between different forms can be difficult because of nonenzymatic oxidation of heme precursors in the urine, the specific laboratory tests chosen, and the presence of combined enzymatic defects.[179,180] ALA and PBG are colorless, yet a characteristic of porphyria is the dark burgundy discoloration of urine after standing in sunlight. This discoloration relates to porphyrin pigments that exist in excess because heme synthesis is incompletely blocked and porphyrins are formed by nonenzymatic oxidation of heme precursors in the urine, both within the bladder and with photooxidation.[181,182] In the laboratory, all porphyrinogens are oxidized to porphyrins, making the distinction between coproporphyria and variegate porphyria difficult. Enzyme determinations are used to precisely identify the specific defect.[182] For example, the partial metabolic defect associated with AIP occurs between PBG and uroporphyrin with decreased porphobilinogen deaminase (uroporphyrinogen I-synthetase).[182]

TREATMENT Treatment of patients with porphyric neuropathy includes avoidance of precipitants and institution of supportive measures similar to those described for the Guillain-Barré syndrome. These include sensible physiologic principles of fluid management and respiratory support.

Medical. A high carbohydrate load is used to reverse the fasting state, and reduction in this load, such as when intravenous glucose administration is discontinued, has been associated with acute relapse. Adequate carbohydrate intake is important, with 300 to 500 g glucose per day required.[183] Hydration is important unless there is evidence of the syndrome of inappropriate antidiuretic hormone (SIADH); serum electrolytes should be monitored and hyponatremia avoided if possible. Narcotic analgesia may be required for pain control; phenothiazines and chloral hydrate have been used successfully for nausea and vomiting.[183] Persistent tachycardia or unstable hypertension is best controlled with medications such as propranolol that have a short half-life.[183] Hematin is used to compensate for the inadequate heme synthesis. Direct treatment of the underlying disorder involves administration of an end product of the abnormal metabolic pathway, resulting in feedback inhibition of heme synthesis.[181] Hematin, a hydroxide of heme, is thought to supplement the depleted hepatic intracellular heme pool, suppressing hepatic ALA synthetase and reducing the production of porphyrins and porphyrin precursors formed prior to the enzymatic block.[181,183] It is administered intravenously at a dosage of 1 to 4 mg/kg a day for days to weeks, depending upon clinical response. Urinary porphobilinogen excretion can be used to assess biochemical response.

Assisted ventilation. Considerations related to general anesthesia are similar to those discussed for Guillain-Barré syndrome, and are related primarily to respiratory insufficiency and possible dysautonomia. In addition, use of sedatives such as phenobarbital has been associated with precipitation of porphyria and should be avoided. A complete listing of all drugs and medications associated with precipitation of porphyria is beyond the scope of this chapter. Standard texts should be consulted prior to use of any medication not known to be safe for use in a porphyria patient.[181] Fasting is one of the provocative factors associated with acute attacks, and carbohydrates are known to suppress ALA synthetase activity.

GENERAL ANESTHESIA CONSIDERATIONS   The anesthesiologist is more likely to be involved with the patient with porphyria before rather than after the problem is identified (other than in association with care provided in the intensive care unit). In fact, presentation with recurrent episodes of abdominal pain resulting in abdominal exploration is considered common. It is only after surgical exploration that the classical syndrome of abdominal pain, psychosis, and neuropathy develops, perhaps in association with anesthetic agents or in association with other medications administered during the hospitalization.

Critical Illness Polyneuropathy

Anesthesiologists are likely to encounter patients who develop critical illness polyneuropathy (CIP) because it develops in the critical care setting, typically in association with prolonged assisted ventilation. Onset of severe weakness in the critically ill patient has many causes, but most involve new onset neuromuscular disease.[184] Less commonly, previously unrecognized disorders such as myasthenia gravis or porphyric neuropathy are unmasked or precipitated by infection, nutritional deficiency, or medications.[184] Guillain-Barré syndrome occasionally follows surgery or develops in the critical care setting in the course of an unrelated illness. More frequently, a polyneuropathy develops in the critical care setting that is atypical of Guillain-Barré syndrome because the underlying pathophysiology involves axonal loss, not demyelination.[28,184] CIP was first described by Bolton and colleagues, in association with intensive care unit stays exceeding one week, multiorgan failure, and sepsis.[28] The polyneuropathy is characterized by a flaccid, areflexic quadri-

paresis. It frequently is unrecognized initially because of the severity of the underlying systemic disease, the presence of an associated encephalopathy, or medical sedation. Typically, failure to wean from the ventilator leads to further evaluations that identify the diffuse weakness and areflexia.

Nerve conduction studies in CIP demonstrate low-amplitude sensory and motor responses. Motor abnormalities may be present to a greater degree than sensory abnormalities. Needle electromyography of skeletal muscles demonstrates neurogenic changes characterized by fibrillation potentials and decreased motor unit recruitment. Occasionally, no motor units can be activated. Tests of neuromuscular transmission, including repetitive motor nerve stimulation studies, are unremarkable, assuming a motor response is available for testing. Morphology confirms a severe sensorimotor polyneuropathy of the axonal type.[28] While the cause remains uncertain, nutritional factors may play a role in development of the polyneuropathy. The natural course in surviving patients is progressive improvement over months.

CIP must be differentiated from persistent paralysis after use of long-term neuromuscular blocking agents such as vecuronium. Persistent paralysis in some patients has been associated with metabolic acidosis, elevated plasma magnesium concentrations, and the presence of 3-desacetylvecuronium, an active metabolite of vecuronium producing persistent neuromuscular blockade.[29] Electrodiagnostic evaluation of the patient shows impaired neuromuscular transmission as opposed to a polyneuropathy or myopathy with a decremental response to repetitive motor nerve stimulation. CIP also resembles the acute quadriplegic myopathy syndrome, although there are distinguishing features. In the quadriplegic myopathy syndrome, sensory amplitudes are normal or near normal, motor unit recruitment is markedly increased with a near-full interference pattern in spite of severe weakness (electromechanical dissociation), and weakness presents after use of neuromuscular blocking and corticosteroid medications.[185]

Other Types of Polyneuropathy

Evaluation of all polyneuropathies encountered by the anesthesiologist is beyond the scope of this chapter, and those of greatest importance are associated with respiratory failure or dysautonomia, as described above. Fortunately, patients having polyneuropathies with those characteristics are uncommon. Far more common are patients with mild generalized sensorimotor polyneuropathy, such as associated with diabetes mellitus or nutritional disorders including excessive ethanol use, whose operation is unrelated to their polyneuropathy. The anesthesiologist probably evaluates patients with such polyneuropathies daily.

Of particular concern is whether patients who have a mild polyneuropathy are at greater risk of developing a compressive mononeuropathy or plexopathy than patients who do not have an underlying polyneuropathy. While controversial, the general consensus is that these patients probably are at greater risk for compressive injury. This is discussed in greater detail in the section on predisposing factors for compressive nerve injuries. There is one group of patients for whom there is no controversy regarding the increased risk. These patients have a familial predilection to compressive mononeuropathy referred to as "hereditary neuropathy with liability to pressure palsy" (HNPP).[186,187] This neuropathy is sometimes referred to as "tomaculous" neuropathy because of abnormal axonal swellings resembling sausages on sural nerve biopsy. HNPP can be identified genetically if there is suspicion of its presence. The typical presentation is that of a mononeuropathy multiplex acquired over many years. When identified, extraordinary care must be taken during any surgical procedure to avoid focal compression. In general, however, conventional techniques for avoiding compressive neuropathy or plexopathy are considered sufficient, and the best rule is to assume that all anesthetic patients have an underlying polyneuropathy and treat them similarly.

MOTOR NEURON DISEASE

The term *motor neuron disease* (MND) suggests diffuse, painless degeneration of the motor neurons without sensory involvement. These disorders range from intrauterine onset with lower motor neuron degneration only (Werdnig-Hoffman disease) to adult-onset upper and lower motor neuron degeneration with wasting, fasciculations, and hyperreflexia (amyotrophic lateral sclerosis).

Amyotrophic Lateral Sclerosis

Amyotrophic lateral sclerosis (ALS), commonly referred to as "Lou Gehrig disease," is an adult-onset form of progressive motor neuron disease having a prevalence of approximately 5 per 100,000. It is of unknown causation.

CLINICAL FEATURES   The ALS form of motor neuron disease is defined as degeneration of the upper motor neurons (causing hyperreflexia, spasticity, "pseudobulbar" affect) as well as the lower motor neurons (causing weakness, wasting, and fasciculations). Certainty in diagnosis requires diffuse abnormality and exclusion of other conditions that can mimic this disorder such as lymphoma, viral infection, and spinal degenerative disease (e.g., cervical spondylosis). Diagnostic criteria vary, but the diagnosis becomes more certain with more diffuse involvement, which often

includes bulbar and respiratory muscles. Most commonly ALS is sporadic, though familial and geographic clusters are known. In spite of numerous theories, the sporadic form is of unknown cause. In some familial cases, association with specific enzyme abnormalities[188,189] and toxin or other exposure in geographic clusters have suggested possible mechanisms.[190,191]

Weakness is the primary symptom of ALS. If disease onset is bulbar, then dysarthria and dysphagia are early symptoms. Purely upper motor neuron presentation leads to spasticity and hyperreflexia without extremity wasting or fasciculation, but importantly no sensory change or pain.

DIAGNOSTIC TESTING   The clinical examination, documenting upper motor neuron findings along with muscle bulk loss and fasciculations, is most important in diagnosing this condition. EMG is helpful in excluding other conditions (myasthenia gravis, polyneuropathy) and to document the extent of denervation and reinnervation. Other testing is designed to exclude "mimicking" disorders. Thyroid and parathyroid function, serum calcium, serum protein electrophoresis, and measurement of antibodies toward the GM1 (possibly associated with conduction block neuropathy) may be helpful.[192] If evidence of motor axon degeneration is confined to a discrete (e.g., cervical) region, MRI may be required to exclude local pathology as a cause of the lower motor neuron change and distal hyperreflexia.

TREATMENT   Treatment is symptomatic. Weak muscles often require splinting or bracing, such as an ankle-foot orthosis (AFO) to treat foot drop. Excessive emotional lability is often treated with tricyclic antidepressants or lithium; excessive oral secretions are treated with glycopyrrolate or other anticholinergic medications. Many patients required relief of cramps, with quinine and phenytoin most effective in our experience. As progressive bulbar dysfunction leads to aspiration and inadequate nutrition, feeding gastrostomy is often required; this may be performed with local anesthetic. Some patients elect to undergo tracheotomy and artificial ventilation.

Many therapeutic trials have been based on suspected etiologies (e.g., supplementation of trophic factors, intense immunosuppression), but to date few therapies have shown promise in potentially altering the course of this disease. Currently, medications thought to inhibit effects of glutamate on the motor neuron, and supplementation of specific trophic factors are under intense review.

General Anesthesia Considerations

The patient with MND of any form may have weakness of bulbar and ventilatory muscles, of most importance after intubation and mechanical ventilation. Preoperative pulmonary function testing is required to determine the possibility of successful weaning. Patients with the ALS form of MND have difficulties with spasticity, hyperreflexia, and frequent involvement of the bulbar musculature. Patients with motor neuropathy may show prolonged and excessive responses to nondepolarizing muscle relaxants, similar to patients with myasthenia gravis, as the immature, reinnervated motor units have a reduced safety margin of neuromuscular transmission. They are also vulnerable to hyperkalemia with cardiac arrest after administration of succinylcholine.[193] Thus, subclinical bulbar or diaphragm weakness may become apparent only after administration of nondepolarizing neuromuscular blocking agents. These patients often experience sialorrhea, leading to anticholinergic treatment for secretion control. Excessive secretions may pose further difficulty in ALS patients at the time of extubation.

Neuromuscular Consequences of General Anesthesia

There are numerous potential neuromuscular consequences of general anesthesia in patients without preexisting neuromuscular disease. The most obvious consequences relate to potential compressive or stretch injuries in anesthetized patients, although other considerations, including systemic hypotension and ischemia or direct effects of anesthetic agents upon muscle tissue, are important. During anesthesia, the neuromuscular system is vulnerable to injury at all levels, from the anterior horn cell to muscle fibers. This section reviews clinical and pathophysiologic information relative to anesthetic injuries for the different levels, and also reviews several idiopathic neuromuscular disorders that occasionally mimic anesthesia complications.

PERIPHERAL NERVE INJURY

Peripheral nerve or plexus injuries are among the most common potential neurological consequences of prolonged immobilization or altered consciousness. A review of the American Society of Anesthesiologists Closed Claims Study database by Kroll and associates indicated that 15 percent of anesthesia-related problems that led to litigation were attributed to peripheral nervous system injuries involving individual nerves, the brachial plexus, or lumbosacral nerve roots.[194] Surprisingly, the exact mechanism of injury was unclear for a large proportion of cases despite intensive investigation. Because of the importance of these injuries, the potential mechanisms of injury are reviewed and several common examples presented.

CHARACTERISTICS

Injury to individual peripheral nerves or more proximal lesions within the plexus is an obvious potential neuromuscular complication of general anesthesia, although modern techniques of limb protection and support have substantially reduced the incidence. For all practical purposes, injuries directly attributable to general anesthesia appear immediately postoperatively, as soon as the patient's level of consciousness permits identification. Persistent sedation, development of a pure motor abnormality such as foot drop in a bed-confined patient, or partial, mild involvement of an individual nerve in a critically ill patient occasionally delays recognition. Nevertheless, delayed recognition is relatively uncommon.

Injury of any consequence to a mixed sensorimotor peripheral nerve produces paralysis of muscles innervated by the involved nerve and sensory loss in the distribution of the sensory fibers. Large myelinated sensory fibers are among the most vulnerable to compression injuries and are typically associated with unpleasant or painful dysesthesias and sensory loss. Nevertheless, there may be asymptomatic peripheral abnormalities apparent using nerve conduction studies during the postoperative period.[195] An exception to the idea of immediate onset of a compressive mononeuropathy occurs in association with a compartment syndrome, where muscle injury results in a progression of edema, increased pressure, and additional muscle injury, eventually producing nerve ischemia over a period of hours.[196] A similar chain of events may evolve at the level of the partially injured peripheral nerve, producing a "microcompartment" syndrome with progressive neuron dysfunction over a period of hours to days.[197]

Additional exceptions to the concept of maximum impairment at onset are associated with problems unrelated or indirectly related to anesthesia. Examples include late development of a hematoma or local edema compressing a nerve, perhaps associated with an indwelling line or anticoagulation treatment. Similarly, development of an ulnar neuropathy during the convalescent period after an operation frequently results from focal compression of the nerve at the elbow in a bed- or chair-confined patient. Development of a compressive neuropathy during an operation does not always indicate neglect, as occasional patients present with isolated mononeuropathy first apparent upon awakening in their own bed, independent of sedation or intoxication. Typically, these mononeuropathies are mild and rapidly resolve, as do most mononeuropathies related to anesthetic complications. The exceptions are those injuries associated with extensive or complete axonal loss.

In most patients with a persistent impairment associated with a mononeuropathy or plexopathy, a combination of conduction block and axonal degeneration exists. Typically, an initial complete impairment is replaced by partial function. Recovery usually is more rapid than experienced by patients with nerve infarction, because the presence of even a single viable motor axon is associated with axonal sprouting, whereby surviving motor axons sprout and reinnervate a portion of the denervated muscle fibers. This process begins within weeks of injury. In time, with axonal regeneration there is a process of shedding and reinnervating existing muscle fibers until motor units approach or return to normal.

MECHANISMS AND CLASSIFICATION OF NERVE INJURY

Several mechanisms exist to explain peripheral nerve injuries associated with general anesthesia, and most involve ischemia or mechanical distortion of nerve axons resulting from direct compression or stretch, usually over an extended time period. Nerve injury also may be related to more severe trauma, including inadvertent laceration, abrupt stretch with disruption of neuronal tissue, focal crush from a tourniquet, or even physical injury related to cooling or freezing of nerve tissue. Most anesthesia-associated injuries presumably relate to compression producing ischemia and mechanical distortion of nerve axons, without actual nerve crush, but the role of nerve stretch in the anesthetized, paralyzed patient is difficult to assess. A limited number of pathophysiologic changes are relevant to the clinical evaluation of nerve injury. These changes include metabolic or physiologic abnormalities that alter nerve conduction, demyelination and remyelination, and axonal degeneration. The pathophysiology of different types of injury is well described.

Classification

One classification used to describe the functional conditions associated with injured nerves was proposed by Seddon, and it has been extended to incorporate the underlying pathophysiology.[198,199] The mildest category, neurapraxia, is associated with a brief period of sensory and motor dysfunction distal to the lesion that resolves completely within hours to weeks (occasionally months).[199,200] Neurapraxia is attributed to a physiologic interruption of neural transmission without demonstrable axonal damage. There may be focal demyelination and remyelination in the vicinity of compression, although no underlying physical alteration of nerve is required to produce transient conduction block. Nerve conduction testing of a neurapraxic lesion demonstrates conduction failure across the lesion and normal sensory and motor responses with nerve stimulation distal to the lesion, long after the responses would have disappeared if the axons had been interrupted. Needle electromyography demonstrates an absence or decreased number of voluntary motor units without findings suggestive of muscle fiber degeneration, even when the impairment persists for weeks.

Axonotmesis refers to a nerve lesion associated with complete or partial axonal degeneration distal to the focal lesion, but without injury to the epineurium or interruption of supportive tissue.[198,199] Neurotmesis indicates nerve transection, with complete axonal loss and disruption of supportive connective tissue structures at the site of the lesion.[198,199,201] These two types of injury are difficult to distinguish electrophysiologically because the primary neuropathologic abnormality is disruption of the neuronal tissue with complete distal axonal degeneration.[201] Conditions associated with axonotmesis include nerve infarction from focal compression, crush, stretch, embolism, or vasculitis. Lesions associated with completed axonal degeneration produce sensory loss and muscle paralysis in the distribution of the peripheral nerve, and the prognosis for recovery differs from neurapraxic lesions. Because the distal axon is separated from the nutritive cell body, there is subsequent degeneration of the distal axon and breakdown of the myelin sheath (Wallerian degeneration).[200] Changes also occur in the proximal stump of a transected nerve, extending for a short distance, as well as in the cell body, where active synthesis of cytoskeletal axon components is associated with swelling.[199] If the transection occurs very close to the cell body, there is central chromatolysis and even cell death.

Landau demonstrated that muscle contraction to nerve stimulation distal to transection persists for several days after transection, and it was later recognized that sensory and motor evoked responses also remain normal for several days when the nerve is stimulated distal to the transection, although voluntary activity is absent.[202] Sensory and motor evoked responses disappear, however, in about one week.[203,204] Needle electromyography demonstrates an absence of voluntary motor units, and fibrillation potentials (spontaneous discharge of individual muscle fibers) appear 1 to 4 weeks after transection, depending upon proximity of the muscle to the lesion (Fig. 13-8).[203] These spontaneous discharges reflect muscle fiber hypersensitivity to acetylcholine (ACh), associated with proliferation and migration of extrajunctional acetylcholine receptors.[205] Partial or incomplete axonal degeneration produces a partial sensory loss and reduced voluntary activity with decreased (instead of absent) sensory and motor responses. Conduction along intact axons remains normal. Abnormal spontaneous activity appears in denervated muscle fibers.

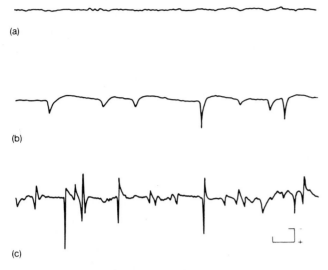

(a)

(b)

(c)

Figure 13-8 Needle EMG recordings from muscle at rest. *a.* Normal muscle with no evidence of abnormal spontaneous activity. *b.* Abnormal spontaneous activity consisting of positive waves. *c.* Abnormal spontaneous activity consisting of fibrillation potentials and occasional positive waves. Calibration: 10 ms and 50 μV. (Modified with permission from Bromberg MB, Albers JW: Electromyography in idiopathic myositis. *Mt Sinai J Med* 55:459, 1988.)

Recovery of axonal lesions is delayed and frequently incomplete. Lesions associated with interruption of supportive connective tissue typically require surgical repair with apposition to the distal stump to promote orderly axonal regeneration down the nerve.[30] When connective tissue is uninvolved, as in most ischemic or crush injuries, the prognosis for recovery is better, particularly for distal nerve lesions, as compared with more proximal lesions that are far removed from the innervation site. The most important prognostic factor for recovery is the presence of any viable fibers within the injured nerve, because these surviving fibers develop collateral sprouts that reinnervate some denervated muscle fibers, producing large motor units.[206] Although the total number of motor units is reduced, the increased size of individual motor units results in improved strength. Regenerating axons produced new motor units by reinnervating muscle fibers shed by abnormally large motor units.[207] Nerve regeneration, even when complete, is associated with abnormalities in the internodal length after remyelination, and patients with intact function typically have electrodiagnostic residua of their previous injury.

Most peripheral injuries are characterized by a combination of physiologic block, focal demyelination and remyelination, and varying degrees of axonal degeneration. It is sometimes difficult or impossible to clinically predict the extent of the lesion, particularly when the neurologic impairment is substantial. However electrodiagnostic testing, sometimes performed se-

quentially, is very useful in defining the underlying pathophysiology.[208] Because most anesthesia-associated injuries involve nerve ischemia and mechanical compression of neuronal tissue, with or without crush injury, these two mechanisms will be discussed separately, recognizing that they share common elements.[209]

Nerve Ischemia

Arteries adjacent to peripheral nerves provide blood supply by numerous small branches that enter the nerve though the epineurium and perineurium, forming an intricate capillary plexus throughout the nerve.[198] This highly redundant blood supply with extensive anastomoses provides protection to individual nerves from focal ischemia such as related to microembolization. In addition, the peripheral nervous system is relatively resistant to ischemia compared with the central nervous system. With complete ischemia, paralysis and sensory loss appear within minutes to slightly over one hour, depending upon a variety of conditions including temperature and the presence of coexistent nerve pressure.[200,204] Ischemia produces demonstrable electrophysiologic block of nerve conduction across the ischemic range.[200] Clinical and electrophysiologic dysfunction, however, is transient if the period of ischemia is limited, and it is well established that the limb can be rendered ischemic for as long as 4 to 6 h, such as in orthopedic procedures using a limb tourniquet, without demonstrable structural damage or permanent clinical impairments. The transient impairment is the clinical correlate of neurapraxia. Nevertheless, the effects of nerve ischemia depend upon the duration of ischemia; and pressure insufficient to mechanically disrupt the nerve but sufficient to cause prolonged ischemia will eventually produce neuronal infarction with axonal degeneration distal to the site of injury, identical with that associated with nerve crush. Because extraneural pressures exceeding systemic blood pressure impair nerve blood flow, patients with prolonged hypotension may be particularly susceptible.

An experimental model of ischemia that produced alterations independent of compression was developed by Dyck and associates.[210] They demonstrated that 24 h after microsphere embolization of rat sciatic nerve capillaries there was histologic evidence of a central fascicular ischemic core of nerve injury. Fibers entering the ischemic core showed reproducible features of acute ischemia. Changes at the edge of the core included a transition from normal appearance to dark axons with organelle accumulation, swollen axons with thin myelin or demyelination, and attenuated axons. More distally, myelinated fibers demonstrated axonal degeneration and myelin collapse at the center of the ischemic core, with a more normal appearance at the edge of the core. The degenerating axons were interpreted to represent Wallerian degeneration with axonal discontinuity. Because organelle accumulation and axonal swelling were the earliest lesions, it was inferred that hypoxia caused axonal stasis as a primary event and that surviving but swollen and attenuated axons were associated with the subsequent demyelination and remyelination known to occur in ischemic lesions.[210,211] This study provided experimental evidence suggesting selective vulnerability of axons to acute ischemia. Depending on the severity of ischemia, fibers underwent axonal degeneration or a transitory structural alteration without degeneration that consisted of axonal changes and secondary demyelination.[210]

Nerve Compression

The resulting impairments associated with nerve compression, crush, or stretch are similar to those of ischemia, and although mechanisms differ, ischemic injury may be a contributing factor in all compressive injuries. Several levels of physiologic and histologic impairment are associated with experimental nerve compression.[212–216]

Using an experimental model that utilized a small compression cuff placed around an isolated nerve, Ochoa and Gilliatt and their associates demonstrated that the initial response to focal compression was slowing of conduction, followed by progressive amounts of conduction block prior to axonal disruption.[212,213,216] Focal ischemia contributed to the earliest reversible physiologic dysfunction without producing identifiable structural abnormality. With continued compression, there was histologic evidence of intussusception or telescoping of the paranodal myelin under the adjacent myelin sheath at the proximal and distal edges of the cuff. This intussusception represents a mechanical disruption that occludes the nodes of Ranvier, thereby obstructing the sodium channels and decreasing or obliterating the resultant ionic currents associated with saltatory conduction. It is likely that mechanical and ischemic factors contribute to the initial dysfunction with external nerve pressure, although the mechanical distortion best explains the resultant conduction block, with compression of intraneural vessels playing a secondary role.[212,216] Regardless of the relative contribution of each, the effects of mechanical compression and ischemia are most evident for large myelinated fibers.[217] Experimental models of nerve compression show that even at low levels of compression known to induce ischemia there is some mechanical distortion of the nerve trunk, and that the magnitude and duration of compression both contribute to the degree of nerve injury.[218] With continued compression, there is progressive involvement to include the small nerve fibers, and

eventually there is histologic evidence of paranodal demyelination and axonal degeneration.

Nerve Stretch

Pure peripheral nerve stretch injuries occur in acute trauma,[219] although the relationship to anesthesia-associated injury is less clear. Peripheral nerves are viscoelastic tissues with measurable mechanical properties.[220] Stretch causes morphologic and functional changes, including nonlinear stress-strain characteristics when the nerve is placed under tension.[221] With progressively increasing tension and stretch beyond physiologic limits, the perineurium ruptures while the epineurium is still intact.[221,222] The conditions under which this occurs are variable, representing the time-dependent viscoelastic behavior of peripheral nerves and factors influenced by the presence or absence of nerve branches and fibrosis.[220,221]

Experimental studies suggest that sustained increases in tension adversely affect the electrophysiologic properties of nerve, and altered conduction results from even a small stretch of 6 percent beyond the in situ length of the nerve, or stress less than 10 percent of the ultimate strength of the nerve.[221] For example, a 5 percent elongation of rabbit sciatic nerve demonstrated no electrodiagnostic or histologic changes, but elongation of just beyond 10 percent was associated with a markedly reduced blood flow and demonstrable partial axonal degeneration after 2 h of elongation.[223] Similar studies, also of rabbit sciatic nerve, showed that 2 h of graded strain producing an 8 percent stretch had no effect upon the electrophysiologic activity, whereas 15 percent strain caused a 99 percent loss of amplitude.[224] Factors related to the speed of stretch also are important.[225]

Peripheral nerve stretch injuries often are associated with poor recovery, related to the character and the extent of structural nerve trunk alterations.[226] Using an in vivo rat model of nerve stretch injury, Spiegel and associates found that nerves stretched but not reaching mechanical failure showed variable amounts of axonal degeneration and demonstrated excellent recovery within 2 to 3 weeks. Conversely, nerves stretched through mechanical failure were permanently deformed, with rupture of the perineurium and the epineurium and widespread axonal degeneration. Nevertheless, even conditions associated with severe pathologic changes demonstrated significant improvement by the end of the trial, suggesting that if nerve continuity is preserved, substantial recovery is possible following severe nerve stretch lesions.[226]

In the context of anesthesia-associated nerve injuries, it is likely that the effects of nerve stretch coexist with increased nerve pressure, resultant compression, and ischemia. Stretch producing true disruption of neuronal tissue occurs in severe physical trauma such as a motor vehicle accident or when neural tissue is extended beyond its physiologic limit. Peripheral nerves are relatively compliant, but they are vulnerable to stretch injury when pulled across immobile objects or beyond nonphysiologic distances in the unconscious, paralyzed patient who has no local protective reflexes. The relationships among ischemia, compression, and stretch injuries are complex and interrelated.[209,227–229] For example, experimental evaluation of nerve blood flow demonstrates that, on average, stretching of about 15 percent obliterates blood flow in the stretched nerve, as does compression by pressures of 60 to 80 percent of the mean arterial pressure.[230]

Predisposing Factors

There is limited epidemiologic information to indicate whether certain patients are at increased risk for ischemic or compressive nerve injuries.[200,209] It is possible that prolonged hypotension increases the risk of an ischemic nerve injury, although neither the duration nor the magnitude of hypotension necessary to produce a substantial increase in risk is known. Because of the long period of time that a nerve can be rendered anoxic without permanent injury, hypotension must be considered a theoretical risk factor. More important, patients with an underlying nerve disease with a reduced number of viable axons have a reduced safety factor and are likely more vulnerable to injury.[200,209,231] The concept that "patients with sick nerves are vulnerable to injury" is attractive, but difficult to demonstrate, even in conditions like diabetic neuropathy. For example, it is known that patients with diabetic neuropathy have an increased frequency of asymptomatic median mononeuropathies at the wrist, yet it is unclear whether this finding is related to the diabetic neuropathy or other factors, such as obesity. In patients with diabetic neuropathy, comparison of patients who have electrodiagnostic evidence of a median neuropathy at the wrist with remaining patients does not demonstrate any significant differences in lower-extremity nerve conduction studies, arguing against the suggestion that an increasing degree of polyneuropathy increases the risk of developing a focal mononeuropathy.[231]

Patients at known increased risk for compressive neuropathy include those who are extremely thin or cachexic.[200] Weight loss involving catabolism of body fat is associated with loss of the protective fat layers, including subcutaneous and epineurial fat. This loss of protection makes these patients particularly vulnerable to compressive neuropathy any time, but particularly when rendered unconscious or sedated. This period of increased risk includes the convalescent period after any illness.

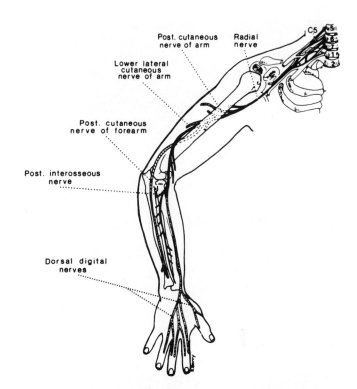

Figure 13-9   Course and important branches of the radial nerve. [Modified with permission from Fisher MA: Other mononeuropathies of the upper extremities. In Brown WF, Bolton CF (eds): *Clinical Electromyography,* 2d ed. Boston, Butterworth-Heinemann, 1993:271–304.]

SELECTED EXAMPLES OF MONONEUROPATHY

A discussion of surgical positioning is beyond the scope of this chapter, as is discussion of all possible compressive mononeuropathies. However, a few examples are discussed below, to highlight important identifying features and risk factors.

RADIAL NERVE   The radial nerve originates from the posterior cord of the brachial plexus and is vulnerable to external compression in the spiral groove of the lower humerus (Fig. 13-9).[198] It innervates extensor muscles of the arm and carries sensory information from much of the dorsal arm and hand. *Saturday night palsy* and *honeymoon palsy* are terms used to describe acute-onset radial mononeuropathy that emphasize the compressive nature of the lesion. Both occur during sleep or decreased consciousness, one with the arm draped over the back of a chair and the other with a bed partner's head cradled in the outstretched arm. Upon awakening, there is wrist and finger extensor weakness or paralysis and sensory loss over the dorsum of the hand. Localization to the spiral groove is helped by demonstrating normal triceps function, because the nerve branch supplying the triceps muscle comes off above the spiral groove.[232] Injection injuries involving the radial nerve are associated with abrupt

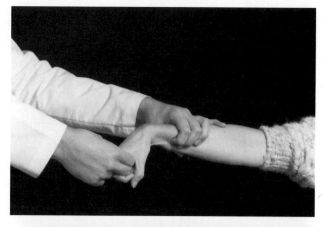

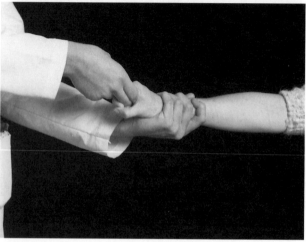

Figure 13-10 Support of the wrist in the evaluation of grip strength in patients with radial mononeuropathy. *Top:* Apparent weakness of grip due to improper support. *Bottom:* Normal grip strength after supporting wrist. [Reproduced with permission from Albers JW, Bromberg MB: Neuromuscular emergencies. In Schwartz GR (ed): *Principles and Practice of Emergency Medicine*, 3d ed. Philadelphia, Lea & Febiger, 1992, vol 1, pp 1544–1573.]

in the vicinity of the elbow, and precise localization requires electrodiagnostic testing.

ULNAR NERVE   The ulnar nerve is vulnerable to compression at the elbow, where it is protected partially by the ulnar groove (Fig. 13-11). The cubital tunnel at the elbow is formed by the medial epicondyle and the olecranon and covered by the flexor carpi ulnaris muscle aponeurosis and the ulnar collateral ligament.[234,235] When the forearm is prone and flexed at the elbow, exposure is maximal, particularly in patients with shallow ulnar grooves. Ulnar mononeuropathies are a common complication of surgical procedures, with a retrospective incidence of up to 1 percent.[195] In the American Anesthesiologists Closed Claims Study database, ulnar neuropathy represented one-third of all peripheral injuries and was the most frequent nerve injury leading to litigation.[194] In that study, reviewers judged that the standard of care had been met significantly more often in claims involving nerve damage than in claims not involving nerve damage. The exact mechanism of nerve injury often was unclear and ulnar mononeuropathies frequently occurred without identifiable mechanism.[194] Ulnar nerve lesions associated with anesthesia are reportedly more common in males than in females, but the severity of the lesion appears unrelated to patient age, sex, type of operation, or type or duration of anesthesia.[236] Malposition, however, is an important risk factor in compressive ulnar lesions,

onset of weakness and sensory loss in association with immediate pain, developing while the needle is in situ.[233] The wrist drop associated with a complete radial nerve lesion produces apparent grip weakness because the finger flexors are placed at a mechanical disadvantage (Fig. 13-10). This should not be confused with coincident median or ulnar nerve involvement. Depending upon the degree of axonal degeneration, resolution occurs over days to months, and recovery may be prolonged or incomplete. Surgical reanastomosis may be required if there is extensive neuroma formation. Conservative treatment usually is preferable in compressive lesions.

Lesions of the posterior interosseous branch of the radial nerve produce weakness of wrist and finger extensors, sparing the extensor carpi radialis brevis and longus muscles and sparing sensation. The posterior interosseous syndrome occurs with compression

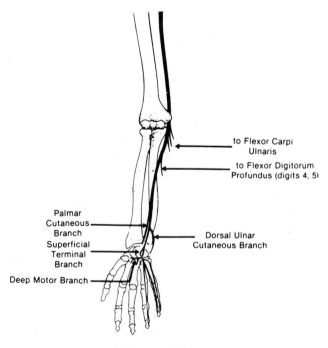

to Flexor Carpi Ulnaris

to Flexor Digitorum Profundus (digits 4, 5)

Palmar Cutaneous Branch

Dorsal Ulnar Cutaneous Branch

Superficial Terminal Branch

Deep Motor Branch

Figure 13-11 Course and important branches of the ulnar nerve. (Modified with permission from Stewart JD: *Focal Peripheral Neuropathies*. New York, Elsevier, 1987:164.)

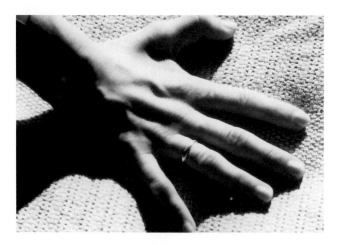

Figure 13-12   Wasting of the ulnar innervated intrinsic hand muscles in a patient with an ulnar mononeuropathy.

and prolonged positioning with the arm in extreme elbow flexion or with surface pressure over the cubital tunnel should be avoided.[237]

Ulnar nerve lesions at the elbow produce elbow pain, nerve tenderness in the ulnar groove, and numbness and weakness involving primarily the hand. Sensory symptoms usually are reported in digits 4 and 5, although examination reveals sparing of medial half of digit 4 (median innervation). Weakness is best demonstrated by finger abduction, examining first dorsal interossei and abductor digiti quinti strength. If the neuropathy is associated with axonal degeneration, atrophy is apparent (Fig. 13-12). Adductor pollicis weakness makes adduction of the thumb against the hand difficult, resulting in activation of the flexor pollicis longus. This produces involuntary flexion of the distal phalanx of the thumb during attempted adduction (Froment's sign) (Fig. 13-13). The flexor carpi ulnaris is frequently innervated by a branch of the ulnar nerve originating above the elbow, and is therefore sometimes spared in lesions at the elbow. The differential diagnosis of a suspected ulnar mononeuropathy includes a C8–T1 radiculopathy or lower-trunk brachial plexopathy. Weakness of median innervated hand muscles excludes an isolated ulnar mononeuropathy. The flexor pollicis brevis muscle is innervated by the median nerve and would be weak in a lower-trunk plexopathy or radiculopathy. The elbow should be examined radiologically if there is suspicion of prior trauma or bony anomaly.

Electrodiagnostic studies are used to localize the problem to the ulnar nerve and identify the level of the lesion, as well as identify a preexisting abnormality.[236,238] Like any suspected mononeuropathy, the most important electrodiagnostic differentiation is between conduction block and axonal degeneration, remembering that definite evidence of axonal loss may not be

apparent for approximately one week after an acute injury. A normal ulnar motor conduction study is shown in Fig. 13-14. The earliest evidence of conduction abnormalities not associated with axonal loss consists of slowing across the elbow (exceeding 20 percent) and loss of amplitude with stimulation proximal to the lesion. An example of a typical ulnar abnormality is shown in Fig. 13-15. This figure is from a study that prospectively evaluated patients before and after coronary artery bypass surgery.[195] Asymptomatic ulnar abnormalities across the elbow were identified in 3 of 20 patients (15 percent). All were electrodiagnostically apparent in the immediate postoperative period, and the prognosis for recovery was excellent. A normal ulnar sensory response with stimulation at the wrist and above the elbow is shown in Fig. 13-16. Note that the sensory studies demonstrate substantial amplitude loss and dispersion with proximal compared with distal stimulation, limiting the usefulness of sensory amplitude measures in localizing a lesion to the elbow. However, because of the predilection of large fibers to compression, distal sensory amplitude and conduction velocity recordings are the most sensitive indicators in defining any compressive neuropathy.

FEMORAL NERVE   The femoral nerve originates from upper lumbar nerve roots and the lumbar plexus (Fig. 13-17). It travels between the psoas and iliacus muscles and passes beneath the inguinal ligament lateral to the femoral artery. The iliacus and quadriceps muscles are innervated by the femoral nerve, and it supplies sensation to the anteromedial thigh and medial leg to the foot. A femoral lesion in the upper

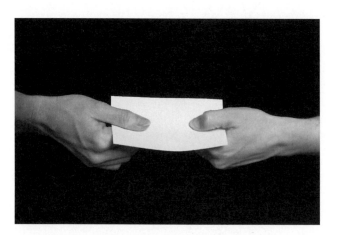

Figure 13-13   Froment's sign in ulnar mononeuropathy. Weakness of left adductor pollicis brevis, resulting in involuntary activation of the flexor pollicis longus during thumb adduction. [Reproduction with permission from Albers JW, Bromberg MB: Neuromuscular emergencies. In Schwartz GR (ed): *Principles and Practice of Emergency Medicine*, 3d ed. Philadelphia, Lea & Febiger, 1992, vol 1, pp 1544–1573.]

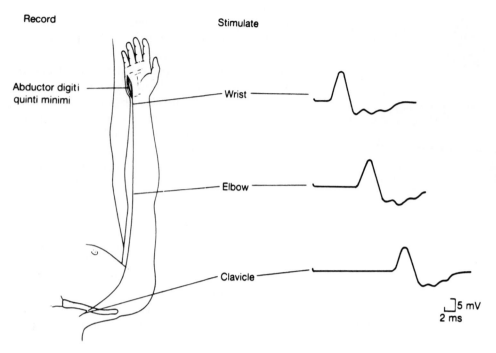

Figure 13-14 Ulnar motor nerve responses recorded following stimulation of the ulnar nerve at the wrist, elbow, and clavicle, recording from the hypothenar muscles. Calibration: 2 ms and 5 mV. [Reprinted with permission from Albers JW, Leonard JA Jr: Nerve conduction studies and electromyography. In Crockard A, et al (eds): *Neurosurgery. The Scientific Basis of Clinical Practice*, 2d ed. Boston, Blackwell Scientific Publications, 1992, vol 2, pp 735–757.]

thigh or at the level of the inguinal ligament produces weakness of knee extension, an absent quadriceps reflex, and diminished sensation in a femoral distribution. There may be very mild weakness of hip flexion, as well, although substantial weakness suggests retroperitoneal involvement of the femoral nerve or lumbar plexus. Thigh adduction is innervated by the obturator nerve and is spared in femoral nerve lesions but present with the plexus or lumbar root lesions.

Perioperative femoral neuropathy has been associated with the lithotomy position, as used in vaginal delivery, exploratory laparoscopy, or radical prostectomy.[239–241] It also has been reported in other situations, including hip arthroplasty or as a result of direct com-

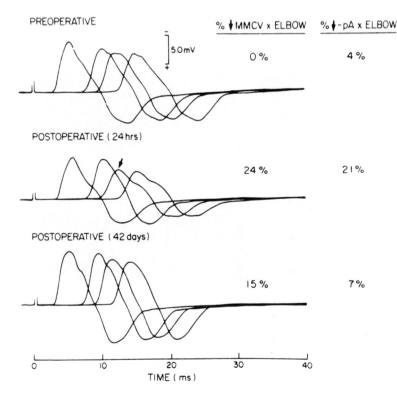

Figure 13-15 Ulnar motor responses recorded from an asymptomatic patient following stimulation of the ulnar nerve at the wrist, elbow, and clavicle, recording from the hypothenar muscles in a patient pre- and postoperatively, where there was a 21 percent reduction in the motor amplitude and a 24 percent reduction in conduction velocity across the elbow relative to the forearm. (Reprinted with permission from Watson BV et al.[195])

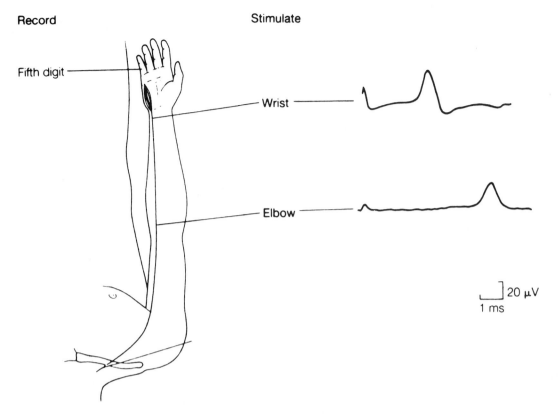

Figure 13-16   Ulnar sensory responses recorded following stimulation of the ulnar nerve at the wrist and above the elbow, recording from the fifth digit. The presence of a normal ulnar response recorded at least one week after clinical onset is inconsistent with a significant compressive ulnar mononeuropathy, because the large sensory fibers are the most sensitive to compression. Calibration: 1 ms and 20 μV. [Reprinted with permission from Albers JW, Leonard JA Jr: Nerve conduction studies and electromyography. In Crockard A, et al. (eds): *Neurosurgery. The Scientific Basis of Clinical Practice,* vol 2, 2d ed. Boston, Blackwell Scientific Publications, 1992:735–757.]

pression from a mechanical pressure clamp.[242,243] Most lesions are attributed to compression of the femoral nerve at the level of the inguinal ligament, but the more proximal portion of the nerve may be injured by stretch associated with excessive hip abduction and external rotation.[241] Onset appears independent of risk factors such as type of pelvic surgery, the presence of systemic illness, or excessive blood loss.[241]

Femoral mononeuropathy may be a sign of serious systemic disease, and prominent iliopsoas involvement, suggesting proximal femoral or lumbar plexus involvement, should promote search for a cause other than isolated compression.[198,241] Hemorrhage into the iliacus muscle may be related to trauma, bleeding disorders, or anticoagulation, producing compression of the nerve in the plexus.[244–246] Retroperitoneal hematoma produces the abrupt onset of inguinal pain which is aggravated by hip motion, anteromedial thigh and leg numbness and paresthesias, knee extensor weakness, and an absent or hypoactive quadriceps reflex.[246] Femoral mononeuropathy occurs in association with retro-peritoneal tumors, herpes zoster, or diabetes mellitus as one form of diabetic amyotrophy.[247]

Evaluation of an isolated femoral neuropathy often requires CT scanning to exclude a structural lesion, such as a hematoma compressing the nerve within the retroperitoneal space (Fig. 13-18). Electrodiagnostic testing localizes the lesion, differentiating a femoral nerve lesion from plexus or root abnormalities. Conduction studies are useful in making side-to-side amplitude comparisons in mild or partial lesions, and sensory recording can be performed on the saphenous nerve, a distal sensory branch of the femoral nerve. The needle examination is particularly important in localizing evidence of partial or complete denervation in femoral innervated muscles, while sparing adjacent muscle of different peripheral nerve but similar nerve root innervation (e.g., thigh adductor muscle innervated by the obturator nerve). The needle examination also is used to identify the presence or absence of iliopsoas muscle involvement, an important finding in locating the lesion at or proximal to the inguinal liga-

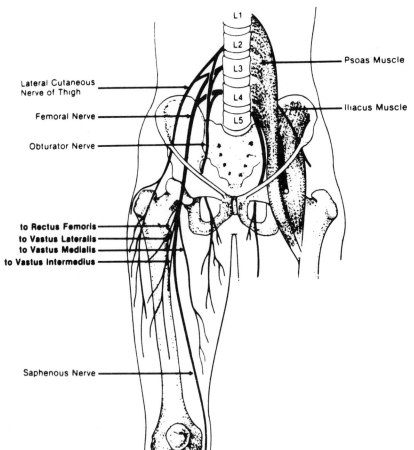

Figure 13-17 Origin, course, and distribution of the femoral nerve. (Modified with permission from Stewart JD: *Focal Peripheral Neuropathies.* New York, Elsevier, 1987:323.)

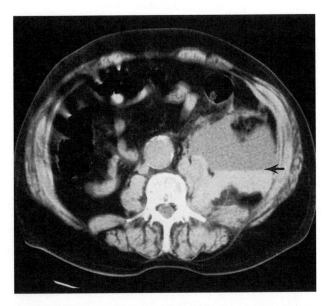

Figure 13-18 CT of hematoma (*arrow*) in femoral neuropathy. Note fluid level. (Courtesy of Isaac R. Francis, University of Michigan Medical Center, Department of Radiology.)

ment. In patients with perioperative femoral lesions unrelated to laceration, the degree of clinical impairment does not reflect prognosis, and patients with complete paralysis often demonstrate full recovery over several days. Conversely, electrodiagnostic evidence of extensive axonal degeneration suggests a poor prognosis.

SCIATIC NERVE The sciatic nerve comprises L4–S2 nerve roots (Fig. 13-19). It includes tibial and peroneal divisions that separate into individual nerves at a variable level in the upper leg. The peroneal component is most lateral, while the tibial component is largest. Sciatic mononeuropathy is exceedingly rare, and most patients with "sciatica" have a radiculopathy. Trauma is the most common cause of sciatic mononeuropathy. This typically includes fracture dislocations of the hip, hip surgery, prolonged compression in an unconscious patient, or intramuscular injections.[198,243,248–250] Sciatic compression within the pelvis by an aneurysm or hematoma occasionally occurs, as does compression within the piriformis muscle, although this is a controversial cause that is exceedingly rare.[251]

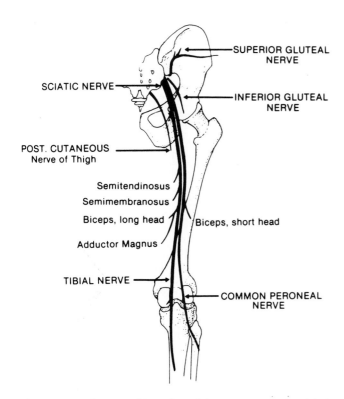

Figure 13-19 Course and branches of the sciatic nerve. (Modified with permission from Stewart JD: *Focal Peripheral Neuropathies.* New York, Elsevier, 1987:323.)

Sciatic mononeuropathy presents with pain and sensory loss in the lower leg and foot (excluding the inner leg), weakness of the leg flexor (hamstring) muscles and all muscles below the knee, and abnormal ankle and hamstring reflexes. The peroneal division is more superficial than the tibial division of the sciatic nerve in the buttock and upper thigh, and it often is preferentially involved in compressive or traumatic injuries.[200] Electrodiagnostic studies are useful in distinguishing a sciatic mononeuropathy from an L5–S1 radiculopathy and are helpful in localizing the lesion along the extent of the nerve. Like most compressive mononeuropathies, isolated sciatic lesions demonstrate partial or complete recovery over time.

PERONEAL NERVE   The peroneal nerve is one component of the sciatic nerve, separating from the tibial nerve in the thigh. It innervaties lower-extremity muscles, including those of foot dorsiflexion and eversion, and it provides sensation to the lateral leg and dorsum of the foot (Fig. 13-20). The peroneal nerve is particularly vulnerable to compression at the head of the fibula, and it is involved as one of the most common anesthesia-associated mononeuropathies.[232] Injury to the common peroneal nerve at this level produces a footdrop with inability to dorsiflex or evert the foot or extend the toes. Just after crossing the fibular head,

the common peroneal nerve divides into its deep and superficial divisions. The deep peroneal nerve is located in the anterior compartment. It innervates foot and toe extensor muscles and provides sensation to the web space between the first and second toes. The deep peroneal nerve may be selectively compressed in an anterior compartment syndrome.[198] The superficial peroneal nerve innervates the foot evertor muscles (peroneus longus and brevis) and provides sensation to the lateral leg.

The most common peroneal mononeuropathy results from focal compression, particularly related to crossed-leg palsy with compression of the nerve between the fibula and the contralateral leg. This can occur during prolonged sitting, such as during recovery from a severe illness when vulnerability may be increased because of weight loss. The peroneal nerve also can be compressed during sleep, anesthesia, pneumatic compression, or coma, or it may be stretched or compressed during prolonged squatting.[252–256] The peroneal nerve occasionally is injured directly by blunt trauma, by laceration, or with fibular fracture.[257] Distal branches may be injured selectively by local trauma (e.g., a component of a cumulative trauma disorder associated with footwear).

It is important to distinguish a peroneal mononeuropathy from an L5 radiculopathy. The most important distinguishing feature is intact foot inversion (posterior tibial muscle) in a peroneal mononeuropathy. The posterior tibial muscle is innervated by the same nerve root as the anterior tibial muscle, but by the posterior

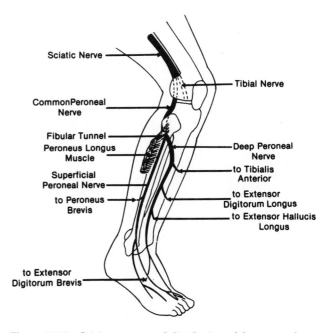

Figure 13-20 Origin, course, and distribution of the peroneal nerve. (Modified with permission from Stewart JD: *Focal Peripheral Neuropathies.* New York, Elsevier, 1987:291.)

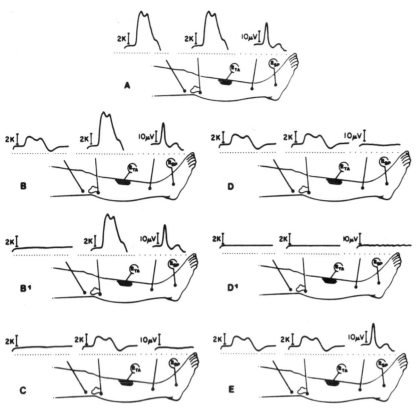

Figure 13-21 Diagrams of peroneal nerve conduction studies in peroneal mononeuropathy. (R_{TA} = peroneal motor response, recording tibialis anterior muscle; R_{SP} = superficial peroneal sensory response.) *A.* Normal. *B* and *B¹.* "Pure" conduction block lesions, partial and complete. *D* and *D¹*, "Pure" axonal degeneration, partial and complete. *C.* Mixed demyelinating, axonal degeneration. *E.* Deep peroneal mononeuropathy. (Proximal latencies not shown to scale.) (Reproduced with permission from Katirji and Wilbourn.[253])

tibial, not the peroneal, nerve. Most patients with compressive peroneal mononeuropathy experience partial or complete recovery. Electrodiagnostic studies are useful in localizing the site of abnormality and determining the extent of axonal damage.[253,258–260] Evidence of involvement of the short head of the biceps femoris muscle in a peroneal lesion localizes the lesion to above the knee. As with all examples of mononeuropathy, electrodiagnostic evidence of extensive axonal degeneration is a poor prognostic sign. Figure 13-21 demonstrates the expected electrodiagnostic findings in several types of peroneal mononeuropathy localized to the knee. In the figure, B and B¹ have the best prognosis for rapid recovery, assuming the lesion is of at least one week duration, because the motor and sensory responses are preserved with distal stimulation, consistent with partial or complete conduction block. Conversely, D¹ has the worst prognosis, because no response is obtainable with surface recordings. In this case, the needle examination would be important, because demonstration of even a single motor unit under voluntary control documents anatomic continuity of the peroneal nerve, and even though the prognosis is poor, improvement can be expected.

PHRENIC NERVE   Cooling or freezing of neural tissue is another form of traumatic injury; it has been implicated in phrenic nerve injury associated with intratho-racic cooling during cardiac surgery. Phrenic nerve injury may occur during cervical or thoracic procedures. Unilateral or bilateral phrenic nerve injury may be present in up to 10 percent of cardiac procedures, with local trauma or hypothermia the most common causation.[261–263]

SELECTED EXAMPLES OF PLEXOPATHY
BRACHIAL PLEXUS   The clinical diagnosis of brachial plexopathy includes identification of muscle involvement in a distribution explained by a specific plexus lesion but not by a radicular or peripheral nerve abnormality (Fig. 13-22).[264] The pattern of sensory loss is a less sensitive indicator of the level of injury. Definitive diagnosis frequently requires EMG evaluation because individual muscles can be investigated for denervation more precisely than allowed by manual muscle testing.

Trauma is a common cause of brachial plexopathy, but numerous examples of nontraumatic plexopathy are associated with systemic lupus, vasculitis, heroin addiction, systemic infection, and vaccination, to name a few.[264–270] Downward shoulder forces, such as a forceful blow in a motor vehicle accident, injure the upper trunk causing weakness of shoulder and proximal arm muscles and sensory loss in a proximal distribution. Upward displacement, as in reaching for a hand hold in a long vertical fall, injures the lower trunk producing hand muscle weakness and sensory loss along the ul-

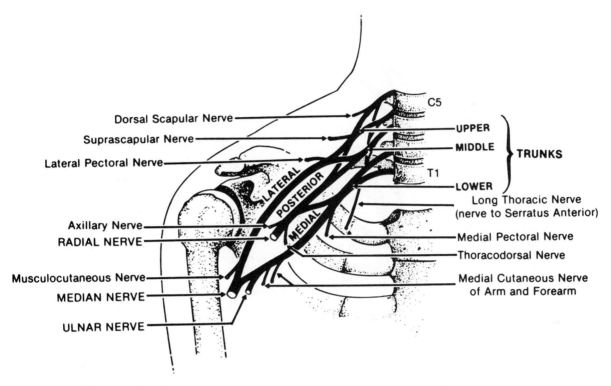

Figure 13-22   Diagram of the brachial plexus showing major branches and nerves derived from it, and bony relationships. For clarity the components of the plexus have been separated and are not drawn to scale. The labels lateral, medial, and posterior refer to the cords of the plexus. (Reproduced with permission from Stewart JD: *Focal Peripheral Neuropathies.* New York, Elsevier, 1987:94.)

nar side of the hand. Extremely forceful injuries can avulse nerve roots, causing permanent deficit. Forceful shoulder and neck contact, as in contact sports, may cause transient burning or stinging of the shoulder, arm, or hands ("burners" or "stingers") which likely reflects transient injury to the brachial plexus. Complex trauma, such as shoulder and clavicular injuries and fractures, stab injuries, and gunshot wounds, can damage the plexus in variable patterns. The classical compressive brachial plexopathy is referred to as "rucksack paralysis" and results from compression of the upper brachial plexus by the straps of a backpack.[271]

Thoracic outlet syndrome is a form of compressive plexopathy associated with substantial diagnostic confusion.[272] There are two forms: a neurogenic form associated with atrophy of hand muscles in a lower trunk distribution and ulnar distribution sensory loss, and a vascular form associated with obstruction of the subclavian artery with signs of Raynaud's phenomenon and emboli to distal limb vessels. Nonspecific limb pain without the aforementioned feature does not represent a true thoracic outlet syndrome, and symptoms occurring with specific arm positions are insufficient to establish the diagnosis of thoracic outlet syndrome. Change or obliteration of the radial pulse and develop-

ment of a supraclavicular bruit with different arm positions are nonspecific findings that are common in the general population and not diagnostic of thoracic outlet syndrome.[272]

In the American Anesthesiologists Closed Claims Study database, brachial plexopathy accounted for 23 percent of all peripheral anesthesia-related nerve injuries leading to litigation.[194] Wilbourne described characteristic forms of compressive brachial plexopathy occurring in association with anesthesia.[264] Upon recovery from anesthesia, usually for an abdominal procedure such as cholycystectomy, the patient experiences weakness of one or occasionally both arms. The neurological impairment may be overlooked in heavily sedated patients in the immediate postoperative period, but is apparent thereafter. Weakness usually is accompanied by paresthesias or numbness, but rarely with pain; an upper trunk distribution is most common, but the entire brachial plexus may be involved.[264] Most patients experience onset of recovery within weeks, suggesting that conduction block is the prominent pathophysiology.[264,273] Prolonged recovery is associated with axonal lesions requiring axonal regeneration and sprouting.

Wilbourne reports that the cause of these immediate-

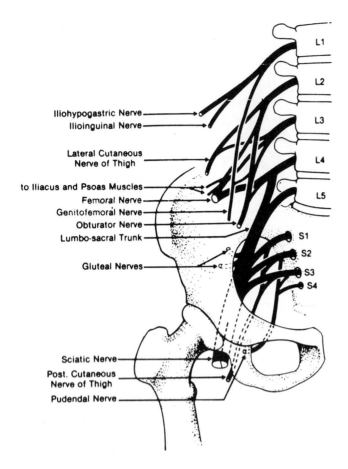

Iliohypogastric Nerve

Ilioinguinal Nerve

Lateral Cutaneous
Nerve of Thigh

to Iliacus and Psoas Muscles

Femoral Nerve

Genitofemoral Nerve

Obturator Nerve

Lumbo-sacral Trunk

Gluteal Nerves

Sciatic Nerve

Post. Cutaneous
Nerve of Thigh

Pudendal Nerve

L1

L2

L3

L4

L5

S1

S2

S3

S4

Figure 13-23 Diagram of the lumbosacral plexus, showing nerves that derive from it and bony anatomic relationships and the nerves. (Reproduced with permission from Stewart JD: *Focal Peripheral Neuropathies*. New York, Elsevier, 1987:253.)

onset plexopathies was originally attributed to a direct effect of anesthesia upon the nervous system.[264] However, the lesion was soon attributed to positioning of the upper limb during surgery, perhaps related to traction on the nerves rather than direct compression.[227,274] A variety of positions have been implicated. The positions most frequently associated with development of brachial plexopathy include a steep or prolonged Trendelenburg, abduction of the arms to greater than 90°, restraint of the arm on an arm board, and flexion of the head to the opposite side.[227,275] Patients undergoing cardiac surgery with medial sternotomy are at special risk for brachial plexopathy, possibly because of the required sternal retraction.[276,277]

LUMBOSACRAL PLEXUS Traumatic lesions of the lumbosacral plexus (Fig. 13-23) are less common than lesions of the brachial plexus, and usually are associated with major pelvic trauma. The most common nontraumatic lumbosacral plexopathy is diabetic amyotrophy, presenting over days with nonspecific proximal

leg pain in diabetic patients (Fig. 13-24). Weakness usually begins days later, and may eventually involve the other leg. The distribution is variable and patchy but includes muscles innervated by the femoral, obturator, or even sciatic nerves. While most lesions are thought to involve the lumbar plexus, there may be localization in some patients to anterior horn cells, nerve roots, the sacral plexus, or even intramuscular branches of motor nerves.[264] The pathology is thought to be ischemic, related to the microangiopathy of diabetes. Most patients will have known diabetes and signs of an underlying polyneuropathy, but a small percentage have painful amyotrophy as the presenting sign of an underlying metabolic disorder. The diagnosis involves exclusion of other causes of plexopathy and documenting the presence of diabetes. Treatment consists of pain and glucose control. The prognosis is good, although recovery is slow; pain subsides over 4 to 6 weeks and strength recovers over 12 to 24 months.[278,279]

Compression or stretch of the lumbosacral plexus has been attributed to operative positioning, commonly in association with compression of the lumbosacral plexus at the pelvic brim during childbirth. Similar presentation may result from L5 nerve root or peroneal nerve involvement.[84] Consideration should be given to retroperitoneal hemorrhage in a new onset lumbosacral plexopathy. Retroperitoneal hemorrhage produces back and abdominal pain with weakness of hip flexion, typically occurring in the setting of hemophilia or anticoagulation therapy.[244] Lumbosacral plexopathy resembling diabetic amyotrophy can present without laboratory evidence of diabetes.[280] Most nondiabetic amyotrophies are idiopathic, but a small percentage

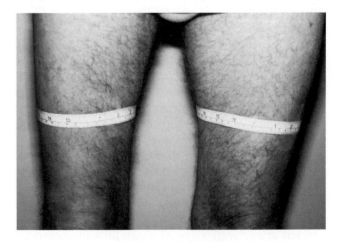

Figure 13-24 Right thigh of a patient with a resolving diabetic amyotrophy demonstrating atrophy 2 months after acute onset of pain and weakness. Examination demonstrated moderate quadriceps and adductor muscle weakness, an absent right quadriceps reflex, and normal sensation. Electrodiagnostic studies localized the lesion to the right lumbar plexus, superimposed on a mild diabetic polyneuropathy.

are associated with an autoimmune disorder and respond to immunosuppressive therapy. This group is suggested by an elevated sedimentation rate.[281]

MUSCLE INJURY

In critically ill patients, particularly those requiring prolonged neuromuscular blockade, high-dose corticosteroids, or extracorporeal membrane oxygenation (ECMO), a number of conditions can lead to muscle weakness and "failure to wean" from the ventilator. Considerations include nerve damage (e.g., critical illness polyneuropathy), muscle damage related to the underlying disorder or its treatment, and persistent neuromuscular junction blockade. For example, patients with renal insufficiency are unable to excrete the active metabolite of vecuronium, leading to drug-induced weakness that may persist for more than 7 days.[29] This condition can be distinguished from a severe medication-induced myopathy (below) by the finding of a decremental response to repetitive motor nerve stimulation. The specific problem of malignant hyperthermia was described earlier.

MYOPATHY RELATED TO PROLONGED NEUROMUSCULAR BLOCKADE

Patients requiring neuromuscular blockade, high-dose corticosteroid treatment (ranging from prednisone 50 to 100 mg daily to methylprednisolone 300 to 1500 mg daily), or both, are at risk of developing a severe, rapidly progressive quadriparesis, occasionally termed *critical illness myopathy* or *acute quadriplegic myopathy.*[27] The CK levels may be normal or elevated in this disorder, and repetitive motor nerve stimulation does not cause a decremental response. Needle EMG typically shows myopathic motor unit change and rapid recruitment of motor units with little force generated, reminiscent of "electromechanical dissociation." Histologic change in affected muscle ranges from atrophy to necrosis to loss of thick myosin filaments (Fig. 13-25).[282] The pathophysiology of these changes is not known, though there is speculation regarding increased susceptibility to steroids in muscle functionally denervated by the neuromuscular blockade and regarding the direct myotoxicity of these agents.[283] Most patients improve or normalize over weeks to months.

ISCHEMIC MYOPATHY

Rhabdomyolysis and subsequent renal failure have been reported independent of malignant hyperthermia in a variety of settings, most commonly in association with use of succinylcholine (an isolated expression of malignant hyperthermia), but also following general anesthesia in a prolonged or exaggerated lithotomy position.[284–287] Most reported patients had minimal muscle destruction, and the presumed cause was ischemic muscle injury. Serum CK increased postoperatively with evidence of myoglobinuria, indicating a risk of muscle injury and potential rhabdomyolysis related to position, independent of other considerations.[286]

NECROTIZING MYOPATHY

Necrotizing myopathy, an acute or subacute onset of painful weakness with necrosis of muscle fibers, is most commonly caused by myotoxins. As these conditions are potentially reversible, their recognition is important. A broad range of medications has been implicated. Lipid-lowering agents, including HMG-CoA reductase inhibitors (particularly when given concurrently with cyclosporin or other immunosuppressants), nicotinic acid, and clofibrate have been associated with necrotizing myopathy.[288,289] The mechanism of muscle damage is unknown; however, there is speculation that the HMG-CoA reductase inhibitors may impair cellular metabolism.[290] Necrotizing myopathy is rarely produced by other medications; however, the potential relationship should be considered whenever subacute myopathy develops. Other commonly encountered toxins producing necrotizing myopathy include substances of abuse such as cocaine, heroin, amphetamines, and alcohol.

SPINAL CORD OR ANTERIOR HORN CELL INJURY

Anterior horn cells are thought to be more vulnerable to injury than adjacent nerve tracts in the spinal cord. This impression is supported by anecdotal patients who develop a central cord syndrome with focal anterior horn cell degeneration but few other findings in association with cervical cord trauma.[291,292] Additional conditions associated with anterior horn cell injury include hypoxia, ischemia (as in complete or partial aortic occlusion), compression, electric shock, and radiation. These associations are of interest to the anesthesiologist in several situations, including, for example, intubation of patients with cervical spondylosis and conditions involving sustained hypotension.

Cervical spondylosis consists of disc degeneration, joint degeneration, and ligamentous hypertrophy and ossification (particularly the posterior longitudinal ligament) producing stenosis of the cervical canal, and it is the most common cause of myelopathy over the age of 55 years.[293] Patients with cervical spondylosis have a restricted cervical range of motion, and excessive cervical motion in the presence of spondylosis is a risk factor for deterioration.[294] Neurologic deterioration after trauma is presumably related to spinal cord compression, although vascular factors, including insuffi-

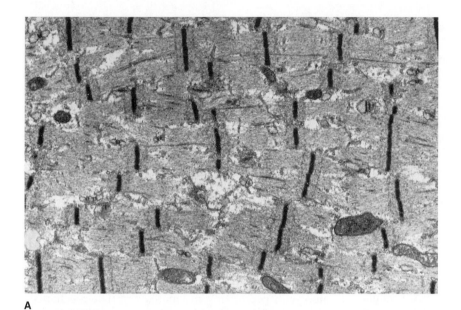

A

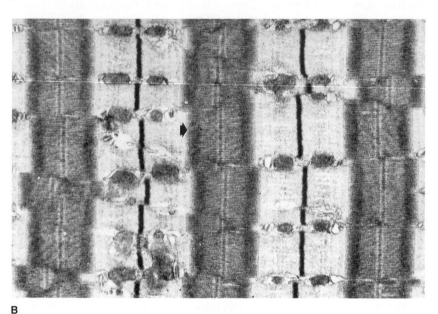

B

Figure 13-25 *A.* Muscle biopsy in acute quadriplegic myopathy. Note loss of myosin and presence of Z bands in muscle from patient with acute quadriplegic myopathy (*upper*). *B.* A normal muscle is shown for comparison. Note normal myosin (*arrow*). (Original electron microscopy magnification ×26,000. Courtesy of Mila Blaivas, University of Michigan Medical Center, Department of Pathology.)

ciency related to stretch of intramedullary vessels and impaired venous drainage, also are implicated in the pathophysiology.[295–298] Pathologic changes in patients with known cervical spondylytic myelopathy include spinal cord atrophy, gray matter degeneration, demyelination, and nerve root scarring.[299,300]

Patients with cervical spondylosis who undergo intubation and general anesthesia will occasionally develop a partial cervical myelopathy, with or without long tract signs. Cervical extension, particularly in the sedated patient with relaxation of volitional guarding mechanisms, may produce cervical movement excessive for these patients, beyond their physiologic limits. It is sometimes difficult to determine whether the lower motor component of the lesion is related to a cervical polyradiculopathy or degeneration of anterior horn

cells, and in some patients a combination undoubtedly exists. It is known that nerve root deformity can be caused as a direct effect of compression in connection with degenerative and traumatic conditions of the spine. Nerve root abnormalities also may relate to changes in the nerve root microcirculation, leading to ischemic injury, intraneural edema, and progressive compression. This can involve the ventral or dorsal roots, and the sequence of compression, ischemia, and edema with increased endoneurial fluid pressure has been associated with a closed-compartment syndrome in nerve roots.[197] Furthermore, it is unclear whether the underlying pathophysiology is ischemia or compression, although most evidence indicates that the effects are additive.[298] The resultant compression of the cervical spinal cord or nerve roots produces weakness and decreased reflexes in the upper extremities, with or without sensory loss. Because destruction of anterior horn cells is associated with axonal degeneration of the motor axons, atrophy develops in weak muscles. Commonly, a component of cervical myelopathy produces lower-extremity hyperreflexia, pathologic reflexes such as Babinski reflexes, and bladder and bowel involvement.[293] Recovery occurs slowly and may be incomplete, and these patients are sometimes thought to have amyotrophic lateral sclerosis, based upon the combination of upper and lower motor neuron abnormalities.

Substantial information is available regarding the effects of prolonged hypotension upon the central nervous system, particularly the brain. Clinical experience suggests that anterior horn cells are less vulnerable to ischemia than cortical neurons, but the additional risk factors that render anterior horn cells more vulnerable to otherwise acceptable levels of ischemia are unknown. Potential risk factors are similar to those of the CNS and include diffuse atherosclerosis, anemia, or preexisting compressive lesions already reducing blood flow to the spinal cord or nerve roots. The resultant effects of distal spinal cord ischemia is best demonstrated by patients with partial aortic occlusion.[301]

Patients with preexisting loss of anterior horn cells may be particularly vulnerable to additional loss because of the reduced safety factor, and because of the potentially increased metabolic load of anterior horn cells that have an increased innervation ratio. Conditions associated with these findings include prior poliomyelitis, degenerative motor neuron disease (e.g., amyotrophic lateral sclerosis), and prior focal myelopathy.

NEUROMUSCULAR DISORDER MIMICKING ANESTHESIA COMPLICATION

Several neurologic disorders present in the perioperative period, suggesting a causal relationship with the procedure or anesthesia. However, several of these disorders are now known to be only indirectly related to the procedure, and not preventable or directly related to faulty technique.

IDIOPATHIC BRACHIAL PLEXOPATHY

Idiopathic brachial plexopathy is characterized by arm and shoulder pain that is followed by weakness and amyotrophy of the shoulder girdle and arm muscles. This syndrome has many names including Parsonage-Turner syndrome, idiopathic brachial plexus neuritis, and cryptogenic brachial plexus neuropathy. It usually begins acutely with severe unilateral neck and shoulder pain.[302-305] Days later weakness develops, most prominently in the proximal arm. Sensory loss is mild. Weeks later atrophy becomes noticeable (Fig. 13-26). Muscles commonly involved include the serratus ante-

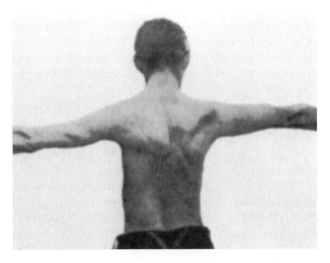

Figure 13-26   Photograph of patient published in 1896 (Lesynsky WM: *New York Med J* 63:469–470, 1896) showing shoulder girdle atrophy following pneumonia, and presumably representing the earliest illustrations of neuralgic amyotrophy (idiopathic brachial plexopathy). [Reproduced with permission from Wilbourn AJ: Brachial plexus disorders. In Dyck PJ, et al (eds): *Peripheral Neuropathy*, 3d ed. Philadelphia, WB Saunders, 1993:911–950.]

rior, supraspinatus and infraspinatus, and deltoid. Idiopathic brachial neuritis has been reported postpartum, following a normal pregnancy and delivery.[306] Bilateral involvement of phrenic nerves occurs, including recurrent isolated alternating phrenic mononeuropathies.[307,308]

About 10% of patients with idiopathic brachial plexopathy in the initial report of Parsonage and Turner had an antecedent surgery.[309] Malmamut and colleagues reported 6 patients who developed symptoms and signs of plexopathy 1 to 13 days postoperatively.[310] The delayed onset of neurologic symptoms and signs, the prominent complaint of shoulder pain, and the multifocal pattern of involvement made a compressive or stretch causation unlikely. Although the cause and pathophysiology of idiopathic plexopathy are unknown, the frequent association with an antecedent immunization, infection, or mild trauma suggests an immune-mediated disorder. The association between surgery and idiopathic plexopathy is speculative, but it also is thought to have an autoimmune basis, analogous to postoperative Guillain-Barré syndrome.[146] One possibility is that the stress of surgery activates an unidentified dormant virus, although confirmation of this hypothesis is lacking. Because postoperative weakness commonly is ascribed to compression of neural tissue occurring as a result of positioning, identification of this disorder is important, in part to prevent unnecessary surgical exploration. The delayed onset helps exclude positioning as the causes. Similarly, the progressive course over days to weeks is inconsistent with a compressive or ischemic cause, as both have maximum impairment at or shortly after onset. The absence of increased prevalence of brachial plexopathy in association with stroke argues strongly against decreased awareness and positioning as common contributing causes.[311]

A diagnosis of idiopathic plexopathy is based upon the clinical and electrodiagnostic distribution of impairment, as well as the presence of an acute painful onset. Examination and laboratory testing should exclude local infection, hematoma, vascular occlusion, and neoplasm. Pain control is an important consideration, and narcotic analgesics initially may be needed during the acute phase. Recovery is usually good; pain subsides in several weeks and strength returns slowly, usually within 12 months, consistent with the rate of reinnervation.[302] Recurrent idiopathic brachial plexopathy, especially if painless, associated with involvement of nerves outside the distribution of the brachial plexus, and with a family history of similar symptoms, suggests an unusual form of familial predisposition to compressive neuropathy.[187]

IDIOPATHIC GUILLAIN-BARRÉ SYNDROME

Approximately 75 percent of patients with Guillain-Barré syndrome report a nonspecific antecedent event within the preceding month before onset of neurological symptoms.[141,142,145,146] A variety of events have been associated with Guillain-Barré syndrome, most commonly a respiratory or gastrointestinal tract infection. For as many as 5 percent of patients, the only antecedent event is a surgical procedure, usually within 1 month of onset.[143,312] The frequency is higher if a longer interval between the surgery and onset is considered, and 8 of 100 patients reported by Winer and associates had a procedure within 3 months of developing Guillain-Barré syndrome.[313] Many, but not all, of the reported operations are complicated by infection, suggesting that infection is the most likely causal event, although others are seemingly uncomplicated.[143] There is no predilection for any specific operation, and there are reports of Guillain-Barré syndrome following neurosurgical, thoracic, abdominal, urologic, and orthopedic procedures.[143] Because operations involving neural tissue are not overrepresented, it seems unlikely that release of neural antigen is the provocative event.[143] The anesthetic agent also seems unrelated to the neurological disorder, as there are anecdotal reports of Guillain-Barré syndrome following administration of general, spinal, and epidural anesthesia.[143,314] The report associating Guillain-Barré syndrome and epidural anesthesia included four patients who developed onset of neurological impairment 1 to 2 weeks after anesthesia.[314] The authors suggested that an interaction between the anesthetic medications and the peripheral nervous system myelin or local trauma to roots may

initiate a cascade of immunologic events that result in the demyelinating neuropathy, although this remains speculative and the association must be rare.[314] Nevertheless, immunologic mechanisms undoubtedly are involved. Importantly, development of Guillain-Barré syndrome is unusual, and at the time of surgery the subsequent development can be neither predicted nor prevented given our current state of knowledge.

MONONEUROPATHY DURING POSTOPERATIVE CONVALESCENCE

During the postoperative convalescence period, patients are typically sedentary and either are confined to bed or spend substantial time in a chair.[198] They are particularly vulnerable to common entrapment mononeuropathies because of prolonged immobilization, often in association with sedative medications. Particularly vulnerable are the radial nerve at the level of the spiral groove, the ulnar nerve at the elbow, and the peroneal nerve at the knee (crossed-leg palsy). In emaciated patients, the sciatic nerve also is vulnerable to compression in the buttock. The radial and sciatic nerves, as well as other peripheral nerves, are also vulnerable to injection injuries in patients receiving frequent intramuscular injections.[30,198,248,315,316]

Nerve Injury Related to Local and Spinal Anesthesia

Local and spinal anesthetic agents are designed to be injected near or into peripheral nerve tissue and, as such, are generally thought to possess no neurotoxic properties.[248,317,318] Nevertheless, nerve injuries occasionally reported after local anesthesia are indistinguishable from injection injuries attributed to medications other than anesthetic agents, raising questions about the possible mechanism of injury. Nerves most commonly involved reflect the location of injection sites, including the sciatic, lateral femoral cutaneous, radial, axillary, and ulnar nerves. Similarly, neurological impairments attributable to a cauda equina syndrome occasionally have been associated with spinal or epidural anesthesia and analgesia, particularly in association with continuous infusion anesthesia.[317,319-321]

CHARACTERISTICS

Peripheral nerve injury resulting from injection is associated with severe pain radiating along the distribution of the involved nerve, occurring immediately during injection.[248,322] The pain is associated with rapid development of sensory and motor impairment, consistent with the distribution of involved sensory and motor fibers. Exceptions exist, however, in which pain is not a prominent feature and in which the neurological symptoms and signs do not appear for minutes to hours after injection. Injury to the cauda equina produces abnormalities referable to one or more lumbosacral nerve roots. The resultant painful radiculopathy or polyradiculopathy is associated with weakness, atrophy, sensory loss, and decreased or absent reflexes in the distribution of the affected nerve roots. Bladder, bowel, and sexual dysfunction are apparent when the lower sacral nerve roots are involved.

POSSIBLE MECHANISMS

Several mechanisms exist to explain nerve injury after injection, and a number of factors are likely involved.[321] Most relate to the direct neurotoxic effects of the injected agent because the concentration is high and the duration of exposure is long, although these factors are not always directly relevant to injection injuries associated with local anesthetic agents. Other mechanisms include direct trauma to nerve fibers by the needle, intrafascicular nerve injection, compression of axons by the injected material, compression by a hematoma related to the injection, or a toxic effect of the medication producing fibrosis or small vessel thrombosis with a delayed secondary effect on nerve.[316,321] These latter considerations also have relevance to injection of local anesthetic agents.

Gentili and associates reported several experimental investigations of nerve injury.[248,323] Following injection of a variety of agents directly into rat sciatic nerve, they found that the exact site of injection was the most crucial factor in predicting resultant axonal degeneration.[248] Injection either around the nerve or into the epineural tissues was not associated with significant axonal degeneration in the majority of cases. In contrast, intrafascicular injection of most medications produced at least partial axonal degeneration in this model of injury. The one exception was intrafascicular injection of normal saline, which did not produce substantial nerve fiber injury. This result argues strongly against a direct mechanical component of nerve injury, and supports the concept that most medications have some neurotoxic potential when placed in direct contact with axons.

These findings would not explain patients in whom the neurologic impairment is not apparent for minutes to hours after injection. In these patients, intrafascicular injection seems unlikely, and a question usually arises about placement of a potentially neurotoxic medication in close proximity to a nerve or other neural tissue. There was evidence in the studies reported by Gentili and associates that injection of some medications around the nerve or into the epineural tissues occasionally produced some degree of nerve fiber damage.[248]

This was observed in association with medications felt to be particularly neurotoxic.[248] It is assumed that migration of an injected neurotoxic medication from its intended location to neural tissue is one explanation for the delayed onset of symptoms and signs (minutes to several hours) occasionally reported by patients after an injection.[316] Other potential mechanisms, such as development of an intraneural or extraneural hematoma or edema with resultant compression of neural tissue, cannot be excluded, but were not observed in the experimental studies.[248]

Gentili and associates also evaluated intrafascicular and extrafascicular injection of local anesthetic agents, with and without epinephrine, using the identical animal model described above.[324] In total, 260 sciatic injections were carried out in 135 animals. Their results indicated that extrafascicular injection did not produce any significant nerve injury or disturbance in the blood-nerve barrier using local anesthetic agents. However, intrafascicular injection was associated with a variable amount of axonal and myelin degeneration, in excess of that associated with injection of normal saline. This study provides further support for the hypothesis that injury is related to a direct toxic effect of the injected medication on nerve tissue in association with breakdown of the blood-nerve barrier, as opposed to direct mechanical trauma. They did not demonstrate evidence of subsequent intrafascicular fibrosis, making this an unlikely explanation for late-onset impairments, remote to an injection.

The mechanisms of peripheral nerve injury associated with local injection seem applicable to nerve root injuries associated with spinal anesthesia.[317,324,325] Lumbar puncture is occasionally associated with meningitis or other complications such as abducen nerve paralysis not directly related to trauma from the needle insertion. Other complications are rare, and direct trauma to nerve roots within the cauda equina must be extremely uncommon, although the American Anesthesiologists Closed Claims Study database revealed that 16 percent of peripheral injuries leading to litigation involved lumbosacral nerve roots.[194] These injuries were associated primarily with regional anesthesia. Direct trauma to the arachnoid, dural, or radicular blood vessels occasionally produces extensive subarachnoid bleeding or even a subdural or epidural hematoma compressing the cauda equina.[326] Postlumbar-puncture back pain and radicular symptoms occur more frequently than overt evidence of radiculopathy, and as many as 13 percent of patients undergoing lumbar puncture alone have radicular pain or paresthesias.[327]

Numerous agents are neurotoxic when injected into the subarachnoid space. This does not have direct application to the anesthesiologist, because spinal and epidural anesthetic agents are not considered neurotoxic, and there are fewer complications with spinal than with general anesthesia.[328] There have been reports of neurologic deficits associated with inadvertent larger-volume injection of local anesthetics into the subarachnoid space during spinal anesthesia, and animal models of subarachnoid injection of local anesthetics have been examined.[329] In these models, paralysis was associated with subpial demyelination and macrophage infiltration. Neurological complications of epidural anesthesia and analgesia are relatively infrequent, and a recent report identified 10 patients who developed lumbosacral radiculopathy or polyradiculopathy after lumbar epidural anesthesia.[321] An additional patient developed a similar neurological impairment after inadvertent subarachnoid injection, and another patient developed a thoracic myelopathy after unintended spinal anesthesia. Most patients experienced mild to moderate neurological deficits involving the L2 nerve roots, although two patients with severe spinal stenosis developed more severe polyradiculopathy, suggesting spinal stenosis as a risk factor.[321] In general, MRI studies were unremarkable, and the prognosis for recovery was good.

A long-term consideration of spinal or epidural anesthesia is development of a chronic arachnoiditis.[326,330–332] The pathogenesis of chronic, progressive arachnoiditis is poorly understood, but it appears to develop in response to a variety of stimuli or irritants, such as the inadvertent introduction of foreign material. However, it also occurs without apparent event or in association with surgery or isolated disc herniation independent of myelography or anesthesia. Patients have been described who developed arachnoiditis with a resultant neurological deficit months to years after spinal or epidural anesthesia, independent of previous lumbar surgery or trauma, infection, or other known causative factors.[331,333] In such patients, arachnoiditis has been attributed to the epidural injection of foreign substances, perhaps related to a subarachnoid hyperergic reaction to the anesthetic agent or contaminants.[333,334] Patients have been described with a pure motor paraplegia following epidural anesthesia.[331,335] The pathophysiology is unclear and may be variable, with spinal cord compression, anterior spinal artery syndrome, or even anterior horn cell involvement being competing hypotheses, although neither cord compression nor spinal artery syndrome is associated with epidural anesthesia.[331] Several older spinal anesthetic agents and extremely high concentrations of procaine or tetracain have been associated with chronic adhesive leptomeningitis or arachnoiditis.[326,336] The neuromuscular manifestation of chronic arachnoiditis is a polyradiculopathy, due to compression or ischemia of the cauda equina.

Summary

Anesthesiology has an important relationship with neurology, in respect to both the central and peripheral nervous systems. Fundamental principles of anesthesia relate to interfering with normal neuromuscular function. As a result, patients with neuromuscular disorders require special consideration during anesthesia because they may have exaggerated or unexpected responses to anesthetic agents or may require medications that influence the choice of anesthetic agent. Examples include patients with myopathy who are susceptible to malignant hyperthermia or patients with impaired neuromuscular transmission who are sensitive to neuromuscular blocking agents. In addition, the peripheral nervous system is particularly vulnerable to injury during anesthesia when normal protective mechanisms are ineffective, independent of any underlying neurological illness. Familiarity with abnormal peripheral nervous system responses allows the anesthesiologist to recognize problems that can be limited by early identification, even when they cannot be predicted in advance. The expanding role of the anesthesiologist in the intensive care unit frequently involves patients with neuromuscular disease, especially those who require respiratory assistance. Most of these patients require intensive care because of a reversible underlying condition such as myasthenia gravis or Guillain-Barré syndrome, but some develop neuromuscular problems such as critical care neuropathy or acute quadriplegic myopathy during treatment. Again, familiarity with the primary neuromuscular disorder improves the quality of care and allows an appropriate combination of preventive and reactive medicine.

Furthermore, the neuromuscular specialist has an important role in the relationship between the patient and the anesthesiologist. Most importantly, this role involves anticipation of potential anesthesia-related problems in patients with neuromuscular disease. As such, the neurologist frequently participates in anesthetic-related medical decisions, including timing of elective operations in patients with neuromuscular disease and postanesthetic extubation. In addition, the neuromuscular specialist occasionally is called upon to identify peripheral nervous system impairments developing during or after anesthesia. The combined training and experience of the anesthesiologist and the neurologist are used to anticipate potential anesthetic problems related to an underlying neuromuscular disease, identify anesthetic-related complications involving the peripheral nervous system, and care for patients with neuromuscular disorders requiring prolonged respiratory assistance.

References

1. Gooch JL, et al: Prolonged paralysis after neuromuscular junction blockade: Case reports and electrodiagnostic findings. *Arch Phys Med Rehabil* 1993; 74:1007.

2. Foldes FF, McNall PG: Myasthenia gravis: A guide for anesthesiologists. *Anesthesiology* 1962; 23:837.

3. Hunter JM: New neuromuscular blocking drugs. *N Engl J Med* 1995; 332:1691.

4. Meyer KC, et al: Prolonged weakness after infusion of atracurium in two intensive care unit patients. *Anesth Analg* 1994; 78:772.

5. Ropper AH: Tips for neurologists who care for patients with mechanical respiratory failure. *Semin Neurol* 1984; 4:497.

6. Ropper AH, Kehne SM: Guillain-Barré syndrome: Management of respiratory failure. *Neurology* 1985; 35:1662.

7. Ropper AH, Kennedy SF: *Neurological and Neurosurgical Intensive Care.* Rockville, MD, Aspen Publishing, 1988.

8. Yang KL, Tobin MJ: A prospective study of indexes predicting the outcome of trials of weaning from mechanical ventilation. *N Engl J Med* 1991; 324:1445.

9. Kennedy SK: Airway management and respiratory support. In Ropper AH, Kennedy SK (eds): *Neurological and Neurosurgical Intensive Care.* Rockville, MD, Aspen Publishing, 1988:55–79.

10. Sorin R, et al: The influence of videofluoroscopy on the management of the dysphagic patient. *Dysphagia* 1988; 2:127.

11. Lingle CJ, Steinbach JH: Neuromuscular blocking agents. *Int Anesthesiol Clin* 1988; 26:288.

12. Thomas ET, Dobkin AB: Untoward effects of muscle relaxant drugs. *Int Anesthesiol Clin* 1972; 10:207.

13. Flacke W: Treatment of myasthenia gravis. *N Engl J Med* 1973; 288:27.

14. Azar I: The response of patients with neuromuscular disorders to muscle relaxants: A review. *Anesthesiology* 1984; 61:173.

15. Cooperman LH: Succinylcholine-induced hyperkalemia in neuromuscular disease. *JAMA* 1970; 213:1867.

16. Karpati G, Waters GV: Adverse anaesthetic reactions in Duchenne dystrophy. In Angeline C, et al (eds): *Muscular Dystrophy Research: Advances and New Trends.* Amsterdam, Excerpta Medica, 1980.

17. Bannister R, et al: Defective cardiovascular reflexes and supersensitivity to sympathomimetic drugs in autonomic failure. *Brain* 1979; 102:163.

18. Kalow W, et al: Epidemiology and inheritance of malignant hyperthermia. *Int Anesthesiol Clin* 1979; 17:119.

19. Guze BH, Baxter LR Jr: Current concepts. Neuroleptic malignant syndrome. *N Engl J Med* 1985; 313:163.

20. Otsu K, et al: Molecular cloning of cDNA encoding the Ca^{2+} release channel (ryanodine receptor) of rabbit cardiac muscle sarcoplasmic reticulum. *J. Biol Chem* 1990; 265:13472.

21. MacLennan DH, et al: The role of the skeletal muscle ryanodine receptor gene in malignant hyperthermia. *Symp Soc Exp Biol* 1992; 46:189.

22. Nelson E, Flewellen EH: The malignant hyperthermia syndrome. *N Engl J Med* 1983; 309:416.

23. Britt BA, Kalow W: Malignant hyperthermia: A statistical review. *Can Anaesth Soc J* 1970; 17:293.

24. Moulds RFW, Denborough MA: Biochemical basis of malignant hyperthermia. *Br Med J* 1974; 2:241.

25. Kolb ME, et al: Dantrolene in human malignant hyperthermia: A multicenter study. *Anesthesiology* 1982; 56:254.

26. Wedel DJ, et al: Clinical effects of intravenously administered dantrolene. *Mayo Clin Proc* 1995; 70:241.

27. Hirano M, et al: Acute quadriplegic myopathy: A complication of treatment with steroids, nondepolarizing blocking agents, or both. *Neurology* 1992; 42:2082.

28. Bolton CF, et al: Polyneuropathy in critically ill patients. *J Neurol Neurosurg Psychiatry* 1984; 47:1223.

29. Serredo V, et al: Persistent paralysis in critical ill patients after long-term administration of vecuronium. *N Engl J Med* 1992; 327:524.

30. Griggs RC, Karpati G: The pathogenesis of dermatomyositis. *Arch Neurol* 1991; 48:21.

31. Arahata K, Engel AG: Monoclonal antibody analysis of mononuclear cells in myopathies. I: Quantitation of subsets according to diagnosis and sites of accumulation and demonstration and counts of muscle fibers invaded by T cells. *Ann Neurol* 1984; 16:193.

32. Arahata K, Engel AG: Monoclonal antibody analysis of mononuclear cells in myopathies. IV: Cell-mediated cytotoxicity and muscle fiber necrosis. *Ann Neurol* 1988; 23:168.

33. Carpenter S, Karpati G: The pathological diagnosis of specific inflammatory myopathies. *Brain Pathol* 1992; 2:13.

34. Carpenter S, et al: Inclusion body myositis: A distinct variety of idiopathic inflammatory myopathy. *Neurology* 1978; 28:8.

35. Horowitz M, et al: Abnormalities of gastric and esophageal emptying in polymyositis and dermatomyositis. *Gastroenterology* 1986; 90:434.

36. Stern R, et al: ECG abnormalities in polymyositis. *Arch Intern Med* 1984; 144:2185.

37. Askari AD, Huettner TL: Cardiac abnormalities in polymyositis/dermatomyositis. *Semin Arthritis Rheum* 1982; 12:208.

38. Lakhanpal S, et al: Pulmonary disease in polymyositis/dermatomyositis: A clinicopathological analysis of 65 autopsy cases. *Ann Rheum Dis* 1987; 46:23.

39. Manchul LA, et al: The frequency of malignant neoplasms in patients with polymyositis-dermatomyositis. A controlled study. *Arch Intern Med* 1985; 145:1835.

40. Plotz PH et al: NIH conference. Myositis: Immunologic contributions to understanding cause, pathogenesis, and therapy. *Ann Intern Med* 1995; 122:715.

41. Behan WM, et al: Cardiac damage in polymyositis associated with antibodies to tissue ribonucleoproteins. *Br Heart J* 1987; 57:176.

42. Dalakas MC: How to diagnose and treat the inflammatory myopathies. *Semin Neurol* 1994; 14:137.

43. Dalakas MC: Current treatment of the inflammatory myopathies. *Curr Opin Rheumatol* 1994; 6:595.

44. DiMauro S, Moraes CT: Mitochondrial encephalomyopathies. *Arch Neurol* 1993; 50:1197.

45. Braakhekke JP, et al: The second wind phenomenon in McArdle's disease. *Brain* 1986; 109:1087.

46. Moufarrej NA, Bertorini TE: Respiratory insufficiency in adult-type acid maltase deficiency. *South Med J* 1993; 86:560.

47. Coleman RA, et al: Glycogen storage disease type III (glycogen debranching enzyme deficiency): Correlation of biochemical defects with myopathy and cardiomyopathy. *Ann Intern Med* 1992; 116:896.

48. Angelini C, et al: Carnitine palmityl transferase deficiency: Clinical variability, carrier detection, and autosomal-recessive inheritance. *Neurology* 1981; 31:883.

49. Argov Z, DiMauro S: Recurrent exertional myalgia and myoglobinuria due to carnitine palmityltransferase deficiency. *Isr J Med Sci* 1983; 19:552.

50. Katsuya H, et al: Postanesthetic acute renal failure due to carnitine palmityl transferase deficiency. *Anesthesiology* 1988; 68:945.

51. Angelini C, et al: Clinical and biochemical aspects of carnitine

deficiency and insufficiency: transport defects and inborn errors of beta-oxidation. *Crit Rev Clin Lab Sci* 1992; 29:217.

52. Luft R: The development of mitochondrial medicine. *Biochim Biophys Acta* 1995; 1271:1.

53. Wallace DC, et al: Mitochondrial DNA mutations in human degenerative diseases and aging. *Biochim Biophys Acta* 1995; 1271:141.

54. Barohn RJ, et al: Recurrent respiratory insufficiency and depressed ventilatory drive complicating mitochondrial myopathies. *Neurology* 1990; 40:103.

55. Folkers K, Simonsen R: Two successful double-blind trials with coenzyme Q10 (vitamin Q10) on muscular dystrophies and neurogenic atrophies. *Biochim Biophys Acta* 1995; 1271:281.

56. Peterson PL: The treatment of mitochondrial myopathies and encephalomyopathies. *Biochim Biophys Acta* 1995; 1271:275.

57. Hoffman EP, et al: Dystrophin: The protein product of the Duchenne muscular dystrophy locus. *Cell* 1987; 51:919.

58. Hoffman EP, Schwartz L: Dystrophin and disease. *Mol Aspects Med* 1991; 12:175.

59. Hoffman EP, Kunkel LM: Dystrophin abnormalities in Duchenne/Becker muscular dystrophy. *Neuron* 1989; 2:1019.

60. Barohn RJ, et al: Gastric hypomotility in Duchenne's muscular dystrophy. *N Engl J Med* 1988; 319:15.

61. Chalkiadis GA, Branch KG: Cardiac arrest after isoflurane anaesthesia in a patient with Duchenne's muscular dystrophy. *Anaesthesia* 1990; 45:22.

62. Griggs RC, et al: Prednisone in Duchenne dystrophy. A randomized, controlled trial defining the time course and dose response. Clinical Investigation of Duchenne Dystrophy Group. *Arch Neurol* 1991; 48:383.

63. Fukunaga H, et al: Long-term follow-up of patients with Duchenne muscular dystrophy receiving ventilatory support. *Muscle Nerve* 1993; 16:554.

64. Motta J, et al: Cardiac abnormalities in myotonic dystrophy. Electrophysiologic and histopathologic studies. *Am J Med* 1979; 67:467.

65. Griggs RC, et al: Cardiac conduction in myotonic dystrophy. *Am J Med* 1975; 59:37.

66. Horowitz M, et al: Gastric and esophageal emptying in dystrophia myotonica. Effect of metoclopramide. *Gastroenterology* 1987; 92:570.

67. Hansotia P, Frens D: Hypersomnia associated with alveolar hypoventilation in myotonic dystrophy. *Neurology* 1981; 31:1336.

68. Mitchell MM et al: Myotonia and neuromuscular blocking agents. *Anesthesiology* 1978; 49:44.

69. Boheimer N, et al: Neuromuscular blockade in dystrophia myotonica with atracurium besylate. *Anaesthesia* 1985; 40:872.

70. Bray RJ, Inkster JS: Anaesthesia in babies with congenital dystrophia myotonica. *Anaesthesia* 1984; 39:1007.

71. Waters DD, et al: Cardiac features of an unusual X-linked humeroperoneal neuromuscular disease. *N Engl J Med* 1975; 293:1017.

72. Griggs RC, et al: Clinical investigation in Duchenne dystrophy: V. Use of creatine kinase and pyruvate kinase in carrier detection. *Muscle Nerve* 1985; 8:60.

73. Hoffman EP, et al: Dystrophinopathy in isolated cases of myopathy in females. *Neurology* 1992; 42:967.

74. Redman JB, et al: Relationship between parental trinucleotide GCT repeat length and severity of myotonic dystrophy in offspring. *JAMA* 1993; 269:1960.

75. Guida M, et al: A molecular protocol for diagnosing myotonic dystrophy. *Clin Chem* 1995; 41:69.

76. Carpenter NJ: Genetic anticipation. Expanding tandem repeats. *Neurol Clin* 1994; 12:683.

77. Lennon VA et al: Experimental autoimmune myasthenia gravis: Cellular and humoral immune responses. *Ann NY Acad Sci* 1976; 274:283.

78. Richman DP, et al: Cellular immunity to acetylcholine receptor in myasthenia gravis: Relationship to histocompatibility type and antigenic site. *Neurology* 1979; 29:291.

79. Drachman DB: Myasthenia gravis. *N Engl J Med* 1994; 330:1797.

80. Lindstrom JM: Pathophysiology of myasthenia gravis: The mechanisms behind the disease. *Adv Neuroimmun* 1994; 1:3.

81. Kurtzke JF, Kurland LT: The epidemiology of neurologic disease. In Joynt RJ (ed): *Clinical Neurology.* Philadelphia, JB Lippincott, 1992:80–88.

82. Vial C, et al: Myasthenia gravis in childhood and infancy. *Arch Neurol* 1991; 48:847.

83. Argov Z, Mastaglia FL: Disorders of neuromuscular transmission caused by drugs. *N Engl J Med* 1979; 301:409.

84. Donaldson JO: *Neurology of Pregnancy.* Philadelphia: WB Saunders Co, 1977:56–65.

85. Stricker RB, et al: Myasthenic crisis. Response to plasmapheresis following failure of intravenous gamma-globulin. *Arch Neurol* 1993; 50:837.

86. Daroff RB: The office Tensilon test for ocular myasthenia gravis. *Arch Neurol* 1986; 43:843.

87. Lindstrom JM, et al: Antibody to acetylcholine receptor in myasthenia gravis. Prevalence, clinical correlates and diagnostic value. *Neurology* 1976; 26:1054.

88. Pestronk A, et al: Measurement of junctional acetylcholine receptors in myasthenia: Clinical correlates. *Muscle Nerve* 1985; 8:245.

89. Vincent A, Newsom-Davis J: Acetylcholine receptor antibody as a diagnostic test for myasthenia gravis: Results in 153 validated cases and 2967 diagnostic assays. *J Neurol Neurosurg Psychiatry* 1985; 48:1246.

90. Kelly JJ Jr, et al: The laboratory diagnosis of mild myasthenia gravis. *Ann Neurol* 1982; 12:238.

91. Drachman DB, et al: Functional activities of autoantibodies to acetylcholine receptors and the clinical severity of myasthenia gravis. *N Engl J Med* 1982; 307:769.

92. Drachman DB, et al: Humoral pathogenesis of myasthenia gravis. *Ann NY Acad Sci* 1987; 505:90.

93. Drachman DB, et al: "Sero-negative" myasthenia gravis: A humorally mediated variant of myasthenia gravis (Abstr). *Neurology* 1987; 37(Suppl 1).

94. Simpson JA: Myasthenia gravis: A new hypothesis. *Scott Med* 1960; 5:419.

95. Oosterhuis HJGH: Clinical aspects. In de Baets MH, Oosterhuis HJGH (eds): *Myasthenia Gravis.* Boca Raton, FL, CRC Press, 1993:13–42.

96. Ozdemir C, Young RR: The results to be expected from electrical testing in the diagnosis of myasthenia gravis. *Ann NY Acad Sci* 1976; 274:203.

97. Massey JM, et al: Sensitivity of diagnostic tests in myasthenia gravis. *Neurology* 1990; 40(Suppl 1):348 (abstr).

98. Stalberg E, et al: Neuromuscular transmission in myasthenia gravis studied with single fibre electromyography. *J Neurol Neurosurg Psychiatry* 1974; 37:540.

99. Borel CO, et al: Ventilatory drive and carbon dioxide response in ventilatory failure due to myasthenia gravis and Guillain-Barré syndrome. *Crit Care Med* 1993; 21:1717.

100. Quera-Salva MA, et al: Breathing disorders during sleep in myasthenia gravis. *Ann Neurol* 1992; 31:86.

101. Drachman DB: Present and future treatment of myasthenia gravis (Editorial). *N Engl J Med* 1987; 316:743.

102. Mendell J: Neuromuscular junction disorders: A guide to diagnosis and treatment. *Adv Neuroimmun* 1994; 1:9.

103. Giang DW: Central nervous system vasculitis secondary to infections, toxins, and neoplasms. *Semin Neurol* 1994; 14:313.

104. McQuillen MP, Leone MG: A treatment carol: Thymectomy revisited (Guest editorial). *Neurology* 1977; 27:1103.

105. Lindberg C, et al: Remission rate after thymectomy in myasthenia gravis when the bias of immunosuppressive therapy is eliminated. *Acta Neurol Scand* 1992; 86:323.

106. Lewis RA, et al: Myasthenia gravis: Immunological mechanisms and immunotherapy. *Ann Neurol* 1995; 37(S1):S51.

107. Dau PC: Plasmapheresis therapy in myasthenia gravis. *Muscle Nerve* 1980; 3:468.

108. Behan PO, et al: Plasma-exchange combined with immunosuppressive therapy in myasthenia gravis. *Lancet* 1979; 2:438.

109. Warmolts JR, Engel WK: Benefit from alternate-day prednisone in myasthenia gravis. *N Engl J Med* 1973; 286:17.

110. Tindall RSA, et al: Preliminary results of a double-blind, randomized, placebo-controlled trial of cyclosporine in myasthenia gravis. *N Engl J Med* 1987; 316:719.

111. Seybold ME, Drachman DB: Gradually increasing doses of prednisone in myasthenia gravis. Reducing the hazards of treatment. *N Engl J Med* 1974; 290:81.

112. Miller RG, et al: Prednisone-induced worsening of neuromuscular function in myasthenia gravis. *Neurology* 1986; 36:729.

113. Hertel G, et al: The treatment of myasthenia gravis with azathioprine. *Muscle Nerve* 1978; 1:343 (abstr).

114. Arsura E, et al: High dose methylprednisolone in myasthenia gravis. *Arch Neurol* 1985; 42:1149.

115. Mertens HG, et al: Effects of immunosuppressive drugs (azathioprine). *Ann NY Acad Sci* 1981; 377:691.

116. Flanagan WM, et al: Nuclear association of a T-cell transcription factor blocked by FK-506 and cyclosporin A. *Nature* 1991; 352:803.

117. Gracey DR, et al: Postoperative respiratory care after transsternal thymectomy in myasthenia gravis. A 3-year experience in 53 patients. *Chest* 1984; 86:67.

118. Gracey DR, et al: Plasmapheresis in the treatment of ventilator-dependent myasthenia gravis patients. Report of four cases. *Chest* 1984; 85:739.

119. Napolitano LM, Chernow B: Guidelines for corticosteroid use in anesthetic and surgical stress. *Int Anesthesiol Clin* 1988; 26:226.

120. Lisak RP, Barchi RL: *Myasthenia Gravis.* Philadelphia, WB Saunders Co, 1982.

121. Bell CF, et al: Atracurium in the myasthenic patient. *Anaesthesia* 1984; 39:961.

122. Hunter JM, et al: Vecuronium in the myasthenic patient. *Anaesthesia* 1985; 40:848.

123. Lennon VA, Lambert EH: Autoantibodies bind solubilized calcium channel-W-conotoxin complexes from small cell lung carcinoma: A diagnostic aid for Lambert-Eaton myasthenic syndrome. *Mayo Clin Proc* 1989; 64:1498.

124. Lambert EH, et al: Myasthenic syndrome occasionally associated with bronchial neoplasm. In Viets HR (ed): *Myasthenia Gravis.* Springfield, IL, Charles C Thomas Publishers, 1961:362–410.

125. Gracey DR, Southorn PA: Respiratory failure in Lambert-Eaton myasthenic syndrome. *Chest* 1987; 91:716.

126. Barr CW, et al: Primary respiratory failure as the presenting symptom in Lambert-Eaton myasthenic syndrome. *Muscle Nerve* 1993; 16:712.

127. Zweifel TJ, Albers JW: Multiple neurologic paraneoplastic syndromes. *Arch Neurol* 1980; 37:315.

128. Guillian-Barré Syndrome Steroid Trial Group: Double-blind trial of intravenous methylprednisolone in Guillain-Barré syndrome. *Lancet* 1993; 341:568.

129. Kiers L, et al: Paraneoplastic anti-neuronal nuclear IgG autoantibodies (Type I) localize antigen in small cell lung carcinoma. *Mayo Clin Proc* 1991; 66:1209.

130. Chalk CH, et al: Response of the Eaton-Lambert myasthenic syndrome to treatment of associated small-cell lung carcinoma. *Neurology* 1990; 40:1552.

131. Cherington M: Guanidine and germine in Eaton-Lambert syndrome. *Neurology* 1976; 26:944.

132. Lundh H, et al: Practical aspects of 3,4-diaminopyridine treatment of the Lambert-Eaton myasthenic syndrome. *Acta Neurol Scand* 1993; 88:136.

133. Bromberg MB, et al: Transient Lambert-Eaton myasthenic syndrome with systemic lupus erythematosus. *Muscle Nerve* 1989; 12:15.

134. Newsome-Davis J, Murray NMF: Plasma exchange and immunosuppressive drug treatment in the Lambert-Eaton myasthenic syndrome. *Neurology* 1984; 34:480.

135. Streib EW, Rothner AD: Eaton-Lambert myasthenic syndrome: Long-term treatment of three patients with prednisone. *Ann Neurol* 1981; 10:448.

136. McEvoy KM: Diagnosis and treatment of Lambert-Eaton myasthenic syndrome. *Neurol Clin* 1994; 12:387.

137. McEvoy KM, et al: 3,4-Diaminopyridine in the treatment of Eaton-Lambert syndrome. *N Engl J Med* 1989; 321:1567.

138. Takano H, et al: Effect of intravenous immunoglobulin in Lambert-Eaton myasthenic syndrome with small-cell lung cancer: Correlation with the titer of anti-voltage-gated calcium channel antibody. *Muscle Nerve* 1994; 17:1073.

139. Bird SJ: Clinical and electrophysiologic improvement in Lambert-Eaton syndrome with intravenous immunoglobulin therapy. *Neurology* 1992; 42:1422.

140. Liang BC, et al: Paraneoplastic pseudo-obstruction, mononeuropathy multiplex, and sensory neuropathy. *Muscle Nerve* 1994; 17:91.

141. Ropper AH: The Guillain-Barré syndrome. *N Engl J Med* 1992; 326:1130.

142. Albers JW, Kelly JJ Jr: Acquired inflammatory demyelinating polyneuropathies; clinical and electrodiagnostic features. *Muscle Nerve* 1989; 12:435.

143. Arnason BGW, Soliven B: Acute inflammatory demyelinating polyradiculopathy. In Dyck PJ, et al (eds): *Peripheral Neuropathy,* 3d ed. Philadelphia, WB Saunders, 1993:1437–1497.

144. Kleyweg RP, et al: The natural history of the Guillain-Barré syndrome in 18 children and 50 adults. *J Neurol Neurosurg Psychiatry* 1989; 52:853.

145. Kaslow RA, et al: Risk factors for Guillain-Barré syndrome. *Neurology* 1987; 37:685.

146. Arnason BG, Asbury AK: Idiopathic polyneuritis after surgery. *Arch Neurol* 1968; 18:500.

147. Soffer D, et al: Clinical features of the Guillain-Barré syndrome. *J Neurol Sci* 1978; 37:135.

148. Kennedy RH, et al: Guillain-Barré syndrome. A 42-year epidemiologic and clinical study. *Mayo Clin Proc* 1978; 53:93.

149. Andersonn T, Siden A: A clinical study of the Guillain-Barré syndrome. *Acta Neurol Scand* 1982; 66:316.

150. Asbury AK, et al: Criteria for diagnosis of Guillain-Barré syndrome. *Ann Neurol* 1978; 3:565.

151. Ropper AH, Weinberg D: Chronic immune demyelinating polyneuropathy (CIDP). *Neurology Chronicle* 1992; 1 (No. 9):1.

152. Barohn RJ, et al: Chronic inflammatory demyelinating polyradiculoneuropathy. *Arch Neurol* 1989; 46:878.

153. Dyck PJ, et al: Chronic inflammatory polyradiculoneuropathy. *Mayo Clin Proc* 1975; 50:621.

154. Simmons Z, et al: Presentation and initial clinical course in patients with chronic inflammatory demyelinating polyradiculoneuropathy: Comparison of patients without and with monoclonal gammopathy. *Neurology* 1993; 43:2202.

155. Cornblath DR, et al: Motor conduction studies in Guillain-

Barré syndrome: Description and prognostic value. *Ann Neurol* 1988; 23:354.

156. Cornblath DR, et al: Conduction block in clinical practice. *Muscle Nerve* 1991; 14:869.

157. The Guillain-Barré Syndrome Study Group: Plasmapheresis and acute Guillain-Barré syndrome. *Neurology* 1985; 35:1096.

158. McKhann GM, et al: Plasmapheresis and Guillain-Barré syndrome: Analysis of prognostic factors and the effect of plasmapheresis. *Ann Neurol* 1988; 23:347.

159. Kleyweg RP, van der Meche FG: Treatment-related fluctuations in Guillain-Barré syndrome after high-dose immunoglobulins or plasma-exchange. *J Neurol Neurosurg Psychiatry* 1991; 54:957.

160. Kleyweg RP, et al: Treatment of Guillain-Barré syndrome with high-dose gammaglobulin. *Neurology* 1988; 38:1639.

161. Parry GJ: Inflammatory demyelinating polyneuropathies: New perspectives in treatment. *Adv Neuroimmun* 1994; 1:9.

162. Dyck PJ, et al: Prednisone improves chronic inflammatory demyelinating polyradiculoneuropathy more than no treatment. *Ann Neurol* 1982; 11:136.

163. Dyck PJ, et al: Plasma exchange in polyneuropathy associated with monoclonal gammopathy of undetermined significance. *N Engl J Med* 1991; 325:1482.

164. Dyck PJ, et al: Plasma exchange in chronic inflammatory demyelinating polyradiculoneuropathy. *N Engl J Med* 1986; 314:461.

165. Wrobel CJ, Watson D: Plasmapheresis in chronic demyelinating polyneuropathy. *N Engl J Med* 1992; 326:1089.

166. Winer JB, Hughes RA: Identification of patients at risk of arrhythmia in the Guillain-Barré syndrome. *Q J Med* 1988; 68:735.

167. Hochman MS, et al: Inappropriate secretion of antidiuretic hormone associated with Guillain-Barré syndrome. *Ann Neurol* 1982; 11:322.

168. van der Meche FGA, Schmitz PIM, Dutch Guillain-Barré Study Group: A randomized trial comparing intravenous immune globulin and plasma exchange in Guillain-Barré syndrome (Review of article). *Neurology Chronicle* 1992; 2:9.

169. Ropper AH, et al: Limited relapse in GBS after plasma exchange. *Arch Neurol* 1988; 45:314.

170. van der Meche FGA, van Doorn PA: Guillain-Barré syndrome and chronic inflammatory demyelianting polyneuropathy: Immune mechanisms and update on current therapies. *Ann Neurol* 1995; 37(S1):S14.

171. Irani DN, et al: Relapse in Guillain-Barré syndrome following human immune globulin therapy. *Neurology* 43:A397, 1993 (abstr).

172. Dyck PJ, et al: A plasma exchange versus immune globulin infusion trial in chronic inflammatory demyelinating polyradiculoneuropathy. *Ann Neurol* 1994; 36:838.

173. Hughes RAC, et al: Controlled trial of prednisolone in acute polyneuropathy. *Lancet* 1978; 1:750.

174. The Dutch Guillain-Barré Study Group: Treatment of Guillain-Barré syndrome with high-dose immune globulins combined with methyprednisolone: A pilot study. *Ann Neurol* 1994; 35:749.

175. Ridley A: Porphyric neuropathy. In Dyck PJ, et al (eds): *Peripheral Neuropathy*, 2d ed. Philadelphia, WB Saunders Co, 1984:1704–1716.

176. Hierons R: Acute intermittent porphyria. *Postgrad Med J* 1967; 43:605.

177. Jedrzejowska H, et al: Morphological changes in the nervous system and muscles in acute intermittent porphyria. *Neuropatol Pol* 1974; 12(1):34.

178. Meyer UA: The porphyrias. In Stanbury JB (ed): *The Metabolic Basis of Inherited Disease*, 5th ed. New York, McGraw-Hill, 1986:1328–1320.

179. Day RS, et al: Coexistent variegate porphyria and porphyria cutanea tarda. *N Engl J Med* 1982; 307:36.

180. Tefferi A, et al: Porphyrias: Clinical evaluation and interpretation of laboratory tests. *Mayo Clin Proc* 1994; 69:289.

181. Moore MR, et al: *Disorders of Porphyrin Metabolism*. New York, Plenum Medical Book Co, 1987:18–155.

182. Meyer UA, et al: Intermittent acute porphyria—demonstration of a genetic defect in porphyrine metabolism. *N Engl J Med* 1972;286:1277.

183. Sack GHJ: Acute intermittent porphyria. *JAMA* 1990; 264:1290.

184. Chad DA, Lacomis D: Critically ill patients with newly acquired weakness: The clinicopathological spectrum (Editorial comment). *Ann Neurol* 1994; 35:257.

185. Rich MM, et al: Distinction between acute myopathy syndrome and critical illness polyneuropathy (Letter comment). *Mayo Clin Proc* 1995; 70:198.

186. Meier C, Moll C: Hereditary neuropathy with liability to pressure palsies. Report of two families and review of the literature. *J Neurol* 1982; 228:73.

187. Felice KJ, et al: Hereditary neuropathy with liability to pressure palsies masquerading as slowly progressive polyneuropathy. *Eur Neurol* 1994; 34:173.

188. Jones CT, et al: Superoxide dismutase mutations in an unselected cohort of Scottish amyotrophic lateral sclerosis patients. *J Med Genet* 1995; 32:290.

189. Orrell RW, deBelleroche JS: Superoxide dismutase and ALS. *Lancet* 1994; 344:1651.

190. Yanagihara R, et al: Calcium and vitamin D metabolism in Guamanian Chamorros with amyotrophic lateral sclerosis and parkinsonism-dementia. *Ann Neurol* 1984; 15:42.

191. Spencer PS, et al: Guam amyotrophic lateral sclerosis-parkinsonism-dementia linked to a plant excitant neurotoxin. *Science* 1987; 237:517.

192. Pestronk A, et al: A treatable multifocal motor neuropathy with antibodies to GM1 ganglioside. *Ann Neurol* 1988; 24:73.

193. Rosenbaum KJ, et al: Sensitivity to nondepolarizing muscle relaxants in amyotrophic lateral sclerosis: Report of two cases. *Anesthesiology* 1971; 35:638.

194. Kroll DA, et al: Nerve injury associated with anesthesia. *Anesthesiology* 1990; 73:202.

195. Watson BV, et al: Early postoperative ulnar neuropathies following coronary artery bypass surgery. *Muscle Nerve* 1992; 15:701.

196. Shields RW Jr, et al: Compartment syndromes and compression neuropathies in coma. *Neurology* 1986; 36:1370.

197. Rydevik BL, et al: Pressure increase in the dorsal root ganglion following mechanical compression. Closed compartment syndrome in nerve roots. *Spine* 1989; 14:574.

198. Stewart JD: *Focal Peripheral Neuropathies*. New York: Elsevier, 1987.

199. Seddon HJ: Three types of nerve injury. *Brain* 1943; 66:236.

200. Sunderland S: *Nerves and Nerve Injuries*, 2d ed. Edinburgh, Churchill Livingstone, 1978.

201. Castaldo JE, Ochoa JL: Mechanical injury of peripheral nerves. Fine structure and dysfunction. *Clin Plast Surg* 1984; 11:9.

202. Landau WM: The duration of neuromuscular function after nerve section in man. *J Neurosurg* 1953; 10:64.

203. Gilliatt RW, Taylor JC: Electrical changes following section of the facial nerve. *Proc R Soc Med* 1959; 52:1080.

204. Gilliatt RW: Physical injury to peripheral nerves. Physiologic and electrodiagnostic aspects. *Mayo Clin Proc* 1981; 56:361.

205. Drachman DB: Pathophysiology of the neuromuscular junction. In Asbury AK, (eds): *Diseases of the Nervous System. Clinical Neurobiology*. Philadelphia, Saunders, 1986:258–259.

206. Wolfart G: Collateral regeneration from residual motor fibers in amyotrophic lateral sclerosis. *Neurology* 1957; 7:124.

207. Ballantyne JP, Hansen S: A quantitative assessment of reinnervation in the polyneuropathies. *Muscle Nerve* 1982; 5:S127.

208. Levin KH: Common focal mononeuropathies and their electrodiagnosis. *J Clin Neurophysiol* 1993; 10:181.

209. Lundborg G, Dahlin LB: The pathophysiology of nerve compression. *Hand Clin* 1992; 8:215.

210. Nukada H, Dyck PJ: Acute ischemia causes axonal stasis, swelling, attenuation, and secondary demyelination. *Ann Neurol* 1987; 22:311.

211. Fowler CJ, Gilliat RW: Conduction velocity and conduction block after experimental ischaemic nerve injury. *J Neurol Sci* 1981; 52:221.

212. Ochoa J, et al: Anatomical changes in peripheral nerves compressed by a pneumatic tourniquet. *J Anat* 1972; 113:433.

213. Ochoa J, et al: Nature of the nerve lesion caused by a pneumatic tourniquet. *Nature* 1971; 233:265.

214. Ochoa J, Marotte L: Nature of the nerve lesion underlying chronic entrapment. *J Neurol Sci* 1973; 19:491.

215. Fowler TJ, Ochoa J: Unmyelinated fibers in normal and compressed peripheral nerves of the baboon. *Neuropathol Appl Neurobiol* 1975; 1:247.

216. Rudge P, et al: Acute peripheral nerve compression in the baboon. *J Neurol Sci* 1974; 23:403.

217. Nitz AJ, Matulionis DH: Ultrastructural changes in rat peripheral nerve following pneumatic tourniquet compression. *J Neurosurg* 1982; 57:660.

218. Dahlin LB, et al: Mechanical effects of compression of peripheral nerves. *J Biomech Eng* 1986; 108:120.

219. Logigian EL, et al: Stretch-induced spinal accessory nerve palsy. *Muscle Nerve* 1988; 11:146.

220. Millesi H, et al: Mechanical properties of peripheral nerves. *Clin Orthop* 1995; 76.

221. Kwan MK, et al: Strain, stress and stretch of peripheral nerve. Rabbit experiments in vitro and in vivo. *Acta Orthop Scand* 1992; 63:267.

222. Rydevik BL, et al: An in vitro mechanical and histological study of acute stretching on rabbit tibial nerve. *J Orthop Res* 1990; 8:694.

223. Hasegawa T: An experimental study on elongation injury of peripheral nerve. *Nippon Seikeigeka Gakkai Zasshi* 1992; 66:1184.

224. Brown R, et al: Effects of acute graded strain on efferent conduction properties in the rabbit tibial nerve. *Clin Orthop* 1993; 296:288.

225. Yamada H: Studies of electrophysiological and morphological changes in the rabbit sciatic nerve under various types of stretch and relaxation. *Nippon Seikeigeka Gakkai Zasshi* 1987; 61:217.

226. Spiegel DA, et al: Recovery following stretch injury to the sciatic nerve of the rat: An in vivo study. *J Reconstr Microsurg* 1993; 9:69.

227. Cooper DE, et al: The prevention of injuries of the brachial plexus secondary to malposition of the patient during surgery. *Clin Orthop* 1988; 228:33.

228. Rydevik B, Lundborg G: Permeability of intraneural microvessels and perineurium following acute, graded experimental nerve compression. *Scand J Plast Reconstr Surg* 1977; 11:179.

229. Lundborg G: Ischemic nerve injury. Experimental studies on intraneural microvascular pathophysiology and nerve function in a limb subjected to temporary circulatory arrest. *Scand J Plast Reconstr Surg Suppl* 1970; 6:3.

230. Ogata K, Naito M: Blood flow of peripheral nerve effects of dissection, stretching and compression. *J Hand Surg [Br]* 1986; 11:10.

231. Albers JW, et al: Frequency of median mononeuropathy in patients with mild diabetic neuropathy in the Early Diabetes Intervention Trial (EDIT). *Muscle Nerve* 1996; 19:140.

232. Haymaker W, Woodhall B: *Peripheral Nerve Injuries. Principles of Diagnosis*. Philadelphia, WB Saunders Co, 1953.

233. Horowitz SH: Iatrogenic causalgia. Classification, clinical findings, and legal ramifications. *Arch Neurol* 1984; 41:821.

234. Kincaid JC: AAEE Minimonograph #31: The electrodiagnosis of ulnar neuropathy at the elbow. *Muscle Nerve* 1988; 11:1005.

235. Miller RG: The cubital tunnel syndrome: Diagnosis and precise localization. *Ann Neurol* 1979; 6:56.

236. Cameron MG, Stewart OJ: Ulnar nerve injury associated with anaesthesia. *Can Anaesth Soc J* 1975; 22:253.

237. Ekerot L: Postanesthetic ulnar neuropathy at the elbow. *Scand J Plast Reconstr Surg* 1977; 11:225.

238. Kincaid JC, et al: The evaluation of suspected ulnar neuropathy at the elbow. *Arch Neurol* 1986; 43:44.

239. Toro OA, Mas A: Femoral neuropathy complicating urologic surgery (Letters to the editor). *Urology* 1991; 38:394 (abstr).

240. Katirji MB, Lanska DJ: Femoral mononeuropathy after radical prostatectomy. *Urology* 1990; 36:539.

241. Hakim MA, Katirji MB: Femoral mononeuropathy induced by the lithotomy position: A report of 5 cases with a review of literature. *Muscle Nerve* 1993; 16:891.

242. Massey EW, Tim RW: Femoral compression neuropathy from a mechanical pressure clamp. *Neurology* 1989; 39:1263.

243. Solheim LF, Hagen R: Femoral and sciatic neuropathies after total hip arthroplasty. *Acta Orthop Scand* 1980; 51:531.

244. Cranberg L: Femoral neuropathy from iliac hematoma. Report of a case. *Neurology* 1979; 29:1071.

245. DeBolt WL, Jordan JC: Femoral neuropathy from heparin hematoma. Report of two cases. *Bull Los Angeles Neurol Soc* 1966; 31:45.

246. Young MR, Norris JW: Femoral neuropathy during anticoagulation therapy. *Neurology* 1976; 26:1173.

247. Calverley JR, Mulder DW: Femoral neuropathy. *Neurology* 1958; 10:963.

248. Gentili F, et al: Clinical and experimental aspects of injection injuries of peripheral nerves. *Le Journal Canadien Des Sciences Neurologiques* 1980; 7:143.

249. McManis PG: Sciatic mononeuropathy during cardiac surgery. *Neurology* 1993; 43:A215(abstr).

250. Dawson DM, Krarup C: Perioperative nerve lesions. *Arch Neurol* 1989; 46:1355.

251. Papadopoulos SM, et al: Unusual cause of "piriformis muscle syndrome." *Arch Neurol* 1990; 47:1144.

252. Kollar RL, Blank NK: Strawberry picker's palsy. *Arch Neurol* 1980; 37:320.

253. Katirji MB, Wilbourn AJ: Common peroneal mononeuropathy: A clinical and electrophysiological study of 116 lesions. *Neurology* 1988; 38:1723.

254. Weber ER, et al: Peripheral neuropathies associated with total hip arthroplasty. *J Bone Joint Surg* 1976; 58A:66.

255. Pittman GR: Peroneal nerve palsy following sequential pneumatic compression. *JAMA* 1989; 261:2201.

256. Lederman RJ, et al: Peripheral nervous system complications of coronary artery bypass graft surgery. *Ann Neurol* 1982; 12:297.

257. Esselman PC, et al: Selective deep peroneal nerve injury associated with arthroscopic knee surgery. *Muscle Nerve* 1993; 16:1188.

258. Brown WF, Watson BV: Quantitation of axon loss and conduction block in peroneal nerve palsies. *Muscle Nerve* 1991; 14:237.

259. Levin KH: Common focal mononeuropathies and their electrodiagnosis. *J Clin Neurophysiol* 1993; 10:181.

260. Pickett JB: Localizing peroneal nerve lesions to the knee by motor conduction studies. *Arch Neurol* 1984; 41:192.

261. DeVita MA, et al: Incidence and natural history of phrenic

neuropathy occurring during open heart surgery. *Chest* 1993; 103:850.

262. Kohorst WR, et al: Bilateral diaphragmatic paralysis following topical cardiac hypothermia. *Chest* 1984; 85:65.

263. Dajee A, et al: Phrenic nerve palsy after topical cardiac hypothermia. *Int Surg* 1983; 68:345.

264. Wilbourn AJ: Brachial plexus disorders. In Dyck PJ, et al (eds): *Peripheral Neuropathy,* 3d ed. Philadelphia, WB Saunders, 1993:911–950.

265. Bloch SL, et al: Brachial plexus neuropathy as the initial presentation of systemic lupus erythematosus. *Neurology* 1979; 29:1633.

266. Challenor YB, et al: Nontraumatic plexitis and heroin addiction. *JAMA* 1973; 225:958.

267. Kidron D, et al: Mononeuritis multiplex with brachial plexus neuropathy coincident with *Mycoplasma pneumoniae* infection. *Eur Neurol* 1989; 29:90.

268. Raz I, et al: Acute bilateral brachial plexus neuritis associated with hypersensitivity vasculitis. A case report and review of literature. *Klin Wochenschr* 1985; 63:643.

269. Cohen MG, Webb J: Brachial neuritis with colitic arthritis (Letter). *Ann Intern Med* 1987; 106:780.

270. Weintraub MI, Chia DT: Paralytic brachial neuritis after swine flu vaccination (Letter). *Arch Neurol* 1977; 34:518.

271. Kraft GH: Rucksack paralysis and brachial neuritis. *JAMA* 1970; 211:300.

272. Cuetter AC, Bartoszek DM: The thoracic outlet syndrome: Controversies, overdiagnosis, overtreatment, and recommendations for management. *Muscle Nerve* 1989; 12:410.

273. Wilbourn AJ, Shields RW: "Classic" post-operative brachial plexopathy: The electrodiagnostic features. *Neurology* 1993; 43:A214(abstr).

274. Britt BA, et al: Positioning trauma. In Orkin FK, Cooperman LH (eds): *Complications in Anesthesia.* Philadelphia, JB Lippincott, 1983:646–670.

275. Kwaan JHM, Rappaport I: Postoperative brachial plexus palsy. *Arch Surg* 1970; 101:612.

276. Graham G, et al: Brachial plexus lesion after medial sternotomy. *J Neurol Neurosurg Psychiatry* 1981; 44:621.

277. Hanson MR, et al: Mechanism and frequency of brachial plexus injury in open-heart surgery. *Ann Thorac Surg* 1983; 36:675.

278. Chokroverty S: Proximal nerve dysfunction in diabetic proximal amyotrophy. *Arch Neurol* 1982; 39:403.

279. Winer JB, et al: A prospective study of acute idiopathic neuropathy. I. Clinical features and their prognostic value. *J Neurol Neurosurg Psychiatry* 1988; 51:605.

280. Evans BA, et al: Lumbosacral plexus neuropathy. *Neurology* 1981; 31:1327.

281. Bradley WG, et al: Painful lumbosacral plexopathy with elevated erythrocyte sedimentation rate: A treatable inflammatory syndrome. *Ann Neurol* 1984; 15:457.

282. al-Lozi MT, et al: Rapidly evolving myopathy with myosin-deficient muscle fibers (See comments). *Ann Neurol* 1994; 35:273.

283. Zochodne DW, et al: Acute necrotizing myopathy of intensive care: Electrophysiological studies. *Muscle Nerve* 1994; 17:285.

284. Bhave CG, et al: Myoglobinuria following the use of succinylcholine. *J Postgrad Med* 1993; 39:157.

285. Goldberg M, et al: Rhabdomyolysis associated with urethral stricture repair: Report of a case. *J Urol* 1980; 124:730.

286. Bildsten SA, et al: The risk of rhabdomyolysis and acute renal failure with the patient in the exaggerated lithotomy position. *J Urol* 1994; 152:1970.

287. Acquarone N, et al: Postanesthetic myoglobinuric renal failure: An isolated expression of malignant hyperthermia. *Nephrol Dial Transplant* 1994; 9:567.

288. Langer T, Levy RI: Acute muscular syndrome associated with administration of clofibrate. *N Engl J Med* 1968; 279:856.

289. Corpier CL, et al: Rhabdomyolysis and renal injury with lovastatin use. Report of two cases in cardiac transplant recipients. *JAMA* 1988; 260:239.

290. Folkers K, et al: Lovastatin decreases coenzyme Q levels in humans. *Proc Natl Acad Sci USA* 1990; 87:8931.

291. Roth EJ, et al: Traumatic center cord syndrome: Clinical features and functional outcomes. *Arch Phys Med Rehabil* 1990; 71:18.

292. Merriam WF, et al: A reappraisal of acute traumatic central cord syndrome. *J Bone Joint Surg (Br)* 1986; 68:708.

293. Krauss WE, McCormick PC: Cervical spondylotic myelopathy. *Semin Neurol* 1993; 13:343.

294. Barnes MP, Saunders M: The effect of cervical mobility on the natural history of cervical spondylotic myelopathy. *J Neurol Neurosurg Psychiatry* 1984; 47:17.

295. Foo D: Spinal cord injury in forty-four patients with cervical spondylosis. *Paraplegia* 1986; 24:301.

296. Hoff JT, Wilson CB: The pathophysiology of cervical spondylotic radiculopathy and myelopathy. *Clin Neurosurg* 1977; 24:474.

297. Nagashima C: Cervical myelopathy due to ossification of the posterior longitudinal ligament. *J Neurosurg* 1972; 37:653.

298. Hukuda S, Wilson CB: Experimental cervical myelopathy: Effects of compression and ischemia on the canine cervical cord. *J Neurosurg* 1972, 37:631.

299. Longley EO, Jones R: Acute trichloroethylene narcosis. *Archives Environ Health* 1963; 7:249.

300. Ogino H, et al: Canal diameter, anteroposterior compression ratio, and spondylotic myelopathy of the cervical spine. *Spine* 1983; 8:1.

301. Larson WL, Wald JJ: Foot drop as a harbinger of aortic occlusion. *Muscle Nerve* 1995; 18:899.

302. Tsairis P, et al: Natural history of brachial plexus neuropathy. Report on 99 patients. *Arch Neurol* 1972; 27:109.

303. Beghi E, et al: Brachial plexus neuropathy in the population of Rochester, Minnesota, 1970–1981. *Ann Neurol* 1985; 18:320.

304. Turner AJW: Acute brachial radiculitis. *Br Med J* 1944; 2:592.

305. England JD, Sumner AJ: Neuralgic amyotrophy: An increasingly diverse entity. *Muscle Nerve* 1987; 10:60.

306. Dumitru D, Liles RA: Postpartum idiopathic brachial neuritis. *Obstet Gynecol* 1989; 73:473.

307. Walsh NE, et al: Brachial neuritis involving the bilateral phrenic nerves. *Arch Phys Med Rehabil* 1987; 68:46.

308. Gregory RP, et al: Recurrent isolated alternating phrenic nerve palsies: A variant of brachial neuritis? *Thorax* 1990; 45:420.

309. Turner AJW, Parsonage MJ: Neuralgic amyotrophy (paralytic brachial neuritis) with special reference to prognosis. *Lancet* 1957; 1:209.

310. Malamut RI, et al: Postsurgical idiopathic brachial neuritis. *Muscle Nerve* 1994; 17:320.

311. Kingery WS, et al: The absence of brachial plexus injury in stroke. *Am J Phys Med Rehabil* 1993; 72:127.

312. Wiederholt WC, et al: The Landry-Guillain-Barré-Strohl syndrome or polyradiculoneuropathy: Historical review, report on 97 patients, and present. *Mayo Clin Proc* 1964; 39:427.

313. Winer JB, et al: A prospective study of acute idiopathic neuropathy. II. Antecedent events. *J Neurol Neurosurg Psychiatry* 1988; 51:613.

314. Steiner I, et al: Guillain-Barré syndrome after epidural anesthesia: Direct nerve root damage may trigger disease. *Neurology* 1985; 35:1473.

315.   Finelli PF, Taylor GW: Unusual injection neuropathy in heroin addict: Case report. *Milit Med* 1977; 142:704.

316.   Geiringer SR, Leonard JA Jr: Injection-related ulnar neuropathy. *Am J Phys Med Rehabil* 1989; 70:705.

317.   Rigler ML, et al: Cauda equina syndrome after continuous spinal anesthesia. *Anesth Analg* 1991; 72:275.

318.   Dripps RD, Vandam LD: Longterm follow up of patients who received 10,098 spinal anesthetics. Failure to discover major neurological sequelae. *JAMA* 1954; 156:1486.

319.   Ross BK, et al: Local anesthetic distribution in a spinal model: A possible mechanism of neurologic injury after continuous spinal anesthesia. *Reg Anesth* 1992; 17:69.

320.   Griffith RW: Complications of continuous spinal anesthesia. *CRNA* 1992; 3:164.

321.   Yuen EC, et al: Neurological complications of lumbar anesthesia and analgesia. *Neurology* 1995; 45:1795.

322.   Braodbent TR, et al: Peripheral nerve injuries from administration of penicillin. *JAMA* 1948; 140:1008.

323.   Gentili F, et al: Peripheral nerve injection injury: An experimental study. *Neurosurgery* 1979; 4:244.

324.   Gentili F, et al: Nerve injection injury with local anesthetic agents: A light and electron microscopic, fluorescent microscopic, and horseradish peroxidase study. *Neurosurgery* 1980; 6:263.

325.   Morton CP, et al: Continuous spinal anesthesia—evolution of a technique. *Ann Acad Med Singapore* 1994; 23:98.

326.   Fishman RA: Clinical examination of cerebrospinal fluid. In *Cerebrospinal Fluid in Diseases of the Nervous System*. Philadelphia, WB Saunders Co, 1980:141–167.

327.   Dripps RD, Vandam LD: Hazards of lumbar puncture. *JAMA* 1951; 147:1118.

328.   Salehi E: The current state of spinal anesthesia in urologic interventions. *Z Urol Nephrol* 1978; 71:397.

329.   Rosen MA, et al: Evaluation of neurotoxicity after subarachnoid injection of large volumes of local anesthetic solutions. *Anesth Analg* 1983; 62:802.

330.   Whisler WW: Chronic spinal arachnoiditis. In Viken PJ, Bruyn GW (eds): *Handbook of Clinical Neurology*, 33d ed. Amsterdam, North Holland Publishing Co, 1978:263–274.

331.   Adriani J, Naragi M: Paraplegia associated with epidural anesthesia. *South Med J* 1986; 79:1350.

332.   Lambert DH: Complications of spinal anesthesia. *Int Anesthesiol Clin* 1989; 27:51.

333.   Sghirlanzoni A, et al: Epidural anesthesia and spinal arachnoiditis. *Anaesthesia* 1989; 44:317.

334.   Boiardi A, et al: Diffuse arachnoiditis following epidural analgesia. *J Neurol* 1983; 230:253.

335.   Skouen JS, et al: Paraplegia following epidural anesthesia. A case report and a literature review. *Acta Neurol Scand* 1985; 72:437.

336.   Reisner LS, et al: Persistent neurologic deficit and adhesive arachnoiditis following intrathecal 2-chloroprocaine injection. *Anesth Analg* 1980; 59:452.

Chapter 14

CEREBROVASCULAR DISEASE

BRADLEY S. BOOP

DAVID G. SHERMAN

Cerebrovascular disease is a concept used to describe processes affecting the cerebral circulation that may produce neurologic dysfunction. Stroke is a generic term applied to the clinical syndrome that results from ischemic or hemorrhagic brain injuries. Because stroke may affect both cognition and physical function, it is among the most feared illnesses of middle to late life. Despite a significant decline in incidence and mortality of stroke in recent decades, it remains the third leading cause of death in the United States after cardiovascular disease and cancer.[1,2] The magnitude of stroke as a health care problem is expected to grow as the number of elderly, and therefore stroke-prone people, is in-

creasing. A majority of stroke victims will survive, but one-third will be severely disabled and another one-third will require some type of rehabilitation.[3–7] Because stroke survivors may live many years with their disability, often requiring skilled nursing care, the cost is enormous: an estimated $20 billion in the United States in 1994.[1] Nevertheless, most strokes are preventable. An increasing number of primary and secondary prevention strategies have had proven benefit in large, randomized, controlled trials in the past two decades. Large trials have demonstrated convincingly that risk factor modification can significantly reduce the risk of ischemic and hemorrhagic cerebrovascular disease. Armed with modern data, it is increasingly important that clinicians recognize stroke as a syndrome with multiple causes. Patients deserve a thorough investigation into the pathophysiology leading to stroke, so that the most appropriate intervention can be offered. While prevention will always remain the most effective way of reducing the impact of stroke, a burgeoning literature about acute stroke interventions has raised hopes that effective therapies will be identified in the near future.

Epidemiology

At current rates, it is estimated that 550,000 strokes will occur each year in the United States, while worldwide an average incidence rate of 114 per 100,000 has been calculated.[8] About one-fourth of strokes in the United States are recurrent, and stroke identifies individuals with a 10 percent per year risk of recurrence. Stroke mortality declined 1 percent per year throughout much of the twentieth century, but in the 1970s and 1980s mortality fell 5 percent per year. This paralleled a reduction in the incidence of ischemic stroke and intracerebral hemorrhage and is likely due to the improved treatment of hypertensive disease. The 30-day mortality from stroke is about 20 percent, and 50 percent mortality is reached by 3 years.[9–13] There is evidence that the decline in stroke incidence and mortality has leveled off.[13–17] Data from the Framingham study identify age as the most important nonmodifiable risk factor for stroke. In that population, the annual incidence for stroke doubled in each successive decade after the age of 35. Atherothrombotic infarction was 1.3 times more frequent in men.[18] Ischemic stroke is a syndrome produced by occlusion of cerebral arteries or veins (Fig. 14-1). It is necessary to classify the cause of stroke in order to identify and understand the varying pathophysiologic mechanisms, and because preventive strategies differ depending on the specific cause.

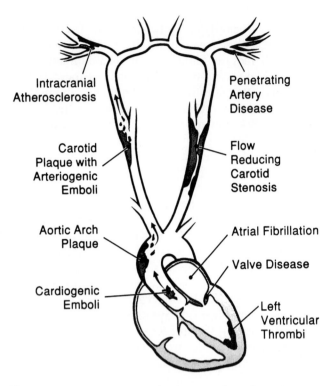

Figure 14-1 Common causes of ischemic stroke and transient ischemic attack. (Courtesy of R. G. Hart et al.[188])

RISK FACTORS

Risk factor identification provides valuable insight into the pathogenesis of cerebrovascular disease, and may lead to prevention of stroke when these risk factors are modified. Large clinical trials continue to identify the relative risk associated with various risk factors for different categories of cerebrovascular disease. However, many risk factors appear to be common to most types of vascular disease. Some of our best data on risk factors for stroke come from the population-based Framingham study (Table 14-1). Hypertension is the most important modifiable risk factor for stroke, and both systolic and diastolic elevations are independently related to atherothrombotic brain infarction (ABI) incidence.[19,20] The relative risk in hypertensive patients compared with normotensive individuals is three times overall. The fraction of risk attributable to hypertension is calculated to be 55 to 65 percent, and trials of treatment of hypertension have reduced stroke by about 50 percent.[21–23] Isolated systolic hypertension is particularly important in the elderly and is associated with a significantly increased risk of stroke.[24] Cigarette smoking compounds the risk of stroke so that an individual who has hypertension and smokes approaches a twenty-fold increase in risk. A normotensive smoker's risk increases with the number of cigarettes smoked, with two-pack-per-day smokers doubling their relative risk of stroke. Cigarette smoking carries an independent risk for ABI, intracerebral

hemorrhage (ICH), and subarachnoid hemorrhage (SAH).[25–27] Heart disease contributes significantly to the risk of ischemic stroke. Left ventricular hypertrophy (by ECG) carried risk in the Framingham study even when the analysis was controlled for age and systolic blood pressure.[18] Prior coronary disease, cardiac failure, and valvular (rheumatic) or nonvalvular atrial fibrillation predispose a patient to ischemic stroke.[28–33] The Stroke Prevention in Atrial Fibrillation (SPAF) investigators identified patients with atrial fibrillation as high risk if previous thromboembolism, recent congestive heart failure, or a history of hypertension or diabetes could be documented.[34,35] Pooled data from a group of Atrial Fibrillation Investigators (AFI) identified patients with age greater than 65 as high risk as well, and confirmed the findings of the SPAF investigators.[36]

Diabetes appears to double the risk for ABI and is a known risk factor for atherosclerosis in general and in the carotid arteries.[37–41] Obesity confers risk via the associated effects on blood pressure, lipids, and glucose intolerance.[42,43] The influence of race on stroke risk is multifactorial and continues to be defined. African-Americans have an excess stroke mortality approaching two times that of whites. Some of the excess mortality is attributable to a higher prevalence of hypertension and decreased access to health care, but about 30 percent of the excess mortality is unexplained.[44] African-Americans also have less extracranial carotid disease than whites.[45–47] Hispanic-Americans have been observed to have ischemic stroke at a

TABLE 14-1
Standardized Multivariate Regression Coefficients for Risk Factors for Atherothrombotic Brain Infarction

	MEN		WOMEN	
Risk Factor	Ages 35–64 Years	Ages 65–94 Years	Ages 35–64 Years	Ages 65–94 Years
Hypertension	0.761[a]	0.426[a]	0.814[a]	0.477[a]
High systolic blood pressure	0.613[a]	0.395[a]	0.629[a]	0.396[a]
High diastolic blood pressure	0.642[a]	0.228[a]	0.615[a]	0.369[a]
Left ventricular hypertrophy[c]	0.113	0.192[d]	0.130[b]	0.228[a]
Cigarette smoking	0.468[a]	0.197[b]	0.090	0.274[a]
High total cholesterol	−0.060	−0.114	0.096	−0.097
Glucose intolerance	0.108	0.115	0.054	0.156[b]
High relative weight	0.266[b]	0.009	0.157	0.195[b]
High hematocrit	0.324[b]	0.105	0.051	−0.098

[a] $p < .001$.

[b] $p < .05$.

[c] Confirmed by electrocardiography.

[d] $p < .01$.

SOURCE: Phillip A. Wolf: In Barnett HJM, et al (eds): *Stroke: Pathophysiology, Diagnosis, and Management.* Churchill-Livingstone Publishers, Oxford, England, 1992, Table 1-2. Reprinted with permission.

younger age, more often have diabetes, and have lacunar type strokes more often. Asians in Japan, China, Korea, and Thailand have a low rate of coronary heart disease but an increased prevalence of stroke.[48] The mortality due to stroke relative to coronary heart disease (CHD) does appear to be falling in Japanese in Hawaii and San Francisco as well as in Japan.[18,49] This may reflect the trend toward a lower salt but higher animal fat diet. It is postulated that this would be accompanied by a fall in hypertension, but an increase in atherosclerosis.[49] Asians also have a higher prevalence of intracranial rather than extracranial atherosclerosis when compared with Western populations.[50]

The link between oral contraceptives and stroke appears to be related to the increased amounts of estrogen in earlier formulations and was most obvious in women who smoked.[51,52] The U-shaped relationship between alcohol consumption and cerebrovascular disease has not been as convincingly demonstrated as it has for coronary heart disease, but it appears that low or moderate consumption offers some protection from stroke while heavy use is associated with an increase in ischemic and hemorrhagic stroke.[53,54]

Geographic variations in stroke rate have been documented in the United States since at least 1940. An ill-defined area of high stroke mortality in the southeastern United States has been called the "stroke belt," but underlying causes remain to be identified.[55–60]

An elevation in blood lipids is associated with atherosclerosis and coronary heart disease. Although the Framingham data did not identify cholesterol as an independent risk factor for stroke, recent clinical trials do. A low total serum cholesterol is associated with increased intracerebral hemorrhage, while at elevated levels an increase in ABI is noted.[49,61] Recent trials provide data indicating that a reduction in LDL cholesterol using hydroxy-methyl-glutaryl CoA antagonists (HMG CoA antagonists or "statins") reverses progression of carotid atherosclerosis and reduces the stroke rate.[62,63] The benefit in stroke reduction remains to be substantiated in trials looking primarily at stroke prevention.

Classification

The syndrome of stroke has many underlying causes. About 85 percent of stroke is ischemic and 15 percent hemorrhagic.[1] Aneurysm and arterial venous malformation as specific causes of hemorrhage will be discussed in another chapter. Ischemic stroke has been subclassified by suspected causation based on clinical and diagnostic data in a number of stroke data banks. Because of differences in methodology, geographic location, improved or new diagnostic tests, and possibly due to a shift in causation over time, it is difficult to compare these different data banks. Despite thorough investigation, stroke causality remains undetermined about 30 percent of the time.[64] During the past 60 years, a trend has been seen toward describing fewer strokes as due to atherosclerosis and toward reporting more as embolic. If embolus from an arterial source is included in the definition of "atherothrombotic" stroke, or ABI, then this likely represents the largest proportion of ischemic stroke at about 40 percent. Cardioembolic stroke represents 15 to 20 percent of stroke, and lacunar stroke another 20 to 25 percent. About 5 percent of stroke is due to a large category of unusual causes including vasculopathies, prothrombotic states, drugs, and myriad rare causes. Depending on the study, how stringent the inclusion criteria are, and how an uncertain diagnosis is categorized, different stroke causes have received emphasis depending on the author.[5,64–70]

Stroke is also classified into a number of time-dependent syndromes. *Transient ischemic attacks* (TIAs) have traditionally been defined as temporary neurologic deficits of sudden onset that resolve within 24 h. Most TIAs last 5 to 15 min, and if symptoms last more than an hour, they are unlikely to resolve by 24 h, and may be associated with evidence of territory appropriate infarction on MRI. The occurrence of TIA is important in identifying a person at high risk for stroke, with 5 percent suffering stroke within several weeks, 12 percent in the first year, and 30 percent at 5 years.[71–73] The risk of stroke goes up significantly to 25 percent over 2 years if a high-grade carotid stenosis is identified.[74] *Amaurosis fugax* or *transient monocular blindness* (TMB) can be thought of as a TIA affecting the retina, and may be caused by emboli from the internal carotid artery. TMB carries a better prognosis than hemispheric TIAs.[73] *Reversible ischemic neurological deficit* (RIND) is a term that has been used to describe a focal ischemic event lasting greater than 24 h, but improving within weeks. For practical purposes, a RIND should be treated the same as a completed stroke. A *progressing stroke* or *stroke in evolution* describes the development of new neurologic deficits usually within 24 h of an initial stroke.[75] It implies extension of an ischemic area to involve adjacent areas of the brain, and should be distinguished from worsening of an existing deficit. Worsening may occur when hemispheric edema develops, usually between 48 to 96 h after stroke onset, but also may be secondary to hypoxia or metabolic disturbances. Progression of stroke is more common in the vertebrobasilar system where it is seen about 40 percent of the time.[76] When stroke symptoms do progress, clinicians are more apt to consider anticoagulation with heparin on the grounds that this could be due to propagation of a thrombus, but any benefit remains unproven. The progression of stroke symptoms does introduce some diagnostic uncertainty, and

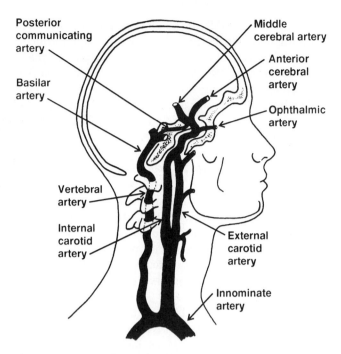

Figure 14-2 Cervical carotid and vertebral arteries.

other processes like hemorrhagic conversion, intracerebral or subdural hematoma, or neoplasia should be considered. A *completed stroke* consists of a stable neurologic deficit present for more than 24 h. The clinical course is less predictable the earlier it is after the onset of an ischemic deficit.

ANATOMY

The clinical stroke syndrome is dependent upon both the pathophysiologic process and the anatomic location of involvement. It is important therefore to review the vascular anatomy. The blood supply to the brain arises from four extracerebral or cervical blood vessels (Figs. 14-2, 14-3)—the paired internal carotid and vertebral arteries. The internal carotid artery has no branches until it enters the skull base. It has been divided into the extracranial, petrosal, cavernous, and supraclinoid portions for the purposes of discussion. There are minor branches within the petrosal and cavernous portions, but the first major branch is the ophthalmic artery with its takeoff in the supraclinoid portion. The internal carotid artery (ICA) then gives off the posterior communicating artery, which supplies the anterior and medial thalamus before joining the posterior cerebral artery. The anterior choroidal artery leaves the ICA just distal to the posterior communicating artery (PCoA) to supply the temporal horn, hippocampus, the posterior limb of the internal capsule, and the basal ganglia. The ICA then bifurcates into the anterior cerebral artery (ACA) and middle cerebral

artery (MCA). The ACA supplies the medial hemisphere back to the parietal lobe. The middle cerebral artery supplies the large lateral convexity of the hemisphere as well as deep white matter and portions of the basal ganglia. Taken together the above circulation is often discussed as the *anterior circulation*. The *posterior circulation* is supplied by the other major cervical vessels: the vertebral arteries, which fuse at the level of the pontomedullary junction to form the single, larger, basilar artery. Because of a variety of changes that occur during fetal development, numerous variations may occur in the vertebrobasilar system. The posterior inferior cerebellar artery usually arises from the intradural segment of the vertebral artery, and variably supplies the lateral medulla and the majority of the inferior cerebellum. The remainder of the cerebellum is supplied by branches usually arising from the basilar artery, the anterior inferior cerebellar artery, and superior cerebellar arteries. In addition to those arteries, the basilar artery supplies critical small branches to the brainstem: the median arteries, and short and long lateral circumferential arteries. Branches are also given to the lateral midbrain before the basilar artery divides into the paired posterior cerebral arteries. The posterior cerebral arteries supply the medial portion of the occipital lobes and give branches to the lateral thalamus. The circle of Willis is an important anastomotic pathway providing for side-to-side and anterior-to-posterior collateral flow (Fig. 14-3). The extracranial blood supply can also provide anastomosis via small leptomeningeal branches.[77]

PATHOPHYSIOLOGY

Occlusion of the major cerebral arteries or their branches can occur because of atherosclerosis, embolization, trauma, or vascular or hematologic disorders. The collateral blood supply becomes increasingly compromised with age in general and if inadequate, focal tissue ischemia may occur. The subsequent cellular events are similar regardless of the precipitating cause. In the case of diffuse hypoxic or ischemic insults as seen with cardiac arrest, a time-dependent pattern of injury occurs which is related to the selective vulnerability of neuronal populations. Thus, laminar necrosis occurs in layers 3, 5, and 6 of the cortex, and necrosis of hippocampal CA-1 and medium-sized striatal neurons as well as cerebellar Purkinje cells is observed.[78] This selective injury may be related to the increased levels of the excitotoxic neurotransmitters glutamate and aspartate in these areas.[79–81] When focal cerebral perfusion fails, metabolic and encephalographic activity stops within 10 s. If the circulation is restored, there is complete recovery of function. If focal ischemia continues, neuronal injury occurs within minutes, and

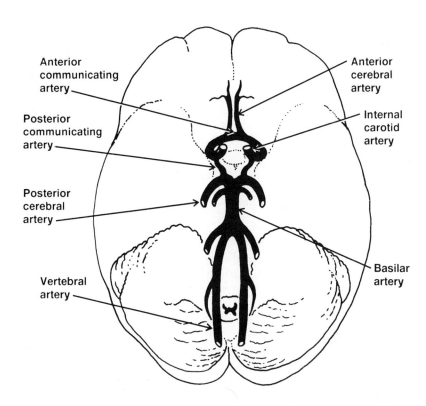

Figure 14-3   Circle of Willis.

increasing numbers of neurons are lost in a time-dependent manner. Focal ischemia lasting more than one hour leads to infarction of neurons, endothelial cells, and glial cells alike within a central core area.[82] The surrounding area, called the *ischemic penumbra*, is defined by hypoperfusion, hypometabolism, and electrical silence on EEG.[83] The neurons are structurally intact and potentially salvageable if perfusion is restored within 6 to 8 h.[84] When regional cerebral blood flow remains inadequate, potentially viable neurons cease production of neurotransmitters, and begin to leak potassium. With continuing ischemia, anaerobic glycolysis produces lactic acidosis and ATP is depleted, leading to energy failure and loss of the sodium/potassium pump. As extracellular potassium accumulates, voltage-dependent calcium channels depolarize. Increased intracellular calcium activity leads to the release of excitatory neurotransmitters like glutamate and aspartate which are felt to be the most important as their levels are increased in the neurons susceptible to ischemic damage and in the extracellular space in ischemic areas.[85,86] The glutamate receptor *N*-methyl-D-aspartate (NMDA) and quisqualate are activated, contributing to a massive influx of calcium which overwhelms mitochondrial oxidative phosphorylation and initiates proteolysis. Calcium influx also activates membrane phospholipases leading to the release of arachidonic acid and other fatty acids. Arachidonic acid is metabolized to the endoperoxides prostaglandin G_2 and prostaglandin H_2 and further to thromboxane A_2, all of which act as platelet aggregators. Endoperoxides also act as free-radical donors, causing further membrane damage. Thus, it appears that the massive influx of calcium heralds terminal events that are probably irreversible.

ATHEROSCLEROSIS

There are a wide variety of vascular and hematologic factors that predispose to focal cerebral ischemia (Tables 14-2, 14-3). By far the most important pathologic process leading to stroke is atherosclerosis either via primary obstruction to flow or from embolization of adherent material. Atherosclerosis is also one underlying cause of cardiac embolic disease. Large-artery atherosclerosis is often discussed separately from small-artery disease because of differences between their

TABLE 14-2
Vascular Causes of Cerebral Ischemia

Atherosclerosis	Drugs
Trauma	Radiation
Aneurysm	Connective tissue diseases
Malformation	(Marfan's, Ehlers-Danlos,
Dissection	pseudoxanthoma elasticum)
Infectious or granulomatous arteritis	Mitochondrial diseases
	Cerebral amyloid angiopathy
Immune-mediated arteritis	

TABLE 14-3
Hematologic Contributors to Ischemia

Polycythemia	Protein C or S deficiency
Thrombocytosis	Homocystinuria
Platelet hyperaggregability	Dysfibrinogenemia
Disseminated intravascular coagulation	Paraproteinemias
Thrombotic thrombocytopenic purpura	Recent infection
	Drugs
Antiphospholipid antibodies	Paraneoplastic
Antithrombin III deficiency	Pregnancy

pathologic appearances. This suggests a difference in pathogenic mechanisms, but the two processes share some common risk factors including hypertension, diabetes, and aging.

LARGE VESSEL ATHEROSCLEROSIS

Large vessel atherosclerosis is a chronic, progressive process beginning with fatty streaks on the intimal surface that may appear as early as childhood. These deposits consist of lipid-laden macrophages and smooth muscle cells. Over years fatty streaks progress, and localized areas of fibrous plaque develop. This is likely in response to endothelial injuries which include mechanical sheer forces, cigarette smoke, hyperlipidemia, and less often elevated homocysteine and radiation. There is increasing evidence that oxidized low-density lipoprotein (LDL) plays an important role in promoting atherogenesis, and possibly in propagating instability in atheroma.[87] The fibrous plaques that develop consist of altered smooth muscle cells, foam cells, lymphocytes, lipid pools, and connective tissue, and are endothelium-lined. Plaques may become complicated by central areas of necrosis, hemorrhage, calcification, and disruption of the endothelium. In response to plaque development, large arteries enlarge and maintain their lumen to some extent until the disease becomes advanced. Arterial obstruction can occur from enlarged atheroma, but the onset of symptoms is often associated with plaque destabilization. Thrombosis may be associated with an underlying plaque ulceration, and can lead to occlusion or embolization of platelet-fibrin aggregates or, more rarely, cholesterol crystals.[88] Secondary intraplaque hemorrhage, the dissection of luminal blood into plaque after endothelial disruption, can lead to increased stenosis, thrombosis, or embolization and the production of symptoms. Primary intraplaque hemorrhage occurs, but its relative importance is not known. Recent autopsy studies suggest that luminal disruption occurs frequently in association with carotid thrombosis.[89,90] The first 2 cm of the internal carotid artery above the carotid bifurcation bears the brunt of atherosclerotic disease and is the most frequent site of thrombosis.[92] The proximal portion of the vertebral arteries is also commonly affected, followed in frequency by the basilar artery, and then disease of other proximal intracranial arteries. There are racial and geographic differences in the sites of atherosclerosis, with African-Americans and Asians having more intracranial disease than white patients of European descent.[90,92]

SMALL VESSEL DISEASE

Small arteries in the brain less than 2 mm in diameter exhibit a different spectrum of pathologic change when compared with large vessels. *Arteriolosclerosis* is a term used to describe a degenerative process in blood vessels of 50 μm or less diameter which lack an internal elastic lamina. These vessels are adversely affected by hypertension, diabetes mellitus, and aging. Smooth muscle fibers become disorganized, and are replaced with concentrically arranged collagen. When associated with lipid deposition, this has been called *lipohyalinosis*.[93] *Fibrinoid necrosis* describes degenerating smooth muscle cells and eosinophilic deposits in the tunica media of perforating arterioles. These degenerative processes can lead to vessel occlusion and a small area of infarction which is called a *lacunar infarct*. Arteriolosclerosis may also lead to formation of microaneurysms which were first implicated in intracerebral hemorrhage by Charcot and Bouchard.[91] Small cerebral blood vessels between 100 μm and 400 μm in diameter may also develop focal deposits of lipid-laden foam cells and fibroblasts similar to large-vessel atheroma and so labeled *microatheroma*. Larger lacunar infarcts are increasingly attributed to microatheroma. Microembolism and hemodynamic insufficiency are other postulated but largely unconfirmed mechanisms of lacunar infarction.[94]

ANGIOPATHY

Nonatherosclerotic disease of blood vessels may also lead to stroke. Aneurysms and vascular malformations are both occasionally associated with ischemic infarcts via thromboembolism. Cerebral vasculitis is a rare cause of stroke. It should be suspected in atypical presentations of stroke, and is usually accompanied by clinical and laboratory signs of systemic inflammatory disease.

Temporal arteritis is a systemic inflammatory disease of unknown causation affecting medium and large elastic arteries. Also known as giant cell arteritis, it is characterized by inflammatory infiltration of the tunica media and the variable presence of multinucleated giant cells within granulomas. Intimal fibrosis and proliferation lead to stenosis and thrombosis. Visual loss occurs when posterior ciliary arteries are occluded, producing anterior ischemic optic neuropathy (AION). The central retinal artery is less often involved. Visual loss is often sudden and is usually monocular. Other common symptoms include focal headache, scalp or temporal tenderness, jaw claudication, polymyalgia rheumatica or other constitutional symptoms, and neuropsychiatric symptoms including confusion or depression. Stroke is uncommon, and most often occurs in the vertebrobasilar system after thrombotic occlusion. Carotid occlusion also occurs, but intracranial arteries are rarely involved, possibly because they lack an organized elastic lamina.[95] Patients are usually over 50 years old, and women have a threefold greater incidence.[96] The erythrocyte sedimentation rate is usually markedly elevated, and there is often a mild normochromic or hypochromic anemia. The diagnosis may be confirmed with temporal artery biopsy, but because involvement is segmental, multiple sections should be made; a negative biopsy does not exclude the diagnosis. Prompt treatment with prednisone 40 mg to 60 mg per day is recommended when the disease is suspected; this will not alter a biopsy obtained within the next week.[97]

Takayasu's arteritis or idiopathic aortitis is similar to temporal arteritis but most often reported in Asia, usually affecting young women. The aorta and its main branches are involved, and stroke has occurred in patients with advanced disease. Constitutional symptoms and an elevated sedimentation rate are common. Treatment is with immunosuppression and reconstructive surgery.[96,98]

Isolated granulomatous angiitis of the central nervous system is distinct from giant cell arteritis, being restricted to the cerebral circulation. An infiltration of lymphocytes, and granulomas with multinucleated giant cells, may involve any portion of the vessel wall. Any cerebral or spinal vessel can be affected, and leptomeningeal arteries are often said to be involved. This rare disorder has ill-defined clinical features, but usually stroke or brain tumor is the initial consideration. Systemic symptoms are uncommon. There are no clear diagnostic criteria, and the diagnosis is most often made after excluding other possibilities, by brain and leptomeningeal biopsy, or at autopsy.[96]

Polyarteritis nodosa is another systemic vasculitis that may affect cerebral blood vessels, but the peripheral nervous system is usually affected first. Medium and small arteries are focally affected by inflammation and necrosis, and visceral angiography may reveal microaneurysms. The diagnosis is supported by sural nerve biopsy, which may reveal a necrotizing vasculitis, and by positive serologic tests for hepatitis B antigen and antineutrophil cytoplasmic antigen (ANCA). Patients may report headache, confusion, or disturbance of mood and may suffer focal or generalized seizures. Stroke is an unusual late complication. Patients treated with immunosuppression may have significant improvement.[94]

Wegener's granulomatosis is a systemic vasculitis with prominent pulmonary and renal involvement. The most common neurologic manifestation is cranial nerve palsy from direct extension of disease from the upper respiratory tract. CNS vasculitis has been reported but stroke is increasingly rare with the institution of cytotoxic and immunosuppressive therapy. Testing for ANCA is sensitive and fairly specific for Wegener's granulomatosis.[96]

INFECTIONS

Any agent producing inflammation of the meninges could theoretically result in infarction. Basilar meningitis, usually caused by tuberculosis, cryptococcosis, or histoplasmosis, may cause inflammation of the proximal middle cerebral artery and its penetrating vessels. This has been labeled *Heubner's arteritis.* Syphilitic arteritis can lead to stroke in addition to the meningovascular symptoms of headache, mental status change, and cranial neuropathy.[99] Herpes ophthalmicus is associated with an intense vasculitis of the intracranial internal carotid artery, and stroke usually occurs weeks after the cutaneous eruption. Angiography may demonstrate segmental narrowing or occlusion, and necropsy reveals a necrotizing vasculitis with thrombosis. Treatment includes acyclovir and immunosuppression and possibly anticoagulation.[100]

DRUGS

Drug abuse is linked to stroke by direct and indirect mechanisms. Intravenous drug abusers may develop bacterial endocarditis with septic emboli or mycotic aneurysm formation. Embolization of talc or starch contaminants may directly produce infarct, or lead to secondary vasculitis and thrombotic infarcts. Oral and IV amphetamine abuse can produce a necrotizing vasculitis and stroke, and amphetamines, cocaine, and phencyclidine can all produce intracranial hemorrhage likely via hypertensive and vasospastic mechanisms.[101]

CEREBRAL AMYLOID ANGIOPATHY

Cerebral amyloid angiopathy (CAA), or congophilic angiopathy, is a disease of microvessels that is associated with lobar hemorrhages in elderly patients, patients with Alzheimer's disease, or younger patients with Down's syndrome, or it presents as one of the familial forms of the disease. As our elderly population becomes larger, and with better control of hypertension, CAA is becoming an increasingly important cause of intracerebral hemorrhage.[102] Pathologically, amyloid protein is found deposited in the media and adventitia of small blood vessels. This eosinophilic hyalin is demonstrated by birefringence on Congo red stain. Two amyloid proteins have been identified in these deposits: cystatin C, which was seen in the hereditary Icelandic type, and a β protein, which is commonly present in senile plaques of Alzheimer's dementia, in Down's syndrome, and in asymptomatic elderly people.[103] The supposed mechanism of hemorrhage is weakening of the vessel wall, possibly with microaneurysmal formation or fibrinoid necrosis.[104] Hemorrhages are lobar, frontal, parietal, or occipital, and involve cortex or subcortical white matter and rarely the deep gray nuclei or cerebellum, and may be multiple. CAA may be associated with 20 percent of nontraumatic hemorrhages in patients older than 70. As many as 50 percent of patients with CAA have clinical evidence of dementia, and 50 percent have Alzheimer's disease pathologically. These patients are at increased risk of hemorrhage during brain surgery, and may be at increased risk from fibrinolytic or anticoagulant therapy. Autosomal dominant forms of the disease are associated with hemorrhage in the third and fourth decade in the Icelandic and Dutch types, respectively.[102]

HEMATOLOGIC CAUSES OF STROKE

An increasing number of hematologic disorders have been implicated in ischemic stroke. Unfortunately, knowledge in the field is incomplete and rapidly evolving, and therefore it is difficult to state with certainty the relative importance of these disorders as a cause of stroke or to recommend rational screening strategies. Hematologic disorders are most often considered in young stroke victims in whom no obvious cause of stroke is apparent, and for this very reason may be underrepresented as contributing causes of stroke in reports on older patients with known cerebrovascular disease. Stroke has been attributed to hematologic disorders about 1 percent of the time overall, and in about 4 to 6 percent of young patients, but these percentages may increase as more complete laboratory screening becomes utilized in investigational settings.[106-108] The discussion of the numerous causes of procoagulable states as listed in Table 14-3 is beyond the scope of this chapter. Available data suggest that specialized screening should be reserved for patients who are less than 50 years of age without an obvious cause for their stroke, those with a personal or a family history of thrombosis, or patients with abnormalities on screening tests including prothrombin time, partial thromboplastin time, platelet count, or hemoglobin and hematocrit. In these select patients, attempts should be made to tailor specialized tests toward identifying disorders suspected on clinical grounds, perhaps with the input

TABLE 14-4
Special Laboratory Studies in Stroke of Unknown Cause[a]

Antithrombin III functional assay	Homocysteine levels
Protein C and S	Hemoglobin electrophoresis for sickle cell disease
Antiphospholipid antibodies, lupus anticoagulant	Sedimentation rate
	ANA

[a] Use as indicated in the text.

of a hematologist or specialist in vascular diseases. Especially when stroke reoccurs without an evident cause, a specialist may feel pressed to pursue special laboratory screening as outlined in Table 14-4. Further clinical studies should be designed to identify the relative importance of these disorders, and to delineate factors that could guide rational laboratory screening.

CARDIAC DISEASE

Emboli to the brain are presumed to arise from a wide variety of sources, including large cerebral vessels, the carotid arteries, aortic arch, or "paradoxically" from the venous system when right-to-left shunting is possible in the heart. *Cardiogenic brain embolism* refers specifically to emboli arising from intracardiac disease, and represents 15 to 20 percent of all ischemic stroke.[5,64-70] A detailed review of cardiac pathology is beyond the scope of this chapter, but the common causes of emboli are presented in Fig. 14-4. Findings associated with cardiogenic embolism are listed in Table 14-5. Although a cardiogenic brain embolism can be the first symptom of heart disease, most often the underlying disorder is evident prior to embolism. This provides the clinician with an opportunity to intervene with effective preventive therapy in many instances.

Certain clinical characteristics are suggestive of a brain embolus. These include a sudden onset of maximal symptoms in an awake patient and the history of cardiac disease or previous systemic embolus. Other features not as specific include headache, seizure, and early symptomatic improvement. Imaging studies most often reveal a large cortical infarct in the MCA or PCA territories. These are most likely to develop hemorrhage after the embolus propagates distally and injured vessels are reperfused.[108,109] Multiple infarcts also suggest cardiogenic embolism, and such an embolus may produce a "cord sign" or "hyperdense MCA" from indwelling embolic material. On angiography performed early, an occluded vessel without other evidence of disease suggests embolus, and serial studies often reveal spontaneous recanalization.

Further cardiac evaluation should be pursued in young patients who are less likely to have atheroscle-

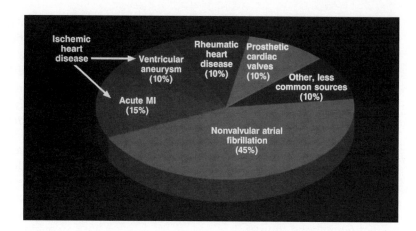

Figure 14-4 Sources of cardiogenic embolism. (Courtesy of R. G. Hart.[65])

TABLE 14-5
Findings Associated with Cardiogenic Embolism

Valvular Diseases
  Rheumatic mitral stenosis
  Prosthetic valves
  Calcific aortic stenosis
  Mitral annulus calcification
  Nonbacterial thrombotic (marantic) endocarditis (associated with malignancy, diffuse intravascular coagulation, antiphospholipid antibodies, and other prothrombotic states)
  Myxomatous mitral valvulopathy with prolapse
  Infective endocarditis
  Inflammatory valvulitis: Libman-Sacks endocarditis, Behçet's disease, syphilis

Myocardial Ischemia with Ventricular Thrombi
  Acute myocardial infarction
  Left ventricular akinesis/aneurysm

Arrhythmias with Atrial Thrombi
  Atrial fibrillation
  Sick sinus syndrome

Nonischemic Dilating Cardiomyopathies

Congenital Heart Disease

Intracardiac Thrombi Related to Prothrombotic States
  Polycystic disease
  Myeloproliferative disorders and thrombocythemia
  Malignancy
  Antiphospholipid antibodies

Cardiac Tumors
  Primary
  Metastatic

Paradoxical Emboli
  Atrial septal defects
  Patent foramen ovale
  Ventricular septal defects
  Pulmonary arteriovenous fistulas

Miscellaneous Sources
  Atrial septal aneurysms
  Postcardiac catheterization and valvuloplasty

SOURCE: Modified from R. G. Hart.[65]

rotic disease, or in older patients who have no obvious source of infarct, or in whom cardiac disease is suggested by history, physical exam, or on screening chest x-ray and electrocardiogram. Echocardiography can provide valuable information in the setting of known cardiac dysfunction. Transesophageal echocardiography (TEE) offers significant technical advantages, including improved resolution and better visualization of the left atrial appendage, mitral valve, and atrial septum. Interest in the aortic arch as a source of embolus has increased since the advent of TEE and its ability to image the arch.[110,111] Further studies should provide information on the utility of TEE in identifying and predicting embolic sources.

Atrial fibrillation deserves special mention as the most common cause of cardiogenic brain embolism. This relatively common disorder affects roughly two million Americans, and its prevalence increases with advancing age.[112] The presence of atrial fibrillation confers a sixfold increase in stroke risk.[113] Autopsy data provide objective evidence that left atrial thrombus is the source of embolic material in the setting of atrial fibrillation.[114] In the past five years, data have become available from five randomized trials investigating the primary prevention of stroke in atrial fibrillation using warfarin.[115–119] Stroke was reduced 68 percent overall in patients randomized to warfarin, and the major bleeding risk was low at about 1 percent in these selected patients who had close follow-up using international normalized ratios (INR) to monitor their anticoagulation. "High-risk" variables were identified and include advancing age, hypertension, previous stroke or TIA, diabetes, and recent heart failure.[35,36] Patients without "high-risk" variables are often referred to as "lone atrial fibrillators" and have about a 1 percent per year risk of stroke compared with greater than 5 percent when risk factors are present.[135] Based on the available data, panels of experts have recommended long-term anticoagulation for patients with atrial fibrillation unless there are contraindications to warfarin, or the patient is under 60 with no "high-risk" variables.[37,113] The risk of stroke in chronic atrial fibrillation now appears to be the same as that for paroxysmal atrial fibrillation.[36,112] Warfarin therapy should be closely monitored with monthly INR determinations with a target INR of 2.0 to 3.0. Patients of advanced age, with previous stroke or hypertension, are at increased risk for intracerebral hemorrhage.[120–123] Because the risk of hemorrhage probably increases with the intensity of anticoagulation, it may be prudent to lower the target INR to 1.5 to 2.5 in these higher-risk patients.[123,124] Pooled data from the atrial fibrillation investigators suggest a 20 percent reduction in stroke in patients with atrial fibrillation taking 325 mg of aspirin per day.[36] Although less effective than warfarin, aspirin is a reasonable alternative in patients with contraindications to warfarin, or in patients with "lone atrial fibrillation." Ongoing studies should more clearly define the role of aspirin, low-dose warfarin, or combinations of the two for atrial fibrillation.

Diagnosis

The diagnosis of cerebrovascular disorders is highly dependent on obtaining a clear history and confirming localization by physical examination (see Table 14-6). The specific underlying cause should be sought especially when the broad differential of ischemic stroke is considered. Toward this goal, the patient's past history and risk factors become important. The patient's ability to provide the history may be significantly impaired by dysarthria, aphasia, symptoms related to the "neglect syndrome," or alterations in consciousness. In those cases, witnesses and family members should be interviewed so that important diagnostic clues are not missed. Effort should be made to time the onset of symptoms and to determine whether symptoms are progressing, fluctuating, or improving. The constellation of symptoms should be defined, and together with physical findings will allow anatomic definition of the clinical syndrome, as discussed later. The activity level of the patient at onset is important, as, in general, thrombosis is associated with rest and embolus with physical activity.[125] Associated symptoms may be diagnostically important and include symptoms of myocardial ischemia or arrhythmia, headache, seizure, or coma.

Myocardial ischemia may occur in up to 11 percent of patients presenting with acute stroke, and stroke is a complication of MI approximately 1 percent of the time.[126,127] Headache is more suggestive of hemorrhage and may be the most prominent symptom of subarachnoid hemorrhage.[128,129] Headache is present in a sizable minority of ischemic stroke patients and is more often reported with embolus or large-vessel thrombosis.[129–132] Seizures are rare in acute ischemic stroke, occurring in about 5 percent of patients. They are slightly more common after intracerebral hemorrhage.[5] Coma is related to processes affecting either both hemispheres or the reticular activating system in the brainstem. For that reason, it is unusual in ischemic stroke unless the basilar artery is occluded. Some presentations are incompatible with the diagnosis of stroke, and some effort should be made toward excluding hysteria, epilepsy, metabolic derangement, infection, and neoplasm. Symptoms unlikely to represent focal ischemia are included in Table 14-7. Uncertainty exists in relating focal ischemia to symptoms occurring in isolation, such as vertigo, dysarthria, dysphagia, or diplopia alone.

The physical exam is important in aiding in localiza-

TABLE 14-6
Symptoms of Focal Brain Ischemia

Carotid System	Vertebrobasilar System	Either
Unilateral weakness or clumsiness	Bilateral	
Unilateral sensory disturbance	Bilateral	
Asphasia or dysarthria	Dysarthria/dysphagia	Dysarthria if alone
Monocular visual loss	Homonymous hemianopia	Homonymous hemianopia alone
	Vertigo, diplopia, ataxia (usually combined with other symptoms)	

tion of cerebrovascular disease and may provide clues regarding causation. The specific implications of certain physical findings are beyond the scope of this chapter, but specific clinical pictures will be covered as part of the clinical syndromes discussion below. The neurovascular examination is a specialized exam that extends beyond the complete neurologic exam. It should include blood pressure in both arms, with seated versus standing pressures. Peripheral and cerebral pulses are assessed by palpation and auscultation. A detailed ophthalmologic exam should include visual field testing and careful examination of the retina for evidence of vascular disease. Examination of the skin can reveal evidence of congenital disorders, vasculitis, and connective tissue disease. Such a diligent exam becomes increasingly important in cases of diagnostic uncertainty.

DIAGNOSTIC TESTS

A rational and time-saving approach is most important for the patient presenting with the acute onset of symptoms of cerebrovascular disease. Panels of experts have now published guidelines for the emergent evaluation of TIA and stroke.[133,134] The goal is to accurately predict the cause of cerebrovascular disease so that appropriate therapy can be initiated as early as possible. A stepwise evaluation is outlined in Table 14-8. The diagnostic evaluation must be tailored to each clinical presentation, but these guidelines provide a logical, general scheme.

CT is often the study of choice for acute presenta-

tions. It is faster and more easily tolerated by the patient and is sensitive for hemorrhage. MRI gives additional information, especially when the posterior fossa is involved, but may not be more sensitive than CT in the first 24 h.[135] After 24 h, MRI has superiority in providing lesion detail and is more sensitive than CT.[136] Magnetic resonance angiography (MRA) is becoming increasingly popular as a screening test for carotid stenosis or dissection, but at present conventional angiography remains the "gold standard." Duplex imaging of the carotid bifurcation is reliable in assessing moderate (greater than 40 percent) to severe stenosis, but may be unreliable in distinguishing a high-grade stenosis from an occlusion. "B mode" imaging with ultrasound has been unreliable in predicting ulceration of carotid plaque.[137] Transthoracic and transesophageal echocardiography can provide important information in the setting of embolic disease, but they are usually reserved for patients with known or suspected cardiac disease, or for young patients who have a higher likelihood of cardiogenic brain embolus. Likewise, Holter monitoring is reserved for patients in whom cardiac dysrhythmia is suspected clinically or by screening ECG. Lumbar puncture is indicated when subarach-

TABLE 14-7
Symptoms Unlikely to Represent Focal Brain Ischemia

Tonic/clonic activity	Scintillating scotoma
Loss of consciousness	Dizziness or giddiness alone
Incontinence	
Sensory march	Confusion or amnesia alone
	Extremity pain

TABLE 14-8
Stepwise Evaluation of Stroke

Step 1 (always)	CBC, platelet count, ESR, PT/PTT VDRL, chemistry profile, lipid profile Urinalysis, Hemoccult ECG CT of the brain
Step II (consider)	Carotid ultrasound Cardiac testing if clinically indicated
Step III (individualize)	MR imaging study MRA or conventional angiography Special coagulation studies Transesophageal echocardiography Lumbar puncture

SOURCE: Modified from R. G. Hart.[65]

noid hemorrhage is suspected clinically, even if the CT appears normal. Lumbar puncture is also indicated when there is evidence of infection or vasculitis. Electroencephalography (EEG) may demonstrate focal abnormalities after acute stroke, but is not a part of the routine diagnostic workup. When the clinical history or lack of diagnostic findings suggests weakness based on a postictal or Todd's paresis from seizure, the EEG contributes supportive information.

Clinical Stroke Syndromes

The definition of ischemic syndromes based on the time course of symptoms has been covered in the section on classification. In addition to the time course, the patient's symptoms and signs aid in predicting the arterial territory involved and the possible mechanism of ischemia.

INTERNAL CAROTID ARTERY SYNDROME

Occlusion of the internal carotid artery (ICA) may occur without symptoms, but more often there are premonitory TIAs or episodes of transient monocular blindness (TMB). The area of infarction after occlusion varies considerably depending on the availability of collateral blood supply. Most often ICA occlusion results in a clinical picture resembling middle cerebral artery (MCA) territory infarction, but the anterior cerebral artery (ACA) territory and less often posterior cerebral artery (PCA) territory may be involved with associated symptoms as described below. Such massive infarctions are often associated with significant brain edema and obtundation of the patient due to the mass effect on the contralateral hemisphere.[125] Infarction in the setting of ICA atherosclerosis may also be due to embolization. This "artery-to-artery" embolization of material may affect individual arterial branches, usually in the MCA territory.

MIDDLE CEREBRAL ARTERY SYNDROME

The picture seen with MCA occlusion is the most common of stroke syndromes. Involvement of motor and sensory cortex near the central sulcus leads to contralateral numbness and weakness of the face, arm, and hand. The optic radiation is affected with inferior division involvement, producing a contralateral homonymous hemianopia. With total MCA occlusion in the dominant hemisphere, global aphasia is observed, but with inferior division occlusion alone, a Wernicke's or receptive aphasia occurs. Ischemia in the territory of the frontal branches produces a Broca's aphasia or expressive aphasia. A total MCA occlusion is often accompanied by gaze deviation toward the side of the lesion and decreased alertness.[125]

ANTERIOR CEREBRAL ARTERY SYNDROME

Anterior cerebral artery occlusion produces variable infarction of the medial frontal and parietal lobes back to the posterior one-fifth of the corpus callosum. The classic syndrome includes contralateral leg and foot weakness with a lesser degree of arm and shoulder weakness and sparing of the face. Sensory loss may be present in this same distribution. When both ACA territories are infarcted, the patient is paraplegic, incontinent of urine, and exhibits abulia or akinetic mutism.[138] Arm and face weakness in the presence of an ACA occlusion is seen with involvement of Heubner's artery supplying the anterior caudate, putamen, and internal capsule. This may also be due to involvement of other deep penetrating branches from the ACA.[139]

POSTERIOR CEREBRAL SYMPTOMS

The two posterior cerebral arteries most often arise from the basilar artery, but about 25 percent of the time, one PCA may arise from a large posterior communicating artery, a finding termed *persistent fetal circulation*.[125] Cortical branch occlusion damages calcarine cortex and the optic radiation, leading to a contralateral homonymous hemianopia. Bilateral occipital infarction will produce blindness at times with the patient denying the visual impairment (cortical blindness or Anton's syndrome).[140] Visual illusions or unformed visual hallucinations may be associated. Prosopagnosia describes a patient's inability to recognize known faces despite being able to describe the face.[141] Palinopsia is also seen with an impaired visual field and consists of persistence of a visual image after an object is gone.[142] With infarction of the dominant parietooccipital lobe, alexia with or without agraphia and color anomia is described. When medial temporal ischemia occurs bilaterally, memory may be severely affected. Thalamic infarction may be followed by severe contralateral pain as numbness resolves, as described by Déjèrine and Roussy. Unilateral midbrain and subthalamic involvement may produce oculomotor paresis, contralateral hemiparesis, ataxia, or hemiballismus.

Basilar artery (BA) occlusion may cause tegmental infarction and coma. Variations of the PCA syndromes may be observed with thrombosis or embolus. The "top of the basilar syndrome," as described by Caplan, can cause altered consciousness, agitation, hallucinations, pupillary constriction and oculomotor abnormalities.[143] Crossed sensory signs or bilateral weakness should suggest brain stem ischemia. Other signs include nystagmus, ophthalmoplegia, ocular bobbing, and pinpoint pupils. Ischemia of vestibular nuclei produces vertigo, nausea, vomiting, and nystagmus. When superior or middle cerebellar peduncle ischemia occurs, ataxia develops.

VERTEBRAL ARTERY OCCLUSION

Vertebral artery occlusion may be asymptomatic, but can produce diverse symptoms referable to medullary ischemia or ischemia in the BA or PCA territories. A lateral medullary infarction produces the most common syndrome, as described by Wallenberg. This occurs most often with vertebral artery occlusion, but posterior inferior cerebellar artery occlusion is also described.[144] The syndrome is usually seen as an incomplete variant. The injured spinothalamic tract, and descending tract and nucleus of the trigeminal nerve cause altered pain and temperature sensation on the ipsilateral face and contralateral hemibody. Ischemia of the vestibular nuclei produces vertigo, oscillopsia, and nystagmus with accompanying nausea. Damaged connections with the cerebellum produce ipsilateral ataxia. The involved sympathetic tract leads to Horner's syndrome, and lower cranial nerve dysfunction produces dysphagia, hoarseness, decreased gag, hiccups, and loss of taste. Cerebellar infarction occurs with occlusion of the vertebral arteries or posterior inferior cerebellar artery. Medial infarcts produce prominent vertigo and nystagmus with gaze deviation to the side of the lesion. Hemispheral lesions produce more appendicular ataxia. Vomiting and dysarthria are common. With larger infarcts, edema may lead to secondary compression of the brain stem. Decompressive surgery may be lifesaving, with minimal permanent deficits.[145]

LACUNES

Lacunar syndromes develop secondary to occlusion of small penetrating arteries arising predominantly from the MCA, but also from other proximal arteries in the circle of Willis. Most common is the *pure motor hemiplegia*, usually caused by infarction of the posterior limb of the internal capsule and producing paralysis of the face, arm, and leg, without other signs. The onset may be stuttering prolonged over hours.[146] Lacunar infarction of the ventral posterior thalamus can produce a purse sensory stroke of the contralateral hemibody. Other syndromes include *clumsy hand dysarthria* and *homolateral ataxia and crural paresis,* both of which occur with lacunar infarction of the brain stem or posterior limb of the internal capsule.

TRANSIENT GLOBAL AMNESIA

Variably attributed to focal ischemia, migraine, and epilepsy, the term *transient global amnesia* was first in-

troduced by Fisher and Adams, but the syndrome was first described by Bender in 1956.[147,148] Criteria were proposed by Caplan and include witnessed amnesia without impaired consciousness, an absence of symptoms or signs of epilepsy, an absence of focal neurologic signs, no history of recent head trauma, and recovery within 24 h.[149] During the episode, cognitive function appears normal, with the exception of the inability to form new memory, and afterward the patient returns to normal but is amnestic for the event. TGA usually occurs in the elderly. Some groups have reported increased risk factors for stroke in these patients, but other groups could not confirm this.[149–153] Migraine and epilepsy are confirmed in a significant minority of cases. At present, it appears that TGA is a syndrome of unknown cause or causes in the majority of cases. The prognosis is good unless the episodes are atypically brief or recurrent, as these patients tended to develop epilepsy. Cerebrovascular disease is manifested at a rate lower than for TIA patients.[153]

Treatment

Because a central core of tissue is irreversibly damaged within minutes of ischemia, the most effective strategy for limiting the impact of stroke will always remain prevention. However, the experimental and clinical identification of a potentially salvageable ischemic penumbra has generated intense investigation of interventions aimed at limiting the damage from infarction once it has occurred. To date there is no acute therapy for stroke proven to alter outcome, but with a burgeoning literature on the subject, expectations are high that such a therapy will be available in the next decade. Early therapy in acute ischemic stroke is aimed at limiting ongoing risk of reinfarction, avoiding extension of infarction, and providing supportive medical care. Arterial hypertension is commonly seen after stroke, but usually blood pressure will return to acceptable levels without treatment. Because the area of ischemia loses autoregulatory function, lowering the blood pressure may cause hypoperfusion and extension of infarction. When the mean arterial pressure exceeds 160 mm of mercury, treatment should be initiated with easily controlled antihypertensive agents.[134] If consciousness is impaired, the airway should be protected and hypoxia should be avoided. Fever and hyperglycemia should be treated or avoided because of a potential for worsening outcome.[134,154] Large infarcts with significant edema, especially in younger patients, may require intervention to reduce intracranial pressure. This is discussed in another chapter. When seizures occur, anticonvulsants should be initiated, but prophylactic administration is not warranted. Swallowing should be assessed early so that aspiration can be prevented. Subcutaneous heparin or external compressive devices should be used in the immobile patient to avoid DVT.[155,156]

ANTIPLATELET THERAPY

Surprisingly, there is currently no information on the efficacy of aspirin or ticlopidine for acute therapy in stroke. An international trial is currently underway. Aspirin has proven effective for secondary prevention of stroke in patients with TIA and stroke and for patients with asymptomatic carotid disease. Risk is reduced overall by about 25 percent in studies of aspirin, in doses ranging from 75 mg to 1300 mg per day.[157] Aspirin is also important for its effect on reducing the significant risk of myocardial infarction in these patients. Because aspirin has a rapid onset of action and a low risk of complications, it is a reasonable therapeutic option immediately after stroke, when full anticoagulation is not indicated.[157] Ticlopidine, on the other hand, takes several days before its full antiplatelet effect is realized. Ticlopidine has been studied in the secondary prevention of stroke after TIA or strokes and appears to be slightly more effective than aspirin, with a 30 percent reduction in stroke risk. Its use is complicated by the drug's side effects, including GI upset, rash, and rarely, neutropenia. This necessitates frequent blood tests after initiation of therapy.[158–160]

Heparin has been used in the setting of acute stroke for decades, but indications for its use are still debated. Heparin did reduce the incidence of early recurrent embolus in a small randomized trial in patients with probable cardiogenic embolus, and no bleeding occurred in the 24 patients on heparin.[161] In other randomized trials of heparin with or without warfarin after completed stroke, no benefit could be proven.[162–167] Because of the risk of hemorrhage in large infarctions, it may be wise to wait several days before beginning heparin in those patients.[169]

Because it is postulated that progressing stroke symptoms may be due to a propagating thrombus, heparin has been offered as an intervention, and some studies suggest benefit.[163,170,171] Particularly when vertebrobasilar thrombosis is suspected, the benefit of heparin may outweigh the risks.[172] However, at least one study has documented a deleterious effect from heparin used in unselected patients with progressing symptoms.[173] Heparin has been advocated as immediate therapy when patients present with TIA until significant carotid stenosis or an embolic source is excluded. This is particularly true in TIA if the frequency is increasing, because of the association with critical carotid stenosis. Although there may be logic to this approach, no definitive data on safety or efficacy of heparin in

TABLE 14-9
Prevention Strategies for Stroke

Primary Prevention
* Detection and control of cerebrovascular risk factors
  —Hypertension (including isolated systolic hypertension)
  —Tobacco smoking, diabetes, hyperlipidemia
* Patient education about TIAs
* Antithrombotic therapy for atrial fibrillation[a]
  —Warfarin unless contraindicated or low-risk
  —Aspirin if warfarin not given
* Asymptomatic carotid disease
  —Sonography and aspirin for bruits
  —Selection for endarterectomy is controversial, best individualized

Secondary Prevention (TIA or prior stroke)
* Cerebrovascular disease (atherosclerosis and penetrating artery disease)
  —Risk factor reduction
  —Antiplatelet agents (aspirin, ticlopidine)
  —Carotid endarterectomy
    Proven beneficial >70% stenosis
    Uncertain benefit 30%–69% stenosis
* Cardiogenic embolism
  —Nonvalvular atrial fibrillation: warfarin INR 2.0–3.0
  —Warfarin for most other cardiac sources[b]

---

[a] See Table 14-10 for specific range of acceptable antithrombotic management. Associated coronary artery disease, sometimes occult, needs attention in management of patients at risk for stroke.

[b] Mechanical prosthetic heart valves require a higher intensity of anticoagulation (INR 2.5 to 4.0), sometimes combined with dipyridamole 75 mg twice a day or aspirin 100 mg per day.

NOTE: TIA = transient ischemic attack; INR = international normalized ratio.

SOURCE: Used with permission from R. G. Hart.[65]

this situation are available. Further studies will be needed to define the optimal use of heparin in ischemic stroke. The use of long-term anticoagulation does have proven benefit for cardiogenic brain embolus, as previously discussed.

THROMBOLYTIC THERAPY

Thrombolytic agents have been used in the treatment of stroke for more than three decades. Their use was significantly complicated with intracerebral hemorrhage and death in the pre-CT era.[174] Renewed interest has now surfaced with improved imaging techniques and data suggesting that an ischemic penumbra might be salvageable with restoration of blood flows.[83,174] In a recent multicenter trial, intravenous tissue plasminogen activator (tPA) was given to patients within 6 h of onset of stroke symptoms.[175] No benefit on outcome was observed using functional scales as an endpoint.

TABLE 14-10
Medical Therapy for Stroke Prevention

Clinical Situation	Recommended Therapy	Acceptable Options
TIA or stroke[a]	Aspirin 325 mg/day[b]	Aspirin 75–1300 mg/day Ticlopidine 250 mg b.i.d.
TIA or stroke during aspirin Rx	Ticlopidine 250 mg b.i.d.	Aspirin 75–1300 mg/day Warfarin INR 2–3
Nonvalvular atrial fibrillation Primary prevention	Warfarin INR 2.0–3.0[c]	Warfarin INR 1.5–3.0 Aspirin 325 mg/day
Secondary prevention	Warfarin INR 2.0–3.0	Warfarin INR 1.5–4.0 Aspirin 325 mg/day
Asymptomatic carotid stenosis	Aspirin 325 mg/day[d]	Aspirin 75–1300 mg
Asymptomatic people >60 years old	No Rx	Aspirin 75–325 mg/day if risk factors

[a] Carotid artery endarterectomy for TIA or minor stroke associated with 70% to 99% ipsilateral stenosis. See text.

[b] Experts disagree about whether > or = 975 mg of ASA offers more benefits than lower doses.

[c] Identification of "low-risk" patients who may not require anticoagulation is controversial; the optimal range in elderly patients (>75 years old) may be lower (1.5–2.5). Patients with mechanical prosthetic heart valve require an INR of 2.5–4.0, often combined with antiplatelet agents.

[d] Selection of patients for carotid endarterectomy is controversial and evolving. See text.

NOTE: TIA = transient ischemic attack; INR = international normalized ratio.

SOURCE: Used with permission from R. G. Hart.[65]

There was no difference in 30-day mortality, but large parenchymal hemorrhages occurred significantly more often in the tPA-treated patients. While thrombolysis may be effective in carefully selected patients, further data from ongoing trials must be awaited.

Ancrod, a thrombin-like enzyme from Malayan pit viper venom, lowers blood viscosity and fibrinogen, induces prostacyclin formation, and may release endogenous tPA from vascular endothelium. In the small studies to date, Ancrod has had a low risk of bleeding complications, and a trend toward improved clinical outcome has been observed.[176–178] A large multicenter trial is now randomizing patients.

OTHER MEDICAL THERAPY

In addition to reperfusion of the ischemic penumbra, cytoprotective drugs may offer some benefit after acute stroke. There are now multiple agents under investigation in human trials, but to date no single agent has demonstrated significant benefit. It is likely that the benefit of cytoprotective drugs will be maximal with administration as early as possible (2 to 3 h after symptoms begin). If these strategies prove beneficial, intense public education about the signs of stroke will be needed to permit such early intervention.

At present the best medical therapy remains prevention through control of risk factors. Treatment of hypertension, the most important treatable risk factor for stroke, can reduce stroke risk on an average of about 40 percent.[22,23] Systolic hypertension is prevalent in elderly

patients and significantly increases their risk for stroke. It had been postulated that treatment in this group might be problematic. However, in the Systolic Hypertension in the Elderly Program, treatment of isolated systolic hypertension in patients older than 60 years of age reduced stroke by 36 percent without producing significant side effects.[24] Smoking cessation has a beneficial impact on stroke, with former smokers approaching the stroke rate of nonsmokers after five years.[27]

LIPID LOWERING

The effectiveness of lipid lowering in primary or secondary prevention of stroke remains unproven, but there is some indication of benefit. In a large recent study, simvastatin, a 3-hydroxy-3-methylglutaric acid coenzyme A (HMG-CoA) reductase inhibitor, was given to patients with coronary artery disease and an elevated total cholesterol greater than 212 mg/dl.[179] A 35 percent reduction in LDL cholesterol was associated with a significant reduction in all causes of mortality, coronary events, and ischemic stroke. Nonembolic stroke was reduced by 50 percent. In a second recent report, a related drug, lovastatin, was shown to reverse progression of mild carotid atherosclerosis in patients with an LDL cholesterol greater than 130 mg/dl at baseline.[187] Other modifiable risk factors include diabetes, a sedentary life-style, oral contraceptive use, and excessive alcohol use. Whether modification of these factors influences the risk of stroke is unknown. Current primary and secondary prevention strategies in specific situations are outlined in Tables 14-9 and 14-10.

SURGICAL THERAPY

Surgical endarterectomy and other surgical options are discussed in another chapter. Carotid endarterectomy (CEA) has proven benefit in patients with TIA and angiographic stenosis greater than 70 percent.[181,182] It should be stressed that the surgeons in these trials were experienced and achieved a perioperative morbidity and mortality rate of 2 to 5 percent. Until recently, data available on CEA for asymptomatic carotid stenosis demonstrated no benefit for stroke and mortality overall.[183–186] The Asymptomatic Carotid Atherosclerotic Study (ACAS) was a large multicenter trial of CEA versus medical therapy for asymptomatic carotid stenosis of greater than 60 percent.[180] This study of 1659 patients confirmed the relatively low risk of stroke in asymptomatic patients, with a rate of about 2 percent per year in the medically treated group. Surgery provided a statistically significant benefit by reducing the risk of stroke to about 1 percent per year. Surgical morbidity and mortality at 30 days was 2.3 percent, with almost half the complications arising from cerebral angiography. The clinical benefit of CEA for asymptomatic carotid stenosis remains in question. The majority of strokes occur because of disease outside the carotid system, and in many instances should not be importantly influenced by CEA (as in cardiogenic brain embolus). Carefully selected patients with as of yet undefined high-risk variables may benefit from CEA in the hands of an expert surgeon. These variables might include the degree of stenosis, type of collateral, presence of ulceration, risk factors for progression, identification of embolic material in the retina, or clinically silent stroke on brain imaging.[188] Extracranial to intracranial bypass was first performed in 1967 by Yasargil.[189] In an international trial published in 1985, no benefit could be identified even after subgroup analysis.[190–192]

References

1. American Heart Association: *Heart and Stroke Facts: 1994 Statistical Supplement.* Dallas, TX, American Heart Association, 1993.
2. Wolf PA, et al: Probability of stroke: A risk profile from the Framingham study. *Stroke* 1991; 22:3312.
3. Dombovy ML, et al: Disability and use of rehabilitation services following stroke in Rochester, Minnesota, 1975–1979. *Stroke* 1987; 18:830.
4. Indredavik B, et al: Benefit of a stroke unit: A randomized controlled trial. *Stroke* 1991; 22:1026.
5. Foulkes MA, et al: The Stroke Data Bank: Design, methods, and baseline characteristics. *Stroke* 1988; 19:547.
6. Bamford J, et al: A prospective study of acute cerebrovascular disease in the community: The Oxfordshire Community Stroke Project—1981–1986. *J Neurol* 1990; 53:16.
7. Dombovy ML: Rehabilitation and the course of recovery after stroke: In Whisnant JP (ed): *Stroke: Populations, Cohorts, and Clinical Trials.* Oxford, England, Butterworth-Heinemann Publishers, 1993:218–237.
8. Terent A: Stroke morbidity: In Whisnant JP (ed): *Stroke: Populations, Cohorts, and Clinical Trials.* Oxford, England, Butterworth-Heinemann Publishers, 1993:37–58.
9. Terent A: Survival after stroke and transient ischemic attacks during the 1970s and 1980s. *Stroke* 1989; 20:1320.
10. Bamford J, et al: The frequency, causes and timing of death within 30 days of a first stroke: The Oxfordshire Community Stroke Project. *J Neurol* 1990; 53:824.
11. Bonita R, et al: Event, incidence and case fatality rates of cerebrovascular disease in Auckland, New Zealand. *Am J Epidemiol* 1984; 120:236.
12. Ward G, et al: Incidence and outcome of cerebrovascular disease in Perth, Western Australia. *Stroke* 1988; 19:1501.
13. Broderick JP, et al: Incidence rates of stroke in the eighties: The end of the decline in stroke? *Stroke* 1989; 20:577.
14. Anderson GL, Whisnant JP: A comparison of trends in mortality from stroke in the United States and Rochester, Minnesota. *Stroke* 1982; 13:804.
15. Cooper R, et al: Slowdown in the decline of stroke mortality in the United States, 1978–1986. *Stroke* 1990; 21:1274.
16. McGovern PG, et al: Trends in mortality, morbidity, and risk factor levels for stroke from 1960 through 1990. *JAMA* 1992; 268:753.
17. Whisnant JP: The decline of stroke. *Stroke* 1984; 15:160.
18. Wolf PA, et al: Epidemiology of stroke. In: Barnett HJM, et al (eds): *Stroke: Pathophysiology, Diagnosis, and Management*, 2d ed. Oxford, England, Churchill-Livingstone, 1992.
19. Rutan GH, et al: A historical perspective of elevated systolic vs. diastolic blood pressure from an epidemiological and clinical trial viewpoint. *J Clin Epidemiol* 1989; 42:663.
20. Fisher CM: The ascendancy of diastolic blood pressure over systolic. *Lancet* 1985; 2:1349.
21. Deubner DC, et al: Attributable risk, population attributable risk, and population attributable fraction of death associated with hypertension in a biracial population. *Circulation* 1975; 52:901.
22. Collins R, et al: Blood pressure, stroke and coronary heart disease. Part 2: Short-term reductions in blood pressure: Overview of randomized drug trials in their epidemiological context. *Lancet* 1990; 335:827.
23. Dahlof B, et al: Morbidity and mortality in the Swedith Trial in Old Patients with Hypertension (STOP-Hypertension). *Lancet* 1991; 338:1281.
24. Colandrea MA, et al: Systolic hypertension in the elderly: An epidemiologic assessment. *Circulation* 1970; 41:239.
25. Abbott RD, et al: Risk of stroke in male cigarette smokers. *N Engl J Med* 1986; 315:717.
26. Colditz GA, et al: Cigarette smoking and risk of stroke in middle-aged women. *N Engl J Med* 1988; 318:937.
27. Wolf PA, et al: Cigarette smoking as a risk factor for stroke: The Framingham Study, *JAMA* 1988; 259:1025.
28. Kannel WB, et al: Manifestations of coronary disease predisposing to stroke: The Framingham study. *JAMA* 1983; 250:2942.
29. Komad MS, et al: Myocardial infarction and stroke. *Stroke* 1984; 34:1403.
30. Parkin TW, et al: Cerebral complications of cardiovascular disease. *Med Clin North Am* 1958; 42:917.
31. Wolf PA, et al: Epidemiological assessment of chronic atrial

fibrillation and risk of stroke: The Framingham study. *Neurology* 1978; 28:973.

32. Rodstein M, et al: Nonvalvular atrial fibrillation and strokes in the aged. *J Insur Med* 1989; 21:192.

33. Halperin JL, Hart RG: Atrial fibrillation and stroke: New ideas, persisting dilemmas. *Stroke* 1988; 19:937.

34. The Stroke Prevention in Atrial Fibrillation Investigators: Predictors of thromboembolism in atrial fibrillation: Clinical features of patients at risk. *Ann Intern Med* 1992; 116:1.

35. The Stroke Prevention in Atrial Fibrillation Investigators: Predictors of thromboembolism in atrial fibrillation: Echocardiographic features of patients at risk. *Ann Intern Med* 1992; 116:6.

36. Atrial Fibrillation Investigators: Risk factors for stroke and efficacy of antithrombotic therapy in atrial fibrillation: Analysis of pooled data from five randomized controlled trials. *Arch Intern Med* 1995; 154:1449.

37. Dyken M, et al: Risk factors in stroke—a statement for physicians by the Subcommittee on Risk Factors and Stroke by the Stroke Council. *Stroke* 1984; 15:1105.

38. Mortel KF, et al: Diabetes mellitus as a risk factor for stroke. *South Med J* 1990; 83:904.

39. Aronow WS, et al: Risk factors for atherothrombotic brain infarction in persons over 62 years of age in a long-term health care facility. *J Am Geriatr Soc* 1987; 35:1.

40. Prati P, et al: Prevalence and determinants of carotid atherosclerosis in a general population. *Stroke* 1992; 23:1705.

41. Yasaka M, et al: Distribution of atherosclerosis and risk factors in atherothrombotic occlusion. *Stroke* 1993; 24:206.

42. Must A, et al: Long-term morbidity and mortality of overweight adolescents. A follow-up of the Harvard growth study of 1922–1935. *N Engl J Med* 1992; 327:1350.

43. Folsom AR, et al: Incidence of hypertension and stroke in relation to body fat distribution and other risk factors in older women. *Stroke* 1990; 21:701.

44. Otten MW, et al: The effect of known risk factors on the excess mortality of black adults in the United States. *JAMA* 1990; 263:845.

45. Gillum RF: Stroke in blacks. *Stroke* 1988; 19:1.

46. Kittner SJ, et al: Black-white differences in stroke incidence in a national sample: The contribution of hypertension and diabetes mellitus. *JAMA* 1990; 264:1267.

47. Gorelick PB, et al: Racial differences in the distribution of anterior circulation occlusive disease. *Neurology* 1984; 34:54.

48. Li S, et al: Cerebrovascular disease in the People's Republic of China: Epidemiologic and clinical features. *Neurology* 1985; 35:1708.

49. Konishi M, et al: Associations of serum total cholesterol, different types of stroke, and stenosis, distribution of cerebral arteries. The Akita Pathology Study. *Stroke* 1993; 24:954.

50. Kagan A, et al: Factors related to stroke incidence in Hawaiian Japanese men: The Honolulu Heart Study. *Stroke* 1980; 11:14.

51. Stampfer MJ, et al: A prospective study of past use of oral contraceptive agents and risk of cardiovascular diseases. *N Engl J Med* 1988; 319:1313.

52. Stadel BV: Oral contraceptives and cardiovascular disease. *N Engl J Med* 1981; 288:672.

53. Lee TK, et al: Impact of alcohol consumption and cigarette smoking on stroke among the elderly in Taiwan. *Stroke* 1995; 26:790.

54. Gorelick PB: The status of alcohol as a risk factor for stroke. *Stroke* 1989; 12:1607.

55. Casper ML, et al: The Shifting Stroke Belt. Changes in the geographic pattern of stroke mortality in the United States, 1962 to 1988. *Stroke* 1995; 26:755.

56. Lanska DJ, Peterson PM: Effects of interstate migration on the geographic distribution of stroke mortality in the United States. *Stroke* 1995; 26:554.

57. Lanska DJ, Kuller LH: The geography of stroke mortality in the United States and the concept of a Stroke Belt. *Stroke* 1995; 26:1145.

58. Howard G, Howard VJ: The end of the Stroke Belt? It may be too early to declare victory. *Stroke* 1995; 26:1150.

59. Howard G, et al: Is the Stroke Belt disappearing? An analysis of racial, temporal, and age effects. *Stroke* 1995; 26:1153.

60. Lanska DJ, Peterson PM: Geographic variation in the decline of stroke mortality in the United States. *Stroke* 1995; 26:1159.

61. Iso H, et al: MRFIT Research Group. Serum cholesterol levels and six-year mortality from stroke in 350,977 men screened for the Multiple Risk Factor Intervention Trial. *N Engl J Med* 1989; 320:904.

62. Scandinavian Simvastatin Survival Study: Randomized trial of cholesterol lowering in 4444 patients with coronary heart disease: The Scandinavian Simvastatin Survival Study (4S). *Lancet* 1994; 344:1383.

63. Furberg CD, et al: Effect of Lovastatin on early carotid atherosclerosis and cardiovascular events. *Circulation* 1994; 90:1679.

64. Yatsu FM, et al: Community hospital-based stroke programs: North Carolina, Oregon, and New York: Goals, objectives, and data collection procedures. *Stroke* 1986; 17:276.

65. Hart RG: Cardiogenic embolism to the brain. *Lancet* 1992; 339:589.

66. Sacco RL, et al: Infarcts of undetermined cause: The NINCDS Stroke Data Bank. *Ann Neurol* 1989; 25:382.

67. Bogousslavsky J, et al: The Lausanne Stroke Registry: Analysis of 1,000 consecutive patients with first stroke. *Stroke* 1988; 19:1083.

68. Anderson CS, et al: Ascertaining the true incidence of stroke: Experience from the Perth Community Stroke Study. *Med J Aust* 1993; 158:80.

69. Kojima S, et al: Prognosis and disability of stroke patients after 5 years in Akita, Japan. *Stroke* 1990; 21:72.

70. Bamford J, et al: A prospective study of acute cerebrovascular disease in the community: The Oxfordshire Community Stroke Project 1981–86. 1. Methodology, demography and incident cases of first-ever stroke. *J Neurol Neurosurg Psychiatry* 1988; 51:1373.

71. Heyman A, et al: Risk of ischemic heart disease in patients with TIA. *Neurology* 1984; 34:626.

72. Sandercock PAG: Recent developments in the diagnosis and management of patients with transient ischaemic attacks and minor ischaemic stroke. *Quart J Med* 1991; 286:101.

73. Dennis M, et al: Prognosis of transient ischemic attacks in the Oxfordshire Community Stroke Project. *Stroke* 1990; 21:848.

74. North American Symptomatic Carotid Endarterectomy Trial Collaborators: Beneficial effect of carotid endarterectomy in symptomatic patients with high-grade carotid stenosis. *N Engl J Med* 1991; 325:445.

75. Jones JR, Jr., Millikan CH: Temporal profile (clinical course) of acute carotid system cerebral infarction. *Stroke* 1976; 7:64.

76. Jones HR, et al: Temporal profile (clinical course) of acute carotid system cerebral infarction. *Stroke* 1980; 11:173.

77. Adams RD, Victor M: Cerebrovascular Diseases: In Day W, Navrozov M (eds): *Principles of Neurology,* 4th ed. New York, McGraw-Hill, 1989:617–692.

78. Rorke LB. Perinatal brain damage: In Adams JH, Duchen LW (eds): *Greenfield's Neuropathology,* 5th ed. New York, Oxford University Press, 1992:676–678.

79. Coyle JT, et al: Excitatory amino acid neurotoxins: Selectivity, specificity, and mechanisms of action. *Neurosci Res Prog Bull* 1981; 19:331.

80. Benveniste H, et al: Elevation of the extracellular concentra-

tions of glutamate and aspartate in rat hippocampus during transient cerebral ischemia monitored by intracerebral microdialysis. *J Neurochem* 1984; 43:1369.

81. Choi DW, et al: Glutamate neurotoxicity in cortical cell culture. *J Neurosci* 1987; 7:357.

82. Pulsinelli W, et al: Temporal profile of neuronal damage in a model of transient forebrain ischemia. *Ann Neurol* 1992; 339:533.

83. Astrup J, et al: Threshold in cerebral ischemia: The ischemic penumbra. *Stroke* 1981; 12:723.

84. Pulsinelli W: Pathophysiology of acute ischemic stroke. *Lancet* 1992; 339:533.

85. Milde LN: Pathophysiology of ischemic brain injury. *Crit Care Clin* 1989; 5:729.

86. Choi D: Methods for antagonizing glutamate neurotoxicity. *Cerebrovasc Brain Metab Rev* 1990; 2:105.

87. Kugiyama K, et al: Impairment of endothelium-dependent arterial relaxation by lysolecithin in modified low-density lipoproteins. *Nature* 1990; 344:160.

88. Adams HP, Gross CE: Embolism distal to stenosis of the middle cerebral artery. *Stroke* 1981; 12:228.

89. Masawa N, et al: Three dimensional morphologic analysis of thrombotic occlusive arteries in autopsies of atherosclerotic cerebral infarction. *Stroke* 1990; 21:1.

90. Ogata J, et al: Rupture of atheromatous plaque as a cause of thrombotic occlusion of stenotic internal carotid artery. *Stroke* 1990; 21:1740.

91. Weller RO: Spontaneous intracranial hemorrhage. In Adams JH, Duchen LW (eds): *Greenfield's Neuropathology*, 5th ed. New York, Oxford University Press, 1992:275–277.

92. Graham DI: Hypoxia and vascular disorders. In Adams JH, Duchen LW (eds): *Greenfield's Neuropathology*, 5th ed. New York, Oxford University Press, 1992:213–215.

93. Fisher CM: Lacunes, small deep cerebral infarcts. *Neurology* 1965; 15:774.

94. Futrell N, Millikin C: The fallacy of the lacune hypothesis. *Stroke* 1990; 21:1251.

95. Huston KA, Hunder GG: Giant cell (cranial) arteritis: A clinical review. *Am Heart J* 1980; 100:99.

96. Petty GW, Mohr JP: Stroke in the setting of collagen vascular disease. In Barnett HJM, et al (eds): *Stroke: Pathophysiology, Diagnosis, and Management*, 2d ed. New York, Churchill-Livingstone, 1992:691–720.

97. Machado EBV, et al: Trends in incidence and clinical presentation of temporal arteritis in Olmstead County, Minnesota, 1950–1985. *Arthritis Rheum* 1088; 31:745.

98. Hall S, et al: Takayasu arteritis: A study of 32 North American patients. *Medicine* 1985; 64:89.

99. Burke JM, Schaberg DR: Neurosyphilis in the antibiotic era. *Neurology* 1985; 35:1368.

100. Gasperetti C, Son SK: Contralateral hemiparesis following herpes zoster ophthalmicus. *J Neurol Neurosurg Psychiatry* 1985; 48:338.

101. Kaku DA, Lowenstein DH: Emergence of recreational drug use as a major risk factor for stroke in young adults. *Ann Intern Med* 1990; 113:821.

102. Vinters HV: Cerebral amyloid angiopathy: A critical review. *Stroke* 1987; 18:311.

103. Maruyanna K, et al: Immunohistochemical characterization of cerebrovascular amyloid in 46 autopsied cases using antibodies to β protein and cystatin C. *Stroke* 1990; 21:397.

104. Vonsattel JP, et al: Coincidence of fibrinoid necrosis with amyloid angiopathy as the cause of cerebral hemorrhage (Abstract). *J Neuropath Exp Neurol* 1984; 43:316.

105. Hart RG, Kanter MC: Hematologic disorders and ischemic stroke—A selective review. *Stroke* 1990; 21:1111.

106. Hart RG, et al: Diagnosis and management of ischemic stroke: Selected controversies. *Curr Probl Cardiol* 1983; 8:43.

107. Adams HP, et al: Nonhemorrhagic cerebral infarction in young adults. *Arch Neurol* 1986; 43:793.

108. Cerebral Embolism Task Force: Cardiogenic brain embolism. *Arch Neurol* 1986; 43:71.

109. Fisher CM, Adams RD: Observations on brain embolism with special reference to hemorrhagic infarction. In Furlan AJ (ed): *The Heart and Stroke: Exploring Mutual Cardiovascular Issues.* New York, Springer-Verlag, 1987:17.

110. Amarenco P, et al: Atherosclerotic disease of the aortic arch and the risk of ischemic stroke. *N Engl J Med* 1994; 331:1474.

111. Barbut D, et al: Cerebral emboli detected during bypass surgery are associated with clamp removal. *Stroke* 1994; 25:2398.

112. Hart RG, Halperin JL: Atrial fibrillation and stroke: Revisiting the dilemmas. *Stroke* 1994; 25:1337.

113. Laupacis A, et al: Antithrombotic therapy in atrial fibrillation. *Chest* 1992; 102:426S.

114. Aberg H: Atrial fibrillation. I. A study of atrial thrombosis and systemic embolism in a necropsy material. *Acta Med Scand* 1969; 185:373.

115. Stroke Prevention in Atrial Fibrillation Investigators: Preliminary report of the Stroke Prevention in Atrial Fibrillation study. *N Engl J Med* 1990; 322:863.

116. Petersen P, et al: Placebo-controlled, randomized trial of warfarin and aspirin for prevention of thromboembolic complications in chronic atrial fibrillation: The Copenhagen AFASAK study. *Lancet* 1989; 175.

117. Connolly SJ, et al: Canadian Atrial Fibrillation Anticoagulation (CAFA) Study. *J Am Coll Cardiol* 1991; 18:349.

118. Ezekowitz MD, et al, for the Veterans Affairs SPINAF Investigators: Warfarin in the prevention of stroke associated with nonrheumatic atrial fibrillation. *N Engl J Med* 1992; 1406.

119. Boston Area Anticoagulation Trial for Atrial Fibrillation Investigators: The effect of low-dose warfarin on the risk of stroke in nonrheumatic atrial fibrillation. *N Engl J Med* 1990; 323:1505.

120. Snyder M, Renaudin J: Intracranial hemorrhage associated with anticoagulation therapy. *Surg Neurol* 1977; 7:31.

121. Hylek EM, Singer DE: Risk factors for intracranial hemorrhage in outpatient taking warfarin. *Ann Intern Med* 1994; 120:897.

122. Dawson I, et al: Ischemic and hemorrhagic stroke in patients on oral anticoagulants after reconstruction for chronic lower limb ischemia. *Stroke* 1993; 24:1655.

123. Hart RG, et al: Oral anticoagulants and intracranial hemorrhage. *Stroke* 1995; 26:1471.

124. Wintzen AR, et al: The risk of intracerebral hemorrhage during oral anticoagulant treatment: A population study. *Ann Neurol* 1984; 16:533.

125. Sherman DG, Easton JD: Clinical syndromes of brain ischemia. In Wilkins (ed): *Neurosurgery*, 2d ed. New York, McGraw-Hill, 1995.

126. Norris JW, et al: Serum cardiac enzymes in stroke. *Stroke* 1979; 10:548.

127. Hess DC, et al: Coronary artery disease, myocardial infarction, and brain embolism. *Neurol Clin* 1993; 11:399.

128. Adams HP, et al: The clinical spectrum of aneurysmal subarachnoid hemorrhage. *J Stroke Cerebrovasc Dis* 1991; 1:3.

129. Gorelick PB, et al: Headache in acute cerebrovascular disease. *Neurology* 1986; 36:1445.

130. Portenoy RK, et al: Heachache in cerebrovascular disease. *Stroke* 1984; 15:1009.

131. Mohr JP, et al: The Harvard Cooperative Stroke Registry: A prospective registry. *Neurology* 1978; 28:754.

132. Ramirez-Lassepas M, et al: Can embolic stroke be diagnosed on the basis of neurologic clinical criteria? *Arch Neurol* 1987; 44:87.

133. Feinberg WM: Guidelines for management of transient ischemic attacks. For the Ad Hoc Committee on Guidelines for the Management of Transient Ischemic Attacks of the Stroke Council, American Heart Association. *Stroke* 1994; 25:1320.

134. Adams HP, et al: Guidelines for management of patients with acute ischemic stroke. *Circulation* 1994; 90:1588.

135. Mohr JP, et al: MR vs CT imaging in acute stroke. *Proc International Conf Stroke Cerebral Circulation, 1992.*

136. DeWitt JD: Clinical use of NMR imaging in stroke. *Stroke* 1986; 17:328.

137. Hennerici M, et al: Sonography in the diagnosis of cerebrovascular diseases. In Barnett HJM (ed): *Stroke: Pathophysiology, Diagnosis, and Management*, 2d ed. New York, Churchill-Livingstone, 1992.

138. Freeman FR: Akinetic mutism and bilateral anterior cerebral artery occlusion. *J Neurol Neurosurg Psychiatry* 1971; 34:693.

139. Dunker RO, Harris AB: Surgical anatomy of the proximal anterior cerebral artery. *J Neurosurg* 1976; 44:359.

140. Symonds C, Mackenzie I: Bilateral loss of vision from cerebral infarction. *Brain* 1957; 80:415.

141. Damasio A, et al: Prosopagnosia: Anatomic basis and behavioral mechanisms. *Neurology* (NY) 1982; 32:331.

142. Bender MB, et al: Palinopsia. *Brain* 1968; 91:321.

143. Caplan LR: "Top of the basilar" syndrome. *Neurology* (NY) 1980; 30:72.

144. Fisher CM, et al: Lateral medullary infarction: The pattern of vascular occlusion. *J Neuropathol Exp Neurol* 1961; 20:323.

145. Heros R: Cerebellar hemorrhage and infarction. *Stroke* 1982; 13:106.

146. Fisher CM: Lacunar strokes and infarcts: A review. *Neurology* (NY) 1982; 32:871.

147. Fisher CM, Adams RD: Transient global amnesia. *Am Neurol Assoc* 1958; 83:143.

148. Feur D, Weinberger J: Extracranial carotid artery in patients with transient global amnesia: Evaluation by real-time B-mode ultrasonography with duplex doppler flow. *Stroke* 1987; 18:951.

149. Caplan IR: Transient global amnesia. In Vinken PG, et al (eds): *Handbook of Neurology*, vol 45. Amsterdam, Elsevier Science Publishers, 1985:205–218.

150. Mathew NT, Meyer JS: Pathogenesis and natural history of transient global amnesia. *Stroke* 1975; 5:303.

151. Shuping JR, et al: Transient global amnesia. *Ann Neurol* 1980; 7:281.

152. Kushner MJ, Hauser WA: Transient global amnesia: A control study. *Ann Neurol* 1985; 18:684.

153. Hodges JR, Warlow CP: Syndromes of transient amnesia: Towards a classification. A study of 153 cases. *J Neurol Neurosurg Psychiatry* 1990; 53:834.

154. Ameriso SF, et al: Immunohematologic characteristics of infection-associated cerebral infarction. *Stroke* 1991; 22:1004.

155. Turpie AGG, et al: A low-molecular-weight heparinoid compared with unfractionated heparin in the prevention of deep vein thrombosis in patients with acute ischemic stroke. A randomized, double-blind study. *Ann Intern Med* 1992; 117:353.

156. Black MMc, et al: External pneumatic calf compression reduces deep venous thrombosis in patients with ruptured intracranial aneurysms. *Neurosurg* 1986; 18:25.

157. Antiplatelet Trialists Collaboration: Collaborative overview of randomized trials of antiplatelet treatment, Part 1. *Br Med J* 1994; 308:81.

158. Hass WK, et al: A randomized trial comparing ticlopidine hydrochloride with aspirin for the prevention of stroke in high-risk patients. *N Engl J Med* 1989; 321:501.

159. Gent M, et al: The Canadian-American Ticlopidine Study (CATS) in thromboembolic stroke. *Lancet* 1989; 1:1215.

160. Albers GW: Role of ticlopidine for prevention of stroke. *Stroke* 1992; 23:912.

161. Cerebral Embolism Study Group: Immediate anticoagulation of embolic stroke: A randomized trial. *Stroke* 1983; 14:668.

162. Duke RJ, et al: Intravenous heparin for the prevention of stroke progression in acute partial stable stroke. A randomized controlled trial. *Ann Intern Med* 1986; 105:825.

163. Baker RN, et al: Anticoagulant therapy in cerebral infarction. *Neurology* 1962; 12:823.

164. Enger E, Royesen S: Long-term anticoagulant therapy in patients with cerebral infarction: A controlled clinical study. *Acta Med Scand* 1965; 38(Suppl):1.

165. Hill AB, et al: Cerebrovascular disease: Trial of long-term anticoagulant therapy. *Br Med J* 1962; 2:1003.

166. Howard FA, et al: Survival following stroke. *JAMA* 1963; 183:921.

167. Marshall J, Shaw DA: Anticoagulant therapy in acute cerebrovascular accidents. A controlled trial. *Lancet* 1960; 1:995.

168. Cerebral Embolism Study Group: Cardioembolic stroke, immediate anticoagulation and brain hemorrhage. *Arch Intern Med* 1987; 174:636.

169. Hart RG, Pearce LA: In vivo antithrombotic effect of aspirin: Dose versus nongastrointestinal bleeding. *Stroke* 1993; 24:138.

170. Carter AB: Anticoagulant treatment in progressing stroke. *Br Med J* 1961; 5244:70.

171. Fisher CM: Anticoagulant therapy in cerebral thrombosis and cerebral embolism. A national cooperative study, interim report. *Neurology* 1961; 11:119.

172. Fisher CM: The "herald hemiparesis" of basilar artery occlusion. *Arch Neurol* 1988; 45:1301.

173. Haley EC Jr, et al: Failure of heparin to prevent progression in progressing ischemic infarction. *Stroke* 1988; 19:10.

174. Warlow JM, Warlow CP: Thrombolysis in acute ischemic stroke: Does it work? *Stroke* 1992; 23:1826.

175. Hacke W, et al: Intravenous thrombolysis with recombinant tissue plasminogen activation for acute hemispheric stroke: The European Cooperative Stroke Study (ECASS). *JAMA* 1995; 274:1017.

176. Hossman V, et al: Controlled trial of Ancrod in ischemic stroke. *Arch Neurol* 1983; 40:803.

177. Olinger CP, et al: Use of Ancrod in acute or progressing ischemic cerebral infarction. *Ann Emerg Med* 1988; 17:1208.

178. Pollak VE, et al: Ancrod causes rapid thrombolysis in patients with acute stroke. *Am J Med Sci* 1990; 299:319.

179. Scandinavian Simvastatin Survival Study Group: Randomized trial of cholesterol lowering in 4444 patients with coronary heart disease: The Scandinavian Simvastatin Survival Study (4S). *Lancet* 1994; 344:1383.

180. Executive Committee for the ACAS: Endarterectomy for asymptomatic carotid artery stenosis. *JAMA* 1995; 273:1421.

181. North American Symptomatic Carotid Endarterectomy Trial Collaborators: Beneficial effect of carotid endarterectomy in symptomatic patients with high-grade carotid stenosis. *N Engl J Med* 1991; 325:445.

182. European Carotid Surgery Trialists' Collaborative Group: MRC European carotid surgery trial: Interim results for symptomatic patients with severe (70–99%) or with mild (0–29%) carotid stenosis. *Lancet* 1991; 337:1235.

183. Mayberg MR, et al: Carotid endarterectomy and prevention of cerebral ischemia in symptomatic carotid stenosis. *JAMA* 1991; 266:3289.

184. The CASA/NOVA Study Group: Carotid surgery versus medical therapy in asymptomatic carotid stenosis. *Stroke* 1991; 22:1229.

185. Mayo Asymptomatic Carotid Endarterectomy Study Group: Results of a randomized controlled trial of carotid endarterec-

tomy for asymptomatic carotid stenosis. *Mayo Clin Proc* 1992; 67:513.

186. Hobson RW II, et al: Efficacy of carotid endarterectomy for asymptomatic carotid stenosis. *N Engl J Med* 1993; 328:221.

187. Furberg CD, et al: Effect of lovastatin on early carotid atherosclerosis and cardiovascular events. *Circulation* 1994; 90:1679.

188. Hart RG, et al: What's new in stroke? *Tex Med* 1995; 91:46.

189. Yasargil MG (ed): *Microsurgery Applied to Neurosurgery.* Stuttgart, Georg Thieme, 1969:105–115.

190. EC/IC Bypass Study Group: Failure of extracranial-intracranial arterial bypass to reduce the risk of ischemic stroke: Results of an international randomized trial. *N Engl J Med* 1985; 313:1191.

191. EC/IC Bypass Study Group: International cooperative study of extracranial/intracranial arterial anastomosis (EC/IC Bypass Study): Methodology and entry characteristics. *Stroke* 1985; 16:397.

192. Barnett HJM: Stroke prevention by surgery for symptomatic disease in carotid territory. *Neurol Clin* 1992; 10:281.

Chapter 15 _____

CHEMICAL NEUROTRANSMISSION

ROGER L. ALBIN

KIRK A. FREY

The unique feature of the central nervous system (CNS) is its ability to process and analyze large volumes of information. Underlying this properly are a series of morphologic and functional specializations that reflect the dedication of the CNS to information processing. Neurotransmitters and neurotransmitter receptors are particularly important examples of such specialization. While all cells use the general hormone-receptor interaction for intercellular information transfer, the complexity of these interactions reaches its peak within the CNS, and neurons exhibit characteristic morphologic and biochemical features to channel and control information transfer. The synapse is the characteristic morphologic specialization of neurons used to channel information transfer. The CNS is characterized also by the presence of a large number of molecules that function as neurotransmitters and an even larger number of receptors for these molecules.[1] Different types of neurotransmitters and neurotransmitter receptors are not indiscriminately distributed throughout the CNS. Rather, neurotransmitters and receptors are associated with specific cell types and systems of the CNS in very complex patterns of organization.

The richness of neurotransmitter and neurotransmitter receptor organization is of great practical significance. Cells, including neurons, possess a limited number of mechanisms for transduction of signals transmitted by neurotransmitters (or other signal / hormone molecules). Consequently, pharmacologic targeting of signal transductions processes runs the risk of interfering with mechanisms shared by many organs, resulting in lack of specificity of desired response. To a large extent, the specificity of information transfer resides at the level of specific synapses with specific neurotransmitter receptors and neurotransmitters. The great variety of neurotransmitters and neurotransmitter receptors, and their differential distribution within the CNS, offers the hope of being able to target CNS and cellular processes with considerable specificity and a very high therapeutic index. While much of neuropharmacology was discovered empirically (anesthetics being the most notable example), future important innovations are likely to be based on scientific understanding of neurotransmitters, neurotransmitter receptors, and their functions.

The Synapse

STRUCTURE

The distinct morphology and function of neurons, in comparison with the cells of other mammalian organs, have attracted the attention of numerous investigators. Our current understanding of the communication between neurons and the physical and biochemical specializations underlying synaptic transmission is derived from parallel anatomic, electrophysiologic, and neurochemical lines of evidence. Frequently, seminal observations have been made in peripheral tissues and synapses, including the amphibian neuromuscular junction and the electric organ of the eel *Torpedo californicus*. Where possible, the critical features of these systems have been redemonstrated in central nervous system synapses; however, the simplicity and homogeneity of the peripheral systems has allowed detailed studies not possible in the brain.

The detailed cellular architecture of the mammalian brain was extensively described by Ramon y Cajal, on the basis of silver-impregnated tissues demonstrating the shapes of entire neurons, including cell bodies as well as attached dendritic and axonal processes. It is now well-appreciated that much of the interneuronal communication takes place in synaptic connections between presynaptic axonal swellings (presynaptic terminals) and dendrites of postsynaptic neurons (Fig.

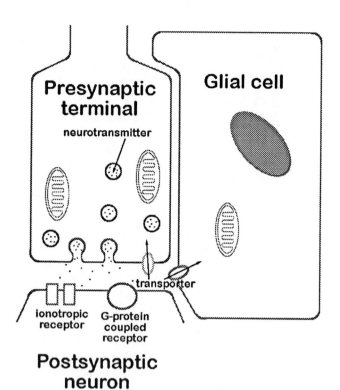

Figure 15-1 Generic synapse, illustrating a presynaptic terminal containing mitochondria, synaptic vesicles, and vesicles undergoing docking and release of neurotransmitters. The postsynaptic element contains both ionotropic and metabotropic receptors. Neurotransmitter transporters are present on both the presynaptic terminal and the membrane of an associated glial cell to terminate neurotransmitter action by removal from the synaptic cleft and to recycle neurotransmitter into the presynaptic terminal. These transporters may be uniquely expressed by the presynaptic terminal or may be uniquely expressed by surrounding astroglia or be shared by neurons and glia.

15-1). In addition to these classic axodendritic synapses, axosomatic and axoaxonic synaptic contacts are described. Ultrastructural studies of synapses at the level of electron microscopic resolution reveal additional specializations associated with synaptic regions. The presynaptic terminal contains abundant mitochondria, which are virtually excluded from the myelinated portions of the axon. Collections of microvesicles, termed *synaptic vesicles*, are identified in association with thickenings of the presynaptic terminal plasma membrane, representing neurotransmitter-containing vesicles and specialized membrane docking zones and calcium channels for exocytotic release, respectively. The postsynaptic membrane is often similarly thickened or more electron-dense than extrasynaptic or nonneuronal plasma membrane, presumably reflecting increased concentration of membrane-spanning chemical transducers (receptor proteins and related "second-messenger" enzymes).

Anatomic identification of central nervous system synapses has been extensively buttressed by biochemical analyses of tissue fractions enriched in synaptic terminals. If freshly obtained brain tissue is homogenized in isotonic buffer, the smallest processes of the neuron are distracted from the cell body and often reseal at the sheared ends. The resulting subcellular particles consist of presynaptic terminals, with or without attached postsynaptic components, termed *synaptosomes*. After homogenization, fractions enriched in synaptosomes can be obtained by differential centrifugation employing both size and density features to separate them from nuclei, myelin, and free cytosolic components. Synaptosomal fractions demonstrate enrichment in biochemical markers of mitochondria as well as neurotransmitter receptors and second-messenger enzymes. Under appropriate conditions, metabolically intact synaptosomes may be obtained that retain active biochemical specializations for synthesis, storage, release, and often postsynaptic transduction of neurotransmitters. Thus, many important aspects of chemical neurotransmission in the mammalian brain have been investigated in detail using synaptosomes.

The essential biochemical feature of a presynaptic nerve terminal is that it contain the chemical "first messenger," the neurotransmitter. Minimal requirements for a putative neurotransmitter are that it must (1) be present in presynaptic nerve terminals; (2) be released on depolarization of the terminal; (3) interact with a postsynaptic signal transducer ("receptor"); and (4) have a mechanism for termination of its action on the postsynaptic cell.[1] There are numerous chemical neurotransmitters in mammalian brain identified to date. They consist largely of small molecules including monoamines, acetylcholine, and amino acids and of peptides. It was originally hypothesized that individual neurons each used a single neurotransmitter; however, available evidence at this time suggests that this may be the exception rather than the rule. It is common for neurons to cosynthesize and release one nonpeptide and an additional peptide transmitter.

METABOLIC ASPECTS OF NEUROTRANSMISSION

An essential feature of presynaptic terminals is that they possess the necessary enzymatic specializations for synthesis and concentration of neurotransmitter. Most often, presynaptic terminals are endowed with specific transport proteins to enhance movement of biosynthetic neurotransmitter precursors or of the transmitters themselves from extracellular space into the cytoplasm. Frequently, expression of these transporters is specific to nerve terminals, and may serve to identify their presence in biochemical assays. Enzymes that synthesize neurotransmitters from available precursors are often specific to this process, and thus also expressed only by the appropriate nerve terminals.

A general feature of axodendritic synapses is their absence of myelination and large surface area-to-volume ratio. This provides maximal contact area for interaction between neurons, but imposes great metabolic energy demands on both pre- and postsynaptic processes. Not only is energy required for the synthesis, storage, release, and reuptake of neurotransmitter, but considerable energy is expended to restore electrochemical cation gradients dissipated during presynaptic nerve terminal depolarization. Postsynaptic responses mediated by excitatory cation channels as well as the production of enzyme-linked second messengers are additionally energy requiring. Given the small size of presynaptic terminals and processes of dendritic trees, the need for metabolic energy in the form of ATP per unit cytoplasmic volume in regions of dense synaptic connections exceeds that of neuronal cell bodies, and greatly exceeds the needs of white matter tracts, where ion fluxes are constrained by myelination. Thus, synapses are richly endowed with mitochrondria. Measures of cerebral energy production from glucose with the 2-deoxyglucose method confirm highest metabolic activity in regions of synaptic neuropil.

TRANSMITTER STORAGE AND RELEASE

After synthesis, neurotransmitters are stored and released from intraneuronal synaptic vesicles, providing means for protection of transmitter from further metabolism and for biochemical regulation of the efficacy of transmitter release. In the instances of small molecule neurotransmitters such as the biogenic amines and acidic amino acids, synaptic vesicles are endowed with transporters that move transmitter from cytoplasm to the interior of the vesicle. These transporters are structurally and biochemically distinct from the synaptic membrane uptake and reuptake transporters for neurotransmitters and precursors, and permit the recycling of vesicles within the nerve terminal after exocytotic transmitter release. In addition to the transporter proteins, synaptic vesicles have a number of specialized proteins involved in intracellular trafficking and partitioning of the vesicle between a storage pool and an activity cycling, releasable pool. Additional specialized vesicle proteins are necessary for the docking and fusion of presynaptic vesicles with plasma membrane specializations for calcium-mediated exocytosis of transmitter triggered by nerve terminal depolarization.

Like postsynaptic dendrites and neuronal cell bodies, presynaptic nerve terminals generally possess a range of neurotransmitter receptors. It is common for terminals to express receptors for the neurotransmitter(s) they employ. In this instance, the receptors often function to regulate the intrasynaptic concentration of neurotransmitter by providing feedback to the presynaptic terminal. Presynaptic terminals often receive synaptic input from other neurons, mediating presynaptic inhibition and facilitation of transmitter release on a polysynaptic basis as well.

INACTIVATION MECHANISMS

The action of neurotransmitters in the synaptic cleft is most often terminated by one of two processes: reuptake or metabolism. As noted previously, many types of presynaptic terminals have specific uptake transporters which move extracellular transmitter to the neuronal cytoplasm. These transporters serve not only to conserve and recycle a portion of a released neurotransmitter, but to terminate its action by reducing its intrasynaptic levels. In some cases, transporters are also expressed by glia surrounding synapses, providing an additional sink for removal of neurotransmitter from the synaptic cleft. These transporters may be identical with those expressed by the presynaptic terminal or may be related protein specific to glia. Many neurotransmitters are readily metabolized by membrane-associated or cytoplasmic enzymes within both neurons and glia. In some instances, the metabolic enzymes appear specifically suited and distributed to regulate the action of a particular neurotransmitter. Both transmitter reuptake transporters and metabolic enzymes are targeted by therapeutic drugs which presumably alter intrasynaptic transmitter levels and their regulation, as discussed in subsequent sections.

RECEPTOR TYPES

Neurotransmitter receptors can be divided into two broad categories: those that exert their actions by direct activation of ion channels, and those whose actions are mediated by activation of other cellular signaling proteins (Fig. 15-2). In the former case, ionotropic receptors are composed of heteromeric proteins which form both the receptor and the ion channel. In the latter case, receptors are single proteins whose effects are mediated by activation of other membrane-bound proteins, the so-called GTP-binding proteins (G proteins, see below). While at least two families of G-protein-coupled receptors exist, these receptor proteins have a characteristic tertiary structure with a 7 transmembrane domain motif. The ionotropic receptors generally exert their effects on a very rapid time scale with effects occurring within milliseconds, while the time course of G-protein-coupled receptor effects is in the seconds to minutes range. It should be emphasized that a given neurotransmitter may possess receptors

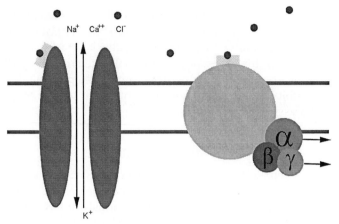

Figure 15-2   Neurotransmitters can activate both ionotropic and G protein (metabotropic) coupled receptors. The former are heteromeric complexes whose activation leads to ion flux and alterations in membrane potential while the latter are single proteins whose activation leads to the activation of specific GTP-coupled proteins that act as signal transducers. α-β-γ complex is the heterotrimeric G-protein complex responsible for signal transduction.

in both categories. Glutamate, GABA, serotonin, acetylcholine, and ATP are all neurotransmitters that possess both ionotropic and G-protein-coupled receptors. For a given neurotransmitter, both ionotropic and G-protein-coupled receptors may be represented at synapses utilizing that neurotransmitter, giving rise to very complex patterns of synaptic effects.

SIGNAL TRANSDUCTION MECHANISMS

G PROTEINS

G-protein-coupled receptors transduce biologic signals by activation of a class of membrane-associated proteins that bind GTP or GDP, and have GTPase activity. The G proteins are heterotrimers consisting of α, β, and γ subunits.[2,3] G-protein trimers exist in a free state with GDP bound to the α subunit. Ligand-receptor interaction leads to association of the G-protein complex and substitution of GTP for GDP. Following GTP binding, the G-protein complex dissociates from the receptor and the α subunit dissociates from the $\beta\gamma$ subunits, the latter remaining associated with each other. Both the dissociated α and $\beta\gamma$ subunits then interact with a variety of other proteins to generate second messengers and modulate cellular function. The process is terminated by hydrolysis of GTP to GDP and reassociation of all three subunits, regenerating the original heterotrimers with GTP hydrolysis thermodynamically driving the whole cycle.

The free α monomers and $\beta\gamma$ dimers regulate cAMP and cGMP production, phosphoinositide signaling, phosphodiesterase activity, the generation of eiconsanoids, and ion channel function. Not surprisingly, there are subtypes of α, β, and γ subunits. There are a particularly large number of α subunit subtypes, each with its own unique pattern of regional/cellular distribution and specific biochemical characteristics. Accompanied by heterogeneity of β and γ subunits, there is clearly great potential variation in the nature of G-protein signaling.

CYCLIC AMP

One of the primary second messengers of all eukaryotic cells is cyclic adenosine monophosphate (cAMP). cAMP is synthesized from ATP by a family of membrane-bound adenylyl cyclases.[4,5] At least four forms of adenylyl cyclase exist, with differing patterns of regional expression and regulatory properties. G-protein α and $\beta\gamma$ subunits are crucial regulators of adenylyl cyclase activity, producing both activation or inhibition of adenylyl cyclases, effects varying with the specific types of adenylyl cyclase and G-protein subunit subtypes. cAMP influences a wide variety of cellular processes, primarily by modulating the activity of cAMP-dependent protein kinases (Fig. 15-3). These kinases in turn can influence a bewilderingly broad set of activities varying from fairly rapid (hundreds of milliseconds latency) effects on ion channels to regulation of gene transcription, which operates over a much longer time course. cAMP may also directly modulate important functions; for example, some ion channels are directly modulated by cAMP without the intermediary step of kinase actions. cAMP levels are also regulated by modulation of catabolism, with specific phosphodiesterases converting cAMP to 5'-AMP. There are a family of cAMP phosphodiesterases, and their activity is regulated by G-protein subunits.

CYCLIC GMP

The role of cyclic guanosine monophosphate (cGMP) has many similarities to, and some major differences with, that of cAMP. Like cAMP, cGMP is an important second messenger with multiple actions, including activation of cGMP-dependent protein kinases, regulation of phosphodiesterases, and modulation of ion channel activity. cGMP is degraded by a family of specific phosphodiesterases whose activity is regulated by G-protein subunits. The functional roles and mechanisms of action of cGMP are less explored than those of cAMP. Major differences from the cAMP cascade

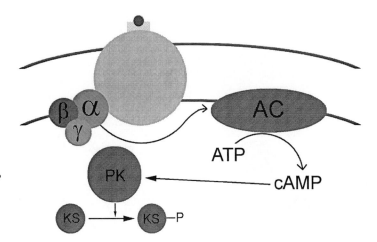

Figure 15-3 The cAMP cascade. A specific G-protein-coupled receptor leads to activation of G proteins (α-β-γ) which stimulate (or inhibit) adenylyl cyclase (AC). The resulting cAMP has many effects, including direct modulation of ion channels but primarily activates cAMP-dependent protein kinases (PKs) that phosphorylate a wide variety of proteins (kinase substrates, KS).

lie in the nature and regulation of the guanylyl cyclases responsible for synthesizing cGMP.

There are two major forms of guanylyl cyclases, a membrane-bound form and a cytosolic form.[6] The membrane-bound forms possess extracellular receptor domains that are activated by the atrial natriuetic peptide (ANP) family of peptides, and members of this family are found in the CNS. The cytosolic forms of guanylyl cyclase are activated by the neuromodulator gas nitric oxide (see below) in a calcium-dependent fashion.

PHOSPHOINOSITIDES
Phosphoinositides, a class of inositol-containing membrane phospholipids, have emerged as important second messengers within the CNS and other organ systems.[7] Activation of a large number of neurotransmitters, including muscarinic cholinergic, adrenergic, serotonergic, histaminergic, glutamateric, and a variety of neuropeptides can activate this signaling cascade. Receptors coupled to the phosphoinositide cascade initiate signaling via activation of G proteins that stimulate the membrane-bound enzyme phospholipase C to cleave phosphatidylinositol-4,5-bisphosphate (PIP$_2$) to form diacylglycerol (DAG) and D-*myo*-inositol-1,4,5-trisphosphate (IP$_3$). Both of these products are important second messengers (Fig. 15-4). DAG activates an important family of regulatory enzymes, the protein kinase Cs (PKCs), which can phosphorylate many important substrate proteins. IP$_3$ diffuses within the cell to bind to specific receptors on the endoplasmic reticulum to regulate intracellular calcium. The IP$_3$ receptor forms a ligand gated calcium channel on the endoplasmic reticulum whose activation releases calcium into the cytosol. This free intracellular calcium has potentially profound and pleiotropic effects on cellular function, including activation of the signaling protein calmodulin which regulates the function of many other proteins, activation of both protein kinases

and protein phosphatases, regulation of ion channels, and regulation of other intracellular calcium pools. IP$_3$ action is terminated by several cytosolic and membrane-bound enzymes that metabolize IP$_3$ to a variety of derivatives. Further metabolism leads to the regeneration of free inositol and its availability for recycling into membrane phosphoinositides.

Neurotransmitter Systems

GLYCINE
The simple amino acid glycine is an important inhibitory neurotransmitter in some regions of the CNS. Glycine participates in a number of metabolic pathways including protein synthesis, nucleotide synthesis, and glutathione production. There is no specific dedicated metabolic pathway for production of neurotransmitter glycine. Most brain glycine is probably synthesized de novo from glucose, and the immediate precursor of glycine is serine. The latter is converted into glycine by serine hydroxymethyltransferase (SHMT), which requires tetrahydrofolate, pyridoxal phosphate, and magnesium as cofactors. SHMT is ubiquitously and uniformly distributed throughout the CNS and does not seem to be enriched in glycinergic neurons. Glycine can be catabolized via a variety of metabolic pathways, and there does not seem to be any preferential pathway for degradation of neurotransmitter glycine. The neurotransmitter actions of glycine are terminated by a high-affinity glycine transporter responsible for removing glycine from the synaptic cleft.

As a neurotransmitter, glycine has a relatively restricted distribution and is an important inhibitor within the spinal cord and some brain stem regions. In the spinal cord, glycine is preferentially used by inhibitory interneurons that are important regulators of spinal cord function. Glycinergic neurons appear to play a very limited role in the forebrain. Interestingly,

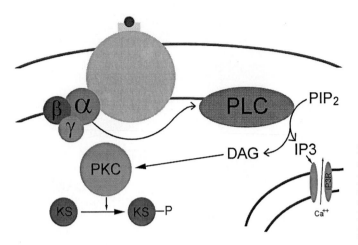

Figure 15-4 The inositol phospholipid cascade. Specific G-protein-coupled receptors activate G proteins (Gq, α-β-γ) that stimulate phospholipase C (PLC) hydrolysis of PIP$_2$ to IP$_3$ and DAG. IP$_3$ acts at specific receptors (IP$_3$R) on the endoplasmic reticulum to release Ca^{2+} from intracellular stores, and DAG activates specific protein kinases (protein kinase C, PKC) that phosphorylate substrate proteins (kinase substrates, KS).

while glycine receptors have a restricted distribution, the glycine transporter is widely distributed throughout the CNS.

Glycine exerts its inhibitory role by activation of a specific ligand gated ionotropic receptor.[8,9] This receptor was originally defined on the basis of electrophysiologic and pharmacologic studies, and analysis of receptor function was facilitated by the discovery that strychnine is a potent antagonist of glycine receptor function. Glycine receptor activation produces a chloride current that hyperpolarizes neurons, and the accompanying increase in membrane conductance tends to "shunt" excitatory currents, magnifying the inhibitory effect of glycine receptor activation. The glycine receptor was subsequently isolated and purified using strychnine analogue affinity chromatography, which permitted molecular cloning of the glycine receptor. Molecular studies revealed that the glycine receptor is probably a pentamer composed of two different types of subunits: α and β. The predicted stoichiometry is 3α and 2β subunits with each individual subunit spanning the neuron membrane and grouped around a central pore that is the physical ion channel.

The α and β subunits possess significant homology, and hydropathy analysis predicts proteins with extended extracellular amino termini, four transmembrane domains, and large intracytoplasmic loops between the third and fourth transmembrane domains. Sequence similarity, the predicted tertiary structure of the subunits, and the probable assembly into a pentamer, all indicate that glycine receptors belong to a superfamily of receptors whose other members include the nicotinic cholinergic receptor, GABA$_A$ receptors and the 5-HT$_3$ (serotonin) receptor. Subsequent molecular cloning studies revealed the existence of a family of α subunits, with four cloned to date. Alternative splicing of α subunit transcripts also contributes to the diversity of glycine receptor expression. There appears to be only one β subunit type. The α subunit appears

to contain the glycine and strychnine binding sites, and the different types of α subunits are important determinants of receptor properties, with α subunit subtype expression influencing the sensitivity of receptors to strychnine and their electrophysiologic properties. Glycine receptor subunit subtypes each have a unique distribution within the CNS, and the degree of expression of α subunit subtypes varies in the course of normal development.

Recent studies have shown that glycine receptor abnormalities are involved in the pathogenesis of some rare genetic disorders. Point mutations of the α_1 subunit are known to give rise to familial hyperekplexia, a human disorder characterized by exaggerated startle responses.[10] Murine homologues of this disorder have also been described with both α_1 and β subunit mutations.[11,12]

γ-AMINOBUTYRIC ACID

γ-Aminobutyric acid (GABA) is the most important inhibitory neurotransmitter of the CNS. Unlike glycine or glutamate (see below), GABA functions uniquely as a neurotransmitter with dedicated pathways for synthesis and catabolism. Most GABA derives ultimately from glucose metabolized via the Krebs cycle into α-ketoglutarate and then converted into glutamate as the immediate precursor of GABA. Glutamate undergoes decarboxylation via the cytosolic enzyme glutamic acid decarboxylase (GAD) to form GABA.[13] GAD is uniquely expressed by GABAergic neurons; biochemical and immunohistochemical assays of GAD distribution have been instrumental in identifying GABAergic neurons and pathways of the CNS. Two separate genes encode forms of GAD distinguished by molecular weight and some enzymologic features—GAD$_{65}$ and GAD$_{67}$. These two forms of GAD are largely coexpressed within the same neurons but differ somewhat in terms of subcellular distribution and regulation of enzyme activity. The functional significance of these differences is not known.

Another interesting aspect of GABA metabolism is the fact that GABA catabolizing pathways act to indirectly maintain cellular GABA levels. The catabolic enzyme for GABA is GABA α-oxoglutarate transaminase (GABA-T), a mitochondrially located protein expressed by both neurons and glia. GABA-T transforms GABA to succinic semialdehyde and in the process converts α-ketoglutarate to glutamate, the immediate precursor of GABA. Ancillary to this so-called GABA "shunt" are two additional pathways potentially involved in GABA metabolism. Succinic semialdehyde is converted by succinic semialdehyde dehydrogenase into succinic acid which can enter the Krebs cycle. In addition, the major mechanism for inactivation of synaptic GABA is reuptake via high-affinity GABA transporters. These transporters are expressed by both neurons and glia. Within glia, GABA-T converts GABA to glutamate which is subsequently converted by glutamine synthase to glutamine. Glutamine can then diffuse into the extracellular space and be transported into neurons where glutaminase converts it to glutamate, where it may be used as a precursor for GABA synthesis.

Manipulation of GABA pathways has been targeted successfully to produce clinically useful compounds. The novel anticonvulsant vigabatrin is the product of a systematic effort to develop drugs that specifically inhibit GABA-T, and the efficacy of vigabatrin is probably based on its ability to raise synaptic GABA levels. Inhibition of the GABA transporter is another strategy pursued presently by the pharmaceutical industry to produce novel anticonvulsants.

There are many GABAergic neurons within the CNS. GABAergic interneurons constitute approximately 20 percent of the neurons in the cortical mantle, and GABAergic interneurons can be found within virtually all other CNS regions. These inhibitory interneurons are known to be very important in shaping the behavior of surrounding neurons. Some important interregional projection systems use GABA as their primary neurotransmitter, including the output projections of the striatum, the pallidothalamic and nigrothalamic projections, and the Purkinje cell output from the cerebellar cortex to the deep cerebellar nuclei.

GABA interacts with two types of receptors to induce biologic effects—the $GABA_A$ and $GABA_B$ receptors. The $GABA_A$ receptor is the predominant mediator of fast synaptic inhibition and, like the glycine receptor, is a ligand gated chloride channel whose activation produces hyperpolarization and increased membrane conductance.[14] The $GABA_A$ receptor belongs to the same superfamily of receptors as the glycine, nicotine cholinergic, and $5-HT_3$ receptors. In addition to signifi-

cant sequence similarity, $GABA_A$ receptors are probably composed of five subunits in a pentameric configuration surrounding a central pore, and each subunit is predicted to have a similar tertiary structure with four transmembrane domains. As with the glycine receptor, there are multiple types of subunits; to date 6 α, 4 β, 3 γ, 1 δ and 2 ρ subunits have been cloned. Further heterogeneity exists because one of the β and one of the γ subunits have alternative splice variants. Given a probable pentameric configuration and the large number of subunit subtypes, there are thousands of potential $GABA_A$ receptor isoforms. It is highly likely that only a restricted number of the potential combinations exist in vivo. Studies of $GABA_A$ receptor subunit expression indicate that different subunit subtypes have unique, though sometimes overlapping, patterns of expression both across and within CNS regions. Within individual neurons, it is thought that there are favored combinations of subunit subtypes. The identification of the combinations composing native $GABA_A$ receptors is a very active area of investigation.

$GABA_A$ receptors possess a very complex pharmacology. The $GABA_A$ receptor exemplifies ligand gated ionophores with multiple sites for receptor regulation. The receptor possesses two agonist binding sites for GABA itself, and pharmacologists have identified a number of agonist and antagonist compounds active at these sites. The prototype competitive antagonist is bicuculline. In addition, there are several sites that allosterically modify the ability of $GABA_A$ receptors to respond to GABA. These include a site for barbiturates, which act to enhance GABA evoked currents, a so-called convulsant site for picrotoxins and related compounds that act to inhibit receptor function, a neurosteroid site where compounds such as alphaxalone act to potentiate receptor function, and a zinc site, where divalent cations act to inhibit receptor function. The most clinically important site is the benzodiazepine site. Classical benzodiazepines act at this site to enhance the action of GABA. Additional compounds have been described as benzodiazepine antagonists, of which the prototype is flumazenil, and yet another class of compounds that act as inverse agonists, such as the β-carbolines. More recent pharmacologic studies established the existence of benzodiazepine receptor subtypes, the existence of GABA receptors insensitive to classical benzodiazepines but sensitive to so-called atypical benzodiazepines such as RO 15-4513, and even receptors insensitive to benzodiazepines.

One of the exciting results of cloning $GABA_A$ receptor subtypes has been increased understanding of the complex pharmacology exhibited by $GABA_A$ receptors. Action of GABA, barbiturates, and picrotoxins requires the presence of both α and β subunits, but heterologous expression of α and β combinations alone produces benzodiazepine-insensitive receptors. Studies of recombinant receptors have shown that the presence of a γ subunit is necessary for benzodiazepine sensitivity. The α subunit composition markedly influences the benzodiazepine response properties of receptors. For example, pharmacologic studies prior to the cloning of GABA$_A$ receptor subunits demonstrated the existence of two types of benzodiazepine receptors, type I and type II, differentiated by affinity for compounds such as zolpidem. The presence of an α_1 subunit confers sensitivity to type I specific compounds, while the presence of α_2, α_3, or α_5 subunits confers sensitivity to type II compounds. The presence of α_6 subunits, which are uniquely expressed by cerebellar granule cells, confers sensitivity to RO 15-4513, and α_4 subunit expression may be responsible for benzodiazepine-insensitive GABA$_A$ receptors. Varying the β receptor subunit seems to produce more subtle effects on GABA sensitivity and receptor kinetics. The role of the δ subunit remains to be clarified and ρ subunits are expressed solely within the retina where they may be involved in the formation of a GABA$_A$-like GABA$_C$ receptor.

While the composition of native GABA$_A$ receptors remains to be determined it is likely that different isoforms will have different properties, raising the possibility that development of isoform-specific drugs will be feasible. Given the additional fact that subunits have unique patterns of expression across and within brain regions, some native isoforms may have expression restricted to specific CNS neuron populations, and isoform-specific drugs could possess exceptionally high therapeutic indices.

The other major GABA receptor is the GABA$_B$ receptor, a G-protein-coupled receptor linked to a variety of effector mechanisms.[16] GABA$_B$ receptors are known to inhibit adenylyl cyclase, potentiate the stimulation of adenylyl cyclase produced by other neurotransmitters, inhibit neuronal voltage-dependent calcium channels, and activate some neuronal potassium channels. Less is known about GABA$_B$ receptor function, but postsynaptic GABA$_B$ receptor activation does produce a degree of membrane hyperpolarization while presynaptic GABA$_B$ receptor activation inhibits neurotransmitter release. One clinically useful drug, baclofen, is known to be a specific GABA$_B$ receptor agonist. Thalamic GABA$_B$ receptor activation is thought to be a component of the pathophysiology of absence epilepsy, and GABA$_B$ receptors are now targets of development as novel anticonvulsants.[17]

GLUTAMATE

The amino acid glutamate is thought to be the predominant excitatory neurotransmitter of the CNS.[18] Virtually all CNS neurons express receptors for glutamate, and glutamate is the primary neurotransmitter of a majority of CNS neurons. As for glycine, there are no dedicated pathways for synthesis and degradation of neurotransmitter glutamate. Instead, neurotransmitter glutamate is probably drawn from pools of glutamate used to satisfy other metabolic and synthetic needs. Inactivation of synaptic glutamate takes place via high-affinity glutamate transporters located on both glia and neurons that remove glutamate from the extracellular space. Glia play a key role in glutamate metabolism, both by virtue of participating in glutamate uptake from the synaptic cleft and by converting glutamate to glutamine for recycling back to nerve terminals where it can participate in neurotransmission, either as glutamate itself or as a precursor for GABA (see above).

While the consensus is that glutamate is the primary excitatory amino acid neurotransmitter, it is possible that related molecules may play a role in excitatory amino acid neurotransmission. Aspartate, cysteine sulfinic acid, and some dipeptides have also been suggested to be endogenous neurotransmitters active at glutamate receptors. The best single piece of evidence that glutamate itself is the primary excitatory amino acid neurotransmitter is the fact that glutamate is the highly preferred substrate of the transporter responsible for concentrating excitatory amino acids within synaptic vesicles.[19] Nonetheless, it is possible that some of these other candidate molecules could play a role in neurotransmission in some brain regions. There are also glia-derived molecules such as homocysteic acid and the endogenous tryptophan metabolites quinolinic acid and kynurenic acid that possess significant activity at glutamate receptors.[20] These compounds could play a role in physiologic signaling and could be involved in some pathophysiologic processes (see Chap. 16, Excitotoxicity).

Among the neuronal systems documented to use glutamate as their primary neurotransmitter are corticofugal neurons, including the corticospinal, corticobulbar, corticostriatal, and corticothalamic pathways. Corticocortical neurons also use glutamate as their primary neurotransmitter, as to thalamocortical afferents. Other important systems using glutamate as a neurotransmitter include the olivocerebellar and pontocerebellar pathways, cerebellar granule cells, and primary sensory afferents.

Glutamate produces its synaptic effects by interacting with a variety of glutamate (or excitatory amino acid) receptors. Like GABA, serotonin, and acetylcholine, glutamate activates both ionotropic and G-protein-coupled receptors, the latter referred to as metabotropic glutamate receptors (mGluRs). Pharmacologic studies based on the use of selective agonists suggested the existence of three classes of ionotropic glutamate receptors termed α-amino-3-hydroxy-5-methyl-4-

isoxazole-proprionic acid (AMPA) receptors, kainic acid (KA) receptors, and *N*-methyl-D-asparate (NMDA) receptors. This agonist-based classification scheme was initially somewhat controversial but has been largely vindicated by molecular cloning studies. As with GABA_A receptors, molecular cloning has revealed previously unsuspected heterogeneity. Another interesting result of molecular cloning is the realization that ionotropic glutamate receptors are not members of the receptor superfamily comprising glycine, GABA_A, and nicotinic cholinergic receptors. Ionotropic glutamate receptors lack significant sequence homology with the GABA_A superfamily, and recent studies indicate that glutamate receptor proteins have a markedly different tertiary structure with a large N-terminus and 3, rather than 4, transmembrane domain.[21,22]

Cloning studies have shown that each class of ionotropic glutamate receptor comprises a number of subunit subtypes that preferentially assemble within their own family to produce functional receptors.[23-27] The AMPA receptor family comprises 4 subunit subtypes termed GluR1–4, all of which have a unique regional distribution within the brain. While expression of homomers produces functional AMPA receptors, in vivo or native AMPA receptors are thought to be heteromers. The precise subunit composition of heteromers significantly influences the physiologic properties of AMPA receptors. AMPA receptors lacking a GluR2 subunit are permeated by both monovalent cations and calcium, while addition of GluR2 subunits blocks calcium permeability. Native AMPA receptors are generally not calcium-permeable, and most in vivo AMPA receptors are assumed to contain GluR2 subunits, though their stoichiometry is not known. Additional AMPA receptor heterogeneity is conferred by the existence of splice variants of all 4 AMPA subunit mRNAs. Whimsically termed *flip* and *flop*, the expression of splice variants is regulated in the course of normal brain development, and splice variants differ in sensitivity to agonists and kinetic properties. Another remarkable feature of AMPA receptors is the existence of RNA editing of GluR2 subunits. The ion selectivity of GluR2 subunits is controlled by a single amino acid at a site within one of the probable transmembrane domains. In GluR1 and GluR3, this is occupied by a glutamine and in GluR2, by an arginine. Experimental site-directed mutagenesis of GluR2 with subsitution of glutamine for arginine at this site results in calcium-permeable GluR2 subunits. Sequencing of GluR2 genomic DNA disclosed a codon for glutamine at this crucial position, while the mature GluR mRNA has an arginine codon, indicating that this codon is posttranscriptionally modified from a glutamine codon to an arginine codon. The pharmacology of AMPA receptors is relatively straightforward, with small groups of competitive agonists and antagonists identified. There are indications that some allosteric sites of potential clinical usefulness exist as well. AMPA receptors possess a zinc site whose activation potentiates receptor activation and a site for 2,3-benzodiazepine compounds whose activation inhibits receptor function. AMPA receptor activation is implicated in the pathogenesis of hypoxic/ischemic brain injury, and AMPA receptor antagonists may prove useful in mitigating the effects of focal and global ischemia.

Molecular cloning has also revealed the existence of several KA receptor subunits. Five subunits have been identified to data, termed GluR5, 6, 7 and KA1, 2. These subunits probably form heteromers in vivo to produce functional KA receptors. As with AMPA receptors there are presumed to be preferential combinations of subunits with somewhat different physiologic properties. KA subunit subtypes all have unique regional distributions, and the properties of KA receptors probably vary across regions as a function of which KA receptor subunit subtypes are expressed with given neurons and regions. RNA editing and alternative splicing also occur with some KA receptor subunits, and the RNA editing is even more complicated than in AMPA/GluR2 subunits. The involved KA subunits possess two edited sites, and these sites are differentially edited in the course of normal development and across regions, providing another source of KA receptor heterogeneity.

The last class of ionotropic glutamate receptors are the NMDA receptors. In addition to pharmacology, these receptors have several features that distinguish them from AMPA and KA receptors. Unlike most AMPA and KA receptors, all NMDA receptors are permeated by calcium in addition to sodium and potassium. This property allows NMDA receptors to influence profoundly the regulation of signal transduction and other intracellular processes. NMDA receptor activation also has a slower time course of activation and inactivation than AMPA or KA receptors. Whereas AMPA and KA currents are generated very rapidly and decay over the course of tens of milliseconds, NMDA currents have a time course of activation and inactivation in the hundreds of milliseconds range. A last unique property is the voltage-dependent nature of NMDA receptor activation. At normal resting membrane potential, the pores of NMDA receptors are physically blocked by magnesium ions. With membrane depolarization, magnesium ions cease to occlude pores, and upon agonist binding, NMDA receptor/ionophore complexes can flux calcium and monovalent cations. Consequently, NMDA receptors are probably activated only when there is a coincidence of membrane depolarization (most commonly from activation of AMPA and/or KA receptors) and sufficient ambient glutamate to interact with the agonist binding site. NMDA receptors also possess multiple allosteric sites for modulation of receptor function. In addition to the agonist glutamate site, there is also a so-called coagonist site for glycine, whose occupation is obligatory for receptor activation. Ambient extracellular glycine levels are probably sufficiently high to saturate this site under normal conditions, and this site is probably not one of normal physiologic regulation of NMDA receptor function. Some compounds, however, have been developed that interact with this glycine site, and NMDA/glycine antagonists may be clinically useful in the treatment of seizures and to prevent excitotoxic insult (see Chap. 16). Other sites which possess endogenous ligands are sites for zinc, activation of which inhibits receptor function, and another site for polyamines, whose activation potentiates receptor activation. Another site of considerable pharmacologic interest is the dissociative anesthetic or phencyclidine site. This site is probably within the channel formed by receptors, and this class of compounds produces open channel blockade of receptor function. Some of the clinical effects of these compounds are mediated by their action at NMDA receptors. All of these NMDA receptor-associated sites are the targets of drug development to produce clinically useful NMDA receptor antagonists.

Molecular cloning has revealed the existence of two types of NMDA receptor subunits. NMDAR1 forms homomeric functional receptors possessing all the functional properties of NMDA receptors. Several splice variants of NMDAR1 have been described with differences in pharmacologic characteristics and marked differences in regional/neuronal expression. A second class of NMDA receptor subunits are termed NMDAR2A, B, C, D. When expressed as homomers or as NMDAR2 heteromers, this class of subunits has no receptor activity. When expressed with NMDAR1, however, functional receptors result, and the combination of NMDAR1-NMDAR2X produces receptors with larger currents than NMDAR1 homomers. NMDAR2 subunits each possess unique regional patterns of expression within the CNS, and the various NMDAR1-NMDAR2X combinations exhibit differences in kinetic and pharmacologic properties, resulting in considerable variation in NMDA receptors between regions and specific types of neurons.

The voltage dependency, relatively slow time course of activation and inactivation, and calcium permeability of NMDA receptors confer properties intermediate between the very fast neurotransmission mediated by other ligand gated ionophores and the G-protein-coupled receptors whose chief effects are slower and more chronic modulation of neuronal functions. NMDA receptors are suggested to function as "molecular coinci-dence detectors," since their activation requires the simultaneous presence of membrane depolarization and agonist occupancy of the glutamate site. Their relatively prolonged duration of opening and calcium permeability allow them to influence intracellular calcium, a key modulator of many cellular processes, and to trigger potentially long duration changes in neuronal function. Activation of NMDA receptors appears to be a crucial event in the phenomenon of long-term potentiation (LTP), an increasing feature of neurotransmission best described at certain hippocampal synapses.[28] In LTP, specific patterns of relatively high-frequency neurotransmission produce long-lasting increases in synaptic efficiency. There is great interest in LTP as a potential synaptic substrate of learning, memory, and other forms of neuronal plasticity. While a number of forms of LTP have been described, some forms require NMDA receptor activation for induction of long-lasting increases in synaptic efficiency. The coincidence of glutamate release by afferent terminals and postsynaptic depolarization by AMPA and/or KA receptors is thought to lead to calcium influx via NMDA receptors and consequent long-lasting changes in neuronal function.

The final group of glutamate receptors are the G-protein-coupled class of glutamate receptors (mGluRs).[29] These receptors belong to their own family of G-protein-coupled receptors; they share the 7 transmembrane domain motif of other G-protein-coupled receptors but have relatively little homology in terms of primary structure and some unique features of tertiary structure. As with other G-protein-coupled receptors, mGluRs are coupled to several signal transduction mechanisms. These include stimulation of the IP_3/DAG cascade, inhibition of adenylyl cyclase, potentiation of the stimulation of adenylyl cyclase by other neurotransmitters, and modulation of ion channels. The pharmacology of mGluRs is still in its infancy.

Molecular cloning has revealed the existence of eight mGluR subtypes, presently partitioned into three subclasses on the basis of sequence homology, pharmacology, and interaction with specific signal transduction mechanisms. Type I mGluRs (mGluR1 and mGluR5) are linked to stimulation of phospholipase C and the IP_3/DAG cascade, and the most potent agonist is quisqualate. Type II (mGluR2 and mGluR3) and Type III (mGluR4, mGluR6, mGluR7, and mGluR8) mGluRs are both linked to inhibition of adenylyl cyclase, but IS,3R-ACPD is a potent agonist for type II mGluRs, while L-AP4 selectively activates type III mGluRs. Each mGluR subtype has a unique regional and cellular distribution. mGluR6, for example, is uniquely expressed by retinal bipolar cells, and mGluR3 is expressed by both neurons and glia in some regions. Alternative splicing of mGluR1 and mGluR5 confers somewhat different properties on the resulting iso-forms, and splice variants have unique regional distributions, adding further to mGluR heterogeneity.

MONOAMINES

Many biochemical, pharmacologic, and neuroanatomic features of neurons employing dopamine (DA), norepinephrine (NE), and serotonin (5-hydroxytryptamine, 5HT) provide a common frame for discussion. It is characteristic of all three systems that there are discrete, brain stem nuclear origins leading to widespread rostrocaudal projections throughout the CNS. In addition, the specific aspects of individual monoamine neurotransmitter metabolism closely parallel one another with identical enzymes and transporters for some steps in the production and storage of the different monamine neurotransmitters.

Biosynthesis of the monoamine transmitters is from amino acid precursors (tyrosine for DA and NE, tryptophan for 5HT), which are transported across the blood-brain barrier endothelia and into the neuron by the large neutral amino acid carrier system. Initial metabolism is by hydroxylation; tyrosine to L-dopa or tryptophan to 5-hydroxytryptophan, catalyzed by tyrosine hydroxylase (TH) and tryptophan hydroxylase, respectively. The activities of these synthetic enzymes are specific for the presence of monoaminergic neurons, and each serves as a key regulatory point in the synthesis of either catecholamines (DA and NE) or serotonin, since the activities of TH and tryptophan hydroxylase are each rate-limiting for neurotransmitter synthesis. The activity and stability of TH are regulated by its state of phosphorylation, under the negative feedback control of presynaptic dopamine receptors. Thus, elevated demand for DA release may be biochemically translated to a parallel increase in the rate of its synthesis.

After hydroxlation, both L-dopa and 5-hydroxytryptophan are next decarboxylated to form DA and 5HT, respectively. The enzyme responsible for this step in catecholaminergic neurons, dopa decarboxylase, is indistinguishable from that in serotonin and other monoaminergic neurons, and is probably identical with the aromatic amino acid decarboxylase which is distributed widely in nonneural cells. Thus, although requisite for transmitter synthesis, decarboxylase enzymes are not substrate-specific, nor are they indicators of monoaminergic neuronal populations. In noradrenergic neurons, dopamine is further metabolized to norepinephrine by the action of doapmine-β-hydroxylase. This enzyme activity is unique to noradrenergic and adrenergic neurons in the CNS, in the sympathetic PNS, and in adrenal medullary chromaffin cells.

The monoamine transmitters are accumulated from the neuronal cytoplasm into synaptic vesicles by active transport. The vesicular monoamine transporters (VMAT) have been successfully isolated and cloned, revealing the existence of two isoforms, VMAT1 and VMAT2.[30] Both are highly homologous and share considerable similarity with the vesicular acetylcholine transporter (see below) as well. VMAT2 is the transporter found in monoaminergic neurons, including serotonergic, dopaminergic, and noradrenergic cells. VMAT1 is localized to adrenal chromaffin cells and has a distinct pharmacologic profile in comparison with VMAT2. While both VMAT1 and VMAT2 are inhibited almost irreversibly by reserpine, tetrabenazine (used in Europe to treat chorea and other hyperkinetic movement disorders) is a very-high-affinity competitive inhibitor of VMAT2 and a weak inhibitor of VMAT1 activity.

After exocytotic release into the synaptic cleft, the monoamine transmitters are inactivated largely through the actions of transmitter-specific, presynaptic transmembrane reuptake transporters. These transporters reaccumulate transmitter into the presynaptic neural cytoplasm, not only participating in termination of synaptic neurotransmitter effect, but contributing substantially to recycling of monoamines into neurotransmitter pools. The presynaptic reuptake transporters are biochemically and structurally distinct from the vesicular transporters. The vesicular transporters derive energy for transmitter concentration from a transvesicular electrochemical proton gradient, while the reuptake sites are sodium countertransporters. Specific DA, NE, and 5-HT reuptake transporters have been isolated on the basis of molecular cloning techniques. Each of the expressed reuptake sites demonstrates considerable selectivity for only one of the monoamines. This selectivity provides a biochemical mechanism for the exclusion of NE and 5-HT from DA presynaptic terminals.

In addition to presynaptic reuptake, the monoamine neurotransmitters are degraded via the actions of two enzymes: catechol-O-methyl transferase (COMT) and monoamine oxidase (MAO). COMT is located in a wide variety of cells and is presumably involved in the metabolism of catechols and related biochemicals outside of monoaminergic neurons. MAO is associated with mitochrondrial membranes and exists in two isoforms, designated types A (MAO-A) and B(MAO-B). The isoforms have distinct cellular expression and pharmacology. MAO-A has higher affinity for 5HT and NE than for DA, and in some species appears to be preferentially associated with dopaminergic and other monoaminergic neurons. MAO-B is expressed at high levels by nonneural cells, particularly astrocytes. The suicide substrate inhibitors clorgyline and deprenyl preferentially alkylate and inactivate MAO-A and MAO-B, respectively. The oxidative metablism of monoamines, particularly by MAO-B, has been the subject of intensive investigation in neurodegenerative syndromes such as Parkinson's and Alzheimer's diseases, since the neurotoxic effect of the dopaminergic neuronal protoxin MPTP has been shown to require metabolism to the reactive species MPP$^+$ via the action of MAO-B. Unfortunately, current evidence does not support the role of MAO-B metabolites in the development and progression of the neurodegenerative human diseases.

Beyond the general features described above, there are specific aspects of the individual dopaminergic, serotonergic, noradrenergic, and other monoamine systems, as described in the following sections.

DOPAMINE

Dopamine neurons and projections in the mammalian central nervous system are few and relatively discrete in distribution. The predominant population of dopaminergic neurons resides in the ventral midbrain, consisting of the substantia nigra pars compacta and the adjacent ventral tegmental area. Projections from the nigra, through the medial forebrain bundle, terminate predominantly within the striatum of the ipsilateral hemisphere; there may be a smaller contralateral (crossed) projection as well. Ascending projections from the ventral tegmental area innervate the anteromesial aspect of the striatal complex, particularly the nucleus accumbens septi. Terminals of these projections additionally innervate other aspects of the basal ganglia, including the olfactory tubercle as well as the amygdala, cerebral cortex, and hippocampal formation. Minor populations of dopaminergic interneurons are identified within the retina, the olfactory bulb, and hypothalamus. Dopamine neurons in the arcuate nucleus of the hypothalamus project to the pituitary and regulate the secretion of prolactin.

Biochemical markers which distinguish dopaminergic nerve terminals from those of other monoaminergic neurons include TH enzyme activity and the presynaptic DA reuptake transporter. The former is not entirely specific, since TH is expressed both in DA and in NE neurons. The presynaptic DA reuptake site, however, is unique to the DA neuronal phenotype. Several drugs in clinical and research use bind to and block the transporter, providing opportunity for clinical interventions and for binding assays to determine presynaptic terminal distribution. The anticholinergic benztropine has low affinity for the transporter, methylphenidate and amphetamine have higher affinity, while the investigational drugs mazindol and nomifensine have highest (nanomolar) affinity for the DA and for the distinct, but related NE presynaptic reuptake transporters. Cocaine and its structural relative WIN 35,428 also bind to the DA reuptake site with very high affinity and additionally interact with the related 5HT reuptake site. The ligands with best selectivity for DA over NE and 5HT presynaptic reuptake sites are from the GBR series, including GBR 12935 and GBR 12909.

Dopamine receptors are most abundant in the striatum (including caudate, putamen, accumbens, and olfactory tubercle) and in the anterior pituitary. Smaller populations are identified in the cerebral cortex and other forebrain regions receiving innervation listed above. Molecular biologic studies reveal that the prior pharmacologic partitioning of dopamine receptors into D1 and D2 types, on the basis of selective binding and differential agonist effects on adenylate cyclase activity, does not account for the full complexity of dopamine receptors expressed in the mammalian brain. There are five distinct dopamine receptor genes, designated d1 through d5, each of which belongs to the 7-transmembrane-G-linked receptor superfamily.[31] As such, the dopamine receptors are involved in "slow" neuromodulatory transmission. The D1 receptors defined pharmacologically consist of the d1 and d5 molecular subtypes, and are linked to stimulation of adenylyl cyclase. The d1 receptor is found postsynaptically in the striatum and cerebral cortex. d5 receptor distribution is less well characterized, but mRNA hybridization studies suggest that neurons in the striatum, thalamus, and hippocampus may express the site. The D2 pharmacologic receptors correspond to the d2, d3, and d4 molecular subtypes, and are linked to inhibition of adenylyl cyclase. The most abundant striatal receptor is d2, which is located postsynaptically on striatal neurons and terminals as well as on presynaptic dopaminergic terminals, functioning as an autoreceptor. The d3 receptor subtype is concentrated postsynaptically in the limbic ventral striatum and is found at lower levels in the dorsal striatum, cerebral cortex, hippocampus, amygdala, and cerebellum. Preliminary studies suggest that the d4 subtype is found diffusely throughout the forebrain, including the striatum and cerebral cortex, at relatively low expression levels. Much of the evidence for an important role of dopamine in psychosis and in extrapyramidal movement disorders comes from clinical observations that classical antipsychotic drugs such as chlorpromazine and haloperidol occupy a substantial fraction of D2 receptors at their empirically determined therapeutic dosages, and that parkinsonism is a frequent complicating side effect of antipsychotic treatment, particularly in elderly patients. Recent evidence from the discovery of the "atypical" neuroleptic clozapine suggests that antipsychotic drug effects may not necessitate blockade of all D2-type receptors. Clozapine is effective in treatment of schizophrenia at doses that may preferentially block the d4 (and perhaps d3) versus the d2 subtype, and it does not produce worsening of extrapyramidal symptoms even in patients with Parkinson's disease. Thus, extrapyramidal motor effects may be predominantly modulated by dorsal striatal d2 receptors, while antipsychotic drugs may exert therapeutic effects on limbic d3 or on striatal and cortical d4 receptor sites.

NOREPINEPHRINE

Noradrenergic neurons in the central nervous system are found in the dorsal pons in the locus ceruleus (LC) and scattered in the ventrolateral brainstem tegmentum. Projections from these nuclei ascend to innervate almost all forebrain structures, including the cerebral cortex and hippocampus, the basal ganglia, and thalamus, and are particularly concentrated in the ventral thalamus and hypothalamus. Additional projections from the LC innervate brain stem and cerebellum, and descending projections terminate in the spinal cord. Thus, with a few areas of relative concentration, NE neurons from the pons project diffusely throughout the neuroaxis. Additional minor cell groups in the pons and medulla are putatively adrenergic (employing epinephrine as a transmitter), based on additional localization of the enzyme phenethanolamine-N-methyltransferase in the cell body. The adrenergic neurons are interspersed within the ventrolateral tegmental NE neurons and are concentrated in the nucleus of the solitary tract (nST). Projections from these putative adrenergic neurons appear restricted to hypothalamic and brain stem sites, including innervation of the dorsal vagal nucleus by nST terminals. In part related to the very widespread distribution of NE innervation, it has been difficult to establish clear behavioral correlates of NE action in the brain. There is evidence that some symptomatic aspects of the affective disorders, including depression and anxiety, may be in part mediated by NE; however, emerging data implicate 5HT to an equivalent or greater extent in these instances.

Specific markers that distinguish NE neurons and presynaptic terminals are TH enzyme activity (shared by DA neurons as well, see above), dopamine-β-hydroxylase activity, and the presynaptic NE reuptake site. The reuptake site is blocked by several drugs including tricyclic antidepressants, methylphenidate, and cocaine, as well as by investigational ligands such as nomifensine and mazindol. The agent with highest selectivity for NE over the 5HT and DA transporters is nisoxitine, although its lipophilic character and the low abundance of NE reuptake sites in most brain regions have limited development of a quantitative binding assay.

Receptors for NE are of three classes: α_1, α_2, and β.[32] All three groups are of the G-protein-linked 7-transmembrane receptor superfamily, indicating a neuromodulatory role for NE in the brain. Available drugs and research assay ligands discriminate the classes of NE receptors from one another, and provide some clues to the existence of heterogeneity of sites within the identified classes. However, as in the instances of many molecularly defined receptor families, available ligands do not adequately discriminate the individual members of the three classes. RNA hybridization studies have been employed to map the distributions of cells and neurons expressing NE receptor mRNA, but detailed analyses of receptor protein distributions using specific immunochemistry and ligand binding will be needed for comprehensive understanding of receptor distributions and function in the brain. The α_1 class of receptors consists of three identified subtypes, designated α_{1A} through α_{1C} (α_{1A}, α_{1B}, and α_{1D} in an alternative nomenclature), each of which has a subnanomolar affinity for the drug prazosin. All apparently favor coupling to the Gq effector protein with resulting activation of phospholipase C, increasing a Ca^{2+} channel conductance after α_{1A} stimulation and stimulating inositol phospholipid turnover after activation of α_{1B} and α_{1C} receptors. The α_2 receptors consist of subtypes designated α_{2A} through α_{2C}, which couple to the effector protein Gi, resulting in inhibition of adenylyl cyclase. They are identified by nanomolar affinity for the drugs yohimbine and rauwolscine, and are a presumed site of action of the α_2 agonist drug clonidine. In addition to serving at postsynaptic sites, the α_{2C} receptor functions as an inhibitory autoreceptor on NE neurons, including central nervous system terminals in the cerebral cortex. The β receptors, characterized by high-affinity interaction with propranolol, consist of the β_1 through β_3 subtypes, each of which appears to preferentially couple through Gi to the inhibition of adenylate cyclase activity. There are molecular hybridization and radioligand binding data to suggest that all nine of the NE receptors are expressed in mammalian brain; however, the detailed mapping of individual subtypes is presently unestablished, and awaits the development and application of selective ligands or receptor-specific antibodies.

SEROTONIN

The distribution of serotonergic neurons in the mammalian brain is restricted to nuclei within the midline brain stem tegmentum, predominantly within the reticular formation of the midbrain and pons. These neurons send ascending projections to the forebrain, terminating diffusely in the cerebral cortex and hippocampus, the basal ganglia, thalamus, hypothalamus, and the cerebellum. Medullary reticular formation serotonin neurons project caudally to other medullary nuclei and to the spinal cord. The anatomic features of the serotonergic system are quite similar to, and overlapping with, those of the noradrenergic system.

Owing in part to the widespread distribution of serotonergic innervation, anatomy alone does not suggest particular clinical or behavioral effects that might be mediated by 5HT. However, a rich psychopharmacologic literature provides insight into a number of potential 5HT actions. Serotonergic effects on higher sensory processing and perception are suggested by the actions of the hallucinogen LSD, which stimulates a subset of 5HT receptors and alters activity in the raphe neurons. Similar effects were historically reported following ergot poisoning which is, again, attributable to interactions between the ergot alkaloids and 5HT receptors. More recently, actions of "atypical" antipsychotics have been attributed to blockade of 5HT receptor subsets, rather than to DA receptor antagonism alone. Aspects of affective psychiatric syndromes including depression, anxiety, and obsessive-compulsive disorder may prominently involve 5HT systems since new selective 5HT reuptake inhibitors are at least as efficacious in these settings as the pharmacologically less-specific tricyclic antidepressants. Finally, a role for antinociceptive aspects of 5HT transmission is suggested by cellular physiologic studies which indicate that descending 5HT fibers may influence the spinal processing and central conduction of painful sensory stimuli. The clinical benefit of tricyclic antidepressants in chronic somatic pain syndromes is attributed in part to modulation of this system.

As in the instances of DA and NE neurons, there are specific biochemical markers that serve to distinguish 5HT neurons and synapses from those of other monoaminergic cells. The enzyme tryptophan hydroxylase, although analogous to tyrosine hydroxylase in its action, is a distinct protein with unique substrate specificity, preferring conversion of tryptophan to 5-hydroxytryptophan (5HTP) over metabolism of tyrosine. There is also preliminary evidence suggesting that 5HTP conversion to 5HT may be mediated by a decarboxylase distinct from dopa decarboxylase. Finally, in parallel with the previously discussed monoamine synapses, there is a unique presynaptic 5HT reuptake site, which favors transport of 5HT over other monoamines. Serotonin reuptake is inhibited by most of the tricyclic antidepressants; however, they are not specific for the 5HT site, demonstrating variable cross-inhibition of the NE reuptake site as well. Highly selective 5HT reuptake inhibitors have been recently introduced for treatment of depression, including fluoxetine, sertraline, and paroxetine.

Serotonin receptors are more numerous and varied in their functional coupling than are the receptors for the other monoamine transmitters.[33] To date, over 25 putative 5HT receptors have been cloned from a variety of species. Some of the complexity of the present nomenclature likely results from differing designations of cognate receptor clones isolated from different species; however, the diversity of 5HT receptors within individual species still exceeds that of the other monoaminergic receptors. Serotonin receptors are presently classified into seven classes, designated 5HT1 through 5HT7. As in the instances of the DA and NE receptors, this diversity is recognized on the basis of multiple genes and mRNA species encoding the various receptors, rather than by ligand binding assays or immunochemical methods for distinguishing the receptor proteins themselves. The 5HT1 receptor family consists of sites designated 5HT1A, 5HT1B, 5HT1D, 5HT1E, and 5HT1F. They preferentially couple to the Gi protein, resulting in reduction of adenylyl cyclase activity. The anxiolytic activity of the nonbenzodiazepine buspirone is attributed to partial agonist activity at the 5HT1A receptor, and the recently introduced migraine abortive sumatriptan is an agonist at the 5HT1D through 5HT1F receptor sites. The 5HT2 family consists of three subtypes, designated 5HT2A through 5HT2C, all of which preferentially couple via Gq to stimulate inositol phospholipid turnover. The 5HT3 receptor is unique in that it is a ligand-gated ion channel, structurally related to the nicotinic ACh and $GABA_A$ receptors, rather than the 7-transmembrane G-protein-linked superfamily to which all other identified 5HT receptors belong. The 5HT3 receptor is a cation channel, mediating depolarization and neuronal excitation on activation similar to the nicotinic ACh receptors. It is blocked by the novel, centrally acting, antiemetic ondansetron. The 5HT4, 5HT6, and 5HT7 receptors are each represented at present by single genes, and the expressed proteins all preferentially couple to Gs, resulting in increased adenylyl cyclase activity upon stimulation. The 5HT5 receptor family consists of three subtypes, 5HT5A through 5HT5C, which have yet unidentified chemical effector linkages. Most, if not all, 5HT receptors are likely to be expressed in the mammalian brain, on the basis of mRNA analyses. However, the precise cellular localizations and functions of individual subtypes are not yet elucidated.

HISTAMINE

The role of histamine as a transmitter in the central nervous system has been controversial for many years. In part, difficulty in clearly establishing its role has been the recognition that a substantial portion of brain histamine content is attributable to perivascular mast cells, rather than to neural elements. Recently, compelling evidence for histaminergic neurons and projections has been obtained from converging lines of evidence.[34] Mechanical lesions of the medial forebrain bundle result in substantial reductions of forebrain histamine. Immunochemical mapping studies, with antibodies directed against histamine itself or the synthetic enzyme histadine decarboxylase, indicate dense fiber staining in the hypothalamic regions as well as an apparent histaminergic fiber projection ascending from posterior hypothalamic neurons through the ipsilateral median forebrain bundle.

Histamine receptors are presently designated H1, H2, and H3, and are presumably all expressed in mammalian brain. The H1 receptor stimulates inositol phospholipid turnover via Gq linkage, while the H2 receptor couples to Gs, increasing adenylyl cyclase activity upon activation. The H3 receptor apparently functions as an inhibitory presynaptic autoreceptor, but its second-messenger linkage is not yet established.

ACETYLCHOLINE

The first discovered neurotransmitter was acetylcholine (ACh), identified by Otto Loewi by virtue of its effects on isolated frog heart preparation after stimulation of the vagus nerve. In addition to serving as the neurotransmitter at the vertebrate neuromuscular junction, ACh is the primary neurotransmitter of the parasympathetic autonomic nervous system. In the CNS, ACh is used by a minority of neurons, constituting several discrete projection systems and a few interneuronal populations. Despite its limited prevalence at CNS synapses, ACh is involved in many critical aspects of brain function. However, the more abundant and "pure" preparations of cholinergic neurons obtainable from autonomic ganglia, neuromuscular junctions, and the electric organ of the eel *Torpedo californicus* have led to the discovery of most of the cholinergic biochemistry and pharmacology principles from these peripheral tissues. More recent studies have permitted verification of the key aspects of cholinergic transmission within the CNS as well.

The distribution of cholinergic neurons in the mammalian nervous system includes discrete spinal cord and brain stem nuclei where lower motor neurons and preganglionic sympathetic and parasympathetic neurons are concentrated. In addition to these neurons, the postganglionic parasympathetic neurons are cholinergic. CNS cholinergic neurons are located in two brain stem nuclei, the pontine laterodorsal tegmental nucleus (ldtn) and the peduculopontine tegmental nucleus (ppn). These brain stem nuclei provide cholinergic projections terminating in the thalamus, hypothalamus, the basal forebrain, the superior colliculus, and caudal brain stem. A second cholinergic projection system is composed of the basal forebrain nuclei, including the nucleus basalis of Meynert (nbM), the diagonal band of Broca (ndB), and the medial septal nucleus

(ms). These nuclei project to the cerebral cortex including neocortices, the hippocampal formation, entorhinal and pyriform cortices, and the olfactory bulb. Finally, there is a substantial population of local cholinergic interneurons in the striatum (caudate, putamen, nucleus accumbens, and olfactory tubercle) and probably minor populations within the hippocampus and cerebral neocortices.

The known CNS cholinergic neurons and projections are associated with a number of clinicopathologic functions. Ascending brain stem cholinergic projections are implicated in the regulation of sleep and arousal.[35] The basal forebrain projection system is hypothesized to play an important role in normal memory and cognition, and is implicated in some of the deficits seen in Alzeheimer's disease, where biochemical analyses demonstrate neocortical and limbic presynaptic cholinergic deficits.[36] The intrinsic striatal cholinergic neurons are involved in regulation of the release of dopamine and its effects on the principal striatal output neurons. There is clinical evidence for a role of striatal cholinergic mechanisms in movement, particularly in Parkinson's disease, where hyperactivity in the cholinergic striatal neurons may underlie the characteristic resting tremor.

Cholinergic synapses are characterized by several unique biochemical pathways underlying the metabolism of ACh. The key enzyme activity in ACh biosynthesis is cholineacetyltransferase (ChAT), which catalyzes the condensation of choline and acetylCoA. Regional brain ChAT activity is nearly synonymous with the presence of presynaptic cholinergic terminals; the enzyme is found exclusively in cholinergic neurons and in the placenta, where its physiologic role is unknown. Choline for ACh synthesis is derived from a minor tissue pool with very high turnover rate in the presynaptic nerve terminal. Active transmembrane transport mediated by a sodium-choline countertransporter is responsible for uptake of choline from the extracellular space into the transmitter pool within nerve terminals. This high-affinity choline uptake (HAChU) transporter is distinct from lower-affinity, sodium-independent choline transporters found in peripheral tissues, in the endothelia of the blood-brain barrier, and additionally in neurons and glia. The HAChU transporter is selectively inhibited by the drug hemicholinium-3, and is uniquely expressed by cholinergic neurons. The source of acetylCoA for ACh synthesis is uncertain, since ChAT and the ACh it produces are cytosolic, yet most acetylCoA is produced in mitochondria. There is some evidence suggesting generation of acetylCoA via the action of a cytoplasmic ATP-citrate lyase in cholinergic neurons to provide the required activated precursor for ACh synthesis.

Following synthesis, ACh is sequestered via active transport in presynaptic vesicles. The vesicular ACh transporter (VAT) has been recently isolated and cloned.[37] It is closely related to the vesicular monoaminergic transporters, not only in the amino acid composition of many segments, but in the nucleic acid sequence of the encoding gene as well. The predicted protein has 12 transmembrane spanning segments, with potential sites for posttranslational phosphorylation and glycosylation. Functional activity of the VAT is inhibited by the drug vesamicol, which binds to VAT, inhibits its transport activity, and whose structural derivatives provide bases for ligand binding assays of VAT density.

Following exocytotic release of vesicular ACh into the synaptic cleft, transmitter is inactivated at cholinergic synapses by the action of the hydrolytic enzyme acetylcholinesterase (AChE). Much of the extracellular choline produced by the action of AChE is reaccumulated into the presynaptic cholinergic nerve terminal by the HAChU transporter. Thus, the combined actions of AChE and HAChU at cholinergic synapses result in the recycling of choline within the ACh neurotransmitter pool. The biochemical importance of this mechanism is underscored by the tight regulation of HAChU and its relationship to ACh synthesis. HAChU is the rate-limiting step in overall synthesis of ACh, and its activity is readily altered by conditions which increase or decrease ACh turnover. Moment-to-moment regulation of the transporter activity appears to result from modifying the number of transporter sites. Action of phospholipase A_2 in presynaptic cholinergic terminals results in a rapid increase in the maximal rate of choline transport and in a parallel increase in the number of transporters determined by the binding of the radiolabeled inhibitor [3H]hemicholinium-3. Thus, there appears to be a pool of cryptic, inactive transporters which can be readily recruited without the delay associated with protein synthesis.

The postsynaptic effects of ACh are transduced by two distinct families of receptors, the nicotinic and muscarinic receptors. The former are ligand-gated cation channels, as are the nicotinic receptors found in peripheral autonomic synapses and at the neuromuscular junction.[38] Nicotinic receptors are heteropentamers of related protein subunits. Distinct genes encode multiple individual members of four-unit families, demonstrating greater within- than between-family structural similarity. Each subunit has a predicted structure which spans the plasma membrane four times, resembling members of the $GABA_A$ and glutamate receptor gated channel subunit families. Functional nicotinic receptor pentamers consist of two α subunits in combination with three from the β, γ, and δ subunit groups; the predominant central neuronal receptor is composed of α_4 and β_2 subunits. When assembled and inserted in the membrane, these heteropentamers serve as ACh-gated cation channels, permitting the passage of sodium and, to lesser extent, potassium ions when stimulated. Nicotinic receptors in the brain, as in the periphery, mediate typical "fast" excitatory neurotransmission. Brain nicotinic receptors are expressed at relatively low levels in comparison with muscarinic receptors. Highest concentrations of nicotinic receptors are found in discrete brain stem nuclei and throughout the thalamus; lower levels are identified in the cerebral cortex and hippocampal formation, where at least some may serve as presynaptic autoreceptors, facilitating further ACh release when activated. Cerebral cortical nicotinic receptors are found reduced in some neurodegenerative disorders, including Alzheimer's and Parkinson's diseases, perhaps related to pathology in presynaptic cholinergic terminals.

The most abundant ACh receptors in the mammalian brain are the five muscarinic ACh receptors (MAChRs).[39] In distinction to nicotinic receptors, MAChRs are members of the G-protein-linked, 7-transmembrane receptor superfamily. They activate "slow" postsynaptic neuromodulatory responses, mediated by chemical second-messenger pathways. Molecular cloning studies have identified distinct genes encoding the receptors designated m1 through m5. In situ mRNA hybridization and immunochemical methods have localized m1, m2, and m4 receptors in major cholinergic projections and synapses. The m3 and m5 receptors in brain have been more difficult to study, owing to lower levels of expression than the other subtypes. The muscarinic receptors are coupled preferentially to distinct biochemical effector pathways, with the m1, m3, and m5 subtypes coupled via the Gq protein to the stimulation of inositol phospholipid turnover. The m2 and m4 subtypes are linked preferentially via Gi to the inhibition of adenylate cyclase activity. In addition to activating different biochemical second messengers, distinct brain regional distributions of MAChR subtypes may serve selectivity of ACh actions. The m1 subtype is predominantly expressed in the forebrain, with highest levels in the striatum, cerebral cortex, and hippocampus. The m2 receptor is distributed throughout the neuroaxis, including the diencephalon, brain stem, and cerebellum. It is highest in concentration and enrichment in the nuclei of cranial motor nuclei, and serves as an inhibitory presynaptic autoreceptor on basal forebrain projections to the cerebral cortex and hippocampus. The m4 receptor is found at highest levels in the striatum, where it may account for as much as 50 percent of the total

TABLE 15-1
An Incomplete List of Neuropeptides

ACTH	Neurotensin
Angiotensin	Neuropeptide Y
Atrial natriuretic polypeptide	Opioid peptides
Calcitonin and calcitonin gene-related product	Oxytocin
	Somatostatin
Cholecystokinin	Tachykinins
Corticotropin-releasing factor	Thyrotropin-releasing hormone
Galanin	Vasoactive intestinal polypeptide
Gonadotropin-releasing hormone	
	Vasopression

MAChR. It is additionally found throughout the cerebral cortex and hippocampus, and at lower levels in the diencephalon.

NEUROPEPTIDES

One of the most important discoveries in neuroscience of the past 20 years was the realization that numerous peptides play neurotransmitter/neuromodulator roles within the CNS (Table 15-1). Several families of peptide neurotransmitters/hormones are represented within the CNS, and all have certain basic features in common. First of all, these neuropeptides are never the sole neurotransmitter of their neuronal populations. In every known case, neuropeptides are expressed in neurons that also use another neurotransmitter—glutamate, GABA, monoamines, acetylcholine. Indeed, more than one type of neuropeptide may be expressed by a given type of neuron. The coexistence of numerous neurotransmitter molecules within a single neuron demonstrates that neurotransmission, even at the level of a single synapse, probably has a formidably complex character. There is also evidence that conventional neurotransmitters and neuropeptides may be at least partially segregated within different pools of synaptic vesicles and be released under somewhat different conditions, for example, differing frequencies of neuron stimulation. Most neuropeptides interact with G-protein-coupled receptors and modulate signal transduction mechanisms. In contrast to conventional neurotransmitters, which are synthesized in nerve terminals, neuropeptides are synthesized largely in the perikarya and transported like other peptides to the nerve terminal. Also unlike the conventional neurotransmitters, the physiologic functions of many neuropeptides are relatively undefined, though interaction with G-protein-coupled receptors indicates that pleiotropic effects are likely.

The opioid neuropeptides are good examples of this type of neurotransmitter.[40-43] These neuropeptides are the product of three different genes—the proopiomelanocortin (POMC), proenkephalin, and prodynorphin genes. Posttranslational processing produces a variety of gene products. POMC mRNA is processed to produce ACTH, the melanocyte-stimulating hormone (MSH), lipotropins, and the endorphins. The predominant product(s) vary between neuronal populations expressing the POMC gene. Similar phenomena have been documented for the proenkephalin and prodynorphin genes; each of these gene transcripts undergoes neuron-specific posttranslational processing to produce specific peptides. Not surprisingly, the different final products of this process have differing regional/neuronal distribution across the CNS.

Adding to the complexity of opioid peptide neurotransmission is the existence of multiple classes of receptors. Three different types of opioid receptors (μ, κ, and δ) have been defined on the basis of pharmacologic and molecular cloning studies. The different opioid peptides vary in their affinities for opioid receptor classes, and these receptors have their own unique patterns of distribution and varying linkage to signal transduction mechanisms within the CNS. Other neuropeptide families display similar heterogeneity of peptide processing and receptor classes. New neuropeptides and neuropeptide receptors continue to be discovered, and it is certain that the complexity of this field will increase in the foreseeable future.

ADENOSINE TRIPHOSPHATE

In addition to its vital roles as the chief intermediary of intracellular energy transfer and substrate for nucleic acid synthesis, adenosine triphosphate (ATP) has emerged as an important neurotransmitter.[44-46] ATP is probably not the primary neurotransmitter of any neurons within the CNS. Like neuropeptides, it probably functions as a cotransmitter in neurons possessing other primary neurotransmitters. ATP appears to be packaged in synaptic vesicles along with other neurotransmitters and is released with exocytosis. Its removal from the synaptic cleft is a relatively complex process in which a series of membrane-associated ectoenzymes convert ATP to adenosine, which also interacts with its own set of receptors (see below), and adenosine is removed from the cleft by a high-affinity transporter.

Several different ATP receptors have been described, with both G-protein-coupled and ionotropic receptors activated by ATP. These P_2 receptors, so-called because the original classification system distinguished between adenosine-activated purine$_1$ (now A_x) and ATP-activated purine$_2$ receptors, have been linked to a multiplicity of functions. G-protein-coupled P$_2$ receptors are linked to stimulation of phospholipase C with activation of the IP$_3$/DAG cascade, inhibition of adenylyl cyclase, activation of other phospholipases, and modulation of ion channels. The ionotropic ATP receptors form their own novel family of ligand gated and cation permeable ionophores and have distinctive structure consisting of two putative transmembrane domains joined by an extracellular loop. The ionotropic P$_2$ receptors are permeated by calcium as well as other cations, and P$_2$ receptors activation is another potential mechanism to regulate intracellular free calcium, with all its attendant consequences. The functional role(s) of these ionotropic receptors are not yet fully explored.

Unconventional Neuromodulators

NITRIC OXIDE

The simple gas nitric oxide (NO) is an important neuromodulator within the CNS.[47,48] Nitric oxide is synthesized by nitric oxide synthase (NOS) from arginine. Three distinct forms of NOS have been defined. One was originally defined in immune cells, a second in vascular endothelium, and a third in neurons. Activation of the neuronal and endothelial forms are dependent on binding of calcium/calmodulin, while the immune form is calcium-independent. In neurons, increased intracellular calcium, particularly that induced by activation of NMDA receptors, results in NOS activation. The resulting NO can diffuse through membranes, and while NO has a very short biologic half-life, on the order of a few seconds, its high diffusion coefficient means that its effective radius of action may be in the hundreds of microns. The signal transduction mechanisms for NO action are not completely known, but it is clear that one important mechanism mediating NO effects is cGMP generation. NO potently activates cytosolic guanylyl cyclase, and activation of cGMP-dependent protein kinases is presumed to be a major mediator of NO effects.

Because of its ability to cross membranes and probable large radius of action, NO is not a conventional neurotransmitter but probably acts in a paracrine manner, allowing a neuron to potentially influence many cells in its surrounding area. There has been considerable interest, for example, in the idea that NO may function as a "retrograde" messenger between the postsynaptic and presynaptic components of a synapse, allowing the postsynaptic cell to feedback information to the afferent terminal. There is also considerable interest in NO in terms of the pathophysiology of neuronal death in both acute and chronic neurologic disease. NO has been suggested to be a mediator of excitotoxic neuronal death. In vitro experiments using cultured neurons and some work with in vivo models of hypoxia/ischemia have suggested a role for NO in neuronal death. In both paradigms, NOS inhibitors have shown substantial protective effect, but these results are controversial and contradictory results have been published. Part of the contradiction may lie in the imperfect nature of presently available NOS inhibitors, which inhibit both neuronal NOS and endothelial NOS. Inhibition of the latter leads to diminished cerebral blood flow and exacerbation of neuronal death in vivo. Recent work with a putatively more selective inhibitor and also work with genetically engineered animals devoid of either neuronal NOS or endothelial NOS activity do suggest that NO may be a mediator of neuronal death in hypoxia/ischemia.[49]

ADENOSINE

Like NO, adenosine has unusual release properties. Neurons appear to release adenosine as a function of cellular activity; the more active the neuron, the more adenosine released into the extracellular space. As described above (see ATP), synaptic adenosine is removed from the extracellular space by a high-affinity transporter. Four types of adenosine receptors have been definitively characterized: A$_1$, A$_{2a}$, A$_{2b}$, and A$_3$.[50] These receptors belong to the G-protein-coupled class of receptors but the degree and character of CNS expression vary markedly. A$_1$ receptors are widely distributed in the CNS, while A$_{2a}$ receptors are expressed very densely in the striatum but to a much lesser extent in other brain regions. A$_{2b}$ receptors are expressed at very low levels, if at all, in the CNS, while A$_3$ receptors are probably expressed in human brain with an unknown distribution. All adenosine receptors modulate adenylyl cyclase. A$_1$ and A$_3$ receptors inhibit adenylyl cyclase, while A$_{2a}$ and A$_{2b}$ receptors stimulate adenylyl cyclase. Adenosine receptors are probably important modulators of neurotransmitter release, acting by modulation of neuronal calcium channel activity. Adenosine also plays an important role in the regulation of cerebral blood flow, and adenosinergic agents are the subject of considerable drug development research for treatment of stroke and other applications.

OTHER UNCONVENTIONAL NEUROMODULATORS

Other molecules within the brain, while not strictly neurotransmitters, may function as significant neuromodulators. One possible modulator is the metal cation zinc, which is stored in synaptic vesicles of glutamatergic neurons, released with exocytosis, and probably attains concentrations within the synaptic cleft in the micromolar range.[51] As described above, zinc interacts with NMDA, AMPA, and GABA$_A$ receptors and may be an important endogenous modulator of these receptors.

Neurosteroids are another potentially important endogenous modulator of GABA$_A$ receptors.[52] These compounds are synthesized by glia from progesterone and could have a profound effect on GABA$_A$ receptor function. Similarly, polyamines are endogenously produced in brain and markedly influence NMDA receptor function. These sites are targets of further drug development. Other molecules will undoubtedly be characterized that serve as neuromodulators within the CNS.

References

1.   Cooper et al: *The Biochemical Basis of Neuropharmacology.* New York, Oxford University Press, 1991.

2.   Strader CD, et al: Structure and function of G protein-coupled receptors. *Annu Rev Biochem* 1994; 63:101.

3.   Neer EJ: Heterotrimeric G proteins: Organizers of transmembrane signals. *Cell* 1995; 80(2):249.

4.   Cooper DM, et al: Adenylyl cyclases and the interaction between calcium and cAMP signaling. *Nature* 1995; 374(6521):421.

5.   Walsh DA, Van Patten SM: Multiple pathway signal transduction by the cAMP-dependent protein kinase. *FASEB J* 1994; 8:1221.

6.   Coy MF: cGMP: The wayward child of the cyclic nucleotide family. *TINS* 1991; 14(7):293.

7.   Fisher SK, et al: Inositol lipids and signal transduction in the nervous system: An update. *J Neurochem* 1992; 58(1):18.

8.   Bechade C, et al: The inhibitory neuronal glycine receptor. *Bioessays* 1994; 16(10):735.

9.   Betz H, et al: Structure, diversity, and synaptic localization of inhibitory glycine receptors. *J Physiol(Paris)* 1994; 88(4):243.

10.   Shiang R, et al: Mutations in the alpha 1 subunit of the inhibitory glycine receptor cause the dominant neurologic disorder, hyperekplexia. *Nat Genet* 1993; 5(4):351.

11.   Buckwalter MS, et al: A frameshift mutation in the mouse alpha 1 glycine receptor gene (Glra 1) results in progressive neurological symptoms and juvenile death. *Hum Mol Genet* 1994; 3(11):2025.

12.   Ryan SG, et al: A missense mutation in the gene encoding the alpha 1 subunit of the inhibitory glycine receptor in the spasmodic mouse. *Nat Genet* 1994; 7(2):131.

13.   Martin DL, Rimvall K: Regulation of gamma-aminobutyric acid synthesis in the brain. *J Neurochem* 1993; 60(2):395.

14.   Macdonald RL, Olsen RW: GABA$_A$ receptor channels. *Annu Rev Neurosci* 1994; 17:569.

15.   Luddens H, et al: GABA$_A$/benzodiazepine receptor heterogeneity: Neurophysiological implications. *Neuropharmacology* 1995; 34:245.

16.   Bowery NG: GABA$_B$ receptor pharmacology. *Annu Rev Pharmacol Toxicol* 1993; 33:109.

17.   Hosford DA, et al: The role of GABA$_B$ receptor activation in absence seizures of lethargic (1h/1h) mice. *Science* 1992; 257(5068):398.

18.   Orrego F, Villanueva S: The chemical nature of the main central excitatory transmitter: A critical appraisal based upon release studies and synaptic vesicle localization. *Neuroscience* 1993; 56(3):539.

19.   Winter HC, Ueda T: Glutamate uptake system in the presynaptic vesicle: Glutamic acid analogs as inhibitors and alternate substrates. *Neurochem Res* 1993; 18(1):79.

20.   Stone TW: Neuropharmacology of quinolinic and kynurenic acids. *Pharmacol Rev* 1993; 45(3):309.

21.   Stern-Bach Y, et al: Agonist selectivity of glutamate receptors is specified by two domains structurally related to bacterial amino acid-binding proteins. *Neuron* 1994; 13(6):1345.

22.   Hollmann M, et al: N-Glycosylation site tagging suggests a three transmembrane domain topology for the glutamate receptor GluR1. *Neuron* 1994; 13(6):1331.

23.   Hollmann M, Heinemann S: Cloned glutamate receptors. *Ann Rev Neurosci* 1994; 17:31.

24.   Nakanishi S: Molecular diversity of glutamate receptors and implications for brain functions. *Science* 1992; 258(5082):597.

25.   Seeburg PH: The TINS/TIPS Lecture. The molecular biology of mammalian glutamate receptor channels. *Trends Neurosci* 1993; 16(9):359.

26.   Bettler B, Mulle C: AMPA and kainate receptors. *Neuropharmacology* 1995; 34:123.

27.   Zukin RS, Bennett MVL: Alternatively spliced isoforms of the NMDAR1 receptor subunit. *Trends Neurosci* 1995; 18:306.

28.   Bliss TVP, Collingridge GL: A synaptic model of memory: Long-term potentiation in the hippocampus. *Nature* 1993; 361:31.

29.   Pin J-P, Duvoisin R: The metabotropic glutamate receptors: Structure and function. *Neuropharmacology* 1995; 34:1.

30.   Erickson JD, Eiden LE: Functional identification and molecular cloning of a human brain vesicle monoamine transporter. *J Neurochem* 1993; 61:2314.

31.   Sibley DR, Monsma FJ: Molecular biology of dopamine receptors. *Trends Pharmacol Sci* 1992; 13:61.

32.   Hieble JP, et al: Alpha- and beta-adrenoceptors: From the gene to the clinic. 1. Molecular biology and adrenoceptor subclassification. *J Med Chem* 1995; 38:3415.

33.   Peroutka SJ: Molecular biology of serotonin (5-HT) receptors. *Synapse* 1994; 18:241.

34.   Hill SJ: Distribution, properties, and functional characteristics of three classes of histamine receptor. *Pharmacol Rev* 1990; 42:45.

35.   Quattrochi JJ, et al: Mapping neuronal inputs to REM sleep induction sites with carbachol-fluorescent microspheres. *Science* 1989; 245:984.

36.   Coyle JT, et al: Alzheimer's disease: A disorder of cortical cholinergic innervation. *Science* 1983; 219:1184.

37.   Roghani A, et al: Molecular cloning of a putative vesicular transporter for acetylcholine. *Proc Natl Acad Sci USA* 1994; 91:10620.

38.   Sargent PB: The diversity of neuronal nicotinic acetylcholine receptors. *Annu Rev Neurosci* 1993; 16:403.

39.   Hulme EC, et al: Muscarinic receptor subtypes. *Annu Rev Pharmacol Toxicol* 1990; 30:633.

40.   Herz A (ed): *Opioids* I. New York, Springer-Verlag, 1993.

41.   Simon E: Opioid receptors and endogeneous opioid peptides. *Med Res Rev* 1991; 11:357.

42.   Reisine T: Opiate receptors. *Neuropharmacology* 1995; 34:463.

43.   Mansour A, et al: Opioid-receptor mRNA expression in the rat CNS: Anatomical and functional implications. *Trends Neurosci* 1995; 18:22.

44.   Zimmerman H: Signaling via ATP in the nervous system. *Trends Neurosci* 1994; 17:420.

45.   Suprenant A, et al: P2X receptors bring new structure to ligand gated ion channels. *Trends Neurosci* 1995; 18:224.

46.   Barnard EA, et al: G protein-coupled receptors for ATP and

other nucleotides: A new receptor family. *Trends Pharmacol Sci* 1994; 5(3):67.

47. Garthwaite J, Boulton CL: Nitric oxide signaling in the central nervous system. *Annu Rev Physiol* 1995; 57:683.

48. Dawson TM, et al: Nitric oxide: Cellular regulation and neuronal injury. *Prog Brain Res* 1994; 103:365.

49. Huang Z, et al: Effects of cerebral ischemia in mice deficient in neuronal nitric oxide synthase. *Science* 1994; 265:1883.

50. Dalziel HH, Westfall DP: Receptors for adenine nucleotides and nucleosides: Subclassification, distribution, and molecular characterization. *Pharmacol Rev* 1994; 46(4):449.

51. Frederickson CJ: Neurobiology of zinc and zinc-containing neurons. *Int Rev Neurobiol* 1989; 31:145.

52. Majewska MD: Neurosteroids: Endogenous bimodal modulators of the GABA$_A$ receptor. Mechanism of action and physiological significance. *Prog Neurobiol* 1992; 38(4):379.

EXCITOTOXICITY

M. FLINT BEAL

Excitotoxicity refers to neuronal death caused by activation of excitatory amino acid receptors. Several lines of evidence have linked excitotoxicity to the pathogenesis of both acute and chronic neurologic diseases. The initial observation that glutamate was neurotoxic was that of Lucas and Newhouse, who found that administration of glutamate to mice resulted in retinal degeneration.[1] Subsequent studies by Olney and colleagues linked neurotoxicity to the activation of excitatory amino acid receptors, and the term *excitotoxin* was coined.[2] Further advances were those of Rothman, linking release of excitatory amino acids to anoxic cell death in hippocampal cultures,[3] and of Choi, linking calcium influx to delayed cell death caused by excitatory amino acids.[4] More recent work has linked activation of excitatory amino acid receptors to free radical generation and nitric oxide, both of which may lead to oxidative stress.[5,6] A role for excitatory amino acids in acute neurologic diseases such as stroke, trauma, and hypoglycemia has received strong support. A possible role of excitotoxicity in chronic neurologic diseases has been supported by both studies in animal models and recent work with a glutamate release inhibitor in amyotrophic lateral sclerosis.

Molecular Biology of Excitatory Amino Acid Receptors

Excitatory amino acid receptors were initially classified pharmacologically into four distinct classes of binding sites in mammalian brain, named according to the agonists: α-amino-3-hydroxy-5-methyl-4-isoxazolepropionic acid (AMPA), kainate, N-methyl-D-aspartate (NMDA), and the quisqualate-sensitive metabotropic site.[7,8] AMPA and kainate sites mediate conventional fast synaptic transmission through an ionotrophic channel. The NMDA sites regulate Ca^{2+} and Na^+ influx, are gated by Mg^{2+}, and have been implicated in both learning and synaptic plasticity. The metabotropic site acts through G proteins either to activate phospholipase C or to decrease cyclic AMP.

Receptor proteins representing each of the major excitatory amino acid receptors have been cloned and sequenced. The AMPA, kainate, and NMDA receptors are members of the superfamily of ion-gated ligand channels. All known members are heterooligomers composed of several subunits. Four subunits of approximately 900 amino acids in length with four membrane-spanning regions were initially identified as AMPA receptors (GluR1–4).[9–12] Each subunit has a unique distribution in brain. There are alternatively spliced subunits termed "flip" and "flop" isoforms.[13] Subsequent studies identified kainate subunits (GluR5–7, KA1, KA2),[14–16] which participate in the formation of high-affinity kainate receptors. KA2 forms active heteromeric channels when expressed with GluR5. These subunits are localized to neurons in the hippocampus where they frequently colocalize with NMDA subunits.[17]

A subunit for the NMDA receptor termed NMDAR1 was initially cloned and sequenced in 1991.[18] This 938-amino-acid protein has about 25 percent homology to the AMPA and kainate subunits. This receptor when expressed shows appropriate agonist and antagonist pharmacology, a glycine coagonist site, calcium permeability, zinc inhibition, and voltage-dependent block by Mg^{2+}. Subsequently four further NMDA subunits (NR2A–D) were cloned.[19–21] Expression of these subunits with the initial subunit to form heteromeric complexes results in NMDA receptor channels of high activity. These complexes show unique distributions in the brain, and differences in gating behavior, affinities for agonists, and sensitivity to antagonists. NR2A is widely distributed in the brain, while NR2B is expressed only in the forebrain and NR2C is found predominantly in the cerebellum.

The metabotropic excitatory amino acid receptor family encodes subunits termed mGluR1–7.[22,23] Two subunits (mGluR1 and mGluR5) are linked by a G protein to phospholipase C, which generates inositol phosphate, which then release calcium from intracellular stores. The proteins have 1199 amino acids and appear to have 7 transmembrane domains. The remaining metabotropic glutamate receptors are linked to inhibition of cAMP formation.

The cloned AMPA receptors vary in their calcium permeability. GluR1, GluR3, and GluR4 all display strong inwardly rectifying current-voltage and calcium permeability.[24] In contrast, GluR2 has a linear current-voltage relation, and when coexpressed with other subunits it suppresses their strong inward rectification, and abolishes their calcium permeability. An arginine to glutamine mutation changes the rectification and confers calcium permeability to GluR2.[25,26] The gene sequence codes for glutamine, but this is changed to arginine as a result of RNA editing.[27]

A similar amino acid sequence results in an asparagine at amino acid 598 in NMDAR1. A mutation of the asparagine to glutamine results in decreased calcium permeability.[28,29] The consequences of this mutation for excitotoxicity have recently been examined in nonneuronal kidney cells which express NMDA receptors following transfection.[30,31] Following expression of NMDA receptors in these cells they undergo cell death, which is blocked by NMDA antagonists. Transfected cells expressing the mutated NMDA receptor, which conducts less Ca^{2+}, are less vulnerable to cell death. In these cells heterodimers expressing NMDAR1 with NR2A show more cell death than those with NR2B, and those with NR2C are resistant to cell death.[30]

The NMDA receptor is also regulated by extracellular pH, which may be important during seizures and ischemia. Protons inhibit the receptor by interacting with the NMDAR1 subunit, and polyamines potentiate receptor function by relief of the tonic proton inhibition. A single amino acid (lysine 211) was identified in exon 5, which mediates the pH sensitivity and polyamine relief of tonic inhibition, indicating that it serves as a pH sensitive constitutive modulator of NMDA receptor function.[32]

These findings provide experimental evidence that alterations in the amino acid sequences of excitatory amino acid subunits could alter calcium permeability or other properties which could then lead to excitotoxicity. Improved knowledge of the pharmacology and distribution of excitatory amino acids may also lead to the development of improved receptor antagonists for the treatment of neurologic disease.

Cellular Mechanisms of Excitotoxicity

CALCIUM

An important advance in clarifying mechanisms of excitotoxicity was Choi's finding that delayed glutamate neurotoxicity was calcium-dependent.[4] Subsequent studies showed that calcium load in cultured cortical neurons correlates with subsequent neuronal degeneration,[33,34] whereas intracellular calcium concentrations do not.[35] This supports the idea that much of the glutamate-induced Ca^{2+} load is sequestered into mitochondria rather than free in the cytoplasm. Recent evidence has shown that mitochondria and Na^+/Ca^{2+} exchange, which is the major means of efflux of mitochondrial Ca^{2+}, buffer glutamate-induced calcium loads in cultured cortical neurons.[36,37] The increases in mitochondrial calcium also lead to metabolic dysfunction, as shown by a lowering in intracellular pH.[37]

Randall and Thayer showed that there are three phases of change in intracellular calcium preceding cell death in cultured hippocampal neurons.[38] There is an initial phase of increased intracellular calcium lasting 5 to 10 min followed by a latent phase of approximately 2 h in which calcium returns to normal. The third phase consists of a gradual sustained rise in intracellular sodium that reaches a plateau associated with cell death. Tymianski and associates showed that cell-permeant Ca^{2+} chelators reduced excitotoxic cell injury.[39] These authors also demonstrated "source specificity" of the Ca^{2+} load, showing the Ca^{2+} entering through the NMDA channel was more toxic than that entering through other sources.[40] This observation is consistent with the earlier work of Choi and colleagues demonstrating that the NMDA receptor mediates most of the excitotoxic effects of glutamate.[4] It has been suggested that Ca^{2+} influx by the NMDA receptor may have access to proteins or compartments that make this Ca^{2+} more efficacious in producing cell death. One possible compartment is the mitochondria. The release of calcium from intracellular stores may also contribute to excitotoxicity.[41,42]

The means by which increased intracellular calcium leads to cell death may involve several mechanisms. These include activation of protein kinases, phospholipases, nitric oxide synthase, proteases, and endonucleases, inhibition of protein synthesis, mitochondrial damage, and free radical generation.[43] Evidence to support or refute these various possibilities is limited, particularly in vivo. Kainic acid neurotoxicity is associated with activation of calpain in vivo.[44] Furthermore, calpain inhibitors reduce AMPA-induced neurotoxicity in vitro, although they are not effective against glutamate toxicity.[45,46] Calpain inhibitors show efficacy in a gerbil model of global ischemia and in models of focal ischemia in rats.[47-49] Following excitotoxic activation of the NMDA receptor there is inhibition of calcium/calmodulin kinase II activity in cultured hippocampal neurons.[50] On the other hand, a specific inhibitor of calcium/calmodulin kinase II protects against NMDA-

and hypoxia/hypoglycemia-induced cell death in cultured cortical neurons.[51]

FREE RADICALS

The initial report linking free radicals to excitotoxicity was that of Dykens, who showed that kainate-induced damage to cerebellar neurons could be attenuated by superoxide dismutase, allopurinol, and hydroxyl radical scavengers such as mannitol.[52] Other studies showed that glutathione depletion exacerbates excitotoxicity while the free radical scavengers α-tocopherol, ascorbic acid, and ubiquinone show neuroprotective effects.[53-55] The 21-aminosteroids and α-phenyl-*N-tert*-butylnitrone which scavenge free radicals also protect against excitotoxicity in vitro. The vitamin E analogue trolox protects cultured neurons from AMPA toxicity.[56] Cultured cortical neurons which overexpress superoxide dismutase are resistant to both glutamate- and ischemia-induced neurotoxicity.[57]

Direct evidence linking excitotoxicity to free radical generation comes from studies using electron paramagnetic resonance which show that NMDA dose-dependently increases superoxide formation in cultured cerebellar neurons.[6] The effects are blocked by NMDA antagonists or removing extracellular Ca^{2+}. This is consistent with the recent findings of Dykens that exposure of isolated cortical mitochondria to 2.5 μM Ca^{2+}, which is similar to concentrations that occur in the setting of excitotoxicity, leads to free radical generation.[58] In synaptosomes NMDA, kainic acid, and AMPA all stimulate free radical generation.[59] Electron paramagnetic resonance also showed generation of free radicals in vivo following systemic administration of kainic acid.[60]

Direct evidence linking increases in intracellular calcium to mitochondrial production of reactive oxygen species has been obtained in vitro.[61,62] Dugan and colleagues used the oxidation-sensitive dye dihydrorhodamine 123 with confocal microscopy to demonstrate that exposure to NMDA, but not kainate, ionomycin, or elevated potassium, led to oxygen radical production in cultured neurons.[61] This was confirmed by studies using electron paramagnetic resonance. The increase in oxygen radical production was blocked by inhibitors of mitochondrial electron transport and mimicked by an uncoupler of electron transport. In contrast, inhibitors of nitric oxide synthase and arachidonic acid metabolism had no effect. Reynolds and Hastings used the oxidation-sensitive dye dichlorodihydrofluorescein to study the effects of glutamate in neuronal cultures.[62] Glutamate at excitotoxic concentrations caused localized areas of increased fluorescence at the margins of the cell body which were dependent on NMDA receptor activation and calcium entry,

and which were blocked by an uncoupler of mitochondrial electron transport. These two studies therefore suggest a critical role of Ca^{2+}-dependent uncoupling of neuronal mitochondrial electron transport in the production of reactive oxygen species following glutamate exposure.

We recently examined the relationship of excitotoxicity to free radical production in vivo.[63] We showed that malonate, which produces excitotoxic lesions, leads to increased hydroxyl radical generation as assessed by the salicylate trapping method. The free radical spin trap *N-tert*-butyl-α (2-sulfophenyl)-nitrone (S-PBN) attenuated both hydroxyl radical generation and neurotoxicity. It also attenuated striatal lesions produced by NMDA, AMPA, and kainate. These findings provide direct in vivo evidence for a role of free radicals in excitotoxicity.

NITRIC OXIDE

The role of nitric oxide in excitotoxicity is under intense investigation. Dawson and colleagues originally demonstrated that nitric oxide synthase inhibitors and hemoglobin, which scavenges nitric oxide, block glutamate neurotoxicity in vitro.[5] They subsequently showed that pretreatment of cultures with quisqualate, which preferentially kills nitric oxide synthase neurons, blocks glutamate neurotoxicity in the cultures.[64] Subsequent studies, however, have been controversial, with several groups reporting that inhibition of nitric oxide synthase had no effect on excitotoxicity in vitro.[65-69] Excitotoxicity can occur in the absence of nitric oxide synthase, since cultured kidney neurons which lack the enzyme show excitotoxicity when transfected with NMDA receptors.[30]

Initial studies of the effects of inhibition of nitric oxide synthase on NMDA-induced excitotoxicity in vivo were also conflicting.[70,71] Similar problems were encountered in studies of focal ischemia. This appears to be due to the nonspecificity of the nitric oxide synthase inhibitors utilized, which have effects on both the neuronal and endothelial isoforms, leading to vascular effects.[72] Recent evidence strongly favoring a role of neuronal nitric oxide synthase in focal ischemic lesions has come from studies showing that lesions are attenuated in mice with a knockout of the enzyme.[72]

Several studies showed that 7-nitroindazole is a relatively specific inhibitor of the neuronal isoform of nitric oxide synthase in vivo. It has no effects on blood pressure or on acetylcholine-induced vasorelaxation.[9,73,74] 7-Nitroindazole reduces focal ischemic lesions.[74] We found that it significantly attenuated excitotoxicity produced by NMDA but not by AMPA or kainate.[75] This is consistent with the in vitro observations of Dawson and colleagues[5,64] and suggests that Ca^{2+} influx via the NMDA receptor leads to activation of neuronal nitric oxide synthase.

Excitotoxic Mechanisms in Acute Neurologic Disease

Direct evidence for the role of excitatory amino acids in human neurologic disease came from observations concerning domoic acid neurotoxicity. In 1987, on Prince Edward Island in Canada, a number of individuals consumed mussels contaminated with domoic acid, a potent agonist of the kainic acid subtype of excitatory amino acid receptors.[76] Many of the afflicted patients developed an encephalopathy with complex partial seizures and memory disturbance. Older individuals were particularly susceptible, consistent with experimental evidence showing age-dependent susceptibility to kainate toxicity. Several deaths occurred and necropsy findings showed a loss of neurons in the CA3 field of the hippocampus, which has large numbers of kainic acid receptors.[76,77]

A compelling case for a role of excitotoxicity in stroke has been made based on observations in experimental animals. These studies show that experimental models of stroke are associated with increased glutamate in the extracellular fluid, and that it is attenuated by glutamatergic denervation or by glutamate antagonists.[78] Levels of extracellular glutamate measured by microdialysis are in the range known to be neurotoxic in vitro. The distribution of ischemic cell changes corresponds roughly with that of NMDA receptors; however, cerebellar Purkinje cells which are vulnerable are devoid of NMDA receptors. The Purkinje cells have AMPA receptors and may be particularly vulnerable because the receptors undergo less complete desensitization to AMPA than those of other cerebellar neurons.[79] Both competitive and noncompetitive NMDA antagonists are effective in focal models of ischemia but show little effect in global models of ischemia. In global models of ischemia non-NMDA antagonists are effective.[80] The experimental studies are sufficiently promising that a number of excitatory amino acid receptor antagonists are currently being tested in human stroke trials.[81,82]

The role of excitotoxicity in head trauma has also received considerable experimental support. Concussive brain injury results in marked increases in extracellular glutamate concentrations.[83] MK-801 attenuates focal brain edema following fluid-percussion brain injury in rats and results in improved brain metabolic status.[84] Dextromethorphan attenuates declines in magnesium and brain bioenergetics following trauma.[85] Similarly, kynurenate and indole-2-carboxylic acid reduce cerebral edema and improve cognitive and motor dysfunction induced by trauma.[86] A recent study showed that kynurenate protects against hippocampal cell loss induced by fluid-percussion injury.[87] Clinical studies of excitatory amino acid antagonists in head trauma in man are under way. Initial results have shown that they reduce increased intracranial pressure. Substantial experimental evidence has also demonstrated that hypoglycemia-induced brain damage is attenuated by NMDA antagonists.[88]

Slow Excitotoxicity

The role of excitotoxicity in neurodegenerative diseases is speculative. In these diseases there is no evidence for an increase in glutamate concentrations, with the exception of glutamate in the CSF in amyotrophic lateral sclerosis (ALS) patients. Furthermore increases in glutamate concentrations by themselves may not be sufficient to cause excitotoxicity.[89] A search for increases in concentrations of other endogenous excitotoxins such as quinolinic acid has been unsuccessful.[90] The concept of slow or weak excitotoxicity has therefore been proposed.[43,91] One possibility to account for this would be a receptor abnormality that could lead to increased calcium influx.

Another possibility is that slow excitotoxicity could occur as a consequence of an impairment in energy metabolism. This could occur by a variety of mechanisms including genetic mutations in mitochondrial electron transport or Krebs cycle enzymes. Another possibility would be oxidative damage to components of the electron transport chain or mitochondrial membranes. The possibility that impaired energy metabolism could result in excitotoxicity was originally demonstrated by the work of Novelli and coworkers.[92] They showed that inhibitors of oxidative phosphorylation or Na-K$^+$ ATPase allowed glutamate to become neurotoxic at concentrations that ordinarily exhibited no neurotoxicity. This was felt to be due to a reduction in ATP leading to partial neuronal depolarization. This may then lead to relief of the voltage-dependent Mg^{2+} block of the NMDA receptor, leading to persistent receptor activation by ambient levels of glutamate.

Consistent with this possibility, Zeevalk and Nicklas showed that partial energy impairment in cultured chick retina either with iodoacetate (a glycolysis inhibitor) or with cyanide (an inhibitor of oxidative phosphorylation) leads to NMDA receptor activation and excitotoxicity in the absence of any increase in extracellular concentrations of glutamate.[93] Furthermore, graded titration of membrane potential with potassium mimicked the toxicity produced by graded metabolic inhibition.[94] Potassium channel activators, which hyperpolarize the cell membrane, can block excitotoxicity in vitro.[95] Inhibitors of the sodium-potassium ATPase produce lesions in rat substantia nigra and striatum.[96] Other studies showed that metabolic inhibition in hippocampal slices not only increased depolarization in response to glutamate, but also inhibited neuronal repolarization.[97] This could be a consequence of mitochondrial uptake of calcium, which then further impairs mitochondrial function and ATP production. A study of cultured fibroblasts from patients with the mitochondrial disorder *mitochondrial encephalopathy, lactic acidosis, and strokes* (MELAS) showed impaired calcium buffering.[98] There is therefore a complex interrelationship between excitotoxicity and mitochondrial function, in that mitochondrial dysfunction can lead to excitotoxicity which then further impairs mitochondrial function. We have recently carried out a series of studies of the effects of mitochondrial toxins in animals which have further validated these concepts in vivo.

Excitotoxicity and Neurodegenerative Diseases

The role of excitotoxicity in neurodegenerative diseases is based on circumstantial evidence. Some of the best evidence is for a role of excitotoxicity in Huntington's disease (HD). Initial observations showed that kainic acid striatal lesions could mimic many of the neuropathologic features of HD.[99,100] They, however, do not spare striatal interneurons containing the histochemical marker NADPH-diaphorase which are spared in HD.[101,102] We and others subsequently showed that quinolinic acid and other NMDA agonists produce an improved animal model, since they result in relative sparing of NADPH-diaphorase neurons.[103,104] The relative sparing is much more dramatic with chronic striatal lesions, in which there is striatal shrinkage.[105,106] Parvalbumin neurons, which are spared in HD, are relatively preserved by NMDA agonists, but preferentially vulnerable to kainate.[106–108] In primates, quinolinic acid produces striking sparing of NADPH-diaphorase neurons as well as an apomorphine-inducible movement disorder.[109]

Further support for an NMDA excitotoxic process comes from studies of NMDA receptors in HD postmortem tissue. If the neurons containing these receptors are preferentially vulnerable, one would expect a depletion of NMDA receptors. This was shown to be the case in HD striatum[110,111] as well as in the striatum of an asymptomatic at-risk patient, who showed a 50 percent depletion of NMDA receptors, suggesting that this occurs early in the disease process.[112]

The case for a role of excitotoxicity in Parkinson's disease (PD) is based on two observations. There is a loss of NMDA receptors in PD substantia nigra with a lesser reduction of AMPA sites and no change in metabotropic sites.[113] Furthermore, several studies have suggested that the toxicity of 1-methyl-4-phenyl-1,2,3,6-tetrahydropyridine (MPTP), which models PD, is reduced by excitatory amino acid antagonists. The initial report was that of Turski and colleagues who showed that 1-methyl-4-phenylpyridinium (MPP$^+$) neurotoxicity in the substantia nigra was attenuated by excitatory amino acid antagonists, although this was later disputed by Sonsalla and colleagues.[114,115] Subsequent studies of attenuation of MPTP neurotoxicity in mice by excitatory amino acid antagonists have been conflicting, however. Two studies in primates showed neuroprotective effects.[116,117]

The case for excitotoxicity in ALS is based on three lines of evidence. First, activity of the glutamate-metabolizing enzyme glutamate dehydrogenase was reported to be reduced in leukocytes of ALS patients.[118,119] This finding, however, appears to be found in a variety of neurological disorders and is not specific to ALS. Second, glutamate concentrations may be increased in both plasma and CSF of ALS patients.[119,120] Rothstein and colleagues found reduced synaptosomal glutamate uptake in ALS postmortem tissue, and more recently showed reductions in the astrocytic glutamate transporter.[121] Lastly, ingestion of beta-N-oxalyl-amino-L-alanine may play a role in lathyrism,[122] and alpha-amino-beta-methylamino-propionic acid (BMAA), which is found in cycads, was linked to the Western Pacific form of ALS.[123] Findings of reduced numbers of NMDA receptors and increases in kainic acid receptors are further evidence supporting a role of excitotoxicity in ALS.[124–126] Studies in organotypic cultures of spinal cord showed that selective inhibition of glutamate transport results in slow degeneration of motor neurons over several weeks, which is blocked by antagonists of non-NMDA glutamate receptors.[127]

A possible role of excitotoxicity in Alzheimer's disease (AD) has been proposed. The toxicity of β-amyloid in cell culture is enhanced both by glutamate and by glucose deprivation.[128–130] A loss of NMDA receptors was found in AD cerebral cortex and hippocampus.[131,132] Glutamatergic neurons are prone to neurofibrillary tangles,[133] and tangles are localized to neurons involved in corticocortical pathways, which are known to utilize glutamate as a transporter.[134,135] Considerable evidence also exists in AD for a defect in energy metabolism which could render cells more vulnerable to secondary excitotoxicity.[136]

Secondary Excitotoxicity Due to Mitochondrial Toxins

A number of mitochondrial toxins are available which have been used to model neurodegenerative diseases.

Some of these compounds can produce selective neuronal degeneration which can model neurodegenerative diseases. Furthermore, studies of these toxins have supported the notion that impairment of energy metabolism can lead to secondary excitotoxic neuronal injury.

AMINOOXYACETIC ACID

Aminooxyacetic acid is a nonselective inhibitor of transaminases, including kynurenine transaminase, GABA transaminase, and aspartate transaminase.[137,138] Aminooxyacetic acid injections lead to a depletion of ATP, which most likely is due to inhibition of aspartate transaminase, an essential component of the malate-aspartate shunt across mitochondrial membranes. This shuttle is the predominant means of moving NADH from the cytoplasm to mitochondria for oxidation. Inhibition of aspartate transaminase in brain slices and synaptosomes results in decreased oxygen consumption and ATP generation.[139-141] Consistent with an effect on energy metabolism we found that pretreatment with either coenzyme Q_{10} or 1,3-butanediol, which can improve ATP generation, could attenuate striatal lesions produced by aminooxyacetic acid.[142] The lesions are blocked by NMDA antagonists.

The lesions are not caused by direct excitatory amino acid receptor activation since aminooxyacetic acid has no direct depolarizing effects in either hippocampal slices or cultured striatal neurons.[137,143] The lesions spare NADPH-diaphorase neurons, consistent with an NMDA-receptor-mediated excitotoxic process.[137] Lesions in the hippocampus and in neonatal rats are also blocked by NMDA receptor antagonists.[143,144]

MALONATE

Malonate is a reversible inhibitor of succinate dehydrogenase.[145] Succinate dehydrogenase plays a central role both in the tricarboxylic acid cycle and as part of complex II of the electron transport chain. We and others have recently examined the effects of intrastriatal injections of malonate in rats.[146,147] Intrastriatal injections of malonate produced dose-dependent excitotoxic lesions which were attenuated by both competitive and noncompetitive NMDA antagonists. Coinjection with succinate blocks the lesions, consistent with an effect on succinate dehydrogenase.[148] Recent work showed that coinjection of subtoxic malonate with nontoxic concentrations of NMDA, AMPA, and L-glutamate produced large lesions, showing that metabolic inhibition can exacerbate both NMDA- and non-NMDA-receptor-mediated excitotoxicity in vivo.[147] An NMDA antagonist reduced the glutamate toxicity by 40 percent but a non-NMDA antagonist had no effect, suggesting that

the NMDA receptor may play a major role in situations of metabolic compromise in vivo.

Malonate lesions were accompanied by a significant reduction in ATP levels and a significant increase in lactate in vivo as shown by chemical shift magnetic resonance imaging.[149,150] Furthermore, we showed that pretreatment with coenzyme Q_{10} or nicotinamide, which blocks malonate-induced ATP depletions, blocked the lesions.[150] Histologic studies showed that the lesions spare both NADPH-diaphorase neurons and somatostatin concentrations, consistent with observations in HD.[146,149] The lesions are strikingly age-dependent, and in vivo magnetic resonance imaging shows a significant correlation between increasing lesion size and lactate production.[149]

3-NITROPROPIONIC ACID

3-Nitropropionic acid is a naturally occurring abundant plant toxin and mycotoxin that is associated with neurological illnesses in grazing animals and humans.[151] Ingestion in livestock results in hindlimb weakness, knocking together of the hindlimbs while walking, and goose stepping. Outbreaks of illness in man occurred in China after ingestion of mildewed sugar cane that contained the fungus *Arthrinium*. The illness is characterized by initial gastrointestinal disturbance followed by encephalopathy with stupor and coma. Patients who recover have delayed onset of nonprogressive dystonia 7 to 40 days after regaining consciousness. The patients also show facial grimacing, torticollis, dystonia, and jerklike movements. Computed tomography scans show bilateral hypodensities in the putamen and, to a lesser extent, in the globus pallidus.

3-Nitropropionic acid (3-NP) is an irreversible inhibitor of succinate dehydrogenase, which is part of both the tricarboxylic acid cycle and the electron transport chain.[152,153] In vitro studies showed that 3-NP has no direct depolarizing effects on neurons in hippocampal slices.[154] Rather it leads to hyperpolarization by activation of ATP-sensitive potassium channels. Studies in cortical explants showed that 3-NP produces cellular ATP depletion and neuronal damage by an excitotoxic mechanism.[155] Pathologic changes were significantly attenuated by pretreatment with excitatory amino acid antagonists. Similarly, in primary mesencephalic cultures, MK-801 attenuated 3-NP toxicity to dopaminergic neurons.[156] In cultured cerebellar neurons, 3-NP produces neurotoxicity which is delayed but not prevented by the competitive NMDA antagonist 2-amino-5-phosphonovaleric acid.[157] In cultured striatal and cortical neurons 3-NP neurotoxicity was unaffected by glutamate antagonists, but was reduced by the macromolecular synthesis inhibitors cycloheximide, emetine, or actinomycin D, consistent with apoptotic cell death.[158] Exposure to 3-NP also produced cell body shrinkage and DNA fragmentation on agarose gels, suggesting apoptotic cell death.

Studies in mice of 3-NP toxicity showed damage in the striatum and CA1 field of the hippocampus.[159] Ultrastructural studies showed dendrosomatic swelling, chromatin clumping, and mitochondrial swelling considered to be consistent with an excitotoxic injury. There were no effects on blood pressure or arterial oxygen levels.[160]

We found that intrastriatal injections of 3-NP in rats produced dose-dependent lesions with neuronal loss and gliosis.[161] There were depletions of ATP and focal increases in lactate in the basal ganglia. The lesions were strikingly age-dependent, with much larger lesions in young adult and adult animals than in juvenile animals, which has been confirmed by others. The age-dependence correlated directly with the degree of increase in lactate concentrations following administration of a uniform dose of 3-NP to animals of various ages.

Subacute systemic administration of 3-NP resulted in the development of motor slowing and dystonic posturing, which has been confirmed by other authors.[162] There were large symmetric lesions in the basal ganglia which were nonselective in that Nissl and NADPH-diaphorase neurons were equally vulnerable. The lesions were accompanied by focal accumulations of lactate in the basal ganglia as shown by magnetic resonance spectroscopy. The lactate accumulations preceded lesions detectable with T_2-weighted imaging.

Consistent with an excitotoxic mechanism, the lesions are attenuated by prior decortication or treatment with lamotrigine, which blocks glutamate release. Turski and Ikonomidou showed that the AMPA antagonist 6-nitro-7-sulfanobenzo(F)quinoxaline-2,3-dione (NBQX) could block the lesions.[163] Microdialysis studies showed that there was no significant increase in extracellular glutamate concentrations after administration of neurotoxic doses of 3-NP, which resulted in twofold increases in lactate.[162] These results are therefore consistent with 3-NP inducing secondary excitotoxicity by making neurons more vulnerable to endogenous levels of glutamate. Furthermore, in vivo ^{3}H-MK-801 receptor autoradiography showed that systemic administration of 3-NP was associated with activation of NMDA receptors.[164]

Chronic low-dose administration of 3-NP over 1 month by subcutaneous osmotic pumps produced subtle lesions in the dorsolateral striatum in which there was neuronal loss, gliosis, and sparing of NADPH-diaphorase neurons, similar to findings in HD.[162] This finding was confirmed using in situ hybridization for somatostatin mRNA which was preserved as com-pared with both substance P and enkephalin mRNA.[164] Dopamine terminals were preserved with lower doses of 3-NP as shown by ^{3}H-mazindol autoradiography.

To investigate the mechanism of the lesions we administered 3-NP to transgenic mice overexpressing the enzyme superoxide dismutase as compared with littermate controls.[165] In the animals overexpressing superoxide dismutase 3-NP neurotoxicity was significantly attenuated. Furthermore 3-NP-induced increases in hydroxyl radical generation and 3-nitrotyrosine, a marker for peroxynitrite-induced damage, were significantly attenuated in the mice overexposing superoxide dismutase. These findings suggest that oxidative damage, perhaps mediated by peroxynitrite, plays a role in 3-NP toxicity.

We extended our studies to nonhuman primates to attempt to produce chorea, the cardinal clinical feature of HD.[161] Following 3 to 6 weeks of 3-NP administration, apomorphine induced a movement disorder closely resembling that seen in HD. The animals showed orofacial dyskinesia, dystonia, dyskinesia of the extremities, and choreiform movements. Both a clinical rating scale and quantitative analysis of individual movement velocities confirmed that 3-NP-treated animals had a significant increase in choreiform and dystonic movements. More prolonged 3-NP treatment in two additional primates resulted in spontaneous dystonia and dyskinesia accompanied by lesions in the caudate and putamen seen on magnetic resonance imaging.

Histologic evaluation showed changes reminiscent of HD with a depletion of Nissl-stained and calbindin-stained neurons, yet sparing of NADPH-diaphorase and large neurons. There were proliferative changes in the dendrites of spiny neurons on Golgi studies, and preservation of the striosomal organization of the striatum, similar to changes in HD. Lastly there was sparing of the nucleus accumbens. These findings therefore show that 3-NP neurotoxicity in primates can replicate many of the characteristic features of HD, strengthening the possibility that slow excitotoxicity might be involved in its pathogenesis.

Therapeutic Directions

EXCITATORY AMINO ACID ANTAGONISTS

If excitotoxicity plays a role in neurologic diseases, then it should be possible to prevent neurologic damage with glutamate release blockers or with excitatory amino acid antagonists. Several compounds have been developed that are sodium channel blockers and block glutamate release. One such compound is lamotrigine, which has been approved for use as an antiepileptic in humans.[130] In rat brain cortical slices it inhibits glutamate release. It is neuroprotective against kainate striatal lesions and against MPTP dopaminergic neurotoxicity in vivo.[166-168] We found that it attenuates malonate, MPP+, and 3-NP neurotoxicity.[149]

Several analogues of lamotrigine show efficacy in models of cerebral ischemia. The related compounds BW1003C87 and BW619C89 decrease ischemia-induced glutamate release and infarct volumes following middle cerebral artery occlusion.[166,169,170] BW1003C87 is also effective in global ischemia.[171]

Riluzole is another compound which blocks glutamate release in hippocampal slices in vitro and in the cat caudate nucleus in vivo.[172,173] It has significant neuroprotective effects in both focal and global models of cerebral ischemia.[174,175] It protects against MPTP-induced decreases in dopamine levels in mice.[176] Of great interest it was recently shown to slow the progression of ALS.[177]

The approach of using glutamate release blockers, therefore, appears to be very promising. In our hands in vivo and in a model of glutamate-induced cortical lesions in vitro, these compounds show equal or better efficacy than glutamate receptor antagonists.[178] These compounds also appear to be well tolerated in man.

A large number of compounds that modulate NMDA receptors have been developed. These compounds include competitive antagonists for the glutamate binding site, noncompetitive antagonists which bind to the ion channel, glycine site antagonists, and polyamine site antagonists.[179,180] Compounds from all of these classes are highly effective in experimental models of stroke, epilepsy, and traumatic brain injury. Among the most potent competitive NMDA antagonists are cis-4-phosphono-methyl-2-piperidine-carboxylic acid (CGS 19755) and D-3 (2-carboxypiperazin-4-yl) propenyl-1-phosphonic acid (D-CPPene). Agents such as MK-801, CNS 1102, and phencyclidine interact with a site within the ion channel to produce a noncompetitive blockade of glutamate. Agents such as 7-chloro-kynurenic acid, 3-amino-1-hydroxy-2-pyrrolidone (HA 966), and ACEA 1021 attenuate NMDA receptor function by blocking the site through which glycine allosterically enhances NMDA receptor function.[181] Another allosteric regulatory site is the polyamine site at which compounds such as ifenprodil appear to act. In addition recent work has led to the developmental of several non-NMDA receptor antagonists such as NBQX. Non-NMDA antagonists are particularly effective in preventing hippocampal damage in global models of ischemia.[80,182] One concern, however, is that they result in widespread reductions in cerebral glucose utilization in experimental animals.[183]

MK-801 has shown efficacy in both cat and rat models of permanent middle cerebral artery occlusion. The extent of reduction in infarct size ranges from 40 to 65

percent.[184-186] In most studies the caudate nucleus is not protected. Gill and others showed that maximal infarct reduction of 60 percent was achieved with plasma MK-801 concentrations of 19 ng/ml. Higher levels led to less protection, which may have been due to hypotension.[187] Protection is less effective in strains of rats such as spontaneous hypertensive rats, which have fewer collaterals.[188] CNS 1102 administered 1 h after ischemia reduced infarct volume by over 50 percent and improved neurological outcome.[189] Dextrorphan showed efficacy in rabbits after 1 h of multiple vessel occlusions, and dextromethorphan was effective when administered 1 h after the onset of focal ischemia.[190,191]

In focal ischemia, rats with permanent middle cerebral artery occlusion showed a 70 to 80 percent reduction in infarct area when given CGS 19755 5 min before or 5 min after vascular occlusion.[192] The competitive antagonist D-CPPene reduced cortical infarct volume by more than 75 percent when therapy was begun prior to permanent MCA occlusion in cats, but had no effect if therapy was delayed for 1 h.[193] Ifenprodil reduced infarct volume by 40 percent in a cat middle cerebral artery occlusion model.[194] A glycine site antagonist (L-687,414) produced a 41 percent decrease in cortical infarct volume in a rat model of focal ischemia.[195] Another glycine antagonist, ACEA 1021, produced a 35 percent reduction in infarct volume in focal ischemia but was ineffective in global ischemia.[196]

As noted above, NBQX is effective in models of global ischemia in which NMDA antagonists are typically ineffective. NBQX has efficacy in focal ischemia models. In a rat permanent middle cerebral artery occlusion model, NBQX reduced infarct volume by 25 percent.[197] Similarly delayed treatment at 90 min produced a 25 percent protection in a middle cerebral artery occlusion model in spontaneously hypertensive rats.[198]

The major concern regarding the use of NMDA antagonists in humans is that they may exert adverse behavioral side effects. NMDA receptors play a critical role in learning and memory, and some noncompetitive NMDA antagonists such as phencyclidine can produce psychotomimetic effects in humans.[199,200] Initial phase II studies of both a competitive NMDA antagonist (CGS 19755) and a noncompetitive NMDA antagonist (dextrorphan) showed significant psychoactive effects at therapeutic doses.[81,82] As many as 50 percent of the patients experienced agitation, somnolence, or hallucinations. It is as yet uncertain whether similar effects are associated with all NMDA antagonists. Some NMDA antagonists such as memantine appear to be well tolerated in humans.[179] It is possible that lower-affinity NMDA antagonists which block and unblock the receptor more rapidly may exhibit less toxicity.[179,201] A potential advantage of noncompetitive

NMDA antagonists is that they are use-dependent. They increase their block of NMDA receptors proportionately with glutamate concentrations, which may be advantageous under conditions of excessive glutamate release. Both glycine site antagonists and polyamine site antagonists may also exhibit less behavioral toxicity.

Both competitive and noncompetitive NMDA antagonists have been reported to attenuate MPP^+ and MPTP neurotoxicity in mice and rats; however, this has been controversial.[114,115,202,203] Two studies in primates using MK-801 and the competitive NMDA antagonist 3-(2-carboxylpiperazin-4-yl)1-propenyl-1-phosphoric acid (CPP) showed protection against MPTP neurotoxicity in primates.[116,117] In our studies both competitive and noncompetitive antagonists were neuroprotective against aminooxyacetic acid, malonate, and 3-acetylpyridine neurotoxicity.[137,149,204] The non-NMDA antagonist NBQX protects against 3-NP neurotoxicity.[163]

FREE RADICAL SCAVENGERS

As discussed above, there is now substantial evidence linking excitotoxicity to free radical generation. A number of studies showed that a variety of free radical scavengers can attenuate excitotoxicity in vitro.[205,206] There, however, is very limited in vivo evidence. One promising approach is to use free radical spin traps such as α-phenyl-N-tert-butyl-nitrone (PBN), N-tert-butyl-α-(2-sulfophenyl)-nitrone (S-PBN), and 5,5-dimethyl-1-pyroline-N-oxide (DMPO). These compounds react with free radicals to form more stable adducts. They are widely used to detect the generation of free radicals using electron paramagnetic resonance. Following systemic administration, PBN is widely distributed in all tissues, with a plasma half-life of about 12 hours.[207] It appears to be concentrated in mitochondria. PBN is effective in reducing ischemia-reperfusion injury in gerbils,[208,209] focal ischemia in rats,[210] and oxidative damage to proteins in aged gerbils.[211]

We found that pretreatment with S-PBN significantly attenuates striatal excitotoxic lesions in rats produced by N-methyl-D-aspartate, kainic acid, and AMPA.[63] In a similar manner striatal lesions produced by malonate were dose-dependently blocked by S-PBN. Lesions produced by MPP^+ and 3-acetylpyridine were also protected. DMPO administration protects against systemic administration of 3-NP. The neuroprotective effects of S-PBN were additive with MK-801 against both malonate and 3-acetylpyridine neurotoxicity. This suggests that a combination of compounds acting at sequential steps in the excitotoxic cascade might have improved efficacy. An advantage of this approach is that one might be able to use lower doses of compounds to avoid behavioral toxicity. S-PBN has no effects on malonate-induced ATP depletions or on spontaneous striatal electrophysiologic activity, showing that it does not act at excitatory amino acid receptors. It does, however, attenuate malonate-induced increases in hydroxyl radical generation.

Another group of compounds that show promise as free radical scavengers are the 21-aminosteroids or lazeroids, which can attenuate glutamate toxicity in vitro.[212] They are effective in both ischemic neuronal damage and experimental head injury in mice.[213–215] They produce dose-dependent neuroprotection in a rat model of focal ischemia.[216] Dihydrolipoate is an antioxidant that is well tolerated in humans and is effective in experimental models of stroke and against malonate- and NMDA-induced striatal lesions.[217,218]

A potential therapeutic advantage of free radical spin traps such as PBN and S-PBN is that they appear to have a much improved therapeutic window. Most studies of either focal sichemia or excitotoxic lesions showed a maximal therapeutic window (the time in which one can administer therapy after the insult and still achieve efficacy) of 1 to 2 hours. PBN, however, was reported to exert neuroprotective effects when administered as long as 12 hours after focal ischemic insult.[210] In another study PBN showed efficacy when administered at 3 hours after a middle cerebral artery occlusion.[219] We found that S-PBN showed efficacy when administered up to 6 hours after malonate injections in rat striatum.[220]

NITRIC OXIDE SYNTHASE INHIBITORS

As discussed above, there is evidence linking excitotoxicity to nitric oxide generation. Results using nonselective nitric oxide synthase (NOS) inhibitors, however, have been controversial. The absence of consensus may be due to the prior lack of inhibitors with specificity for the various isoforms of the enzyme. The three isoenzymes are the constitutive neuronal and endothelial isoforms and the inducible form localized to macrophages. An initial report showed that L-nitroarginine at 1 mg/kg reduced infarct volume in a mouse model of focal cerebral ischemia.[221] The same dosing regimen was effective in reducing size following middle cerebral artery occlusion in rats.[222] Other studies showed that NOS inhibition reduced caudate injury in cats following focal ischemia, although there was no effect on cortical infarct volume.[223] In contrast, several studies showed that inhibition of NOS increased infarct volume following focal ischemia in rats.[224–226] These studies generally used higher doses of NOS inhibitors, which will inhibit endothelial NOS, leading to vasoconstriction and reduced cerebral perfusion. Consistent with this effect NOS donors increase blood flow and reduce brain damage in focal ischemia.[227] These findings have been clarified by the observation that low doses of NOS inhibitors are neuroprotective, whereas higher doses are ineffective in the mouse focal ischemic model, consistent with adverse vascular effects at higher dose levels.[228] Similar controversy exists concerning neuroprotective effects of NOS inhibition on survival of hippocampal CA1 neurons following global ischemia,[229–231] with more consistent protection with lower dosage of NOS inhibitors.[232] Strong evidence for a role of the neuronal isoform of NOS in focal ischemia came from studies in mice with a knockout of the neuronal isoform of NOS. These mice show a significant attenuation in the size of focal ischemic lesions.[72]

Improved inhibitors of NOS have recently been described. One of these is 7-nitroindazole (7-NI), which is a relatively specific inhibitor of the neuronal isoform of NOS in vivo.[9] In vivo studies showed no effects on blood pressure and on endothelium-dependent and acetycholine-induced blood vessel relaxation. 7-NI is effective against focal ischemic lesions in vivo.[74]

We found that 7-NI significantly attenuated NMDA striatal excitotoxic lesions, but not those induced by kainic acid or AMPA.[75] 7-NI dose-dependently reduced striatal malonate lesions, and the protection was reversed by L-arginine but not by D-arginine. 7-NI produced nearly complete protection against lesions produced by systemic administration of 3-NP. 7-NI protected against malonate-induced decreases in ATP and increases in lactate. Its effects were not mediated by excitatory amino acid receptors since it had no effect on spontaneous electrophysiologic activity in the striatum in vivo. One mechanism by which NO• is thought to mediate its toxicity is by interacting with superoxide to form peroxynitrite which then may nitrate tyrosine residues. 7-NI attenuated increase in hydroxyl radical and 3-nitrotyrosine generation in vivo, which may be a consequence of peroxynitrite formation. We also found that 7-NI dose-dependently protected against MPTP-induced dopaminergic toxicity in mice.[63] 7-NI also attenuated increases in striatal 3-nitrotyrosine induced by MPTP. Another study showed that inhibition of NOS with the nonselective inhibitor nitro-L-arginine reduced MPP$^+$-induced increases in hydroxyl radical generation and showed mild protection against MPTP-induced depletions of dopamine.

Conclusions

A role of excitotoxicity in acute neurologic diseases is strongly supported by experimental studies. The role of excitotoxicity in neurodegenerative diseases is more speculative, but evidence favoring this possibility continues to accrue. There is now strong evidence linking excitotoxicity to both free radical and nitric oxide generation. Therapeutic studies in animals have firmly established the efficacy of excitatory amino acid antagonists in models of focal cerebral ischemia and head trauma. Recent studies have also shown efficacy of free radical scavengers and neuronal NOS inhibitors. These studies are now being extended to therapeutic trials in man. These studies should definitively establish the role of excitotoxicity in neurologic illnesses.

References

1. Lucas DR, Newhouse JP: The toxic effect of sodium L-glutamate on the inner layers of the retina. *Arch Ophthalmol* 1957; 58:193.
2. Olney JW: Brain lesions, obesity and other disturbances in mice treated with monosodium glutamate. *Science* 1969; 164:719.
3. Rothman SM: Synaptic release of excitatory amino acid neurotransmitter mediates anoxic neuronal death. *J Neurosci* 1984; 4:1884.
4. Choi DW: Ionic dependence of glutamate neurotoxicity and cortical cell culture. *J Neurosci* 1987; 7:369.
5. Dawson VL, et al: Nitric oxide mediates glutamate neurotoxicity in primary cortical cultures. *Proc Natl Acad Sci USA* 1991; 88:6368.
6. Lafon-Cazal M, et al: NMDA-dependent superoxide production and neurotoxicity. *Nature* 1993; 364:535.
7. Monaghan DT, et al: The excitatory amino acid receptors: Their classes, pharmacology, and distinct properties in the function of the central nervous system. *Annu Rev Pharmacol Toxicol* 1989; 29:365.
8. Young AB, Fagg GE: Excitatory amino acid receptors in the brain: Membrane binding and receptor autoradiographic approaches. *Trends Pharm Sci* 1990; 11:126.
9. Babbedge RC, et al: Inhibition of rat cerebellar nitric oxide synthase by 7-nitroindazole and related substituted indazoles. *Br J Pharmacol* 1993; 110:225.
10. Boulter J, et al: Molecular cloning and functional expression of glutamate receptor subunit genes. *Science* 1990; 249:1033.
11. Hollmann M, et al: Cloning by functional expression of a member of the glutamate receptor family. *Nature* 1989; 343:643.
12. Kleinanen K, et al: A family of AMPA-selective glutamate receptors. *Science* 1990; 249:556.
13. Sommer B, et al: Flip and flop: A cell-specific functional switch in glutamate-operated channels of the CNS. *Science* 1990; 249:1580.
14. Ejeberg J, et al: Cloning of a cDNA for a glutamate receptor subunit activated by kainate but not AMPA. *Nature* 1991; 351:745.
15. Herb A, et al: The KA-2 subunit of excitatory amino acid receptors shows widespread expression in brain and forms ion channels with distantly related subunits. *Neuron* 1992; 8:775.
16. Werner P, et al: Cloning of a putative high-affinity kainate receptor subunit activated by kainate but not AMPA. *Nature* 1991; 351:745.
17. Siegel SJ, et al: Distribution of the excitatory amino acid receptor subunits GluR2(4) in monkey hippocampus and colocalization with subunits GluR5-7 and NMDAR1. *J Neurosci* 1995; 15:2707.
18. Moriyoshi K, et al: Molecular cloning and characterization of the rat NMDA receptor. *Nature* 1991; 354:31.
19. Meguro H, et al: Functional characterization of a heteromeric

NMDA receptor channel expressed from cloned cDNAs. *Nature* 1992; 357:70.

20. Monyer H, et al: Heteromeric NMDA receptors: Molecular and functional distinction of subtypes. *Science* 1992; 256:1217.

21. Kutsuwada T, et al: Molecular diversity of the NMDA receptor channel. *Nature* 1992; 358:36.

22. Houamed KM, et al: Cloning, expression and gene structure of a G-protein-coupled glutamate receptor from rat brain. *Science* 1991; 252:1318.

23. Tanabe Y, et al: A family of metabotropic glutamate receptors. *Neuron* 1922; 8:169.

24. Hollmann M, et al: Ca^{2+} permeability of Ka-AMPA-gated glutamate receptor channels depends on subunit composition. *Science* 1991; 252:851.

25. Hume RI, et al: Identification of a site in glutamate receptor subunits that controls calcium permeability. *Science* 1991; 253:1028.

26. Verdoorn TA, et al: Structural determinants of ion flow through recombinant glutamate receptor channels. *Science* 1991; 252:1715.

27. Sommer B, et al: RNA editing in brain controls a determinant of ion flow in glutamate-gated channels. *Cell* 1991; 67:11.

28. Burnashev N, et al: Control by asparagine residues of calcium permeability and magnesium blockade in the NMDA receptor. *Science* 1992; 257:1415.

29. Sakurada K, et al: Alteration of Ca^{2+} permeability and sensitivity to Mg^{2+} and channel blockers by a single amino acid substitution in the *N*-methyl-D-aspartate receptor. *J Biol Chem* 1993; 268:410.

30. Anegawa NJ, et al: Transfection of *N*-methyl-D-aspartate receptors in a nonneuronal cell line leads to cell death. *J Neurochem* 1995; 64:2004.

31. Cik M, et al: Expression of NMDAR1-1a(N598Q)/NMDAR2A receptors results in decreased cell mortality. *Eur J Pharmacol* 1994; 266:R1.

32. Traynelis SF, et al: Control of proton sensitivity of the NMDA receptor by RNA splicing and polyamines. *Science* 1995; 268:973.

33. Hartley DM, et al: Glutamate receptor-induced $^{45}Ca^{2+}$ accumulation in cortical cell culture correlates with subsequent neuronal degeneration. *J Neurosci* 1993; 13:1993.

34. Eimerl S, Schramm M: The quantity of calcium that appears to induce neuronal death. *J Neurochem* 1994; 62:1223.

35. Witt M-R, et al: Complex correlation between excitatory amino acid-induced increase in the intracellular Ca^{2+} concentration and subsequent loss of neuronal function in individual neocortical neurons in culture. *Proc Natl Acad Sci USA* 1994; 91:12303.

36. White RJ, Reynolds IJ: Mitochondria and Na^+/Ca^{2+} exchange buffer glutamate-induced calcium loads in cultured cortical neurons. *J Neurosci* 1995; 15:1318.

37. Wang GJ, et al: Glutamate-induced intracellular acidification of cultured hippocampal neurons demonstrates altered energy metabolism resulting from Ca^{2+} loads. *J Neurophysiol* 1994; 72:2563.

38. Randall RD, Thayer SA: Glutamate-induced calcium transient triggers delayed calcium overload and neurotoxicity in rat hippocampal neurons. *J Neurosci* 1992; 12:1882.

39. Tymianski M, et al: Cell-permeant Ca^{2+} chelators reduce early excitotoxic and ischemic neuronal injury in vitro and in vivo. *Neuron* 1993; 11:221.

40. Tymianski M, et al: Source specificity of early calcium neurotoxicity in cultured embryonic spinal neurons. *J Neurosci* 1993; 13:2085.

41. Frandsen A, Schousboe A: Dantrolene prevents glutamate cytotoxicity and Ca^{2+} release from intracellular stores in cultured cerebral cortical neurons. *J Neurochem* 1991; 56:1075.

42. Lei SZ, et al: Blockade of NMDA receptor-mediated mobilization of intracellular Ca^{2+} prevents neurotoxicity. *Brain Res* 1992; 598:196.

43. Beal MF: Does impairment of energy metbolism result in excitotoxic neuronal death in neurodegenerative illnesses? *Ann Neurol* 1992; 31:119.

44. Siman R, Noszek JC: Excitatory amino acids activate calpain I and induce structural protein breakdown in vivo. *Neuron* 1988; 1:279.

45. Caner H, et al: Attenuation of AMPA-induced neurotoxicity by a calpain inhibitor. *Brain Res* 1993; 607:354.

46. Manev H, et al: Glutamate neurotoxicity is independent of calpain 1 inhibition in primary cultures of cerebellar granule cells. *J Neurochem* 1991; 57:1288.

47. Bartus RT, et al: Postischemic administration of AK275, a calpain inhibitor, provides substantial protection against focal ischemic brain damage. *J Cereb Blood Flow Metab* 1994; 14:537.

48. Hong S-C, et al: Neuroprotection with a calpain inhibitor in a model of focal cerebral ischemia. *Stroke* 1994; 25:663.

49. Lee KS, et al: Inhibition of proteolysis protects hippocampal neurons from ischemia. *Proc Natl Acad Sci USA* 1991; 88:7233.

50. Churn SB, et al: Excitotoxic activation of the NMDA receptor results in inhibition of calcium/calmodulin kinase II activity in cultured hippocampal neurons. *J Neurosci* 1995; 15:3200.

51. Hajimohammadreza I, et al: A specific inhibitor of calcium/calmodulin-dependent protein kinase-II provides neuroprotection against NMDA- and hypoxia/hypoglycemia-induced cell death. *J Neurosci* 1995; 15:4093.

52. Dykens JA, et al: Mechanisms of kainate toxicity to cerebellar neurons in vitro is analogous to reperfusion tissue injury. *J Neurochem* 1987; 49:1222.

53. Bridges RJ, et al: Increased excitotoxic vulnerability of cortical cultures with reduced levels of glutathione. *Eur J Pharmacol* 1991; 192:199.

54. Favit A, et al: Ubiquinone protects cultured neurons against spontaneous and excitotoxin-induced degeneration. *J Cereb Blood Flow Metab* 1992; 12:638.

55. Majewska MD, Bell JA: Ascorbic acid protects neurons from injury induced by glutamate and NMDA. *NeuroReport* 1990; 1:94.

56. Chow HS, et al: Trolox attenuates cortical neuronal injury induced by iron, ultraviolet light, glucose deprivation, or AMPA. *Brain Res* 1994; 639:102.

57. Chan PH, et al: Reduced neurotoxicity in transgenic mice overexpressing human copper-zinc-superoxide dismutase. *Stroke* 1990; 21:11180.

58. Dykens JA: Isolated cerebral and cerebellar mitochondria produce free radicals when exposed to elevated Ca^{2+} and Na^+: Implications for neurodegeneration. *J Neurochem* 1994; 63:584.

59. Bondy SC, Lee DK: Oxidative stress induced by glutamate receptor agonists. *Brain Res* 1993; 610:229.

60. Sun AY, et al: The biochemical mechanisms of the excitotoxicity of kainic acid. Free radical formation. *Mol Chem Neuropathol* 1992; 17:51.

61. Dugan LL: Mitochondrial production of reactive oxygen species in cortical neurons following exposure to *N*-methyl-D-aspartate. *J Neurosci* 1995; 15:6377.

62. Reynolds IJ, Hastings TG: Glutamate induces the production of reactive oxygen species in cultured forebrain neurons following NMDA receptor activation. *J Neurosci* 1995; 15:3318.

63. Schulz JB, et al: Involvement of free radicals in excitotoxicity in vivo. *J Neurochem* 1995; 64:2239.

64. Dawson VL, et al: Mechanisms of nitric oxide mediated neurotoxicity in primary brain cultures. *J Neurosci* 1993; 13:2651.

65. Demerle-Pallardy, et al: Absence of implication of L-arginine/nitric oxide pathway in neuronal cell injury induced by

L-glutamate or hypoxia. *Biochem Biophys Res Commun* 1991; 181:456.

66. Hewett SJ, et al: Inhibition of nitric oxide formation does not protect murine cortical cell cultures from *N*-methyl-methyl-D-aspartate neurotoxicity. *Brain Res* 1993; 625:337.

67. Pauwels P, Leysen JE: Blockade of nitric oxide formation does not prevent glutamate-induced neurotoxicity in neuronal cultures from rat hippocampus. *Neurosci Lett* 1992; 143:27.

68. Puttfarcken PS, et al: Dissociation of nitric oxide generation and kainate-mediated neuronal degeneration in primary cultures of rat cerebellar granule cells. *Neuropharmacology* 1992; 31:565.

69. Regan RF, et al: NMDA neurotoxicity in murine cortical cell cultures is not attenuated by hemoglobin or inhibition of nitric oxide synthesis. *Neurosci Lett* 1993; 153:53.

70. Moncada C, et al: Effect of NO synthase inhibition on NMDA- and ischaemia-induced hippocampal lesions. *NeuroReport* 1992; 3:530.

71. Lerner-Natoli M, et al: Chronic NO synthase inhibition fails to protect hippocampal neurones against NMDA toxicity. *NeuroReport* 1992; 3:1109.

72. Huang Z, et al: Effects of cerebral ischemia in mice deficient in neuronal nitric oxide synthase. *Science* 1994; 265:1883.

73. Moore PK, et al: Characterization of the novel nitric oxide synthase inhibitor 7-nitroindazole and related indazoles: Antinociceptive and cardiovascular effects. *Br J Pharmacol* 1993; 110:219.

74. Yoshida T, et al: The NOS inhibitor, 7-nitroindazole, decreases focal infarct volume but not the response to topical acetylcholine in pial vessels. *J Cereb Blood Flow Metab* 1994; 14:924.

75. Schulz JB, et al: Inhibition of neuronal nitric oxide synthase (NOS) protects against neurotoxicity produced by 3-nitropropionic acid, malonate, and MPTP. *Soc Neurosci Abstr* 1994; 20:1661.

76. Teitelbaum J-S, et al: Neurologic sequelae of domoic acid intoxication due to ingestion of contaminated mussels. *N Engl J Med* 1990; 322:1781.

77. Cendes F, et al: Temporal lobe epilepsy caused by domoic acid intoxication: Evidence for glutamate receptor-mediated excitotoxicity in humans. *Ann Neurol* 1995; 37:123.

78. McCulloch J: Glutamate receptor antagonists in cerebral ischemia. *J Neural Transm* 1994; 43:71.

79. Brorson JR, et al: AMPA receptor desensitization predicts the selective vulnerability of cerebellar Purkinje cells to excitotoxicity. *J Neurosci* 1995; 15:4515.

80. Sheardown MJ, et al: 2,3-Dihydroxy-6-nitro-7-sulfamoyl-benzoic (F) quinoxaline: A neuroprotectant for cerebral ischemia. *Science* 1990; 247:571.

81. Albers GW, et al: Safety, tolerability, and pharmacokinetics of the *N*-methyl-D-aspartate antagonist dextrorphan in patients with acute stroke. *Stroke* 1995; 26:254.

82. Grotta J, et al: Safety and tolerability of the glutamate antagonist CGS 19755 (Selfotel) in patients with acute ischemic stroke. *Stroke* 1995; 26:602.

83. Katayama Y, et al: Massive increases in extracellular potassium and the indiscriminate release of glutamate following concussive brain injury. *J Neurosurg* 1990; 73:889.

84. McIntosh TK, et al: Effect of noncompetitive blockade of *N*-methyl-D-aspartate receptors on the neurochemical sequelae of experimental brain injury. *J Neurochem* 1990; 55:1170.

85. Golding EM, Vink R: Efficacy of competitive vs noncompetitive blockade of the NMDA channel following traumatic brain injury. *Mol Chem Neuropathol* 1995; 24:137.

86. Smith DH, et al: Effects of the excitatory amino acid receptor antagonists kynurenate and indole-2-carboxylic acid on be-

havioral and neurochemical outcome following experimental brain injury. *J Neurosci* 1993; 13:5383.

87. Hicks RR, et al: Kynurenate is neuroprotective following experimental brain injury in the rat. *Brain Res* 1994; 655:91.

88. Wieloch T: Hypoglycemia-induced neuronal damage prevented by an *N*-methyl-D-aspartate antagonist. *Science* 1985; 230:681.

89. Massieu L, et al: Accumulation of extracellular glutamate by inhibition of its uptake is not sufficient for inducing neuronal damage: An in vivo microdialysis study. *J Neurochem* 1995; 64:2262.

90. Heyes MP, et al: Regional brain and cerebrospinal fluid quinolinic acid concentrations in Huntington's disease. *Neurosci Lett* 1991; 122:265.

91. Albin RL, Greenamyre JT: Alternative excitotoxic hypotheses. *Neurology* 1992; 42:733.

92. Novelli A, et al: Glutamate becomes neurotoxic via the *N*-methyl-D-aspartate receptor when intracellular energy levels are reduced. *Brain Res* 1988; 451:205.

93. Zeevalk GD, Nicklas WJ: Chemically induced hypoglycemia and anoxia: Relationship to glutamate receptor-mediated toxicity in retina. *J Pharmacol Exp Ther* 1990; 253:1285.

94. Zeevalk GD, Nicklas WJ: Mechanisms underlying initiation of excitotoxicity associated with metabolic inhibition. *J Pharmacol Exp Ther* 1991; 257:870.

95. Abele AE, Miller RJ: Potassium channel activators abolish excitotoxicity in cultured hippocampal pyramidal neurons. *Neurosci Lett* 1990; 115:195.

96. Lees GJ, Leong W: The sodium-potassium ATPase inhibitor ouabain is neurotoxic in the rat substantia nigra and striatum. *Neurosci Lett* 1995; 188:113.

97. Riepe MW, et al: Failure of neuronal ion exchange, not potentiated excitation, causes excitotoxicity after inhibition of oxidative phosphorylation. *Neurosci* 1995; 64:91.

98. Moudy AM, et al: Abnormal calcium homeostasis and mitochondrial polarization in a human encephalomyopathy. *Proc Natl Acad Sci USA* 1995; 92:729.

99. Coyle JT, Schwarcz R: Lesions of striatal neurons with kainic acid provide a model for Huntington's chorea. *Nature* 1976; 263:244.

100. McGeer EG, McGeer PL: Duplication of biochemical changes of Huntington's chorea by intrastriatal injections of glutamic and kainic acids. *Nature* 1976; 263:517.

101. Dawbarn D, et al: Survival of basal ganglia neuropeptide Y-somatostatin neurons in Huntington's disease. *Brain Res* 1985; 340:251.

102. Ferrante RJ, et al: Selective sparing of a class of striatal neurons in Huntington's disease. *Science* 1985; 230:561.

103. Beal MF, et al: Differential sparing of somatostatin-neuropeptide Y and cholinergic neurons following striatal excitotoxic lesions. *Synapse* 1989; 3:38.

104. Beal MF, et al: Replication of the neurochemical characteristics of Huntington's disease with quinolinic acid. *Nature* 1986; 321:168.

105. Beal MF, et al: Chronic quinolinic acid lesions in rats closely mimic Huntington's disease. *J Neurosci* 1991; 11:1649.

106. Bazzett TJ, et al: Chronic intrastriatal quinolinic acid produces reversible changes in perikaryal calbindin and parvalbumin immunoreactivity. *Neuroscience* 1994; 60:837.

107. Harrington KM, Kowall NW: Parvalbumin immunoreactive neurons resist degeneration in Huntington's disease striatum. *Exp Neurol* 1991; 50:309.

108. Waldvogel HJ, et al: Differential sensitivity of calbindin and parvalbumin immunoreactive cells in the striatum to excitotoxins. *Brain Res* 1991; 546:329.

109. Ferrante RJ, et al: Excitotoxin lesions in primates as a model

for Huntington's disease. Histologic and neurochemical characterization. *Exp Neurol* 1993; 119:46.

110. Dure LS, et al: Excitatory amino acid binding sites in the caudate nucleus and frontal cortex of Huntington's disease. *Ann Neurol* 1991; 30:785.

111. Young AB, et al: NMDA receptor losses in putamen from patients with Huntington's disease. *Science* 1988; 241:981.

112. Albin RL, et al: Abnormalities of striatal projection neurons and *N*-methyl-aspartate receptors in presymptomatic Huntington's disease. *N Engl J Med* 1990; 322:1293.

113. Difazio MC, et al: Glutamate receptors in the substantia nigra of Parkinson's disease brains. *Neurology* 1992; 42:402.

114. Sonsalla PK, et al: MK-801 fails to protect against the dopaminergic neuropathology produced by systemic 1-methyl-4-phenyl-1,2,3,6-tetrahydropyridine in mice or intranigral 1-methyl-4-phenylpyridinium in rats. *J Neurochem* 1992; 58:1979.

115. Turski L, et al: Protection of substantia nigra from MPP^+ neurotoxicity by *N*-methyl-D-aspartate antagonists. *Nature* 1991; 349:414.

116. Lange KW, et al: The competitive NMDA antagonist CPP protects substantia nigra neurons from MPTP-induced degeneration in primates. *Naunyn Schmiedebergs Arch Pharmacol* 1993; 348:586.

117. Zuddas A, et al: MK-801 prevents 1-methyl-4-phenyl-1,2,3,6-tetrahydropyridinine-induced Parkinsonism in primates. *J Neurochem* 1992; 59:733.

118. Malessa S, et al: Amyotrophic lateral sclerosis: Glutamate dehydrogenase and transmitter amino acids in the spinal cord. *J Neurol Neurosurg Psychiatry* 1991; 54:984.

119. Plaitakis A, et al: The neuroexcitotoxic amino acids glutamate and aspartate are altered in the spinal cord and brain in amyotrophic lateral sclerosis. *Ann Neurol* 1988; 24:446.

120. Rothstein JD, et al: Abnormal excitatory amino acid metabolism in amyotrophic lateral sclerosis. *Ann Neurol* 1990; 28:18.

121. Rothstein JD, et al: Decreased glutamate transport by the brain and spinal cord in amyotrophic lateral sclerosis. *N Engl J Med* 1992; 362:1464.

122. Spencer PS, et al: Lathyrism: Evidence for role of the neuroexcitatory aminoacid BOAA. *Lancet* 1986; 1:1066.

123. Spencer PS, et al: Guam amyotrophic lateral sclerosis–Parkinsonism-dementia linked to a plant excitant neurotoxin. *Science* 1987; 237:517.

124. Shaw PJ, et al: Non-NMDA receptors in motor neuron disease (MND): A quantitative autoradiographic study in spinal cord and motor cortex using [^{3}H]CNQX and [^{3}H]kainate. *Brain Res* 1994; 655:186.

125. Krieger C, et al: Amyotrophic lateral sclerosis: Quantitative autoradiography of [^{3}H]MK-801/NMDA binding sites in spinal cord. *Neurosci Lett* 1993; 159:191.

126. Allaoua H, et al: Alterations in spinal cord excitatory amino acid receptors in amyotrophic lateral sclerosis patients. *Brain Res* 1992, 579:169.

127. Rothstein JD, et al: Chronic inhibition of glutamate uptake produces a model of slow neurotoxicity. *Proc Natl Acad Sci USA* 1993; 90:6591.

128. Copani A, et al: β-Amyloid increases neuronal susceptibility to injury by glucose deprivation. *NeuroReport* 1991; 2:763.

129. Koh J-Y, et al: β-Amyloid protein increases the vulnerability of cultured cortical neurons to excitotoxic damage. *Brain Res* 1990; 533:315.

130. Mattson MP, et al: β-Amyloid peptides destabilize calcium homeostasis and render human cortical neurons vulnerable to excitotoxicity. *J Neurosci* 1992; 12:376.

131. Greenamyre JT, et al: Alterations in L-glutamate binding in Alzheimer's and Huntington's disease. *Science* 1985; 227:1496.

132. Greenamyre JT, et al: Dementia of the Alzheimer type: Changes in hippocampal L-[^{3}H] glutamate binding. *J Neurochem* 1987; 48:543.

133. Kowall NW, Beal MF: Glutamate-, glutaminase-, and taurine-immunoreactive neurons develop neurofibrillary tangles in Alzheimer's disease. *Ann Neurol* 1991; 29:162.

134. Rogers J, Morrison JH: Quantitative morphology and regional laminar distributions of senile plaques in Alzheimer's disease. *J Neurosci* 1985; 5:2801.

135. Pearson RCA, et al: Anatomical correlates of the pathological changes in the neocortex in Alzheimer's disease. *Proc Natl Acad Sci USA* 1985; 82:4531.

136. Beal MF: Mechanisms of excitotoxicity in neurologic diseases. *FASEB J* 1992; 6:3338.

137. Beal MF, et al: Aminooxyacetic acid results in excitoxin lesions by a novel indirect mechanism. *J Neurochem* 1991; 57:1068.

138. Urbanska E, et al: Aminooxyacetic acid produces excitotoxic lesions in the rat striatum. *Synapse* 1991; 9:129.

139. Cheeseman AJ, Clark JB: Influence of the malate-aspartate shuttle on oxidative metabolism in synaptosomes. *J Neurochem* 1988; 50:1559.

140. Kauppinen RA, et al: Aminooxyacetic acid inhibits the malate-aspartate shuttle in isolated nerve terminals and prevents the mitochondria from utilizing glycolytic substrates. *Biochim Biophys Acta* 1987; 930:173.

141. Fitzpatrick SM, et al: Use of β-methylene-D,L-aspartate to assess the role of aspartate amino-transferase in cerebral oxidative metabolism. *J Neurochem* 1983; 41:1370.

142. Brouillet E, et al: Aminooxyacetic acid striatal lesions are blocked by energy repletion. *Neurosci Lett* 1994; 177:58.

143. McMaster OG, et al: Focal injection of aminooxyacetic acid produces seizures and lesions in rat hippocampus: Evidence for mediation by NMDA receptors. *Exp Neurol* 1991; 113:378.

144. McDonald JW, Schoepp DD: Aminooxyacetic acid produces excitotoxic brain injury in neonatal rats. *Brain Res* 1991; 624:239.

145. Webb JL: *Enzyme and Metabolic Inhibitors.* New York, Academic Press, 1966.

146. Beal MF, et al: Age-dependent striatal excitotoxic lesions produced by the endogenous mitochondrial inhibitor malonate. *J Neurochem* 1993; 61:1147.

147. Greene JG, et al: Inhibition of succinate dehydrogenase by malonic acid produces an "excitotoxic" lesion in rat striatum. *J Neurochem* 1993; 61:1151.

148. Greene JG, Greenamyre JT: Exacerbation of NMDA, AMPA, and L-glutamate excitotoxicity by the succinate dehydrogenase inhibitor malonate. *J Neurochem* 1995; 64:2332.

149. Henshaw R, et al: Malonate produces striatal lesions by indirect NMDA receptor activation. *Brain Res* 1994; 647:161.

150. Beal MF, et al: Coenzyme Q_{10} and nicotinamide block striatal lesions produced by mitochondrial toxin malonate. *Ann Neurol* 1994; 36:882.

151. Ludolph AC, et al: 3-Nitropropionic acid–exogenous animal neurotoxin and possible human striatal toxin. *Can J Neurol Sci* 1991; 18:492.

152. Alston TA, et al: 3-Nitropropionate, the toxic substance of *Indigofera*, is a suicide inactivator of succinate dehydrogenase. *Proc Natl Acad Sci USA* 1977; 74:3767.

153. Coles CJ, et al: Inactivation and succinate dehydrogenase by 3-nitropropionate. *J Biol Chem* 1979; 254:5161.

154. Riepe M, et al: Inhibition of energy metabolism by 3-nitropropionic acid activates ATP-sensitive potassium channels. *Brain Res* 1992; 586:61.

155. Ludolph AC, et al: 3-Nitropropionic acid decreases cellular energy levels and causes neuronal degeneration in cortical explants. *Neurodegeneration* 1992; 1:155.

156. Zeevalk GD, et al: NMDA receptor involvement in toxicity to

dopamine neurons in vitro caused by the succinate dehydrogenase inhibitor 3-nitropropionic acid. *J Neurochem* 1995; 64:455.

157. Weller M, Paul SM: 3-Nitropropionic acid is an indirect excitotoxin to cultured cerebellar granule neurons. *Eur J Pharmacol* 1993; 248:223.

158. Behrens MI, et al: 3-Nitropropionic acid induces apoptosis in cultured striatal and cortical neurons. *NeuroReports* 1995; 6:545.

159. Gould DH, Gustine DL: Basal ganglia degeneration, myelin alterations, and enzyme inhibition in mice by the plant toxin 3-nitropropionic acid. *Neuropathol Appl Neurobiol* 1982; 8:377.

160. Hamilton BF, Gould DH: Correlation of morphologic brain lesions with physiologic alterations and blood-brain barrier impairment in 3-nitropropionic acid toxicity in rats. *Acta Neuropathol* 1987; 74:67.

161. Brouillet E, et al: Chronic administration of 3-nitropropionic acid induced selective striatal degeneration and abnormal choreiform movements in monkeys. *Soc Neurosci Abstr* 1993; 19:409.

162. Beal MF, et al: Neurochemical and histologic characterization of excitotoxic lesions produced by the mitochondrial toxin 3-nitropropionic acid. *J Neurosci* 1993; 13:4181.

163. Turski L, Ikonomidou H: Striatal toxicity of 3-nitropropionic acid prevented by the AMPA antagonist NBQX. *Soc Neurosci Abstr* 1994; 20:1677.

164. Wullner U, et al: 3-Nitropropionic acid toxicity in the striatum. *J Neurochem* 1994; 63:1772.

165. Beal MF, et al: 3-Nitropropionic acid neurotoxicity is attenuated in copper/zinc superoxide dismutase transgenic mice. *J Neurochem* 1995; 65:919.

166. Leach MJ, et al: BW619C89, a glutamate release inhibitor, protects against focal cerebral ischemic damage. *Stroke* 1993; 24:1063.

167. McGeer EG, Zhu SG: Lamotrigine protects against kainate but not ibotenate lesions in rat striatum. *Neurosci Lett* 1990; 112:348.

168. Jones-Humble SA, et al: The novel anticonvulsant lamotrigine prevents dopamine depletion in C57 black mice in the MPTP animal model of Parkinson's disease. *Life Sci* 1994; 54:245.

169. Graham SH, et al: Limiting ischemic injury by inhibition of excitatory amino acid release. *J Cereb Blood Flow Metab* 1993; 13:88.

170. Graham SH, et al: Neuroprotective effects of a use-dependent blocker of voltage-dependent sodium channels, BW619C89, in rat middle cerebral artery occlusion. *J Pharmacol Exp Ther* 1994; 269:854.

171. Lekiefre D, Meldrum BS: The pyrimidine-derivative, BW1003C87, protects CA1 and striatal neurons following transient severe forebrain ischaemia in rats. *Neuroscience* 1993; 56:93.

172. Cheramy A, et al: Riluzole inhibits the release of glutamate in the caudate nucleus of the cat in vivo. *Neurosci Lett* 1992; 147:209.

173. Martin D, et al: The neuroprotective agent riluzole inhibits release of glutamate and aspartate from slices of hippocampal area CA1. *Eur J Pharmacol* 1993; 250:473.

174. Malgouris C, et al: Riluzole, a novel antiglutamate, prevents memory loss and hippocampal neuronal damage in ischemic gerbils. *J Neurosci* 1989; 9:3720.

175. Pratt J, et al: Neuroprotective actions of riluzole in rodent models of global and focal cerebral ischemia. *Neurosci Lett* 1992; 140:225.

176. Boireau A, et al: Riluzole and experimental parkinsonism: Antagonism of MPTP-induced decrease in central dopamine levels in mice. *NeuroReport* 1994; 5:2657.

177. Bensimon G, et al: A controlled trial of riluzole in amyotrophic lateral sclerosis. *N Engl J Med* 1994; 330:585.

178. Fujisawa H, et al: Pharmacological modification of glutamate neurotoxicity in vivo. *Brain Res* 1993; 629:73.

179. Lipton SA, Rosenberg PA: Excitatory amino acids as a final common pathway for neurologic disorders. *N Engl J Med* 1994; 330:613.

180. McCulloch J: Excitatory amino acid antagonists and their potential for the treatment of ischaemic brain damage in man. *Br J Clin Pharmacol* 1992; 34:106.

181. Newell DW, Malouf BAT: Glycine site NMDA receptor antagonists provide protection against ischemia-induced neuronal damage in hippocampal slice cultures. *Brain Res* 1995; 675:38.

182. Bullock R, et al: Neuroprotective effect of the AMPA receptor antagonist LY-293558 in focal cerebral ischemia in the cat. *J Cereb Blood Flow Metab* 1994; 14:466.

183. Browne SE, McCulloch J: AMPA receptor antagonists and local cerebral glucose utilization in the rat. *Brain Res* 1994; 641:10.

184. Ozyurt E, et al: Protective effect of the glutamate antagonist MK-801 in the focal cerebral ischemia in the cat. *J Cereb Blood Flow Metab* 1988; 8:138.

185. Park CK, et al: Focal cerebral ischaemia in the cat: Treatment with the glutamate antagonist MK-801 after induction of ischaemia. *J Cereb Blood Flow Metab* 1988; 8:757.

186. Park CK, et al: The glutamate antagonist MK-801 reduces focal ischemic brain damage in the rat. *Ann Neurol* 1988; 24:543.

187. Gill R, et al: The neuroprotective action of dizocilpine (MK-801) in the rat middle cerebral artery occlusion model of focal ischaemia. *Br J Pharmacol* 1991; 103:2030.

188. Roussel S, et al: Effect of MK-801 on focal brain infarction in normotensive and hypersensive rats. *Hypertension* 1992; 19:40.

189. Meadows M-E, et al: Delayed treatment with a noncompetitive NMDA antagonist CNS-1102, reduces infarct size in rats. *Cerebrovasc Dis* 1994; 4:26.

190. Steinberg GK, et al: Neuroprotection following focal cerebral ischaemia with the NMDA antagonist dextromethorphan, has a favorable dose response profile. *Neurol Res* 1993; 15:174.

191. Steinberg GK, et al: Dextromethorphan protects against cerebral injury following transient focal ischemia in rabbits. *Stroke* 1988; 19:1112.

192. Simon R, Shiraishi K: N-Methyl-D-aspartate antagonist reduces stroke size and regional glucose metabolism. *Ann Neurol* 1990; 27:606.

193. Chen M, et al: Evaluation of a competitive NMDA antagonist (D-CPPene) in feline focal cerebral ischemia. *Ann Neurol* 1991; 30:62.

194. Gotti B, et al: Ifenprodil and SL-82.0715 as cerebral antiischemic agents. 1. Evidence of efficacy in models of focal cerebral ischemia. *J Pharmacol Exp Ther* 1988; 247:1211.

195. Gill R, et al: The neuroprotective effect of the glycine site antagonist 3R-(+)-cis-4-methyl-HA966 (L-687,414) in a rat model of focal ischemia. *J Cereb Blood Flow Metab* 1995; 15:197.

196. Warner DS, et al: In vivo models of cerebral ischemia: Effects of parenterally administered NMDA receptor glycine site antagonists. *J Cereb Blood Flow Metab* 1995; 15:188.

197. Gill R, et al: The neuroprotective actions of 2,3-dihydroxy-6-nitro-7-sulfamoyl-benzo(F)quinoxaline (NBQX) in a rat focal ischaemia model. *Brain Res* 1992; 580:35.

198. Xue D, et al: Delayed treatment with AMPA, but not NMDA, antagonists reduces neocortical infarction. *J Cereb Blood Flow Metab* 1994; 14:251.

199. Koek W, Koek CC: Selective blockade of N-methyl-D-aspartate (NMDA)-induced convulsions by NMDA antagonists and putative glycine antagonists: Relationship with phencyclidine-like behavioral effects. *J Pharmacol Exp Ther* 1990; 252:349.

200. Morris RGM, et al: Selective impairment of learning and blockade of LTP by an NMDA receptor antagonist AP5. *Nature* 1986; 319:774.

201. Rogawski MA: Therapeutic potential of excitatory amino acid antagonists: Channel blockers and 2,3-benzodiazepines. *TIPS* 1993; 14:325.

202. Kupsch A, et al: Do NMDA receptor antagonists protect against MPTO-toxicity? Biochemical and immunocytochemical analyses in black mice. *Brain Res* 1992; 592:74.

203. Brouillet E, Beal MF: NMDA antagonists partially protect against MPTP induced neurotoxicity in mice. *NeuroReport* 1993; 4:387.

204. Schulz JB, et al: 3-Acetylpyridine produces age-dependent excitotoxic lesions in rat striatum. *J Cereb Blood Flow Metab* 1994; 14:1024.

205. Lafon-Cazal M, et al: Nitric oxide, superoxide and peroxynitrite: Putative mediators of NMDA-induced cell death in cerebellar granule cells. *Neuropharmacology* 1993; 32:1259.

206. Yue T-L, et al: Neuroprotective effects of phenyl-*t*-butyl-nitrone in gerbil brain ischemia and in cultured rat cerebellar neurons. *Brain Res* 1992; 574:193.

207. Chen G, et al: Excretion, metabolism and tissue distribution of a spin trapping agent, α-phenyl-*N*-tert-butyl-nitrone (PBN) in rats. *Free Radic Res Commun* 1990; 9:3.

208. Oliver CN, et al: Oxidative damage to brain proteins, loss of glutamine synthetase activity, and production of free radicals during ischemia/reperfusion-induced injury to gerbil brain. *Proc Natl Acad Sci USA* 1990; 87:5144.

209. Phillis JW, Clough-Helfman C: Protection from cerebral ischemia injury in gerbils with spin trap agent *N*-tert-butyl-α-phenylnitrone. *Neurosci Lett* 1990; 116:31.

210. Cao X, Phillis JW: α-Phenyl-*tert*-butyl-nitrone reduces cortical infarct and edema in rats subjected to focal ischemia. *Brain Res* 1994; 644:367.

211. Carney JM, et al: Reversal of age-related increase in brain protein oxidation, decrease in enzyme activity, and loss in temporal and spatial memory by chronic administration of the spin-trapping compound *N*-tert-butyl-α-phenylnitrone. *Proc Natl Acad Sci USA* 1991; 88:3633.

212. Monyer H, et al: 21-Aminosteroids attenuate excitotoxic neuronal injury in cortical cell cultures. *Neuron* 1990; 5:121.

213. Hall ED: Cerebral ischemia, free radicals and antioxidant protection. *Biochem Soc Trans* 1988; 21:334.

214. Hall ED, et al: Effects of the 21-aminosteroid U74006F on experimental head injury in mice. *J Neurosurg* 1988; 68:456.

215. Hall ED, Yonkes PA: Attenuation of postischemic cerebral hypoperfusion by the 21-amino steroid U74006. *Stroke* 1988; 19:340.

216. Park CK, Hall ED: Dose-response analysis of the effect of 21-aminosteroid tirilazad mesylate (U-74006F) upon neurological outcome and ischemic brain damage in permanent focal cerebral ischemia. *Brain Res* 1994; 645:157.

217. Prehn JHM, et al: Dihydrolipoate reduces neuronal injury after cerebral ischemia. *J Cereb Blood Flow Metab* 1992; 12:78.

218. Greenamyre JT, et al: The endogenous cofactors, thioctic acid and dihydrolipoic acid, are neuroprotective against NMDA and malonic acid lesions of striatum. *Neurosci Lett* 1994; 171:17.

219. Zhao Q, et al: Delayed treatment with the spin trap alpha-phenyl-*n*-tert-butyl nitrone (PBN) reduces infarct size following transient middle cerebral artery occlusion in rats. *Acta Physiol Scand* 1994; 152:349.

220. Schulz JB, et al: Improved therapeutic window for treatment of histotoxic hypoxia with a free radical spin trap. *J Cereb Blood Flow Metab* 1995; 15:948.

221. Nowicki JP, et al: Nitric oxide mediates neuronal death after focal ischemia in the mouse. *Eur J Pharmacol* 1991; 204:339.

222. Nagafuji T, et al: Blockade of nitric oxide formation by N^{W}-nitro-L-arginine mitigates ischemic brain edema and subsequent cerebral infarction in rats. *Neurosci Lett* 1992; 147:159.

223. Nishikawa T, et al: Nitric oxide synthase inhibition reduces caudate injury following transient focal ischemia in cats. *Stroke* 1994; 25:877.

224. Dawson DA, et al: Inhibition of nitric oxide synthesis does not reduce infarct volume in a rat model of focal cerebral ischaemia. *Neurosci Lett* 1992; 142:151.

225. Kuluz JW, et al: The effect of nitric oxide synthase inhibition on infarct volume after reversible focal cerebral ischemia in conscious rats. *Stroke* 1993; 24:2023.

226. Yamamoto S, et al: Inhibition of nitric oxide synthesis increases focal ischemic infarction in rat. *J Cereb Blood Flow Metab* 1992; 12:717.

227. Zhang F, et al: Nitric oxide donors increase blood flow and reduce brain damage in focal ischemia: Evidence that nitric oxide is beneficial in the early stages of cerebral ischemia. *J Cereb Blood Flow Metab* 1994; 14:217.

228. Carreau A, et al: Neuroprotective efficacy of N-nitro-L-arginine after focal cerebral ischemia in the mouse and inhibition of cortical nitric oxide synthase. *Eur J Pharmacol* 1994; 256:241.

229. Buchan AM, et al: Failure to prevent selective CA1 neuronal death and reduce cortical infarction following cerebral ischemia with inhibition of nitric oxide synthase. *Neuroscience* 1994; 61:1.

230. Caldwell M, et al: N^{G}-Nitro-L-arginine protects against ischaemic-induced increases in nitric oxide and hippocampal neurodegeneration in the gerbil. *Eur J Pharmacol* 1994; 260:191.

231. Sancesario G, et al: Nitric oxide inhibition aggravates ischemic damage of hippocampal but not of NADPH neurons in gerbils. *Stroke* 1994; 25:436.

232. Shapira S, et al: Dose-dependent effect of nitric oxide synthase inhibition following transient forebrain ischemia in gerbils. *Brain Res* 1994; 668:80.

Chapter 17

RESUSCITATION OF THE ISCHEMIC BRAIN

PETER SAFAR

Definitions

Cerebral *protection* (pretreatment) and *preservation* (intrainsult treatment) before and during (anticipated) cerebral ischemia are important factors in the anesthetic management of neurosurgical patients. This chapter primarily concerns cerebral *resuscitation* from the temporary, complete global brain ischemia (GBI) of *cardiac arrest*. Resuscitation is treatment to reverse the insult and support recovery. Resuscitation is relevant to neuroanesthesiologists when a cerebral ischemic insult unexpectedly occurs unprotected. Focal cerebral ischemic insults during or after intracranial surgery are not uncommon; they may represent incomplete or complete, temporary or permanent lesions of focal brain ischemia (FBI). GBI may occur during surgery either deliberately, when controlled hypotension is used, or accidentally, when surgery or anesthesia causes severe hypo-

tension or cardiac arrest. Also, neuroanesthesiologists should know about novel potentials for cerebral resuscitation from cardiac arrest because they are often consulted on such cases outside the realm of neurosurgery.[1,2] Finally, the mechanisms of encephalopathy and treatment potentials for FBI or traumatic brain injury (TBI) have some features in common with those after GBI. The multifactorial pathogenesis of TBI includes ischemia. Because temporary GBI is a more reproducible insult, results of GBI studies are important.

Temporary, severe hypotension of mean arterial pressure (MAP = 30 to 60 mmHg) can be tolerated by the normal brain, but even mild hypotension can cause permanent brain damage when it occurs in a state of asphyxiation (hypoxemia with or without hypercapnia) or in a patient with atherosclerotic cerebral arteries that fail to go into autoregulatory vasodilation with hypotension.

Management of TBI is covered in Chap. 34 and neurologic intensive care in Chap. 36. Much of what applies to cerebral resuscitation from GBI is relevant for neurosurgery under temporary, profound hypothermic circulatory arrest. The latter represents the entire sequence of protection-preservation-resuscitation, which we like to call "suspended animation." Some thoughts on these noncardiac arrest topics are briefly summarized at the end of this chapter.

One must differentiate between the temporary, complete GBI of cardiac arrest (the subject of this chapter); the permanent, complete GBI of panorganic death without resuscitation; the temporary, incomplete GBI of shock states; the incomplete FBI (in the penumbra) (permanent without treatment and temporary with treatment) of ischemic stroke (e.g., cerebral embolism); a variety of unifocal, multifocal, or global ischemic components of TBI; and a variety of toxic brain insults. Treatments that are effective for protection-preservation during an insult are not necessarily effective for resuscitation from an insult. Treatments that are effective during incomplete ischemia are not necessarily effective after complete ischemia.

One must further differentiate between ischemic hypoxia or anoxia caused by reduced cerebral blood flow (CBF); hypoxic hypoxia caused by low arterial P_{O_2} (Pa_{O_2}); and anemic hypoxia caused by very low hemoglobin levels [low hematocrit (Hct) or carbon monoxide poisoning]. One must also differentiate between *process* variables during and early after the insult, such as electroencephalographic activity (EEG), CBF, or cerebral metabolic rates for oxygen, glucose, or lactate ($CMRO_2$, CMRG, CMRL); and the much more important *outcome* variables after maturing of the postischemic encephalopathy over at least 3 days, perhaps weeks. Outcome should be determined in terms of permanent dysfunction and morphologic damage. The

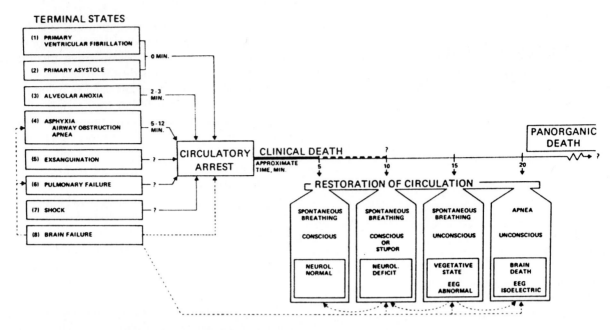

Figure 17-1 Diagram of circulatory arrests and their reversibility. Flow chart illustrates diagrammatically the development of circulatory arrest—suddenly [terminal states 1 (ventricular fibrillation), or 2 (primary asystole)]; over minutes (terminal states 3–5); or protracted (terminal states 6–8). "Clinical death" is defined as "total circulatory arrest with potential reversibility to complete recovery, including brain function." Duration of reversible clinical death depends on terminal state, resuscitation, and postresuscitation syndrome. After restoration of circulation, various possible outcomes. (Reproduced by permission from Safar P: The pathophysiology of dying and reanimation. In Schwartz G, et al (eds): *Principles and Practice of Emergency Medicine*. Philadelphia, WB Saunders, 1985:2–41.)

latter is presently still the most reliable proof of nonviability of cerebral tissue.

In ischemic insults like cardiac arrest [sudden cardiac death (SCD)] (Figs. 17-1 and 17-2) one must further differentiate between the many different mechanisms leading to cardiac arrest, such as asphyxia, exsanguination, ventricular fibrillation (VF), and electromechanical dissociation (EMD) [=pulseless electric activity (PEA)]-asystole. One must differentiate between cardiac arrest (no-flow) time and cardiopulmonary resuscitation (CPR) (low-flow) time.

Reversal of cardiac arrest calls for cardiopulmonary-cerebral resuscitation (CPCR) in three phases (the "chain of survival"), which consists of basic-, advanced-, and prolonged life support (BLS-ALS-PLS).[2] When initiated outside the hospital, the chain of resuscitation steps (BLS-ALS-PLS) is to be delivered throughout another chain, the emergency medical services (EMS) delivery system, from scene via transportation to the hospital's emergency department (ED), operating room (OR), and intensive care unit (ICU).[3] Each chain is only as effective as its weakest link.

When talking about therapeutic or accidental *hypothermia* (see below), one must differentiate between temperature levels, such as normothermia (37° to 38°C), mild hypothermia (34° to 36°C), and moderate (28° to

32°C), deep (10° to 20°C), profound (5° to 10°C), or ultraprofound hypothermia (<5°C). One must further differentiate between temperature monitoring sites such as brain temperature in terms of intracerebral (Tcer), intraventricular (Tiv), epidural (Tep), tympanic membrane (Tty), or nasopharyngeal temperature (Tnp); and core temperatures in terms of esophageal (Tes), central venous (Tcv), pulmonary artery (Tpa), rectal (Tr), and urinary bladder temperature (Tu). Again, one must differentiate between protective-preservative versus resuscitative hypothermia, and state the methods of cooling, duration of hypothermia, and mode of rewarming.

Importance

The *socioeconomic* (epidemiologic) importance of neurologic surgery, anesthesia, and life support is covered in Chaps. 1 and 34 through 38. The importance of attempts at mitigating any type of cerebral insult is obvious because survival in persistent vegetative state (PVS) is an enormous burden to society, and conscious survival with partial paralysis, aphasia, mental and cognitive disturbances, or other deficits, is not only a burden to family and friends, but also torture for the

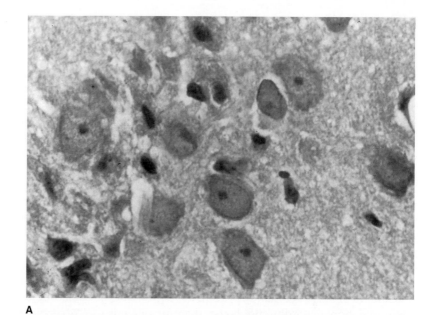

A

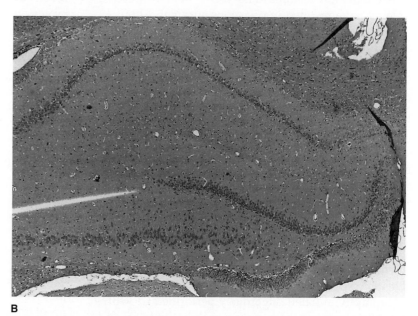

B

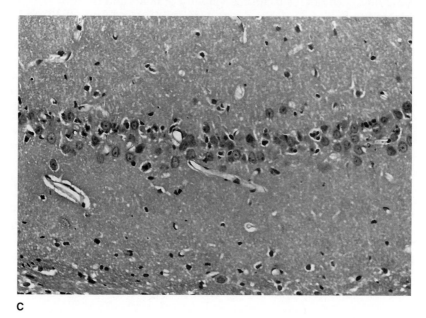

C

Figure 17-2 Morphologic changes of cerebral neurons 3 to 5 days postarrest. *A.* Typical ischemia-induced death of neurons (eosinophilic shrunken cytoplasm and pyknotic nucleus), side-by-side with morphologically normal neurons; ×400. *B.* Normal rat hippocampus; ×40. *C.* Abnormal rat hippocampus 72 h after asphyxiation of 8 min, with loss of normal neurons in the Ca-1 region (selectively vulnerable zone); ×100. (Courtesy of A. Radovsky, Ph.D., D.V.M., I.R.R.C., University of Pittsburgh.)

patients themselves. Billions of dollars are spent each year in the United States on the care of such patients. The *clinical* importance of resuscitation from GBI goes beyond the cases of cardiac arrest. Resuscitation and intensive care life support for the whole organism should always focus on the brain. The *scientific* importance of research into cerebral resuscitation from temporary GBI is considerable because this most controllable insult gives clues and permits extrapolation for treatment potentials also for the more variable and more complex insults of shock, FBI, and TBI.

Current attempts at implementing CPR[1] or CPCR guidelines[2] through community-wide EMS systems[3] have so far yielded suboptimal results.[4-11] At present, among prehospital or in-hospital CPR attempts outside special care units, fewer than 50 percent have spontaneous circulation restored, and fewer than 10 percent overall have resulted in conscious survival. About 10 to 30 percent of long-term survivors have some permanent brain damage.[5-9] The main problems seem to be delayed, suboptimal application of recommended CPR and preexisting disease.

In 1961, the CPCR system was assembled[12] as step A (airway control),[13] step B (breathing control),[14-16] and step C (circulation support)[17] (phase I, BLS[18,19]); followed by steps D, E, and F (drugs and fluids, electrocardiography, and fibrillation treatment (phase II, ALS[2,20,21]); and G (gauged), H (humanized = brain-oriented), I (intensive care) (phase III, brain-oriented PLS[22-24]). Cerebral resuscitation[2,12] starts with optimizing BLS. Brain orientation, expressed in the extension of CPR to CPCR,[2,12] was readily adopted by international guidelines in the 1970s,[2] but has not yet been included in the national guidelines of the American Heart Association.[1]

Promptly initiated, vigorously performed CPR-BLS (low-flow) can often sustain the viability of heart and brain even during prolonged transport.[1,25-27] Reducing the response time of mobile ICU ambulances to less than 10 min is usually not feasible.[4] The currently quoted maximal period of normothermic no-flow that is consistently reversible to complete recovery of cerebral function and structure is 4 to 5 min.[28-31] If that were extended to 10 min (this author's goal since 1970), an estimated 100,000 additional lives could be saved in the United States every year with good neurologic outcome (personal communication, M. Eisenberg, MD, University of Washington, Seattle, 1992).

Several new therapies have been shown to improve (but not to normalize) cerebral outcome in animal models of normothermic cardiac arrest (no-flow) of 10 to 12 min. These benefits have not yet been documented in controlled patient trials. A single penicillin-like "magic bullet," with a unifactorial breakthrough effect, may never be found, because the postischemic-anoxic encephalopathy (i.e., the cerebral postresuscitation syndrome) is complex and multifactorial.[31-43] This complexity calls for the design and evaluation of mechanism-specific multifaceted combination treatments.[33] Optimism is justified because most (but not all) cerebral neurons,[37-44] and cardiac myocytes,[45-47] can tolerate up to 20 min of complete normothermic ischemic anoxia in vivo. A few multifocal necroses in the brain can prevent human mentation, whereas loss of up to 40 percent of cardiac myocytes may not significantly impair cardiac function. Normothermic no-flow of up to 20 min can be reversed to cardiovascular survival[46] and recovery of cerebral oxygen metabolism,[29] apparently without permanent damage to nuclear DNA of most cerebral neurons.[48] This is now being reexamined (see below). Normothermic no-flow of 5 to 20 min reversed by standard or CPR, however, is still followed by various degrees of permanent multifocal brain damage.[30,46,47,49-61] Again, optimism is justified because a clinically realistic physical combination treatment has recently achieved complete functional recovery in dogs after 11 min of normothermic cardiac arrest (no-flow).[61]

History

CARDIOPULMONARY RESUSCITATION

Occasional attempts to reverse airway obstruction, cessation of breathing, and coma have been made since prehistoric times; however, pulselessness (cardiac arrest) was not recognized until the Renaissance.[62] The early history of CPR has many sparks that failed to benefit patients over centuries probably because of lack of communication and collaboration between laboratory researchers, clinicians, and rescuers. Scientific proof of the efficacy of modern resuscitation measures, many of which are outgrowths of findings in the nineteenth century provoked by the discovery of general anesthesia in the 1840s, did not occur until the 1950s.[12-21]

The recent history of modern CPR shows a series of landmark developments during the past 30 years:

- Proof that ventilation with the operator's exhaled air is physiologically sound.[14]
- Proof in curarized adult human volunteers without tracheal tube that soft-tissue obstruction of the upper airway in unconscious patients can be prevented or corrected by backward tilt of the head, forward displacement of the mandible, and opening of the mouth.[13]
- Mouth-to-mouth (nose) ventilation is superior to manual chest-pressure arm-lift methods.[15]
- Proof of the ventilatory superiority of mouth-to-

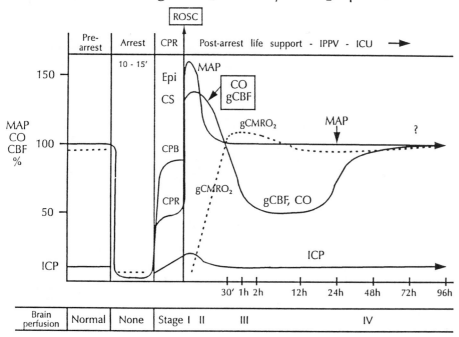

Figure 17-3 Diagram of postcardiac arrest reperfusion failure in brain and extracerebral organs. Reperfusion failure in brain (proven) and extracerebral organs (suspected) after ventricular fibrillation (VF) cardiac arrest and CPR or cardiopulmonary bypass (CPB) for restoration of spontaneous circulation (ROSC). After no-flow of 10 to 15 min, despite control of normal mean arterial pressure (MAP), global cerebral blood flow (gCBF) and cardiac output (CO) go through four postarrest stages: stage I, multifocal no-reflow (which may be overcome with high reperfusion pressure); stage II, brief diffuse global hyperemia, with mild transient intracranial pressure (ICP) rise; stage III, delayed protracted global hypoperfusion (with normal ICP) accompanied by normal or supranormal global cerebral O_2 uptake ($gCMR_{O_2}$) between about 2 h and 12 h postarrest (mismatching); and stage IV, outcome (resolution), which is still unclear. IPPV, intermittent positive-pressure ventilation.

mouth ventilation over the manual chest-pressure arm-lift methods in children.[16]

- Rediscovery, laboratory documentation, and the first clinical proof of the efficacy of external cardiac (chest) compressions for artificial circulation.[17]
- Combining steps A (head-tilt, jaw-thrust), B (positive pressure ventilation), and C (external cardiac compressions) into BLS.[18,19]
- First successful electric defibrillation of a human heart via thoracotomy.[20]
- First successful external electric defibrillation and pacing of a human heart.[21]
- Concept of "the heart too good to die" (reversible sudden cardiac death) (Beck, 1960).
- Concept of "the brain too good to die" (Safar, 1970).
- Development of cardiac arrest-CPCR models in animals high on the phylogenetic scale.[38,39,57-61,63-68]

CEREBRAL RESUSCITATION

For almost 100 years before 1970, some pathologists, neurosurgeons, neurologists and (since the 1950s) neuroanesthesiologists studied the brain after operative trauma, accidental trauma, intracranial hemorrhage, or focal ischemia (stroke). Present cerebral resuscitation researchers stand on the shoulders of pioneers in therapeutic cerebral hypothermia of the 1950s and 1960s. Neuropathologists documented post-GBI delayed death of scattered neurons in the 1960s (see Fig. 17-

2). Concerning polytrauma and shock (i.e., incomplete global ischemia), which have been thoroughly studied for extracerebral organ failure since the 1960s, the brain remains relatively unexplored.

In 1970, systematic laboratory and clinical research programs were initiated into cerebral resuscitation from temporary GBI[40,50-53] and cardiac arrest.[5,12,31,33-38,49] Hossmann and colleagues[40-43] showed that the majority of cerebral neurons (by far not all) in cats or monkeys can tolerate up to 60 min of complete normothermic GBI, in terms of recovery of EEG activity and protein synthesis—provided reperfusion is good. In 1971, we documented the delayed postarrest protracted cerebral hypoperfusion in dogs.[66,67] We postulated that this hypoperfusion had to be overcome to improve outcome (Fig. 17-3).[49,50]

In the mid-1970s, the first reproducible large animal outcome models of prolonged GBI or cardiac arrest and long-term intensive care were initiated.[63-65,68] They are needed to let the encephalopathy mature over at least 3 days. Since the 1970s, research into cerebral resuscitation from various ischemic insults has been greatly expanded by several groups, which has revealed the increasingly complex molecular and cellular mechanisms of postischemic encephalopathies (Fig. 17-4). How to prevent delayed postarrest dying of vulnerable neurons remains the challenge.

Moderate resuscitative (postinsult) hypothermia (30°C) introduced in the 1950s[69-82] was given up three

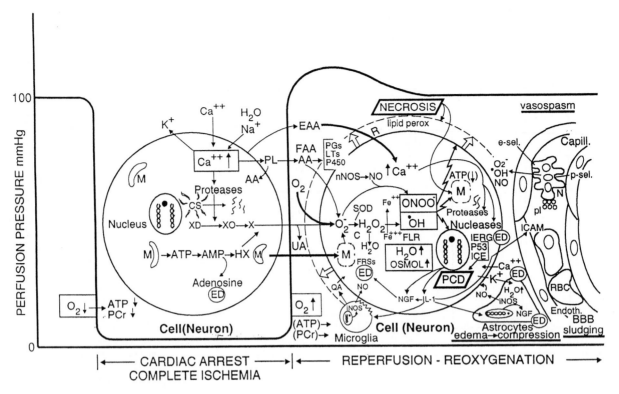

Figure 17-4 *How cerebral neurons die after temporary ischemia.* Diagram of the very complex, partially hypothesized biochemical cascades in vital organ cells (e.g., cerebral neurons) during and after cardiac arrest. Normally, intracellular ($[Ca^{2+}]_i$) to extracellular ($[Ca^{2+}]_e$) calcium gradient is 1:10,000 (i.e., 0.1 μmol: 1 mmol). Calcium regulators include calcium/magnesium ATPase, the endoplasmic reticulum (ER), mitochondria (M), and arachidonic acid (AA). With stimulation, different cell types respond with an increase in $[Ca^{2+}]_i$ because of release of bound Ca^{2+} in the ER, and influx of $[Ca^{2+}]_e$, or both.

During sudden, complete ischemic anoxia (cardiac arrest) (*left side*), oxygen stores in the brain are consumed in about 15 s. The level of energy [phosphocreatine (PCr) and adenosine triphosphate (ATP)] decreases to near zero in all tissues at different rates, depending on stores of oxygen and substrate; it is fastest in the brain (about 5 min), and slower in the heart and other vital organs. This energy loss causes membrane pump failure, which causes a shift of sodium (Na^+) ions, water (H_2O), and (Ca^{2+}) from the extracellular into the intracellular space (cytosolic edema); and potassium (K^+) leakage from the intracellular into the extracellular space. Increase in $[Ca^{2+}]_i$ activates phospholipase A_2, which breaks down membrane phospholipids (PL) into free fatty acids (FAA), particularly AA. Increase in $[Ca^{2+}]_i$ also activates proteolytic enzymes, such as calpain, which may disrupt the cytoskeleton (CS) and possibly the nucleus. In mitochondria, hydrolysis of ATP to adenosine monophosphate (AMP) leads to an accumulation of hypoxanthine (HX). Increased $[Ca^{2+}]_i$ may enhance conversion of xanthine dehydrogenase (XD) to xanthine oxidase (XO), priming the neuron for the production of the oxygen free radical (O_2^-), although this pathway is of questionable importance in neurons. X, xanthine; UA, uric acid. Excitatory amino acid neurotransmitters (EAA), particularly glutamate and aspartate, increase in extracellular fluid. Increased $[EAA]_e$ activates *N*-methyl-D-aspartate (NMDA) and non-NMDA receptors (R), thereby increasing calcium and sodium influx and mobilizing stores of $[Ca^{2+}]_i$. Increased extracellular potassium activates EAA receptors by membrane depolarization.

Glycolysis during hypoxia results in anaerobic metabolism and lactic acidosis, until all glucose is used (in the brain, during anoxia after about 20 min). This lactic acidosis, plus inability to wash out CO_2, results in a mixed tissue acidosis that adversely influences neuronal viability. The net effect of acidosis on the cascades during and after ischemia is not clear. Mild acidosis may actually attenuate NMDA-mediated $[Ca^{2+}]_i$ accumulation. Without reoxygenation, cells progress via first reversible, later irreversible, structural damage to necrosis of all neurons or myocytes, homogeneously, at specific rates for different cell types.

During reperfusion and reoxygenation (*right side*), lactate and molecular breakdown products can create osmotic edema and rupture of organelles and mitochondria. Recovery of ATP and PCr and of the ionic membrane pump may be hampered by hypoperfusion as a result of vasospasm, cell sludging, adhesion of neutrophils (granulocytes) (N), and capillary compression by swollen

Figure 17-4 (*Continued*)   astrocytes, which also help to protect neurons by absorbing extacellular potassium. Capillary [blood-brain barrier (BBB)] leakage results in interstitial (vasogenic) edema. Increased concentrations of at least four free radical species that break down membranes and collagen, worsen the microcirculation, and possibly also damage the nucleus may be formed: superoxide (O_2^-) leading to hydroxyl radical ($\cdot OH$) (via the iron-catalyzed $Fe^{3+} \rightarrow Fe^{2+}$, Haber-Weiss/Fenton reaction); free lipid radicals (FLR); and peroxynitrite ($OONO^-$). O_2^- may be formed from several sources: (a) directly from AA metabolism by cyclooxygenase; (b) by the previously described XO system; (c) via quinone-mediated reactions within and outside the electron transport chain (from M); and (d) by activation of NADPH-oxidase in accumulated neutrophils in the microvasculature or after diapedesis into tissue. Increased O_2^- leads to increased hydrogen peroxide (H_2O_2) production as a result of intracellular action of superoxide dismutase (SOD). H_2O_2 is controlled by intracellular catalase (c). Increased O_2 further leads to increased $\cdot OH$ because of conversion of H_2O_2 to $\cdot OH$, via the Haber-Weiss/Fenton reaction, with iron liberated from mitochondria. This reaction is promoted by acidosis: $\cdot OH$ and $OONO^-$ damage cellular lipids, proteins, and nucleic acids.

Also, AA increases activity of the cyclooxygenase pathways to produce prostaglandins (PGs), including thromboxane A_2, the lipoxygenase pathway, to produce leukotrienes (LTs); and the cytochrome P-450 pathway. These products can act as neurotransmitters and signal transducers in neuron and glia, and can activate thrombotic and inflammatory pathways in the microcirculation. Inflammatory reactions after ischemia occur in extracerebral organs, focal brain ischemia, or brain trauma; but so far, they have not been proven after temporary complete GBI. Neuronal injury can signal interleukin 1 and other cytokines to be produced and trigger endogenous activation of microglia, with additional injury. QA, quinolinic acid. In addition, tissue or endothelial injury—particularly associated with necrosis—can signal the endothelium to produce adhesion molecules (intracellular [ICAM], *a*-selectin, *p*-selectin), cytokines, chemokines, and other mediators, triggering local involvement of systemic inflammatory cells in an interaction between blood and damaged tissue.

Reoxygenation restores ATP through oxidative phosphorylation, which may result in massive uptake of $[Ca^{2+}]_i$ into mitochondria, which are swollen from increased osmolality. Thus, mitochondria loaded with bound Ca^{2+} may self-destruct by rupturing and releasing free radicals. Increased $[Ca^{2+}]_i$ by itself and by triggering free radical reactions may result in lipid peroxidation, leaky membranes, and cell death. Neuronal damage can be caused, in part, by increased $[EAA]_e$ (excitotoxicity), resulting in increased $[Ca^{2+}]_i$. During reperfusion, $[Ca^{2+}]_i$ and increased $[EAA]_e$ normalize. Their contribution to ultimate death of neurons is more likely through the cascades they have triggered during ischemia.

During ischemia and subsequent reperfusion, loading of cells and maldistribution in cells of calcium is believed to be the key trigger common to the development of cell death. This calcium loading signals a wide variety of pathologic processes. Proteases, lipases, and nucleases are activated, which may contribute to activation of genes or gene products (i.e., interleukin-converting enzyme, ICE or P53) critical to the development of programmed cell death (PCD, i.e, apoptosis); or inactivation of genes or gene products normally inhibiting this process. Activation of neuronal nitric oxide synthase (nNOS) by calcium can lead to production of NO, which can combine with superoxide to generate peroxynitrite ($OONO^-$). $OONO^-$ and $\cdot OH$ both can lead to DNA injury and PCD, or protein and membrane peroxidation and necrosis, respectively. Nerve growth factor (NGF), nuclear immediate early response genes (IERG) such as heat shock protein, free radical scavengers (FRSs), adenosine, and other endogenous defenses (ED) work to lessen the damage.

The relative influences on ultimate nonviability of neurons depend on ischemia time. After short arrests, excitotoxicity may be a dominant factor; longer ischemia may trigger apoptosis; and very long arrests and reperfusion are followed by membrane damage, in part due to free radical reactions.

Treatment potentials must be multifaceted during ischemia (protection-preservation) and during and after reperfusion (resuscitation), because of the many pathogenic factors above. With the above rationale, at this time, treatment potentials include hypertensive reperfusion; cerebral blood flow promotion by hypertension, hemodilution, normocapnia, and osmotherapy; hypothermia (which reduces oxygen demand and mitigates or slows down most of the above reactions); and superoxide dismutase (SOD), catalase, deferoxamine, calcium entry blockers, xanthine oxidase inhibitors, intracellular buffers, corticosteroids (membrane stabilizers), aminosteroids ("lazaroids," lipid peroxidation inhibitors), a combination of NMDA and non-NMDA EAA receptor blockers, selective inducible NOS (iNOS) inhibitors and gene therapy. (Designed in 1995 by P. Safar, M.D., and P. Kochanek, M.D., with input from N. Bircher, M.D., and J. Severinghaus, M.D. Based on a previous diagram and legend by P. Safar, M.D., R. Basford, Ph.D., and L. Ernster, Ph.D.)

decades ago. The discovery in the late 1980s that mild hypothermia (34°C), which is safer, has protective[46] and resuscitative effects on the brain after cardiac arrest in dogs[57-61] and after forebrain ischemia in rats (see below) has rekindled widespread hypothermia research in the 1990s. Now, cerebral resuscitation from cardiac arrest remains at the cutting edge of reanimatology. This is the topic of this chapter.

The main "incremental risk" of increasingly effective CPCR methods is survival with severe brain damage. Since the mid-1960s, the topics of brain death determination and certification and letting patients in a PVS die (passive euthanasia) have assumed increasing socioeconomic importance.

Research Approaches

LABORATORY RESEARCH

Steps A and B of BLS were developed and documented in curarized human volunteers.[13-16] Step C by open chest CPR,[20,83-94] closed chest CPR,[17,18,84,87,95,96] or closed chest emergency cardiopulmonary bypass (CPB)[97-107] was first documented in canine models and patients with cardiac arrest. Mechanisms of dying and their reversibility[36] have been studied with acute (<12 h) or short-term (12 to 24 h) models in large animals of VF, asphyxiation,[96] exsanguination,[32] hyperthermia,[108,109] accidental hypothermia,[110] drowning,[111] and other insults.[63-65,112,113] Cerebral outcome, however, can be determined best with long-term (3 days or longer) models in animals high on the phylogenetic scale. We developed the first such outcome models in monkeys with GBI by high pressure neck tourniquet.[68] Use of expensive monkeys was given up because our highly reproducible dog models of prolonged cardiac arrest, in which extracerebral variables are controlled by postarrest intensive care, are now available.[30,54,57-61,65,103]

Only after the postischemic encephalopathy has "matured" is outcome evaluation meaningful in terms of overall performance categories [OPC 1 (best) to 5 (death)], including behavior, neurologic deficit scores [NDS 0 percent (normal) to 100 percent (brain death)], and histopathologic damage scores (HDS) of the whole brain (see Fig. 17-2).[30,50,61,68] Early postarrest EEG recovery patterns in animals are consistent,[43,114,115] but do not correlate with functional outcome.[51,53,54,57,68]

Models of ischemia of the head only,[51-53,68] of occlusion of the ascending aorta,[113] of cerebrospinal fluid (CSF) brain compression,[116-118] or of potassium arrest[119] are all less clinically relevant than cardiac arrest models.[27,30,46,54,56-65] Dogs have a large blood volume and large vessels, allowing for monitoring and life support. Our extensive experience through the 1970s and 1980s led us to propose ten goals for such outcome models (Table

TABLE 17-1

Requirements for Controlled Large Animal Outcome Models of CPCR

1. All animals same subspecies, sex, age, weight
2. Insult sufficiently moderate to allow mitigation of brain damage (e.g., by mild precooling)
3. Arrest reversal with controlled perfusion pressure, without adding variable low-flow states
4. Chance minimized by concurrent randomized controls
5. Life support standardized, using same team, stringent controls of physiologic variables that can influence cerebral and overall outcome
6. Brain temperature (at least core temperature) controlled within ± 0.5°C before, during, and after arrest
7. Intensive care for at least 72 h postarrest to final evaluation, to allow maturation of cerebral changes while controlling extracerebral variables
8. All control experiments within protocol result in survival with brain damage
9. Postarrest deaths prior to 72 h excluded from neurologic outcome evaluation if due to extracerebral complications, but primary brain deaths included
10. Bias avoided as feasible by placebo controls, blinded outcome evaluation by same person or several persons with minimal interobserver variability

17-1).[37] All these goals were first met by a canine model of VF 12.5-min no-flow, resuscitation by brief CPB, controlled intermittent positive-pressure ventilation (IPPV) to 20 h, and intensive care to 96 h[61,103]; they were also met by a similar canine model of VF of 10 min and external CPR.[54,58,64,65,87] The principles of our dog models have recently been applied to porcine cardiac arrest models.[120-123] These have been used for short-term cardiovascular studies, but no porcine model has yet been documented that fulfills all our present goals for cerebral resuscitation *outcome* research (see Table 17-1).

The currently available dog outcome model with greatest reproducibility that honors all ten of our goals (see Table 17-1)[61,124] is that of VF 11-min (no-flow), reperfusion by brief low-flow CPB (simulating low-flow CPR), IPPV to 20 h, and intensive care to 96 h. This model is clinically realistic. With standard life support (controls), all animals within protocol achieved restoration of spontaneous circulation (ROSC) within 2 min and survived to 96 h with severe brain damage.

Hearts in smaller animals tend to defibrillate themselves. Cats tend to convulse.[125] Rabbits[126-128] have delicate lungs, and no cerebral outcome data are available in the literature. The widely used incomplete forebrain ischemia models in rats[112,129,130] include neither ischemia of the brainstem nor heart failure, nor intoxication from postischemic extracerebral organs—all features of cardiac arrest. These rat models, however, have been useful for elucidating cerebral ischemic mechanisms and for screening the potential of some brain-oriented treatments. Unfortunately, results in such rat studies have sometimes differed from those in larger animals and patients. A rat cardiac arrest outcome model is clinically more realistic than the rat forebrain ischemia model because total circulatory arrest is more injurious to the whole organism.[131-134] An asphyxial cardiac arrest rat model, with 1 h of IPPV and 3 or more days' survival (with functional and histologic outcome evaluation) proved feasible.[133] In rats, the CA-1 region of the hippocampus seems most vulnerable (see Fig. 17-2), but other areas (neocortex, cerebellum, basal ganglia) are equally vulnerable in higher species. Rats allow for at least short-term control of cardiovascular-pulmonary variables. For clinically relevant neurologic and overall outcome documentation, however, rats are too low on the phylogenetic scale.

Mice and gerbils, even lower on the phylogenetic scale, have vessels and blood volume too small to permit any control of extracerebral variables, and they tend to convulse. In vitro studies lack the milieu of the whole organism, which influences neuronal viability. Brain slice preparations[135] might be explored for real-time observations of neuronal recovery from ischemic anoxia and reoxygenation. Nerve cell cultures[136] lack the glial matrix, but can answer basic questions under various physical and pharmacologic influences.

CLINICAL RESEARCH

To study large numbers of patients, it is necessary to conduct multicenter studies. The first controlled randomized clinical study of cardiac arrest and CPCR was initiated by Safar in 1979 and is ongoing (Table 17-2).[5-7,137-142] Investigators in 20 hospitals in seven countries have studied a progression of hypotheses. The first concerned the effect of postarrest thiopental loading [Brain Resuscitation Clinical Trial (BRCT) I, 1979–1984][5,137]; the second, calcium entry blocker therapy (BRCT II, 1984–1989)[6,138,139]; and the third, titrated high-dose epinephrine (BRCT III, 1989–1994).[7,140] The methods developed in Glasgow for the evaluation of coma[143] and outcome[144] after brain trauma have been modified for use after cardiac arrest (Tables 17-3 and 17-4).[2] The large data base has proved valuable in exploring many other disease and treatment-related clues or hypotheses.[145-152] The study mechanism (Tables 17-2 to 17-5)[138-140] has been adopted by other clinical trials[153-155] and for international evaluation of CPR cases.[10,11]

The BRCT I and II studies did not reveal a statistically significant greater proportion (of all subjects combined) of survivors with good cerebral function in the treatment group,[5,6] although these treatments were effective in large animal outcome models.[51,54] Subgroup

TABLE 17-2
Requirements for Controlled Clinical Outcome Studies of CPCR

1. Goal, question(s), hypotheses
2. Case selection (criteria for inclusion and exclusion)
   Assumptions and sample size estimate
3. Recruiting investigators, hospitals, EMS systems
   influence over entire life support chain
   (Prehospital-transportation ED-OR-ICU)
4. Institutional review board approval
   Start CPCR under emergency exception to consent
   When feasible, obtain consent to continue
5. Concurrent or immediate retrospective estimation of arrest (no-flow) time; CPR (low-flow) time; prearrest and postarrest hypoxia (hypotension) times
6. CPR BLS-ACLS-PLS by protocol throughout the life support chain
7. Monitoring early recovery with coma scoring
8. Monitoring outcome to 6 months with overall performance category 1–5 and cerebral performance category 1–5
9. Monitoring risks (side effects)
10. Overall analysis, subgroup analysis
    Evaluation, interpretation

data, however, suggested some benefit.[5,6,139] We learned about the limitations of randomized clinical outcome trials of novel therapies through these studies.[139] Those limitations include the problem that minor or infrequent benefit may not be detected, even with randomization of large numbers, because of the enormous variability in numerous unknown or uncontrollable factors that influence outcome. Despite standardized protocols, there may still be variability in the timing of life support measures and the titration and skill of their administration. On entering patients into a CPCR study, the selection within seconds of only those cases who are within the therapeutic window is impossible. Subgroup analyses might be revealing,[5-7,139,155] but creation of subgroups by postrandomization characteristics is considered unreliable and may be misleading.[156] There is no known method to overcome this problem (see discussion of research initiatives below). Other disadvantages include the high cost and necessity to test a novel treatment's effects against variable combinations of "standard" therapies. It may be impossible to statistically document anything less than a consistent breakthrough effect, which may never be found. These limitations and others also seem to prevail in randomized clinical trials of novel drug treatments after FBI or TBI. The advantages of randomized clinical trials over outcome studies in large animals include the ability to test feasibility and risk factors in sick people.

TABLE 17-3
Glasgow Coma Score[143] and Pittsburgh Brain Stem Scale[2,6] for Early Postarrest Evaluation of Patients

Glasgow Coma Score (GCS)		Pittsburgh Brain Stem Score (PBSS)		
If patient is under the influence of anesthetics, sedatives, or neuromuscular blockers, give best estimate of each item. Write number in box to indicate status at time of this examination.		Add to GCS (A, B, C)		
		Lash reflex present	yes = 2	
		(either side)	no = 1 ☐	
(A) *Eye Opening*		Corneal reflex present	yes = 2	
Spontaneous	= 4	(either side)	no = 1 ☐	
To speech	= 3	Doll's eye or iced water calorics reflex present	yes = 5	
To pain	= 2	(either side)	no = 1	
None	= 1 ☐	Right pupil reacts to light	yes = 2	
			no = 1 ☐	
(B) *Best Motor Response*		Left pupil reacts to light	yes = 2	
(extremities of best side)			no = 1 ☐	
Obeys	= 6	Gag or cough reflex present	yes = 2	
Localizes	= 5		no = 1 ☐	
Withdraws	= 4	Total PBSS	☐	
Abnormal flexion	= 3	(best PBSS = 15)		
Extends	= 2	(worst PBSS = 6)		
None	= 1 ☐	Patient condition at time of examination:		
(C) *Best Verbal Response*		Check all that apply.		
(if patient intubated, give best estimate)		☐ Anesthesia/heavy sedation		
Oriented	= 5	☐ Paralysis (partial or complete neuromuscular blockade)		
Confused conversation	= 4	☐ Intubation		
Inappropriate words	= 3	☐ None of the above		
Incomprehensible				
sounds	= 2			
None	= 1 ☐			
Total GCS				
(best GCS = 15)	☐			
(worst GCS = 3)				

SOURCE: Reproduced by permission from Teasdale and Jennett[143] and Brain Resuscitation Study Group (BRGT).[2,6]

Pathophysiology

The temporary complete GBI of cardiac arrest can occur instantly, as in VF; over minutes, as in asphyxiation or exsanguination; or over hours, as in shock or hypoxemia (see Fig. 17-1).[36] Sudden cardiac death and resuscitation create a cerebral insult that is often caused by the initial no-flow, followed by the incomplete ischemia of CPR (low-flow), and after ROSC, by the postresuscitation disease[32] or syndrome[36] in vital organs, despite controlled normotension.

In normal brain, autoregulation maintains global cerebral blood flow (CBF) of about 50 ml/100 g brain per min, despite cerebral perfusion pressures (CPP) [i.e., MAP minus intracranial pressure (ICP)] changing between 50 and 150 mmHg. When CPP decreases below 50 mmHg, CBF decreases. During incomplete ischemia (e.g., shock or VF with external CPR), the viability of normal neurons seems threatened by CPP less than about 30 mmHg,[157,158] CBF less than 15 ml/100 g of brain per min,[159] or cerebral venous P_{O_2} of less than 20 mmHg.[159–161] The brain apparently tolerates low-flow (e.g., global CBF 10 percent of normal, i.e., 5 ml/100 g of brain per min) better than no flow[162]; however, trickle flow (CBF <10 percent normal) can sometimes be worse than no-flow.[163]

With sudden circulatory arrest at normothermia, loss of brain O_2 stores[29,164] and unconsciousness[165] occur within 10 to 20 s. For complete reversibility, the 4- to 5-min limit concept[28] is supported by evidence that brain glucose and adenosine triphosphate (ATP) stores are depleted[166,167] and the membrane pump arrested[164,168] within 3 to 5 min of complete ischemic anoxia. In dog outcome experiments, VF no-flow of 1 or 2 min resulted in complete functional recovery and normal brain histology, whereas VF no-flow of 5 min[30] or asphyxial asystole of only 2 min[169,170] resulted in complete functional recovery, but with mild histologic damage in vulnerable regions.[39] The 4- to 5-min limit is being challenged by the occasional survival without severe neurologic deficit after apparently normothermic no-flow of 10 to 20 min in dogs[46,103] or patients.[145] Normothermic no-flow of 60 min was survived by one cat,[42] but with abnormal behavior and histologic brain dam-

TABLE 17-4
Overall[144] and Cerebral Performance Categories[2,6] for Outcome Evaluation of Patients

Cerebral Performance Category (CPC)	Check one	Overall Performance Category (OPC)	Check one
Evaluate only cerebral performance capabilities		Reflects cerebral *plus* noncerebral status. Evaluate actual overall performance	
CPC 1. *Good cerebral performance* Conscious, alert, normal cerebral function. May have minor psychologic or neurologic deficits that do not significantly compromise cerebral or physical function.		OCP 1. *Good overall performance* Conscious, alert, capable of normal life. Good cerebral performance (CPC 1) plus slight or no functional disability from noncerebral organ system dysfunction.	☐
CPC 2. *Moderate cerebral disability* Conscious, alert, normal cerebral function for activities of daily life (e.g., dress, travel by public transportation, food preparation). May have hemiplegia, seizures, ataxia, dysarthria, dysphasia, or permanent memory or mental changes.	☐	OPC2. *Moderate overall disability* Conscious, alert. Moderate cerebral disability alone (CPC 2) or moderate disability from noncerebral organ system dysfunction alone or both. Performs independent activities of daily life (dress, travel, food preparation) or able to work in part-time sheltered environment. Disabled for competitive work.	☐
CPC 3. *Severe cerebral disability* Conscious, has at least limited cognition. Dependent on others for daily support (i.e., institutionalized or at home with exceptional family effort) because of impaired brain function. Includes wide range of cerebral abnormalities, from ambulatory patients who have severe memory disturbance or dementia precluding independent existence to paralyzed patients who can only communicate with their eyes (e.g., the locked-in syndrome).	☐	OPC 3. *Severe overall disability* Conscious. Severe cerebral disability alone (CPC 3) or severe disability from noncerebral organ system dysfunction alone or both. Dependent on others for daily support.	☐
CPC 4. *Coma/vegetative state* Not conscious, unaware of surroundings, *no cognition.* No verbal or psychologic interaction with environment. May appear awake because of spontaneous eye opening or sleep-wake cycle. Includes all degrees of unresponsiveness that are neither CPC 3 (conscious) nor CPC 5 (coma that satisfies brain death criteria).	☐	OPC 4. *Coma/vegetative state* Definition same as CPC 4.	☐
CPC 5. *Brain death* (with beating heart) or *death* (without beating heart). Apnea, areflexia, "coma," EEG silence.	☐	OPC 5. *Death* (without beating heart) Apnea, areflexia, "coma," no pulses (see text).	☐
CPC A. *Anesthesia* (CNS depressant) Uncertain as to above categories because of anesthetic, other CNS depressant drug or relaxant effects.	☐	OPC A. *Anesthesia* (CNS depressant) Uncertain as to above categories because of anesthetic, other CNS depressant drug, or relaxant effects.	☐

CPC Time achieved ☐ ☐ ☐		
Hour Minute		

OPC Time achieved ☐ ☐
Hour Minute

Compared with baseline status before the insult, the patient's intellectual functions *now* are (check one in each column):

	Patient opinon	Family opinion	Examiner opinion
Unchanged (1)	☐	☐	☐
Worsened (2)	☐	☐	☐
Unsure (3)	☐	☐	☐
Other or unable to determine (4)	☐	☐	☐

Explain _____

SOURCE: Reproduced by permission from Jennett and Bond[144] and Safar and Bircher.[2]

age. Undoubtedly, multiple factors, some understood (e.g., mild hypothermia, see below) and others as yet unknown, explain these discrepancies.

During complete cerebral ischemia, calcium shifts,[29,164,171,172] brain tissue lactic acidosis,[173] and increases in the brain of free fatty acids,[174] osmolality,[175] and extracellular concentration of excitatory amino acids (particularly glutamate and aspartate)[176–178] set the stage for reoxygenation injury (see Fig. 17-4). These mechanisms seem partially responsible for the selective vulnerability of some neurons in certain regions, such as the hippocampus, neocortex, and cerebellum. Greater cerebral lactic acidosis with incomplete ischemia[173] or prearrest hyperglycemia[179] is followed by greater histologic brain damage. Brain acidosis caused by high CO_2 without tissue hypoxia seems to be well tolerated.[180,181]

What is the *multifactorial pathogenesis* of the postcardiac arrest encephalopathy? After normothermic no-flow of 10 to 20 min and reperfusion, at least eight secondary derangements might be considered: Mainly (1) the loss of brain energy charge; (2) ion pump

TABLE 17-5
Brain-Oriented Standard Basic-Advanced-Prolonged Life Support (for references, see text)

BLS-ALS

Teach life-supporting first aid to lay public, including immediate vigorous CPR BLS steps A-B-C

Suggest to resuscitate when possible with head cooled (snow)

Minimize arrest time with earliest automatic external defibrillation by laypersons

Increase perfusion pressure during external CPR with early (intratracheal) epinephrine

Use titrated high-dose epinephrine

Explore prolonged mechanical external CPR

Correct base deficit empirically

In ALS-resistant cases, switch to open chest CPR or CPB

Give brief hypertensive bout (systolic arterial pressure 150–200 mmHg on restoration of spontaneous circulation, with epinephrine, norepinephrine, or dopamine, followed by control of normotension or mild hypertension with fluid and titrated infusion of dopamine, dobutamine, or other cardiovascular drugs

Infuse Ringer's solution IV during and following ALS

Check blood glucose level and keep it at 100–200 mg/dl

Give glucose load IV if prearrest coma or seizures

Prolonged Life Support (PLS) (throughout coma)

After hypertensive bout, control normotension or mild hypertension, normoxia, normocarbia

Control arterial base deficit at ± 5 mmol/l

Monitor brain temp. (Tty or Tnp) and core temperature (Tpa or Tcv or Tes)

  Explore feasibility of mild (34°C) resuscitative cerebral hypothermia induced as early and as rapidly as feasible (see Table 17-7) (optimal duration of mild hypothermia not known)

  Prevent or correct even mild hyperthermia

Immobilize with softening doses of relaxant

Sedate (e.g., with titrated IV diazepam or barbiturate), control seizures (e.g., with diazepam-phenytoin)

Give fluid load about 10 ml/kg

Conduct hemodynamic monitoring as feasible to guide administration of drugs and fluids

Keep hematocrit at 30–35%; electrolytes normal; plasma COP 15 mmHg; serum osmolality 280–330 mosm/l

Give fluids IV; no dextrose in H_2O; give dextrose 5% or 10% in NaCl 0.25% or 0.5% (e.g., 50 ml/kg/24 h)

Maintain fluid balance; acid–base balance; alimentation

Use standard intensive care life support including head slightly elevated; turn trunk side to side

failure; and (3) acidosis are fairly quickly restored.[29,42,66,164,168,182,183] The remaining cerebral postresuscitation syndrome seems to consist of the remaining five components[37]; (4) perfusion failure (see Fig. 17-3); (5) reoxygenation injury with chemical cascades to cell necrosis (see Fig. 17-4); (6) extracerebral organ derangements; and (7) blood derangements due to stasis. The eighth possible derangement, postarrest inflammatory processes, which are proven to occur after TBI or FBI,[184–187] have not been investigated after cardiac arrest.

Although ICP remains normal, after survivable cardiac arrest up to 15 min,[66–68,188] extracellular-to-intracellular fluid and electrolyte shifts occur early during ischemia (cytotoxic edema).[66,164,182] Vasogenic edema may form late after reperfusion, at least following prolonged ischemia.[43,68,189–191] Starting at about 24 h after arrest, irreversible morphologic changes can be seen by light microscopy in some neurons scattered throughout the brain (see Fig. 17-2).[30,68,169] Electron microscopy may also miss affected areas.

Perfusion failure (see Fig. 17-3) (i.e., CBF changes during normotensive reperfusion after at least 10 min of no-flow) seems to progress through four stages:

1. Multifocal no-reflow, which occurs immediately,[32,192,193] and seems to be readily overcome by normotensive or hypertensive reperfusion.[193–195]

2. Transient global "reactive" hyperemia (vasoparalysis), which lasts 15 to 30 min.[66,67,194–198]

3. Delayed, prolonged global[66,67,196] and multifocal hypoperfusion,[194,195,197] evident from about 2 to 12 h after arrest. Global CBF is reduced to about 50 percent of baseline; global CMR_{O_2} returns to or above baseline values,[66,67,183,194–196] and cerebral venous P_{O_2} may decrease to less than the critical level of 20 mmHg, reflecting inadequate O_2 delivery in relation to O_2 uptake.[188,198]

4. Late resolution when either normal global CBF and CMR_{O_2} (and consciousness) are restored,[194] or both remain low (with coma),[199] or there is delayed secondary hyperemia.[183,200–205] The latter, we hypothesize, could be associated with a drastic decrease in oxygen uptake and the clinical picture of brain death.[203–205]

The pathogenesis of the third stage (protracted hypoperfusion) needs clarification; vasospasm,[195] edema,[187–191] and blood cell aggregates[186,206] are possibilities.

Reoxygenation, although essential and effective in restoring energy charge, also might provoke chemical cascades (involving free iron, free radicals, calcium shifts, acidosis, excitatory amino acids, and catecholamines) that result in lipid peroxidation of membranes,[114,172,177,206–218] and DNA damage (see Fig. 17-4).[219–221] These cascades have been partially documented in vitro and in extracerebral organs, but have not been documented convincingly in brain in vivo. The optimal P_{O_2} and rate of reoxygenation during resuscitation need to be determined.[114] During ischemia, the increased lactic acid[173] and excitatory amino acids[176] are rapidly washed out with reperfusion, and ionic balance is partially restored.[164] Although there might be a delayed postarrest increase in total brain calcium,[217] treatable surges in brain intracellular calcium or glutamate release after arrest remain to be documented. Some of these molecular changes could be merely epiphenomena of permanent brain damage, whereas others might explain why dying neurons and dying cardiac myocytes can be found side by side with surviving cells (see Fig. 17-2).

Present research interests include how selectively vulnerable neurons die alongside of surviving neurons, predominantly in the CA-1 region of the hippocampus, neocortex, and cerebellum. There is a possibility that temporary, complete ischemia can damage DNA and thereby trigger programmed cell death (PCD) of some (scattered) and not other neurons, that is, "apoptosis" (in Greek, "falling apart") of membranes.[219-221] This would differ from inducing primary necrotizing processes that would affect membranes first and most neurons equally.

Extracerebral derangements can worsen cerebral outcome.[32] Cardiac arrest in patients with previously sick hearts often is followed by recurrent VF or cardiovascular-pulmonary failure.[5-7] Cardiac arrest in previously healthy dogs is followed by delayed reduction in cardiac output despite controlled normotension.[47,54] Postarrest pulmonary edema can be prevented by prolonged controlled ventilation.[47] Intoxication of the brain from postischemic viscera has been suggested,[32] but convincing documentation is lacking.[222,223] After no-flow of 10 min in healthy dogs, neither intravascular coagulation nor pulmonary failure nor prolonged renal or hepatic malfunction appears to occur.[47,222,223]

Blood derangements might include aggregates of polymorphonuclear leukocytes and macrophages that might obstruct capillaries, release free radicals, and damage endothelium.[184-186,224] Their role after cardiac arrest has not been clarified. Macrovascular clotting apparently does not occur during 20 min of normothermic no-flow.[99] Endothelium-derived nitrogenous vasodilators, which seem to play a role in sepsis,[225,226] have not been conclusively studied after cardiac arrest. The role of inflammatory mediators[224] in permanent brain damage after cardiac arrest has not been investigated.

Therapeutic Considerations for Cardiac Arrest

STANDARD BRAIN-ORIENTED LIFE SUPPORT

Brain-oriented BLS-ALS-PLS guidelines[1,2] should be modified (see Table 17-5). Steps A and B (with or without a tracheal tube) are as important as step C. Coma in humans invariably causes upper airway obstruction unless there is backward tilt of the head (sometimes jaw thrust and open mouth are also needed).[13] Asphyxial cardiac arrest appears to cause brain damage more rapidly than VF.[39,169,170] In asphyxiation that leads to EMD-asystole rather than VF, steps A-B-C alone may restore a pulse.[96] For direct exhaled air ventilation on a stranger, a pocket-size face shield may be used. Health professionals should use a valved O_2 mask or other adjunct.[2] Even patients with sudden VF may have suffered deoxygenation before arrest. The C-A-B sequence

is physiologically sound only in sudden VF in well oxygenated patients. Pa_{O_2} remains normal for 20 min of sudden no-flow, but decreases after 20 s of chest compressions only.[226a] Minimizing arrest time and CPR time with earliest defibrillation[227] and other ALS measures[1,2] to achieve rapid ROSC is more important for brain and heart than the details of prolonged steps A-B-C.

Attempts to increase perfusion pressures through heart and brain during external CPR steps A-B-C with simultaneous ventilation[18,228] have not resulted in clear documentation of improved outcomes in patients.[229] Intermittent abdominal compression (IAC) CPR,[230] active compression-decompression (ACD) CPR,[231] or vest CPR[232] can improve blood flow. In dogs, sustained abdominal compression can promote liver rupture[233] and increase ICP.[234] For ROSC-resistant cases, use of prolonged mechanical chest compression and ventilation[235,236] can generate more consistent O_2 delivery and would free the hands of rescuers for cerebral resuscitation measures.

Standard external CPR in dogs, if started immediately on arrest, can sustain normal brain ATP and intracellular pH even with low perfusion pressures and despite systemic acidosis.[237] After no-flow of 6 min, however, during idealized external CPR with CPP of 70 mmHg and normal CBF, without ROSC, full restoration of ATP was not possible during external CPR.[238] Thus, even after short arrests, reperfusion with abovenormal perfusion pressure is ultimately needed, not only to overcome the no-reflow phenomenon,[192-195] but also to restore ATP. In a dog model with ultimate ROSC, however, even after VF 10-min no-flow, vigorous external CPR followed by ROSC and a hypertensive bout preserved brain viability compared with continued no-flow of the same duration.[27]

Epinephrine[239-243] should be given early intratracheally or intravenously during CPR steps A-B-C to increase perfusion pressures through heart and brain. Higher doses of epinephrine than previously recommended[1] enhance ROSC,[2,7,120,153] but more than needed can produce post-ROSC cardiac damage.[134] Optimal epinephrine doses for short versus long arrest times need clarification.

In a recent large multicenter clinical outcome study of CPCR in 1989 to 1994 (BRCT III),[7] escalating highdose epinephrine (5 to 15 mg in adults) achieved overall higher ROSC rates compared with standard 1-mg doses. Overall survival rates and the proportion of patients who achieved good cerebral outcome were equally poor in both groups; however, epinephrine was given very late in most patients.

Other α-receptor agonists have not been proven to be superior.[121,122,239-241] Vigorous VF is easier to convert to a perfusing heartbeat than is fading VF. This author suggests that the first dose of epinephrine might best be proportional to the estimated arrest time (e.g., 1 mg/70 kg for every estimated minute of arrest beyond 3 min), followed by titration according to response. Sympathomimetic amines help the brain to recover by increasing perfusion pressure, but their subtle metabolic (neurotransmitter) effect on recovery of postischemic neurons needs to be studied. In exsanguination cardiac arrest to PEA, retrograde intraaortic infusion of warm oxygenated blood with epinephrine (a method not readily available) can restart the heart without the need for heart message[32]; this method is also effective in rats with exsanguination or normovolemic asphyxial cardiac arrest.[244]

Buffer therapy[96,133,173,239,245-254] depends on arrest and CPR times and use of epinephrine. Metabolic acidemia (base deficit) should be corrected because proper acid-base balance improves cardiovascular resuscitability and early cerebral recovery in dogs[245,246]; after VF no-flow of 5 min in dogs, metabolic acidemia is mild and transient; early $NaHCO_3$ administration seems neither harmful nor beneficial. After longer arrest or CPR times (unwitnessed arrest), ROSC is enhanced by epinephrine plus $NaHCO_3$ 1 mmol/kg intravenously during CPR, followed by correction of monitored base deficit greater than about 5 mmol/liter. $NaHCO_3$ produces a transient CO_2 load that worsens the arrest-induced myocardial hypercarbia,[248] which could depress cardiac resuscitability.[249,250] This $NaHCO_3$-induced hypercarbia is mild, transient, and harmless for the heart when used with epinephrine and controlled with hyperventilation, and it does not seem to be harmful to the brain.[245,246]

Intensive care calls for brain-oriented prolonged postarrest life support, for which our guidelines have changed slightly[38] (see Table 17-5). For control of MAP early postarrest, a titrated intravenous infusion of epinephrine or norepinephrine may be more effective than infusion of phenylephrine, dopamine, or dobutamine, the latter being perhaps preferred later. In cardiac failure late postarrest, a spectrum of possibilities, from titrated dobutamine or norepinephrine to assisted circulation with CPB or aortic balloon pumping, is available for trial. Throughout coma, controlled ventilation to at least 12 h postarrest seems desirable to combat cardiovascular-pulmonary failure. To control "fighting" with the ventilator, I favor use of only low (softening, not apneic) doses of a relaxant to allow for monitoring of neurologic recovery. A hypnotic or narcotic should be titrated intravenously to control hypertension and mydriasis (sympathetic discharge). Corticosteroid therapy is controversial.[148] Postarrest optimal Pa_{O_2} levels, Pa_{CO_2} levels, buffer for base deficit control, and osmotherapy are not yet clarified.

Optimal blood glucose levels after cardiac arrest remain to be clarified.[255] Prolonged hypoglycemia (blood glucose <50 mg/dl) is deleterious to the brain.[164] Severe hyperglycemia before and during global cerebral ischemia in animal models seems to worsen neurologic damage,[164,179] most likely because it increases brain lactic acidosis,[173] which decreases brain pH. During and after CPR, there is usually a spontaneous moderate hyperglycemic response. Three animal studies showed worsened outcome with intravenous glucose during or after reperfusion[256-258]; and two studies suggest improved neuronal recovery with hyperglycemia in focal ischemia[259] or hypoxia.[260] After asphyxial cardiac arrest in a recent rat study by our group, moderate postarrest *hyperglycemia* by glucose administration *plus insulin* improved functional and histologic cerebral outcome over glucose alone, insulin alone, or no treatment.[261] In prehospital CPR cases, high blood glucose levels on hospital arrival correlated with poor neurologic recovery[262]; however, most of these hyperglycemic patients were diabetic.[263] High glucose levels correlated with the duration of CPR attempts.[263] Immediately after acute stroke, hyperglycemia might be helpful[259] but more likely would be harmful.[255,264] Because sudden coma can be caused by hypoglycemia, routine withholding of intravenous glucose postarrest is debatable. We currently recommend reperfusion without added glucose and postarrest monitoring and titration of blood glucose levels at 100 to 200 mg/dl. In suspected hypoglycemia, an immediate emergency blood glucose test should be followed by glucose infusion if indicated.

TREATMENT WITH OUTCOME BENEFIT DOCUMENTED

IMPROVING CEREBRAL O_2 DELIVERY

In arrests in which external CPR-ALS attempts of longer than 5 min fail to restore stable spontaneous normotension (usually patients with acute myocardial infarction), artificial circulation methods that are physiologically more powerful may be tried. Chest compressions raise venous (right atrial) pressure peaks almost as high as arterial pressure peaks[88] and increase ICP,[234,265] thus usually causing very low cerebral and myocardial perfusion pressures.[84-89,102,128,266] Open chest CPR does not raise right atrial pressure, provides better cerebral and coronary perfusion pressures and flows than does external CPR in animals[86,89,90] and patients,[85] and achieves better outcome in dogs.[87,89,90] When applied promptly in operating room arrests, open chest CPR, which was introduced clinically around 1900,[62] yielded (until 1960) good clinical outcome results.[83] In recent clinical comparisons, the switch from external to open chest CPR has not yet been shown to improve outcome,[91] probably because open chest CPR was initiated too late. Physician teams that are adequately trained should consider switching to open chest CPR very early, not only in victims of trauma,[1,2] and perhaps even outside the hospital. Bystanders have not objected when open chest CPR was tried in the field.[92] In such prehospital trials, failure by external CPR-ALS of over 20 to 30 min to achieve ROSC was followed by open chest CPR achieving ROSC (personal communication, L. Corne, Brussels, 1995). After such prolonged low CBF by external CPR, awakening cannot be expected. If the stunned heart cannot be started, even with open chest CPR, prolonged direct heart compressions can be performed with a mechanical device.[93] A method of minimally invasive direct heart compression, not requiring thoracotomy, is being evaluated.[94] Open chest CPR can be initiated rapidly and serve as a bridge to long-term CPB and definitive cardiac repair.[46]

For cardiac arrest, emergency CPB [i.e., venoarterial pumping via an oxygenator (without the need for thoracotomy)] was tried in dogs[97] and in patients[98] in the 1970s, but not pursued. Because CPB provides full control over blood pressure, flow, composition, and temperature, Safar and colleagues initiated its systematic evaluation during the 1980s with eight cardiac arrest outcome studies in dogs.[103] CPB provided greater cardiovascular resuscitability than CPR-ALS and thereby improved cerebral recovery.[27,99–104] In dog cardiac arrest models, brief CPB provides controlled reperfusion that results in more reproducible outcome.[30,103] CPB is now being tried in hospital emergency departments; however, late initiation of CPB and the excessive time (>10 min) taken for cannulation of femoral vessels have led to relatively disappointing results thus far.[105,106] CPB might be initiated more rapidly via thoracotomy. Improvement should be sought by experimenting with more rapid vessel cannulation methods and by providing ambulance physicians with a portable CPB device for initiation in the prehospital setting.[107] A simplified initiation of intraarterial resuscitation, in need of further development and evaluation, is insertion of an aortic balloon (e.g., via femoral artery) to increase coronary and cerebral perfusion pressures during sternal compressions.[267–270]

Prolonged emergency CPB[103–107] or open chest mechanical cardiac massage[93] (for hours to days) could give the stunned heart a chance to recover from reversible cardiac failure or could be a bridge to coronary angioplasty, bypass procedure, left ventricular assist device, or emergency heart replacement.[46,105,271] When brain death is determined during CPB, it could become a bridge to organ donation.

HYPERTENSIVE HEMODILUTION   In a dog model of VF 12 min no-flow and external CPR, an immediate post-CPR combination of norepinephrine-induced hypertension, intracarotid hemodilution with dextran 40, and heparinization improved outcome.[49] The effects of

heparinization and thrombolytic therapy immediately after cardiac arrest remain to be clarified.[272] In a recent dog outcome study, a *brief* hypertensive bout (MAP of 150 to 200 mmHg for 1 to 5 min) followed by controlled normotension abolished evidence of immediate no-reflow[194,195] and correlated with improved neurologic and brain histologic outcome.[50] After ROSC in patients, brief hypertension correlates with a good cerebral outcome and hypotension correlates with a poor cerebral outcome.[273,274] *Prolonged* severe hypertension late postarrest might not be tolerated by the ischemic heart and can worsen vasogenic cerebral edema.[275] Postischemic cerebral hypoperfusion could be prevented by hypertensive reperfusion plus normovolemic hemodilution with plasma substitute to a Hct of 20 percent.[195] The effect of such hemodilution alone on outcome is uncertain,[50,276] possibly because Hct values less than 30 percent can reduce arterial O_2 content below that compensated for by increased flow, and thus decrease O_2 delivery.[277]

Further *support of hypertensive reperfusion* can be found in papers documenting this treatment's ability to overcome the immediate no-reflow phenomenon,[193–195] to open highly resistant areas of the cerebral microcirculation,[193] to improve EEG recovery after prolonged GBI in cats,[41–43] and to have a variety of other positive physiologic effects in acute animal models.[50,120,278,279] Induced hypertension has not undergone a formal clinical trial. Nevertheless, I recommended for clinical use now, a hypertensive bout following ROSC. Indeed, this often occurs spontaneously, as a result of prior epinephrine administration; if not, it should be induced as early as possible after ROSC, by using a titrated infusion of vasopressor. In animals, norepinephrine proved more effective than other vasopressors. Aiming for a systolic arterial pressure of about 200 mmHg for 1 to 5 min seems reasonable. After reperfusion, a combination of Hct 30 percent, Pa_{CO_2} 40 mmHg, plus titrated moderate hypertension seems more beneficial for the brain than Hct 40 percent, Pa_{CO_2} 30 mmHg, and normotension.[61]

CALCIUM ENTRY BLOCKERS
Calcium entry blockers may benefit the postischemic brain through vasodilation, blocking further calcium loading of neurons after the arrest and suppressing cascades from noxious mediators within blood elements.[6,54,55,213,280] Stimulated by a publication of Siesjo[164] and suggestions by White and colleagues[281] that calcium entry blockers might improve postarrest CBF and 24-h recovery,[282] the Pittsburgh group conducted the first cardiac arrest study of long-term cerebral outcome (in dogs) that documented the ability of a calcium entry blocker (lidoflazine), given immediately after arrest, to mitigate neurologic deficit and brain histologic dam-

TABLE 17-6
Calcium Entry Blocker Therapy After Cardiac Arrest:
Suggestion of Clinical Benefit

A. Multicenter clinical trial of lidoflazine therapy[6,139]
   Total groups with good cerebral outcome (CPC 1,2)—
     with placebo 23% ($n = 257$)
     with lidoflazine 24% ($n = 259$; NS)
   Subgroups without postarrest hypotension or rearrest with
     good cerebral outcome (CPC 1,2)—
      with placebo 29% ($n = 103$)
      with lidoflazine 46% ($n = 79$; $p = .02$)
     (Subgroup selection after randomization)
B. Unicenter clinical study of nimodipine therapy[155]
   Total groups with good cerebral outcome (CPC 1,2)—
     with placebo 36% ($n = 80$)
     with nimodipine 40% ($n = 75$; NS)
   Subgroups with ACLS attempts for longer than 10 min with
     good cerebral outcome (CPC 1,2)—
      with placebo 8% ($n = 26$)
      with nimodipine 47% ($n = 17$) ($p < .05$)

age and improve cardiac output to 96 h after arrest.[54] Subsequently, the same positive outcome results were obtained with early postarrest nimodipine therapy in the neck-tourniquet monkey model of the Pittsburgh group[68] introduced by Gisvold to colleagues at the Mayo Clinic.[55] Two negative 48-h outcome studies of postarrest lidoflazine therapy, one in dogs[283] and one in monkeys,[284] are unconvincing. Dog studies of nimodipine given before arrest or after arrest, with CBF or 48-h outcome models, gave variable results.[285,286] Different details in modeling might explain the failure of nimodipine to improve neurologic or histologic damage in cats.[287]

In the first clinical trial of calcium entry blocker therapy (BRCT II),[6,138] lidoflazine was used, because at that time it was the only such drug for which cerebral outcome data in animals had been reported.[54,282] It also had a cardiovascular benefit in dogs[288] and was well tolerated by cardiac patients.[289] In the cardiac arrest study, the lidoflazine group did not have a significantly higher proportion of patients overall with good cerebral outcome than the placebo group.[6] Among subgroups of patients without postarrest hypotension or rearrest, however, a significantly higher proportion achieved good cerebral outcome in the lidoflazine group (Table 17-6).[139] Unavoidably, this finding is based on selection by postrandomization characteristics. Lidoflazine after cardiac arrest in patients was associated with a higher incidence of postarrest hypotension or recurrent VF,[6] which would make its routine clinical use after cardiac arrest unwise.

A clinical study of nimodipine in Helsinki also failed to show a statistically significant overall improvement, whereas a subgroup with prolonged CPR times had a significantly higher proportion with good cerebral

outcome with nimodipine[155] (see Table 17-6). Lidoflazine- or nimodipine-induced postarrest hypotension must and can be controlled by titrated vasopressor therapy.[6,155] A European multicenter cardiac arrest study of nimodipine has been discontinued (personal communication, R. Roine, MD, Helsinki, Finland, 1992). Nimodipine mitigates postarrest reduction in CBF in patients,[290] decreases infarct size in stroke,[291] and controls vasospasm after subarachnoid hemorrhage in patients.[292] Intravenous administration of nimodipine in pigs[123] or diltiazem in dogs[293] *during* CPR steps A-B-C did not offset the beneficial effect of epinephrine on perfusion pressure and even enhanced initiation of heartbeat. Although nimodipine is not available in the United States for intravenous administration, it could be given via gastric tube during CPR immediately after intubation. The effects of available calcium entry blockers that do not produce hypotension on outcome after cardiac arrest in dogs deserve study.

Convincing data on use of flunarizine,[294–296] nicardipine,[297,298] verapamil,[299–301] nifedipine,[300] diltiazem,[302] or other calcium entry blockers[303–308] after cardiac arrest are lacking because of unreliable models, small numbers, or questionable experimental design. A recently completed European clinical study of flunarizine after cardiac arrest reportedly found no significant benefit (personal communication, R. Schroeder, MD, Berlin, Germany, 1992). Conceptually, new (neuron-specific, N-type) calcium entry blockers are now becoming available for laboratory and clinical evaluation.[171,303,304] One, although found effective in a rat forebrain ischemia model,[304] and after focal ischemia[305,306] did not improve cerebral outcome in a series of several cardiac arrest outcome studies in our dog model.[307,308]

HYPOTHERMIA

Moderate therapeutic hypothermia (28° to 32°C) induced *before* circulatory arrest *protects* the brain *during* noflow of up to 20 min.[69–72] *Deep* hypothermia (15° to 25°C) causes VF or asystole but, when induced and reversed by CPB, protects the brain during even longer circulatory arrests.[309–315] The seemingly "miraculous" recoveries after ice water drowning of 40 min or longer[316–318] may occur because the brain can reach protective hypothermic levels during asphyxiation before the heart stops.[99,319] This is in contrast to severe brain damage after even brief normothermic asphyxiation cardiac arrest[38,170] or normothermic drowning.[317,320,321] In dogs, prearrest induction of *profound* hypothermia (below 10°C) for preservation can protect the brain for over 1 h of total circulatory arrest, even when induced during hemorrhagic shock.[315]

Induction of hypothemia causes risky shivering, vasoconstriction, and thermogenesis, which must be blocked by the insult-generated CNS depression or drugs (poikilothermia) to make hypothermia "therapeutic" and safe. Prolonged hypothermia can cause infections and coagulopathies.[70] Deep-profound hypothermia causes myocardial depression, hypotension, arrhythmias, and cardiac arrest and potentially causes multifocal ischemia from reduced microcirculation.

Moderate hypothermia induced immediately *after* the insult, first studied in the 1950s, showed benefit in dog models of FBI[73] or brain contusion,[74] but yielded unconvincing results after cardiac arrest in dogs[77,78] and patients.[79, 80] It was discontinued, probably because it caused problems in clinical management, shivering, arrhythmias, and, in cases of prolonged cooling, coagulopathy and pulmonary infection.[70,322]

In the 1980s, Safar and others revived investigation of resuscitative hypothermia for cardiac arrest using reliable animal outcome models. Moderate hypothermia (30°C) gave borderline benefit for the brain,[53,56] but had side effects for the heart.[56] In 1987, Hossmann[43] reported that in cats with GBI there was a correlation between *mild* (unintentional) precooling and enhanced EEG recovery, and Safar[46,103] discovered a correlation between good cerebral outcome and *mild* (unintentional) hypothermia (34° to 36°C) present at the onset of VF in dog models. This led to a systematic series of five cardiac arrest outcome studies in dogs from 1988 to 1994 (Fig. 17-5), of *mild resuscitative* cerebral hypothermia (34°C), induced *immediately after* reperfusion and maintained for 2 or 12 h.[57-61]

In the *first* study,[57] VF 12.5-min no-flow was accompanied by head immersion in iced water (which reduced brain temperature by only 1°C) and followed by reperfusion cooling with brief CPB to 34°C. Functional and morphologic brain outcome variables were significantly improved in the hypothermic groups.

In the *second* study,[58] VF 10-min no-flow was reversed by standard external CPR; mild hypothermia induced within 5 to 10 min after reperfusion achieved the same significant improvement as in the first study. Cooling was performed with a clinically feasible but complex combination of head-neck-trunk surface cooling, plus cold fluid loads administered intravenously, intragastrically, and nasopharyngeally.

In the *third* study,[59] VF 12.5-min no-flow, brief CPB, and immediate mild (34°C) or moderate (to 30°C) hypothermia improved functional and morphologic brain outcome, but deep postarrest hypothermia (to 15°C with CPB) did not improve function and worsened brain histology. This contrasts with the greater brain protection (with prearrest induction) achieved with deep versus moderate hypothermia.[309-315] Moderate or deep postarrest hypothermia also worsened necrotic foci in the myocardium. It could worsen reperfusion.

In the *fourth* study,[60] with the same model as the first study, a 15-min delay in the initiation of mild cooling after normothermic reperfusion did not improve functional outcome, although a statistically significant decrease was seen in histologic damage scores of the brain in spite of the 15-min delay.

In the *fifth* study,[61] a combination treatment, including mild hypothermia for 12 h and CBF promotion, led to the best outcome yet encountered in dogs (see below, Combination Treatments).

Mild cooling in all five studies caused no cardiovascular or other side effects. In studies 1 to 4, however, even dogs with complete functional recovery had some histologic brain damage after 10 to 12 min of no-flow. We also found mild protective or resuscitative hypothermia reduced brain damage in our asphyxial cardiac arrest rat model.[323]

Simultaneously and independently, investigative groups in Miami,[324,325] Lund,[326] and Detroit[327,328] documented the ability of mild resuscitative hypothermia to reduce hippocampal histologic damage in the rat or cat brain after (incomplete) GBI. Postinsult mild to moderate hypothermia has also been shown to be beneficial after experimental focal ischemia in dogs[73] and rats,[329] after experimental brain contusion in dogs[75] and rats,[330] after epidural brain compression (brain trauma) in dogs,[331,332] and after severe hemorrhagic shock in rats.[333-335] For prevention of posttraumatic intracranial hypertension, which can lead to herniation and brain death, moderate hypothermia (31°C) was more effective than mild hypothermia (35°C).[331]

The *mechanism* of protection and resuscitation by mild hypothermia must be multifactorial[57] because its ability to reduce $CMRO_2$ by about 7 percent per degree centigrade alone (in the absence of shivering) in normal animals[71] or humans[336] cannot explain it. The temperature coefficient Q10 expresses $CMRO_2$ at one temperature divided by $CMRO_2$ at 10°C lower. A Q10 of 2 expresses a 50 percent reduction in $CMRO_2$, as it occurs in the normal brain between about 38°C and 28°C. Then, with artificial circulation, a Q10 of 5 expresses a reduction in $CMRO_2$ from 50 percent to 10 percent between 28°C to 18°C. The latter is caused by depression of basal metabolism.

After cardiac arrest, however, mild hypothermia seems to have no significant effect on CBF and $CMRO_2$.[188,337] We reviewed and referenced the multifactorial potentially beneficial effects in a previous publication.[57] They include preservation of ATP,[166,167] mitigation of abnormal ion fluxes,[168] reduced lactacidosis,[327] reduced free fatty acid production, and reduced excitatory neurotransmitter release,[325] slowing of destructive enzymatic reactions by 1.5 percent per degree centigrade (Arrhenius' equation), protection of lipoprotein membrane integrity (assumed), reduced edema, reduced leukotrienes,[338] improved glucose utilization, and slowing of free radical reactions.[339]

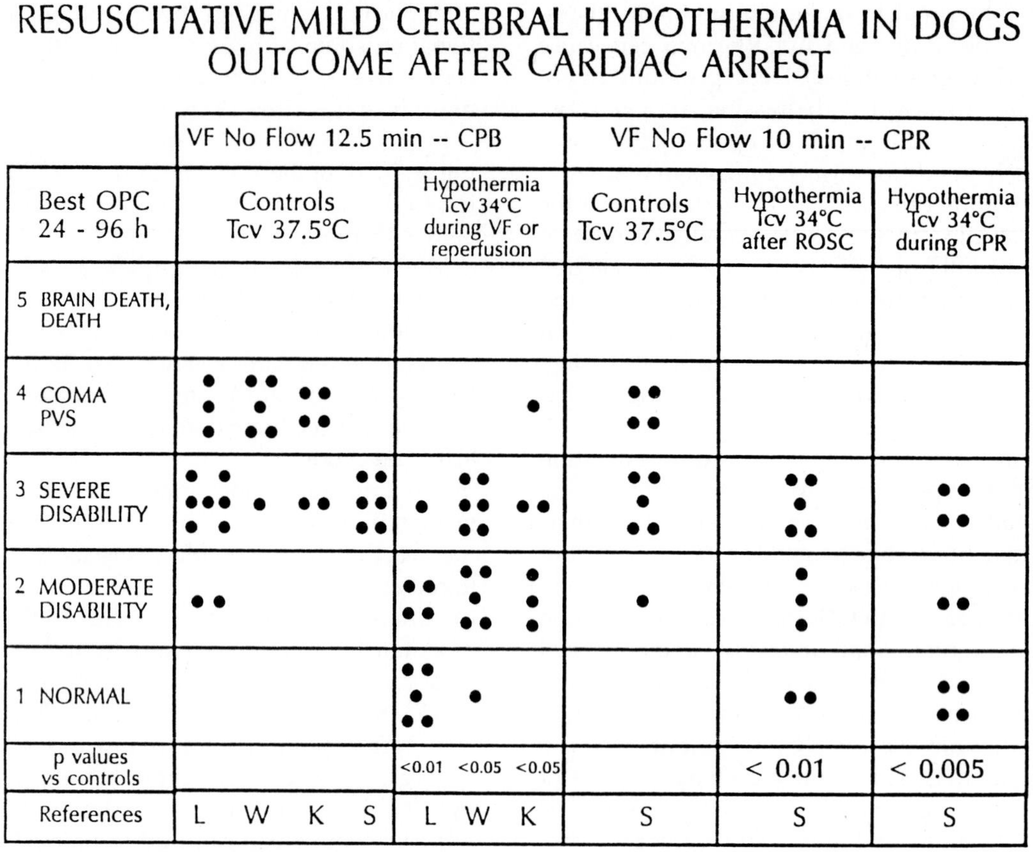

RESUSCITATIVE MILD CEREBRAL HYPOTHERMIA IN DOGS OUTCOME AFTER CARDIAC ARREST

Best OPC 24 - 96 h	VF No Flow 12.5 min -- CPB		VF No Flow 10 min -- CPR		
	Controls Tcv 37.5°C	Hypothermia Tcv 34°C during VF or reperfusion	Controls Tcv 37.5°C	Hypothermia Tcv 34°C after ROSC	Hypothermia Tcv 34°C during CPR
5 BRAIN DEATH, DEATH					
4 COMA PVS	• •• •• • • • • •	•	•• ••		
3 SEVERE DISABILITY	•• •• ••• •• •• •• ••	• •• •• •• •• ••	•• • ••	•• • ••	•• ••
2 MODERATE DISABILITY	••	•• •• •• • ••	•	• • •	••
1 NORMAL		•• • • ••		••	•• ••
p values vs controls		<0.01 <0.05 <0.05		< 0.01	< 0.005
References	L W K S	L W K	S	S	S

Figure 17-5 Improved cerebral and overall outcome after ventricular fibrillation (VF) cardiac arrest in reliable dog outcome models with immediate postarrest (resuscitative) mild cerebral hypothermia (34°C); cooling induced within 15 min of reflow. Each dot represents one experiment with 72 or 96 h postarrest intensive care. Overall performance categories (OPCs) as follows. *Left.* Control experiments after VF no-flow 12.5 min and CPB achieved severe disability or coma (OPC 3 or 4) in 28 of 30 experiments. *Right.* Control experiments after VF no-flow 10 min and external CPR achieved OPC 3 or 4 in 9 of 10 experiments. No controls achieved OPC 1 or OPC 5 (reliable models). Mild early postarrest hypothermia increased significantly the proportion of experiments with good outcome (OPC 1 or 2) in all four studies. Data from: L,[57] S,[58] W,[59] K.[60] Data from a fifth mild hypothermia study not shown.[61]

A recent rat study opened the possibility of mild resuscitative hypothermia of 4 h merely postponing an inevitable late loss of neurons.[340] It would be disappointing, but still provide time for additional treatments. A gerbil study of post-ischemic mild hypothermia over 24 h found permanent benefit.[341,342] The possibility of hypothermia mitigating "apoptosis" (acceleration of naturally programmed cell death), triggered by ischemic DNA damage, remains to be examined in cardiac arrest studies.

Clinical implementation must consider that mild hypothermia (34°C) benefits the brain, moderate hypothermia (28° to 30°C) might induce VF, and mild cerebral *hyper*thermia (which can occur in brain-injured patients even with normal core temperature) is deleterious for the injured brain in rats.[343] Therefore, I recommend that all comatose patients should have monitoring and control of brain temperature (Tty or Tnp), as well as heart temperature (Tes, Tcv, Tpa, or Tu). Shivering and vasospasm, if not absent because of postanoxic coma, should be prevented with muscle relaxant and diazepam or barbiturate. Clinical methods for rapidly inducing mild cerebral hypothermia in any acutely comatose patient, outside and inside hospitals, are now under development (Table 17-7).[57,109,344–347] Peritoneal cooling looks promising[61,346] (see below). Although the safe and effective temperature level seems to be about 33° to 35°C, the optimal duration of mild hypothermia is uncertain. Although a 15-min delay decreased the effectiveness,[60] even much later induction of mild cooling might have some beneficial effect.[348] Isolated brain cooling is feasible in children.[349,350]

TABLE 17-7
Mild Resuscitative Cerebral Hypothermia for Comatose Patients:
Clinical Cooling Methods (for references, see text)

A. Indications:
    Immediate cooling after cardiac arrest
    Early cooling after traumatic brain injury (TBI)
    Early cooling after severe stroke (FBI)

B. Temperature control:
    Core temperature monitoring to prevent heart-endangering temperature lower than 30°C
    (Monitor Tes, Tpa, Tcv, or Tb)
    Cerebral temperate monitoring to achieve brain-saving temperature of 34°C (32°C after TBI)
    (Monitor Tty or Tnp as noninvasive brain temperature)
    In cases of brain trauma, monitor brain temperature with ICP probe

C. Rapid brain cooling methods:

	RANKED	
	by Feasibility to initiate	by Speed to reach Cerebral T 34°C
Head-neck (trunk) ice, fanning surface	1	6
Nasopharyngeal	2	5
Eosophagogastric	2	5
IV cold infusion	2	5
Peritoneal cold lavage	3	3
Venovenous shunt with pump, heat exchanger	4	4
Arteriovenous shunt, heat exchanger	4	4
Intracarotid cold flush	5	1
Cardiopulmonary bypass, heat exchanger	6	1
Whole body ice water immersion	6	2

COMBINATION TREATMENTS

Our goal of consistent reversibility of VF 10-min normothermic no-flow to complete functional recovery with histologically normal brains has not yet been achieved with mild resuscitative hypothermia alone; therefore, adjunctive treatments need evaluation. The first dog study that showed that any treatment after cardiac arrest can improve outcome was with a normothermic CBF-promoting combination.[49] The model we used at that time did not meet our present goals (see Table 17-1). Combining moderate hypothermia with specific drugs resulted in some improvement of outcome after GBI in monkeys.[53] Various single-drug treatments have not yielded beneficial effects on neurologic outcome (see next section), except for mild benefit from some calcium entry blockers, which exert multiple therapeutic effects.[6,54,55,139,155]

In pursuit of the hypothesis that etiology-specific combination treatments would be most effective in improving outcome, we recently conducted six series of exploratory experiments with combination treatments.[351] This led to a definitive randomized outcome study in dogs with VF no-flow of 11 min and a clinically realistic but with CPB-controlled, reperfusion method that simulates the low O_2 delivery produced by external CPR.[61,352] We compared a control group 1 of eight dogs (normothermic standard therapy) with a combination treatment group 2, which received mild hypothermia by head-neck-surface cooling plus peritoneal instillation of cold Ringer's solution to keep brain temperature 34°C from 11 min to 12 h after reperfusion. In addition, group 2 received CBF promotion[50,195] by induced moderate hypertension (MAP 110 to 140 mmHg) to 4 h, colloid (dextran 40)-induced reduction of Hct from 40 to 30 percent for 12 h, and Pa_{CO_2} of 40 mmHg (instead of 30 mmHg in control group 1) from 3 h to 20 h.[61] At 96 h after resuscitation, all eight dogs in control group 1 remained severely damaged, whereas six of eight dogs in treatment group 2 had recovered to functional normality. The histopathologic damage scores in the treatment group were the lowest ever achieved.[61] Final 96-h overall performance category, neurologic deficit scores, and brain histopathologic damage scores showed highly significant group differences ($p < .001$). Also significant was the difference between the outcome in treatment group 2 of this study versus outcomes in previous studies in the same model with comparable insult, with CBF promotion alone[50] or mild hypothermia alone.[60] The control group had the same severe outcome results as occurred in 50 control experiments with a comparable insult and the same model in the past.[30,50,60,103,124] We recommend clinical trials of a combination treatment protocol based on (but not exactly like) that of experimental group 2 in this study.[61]

In this same study,[61] we simultaneously randomized a third group, which received the same treatment protocol as group 2 plus six inexpensive available drugs to counteract various steps in the necrotizing cascades (see Fig. 17-4).[352] These drugs were deferoxamine, ascorbic acid (a free radical scavenger), $MgSO_4$ (a calcium entry blocker), methylprednisolone, thiopental, and phenytoin. Outcomes in group 3 were worse than those in group 2 for unknown reasons. We suspect the hypotensive effects of $MgSO_4$ and thiopental, which increased the norepinephrine requirement. Subsequently, adding only thiopental loading to the group 2 treatment protocol did not abolish the few remaining histologic lesions.[352] Several other combinations of drugs have seemed promising in short-term models,[353] but have not yet been documented in large animal outcome studies.

TREATMENTS WITH UNPROVEN OUTCOME BENEFIT

Barbiturate loading improved outcome after experimental focal ischemia[354,355] or incomplete global ischemia[356] and had several potentially beneficial effects,[357] including reduction of active cerebral metabolism, which might be beneficial in postarrest multifocal hypoperfusion (multifocal incomplete ischemia),[194,197] and reduction of ICP.[358] In 1976, the Pittsburgh group evaluated the efficacy of barbiturate loading after GBI in monkeys[51] using the first long-term intensive care model[68] and found a significant reduction in postarrest neurologic deficit and morphologic brain damage. Because no other reliable animal outcome model was available at the time, a second (somewhat different) study in monkeys was conducted,[52] which failed to duplicate the outcome benefit of the first. Subsequent studies by others also gave mixed results.[359,360] Because of the uncontrolled clinical use of barbiturate loading at the time and promising feasibility trials,[145] a multicenter clinical trial was conducted.[5] Overall, outcome results were statistically negative, but subgroups with long arrest or CPR times showed a trend toward better cerebral outcome after thiopental treatment.[5] Recently, a preliminary reevaluation of thiopental loading after 12.5-min VF cardiac arrest in dogs gave encouraging results,[351] but in a following definitive dog study, this treatment did not prevent the slight histologic damage remaining after VF 11-min no-flow followed by CBF promotion and mild hypothermia.[352] At present, titrated barbiturate therapy for resuscitation after cardiac arrest or GBI remains optional, for FBI or TBI see below.

Phenytoin reduces deleterious ion shifts in hypoxia; trials for protection[361] and resuscitation[362] have had suggestive positive results. Phenytoin deserves reevaluation in a reliable model (see Table 17-1).

Anti-reoxygenation injury cocktails based on mechanistic rationale (see Fig. 17-4) in animals improved postarrest CBF[114] or recovery of EEG or evoked potentials,[115,214] but failed to improve outcome.[347,363-366] One anti-reoxygenation injury cocktail seemed slightly beneficial in a dog model of asphyxial cardiac arrest but not after VF arrest, whereas a calcium entry blocker was effective after VF arrest but not after the more injurious asphyxial arrest.[366] Another cocktail of six drugs made outcome worse.[351] The local anesthetic *lidocaine*, given in an external CPR model in dogs after ROSC in maximal subconvulsive doses, did not improve outcome (T. M. Hoel and P. Safar, unpublished data, 1990).

The *excitatory neurotransmitter NMDA receptor blocker* MK-801, an anti-epileptic drug, gave seemingly positive results in FBI and GBI models[178,367,368]; these studies were flawed, however, by inadvertent mild hypothermia caused by the drug. MK-801 did not improve cerebral outcome when brain temperature was well controlled in a dog model of VF,[369] a gerbil model,[370] or a primate model.[371] Also, MK-801 depresses breathing.[369] The AMPA/kainate receptor blocker NBQX looks more promising.[372,373]

The *aminosteroid* ("lazaroid") U74006F (trilizad) seemed to be effective in animal models of trauma and focal ischemia.[374,375] U74006F did not change postarrest CBF and metabolism[376] and did not improve outcome in a rat forebrain ischemia model.[377] Pretreatment with U74006F improved neurologic outcome after global ischemia in dogs.[378,379] Resuscitative treatment after cardiac arrest remains to be studied. Aminosteroids have the advantage over calcium entry blockers of supporting rather than suppressing perfusion pressure and cardiac output, which are critical and labile after ROSC.

Visceral damage after arrests of 10 to 12 min seems mild and transient,[222] which might explain the failure of gut sterilization or hemabsorption to improve cerebral outcome.[223]

TREATMENTS TO BE EVALUATED

For resuscitation from cardiac arrest, the search should begin with reoxygenation methods. To improve initial O_2 delivery over that provided by external CPR by bystanders, a totally new (still elusive) approach is needed. Basic life support should not require the use of devices. Optimal initial high versus normal Pa_{O_2}, as well as benefit from later hyperbaric oxygenation, which appears promising,[380] needs clarification.

Clinical trials of the currently best documented and most effective combination treatment, namely, mild hypothermia with or without CBF promotion,[61] can and should be introduced in various centers immediately, at least to establish feasibility and side effects. Various cooling methods (see above) should be tried. Hypothermia should be studied to determine optimal duration, control of shivering, and methods of rewarming. The possibility of mild hypothermia causing merely a delay in the development of ultimate brain damage[340] (once triggered, irreparable "apoptosis") (see above) deserves evaluation in reliable cardiac arrest models, with follow-up over months.

Although VF 11-min no-flow has recently been reversed to complete functional recovery with a physical combination treatment after arrest,[61] an attempt to achieve a histologically "clean" brain, will require pharmacologic cocktails based on good rationale (see Fig. 17-4). Slight protective-preservation effects of some anesthetics[381,382] (Chap. 18) justify their evaluation *after* GBI.

A new approach to the systematic development of additional pharmacologic combination treatments is needed.[307] The selection of drugs should be based on preliminary data of pharmacologic and physiologic mechanisms (in vitro; in normal organisms; in rodent ischemia models) and on serendipity.[35,383–387] Ideally, the effects of various doses of promising pharmacologic agents on overall, cardiac, and cerebral outcome should be compared, perhaps first in an inexpensive cardiac arrest outcome model in rats.[133] There should be data on pharmacodynamics, including brain penetration. Side effects of deliberate overdose in normal large animals should be evaluated.[307] Treatments with promising but not reproducible outcome results in past unreliable models and good mechanistic rationale should be reevaluated. Finally, single and multifaceted therapies, initiated during and continued after resuscitation in a clinically feasible form, should be evaluated in a reproducible large animal outcome model (see Table 17-1). Positive effects on the rat hippocampus after incomplete forebrain ischemia do not predict similar benefit in dogs after cardiac arrest.

Increasing cerebral O_2 delivery postarrest to maximize O_2 uptake, an approach found beneficial after shock[388] or in stunned myocardium,[389] might be achieved by a titrated combination of hemodilution with stroma-free hemoglobin or fluorocarbon solution, hypertension, vasodilation, osmotherapy, or hyperbaric O_2. Simultaneous depression of CNS activity and metabolism might further improve O_2 delivery/demand ratio (e.g., mild hypothermia, barbiturate, phenytoin, diazepam, chlorpromazine, narcotic, local anesthetic, isoflurane). All these could be titrated with respect to mixed cerebral venous O_2 values, that is, sagittal sinus blood in animals or superior jugular bulb blood in humans.

Once there is evidence of a late postarrest surge in excitotoxicity, infusions of new NMDA and AMPA antagonists should be evaluated, and various other antiepileptic drugs and anesthetics reevaluated. Once there are data in the brain concerning free radical reactions during and after reperfusion, an increase in intracellular calcium, or an inflammatory response, the following might be tried: antireoxygenation injury cocktails including mega doses of ascorbate[391]; penetrating superoxide dismutase conjugated with polyethylene glycol or with liposomal inclusion[392]; an improved iron chelator[351]; improved calcium entry blockers; antilipid peroxidation aminosteroids; and anticomplement therapy.[393,394] If specific blood elements are identified as culprits, specific antagonists (e.g., prostacyclin-indomethacin-heparin),[184,185] blood detoxification methods (leukapheresis, hemabsorption, plasmapheresis, total blood exchange),[223] and heparinization-thrombolysis[49,272,276] might be tried in new, improved outcome models. There is potential to increase ATP by modifying substrate, such as with fructose biphosphate,[126,395] and to promote late reparative processes,[396] such as with titrated administration of insulin (irrespective of its effect on blood glucose levels).[261,397] The injured brain may first need sedation, but later stimulation.[396] Finally, once we have learned how cerebral neurons die later after reperfusion from ischemic insults, protective and resuscitative DNA-modifying treatment trials might be conducted to study ways to prevent PCD.[398–400]

Evaluation of outcome after single drugs, which are to be selected with good rationale, in different doses, followed by escalating combinations with other drugs will make the systematic development of an optimal combination treatment an unavoidably tedious process.

Resuscitation from Focal Brain Ischemia

Each year, FBI (i.e., ischemic stroke)[401] occurs outside the operating room in approximately 230,000 Americans. Most of these cases represent a form of FBI with permanent, complete ischemia in the necrotic focus, plus incomplete ischemia in the surrounding penumbra zone. Transient ischemic attacks (TIAs) occur in an additional 68,000 Americans each year. The majority of those attacks involve pathology of the extracranial cerebral arteries, a condition that is of major concern to neuroanesthesiologists (Chaps. 14 and 27). In about 15 percent of ischemic stroke patients, cerebral emboli travel from the heart into the middle cerebral artery (MCA). Treatment for these patients has been until recently unjustifiably conservative, consisting mostly of observation. This approach can be explained in part by the reluctance of neurologists to let rescuers diagnose or suspect FBI in the field; to have anesthesiologists-intensivists use risky therapy such as barbiturate anesthesia and hypothermia on conscious patients; and to use thrombolysis because of fear to provoke cerebral hemorrhage. This author considers this conservatism unjustified because of the devastating effect of massive MCA occlusion, particularly in the dominant hemisphere, on the quality of survival. Moreover, when untreated, some patients with FBI develop brain swelling to the point of herniation, apnea, and death.

This author has promoted since the 1960s, when modern external CPR was introduced, a resuscitative approach to sudden ischemic stroke, with the same urgency and activism directed at attempts to save cerebral neurons after cardiac arrest. Only recently have prehospital emergency physicians begun to consider blood pressure control and other measures in suspected stroke patients. Hospital-based physicians are beginning to study and introduce (still often too late) various special physical and pharmacologic treatments to increase regional CBF in the partially ischemic penumbra zone, thereby reducing infarct size and neurologic deficit. Some are exploring the use of intravenous tissue plasminogen activator (tPA) therapy,[402,403] thrombolysis directly into the MCA, and infarctectomy (H. Yonas, Pittsburgh, unpublished data). Extracranial to intracranial bypass surgery as an emergency procedure is controversial. A major prospective randomized trial gave no significantly positive results.[404]

Without anesthetics, a low-flow penumbra zone can have its regional CBF reduced from a normal of about 50 to 15 ml/100 g per min, a threshold level for EEG failure. The threshold for energy failure threatening viability of neurons, is about 10 ml/100 g per min. Normally, about half of cerebral O_2 uptake is for active metabolism (which can be silenced by high doses of barbiturate), whereas the other half, the basal metabolism, is for maintenance of cell viability (integrity), which can be reduced even by mild hypothermia and silenced by profound hypothermia.[405] Narcotics can reduce $CMRO_2$ and CBF (in parallel) only in large doses.

The therapeutic time window for ischemic FBI is not 6 h, but probably 10 to 20 min for normothermic no-flow in the focus that is to become necrotic, and about 1 h for the penumbra zone. Several special treatments, if applied immediately, can diminish infarct size at least in experimental MCA occlusion in various animal species. These treatments, which have not been transferred to clinical trials, are induced hypertension, hemodilution, hypothermia, vasodilation, barbiturate, and isoflurane. Conclusions from the experimental results have sometimes been contradictory, which is easily explained by differences in details of experimental pro-

tocols. Several of the above treatments, however, could be induced in the emergency room without delay, and perhaps even in the prehospital arena, particularly by EMS systems with physicians experienced with resuscitation going to the scene.

Moderate *hypertension*, induced by vasopressor, with or without volume expansion, early after MCA occlusion reduced infarct size in various animal models, and increased regional CBF in patients.[406-410] Induced hypertension is an established treatment for vasospasm associated with subarachnoid hemorrhage, as after aneurysm clipping surgery.[410] Hypertension induced late does not reduce infarct size and may provoke hemorrhage when the blood-brain barrier is already damaged.

The case for *hemodilution* reducing blood viscosity and increasing microcirculation in the penumbra zone is based on many experimental studies, which have been reviewed.[411] The degree of hemodilution is critical. Hypervolemic hemodilution seems more beneficial than normovolemic or hypovolemic hemodilution.[412] In dogs, oxygen transport to the whole body is maintained through increased flow, as the arterial O_2 content declines with hemodilution to a critical level of Hct 25 percent.[277] Hypervolemic hemodilution to Hct of 30 percent with colloid plasma substitute in patients with FBI has improved neurologic function and CBF.[413-416]

Controlled *hyperventilation*, suggested for FBI to create a "reverse steal effect" (constricting normal vessels and donating blood to the penumbra zone), has been effective in reducing infarct size when used prophylactically before MCA occlusion,[417] but not if begun after ischemia.[418,419]

Hypothermia, with its ability to reduce brain oxygen needs and to suppress membrane damaging cascades (see Fig. 17-4) (see hypothermia for cardiac arrest, above), is probably the most potent protective-preservative and resuscitative mechanism for FBI. A prerequisite is sufficient anesthesia and paralysis to create pharmacologic poikilothermia without shivering or vasospasm. The lower the temperature the more protection and preservation that can be achieved. Deep cooling after ischemia, however, might worsen outcome.[59] Since the lower temperatures are risky for the cardiovascular system, hypothermia has not until recently entered the FBI treatment scene. Moderate hypothermia (30°C) induced 1 h after MCA in dogs, even if brief, diminished infarct size.[73] Mild hypothermia (34°C), which is risk free, has been shown in rats to reduce infarct size.[329] This mild hypothermia treatment deserves clinical trials.

Barbiturate therapy before or after FBI, despite its somewhat confusing and contradictory data after GBI, has strong support from experiments that showed reduced infarct size in dogs[355] and monkeys,[354] with large doses of barbiturate, even when given after FBI. Among anesthetics, barbiturates offer the most protection,[420-425] but not always.[426] Pentobarbital reduces edema.[423]

Strangely, controlled clinical trials of barbiturate therapy in FBI are lacking. To reproduce the benefit seen in animal models,[354,355] the EEG has to be depressed to burst suppression pattern, which requires intravenous thiopental 5 to 10 mg/kg followed by a continuous infusion of 3 to 5 mg/kg per h. This may not be tolerated by the cardiovascular system of elderly people. Thiopental 40 mg/kg (i.e., burst suppression doses), in patients undergoing open heart surgery with CPB who are expected to develop (subtle) multifocal infarcts, was followed by less neurologic dysfunction than seen in untreated controls.[419] Such large barbiturate doses, however, require much pharmacologic cardiovascular support.

Isoflurane, in contrast to other inhalation anesthetics, can at 2 minimum alveolar concentration (MAC) (2.5%) silence the EEG without depressing blood pressure.[401] With comparable MAP, temporary focal ischemia in monkeys has reduced infarct size by isoflurane when induced before and maintained during FBI.[427] Various general anesthetics which depress active CMR_{O_2}[405] might benefit the penumbra of FBI with low CBF[428,429] (Chap. 18).

Vasodilation can be achieved with sodium nitroprusside[430] or nimodipine (or other calcium entry blockers). Nimodipine has undergone three controlled studies in patients with vasospasm after subarachnoid hemorrhage[431-433] and has significantly improved outcome. In animal studies, pretreatment with nimodipine before FBI attenuated the decreasing CBF and reduced infarct size.[434-436] In patients with acute stroke, long-term oral nimodipine (120 mg/day) resulted in significantly lower mortality and morbidity.[437,438] If vasodilation seems to enhance cerebral edema,[439] concomitant osmotherapy or hypothermia is indicated. Other drugs, which, like calcium entry blockers, have multifaceted potentially beneficial effects besides vasodilation, such as the aminosteroid (lazaroid) trilazad, are under investigation for FBI in patients at this time.

Resuscitation from Traumatic Brain Injury

Traumatic brain injury (TBI) (Chap. 34) includes cerebral multifocal ischemia.[386] TBI occurs in over 400,000 persons per year in the United States, as a result of motor vehicle accidents, falls, guns, and other insults. Almost 40,000 Americans die early and another 40,000 remain severely dysfunctional each year as a result of TBI.[440,441] Modern cerebral resuscitation from severe TBI

with coma, that is, with a Glasgow coma score less than 8 (best 15, worst 3) (see Table 17-3), should include extra- and intracranial measures, starting immediately after impact in the field and continuing to recovery of consciousness. A realistic therapeutic goal is twofold: (1) to reduce acute mortality due to acute or delayed brain swelling and herniation from edema or hyperemia, resulting in apnea and cardiovascular collapse (often on days 2 to 3); and (2) to reduce morbidity by mitigating or preventing secondary tissue damage beyond the mechanically destroyed tissue, due to inflammatory and other cascades, following the initial insult.

In contrast to GBI with its predictable pathophysiology, TBI encompasses a large variety of multifocal insults. The *primary insult* may include skull fractures, focal mass lesions (e.g., subdural, epidural, or intracerebral hematoma; hemorrhagic contusions), or diffuse axonal injury (DAI). Contusions result in necrotic foci, penumbra zones of potentially recuperable tissue, and distant effects on neurons, such as the CA-3 region of the hippocampus, even far away from the contusion.[442]

The *secondary derangements* in the brain can include any of the molecular and cellular tissue reactions identified for cardiac arrest (see above) (see Fig. 17-4) and in addition, the mechanical destruction of tissue with rupture of cell membranes and blood-brain barrier, free heme which is neurotoxic,[443] glutamate release,[444] and a pronounced delayed inflammatory response of cytokines,[187] which upregulate nerve growth factor.[445,446] The secondary derangements outside the brain that can add injury to the brain include arterial hypotension,[447,448] hypoxemia,[449,450] hypercapnia,[451] hyperthermia (even mild),[343] and increased cerebral venous pressure. The latter is an often ignored secondary insult caused by "bucking" during or after tracheal intubation or neck vein compression by malpositioning of the head. Although the normal brain, in normal life activities, can tolerate large temporary increases in ICP, Pa_{CO_2}, or temperature (to 41°C), injured brain can suffer irreversible additional damage from mild transient ICP rise, mild hypercapnia, or even mild hyperthermia.

Neurologic and radiologic examination and indications for emergency craniotomy are beyond the scope of this chapter. Intracranial hematomas should be evacuated immediately.

Management[452-465] should begin immediately after impact and aim at mitigating brain swelling from a mix of vasogenic (extracellular) and cytotoxic (intracellular) edema (which cause compression ischemia) or hyperemia due to local vasoparalysis. These derangements occur in a variable, unpredictable mix, resulting in progressively increasing ICP with possible herniation.[331,332] Global and regional CBF after closed brain trauma in animals and patients might cause an extremely brief period of hyperemia,[456] followed by hypoperfusion for 1 to 2 days,[203,204] after which delayed hyperemia[203] and increased cerebral blood volume,[457] with low $CMRO_2$ (vasoparalysis and coma) can lead to ICP rise and death.[202–204,458]

Management should begin at the scene with step A for impact coma, that is, backward tilt of the head and jaw thrust; and step B for impact apnea,[459,460] that is, mouth-to-mouth (in trismus mouth-to-nose) ventilation. When health professionals arrive, intubation can be difficult; bucking and even brief periods of hypoxemia and hypercarbia (asphyxiation) must be avoided using skillful, rapid, and smooth tracheal intubation.[2,461] The impact-induced sympathetic discharge may also be harmful.[462] Brain-oriented intensive care life support should appreciate that not only extracerebral derangements can add injury to the brain, but also the reverse may be the case, that is, TBI can influence extracerebral variables, mostly through damage of hypothalamus and the pituitary.

Management should include ICP monitoring and control. This according to guidelines[454] should keep monitored ICP below a threshold of 20 to 25 mmHg, with the following sequential actions: (1) CSF drainage; (2) head elevation 30°; (3) paralysis and controlled ventilation with mild hyperventilation (prophylactic severe hyperventilation is not recommended[463]); (4) osmotherapy (mannitol in intermittent boluses of 0.25 to 1.0 g/kg); (5) seizure control; (6) barbiturate (thiopental) titrated for transient ICP control and seizure control; and (7) mild (34°C) to moderate (30°C) *hypothermia*.[330–332] Systolic arterial pressure should not be allowed to decrease below 90 mmHg, and CPP (MAP − ICP) should be maintained at a minimum of 70 mmHg. Brief hyperventilation may be necessary when there is acute neurologic deterioration, or for longer periods, when ICP increase is refractory to CSF drainage and osmotherapy. Global cerebral hypoxia might be combatted, as guided by keeping mixed cerebral venous (superior jugular bulb) O_2 saturation ≥50% ($P_{O_2} > 20$ mmHg).

Therapeutic hypothermia for TBI is based on studies of Rosomoff and colleagues in the 1950s in dogs with brain contusion,[71–76] and on pioneering work by Albin and White that found hypothermia effective in experimental spinal cord injury.[464,465] Early post-TBI mild to moderate hypothermia sustained for 12 to 24 h suppresses the inflammatory reactions[466] and protects the brain against ischemia by decreasing cerebral metabolism and against many deleterious chemical reactions (see above). Hypothermia specifically may control ICP rise when caused by an increase in cerebral blood volume. Mild hypothermia is less effective than moderate hypothermia in preventing lethal ICP rise after experimental brain trauma in dogs.[331] Documentation of the benefit of early (not immediate) hypothermia induced after TBI in patients is underway.[467]

Cerebral Protection-Preservation-Resuscitation and Suspended Animation

Prophylactic (protective) measures against anticipated GBI or FBI have been mentioned under FBI above. In general, special treatments for GBI found to protect-preserve the brain during low O_2 delivery may not necessarily improve outcome when initiated for resuscitation from an unprotected ischemia. In general, the lower the level of hypothermia *during* ischemia, the better its protective effect, but *after* a normothermic insult deep hypothermia for resuscitation may be harmful,[59] whereas mild resuscitative hypothermia is more effective than moderate resuscitative hypothermia.[57–61] Finally, although mild resuscitative hypothermia may merely slow the secondary damage, mild protective-preservative hypothermia gives a permanent neuron-saving effect.[340]

For neurosurgery, safe prophylactic protection-preservation against anticipated FBI or GBI, particularly low-flow (shock) states, seems to be best provided by anesthesia with thiopental to EEG burst suppression or with isoflurane 2 MAC plus mild hypothermia, which is safe. Cerebral protection against global temporary no-flow states (cardiac arrest) is best provided by safe mild-to-moderate hypothermia, which requires pharmacologic poikilothermia to block shivering, vasoconstriction, and thermogenesis. This requires some anesthesia plus neuromuscular blockade. Even after mild hypothermia, during rewarming and recovery from general anesthesia, shivering can occur and should also be suppressed.[468]

During normal circulation, deep brain and core (heart) temperature quickly equilibrate. A slight temperature gradient (brain 1° to 2°C cooler than the heart) can be maintained by added head-neck-surface cooling. To maintain safe spontaneous circulation, core temperature should be maintained at 30°C or above and to provide cerebral protection, brain temperature should be maintained at 34°C or less, the lower the more protective. Below 30°C, because of cold-induced cardiac arrest usually at 20° to 25°C, protection-preservation with hypothermia requires CPB for induction and resuscitation-rewarming. Deep (15° to 20°C) or profound hypothermic circulatory arrest (<10°C) (DHCA, PHCA) has been in use for selected cardiac or intracranial operations for three decades.[69,70,309,469] CPB-induced deep hypothermia protects the brains in dogs and humans for up to about 30 min no-flow, whereas profound hypothermia protects for up to about 60 min no-flow.[309,315] The latter has been documented recently in dogs in terms of not only complete functional recovery, but also histologically "clean" brains.[315]

A new field of resuscitation research is "suspended animation for delayed resuscitation," a concept introduced by P. Safar and R. Bellamy in 1984, primarily to try and save rapidly exsanguinating combat casualties.[470] My definition of suspended animation is as follows: "Protection and preservation of the whole organism during prolonged (≥ 1 h) clinical death for transport and resuscitative surgery (or otherwise infeasible elective surgical repair), without pulse, followed by delayed resuscitation to complete recovery without brain damage." The circulatory arrest would be induced by the insult itself or protective-preservative therapy (drugs plus hypothermia), which still needs to be worked out. Suspended animation, which means tolerance of prolonged tissue anoxia without blood flow, must be differentiated from hibernation, which is hypothermia without tissue anoxia and with sustained low blood flow and low metabolism.

In 1988, we started dog studies on suspended animation during hemorrhage.[310–315] These studies relied on hypothermia induced and reversed with emergency (portable) CPB. In study #1,[310] we found the limit for DHCA with Tty 15°C to be 60 min, which is clinically accepted as the safe limit for DHCA when used in cardiac surgery. The preceding normothermic hemorrhagic shock of 40 mmHg for 30 min did not add injury. In study #2,[311] we found that PHCA provided better outcome than DHCA. PHCA of 2 h allowed survival, but with some histologic brain damage. In study #3,[312] we used the University of Wisconsin organ preservation solution for blood washout before stasis under PHCA of 2 h. It offered no additional benefit for the brain, but some benefit for the heart. This suggests that some of these interventions will have different effects on different organs. In study #4,[313] we induced PHCA of 2 h with CPB, using a heparin-bonded circuit without systemic anticoagulation. We achieved the same results in terms of neurologic outcome and had no thrombotic complications. In study #5,[314] we found a hint that moderate hemodilution to Hct 20 percent at the time of PHCA of 2 h may be better than total blood washout with Hct 5 percent or less. In our initial studies, we wanted to use severe hemodilution to prevent blood from sludging during the period of circulatory arrest at these very low temperatures. The optimal Hct needs to be determined. In study #6,[315] we found histologically new data. In the above dog model, after normothermic hemorrhagic shock with MAP 40 mmHg for 60 min (not 90 min), PHCA for 60 min (not 90 min) could be reversed to complete functional recovery with histologically "clean" brains. Detailed search for ischemic neuronal changes in 19 brain regions found no

changes after arrest of 2 h. Much research is needed to extend the 1-h limit of PHCA and to induce suspended animation without CPB in the field.

Certain complex operations on the brain have been performed electively under DHCA or PHCA, induced and reversed by CPB.[474] Bloodless brain operations have also been tried without PHCA, with blood washout and continued asanguinous low-flow perfusion by CPB, using special crystalloid solution mixtures of extracellular (for induction and reversal) and intracellular compositions (for low-flow).[471–473] At about 5 to 10°C, 2 to 3 h of asanguinous low-flow was tolerated.

The experiences with emergency PHCA in dogs are making practical use of the earlier pioneering observations by White and Albin[474] who demonstrated electric and metabolic recovery of the totally isolated brain after 4 h of no-flow at 2°C. *Normothermic* induction of suspended animation under emergency conditions in the field, without CPB, is a challenge for future research. Lessons might be learned from anoxia-tolerant animals,[475] from "pharmacologic" hibernation,[476] and from studies of ways to stabilize membranes during hypoxia by preventing calcium influx[477,478] or by hyperpolarizing.[479] Membrane protection during no-flow (metabolic silence) will require more than active CMR_{O_2} depression by anesthetics (Chap. 18).

The additional measures to be evaluated include attempts to zero basal metabolic O_2 requirements by reducing brain temperature further to just above crystal formation. A pharmacologic (normothermic) induction of suspended animation could lead to spontaneous exposure cooling, and as soon as feasible to CPB-induced (and reversed) ultra-PHCA. One would have to tailor the solutions for suspended animation versus reperfusion-rewarming patterns, which would optimize recovery of the brain and entire organism after circulatory arrest longer than 1 h.

Prediction of Cerebral Outcome

When not to start (inexpensive) emergency resuscitation is less crucial than when to stop (expensive) prolonged life support.[2] Ideally, CPCR should not be permitted to result in long-term survival with persistent severe brain damage. Cerebral resuscitation research should continue to include studies on how to predict with certainty, early after the insult, severe permanent brain damage with consciousness (CPC 3) or PVS (CPC 4) (see Table 17-4). Discontinuance of all life support in cases of PVS, including artificial airway, ventilation, feeding, hydration, antibiotics, and emergency surgery, is ethically justified.[480–483]

Determination and certification of whole brain death (which is only possible hours to days after restoration of normotension), followed by discontinuance of artificial ventilation, does not present dilemmas. No one certified "brain dead," according to brain death certification guidelines, has yet recovered. PVS is cerebral (supratentorial) death (apallic syndrome), without destruction of brain stem and medulla, that is, with continued spontaneous breathing. This state might, however, also be called "death."[483,484] Determination with 100 percent certainty of the irreversibility of a vegetative state is not always possible. To our knowledge, after cardiac arrest and no purposeful response to stimuli for 1 to 2 weeks (in the absence of hypotension, hypothermia, CNS depressants, or relaxants), complete cerebral recovery has not been reported. Certain clinical and laboratory measurements on day 3 after cardiac arrest permit prognostication of PVS with near certainty in the majority (but not all) cases of postcardiac arrest coma.[2,147,154] In one recent study, incomplete recovery of somatosensory evoked potentials early after cardiac arrest correlated with poor cerebral outcome.[485] In another recent study, we were able to confirm various observations of the past, that fixed pupils or no purposeful response to painful stimuli on day 3 after cardiac arrest correlates with PVS, seemingly with 100 percent certainty.[147]

The correlation with severity of insult and with poor neurologic outcome of creatine-kinase BB and lactate dehydrogenase peaks in the CSF 2 to 3 days after arrest, in animals[169] and patients,[146,152] makes such tests potentially valuable adjuncts for decision making. CBF and metabolism correlations with outcome appear promising. In posttraumatic coma, reliable early prognostication is not possible, even with the aid of CSF analysis.

Conclusions and Recommendations

Since the National Conference on CPR and Emergency Cardiac Care in 1992,[1] CPCR research has yielded much new information of scientific importance and documentation of several promising new therapies, but no documentation yet of a maximally reproducibly effective CPCR protocol in patients. This is underscored by the single addition of hypertensive reperfusion in the 1992 guidelines.[1] Reasons for the lack of a cerebral resuscitation breakthrough so far include the multifactorial complexity of the cerebral postresuscitation syndrome, the unreliability until recently of most laboratory models, inadequate funding of reliable outcome models in high animal species, and the limitations of clinical trials.

For *clinicians,* I recommend:

1. A brain orientation of standard CPR BLS, ALS, and PLS (see Table 17-5)
2. For cases resistant to external CPR-ALS, clinical feasibility and ROSC trials of improved external CPR methods and of an early switch to open chest CPR or emergency CPB
3. Further clinical feasibility and side effect trials of therapy with available calcium entry blockers (also started during CPR)
4. Clinical feasibility and side effect trials of the physical combination treatment of CBF promotion and mild hypothermia, the most effective cerebral resuscitation protocol yet in dogs.[61]

For *researchers,* I recommend[486] that projects be carried out at multiple levels—molecular, cellular, organ systems, organisms (from rats via a high animal species to humans), and the community level. One or more research teams with experience in cardiac arrest outcome models in large animals in an animal ICU (see Table 17-1) should be securely funded for ongoing research. This would be more cost effective than jumping from rat studies to multicenter randomized clinical trials, which have so far yielded inconclusive outcome results.

Mechanism-oriented studies in low species or in vitro, although scientifically important, are only preliminary and adjunctive to the decisive outcome-oriented studies in whole organisms high on the phylogenetic scale. Some of the greatest breakthroughs in medicine, such as anesthesia, antibiotics, insulin, and cortisone, occurred without knowledge of the molecular mechanisms of these treatments.

Treatment potentials to be researched could be ranked for evaluation according to their scientific (theoretical, mechanism-oriented) importance, as well as clinical and socioeconomic (practical, patient outcome-oriented) importance and feasibility (likelihood of finding important results). A combination of these rankings might guide funding priorities.

The U.S. Food and Drug Administration must recognize the limitations of randomized clinical trials and rat studies and the importance of CPCR research with large animal outcome models. Clinical resuscitation research is only possible with waiving of prospective consent for entering patients.[141,142,487] This proved feasible and acceptable and must be legalized, provided the incremental (relative) risk is low and the study is approved by an institutional peer review board. Trials should include assessment of acceptance by prehospital and in-hospital providers. Cases of coma without pulselessness should also be evaluated.

The multifactorial pathogenesis of the postresuscitation syndrome also calls for more than one agent, namely, the need to evaluate combination treatments. The transfer to patients of novel CPCR methods found effective in large animal outcome models should begin in community EMS systems that incorporate ongoing evaluations of CPR cases. Clinical feasibility and side effects trials are needed in patients with sick hearts.

I recommend something potentially controversial. Novel treatments that are simple and inexpensive and that significantly improved overall and cerebral outcome (without undesirable side effects) in two or three reliable reproducible large animal outcome studies should have safety and feasibility tested in clinical trials (Table 17-1). If found safe and economically feasible in sick people, such treatments should be approved for general clinical use without insisting on statistical documentation of "benefit" in expensive, time-consuming randomized clinical outcome trials. The latter cannot discriminate between the ability of a treatment to mitigate brain damage in selected cases and the absence of any treatment effect. For novel expensive treatments with risks, there is still no substitute for a randomized clinical trial to document a (breakthrough) benefit. The ability to reveal benefit in some cases should be increased by excluding a priori hopeless cases and immediately reversible arrests and including only skilled, specially trained resuscitating teams. Continuance of clinical trial mechanisms as "case registries" is also valuable for the ongoing community-wide evaluation of CPCR delivery.

A comprehensive approach should be directed toward achieving *consistent* reversibility after a 10-min period of normothermic no-flow in patients. This requires one or more goal-oriented, systematic, multidisciplinary, international, multicenter programs, securely funded by a society that recognizes the challenges and potentials summarized in this review, and considers saving "hearts (C. Beck) and brains (P. Safar) too good to die" as a challenge as great as that which impelled the Manhattan project.

The goal of cerebral resuscitation research is to help an increasing proportion of people stricken with an unexpected terminal state or clinical death to complete full lives with healthy minds, to restore *"mens sana* in *corpore sano"* (Decimus Iunius Juvenalis, Roman poet and satirist, about A.D. 100).

Acknowledgments

I am grateful for valuable input from Drs. N. Abramson, R. Basford, N. Bircher, C. Brown, R. Cummins, R. Eisenberg, S. Eleff, L. Ernster, M. Ginsberg, K.-A. Hossmann, P. Kochanek, N. Paradis, J. W. Severinghaus, M. L. Smith (for B. Siesjo), and R. Traystman. I also thank Francie Siegfried for editoral assistance and Fran Mistrick for help in preparing the manuscript.

References

1. American Heart Association: Guidelines for cardiopulmonary resuscitation and emergency cardiac care. *JAMA* 1992; 268:2171.

2. Safar P, Bircher N: *Cardiopulmonary Cerebral Resuscitation: Guidelines by the World Federation of Societies of Anesthesiologists (WFSA)*, 3d ed. Philadelphia, W. B. Saunders, 1988.

3. American Society of Anesthesiologists, Committee on Acute Medicine: Community-wide emergency medical services. *JAMA* 1968; 204:595.

4. Eisenberg MS, et al: Cardiac arrest and resuscitation: A tale of 29 cities. *Ann Emerg Med* 1990; 19:179.

5. Brain Resuscitation Clinical Trial I Study Group, Abramson NS, et al: Randomized clinical study of thiopental loading in comatose survivors of cardiac arrest. *N Engl J Med* 1986; 314:397.

6. Brain Resuscitation Clinical Trial II Study Group, Abramson NS, et al: A randomized clinical study of a calcium-entry blocker (lidoflazine) in the treatment of comatose survivors of cardiac arrest. *N Engl J Med* 1991; 324:1225.

7. Brain Resuscitation Clinical Trial III Study Group, Abramson NS, et al: A randomized clinical trial of high dose epinephrine during cardiac arrest. *Crit Care Med* 1995; 23:A178 (abstr).

8. Longstreth WT, et al: Neurologic recovery after out of hospital cardiac arrest. *Ann Intern Med* 1983; 98:588.

9. Levy DE, et al: Predicting outcome from hypoxic-ischemic coma. *JAMA* 1985; 253:1420.

10. Cummins RO, et al: Improving survival from sudden cardiac arrest: The "chain of survival" concept. *Circulation* 1991; 83:1832.

11. Cummins R, et al: Recommended guidelines for uniform reporting of data from out-of-hospital cardiac arrest: The Utstein style. *Circulation* 1991; 84:960.

12. Safar P (Chairman): International Symposium (1962) on Resuscitation: Controversial aspects. *Anesthesiology and Resuscitation Monograph Series,* vol 1. Heidelberg, Springer-Verlag, 1963.

13. Safar P, et al: Upper airway obstruction in the unconscious patient. *J Appl Physiol* 1959; 14:760.

14. Elam JO, et al: Artificial respiration by mouth-to-mask method. A study of the respiratory gas exchange of paralyzed patients ventilated by operator's expired air. *N Engl J Med* 1954; 250:749.

15. Safar P, et al: A comparison of the mouth-to-mouth and mouth-to-airway methods of artificial respiration with the chest-pressure arm-lift methods. *N Engl J Med* 1958; 258:671.

16. Gordon AS, et al: Mouth-to-mouth versus manual artificial respiration for children and adults. *JAMA* 1958; 167:320.

17. Kouwenhoven WB, et al: Closed-chest cardiac massage. *JAMA* 1960; 173:1064.

18. Harris LC, et al: Ventilation-cardiac compression rates and ratios in cardiopulmonary resuscitation. *Anesthesiology* 1967; 28:806.

19. Safar P, et al: Ventilation and circulation with closed chest cardiac massage in man. *JAMA* 1961; 176:574.

20. Beck CS, et al: Ventricular fibrillation of long duration abolished by electric shock. *JAMA* 1947; 135:985.

21. Zoll PM, et al: Termination of ventricular fibrillation in man by externally applied electric countershock. *N Engl J Med* 1956; 254:727.

22. Holmdahl MH: Respiratory care unit. *Anesthesiology* 1962; 23:559.

23. Safar P, et al: Intensive care unit. *Anaesthesia* 1961; 16:275.

24. Society of Critical Care Medicine (SCCM) (USA): Guidelines for organization of critical care units. *JAMA* 1972; 222:1532.

25. Wilder RJ, et al: Cardiopulmonary resuscitation by trained ambulance personnel. *JAMA* 1964; 190:531.

26. Stept WJ, Safar P: Cardiac resuscitation following two hours of cardiac massage and 42 countershocks. *Anesthesiology* 1966; 27:97.

27. Angelos M, et al: External cardiopulmonary resuscitation preserves brain viability after prolonged cardiac arrest in dogs. *Am J Emerg Med* 1991; 9:436.

28. Cole SL, Corday E: Four-minute limit for cardiac resuscitation. *JAMA* 1956; 161:1454.

29. Siesjo BK: Mechanisms of ischemic brain damage. *Crit Care Med* 1988; 16:954.

30. Radovsky A, et al: Regional prevalence and distribution of ischemic neurons in dogs' brains 96 hours after cardiac arrest of 0-20 minutes. *Stroke* 1995; 26:2127.

31. Plum F (ed): The clinical problem: How much anoxia-ischemia damages the brain? Symposium on Brain Ischemia. *Arch Neurol* 1973; 29:259.

32. Negovsky VA: Postresuscitation disease. *Crit Care Med* 1988; 16:942.

33. Safar P (ed): Brain resuscitation. Special Symposium Issue. *Crit Care Med* 1978; 6:199.

34. Safar P, et al (eds): International resuscitation research symposium on the reversibility of clinical death. *Crit Care Med* 1988; 16:919.

35. Safar P, et al (eds): Future Directions for Resuscitation Research. *Crit Care Med* 1996; 24:52 (suppl).

36. Safar P, Bircher N: The pathophysiology of dying and reanimation. In Schwartz GR, et al (eds): *Principles and Practice of Emergency Medicine*, 3d ed, vol 1. Philadelphia, Lea & Febiger, 1992:3–41.

37. Safar P: Cerebral resuscitation after cardiac arrest: A review. *Circulation* 1986; 74(suppl IV):IV–138.

38. Safar P: The prevention and therapy of postresuscitation neurologic dysfunction and injury. In Paradis N (ed): *Cardiac Arrest*. Baltimore, Williams & Wilkins, 1996: chap. 49.

39. Safar P: Asphyxial sudden death. In Paradis N (ed): *Cardiac Arrest*. Baltimore, Williams & Wilkins, 1996, chap 39.

40. Hossmann K-A, Sato K: Recovery of neuronal function after prolonged cerebral ischemia. *Science* 1970; 168:375.

41. Hossmann KA, et al: The role of cerebral blood flow for the recovery of the brain after prolonged ischemia. *Z Neurol* 1973; 204:281.

42. Hossmann K-A, et al: Recovery of integrative central nervous function after one hour global cerebro-circulatory arrest in normothermic cat. *J Neurol Sci* 1987; 77:305.

43. Hossmann KA: Resuscitation potentials after prolonged global cerebral ischemia in cats. *Crit Care Med* 1988; 16:964.

44. Ames A III, Nesbett FB: Pathophysiology of ischemic cell death. I. Time of onset of irreversible damage; importance of the different components of the ischemic insult. *Stroke* 1983; 14:219.

45. Jennings RB et al: Complete global myocardial ischemia in dogs. *Crit Care Med* 1988; 16:988.

46. Safar P: Resuscitation from clinical death: Pathophysiologic limits and therapeutic potentials. *Crit Care Med* 1988; 16:923.

47. Cerchiari EL, et al: Cardiovascular function and neurologic outcome after cardiac arrest in dogs. The cardiovascular postresuscitation syndrome. *Resuscitation* 1993; 25:9.

48. White BC, et al: Brain nuclear DNA survives cardiac arrest and reperfusion. *Free Radical Biol Med* 1991; 10:125.

49. Safar P, et al: Amelioration of brain damage after 12 minutes cardiac arrest in dogs. *Arch Neurol* 1976; 33:91.

50. Sterz F, et al: Hypertension with or without hemodilution after cardiac arrest in dogs. *Stroke* 1990; 21:1178.

51. Bleyaert AL, et al: Thiopental amelioration of brain damage after global ischemia in monkeys. *Anesthesiology* 1978; 49:390.

52. Gisvold SE, et al: Thiopental treatment after global brain ischemia in pigtail monkeys. *Anesthesiology* 1984; 60:88.

53. Gisvold SE, et al: Multifaceted therapy after global brain ischemia in monkeys. *Stroke* 1984; 15:803.

54. Vaagenes P, et al: Amelioration of brain damage by lidoflazine after prolonged ventricular fibrillation cardiac arrest in dogs. *Crit Care Med* 1984; 12:846.

55. Steen PA, et al: Nimodipine improves outcome when given after complete cerebral ischemia in primates. *Anesthesiology* 1985; 62:406.

56. Leonov Y, et al: Moderate hypothermia after cardiac arrest of 17 minutes in dogs. Effect on cerebral and cardiac outcome. A preliminary study. *Stroke* 1990; 21:1600.

57. Leonov Y, et al: Mild cerebral hypothermia during and after cardiac arrest improves neurologic outcome in dogs. *J Cereb Blood Flow Metab* 1990; 10:57.

58. Sterz F, et al: Mild hypothermic cardiopulmonary resuscitation improves outcome after prolonged cardiac arrest in dogs. *Crit Care Med* 1991; 19:379.

59. Weinrauch V, et al: Beneficial effect of mild hypothermia and detrimental effect of deep hypothermia after cardiac arrest in dogs. *Stroke* 1992; 23:1454.

60. Kuboyama K, et al: Delay in cooling negates beneficial effect of mild resuscitative hypothermia after cardiac arrest in dogs. *Crit Care Med* 1993; 21:1348.

61. Safar P, et al: Improved cerebral resuscitation from cardiac arrest in dogs with mild hypothermia plus blood flow promotion. *Stroke* 1996; 27:105.

62. Safar P: History of cardiopulmonary-cerebral resuscitation. In Kaye W, Bircher N (eds): *Cardiopulmonary Resuscitation*. New York, Churchill Livinstone, 1989:1–53.

63. Safar P: Long-term animal outcome models for cardiopulmonary-cerebral resuscitation research. *Crit Care Med* 1985; 13:936.

64. Safar P, et al: Long-term animal models for the study of global brain ischemia. In Wauquier A, et al (eds): *Protection of Tissues Against Hypoxia*. Amsterdam, Elsevier, 1982:147–170.

65. Safar P, et al: Systematic development of cerebral resuscitation after cardiac arrest. Three promising treatments: Cardiopulmonary bypass, hypertensive hemodilution and mild hypothermia. In Balthman A (ed): *Causes and Mechanisms of Secondary Brain Damage. Acta Neurochir* 1993; 57:110.

66. Lind B, et al: Total brain ischemia in dogs. Cerebral physiologic and metabolic changes after 15 minutes of circulatory arrest. *Resuscitation* 1975; 4:97.

67. Snyder JV, et al: Global ischemia in dogs: Intracranial pressures, brain blood flow and metabolism. *Stroke* 1975; 6:21.

68. Nemoto EM, et al: Global brain ischemia: A reproducible monkey model. *Stroke* 1977; 8:558.

69. Bigelow WG, et al: Hypothermia: Its possible role in cardiac surgery. *Ann Surg* 1950; 132:849.

70. Dripps RD, (ed): *The Physiology of Induced Hypothermia*. Washington, DC, National Academy of Sciences, 1956.

71. Rosomoff HL, Holaday BA: Cerebral blood flow and cerebral oxygen consumption during hypothermia. *Am J Physiol* 1954; 179:85.

72. Rosomoff HL: Hypothermia and cerebral vascular lesions. I. Experimental interruption of the middle cerebral artery during hypothermia. *J Neurosurg* 1956; 13:244.

73. Rosomoff HL: Hypothermia and cerebral vascular lesions. II. Experimental middle cerebral artery interruption followed by induction of hypothermia. *Arch Neurol Psychiatry* 1957;78:454.

74. Rosomoff HL: Protective effects of hypothermia against pathological processes of the nervous system. *Ann N Y Acad Sci* 1959; 80:475.

75. Rosomoff HL, et al: Experimental brain injury and delayed hypothermia. *Surg Gynecol Obstet* 1960; 110:27.

76. Rosomoff HL, Safar P: Management of the comatose patient. In Safar P, (ed): *Respiratory Therapy*. Philadelphia, FA Davis, 1965:244–258.

77. Wolfe KB: Effect of hypothermia on cerebral damage resulting from cardiac arrest. *Am J Cardiol* 1960; 6:809.

78. Zimmerman JM, Spencer FC: The influence of hypothermia on cerebral injury resulting from circulatory occlusion. *Surg Forum* 1959; 10:216.

79. Benson DW, et al: The use of hypothermia after cardiac arrest. *Anesth Analg* 1958; 38:423.

80. Ravitch MM, et al: Lighting stroke. Recovery following cardiac massage and prolonged artificial respiration. *N Engl J Med* 1961; 264:36.

81. White RJ: Hypothermic preservation and transplantation of brain. *Resuscitation* 1975; 4:197.

82. Albin MS, et al: Spinal cord hypothermia by localized perfusion cooling. *Nature* 1966; 210:1059.

83. Stephenson HE Jr, et al: Some common denominators in 1200 cases of cardiac arrest. *Ann Surg* 1953; 137:731.

84. Redding J, Cozine R: A comparison of open-chest and closed-chest cardiac massage in dogs. *Anesthesiology* 1961; 22:280.

85. Del Guercio LRM, et al: A comparison of blood flow during external and internal cardiac massage in man. *Circulation* 1965; 31(suppl 1):1171.

86. Bircher N, Safar P: Manual open-chest cardiopulmonary resuscitation. *Ann Emerg Med* 1984; 13:770.

87. Bircher NG, Safar P: Cerebral preservation during cardiopulmonary resuscitation in dogs. *Crit Care Med* 1985; 13:185.

88. MacKenzie GJ, et al: Hemodynamic effects of external cardiac compression. *Lancet* 1964; i:1342.

89. Byrne D, et al: External vs. internal cardiac massage in normal and chronically ischemic dogs. *Am Surg* 1980; 46:657.

90. Arai T, et al: Cerebral blood flow during conventional, new and open chest CPR in dogs. *Resuscitation* 1984; 12:147.

91. Geehr EC, et al: Failure of open-heart massage to improve survival after prehospital nontraumatic cardiac arrest. *N Engl J Med* 1986; 314:1189 (letter).

92. Mullie A, et al: Open chest cardiopulmonary resuscitation in the prehospital environment. Proceedings 9th World Congress of Anaesthesiologists, May 1988. Washington, DC, vol I:A0317 (abstr).

93. Anstadt MP, et al: Direct mechanical ventricular actuation for cardiac arrest in humans: clinical feasibility trial. *Chest* 1991; 100:86.

94. Buckman RF, et al: Direct cardiac massage without major thoracotomy: Feasibility and systemic blood flow. *Resuscitation* 1995; 29:237.

95. Redding J, Pearson JW: Resuscitation from ventricular fibrillation. *JAMA* 1968; 203:255.

96. Redding JS, Pearson JW: Resuscitation from asphyxia. *JAMA* 1962; 182:283.

97. Bozhiev AA, et al: Peculiar features of resuscitation with the use of extracorporeal circulation. *Kardiologiia* 1976; 14:101 (in Russian).

98. Mattox KL, Beall AC: Resuscitation of the moribund patient using portable cardiopulmonary bypass. *Ann Thorac Surg* 1976; 22:436.

99. Tisherman S, et al: Resuscitation of dogs from cold-water submersion using cardiopulmonary bypass. *Ann Emerg Med* 1985; 14:389.

100. Pretto E, et al: Cardiopulmonary bypass after prolonged cardiac arrest in dogs. *Ann Emerg Med* 1987; 16:611.

101. Levine R, et al: Improved outcome after cardiac arrest in dogs using emergency cardiopulmonary bypass. *Am J Emerg Med* 1986; 4:419.

102. Angelos M, et al: A comparison of cardiopulmonary resuscitation with cardiopulmonary bypass after prolonged cardiac arrest in dogs: Reperfusion pressures and neurologic recovery. *Resuscitation* 1991; 21:121.

103. Safar P, et al: Emergency cardiopulmonary bypass for resuscitation from prolonged cardiac arrest. *Am J Emerg Med* 1990; 8:55.

104. Martin G, et al: Cardiopulmonary bypass vs CPR as treatment for prolonged canine cardiopulmonary arrest. *Ann Emerg Med* 1987; 16:628.

105. Tisherman SA, et al: Cardiopulmonary-cerebral resuscitation: Advanced and prolonged life support with emergency cardiopulmonary bypass. *Acta Anaesth Scand* 1990; 94:63.

106. Tisherman S, et al: Clinical feasibility of emergency cardiopulmonary bypass for external CPR-refractory prehospital cardiac arrest. *Resuscitation* 1994; 28:S5 (abstr 071).

107. Klain M, et al: Portable cardiopulmonary bypass system for resuscitation. In *Cardiovascular Science & Technology: Basic & Applied, I. Proceedings*. Louisville, Oxymoron Press, 1989: 318–320.

108. Sassano J, et al: Hyperthermic cardiac arrest in monkeys. *Crit Care Med* 1981; 9:409.

109. Eshel GM, et al: Evaporative cooling as an adjunct to ice bag use after resuscitation from heat-induced arrest in a primate model. *Pediatr Res* 1990; 27:264.

110. Steinman AM: Cardiopulmonary resuscitation and hypothermia. *Circulation* 1986; 74(suppl IV):IV29.

111. Redding J, et al: Resuscitation from drowning. *JAMA* 1961; 178:1136.

112. Ginsberg MD: Models of cerebral ischemia in the rodent. In Schurr A, Rigor BM (eds): *Cerebral Ischemia and Resuscitation*. Boca Raton, Fla, CRC Press, 1990:1–25.

113. Lind B, et al: A review of total brain ischaemia models in dogs and original experiments on clamping the aorta. *Resuscitation* 1975; 4:19.

114. Cerchiari EL, et al: Protective effects of combined superoxide dismutase and deferoxamine on recovery of cerebral blood flow and function after cardiac arrest in dogs. *Stroke* 1987; 18:869.

115. Cerchiari EL, et al: Effects of combined superoxide dismutase and deferoxamine on recovery of brain stem auditory evoked potentials and EEG after asphyxial cardiac arrest in dogs. *Resuscitation* 1990; 19:25.

116. Lanier WL, et al: Post-ischemic neurologic recovery and cerebral blood flow using a compression model of complete "bloodless" cerebral ischemia in dogs. *Resuscitation* 1988; 16:271.

117. Michenfelder JD, Milde JH: Postischemic canine cerebral blood flow appears to be determined by cerebral metabolic needs. *J Cereb Blood Flow Metab* 1990;10:71.

118. Sieber FE, et al: Global incomplete cerebral ischemia produces predominantly cortical neuronal injury. *Stroke* 1995; 26:2091.

119. Blomqvist P, Wieloch T: Ischemic brain damage in rats following cardiac arrest using a long-term recovery model. *J Cereb Blood Flow Metab* 1985; 5:420.

120. Brown CG, et al: Comparative effect of graded doses of epinephrine on regional brain blood flow during CPR in a swine model. *Ann Emerg Med* 1986; 15:1138.

121. Brown CG, et al: The effect of norepinephrine versus epinephrine on regional cerebral blood flow during cardiopulmonary resuscitation. *Am J Emerg Med* 1989; 7:278.

122. Lindner KH, et al: Effects of epinephrine and norepinephrine on cerebral oxygen delivery and consumption during open-chest CPR. *Ann Emerg Med* 1990; 19:249.

123. Schindler I, et al: Effects of nimodipine administration during cardiopulmonary resuscitation in pigs. *Eur J Anesth* 1992; 9:411.

124. Safar P, et al: Reproducible cardiac arrest-intensive care outcome models in dogs for comparing insults and cerebral resuscitation potentials. Resuscitation 1994; 28:S20 (abstr).

125. Todd MM, et al: Ventricular fibrillation in the cat: A model for global cerebral ischemia. *Stroke* 1981; 12:808.

126. Farias LA, et al: Prevention of ischemic-hypoxic brain injury and death in rabbits with fructose-1,6-diphosphate. *Stroke* 1990; 21:606.

127. Pluta R: Resuscitation of the rabbit brain after acute complete ischemia lasting up to one hour: Pathophysiological and pathomorphological observations. *Resuscitation* 1987; 15:267.

128. Lee SK, et al: Effect of cardiac arrest time on the cortical cerebral blood flow during subsequent standard external cardiopulmonary resuscitation in rabbits. *Resuscitation* 1989; 17:105.

129. Pulsinelli W, et al: Temporal profile of neuronal damage in a model of transient forebrain ischemia. *Ann Neurol* 1982; 11:491.

130. Smith ML, et al: Models for studying long-term recovery following forebrain ischemia in the rat. A two vessel occlusion model. *Acta Neurol Scand* 1984; 69:385.

131. Hendrickx H, et al: Asphyxia, cardiac arrest and resuscitation in rats. I. Short-term recovery. *Resuscitation* 1984; 12:97.

132. Hendrickx HHL, Safar P, Miller A: Asphyxia, cardiac arrest and resuscitation in rats. II. Long-term behavioral changes. *Resuscitation* 1984;12:117.

133. Katz L, et al: Outcome model of asphyxial cardiac arrest in rats. *J Cereb Blood Flow Metab* 1995; 15:1032.

134. Neumar RW, et al: Epinephrine and sodium bicarbonate during CPR following asphyxial cardiac arrest in rats. *Resuscitation* 1994; 29:249.

135. Krnjevic K, Lebond J: Anoxia reversibility suppresses neuronal Ca currents in rat hippocampal slices. *Can J Physiol Pharmacol* 1987; 65:2157.

136. Choi DW: Limitations of in vitro models of ischemia. In Meldrum BS (ed): *Current and Future Trends in Anticonvulsants, Anxiety and Stroke Therapy.* New York, Wiley-Liss, 1990: 291–299.

137. Brain Resuscitation Clinical Trial I Study Group, Kelsey SK, et al: Randomized clinical study of cardiopulmonary resuscitation: Design, methods and patient characteristics. *Am J Emerg Med* 1986; 4:72.

138. Brain Resuscitation Clinical Trial II Study Group, Kelsey SF, et al: A randomized clinical trial of calcium entry blocker administration to comatose survivors of cardiac arrest. Design, methods, and patient characteristics. *Control Clin Trials* 1991; 12:525.

139. Abramson NS, et al: Simpson's paradox and clinical trials: What you find is not necessarily what you prove. *Ann Emerg Med* 1992; 21:1480.

140. Abramson NS: Clinical trials of brain resuscitation after cardiac arrest. A review. *Acta Anaesth Scand* 1991; 96:54.

141. Abramson NS, et al: Deferred consent: Use in clinical resuscitation research. *Ann Emerg Med* 1990;19:781.

142. Abramson NS, et al: Deferred consent. A new approach for resuscitation research on comatose patients. *JAMA* 1986; 255:2466.

143. Teasdale G, Jennett B: Assessment of coma and impaired consciousness. A practical scale. *Lancet* 1974; 2:81.

144. Jennett B, Bond M: Assessment of outcome after severe brain damage: A practical scale. *Lancet* 1975; 1:480.

145. Breivik H, et al: Clinical feasibility trials of barbiturate therapy after cardiac arrest. *Crit Care Med* 1978; 6:228.

146. Edgren E, et al: Cerebral spinal fluid markers in relation to outcome in patients with global cerebral ischemia. *Crit Care Med* 1983; 11:4.

147. Edgren E, et al: Assessment of neurological prognosis in comatose survivors of cardiac arrest. *Lancet* 1994; 343:1055.

148. Jastremski M, et al: Glucocorticoid treatment does not improve neurological recovery following cardiac arrest. *JAMA* 1989; 262:3427.

149. Mullie A, et al: Monitoring of cerebro-spinal fluid enzyme levels in postischemic encephalopathy after cardiac arrest. *Crit Care Med* 1981; 9:399.

150. Rogove HJ, et al: Old age does not negate good cerebral outcome after cardiopulmonary resuscitation: Analyses from the brain resuscitation clinical trials. *Crit Care Med* 1995; 23:18.

151. Safar P: Future aspects of cardiopulmonary-cerebral resuscitation. Including hypothermia and cardiopulmonary bypass. *Acta Anaesth Scand* 1991; 96:18.

152. Vaagenes P, et al: The use of cytosolic enzyme increase in cerebrospinal fluid of patients resuscitated after cardiac arrest. *Am J Emerg Med* 1994; 12:21.

153. Brown CG, et al: A comparison of standard-dose and high-dose epinephrine in cardiac arrest outside the hospital. *N Engl J Med* 1992; 327:1051.

154. Mullie A, et al: Predictive value of Glasgow coma score for awakening after out-of-hospital cardiac arrest. *Lancet* 1988; i:137.

155. Roine RO, et al: Nimodipine after resuscitation from out-of-hospital ventricular fibrillation: A placebo-controlled, double-blind randomized trial. *JAMA* 1990; 264:3171.

156. Yusuf S, et al: Analysis and interpretation of treatment effects in subgroups of patients in randomized clinical trials. Special Communication. *JAMA* 1991; 266:93.

157. Kovach AGB, Sandor P: Cerebral blood flow and brain function during hypotension and shock. *Ann Rev Physiol* 1976; 38:571.

158. Bar-Joseph G, et al: Monkey model of severe volume-controlled hemorrhagic shock with resuscitation to outcome. *Resuscitation* 1991; 22:27.

159. Symon L: Flow thresholds in brain ischemia and the effects of drugs. *Br J Anaesth* 1985; 57:34.

160. Robertson CS, et al: Cerebral arterial venous oxygen difference as an estimate of cerebral blood flow in comatose patients. *J Neurosurg* 1989; 70:222.

161. Thews G: Implications to physiology and pathology of oxygen diffusion at the capillary level. In Schade JP, McMenemey WH (eds): *Selective Vulnerability of the Brain in Hypoxemia.* Philadelphia, FA Davis, 1963:27–35.

162. Steen PA, Michenfelder JD, Milde JH: Incomplete versus complete cerebral ischemia: Improved outcome with a minimal blood flow. *Ann Neurol* 1979; 6:389.

163. Rehncrona S, et al: Recovery of brain mitochondrial function in the rat after complete and incomplete cerebral ischemia. *Stroke* 1979; 10:437.

164. Siesjo BK: Cell damage in the brain: A speculative synthesis. *J Cereb Blood Flow Metab* 1981; 1:155.

165. Rossen R, et al: Acute arrest of cerebral circulation in man. *Arch Neurol* 1943; 50:510.

166. Kramer RS, et al: The effect of profound hypothermia on preservation of cerebral ATP content during circulatory arrest. *J Thorac Cardiovasc Surg* 1968; 56:599.

167. Michenfelder JK, Theye RA: The effects of anesthesia and hypothermia on canine cerebral ATP and lactate during anoxia produced by decapitation. *Anesthesiology* 1970; 33:430.

168. Astrup J, et al: The increase in extracellular potassium concentration in the ischemic brain in relation to the preischemic functional activity and cerebral metabolic rate. *Brain Res* 1980; 199:61.

169. Vaagenes P, et al: Brain enzyme levels in CSF after cardiac

arrest and resuscitation in dogs: Markers of damage and predictors of outcome. *J Cereb Blood Flow Metab* 1988; 8:262.

170. Vaagenes P, et al: Differences in the effects of CNS treatments after ventricular fibrillation (VF) vs. asphyxiation (A) cardiac arrest (CA) in dog models. *Crit Care Med* 1988; 16:447 (abstr).

171. Miller RJ: Multiple calcium channels and neuronal function. *Science* 1987; 235:46.

172. Schanne FAX, et al: Calcium dependence of toxic cell death: A final common pathway. *Science* 1979; 206:700.

173. Rehncrona S, et al: Excessive cellular acidosis: An important mechanism of neuronal damage in the brain? *Acta Physiol Scand* 1980; 110:425.

174. Nemoto EM, et al: Free fatty acid liberation in the pathogenesis and therapy of ischemic brain damage. In Bazan NG, et al (eds): *Advances in Neurochemistry, Neurochemistry Correlates of Cerebral Ischemia,* vol 7. New York, Plenum Press, 1992:183–218.

175. Bandaranayke NM, et al: Rat brain osmolality during barbiturate anesthesia and global brain ischemia. *Stroke* 1978;9:249.

176. Benveniste H: The excitotoxin hypotheses in relation to cerebral ischemia. Cerebrovasc Brain Metab Rev 1991; 3:213.

177. Globus MYT, et al: Excitotoxic index—A biochemical marker of selective vulnerability. *Neurosci Lett* 1991; 127:39.

178. Rothman SM, Olney JW: Glutamate and the pathophysiology of hypoxic-ischemic brain damange. *Ann Neurol* 1986; 19:105 (review).

179. Ginsberg MD, et al: Deleterious effect of glucose pretreatment on recovery from diffuse cerebral ischemia in the cat. *Stroke* 1980; 11:347.

180. Frumin MJ, et al: Apneic oxygenation in man. *Anesthesiology* 1959; 20:789.

181. Holmdahl MH: Pulmonary uptake of oxygen, acid-base metabolism, and circulation during prolonged apnea. *Acta Chir Scand (Suppl)* 1956; 212:1.

182. VanHarreveld A, Ochs S: Cerebral impedance changes after circulatory arrest. *Am J Physiol* 1957; 187:180.

183. Singh NC, et al: Uncoupled cerebral blood flow and metabolism after severe global brain ischemia in rats. *J Cereb Blood Flow Metab* 1992; 12:802.

184. Hallenbeck JM, et al: Prostaglandin I_2, indomethacin, and heparin promote postischemic neuronal recovery in dogs. *Ann Neurol* 1982; 12:145.

185. Kochanek PM, et al: Indomethacin, prostacyclin and heparin improve postischemic cerebral blood flow without affecting early postischemic granulocyte accumulation. *Stroke* 1987; 18:634.

186. Kochanek PM, Hallenbeck JM: Polymorphonuclear leukocytes and monocytes-macrophages in the pathogenesis of cerebral ischemia and stroke. A review. *Stroke* 1992; 23:1267.

187. Kochanek PM, et al: Severe traumatic brain injury in children: Pathobiology, management, and controversies. In: *Current Concepts in Critical Care.* Anaheim, CA: Society of Critical Care Medicine, 1995; 153–170.

188. Oku K, et al: Mild hypothermia after cardiac arrest in dogs does not affect postarrest multifocal cerebral hypoperfusion. *Stroke* 1993; 24:1590.

189. Dietrich WD, et al: Histopathological and hemodynamic consequence of complete vs. incomplete ischemia in the rat. *J Cereb Blood Flow Metab* 1987; 7:300.

190. Dietrich WD, et al: Interrelationships between increased vascular permeability and acute neuronal damage following temperature-controlled brain ischemia in rats. *Acta Neuropathol* 1991; 81:615.

191. Klatzo I: Brain edema following brain ischemia and the influence of therapy. *Br J Anaesth* 1985; 57:18.

192. Ames A III, et al: Cerebral ischemia. II. The no-reflow phenomenon. *Am J Pathol* 1968; 52:437.

193. Nemoto EM, et al: Regional brain P_{O_2} after global ischemia in monkeys: Evidence for regional differences in critical perfusion pressures. *Stroke* 1979; 10:44.

194. Sterz F, et al: Multifocal cerebral blood flow by Xe-CT and global cerebral metabolism after prolonged cardiac arrest in dogs: Reperfusion with open-chest CPR or cardiopulmonary bypass. *Resuscitation* 1992; 24:27.

195. Leonov Y, et al: Hypertension with hemodilution prevents multifocal cerebral hypoperfusion after cardiac arrest in dogs. *Stroke* 1992; 23:45.

196. Kofke WA, et al: Monkey brain blood flow and metabolism after global brain ischemia and post-insult thiopental therapy. *Stroke* 1979; 10:554.

197. Kagstroem E, et al: Local cerebral blood flow in the recovery period following complete cerebral ischemia in the rat. *J Cereb Blood Flow Metab* 1983; 3:170.

198. Oku K, et al: Cerebral and systemic arteriovenous oxygen monitoring after cardiac arrest. Inadequate cerebral oxygen delivery. *Resuscitation* 1994; 27:141.

199. Shalit MN, et al: The blood flow and oxygen consumption of the dying brain. *Neurology* 1970; 20:740.

200. Beckstead JE, et al: Cerebral blood flow and metabolism in man following cardiac arrest. *Stroke* 1978; 9:569.

201. Cohan SL, et al: Cerebral blood flow in humans following resuscitation from cardiac arrest. *Stroke* 1989; 20:761.

202. Obrist WD, et al: Relation of cerebral blood flow to neurological status and outcome in head-injured patients. *J Neurosurg* 1979; 51:292.

203. Obrist WD, et al: Cerebral blood flow and metabolism in comatose patients with acute head injury. *J Neurosurg* 1984; 61:241.

204. Obrist WD, et al: Time course of cerebral blood flow and metabolism in comatose patients with acute head injury. *J Cereb Blood Flow Metab* 1993; 13(suppl 1):S571 (abstr).

205. Darby JM, et al: Xenon-enhanced computed tomography in brain death. *Arch Neurol* 1987; 44:551.

206. Hossmann V, et al: Effect of intravascular platelet aggregation on blood recirculation following prolonged ischemia of the cat brain. *J Neurol* 1980; 222:159.

207. Babbs CF: Role of iron ions in the genesis of reperfusion injury following successful cardiopulmonary resuscitation: Preliminary data and biochemical hypothesis. *Ann Emerg Med* 1985; 14:777.

208. Bulkley GB: The role of oxygen free radicals in human disease processes. *Surgery* 1983; 94:407.

209. Ernster L: Biochemistry of reoxygenation injury. *Crit Care Med* 1988; 16:947.

210. Fridovich I: Superoxide radical: An endogenous toxicant. *Ann Rev Pharmacol Toxicol* 1983; 23:239.

211. Globus MYT, et al: Direct evidence for acute and massive norepinephrine release in the hippocampus during transient ischemia. *J Cereb Blood Flow Metab* 1989; 9:892.

212. McCord JM: Oxygen-derived free radicals in postischemic tissue injury. *N Engl J Med* 1985; 312:159.

213. Siesjo BK, Bengtsson F: Calcium fluxes, calcium antagonists, and calcium-related pathology in brain ischemia, hypoglycemia, and spreading depression: A unifying hypothesis. *J Cereb Blood Flow Metab* 1989; 9:127.

214. Traystman RJ, et al: Oxygen radical mechanisms of brain injury following ischemia and reperfusion. *J Appl Physiol* 1991; 71:1185.

215. Kontos HA: Oxygen radicals in CNS damage. Review article. *Chem Biol Interactions* 1989; 72:229.

216. White BC, et al: Brain injury by ischemic anoxia—hypothesis. A tale of two ions? *Ann Emerg Med* 1984; 13:862.

217. Deshpande JK, et al: Calcium accumulation and neuronal damage in the rat hippocampus following cerebral ischemia. *J Cereb Blood Flow Metab* 1987; 7:89.

218. Zar H, et al: Postischemic hepatic endothelial injury and lipid peroxidation (LP) are decreased by mild hypothermia (MHT). *Anesthesiology* 1984; 81:A851 (abstr).

219. MacManus JP, et al: Global ischemia can cause DNA fragmentation indicative of apoptosis in rat brain. *Neurosci Lett* 1993; 164:89.

220. Crumrine RC, et al: Attenuation of p53 expression protects against focal ischemic damage in transgenic mice. *J Cereb Blood Flow Metab* 1994; 14:887.

221. Nitatori T, et al: Delayed neuronal death in the CA 1 pyramidal cell layer of the gerbil hippocampus following transient ischemia is apoptosis. *J Neurosci* 1995; 15:1001.

222. Cerchiari EL, et al: Visceral hematologic and bacteriologic changes and neurologic outcome after cardiac arrest in dogs. The visceral post-resuscitation syndrome. *Resuscitation* 1993; 25:119.

223. Sterz F, et al: Detoxification with hemabsorption after cardiac arrest does not improve neurologic recovery. Review and outcome study in dogs. *Resuscitation* 1993; 25:137.

224. Baethmann A, et al: Mediators of brain edema and secondary brain damage. *Crit Care Med* 1988; 16:972.

225. Furchgott RF, Vanhoutte PM: Endothelium derived relaxing and contracting factors. *FASEB J* 1989; 3:2007.

226. Fink MP (ed): Nitric oxide. *New Horizons* 1994; 3:1.

227. Cummins RO, et al: Automatic external defibrillators used by emergency medical technicians: A controlled clinical trial. *Crit Care Med* 1985; 13:945.

228. Chandra N, et al: Simultaneous chest compression and ventilation at high airway pressure during cardiopulmonary resuscitation. *Lancet* 1980; 1:175.

229. Krischer JP, et al: Comparison of prehospital conventional and simultaneous compression-ventilation cardiopulmonary resuscitation. *Crit Care Med* 1989; 17:1263.

230. Sack JB, et al: Survival from in-hospital cardiac arrest with interposed abdominal counter pulsation during CPR. *JAMA* 1992; 267:379.

231. Cohen TJ, et al: A comparison of active compression-decompression cardiopulmonary resuscitation with standard cardiopulmonary resuscitation for cardiac arrests occurring in the hospital. *N Engl J Med* 1993; 329:1918.

232. Halperin HR, et al: Vest inflation without simultaneous ventilation during cardiac arrest in dogs. Improved survival from prolonged CPR. *Circulation* 1986; 74:1407.

233. Redding JS: Abdominal compression in CPR. *Anesth Analg* 1971; 50:668.

234. Bircher N, Safar P: Comparison of standard and "new" closed-chest CPR and open-chest CPR in dogs. *Crit Care Med* 1981; 9:384.

235. Barkalow CE: Mechanized cardiopulmonary resuscitation: Past, present, and future. *Am J Emerg Med* 1984; 2:262.

236. Wik L, et al: Survival after cardiac arrest with prolonged manual vs mechanical external cardiopulmonary resuscitation (CPR) in dogs. *Crit Care Med* 1993; 21:S191 (abstr).

237. Eleff SM, et al: Brain bioenergetics during cardiopulmonary resuscitation in dogs. *Anesthesiology* 1992; 76:77.

238. Eleff SM, et al: Sodium, ATP and intracellular pH transients during reversible complete ischemia of dog cerebrum. *Stroke* 1991; 22:233.

239. Redding JS: Drug therapy during cardiac arrest. In Safar P, Elam J (eds): *Advances in Cardiopulmonary Resuscitation*. New York, Springer-Verlag, 1977:87.

240. Ornato JP: Use of adrenergic agonists during CPR in adults. *Ann Emerg Med* 1993; 22:411 (review).

241. Otto CW: Cardiovascular pharmacology II: The use of catecholamines pressor agents, digitalis, and corticosteroids in CPR and emergency cardiac care. *Circulation* 1986; 74(suppl IV):80.

242. Paradis NA, Koscove EM: Epinephrine in cardiac arrest: A critical review. *Ann Emerg Med* 1990; 19:1288.

243. Schleien CL, et al: Effect of epinephrine on cerebral and myocardial perfusion in an infant animal preparation of cardiopulmonary resuscitation. *Circulation* 1986; 73:809.

244. Ebmeyer U, et al: Intra-aortic (IA) vs. intravenous (IV) epinephrine for cardiopulmonary resuscitation in rats. *Anesthesiology* 1992; 77:A291 (abstr).

245. Vukmir RB, et al: Sodium bicarbonate may improve outcome in dogs with brief or prolonged cardiac arrest. *Crit Care Med* 1995; 23:515.

246. Bircher NG: Sodium bicarbonate improves cardiac resuscitability, 24 hour survival and neurologic outcome after 10 minutes of cardiac arrest in dogs. *Anesthesiology* 1991; 75:A246 (abstr).

247. Bishop RL, Weisfeldt ML: Sodium bicarbonate administration during cardiac arrest. Effect on arterial pH, PCO_2, and osmolality. *JAMA* 1976; 235:506.

248. Weil MH, et al: Difference in acid-base state between venous and arterial blood during cardiopulmonary resuscitation. *N Engl J Med* 1986; 315:153.

249. Grundler W, et al: Arteriovenous carbon dioxide and pH gradients during cardiac arrest. *Circulation* 1986; 74:1071.

250. von Planta I, et al: Hypercarbic acidosis reduces cardiac resuscitability. *Crit Care Med* 1991; 19:1177.

251. von Planta M, et al: Pathophysiologic and therapeutic implications of acid-base changes during CPR. AHA CPR Conference 1992. *Ann Emerg Med* 1992; 22:404.

252. Berenyi KJ, et al: Cerebrospinal fluid acidosis complicating therapy of experimental cardiopulmonary arrest. *Circulation* 1975; 52:319.

253. Gotoh F, et al: Cerebral effects of hyperventilation in men. *Arch Neurol* 1975; 12:410.

254. Wiklund L, et al: Clinical buffering of metabolic acidosis: Problems and a solution. *Resuscitation* 1985; 12:279.

255. Sieber FE, Traystman RJ: Special issues, glucose and the brain. *Crit Care Med* 1991; 20:104.

256. D'Alecy LG, et al: Dextrose containing intravenous fluid impairs outcome and increases death after eight minutes of cardiac arrest and resuscitation in dogs. *Surgery* 1986; 100:505.

257. Lanier WL, et al: The effects of dextrose infusion and head position on neurologic outcome after complete cerebral ischemia in primates: Examination of a model. *Anesthesiology* 1987; 66:39.

258. Luncy EF, et al: Infusion of 5% dextrose increases mortality and morbidity following six minutes of cardiac arrest in resuscitated dogs. *J Crit Care* 1987; 2:4.

259. Ginsberg MD, et al: Hyperglycemia reduces the extent of cerebral infarction in rats. *Stroke* 1987; 18:570.

260. Schurr A, et al: Increased glucose improves recovery of neuronal function after cerebral hypoxia in vitro. *Brain Res* 1987; 421:135.

261. Katz LM, et al: Dextrose plus insulin after cardiac arrest (CA) improves cerebral outcome in rats. *Acad Emerg Med* 1995; 2:381 (abstr).

262. Longstreth WT Jr, Inui TS: High blood glucose level on hospital admission and poor neurological recovery after cardiac arrest. *Ann Neurol* 1984; 15:59.

263. Longstreth WT Jr, et al: Neurologic outcome and blood glucose levels during out-of-hospital cardiopulmonary resuscitation. *Neurology* 1986; 36:1186.

264. Pulsinelli WA et al: Increased damage after ischemic stroke

in patients with hyperglycemia with or without established diabetes mellitus. *Am J Med* 1983; 74:540

265. Rogers MC, et al: Effects of closed-chest cardiac massage on intracranial pressure. *Crit Care Med* 1979; 7:454.

266. Ditchey RV, et al: Relative lack of coronary blood flow during closed-chest resuscitation in dogs. *Circulation* 1982; 66:297.

267. Paradis N, et al: Intra-aortic epinephrine and perfusion pressures during ACLS and selective aortic perfusion and oxygenation. *Crit Care Med* 1994; 22:A224 (abstr).

268. Rubertsson S, et al: Influence of intra-aortic balloon occlusion on hemodynamics and survival after cardiopulmonary resuscitation in dogs. *Anesthesiology* 1995; 83:A254 (abstr).

269. Tang W, et al: Augmented efficacy of external CPR by intermittent occlusion of the ascending aorta. *Circulation* 1993; 88(part 1):1916.

270. Manning JE: Selective aortic arch perfusion during cardiac arrest. *Ann Emerg Med* 1992; 21:1058.

271. Griffith BP: Some futuristic possibilities for resuscitation. *Crit Care Med* 1988; 16:1007.

272. Eisenberg MS, et al: Thrombolytic therapy. *Ann Emerg Med* 1993; 22:417 (review).

273. Martin DR, et al: Relation between initial post-resuscitation systolic blood pressure and neurologic outcome following cardiac arrest. *Ann Emerg Med* 1993; 22:206 (abstr).

274. Spivey WH, et al: Correlation of blood pressure with mortality and neurologic recovery in comatose postresuscitation patients. *Ann Emerg Med* 1991; 20:453 (abstr).

275. Bleyaert AL, et al: Augmentation of post-ischemic brain damage by severe intermittent hypertension. *Crit Care Med* 1980; 8:41.

276. Lin SR, et al: The effect of combined dextran and streptokinase on cerebral function and blood flow after cardiac arrest: An experimental study on the dog. *Invest Radiol* 1978; 13:490.

277. Takaori M, Safar P: Treatment of massive hemorrhage with colloid and crystalloid solution. *JAMA* 1967; 199:297.

278. Iannotti F, Hoff J: Ischemic brain edema with and without reperfusion: An experimental study in gerbils. *Stroke* 1983; 14:562.

279. Ito U, et al: Transient appearance of "no-reflow" phenomenon in Mongolian gerbils. *Stroke* 1980; 11:517.

280. Van Reempts J, Borgers M: Ischemic brain injury and cell calcium: Morphologic and therapeutic aspects. *Ann Emerg Med* 1985; 14:736.

281. White BC, et al: Effect of flunarizine on canine cerebral cortical blood flow and vascular resistance post cardiac arrest. *Ann Emerg Med* 1982; 11:119.

282. Winegar CP, et al: Early amelioration of neurologic deficit by lidoflazine after fifteen minutes of cardiopulmonary arrest in dogs. *Ann Emerg Med* 1983; 12:471.

283. Fleischer JE, et al: Effect of lidoflazine on cerebral blood flow and neurologic outcome when administered after complete cerebral ischemia in dogs. *Anesthesiology* 1987; 66:304.

284. Fleischer JE, et al: Lidoflazine does not improve neurologic outcome when administered after complete cerebral ischemia in primates. *J Cereb Blood Flow Metab* 1987; 7:366.

285. Steen PA, et al: Nimodipine improves cerebral blood flow and neurologic recovery after complete cerebral ischemia in the dog. *J Cereb Blood Flow Metab* 1983; 3:38.

286. Steen PA, et al: Cerebral blood flow and neurologic outcome when nimodipine is given after complete cerebral ischemia in the dog. *J Cereb Blood Flow Metab* 1984; 4:82.

287. Tateishi A, et al: Nimodipine does not improve neurologic outcome after 14 minutes of cardiac arrest in cats. *Stroke* 1989; 20:1044.

288. Flameng W, et al: Cardioprotective effects of lidoflazine during 1-hour normothermic global ischemia. *Circulation* 1981; 64:796.

289. Flameng W, et al: Myocardial protection in open-heart surgery. In Waquier A, et al (eds): *Protection of Tissues against Hypoxia.* New York, Elsevier, 1982:403.

290. Forsman M, et al: Effects of nimodipine on cerebral blood flow and cerebrospinal fluid pressure after cardiac arrest: Correlation with neurologic outcome. *Anesth Analg* 1989; 68:436.

291. Gelmers HJ, et al: A controlled trial of nimodipine in acute ischemic stroke. *N Engl J Med* 1988; 318:203.

292. Allen GS, et al: Cerebral arterial spasm—A controlled trial of nimodipine in patients with subarachnoid hemorrhage. *N Engl J Med* 1983; 308:619.

293. Capparelli EV, et al: Diltiazem improves resuscitation from experimental ventricular fibrillation in dogs. *Crit Care Med* 1992; 20:1140.

294. Edmonds HL, et al: Improved short-term neurological recovery with flunarizine in a canine model of cardiac arrest. *Am J Emerg Med* 1985; 3:150.

295. Kumar K, et al: Effect of flunarizine on global brain ischemia in the dog: A quantitative morphologic assessment. *Exp Neurol* 1987; 97:115.

296. Newberg LA, et al: Failure of flunarizine to improve cerebral blood flow or neurologic recovery in a canine model of complete cerebral ischemia. *Stroke* 1984; 15:666.

297. Grotta JC, et al: Efficacy and mechanism of action of a calcium channel blocker after global cerebral ischemia in rats. *Stroke* 1988; 19:447.

298. Sakabe T, et al: Nicardipine increases cerebral blood flow but does not improve neurologic recovery in a canine model of complete cerebral ischemia. *J Cereb Blood Flow Metab* 1986; 6:684.

299. Lanza RP, et al: Lack of efficacy of high-dose verapamil in preventing brain damage in baboons and pigs after prolonged partial cerebral ischemia. *Am J Emerg Med* 1984; 2:481.

300. Schwartz AC: Neurological recovery after cardiac arrest: Clinical feasibility trial of calcium blockers. *Am J Emerg Med* 1985; 3:1.

301. Vaagenes P, et al: The effect of lidoflazine and verapamil on neurologic outcome after 10 minutes ventricular fibrillation cardiac arrest in dogs. *Crit Care Med* 1984; 12:228 (abstr).

302. Lindner KH, et al: Effects of diltiazem on oxygen delivery and consumption after asphyxial cardiac arrest and resuscitation. *Crit Car Med* 1992; 20:650.

303. Fleischer JE, et al: Effects of levemopamil on neurologic and histologic outcome after cardiac arrest in cats. *Crit Care Med* 1992; 29:126.

304. Valentino K, et al: A selective N-type calcium channel antagonist protects against neuronal loss after global cerebral ischemia. *Proc Natl Acad Sci USA* 1993; 90:7894.

305. Zhao Q, et al: The ω-conopeptide SNX-111, an N-type calcium channel blocker, dramatically ameliorates brain damage due to transient focal ischaemia. *Acta Physiol Scand* 1994; 150:459.

306. Buchan AM, et al: A selective N-type Ca^{2+}-channel blocker prevents CA1 injury 24 hours following severe forebrain ischemia and reduces infarction following focal ischemia. *J Cereb Blood Flow Metab* 1994; 14:903.

307. Sim K, et al: Systematic evaluation of promising new cerebral resuscitation drugs for use after cardiac arrest. *Resuscitation* 1994; 28:S36.

308. Xiao F, et al: Beneficial effects of neuron-specific calcium entry blocker SNX-111 on cerebral outcome after forebrain ischemia in rats, but not after ventricular fibrillation (VF) cardiac arrest (CA) in dogs. *Resuscitation* 1994; 28:S36.

309. Connolly JE, et al: Bloodless surgery by means of profound hypothermia and circulatory arrest. *Ann Surg* 1965; 162:274.

310. Tisherman SA, et al: Therapeutic deep hypothermic circulatory

arrest in dogs: A resuscitation modality for hemorrhagic shock with 'irreparable' injury. *J Trauma* 1990; 30:836.

311. Tisherman SA, et al: Profound hypothermia (<10°C) compared with deep hypothermia (15°C) improves neurologic outcome in dogs after two hours' circulatory arrest induced to enable resuscitative surgery. *J Trauma* 1991; 31:1051.

312. Tisherman SA, et al: Profound hypothermia does, and an organ preservation solution does not, improve neurologic outcome after therapeutic circulatory arrest of 2 h in dogs. *Crit Care Med* 1991; 19:S89.

313. Tisherman S, et al: Cardiopulmonary bypass without systemic anticoagulation for therapeutic hypothermic circulatory arrest during hemorrhagic shock in dogs. *Crit Care Med* 1992; 20:S41 (abstr).

314. Tisherman S, et al: Therapeutic hypothermic circulatory arrest to enable resuscitative surgery for uncontrollable hemorrhage in dogs ("suspended animation"). *Resuscitation* 1994; 28:S14 (abstr).

315. Capone A, et al: Complete recovery after normothermic hemorrhagic shock and profound hypothermic circulatory arrest of 60 minutes in dogs. *J Trauma* 1996; 40:388.

316. Siebke H, et al: Survival after 40 minutes submersion without cerebral sequelae. *Lancet* 1975; I:1275.

317. Conn AW, et al: Cerebral resuscitation in near-drowning. *Paediatr Clin North Am* 1979; 4:691.

318. Bolte RG, et al: The use of extracorporeal rewarming in a child submerged for 66 minutes. *Stroke* 1988; 260:377.

319. Alfonsi G, et al: Cold water drowning and resuscitation in dogs. *Anesthesiology* 1982; 57:A80 (abstr).

320. Frates RC Jr: Analysis of predictive factors in the assessment of warm-water near-drowning in children. *Am J Dis Child* 1981; 135:1006.

321. Quan L, et al: Ten-year study of pediatric drownings and near-drownings in King County, WA: Lessons in injury prevention. *Pediatrics* 1989; 83:1035.

322. Steen PA, et al: Detrimental effect of prolonged hypothermia in rats and monkeys with and without regional cerebral ischemia. *Stroke* 1979; 10:522.

323. Xiao F, et al: Mild protective and resuscitative cerebral hypothermia improves outcome after asphyxial cardiac arrest in rats. *Resuscitation* 1994; 28:S21 (abstr).

324. Busto R, et al: Postischemic moderate hypothermia inhibits CA1 hippocampal ischemic neuronal injury. *Neurosci Lett* 1989; 101:299.

325. Busto R, et al: Effect of mild hypothermia on ischemia-induced release of neurotransmitters and free fatty acids in rat brain. *Stroke* 1989; 20:904.

326. Boris-Moller F, et al: Effects of hypothermia on brain ischemia: A comparison of intraischemic and postischemic hypothermia *J Cereb Blood Flow Metab* 1989; 9:S276 (abstr).

327. Chopp M, et al: The metabolic effects of mild hypothermia on global cerebral ischemia and recirculation in the cat: Comparison to normothermia and hyperthermia. *J Cereb Blood Flow Metab* 1989; 9:141.

328. Chopp M, et al: Mild hypothermic intervention after graded ischemic stress in rats. *Stroke* 1991; 22:37.

329. Morikawa E, et al: The significance of brain temperature in focal cerebral ischemia: Histopathological consequences of middle cerebral artery occlusion in the rat. *J Cereb Blood Flow Metab* 1992; 12:380.

330. Clifton GL, et al: Marked protection by moderate hypothermia after experimental traumatic brain injury. *J Cereb Blood Flow Metab* 1991; 11:114.

331. Pomeranz S, et al: The effect of resuscitative moderate hypothermia following epidural brain compression on cerebral damage in a canine outcome model. *J Neurosurg* 1993; 79:241.

332. Ebmeyer U, et al: Moderate resuscitative hypothermia after brain trauma (simulated epidural hematoma) in a new intensive care outcome model in dogs. *Resuscitation* 1994; 28:S13 (abstr).

333. Crippen D, et al: Improved survival of hemorrhagic shock with oxygen and hypothermia in rats. *Resuscitation* 1991; 21:271.

334. Leonov Y, et al: Extending the golden hour of volume controlled hemorrhagic shock in awake rats with oxygen plus moderate hypothermia. *Acad Emerg Med* 1995; 2:401 (abstr).

335. Kim SH, et al: Hypothermic (Hth) minimal fluid resuscitation (FR) extends the golden hour of uncontrolled hemorrhagic shock (UHS) in new outcome model in rats. *Acad Emerg Med* 1995; 2:364 (abstr).

336. Stone HH, et al: The effect of lowered body temperature on the cerebral hemodynamics and metabolism of man. *Surg Gynecol Obstet* 1956; 103:313.

337. Kuboyama K, et al: Mild hypothermia after cardiac arrest in dogs does not affect postarrest cerebral oxygen uptake/delivery mismatching. *Resuscitation* 1994; 27:231.

338. Dempsey AJ, et al: Moderate hypothermia reduces postischemic edema development and leukotriene production. *Surgery* 1987; 21:177.

339. Baiping L, et al: Effect of moderate hypothermia on lipid peroxidation in canine brain tissue after cardiac arrest and resuscitation. *Stroke* 1994; 25:147.

340. Dietrich WD, et al: Intraischemic but not postischemic brain hypothermia protects chronically following global forebrain ischemia in rats. *J Cereb Blood Flow Metab* 1993; 13:541.

341. Colbourne F, Corbett D: Delayed and prolonged postischemic hypothermia is neuroprotective in the gerbil. *Brain Res* 1994; 654:265.

342. Colbourne F, Corbett D: Delayed postischemic hypothermia: A six-month survival study using behavioral and histological assessments of neuroprotection. *J Neurosci* 1995; 15:7250.

343. Sternau LL, et al: Ischemia-induced neurotransmitter release: Effects of mild intraischemic hyperthermia. In Globus MYT, Dietrich WD (eds): *Role of Neurotransmitters in Brain Injury.* New York, Plenum Press, 1992.

344. White RJ: Cerebral hypothermia and circulatory arrest. Review and commentary. *Mayo Clin Proc* 1978; 53:450.

345. Wolfson SK, et al: Preferential cerebral hypothermia for circulatory arrest. *Surgery* 1965; 57:846.

346. Xiao F, et al: Peritoneal cooling for mild cerebral hypothermia after cardiac arrest in dogs. *Resuscitation* 1995; 30:51.

347. Marion DW, et al: Resuscitative hypothermia. *Crit Care Med* 1996; 24:581.

348. Coimbra C, Wieloch T: Hypothermia ameliorates neuronal survival when induced 2 hours after ischaemia in the rat. *Acta Physiol Scand* 1992; 146:543.

349. Gelman B, et al: Selective brain cooling in infant piglets after cardiac arrest and resuscitation. *Crit Care Med* 1996; 24:1009.

350. Safar P, et al: Selective brain cooling after cardiac arrest. *Crit Care Med* 1996; 24:911.

351. Ebmeyer U, et al: Effective combination treatment for cerebral resuscitation from cardiac arrest in dogs. Exploratory studies. *Resuscitation* 1994; 28:S20 (abstr P57).

352. Xiao F, et al: Mild hypothermia plus cerebral blood flow promotion, but not drugs, give complete functional recovery after 11 minute cardiac arrest in dogs. *Crit Care Med* 1995; 23:A179 (abstr).

353. Koehler R, et al: Global neuronal ischemia and reperfusion. In Paradis NA, et al (eds): *Cardiac Arrest, The Pathophysiology and Therapy of Sudden Death.* Baltimore, Williams & Wilkins, 1996.

354. Michenfelder JD, et al: Cerebral protection by barbiturate anes-

thesia. Use after middle cerebral artery occlusion in Java monkeys. *Arch Neurol* 1976; 33:345.

355. Smith AL, et al: Barbiturate protection against cerebral infarction. *Stroke* 1974; 5:1.

356. Yatsu FM, et al: Experimental brain ischemia: Protection from irreversible damage with a rapid-acting barbiturate (methohexital). *Stroke* 1972; 3:726.

357. Safar P: Amelioration of postischemic brain damage with barbiturates. *Stroke* 1980; 11:565.

358. Shapiro HM: Intracranial hypertension. Therapeutic and anesthetic considerations. *Anesthesiology* 1975; 43:445.

359. Snyder BD, et al: Failure of thiopental to modify global anoxic injury. *Stroke* 1979; 10:135.

360. Steen PA, et al: No barbiturate protection in a dog model of complete cerebral ischemia. *Ann Neurol* 1979; 5:343.

361. Aldrete JA, et al: Effect of pretreatment with thiopental and phenytoin on postischemic brain damage in rabbits. *Crit Care Med* 1979; 7:466.

362. Cullen JP, et al: Protective action of phenytoin in cerebral ischemia. *Anesth Analg* 1979; 58:165.

363. Forsman M, et al: Superoxide dismutase and catalase failed to improve neurologic outcome after complete cerebral ischemia in the dog. *Acta Anaesth Scand* 1988; 32:152.

364. Reich H, et al: Failure of a multifaceted anti-reoxygenation injury (RI) therapy to ameliorate brain damage after ventricular fibrillation (VF) cardiac arrest (CA) of 20 minutes in dogs. *Crit Care Med* 1988; 16:387 (abstr).

365. White BC, et al: Effect on biochemical markers of brain injury of therapy with deferoxamine or superoxide dismutase following cardiac arrest. *Am J Emerg Med* 1988; 6:569.

366. Vaagenes P, et al: Outcome trials of free radical scavengers and calcium entry blockers after cardiac arrest in two dog models. *Ann Emerg Med* 1986; 15:665 (abstr).

367. Gill R, et al: Systemic administration of MK-801 protects against ischemia induced hippocampal neuro-degeneration in the gerbil. *J Neurosci* 1987; 7:3343.

368. Park C, et al: Focal cerebral ischemia in the cat: Treatment with glutamate antagonist MK-801 after induction of ischemia. *J Cereb Blood Flow Metab* 1988; 8:757.

369. Sterz F, et al: Effect of excitatory amino acid receptor blocker MK-801 on overall, neurologic, and morphologic outcome after prolonged cardiac arrest in dogs. *Anesthesiology* 1989; 71:907.

370. Buchan A, Pulsinelli WA: Hypothermia but not the *N*-methyl-p-aspartate antagonist MK-801, attenuates neuronal damage in gerbils subjected to transient global ischemia. *J Neurosci* 1990; 10:311.

371. Lanier WL, et al: The effects of dizocilpine maleate (MK-801), an antagonist of the *N*-methyl-D-aspartate receptor, on neurologic recovery and histopathology following complete cerebral ischemia in primates. *J Cereb Blood Flow Metab* 1990; 10:252.

372. Sheardown MJ, et al: 2,3-Dihydroxy-6-nitro-7-sulfamoyl-benzo(F)quinoxaline; A neuroprotectant of cerebral ischemia. *Science* 1990; 247:571.

373. Buchan AM, et al: Failure of the lipid peroxidation inhibitor, U74006F, to prevent postischemic selective neuronal injury. *J Cereb Blood Flow Metab* 1992; 12:250.

374. Braughler JM, Pregenzer JF: The 21-aminosteroid inhibitors of lipid peroxidation: Reactions with lipid peroxyl and phenoxy radicals. *Free Radical Biol Med* 1989; 7:125.

375. Hall ED, et al: Effects of the 21-aminosteroid U74006F on experimental head injury in mice. *J Neurosurg* 1988; 68:456.

376. Sterz F, et al: Effects of U74006F on multifocal cerebral blood flow and metabolism after cardiac arrest in dogs. *Stroke* 1991; 22:889.

377. Buchan AM, et al: Failure of the lipid peroxidation inhibitor,

U74006F, to prevent postischemic selective neuronal injury. *J Cereb Blood Flow Metab* 1992; 12:250.

378. Natale JE, et al: Effect of the aminosteroid U74006F after cardiopulmonary arrest in dogs. *Stroke* 1988; 19:1371.

379. Perkins WJ, et al: Pretreatment with U74006F improves neurologic outcome following complete cerebral ischemia in dogs. *Stroke* 1991; 22:902.

380. Iwatsuki N, et al: Hyperbaric oxygen combined with nicardipine administration accelerates neurologic recovery after cerebral ischemia in a canine model. *Crit Care Med* 1994; 22:858.

381. Warner D, et al: The effect of isoflurane on neuronal necrosis following near-complete forebrain ischemia in the rat. *Anesthesiology* 1986; 64:19.

382. Church J, et al: The neuroprotective effect of ketamine and MK-801 after transient cerebral ischemia in rats. *Anesthesiology* 1988; 69:702.

383. Safar P, et al: Recommendations for future research on the reversibility of clinical death. *Crit Care Med* 1988; 16:1077.

384. Vaagenes P, et al: Cerebral resuscitation from cardiac arrest: Pathophysiologic mechanisms. *Crit Care Med* 1996; 24:557.

385. Gisvold S, et al: Cerebral resuscitation from cardiac arrest. Treatment potentials. *Crit Care Med* 1996; 24:569.

386. Rosomoff HL, et al: Resuscitation from severe brain trauma. *Crit Care Med* 1996; 24:548.

387. Ebmeyer U, et al: Concluding comments. *Crit Care Med* 1996; 24:595.

388. Shoemaker WC: Diagnosis and therapy of shock syndromes. In Shoemaker WC, et al (eds): *Textbook of Critical Care*, Philadelphia, WB Saunders, 1985:85.

389. Stahl LD, et al: Selective enhancement of function of stunned myocardium by increased flow. *Circulation* 1986; 74:843.

390. Hallenbeck J, Kochanek P: Inflammatory responses in cerebral ischemia. Role of leukocytes. In Bogousslavsky J, Ginsberg M (eds): *Cerebrovascular Disease*. Cambridge, Blackwell Science, 1995:chap 35.

391. Eddy L, et al: A protective role for ascorbate in induced ischemic arrest associated with cardiopulmonary bypass. *J Appl Cardiol* 1990; 5:409.

392. Imaizumi S, et al: Liposome-entrapped superoxide dismutase reduces cerebral infarction in cerebral ischemia in rats. *Stroke* 1990; 21:1312.

393. Weisman HF, et al: Soluble human complement receptor type 1: In vitro inhibitor of complement suppressing post-ischemic myocardial inflammation and necrosis. *Science* 1990; 249:146.

394. Kaczorowski SL, et al: Effect of soluble complement receptor-1 on neutrophil accumulation after traumatic brain injury in rats. *J Cereb Blood Flow Metab* 1995; 15:860.

395. Gregory GA, et al: Fructose-1,6-bisphosphate reduces ATP loss from hypoxic astrocytes. *Brain Res* 1990; 516:310.

396. Gurvitch AM: Role of neurophysiological mechanisms in post-resuscitation pathology and postresuscitation restoration of CNS functions. *Minerva Anesth* 1994; 60:501.

397. Voll CL, Auer RN: Insulin attenuates ischemic brain damage independent of its hypoglycemic effects. *J Cereb Blood Flow Metab* 1991; 11:1006.

398. White BC, et al: Brain mitochondrial DNA is not damaged by prolonged cardiac arrest or reperfusion. *J Neurochem* 1992; 58:1716.

399. Nitatori T, et al: Delayed neuronal death in the CA 1 pyramidal cell layer of the gerbil hippocampus following transient ischemia is apoptosis. *J Neurosci* 1995; 15:1001.

400. Chen J, et al: Bcl-2 is expressed in neurons that survive focal ischemia in the rat. *Neurol Rept* 1995; 6:394.

401. Gelabert HA, Moore WS: Occlusive cerebrovascular disease. Medical and surgical considerations. In Cottrell JE, Smith DS

(eds): *Anesthesia and Neurosurgery*. St. Louis, CV Mosby, 1994:448.

402. Meyer JS, et al: Anticoagulants plus streptokinase therapy in progressive stroke. *JAMA* 1964; 189:373.

403. The National Institute of Neurological Disorders and Stroke, rt-PA Stroke Study Group: Tissue plasminogen activator for acute ischemic stroke. *N Engl J Med* 1995; 333:1581.

404. EC/IC Bypass Study Group: Failure of extracranial-intracranial arterial bypass to reduce the risk of ischemic stroke: Results of an international randomized trial. *N Engl J Med* 1985; 313:1191.

405. Nemoto EM, et al: Compartmentation of whole brain blood flow and oxygen and glucose metabolism in monkeys. *J Neurosurg Anesth* 1994; 6:170.

406. Hayashi S, et al: Beneficial effects of induced hypertension on experimental stroke in awake monkeys. *J Neurosurg* 1984; 60:51.

407. Hope DT, et al: Restoration of neurological function with induced hypertension in acute experimental cerebral ischemia. *Acta Neurol Scand Suppl* 1977; 64:506.

408. Wise G, et al: The treatment of brain ischemia with vasopressor drugs. *Stroke* 1972; 3:135.

409. Hoff JT: Cerebral circulation. *J Neurosurg* 1986; 65:579.

410. Muizelaar JP, Becker DP: Induced hypertension for the treatment of cerebral ischemia after subarachnoid hemorrhage. Direct effect on cerebral blood flow. *Surg Neurol* 1986; 25:317.

411. Heros RC, Korosue K: Hemodilution for cerebral ischemia. *Curr Concepts Cerebrovasc Dis Stroke* 1988; 23:31.

412. Kusunoki M, et al: Effects of hematocrit variations on cerebral blood flow and oxygen transport in ischemic cerebrovascular disease. *J Cereb Blood Flow Metab* 1981; 1:413.

413. Wood JH, et al: Hypervolemic hemodilution in experimental focal cerebral ischemia. Elevation of cardiac output, regional cortical blood flow, and ICP after intravascular volume expansion with low molecular weight dextran. *J Neurosurg* 1983; 59:500.

414. Wood JH et al: Failure of intravascular volume expansion without hemodilution to elevate cortical blood flow in region of experimental focal ischemia. *J Neurosurg* 1982; 56:80.

415. Kassell NF, et al: Treatment of ischemic deficits from vasospasm with intravascular volume expansion and induced arterial hypertension. *Neurosurgery* 1982; 11:337.

416. Grotta JC, et al: Baseline hemodynamic state and response to hemodilution in patients with acute cerebral ischemia. *Stroke* 1985; 16:790.

417. Soloway M, et al: The effect of hyperventilation on subsequent cerebral infarction. *Anesthesiology* 1968; 29:975.

418. Soloway M, et al: Effect of delayed hyperventilation on experimental cerebral infarction. *Neurology* 1971; 21:479.

419. Yamaguchi T, et al: Effects of hyperventilation with and without carbon dioxide on experimental cerebral ischemia and infarction. *Brain* 1972; 95:123.

420. Steen PA, et al: Hypothermia and barbiturates: Individual and combined effects on canine cerebral oxygen consumption. *Anesthesiology* 1983; 58:517.

421. Hoff JT, et al: Barbiturate protection from cerebral infarction in primates. *Stroke* 1975; 6:28.

422. Black KL, et al: Delayed pentobarbital therapy of acute focal cerebral ischemia. *Stroke* 1978; 9:245.

423. Selman WR, et al: Barbiturate-induced coma therapy for focal cerebral ischemia, effect after temporary and permanent MCA occlusion. *J Neurosurg* 1981; 55:220.

424. Hoff JT, et al: Pentobarbital protection from cerebral infarction without suppression of edema. *Stroke* 1982; 13:623.

425. Nussmeier NA, et al: Neuropsychiatric complications after cardiopulmonary bypass: Cerebral protection by a barbiturate. *Anesthesiology* 1986; 64:165.

426. Gelb AW, et al: A prophylactic bolus of thiopental does not protect against prolonged focal cerebral ischemia. *Can Anaesth Soc J* 1986; 33:173.

427. Milde LN, et al: Comparison of the effects of isoflurane and thiopental on neurologic outcome and neutropathology following temporary focal cerebral ischemia in primates. *Anesthesiology* 1988; 69:905.

428. Warner D, et al: Low-dose pentobarbital reduces focal ischemic infarct volume in a magnitude similar to burst suppression. *J Neurosurg Anesth* 1995; 7:303 (abstr).

429. Warner D, et al: Reversible focal ischemia in the rat: Effects of halothane, isoflurane and methohexital anesthesia. *J Cereb Blood Flow Metab* 1991; 11:794.

430. Henriksen L, et al: Controlled hypotension with sodium nitroprusside: Effects on cerebral blood flow and cerebral venous blood gases in patients operated for cerebral aneurysms. *Acta Anesthesiol Scand* 1983; 27:62.

431. Allen GS, et al: Cerebral arterial spasm—A controlled trial of nimodipine in patients with subarachnoid hemorrhage. *N Engl J Med* 1983; 308:619.

432. Philippon J, et al: Prevention of vasospasm in subarachnoid hemorrhage. A controlled study with nimodipine. *Acta Neurochir* 1986; 82:110.

433. Petruk KC, et al: Nimodipine treatment in poor-grade aneurysm patients: Results of a multicenter double-blind placebo-controlled trial. *J Neurosurg* 1988; 68:505.

434. Mohamed AA, et al: Effect of pretreatment with calcium antagonist nimodipine on local cerebral blood flow and histopathology after middle cerebral artery occlusion. *Ann Neurol* 1986; 18:705.

435. Gotoh O, et al: Nimodipine and the haemodynamic and histopathological consequences of middle cerebral artery occlusion in the rat. *J Cereb Blood Flow Metab* 1986; 6:321.

436. Barnett GH, et al: Effects of nimodipine on acute focal cerebral ischemia. *Stroke* 1986; 17:884.

437. Gelmers HJ: The effects of nimodipine on the clinical course of patients with acute ischaemic stroke. *Acta Neurol Scand* 1984; 69:232.

438. Gelmers HJ, et al: A controlled trial of nimodipine in acute ischemic stroke. *N Engl J Med* 1988; 318:203.

439. Harris RJ, et al: The effects of a calcium antagonist, nimodipine, upon physiological responses of the cerebral vasculature and its possible influence upon focal cerebral ischaemia. *Stroke* 1982; 13:759.

440. Foulkes M, et al: The traumatic coma data bank: Design, methods, and baseline characteristics. *J Neurosurg* 1991; 75(suppl):S8.

441. Kalsbeek WD, et al: The National Head and Spinal Cord Injury Survey: Major findings. *J Neurosurg* 1980; 53(suppl 5):19.

442. Smith DH, et al: A model of parasagittal controlled cortical impact in the mouse: Cognitive and histopathologic effects. *J Neurotrauma* 1995; 12:169.

443. Dunford HB: Free radicals in iron containing systems. *Free Radic Biol Med* 1987; 3:405.

444. Palmer AM, et al: Traumatic brain injury induced excitotoxicity assessed in a controlled cortical impact model. *J Neurochem* 1993; 61:2015.

445. DeKosky ST, et al: Interleukin-1 receptor antagonist suppresses neurotrophin response in injured rat brain. *Ann Neurol* 1996; 39:123.

446. DeKosky ST, et al: Upregulation of nerve growth factor following cortical trauma. *Exp Neurol* 1995; 130:173.

447. Marion DW, et al: Acute regional cerebral blood flow changes caused by severe head injury. *J Neurosurg* 1991; 74:407.

448. Kohi YM, et al: Extracranial insults and outcome in patients with acute head injury—relationship to the Glasgow Coma Score. *Injury* 1984; 16:25.

449. Ishige N, et al: The effect of hypoxia on traumatic head injury in rats: Alterations in neurologic function, brain edema, and cerebral blood flow. *J Cereb Blood Flow Metab* 1987; 6:759.

450. Clark RSB, et al: Neuropathologic effects of hypoxemia after moderate-severe controlled cortical impact injury in rats. 14th Annual Meeting of the Neurotrauma Society, Washington, DC, November 15–16, 1996, (abstr) in press.

451. Andersen BJ, et al: Effect of post-traumatic hypoventilation on cerebral energy metabolism. *J Neurosurg* 1988; 68:601.

452. White RJ, Likavec MJ: The diagnosis and initial management of head injury. *N Engl J Med* 1992; 327:1507.

453. McIntosh TK: Novel pharmacologic therapies in the treatment of experimental traumatic brain injury: A review. *J Neurotrauma* 1993; 10:215.

454. Bullock R, et al: *Guidelines for the Mangement of Severe Head Injury.* Joint Section on Neurotrauma and Critical Care. New York, The Brain Trauma Foundation, 1995.

455. Tsubokawa T, et al: *Neurochemical Monitoring in the Intensive Care Unit.* Heidelberg, Springer-Verlag, 1994.

456. Muir JK, et al: Continuous monitoring of posttraumatic cerebral blood flow using laser-doppler flowmetry. *J Neurotrauma* 1992; 9:355.

457. Bouma GJ, et al: Cerebral blood volume in acute head injury: Relationship to CBF and ICP. In Avezaath CJJ (ed): *Intracranial Pressure VIII.* Berlin/Heidelberg, Springer-Verlag, 1992: 529–534.

458. Yoshino A, et al: Dynamic changes in local cerebral glucose utilization following cerebral concussion in rats: Evidence of a hyper- and subsequent hypometabolic state. *Brain Res* 1991; 561:106.

459. Gennarelli TA, et al: Physiological response to angular acceleration of the head. In Grossman RG, Gildenberg PL (eds): *Head Injury, Basic and Clinical Aspects.* New York, Raven Press, 1982:129–140.

460. Levine JE, Becker DP: Reversal of incipient brain death from head injury apnea at the scene of accident. *N Engl J Med* 1979; 301:109.

461. Stept WJ, Safar P: Rapid induction/intubation for prevention of gastric content aspiration. *Anesth Analg* 1970; 49:633.

462. Rosner MJ, et al: Mechanical brain injury: The symphoadrenal response. *J Neurosurg* 1984; 61:76.

463. Forbes ML, et al: Hyperventilation early after controlled cortical impact augments neuronal death in CA3 hippocampus. 14th Annual Meeting of the Neurotrauma Society, Washington, DC, November 15–16, 1996, (abstr), in press.

464. Albin MS, et al: Study of functional recovery produced by delayed localized cooling after spinal cord injury in primates. *J Neurosurg* 1968; 29:113.

465. Albin MS: Resuscitation of the spinal cord. *Crit Care Med* 1978; 5:270.

466. Marion DW, et al: The use of moderate therapeutic hypother-mia for patients with severe head injuries: A preliminary report. *J Neurosurg* 1993; 79:354.

467. Goss JR, et al: Hypothermia attenuates the normal increase in interleukin-1β RNA and nerve growth factor following traumatic brain injury in the rat. *J Neurotrauma* 1995; 12:159.

468. Baker KZ, et al: Deliberate mild intra-operative hypothermia for craniotomy. *Anesthesiology* 1994; 81:361.

469. Baumgartner WA, et al: Reappraisal of cardiopulmonary bypass with deep hypothermia and circulatory arrest for complex neurosurgical operations. *Surgery* 1983; 94:242.

470. Bellamy R, et al: Future directions for resuscitation research: 4. Suspended animation for delayed resuscitation. *Crit Care Med* 1996; 24:524.

471. Newburger JW, et al: A comparison of the perioperative neurologic effects of hypothermic circulatory arrest versus low-flow cardiopulmonary bypass in infant heart surgery. *N Engl J Med* 1993; 329:1057.

472. Taylor MJ, et al: A new solution for life without blood: Asanguinous low flow perfusion of a whole-body perfusate during 3 hours of cardiac arrest and profound hypothermia. *Circulation* 1995; 91:431.

473. Elrifai AM, et al: Blood substitution: An experimental study. *Journal of Extra-Corporeal Technology* 1992; 24:58.

474. White RJ, et al: Prolonged whole brain refrigeration with electrical and metabolic recovery. *Nature* 1966; 209:1320.

475. Hochochka PW, et al (eds): *Surviving Hypoxia. Mechanisms of Control and Adaptation.* Boca Raton, FL CRC Press, 1993.

476. Laborit H, Huguenard P: *Practice of Hibernation Therapy in Surgery and Medicine* (French). Paris, Masson, 1954.

477. Bickler PE, et al: Developmental changes in intracellular calcium regulation in rat cerebral cortex during hypoxia. *J Cereb Blood Flow Metab* 1993; 13:811.

478. Bickler PE, Hansen BM: Causes of calcium accumulation in rat cortical brain slices during hypoxia and ischemia: Role of ion channels and membrane damage. *Brain Res* 1994; 665:269.

479. Cohen NM, et al: Is there an alternative to potassium arrest? *Ann Thorac Surg* 1995; 60:858.

480. Grenvik A, et al: Cessation of therapy in terminal illness and brain death. *Crit Care Med* 1978; 6:284.

481. Wanzer SH, et al: The physician's responsibility toward hopelessly ill patients: *N Engl J Med* 1984; 310:955.

482. Wanzer SH, et al: The physician's responsibility toward hopelessly ill patients, a second look. *N Engl J Med* 1989; 320:844.

483. Safar P: The physician's responsibility towards hopelessly critically ill patients. Ethical dilemmas in resuscitation medicine. *Acta Anaesth Scand* 1991; 35(suppl 96):147.

484. Youngner SJ, Bartlett ET: Human death and high technology: The failure of the whole-brain formulations. *Ann Intern Med* 1983; 99:252.

485. Madl C, et al: Early prediction of individual outcome after cardiopulmonary resuscitation. *Lancet* 1993; 341:855.

486. Safar P: Resuscitation medicine research: Quo vadis. *Ann Emerg Med* 1996; 27:542.

487. Biros MH, et al: Informed consent in emergency research. Consensus statement from Coalition Conference of Acute Resuscitation and Critical Care. *JAMA* 1995; 273:1283.

Chapter 18

EFFECTS OF ANESTHETIC AGENTS AND TEMPERATURE ON THE INJURED BRAIN

DAVID S. WARNER

INTRAVENOUS AGENTS
    Barbiturates
    Propofol
    Etomidate
    Opioids
    Ketamine
INHALATIONAL AGENTS
    Volatile Anesthetics
    Nitrous Oxide
HYPOTHERMIA
    Introduction
    Laboratory Evidence of Hypothermia Protection
    Mechanisms of Hypothermia Protection
    Human Evidence of Hypothermia Protection
    Practical Considerations for Hypothermia Protection
HYPERTHERMIA

Numerous neurosurgical procedures present risk of ischemic or traumatic injury to the brain and spinal cord. For decades, it has been the pursuit of neuroanesthesiologists and neurosurgeons to understand how these injuries occur and what therapy might provide protection against insults such as occlusion of major intracranial vessels, intracranial hypertension, retractor pressure, emboli, or excision of eloquent areas of brain.

Originally, a rather simplified approach to the problem consisted of examination of drug or therapeutic effects variables including cerebral blood flow (CBF), cerebral metabolic rate (CMR), and intracranial pressure (ICP). Indisputably, things done by anesthesiologists were found to affect these variables, sometimes in substantial ways. It could only be presumed, in the absence of appropriate human outcome studies, that such phenomena were either injurious or beneficial to the patient. Around these concepts and information, neuroanesthetic practice was defined.

Even to date, the subspecialty of neuroanesthesia operates in a void of human outcome studies that would provide definitive guidance in decisions including choice of anesthetic, management of blood pressure and temperature, importance of CBF, CMR, or ICP changes, and utility of electrophysiologic monitoring.

However, both accumulated clinical experience and a rapidly evolving basic science dedicated to these questions allows an increasingly rational basis for management of patients during neurosurgical procedures. Included in this domain is the field of brain protection. This chapter catalogues such advances and presents some recommendations that might reduce neurologic morbidity resulting from intraoperative events through the use of clinically available pharmacologic agents and manipulations of brain temperature.

Intravenous Agents

BARBITURATES

Barbiturates have been the most thoroughly investigated anesthetic agents with respect to effects on the injured brain. Despite this, major issues remain regarding mechanisms of action, efficacy, and indications for use in the perioperative environment.

The idea that barbiturates provide unique protection dates back to at least the mid-1960s. Two studies provided impetus for thorough investigation of the effects of these compounds on ischemic brain. In the first, it was reported that patients had better neurologic outcome if carotid endarterectomy was performed with general as opposed to local anesthesia.[1] That study had numerous methodologic deficiencies and the issue regarding an ideal anesthetic state for carotid endarterectomy is still far from settled. However, the investigators asked an important question regarding what aspect of general anesthesia might be accountable for the presumed neuroprotective benefit. Accordingly, a canine study was performed in which dogs had improved outcomes from transient complete global ischemia if administered pentobarbital before the insult.[2] This observation was consistent with recognition that barbiturates cause major reduction in CMR with a maximal effect being obtained coincident with onset of encephalographic (EEG) burst suppression.[3] Numerous studies followed this work looking at both physiologic and outcome effects of this class of drugs. Early reports supported the concept that barbiturates reduced global ischemic brain damage.[4,5] More rigorous studies performed since then have consistently failed to find benefit.[6–9]

One experiment was critical in providing a theoretical basis for predicting which types of ischemic injury might benefit from barbiturate therapy. Dogs were assigned to either no thiopental or EEG burst suppression doses of the drug.[10] Animals were then subjected to either acute hemorrhagic shock (which was insufficiently severe to ablate EEG activity) or anoxia (which ablated all EEG activity). In all cases, cortical high-energy phosphate stores were examined during the insult. In those cases where the insult caused loss of EEG activity, thiopental had no effect on the rate of high-energy phosphate depletion. In contrast, if the insult allowed continued EEG activity, thiopental slowed depletion of adenosine triphosphate (ATP). From this it was concluded that barbiturates provide protection by suppressing EEG activity and thus energy requirements. Therefore, only in those conditions where the insult allows persistent EEG activity will there be opportunity for barbiturates to provide protection. Indeed, the bulk of laboratory studies finding barbiturate protection have studied focal ischemic results. Presumably, EEG activity persists in the ischemic penumbra, which can be suppressed by barbiturates. In contrast, during global ischemic insults where EEG isoelectricity is typical, barbiturates have proven to be of little value.

This concept is heavily dependent on the belief that the principle mechanism of action by which barbiturates reduce injury is by virtue of the reduction in CMR. If so, one would predict that a dose-dependent reduction in ischemic damage can be observed as a function of the magnitude of CMR reduction afforded by drug therapy. Two early studies examined a dose-response relationship between barbiturate therapy and outcome from focal cerebral ischemia but were inappropriately designed to evaluate the CMR reduction hypothesis. In the first, baboons were subjected to permanent middle cerebral artery (MCA) occlusion (MCAO) while anesthetized with either 1.2% halothane or three different doses of pentobarbital (60, 90, or 120 mg/kg).[11] The EEG was recorded and showed persistent isoelectricity when the pentobarbital dose exceeded 50 mg/kg. Thus, the EEG was quiescent in all three pentobarbital groups. Doses less than those required for EEG quiescence were not examined. In the second study, dogs were subjected to permanent MCAO.[12] One hour after onset of ischemia animals were assigned to receive varying doses of pentobarbital (10 to 80 mg/kg). The control group was nonconcurrent, which consisted of halothane anesthetized animals used in a different study. A dose-dependent reduction in infarct size was observed with maximal effect at 20 mg/kg. However, temperature was not monitored or controlled at any site in the body and no attempt was made to provide mechanical ventilation in any of the groups. Further, EEG was not monitored. Therefore, it is impossible to discern what, if any, relationship was present between the neuroprotective effect of the drug and the effect on the EEG/CMR.

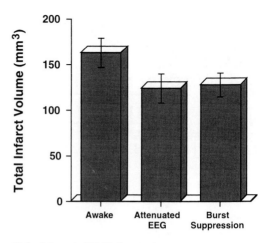

Figure 18-1 Mean ± SEM infarct volumes in rats maintained awake or anesthetized with pentobarbital so as to produce an attenuated EEG or EEG burst suppression during 90 min of temporary MCAO. Low-dose pentobarbital resulted in a 25 percent reduction in total infarct volume compared to awake rats. A larger dose of pentobarbital provided no additional benefit. (Reproduced with permission from Warner and coworkers.[13])

More recently a rat MCAO model was used to examine this issue.[13] Rats were assigned to undergo 90 min of ischemia while either awake or when administered pentobarbital in a dose sufficient to cause mild EEG attenuation or burst suppression. Both barbiturate groups showed a similarly reduced infarct size compared to awake animals but the magnitude of reduction was small (Fig. 18-1). These data suggest that either the difference in CMR reduction provided by the larger dose of pentobarbital was unimportant or instead that other properties of barbiturates are critical in providing the observed protection and those properties provide maximal efficacy at substantially lower doses than are required to elicit EEG burst suppression.

The efficacy of barbiturates in human trials has been disappointing. Patients suffering from head injury, while exhibiting improved control of ICP, did not experience improved neurologic outcome when administered barbiturate-induced EEG quiescence during the acute stage of their illness.[14] Survivors of cardiac arrest faired no better when administered thiopental after recovery of spontaneous circulation. In such patients the EEG was not monitored but would be presumed to have recovered some activity that would have been amenable to barbiturate reduction in CMR.[15] In patients undergoing coronary artery bypass grafting, again no benefit was observed in patients administered thiopental to the end point of EEG burst suppression.[16] Although some neurologic injury associated with cardiopulmonary bypass can be attributed to global hypoperfusion, it has since become clear from the use of transcranial ultrasonography that those patients are exposed to a substantial number of cerebral embolic events that would be expected to cause focal ischemic challenges,[17] again providing an opportunity for barbiturate-induced reduction in CMR. Nussmeier and colleagues did observe a beneficial effect of thiopental on neurologic outcome from valvular heart surgery.[18] This is perhaps our best evidence that barbiturates can reduce ischemic brain damage under specific operative conditions,[19] but currently stands alone with respect to human data in supporting the use of barbiturates as neuroprotective agents. Although barbiturates remain perhaps the best of the currently available pharmacologic agents for treatment of intraoperative cerebral ischemia, it is fortunate that alternative pharmacologic approaches to brain protection / resuscitation are being aggressively pursued where protection depends on mechanisms of action other than simple CMR suppression.

Clinically it is common practice to administer barbiturates (or other CMR-reducing agents) to the end point of EEG isoelectricity, which is consistent with obtaining maximal CMR reduction. However, it is more likely this end point has become accepted because it is discrete and can be readily interpreted from an EEG monitor. Rats do not show a dose-dependent protective response to high-dose barbiturate therapy. If barbiturates are to remain as drugs of choice for neuroprotection, then definition of a dose-response relationship for their efficacy must occur. Clearly with processed EEG signals, it is now feasible to determine optimal dosing for these compounds.

In conclusion, barbiturates remain the drug of choice when pharmacologic brain protection is desired. However, the benefit is likely to be small and this must be weighed against the cost of a delayed emergence from anesthesia in the postoperative period.

PROPOFOL

Propofol was introduced as an induction and maintenance anesthetic in the late 1980s. The elimination half-life for propofol is shorter than for thiopental or pentobarbital. It has been proposed that perhaps propofol might be a superior agent because a more rapid emergence from burst suppression levels of anesthesia can be obtained.

Propofol has cerebrovascular and metabolic properties similar to barbiturates. Increasing doses of the drug result in decreasing CBF and CMR.[20–23] Initial reports indicated that propofol, while capable of reducing ICP, also reduced cerebral perfusion pressure (CPP) to a substantial degree, principally because of reductions in mean arterial pressure (MAP).[24] Subsequent work demonstrated that reduced doses given over a longer interval allow preservation of adequate CPP.[25] Two large prospective trials examining patients undergoing

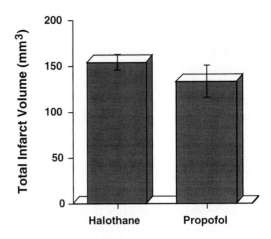

Figure 18-2   Cerebral infarct volumes as determined 96 h after reperfusion for rats anesthetized with either an EEG burst suppression dose of propofol or 0.5 MAC halothane during 90 min of MCAO. There was no statistical difference between groups. (Reproduced with permission from Ridenour and coworkers.[32])

craniotomy found propofol-based anesthesia provides satisfactory hemodynamic and recovery profiles.[26,27] Given these findings, propofol would seem to be well suited for use during neurosurgery for the purpose of providing anesthesia.

With respect to neuroprotective effects, propofol has properties other than CMR depression that provide a theoretical basis for expecting positive results. Propofol is a glutamate antagonist at the *N*-methyl-D-aspartate (NMDA) receptor, which might reduce excitotoxicity.[28] In addition, recent work indicates that γ-aminobutyric acid (GABA)ergic compounds improve outcome in ischemia preparations.[29,30]

Two studies have directly examined the neuroprotective effects of propofol against ischemic insults. In the first, propofol-anesthetized rats subjected to hemispheric incomplete ischemia had better outcomes than did rats anesthetized with nitrous oxide and fentanyl.[31] In the second study, rats receiving sufficient propofol to result in EEG burst suppression had similar outcomes from temporary MCAO as did those anesthetized with 0.5 minimum alveolar concentration (MAC) halothane[32] (Fig. 18-2). In the latter case, it is now unfortunate in retrospect that halothane was chosen as the comparator. Given the strong protective effect of halothane against focal ischemia in the rat as discussed below,[33] it is no longer reasonable to conclude that propofol offered no protective advantage in this model. This is an excellent example of a situation in which the neuroprotective properties of an anesthetic must be examined in a model that allows direct comparison of outcome against the awake state. At present, we can only conclude that propofol is as efficacious as halothane. What remains undefined is if propofol offers any unique neuroprotective benefits that would indicate it as a drug of choice as opposed to other available compounds. Like most other compounds, the neuroprotective properties of propofol have not been held to the same scrutiny in humans as have the barbiturates. Accordingly, use of this agent for intraoperative neuroprotection remains speculative.

ETOMIDATE

Etomidate is yet another intravenous anesthetic that exhibits cerebrovascular and metabolic properties similar to barbiturates.[34] Increasing doses of the drug result in decreasing CBF and CMR.[35–37] Again the proposed advantage from this drug is a more rapid elimination. This should allow earlier performance of a neurologic examination in the postoperative period in patients who are administered a dose sufficient to cause sustained EEG burst suppression.

Etomidate has been championed by some as an intraoperative neuroprotectant.[38] Despite this, etomidate has only been partially examined as a neuroprotective agent in laboratory animals and the little human work done with this drug has provided unconvincing evidence regarding efficacy. For example, one series of patients underwent giant intracranial aneurysm clipping under etomidate-induced EEG burst suppression resulting in a 71 percent incidence of good outcome.[39] However, no control group was examined to provide comparison.

Evidence indicates that etomidate reduces extracellular glutamate accumulation during global ischemia and that this relates to a small reduction in the number of neurons showing histologic damage.[40,41] Etomidate has recently been found to offer only transient benefit over isoflurane in dogs subjected to temporary hindbrain ischemia.[42] In contrast, although long-term outcome was not assessed, etomidate and isoflurane both offered inferior protection to thiopental in rats undergoing temporary focal ischemia followed by 2 h of reperfusion.[43]

Numerous human studies have demonstrated that etomidate reduces ICP in both normal brain and brain with reduced compliance.[44–46] Concern remains regarding the suppression of steroidogenesis by etomidate,[47] but in neurosurgical patients already undergoing high-dose steroid therapy this may be unimportant. Finally, recent work has suggested that although etomidate causes reduced ICP in patients with refractory intracranial hypertension, renal toxicity may result from prolonged infusions of the drug (most likely attributable to the vehicle).[48] Together, available information argues that etomidate is not indicated as a drug of choice for neuroprotective purposes.

OPIOIDS

Opioid-based anesthesia remains a mainstay for neurosurgical procedures. This probably has arisen from the stable hemodynamics and predictable emergence that can be obtained. Further, early work showed that opioids were generally devoid of substantive effects on CBF, CMR, or ICP.[49–52] In fact, one school held that pure high-dose opioid anesthesia provided an ideal neuroanesthetic.[53] However, later work in humans undergoing supratentorial craniotomy or suffering from head injury questioned this suggestion. Patients undergoing craniotomy exhibited increased ICP and decreased CPP when administered induction doses of fentanyl, sufentanil, or alfentanil.[54] Numerous similar studies followed with inconsistent findings except that if opioids cause an increase in ICP, that increase is small (i.e., <10 mmHg) and transient.[55–61]

Close examination of this isssue has provided some insight into the probable mechanism for opioid-induced ICP changes. It has been suggested that ICP changes can be explained by an autoregulatory response to decreased MAP. Werner and colleagues provided convincing evidence to support this concept.[62] In their study, 3 μg/kg sufentanil was administered to head trauma patients. ICP was measured while transcranial Doppler ultrasonography was used to estimate CBF. Attempts were made to maintain MAP at baseline by phenylephrine infusion. In patients in whom MAP was successfully maintained near baseline, ICP did not change. In patients in whom MAP did decrease, ICP became increased. In either case, CBF velocity did not change consistent with preservation of autoregulation. It can be construed from these data that patients with low cerebral compliance exhibit increased ICP due to increased blood volume occurring because of a vasodilatory response to decreased MAP. It thus seems unlikely that ICP increases occurring in response to opioid administration are attributable to anything other than decreased MAP, an expected effect from virtually all anesthetic agents. If an ICP response to opioid infusion is undesired, then effort must be made to control blood pressure.

With respect to opioid effects on ischemic pathophysiology, less is known. In general, opioids have been considered to be inert. However, some evidence presented in the 1980s argued that naloxone therapy might provide some benefit against ischemic injury although this has been questioned and, in fact, is rarely practiced.[63] Other work has shown that opioids, if administered in sufficient doses, can cause electroconvulsive activity in laboratory animals.[64] If this is allowed to persist, despite adequate oxygenation, neuronal injury will occur.[65] It is known that an exaggerated metabolic demand is posed by opioid-induced seizures.[66] It could be postulated that this would result in a more rapid

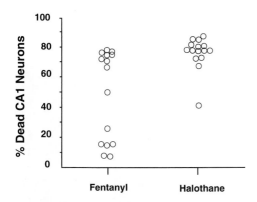

Figure 18-3   Percent dead neurons in the CA1 sector of the rat hippocampus observed 7 days after 10 min of transient global ischemia. Rats were anesthetized during ischemia with either 400 μg/kg fentanyl or 0.5 MAC halothane. A mild protective effect of fentanyl is observed in this model (Morimoto and Warner, unpublished data).

depletion of intracellular energy stores and consequently worsened ischemic outcome. Evidence for this is marginal to date. In contrast, in rats undergoing acute spinal cord ischemia, fentanyl has actually been found to reduce injury.[67] Recent work in our laboratory suggests that this is also the case for cerebral tissue (Fig. 18-3). Regardless, the vast number of neurosurgical procedures performed with opioid-based anesthesia speaks strongly for the value of these agents when all factors are considered.

KETAMINE

Ketamine has never been a favorite drug of neuroanesthesiologists. This is attributable to early reports regarding increases in ICP in patients with intracranial hypertension.[68] In addition, neuroanesthesia requires a rapid predictable emergence. The dissociative nature of ketamine when used as the sole anesthetic as well as emergence delirium make this drug inferior to alternative agents. However, interest in ketamine has resurged because of its mechanism of action, which is principally attributable to noncompetitive antagonism of the glutamatergic NMDA receptor.[69–71] Other compounds that have similar effects have been shown to afford significant neuroprotection in animal models of ischema.[72] If ketamine shared the same properties, the clinical availability of ketamine would make the drug attractive at least in limited doses. Several studies have examined this issue. However, the results have been mixed. One report showed a weak protective effect for ketamine in rat global ischemia,[73] whereas another study showed protection in rat hemispheric ischemia.[74] The positive findings are somewhat troubling, however, because NMDA antagonists are generally ineffective against global ischemia and others have failed to

find a protective effect in similar models.[75,76] Another study examined the effect of ketamine in a rat MCAO model.[77] Ketamine was as efficacious as halothane. Ketamine has been shown to be protective against percussion head injury in the rat consistent with several other NMDA antagonists.[78–80] Finally, in a rat model of spinal cord ischemia ketamine resulted in a poorer neurologic outcome than was observed in rats anesthetized with either isoflurane or fentanyl/nitrous oxide.[81] As a result, the ICP and emergence effects of ketamine continue to outweigh the unconvincing neuroprotection profile for this agent. Ketamine therefore remains an infrequently used drug in neuroanesthesia.

Inhalational Agents

VOLATILE ANESTHETICS

HALOTHANE

Halothane was introduced to clinical practice in the mid-1950s and was soon hailed as an excellent agent for use during craniotomy. As stated by Schapira in 1964 "halothane has been used for years for neuroanesthesia and has proved to be a nearly ideal agent for this purpose."[82] This statement was made on the basis of clinical experience rather than from measurement of specific neurophysiologic values. In the same era, continuous measurement of ICP was just becoming clinically available.[83] One of the early reports regarding intraoperative ICP events concerned the effects of halothane.[84] Jennett and colleagues reported data on two patients undergoing anesthesia for tumor resection. These patients had marked increases in ICP when halothane was added to the respiratory gas mixture. This ICP increase was readily reversed when halothane was discontinued. In both patients, normocapnia had been ensured by controlled ventilation. It was recommended that halothane not be used in this patient population. The type of dichotomy seen between the clinical experience of Schapira and the physiologic measurements made by Jennett and coworkers continues to raise debate regarding choice of anesthetic for craniotomy. Nevertheless, the use of halothane was appreciably decreased after the reports by Jennett and associates until it was observed that halothane could be administered without causing a substantial increase in ICP, but only if given after hyperventilation had been well established.[85] This cumbersome aspect of halothane administration as well as reports (discussed below) regarding adverse effects of the drug during ischemic conditions,[86] left clinicians desiring better drugs to provide anesthesia in neurosurgical patients.

At approximately the same time that halothane had become a standard anesthetic agent, it was being recognized that barbiturates had a role during neurosurgery as cerebral protective agents. One study examined the effects of different doses of halothane or barbiturates on lesion size resulting from MCAO in the dog.[86] In contrast to thiopental, light halothane anesthesia (about 0.8%) offered no advantage over the awake state, whereas deep halothane anesthesia (about 1.9%) caused substantial worsening of outcome. Although this work was state of the art science at the time of publication, numerous methodologic concerns would probably preclude publication of such a study in the current era. Problems included a small sample size, failure to regulate brain temperature or plasma glucose, and failure to control duration of anesthetic exposure between different drugs. However, this work, in concert with observations that large doses of halothane caused metabolic toxicity,[87] effectively "killed" the agent as one having potential for providing intraoperative neuroprotection.

More recent work has questioned that conclusion. Several in vitro studies have demonstrated that volatile anesthetics possess potent antagonism of glutamatergic neurotransmission at the NMDA receptor. Administration of halothane results in reduced Ca^{2+} influx in synaptosomes stimulated with the glutamate agonist NMDA.[88] Further, in patch clamp studies, both halothane and isoflurane inhibited calcium influx induced by glutamate in isolated neurons.[89] Halothane also inhibited the cytotoxic effects of the noncompetitive NMDA receptor antagonist MK-801.[90] This effect was speculated to be due to up-regulation of inhibition from GABAergic afferents.

To examine if halothane also provides protection in vivo when brain temperature is strictly controlled, rats undergoing temporary MCAO had a 46 percent reduction in infarct size if administered 1 MAC halothane as opposed to being awake during the insult (Fig. 18-4).[33] Another study demonstrated improved histologic/neurologic outcome in halothane- (as opposed to nitrous oxide-) anesthetized rats exposed to incomplete hemispheric ischemia.[91] Although halothane has largely been discarded from clinical practice in the favor of isoflurane, which is essentially devoid of hepatotoxicity and arrythmogenicity, the above information suggests that neuroprotective properties of anesthetic agents in general should continue to undergo careful scrutiny as advances are made in laboratory models and understanding of the basic pathomechanisms of ischemic injury.

ISOFLURANE

When isoflurane was first introduced for neuroanesthesia, considerable enthusiasm for its use emerged. First, the ICP effects of isoflurane appeared to be more manageable than was the case for halothane. Rather than having to precede administration of the drug with

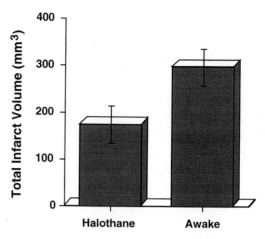

Figure 18-4 Total infarct volumes (mean ± SEM) in rats undergoing 90 min of MCAO and 4-day recovery. In both awake and halothane-anesthetized rats, brain temperature was maintained at 38.0°C during the ischemic insult and early reperfusion period. Mean infarct volume was reduced by 46 percent in the anesthetized rats. (Reproduced with permission from Warner and coworkers.[33])

hyperventilation, onset of isoflurane administration and hyperventilation could be simultaneous without appreciable increases in ICP occurring.[92] In vivo cerebrovascular dilating effects of isoflurane were less than halothane,[93] although in vitro direct effects of halothane and isoflurane were similar.[94] Most importantly, isoflurane provided barbiturate-like reductions in CMR.[95] This property was available in clinically relevant doses, which distinguished isoflurane again from halothane.[96] Preliminary studies suggest that these properties were likely to result in in vivo neuroprotection against ischemic insults.[97] Because of the relatively rapid elimination for isoflurane (as opposed to barbiturates), it was hoped that isoflurane could be administered intraoperatively providing "neuroprotection insurance" while allowing rapid emergence from neuroanesthesia so that neurologic examinations could be readily performed.

Several studies were then performed that examined the potential for isoflurane to reduce ischemic brain damage in comparison to other available anesthetic regimens. Nehls and colleagues subjected baboons to temporary MCAO while anesthetized with either EEG burst suppression doses of isoflurane or thiopental or instead a nitrous oxide/fentanyl anesthetic.[98] Isoflurane was inferior to thiopental but similar to nitrous oxide/fentanyl with respect to resultant infarct size and neurologic function. Warner and coworkers performed a similar study wherein rats were subjected to transient MCAO during either halothane, isoflurane, or pentobarbital anesthesia (Fig. 18-5).[99] Although a small superiority was observed for the barbiturate, the two volatile anesthetics provided similar protection.

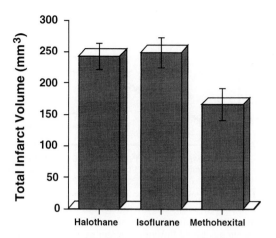

Figure 18-5   Cerebral infarct volumes (mean ± SEM), as determined by triphenyl tetrazolium chloride staining 96 h after reperfusion from 90 min MCAO, for rats anesthetized with EEG burst suppression doses of methohexital or isoflurane or 1.3 MAC halothane. Infarct volume for methohexital-treated rats was significantly less than observed for isoflurane ($p < .03$) or halothane ($p < .04$) anesthesia, between which infarct volumes were not different. (Reproduced with permission from Warner and coworkers.[99])

Finally, Gelb and associates examined primates undergoing MCAO combined with induced hypotension attempting to simulate a vascular occlusive event during intracranial aneurysm surgery. Again halothane and isoflurane offered similar outcomes.[100]

Human studies also examined the issue regarding the relative neuroprotective potential of isoflurane. A large series of patients undergoing carotid endarterectomy at the Mayo Clinic were administered either halothane, enflurane, or isoflurane anesthesia.[101] The EEG and CBF were measured during carotid cross clamping. Patients who had received isoflurane had the lowest incidence of EEG changes. Further, when EEG changes did occur, the CBF threshold for this response was substantially lower in patients anesthetized with isoflurane as opposed to the other two agents. This study was criticized for several reasons, the most important of which was the retrospective nature of the study design. The importance of this is that patients had received the different drugs over different eras of drug development such that those who had received halothane were studied approximately 10 years earlier than those who had received isoflurane. However, a later prospective study validated the relatively low flow threshold for ischemic EEG changes during isoflurane anesthesia.[102] Further, when rats were subjected to abrupt onset of cardiac arrest, onset of terminal depolarization was more rapid during halothane as opposed to isoflurane anesthesia.[103] However, these electrophysiologic differences have been difficult to document as having value with respect to neurologic outcome. In the retrospective Mayo Clinic carotid endarterectomy series, neurologic outcome was similar for the three anesthetic regimens.[101]

Isoflurane has become widely accepted as the agent of choice when a volatile anesthetic is to be selected for neuroanesthesia. This is most likely attributable to its general popularity as an anesthetic rather than due to unique characteristics regarding its effect on the brain. Probably in response to the initial enthusiasm for this drug to provide superlative neuroprotection, a backlash in opinion has occurred that has questioned the basic theoretical reasons why isoflurane should provide protection. This certainly is healthy for our discipline because more is now known about the interaction between anesthetics and the brain than simple issues regarding effects on CMR. Isoflurane has been successfully used in a great number of neurosurgical procedures and its value has been enormous. What is yet to be done, is to more carefully examine the effects of this drug on ischemic pathophysiology in the context of other advances in the field of neuroscience. For example, isoflurane has recently been shown to be a potent inhibitor of glutamate receptor-mediated calcium influx in brain slices resulting in reduced accumulation of lactate dehydrogenase, a marker of cell death.[104]

SEVOFLURANE

Like isoflurane, sevoflurane is capable of producing EEG burst suppression at clinically relevant doses. In fact the CBF, ICP, and CMR profile for the two drugs is remarkably similar.[105-110] Little is known regarding its neuroprotective potential. One study has been performed that compared sevoflurane and halothane anesthesia to an awake state during transient focal ischemia in the rat.[111] Although both sevoflurane and halothane exhibited a marked and similar reduction in infarct size, brain temperature in the awake animals was not controlled leaving open the possibility that the protective effect of sevoflurane was attributable only to effects on brain temperature. Further work with this compound is required before a conclusion regarding its role in neuroanesthesia can be made.

DESFLURANE

Desflurane offers unique advantage over other volatile anesthetic agents with respect to its low blood solubility allowing a demonstrably more rapid emergence from anesthesia, which might provide benefit in neurosurgery.[112,113] Unfortunately, early work with neurosurgical patients left a confusing answer regarding the effect of desflurane on ICP. The original study designed to examine this issue was performed without a control group. In that study desflurane caused an insidious increase in cerebrospinal fluid (CSF) pressure over a 45-min exposure to the drug.[114] Later work suggested that this was different from isoflurane-treated patients, but the patients were not studied contemporaneously and thus this issue is unresolved.[115] Work by Artru has proposed that the effects of desflurane on CSF formation and adsorption might account for the ICP increase. However, direct examination of this failed to reveal such an effect.[116] Desflurane has similar EEG, CBF, and CMR effects as does isoflurane.[117–121] The effect of this drug on ischemic brain has not been examined.

NITROUS OXIDE

Nitrous oxide remains a frequently used agent during neurosurgical procedures. Despite attempts to encourage abandonment of the use of this drug, the properties of nitrous oxide make it a valuable adjunct in neuroanesthesia. The principal benefit of nitrous oxide is the rapid elimination half-life. In cases where only modest noxious stimulation is present, the relatively low potency is offset by the ability to allow rapid emergence. Its widespread use speaks strongly for the importance of this drug in neuroanesthesia. However, not all of the properties of nitrous oxide make it an ideal agent for neuroanesthesia and the neuroanesthetist should be aware of these considerations.

The drug has been associated with expansion of closed gas spaces, which might have bearing under conditions of pneumocephalus.[122,123] A recent examination of postoperative computed tomography (CT) scans showed that pneumocephalus is a common finding until approximately 2 weeks after a craniotomy.[124] Thus patients undergoing repeat craniotomy within this interval might benefit from the use of alternative anesthetics until the dura is opened.

Another concern is the effect of nitrous oxide on CBF and ICP. Studies examining the ICP effects have produced variable results although the preponderance of evidence indicates that under conditions of decreased intracranial compliance nitrous oxide will enhance intracranial hypertension.[125–128] More consistent results have been obtained with respect to the CBF effects of nitrous oxide. When nitrous oxide is used alone, CBF is substantially increased.[129,130] Concomitant with this, a modest increase in metabolic rate occurs. When used in combination with volatile anesthetics a similar increase in CBF occurs. In fact, animal studies have shown that equal MAC concentrations of nitrous oxide result in greater increases in CBF than do either halothane or isoflurane[131] (Fig. 18-6). This effect was not attributable to changes in metabolic rate.[132] Three human studies have since confirmed this CBF finding.[133–135] Although direct in vitro comparisons of the vasodilatory activity of nitrous oxide versus volatile anesthetics have not been performed, it is reasonable

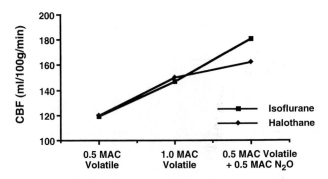

Figure 18-6 Cerebral blood flow as a function of depth of anesthesia for rats anesthetized with isoflurane or halothane in the presence or absence of nitrous oxide. For both volatile anesthetic agents, blood flow was greater at a depth of anesthesia equal to 1 MAC when that depth of anesthesia was achieved with the coadministration of nitrous oxide as opposed to administration of the volatile anesthetic alone. (Reproduced with permission from Hansen and coworkers.[131])

to conclude that this drug should be considered as a potent cerebrovasodilator. When confronted with a swollen brain, it might be most appropriate to discontinue nitrous oxide administration before discontinuing volatile agents both because of the above findings as well as the fact that nitrous oxide will be cleared more rapidly. This may provide the most prompt reduction of pharmacologic increases in brain blood volume.

With respect to ischemia, there is incomplete agreement regarding the effects of nitrous oxide although in general the drug appears to be relatively inert. Only a few studies have directly examined this issue. Rats subjected to incomplete hemispheric ischemia have consistently experienced worsened outcome when receiving nitrous oxide only as opposed to rats more deeply anesthetized with a variety of anesthetic agents.[91,136] It is unclear whether this can be attributed to the physiology of light anesthesia or to nitrous oxide itself. In contrast, rats subjected to 10 min of near-complete forebrain ischemia faired equally well when anesthetized with nitrous oxide alone or burst suppression doses of isoflurane.[137] There has been the suggestion that nitrous oxide may reduce the neuroprotective benefit from barbiturates.[138] This presumably would be the result of neuronal activation induced by an increase in metabolic rate caused by the gas. However, when this question was specifically addressed in pentobarbital-anesthetized rats underoing temporary focal cerebral ischemia, neither histologic nor neurologic outcome were altered by the coadministration of nitrous oxide (Fig. 18-7).[139] This probably is a rhetorical question, however, because in most cases where barbiturate protection would be employed, use of a high fraction inspired oxygen would also seem prudent.

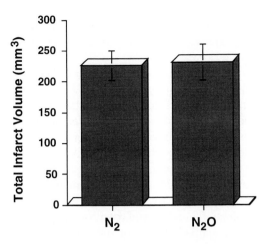

Figure 18-7   Cerebral infarct volume for rats undergoing 90 min of MCAO while anesthetized with burst suppression doses of methohexital in the presence 70% nitrogen or 70% nitrous oxide mixed with 30% oxygen in the respiratory gas mixture. No difference between groups was observed. (Reproduced with permission from Warner and coworkers.[139])

Hypothermia

INTRODUCTION

Hypothermia as a strategy for intraoperative neuroprotection has been recognized by neuroanesthesiologists for decades. In large part it was abandoned early because it was thought that the principal mechanism by which hypothermia protects is by reduction in CMR. This implied that deep levels of hypothermia are necessary to provide meaningful benefit. Accordingly, cardiopulmonary bypass would be essential to avoid complications of arrhythmia and coagulopathy. Besides logistical issues, bypass also requires administration of heparin, which considerably increases the complexity of performing surgery on the brain.

Largely by accident it has become evident that mild levels of hypothermia can provide substantial and lasting protection in laboratory animals. Active investigation is now defining the relevance of these findings to the human condition. Further, advances in animal modeling have allowed clearer definition of mechanisms of hypothermic brain protection as well as limitations regarding efficacy. The discussion below outlines these developments.

LABORATORY EVIDENCE OF HYPOTHERMIA PROTECTION

The development of rodent models of cerebral ischemia was crucial to this issue. Those models provided opportunity for thorough examination of factors influencing ischemic outcome using disease-free, ge-

netically consistent, and low-cost subjects. Dramatic reduction in neural injury was observed when brain temperature was reduced by only 3° to 5°C in models of focal ischemia,[140–142] global ischemia,[143,144] brain trauma,[145,146] or status epilepticus.[147]

Anesthesiologists promptly recognized the logical extension that mild hypothermia might also be beneficial in the care of patients at risk for perioperative ischemic insults. Mild hypothermia is easy to induce in the anesthetized patient and presumably the risk associated with this practice is small, particularly if the patient is rewarmed before emergence from anesthesia. Second, anesthesiologists were beginning to recognize the improbable benefit from anesthetic agents that purportedly offer ischemia protection simply by reduction of CMR. Thus, alternative therapies were actively being sought. This was most clearly demonstrated by Sano and colleagues who observed that histologic outcome from global ischemia was poor and similar for halothane- and isoflurane-anesthetized rats (despite large differences in CMR). In contrast, virtually all damage was inhibited by reducing brain temperature by only 3°C (small effect on CMR).[144] Work such as this has caused those caring for patients with acute cerebral insults to seriously consider application of mild hypothermia as a tool for improving outcome.

Evidence also suggests that postischemic hypothermia is protective. Original work indicated that the therapeutic window may persist for only 30 min after reperfusion of the brain.[148] Later work indicates that the window for onset of hypothermia may extend up to 12 h after reperfusion. This is true, however, only if the duration of hypothermia lasts at least several hours.[149]

There also has been some discussion as to whether hypothermia truly offers protection or instead causes only a delay in the cascade of pathophysiologic events that ultimately results in a similar outcome as observed for nomothermic comparators. Indeed, the majority of laboratory studies that examined hypothermic protection have only evaluated animals as far out as several days after the ischemic event. Others who have examined animals at weeks to months after ischemia have observed that long-term hypothermic protective effects against histologic changes become small if the duration of hypothermia is 12 h or less.[150,151] Perhaps the definitive study has recently been performed.[152] Gerbils with appropriate monitoring of brain temperature were exposed to mild hypothermia for 24 h after global ischemia. Examination of histologic and neurologic changes at 6 months revealed a persistent benefit from hypothermia. The clinical relevance of this is unknown. The data suggest, however, that should postischemic hypothermia be used, prolonged intervals (up to 24 h) may be required to obtain lasting benefit.

MECHANISMS OF HYPOTHERMIA PROTECTION

For several decades it was thought that the predominant mechanism by which hypothermia caused protection was by virtue of its effects on CMR. This has been called into question because mild hypothermia offers potent neuroprotection although CMR is only minimally reduced. Other cellular and biochemical effects better explain how hypothermia protects. For example, during an ischemic insult, extracellular concentrations of glutamate become massively increased. Such increases in glutamate are believed to initiate an excitotoxic cascade ultimately resulting in cell death. Mild hypothermia effectively blocks this increase in glutamate.[153–155] The mechanism for this is unknown. What is becoming clear is that the postsynaptic consequences may be important. One postsynaptic glutamate receptor type (NMDA) is coupled with a calcium channel. Because there is an approximate 10,000 : 1 gradient between extracellular and intracellular calcium, intracellular calcium is tightly regulated. Energy failure is associated with a large influx of calcium. In vitro studies have shown that mild hypothermia reduces calcium influx.[104,156] Presumably, such an effect causes decreased opportunity for intracellular calcium to accumulate to concentrations sufficient to exert toxic effects.

Undoubtedly there are also numerous generalized effects of hypothermia on intracellular enzymatic activity. Mild reductions in brain temperature, while having no effect during the early recirculation interval,[157] hasten recovery of protein synthesis several hours after reperfusion.[158] However, specific effects are also being defined. Protein kinase C (PKC), an enzyme involved in regulating neuronal excitability and neurotransmitter release, is activated in response to an increase in cytosolic calcium. Hypothermia diminishes membrane-bound PKC activity in selectively vulnerable regions of the postischemic brain.[159]

Nitric oxide synthase activity in the ischemic brain is also suppressed by hypothermia.[160] It is not clear, however, whether this is beneficial or detrimental because of the variability in results obtained when nitric oxide synthase inhibitors are examined in outcome models of ischemia.[161] If nitric oxide or other free radical mechanisms are germane to the pathogenesis of neuronal death, then the effects of hypothermia are again relevant. Hypothermia has been demonstrated to reduce accumulation of lipid peroxidation products and the consumption of free radical scavengers in ischemic brain.[162,163]

Other information is available regarding free radical effects of hypothermia. Using two different models of brain injury (global ischemia or traumatic brain injury), Globus and colleagues have demonstrated that free radical production persists for at least several hours after reperfusion.[164,165] The quantity of free radical generated is reduced to almost normal values by moderate hypothermia.

Perhaps of greatest interest are the electrophysiologic effects of hypothermia during focal ischemia. If monitored for direct current potential, tissue in the ischemic penumbra shows recurrent episodes of depolarization that have been associated with transient intervals of tissue hypoxia and depression of electrical activity.[156] If such events can be considered as insults secondary to the primary etiology of ischemia, then the observation that hypothermia greatly diminishes the frequency of such depolarizations provides an additional mechanistic basis for its protective effects.[167]

HUMAN EVIDENCE OF HYPOTHERMIA PROTECTION

Evidence that profound reduction of brain temperature can reduce injury resulting from prolonged intervals of ischemia seems strong. Perhaps the most convincing example was provided by Silverberg and coworkers, who reported that adults undergoing cardiopulmonary bypass for cerebral aneurysm clipping were capable of sustaining up to 1 h of circulatory arrest when core temperature was reduced to approximately 20°C.[168]

Although an extension from laboratory models to human efficacy for mild or moderate hypothermia may seem intuitive, it is not that simple. For example, there is not uniform agreement that even deep hypothermia is of value in cardiac surgery where considerable experience already has been had. The incidence of frank stroke was not different in a population of 1732 patients randomized to either "warm" (core temperature, 33° to 37°C) or "cold" (25° to 30°C) groups during coronary artery bypass grafting.[169] Even if hypothermia is efficacious, other factors involved with the surgical technique may have overshadowing importance such as the use of cardiac standstill versus low-flow bypass in pediatric heart surgery.[170] No data exist with respect to neurosurgical procedures, but it seems obvious that hypothermia will not protect against a variety of iatrogenic events including excision of an eloquent area of the brain. However, of greatest relevance to the use of mild hypothermia in the neurosurgical patient were three reports made almost simultaneously in 1993. All three studies were only preliminary trials because of small sample size. Nevertheless, either a clear benefit or a trend toward benefit was observed in patients being rendered mildly hypothermic in the acute phase after head injury.[171–173]

Until studies are performed that examine outcome in neurosurgical patients the clinician must decide to use mild intraoperative hypothermia in the presence of sound animal evidence for efficacy but in the absence of direct human data to support that practice. Fortunately, as far as it is known, the risk associated with use of mild hypothermia is small. In a recent poll taken from members of the Society of Neurosurgical Anesthesia and Critical Care, 40 percent of clinicians practiced induced hypothermia in patients undergoing cerebral aneurysm surgery.[174]

PRACTICAL CONSIDERATIONS FOR HYPOTHERMIA PROTECTION

If one accepts that mild hypothermia is indicated in either the intraoperative period or intensive care environment, then several questions regarding the method of cooling and monitoring of temperature arise. For example, during craniotomy, the brain is differentially exposed to ambient temperature. Despite core normothermia, some regions of the brain may undergo substantial cooling while other regions will not. Because it is difficult to define exactly which regions are at greatest risk (i.e., tissue under a retractor versus tissue distal to a cerebral artery potentially undergoing occlusion), it is virtually impossible to use core temperature to accurately define ideal conditions for specific tissue at risk. Some work has been done to relate brain temperature to core temperature, but most data are derived from the cardiopulmonary bypass literature. For example, Stone and colleagues directly measured cortical surface temperature during cooling and rewarming for circulatory arrest in cerebral aneurysm surgery.[175] Temperature from other measurement sites (e.g., nasopharynx, tympanic membrane, etc.) often varied by 2° to 3°C from brain temperature during various stages of cooling and rewarming. Although such differences might be negligible during profound hypothermia, when mild hypothermia is in question, such errors constitute the full therapeutic range. Others have examined the effects of various methods of cooling on brain temperatures of patients in intensive care units. Intraventricular thermistors were used to compare brain temperature against rectal temperature.[176] During normothermia, rectal temperature underestimated brain temperature by as much as 2° to 3°C although most often values were within 0.5°C. When attempts were made to specifically reduce brain temperature to 34°C, rectal temperature values (while tracking brain temperature) were often at variance from the brain by 1° to 2°C.[176] The same study also showed that brain temperature in the comatose patient was surprisingly resistant to efforts of cooling and that only intensive total body surface cooling combined with pharmacologic therapy was effective in achieving that result. These data would suggest a role for either intracranial pressure monitors or ventriculostomy drains with incorporated thermistors to be made commercially available if induced hypothermia is to become routine practice and if maximal efficacy is desired.

With respect to craniotomy, it therefore remains to be decided what end point is ideal for induced hypothermia. An additional concern in the patient undergoing craniotomy is the practicality of cooling and rewarming in an interval of only several hours. One investigation has examined this practice and found that indeed it is feasible to achieve core temperatures of about 34°C but that full rewarming to normothermia before emergence from anesthesia is unlikely.[177] As expected, rewarming was most easily accomplished in adult patients with a low body surface area. Overall, a rewarming rate of 0.7 ± 0.6°C/h was obtained using standard surface rewarming techniques.

Mild hypothermia is not known to be associated with the life-threatening complications found with deep hypothermia (e.g., coagulopathy, arrhythmia). Nevertheless, several factors have potential relevance to patient outcome and may influence the decision whether to use this technique. During emergence from anesthesia, myocardial ischemia may occur in patients who develop shivering in response to incomplete recovery to normothermia. To date, this has not been associated with an increased incidence of myocardial infarction. However, the incidence of electrocardiographic ischemic changes is nearly tripled when peripheral vascular patients are allowed to begin recovery from anesthesia with core temperatures less than 34.5°C.[178] Follow-up work in a similar patient population has shown that hypothermic patients exhibit greater peripheral vasoconstriction, increased norepinephrine concentrations, and higher blood pressures in the early postoperative period.[179]

Mild hypothermia may also alter the dose of anesthetic required. Volatile anesthetic MAC is known to decrease with decreases in temperature.[180] The fall in MAC with temperature has been shown to be rectilinear over the range of 39° to 20°C in the goat. At 20°C, hypothermia provides a sufficient state of anesthesia in and of itself.[181] However, it is unlikely that the effect on MAC is clinically relevant at temperatures of 33° to 35°C. In contrast, the MAC for nitrous oxide appears largely resistant to the effects of body temperature.[182]

The duration of action of muscle relaxants is likely to be increased by mild hypothermia. For example a twofold increase in the duration of action of vecuronium has been documented when body temperature is reduced from 36.8° to 34.4°C.[183] The cause for this is unknown although it is clear that it is not attributable to changes in a plasma concentration-effect relationship.[184] At the same time, neostigmine-induced reversal of neuromuscular blockade may be enhanced at lower temperatures.[185]

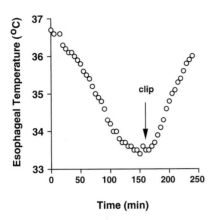

Figure 18-8 Example of intraoperative esophageal temperature profile during induced hypothermia and rewarming in a patient undergoing cerebral aneurysm clipping.

Three concerns remain for complications from induced mild hypothermia. First, it is well known that significant coagulopathies become manifest at temperatures less than 30°C. However, within the range of mild hypothermia, clinical evidence of coagulopathies in neurosurgical patients has been absent.[171–173,186] Second, there is some concern that mild hypothermia may suppress the immune system, allowing a greater chance of infection. Although animal evidence supports the contention that hypothermia during anesthesia may increase risk of dermal wound infection,[187] an increase in infections was not noted in any of the three trials of mild hypothermia in head-injured patients.[171–173] Finally, there is concern that rapid intraoperative rewarming may increase the risk of thermal injury to the patient. Indeed, burns from warming devices used during anesthesia constitute about 1 percent of anesthesia malpractice claims in the United States.[188] These cases were not those that used induced hypothermia and active rewarming but instead were simply those where an attempt was being made to maintain normothermia. Most of these injuries were attributable to placing heated saline bottles adjacent to the skin.

The short interval between completion of the high-risk phase of a neurosurgical procedure (e.g., temporary vascular occlusion during aneurysm clipping) and emergence from anesthesia requires that aggressive rewarming techniques be used (Fig. 18-8). The most appropriate approach to rewarming from induced hypothermia has not yet been defined. However, it seems reasonable that the simultaneous use of multiple heating devices including warmed intravenous fluid, forced air heating blankets, circulating warmed water blankets, and heated humidified inspiratory gases should be efficacious, but require the temperature of no single device to increase to the level where the risk of thermal injury is present.

Hyperthermia

Another series of laboratory-based observations have been made in recent years, which have relevance to intraoperative neuroprotection. Hyperthermia causes adverse effects on both pathophysiologic processes as well as histologic/neurologic outcome from brain ischemia or trauma. The first observation was made by Busto and colleagues who showed in the rat that increasing brain temperature from 36° to 39°C during global ischemia caused an approximate 50 percent increase in neuronal injury.[143] This observation has been repeated by others.[189] Perhaps the most convincing data regarding global ischemia come from a canine study conducted by Wass and coworkers.[190] Dogs were subjected to transient global ischemia with brain temperature held at 37.0°, 38.0°, or 39.0°C. Normothermic animals (37.0°C) were left essentially neurologically normal by the ischemic insult. In contrast, hyperthermic animals (39.0°C) were either comatose or died.

With respect to focal ischemia a similar pattern emerges. Infarct volumes in rats undergoing transient middle cerebral artery occlusion were almost tripled when brain temperature was increased from 37.0° to 40.0°C.[167] Work in our own laboratory has demonstrated that an increase in brain temperature by as little as 1.2°C from normothermic values is sufficient to double the size of the resultant infarct (Fig. 18-9).[111]

The mechanistic basis for this potent adverse effect of hyperthermia is not entirely worked out, but some clues have been provided. Glutamate release in the penumbra of a rat focal ischemic lesion is increased by about tenfold when brain temperature is increased

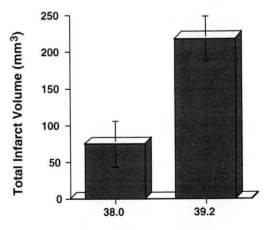

Figure 18-9 Total infarct volumes (mean ± SEM) in normothermic (38.0°C) or hyperthermic (39.2°C) halothane-anesthetized rats after 90 min of MCAO and a 96-h reperfusion interval. (Reproduced with permission from Warner and coworkers.[111])

from 37.0° to 39.0°C.[191] The frequency of spontaneous depolarizations occurring in the ischemic penumbra is also markedly increased during mild hyperthermia. In both head injury and ischemia models, mild hyperthermia increases the rate of free radical formation.[164,165]

While debate continues regarding the efficacy and role for mild hypothermia as a strategy for intraoperative neuroprotection, there is little disagreement that mild hyperthermia presents an adverse challenge to the injured brain. It is imperative that hyperthermia be guarded against in the anesthetized patient at risk for ischemic complications.

References

1. Wells B, et al: Increased tolerance to cerebral ischemia produced by general anesthesia during temporary carotid occlusion. *Surgery* 1963; 54:216.

2. Goldstein A, et al: Increased tolerance to cerebral anoxia by pentobarbital. *Arch Int Pharmacodyn* 1966; 161:138.

3. Michenfelder J: The interdependency of cerebral function and metabolic effects following massive doses of thiopental in the dog. *Anesthesiology* 1974; 41:231.

4. Yatsu F, et al: Experimental brain ischemia: Protection from irreversible damage with a rapid acting barbiturate (methohexital). *Stroke* 1972; 3:726.

5. Bleyaert A, et al: Thiopental amelioration of brain damage after global ischemia in monkeys. *Anesthesiology* 1978; 49:390.

6. Steen P, et al: No barbiturate protection in a dog model of complete cerebral ischemia. *Ann Neurol* 1979; 5:343.

7. Snyder B, et al: Failure of thiopental to modify global anoxic injury. *Stroke* 1979; 10:135.

8. Todd M, et al: The neurologic effects of thiopental therapy following experimental cardiac arrest in cats. *Anesthesiology* 1982; 57:76.

9. Gisvold S, et al: Thiopental treatment after global brain ischemia in pigtailed monkeys. *Anesthesiology* 1984; 60:88.

10. Michenfelder JD, Theye R: Cerebral protection by thiopental during hypoxia. *Anesthesiology* 1973; 39:510.

11. Hoff, J, et al: Barbiturate protection from cerebral infarction in primates. *Stroke* 1975; 6:28.

12. Corkill G, et al: Dose dependency of the post-insult protective effect of pentobarbital in the canine experimental stroke model. *Stroke* 1978; 9:10.

13. Warner D, et al: Lose-dose pentobarbital reduces focal ischemic infarct volume in a magnitude similar to burst suppression. *J Neurosurg Anesth* 1995; 7:303 (abstr).

14. Ward J, et al: Failure of prophylactic barbiturate coma in the treatment of severe head injury. *J Neurosurg* 1985; 62:383.

15. Brain Resuscitation Clinical I Study Group: Randomized clinical study of thiopental loading in comatose survivors of cardiac arrest. *N Engl J Med* 1986; 314:397.

16. Zaidan J, et al: Effect of thiopental on neurologic outcome following coronary artery bypass grafting. *Anesthesiology* 1991; 74:406.

17. Padayachee T, et al: The detection of microemboli in the middle cerebral artery during cardiopulmonary bypass: A transcranial Doppler ultrasound investigation using membrane and bubble oxygenators. *Ann Thorac Surg* 1987; 44:298.

18. Nussmeier N, et al: Neuropsychiatric complications after cardiopulmonary bypass: Cerebral protection by a barbiturate. *Anesthesiology* 1986; 64:165.

19. Michenfelder J: A valid determination of barbiturate-induced brain protection in man—At last. *Anesthesiology* 1986; 64:140.

20. Vandesteene A, et al: Effect of propofol on cerebral blood flow and metabolism in man. *Anaesthesia* 1988; 43:42.

21. Dam M, et al: The effects of propofol anesthesia on local cerebral glucose utilization in the rat. *Anesthesiology* 1990; 73:499.

22. Alkire M, et al: Cerebral metabolism during propofol anesthesia in humans studied with positron emission tomography. *Anesthesiology* 1995; 82:393.

23. Newman M, et al: Cerebral physiologic effects of burst suppression doses of propofol during nonpulsatile cardiopulmonary bypass. *Anesth Analg* 1995; 81:452.

24. Herregods L, et al: Effect of propofol on elevated intracranial pressure. Preliminary results. *Anaesthesia* 1988; 43:107.

25. Ravussin P, et al: Effect of propofol on cerebrospinal fluid pressure and cerebral perfusion pressure in patients undergoing craniotomy. *Anaesthesia* 1988; 43:37.

26. Ravussin P, et al: Propofol vs. thiopental-isoflurane for neurosurgical anesthesia: Comparison of hemodynamics, csf pressure, and recovery. *J Neurosurg Anesth* 1991; 2:85.

27. Todd M, et al: A prospective comparative trial of three anesthetics for supratentorial craniotomy: Fentanyl/propofol, isoflurane/N₂O, and fentanyl/N₂O. *Anesthesiology* 1993; 78:1005.

28. Orser B, et al: Inhibition by propofol (2,6 di-isopropylphenol) of the N-methyl-D-aspartate subtype of glutamate receptor in cultured hippocampal neurones. *Br J Pharmacol* 1995; 116:1761.

29. Globus M, et al: Excitotoxic index—A biochemical marker of selective vulnerability. *Neurosci Lett* 1991; 127:39.

30. Schwartz R, et al: Diazepam, given postischemia, protects selectively vulnerable neurons in the rat hippocampus and striatum. *J Neurosci* 1995; 15:529.

31. Kochs E, et al: The effects of propofol on brain electrical activity, neurologic outcome, and neuronal damage following incomplete ischemia in rats. *Anesthesiology* 1992; 76:245.

32. Ridenour T, et al: Comparative effects of propofol and halothane on outcome from temporary middle cerebral artery occlusion in the rat. *Anesthesiology* 1992; 76:807.

33. Warner D, et al: Halothane reduces focal ischemic injury in the rat when brain temperature is controlled. *Anesthesiology* 1995; 82:1237.

34. Milde L, et al: Cerebral functional, metabolic, and hemodynamic effects of etomidate in dogs. *Anesthesiology* 1985; 63:371.

35. Cold G, et al: CBF and CMRO₂ during continuous etomidate infusion supplemented with nitrous oxide and fentanyl in patients with supratentorial cerebral tumor. A dose response study. *Acta Anaesthesiol Scand* 1985; 29:490.

36. Cold G, et al: Changes in CMRO₂, EEG, and concentration of etomidate in serum and brain tissue during craniotomy with continuous etomidate. *Acta Anaesthsiol Scand* 1986; 30:159.

37. Renou A, et al: Cerebral blood flow and metabolism during etomidate anaesthesia in man. *Br J Anaesth* 1978; 50:1047.

38. Batjer H: Cerebral protective effects of etomidate—Experimental and clinical aspects. *Cerebrvasc Brain Metab Rev* 1993; 5:17.

39. Batjer H, et al: Use of etomidate, temporary arterial occlusion, and intraoperative angiography in surgical treatment of large and giant cerebral aneurysms. *J Neurosurg* 1988; 68:234.

40. Sano T, et al: A comparison of the cerebral protective effects of etomidate, thiopental, and isoflurane in a model of forebrain ischemia in the rat. *Anesth Analg* 1993; 76:990.

41. Patel P, et al: Etomidate reduces ischemia-induced glutamate release in the hippocampus in rats subjected to incomplete forebrain ischemia. *Anesth Analg* 1995; 80:933.

42. Guo J, et al: Limited protective effects of etomidate during brainstem ischemia in dogs. *J Neurosurg* 1995; 82:278.

43. Cole D, et al: The effect of thiopental, isoflurane, and etomidate on focal cerebral ischemic injury in rats. *J Neurosurg Anesth* 1993; 5:285 (abstr).

44. Cunitz G, et al: Comparative investigations on the influence of etomidate thiopentone and methohexitone on the intracranial pressure of the patient. *Anaesthesia* 1978; 27:64.

45. Moss E, et al: Effect on etomidate on intracranial pressure and cerebral perfusion pressure. *Br J Anaesth* 1979; 51:347.

46. Modica P, Tempelhoff R: Intracranial pressure during induction of anaesthesia and tracheal intubation with etomidate-induced EEG burst suppression. *Can J Anaesth* 1992; 39:236.

47. Fragen R, et al: Effects of etomidate on hormonal responses to surgical stress. *Anesthesiology* 1984; 61:652.

48. Levy M, et al: Propylene glycol toxicity following continuous etomidate infusion for the control of refractory cerebral edema. *Neurosurgery* 1995; 37:393.

49. Michenfelder J, Theye R: Effects of fentanyl, droperidol, and innovar on canine cerebral metabolism and blood flow. *Br J Anaesth* 1971; 43:630.

50. Moss E, et al: Effects of fentanyl on intracranial pressure and cerebral perfusion pressure during hypocapnia. *Br J Anaesth* 1978; 50:779.

51. Safo Y, et al: Effects of fentanyl on local cerebral blood flow in the rat. *Acta Anaesthesiol Scand* 1985; 29:594.

52. Keykhah M, et al: Effects of sufentanil on cerebral blood flow and oxygen consumption. *Anesthesiology* 1982; 57:A248.

53. Shupak R, et al: High dose sufentanil vs fentanyl anesthesia in neurosurgery. *Anesthesiology* 1982; 57:A350.

54. Marx W, et al: Sufentanil, alfentanil, and fentanyl: Impact on cerebrospinal fluid pressure in patients with brain tumors. *J Neurosurg Anesth* 1989; 1:3.

55. Weinstabl C, et al: Effect of sufentanil on intracranial pressure in neurosurgical patients. *Anaesthesia* 1991; 40:837.

56. Mayer N, et al: Impact of sufentanil on intracranial dynamics in neurosurgical ICU patients. *Anesthesiology* 1989; 71:A1138.

57. Herrick I, et al: Effects of fentanyl, sufentanil, and alfentanil on brain retractor pressure. *Anesth Analg* 1991; 72:359.

58. Markovitz B, et al: Effects of alfentanil on intracranial pressure in children undergoing ventriculoperitoneal shunt revision. *Anesthesiology* 1992; 76:71.

59. Moss E: Alfentanil increases intracranial pressure when intracranial compliance is low. *Anaesthesia* 1992; 47:134.

60. Hanowell L, et al: Alfentanil administered prior to endotracheal suctioning reduces cerebral perfusion pressure. *J Neurosurg Anesth* 1993; 5:31.

61. Albanese J, et al: Sufentanil increases intracranial pressure in patients with head trauma. *Anesthesiology* 1993; 79:493.

62. Werner C, et al: Effects of sufentanil on cerebral hemodynamics and intracranial pressure in patients with brain injury. *Anesthesiology* 1995; 83:721.

63. Hamilton A, et al: Contrasting actions of naloxone in experimental spinal cord trauma and cerebral ischemia: A review. *Neurosurgery* 1985; 17:845.

64. Chugani H, et al: Opioid-induced epileptogenic phenomena: Anatomical, behavioral, and electroencephalographic features. *Ann Neurol* 1984; 15:361.

65. Kofke W, et al: Alfentanil-induced hypermetabolism, seizure, and histopathology in rat brain. *Anesth Analg* 1992; 75:953.

66. Tommasino C, et al: Fentanyl-induced seizures activate subcortical brain metabolism. *Anesthesiology* 1984; 60:283.

67. Cole D, et al: Halothane, fentanyl/nitrous oxide, and spinal lidocaine protect against spinal cord injury in the rat. *Anesthesiology* 1989; 70:967.

68. List W, et al: Increased cerebrospinal fluid pressure after ketamine. *Anesthesiology* 1972; 36:98.

69. Thomson A, et al: An *N*-methylaspartate receptor-mediated synapse in rat cerebral cortex: A site of action of ketamine? *Nature* 1985; 313:479.

70. Yamamura T, et al: Is the site of action of ketamine anesthesia the *N*-methyl-D-aspartate receptor? *Anesthesiology* 1990; 72:704.

71. Irifune M, et al: Ketamine-induced anesthesia involves the *N*-methyl-D-aspartate receptor-channel complex in mice. *Brain Res* 1992; 596:1.

72. Park C, et al: Focal cerebral ischaemia in the cat: Treatment with the glutamate antagonist MK-801 after induction of ischaemia. *J Cereb Blood Flow Metabol* 1988; 8:757.

73. Church J, et al: The neuroprotective effect of ketamine and MK-801 after transient cerebral ischemia in rats. *Anesthesiology* 1988; 69:702.

74. Hoffman W, et al: Ketamine decreases plasma catecholamines and improves outcome from incomplete cerebral ischemia in rats. *Anesthesiology* 1992; 76:755.

75. Jensen M, Auer R: Ketamine fails to protect against ischaemic neuronal necrosis in the rat. *Br J Anaesth* 1988; 61:206.

76. Church J, Zeman S: Ketamine promotes hippocampal CA1 pyramidal neuron loss after a short-duration ischemic insult in rats. *Neurosci Letters* 1991; 123:65.

77. Ridenour T, et al: Effects of ketamine on outcome from temporary middle cerebral artery occlusoin in the spontaneously hypertensive rat. *Brain Res* 1991; 565:116.

78. Smith D, et al: Magnesium and ketamine attenuate cognitive dysfunction following experimental brain injury. *Neurosci Lett* 1993; 157:211.

79. Shapira Y, et al: Ketamine alters calcium and magnesium in brain tissue following experimental head trauma in rats. *J Cereb Blood Flow Metab* 1993; 13:962.

80. Shapira Y, et al: Therapeutic time window and dose response of the beneficial effects of ketamine in experimental head injury. *Stroke* 1994; 25:1637.

81. Grissom T, et al: The effect of anesthetics on neurologic outcome during the recovery period of spinal cord injury in rats. *Anesth Analg* 1994; 79:66.

82. Schapira M: Evolution of anesthesia for neurosurgery. *N Y State J Med* 1964; 1301.

83. Lundberg N: Continuous recording and control of ventricular fluid pressure in neurosurgical practice. *Acta Psychiatr Scand* 1960; 36(suppl) 149:1.

84. Jennett W, et al: The effect of halothane on intracranial pressure in cerebral tumors: Report of two cases. *J Neurosurg* 1967; 26:270.

85. Adams R, et al: Halothane, hypocapnia, and cerebrospinal fluid pressure in neurosurgery. *Anesthesiology* 1972; 37:510.

86. Smith A, et al: Barbiturate protection in acute focal cerebral ischemia. *Stroke* 1974; 5:1.

87. Michenfelder J, Theye R: In vivo toxic effects of halothane on canine cerebral metabolic pathways. *Am J Physiol* 1975; 229:1050.

88. Aronstam R, et al: Volatile anesthetics inhibit NMDA-stimulated ^{45}Ca uptake by rat brain microvesicles. *Neurochem Res* 1994; 19:1515.

89. Yang J, Zorumski C: Effects of isoflurane on *N*-methyl-D-aspartate gated ion channels in cultured rat hippocampal neurons. *Ann N Y Acad Sci* 1991; 625:287.

90. Ishimaru M, et al: Halothane prevents MK-801 neurotoxicity in the rat cingulate cortex. *Neurosci Lett* 1995; 193:1.

91. Baughman V, Hoffman W: Neurologic outcome in rats following incomplete cerebral ischemia during halothane, isoflurane, or N$_2$O. *Anesthesiology* 1988; 69:192.

92. Adams R, et al: Isoflurane and cerebrospinal fluid pressure in neurosurgical patients. *Anesthesiology* 1981; 54:97.

93. Drummond J, et al: A comparison of the direct cerebral vasodi-

lating potencies of halothane and isoflurane in the New Zealand white rabbit. *Anesthesiology* 1986; 65:462.

94. Jensen N, et al: A comparison of the vasodilating effects of halothane and isoflurane on the isolated rabbit basilar artery with and without intact endothelium. *Anesthesiology* 1992; 76:624.

95. Newberg L, et al: The cerebral metabolic effects of isoflurane at and above concentrations that suppress cortical electrical activity. *Anesthesiology* 1983; 59:23.

96. Theye R, Michenfelder J: The effect of halothane on canine cerebral metabolism. *Anesthesiology* 1968; 29:1113.

97. Newberg L, Michenfelder J: Cerebral protection by isoflurane during hypoxemia or ischemia. *Anesthesiology* 1983; 59:29.

98. Nehls D, et al: A comparison of the cerebral protective effects of isoflurane and barbiturates during temporary focal ischemia in primates. *Anesthesiology* 1987; 66:453.

99. Warner D, et al: Reversible focal ischemia in the rat: Effects of halothane, isoflurane and methohexital anesthesia. *J Cereb Blood Flow Metab* 1991; 11:794.

100. Gelb A, et al: Primate brain tolerance to temporary focal cerebral ischemia during isoflurane- or sodium nitroprusside-induced hypotension. *Anesthesiology* 1989; 70:678.

101. Michenfelder J, et al: Isoflurane when compared to enflurane and halothane decreases the frequency of cerebral ischemia during carotid endarterectomy. *Anesthesiology* 1987; 67:336.

102. Messick JJ, et al: Correlatoin of regional cerebral blood flow (rCBF) with EEG changes during isoflurane anesthesia for carotid endarterectomy: Critical rCBF. *Anesthesiology* 1987; 66:344.

103. Verhaegen M, et al: A comparison of cerebral ischemic flow thresholds during halothane/N_2O and isoflurane/N_2O anesthesia in rats. *Anesthesiology* 1992; 76:743.

104. Bickler P, et al: Effects of isoflurane and hypothermia on glutamate receptor-mediated calcium influx in brain slices. *Anesthesiology* 1994; 81:1461.

105. Scheller M, et al: Effects of sevoflurane on cerebral blood flow, cerebral metabolic rate for oxygen, intracranial pressure, and the electroencephalogram are similar to those of isoflurane in the rabbit. *Anesthesiology* 1988; 68:548.

106. Scheller M, et al: Cerebral effects of sevoflurane in the dog: Comparison with isoflurane and enflurane. *Br J Anaesth* 1990; 65:388.

107. Kitaguchi K, et al: Effects of sevoflurane on cerebral circulation and metabolism in patients with ischemic cerebrovascular disease. *Anesthesiology* 1993; 79:704.

108. Takahashi H, et al: Sevoflurane does not increase intracranial pressure in hyperventilated dogs. *Br J Anaesth* 1993; 71:551.

109. Fujibayashi T, et al: Brain energy metabolism and blood flow during sevoflurane and halothane anesthesia: Effects of hypocapnia and blood pressure fluctuations. *Acta Anaesthesiol Scand* 1993; 37:806.

110. Osawa M, et al: Effects of sevoflurane on central nervous system electrical activity in cats. *Anesth Analg* 1994; 79:52.

111. Warner D, et al: Sevoflurane and halothane reduce focal ischemic brain damage in the rat: Possible influence on thermoregulation. *Anesthesiology* 1993; 79:985.

112. Smiley R, et al: Desflurane and isoflurane in surgical patients: Comparison of emergence time. *Anesthesiology* 1991; 74:425.

113. Bennett J, et al: Elderly patients recover more rapidly from desflurane than from isoflurane anesthesia. *J Clin Anesth* 1992; 4:378.

114. Muzzi D, et al: The effect of desflurane on cerebrospinal fluid pressure in neurosurgical patients. *J Neurosurg Anesth* 1990; 2:214.

115. Muzzi D, et al: The effect of desflurane and isoflurane on cerebrospinal fluid pressure in humans with supratentorial mass lesions. *Anesthesiology* 1992; 76:720.

116. Artru A: Rate of CSF formation, resistance to reabsorption of CSF, brain tissue water content and electroencephalogram during desflurane anesthesia in dogs. *J Neurosurg Anesth* 1993; 5:297(abstr).

117. Lutz L, et al: The cerebral functional, metabolic, and hemodynamic effects of desflurane in dogs. *Anesthesiology* 1990; 73:125.

118. Rampil I, et al: The electroencephalographic effects of desflurane in humans. *Anesthesiology* 1991; 74:434.

119. Rampil I, et al: No EEG evidence of acute tolerance to desflurane in swine. *Anesthesiology* 1991; 74:889.

120. Milde L, Milde J: The cerebvral and systemic hemodynamic and metabolic effects of desflurane-induced hypotension in dogs. *Anesthesiology* 1991; 74:513.

121. Ornstein E, et al: Desflurane and isoflurane have similar effects on cerebral blood flow in patients with intracranial mass lesions. *Anesthesiology* 1993; 79:498.

122. Artru A; Nitrous oxide plays a direct role in the development of tension pneumocephalus intraoperatively. *Anesthesiology* 1982; 57:59.

123. Raggio J, et al: Expanding pneumocephalus due to nitrous oxide anesthesia: Case report. *Neurosurgery* 1979; 4:261.

124. Reasoner D, et al: The incidence of pneumocephalus after supratentorial craniotomy—Observations on the disappearance of intracranial air. *Anesthesiology* 1994; 80:1008.

125. Henriksen H, Jorgensen P: The effect of nitrous oxide on intracranial pressure in patients with intracranial disorders. *Br J Anaesth* 1973; 45:485.

126. Domino K, et al: Effect of nitrous oxide on intracranial pressure after cranialdural closure in patients undergoing craniotomy. *Anesthesiology* 1992; 77:421.

127. Jung R, et al: Isoflurane and nitrous oxide—Comparative impact on cerebrospinal fluid pressure in patients with brain tumors. *Anesth Analg* 1992; 75:724.

128. Phirman J, Shapiro H: Modification of nitrous oxide-induced intracranial hypertension by prior induction of anesthesia. *Anesthesiology* 1977; 46:150.

129. Pelligrino D, et al: Nitrous oxide markedly increases cerebral cortical metabolic rate and blood flow in the goat. *Anesthesiology* 1984; 60:405.

130. Deutsch G, Samra S: Effects of nitrous oxide on global and regional cortical blood flow. *Stroke* 1990; 21:1293.

131. Hansen T, et al: Effects of nitrous oxide and volatile anesthetics on cerebral blood flow. *Br J Anaesth* 1989; 63:290.

132. Reasoner D, et al: Effects of nitrous oxide on cerebral metabolic rate in rats anaesthetized with isoflurane. *Br J Anaesth* 1990; 65:210.

133. Algotsson L, et al: Effects of nitrous oxide on cerebral haemodynamics and metabolism during isoflurane anaesthesia in man. *Acta Anaesthesiol Scand* 1992; 36:46.

134. Lam A, et al: Nitrous oxide-isoflurane anesthesia causes more cerebral vasodilation than an equipotent dose of isoflurane in humans. *Anesth Analg* 1994; 78:462.

135. Strebel S, et al: Nitrous oxide is a potent cerebrovasodilator in humans when added to isoflurane. A transcranial Doppler study. *Acta Anaesthesiol Scand* 1995; 39:653.

136. Baughman V, et al: The interaction of nitrous oxide and isoflurane with incomplete cerebral ischemia in the rat. *Anesthesiology* 1989; 70:767.

137. Warner D, et al: The effect of isoflurane on neuronal necrosis following near-complete forebrain ischemia in the rat. *Anesthesiology* 1986; 64:19.

138. Hartung J, Cottrell J: Nitrous oxide reduces thiopental-induced prolongation of survival in hypoxic and anoxic mice. *Anesth Analg* 1987; 66:47.

139. Warner D, et al: Nitrous oxide does not alter infarct volume in rats undergoing reversible middle cerebral artery occlusion. *Anesthesiology* 1990; 73:686.

140. Onesti S, et al: Transient hypothermia reduces focal ischemic brain damage in the rat. *Neurosurgery* 1991; 29:369.

141. Ridenour T, et al: Mild hypothermia reduces infarct size resulting from temporary but not permanent focal ischemia in the rat. *Stroke* 1992; 23:733.

142. Chen H, et al: The effect of hypothermia on transient middle cerebral artery occlusion in the rat. *J Cereb Blood Flow Metab* 1992; 12:621.

143. Busto R, et al: Small differences in intraischemic brain temperature critically determine the extent of neuronal injury. *J Cereb Blood Flow Metabol* 1987; 7:729.

144. Sano T, et al: A comparison of the cerebral protective effects of isoflurane and mild hypothermia in a model of incomplete forebrain ischemia in the rat. *Anesthesiology* 1992; 76:221.

145. Clifton G, et al: Marked protection by moderate hypothermia after experimental traumatic brain injury. *J Cereb Blood Flow Metab* 1991; 11:114.

146. Dietrich W, et al: Post-traumatic brain hypothermia reduces histopathological damage following concussive brain injury in the rat. *Acta Neuropathol* 1994; 87:250.

147. Lundgren J, et al: Hyperthermia aggravates and hypothermia ameliorates epileptic brain damage. *Exp Brain Res* 1994; 99:43.

148. Busto R, et al: Postischemic moderate hypothermia inhibits CA1 hippocampal ischemic neuronal injury. *Neurosci Lett* 1989; 101:299.

149. Coimbra C, Wieloch T: Moderate hypothermia mitigates neuronal damage in the rat brain when initiated several hours following transient cerebral ischemia. *Acta Neuropathol* 1994; 87:325.

150. Dietrich W, et al: Intraischemic but not postischemic brain hypothermia protects chronically following global forebrain ischemia in rats. *J Cereb Blood Flow Metabol* 1993; 13:541.

151. Colbourne F, Corbett D: Delayed and prolonged post-ischemic hypothermia is neuroprotective in the gerbil. *Brain Res* 1994; 654:265.

152. Colbourne F, Corbett D: Delayed postischemic hypothermia: A six month survival study using behavioral and histologic assessments of neuroprotection. *J Neurosci* 1995; 15:7250.

153. Busto R, et al: Effect of mild hypothermia on ischemia-induced release of neurotransmitters and free fatty acids in rat brain. *Stroke* 1989; 20:904.

154. Patel P, et al: Differential temperature sensitivity of ischemia-induced glutamate release and eicosanoid production in rats. *Brain Res* 1994; 650:205.

155. Illievich U, et al: Effects of hypothermia or anesthetics on hippocampal glutamate and glycine concentrations after repeated transient global cerebral ischemia. *Anesthesiology* 1994; 80:177.

156. Arai H, et al: Effect of low temperature on glutamate-induced intracellular calcium accumulation and cell death in cultured hippocampal neurons. *Neurosci Lett* 1993; 163:132.

157. Bergstedt K, et al: Postischaemic changes in protein synthesis in the rat brain: Effects of hypothermia. *Exp Brain Res* 1993; 95:91.

158. Widmann R, et al: Protective effect of hypothermia on hippocampal injury after 30 minutes of forebrain ischemia in rats is mediated by postischemic recovery of protein synthesis. *J Neurochem* 1993; 61:200.

159. Busto R, et al: Regional alterations of protein kinase C activity following transient cerebral ischemia: Effects of intraischemic brain temperature modulation. *J Neurochem* 1994; 63:1095.

160. Kader A, et al: Effect of mild hypothermia on nitric oxide synthesis during focal cerebral ischemia. *Neurosurgery* 1994; 35:272.

161. Dawson D: Nitric oxide and focal cerebral ischemia: Multiplicity of actions and diverse outcome. *Cerebrovasc Brain Metab Rev* 1994; 6:299.

162. Baiping L, et al: Effect of moderate hypothermia on lipid peroxidation in canine brain tissue after cardiac arrest and resuscitation. *Stroke* 1994; 25:147.

163. Karibe H, et al: Mild intraischemic hypothermia suppresses consumption of endogenous antioxidants after temporary focal ischemia in rats. *Brain Res* 1994; 649:12.

164. Globus M, et al: Detection of free radical activity during transient global ischemia and recirculation: Effects of intraischemic brain temperature modulation. *J Neurochem* 1995; 65:1250.

165. Globus M, et al: Glutamate release and free radical production following brain injury: Effects of posttraumatic hypothermia. *J Neurochem* 1995; 65:1704.

166. Back T, et al: Cortical negative DC deflections following middle cerebral artery occlusion and KCl-induced spreading depression: Effect on blood flow, tissue oxygenation, and electroencephalogram. *J Cereb Blood Flow Metab* 1994; 14:12.

167. Chen Q, et al: Temperature modulation of cerebral depolarization during focal cerebral ischemia in rats: Correlation with ischemic injury. *J Cereb Blood Flow Metab* 1993; 13:389.

168. Silverberg G, et al: Hypothermia and cardiac arrest in the treatment of giant aneurysms of the cerebral circulation and hemangioblastoma of the medulla. *J Neurosurg* 1981; 55:337.

169. Naylor C, et al: Randomised trial of normothermic versus hypothermic coronary bypass surgery. *Lancet* 1994; 343:559.

170. Bellinger D, et al: Developmental and neurologic status of children after heart surgery with hypothermic circulatory arrest or low-flow cardiopulmonary bypass. *N Engl J Med* 1995; 332:549.

171. Clifton G, et al: A phase II study of moderate hypothermia in severe brain injury. *J Neurotrauma* 1993; 10:263.

172. Marion D, et al: The use of moderate therapeutic hypothermia for patients with severe head injuries: A preliminary report. *J Neurosurg* 1993; 79:354.

173. Shiozaki T, et al: Effect of mild hypothermia on uncontrollable intracranial hypertension after severe head injury. *J Neurosurg* 1993; 79:363.

174. Craen R, et al: Current anesthetic practices and use of brain protective therapies for cerebral aneurysm surgery at 41 North American centers. *J Neurosurg Anesth* 1994; 6:303(abstr).

175. Stone J, et al: Do standard monitoring sites reflect true brain temperature when profound hypothermia is rapidly induced and reversed? *Anesthesiology* 1995; 82:344.

176. Mellergård P, Nordström C: Intracerebral temperature in neurosurgical patients. *Neurosurgery* 1991; 28:709.

177. Baker K, et al: Deliberate mild intraoperative hypothermia for craniotomy. *Anesthesiology* 1994; 81:361.

178. Frank S, et al: Unintentional hypothermia is associated with postoperative myocardial ischemia. *Anesthesiology* 1993; 78:468.

179. Frank S, et al: The catecholamine, cortisol, and hemodynamic responses to mild perioperative hypothermia: A randomized clinical trial. *Anesthesiology* 1995; 82:83.

180. Vitez T, et al: Effects of hypothermia on halothane MAC and isoflurane MAC in the rat. *Anesthesiology* 1974; 41:80.

181. Antognini J: Hypothermia eliminates isoflurane requirements at 20°C. *Anesthesiology* 1993; 78:1152.

182. Antognini J, et al: Hypothermia minimally decreases nitrous oxide anesthetic requirements. *Anesth Analg* 1994; 79:980.

183. Heier T, et al: Mild intraoperative hypothermia increases duration of action and spontaneous recovery of vecuronium blockade during nitrous oxide-isoflurane anesthesia in humans. *Anesthesiology* 1991; 74:815.

184. Heier T, et al: Mild intraoperative hypothermia does not change the pharmacodynamics (concentration-effect relationship) of vecuronium in humans. *Anesth Analg* 1994; 78:973.

185. Aziz L, et al: Effect of hypothermia on the in vitro potencies of neuromuscular blocking agents and on their antagonism by neostigmine. *Br J Anaesth* 1994; 73:662.

186. Resnick D, et al: The effect of hypothermia on the incidence of delayed traumatic intracerebral hemorrhage. *Neurosurgery* 1994; 34:252.

187. Sheffield C, et al: Mild hypothermia during isoflurane anesthesia decreases resistance to *E. coli* dermal infection in guinea pigs. *Acta Anaesthesiol Scand* 1994; 38:201.

188. Cheney F, et al: Burns from warming devices in anesthesia: A closed claims analysis. *Anesthesiology* 1994; 80:806.

189. Minamisawa H, et al: The effect of mild hyperthermia and hypothermia on brain damage following 5, 10, and 15 minutes of forebrain ischemia. *Ann Neurol* 1990; 28:26.

190. Wass C, et al: Temperature changes of ≥1 degree Celcius alter functional neurologic outcome and histopathology in a canine model of complete cerebral ischemia. *Anesthesiology* 1995; 83:325.

191. Takagi K, et al: Effect of hyperthermia on glutamate release in ischemic penumbra after middle cerebral artery occlusion in rats. *Am J Physiol* 1994; 266:H1770.

Chapter 19
SEIZURES AND EPILEPSY
LEON S. DURE IV

The physical event defined as a seizure may take many forms, from the well-recognized generalized tonic-clonic convulsion to more subtle changes in behavior such as staring or simple behavior arrest. Seizures taken as a whole may affect up to 10 percent of people at some time of life, and thus are a problem with which physicians, particularly anesthesiologists, are familiar. The remarkable variety of expression is matched only by the myriad of causes associated with ictal events. Despite the multitude of causes and phenotypes for seizures, the common feature is a paroxysmal disturbance of central nervous system synchrony as determined by neurophysiologic examination of cortical activity. This chapter discusses the phenomenology and classification of seizures and epilepsy, as well as some of the more recent therapeutic issues. The bulk of this chapter, however, is comprised of a thorough examination of the neurobiology of seizures, with an emphasis on laboratory models, to provide an understanding of the physiologic underpinnings of ictal phenomena.

Seizure Classification

Before beginning a discussion of the various features associated with seizures, it is important to understand the nosology of seizure types. *Seizures* must be differentiated from *epilepsy*, in that the one is an event and the other is a process. Although a hypoglycemic seizure may have the same clinical presentation as a seizure

caused by idiopathic generalized epilepsy, the causes are presumed to be distinct. In an attempt to classify seizure types on the basis of phenomenology, in 1981 the Commission on Classification and Terminology of the International League Against Epilepsy developed a scheme based on clinical and electrographic determinants (Fig. 19-1), which broadly separated seizures into the categories of partial, generalized, and unclassified.[1] This scheme was generally useful because a distinction between seizures according to the extent of brain involvement provided a framework for the evaluation of etiology and pathogenesis of epilepsy.[2] However, a revised classification was developed in 1989 to better accommodate the clinical phenotypes of epilepsy,[1] which characterizes patients according to epileptic syndromes (Fig. 19-2). By assigning patients to specific syndrome categories, clinical considerations concerning pharmacologic or surgical interventions could be better and more uniformly addressed.[3,4] This revision of classification of seizures and epilepsies represents a marked shift from the purely descriptive to a more pathophysiologic orientation for the understanding of epilepsy. Although more mechanistically organized, the classification criteria of 1989, as was true for the previous scheme, is crucially dependent on the accurate characterization of the patient in question, and it has been suggested that a thorough evaluation is needed to effectively classify individuals with epilepsy.[5]

Epidemiology and Genetics of Seizures

Seizures are a common problem faced by physicians, and epidemiologic studies are vital to understanding the magnitude of the problem. For population-based studies, the most reliable estimates of incidence (the number of new occurrences per unit time in a population) and prevalence (the number of occurrences in a population at a specific time) require that the cohort studied be representative of the population as a whole and that there are no demographic or reporting biases.[6] Some of the seminal epidemiologic surveys of seizures and epilepsy have been performed in Rochester, Minnesota where there is an estimated incidence of 30 to 50/100,000 person-years for epilepsy, a prevalence of 5 to 8/1000 persons, and a lifetime risk of 10 percent for seizures.[7] Age-related estimates of etiology for seizures indicate a prominence of febrile convulsions in the young, with a gradual increase in the incidence of acute symptomatic seizures, idiopathic isolated seizures, and epilepsy.[7,8] In the few studies that exist for developing countries, the epidemiologic and causative factors differ markedly from those of industrialized nations.[9] Although the estimates for prevalence are roughly com-

I. Partial (focal, local) seizures
   A. Simple partial seizures (consciousness not impaired)
      1. With motor symptoms
      2. With somatosensory or special sensory symptoms
      3. With autonomic symptoms
      4. With psychic symptoms
   B. Complex partial seizures (with impaired consciousness)
      1. Beginning as simple partial seizures and progressing to impairment of consciousness
         a. With no other features
         b. With features as in A.1–4
         c. With automatisms
      2. With impairment of consciousness at onset
         a. With no other features
         b. With features as in A.1–4
         c. With automatisms
   C. Partial seizures secondarily generalized
II. Generalized seizures (convulsive or nonconvulsive)
   A. 1. Absence seizures
      2. Atypical absence seizures
   B. Myoclonic seizures
   C. Clonic seizures
   D. Tonic seizures
   E. Tonic-clonic seizures
   F. Atonic seizures
III. Unclassified epileptic seizures

Figure 19-1 Classification of epileptic seizures, International League Against Epilepsy Revision of 1981. (Reprinted with permission.)

parable in many countries, there are strikingly high figures in parts of Nigeria, Tanzania, and among isolated native tribes of Latin America of 20 to 40 epileptics per 1000 persons. Part of the reason for these high prevalences may relate to the relative lack of health care among some of these populations, but the characteristic geographic and cultural isolation of these groups could also reflect a genetic component of epilepsy.[10]

With the current explosion of knowledge in medical genetics and the concomitant development of techniques to explore the human genome, it has become possible to address the hypothesis of a genetic basis for epilepsy. Epidemiologic studies of the causative factors in unprovoked seizures indicate a 2.5-fold increased risk of epilepsy in first-degree relatives,[8,11] and an increased risk of inheritance from epileptic mothers compared with epileptic fathers.[12] In twin studies, concordance for idiopathic generalized epilepsy is 94.7 percent for monozygotic twins, compared with 15.4 percent for dizygotic twins.[13] The basis of these presumed familial tendencies toward epilepsy is as yet unknown, but the degree of risk conferred by heredity is consistent with a probable multifactorial mode of inheritance, perhaps involving a number of genes.

Some epileptic syndromes obey mendelian inheritance, are amenable to linkage analysis,[13–15] and provide a starting point for the elucidation of intrinsic causative factors for seizures. Benign familial neonatal convulsions is an autosomal dominant inherited entity charac-

terized by seizures occurring in the newborn period and resolving by 6 months of age; it has been linked to the long arm of chromosome 20 in a number of families. Progressive myoclonic epilepsy of the Unverricht-Lundborg type (PME or Baltic myoclonus) is transmitted in an autosomal recessive fashion and is a progressive neurodegenerative disorder with prominent seizures, including stimulus-sensitive myoclonus and generalized tonic-clonic seizures. PME has been linked to the long arm of chromosome 21. Other forms of PME, Lafora body disease and the myoclonic epilepsy associated with juvenile Gaucher's disease, do not map to the same locus.[16] The third epilepsy syndrome that has been mapped to a gene is juvenile myoclonic epilepsy (JME), a condition with onset in adolescence characterized by nonprogressive sporadic myoclonus and generalized seizures and linked to chromosome 6. For none of these three conditions is the gene product known, nor how these genes act to produce the clinical phenotype of seizures. Given that there is some clinical similarity between PME and JME, it has been hypothesized that other idiopathic generalized epilepsies such as childhood absence and early childhood myoclonic epilepsy should be investigated for linkage at loci on chromosomes 20 and 6, to determine if genetic heterogeneity is involved in the phenotypic variations of expression for these conditions.[17]

Another area of research in inherited diseases focuses on disorders of mitochondria. These intracellular organelles contain DNA used to express specific en-

1.0 Localization-related (focal, local, partial)
1.1 Idiopathic
   a. Benign childhood epilepsy with centro-temporal spikes
   b. Childhood epilepsy with occipital paroxysms
   c. Primary reading epilepsy
1.2 Symptomatic
   a. Arising from frontal lobes
   b. Arising from parietal lobes
   c. Arising from temporal lobes
   d. Arising from occipital lobes
   e. Arising from multiple lobes
   f. Locus of onset unknown
1.3 Cryptogenic (unknown if idiopathic or symptomatic)
2.0 Generalized
2.1 Idiopathic
   a. Benign familial neonatal convulsions
   b. Benign neonatal convulsions
   c. Benign myoclonic epilepsy of infancy
   d. Childhood absence epilepsy (pyknolepsy)
   e. Juvenile absence epilepsy
   f. Juvenile myoclonic epilepsy
   g. Epilepsy with grand mal (GTCS) on awakening
2.2 Cryptogenic or symptomatic
   a. West syndrome (infantile spasms)
   b. Lennox-Gastaut syndrome
   c. Epilepsy with myoclonic-astatic seizures
   d. Epilepsy with myoclonic absence
2.3 Symptomatic
2.3.1 Nonspecific etiology - Early myoclonic encephalopathy
2.3.2 Specific syndromes
3.0 Undetermined epilepsies
3.1 With generalized and focal seizures
   a. Neonatal seizures
   b. Severe myoclonic epilepsy in infancy
   c. Epilepsy with continuous spike-waves during slow wave sleep
   d. Acquired epileptic aphasia (Landau-Kleffner syndrome)
3.2 Without unequivocal generalized or focal features
4.0 Special syndromes
4.1 Situation-related seizures
   a. Febrile convulsions
   b. Isolated seizures or status epilepticus
   c. Seizures secondary to acute toxic or metabolic insult

Figure 19-2 Classification of epileptic syndromes, International League Against Epilepsy Revision of 1989. (Reprinted with permission.)

zymes, and they are crucial to normal metabolic activity and oxidative phosphorylation.[18] At least one mutation of mitochondrial DNA, a substitution in the tRNA^{Lys} gene, produces the syndrome of myoclonic epilepsy and ragged-red fibers.[19] Although the pathophysiology of these mutations in the causation of diseases is not yet fully understood, some of the features of mitochondropathies make them intriguing candidates for further investigation of the genetic basis of epilepsy. Because the mitochondrial genome is maternally inherited, mutations are more commonly expressed from mother to child. The greater risk of epilepsy in children of epileptic mothers[12] would make

such families attractive candidates for DNA analysis of the mitochondrial genome. The other characteristic of mitochondrial disorders germane to the heredity of epilepsy is the delayed onset. Mitochondria are susceptible to genomic mutations with increasing age,[20] and regional differences are evident in the appearance of these mutations within brain.[21] These findings could help to explain the appearance of "idiopathic" epilepsies later in life.

Laboratory studies of animals with genetically based electrographic and clinical seizures has been of immense value in the characterization and investigation of seizures.[22-25] Increased susceptibility to seizures has been described in dogs, cows, rodents, and chickens, among others.[26] From analyses of these animal models, a number of general principles have been determined, which are relevant to the consideration of the genetic basis of seizures in humans. First, abnormalities on different chromosomes may produce identical seizure phenotypes. Second, mice that are heterozygous for a mutation may show an intermediate phenotype, and homozygous mice with incomplete phenotypic expression also exhibit incomplete mutant gene expression. Third, cross-breeding experiments indicate that multiple genes may be involved in the expression of a mutation, as evidenced by incomplete phenotypes. These principles are important because they mirror what has been observed in human epileptic syndromes with a presumed genetic basis but variable expression.

Clinical Considerations

This section deals primarily with selected aspects of the diagnosis and management of patients with seizures or epilepsy. For more detailed discussions of some of these issues, see Chaps. 6, 21, and 24.

SEIZURE ETIOLOGY

When discussing the etiology of seizures, by definition idiopathic seizures and epileptic syndromes are excluded. Also, it is important to consider nonepileptic paroxysmal events that may be mistaken for seizures, such as syncope, hyperventilation, migrainous phenomenon, or cerebrovascular accident, and to rule out behavioral or psychiatric disturbances,[27,28] because 10 to 25 percent of patients referred to epilepsy centers have diagnoses other than seizures. Appropriate performance of a history and physical examination and judicious use of laboratory and other ancillary services can often rule out other paroxysmal conditions.[29]

Among definable causes of seizures, structural lesions in brain and drugs are two of the most commonly seen by neurologists, internists, and pediatricians.[30,31] In children and occasionally young adults, develop-

TABLE 19-1
The Causes of Seizures

Infant (0–2 years)	Paranatal hypoxia and ischemia
	Intracranial birth injury
	Acute infection
	Metabolic disturbances (hypoglycemia, hypocalcemia, hypomagnesemia, pyridoxine deficiency)
	Congenital malformation
	Genetic disorders
Child (2–12 years)	Idiopathic
	Acute infection
	Trauma
	Febrile convulsion
Adolescent (12–18 years)	Idiopathic
	Trauma
	Drug, alcohol withdrawal
	Arteriovenous malformations
Young adult (18–35 years)	Trauma
	Alcoholism
	Brain tumor
Older adult (>35 years)	Brain tumor
	Cerebrovascular disease
	Metabolic disorders (uremia, hepatic failure, electrolyte abnormality, hypoglycemia)
	Alcoholism

SOURCE: From Dichter MH: The epilepsies and convulsive disorders. In Wilson JD, et al (eds): *Harrison's Principles of Internal Medicine,* 12th ed. New York, McGraw-Hill, 1991:1968, with permission.

mental anomalies and neuronal migration disorders may give rise to seizures,[32] as do the sequelae of perinatal hypoxic-ischemic insults. The pathologic entity of mesial temporal sclerosis is detected either radiographically or in pathologic specimens in over 40 percent of cases in some series,[33,34] but the cause of this lesion is not known. Cerebrovascular accidents commonly cause seizures in adults and occasionally may present as status epilepticus.[35] The other major type of structural lesion producing seizures is neoplastic, which may account for over 15 pecent of seizures in adults.[36] Other, more rare conditions associated with seizures include the neurocutaneous syndromes[37] and metabolic and neurodegenerative syndromes.[38] A summary of the causes of seizures according to age groups can be seen in Table 19-1.

Although the risk of seizures from drugs is low,[39] the number of persons taking various medications makes drug-induced seizures a relatively frequent event. Seizures secondary to medication use may be a side effect of the agent itself, such as occurs with meperidine or radiologic contrast agents, or may relate to a propensity for seizures in a patient and a lowered seizure threshold. The list of drugs reported to have caused seizures is extensive and beyond the scope of this review; the reader is referred to the review of Garcia and

Alldredge.[31] A listing of the drugs used in the treatment of seizures together with the principal therapeutic indications and blood levels can be noted in Table 19-2.

ELECTROENCEPHALOGRAPHY

One of the most important tools for the investigation of seizures and epilepsy is the electroencephalogram (EEG). The EEG is performed by measuring electrical potentials over the scalp, or in rare instances, via electrodes placed intranasally or intracranially to sample specific brain regions. The potentials measured are actually summations of electrical activities in rather large areas of brain, but the use of multiple electrodes in various combinations allows for relatively precise location of abnormal brain activity. Although it has been estimated that almost 4 percent of nonepileptic patients will have an abnormal EEG,[40] the sensitivity of the EEG for the detection of abnormalities in the epileptic population is over 90 percent.[41]

In practice, the EEG seldom records a seizure in progress, but there are recognized patterns of electrical activity which, when coupled with a consistent clinical presentation, are strongly suggestive of an epileptic process. Furthermore, the use of sleep deprivation, photic stimulation, and long-term video monitoring have proven invaluable in the detection of EEG abnormalities.[41,42]

Given that clinical seizures are not often recorded, there has been emphasis on the study of subclinical or "larval" seizures. These paroxysmal electrical events are typically in evidence only on the EEG. Although indicating that an epileptiform process is operant, it has also been speculated that there is a subtle clinical correlate to these episodes, the so-called transient cognitive impairment. In studies of patients with paroxysmal EEGs, there may be associated deficits in the performance of cognitive tasks,[43] which could adversely affect functional abilities, but it is unclear how common this impairment is in the various forms of epilepsy.[44] Further studies of psychomotor performance with simultaneous EEG monitoring are necessary to more clearly elucidate the presence or absence of subclinical effects on cognition associated with various EEG abnormalities.

IMAGING STUDIES

As part of the initial evaluation of the patient with seizures, an imaging study of the brain is often warranted. When a clear etiology for a seizure is present, such as with hypoglycemia or an electrolyte disturbance, no further evaluation may be necessary. However, in the patient with no obvious cause for a seizure or with accompanying neurologic findings, further in-

TABLE 19-2
Drugs Used in the Treatment of Seizures

| Generic Name | Trade Name | USUAL DAILY DOSAGE | | Principal Therapeutic Indications | Serum Half-life, (h) | Effective Blood Level, μg/ml |
		Children	Adults (mg)			
Phenobarbital[a]	Luminal	3–5 mg/kg (8 mg/kg infants)	60–200	Tonic-clonic seizures; simple and complex partial seizures; absence	96 ± 12	10–40
Phenytoin[a]	Dilantin	4–7 mg/kg	300–400	Tonic-clonic seizures; simple and complex partial seizures	24 ± 12	10–20
Carbamazepine	Tegretol	20–30 mg/kg	600–1200	Tonic-clonic seizures; complex partial seizures	12 ± 3	4–10
Primidone	Mysoline	10–25 mg/kg	750–1500	Tonic-clonic seizures; simple and complex partial seizures	12 ± 6	5–15
Ethosuximide	Zarontin	20–40 mg/kg	750–2000	Absence	40 ± 6	50–100
Methsuximide	Celontin	10–20 mg/kg	500–1000	Absence	40 ± 6	40–100
Diazepam	Valium	0.15–2 mg/kg (IV)	10–150	Status epilepticus		
Lorazepam	Ativan	0.1 mg/kg (IV)		Status epilepticus		
ACTH	—	40–60 units/day		Infantile spasms		
Valproic acid	Depakene	30–60 mg/kg	1000–3000	Absence and myoclonic seizures; as an adjunctive drug in tonic clonic and complex partial seizures	8 ± 2	50–100
Clonazepam	Clonopin	0.01–0.2 mg/kg	1.5–20	Absence; myoclonus	18–50	0.01–0.07

[a] Dosages differ in treatment of status epilepticus.
SOURCE: From Adams RD, Victor M: *Principles of Neurology*, 5th ed. New York, McGraw-Hill, 1993, with permission.

vestigation of intracranial causes of seizures is often informative. Computed tomography (CT) and more recently magnetic resonance imaging (MRI) have greatly aided in the diagnosis and management of patients with seizures, providing high-quality assessment of intracranial pathology.[45]

In the acute evaluation of seizures of undetermined etiology, a CT scan may be used with great efficacy to examine evolving or ongoing processes such as neoplasms, hemorrhage, or stroke, or for the detection of intracranial calcifications such as those seen in neurocutaneous syndromes.[37] However, for more subtle manifestations of metabolic abnormalities, trauma, or cerebrovascular accident, the MRI is superior.[45,46] In the case of less emergent evaluations of seizures, the MRI is the study of choice to detect pathologic processes affecting the hippocampal formation or other brain regions.[47] Hippocampal sclerosis is easily demonstrable with high-quality MRI, as are developmental anomalies of brain including holoprosencephaly, schizencephaly, or lissencephaly. Although CT may suggest gray matter heterotopias, a common developmental etiology of seizures, MRI more clearly demonstrates the extent and distribution of such lesions, as well as any associated gyral anomalies.

Magnetic resonance imaging has proven to be a more flexible tool than CT because of the ability to perform magnetic resonance spectroscopy (MRS) and functional MRI (fMRI).[48] MRS provides information on the distribution of *N*-acetylaspartate, creatine, and phosphocreatine, indicating regions of possible neuronal loss or gliosis. fMRI involves the dynamic properties of blood flow in the brain during cognitive tasks, which can be evaluated in real time, allowing for regional mapping of brain function and the detection of regions demonstrating pathologic brain activation.

Finally, single photon emission computed tomography (SPECT) and positron emission tomography (PET) hold great promise in the detailed evaluation of seizure localization.[49] SPECT is essentially a measure of cerebral blood flow, and analysis during a seizure yields valuable data that, when considered concurrently with MRI, provides information on the site of a seizure focus for possible resection. PET scanning is helpful because of its ability to measure various markers of interictal metabolism and is useful in the evaluation of temporal lobe epilepsy. Although usually available only in comprehensive epilepsy centers, the information gleaned from investigations such as SPECT and PET is becoming more necessary as the use of epilepsy surgery increases.

Neurobiology of Seizures

The previous sections have focused on some of the salient features of seizures as they apply to the clinical presentation and evaluation of the condition. To understand the physiologic and biologic aspects of seizures and epilepsy, it is important to consider the functional anatomy of the nervous system as it relates to the electrical derangements that are operant. A fundamental knowledge of neuroanatomy, neuronal circuitry, and neurophysiology is required, and the following section provides an overview of these concepts in the region of the hippocampus, where many seizures originate.

PATHOLOGIC ANATOMY OF EPILEPSY

The majority of information concerning the pathology seen in epilepsy is derived from postmortem and surgical specimens. Interestingly, in postmortem brains from epileptics with both partial and generalized seizure disorders, hippocampal pathology demonstrates atrophy and neuronal loss in granule cells of the dentate gyrus (DG) and pyramidal cells of the cornu Ammonis (CA).[50] Hippocampal sclerosis, which is the term used to describe this atrophy and associated gliotic change, has been found in a large number of pathologic specimens from epilepsy surgery[34] and is also seen radiographically in nonsurgical candidates (see above). The specificity of hippocampal sclerosis in regard to the pathogenesis of seizures is significant because of its simultaneous occurrence with other brain lesions, the so-called dual pathology. It has been questioned, therefore, whether hippocampal sclerosis is a cause or an effect of seizures.[51–53] It may be the primary lesion, or it may be induced by extrahippocampal pathology, but in any event, it remains crucial to the expression of seizures and has been a focus of intensive investigation into the pathogenesis of epilepsy.

Hippocampal anatomy consists of a trisynaptic excitatory pathway, with projections from the entorhinal cortex exciting granule cells of the DG, which in turn project to the CA3 subfield via mossy fibers. CA3 projections are directed to CA1 by way of the Schaffer collaterals, and CA1 neurons project to extrahippocampal structures and hippocampal-related structures such as the subiculum and entorhinal cortex. Inhibitory modulation of excitatory neurotransmission is presumed to be provided by the neurotransmitter γ-aminobutyric acid (GABA), and it has long been postulated that seizures arise secondary to an imbalance between the excitatory and inhibitory pathways.[54,55] It has been demonstrated electrophysiologically that CA3 neurons are associated with interictal spiking and CA1 neurons are related to the origin of ictal events, but the role of the DG is less clear.[56] Morphologically, Golgi impregnation of the human hippocampus from epileptics has demonstrated reorganization and loss of dendritic and axonal profiles[57,58] in regions of the hippocampus, suggesting that a dynamic process is involved in the creation of an epileptic focus.

KINDLING AND OTHER ANIMAL MODELS OF EPILEPSY

One example of an experimental process that produces an epileptic lesion is the phenomenon of kindling. First described in 1969 by Goddard,[59] kindling refers to the technique of inducing a permanent epileptic state by the administration of repeated subclinical electrical stimulations to brain over time. In multiple experimental paradigms involving different species, kindling produced a susceptibility to spontaneous electrical seizures and had apparent relevance to complex partial epilepsy in humans.[60,61] Kindling represents a phenomenon of seizure focus activation that may be remote from the site of electrical stimulation, a situation similar to the "dual pathology" noted in human pathologic specimens.

The mechanism of kindling is not completely understood, and microscopic examination in kindled animals has failed to demonstrate pathology comparable to human epilepsy. However, it has been reported that kindling may induce changes in neurotransmitter pharmacology of the N-methyl-D-asparate receptor (NMDA) (see below), which predispose hippocampal neurons to ictal bursts.[53] Detailed neurophysiologic and neurochemical analysis of kindling in hippocampus will undoubtedly lead to further understanding of the role that neuronal circuits play in the generation of seizures.[62]

A number of other animal models have been extremely useful in the study of seizures. As mentioned previously, genetic strains of various species with epilepsy have proven informative in the determination of neurochemical abnormalities associated with seizures and epilepsy.[63] Genetically epilepsy-prone animals demonstrate a lowered threshold to electrical and chemical stimulants and serve as models for the assessment of anticonvulsant drugs.[64] However, despite a phenotypic similarity to various seizure types in humans, incuding partial, complex partial, and generalized epilepsies, these animal models have some limitations with regard to variations in pathology and clinical responses to anticonvulsants.

Another type of animal model is derived from the application or administration of toxic agents that produce seizures. Such agents include penicillin, alumina hydroxide,[24] cobalt chloride,[65] kainic acid,[66–70] pentylenetetrazole,[71] and bicuculline.[72,73] Although these paradigms most often produce an acute syndrome of seizure activity, the focal application of these toxins can produce a sustaining epileptic focus that results in a syndrome similar to a chronic epilepsy.[74]

EXCITATORY AMINO ACIDS (EAAs) IN SEIZURES AND EPILEPSY

The most prevalent excitatory neurotransmitters in brain include the amino acids glutamate and aspartate.[75,76] Evidence for EAA involvement in seizures and epilepsy comes from animal models of seizure propagation using agonists such as kainic acid[67,70,77] and is consistent with the hypothesis that there is an imbalance of excitatory and inhibitory influences in hippocampus in epilepsy. Part of the pathology of EAA agonists is derived from excitotoxic neuronal loss secondary to EAA neurotransmission, which has in itself been hypothesized to contribute to the pathogenesis of epilepsy.[78,79] Investigation of EAA receptors has identified a number of pharmacologically distinct subtypes depending on differential binding affinities of glutamate analogues.[80–83] From these studies, EAA receptors have been subdivided into NMDA, quisqualate, and kainate receptors. Quisqualate receptors have been further delineated by their association with either ion channels (AMPA receptors) or second messenger systems (metabotropic receptors).[84,85] Of these receptor types, the NMDA receptor is of great significance in the pathogenesis of seizures. NMDA receptors are linked to voltage-gated ionic channels that regulate calcium conductance and are crucial to the expression of hippocampal kindling (see above). Extrahippocampal neuropathology of seizures secondary to kainic acid is ameliorated by NMDA receptor blockade,[86] indicating an interaction of NMDA and non-NMDA receptor transmission in this model of neurotoxicity. These findings have led to reevaluation of traditional anticonvulsants with regard to their effects on the NMDA receptor complex and a search for therapeutic agents directed specifically toward NMDA receptors.[87–89]

The investigation of the role of EAA receptors in epilepsy has developed a new layer of complexity since the discovery of the genes that code for the various EAA receptor subtypes.[90–96] All of the EAA receptors except metabotropic quisqualate receptors are heteromeric and are comprised of various combinations of these gene products. Analyses of mRNA expression of these various genes demonstrate distinct and specific regional distributions of various EAA subunits,[95,97–99,100–102] which indicate that the spectrum of pharmacologically and anatomically distinct EAA receptors is extremely broad. Furthermore, it has been shown that subunit composition of EAA receptors changes in the hippocampus after excitotoxic, epileptogenic lesions, suggesting that there is an alteration of hippocampal receptors that may influence the chronic expression of seizures in animal models.[103,104]

Another amino acid implicated in the pathogenesis of seizures and epilepsy is taurine, a putative inhibitory neurotransmitter. Taurine may be important because of its reciprocal relationship to glutamate with regard to relative tissue concentrations.[105] Taurine levels in tissues are primarily derived from dietary sources, and there are no endogenous metabolic pathways for taurine synthesis in brain. Nevertheless, glutamate levels in neurosurgical specimens from human epileptics are higher than in controls, again illustrating the possibility of an excitation/inhibition imbalance, and taurine levels are decreased in models of epilepsy. A possible anticonvulsant effect of taurine has been postulated,[106] and taurine loss in epilepsy is perhaps related to aberrant compartmentation of neutral amino acids.[107] However, long-term trials of the anticonvulsant properties of taurine have not been promising.[108]

GABA AND ITS ROLE IN EPILEPSY

Seizures are postulated to be a result of either excessive excitatory or decreased inhibitory influences in brain, possibly resulting in either a propensity for ictal phenomenon or in a frank epileptogenic state.[109] GABA is linked to an ionic chloride channel and is thought to decrease neuronal excitability when activated. In certain animal models of epilepsy, diminished GABAergic tone may enhance the phenotype,[110] and there are reports of decreased amounts of glutamic acid by dehydrogenase, the enzyme responsible for GABA formation, in human epileptic brain.[106]

The trisynaptic pathway of excitatory neurotransmission in the hippocampus as described above is subject to inhibitory modulation by GABA in basket cells. In animal models of hippocampal seizures, it has been demonstrated electrophysiologically that there is a loss of GABA-mediated recurrent inhibition in dentate granule cells, resulting in hyperexcitability and presumably a tendency toward epileptic discharges.[111,112] However, GABAergic basket cells are preserved, which has led to the "dormant basket cell" hypothesis.[53] This theory postulates that recurrent inhibition acting on DG granule cells is mediated by excitatory impulses from axon collaterals of granule cells to the GABA-containing basket cells and similar excitation from mossy cells. If mossy cells are lost, the resultant decrease in basket cell excitation would result in a net loss of GABA-mediated inhibition to the DG granule cells. Another theory of DG hyperexcitability concerns the phenomenon of mossy fiber rearrangements, or sprouting, which occurs in both animal models and in human epilepsy.[113,114] Sprouting is observed in mossy fiber projections to CA3, and a loss of mossy cell afferents with a concomitant overrepresentation of DG granule cell afferents could shift the balance more toward excitation and epileptogenesis. Further work in both animal models and human tissue specimens is clearly necessary to resolve the issues of hippocampal hyperexcitability and the role of GABA.

Neurotransmission of GABA is also important in the substantia nigra (SN) with regard to seizure expression. Although not considered a site of epileptogenesis, the SN has been implicated as a possible gating mechanism for ictal discharges within the brain. Chemical ablations of GABAergic efferents from SN or frank SN lesions lower seizure threshold, and augmentation of GABAergic tone by administration of GABA transaminase inhibitors raises the threshold for seizure expression.[115,116] It is as yet unclear how this alteration in epileptogenesis is mediated, but the widespread projections of SN to thalamus and the basal ganglia suggest a modulatory role.

BIOGENIC AMINES AND SEIZURES

The biogenic amines dopamine, norepinephrine, and serotonin are neurotransmitters synthesized in discrete midbrain and brainstem nuclei and have widespread efferent projections from these nuclei to the cortex and hippocampus. Their role in neurotransmission is modulatory,[117] which could presumably affect the imbalance in excitatory activity hypothesized to occur in epilepsy. Clinical evidence for such an effect comes from the increased risk for seizures observed in the setting of psychiatric depression treated with nonmonamine oxidase inhibitor antidepressants.[118] These agents, although certainly not specific for dopamine, norepinephrine, or serotonin, have the general effect of decreasing the neurochemical activity of biogenic amines, which parallels their propensity for epileptogenesis. Furthermore, in pathologic specimens from human epileptic brains, a decrease in tyrosine hydroxylase activity has been described.[106] The action of tyrosine hydroxylase is the rate-limiting step in catecholamine biosynthesis, and a decrease in activity could result in diminishment of dopamine and norepinephrine.

Concordant data concerning alterations in norepinephrine come from the epilepsy-prone rat, a genetic model of seizures. In these animals, norepinephrine concentrations are diminished in multiple brain regions, which is not a consequence of seizures.[119] Norepinephrine abnormalities are also seen in toxin-induced animal models of epilepsy, including that induced by metallic cobalt,[65] where there is evidence of a denervation supersensitivity to norepinephrine and an up-regulation of β adrenoreceptors, and in kindling, which increases norepinephrine turnover.[120] These investigations would indicate that depletion of norepinephrine is somehow epileptogenic or predisposes to epilepsy. One genetic animal model of chronic epilepsy, the tottering mouse, is in seeming conflict with the notion of norepinephrine depletion contributing to seizures.[121] This strain of mouse is characterized by a marked norepinephrinergic hyperinnervation of forebrain. It is unclear in this mouse how the increase in norepinephrine relates to the development of seizures, because this may be a compensatory phenomenon and not a primary lesion. With regard to other biogenic amines, dopamine and serotonin may exert some anticonvulsant effects, but data from various animal models are somewhat conflicting, and more study is needed.[63,122,123]

OTHER INFLUENCES ON SEIZURES AND EPILEPSY

During repeated seizures and in experimental status epilepticus in animals, there is a persistent activation of transcription factors,[124–126] which is only one aspect of the many metabolic changes that occur in epilepsy. The previous discussion has concerned many of the more common studies of neurobiologic phenomenon in epilepsy. This section deals with other neurochemical features that affect the expression of seizures.

Adrenocorticotropin hormone (ACTH) and steroid hormones have been used effectively, primarily to treat infantile spasms, but they have also been useful for other seizure disorders.[127–129] The basis for their efficacy in the treatment of seizures is unknown, but animal studies have demonstrated significant anticonvulsant activity with ACTH in kindling and electroshock paradigms.[128–131] Dexamethasone has been used to affect gene expression and second messenger systems in animal models,[132] and corticotropin-releasing factor (CRF) has caused status epilepticus in immature rats, suggesting a possible role of hormones in brain maturation and epileptogenesis.[133] In animals undergoing adrenalectomy, there is a progressive loss of dentate granule cells in the hippocampus,[134,135] perhaps indicating a trophic role for ACTH and steroids.

Investigations of CRF, which stimulates ACTH release, have also revealed a relationship with endogenous opiopeptides. Naloxone, which blocks endogenous opiates, partially attenuates electrographic responses in CRF-induced status epilepticus,[136] indicating a role for β endorphin in seizures. Another opiopeptide, dynorphin A, is released at mossy fiber terminals and has naloxone-resistant effects on seizure propagation, which suggests a nonopioid effect of this neuropeptide.[137] However, in various animal models, both pro- and anticonvulsant actions of the opiopeptides[138] have made their characterization problematic, but they remain an interesting area of epilepsy research.

Conclusion

An interpretation of the phenomena of seizures and epilepsy may be accomplished on various levels (clinical, psychological, neurobiologic, pathologic, etc.). This chapter has provided an overview of seizures, but one more directed toward neurochemical and neurobiologic perspectives. Ictal events are of great clinical significance because of their ubiquity and deleterious effects on the central nervous system. Although descriptive characterizations have provided a framework, it will be the incorporation of modern neuroscientific methods that ultimately produces a focused understanding of seizures and epilepsy in man.

References

1. Commission on Classification and Terminology of the International League Against Epilepsy: Proposal for revised classification of epilepsies and epileptic syndromes. *Epilepsia* 1989; 30:389.
2. Dreifuss FE, Henriksen O: Classification of epileptic seizures and the epilepsies. *Acta Neurol Scand Suppl* 1992; 140:8.
3. Dreifuss FE: The epilepsies: Clinical implications of the international classification. *Epilepsia* 1990; 31:S3.
4. Vassella F: Seizure types and epileptic syndromes. *Eur Neurol* 1994; 34:3.
5. Farrell K: Classifying epileptic syndromes: Problems and a neurobiologic solution. *Neurology* 1993; 43:S8.
6. Sander JW, Shorvon SD: Incidence and prevalence studies in epilepsy and their methodological problems: A review. *J Neurol Neurosurg Psychiatry* 1987; 50:829.
7. Hauser WA, et al: The incidence of epilepsy in Rochester, Minnesota, 1935–1984. *Epilepsia* 1993; 34:453.
8. Annegers JF: Epidemiology and genetics of epilepsy. *Neuro Clin North Am* 1994; 12:15.
9. Senanayake N, Roman GC: Epidemiology of epilepsy in developing countries. *Bull World Health Organ* 1993; 71:247.
10. Jilek-Aall L, et al: Clinical and genetic aspects of seizure disorders prevalent in an isolated African population. *Epilepsia* 1979; 20:613.
11. Annegers JF, et al: Risk of recurrence after an initial unprovoked seizure. *Epilepsia* 1986; 27:43.
12. Ottman R, et al: Higher risk of seizures in offspring of mothers than fathers with epilepsy. *Am J Hum Genet* 1988; 43:257.
13. Lindhout D, et al: In search for genes predisposing to epilepsy: Motives and methods. *Acta Neurol Scand Suppl* 1992; 140:51
14. Gardiner RM: Genes and epilepsy. *J Med Genet* 1990; 27:537.
15. Treiman LJ: Genetics of epilepsy: An overview. *Epilepsia* 1993; 34:S1.
16. Delgado-Escueta, AV, et al: Progress in mapping human epilepsy genes. *Epilepsia* 1994; 35(suppl 1):S29.
17. Delgado-Escueta AV, et al: Gene mapping in the idiopathic generalized epilepsies: Juvenile myoclonic epilepsy, childhood absence epilepsy, epilepsy with grand mal seizures, and early childhood myoclonic epilepsy. *Epilepsia* 1990; 31:S19.
18. Schapira AHV: Mitochondrial cytopathies. *Curr Opin Neurobiol* 1993; 3:760.
19. Wallace DC, et al: Mitochondrial DNA mutations in epilepsy and neurological disease. *Epilepsia* 1994; 35(suppl 1):S43.
20. Cortopassi GA, Arnheim, N: Detection of a specific mitochondrial DNA deletion in tissues of older humans. *Nucleic Acids Res* 1990; 18:6927.
21. Corral-Debrinski M, et al: Mitochondrial DNA deletions in human brain: Regional variability and increase with advanced age. *Nat Genet* 1992; 2:324.
22. Noebels JL: Mutational analysis of inherited epilepsies. *Adv Neurol* 1986; 44:97.
23. Faingold CL: The genetically epilepsy-prone rat. *Gen Pharmacol* 1988; 19:331.
24. Fisher RS: Animal models of the epilepsies. *Brain Res Brain Res Rev* 1989; 14:245.
25. Buchhalter JR: Animal models of inherited epilepsy. *Epilepsia* 1993; 34:S31.
26. Dreifuss FE: *Pediatric Epileptology.* Boston, PSG Inc., 1983:17.
27. Morrell MJ: Differential diagnosis of seizures. *Neurol Clin North Am* 1993; 11:737.
28. Pacia SV, et al: The prolonged QT syndrome presenting as epilepsy: A report of two cases and literature review. *Neurology* 1994; 44:1408.
29. Golden GS: Nonepileptic paroxysmal events in childhood. *Pediat Clin North Am* 1992; 39:715.
30. Ettinger AB: Structural causes of epilepsy. Tumors, cysts, stroke, and vascular malformations. *Neurol Clin North Am* 1994; 12:41.
31. Garcia PA, Alldredge BK: Drug-induced seizures. *Neurol Clin North Am* 1994; 12:85.
32. Raymond AA, et al: Subependymal heterotopia: A distinct neuronal migration disorder associated with epilepsy. *J Neurol Neurosurg Psychiatry* 1994; 57:1195.
33. Bruton CJ: *The Neuropathology of Temporal Lobe Epilepsy.* New York, Oxford University Press, 1988:158.
34. Jay V, Becker LE: Surgical pathology of epilepsy: A review. *Pediatr Pathol* 1994; 14:731.
35. Gupta SR, et al: Postinfarction seizures. A clinical study. *Stroke* 1988; 19:1477.
36. Dam AM, et al: Late-onset epilepsy: Etiologies, types of seizure, and value of clinical investigation, EEG, and computerized tomography scan. *Epilepsia* 1985; 26:227.
37. Kotagal P, Rothner AD: Epilepsy in the setting of neurocutaneous syndromes. *Epilepsia* 1993; 34:S71.
38. Cohen BH: Metabolic and degenerative diseases associated with epilepsy. *Epilepsia* 1993; 34:S62.
39. Porter J, Jick H: Drug-induced anaphylaxis, convulsions, deafness, and extrapyramidal symptoms. *Lancet* 1977; 1(8011):587.
40. Gastaut H, Tassinari CA: EEG in diagnosis, prognosis and treatment of epilepsy. In Gastaut H (ed): *Handbook of Electroencephalography and Clinical Neurophysiology.* Amsterdam, Elsevier, 1975:65–104.
41. Jallon P: Electroencephalogram and epilepsy. *Euro Neurol* 1994; 34:18.
42. Logar C, et al: Role of long-term EEG monitoring in diagnosis and treatment of epilepsy. *Eur Neurol* 1994; 34:29.
43. Binnie CD, Marston D: Cognitive correlates of interictal discharges. *Epilepsia* 1992; 33:S11.
44. Aldenkamp AP, Gutter T, Beun AM: The effect of seizure activity and paroxysmal electroencephalographic discharges on cognition. *Acta Neurol Scand Suppl* 1992; 140:111.
45. Radue EW, Scollo-Lavizzari G: Computed tomography and magnetic resonance imaging in epileptic seizures. *Eur Neurol* 1994; 34:55.
46. Yaffe K, et al: Reversible MRI abnormalities following seizures. *Neurology* 1995; 45:104.

47. Kuzniecky RI: Magnetic resonance imaging in developmental disorders of the cerebral cortex. *Epilepsia* 1994; 35:S44.

48. Jackson GD: New techniques in magnetic resonance and epilepsy. *Epilepsia* 1994; 35:S2.

49. Spencer SS: The relative contributions of MRI, SPECT, and PET imaging in epilepsy. *Epilepsia* 1994; 35:S72.

50. Dam AM: Hippocampal neuron loss in epilepsy and after experimental seizures. *Acta Neurol Scand* 1982; 66:601.

51. McNamara JO: The neurobiological basis of epilepsy. *Trends Neurosci* 1992; 15:357.

52. McNamara JO, et al: Recent advances in understanding mechanisms of the kindling model. *Adv Neurol* 1992; 57:555.

53. McNamara JO: Cellular and molecular basis of epilepsy. *J Neurosci* 1995; 14:3413.

54. Snead OC: On the sacred disease: The neurochemistry of epilepsy. *Int Rev Neurobiol* 1983; 24:93.

55. Wheal HV: Function of synapses in the CA1 region of the hippocampus: Their contribution to the generation or control of epileptiform activity. *Comp Biochem Physiol A* 1989; 93:211.

56. Lothman EW: Functional anatomy: A challenge for the decade of the brain. *Epilepsia* 1991; 32:S3.

57. Scheibel AB: Morphological correlates of epilepsy: Cells in the hippocampus. *Adv Neurol* 1980; 27:49.

58. Babb TL, Brown WJ: Neuronal, dendritic, and vascular profiles of human temporal lobe epilepsy correlated with cellular physiology in vivo. *Adv Neurol* 1986; 44:949.

59. Goddard GV, et al: A permanent change in brain function resulting from daily electrical stimulation. *Exp Neurol* 1969; 25:295.

60. Majkowski J: Kindling: A model for epilepsy and memory. *Acta Neurol Scand Suppl* 1986; 109:97.

61. McNamara JO: Kindling model of epilepsy. *Adv Neurol* 1986; 44:303.

62. Lopes da Silva FH, et al: Epileptogenesis as a plastic phenomenon of the brain, a short review. *Acta Neurol Scand Suppl* 1992; 140:34.

63. Jobe PC, Laird HE: Neurotransmitter abnormalities as determinants of seizure susceptibility and intensity in the genetic models of epilepsy. *Biochem Pharmacol* 1981; 30:3137.

64. Löscher W, Meldrum BS: Evaluation of anticonvulsant drugs in genetic animal models of epilepsy. *Federation Proceedings* 1984; 43:276.

65. Bregman B, et al: Chronic cobalt-induced epilepsy: Noradrenaline ionophoresis and adrenoceptor binding studies in the rat cerebral cortex. *J Neural Transm* 1985; 63:109.

66. Ben-Ari Y: The role of seizures in kainic acid induced brain damage. In Fuxe K, et al (eds): *Excitotoxins.* New York, Plenum Press, 1984; 184–198.

67. Ben-Ari Y: Limbic seizure and brain damage produced by kainic acid: Mechanisms and relevance to human temporal lobe epilepsy. *Neuroscience* 1985; 14:375.

68. Berger ML, et al: Effect of seizures induced by intra-amygdaloid kainic acid on kainic acid binding sites in rat hippocampus and amygdala. *J Neurochem* 1986; 47:720.

69. Nayel M, et al: Experimental limbic epilepsy: Models, pathophysiologic concepts, and clinical relevance. *Clev Clin J Med* 1991; 58:521.

70. Sperk G: Kainic acid seizures in the rat. *Prog Neurobiol* 1994; 42:1.

71. Ingvar M, et al: Metabolic, circulatory, and structural alterations in the rat brain induced by sustained pentylenetetrazole seizures. *Epilepsia* 1984; 25:191.

72. Morrisett RA, et al: Status epilepticus is produced by administration of cholinergic agonists to lithium-treated rates: Comparison with kainic acid. *Exp Neurol* 1987; 98:594.

73. Williams MB, Jope RS: Circadian variation in rat brain AP-1 DNA binding activity after cholinergic stimulation: Modulation by lithium. *Brain Res Mol Brain Res* 1996; in press.

74. Lothman EW, Bertram EH III: Epileptogenic effects of status epilepticus. *Epilepsia* 1993; 34(Suppl 1): S59.

75. Young AB, Fagg GE: Excitatory amino acid receptors in the brain: Membrane binding and receptor autoradiographic approaches. *Trends Pharmacol Sci* 1990; 11:126.

76. Albin RL, et al: Excitatory amino acidergic pathways and receptors in the basal ganglia. *Amino Acids* 1991; 1:339.

77. Sperk G, et al: Kainic acid induced seizures, neurochemical and histopathological changes. *Neuroscience* 1983; 10:1301.

78. Olney JW: Excitatory transmitters and epilepsy-related brain damage. *Int Rev Neurobiol* 1985; 27:337.

79. Olney JW, et al: Excitotoxic mechanisms of epileptic brain damage. *Adv Neurol* 1986; 44:857.

80. Greenamyre JT, et al: Quantitative autoradiography of L-[3H]glutamate binding to rat brain. *Neurosci Lett* 1983; 37:155.

81. Greenamyre JT, et al: Quantitative autoradiographic distribution of L-[3H]glutamate-binding sites in rat central nervous system. *J Neurosci* 1984; 4:2133.

82. Cha JH, et al: Properties of quisqualate-sensitive L-[3H]glutamate binding sites in rat brain as determined by quantitative autoradiography. *J Neurochem* 1988; 51:469.

83. Greenamyre JT, Young AB: Synaptic localization of striatal NMDA, quisqualate and kainate receptors. *Neurosci Lett* 1989, 101:133.

84. Conn PJ, Desai MA: Pharmacology and physiology of metabotropic glutamate receptors in mammalian central nervous system. *Drug Dev Res* 1991; 24:207.

85. Schoepp DD, Conn, PJ: Metabotropic glutamate receptors in brain function and pathology. *Trends Pharmacol Sci* 1993; 14:13.

86. Clifford DB, et al: Ketamine, phencyclidine, and MK-801 protect against kainic acid-induced seizure-related brain damage. *Epilepsia* 1990; 31:382.

87. Meldrum B: Possible therapeutic applications of antagonists of excitatory amino acid neurotransmitters. *Clin Sci* 1985; 68:113.

88. Rogawski MA: The NMDA receptor, NMDA antagonists and epilepsy therapy. *Drugs* 1922; 44:279.

89. Chapman AG, Meldrum BS: Excitatory amino acid antagonists and epilepsy. *Biochem Soc Trans* 1993; 21:106.

90. Keinanen K, et al: A family of AMPA-selective glutamate receptors. *Science* 1990; 249:556.

91. Sommer B, et al: Flip and flop: A cell-specific functional switch in glutamate-operated channels of the CNS. *Science* 1990; 249:1580.

92. Moriyoshi K, et al: Molecular cloning and characterization of the rat NMDA receptor. *Nature* 1991; 354:31.

93. Nakanishi S: Molecular diversity of glutamate receptors and implications for brain function. *Science* 1992; 258:597.

94. Sugihara H, et al: Structures and properties of seven isoforms of the NMDA receptor generated by alternative splicing. *Biochem Biophys Res Commun* 1992; 185:826.

95. Wisden W, Seeburg PH: A complex mosaic of high-affinity kainate receptors in rat brain. *J Neurosci* 1993, 13:3582.

96. Okamoto N, et al: Molecular characterization of a new metabotropic glutamate receptor mGluR7 coupled to inhibitory cyclic AMP signal transduction. *J Biol Chem* 1994, 269:1231.

97. Monyer H, et al: Heteromeric NMDA receptors: Molecular and functional distinction of subtypes. *Science* 1992; 256:1217.

98. Tanabe Y, et al: A family of metabotropic glutamate receptors. *Neuron* 1992; 8:169.

99. Standaert DG, et al: Alternatively spliced isoforms of the NMDAR1 glutamate receptor subunit: Differential expression in the basal ganglia of the rat. *Neurosci Lett* 1993; 152:161.

100. Standaert DG, et al: Organization of N-methyl-D-aspartate glu-

tamate receptor gene expression in the basal ganglia of the rat. *J Comp Neurol* 1994; 343:1.

101. Testa CM, et al: Metabotropic glutamate receptor mRNA expression in the basal ganglia of the rat. *J Neurosci* 1994; 14:3005.

102. Testa CM, et al: Differential expression of mGluR5 metabotropic glutamate receptor mRNA by rat striatal neurons. *J Comp Neurol* 1995; 354:241.

103. Pollard H, et al: Alterations of the GluR-B AMPA receptor subunit flip/flop expression in kainate-induced epilepsy and ischemia. *Neuroscience* 1993; 57:545.

104. Friedman LK, et al: Kainate-induced status epilepticus alters glutamate and GABA$_A$ receptor gene expression in adult rat hippocampus: An in situ hybridization study. *J Neurosci* 1994; 14:2697.

105. van Gelder NM: Taurine, the compartmentalized metabolism of glutamic acid, and the epilepsies. *Can J Physiol Pharmacol* 1978; 56:362.

106. Sherwin AL, van Gelder NM: Amino acid and catecholamine markers of metabolic abnormalities in human focal epilepsy. *Adv Neurol* 1986; 44:1011.

107. van Gelder NM: Glutamic acid in nervous tissue and changes of the taurine content: Its implication in the treatment of epilepsy. *Adv Biochem Psychopharmacol* 1981; 29:115.

108. Durelli L, Mutani R: The current status of taurine in epilepsy. *Clin Neuropharmacol* 1983; 6:37.

109. Meldrum BS: Excitatory amino acid transmitters in epilepsy. *Epilepsia* 1991; 32:S1.

110. Meldrum, BS: GABAergic mechanisms in the pathogenesis and treatment of epilepsy. *Br J Clin Pharmacol* 1989; 27:3S.

111. Sloviter RS: "Epileptic" brain damage in rats induced by sustained electrical stimulation of the perforant path. I. Acute electrophysiological and light microscopic studies. *Brain Res Bull* 1983; 10:675.

112. De Deyn PP, et al: Epilepsy and the GABA-hypothesis a brief review and some examples. *Acta Neurol Belg* 1990; 90:65.

113. Moshe SL, et al: Experimental epilepsy: Developmental aspects. *Cleve Clin J Med* 1989; 56:S92.

114. Sutula T, et al: Mossy fiber synaptic reorganization in the epileptic human temporal lobe. *Ann Neurol* 1989; 26:321.

115. Gale K: Mechanisms of seizure control mediated by gamma-aminobutyric acid: Role of the substantia nigra. *Federation Proceedings* 1985; 44:2414.

116. Gale K: GABA and epilepsy: Basic concepts from preclinical research. *Epilepsia* 1992; 33:S3.

117. Cooper JR, et al: *The Biochemical Basis of Neuropharmacology.* New York, Oxford University Press, 1991:203.

118. Trimble M: Non-monoamine oxidase inhibitor antidepressants and epilepsy: A review. *Epilepsia* 1978; 19:241.

119. Jobe PC, et al: Noradrenergic abnormalities in the genetically epilepsy-prone rat. *Brain Res Bull* 1994; 35:493.

120. Chauvel P, Trottier S: Role of noradrenergic ascending system in extinction of epileptic phenomena. *Adv Neurol* 1986; 44:475.

121. Kostopoulos GK: The tottering mouse: A critical review of its usefulness in the study of the neuronal mechanisms underlying epilepsy. *J Neural Trans Suppl* 1992; 35:21.

122. Browning RA: Role of the brain-stem reticular formation in tonic-clonic seizures: Lesion and pharmacological studies. *Federation Proceedings* 1985; 44:2425.

123. Ferrendelli JA: Roles of biogenic amines and cyclic nucleotides in seizure mechanisms. *Adv Neurol* 1986; 44:393.

124. Pennypacker KR, et al: Prolonged expression of AP-1 transcription factors in the rat hippocampus after systemic kainate treatment. *J Neurosci* 1994; 14:3998.

125. Williams MB, Jope RS: Distinctive rat brain immediate early gene responses to seizures induced by lithium plus pilocarpine. *Brain Res Mol Brain Res* 1994; 25:80.

126. Unlap T, Jope RS: Diurnal variation in kainate-induced AP-1 activation in rat brain: Influence of glucocorticoids. *Brain Res. Mol Brain Res* 1995; 28:193.

127. Snead OC III, et al: ACTH and prednisone in childhood seizure disorders. *Neurology* 1983; 33:966.

128. Goldman H, et al: ACTH-related peptides, kindling and seizure disorders. In Nerozzi D, et al (eds): *Hypothalamic Dysfunction in Neuropsychiatric Disorders.* New York, Raven Press, 1987: 317–327.

129. Holmes GL: Effect of non-sex hormones on neuronal excitability, seizures, and the electroencephalogram. *Epilepsia* 1991; 32(suppl 6):S11.

130. Goldman H, Berman, RF: Reduction of amygdaloid kindled seizures by an analog of ACTH/MSH. *Peptides* 1984; 5:1061.

131. Croiset G, De Wied D: ACTH: A structure-activity study on pilocarpine-induced epilepsy. *Eur J Pharmacol* 1992; 229:211.

132. Unlap T, Jope RS: Dexamethasone attenuates kainate-induced AP-1 activation in rat brain. *Brain Res Mol Brain Res* 1994; 24:275.

133. Baram TZ, Ribak CE: Peptide-induced infant status epilepticus causes neuronal death and synaptic reorganization. *Neuroreport* 1995; 6:277.

134. Sloviter RS, et al: Selective loss of hippocampal granule cells in the mature rat brain after adrenalectomy. *Science* 1989; 243:535.

135. Sloviter RS, et al: Adrenalectomy-induced granule cell degeneration in the rat hippocampal dentate gyrus: Characterization of an in vivo model of controlled neuronal death. *J Comp Neurol* 1993; 330:324.

136. Ortolani E, et al: Neuropeptides and seizures: An experimental model on the possible relationships among C.R.F., ACTH and endorphinic system. In Nerozzi D, et al (eds): *Hypothalamic Dysfunction in Neuropsychiatric Disorders.* New York, Raven Press, 1987:329–334.

137. Shukla VK, Lemaire S: Central non-opioid physiological and pathophysiological effects of dynorphin A and related peptides. *J Psychiatry Neurosci* 1992; 17:106.

138. Ramabadran K, Bansinath M: Endogenous opioid peptides and epilepsy. *Int J Clin Pharmacol Therapy Toxicol* 1990; 28:47.

Chapter 20

SEIZURE ACTIVITY AND ANESTHETIC AGENTS AND ADJUVANTS

IAN A. HERRICK

It may seem rather curious therefore that from time to time patients develop convulsions while receiving an anaesthetic. . . . However, convulsions have been reported as occurring under the influence of most drugs which have been used as general anaesthetic agents and no generally accepted explanation has so far been advanced to explain their occurrence.[1]

Eloquently summarizing the state of knowledge pertaining to convulsions reported in association with halothane anesthesia in 1966, this statement by Smith and colleagues remains valid 30 years later. Neuroexcitatory movements that occur in the perioperative period have interested anesthesiologists for many years. Perioperative seizures were described in association with ether anesthesia[2,3] and more recently have been re-

ported in association with a variety of modern anesthetic drugs. Desite a marked expansion of the case report literature related to perioperative neuroexcitatory movements, a definitive explanation remains elusive. This chapter reviews neuroexcitatory movements associated with anesthesia and discusses the current state of knowledge regarding the etiology of these phenomena.

Several factors confound the development of a coherent understanding of the role of anesthetic agents in the sporadic generation of convulsions and other neuroexcitatory phenomena. First, perioperative convulsions are rare events; thus, many of the documented episodes involve case reports. The case report literature describes a wide variety of neuroexcitatory movements that include muscular twitching or jerking, myoclonic and dystonic movements, and tonic or clonic convulsive movements. Such phenomena are often loosely classified as "seizures" or "convulsions." However, it remains unclear whether these various movements share a common etiology. On this basis, with the exception of reports that include electroencephalographic (EEG) documentation of epileptiform activity (and possibly reports involving clear descriptions of clinical tonic-clonic convulsions), the term neuroexcitatory movements more appropriately describes the broad spectrum of abnormal movements reported in association with anesthesia.

Second, few reports include EEG documentation. Furthermore, many of the EEG reports that accompany case reports were obtained after the neuroexcitatory activity had ceased. In addition, with the exception of studies involving epileptic patients during electrocortography (ECoG), EEG reports involve scalp recordings that may fail to detect deep cortical and subcortical seizure activity.

Third, the temporal relationship between the administration of anesthesia and the occurrence of neuroexcitatory phenomena is diverse. Most episodes are reported to commence during the intraoperative and early postoperative periods. However, in some cases onset was delayed for several days after anesthesia. Arguments favoring an etiologic role for anesthetic drugs in the development of late postoperative neuroexcitatory phenomena become less convincing as the temporal relationship to anesthesia widens.

Fourth, elucidation of the etiology of neuroexcitatory movements is complicated by the fact that anesthetic drugs are typically not administered in isolation. Attempts to assign proconvulsant activity to a specific drug within a multidrug anesthetic regimen often generate controversy.

Finally, reports of perioperative neuroexcitatory phenomena involve epileptic and nonepileptic patients. Based on our limited understanding of the mechanisms underlying the generation of these periop-

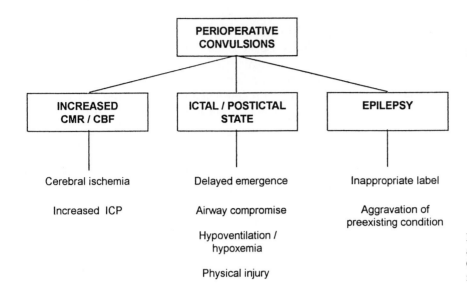

Figure 20-1 Summary of clinical concerns associated with perioperative convulsions. CBF, cerebral blood flow; CMR, cerebral metabolic rate; ICP, intracranial pressure.

erative movements, it is unclear whether data derived from one group of patients are applicable to the other. (See also Chaps. 6, 7, 12, 15, 16, 19, 21, and 23.)

Clinical Implications

Neuroexcitatory movements have been reported in association with most general anesthetics. However, these phenomena appear to cluster more prominently around certain drugs. Clinical interest in perioperative neuroexcitatory movements is related to the assumption that such phenomena share common or similar etiologic mechanisms that reflect the proconvulsant potential of the anesthetic drugs. Based on this assumption, several clinical implications follow (Fig. 20-1).

First, the development of perioperative convulsions may result in an increase in cerebral metabolism, blood flow and intracranial pressure. The use of proconvulsant anesthetic drugs may pose a hazard to patients who are at risk of developing perioperative cerebral ischemia or intracranial hypertension.

Second, the ictal or postictal state associated with the development of perioperative convulsions may delay emergence from anesthesia, may compromise ventilation or protective airway reflexes, and may pose a risk of physical injury to the patient or attending health care personnel.

Third, concern arises that the use of proconvulsant drugs may aggravate preexisting epilepsy.

Fourth, the possibility exists that patients who experience perioperative neuroexcitatory phenomena, particularly convulsions, will be inappropriately labeled as epileptic or potentially epileptic.

Inhalational Anesthetics

Neuroexcitatory movements, including convulsions, have been reported in association with most of the inhalational anesthetics. Based on investigations of halogenated ethers as potential general anesthetics, the proconvulsant properties and the anesthetic effects associated with these compounds have been reported to be prominently influenced by the degree of halogen (especially fluoride) substitution.[4] Increasing substitution of fluoride atoms results in a progression of pharmacologic effects from anesthesia through proconvulsant properties to lack of either effect with full fluorination. Although this relationship has been recognized for many years. it does not entirely explain the proconvulsant properties of some halogenated ethers. Flurothyl (Indoklon) is a proconvulsant fluorinated ether marketed briefly in the 1960s as a pharmacologic alternative to electroconvulsive therapy (ECT).[5] Although flurothyl is a potent proconvulsant with minimal anesthetic properties, its structural isomer, iso-Indoklon, has anesthetic properties devoid of proconvulsant effects.[6] Similarly, enflurane and isoflurane possess markedly different proconvulsant properties, despite being structural isomers.

NITROUS OXIDE

Withdrawal seizures have been reported in mice after exposure to normobaric and hyperbaric nitrous oxide (N_2O) and myoclonic movements have been reported in humans under similar circumstances.[7-10] Nevertheless, ECoG studies in epileptic patients administered N_2O alone or in combination with enflurane have not revealed evidence of proconvulsant (nor anticonvulsant) activity.[11,12] The administration of N_2O alone (60%) attenuates, but does not abolish, status epilepticus.[13]

In contrast, one case report has been described involving the precipitation of seizure-like movements (without EEG documentation) in a child who received N_2O alone.[4,14] N_2O has also been included in the anesthetic regimens associated with many case reports involving convulsions during halothane, isoflurane, and enflurane anesthesia. On this basis, it has been suggested that the use of N_2O may be responsible for perioperative convulsions reported in association with isoflurane-N_2O anesthesia.[15,16]

Although definitive verification is lacking, the available evidence suggests that N_2O does not possess significant proconvulsant properties. A possible facilitatory role cannot be excluded (when administered concomitantly with another anesthetic), but the long-standing safety record and enormous clinical experience with this drug support the belief that its proconvulsant potential must be very low.[17]

HALOTHANE AND ISOFLURANE

Halothane and isoflurane are considered together because the data for these agents are similar. Each drug possesses potent anticonvulsant properties and each agent has been used to successfully terminate status epilepticus.[18-21] Nevertheless, occasional case reports involving perioperative seizures have been published in relation to both halothane and isoflurane anesthesia. Smith reported intraoperative seizures during N_2O-halothane anesthesia in two young children undergoing urologic procedures. However, in neither case was EEG documentation available.[1] Millar reported convulsions in a young adult during the early postoperative period after halothane-N_2O anesthesia.[22] The case report was complicated by a history of a remote head injury. Steen and Michenfelder discussed a case report involving a child who convulsed during halothane-N_2O anesthesia.[4,14] However, a subsequent convulsion was precipitated by exposure to N_2O alone but not to halothane alone.

Three cases of seizures associated with isoflurane have been reported. Two cases involve tonic-clonic seizure activity during isoflurane-N_2O anesthesia.[23,24] One of these cases[24] involved an otherwise healthy adult patient who developed tonic-clonic seizure activity intraoperatively on two occasions. Intraoperative EEG recording was performed during the second anesthetic administered, in an identical manner, using a mask induction with N_2O and isoflurane. EEG seizure activity was documented during the intraoperative convulsion (Fig. 20-2). The third case involved a patient who developed myoclonic movements in the recovery

room about 20 min following isoflurane-N_2O anesthesia. The myoclonic activity persisted for about 2 h.[25]

These case reports, particularly those associated with isoflurane, have been criticized on the basis that N_2O was included in the anesthetic regimen in each case. It has been suggested that N_2O rather than isoflurane or halothane may have been responsible for the intraoperative seizure activity.[15,16] However, little support exists for a significant proconvulsant role associated with N_2O. Overall, reports of perioperative convulsions associated with the administration of isoflurane or halothane are remarkably scarce and little evidence suggests that these agents pose a significant risk of perioperative seizures in either epileptic or nonepileptic patients.

ENFLURANE

Enflurane probably represents the most widely recognized proconvulsant anesthetic drug in current clinical use. Numerous studies, in both animals and humans, have demonstrated EEG polyspike and wave activity during enflurane anesthesia.[12,26-28] Several of these studies also reported myoclonic-like muscle jerking associated with epileptiform EEG activity.[26,27] Enflurane-induced seizure activity typically occurs at inspired enflurane concentrations of 2 to 2.5 vol% and is exacerbated by concomitant hyperventilation. Increasing the inspired enflurane concentration ultimately results in EEG burst suppression (Fig. 20-3).[12]

Enflurane has been used during cortical resection for refractory epilepsy to activate epileptic foci although the specificity of this effect remains controversial.[21,29,30] Evidence from depth electrode studies in animals suggests that enflurane-induced seizures originate in subcortical structures.[31] Increased hippocampal glucose metabolism in rats during enflurane-induced seizures has been suggested to support this possibility.[32] However, these findings remain controversial because they have also been reported in association with a variety of other anesthetic drugs that lack proconvulsant properties.[33] A recent study in cats compared somatically stimulated seizures during deep enflurane anesthesia with lidocaine-induced convulsions.[33] The sensorimotor cortex was reported to be essential for the development of somatically triggered seizures during enflurane anesthesia but not for lidocaine-induced convulsions. These results suggest a cortical (rather than subcortical) origin for seizures associated with enflurane anesthesia.

In addition to enflurane's documented potential for producing seizure activity during anesthesia, multiple cases of postoperative neuroexcitatory movements, including convulsions, have been reported following enflurane anesthesia.[34-41] The majority of these reports

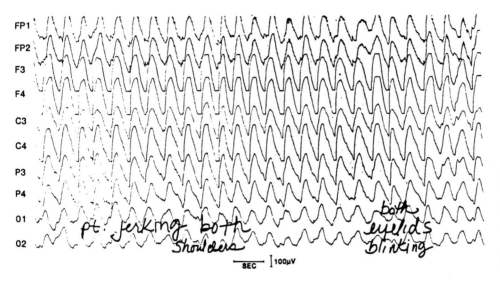

Figure 20-2   Electroencephalographic recording associated with clinical convulsive activity during isoflurane-nitrous oxide anesthesia. (Reproduced with permission from Poulton and Ellingson.[24])

involve nonepileptic patients and EEG documentation of seizure activity is not available. Most case reports describe tonic-clonic convulsive movements, but 20 to 25 percent of the cases involve myoclonic or dystonic type movements. Onset of neuroexcitatory movements commonly occurs early in the postoperative period, typically within 1 to 2 h after emergence. However, in some case reports convulsions commenced several hours and even several days after enflurane anesthesia.

Despite the relative abundance of case reports of postoperative neuroexcitatory movements following enflurane anesthesia (compared to isoflurane or halo-

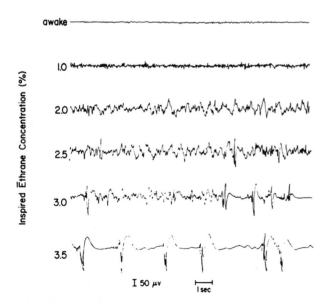

Figure 20-3   Electroencephalographic patterns associated with increasing inspired concentrations of enflurane at normocapnia (Pa_{CO_2} = 35 to 39 mmHg). (Reproduced with permission from Neigh and coworkers.[12])

thane), the etiologic basis for these phenomena and their clinical significance remain controversial. Burchiel and coworkers[27] studied the intraoperative and postoperative EEG effects of enflurane in 12 nonepileptic volunteers and reported nonepileptiform EEG abnormalities persisting for 6 to 30 days following enflurane anesthesia. All 12 patients had decreased alpha activity, 8 patients had persistent intermittent posterior rhythmic delta activity, and 6 had increased amplitude and frequency of benign preanesthetic focal EEG findings. Although 6 of the 12 patients developed EEG seizure activity during enflurane anesthesia, none demonstrated evidence of postanesthetic epileptiform EEG activity. No correlation was found between the development of EEG seizure activity during anesthesia and the occurrence or duration of postanesthesia EEG abnormalities. Burchiel and colleagues also investigated EEG abnormalities following halothane anesthesia in 7 healthy volunteers.[42] EEG abnormalities similar to those observed with enflurane were reported. Compared to enflurane, halothane-induced postoperative EEG abnormalities were more pronounced and included transient spikes, but resolved more rapidly over 7 to 14 days compared to enflurane. Consistent with the results for enflurane, no evidence of epileptiform activity was noted in the postanesthetic period.

Opitz and coworkers[43] reported experience providing anesthesia for 1172 patients with epilepsy, including 345 who received enflurane. In a subgroup of 45 patients[44] who underwent intraoperative EEG monitoring, these investigators reported that the incidence of EEG epileptiform activity was lower during enflurane anesthesia compared to preanesthetic EEG recordings obtained during both wakefulness and physiologic sleep. They also reported no clinical seizures in the early postoperative period and no evidence of any change in seizure pattern during a subsequent 6-week follow-up.

Enflurane possesses anticonvulsant properties in animal models and in humans and has been used to terminate status epilepticus in children.[44,45] Enflurane has a documented capacity for producing EEG seizure activity when administered in high doses especially with concomitant hyperventilation. The effect appears to occur in both epileptic and nonepileptic patients. Although case reports of postoperative neuroexcitatory movements are more numerous following enflurane anesthesia compared to halothane or isoflurane, such case reports remain rare and a definitive etiologic role for enflurane remains to be established. The use of enflurane does not appear to pose a significant risk of postoperative seizures in either epileptic or nonepileptic patients, particularly in view of current anesthesia practice patterns that tend to use low anesthetic concentrations combined with neuromuscular blockade. Nevertheless, given the availability of less controversial and equally efficacious drugs such as isoflurane or halothane, most clinicians prefer to avoid enflurane in epileptic patients.

DESFLURANE AND SEVOFLURANE

Clinical or EEG-documented seizure activity has not been reported in humans in association with either desflurane or sevoflurane.[46-49] The pro- and anticonvulsant properties of both drugs have not been extensively investigated. EEG patterns associated with increasing depth of desflurane anesthesia are reported to be similar to isoflurane and this drug is anticipated to demonstrate similar anticonvulsant properties.

Sevoflurane has been less extensively studied. EEG suppression, leading to a burst-suppression pattern, occurs with increasing sevoflurane concentrations. Epileptiform activity has not been reported in humans. Osawa and colleagues reported somatically stimulated seizure activity originating in deep cortical structures (amygdala and hippocampus) and spontaneous spike generation at high sevoflurane concentrations (5%) in cats.[50] These results have been interpreted as suggesting that the proconvulsant potential of sevoflurane may reside intermediate to that of enflurane and isoflurane.

Figures 20-4 and 20-5 list the anesthetic drugs associated with intraoperative and postoperative neuroexcitatory phenomena.

Intravenous Anesthetic Drugs

BARBITURATES

Derivatives of barbituric acid possess both proconvulsant and anticonvulsant properties depending on the nature of the substitution groups attached to the barbituric acid ring. Convulsant properties appear to correlate with substitution at the C_5 position with groups containing six or more carbon atoms or with increasing alkylation of the nitrogen atoms in the barbiturate ring.[51]

Thiopental has potent anticonvulsant properties and has long been a useful drug in the management of seizures, including status epilepticus. Proconvulsant activity has not been reported in association with the administration of thiopental during anesthesia. Thiopental, administered in small doses, has been used to activate spike activity during the EEG investigation of patients with temporal lobe epilepsy. However, the mechanism of action associated with this application is thought to relate to the induction of narcosis similar to the activation of interictal spike activity observed with the onset of natural sleep.[52]

Convulsions were commonly observed after administration of early formulations of methohexital. Subsequent elimination of proconvulsant isomers has markedly reduced the convulsant properties associated with this drug.[4] Methohexital has been reported, and used clinically, to activate EEG seizures in patients with temporal lobe epilepsy.[53-55] However, in its current formulation, this proconvulsant activity appears to be restricted to patients with this condition. A study comparing the EEG effects of methohexital in patients with psychomotor seizures or generalized epilepsy and nonepileptic patients demonstrated activation of seizure foci in 72 percent of patients with temporal lobe epilepsy but no evidence of epileptiform activity in nonepileptic patients nor in patients with generalized seizures.[56]

BENZODIAZEPINES

The benzodiazepines, like thiopental, have potent anticonvulsant properties and are widely used to treat seizures both acutely and chronically. Benzodiazepines, particularly diazepam and lorazepam, which are the most extensively studied (as well as midazolam), are considered first-line drugs in the management of status epilepticus.[57] Seizure activity has not been reported in association with any of the benzodiazepines during or following anesthesia. Several nonanesthesia-related cases of diazepam-induced status epilepticus have been reported in patients with epilepsy but these appear to be restricted to children with Lennox-Gastaut syndrome.[58,59]

KETAMINE

Ketamine, a derivative of phencyclidine (PCP), produces an anesthetic state termed "dissociative anesthe-

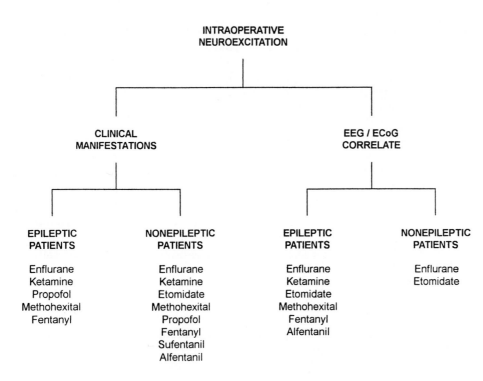

Figure 20-4 Anesthetic drugs associated with intraoperative neuroexcitatory phenomena. Drugs are classified based on reported clinical manifestations (e.g., tremors, myoclonus, dystonic movements, and tonic-clonic convulsions) or the availability of electroencephalographic (EEG) or electrocortographic (ECoG) evidence of epileptiform activity. Anesthetic drugs associated with reports involving epileptic and nonepileptic patients are listed separatedly.

sia." PCP was originally developed in 1957 as a dissociative anesthetic but was withdrawn due to a convulsant tendency and a high incidence of psychotic reactions.[4,60] Ketamine has less potent hallucinogenic and convulsant properties. Nevertheless, considerable evidence suggests an association of ketamine with neuroexcitatory movements and proconvulsant activity.

In nonepileptic humans, neuroexcitatory movements are common after the administration of ketamine. Opisthotonos and extensor spasms in infants[61] and a tonic-clonic seizure in an adult[62] have been re-

ported following ketamine administration. However, EEG documentation of electrical seizure activity associated with ketamine is lacking in nonepileptic patients.

Among epileptic patients, ketamine reportedly activates epileptogenic foci. During ECoG, seizure activity has been consistently demonstrated after the intravenous administration of ketamine, 2 to 4 mg/kg.[11] The onset of seizure activity has been correlated with peak plasma levels of ketamine and has been reported to originate in the hippocampus and amygdala. Based on depth electrode studies, electrical seizure activity was

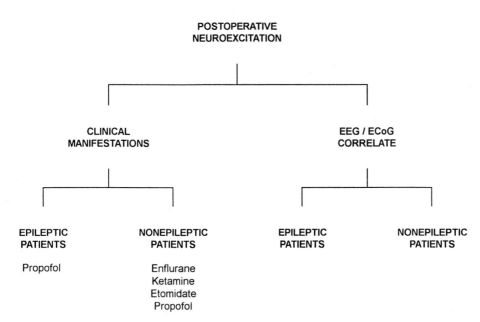

Figure 20-5 Anesthetic drugs associated with postoperative neuroexcitatory phenomena classified on the basis of reported clinical manifestations or electroencephalographic (EEG) or electrocortographic (ECoG) evidence of epileptiform activity. Anesthetic drugs associated with reports involving epileptic and nonepileptic patients are listed separately.

reported to propagate widely to subcortical structures, but only seizure propagation, which included the thalamus or cerebral cortex, was associated with clinical convulsive activity (tonic-clonic or muscular jerking movements). Based on these findings, it has been suggested that scalp EEG recordings may fail to detect hippocampal and subcortical seizure activity induced by ketamine.[11]

Depth and cortical electrode studies in cats have demonstrated that anesthetic doses of ketamine produce a hypersynchronous EEG pattern with spikes associated clinically with bizarre posturing and catalepsia.[60,63] Electrical seizure activity was reported to originate in hippocampal and subcortical structures. Winters has argued that the neuroexcitatory effects seen in cats are also applicable to nonepileptic humans.[64]

Despite the foregoing considerations, considerable evidence, in several experimentally induced seizure models in animals, indicates that ketamine also possesses significant anticonvulsant properties.[65] In addition, successful termination of status epilepticus has been reported after the administration of ketamine in humans.[66]

The proconvulsant and anticonvulsant properties of ketamine are dose dependent. Anticonvulsant effects predominate at subanesthetic doses, whereas somewhat higher anesthetic doses are proconvulsant. A large body of experimental evidence suggests that some of the central effects of ketamine and other PCP-like drugs (e.g., psychotomimetic actions, anticonvulsant properties) are mediated through antagonism at the *N*-methyl-D-aspartate (NMDA) subclass of excitatory amino acid (EEA) receptor.[65] A strong correlation has been reported between the anticonvulsant potency of a wide variety of PCP-like drugs, including ketamine, and their potency as NMDA antagonists. Furthermore, NMDA antagonism occurs at subanesthetic doses. Unfortunately, because these effects occur at subanesthetic doses, NMDA antagonism does not adequately explain the general anesthetic properties associated with this class of drugs. Similarly, an etiologic basis for the proconvulsant properties observed at anesthetic doses also remains elusive.

ETOMIDATE

Neuroexcitatory movements are commonly associated with etomidate anesthesia. These abnormal movements include tremor, dystonia, generalized convulsions, and particularly, myoclonus. Although neuroexcitatory phenomena occur most commonly during induction, similar activity has also been reported during emergence and in the early postoperative pe-

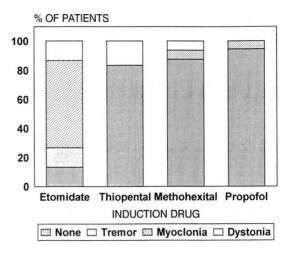

% OF PATIENTS

Figure 20-6 Incidence of neuroexcitatory movements during induction of anesthesia using etomidate (0.3 mg/kg), thiopental (4 mg/kg), methohexital (1.5 mg/kg), or propofol (2 mg/kg). (Reproduced with permission from Reddy and coworkers.[72])

riod.[67-70] In most cases neuroexcitatory movements are of short duration (a few minutes) but myoclonus persisting for 2.5 h after anesthesia has been reported.[67] Convulsions (focal and generalized) have also been reported in patients receiving long-term etomidate infusions for sedation during mechanical ventilation.[71] Most case reports involve nonepileptic patients and none have included EEG documentation during the convulsive activity.

Neuroexcitatory movements have been reported to occur in 60 to 87 percent of patients receiving etomidate anesthesia. In nonepileptic patients, Reddy and coworkers[72] reported a higher incidence of neuroexcitatory movements during induction of anesthesia with etomidate (86.6 percent) compared to thiopental (16.6 percent), methohexital (12.5 percent) or propofol (5.5 percent) (Fig. 20-6). Myoclonus accounted for 69 percent of the neuroexcitatory activity. Several patients developed generalized myoclonic seizures, but simultaneous scalp EEG recordings failed to detect seizure activity. However, multiple EEG spikes were observed in 22 percent of patients who experienced focal or multifocal myoclonus. None of the other induction drugs were associated with EEG evidence of epileptiform activity. EEG-documented seizure activity has also been observed in 20 percent of a series of more than 30 nonepileptic patients receiving etomidate for induction of anesthesia for cardiac surgery.[73] In contrast, Ghoneim and Yamada failed to detect EEG epileptiform activity during etomidate-induced myoclonic activity.[74]

Etomidate also activates seizure activity among epileptic patients during ECoG[69,75,76] and during scalp EEG.[43,44] Several investigators have suggested that the administration of etomidate should be avoided, or used cautiously, in patients with preexisting epilepsy presenting for nonepilepsy-related surgery.[69,70,72,76]

Myoclonus represents a prominent feature of etomidate neuroexcitation. Reddy and coworkers[72] have suggested that myoclonic activity associated with etomidate anesthesia is likely subcortical in origin and have postulated that brainstem structures (e.g., red nucleus, vestibular nucleus, reticular formation, and cerebellar dentate nucleus) may be involved. Modica and colleagues,[77] citing evidence based on electromyographic studies, have suggested that some neuroexcitatory movements associated with etomidate may be spinal in origin.

PROPOFOL

Propofol is the most recent anesthetic agent to be thrust into the proconvulsant versus anticonvulsant controversy. Numerous reports of neuroexcitatory phenomena associated with propofol anesthesia have renewed speculative interest in potential neuroexcitatory mechanisms and their clinical significance.[78,79]

Following the introduction of propofol into clinical practice in 1986, sporadic case reports involving neuroexcitatory phenomena were reported. By 1989, although a definitive causal relationship had not been established, evidence indicting propofol as the most likely cause was sufficient to prompt the Committee on the Safety of Medicines in the United Kingdom to issue an advisory warning of the possible link between perioperative seizures and propofol administration.[80]

A wide variety of neuroexcitatory movements have been reported in association with propofol administration including muscular twitching, tremors, myoclonus, opisthotonos, and other dystonic posturing and tonic-clonic convulsions.[81-98] Case reports involve both epileptic and nonepileptic patients. Although a few case reports document such phenomena during induction, the majority of reports involve neuroexcitatory movements that commence either during emergence or in the early postoperative period (within a couple of hours following emergence). This likely accounts for the low incidence of neuroexcitatory phenomena observed by Reddy and colleagues[72] during propofol induction. In most cases the condition resolves spontaneously in less than an hour. However, cases involving delayed onset of up to 5 days have been reported,[89] and one case report described recurrent tonic-clonic seizures and opisthotonic attacks associated with apnea that occurred intermittently for 23 days after propofol-N_2O-enflurane anesthesia in a healthy 29-year-old woman.[82]

Despite numerous case reports describing neuroexcitatory movements associated with the administration of propofol, many studies have reported that propofol is also a potent anticonvulsant. Among epileptic patients undergoing ECoG with depth electrodes, bolus doses of propofol reportedly suppress interictal epileptiform activity.[99,100] Using sedative infusions, Samra and coworkers[101] reported a high degree of individual variability in the ECoG response to propofol, but overall, no significant change in epileptogenic activity was observed. Our own experience using propofol sedation during cortical resection for refractory epilepsy demonstrated no significant effect on interictal ECoG spike frequency but a significantly lower incidence of intraoperative seizures compared to neurolept analgesia (fentanyl and droperidol).* Similarly, EEG interictal epileptiform activity was either unchanged or depressed among epileptic patients administered propofol sedation during dental surgery.[102] In contrast, during cortical resection, ECoG activation of epileptiform activity has been reported in three patients following the administration of propofol.[103]

Propofol effectively terminates status epilepticus in both humans and animal models.[104-106] Furthermore, propofol markedly decreases the duration of seizure activity during ECT.[107-109] In rat models, anesthetic doses of propofol have prevented lidocaine-induced seizures, and subanesthetic doses have increased the seizure threshold.[110] Similarly, propofol offers protection comparable to thiopental against pentylenetetrazol and electroshock-induced seizures in mice.[111] Ahmad and Pleuvry[112] have reported in studies in mice that propofol exhibits anticonvulsant activity against bicuculline, kainic acid, and N-methyl-DL-aspartic acid-induced seizures. This anticonvulsant effect could be abolished by proconvulsant doses of fentanyl and meperidine (pethidine). Proconvulsant doses of fentanyl and meperidine in this model were low (15 μg/kg and 0.5 mg/kg, respectively), suggesting that concomitantly administered opioids may play an important role in the generation of neuroexcitatory phenomena associated with propofol.

An interesting feature of reports of propofol-induced neuroexcitation is the relatively high incidence of opisthotonic movements. Although opisthotonos has been reported in association with other anesthetic drugs, its occurrence appears to be a relatively common feature of propofol-induced neuroexcitation, either independently or in association with myoclonus or tonic-clonic convulsions. Ries and coworkers[97] have reviewed case reports of propofol-induced opisthotonos and have suggested a spinal-mediated mechanism involv-

---

* Herrick IA, Craen RA, Gelb AW, et al. Propofol sedation during awake craniotomy for seizures: effects on electrocortography. *Anesth Analg* 1996; 82:S173.

ing acute desensitization of γ-aminobutyric acid (GABA)ergic and glycinergic (inhibitory receptor) pathways. These authors also caution against the use of antiepileptic drugs such as carbamazepine or phenytoin in the treatment of opisthotonos, suggesting that these drugs may aggravate such movements.

OPIOIDS

FENTANYL, SUFENTANIL, AND ALFENTANIL

Several case reports have described myoclonic and tonic-clonic convulsive movements following the administration of fentanyl (100 to 2500 μg), sufentanil (75 to 600 μg), and alfentanil (1500 μg) among nonepileptic patients during anesthesia.[113–121] Two of these reports involving fentanyl[117] and sufentanil[118] failed to detect seizure activity during simultaneous scalp EEG recording. In most cases successful termination of convulsive activity followed the administration of thiopental or diazepam.

The etiology of neuroexcitatory movements associated with these drugs remains speculative. Investigations evaluating the scalp EEG effects of high-dose opioids during cardiac anesthesia have generally reported no evidence of epileptiform activity.[122] Although Sebel and colleagues[123] reported isolated spike waves during high-dose fentanyl anesthesia, other investigators have not substantiated these findings. Murkin and coworkers[124] reported some minor movements (e.g., limb flexion) associated with the onset of truncal rigidity during high-dose fentanyl (50 or 150 μg/kg) induction of anesthesia. These movements were not associated with scalp EEG epileptiform activity and occasional spike waves observed were attributed to artifact.

In contrast, several investigators have documented the activation of epileptiform activity during ECoG in epileptic patients. Tempelhoff and associates[125] reported that moderate doses of fentanyl (18 to 36 μg/kg) consistently activated electrical seizure activity originating in perihippocampal electrodes among patients undergoing temporal lobectomy for refractory epilepsy. In half of these patients seizure activity began in the temporal lobe contralateral to site of surgery. Similarly, Cascino and coworkers[126] have reported ECoG mesial temporal (hippocampal) epileptiform activation, including seizure activity, following moderate doses of alfentanil (50 μg/kg) in patients with intractable epilepsy. Extratemporal epileptiform activation was not observed. Studies in rats have also demonstrated limbic seizures after the administration of fentanyl or alfentanil.[127,128]

The significance of these contrasting results remains uncertain. Case reports of neuroexcitatory phenomena associated with these opioids involve nonepileptic patients, whereas human investigations documenting

electrical epileptiform activity involve patients with intractable complex partial epilepsy. It is possible that the basis for these phenomena differ mechanistically among epileptic versus nonepileptic patients. Contrasting studies also differ with respect to the doses of opioid administered (moderate dose versus high dose), suggesting that differences in observed epileptiform activity may be dose dependent. Studies that reported no evidence of electrical seizure activity used scalp EEG monitoring; thus, it is possible that these studies failed to detect seizure activity originating in subcortical structures.

MORPHINE

Morphine does not appear to be associated with neuroexcitatory phenomena when administered intravenously at clinically appropriate doses. During high-dose intravenous morphine administration (≥1.0 mg/kg) for induction of anesthesia for cardiac surgery, Smith and colleagues[122] observed no EEG epileptiform activity. Morphine can induce seizures following intracerebroventricular injection or peripheral systemic administration in animal seizure models. However, systemically administered doses required to induce seizures are many times higher than those used clinically, in the absence of other convulsant manipulations (e.g., concomitant administration of pentylenetetrazol or kainic acid).[129] Modica and coworkers[17] discuss two case reports[130,131] of seizures associated with the administration of morphine in humans. One case involved a tonic-clonic seizure following 20 mg intramuscular morphine and 0.4 mg scopolamine administered to a 14-year-old boy. The second case involved a tonic-clonic seizure reported in a 30-year-old epileptic patient 6 h after the epidural administration of 3 mg morphine. Despite these two case reports, the vast majority of evidence in both animals and humans, as well as enormous clinical experience, suggests that morphine is essentially devoid of proconvulsant activity and neuroexcitatory effects at clinically relevant doses.

MEPERIDINE

Neuroexcitatory phenomena have not been reported in association with the acute administration of clinically appropriate doses of meperidine. Although not extensively studied, the EEG response to intravenous administration of high-dose meperidine (400 mg) has been reported to be similar to that associated with morphine.[132] Like morphine, meperidine administered intravenously in very high doses, exceeding those used clinically, produces seizures in dogs. However, in contrast to morphine, the therapeutic margin between the effective dose for surgical anesthesia versus the induction of seizure activity was 2.2 times lower for meperidine.[17,133] In the perioperative setting, doses of meperidine used in conjunction with anesthesia do not appear to cause neuroexcitatory effects.

Neuroexcitation manifesting as myoclonus, tremors, and seizures is well documented in association with chronic meperidine administration. These neuroexcitatory effects are attributed to the accumulation of normeperidine, a neurotoxic metabolite of meperidine with a long half-life. Susceptibility to normeperidine neurotoxicity appears to be increased by factors that enhance biotransformation (e.g., concurrent administration of phenothiazines or anticonvulsants such as phenytoin or phenobarbital), disease processes that impair normeperidine excretion (e.g., renal failure), and diseases associated with escalating drug requirements (e.g., cancer, sickle cell disease).

OPIOIDS AND EPILEPSY

Opioid peptides (endogenous opioids) have long been recognized as important neurotransmitters and neuromodulators, particularly in the limbic system. Initial observations, in the late 1970s, that the intraventricular administration of enkephalins and β endorphin in rats resulted in EEG seizure activity originating in limbic structures generated intense interest and speculation on the potential role of these substances in epilepsy. Although our understanding of the function of endogenous opioids in epilepsy is far from complete, a general concept of their role is emerging.[129,134-136] The effect of opioid peptides on neuronal activity appears to be inhibitory throughout the central nervous system (CNS) with the exception of the limbic system. Anticonvulsant effects associated with endogenous opioids have been firmly established in a variety of animal models and are believed to involve neuronal hyperpolarization. Seizures appear to activate peptide opioid production and release and current opinion suggests that these substances contribute to the termination of seizure activity. Intrinsic to the hippocampus, opioid peptides appear to induce neuronal (pyramidal cell) excitation through presynaptic inhibition of inhibitory interneurons. Thus, depending on the site of action and the experimental conditions, peptide opioids appear to possess both proconvulsant and anticonvulsant properties.

Interest has also been focused on the epileptogenic effects of nonpeptide opioids (particularly morphine). Drugs such as morphine can induce seizure activity in a variety of animal models under appropriate conditions (very high doses). However, it is unclear whether these effects are mediated through similar mechanisms to the peptide opioids. Tortella[137] has noted that distinct differences exist between the EEG epileptiform effects produced by peptide versus nonpeptide opioids. Endogenous opioid-induced seizures can be completely antagonized with naloxone, occur at doses that are lower than those needed to produce analgesia, and are typically not associated with clinically apparent convulsive activity. In contrast, nonpeptide opioid (morphine)-induced EEG seizures are not antagonized, or are incompletely antagonized, by naloxone, occur only at doses that are several times higher than those needed to produce analgesia, and are invariably associated with behavioral manifestations of convulsive activity. On this basis, opioid-induced seizures have been suggested to involve several opioid receptor systems as well as nonreceptor-mediated mechanisms depending on the dose, the route of opioid administration, and the experimental conditions.[129]

The implications of these observations to the clinical occurrence of neuroexcitatory phenomena associated with the administration of opioids in the perioperative setting is unclear. It may, however, be more than coincidence that clinical documentation of electrical seizure activity associated with opioid administration in humans is available only among patients with temporal lobe epilepsy. Whether neuroexcitatory phenomena observed in nonepileptic patients is mediated via epileptiform or nonepileptiform mechanisms remains entirely conjectural.

Local Anesthetics and Ancillary Anesthetic Agents

LOCAL ANESTHETICS

Local anesthetics possess both proconvulsant and anticonvulsant properties. In contrast to many of the general anesthetic drugs, proconvulsant properties associated with local anesthetics occur at toxic doses. CNS toxicity associated with local anesthetic drugs parallels their intrinsic anesthetic potency.[138]

Neuroexcitatory movements often precede local anesthetic-induced convulsions and typically manifest as shivering and muscular twitching and tremors, which often involve the face and distal extremities. However, the occurrence of such neuroexcitatory phenomena before convulsive activity is inconsistent and likely relates to the dose and rate of administration. Local anesthetic-induced convulsions are typically clonic or tonic-clonic in nature and originate, based on studies involving both animals and humans, in the limbic system (amygdala and hippocampus).[138-142]

At clinically appropriate doses, local anesthetics possess anticonvulsant activity.[77] Subtoxic doses of lidocaine have been used to terminate status epilepticus and both lidocaine and procaine have been reported to prevent, or reduce, ECT-induced seizures in humans.[143]

Local anesthetics block neural transmission by blockade of sodium channels, thereby increasing the threshold for generation of action potentials. At low doses, the result is a neuronal stabilizing effect that is believed to account for the anticonvulsant properties of these drugs. At neurotoxic doses, neuroexcitation, including convulsions, result from the differential blockade of inhibitory pathways in the brain. This differential blockade permits unopposed activity in facilitatory (excitatory) pathways leading to convulsions. At higher doses, conduction in both the inhibitory and facilitatory pathways is impaired, resulting in a state of generalized CNS depression.[138,144]

DROPERIDOL

Consistent with other neuroleptic drugs, droperidol, a butyrophenone, lowers the seizure threshold.[145,146] The mechanism of this effect is believed to relate to dopamine antagonism. Dopaminergic projections from the substantia nigra are postulated to play a role in the control of cortical excitability and substantia nigra–mediated seizure inhibition, in some hippocampal seizure models, can be blocked by haloperidol.[147]

Caution has been advised when administering these drugs to patients with untreated epilepsy.[145] However, neuroexcitatory phenomena do not appear to be associated with the administration of droperidol in relation to anesthesia. Despite extensive experience among epileptic patients in whom neurolept analgesia has been used preferentially for conscious sedation during cortical resection for intractable epilepsy, no cases involving seizures related directly to the administration of droperidol have been reported.

The possibility that antipsychotic medications may lower the threshold for anesthetic-induced neuroexcitatory effects has been suggested recently. Vohra[41] reported data on a nonepileptic, schizophrenic patient receiving antipsychotic medications (flupenthixol and chlorpromazine) who experienced a seizure (EEG documentation not available) following emergence from enflurane-N_2O anesthesia. Because inspired concentrations of enflurane were relatively low (1 to 1.5 vol%), these authors speculate that the concomitant administration of antipsychotic agents may have contributed to the development of tonic-clonic seizure activity.

FLUMAZENIL

Flumazenil is a benzodiazepine antagonist recently released in North America for reversing the sedative effects of benzodiazepines.[148,149] The mechanism of action involves the benzodiazepine receptor site on the $GABA_A$ receptor-chloride channel complex where it competitively inhibits the binding of agonists. In relation to anesthesia, flumazenil has been used to hasten recovery from the effects of benzodiazepines administered as a component of general anesthesia or con-

scious sedation. It has also been used extensively for the treatment of benzodiazepine overdose.

Neuroexcitatory phenomena, especially seizures, have been reported in association with the administration of flumazenil, presumably related to antagonism of the anticonvulsant effects of benzodiazepines. Reviewing 43 case reports of seizures following flumazenil administration, Spivey[150] reported 88.2 percent of the seizures were single or multiple, 9.3 percent involved status epilepticus, and 2.3 percent consisted of twitching and jerking movements. Seizures occurred in a variety of settings. The most common situation (47 percent of case reports) involved the administration of flumazenil for treatment of mixed overdoses, which included a benzodiazepine and a proconvulsant drug, particularly cyclic antidepressants. Other co-administered proconvulsant drugs included cocaine, heroin, cyclosporine, isoniazid, methaqualone, and propoxyphene. Other circumstances associated with seizures included the administration of flumazenil to: (1) patients who had recently received benzodiazepines for the treatment of seizure disorders (16 percent), (2) patients receiving benzodiazepines with an underlying medical cause for seizures (12 percent), (3) patients with a history of chronic benzodiazepine use or abuse treated for acute benzodiazepine overdose (7 percent), (4) patients receiving benzodiazepines during conscious sedation (5 percent), and (5) patients in whom no clear correlation was found between seizures and the reversal of benzodiazepine effects (14 percent). No correlation was found between the dose of flumazenil and the development of seizures. The two case reports involving patients receiving conscious sedation consisted of nonepileptic adult patients (one had a history of febrile convulsions in infancy) who experienced seizures following small intravenous doses of flumazenil (0.5 and 0.6 mg). Overall, 14 percent of patients required no pharmacologic treatment for these seizures. Among the patients who were treated, most seizures responded to standard anticonvulsant drugs such as barbiturates, benzodiazepines, or phenytoin.[148,150]

Paradoxically, flumazenil has also been reported to possess anticonvulsant activity. Scollo-Lavizzari reported a marked reduction in EEG-monitored epileptiform activity among epileptic patients administered flumazenil intravenously (2.5 mg) or orally (10 to 90 mg/day).[151,152]

Management of Anesthetic-Induced Neuroexcitatory Phenomena

In most cases, neuroexcitatory movements associated with anesthesia are benign and self-limited. Observation and supportive care are typically appropriate including the provision of supplemental oxygen, maintenance of an adequate airway, ventilation and secure intravenous access, protection from physical injury, and reassurance, if the patient is conscious. Because of the sporadic nature of these events, efforts to arrange investigations (particularly EEG recording), while neuroexcitatory activity persists, deserve consideration.

Pharmacologic intervention is largely empirical with conflicting evidence in the case report literature regarding the efficacy of many drugs. Although it is difficult to draw firm conclusions, in general, tonic-clonic seizures (if treated) appear to be responsive to standard anticonvulsants such as thiopental or diazepam. Myoclonic and dystonic movements (primarily opisthotonos) are less consistently responsive to treatment. The combination of opisthotonos and tonic-clonic convulsive movements appears to occur exclusively in association with propofol. These neuroexcitatory phenomena are seen in a recurrent, cyclic pattern and are relatively unresponsive to conventional therapy. Ries and coworkers[97] reviewed the case reports of opisthotonos associated with propofol and concluded that thiopental, diazepam, diphenhydramine, and lorazepam are ineffective, or inconsistently effective, at terminating these events. Similarly, these authors have suggested that phenytoin and divalproex sodium also appear to be ineffective and may aggravate the condition. Ries and colleagues[97] have suggested that these findings support the premise that dystonic movements associated with propofol are probably not epileptiform in origin and have speculated that other therapeutic avenues, such as the use of physostigmine or chlormethiazole, deserve consideration. Orser,[78] however, has emphasized that based on our incomplete understanding of the etiologic basis for these phenomena, such treatments remain highly speculative.

Mild, short-lived, neuroexcitatory activity that is self-limited or promptly responsive to pharmacologic intervention does not appear to pose a significant risk to the patient. No evidence suggests that these events, including convulsions, correlate with latent epilepsy. In many cases, uneventful completion of the operation and safe discharge after ambulatory care procedures have been reported. Although management must be individualized, extraordinary interventions do not seem warranted in most cases.

In cases involving prolonged or severe neuroexcitatory activity, especially recurrent episodes of opisthotonic activity following propofol, a more cautious approach to management seems appropriate. The assistance of a neurologist may be helpful (although neurologists are often equally perplexed with respect to the management of these events). Arrangements should be made for observation, or active management, in an appropriate environment until abnormal movements have resolved.

Mechanistic Musings

Our understanding of the mechanisms that underlie neuroexcitatory phenomena associated with anesthesia is far from complete. However, advances in neurophysiology and epileptology and our understanding of the CNS effects of anesthetic drugs demonstrate some interesting parallels.

The focus of intense research, our understanding of the mechanisms of neurotransmission and neuronal ion channel physiology is advancing rapidly. These developments have spurred parallel advances in our understanding of the mechanisms involved in the generation and termination of seizures and our interest in the effects of anesthetic drugs on neurotransmitter-receptor systems.

Proposed at the turn of the century, the Meyer-Overton rule, which demonstrates a linear relationship between anesthetic potency and lipid or oil solubility, has formed the foundation for the long-standing belief that a perturbation of cellular membranes underlies the mechanism of general anesthetic drugs. However, 15 to 20 years ago a similar relationship was shown to exist between general anesthetic potency and potency for inhibiting the enzyme luciferase. This discovery, and subsequent work demonstrating that anesthetic agents competitively block the enzymatic site on luciferase, has renewed interest in the effects of anesthetic drugs on cellular proteins, particularly receptors.[153-155]

General anesthetic drugs interact with a variety of neuronal constituents including voltage-gated ion channels for sodium, potassium, and calcium and the ligand-gated ion channels.[156-159] This latter group includes receptors for acetylcholine (nicotinic), $GABA_A$, glutamate (kainate, AMPA and NMDA subtypes), glycine, and serotonin. The $GABA_A$ and glutamate receptors and their respective ion channels have attracted intense interest because they represent the predominant inhibitory and excitatory fast neurotransmitter systems in the CNS. Given the ubiquitous nature of these neurotransmitters in the mammalian CNS, and their importance in neuroexcitation and inhibition, it is not surprising that they have been postulated to play important roles in the mechanisms of general anesthesia. Some drugs such as the barbiturates and benzodiazepines have been known, for many years, to act as GABAergic agonists. Recent investigations have also demonstrated that many other anesthetic drugs, including propofol, etomidate, and halothane, have agonist activity at $GABA_A$ receptors (Fig. 20-7).[158] Ketamine, as discussed previously, possesses potent NMDA antagonist activity.[65]

Many of these receptor systems and ion channels also play important roles in the generation and termination of seizures. $GABA_A$ agonists, for example, possess anticonvulsant properties (e.g., benzodiazepines,

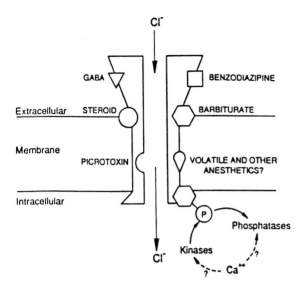

Figure 20-7 Diagram of the GABA$_A$ receptor/chloride channel complex showing proposed sites of action for anesthetic drugs. GABA acting on the extracellular receptor opens the chloride-selective channel. Drugs acting on several distinct sites (barbiturates, benzodiazepines, steroid anesthetics) enhance GABA binding or chloride conductance. Drugs acting at the picrotoxin site block channel conductance. Propofol, etomidate, and the volatile anesthetics also act as agonists, but specific binding sites have not been fully elucidated. Channel kinetics also can be modulated by phosphorylation/dephosphorylation of intracellular regulatory sites, some of which may be calcium dependent. Volatile anesthetics may modulate channel activity via a calcium-dependent mechanism. (Reproduced with permission from Tanelian and coworkers.[157])

In an attempt to explain the neuroexcitatory properties of anesthetic drugs, Winters and coworkers[63] (based on investigations involving ketamine) proposed a schema of general anesthesia (Fig. 20-8) that suggested that the anesthetic state can be achieved either by inducing CNS depression resulting in coma or by inducing a state of CNS excitation resembling catatonia (Fig. 20-8). Drugs such as halothane and thiopental are postulated to produce CNS depression and hence are relatively devoid of neuroexcitatory phenomena. In contrast, drugs such as enflurane and ketamine are postulated to produce a cataleptic anesthetic state characterized by neuroexcitation. In this cataleptic state, EEG burst suppression, which commonly accompanies deep levels of anesthesia, is postulated to represent an excitatory phenomenon which can culminate in epileptiform discharges manifesting clinically in the form of abnormal movements (e.g., myoclonus and seizures). While Winters[63] did not offer a mechanistic explanation for differences in anesthetic states, the concept may continue to be relevant. It is at least conceivable that different anesthetic drugs may differ in their potential for aberrant interactions with neurotransmitter systems.

Several subtypes of glutamate receptors are known to exist and evidence suggests that, at least for the NMDA receptor, the subtypes exist in several isoforms (based on differences in receptor subunit composition) each with differing pharmacologic properties and distributions in the brain.[160,161] Similarly, the GABA$_A$ receptor also exists in a variety of isoforms with different

barbiturates) and GABA$_A$ antagonists produce seizures (e.g., bicuculline). Similarly, EAA receptor pathways (principally glutamate) are believed to play an important role in the initiation and spread of seizures. EEA receptor agonists are strongly epileptogenic and EEA antagonists generally inhibit seizure activity.[135,136]

Whether interactions with neurotransmitters are sufficient to explain the anesthetic properties of general anesthetic drugs remains controversial. However, it seems highly probable that the anticonvulsant properties associated with most anesthetic drugs relate to interactions with neurotransmitters, a situation well documented in the case of benzodiazepines and barbiturates.[135,136] It also seems likely, although as yet unsubstantiated, that similar interactions also underlie neuroexcitatory phenomena reported in association with anesthesia.

Most anesthetic drugs possess well-documented anticonvulsant properties.[17,77] The proconvulsant or neuroexcitatory potential of anesthetic drugs appears to represent an aberrant phenomenon, contrary to the anticipated CNS depressant effects. The aberrant nature of these events is supported by the sporadic nature of their occurrence.

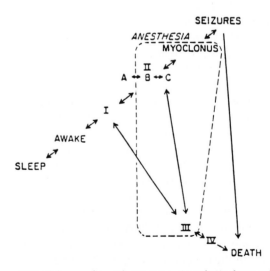

Figure 20-8 Schema of anesthetic states. Anesthetic drugs with neuroexcitatory properties (e.g., ketamine, enflurane) are postulated to produce a cataleptic anesthetic state characterized by neuroexcitation (stage II). Drugs that are devoid of neuroexcitatory properties (e.g., thiopental, halothane) produce an anesthetic state characterized by neurodepression (stage III). (Reproduced with permission from Winters and coworkers.[63])

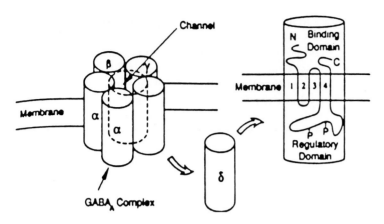

Figure 20-9 Diagram of the GABA$_A$ receptor/chloride channel complex showing subunit composition. Different combinations of subunits, in different stoichiometry, can produce receptors with different binding affinities and channel kinetics. The subunits are differentially expressed in different brain regions. (Reproduced with permission from Tanelian and coworkers.[157])

distributions in the brain and presumably different affinities for agonists and antagonists (Fig. 20-9).[157,159] Although many anesthetic drugs have been shown to possess GABA$_A$ agonist anticonvulsant activity it is possible that interactions with different receptor isoforms produce different effects under appropriate conditions. Paradoxical epileptiform activity has been reported in rats following administration of GABA agonists.[162]

Neurotransmitter-neuroreceptor physiology is extremely complex. Many anesthetic drugs have been reported to affect a variety of neuronal receptors and ion channels (Fig. 20-9).[155,156,158,163,164] The behavior of receptors is also affected by other neurotransmitters and neuropeptides, which act as neuromodulators, influencing the receptor response to agonists. In addition, the neuronal response to receptor activation is not direct but rather reflects the temporal and somatic summation of excitatory and inhibitory inputs.

Our understanding of the neuroexcitatory effects of anesthetic drugs is further confounded by our limited understanding of the behavior of neuronal networks. It is certainly conceivable that neuroexcitatory phenomena derive from differing sensitivities of neuronal systems as opposed to individual neurons. Local anesthetic toxicity exemplifies this concept.[138,144] Local anesthetic-induced convulsions suggest that local anesthetic drugs possess neuroexcitatory properties at toxic doses. Current evidence suggests, however, that local anesthetics are neuroinhibitory at all concentrations. Seizure activity is postulated to result from the differential sensitivity of inhibitory neuron systems. Initial depression of inhibitory systems leads to unopposed activity in the excitatory systems resulting in seizures. Higher concentrations of local anesthetics depress activity in both neuron groups. It is possible that a similar mechanism operates in the case of other anesthetic drugs. The pharmacologic effects of anesthetic drugs may be consistently inhibitory; however, the popula-

tion of neurons or neural systems affected may vary depending on a variety of conditions (e.g., dose, rate of change of brain concentrations, rate of change of local brain concentrations in different areas, the preexisting state of neuronal tone). Superficially, this possibility is supported by the fact that neuroexcitatory phenomena associated with anesthesia appear to be rather sporadic, suggesting that certain specific conditions may be necessary for the expression of neuroexcitation. Furthermore, particularly in the case of etomidate, methohexital, and propofol, such phenomena often occur during induction and emergence rather than during periods of stable deep anesthesia, circumstances under which drug levels are changing rapidly. The recurrent, waxing and waning nature of some of these phenomena suggests that some form of cyclic aberrancy in neuronal activity may be involved.

It is still unclear whether the diverse range of abnormal movements reported in association with different anesthetic drugs, or in association with a single anesthetic drug, share common, or similar, etiologic mechanisms. Although epileptiform activity has been reported in association with some neuroexcitatory events, it is possible, indeed probable, that all of these phenomena are not epileptiform in nature. Besides the cerebral cortex, many other areas of the brain can initiate, or influence the expression of, abnormal movements including the basal ganglia, brainstem structures, and spinal cord. Mechanisms involving brainstem nuclei have been postulated to explain myoclonic movements associated with etomidate[72] and a spinal-mediated mechanism involving desensitization of GABA receptors[97] has been suggested as a possible explanation for opisthotonic movements associated with propofol. The etiologic basis for anesthesia-related neuroexcitatory phenomena remains elusive. Theories attempting to explain these events are largely speculative. However, recent speculative and investigative efforts, seemingly fueled by the introduction of propofol, signal an expanding interest among anesthesiologists to reexamine these phenomena in the light of advances in epileptogenesis and neuroreceptor physiology.

Summary

Neuroexcitatory phenomena associated with anesthesia are not new. Such events have intrigued anesthesiologists for many years and have been reported in association with most of the anesthetic drugs in current use. Nevertheless, case reports tend to cluster around certain drugs. Halothane, isoflurane, benzodiazepines, and thiopental appear to be essentially devoid of neuroexcitatory effects. Enflurane, ketamine, etomidate, and propofol possess significant neuroexcitatory potential. In contrast to seizure activity associated with toxic doses of local anesthetics, neuroexcitation associated with the general anesthetics occurs in the clinical dose range. With the exception of enflurane, which has been documented to produce electrical epileptiform activity at deep levels of anesthesia, neuroexcitatory activity associated with other drugs typically occurs during induction or emergence (including the early postoperative period).

The case report literature does not support a disproportionate risk of neuroexcitatory phenomena among patients with preexisting epilepsy compared to nonepileptic patients. However, for some drugs such as etomidate, ketamine, methohexital, and enflurane, the potential to activate seizures in patients with epilepsy is clearly documented. On this basis, some investigators have suggested that these drugs should be used with caution in this patient populaton. Because seizure activity associated with many of these drugs appears to originate in deep cortical and subcortical structures, consistently detectable only with depth electrode recordings, it is unclear at present whether similar activity also occurs in nonepileptic humans.

The etiologic basis for neuroexcitatory movements associated with anesthesia remains obscure and largely speculative. Some movements correlate with documented electrical epileptiform activity but it is likely that some movements are not epileptiform in nature. Recent advances in neurotransmitter-receptor physiology have led to a major revision of our understanding of the CNS effects of general anesthetic drugs. Epileptologists and anesthesiologists share an interest in the physiology and pharmacology of neuroexcitation and inhibition. Our understanding of the mechanisms underlying anesthesia-related neuroexcitatory phenomena appears to be intimately related to advances in these fields. Collaborative investigations offer a promising future in terms of both the interdisciplinary dissemination of information and the pursuit of parallel research interests.

References

1. Smith PA, et al: Convulsions associated with halothane anaesthesia. Two case reports. *Anaesthesia* 1966; 21:229.
2. Rosenow EC, Tovell RM: Etiology of muscular spasms during general anesthesia. *Am J Surg* 1936; 34:474.
3. Lundy JS: *A Manual of Clinical Anesthesiology.* Philadelphia, WB Saunders, 1942:406–407.
4. Steen PA, Michenfelder JD: Neurotoxicity of anesthetics. *Anesthesiology* 1979; 50:437.
5. Rose L, Watson A: Flurothyl. Experience with an inhalational convulsant agent. *Anaesthesia* 1967; 22:425.
6. Koblin DD, et al: Are convulsant gases also anesthetics? *Anesth Analg* 1981; 60:464.
7. Smith RA, et al: Tolerance to and dependence on inhalational anesthetics. *Anesthesiology* 1979; 50:505.
8. Smith RA, et al: Convulsions in mice after anesthesia. *Anesthesiology* 1979; 50:501.
9. Harper MH, et al: Withdrawal convulsions in mice following nitrous oxide. *Anesth Analg* 1980; 59:19.
10. Hornbein TF, et al: The minimum alveolar concentration of nitrous oxide in man. *Anesth Analg* 1982; 61:553.
11. Ferrer-Allado T, et al: Ketamine-induced electroconvulsive phenomena in the human limbic and thalamic regions. *Anesthesiology* 1973; 38:333.
12. Neigh JL, et al: The electroencephalographic pattern during anesthesia with Ethrane: Effects of depth of anesthesia, $PaCO_2$ and nitrous oxide. *Anesthesiology* 1971; 35:482.
13. Ropper AH, et al: Comparison of isoflurane, halothane, and nitrous oxide in status epilepticus. *Ann Neurol* 1986; 19:98.
14. Krenn J, et al: Ein fall von narkosekrampfen unter stickoxydul-halothan-narkose. *Anaesthetist* 1967; 16:83.
15. Eger EI II: Are seizures caused by nitrous oxide or isoflurane? *Anesthesiology* 1985; 62:697.
16. Frost EAM: Seizures after anesthesia: Identifying the causes. *Anesth Analg* 1987; 66:1053.
17. Modica PA, et al: Pro- and anticonvulsant effects of anesthetics (part I). *Anesth Analg* 1990; 70:303.
18. Ropper AH, et al: Comparison of isoflurane, halothane, and nitrous oxide in status epilepticus. *Ann Neurol* 1986; 19:98.
19. Kofke WA, et al: Isoflurane anesthesia for status epilepticus. *Neurology* 1987; 37(supp 1):89.
20. Fiol ME, et al: Effect of isoflurane (Forane) on intraoperative electrocorticogram. *Epilepsia* 1993; 34:897.
21. Ito BM, et al: Effect of isoflurane and enflurane on the electrocorticogram of epileptic patients. *Neurology* 1988; 38:924.
22. Millar TWP: Convulsions following halothane anaesthesia. *Anaesthesia* 1958; 13:341.
23. Hymes JA: Seizure activity during isoflurane anesthesia. *Anesth Analg* 1985; 64:367.
24. Poulton TJ, Ellingson RJ: Seizure associated with induction of anesthesia with isoflurane. *Anesthesiology* 1984; 61:471.
25. Harrison JL: Postoperative seizures after isoflurane anesthesia. *Anesth Analg* 1986; 65:1235.
26. Libowitz MH, Blitt CD, Dillon JB: Enflurane-induced central nervous system excitation and its relationship to carbon dioxide tension. *Anesth Analg* 1972; 51:355.
27. Burchiel KJ, et al: Relationship of pre- and postanesthetic EEG abnormalities to enflurane-induced seizure activity. *Anesth Analg* 1977; 56:509.
28. Nakakimura K, et al: Metabolic activation of intercortical and

corticothalamic pathways during enflurane anesthesia in rats. *Anesthesiology* 1988; 68:777.

29. Niejadlik K, Galindo A: Electrocorticographic seizure activity during enflurane anesthesia. *Anesth Analg* 1975; 54:722.

30. Flemming DC, et al: Diagnostic activation of epileptogenic foci by enflurane. *Anesthesiology* 1980; 52:431.

31. Kavan EM, et al: Electroencephalographic alterations induced in limbic and sensory systems during induction of anesthesia with halothane, methoxyflurane, diethyl ether, and enflurane (Ethrane). *Br J Anaesth* 1972; 44:1234.

32. Nakakimura K, et al: Metabolic activation of intercortical and corticothalamic pathways during enflurane anesthesia in rats. *Anesthesiology* 1988; 68:777.

33. Kurata J, et al: The cerebral cortex origin of enflurane-induced generalized seizures in cats. *Anesth Analg* 1994; 79:713.

34. Kruczek M, et al: Postoperative seizure activity following enflurane anesthesia. *Anesthesiology* 1980; 53:175.

35. Ng ATH: Prolonged myoclonic contractions after enflurane anaesthesia—A case report. *Can Anaesth Soc J* 1980; 27:502.

36. Jenkins J, Milne AC: Convulsive reactions following enflurane anaesthesia. *Anaesthesia* 1984; 39:44.

37. Yazji NS, Seed RF: Convulsive reaction following enflurane anaesthesia. *Anaesthesia* 1984; 39:1249.

38. Allan MWB: Convulsions after enflurane. *Anaesthesia* 1984; 39:605.

39. Grant IS: Delayed convulsions following enflurane anaesthesia. *Anaesthesia* 1986; 41:1024.

40. Nicoll JMV: Status epilepticus following enflurane anaesthesia. *Anaesthesia* 1986; 41:927.

41. Vohra SB: Convulsions after enflurane in a schizophrenic patient receiving neuroleptics. *Can J Anaesth* 1994; 41:420.

42. Burchiel KJ, et al: Electroencephalographic abnormalities following halothane anesthesia. *Anesth Analg* 1978; 57:244.

43. Opitz A, et al: General anesthesia in patients with epilepsy and status epilepticus. *Adv Neurol* 1983; 34:531.

44. Opitz A, Oberwetter WD: Enflurane or halothane anaesthesia for patients with cerebral convulsive disorders? *Acta Anaesth Scand* 1979; 71:43.

45. Oshima E, et al: Anticonvulsant actions of enflurane on epilepsy models in cats. *Anesthesiology* 1985; 63:29.

46. Young WL: Effects of desflurane on the central nervous system. *Anesth Analg* 1992; 75(suppl):S32.

47. Scheller MS: New volatile anesthetics: Desflurane and sevoflurane. *Semin Anesth* 1992; 11:114.

48. Jones RM, Nay PG: Desflurane. *Anaesth Pharmacol Rev* 1994; 2:51.

49. Koenig HM: What's up with the new volatile anesthetics, desflurane and sevoflurane, for neurosurgical patients? *J Neurosurg Anesth* 1994; 6:229.

50. Osawa M, et al: Effects of sevoflurane on central nervous system electrical activity in cats. *Anesth Analg* 1994; 79:52.

51. Harvey SC: Hypnotics and sedatives. In: Gilman AG, et al (eds): *The Pharmacological Basis of Therapeutics*, 7th ed. New York, MacMillan, 1985:351–353.

52. Engel J Jr: *Seizures and Epilepsy*. Philadelphia, FA Davis, 1989:315–318.

53. Hardiman O, et al: Interictal spike localization with methohexitone: Preoperative activation and surgical-follow-up. *Epilepsia* 1987; 28:335.

54. Wyler AR, et al: Methohexital activation of epileptogenic foci during acute electrocortography. *Epilepsia* 1987; 28:490.

55. Fiol ME, et al: Methohexital (Brevital) effects on electrocortogram may be misleading. *Epilepsia* 1990; 31:524.

56. Musella L, et al: Electroencephalographic activation with intravenous methohexital in psychomotor epilepsy. *Neurology* 1971; 21:594.

57. Working Group on Status Epilepticus. Treatment of convulsive status epilepticus. Recommendations of the Epilepsy Foundation of America's working group on status epilepticus. *JAMA* 1993; 270:854.

58. Tassinari CA, et al: Tonic status epilepticus precipitated by intravenous benzodiazepine in five patients with Lennox-Gastaut syndrome. *Epilepsia* 1972; 13:421.

59. Prior PF, et al: Tonic status epilepticus precipitated by intravenous diazepam in a child with petit mal status. *Epilepsia* 1972; 13:467.

60. Winters WD: Neuropharmacological effects of ketamine: Gross behavior, EEG, unit activity, wake-sleep, kindling, and interactions with diazepam and propranolol. In Domino EF (ed): *Status of Ketamine in Anesthesiology*. Ann Arbor, NPP Books, 1990:261–278.

61. Radnay PA, Badola RP: Generalized extensor spasm in infants following ketamine anesthesia. *Anesthesiology* 1973; 39:459.

62. Thompson GE: Ketamine-induced convulsions. *Anesthesiology* 1972; 37:662.

63. Winters WD, et al: The cataleptic state induced by ketamine: A review of the neuropharmacology of anesthesia. *Neuropharmacology* 1972; 11:303.

64. Winters WD: Epilepsy or anesthesia with ketamine. *Anesthesiology* 1972; 36:309.

65. Church J: The anticonvulsant activity of ketamine and other phencyclidine receptor ligands, with particular reference to N-methyl-D-aspartate receptor mediated events. In Domino EF (ed): *Status of Ketamine in Anesthesiology*. Ann Arbor, NPP Books, 1990:521–540.

66. Sybert JW, Kyff JV: Ketamine treatment of status epilepticus. *Anesthesiology* 1983; 58:203.

67. Laughlin TP, Newberg LA: Prolonged myoclonus after etomidate anesthesia. *Anesth Analg* 1985; 64:80.

68. Goroszeniuk T, et al: Generalized grand mal seizure after recovery from uncomplicated fentanyl-etomidate anesthesia. *Anesth Analg* 1986; 65:979.

69. Krieger W, Koerner M: Generalized grand mal seizure after recovery from uncomplicated fentanyl-etomidate anesthesia. *Anesth Analg* 1987; 66:284.

70. Hansen HC, Drenck NE: Generalized seizures after etomidate anaesthesia. *Anaesthesia* 1988; 43:805.

71. Grant IS, Hutchison G: Epileptiform seizures during prolonged etomidate sedation. *Lancet* 1983; ii:511.

72. Reddy RV, et al: Excitatory effects and electroencephalographic correlation of etomidate, thiopental, methohexital, and propofol. *Anesth Analg* 1993; 77:1008.

73. Krieger W, et al: Seizures with etomidate anesthesia. *Anesth Analg* 1985; 64:1226.

74. Ghoneim MM, Yamada T: Etomidate: A clinical and electroencephalographic comparison with thiopental. *Anesth Analg* 1977; 56:479.

75. Gancher S, et al: Activation of epileptogenic activity by etomidate. *Anesthesiology* 1984; 61:616.

76. Ebrahim ZY, et al: Effect of etomidate on the electroencephalogram of patients with epilepsy *Anesth Analg* 1986; 65:1004.

77. Modica PA, et al: Pro- and anticonvulsant effects of anesthetics (part II). *Anesth Analg* 1990; 70:433.

78. Orser B: Propofol-induced neuroexcitation and receptor desensitization. *Can J Anaesth* 1994; 41:366.

79. Bevan JC: Propofol-related convulsions. *Can J Anaesth* 1993; 40:85.

80. Committee on Safety of Medicines, Current Problems: Propofol—convulsions, anaphylaxis, and delayed recovery from anaesthesia. No. 26, May 1989.

81. Cameron AE: Opisthotonos again. *Anaesthesia* 1987; 42:1124.

82. Hopkins CS: Recurrent opisthotonos associated with anaesthesia. *Anaesthesia* 1988; 43:904.

83. Laycock GJA: Opisthotonos and propofol: A possible association. *Anaesthesia* 1988; 43:257.

84. Jones GW, et al: Propofol, opisthotonos and epilepsy. *Anaesthesia* 1988; 43:905.

85. Au J, et al: Withdrawal syndrome after propofol infusion. *Anaesthesia* 1990; 45:741.

86. Saunders PRI, Harris MNE: Opisthotonos and other unusual neurological sequelae after outpatient anaesthesia. *Anaesthesia* 1990; 45:552.

87. Paech MJ, Storey JM: Propofol and seizures. *Anaesth Intensive Care* 1990; 18:585.

88. Mather SJ: Unusual neurological sequelae. *Anaesthesia* 1990; 45:1096.

89. Thomas JS, Boheimer NO: An isolated grand mal seizure 5 days after propofol anaesthesia. *Anaesthesia* 1991; 46:508.

90. Collier C, Kelly K: Propofol and convulsions—The evidence mounts. *Anaesth Intensive Care* 1991; 19:573.

91. Haynes SR, Best CJ: Opisthotonos and propofol. *Anaesthesia* 1992; 47:442.

92. DeFriez CB, Wong HC: Seizures and opisthotonos after propofol anesthesia. *Anesth Analg* 1992; 75:630.

93. Costello TG, Tyers MR: Propofol and convulsions—Fact or fiction? *Anaesth Intensive Care* 1992; 20:395.

94. deLima JC, et al: Propofol convulsions again? *Anaesth Intensive Care* 1992; 20:396.

95. Gildar J: Another case report of opisthotonos and propofol. *Anesth Analg* 1993; 76:1171.

96. Finley GA, et al: Delayed seizures following sedation with propofol. *Can J Anaesth* 1993; 40:863.

97. Ries CR, et al: Opisthotonos following propofol: A nonepileptic perspective and treatment strategy. *Can J Anaesth* 1994; 41:414.

98. Hughes NJ, Lyons JB: Prolonged myoclonus and meningism following propofol. *Can J Anaesth* 1995; 42:744.

99. Rampil IJ, et al: Propofol sedation may disrupt interictal epileptiform activity from a seizure focus. *Anesth Analg* 1993; 77:1071.

100. Ebrahim ZY, et al: The effect of propofol on the electroencephalogram of patients with epilepsy. *Anesth Analg* 1994; 78:275.

101. Samra SK, et al: Effects of propofol sedation on seizures and intracranially recorded epileptiform activity in patients with partial epilepsy. *Anesthesiology* 1995; 82:843.

102. Oei-Lim VLB, et al: A comparison of the effects of propofol and nitrous oxide on the electroencephalogram in epileptic patients during conscious sedation for dental procedures. *Anesth Analg* 1992; 75:708.

103. Hodkinson BP, et al: Propofol and the electroencephalogram. *Lancet* 1987; 2:1518.

104. MacKenzie SJ, et al: Propofol infusion for control of status epilepticus. *Anaesthesia* 1990; 45:1043.

105. Yanny HF, Christmas D: Propofol infusions for status epilepticus. *Anaesthesia* 1988; 43:514.

106. De Riu PL, et al: Propofol anticonvulsant activity in experimental epileptic status. *Br J Anaesth* 1992; 69:177.

107. Simpson KH, et al: Propofol reduces seizure duration in patients having anaesthesia for electroconvulsive therapy. *Br J Anaesth* 1988; 61:343.

108. Rouse EC: Propofol for electroconvulsive therapy. *Anaesthesia* 1988; 43(suppl):61.

109. Rampton AJ, et al: Comparison of methohexital and propofol for electroconvulsive therapy: Effects on hemodynamic responses and seizure duration. *Anesthesiology* 1989; 70:412.

110. Hartung J, et al: Propofol prevents or elevates the threshold for lidocaine-induced seizures in rats. *J Neurosurg Anesth* 1994; 6:254.

111. Lowson S, et al: Anticonvulsant properties of propofol and thiopentone: Comparison using two tests in laboratory mice. *Br J Anaesth* 1990; 64:59.

112. Ahmad I, Pleuvry BJ: Interaction between opioid drugs and propofol in laboratory models of seizures. *Br J Anaesth* 1995; 74:311.

113. Rao TLK, et al: Convulsions: An unusual response to intravenous fentanyl administration. *Anesth Analg* 1982; 61:1020.

114. Safwat AM, Daniel D: Grand mal seizure after fentanyl administration. *Anesthesiology* 1983; 59:78.

115. Hoien AO: Another case of grand mal seizure after fentanyl administration. *Anesthesiology* 1984; 60:387.

116. Baraka A, Haroun S: Grand mal seizures following fentanyl-lidocaine. *Anesthesiology* 1985; 62:206.

117. Scott JC, Sarnquist FH: Seizure-like movements during a fentanyl infusion with absence of seizure activity in a simultaneous EEG recording. *Anesthesiology* 1985; 62:812.

118. Bowdle TA: Myoclonus following sufentanil without EEG seizure activity. *Anesthesiology* 1987; 67:593.

119. Rosman EJ, et al: Another case of probable seizure after sufentanil. *Anesth Analg* 1987; 66:922.

120. Molbegott LP, et al: Probable seizures after sufentanil. *Anesth Analg* 1987; 66:91.

121. Strong WE, Matson M: Probable seizure after alfentanil. *Anesth Analg* 1989; 68:692.

122. Smith NT, et al: EEGs during high-dose fentanyl-, sufentanil-, or morphine-oxygen anesthesia. *Anesth Analg* 1984; 63:386.

123. Sebel PS, et al: Effects of high-dose fentanyl anesthesia on the electroencephalogram. *Anesthesiology* 1981; 55:203.

124. Murkin JM, et al: Absence of seizures during induction of anesthesia with high-dose fentanyl. *Anesth Analg* 1984; 63:489.

125. Tempelhoff R, et al: Fentanyl-induced electrocorticographic seizures in patients with complex partial epilepsy. *J Neurosurg* 1992; 77:201.

126. Cascino GD, et al: Alfentanil-induced epileptiform activity in patients with partial epilepsy. *J Clin Neurophysiol* 1993; 10:520.

127. Tommasino C, et al: Fentanyl-induced seizures activate subcortical brain metabolism. *Anesthesiology* 1984; 60:283.

128. Kofke WA, et al: Alfentanil-induced hypermetabolism, seizure, and histopathology in rat brain. *Anesth Analg* 1992; 75:953.

129. Ramabadran K, Bansinath M: Endogenous opioid peptides and epilepsy. *Int J Clin Pharmacol Ther Toxicol* 1990; 28:47.

130. Holmes RP: Convulsions following pre-operative medication. *Br J Anaesth* 1968; 40:633.

131. Borgeat A, et al: Grand mal seizure after extradural morphine analgesia. *Br J Anaesth* 1988; 60:733.

132. Pearcy WC, et al: Studies on nitrous oxide, meperidine and levallorphan with unipolar electroencephalography. *Anesthesiology* 1957; 18:310.

133. DeCastro J, et al: Comparative study of cardiovascular, neurological and metabolic side effects of eight narcotics in dogs. *Acta Anaesthesiol Belg* 1979; 30:6.

134. Tortella F: Endogenous opioid peptides and epilepsy: Quieting the seizing brain? *Trends Pharmacol Sci* 1988; 9:366.

135. Johnston MV: Neurotransmitters and epilepsy. In Wyllie E (ed): *The Treatment of Epilepsy: Principle and Practice.* Philadelphia, Lea & Febiger, 1993:111–125.

136. Engel J Jr: *Seizures and Epilepsy.* Philadelphia, FA Davis 1989:41–70.

137. Tortella F, et al: Evidence for mu opioid receptor mediation of enkephalin-induced electroencephalographic seizures. *J Pharmacol Exp Therap* 1987; 240:571.

138. Covino BG: Clinical pharmacology of local anesthetic agents.

In Cousins MJ, Bridenbaugh PO (eds): *Neural Blockade,* 2d ed. Philadelphia, JB Lippincott, 1988:121–123.

139. Usubiaga JE, et al: Local anesthetic-induced convulsion in man. An electroencephalographic study. *Anesth Analg* 1966; 45:611.

140. de Jong RH, Walts LF: Lidocaine-induced psychomotor seizures in man. *Acta Anaesthesiol Scand* 1966; 23(suppl):598.

141. Wagman IH, et al: Effects of lidocaine on the central nervous system. *Anesthesiology* 1967; 28:155.

142. Martin Ingvar MK, Shapiro HM: Selective metabolic activation of the hippocampus during lidocaine-induced pre-seizure activity. *Anesthesiology* 1981; 54:33.

143. Wikinski JA, et al: Mechanisms of convulsions elicited by local anesthetic agents. *Anesth Analg* 1970; 49:504.

144. Strichartz GR, Berde CB: Local anesthetics. In Miller RD (ed): *Anesthesia,* 4th ed. New York, Churchill Livingstone, 1994:510–511.

145. Baldessarini RJ: Drugs and the treatment of psychiatric disorders. In Gilman AG, et al (eds): *The Pharmacological Basis of Therapeutics,* 7th ed. New York, MacMillan, 1985:396.

146. Engel J Jr: *Seizures and Epilepsy.* Philadelphia, FA Davis, 1989:49.

147. Johnston MV: Neurotransmitters and epilepsy. In Wyllie E (ed): *The Treatment of Epilepsy: Principle and Practice.* Philadelphia, Lea & Febiger, 1993:113–114.

148. Hoffman EJ, Warren EW: Flumazenil: A benzodiazepine antagonist: *Clin Pharmacy* 1993; 12:641.

149. Philip BK: Flumazenil. The benzodiazepine antagonist. *Anesthesiol Clin North Am* 1993; 11:799.

150. Spivey WH: Flumazenil and seizures: Analysis of 43 cases. *Clin Ther* 1992; 14:292.

151. Scollo-Lavizzari G: The anticonvulsant effect of the benzodiazepine antagonist, Ro 15-1788: An EEG study in 4 cases. *Eur Neurol* 1984; 23:1.

152. Scollo-Lavizzari G: The clinical anti-convulsant effects of flumazenil, a benzodiazepine antagonist. *Eur J Anaesthesiol Suppl* 1988; 2:129.

153. Franks NP, Lieb WR: What is the molecular nature of general anaesthetic target sites? *Trends Pharmacol Sci* 1987; 8:169.

154. Franks NP, Lieb WR: Mechanisms of general anesthesia. *Environ Health Perspect* 1990; 87:199.

155. Pocock G, Richards CD: Cellular mechanisms in general anaesthesia. *Br J Anaesth* 1991; 66:116.

156. Lees G, et al: Molecular biology and fine structure of ion channels: Potential targets for general anesthetics in the central nervous system. *Anesth Pharmacol Rev* 1994; 2:11.

157. Betz H: Ligand-gated ion channels in the brain: The amino acid receptor superfamily. *Neuron* 1990; 5:383.

158. Tanelian DL, et al: The role of the GABA$_A$ receptor/chloride channel complex in anesthesia. *Anesthesiology* 1993; 78:757.

159. Terrar DA: Structure and function of calcium channels and the actions of anaesthetics. *Br J Anaesth* 1993; 71:39.

160. Kutsuwada T, et al: Molecular diversity of the NMDA receptor channel. *Nature* 1992; 358:36.

161. Stevens CF: On to molecular mechanisms. *Nature* 1992; 358:18.

162. Golden GT, Fariello RG: Epileptogenic action of some direct GABA agonists: Effects of manipulation of the GABA and glutamate systems. In Fariello RG (ed): *Neurotransmitters, Seizures and Epilepsy II.* New York, Raven Press, 1984:237–244.

163. Krnjevic K: Cellular mechanisms of anesthesia. *Ann N Y Acad Sci* 1991; 625:1.

164. Lynch C III, Pancrazio JJ: Snails, spiders, and stereospecificity—Is there a role for calcium channels in anesthetic mechanisms? *Anesthesiology* 1994; 81:1.

Chapter 21

SEIZURE SURGERY
Anesthetic, Neurologic, Neurosurgical, and Neurobehavioral Considerations

DAVY TROP

ANDRÉ OLIVIER

FRANÇOIS DUBEAU

MARILYN JONES-GOTMAN

Historical Perspectives in the Surgical Management of the Epilepsies

This chapter is the result of the efforts of clinician-scientists with diverse backgrounds who share a mutual interest in understanding and treating epileptic conditions. Epilepsy surgery is a complex undertaking that requires equipment and personnel to be found only in epilepsy surgery centers. A central team of practitioners consisting of a neurologist with electroencephalographic expertise, an electrophysiologist, a neuroradiologist versed in morphometrics, a neuropsychologist, and a neuropsychiatrist share the responsibility for selecting potential candidates for active treatment during the preoperative phase. Once accepted, the epileptic patient will be cared for by a team consisting of a neurosurgeon, an anesthesiologist, and an electroencephalographer. The neurosurgeon dealing with seizures will have many skills and a broad expertise in epileptology, electroencephalography, and in the vascular and functional anatomy of the brain. His/her functions extend beyond the technical aspect of the operative procedure and he takes part directly in the preliminary investigations, the decision to operate, the choice of operative modalities, and the follow-up of the patients. Similarly, the anesthesiologist will gain additional knowledge in epileptology, particularly on the aspects of functional anatomy of the brain and the clinical manifestations of epilepsy, the effects of the various antiepileptic medications (AED), the patients condition, the interactions between the AED and the anesthetic drugs, as well as the effects of these agents on consciousness and epileptic activity during the surgical procedure and the perioperative period.

For the last 20 years, few areas in neurosurgery have raised more interest than the field of epilepsy surgery. This is obvious if one considers the many international conferences on epilepsy surgery that have taken place and the large number of multidisciplinary centers recently created to investigate complex cases of epilepsy with a view toward surgical treatment. Many other factors have contributed to the contemporary resurgence of interest in epilepsy surgery, such as the techniques of computer detection of epileptic activity and the outstanding development in brain imaging techniques, namely the appearance of magnetic resonance imaging (MRI) in the mid-1980s. It has also become obvious to workers in the field that all epilepsies cannot be controlled by medication and that in a substantial number of patients even partial medical control of seizures can be obtained only at the price of severe side effects.

Historically, this marked interest in the surgery of epilepsy is not unprecedented. Around 400 B.C. Hippocrates broke away from the superstitious ideas of his time and recognized that epilepsy results from an organic process in the brain. Notwithstanding the teaching of the master, two milleniums later epileptics were still seeking a cure by attending pilgrimages,[1] while some enlightened individuals would consider crude forms of brain surgery as an alternative.[2]

In the early 19th century, a few successful operations were reported by Hernsted in England and Dudley in Kentucky[3,4] with surprisingly large series published a few years later.[5,6] The scientific era of epilepsy surgery began when J. Hughlings Jackson recognized that seizures might originate in a focal area of abnormality in the brain.[7] The first successful operation for an intracranial mass lesion localized solely on the base of ictal symptoms was performed by William Macewen in Glasgow in 1879.[8] However, credit for initiating modern epilepsy surgery is generally given to Victor Horsley, who on May 25th, 1886, excised a posttraumatic cortical scar under general anesthesia from a 22-year-old man.[9,10] Intraoperative decisions were guided by cortical stimulation mapping. In his paper, Horsley discussed the choice of anesthetic, indicating he had not employed ether, fearing it would tend to cause cerebral excitement. Chloroform, on the contrary, produced marked depression.

For a long period thereafter, progress was hampered by the absence of accurate methods to detect brain anomalies, and epilepsy surgery remained confined to the treatment of posttraumatic or postinfectious convulsive seizures, usually of central origin manifested by focal convulsions. The numerous papers dealing with this topic, especially in the German literature, confirm this very high degree of interest. In 1914, Krause published a textbook of surgery containing a large chapter dealing mainly with central epilepsy.[11] The state of knowledge concerning the somatotopic organization of the motor cortex was well summarized in the stimulation map presented by this author. However, the "Horsley operation," as it was called by E. Sach,[12] slowly became obsolete, probably as a result of the paralysis that often resulted from central resections. It was not clear then that an almost certain paralysis could not be traded for an uncertain control of seizures.

Further development in the surgery of epilepsy took place in Germany with Otfried Foerster.[13] By the time Wilder Penfield visited Foerster in 1928, the latter was performing operations under ether anesthesia so that routine stimulation of the brain could be carried out in an attempt to reproduce the patient's seizure pattern and localize the motor centers. Many of these patients were soldiers with sequelae of craniocerebral injuries.[14] In 1930, Foerster and Penfield published a classic paper on posttraumatic epilepsy showing that removal of a meningocerebral scar could cure the epilepsy.[15]

In 1875, Richard Caton, a surgeon from Liverpool, had demonstrated that electrical activity could be measured from animal brains.[16] However, 50 years went by before Hans Berger of Iena published his first report on the electroencephalogram in man in 1929.[17] Foerster, who relied extensively on electrical stimulation of the cortex to elicit manifestations of epilepsy,[13] soon applied the EEG technique to the exposed cortex to identify the epileptic focus.[18] Subsequent work by Gibbs[19–21] and by Jasper[22,23] confirmed the key role of electrophysiologic recordings in providing accurate localization of the origin of epileptogenic electrical activity. It thus became apparent the need for operating under local anesthesia in awake patients, so as not to disturb the EEG recordings.

The next phase of enthusiasm for the surgery of epilepsy was generated by the work of Wilder Penfield in Montreal, especially by the publication of his first series in 1947 and 1950 on temporal lobe epilepsy,[24,25] and by the publication in 1954 of his book with Jasper, *Epilepsy and the Functional Anatomy of the Human Brain.*[26] It is impossible to quote all subsequent papers dealing with temporal lobe surgery using methods and techniques similar to those described by Penfield and co-workers. However, as the series were published, it became obvious that the successes and failures varied markedly from one center to the other. These differences were explained by the diversity of patient selection, operative modalities, evaluation of results, medication withdrawal, and other factors. As time went on, the failure rate became high in many centres, which led to a slow abandonment of operations for epilepsy. There were a few centers where the number of patients operated never decreased, and this included the Montreal Neurological Institute (MNI). The most frequent cause of failure was likely an inadequate identification of the seizure focus due to a lack of expertise in electroencephalography (EEG), resulting in poor patient selection. In Europe, surgery continued to be performed mainly in England by Murray Falconer and his group, and they put great emphasis on the pathologic substratum of surgical epilepsy. In Paris, Talairach and Bancaud,[27–29] placed emphasis on stereotaxic intracranial recording. In the United States, Paul Crandall at UCLA developed and maintained a program of surgery that combined the Paris and Montreal approaches.

An intact level of consciousness and full alertness at the time of electrical stimulation was deemed essential to the successful outcome of the radical treatment of focal epilepsy.[30] Supplementary sedation and analgesia were, however, considered acceptable.[31] A small minority of patients who could not tolerate an awake procedure would receive a modified form of general anesthesia.[31] The hybrid combination of alternated local and general anesthesia during a single operative session turned out to be a formidable procedure for the patient and the anesthesiologist alike. Pharmacologic advances and the introduction of newer anesthetic agents (local anesthetics, neuroleptics, sedative-hypnotics, narcotics, and inhalation agents)[32-35] provided smoother conditions in the operating theater.

The more recent phase of interest for surgery of epilepsy has covered most of the last decade. As indicated above, it is the result of several factors, namely: the development of seizure monitoring by computer techniques[36-38]; the use of intracranial EEG recording, for example, depth electrodes[39,40]; and the revolution brought about in brain imaging and especially the advent of MRI, which revealed clearly otherwise undetectable small epileptogenic lesions. The technical advances in microsurgery developed in the 1970s became applicable to the surgery of epilepsy and further technological development such as the ultrasonic dissector appeared on the scene. While these advances were taking place, there was also a change of attitude toward epilepsy itself, with the realization by neurologists that seizure control by medication is inadequate in a large number of patients and often is obtained at the expense of intellectual function and other side effects.

These changes in attitude and technology led to the creation of a large number of comprehensive epilepsy centers around the world. With the concentrated efforts of numerous specialists within these centers more and more patients with focal seizures were brought to surgery.

Clinical Aspects of Epilepsy

CLASSIFICATION OF EPILEPTIC SEIZURES AND OF THE EPILEPSIES

Efforts to categorize epileptic seizures and syndromes date back to earliest medical literature.[41] The Commission on Classification and Terminology of the International League Against Epilepsy (ILAE) developed a classification system for epileptic seizures based on the clinical characteristics of the seizures and their electroencephalographic (EEG) features.[42] The International Syndrome Classification is also the result of a consensus.[43] Epilepsy syndromes however, include not only the elements described in the classification of epileptic seizures, but also other signs and symptoms occurring together, such as age at onset, etiology, and genetic background. The seizure classification and the classification of epileptic syndromes both refer to a dichotomy between two major classes of seizures and syndromes, one class "generalized," and the other "partial" (focal or local) or, in reference to syndromes, localization-related.[44]

Epileptic seizures are defined as transient clinical events due to excessive and hypersynchronous neu-

ronal activity in the cerebral cortex. This abnormal cellular activity usually results in a paroxysmal disturbance of one or several cerebral functions, and the clinical features relate either to the site of origin of the seizure or correspond to structures indirectly activated by the propagation of the epileptic discharge. These transient functional events may be manifested either by positive, for example, motor, sensory or experiential, or by negative, that is, loss of consciousness or loss of tone. Both usually tend to occur together.

Seizures can occur in a normal brain, triggered by specific factors such as fever, hypoglycemia or an acute infection of the central nervous system (CNS). These attacks are considered occasional when occurring under unusual circumstances, or may be referred to as "neighborhood seizures" if they are related to an acute cerebral insult such as a trauma or infection. If they occur spontaneously with no precipitating factors, and if they are repetitive, then we talk of *epilepsy*. In that circumstance, seizures can occur in an apparently normal brain which has a known tendency to repeated epileptic attacks due to putative genetic or biochemical abnormalities. Recurrent seizures may also occur in a brain that sustains a focal or generalized structural cortical abnormality.[45]

Epilepsy terminology has changed rapidly over a relatively short time. However, many terms and concepts that no longer fit with modern classifications of seizures and epileptic syndromes are still used. For example, the term "grand mal" now refers to "tonic-clonic seizure," a seizure type found in the ILAE seizure classification. Similarly, the term "petit mal" refers to "absence seizure," another seizure type found in the classification. Because of the confusion resulting from the use of these old concepts and definitions, the terms "petit mal" and "grand mal" should no longer be used. Similarly, the term "psychomotor seizure," now defined as a complex partial seizure type, was abandoned, in part to avoid any connotation of a psychiatric disturbance. Recent proposals to improve the classification of seizures have been suggested, reflecting the dynamic and continuous advance in our understanding of seizure symptomatology and mechanisms[46,47] and these continue to be assessed by the commission on classification and terminology of the ILAE.

EPILEPTIC SEIZURES

In the 1981 ILAE classification epileptic seizures are divided into those that are either partial or focal, generalized or unclassified (Table 21-1). The classification emphasizes the clinical features of the seizure that can be used to make hypotheses about the underlying mechanism. The presence of partial seizures implies that the seizures originate in one specific hemispheric site. Simple partial seizures present with an elementary

TABLE 21-1
International Classification of Epileptic Seizures

Partial (focal, local) Seizures

A. Simple partial seizures
    1. With motor signs
    2. With somatosensory or special sensory symptoms
    3. With autonomic symptoms or signs
    4. With psychic symptoms

B. Complex partial seizures
    1. Simple partial onset followed by impairment of consciousness
        a. With no other features
        b. With features as in A. 1–4
        c. With automatisms
    2. With impairment of consciousness at onset
        a. With no other features
        b. With features as in A. 1–4
        c. With automatisms

C. Partial seizures evolving to secondarily generalized seizures
    1. Simple partial seizures evolving to generalized seizures
    2. Complex partial seizures evolving to generalized seizures
    3. Simple partial seizures evolving to complex partial seizures evolving to generalized seizures

Generalized Seizures (convulsive or nonconvulsive)

A. Absence seizures
    1. Typical absences
    2. Atypical absences

B. Myoclonic seizures

C. Clonic seizures

D. Tonic seizures

E. Tonic-clonic seizures

F. Atonic seizures

Unclassified Seizures

SOURCE: From the report of the Commission on Classification and Terminology, *Epilepsia* 1981; 22:489,[42] with permission.

symptomatology owing to the activation of primary cortical areas such as the primary motor or sensory cortex, and primary visual or auditory areas. Partial seizures are classified primarily on the basis of whether or not consciousness is disturbed during the attack. When consciousness is not impaired, the attack is classified as a simple partial seizure. Auras are examples of simple partial seizures, and they often have a high localizing value. They represent subjective sensations described by the patient and indicate activation of a specific group of neurons, usually limited to a small part of one hemisphere. Auras are classified as: somatosensory, visual, olfactory, gustatory, auditory, vertiginous, psychic, autonomic, and abdominal. When consciousness is impaired, the attack is classified as a complex partial seizure. In patients with impairment

of consciousness but sometimes also when awareness is retained, automatisms may occur. These consist of aberrant motor or behavioral, often stereotyped, activity. Examples of this abnormal motor activity include: orofacial automatisms (such as chewing, swallowing, vocalization), expressing fear or anger, gesturing, tapping, patting, wandering, fumbling. In contradistinction to many auras, automatisms have no localizing value. Finally, secondarily generalized seizures are those also described as tonic-clonic convulsions of focal onset (partial seizures evolving to secondarily generalized attacks).

In generalized seizures, clinical and EEG changes translate an epileptic process involving both cerebral hemispheres simultaneously from the onset of the attack. In contrast to partial seizures, the changes here imply early widespread neuronal activation, and there is no evidence for a localized anatomic or functional focus. Consciousness is almost invariably impaired, and this impairment is usually the initial manifestation. Generalized seizures may be convulsive or nonconvulsive, and the motor manifestations are bilateral and more or less symmetric.[48] They are divided into several clinical sub-types (Table 21-1), but any combinations may occur, and atypical forms are frequent, if not the rule. For a more detailed discussion, the reader may refer to comprehensive descriptions.[49–52]

EPILEPSIES AND EPILEPTIC SYNDROMES

A classification of the epileptic seizures should include the description of attacks, the patients main symptom, and a cluster of features grouped to constitute an epileptic syndrome. A seizure is a well-defined event, and its classification depends on an accurate description by both the patient and a reliable witness. The epilepsies are diseases that cause recurrent epileptic seizures. Often, however, these disorders cannot be defined in terms of underlying pathophysiology and etiology. To outline a syndrome is a matter of conceptualization and of interpretation of descriptive data that may have been available but not obviously related to each other.[44] These data include age at onset, etiology, the genetic background, and information from the investigative modalities, such as EEG and imaging.

The International Classification of the Epilepsies and Epileptic Syndromes[43] is based on classic concepts (Table 21-2). First, the epilepsies are divided into those with generalized seizures and epilepsies with partial attacks. Second, the classification groups the epilepsies according to whether they are idiopathic or symptomatic. Idiopathic epilepsies and syndromes are disorders not preceded or occasioned by previous neurologic symptoms or abnormalities. They are defined by age-related onset, clinical and EEG characteristics, and

TABLE 21-2
The International Classification of Epilepsies and Epileptic Syndromes

1. Localization-related (focal, local, partial) epilepsies and syndromes
    1.1. Idiopathic (with age-related onset)
        Benign childhood epilepsy with centro-temporal spikes
        Childhood epilepsy with occipital paroxysms
        Primary reading epilepsy
        Other syndromes may be added in the future
    1.2. Symptomatic
        Chronic progressive epilepsia partialis continua of childhood (Kojewnikow syndrome)
        Seizures characterized by specific modes of precipitation
        Other epilepsies and syndromes based on localization or etiology
    1.3. Cryptogenic
2. Generalized epilepsies and syndromes
    2.1. Idiopathic (age-related)
        Benign neonatal familial convulsions
        Benign neonatal convulsions
        Benign myoclonic epilepsy of infancy
        Childhood absence epilepsy
        Juvenile absence epilepsy
        Juvenile myoclonic epilepsy
        Epilepsy with generalized tonic-clonic seizures on awakening
        Epilepsies with seizures characterized by specific modes of precipitation
        Other generalized idiopathic epilepsies not defined above
    2.2. Cryptogenic and/or symptomatic
        West syndrome (infantile spasms)
        Lennox-Gastaut syndrome
        Epilepsy with myoclonic-astatic seizures
        Epilepsy with myoclonic absences
    2.3. Symptomatic
        2.3.1. Non-specific etiology
            Early myoclonic encephalopathy
            Early infantile epileptic encephalopathy with suppression-bursts
            Other symptomatic generalized epilepsies not defined above
        2.3.2. Specific syndromes
3. Epilepsies and syndromes undetermined whether focal or generalized
    3.1. With both generalized and focal seizures
        Neonatal seizures
        Severe myoclonic epilepsy in infancy
        Epilepsy with continuous spike-waves during slow wave sleep
        Acquired epileptic aphasia (Landau-Kleffner syndrome)
    3.2. Without unequivocal generalized or focal features
4. Special syndromes
    4.1. Situation-related seizures
        Febrile convulsions
        Seizures occuring only in the context of acute metabolic or toxic events
    4.2. Isolated seizures or isolated status epilepticus

SOURCE: Commission on Classification and Terminology, *Epilepsia* 1989; 30:389,[43] with permission.

usually have a genetic background; idiopathic epilepsy often begins early in life, there are as a rule no signs of structural disease or of intellectual retardation, the EEG background is normal, and the condition is at times self-limited. Idiopathic generalized epilepsies are manifested by the association of specific seizure types (for example, absence, myoclonic and/or tonic-clonic seizures) in an infant, a child or adolescent with a normal intellect and no neurologic signs. As with localization-related epilepsies, the idiopathic generalized epilepsies are usually easily treatable, and spontaneous remission often occurs. There is often a strong genetic predisposition, and in some syndromes the responsible epilepsy genes have been identified.[53] The International Classification recognizes a number of syndromes of idiopathic generalized epilepsy. Good examples include childhood absence epilepsy, juvenile absence epilepsy, and juvenile myoclonic epilepsy. Idiopathic localization-related (focal, local, partial) epilepsies are childhood epilepsies with partial seizures and focal EEG abnormalities, without demonstrable anatomic lesions. Patients have neither neurologic nor intellectual deficit, but may have a family history of benign epilepsy. Benign rolandic epilepsy (benign childhood epilepsy with centrotemporal spikes) represents a good example of an idiopathic partial form of epilepsy. Several other types of idiopathic localization-related epilepsies have recently been identified and may well be added to the classification in the near future.[54–56]

Symptomatic epilepsies and syndromes represent the consequences of a known disorder of the CNS. This category includes syndromes of great individual variability, based mainly on anatomic localization, clinical features, seizure types, and etiologic factors; symptomatic epilepsies are often less benign than idiopathic forms, with more frequent neurologic findings and intellectual retardation. The EEG background is usually slow and disorganized, and the condition frequently deteriorates. The syndrome of mesial temporal epilepsy is one example of symptomatic localization-related or lesional epilepsy. In symptomatic generalized epilepsies, epileptic seizures complicate or are the predominant feature of a diffuse specific or nonspecific encephalopathy. Such conditions include: malformations due to abnormal brain development (e.g., neuronal migration disorders, phacomatoses); inborn errors of metabolism; and the progressive myoclonus epilepsies (e.g., ceroid lipofuscinosis, Unverricht-Lündborg disease, Lafora disease, and mitochondrial encephalomyopathies).

A cryptogenic group was also introduced into the classification. This term refers to categories of epilepsies and epileptic syndromes that are presumed to be symptomatic but where etiology remains unknown.

EPIDEMIOLOGY

The prevalence of epilepsy (the total number of patients with epilepsy) was assessed in many different countries, and with only few exceptions the figures appear to be quite comparable.[57] Most studies report a prevalence rate of 5 to 8 per 1000. From a study of prevalence in 1980 in Rochester, Minnesota, Hauser and coworkers[58] extrapolated that approximately 1,700,000 persons in the United States would have epilepsy. The prevalence rates are age-specific: they rise from birth to adolescence, remain constant with advancing age; and show again a slight increase after age 70. According to the Rochester data,[58,59] the risk of epilepsy from birth through age 20 is approximately 1 percent and reaches 3 percent after 70.

Incidence rates for epilepsy (the number of new cases in a population over time) are typically 30 to 50 per 100,000 person-years.[57] The rates are high during infancy and childhood, between 50 to 120 per 100,000, decline thereafter, and remain stable until 60, between 20 to 50 per 100,000, and then rise again after 70, reaching 120 per 100,000 person-years. The incidence of epilepsy among the elderly appears to be increasing as the population of Western countries continues to age.

Incidence rates of epilepsy also vary according to seizure type.[58] Myoclonic seizures have their highest incidence during infancy (40 to 50 per 100,000) and diminish rapidly thereafter. The incidence of absence seizures is high (approximately 10 per 100,000) between ages 1 to 10. Similarly, the incidence of generalized tonic-clonic seizures is high in children younger than 1 year (15 per 100,000), declines at puberty (10 per 100,000), and remains at that level until the rates increase again after 65, (20 to 30 per 100,000). The incidence rate of partial seizures is approximately 20 per 100,000 person-years and remains so until age 65, when the incidence rises to 80 per 100,000. The proportion of new cases of partial seizures rises progressively with age. This is probably explained by the fact that postnatal insults—brain trauma, infections, cerebrovascular disease, and brain tumors—which represent the major causes of symptomatic localization-related epilepsies, greatly increase the incidence of epilepsy in advancing age.

CRITERIA FOR INTRACTABILITY AND SELECTION OF SURGICAL CANDIDATES

Failure of medical therapy in persons with epilepsy is a common phenomenon, recognized in 20 to 30 percent of those affected. Several mechanisms have been suggested to account for its development.[60–63] Seizures may be particularly intractable when they are associated with structural abnormalities, as in mesial temporal sclerosis, or with progressive brain diseases, such as metabolic and degenerative encephalopathies. Some syndromes, although not clearly associated with structural or metabolic disorders, are also predictors of intractability (e.g., West and Lennox-Gastaut syndromes, the severe progressive secondary generalized epilepsies of childhood). However, failure of medical therapy is not only dependent on the type and etiology of epilepsy, and uncontrolled seizures have to be distinguished from exogenous etiologies and potentially modifiable ones. Some patients from the medically intractable group may belong to a subgroup of "inadequately treated epilepsies." Unsatisfactory seizure control may be the consequence of a lack of compliance with prescribed drug regimens, an erratic life-style, or ignorance of the precipitating and triggering factors. Resistance of seizures to medical therapy also may be due to an error on the part of the treating physician, leading to faulty diagnosis and wrong choice of treatment. The resistance may be a result of misdiagnosed, nonepileptic seizures, or unrecognized, progressive brain disease, or a failure to recognize precipitating factors that could have been eliminated. The prescription of improper medication resulting from incorrect diagnosis, inadequate drug dosage, and inappropriate drug combinations are also common errors. Finally, additional intractability may be due to the drugs themselves. Adverse idiosyncratic reactions or unusually poor tolerance to otherwise adequate drug regimens may occasionally contribute to poor seizure control. Frequent assessment of patients with refractory seizures is important, as causative or provocative factors and drug toxicity may remain either latent or unnoticeable for long periods. Improvements in the quality of treatment of epilepsy have significant socioeconomic implications, and patients with medically uncontrolled seizures present a major challenge to physicians.

Surgery for epilepsy is considered when seizures are of sufficient frequency and severity to interfere with an individuals life-style. No particular seizure pattern that can be defined qualifies a seizure patient for presurgical evaluation. Typically, the partial epilepsies are, however, the most medically intractable. Focal resections in patients with intractable epilepsies and well-defined structural brain abnormalities identified as responsible for the generation of seizures[64] have the best outcomes and least morbidity.[65] Mesial-temporal epilepsy, for example, usually responds poorly to antiepileptic drugs (AED), but has an excellent postoperative outcome. On the other hand, patients with secondary generalized epilepsies can in certain circumstances be helped by section of the corpus callosum. There is also no specific age limitation. Patients over 50 can undergo successful seizure surgery, but younger patients are more likely to achieve significant improvement in life-style due to earlier intervention. Neuropsychologic deterioration due to surgery itself is less likely to occur in younger patients.[66,67] Similarly, young children and infants can be considered for surgery when it is apparent that their seizures are refractory to medical treatment. With early intervention, it is hoped that the pathophysiologic damage that occurs, and hence the psychosocial consequences, can be avoided.

Diagnostic Methods for the Selection of Surgical Candidates

NONINVASIVE METHODS

The management of uncontrolled epilepsy is a process dependent on a multidisciplinary and analytic approach. We first need to define whether the epilepsy syndrome is partial or generalized (localized versus diffuse seizure onset), and whether a structural abnormality of the brain exists or not (symptomatic versus idiopathic epilepsy). Then we have to understand which lesions are epileptogenic and whether they are indeed responsible for the generation of the seizures. Finally, we should try to determine the effects of seizures on the brain, and identify the functional and eloquent brain areas.[68] As in many other centers, we perform resective or palliative surgeries on the basis of combined information derived from seizure semiology, EEG abnormalities, neuroimaging, and other tests of cerebral function (Table 21-3). The history-taking process should, in most cases, lead to seizure diagnosis and, therefore, should help in establishing the etiology. A detailed description from a reliable witness is essential. Special attention should be given to factors known to be associated with refractory epilepsy that predispose an individual to seizures, thereby interfering with treatment. These factors include mental development and behavior, early onset of seizure, and the presence of focal or diffuse brain pathology. A history of previous AEDs used should be carefully reviewed, stressing previous drug selection, method of administration, tolerance, interactions, and compliance. Approximately one-third to one-half of patients with epilepsy are noncompliant, often to a detrimental degree.[69] Intensive EEG monitoring, including prolonged EEG/video recording, may be necessary to establish a definite diagnosis.[70] Interictal and ictal activity may help in defining seizure classification and origin, and hence elucidate the nature of the clinical syndrome. Psychogenic seizures are especially common in adults and their identification may be difficult.[71] Prolonged EEG/video monitoring may also be useful when other nocturnal or daytime paroxysmal disorders are suspected.[72] Finally, intensive monitoring may determine whether or not a patient is a suitable candidate for surgical treatment

or whether further invasive monitoring is indicated.[73] Modern neuroimaging techniques further the investigation of many aspects of the underlying pathophysiology of intractable seizures. These imaging studies allow the detection of progressive disease that may require treatment in its own right, not only for the lesion itself but also for the epilepsy. One may identify a resectable epileptogenic lesion or a diffuse or extensive disorder not treatable by surgery. Neuropsychologic assessment in patients with uncontrolled epilepsy allows for a correlation of seizure history variables and may identify adverse drug effects. In epileptic patients considered for surgical treatment, neuropsychologic evaluation aids in determining the site of cerebral dysfunction, provides information that may help predict the effect of the surgery on brain functioning and also may help to evaluate surgical outcome. Finally, such assessment helps delineate a patients specific strengths and weaknesses, allowing guidance for education and employment.

TESTS OF EPILEPTIC ACTIVITY
Electroencephalograpy (EEG)
Electroencephalography remains the gold-standard test for the identification of epileptic activity and, in partial epilepsies, for the definition of epileptogenic zone. The epileptogenic zone represents a theoretical concept that may be defined as the region of the cortex that can generate seizures.[64] Two other related concepts include the "irritative" and the "lesional" zones. The first is defined as the region of cortex that generates interictal epileptiform abnormalities, and the latter as that region of the brain that contains a lesion causing the epilepsy. Understanding of these concepts and of their mutual relationships is essential in defining appropriate presurgical strategies and hence providing effective surgical treatment for the largest number of patients.

We pay a great deal of attention to all electrophysiologic data available for each patient investigated.[74] This includes review of all previous interictal and, when available, ictal EEG recordings performed since the onset of the epileptic disorder. The finding of a stable, well-lateralized interictal epileptic focus may have a high localizing value, especially when combined with congruent information from other sources. During presurgical evaluation, patients often have many EEGs, using the standard 10 to 20 electrode placement and the expanded 10–10 system,[75] sometimes up to 15 tracings or more over a 3-week period. Additional extracranial electrodes are often employed. Sphenoidal electrodes are usually inserted and used during the investigation to improve recording of epileptic activity arising in the inferomesial (mesolimbic) temporal structures.[76–78] Similarly supraorbital or infraorbital

TABLE 21-3
Presurgical Evaluation Protocol at the Montreal Neurological Hospital and Institute

Patients Accepted for Presurgical Investigation

- Patients with uncontrolled, partial seizures associated with impairment of awareness (including those secondarily generalized).
- Patients who continue to have intractable seizures despite optimal medical treatment.
- Patients with seizures associated with a focal lesion, including those with dominant hemisphere involvement, or with origin in motor or sensory cortex.
- Patients showing, on serial EEGs, a localized area of epileptic discharges thought to be responsible for the epileptic attacks.
- Patients with drop attacks, secondary generalized epilepsy and multifocal or shifting EEG epileptiform abnormalities.
- Marked intellectual retardation (FSIQ < 65) and psychiatric disorders, including chronic psychosis, do not represent absolute contraindications to presurgical evaluation and surgical treatment.

Diagnostic Approach

	% of patients
• General diagnostic evaluation	100
Epileptic seizure history (from patient and witnesses)	
Past medical history (etiological, predisposing and precipitating factors)	
Family history	
Psychosocial history	
Physical and neurologic evaluation (phenotype, skin, focal deficits)	
• Extracranial EEG evaluation	
Interictal EEG (wakefulness, sleep)	100
Ictal EEG (spontaneous, after AED withdrawal)	80
Long-term video/EEG monitoring	80
• Intracranial EEG evaluation	
Stereotaxic depth electrodes (usually combined with epidural pegs)	6–14
Electrocorticography (usually with brietal activation)	80
Subdural grids or strips	none
• Neuroimaging	
Qualitative (visual analysis) MR imaging	100
Quantitative (volumetric, morphometric analysis) MR imaging	90–95
MR spectroscopy	50–75
Interictal PET	25
Ictal or peri-ictal SPECT	10
• Tests of cerebral function	
Neuroophtalmologic evaluation (visual fields)	80
Neuropsychological evaluation	100
Intracarotid sodium amobarbital procedure	60
PET activation	10
Peroperative cortical stimulation	25
• Neuropsychiatric evaluation	50

electrodes are often used to improve detection of orbitofrontal epileptic discharges.[79,80] Most patients considered for surgical treatment undergo computerized long-term EEG/video monitoring (telemetry), particularly those in whom the clinical pattern is not clear, when the epileptogenic zone is not well defined or when there is lack of congruence between the interictal EEG findings and anatomic abnormalities. The medication is usually tapered during monitoring, while drug levels are periodically measured. During the past three years, an average of 145 epileptic patients per year underwent prolonged video/EEG monitoring. Mean duration of monitoring was 9.3 days, with an average number of 10.1 seizures (including electrographic attacks) recorded in each patient. Every year 16 of those patients underwent intracranial depth electrode investigation when localization problems could not be clarified by extracranial EEG studies and detailed noninvasive structural and functional imaging tests.

The EEG is used to identify the epileptogenic and irritative zones and to delineate, together with neuroimaging and functional studies, the extent of the epileptic zone that needs to be removed to achieve complete cessation of seizures. Surface EEG recordings provide an overall view of interictal non-epileptiform and epileptiform abnormalities, and of the ictal EEG. Notwithstanding the potential for misleading information, interictal and ictal surface recordings often provide useful lateralizing and localizing data in temporal lobe epilepsy (TLE).[73,81-83] Unifocal or predominantly unifocal interictal spiking may be found in the majority of cases,[83] but, at times, interictal temporal discharges may falsely lateralize a temporal lobe focus[84,85] or even be found in patients with further extratemporal lobe epilepsy.[86] For several reasons that are beyond the scope of this chapter, ictal recordings, when properly analyzed, have the least probability of false localization or lateralization. In approximately 50 percent of patients with intractable TLE, early (within 30 s of ictal onset) theta (4 to 7 Hz) or alpha (8 to 11 Hz) frequency EEG activity could be seen in one temporal region, suggesting the presence of an ipsilateral temporal epileptic focus. Interictal epileptic abnormalities, however, may falsely lateralize or localize the epileptic discharges. Non-localizing ictal surface patterns also may be seen.[81,87,88] The problem is even more complex in extratemporal lobe epilepsy, where only a minority of patients will show evidence of a well-localized surface interictal or ictal EEG pattern. Interictal epileptic abnormalities are often poorly localized, suggesting a widespread, multilobar or multifocal, epileptogenic zone, or, in a significant number of cases, such discharges may be completely absent. For example, in frontal lobe epilepsy, seizures may be poorly localized at onset because they originate from deeper brain structures. Clinical seizures also may occur with no visible ictal EEG correlate, or because of the appearance of widespread epileptiform abnormalities, suggesting again that multilobar or multifocal origin may be impossible to localise. Finally, extratemporal focal epilepsy often presents with different pathways of propagation, even in the same individual, leading to different seizure patterns.[82,89]

Neuroimaging

Technological progress in neuroimaging procedures has considerably modified the approach to diagnosis and treatment of epileptic patients. Development in MRI, magnetic resonance spectroscopy (MRS), functional MRI (fMRI), single photon emission tomography (SPECT), and positron emission tomography (PET) have opened opportunities for localization using these noninvasive procedures (Table 21-4). These new techniques demonstrate the structure of the brain in fine detail, provide information for localization of the epileptogenic zone, enable the investigation of the relationship of functional abnormalities to structural lesions and to electrographic foci, and finally demonstrate functional activity of the brain.[68,90,91]

STRUCTURAL MAGNETIC RESONANCE IMAGING. Magnetic resonance is the anatomic imaging technique with the best resolution. It has been shown to be a reliable and accurate indicator of the common pathologic findings underlying seizure disorders. In temporal lobe epilepsy (TLE), for example, qualitative analysis of MR images allows recognition of hippocampal atrophy, foreign tissue lesions, vascular malformations, developmental or dysgenetic disorders, and cystic or post-traumatic lesions. The majority of patients have defined brain abnormalities, and in some series a specific imaging abnormality was found in over 90 percent of the patients.[92] Moreover, the temporal lobe lesions are usually concordant with the EEG localization. Extratemporal abnormalities are less frequently found, and there is a lower concordance rate with EEG localization. The improvement in resolution has helped, however, in the detection of such structural abnormalities as developmental disorders, hamartomatous lesions, and cortical dysplasias.

The clinical problem of defining hippocampal abnormalities is central in the investigation of patients with intractable TLE. Qualitative (visual analysis) and quantitative (by volumetric and morphometric analysis) measurements of hippocampus have proved reliable in lateralizing hippocampal pathology.[93-99] Visual and quantitative analysis is an excellent method of detecting hippocampal sclerosis (Fig. 21-1). The four main features of hippocampal sclerosis visible on MRI are: (1) unilateral hippocampal atrophy; (2) disruption of internal hippocampal structure (loss of neurons in CA1, CA2 and CA4, and gliosis); (3) increased signal in T2-weighted images (gliosis); and (4) decreased signal in T1-weighted images (gliosis). In some cases, visual analysis may be superior to volumetric techniques because features other than atrophy are considered (e.g., hippocampal sclerosis without hippocampal atrophy). Volumetric techniques (Fig. 21-2) are more sensitive for the detection of atrophy (it allows the measurement of right/left index asymmetry in bilateral hippocampal atrophy) and its anterior-posterior distribution. These studies are more objective, allow measurement of the degree of abnormality as a continuous variable, and therefore are important for research.

MAGNETIC RESONANCE SPECTROSCOPY (MRS). This is a noninvasive technique capable of measuring chemical tissue components during life and contributing to our understanding of cell and energy metabolism. Proton (^{1}H) and phosphorus (^{31}P) MRS techniques provide, like conventional MRI and interictal metabolic PET, a means of identifying abnormalities within the epileptogenic areas and help in the localization of the seizure origin.[100-106] Because MRS provides quantitative measurement of metabolic abnormalities it is also sen-

TABLE 21-4
Comparison of Imaging Techniques

	MRI	MRv	MRS	fMRI	SPECT	PET
Resolution	1–3 mm	1–3 mm	1–3 mm	1–3 mm	10–12 mm	5 mm
Quantitation	No	Yes	Yes	Yes	No	Yes
Measurements						
Interictal	+	+	+	+	+	+
Ictal	−	−	+	+	+	+/−
Function	−	−	−	+	+/−	+
Anatomy	+	+	−	+	−	−
Blood flow	−	−	−	+	+	+
Metabolism	−	−	+	−	−	+
Receptors	−	−	−	−	+	+
Drugs	−	−	?	−	?	+

SOURCE: Adapted from Spencer,[91] with permission.

sitive to bilateral and diffuse pathology that cannot be visualized with conventional MRI.

The data accumulated so far have dealt mainly with interictal epileptic states and therefore with relatively stable pathologic conditions. For example, in vivo ^{1}H MRS techniques have been very successful in measuring N-acetylaspartate (NAA), a compound localized exclusively in neurons and their processes (Fig. 21-3, 21-4). N-Acetylaspartate has been used to reflect the neuronal damage and loss in several disorders, including TLE and extratemporal epilepsies.[107-110] In several studies, the NAA/creatine or NAA/creatine+choline ratio correlated with volume loss as demonstrated by structural MRI in patients with TLE, and the two modalities taken together allow lateralization in over 90 percent of patients.[109] In a small number of these pa-

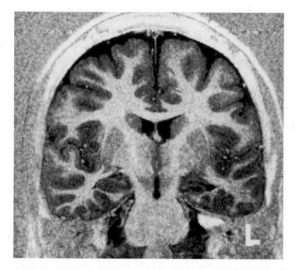

Figure 21-1. Hippocampal sclerosis with hippocampal atrophy. Coronal T1 image showing atrophy and reduced T1 signal from abnormal sclerotic left hippocampus. (Courtesy of Dr. Fernando Cendes.)

tients, MRS was abnormal but conventional MRI was normal. MRS more frequently revealed bilateral asymmetrical damage compared to MRI, even including volumetric studies, suggesting that MRS may be more sensitive than MRI in the evaluation of TLE.[109] Similarly, MRS shows promise in localizing neuronal loss or dysfunction in the epileptogenic areas of patients with extratemporal epilepsy.[110]

MRS also can provide information about transient functional events that occur during seizure or during status epilepticus. Elevated lactate was demonstrated in vivo by ^{1}H MRS in patients with chronic encephalitis and epilepsia partialis continua and this was thought to be due to the seizures and not to the disease itself.[101,108] Phosphocreatine (PCr) and intracellular pH (pHi) fall and inorganic phosphate (P_i) rises during seizures. Youkin and coworkers in 1986[111] were the first to show in epileptic humans that with ^{31}P MRS, the PCr/P_i ratio was transiently decreased during seizures.

FUNCTIONAL MAGNETIC RESONANCE IMAGING (fMRI). Functional magnetic resonance imaging techniques are highly sensitive to hemodynamic alterations, such as cerebral blood flow and cerebral blood volume, and to the changes of blood oxygenation that accompany neuronal activation. These MR studies allow brain function to be visualized, noninvasively, with high spatial and temporal resolution. Moreover, fMRI permits simultaneous structural and functional brain data acquisition, which eliminates the problem of co-registration. This technology can now be used to study the normal physiology of the human brain. Visual, sensory, and motor activation, and speech and even memory localization can be demonstrated with high anatomic and spatial resolution.[112-116] fMRI can be used preoperatively to identify the primary sensory and motor cortical areas. Neurosurgeons attempting to preserve these important regions may be handi-

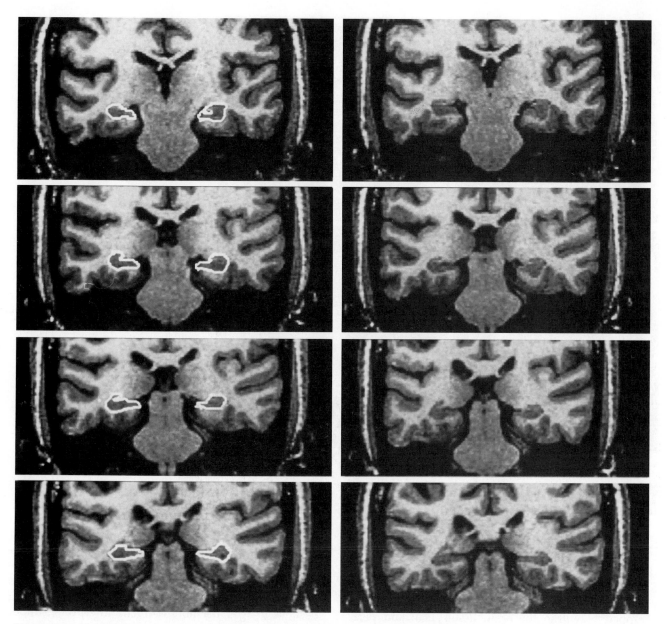

Figure 21-2.   Volumetric measurement of the hippocampus. Measurements in the coronal plane (T1-weighted images), 1 mm thick slices at the level of the body-tail of the hippocampi. The images on the left have the hippocampus outlined for calculation of their volumes using an interactive software program. (Courtesy of Dr. Fernando Cendes.)

capped by the normal variability of these regions, as well as by the reorganization that may follow neurologic disease.[117]

Seizures have long been known to be associated with vascular and oxygenation changes. In 1933, Penfield was the first to report his observations on the changes that occurred during focal seizures during neurosurgical operations. During these attacks, there was a great increase in rCBF and an alteration of capillary and venous oxygenation.[118] These early findings are consistent with more recent reports on the focal changes in blood flow and metabolism associated with sei-

zures.[119–124] Jackson and coworkers,[125] first, and Detre and associates,[126] later, demonstrated that *f*MRI can map subclinical and clinical cortical activation that occurs during partial seizures. They showed that this noninvasive technique can provide excellent temporal and spatial mapping of events that occur in the epileptic brain. There remain technical problems pertaining mainly to the unpredictabililty of occurrence of seizures and the problems that movement artifact cause. Despite this, *f*MRI already has affected the clinical evaluation of patients, the understanding of mechanisms underlying the origin and propagation of sei-

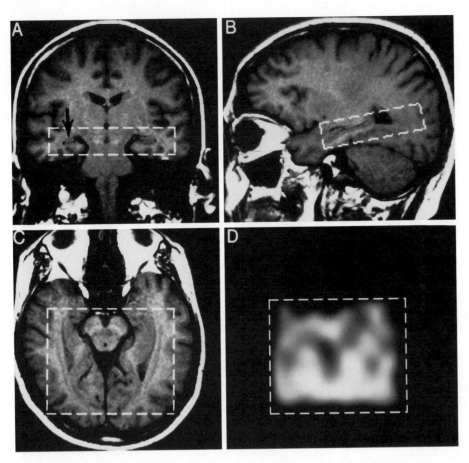

Figure 21-3 Proton magnetic resonance spectroscopic (^{1}H MRS) acquisition technique. *A*, *B*, and *C*. Coronal, sagittal, and axial planes (T1-weighted images) with superimposed regions of interest (ROI) for MRS acquisition. Note the atrophy of the right hippocampus (*arrow*, *A* and *C*). *D*. ^{1}H magnetic resonance spectroscopy (1.5 Tesla) from the left and right temporal lobes (ROI defined at *C*). MRS showed a significant reduction of NAA over both temporal lobes more pronounced on the right side. (Courtesy of Dr Fernando Cendes.)

zures, and the basic investigations of pathophysiologic responses of the brain to seizures.

SINGLE-PHOTON EMISSION COMPUTED TOMOGRAPHY (SPECT).   Blood flow and metabolism increase during seizures and are decreased in the interictal state. SPECT images are created by recording emissions of photons from radiotracers injected intravenously and "trapped"[127] within the brain tissue. Ictal and peri-ictal SPECT is an accurate and sensitive method for localizing epileptic foci in patients with partial, refractory epilepsies.[122,123] The accuracy of these studies in patients with TLE is very high, and ictal SPECT localization power is probably greater than that of any other currently available noninvasive investigational technique, especially in the absence of a structural imaging abnormality.[91] SPECT provides means for demonstrating the localized area of increased or decreased cerebral blood flow (CBF). Interpretation may, however, be difficult and requires knowledge of seizure type, duration, spread, and origin, particularly in extratemporal partial epilepsies, and time of injection with respect to seizure onset and MRI findings.[128,129]

POSITRON EMISSION TOMOGRAPHY (PET).   This technique permits the study of functional brain anatomy

in humans. It provides high resolution, three-dimensional images of various biochemical functions: regional cerebral glucose metabolism [2-(^{18}F)FDG]; blood flow [(^{15}O)O$_2$, (^{15}O)H$_2$O, (^{15}O)CO$_2$, and (^{13}N)NH$_3$], oxygen extraction and metabolism [(^{15}O)O$_2$], receptor localization and kinetics (benzodiazepine, opiate and dopamine receptors); drug distribution; pH; and amino acid transport. PET is not very suitable for ictal imaging because images are more correctly interpreted under steady-state conditions.

Interictal FDG-PET has shown high sensitivity for demonstrating the epileptogenic zone in patients with TLE. FDG-PET demonstrated temporal lobe hypometabolism in 60 to 90 percent of patients.[120,130–134] The hypometabolism is often regional, but may extend outside the temporal lobe and may involve adjacent ipsilateral cortical and subcortical structures. Results have been less revealing in extratemporal frontal and parieto-occipital epilepsies, particularly when no structural lesion could be found on MRI or when no focal EEG abnormalities were present.[135,136] Interictal FDG-PET may be indicated for lateralization or localization of metabolic dysfunction in patients with certain types of secondary generalized epilepsies such as infantile spasms.[137] Interictal studies in those children have revealed the presence of focal metabolic defects, usually

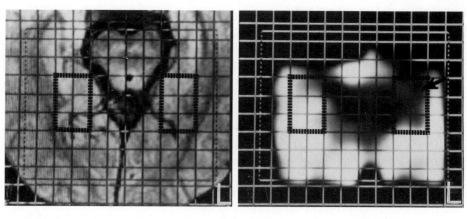

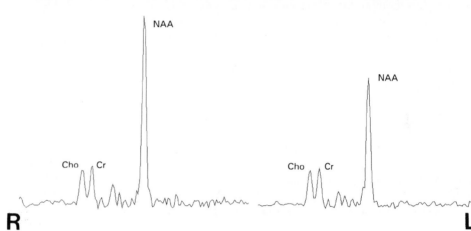

Figure 21-4. ¹H MRS from a patient with left temporal lobe epilepsy. *Top.* Axial image (*left*) showing the position of the ROIs selected for spectroscopy. Axial image (*right*) generated from the resonance intensity of NAA. The ROI for spectroscopic image and the phase-encoding grid are superimposed. Note the reduced NAA resonance intensity over the left temporal lobe (*arrow*). *Bottom.* ¹H magnetic resonance spectra (1.5 Tesla) from the left and right temporal lobes. (Courtesy of Dr. Fernando Cendes.)

representing areas of focal cortical dysplasia. Interictal FDG-PET may also help in selecting intracranial electrode placement sites for invasive interictal and ictal monitoring in patients with refractory partial seizures.[124] Advances in PET quantification and receptor scanning have shown promise with respect to more discrete delineation of the areas of maximal involvement in partial epilepsies. For example, studies with flumazenil (benzodiazepine receptors) both in TLE and extratemporal epilepsy appear to be a promising approach for noninvasive identification of epileptogenic zones.[138-140] These studies showed focal reduction of receptor density in epileptogenic regions compared with FDG-PET studies, revealing more variable and often more diffuse metabolic changes. Finally, preoperative activation PET [(¹⁵O)O₂)] may be used for localization of cerebral function prior to resective surgery, especially when it is performed in or near eloquent cortical areas, such as speech centers or central areas.[141-142]

INVASIVE PREOPERATIVE EVALUATION

By invasive preoperative evaluation, one refers to one of several methods of direct intracranial recording of

the epileptic activity, such as subdural strips or grids or depth electrodes.

The need for intracranial recording in the determination of an epileptogenic focus may have been overemphasized. For instance, in most cases of temporal lobe epilepsy standard electroencephalography combined with sphenoidal electrodes and evidence of mesial sclerosis on MRI will suffice to define the surgical indication. However, there will always be a wide range of indications for intracranial recording. These will be related to the crucial problems of lack of lateralization to one hemisphere and of localization within one hemisphere. It goes without saying that the most fundamental element of seizure localization is its lateralization to one hemisphere. An error of lateralization is the pitfall to be avoided at all cost and this uncertainty and ambiguity can sometimes be clarified only by intracranial recording. Although the progress in brain imaging may already have reduced some indications for intracranial recording, at times these developments have created additional indications for the approach.

INDICATIONS FOR INTRACRANIAL RECORDING
The main purpose of intracranial recording is to further delineate the area of onset and early propagation of

a seizure when this is suspected but not proved by extracranial EEG. It is important to cover the suspected zone of onset by placing electrodes in strategic areas, and to add specific electrodes when the clinical pattern or EEG data suggest another region as the potential site of onset. The idea is to confirm that seizures arise in one area and not in another.

Nowadays a frequent indication for intracranial recording is the lack of spatial congruence between a predominant electrical focus and a lesion suspected of being the primary cause of seizures. This condition can present as an ambiguity of hemispheric lateralization, but more often as a problem of intrahemispheric localization. Intracranial recording can help to solve the dilemma of focus-oriented versus lesion-oriented resection. However, other factors such as the nature of the lesion, the possibility of it being a tumor, or its bleeding potential may take precedence.

In suspected temporal epilepsy, the main indication for intracranial recording has been the bitemporal syndrome.[143–145] This syndrome is characterized by the presence of bilateral and equal amounts of interictal anomalies arising from both temporal areas, the occurrence of a seizure interpreted as originating from the side contralateral to the maximal interictal anomalies, or the recording of seizures with undetermined side of onset, often owing to recording artifacts. In suspected extratemporal epilepsy the main purposes of intracranial recording are the following: (1) lateralization of an uncertain focus (usually frontal); (2) determination of a lead of seizure onset in secondary generalized seizures; (3) determination of seizure onset across the central area in the presence of parieto-centro-frontal discharges; and (4) determination of seizure onset across the Sylvian fissure in the presence of fronto-temporal discharges.

TYPES OF INTRACRANIAL RECORDING
It is not our purpose here to discuss the relative value of the various intracranial methods of recording. Any one of these can be used alone or in combination to solve specific problems. Suffice it to say that the value of the data obtained is totally dependent on a sound working hypothesis and on the accurate topographic identification of the recording sites. Several studies have confirmed the usefulness of these methods.[146–151]

Subdural Strips
Strips are introduced at specific angles through burr holes and directed at various targets. The precise identification of each recording site can now be established with MRI.

Intracranial Grids
Epidural recording with grids to localize the seizure focus has been used extensively by Goldring in the

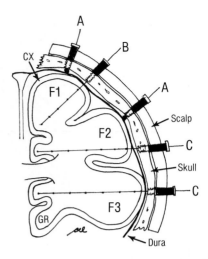

Figure 21-5. Intracranial recording with electrodes placed over the surface of the brain (*A*) or within the depth of the brain (*B* and *C*). (CX = cortex; F1, F2, F3 = first, second, and third frontal gyri; GR = gyrus rectus.)

presurgical investigation of young children.[152] Subdural grids have also been used extensively and have been shown to be useful in determining sites of seizure onset over the convexity of one hemisphere.[153] Their role in problems of lateralization is limited by the need for bilateral craniotomies, which is contraindicated. The MRI correlation technique can now be used to determine precisely the gyral and sulcal positions of the recording or stimulation points.

STEREOELECTROENCEPHALOGRAPHY (SEEG)
Initially developed by Talairach and Bancaud,[27,28] this technique has been further developed at the MNI by the incorporation of DSA, MRI, and PET in stereotactic brain mapping methods.[154] As illustrated in Fig. 21-5, electrodes can now be directed precisely on the surface or within a gyrus or toward any deep structure. Intermediate recording sites can also be identified in relation to buried cortical areas. To call this technique "depth electrodes" is a misnomer, since its purpose is really to provide a tridimensional evaluation of the seizure process, which necessitates placement of electrodes in deep, intermediate, and superficial planes. As is the case for any other intracranial investigation, a well-defined working hypothesis must be developed prior to embarking on such study. This technique has been most useful for solving problems of lateralization and further localization in temporal lobe epilepsy. The placement of intracranial electrodes is done under general anaesthesia. While it was traditionally done with the help of a stereotaxic frame, it can now be carried out with frameless MRI guided stereotaxy.[154–157]

Neuropsychological Procedures

Patients who undergo surgery as a treatment for intractable epileptic seizures receive a neuropsychological evaluation as an integral part of their pre- and postoperative surgical evaluation. The information contributed by a neuropsychological evaluation differs from information derived from other methods of assessment in that neuropsychology measures function, through evaluation of a patient's strengths and weaknesses on a wide range of cognitive tests, while most of the information from other sources is anatomic (neuroimaging) or physiologic (EEG).

Knowledge about function is valuable in several ways. Interpretation of the *pattern of results* on neuropsychological tests provides information about the site of epileptic focus and the focus site is inferred from the type of cognitive dysfunction observed. This information can reinforce data from other sources about the site of the focus, but if in disagreement with other data, the neuropsychological results are especially important for uncovering discrepancies that can provoke further investigation. An otherwise unsuspected atypical cerebral dominance for speech is sometimes exposed in this way, and discrepant or unexpected findings from memory assessment can have a strong and direct impact on surgical management.

Because neuropsychological results show the functional effect of a lesion or of abnormally discharging tissue, they allow evaluation of the impact of epilepsy on a patient's life, and they provide a basis for offering the patient guidance. Preoperative neuropsychological measurements also form a solid basis for evaluating the outcome of surgery with respect to cognitive function by comparing pre- to postoperative performance on the neuropsychological tests. This allows an objective determination of possible changes that can affect a patient's work, schooling or other activities.

PSYCHOLOGICAL TESTING

A basic neuropsychological test battery should sample a wide range of cognitive functions; initial tests should not be tailored for an individual patient too soon in the evaluation because the tests chosen would then be skewed to reflect one's expectations. However, after exploring the whole brain with a comprehensive basic battery, hypotheses about an individual patient can be pursued, with further tests aimed at delineating that patient's cognitive profile more precisely.

Only limited testing may be possible in very low-functioning patients, whose failure on even the easiest cognitive tests reflects a concomitant widespread brain dysfunction. However, cerebral dominance (speech laterality) is frequently in question in such individuals,

and this can be determined with sodium amobarbital testing[157,158] in almost any cooperative patient without respect to intellectual capacity.

Included in a neuropsychological battery should be tests sensitive to function in the frontal and temporal lobes, and to parietal and more posterior regions. The majority of such tests are cognitive, but many neuropsychologists include some somatosensory[159] and motor tests, to evaluate function in somatosensory cortex and in parietal and frontal regions. Specific test instruments will not be discussed here, but have been presented in detail elsewhere.[160]

A basic premise in cognitive evaluations is that the left dominant hemisphere serves primarily verbal functions, and that right hemisphere processes are primarily "nonverbal," involving spatial and perceptual operations, for example. The evaluation aims to explore functions in both hemispheres, and to compare them. Therefore, whenever possible, verbal and nonverbal analogues of a same type of test should be used, as this allows a more direct comparison of function in the two hemispheres.[161,162]

MEMORY ASSESSMENT

A thorough evaluation of memory is particularly important in the assessment of epileptic patients because the majority of surgical candidates have a temporal-lobe focus, and memory is the most salient of temporal-lobe functions. Memory test results provide information about the functional status of the temporal lobes, and such results should also provide detail about a patient's capabilities in different aspects of memory.

The fundamental difference between the two temporal lobes is that the left temporal lobe is involved in memory for verbal material, such as names, word lists, or number sequences, and that the right temporal lobe is involved in memory for material that cannot be verbalized readily, such as faces, places, or abstract designs. This difference between the temporal lobes is exploited in the design of memory tests by devising the tests to be as purely verbal, or purely nonverbal, as possible. Thus, the differences between the hemispheres are maximized by using memory tasks that are polarized into the verbal or nonverbal domain.

A second important factor in testing memory is to use tasks that sample different aspects of learning and memory. For example, because bilateral hippocampal lesions can result in severe memory deficits,[163–168] a thorough memory assessment should explore the viability of each hippocampus. Since it may be that not all memory tests are sensitive to damage in the hippocampus,[169–174] care should be taken to include in a memory-test battery some tests that are believed to be sensitive to hippocampal function. It is also essential that learning tasks, as opposed to one-trial memory tasks, be included in the battery. Learning tasks allow unimpaired individuals to improve with additional exposure to the material to be learned[161]; this increases the difference between people with a true learning or memory deficit and those who do poorly on a first trial for other reasons. Wherever possible, matched tasks that are identical in all ways except for the verbal versus nonverbal nature of the material, should be used. These allow direct comparison of the efficiency of the two hemispheres, even within individual patients.

Several matched memory tasks have become available in recent years[161,162,175,176] and these have often grown out of a previously-existing verbal test for which a nonverbal analogue was later developed. Some matched tasks exist also for assessment of left versus right frontal-lobe function.[177-181] The strategy of using matched tasks to study analogous brain regions in left and right hemispheres adds power to the neuropsychologist's ability to localize dysfunction and to analyze the nature of a patient's deficits.

INTERPRETATION

The interpretation of neuropsychological results is implied in the foregoing discussions. Deficient performance on tests "sensitive to" frontal lobe or temporal lobe damage, in the context of adequate performance on tests that tap function in other brain regions, will be interpreted as indicating focal dysfunction and thus the site of the epileptic focus. The verbal or nonverbal nature of the tests on which deficits were observed will further designate the site of dysfunction as being in the dominant or nondominant hemisphere.

Significant impairments on verbal memory tests are interpreted as reflecting left temporal lobe dysfunction, and impairments on "nonverbal" memory tests point to dysfunction in the right temporal lobe. People who have significant memory deficits for both kinds of material are believed to have bitemporal dysfunction; those patients will usually receive further investigation with an amobarbital procedure.

An individual's pattern of cognitive results tends to be very stable. Although retesting can result in slight rises in scores owing to practice effects, and although there can be some small fluctuations in scores from one testing to another owing to various external factors (such as poor attention after bad news or a bad night, or changes in AEDs), when patients receive many assessments the pattern of strengths and weaknesses remains similar in evaluation after evaluation. Tests performed after a surgical intervention show lowered scores on some measures in the early postoperative period, with a return to preoperative levels on most tests after a few months.[174,182] Big changes in the individual profile are the exception, not the rule, and they signal changes in the patient's condition that should be investigated.

An important exception to the observation that postoperative changes tend to be small occurs in patients whose memory is very good, and who have hippocampal volumes within normal limits: these are the patients who show the most severe memory loss after surgery, if excision has been made from the healthy hippocampus.[183-186]

INTRACAROTID SODIUM AMOBARBITAL PROCEDURE (IAP)

This procedure is an essential part of the preoperative evaluation of most patients who are candidates for surgical treatment of epilepsy. It was originally introduced in North America in the late 1950s by Juhn Wada[158]—hence the frequently used nickname, "Wada Test"—as a means of determining cerebral dominance for speech before a surgical intervention. The IAP is now a basic part of neuropsychological evaluation in most epilepsy centers.

The rationale underlying the IAP is simple: one hemisphere is anesthetized temporarily by injecting a barbiturate, sodium amobarbital, into its ipsilateral internal carotid artery. This allows one to apply simple tests to the awake hemisphere alone; the results of such tests are expected to allow one to predict certain possible sequelae of the proposed surgery.

In many institutions all surgical candidates undergo the procedure; in others, only certain patients receive it, according to specific selection criteria. Patients are usually selected to undergo the test based either on suspicion of atypical speech representation or of possible bitemporal dysfunction.[187] Whether the test is performed to assess speech or evaluate memory, the actual procedure remains the same.

IAP SELECTION CRITERIA FOR SPEECH TESTING

When there is reason to suspect an atypical cerebral organization for language, the IAP is considered necessary because the localization of speech functions might lie in, or too near, the area of planned surgical intervention. Left-handed individuals, those with a strong family history of left-handedness, and people with evidence of early damage in or near speech areas of the left hemisphere fall into this category. Patients whose focus according to anatomic tests is discordant with lateralization designated by functional (cognitive) tests are also candidates for an IAP, because in such cases the mismatch may reflect right-hemisphere speech dominance.

IAP SELECTION CRITERIA FOR MEMORY TESTING

When an IAP is performed because of a suspicion of bitemporal dysfunction, the question can arise in several ways. First, memory impairments observed on both verbal and nonverbal tests given in the basic, noninvasive clinical memory evaluation suggest bitemporal abnormality, as outlined above. Evidence from EEG or neuroimaging pointing to bitemporal abnormality is also grounds for performing an IAP, as is conflicting evidence arising when an EEG focus is clearly in one temporal lobe but the opposite hippocampus is significantly small according to MRI.

TECHNIQUE

Basically, the technique involves injection of sodium amobarbital into one cerebral hemisphere, usually through the internal carotid artery. This anesthetizes the injected hemisphere briefly, during which time the abilities of the awake hemisphere can be tested in isolation. The effect is short, and is usually dissipated after about 6 to 8 min,[188,189] depending on the dosage[190,192] and individual differences.[193] During the hemianesthesia, simple speech and memory tests are performed. Rather elementary tests are used because the effect is short, because patients must perform them with a single hemisphere, and because the basic clinical questions asked by this procedure can be answered adequately with simple tasks.

Neuropsychologists usually administer the cognitive tests. An angiogram is obtained before the IAP to make sure that there is no serious vascular anomaly and to predict the distribution of the drug; this is done by a radiologist, who also injects the amobarbital. The effect of the drug on the brain is monitored by EEG[194,195]; in some institutions this is done online during the test, and in others the EEG is recorded on a computer for playback and blind interpretation by an electroencephalographer afterwards.[188,196,197] The patient's recovery from the hemiplegia that has been induced by amobarbital injection is also monitored to estimate return of function, although this estimate is less satisfactory.[188,198]

COGNITIVE TESTING DURING IAP (SPEECH)

IAP speech tests sample different aspects of language, including serial or automatic speech (counting, reciting days of the week), naming, repetition, spelling, reading, and auditory comprehension.[189,192] Cerebral dominance should not be assessed with a single task because dissociations among types of speech functions are sometimes observed.[157,199,200] Speech tasks should be rotated throughout the period of densest hemianesthesia so that all can be sampled.

Interpretation of the speech tests is most often unambiguous because if the dominant hemisphere is injected the patient will become aphasic while the drug is active, whereas if the nondominant hemisphere is injected the patient will continue talking without significant errors. However, in cases of bilateral speech

representation a range of different patterns may be observed. Some of these are:

- Disruption of all speech functions tested from injection in one hemisphere with minor but significant disruption from injection in the other
- Dissociation of type of disruption (e.g., naming in one hemisphere and comprehension in the other)
- Equal and significant disruption in both hemispheres
- No obvious disruption in either hemisphere

Interpretation of bilateral speech differs among institutions and individuals; consequently, reported incidence of this type of atypical language organization varies widely.[200,201] This is of considerable theoretical interest but it does not impact significantly on patient management because the most crucial practical question (is there significant language function in the hemisphere destined for surgery?) can almost always be answered.

COGNITIVE TESTING DURING IAP (MEMORY)

Memory is tested by presenting new material to be remembered soon after injection of the drug. The idea is that the new material must be processed while only one hemisphere is active. The type of material used might be words or pictures or three-dimensional objects (this varies among epilepsy centers), but items should be simple and easy to perceive. In most centers the final interpretation of memory results is based on the patient's ability to *recognize* later the new material that had been shown during hemianesthesia, because free recall of the material has not been shown to provide reliable results.[202]

Underlying the memory application of the IAP is a basic assumption that while one hemisphere is anesthetized the patient will have to rely on the awake hemisphere to remember material shown while the drug is active. The patient will not remember the material if the awake, noninjected hemisphere is damaged. The crucial test is when the hemisphere of the planned surgery is injected, because in that case the memory function of the hemisphere that will be left intact is being tested. The premise is that in that situation the test should predict how well the patient's memory will function after resection from a temporal lobe.[191]

Another assumption underlying IAP memory tests is that they are addressing the adequacy of hippocampal function specifically.[202] This assumption has been challenged because only the anterior hippocampus is irrigated by the usual internal carotid artery route for amobarbital injection; therefore, selective injections into the posterior cerebral artery[203] or the anterior cerebral artery[204] have been made to ensure irrigation of the hippocampus. However, the hippocampus has been shown to be affected functionally after internal carotid injection by depth electrode EEG recordings that showed slow waves in the hippocampus[196] and by SPECT images that showed hypoperfusion in the hippocampus.[205]

Because of the implications for hippocampal function in patients who fail amobarbital memory tests after injection into the hemisphere of a planned temporal lobe excision, in some centers those patients receive a limited resection that spares hippocampus. In some other centers, surgery is denied altogether to such patients; in still other cases, operation with encroachment on the hippocampus has been offered. Thus, failing an IAP memory test can have important consequences for a patient's surgical management.

Failure of an IAP memory test is defined differently in different centers. Indeed, the way that the IAP memory-test results are interpreted is changing, and the concept of simply passing or failing is becoming infrequent. In many centers the test is used in a more general sense to predict postoperative memory performance, without specific reference to either "failure" or to amnesia.[206,207] It is also used as additional evidence pointing to the side of epileptic focus when injection opposite the supposed focus results in substantially poorer memory performance than when injection was made on the side of focus.[208–210]

SUMMARY AND CONCLUSIONS

Neuropsychological tests are an integral part of preoperative investigations offered to patients being considered for surgical treatment of epilepsy. These tests, which assess cognitive function, add information about the site of cerebral dysfunction and they provide information to patients about their cognitive strengths and weaknesses. This systematic assessment provides an objective basis for comparing an individual's performance over time or before and after medical treatments as well. Results from neuropsychological evaluation contribute to decisions about patient management with respect to feasibility of surgery, extent of surgery, and cognitive outcome after surgery.

Surgical Treatment of the Epilepsies

TIMING OF OPERATION

The timing of surgery is of great importance. In our experience few patients are operated too early and possibly many too late. The majority could have benefited from surgery earlier in life. The important and crucial issue for these patients is to be operated on time, that is, before the terrible impact of their disease on the psychosocial development of a child and on the

quality of life of the adolescent and young adult have manifested themselves fully. Young children with evidence of focal cortical disorders and intractable epilepsy should be considered for surgery as soon as possible, since continuous seizure discharges have a deleterious effect on brain development. An adolescent with complex partial seizures of mesial temporal origin and evidence of mesial sclerosis on MRI should be considered for surgery. Once such a focus is demonstrated there is no need to submit the patient and family to a trying trial of all the new medications available on the market. Over the last several years, there has been a tendency to offer surgery to an older age group of particularly well selected patients presenting with an active temporal lobe epilepsy and clear evidence of ipsilateral unilateral structural damages associated with mesial temporal sclerosis. Our oldest patient who has undergone a temporal resection including amygdalo-hippocampectomy was 63 years old. The duration of the epileptic syndrome does not seem to alter significantly the prognosis for seizure control. Unfortunately, and in spite of the changes in attitude noted above, there are still too many misunderstandings and too much misinformation about the surgery of epilepsy, resulting in too many patients being deprived of a chance of becoming seizure-free, improving their quality of life, and reducing drug intake if not stopping it completely.

WITHDRAWAL OF ANTIEPILEPTIC DRUGS FOR PREOPERATIVE ASSESSMENT

Withdrawal of antiepileptic medication is usually undertaken because the epilepsy has presumably remitted, and a number of factors indicate the likely favorable outcome of drug withdrawal in seizure-free patients. On the other hand, in therapy-resistant patients, withdrawal of AEDs may be undertaken because of lack of efficacy or unacceptable toxicity. In those circumstances one would want to begin with an overlapping new drug regimen and then taper the unsuccessful agent without causing any increase in seizure frequency and disruption in the patients daily activity. Finally, AEDs may be reduced and at times completely withdrawn during the presurgical evaluation of patients with intractable epilepsy. Whatever the conditions, drug withdrawal strategy is essential in order to minimize the risk of recurrence or, in presurgical evaluation, the danger to the patient from major or repeated seizures.

DRUG WITHDRAWAL DURING PRESURGICAL ASSESSMENT

Partial or complete abrupt withdrawal of AEDs is often required to record seizures during video/EEG long-

TABLE 21-5
Effects of Acute AEDs Withdrawal

- *Adverse effects on patients*
  Detrimental partial or generalized seizures[216,218,220]
  Repetitive seizures or status epilepticus[446,451,453]
  Physical injuries
  Psychiatric effects: anxiety, mood disorders, insomnia, psychosis[210,454,455]

- *Effects on seizure activity*
  Increase in seizure frequency[215-222]
  Increase in seizure severity and length[216,220,222,223]
  Occurrence of atypical, novel or false localizing clinical events[230-232]

- *Effects on electroencephalographic activity*
  On interictal spiking rate and localization[215,219,228]
  On ictal localization[221,230-232]

Strategy for Acute AED Withdrawal During Long-term Video/EEG Monitoring

- *Patients on polytherapy*
  1. First consider withdrawing medications with no clinical relevance, no risk of withdrawal seizures (e.g., ethosuximide) or with subtherapeutic blood levels.
  2. Barbiturates and hypnotic-sedative drugs like benzodiazepines, because of their long half-lives may either be tapered very slowly before hospitalization and monitoring, or considered as the last medications to reduce.
  3. CBZ, PHT, GBP, VGB or VAP should be discontinued in stages, by a third or a half every day, during monitoring. Their short half-lives make them more suitable to lead to seizures in a short period of time. In addition, partial seizures should be evoked rather than generalized tonic-clonic seizures. These drugs are more suitable at controlling the latter.
  4. Sequential withdrawal is preferable to simultaneous discontinuation of drugs. Withdraw the ones that you would not like to continue with after surgery.
  5. Stat-doses of short half-life AEDs should be used to control severe or repeated seizures: e.g., lorazepam 1–2 mg po or iv, or CBZ 200–400 po after a generalized tonic-clonic seizure or after three or more complex partial seizures within a 24-h period.
  6. Insomnia should be avoided.
  7. After monitoring, AEDs are reintroduced at their prior dosages. CBZ is often reintroduced gradually to avoid toxicity.

term monitoring. Within a few days, one or more AEDs are partly or completely tapered and, after a typical inpatient monitoring session lasting approximately one week, rapidly reintroduced to their previous dosages. Acute drug withdrawal can affect the patient's clinical status in different ways, can modify interictal and ictal EEG activity, and may also have effects on the seizure characteristics themselves (Table 21-5). Usually, however, seizures that occur during monitoring are assumed to provide reliable localization of an epileptic focus.

ADVERSE EFFECTS OF ACUTE AEDs WITHDRAWAL

Generalized tonic-clonic seizures cause extreme discomfort to patients, families, and hospital staff. In a small but significant number of patients, complications including vertebral compression fractures, shoulder dislocations, and a postictal confusional state occur. Complex partial seizures, particularly those of temporal lobe origin, may also be detrimental to the patients and, particularly if clustered, may cause postictal confusion or psychosis, or may lead to prolonged amnestic states. To reduce the risk of detrimental seizures and the development of status epilepticus we have adopted over the past few years a strategy for acute drug withdrawal during long-term monitoring (Table 21-5). One

tries to balance the necessity for recording an adequate number of habitual seizures in order to obtain reliable localization with the patient's comfort and safety and the concerns of the families and the hospital staff.

Appropriate manipulations of drugs are likely to be useful and safe if: (1) the patient's own response to medications and withdrawal is known; (2) pharmacokinetic and mechanisms of action of drugs are well understood; and (3) if an appropriate protocol is established for safety issues, seizure monitoring, and drug administration. The rate and extent of drug reduction depends largely on the patient's baseline seizure frequency and epileptic syndrome. For example, in patients with frequent daily seizures, a tendency for secondary generalization and a past history of status epilepticus, drug reduction will be slower or may even not be necessary. We often wait 24 h (and even 48 h during invasive monitoring) after the beginning of monitoring before reducing AEDs. Reduction is then sequential and gradual, starting with short-acting drugs and by one-third to one-half of total daily dose. Complete cessation of medication is needed only in a minority of our patients. We often maintain drugs like phenytoin and valproic acid because of their efficacy to control generalized and secondarily generalized seizures. Any unusual clinical event is carefully monitored. For example after a generalized tonic-clonic seizure a patient with usually complex partial seizures, will immediately receive a dose of the withdrawn drug or a bolus of lorazepam orally (p.o.) or intravenously (iv) in order to prevent, as much as possible, a second major event. The same patient will also receive an extra dose of medication if, within a 24-hour period, he/she has three or more habitual complex partial seizures. We closely monitor patients with more severe and widespread brain damage or with bilateral temporal epilepsy, because these patients are more vulnerable and prone to develop acute and chronic psychiatric disorders.[211–214] Monitoring, sensory and sleep deprivation, drug withdrawal, the occurrence of generalized seizures or of repeated attacks—all contribute to circumstances favoring the emergence of psychopathology. In such patients, we reduce medication much more gradually, hypnotic medication is often prescribed to prevent sleep deprivation, and most are followed concomitantly by the consultant psychiatrist. Obviously, there is no standard or routine approach to these management issues, and one should not automatically assume that a specific event needs specific treatment.

EFFECT OF ACUTE AED WITHDRAWAL ON SEIZURE ACTIVITY AND THE EEG

Antiepileptic drugs reduce the frequency and severity of seizures and, conversely, seizure activity is expected to increase after their withdrawal in patients with active epilepsy. The effects of acute withdrawal of most of the conventional AEDs like phenobarbital (PB), primidone (PRI), phenytoin (PHT), carbamazepine (CBZ), and valproate (VPA) have been studied. These studies show that drug withdrawal causes seizures to increase in frequency and duration both during and after withdrawal.[215–224] Seizures also tend to become more severe.[216,220,222,223] For example, patients who never or very rarely have a generalized convulsion may experience them during withdrawal. These effects are sustained as long as drugs are withheld or blood levels of the drugs are subtherapeutic, but the rate of drug withdrawal seems to have little effect on the length, severity, or frequency of clinical attacks. Interestingly, recent studies suggested that there is no rebound or true withdrawal effect, except after withholding benzodiazepines, in particular clonazepam,[224] and barbiturates (in particular the short-acting ones, such as pentobarbital).[225,226] Because of the risks of uncontrolled generalized tonic-clonic seizures, barbiturates and benzodiazepines should be tapered very slowly long before a patient enters the epilepsy monitoring unit.[227] It may even be preferable not to reduce those drugs unless absolutely necessary.

Ludwig and Ajmone-Marsan[228] were the first to show that acute AED withdrawal was associated with an increase in spiking rate in the majority of patients with partial epilepsy. Later, Gotman and collaborators[215,220,229] studied the effect of drug withdrawal on seizure occurrence and interictal spiking. They found that the increase in spiking rate may be due to an increase in seizures rather than to the direct effect of drug withdrawal. The activation may be specific, that is, in the site of the presumed focus, or nonspecific, at a distance from the presumed epileptic focus, either contralaterally, multifocal, bilateral, or generalized.[228,229] The exact mechanisms underlying postictal spike activation and localization during drug withdrawal are still unclear and should not be considered a reliable factor for localization. Atypical, unexpected, or false localizing clinical and EEG seizures have been described during acute drug withdrawal.[230–232] In most cases, they probably represent site(s) of genuine but unsuspected abnormal epileptic activity, indicating multifocal disease rather than a "pure" drug withdrawal effect.[223]

PERIOPERATIVE ISSUES

Cases of hemorrhagic complications thought to be due to valproic acid have been reported, both after neurosurgical or other operations.[233,234] Recently, Spencer and Packey[235] reviewed the literature on VPA and hemorrhagic complications in which thrombocytopenia and thrombasthenia and reduction of fibrinogen or von Willebrand factor have been described.[236–239] One major concern is that hemorrhagic complications may occur regardless of whether the prothrombin time (PT), partial thromboplastin time (PTT), fibrinogen level, and bleeding time are abnormal.[233] In our own center, we usually withdraw VPA at least a week before any invasive surgical procedure, including intracranial depth electrode placement, epilepsy resective surgery, or callosotomy, even if bleeding parameters are normal. Spencer and Packey[235] recommend a check of each of the bleeding parameters, that is, PT, PTT, bleeding time, and fibrinogen level, before surgery. They discontinue VPA if bleeding time is elevated or if platelet count is low. They postpone surgery until all bleeding parameters are normal, which may take two weeks or more.

Another important aspect of perioperative AED management is to maintain stable and therapeutic drug levels in order to avoid, as much as possible, potential seizures and also drug toxicity. A higher rate of toxic events with CBZ was reported, associated with a substantial and rapid rise in the CBZ level early after surgery.[240] Proposed mechanisms include rapid absorption of an accumulated pool from the gastrointestinal tract, drug interactions resulting in slower metabolism of CBZ, difficult oral administration, and decreased elimination. To avoid this problem, Spencer and Packey[235] suggested that on the second, third, and fourth postoperative day the dosage of CBZ be reduced, while following levels and monitoring the patient for toxicity. By the fourth or fifth day, the patients drug dose should return to the presurgical level. Our experience supports these findings. With the exception of VPA, our patients usually receive their habitual drug regimen before and after surgery. They are closely monitored for drug toxicity, and blood levels are measured once during the first postoperative week. Occasionally, we have observed patients with definite CBZ toxicity occurring after the first postoperative week and with therapeutic CBZ and CBZ-10, 11-epoxide levels. They were all receiving polytherapy, most of them more than two AEDs. Reducing CBZ alone usually relieved toxicity. On the other hand, Ojemann described low levels of medication during early postoperative period, and we have also seen that many times. Postoperative seizures, habitual or neighborhood, often occur because of low blood levels. The experience with the new antiepileptic agents is minimal and does not allow specific management guidelines. We, however, apply a protocol similar to the one used with conventional AEDs, taking into account their pharmacologic properties, particularly the half-life, their effects on different seizure types, and their tendency to cause "rebound seizures."

OVERVIEW OF SURGICAL PROCEDURES

Although surgery of epilepsy has attracted interest for over a century, its full recognition as the therapeutic modality of choice in a large number of patients had to wait for such recent developments in technology as computer monitoring, brain imaging, intracranial microsurgery, and the advent of the ultrasonic dissector and neuroanaesthesia.

Numerous specialists, including anesthesiologists, have teamed up with neurosurgeons to develop a combined approach for the investigation of patients, the choice of surgical modalities, the actual surgery, and the evaluation of results. This team approach has created an ever-increasing demand for neurosurgeons and neuroanesthesiologists becoming involved in this field.

IMAGE GUIDED SURGERY

Over the last 4 years, practically all procedures for epilepsy carried out by one (A.O.) of us (more than 300) have been performed by image-guided surgery or frameless stereotaxy.[154,155] This technique uses a pointer (viewing wand) linked to a computer station that displays 3D MRI reconstructions of the brain (Fig. 21-6). This means that once a coregistration of the patient's head with its computer counterpart has been made, the technique can be used to display and project any

point of the cortical anatomy directly on the scalp and to indicate the position of the pointer during the course of the surgery. The applications of this technique have been numerous in the presurgical investigation, during preoperative planning, and during the course of the procedure itself. For instance, at the MNI/MNH, depth electrode implantations are no longer carried out with a stereotaxic frame but by a technique of frameless stereotaxy with a simplified apparatus. It has been used to locate the position of such crucial vascular structures as the superior longitudinal structures and to identify the main cortical landmarks, thus optimizing the size and location of the bone flap. During electrocorticography the sites of epileptic activity and physiologic responses can be identified readily on the computer display, and the data can be easily archived, thus creating a precise brain map and operative record. The procedure has proved invaluable in performing selective removal, such as the selective transcortical amygdalo-hippocampectomy. In this procedure, the exact point of entry in the cortex can be determined together with the optimal angle of approach to the amygdala and hippocampus. The extent of the resection also can be measured. Another frequent and obvious application has been in the removal of small subcortical epileptogenic brain tumors or vascular lesions. The procedure has also been utilized advantageously to perform callosotomy, to display in an optimal fashion the placement of the craniotomy, the actual sites of dissection along the corpus callosum and to show to what extent the corpus callosum has been divided according to a preoperative plan. Finally, the use of this technique has drastically changed our approach to cerebral localization. Indeed, PET scan data obtained by cerebral blood flow activation can now be integrated in the 3D allegro MRI and used in conjunction with the pointer (viewing wand) during the surgery in awake or asleep patients. The technique has been used to locate sensory, motor and speech centers in the process of tumor or epileptic focus removal.

SPECIAL TECHNIQUES

INTRAOPERATIVE ELECTROCORTICOGRAPHY (ECoG)

Intraoperative ECoG is used for two main purposes. The first is to further delineate the extent of the epileptogenic abnormalities. Brief (usually less then 20 min in duration) direct intraoperative ECoG recordings are obtained from the exposed cortical surface with or without acute depth electrode recordings or other technical variations (activation techniques such as hyperventilation and short-acting barbiturates). Standard flexible electrodes with carbon-ball tips are often used for intraoperative monitoring. In our center, most in-

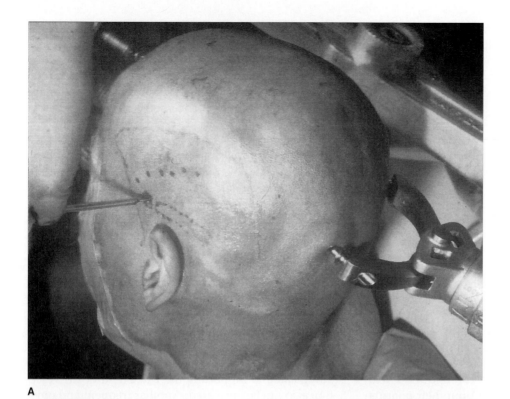

A

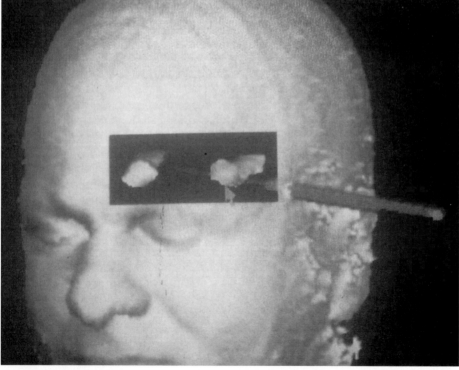

B

Figure 21-6 *A.* In the frameless stereotactic technique a pointer linked to a computer station is used to indicate the position of intracranial structures in relation to the scalp surface. *B.* Display of a 3D reconstruction of head and brain showing the amygdala and hippocampus bilaterally. Note the position of computer pointer which follows movements of the real pointer.

traoperative ECoGs are now performed under general anesthesia, and the technique is used mainly to confirm and more rarely to alter the extent of a predetermined resection. The surgeon uses the preoperative information to demonstrate the epileptogenic zone and lesion, and the intraoperative ECoG to optimize the resection of electrically abnormal tissue. Interictal spiking cortex is, however, not necessarily removed if it includes regions that do not conform to the suspected epileptogenic zone and this is what Theodore Rasmussen used to designate as the "green spikes" versus the "red spikes." Whatever the technique used, intraoperative ECoG aims at improving seizure outcome, if possible. The use of ECoG to assess the completeness of resection is subject to much debate. The intraoperative ECoG provides only a brief sample compared with interictal EEG, and seizures are fortuitously and rarely recorded. In addition, attempts to correlate the ECoG findings with the location of pathologic lesions have not given consistent results. Because of their sources of origin or of their pathways of propagation, spikes may be difficult to classify. For instance, primary spikes (those originating in the region of interest or from the epileptogenic zone) may be difficult to differentiate from projected spikes (those originating outside the region of interest or from other irritative areas). Finally, the technique of EEG monitoring used (e.g., neocortical lateral vs. basal vs. depth electrode recordings in TLE), the level of the patient's alertness (including various stages of sleep or anesthesia), the level of AEDs, and the type of surgical resection, may all alter spiking activity and distribution of interictal epileptiform discharges, further complicating the use and interpretation of the intraoperative ECoG.

The second important purpose of intraoperative ECoG is the identification of essential or eloquent cortical areas using electrical stimulation mapping. Wilder Penfield pioneered mapping cortical functions by electrical stimulation during awake brain operations.[241,242] With this technique, sites essential for motor, sensory, or language function can now be identified. For example, the central area of the brain has a fairly constant sulcal and gyral pattern, and close inspection will often reveal the location of the pre- and postcentral gyri. However, the exact position of the motor and sensory cortices can be determined with precision only by electrical stimulation. Thus, identification of location of eloquent areas by stimulation techniques allows for a more extensive and a safer resection of the epileptogenic lesion and zone while reducing postoperative morbidity. Newer technologies such as fast-flare MRI, PET, and magnetoencephalography may also be used for localizing cognitive functions, and may eventually render cortical stimulation obsolete. The latter, however, still represents the gold standard for cortical map-

ping, and comparative studies with the newer techniques are still necessary. For a more detailed discussion on functional mapping, refer to the reviews of Ojemann and coworkers[243] and of Perrine.[244]

ELECTROCORTICOGRAPHY: METHODOLOGY

The first condition for a worthwhile ECoG is sufficient brain exposure. The areas to be studied should be easily recognizable and reachable. Usually, a combination of 16 electrodes is utilized. The electrode tip is made of a carbon ball supported by a flexible wire. Thus they can be used to record from the cortical surface and from structures deep within a cavity, which is particularly useful in post-resection electrocorticography. The electrodes can be arranged in any bipolar or monopolar montage. Typically, with a temporo-frontal exposure, rows of four electrodes each are disposed over the first and second temporal gyri and along the third and second frontal gyri, with electrodes covering the central area. Flexible subdural electrodes can also be used to record from the temporal pole, the undersurface of the temporal lobe, the fronto-orbital area, or from cortex covered by dura. ECoG provides both diagnostic and prognostic information by further delineating the active zone prior to resection and by showing the areas of residual discharges after cortical removal. Perioperative depth recording from the limbic structures of the temporal lobe (amygdala and hippocampus) is also routinely combined with surface electrocorticography. Such recording is most useful to determine the amount and distribution of subcortical epileptic discharges and their relationships with the surface activity. Electrocorticography is an integral part of cortical mapping by stimulation and serves to detect poststimulation after discharges. The patient's typical auras are frequently obtained by stimulation of the deepest contacts of the depth electrodes. Areas of epileptic activity are indicated with letter tags placed on the cortical surface and physiologic responses are indicated with numbers (Fig. 21-7).

INTRAOPERATIVE CORTICAL MAPPING

The identification of the sensorimotor strip (pre- and postcentral gyri) is an essential step in many cortical resections. It is best determined by electrical stimulation under local anesthesia or sensory evoked potentials under general anesthesia. The constant current generator is equipped with an in-built 1000-ohm resistance and delivers pulses of 2 msec duration at a frequency of 60 Hz. Increasing increments of 0.5 V over the range from 0.5 V to 7.5 V results in stimulations between 0.5 mA and 7.5 mA. Most responses are obtained around 3 volts.[245] The postcentral gyrus is best identified by obtaining sensory responses from the tongue area, which correspond to the lower 2.5 cm of

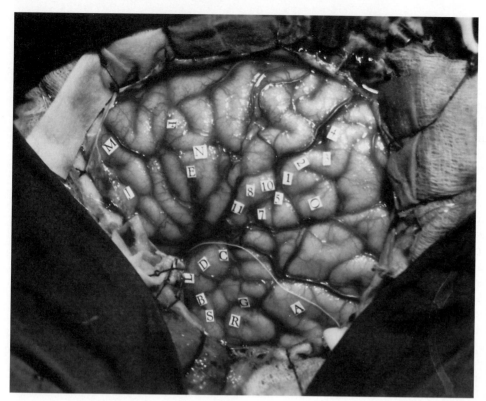

Figure 21-7. Perioperative photograph. The sites of epileptic activity are indicated with letters placed on the cortical surface and positive responses are shown with numbers. L, D, C, B, S, R, G, and A define an area of epileptic activity over the left temporal lobe. Numbers 4, 3, 2, 1, and 5 represent sensory responses over the postcentral gyrus.

the postcentral gyrus, above the Sylvian fissure and behind the central sulcus. Based on these responses, the central sulcus, precentral, and postcentral gyri can be readily identified. Positive responses to stimulation are indicated with numbers, sites of epileptic activity with letters, and negative responses with blanks (Fig. 21-8). If a seizure is induced by stimulation, it is quickly stopped by the intravenous injection of a fast-acting barbiturate.

CORTICAL RESECTIONS

TEMPORAL RESECTIONS

The temporal lobe is by far the most frequent site of surgery of epilepsy. In the MNI series covering the period 1929 through 1980, it represents 56 percent of the total procedures.

The question of modalities and extent of temporal resections was already being discussed in the mid 1950s. A failure rate of the order of 21.5 percent was attributed by Penfield and Jasper,[195] in 1954 to a too-limited resection of the temporal lobe, especially of its internal structures.[26] Based on a series of 81 patients operated over a 3-year period, they suggested the systematic exclusion of the uncus and of the hippocampus.

There are many varieties of tailored resection of the temporal lobe structures, incorporating various extents of the anterior temporal cortex and the amygdalo-hip-

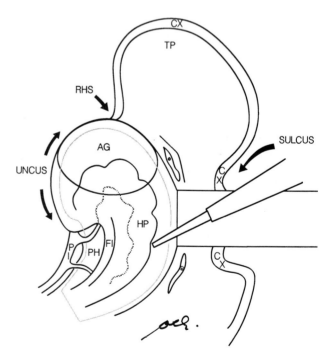

Figure 21-8. Diagram to illustrate the procedure of transcortical selective amygdalo-hippocampectomy. (HP = hippocampus; PH = parahippocampus; AG = amygdala.) The dotted line represents the extent of the resection.

pocampal complex. Extremely rarely is the temporal lobe resected in its entirety. For this reason it is preferable to abandon the terms "temporal lobectomy" or "anterior lobectomy" and to replace them by the term "temporal resection" with its variations, such as cortico-amygdalo-hippocampectomy, cortico-amygdalectomy, or selective amygdalo-hippocampectomy.

CORTICO-AMYGDALO-HIPPOCAMPECTOMY (CAH)

Nowadays the most frequently used surgical procedure for temporal lobe epilepsy still consists of an anterior cortical resection combined with a removal of the amygdala (cortico-amygdalectomy) and of the hippocampus (cortico-amygdalo-hippocampectomy). The cortical resection proper illustrates how such removal is carried out in any region of the brain. It is done by bipolar coagulation of the arachnoid and pia along the first temporal gyrus between the looping opercular branches of the middle cerebral artery. Perforation and opening of the leptomeninges is carried out with the tips of the bipolar coagulator. The tip of an ultrasound dissector is then inserted subpially, and the cortex is fragmented and aspirated. The pia arachnoid is further coagulated and divided with microscissors. Each looping temporal branch is then thoroughly coagulated and divided, leaving enough of a stump at the exit of the Sylvian fissure in case of eventual bleeding. The cortex is removed by the subpial technique, which means that each gyrus is emptied along a pial plane, without leaving any devascularized tissue behind. First an en bloc surface resection of the cortex is performed. In the author's experience with over 800 such procedures, the extent of the cortical resection has varied slightly according to the side of the operation. Thus, on the dominant side, it averages 4.5 cm along the Sylvian fissure and extends to the level of the precentral sulcus but not beyond. On the nondominant side, it averages 5 cm along the Sylvian fissure. Any by-passing artery and its distal territory should be assessed prior to its occlusion. The posterior resection line slopes backward toward the floor of the middle fossa and usually is extended back to a larger obliquely running artery or vein. Following removal of the surface cortex, as much as possible of the amygdala is removed with various extents of hippocampal formation.

This standard temporal removal can be further modified by reducing further the extent of cortical removal and extending the removal of the hippocampal resection.[246] Basically these modalities have much in common and whether the beneficial or side effects are different remains to be established. This also applies to the selective amygdalo-hippocampectomy (Tables 21-6, 21-7).

TABLE 21-6
Outcome of Surgical Treatment

The Following Classification Was Used for All the Patients Operated at the MNH/MNI

Class 1:	Seizure free
Class 2:	Aura only
Class 3:	Maximum of three seizures per year
Class 4:	Over 90% seizure reduction without monthly seizures
Class 5:	60–90% or more seizure reduction, still having monthly seizures, with significant improvement in quality of life.
Improved:	Patients who have benefited from surgical treatment
Class 6:	Less than 60% seizure reduction without significant improvement in the quality of life

SELECTIVE AMYGDALO-HIPPOCAMPECTOMY (SAH)

In 1958, Niemeyer proposed the selective removal of the limbic structures by a transcortical approach through the second temporal gyrus.[247] In 1969, he reported on the microsurgical route to those structures. In the 1970s this procedure was modified by Yasargil, who used a transsylvian approach to reach the hippocampus and amygdala.[248] We have further modified the Niemeyer approach by using a parasulcal transcortical approach.

TRANSCORTICAL AMYGDALO-HIPPOCAMPECTOMY

A 2- to 3-cm incision is made through the second temporal gyrus just below the superior temporal sulcus,

TABLE 21-7
Outcome of Temporal Resections

	ATR	SAH	TR
No. of patients	**458**	**111**	**569**
Class 1 (%)	67	82	74.5
Class 2 (%)	7	6	6.5
Class 3 (%)	10	6	8
Class 4 (%)	8	4	6
Class 5 (%)	5	2	3.5
Improved (%)	**97**	**100**	**98**
Class 6 (%)	3	0	1.5
Reoperation (%)	20	4.5	12.2
Min. yr F/U	1	1	1
Max. yr F/U	23.2	8.3	15.7
Mean yr F/U	7.1	2.5	4.8

NOTE: ATR (CAH): anterior temporal resection including removal of the amygdala and hippocampus; SAH: selective amygdalo-hippocampectomy (temporal left intact); TR: combined ATR & SAH; F/U: follow-up.

and this sulcus is followed down toward the ventricle. This parasulcal approach minimizes manipulation and division of vessels and decreases the amount of cortical contusion resulting from a subarachnoid dissection. The ventricle is approached by a subinsular transsection of the white matter. Once the ventricle is entered, the hippocampal formation and amygdala are removed in accordance with series of clear anatomic landmarks.

TRANSSYLVIAN AMYGDALO-HIPPOCAMPECTOMY

This approach was devised and used extensively by Yasargil.[248,249] The temporal horn is reached through the sylvian fissure. The hippocampus is exposed and resected with a small-bore suction according to the authors. This approach is technically more tedious and entails more manipulation of major arterial trunk than does the transcortical approach. The looping temporal arteries usually limit the extent of the transcortical incision and preclude the use of the ultrasonic dissector.

In our opinion, the selective amygdalo-hippocampectomy is a justified alternative to cortico-amygdalo-hippocampectomy when a clear mesiobasal onset has been demonstrated by adequate recording and by demonstration of mesial sclerosis on MRI. This procedure, however, with its inherent difficulties, cannot entirely replace the anterior cortical resection combined with the amygdalo-hippocampectomy as the standard procedure in temporal lobe epilepsy. The cortico-amygdalo-hippocampectomy with its progressive modification (smaller neocortical removal and larger limbic removal) appears to be a practical compromise that takes into account physiologic, neuropsychological, and technical factors. It can remove a larger volume of epileptogenic brain tissue without causing intellectual or memory deficit.

EXTRATEMPORAL RESECTIONS

Surgery of epilepsy is too often equated with surgery of temporal lobe epilepsy. Indeed, surgical series show that the temporal lobe is by far the most frequent site of surgery for intractable epilepsy. In one of the authors' series of 1275 procedures, operations on the temporal lobe represented 66 percent, while frontal resections represented 11 percent, central 3 percent, parietal 3 percent, and occipital 2 percent. Multilobe resections (often the equivalent of subtotal hemispherectomies) amounted to 2 percent, and callosotomies represented 13 percent. Since 1972, over 200 patients with temporal and extratemporal partial epilepsies were investigated with implantation of depth electrodes.

These differences no doubt reflect the variation in the epileptic threshold of various brain areas. They

TABLE 21-8
Outcome of Frontal and Central Resections

	Frontal	Central	MST
No. of patients	**88**	**33**	**10**
Class 1 (%)	35	38	50
Class 2 (%)	0	0	0
Class 3 (%)	5	3	0
Class 4 (%)	25	19	20
Class 5 (%)	20	19	30
Improved (%)	**85**	**79**	**100**
Class 6 (%)	15	21	0
Min. yr F/U	1	1	1
Max. yr F/U	17	4	3
Mean (year) F/U	6.2	2.5	2

NOTE: MST: multiple subpial transection.

also reflect the difficulty in properly assessing the exact site of origin of seizures outside the temporal lobe, and the reluctance of the surgeon to venture into some of these often more eloquent or more dangerous extratemporal zones. As noted by Rasmussen, epileptogenic lesions outside of the temporal lobe are considerably more varied in extent and geographic configuration than are the more common lesions in the temporal lobe.

There is thus an enormous challenge in tackling the extratemporal epilepsies. Nowhere else than in those extratemporal zones are Rasmussen's triad of questions more difficult to define: (1) Where do the seizures start? (2) How much volume must be involved for the seizure to manifest itself? (3) How much tissue should the neurosurgeon remove in order to obtain a good result? The approach consists essentially in identifying as accurately as possible the epileptogenic area in terms of location and extent and in determining what the optimal cortical removal should be. Various types of extratemporal resections will now be briefly described (Tables 21-8, 21-9).

FRONTAL RESECTION

Based on clinical presentation, brain imaging, and extracranial and intracranial EEG findings, various types of frontal resections can be considered such as the total frontal lobectomy, paramedian removals, fronto-polar removal, lateral convexity removal and central removal.

Large frontal resections in the nondominant hemisphere can be safely carried out in front of the precentral gyri. Clear identification of the motor cortex is absolutely essential and is best accomplished by stimulation under local anesthesia. The posterior orbital cortex and the subcallosal gyrus are usually left alone. On the dominant side, the resection is brought down to

TABLE 21-9
Outcome of Parietal and Occipital Resections

	Parietal	Occipital
No. of patients	**23**	**18**
Class 1 (%)	57	62
Class 2 (%)	0	5
Class 3 (%)	13	11
Class 4 (%)	13	5
Class 5 (%)	13	0
Improved (%)	**96**	**83**
Class 6 (%)	4	17
Min. yr F/U	1	1
Max. yr F/U	20	12.8
Mean F/U	6	5.2

either the middle of the second frontal gyrus or, preferably, to the inferior frontal sulcus. The posterior 2.5 cm of the third frontal gyrus is left alone to avoid speech disturbance. In this region we tend to rely heavily on topography and anatomic landmarks rather than on response to stimulation. Speech interference in the so-called "Broca area" is, in our experience, often negative with currents well above sensory and motor thresholds, and a negative response does not always indicate absence of function. Here also careful analysis of the vascular anatomy is essential. The arterial pattern over the frontal lobe is fairly constant, with a clear watershed zone between the middle and anterior cerebral arteries territories over the second frontal gyrus. Venous drainage is much more variable. The downward drainage to the sylvian veins should be ascertained prior to dividing an ascending frontal vein. In the author's opinion, many cases of transient postoperative dysphasia following frontal resections in the dominant hemisphere are due to venous occlusion of ascending frontal veins draining into the superior longitudinal sinus rather than actual cortical removals.

Paramedian frontal removals including the first frontal gyrus and the "supplementary motor area" located on its mesial surface can extend from the frontal pole to the precentral sulcus. It is crucial that the lateral border of the excision extends at least to the middle of the second frontal gyrus, and preferably even to the inferior sulcus, to avoid postoperative edema secondary to arterial and venous occlusions. The cingulate gyrus is also usually resected. When the cingulate gyrus is resected it is of even greater importance to remove tissue as far laterally as possible over the convexity since interference with arterial feeders in the depth of the calloso-marginal and the pericallosal sulci can occur with subsequent edema of subcortical white mat-

ter. This is especially true if some of the frontal ascending veins have been divided.

Fronto-polar resections involve removal of the pole of the frontal lobe on some extent of its intermediate portion. They are typically carried out in cases of posttraumatic frontal lobe epilepsy with a history of depressed skull fracture, dural laceration, and fronto-polar contusions.

CENTRAL RESECTION

The majority of patients with central area seizure have a fairly stereotyped pattern of seizures. In the vast majority, the attacks are either somatomotor or somatosensory. In some patients, the attacks remain localized, but in most patients a certain portion of the attacks progress to generalized convulsive seizures. Focal status epilepticus and epilepsia partialis continua are particularly common. Resection of the lower central area, including both pre- and postcentral gyri, can be done in cases of focal motor or sensory seizures, even in the dominant hemisphere. This is particularly true if the seizure involves the face early in the attack. The removal can extend up for a distance of close to 3 cm above the sylvian fissure without any deficit as long as the tongue, thumb, and lip area are well identified by stimulation under local anesthesia. Central arteries should be recognized as they exit from the sylvian fissure and should be left intact, especially the central sulcus artery, which is fairly constant and usually found looping over the central operculum before penetrating deep within the lower extent of the central sulcus. It is important also to recognize arteries from the pre- and postcentral sulci, which vascularize the pre- and postcentral gyri and often penetrate into the central sulcus. The resection is best done by emptying those gyri with an ultrasonic dissector set at very low suction parameters and low amplitude of vibration in order to respect the pial banks, including the upper bank of the insula. When no voluntary hand movement is preserved and there is absence of position sense and presence of paresis of the lower limb, the whole central area can be removed without additional neurologic deficits.

PARIETAL RESECTION

Approximately one-half of patients with parietal lobe epilepsy have somatomotor or somatosensory attacks similar to those arising in the central region. Most of the remainder exhibit attacks consisting of unilateral motor or sensory phenomena, with additional features such as dizziness, cephalic sensation, perceptual illusions, informed visual hallucinations, mental confusion, epigastric sensation, dysphasia, or automatism.

Resections in the parietal region are possible only after careful and clear identification of the postcentral gyrus. As for the central region proper, it is of the utmost importance to respect and leave intact any ascending vein to the superior sagittal sinus draining from the central or postcentral sulci. On the dominant side, resections should be limited to the superior parietal lobule and any ascending vein from the inferior parietal lobule should be left intact to avoid speech disturbance. The lower 2 to 3 cm of the postcentral gyrus can be resected without significant deficit. Resection of the hand and foot area of the postcentral gyrus will be followed by a profound proprioceptive deficit. In the nondominant hemisphere, the whole parietal lobe posterior to the postcentral sulcus can be removed without sensorimotor deficit as long as the postcentral gyrus is left intact. A partial visual field deficit can be expected. Careful study of the regional arteriovenous pattern will indicate the position of the intraparietal sulcus, which should be the inferior limit of the resection. The anterior limit is the postcentral sulcus.

Indications for operations in the parietal lobe are few, and these removals are usually based on strong congruence of clinical, imaging, and EEG data. Intracranial recordings may be necessary to determine whether the central area is included in the epileptogenic zone.

OCCIPITAL RESECTION

Occipital lobe seizures manifest themselves by such visual symptoms as transient blindness or visual hallucinations usually characterized by flashes of lights, colored balls and other geometric patterns, which are not organized in complex hallucinations. Progression to contralateral sensorimotor seizures with contraversion of head and eyes is frequent. Surgery on the occipital lobes is done only when there is clear evidence for an occipital focus, usually proved by intracerebral recordings. Most seizures of occipital onset tend to spread to the temporal or parieto-central areas. If the seizure only manifests itself mainly when the temporal lobe is invaded, it is often preferable to proceed with a temporal resection first to avoid the visual deficits that usually follow most occipital resections.

MULTILOBAR RESECTIONS AND HEMISPHERECTOMIES

Multilobar resections usually consist of subtotal hemispherectomies. They are done for large destructive lesions and for epileptic zones that affect more than one lobe of the brain. Rasmussen observed that in these patients even the full battery of recording techniques frequently failed to demonstrate a focal seizure onset in the damaged hemisphere. Removal of various combinations of lobes, such as fronto-temporal, fronto-parietal, or occipito-temporal, frequently is indicated in these patients. Over the last several years we have

preferred to proceed in two stages, that is, limit the initial resection to the most active or most damaged lobe and proceed, one to two years later, with resection of another lobar area if seizures persist.

In patients with congenital hemiplegia or chronic encephalitis that has progressed to the stage of hemiplegia, hemispherectomy usually produces a dramatic arrest of focal motor and generalized convulsive seizures. Total hemispherectomy has, however, been associated with a high rate of morbidity and mortality due to superficial hemosiderosis and hydrocephalus. This led Rasmussen to develop a central disconnection technique, later modified by Villemure, which is equivalent to an "anatomically incomplete but physiologically complete hemispherectomy.[250–252] This operation consists of a large and deep central resection combined with removal of the temporal lobe. All projections, associative and commissural, are thus transected, including fibers of the corpus callosum. The classic hemispherectomy is now rarely carried out in our institution, but we feel that a subtotal hemispherectomy where one-fifth to one-third of the hemisphere is preserved is still frequently indicated and is not associated with delayed hydrocephalus. Appraisal of the preoperative hand deficit is particularly crucial when considering surgery in these patients. No postoperative deficit will occur when the hand barely moves, is spastic, and is kept closed with the elbow flexed. The functional deficit after hemispherectomy will be minimal when there is some useful but diminished hand prehension movement without any individual finger movements. Patients who have hand prehension are likely to lose this ability postoperatively. Patients who have severe limping and are unable to perform foot tapping movements may develop some temporary increased deficit, but usually there is no permanent additional deficit. The potential for further loss of function in the hand or foot must be discussed in depth with the patient and/or family before the surgical procedure. This is especially important in young patients suffering from Rasmussen's chronic encephalitis, in whom the unilateral weakness at the time of surgery may be only partial. The occurrence of a complete hemiplegia to arrest focal seizures should be considered unacceptable except in life-threatening status epilepticus.

Cortical Resection in Chronic Encephalitis

The indication for surgery in chronic encephalitis is to obtain or confirm a diagnosis and/or to decrease seizure frequency. The modalities of cortical resections depend essentially on the clinical picture, more specifically on the degree of deterioration of motor function and the side of hemispheric involvement. Limited resections in the central area and a large resection outside the central area, or a combination of both, are usually ineffective. A subtotal or functional hemispherectomy of the nondominant hemisphere encompassing the whole central area should be done when the patient has no useful left hand and finger movements. A sufficiently large specimen should be obtained for diagnosis. In patients in whom the dominant hemisphere is affected and who have preserved speech and hand function, only a diagnostic brain biopsy is indicated. A functional hemispherectomy should be considered only in cases with involvement of the dominant hemisphere when the motor and speech deficits are severe. A thorough discussion with the patient and/or parents stressing the purpose of the surgery and the permanent and irreversible nature of the deficit is essential in these cases.

Subtotal hemispherectomy or functional hemispherectomy usually produces satisfactory control of seizures. It is uncertain, however, whether this type of operation may be considered even before the disease has caused maximal deficit. Early surgery may reduce additional contralateral neurologic deficits due to the seizures, but the complications of the surgical procedure itself may not be acceptable to the patient and/or the family, despite detailed and repeated explanations.

MULTIPLE SUBPIAL CORTICAL TRANSECTIONS

A technique of subpial vertical cortical transection has been recommended by Morrel and coworkers[253] for patients with epileptic zones located in eloquent areas of the brain. This technique is meant to leave intact the vertical columnar arrangement of the cerebral cortex, preserving most vertical outgoing and incoming fibers, but would prevent spread of seizure discharge in the horizontal plane along a gyrus.

CALLOSOTOMY

This procedure has been used first by Van Wagenen and Herren[254] with encouraging results, but was never fully accepted as a recognized mode of surgical treatment until recently. Bogen[255] reintroduced the procedure in the early 1960s, but again, in spite of its demonstrated effectiveness, the procedure never gained wide popularity. This was most likely due to the fact that the section was not restricted to the corpus callosum only but included most if not all of the forebrain commissures, that is, the corpus callosum in its entirety, the anterior commissure, and at times the massa intermedia of the thalamus. These divisions constituted high-morbidity procedures at a time when the technical facilities were not readily available. We owe to Wilson[256] the introduction of microsurgical techniques in callosotomy in selected cases of intractable epilepsies. Wilson's efforts are probably responsible for the aforementioned resurgence of interest in callosotomy. In recent years, callosotomy has been carried out with increasing frequency in patients with epilepsy who are not candidates for the classic approach, which consists in removing the epileptogenic area. The surgical indications for callosotomy are still debated, but the presence of drop attacks has emerged as the major indication for this procedure.[257-259] A more recent analysis of our material indicated that the drop attacks can be abolished in about 70 percent of patients who have had a callosotomy involving the anterior two-thirds of the corpus callosum.[260] A meticulous technique is most important to avoid several of the side effects or complications not directly due to actual transection of the corpus callosum. The division of the callosum proper is best achieved with the ultrasonic dissector set at a very low parameters of suction and vibration. In this way, it is possible to divide the callosal fibers and leave intact the ependymal veins. Meticulous hemostasis is insured prior to dural closure. If a total callosotomy is planned, we prefer a two-stage approach. For the posterior section, namely the splenium section, a parietal craniotomy is performed. In our experience, division of the anterior two-thirds of the callosum does not give rise to significant hemispheric disconnection, but complete transsection should be considered only in patients with significant mental retardation. The most frequent side effect of anterior callosotomy has been a transient state of mutism.

OUTCOME IN CALLOSOTOMY

We reviewed 44 cases retrospectively, in which microsurgical two-thirds anterior callosotomies were performed for the treatment of drop attacks, often in two stages.[260] The inclusion criteria for surgery consisted of: (1) lack of control of drop attacks with therapeutic serum concentration of antiepileptic drugs for at least three years; (2) seizures were of sufficient frequency or severity leading to injury, deterioration, or both; and (3) no identifiable or resectable focus.

In this series, drop attacks were abolished in 78 percent of the patients following callosotomy. Postoperative complications include four cases of transient mutism, one case of transient hemiparesis, one case of bronchopneumonia, and one case of aseptic meningitis. The mean follow-up was 35 months. It is concluded that microsurgical two-thirds anterior callosotomy can be performed with low morbidity and is a useful procedure for the treatment of drop attacks.

Considerations on Treatment in Childhood

Awareness of the progressive development of personality changes, of psychosocial problems, and of downward social mobility in patients with intractable epilepsy has led to the hope that some of these deficits may be prevented by earlier definitive therapy.[261-263] There was, however, a natural reluctance to perform routine resective surgery for intractable seizures in children, and epilepsy surgery in this age group was until recently a relatively rare procedure, used only in hopeless cases. A greater knowledge of the risk factors and poor long-term cognitive and psychosocial prognosis of chronic childhood epilepsy, a better understanding of the long-term effects of surgery on the developing brain, and also a better understanding of the neuropathologic substrates underlying epileptic syndromes of infancy and childhood, improved protocols for candidate selection.[264-266]

Knowledge of the natural history of the illness in children with epilepsy is clearly needed before considering any epilepsy surgery. Many seizure disorders that occur in children include such age-dependent benign epileptic syndromes as febrile seizures, benign childhood epilepsy with centro-temporal spikes, and childhood epilepsy with occipital paroxysms (see Table 21-2). Typically, these disorders have very little or no long-term side effects, the prognosis is excellent, and there may even be no need for medication, especially if the seizures are nondisabling, nocturnal only, and rare. Idiopathic age-related generalized epilepsies, although usually more serious, often negatively affect the ability of children to function normally, have also a good prognosis for seizure control, and tend to disappear with advancing age. Lesion-related and symptomatic/cryptogenic generalized epilepsies, such as infantile spasms and Lennox-Gastaut syndrome, are serious disorders causing intractable and very disabling seizures. Children affected by these disorders usually show early cognitive impairment, decline in intelligence, and long-term behavioral deficits.

Frequently, a hope may persist in the minds of the parents and treating physicians that the epileptic disorder will remit spontaneously, and one of the major problems in the selection of surgical candidates is to identify precisely those who are likely not to do so. Huttenlocher and co-workers,[267] in an attempt to define criteria for the selection of children for epilepsy surgery, analyzed a cohort of children with seizures refractory to medical therapy; follow-up from onset of seizures varied from five to 20 years. This study showed spontaneous remission of seizures in a significant proportion of children with borderline to normal intelligence compared with those with mental retardation (4 percent vs 1.5 percent per year). Their data suggested that the natural history of intractable seizures in both groups appears to be a slow linear improvement for at least 18 years after onset. Age of onset

and seizure type also seemed to have some effects on outcome. Other predictors of intractability include the lack of initial responsiveness to AED therapy, a high seizure frequency or a history of status epilepticus, failure to achieve normal developmental milestones and an abnormal neurologic examination, and a localization-related symptomatic epilepsy.[268]

A stable habitual seizure pattern that shows, similar to adult patients, no improvement over the years represents a major indication for surgery. Complex partial seizures that develop after prolonged febrile status epilepticus and are related to hippocampal sclerosis represent a good example. Recent MRI studies demonstrated a high incidence of hippocampal sclerosis in chronic childhood TLE, suggesting that this lesion represents an early acquired phenomenon.[269,270] Seizures may be associated with other known very deleterious syndromes. They may have developmental disorders such as Sturge-Weber syndrome, tuberous sclerosis, or the larger group of diffuse or focal cortical migrational defects, acquired diseases such as Rasmussen encephalitis, hemiconvulsions, hemiplegia, epilepsy (HHE) syndrome, and postencephalitic epilepsy. Children with intractable generalized seizures may also be amenable to resective surgery. Advances in imaging technology, particularly PET and MRI, further characterized the basic mechanisms of infantile spasms, or hypsarhythmia, and their management.[137,271-273] Infantile spasms are classified as a generalized seizure disorder (Table 21-2) and, although previously considered as cryptogenic, are now known to be associated with various structural brain anomalies, including focal lesions. When the structural lesion was resected, the generalized seizures ceased.

The progressive deterioration of behavior and cognitive functions in epileptic children clearly represent indications for early surgical intervention. The high number of seizures, at times hundreds each day, known deleterious syndromes, and poor prognosis also lead one to urge consideration of a surgical approach that hopefully may arrest and reverse the pathologic process. The development of pediatric neurology and epileptology has led to a reluctance to accept as inevitable the deterioration that may accompany seizures related to brain lesions.[74] Most children now evaluated at epilepsy centers with a pediatric orientation benefit from the same diagnostic procedures that have been used in adults. Pediatric epilepsy surgery candidates are now best handled by multidisciplinary teams of consultant pediatric, intensivist, neuroanesthesiologist, and surgeon. Even children with difficult to localize nonlesional epileptic seizures may undergo invasive intracranial monitoring and eventually be successfully treated by surgery.[274]

Anesthesia for Epilepsy Surgery

For the last 20 years, surgical interventions for control of epilepsy that traditionally were carried out in awake patients under local anesthesia have been performed in increasing numbers under general anesthesia. The technical advances that allowed for this shift have been presented in the previous sections. Not only has the preoperative evaluation and the selection of surgical candidates improved since the introduction of CT scanning, MRI, PET, SPECT, and measurements of cerebral blood flow, but localization of abnormal epileptogenic foci has benefited greatly from the ability to perform prolonged EEG studies with telemetry and continuous video-recordings. Although these procedures are generally done without anesthesia, such more invasive procedures as stereotactic implantation of depth electrodes and subdural strips and grids will necessarily require anesthetic involvement.

As long as it was considered essential to have the patient awake for the successful outcome of the neurosurgical procedure[30] the mandate of the neuroanesthesiologist was defined in the following terms:

- No medication with a potential to alter the EEG recording should be used.
- Anesthetic agents should not interfere with the electrical stimulation process of the cortex.
- The patient should be alert and cooperative and should participate in verbal and motor testing when indicated.
- The patient should be given sedation and analgesia to tolerate the long craniotomy procedure.
- The anesthesiologist should control adequately sudden bursts of epileptic activity and, if necessary, administer a general anesthetic to permit termination of the procedure.

The number of drugs available at the time limited strongly the capacity of the anesthesiologist to respond to the task.[31,32,35] General anesthesia provides optimal conditions for the surgeon and a stable environment for the patient. A large array of potent agents is now available, making it possible manipulate hemodynamic and respiratory parameters, brain volume, and cerebral perfusion, and interfering minimally with the electrical activity of the brain. The anesthesiologist involved in seizure surgery must maintain great familiarity with the general pharmacologic aspects of drugs and also with their pro- and anticonvulsant properties. The experience gained with the newer intravenous anesthetics and the sedative-hypnotics, for example, propofol, has resulted in the emergence of a mixed form of anesthesia, conscious-sedation anesthesia (CSA), or monitored anesthesia care (MAC).

As an introduction to the anesthetic management of a surgical procedure for epilepsy a short review of electrophysiologic effects of widely used anesthetic agents is presented.

PHARMACOLOGICAL AGENTS

INHALATION AGENTS

Without exception, cerebral activity is affected in a dose-dependent manner, with low doses activating the EEG and larger doses suppressing the activity.[275,276]

Halothane

In keeping with the general pattern, the background alpha frequencies are replaced at 1.2 MAC by fast beta activity. With concentrations increasing to 2.5 MAC, high-amplitude delta activity becomes predominant. Activation of epileptiform spikes is not seen.[277-279] At concentrations that are still clinically useful, suppression of the spike activity has been observed.[280,281]

Enflurane

Enflurane has potent activating properties. At low inspired concentrations, beta activity is present, which is replaced by high-amplitude delta and theta waves as the agent concentration rises. At high concentrations, spike and polyspike activity is produced, with burst suppression and interspaced polyspike activity observed.[278,282,283] Hypercarbia suppresses these activating effects.[282,284,285] Enflurane has been known to produce generalized seizures in patients with no previous history of seizure activity,[286-288] particularly in the presence of severe hypocarbia.[289] Concern has been raised about its use in epileptic patients, but there appears to be no greater risk than in the general population.[290,291] During ECoG, epileptiform discharges outside the area of spontaneous activity were noted,[292] casting serious doubts about the validity of recordings under such conditions. Enflurane has been used as an activating agent during diagnostic mapping procedures.[279,293] Several authors have questioned the practice as the presence of spikes over normal areas were registered.[283,284,294] Recently, a synergistic role of enflurane and neuroleptic drugs in producing seizure activity has been confirmed.[295-297]

Isoflurane

Fast low-voltage EEG activity is observed at low concentrations, with bursts of high-voltage beta activity at 1 MAC. At 1.5 MAC, burst suppression occurs, and isoelectric EEG are noticed at levels in excess of 2 MAC.[277,298,299] Background epileptiform activity may be reduced or suppressed in the presence of low doses of isoflurane.[300,301] Concern regarding the suppression of epileptic activity on the ECoG has been raised,[292,302] but most centers using low concentrations of isoflurane simultaneously with intravenous narcotics have not observed any negative effects.[303,304] Elimination of nitrous oxide, which potentiates the anesthetic effect of isoflurane, and reduction of the inspired concentration to 0.25 percent (less than 0.2 MAC) may minimize the suppressive effects of the agent. Although isoflurane has intrinsically no proconvulsant effect, seizure activity has been reported when it was administered in combination with nitrous oxide.[305,306]

Desflurane

This halogenated ether derived from isoflurane produces EEG changes comparable to those observed with equipotent levels of isoflurane. No proconvulsant activity has been reported. Desflurane suppresses EEG activity significantly, and burst suppression has been observed at 1.25 MAC and higher values.[307]

Sevoflurane

Increases in frequency and amplitude of EEG tracing are observed with low concentrations. At higher concentrations frequency and amplitude decrease. No evidence of epileptiform activity has been observed.[308,309]

Nitrous Oxide

Dose-dependent EEG changes occur at nitrous oxide concentrations above 25 percent.[310] Normal alpha rhythm is replaced by low-amplitude fast activity, and at higher concentrations EEG slowing occurs.[311] Nitrous oxide has no convulsant properties by itself,[310,311] but in combination with other agents potentiation has been noticed.[275,305,306] Gloor[313] has claimed that nitrous oxide may negatively affect the interpretation of ECoG as it can suppress or eliminate spike activity. Several centers will not use nitrous oxide during epilepsy surgery because of the suppressive effect on the ECoG[32,314,315] Others recommend discontinuation of nitrous oxide 30 to 50 min prior to the recording of ECoG to avoid confounding interactions with other agents and to prevent whatever minimal effects might be attributed directly to the agent.[294] We usually prefer to abstain entirely from nitrous oxide, although at times some of us use nitrous oxide even during ECoG, as does Smith.[304] Recent studies in nonepileptic patients[312,316] have indicated that combined with propofol, nitrous oxide will result in activation of alpha and beta waves while on the other hand, decreased alpha and increased delta wave activity has been observed in the presence of isoflurane.[312,316]

INTRAVENOUS ANESTHETIC AGENTS

Barbiturates

Because of their many side effects, most barbiturates are no longer utilized as hypnotics and sedatives. Con-trary to the general trend, all ultrashort barbiturates (thiopental, methohexital, amobarbital) are widely used in anesthesia. Phenobarbital, a long-acting compound, on the other hand, is still prescribed for treatment of epileptic manifestations. After administration of barbiturates, normal alpha rhythm is progressively replaced by fast beta activity[294] and with increasing doses, delta activity appears, succeeded by burst suppression and electric silence. At low concentrations, thiopental has proconvulsant properties and produces paroxysms of spike activity in epileptic patients.[316] At higher doses, it is a potent anticonvulsant drug. Thiopental and pentobarbital have been widely used to treat postoperative seizures[317] and status epilepticus.[318]

Methohexital is a potent activator in patients with temporal lobe or primary generalized epilepsies.[319–321] Recordings of epileptogenic regions in patients with known temporal epilepsy have revealed spikes, polyspikes, and spike-and-wave activity in the face of methohexital activation.[322–324] Although activation may spread outside the area of epileptogenic activity,[325] experience has shown the activation remains principally within the epileptogenic zone.

Amobarbital (in doses utilized for the Wada test) and methohexital, have been observed to produce spiking activation in the hippocampal region.[326] The use of intraoperative activation varies between centers. Barbiturates will induce focal electrographic changes within or adjacent to epileptogenic cortex. Some feel the information to be helpful to circumscribe the zone of resection while others do not share this view.

Propofol

Since its introduction propofol has been at the center of a controversy. Numerous case reports with or without EEG have documented both its pro- and anticonvulsant effects. The evidence has been extensively reviewed by Smith and coworkers[327] and Borgeat and associates.[328] The effects of propofol on EEG are no different from other intravenous sedative hypnotic drugs; the agent induces dose-dependent changes in the EEG. At low infusion rates an increase in beta activity is likely to occur,[329] followed at higher rates by an increase in delta activity[330] and burst suppression.[331] In known epileptics and particularly during seizure surgery, the use of propofol has been controversial. Hodkinson and coworkers[332] reported three instances of spiking activation over brain areas that previously had not displayed epileptic activity. Ebrahim and associates[333] observed profound burst suppression and an increase in beta activity in 17 patients that interfered with the recording of EEG spikes. Drummond and coworkers[334] observed a substantial increase in beta activity in one patient, although the patient appeared to be fully awake. Drummond cautioned that this activity might be sufficient to obscure other underlying EEG patterns. Rampil and associates[335] recommended—particularly if surgical technique depends on intraoperative electrocorticography to optimize focal brain resection—that propofol not be used, at least until the recordings have been completed. In view of the possibility that in some instances epileptiform activity may be evoked outside the sensitive area, Smith and coworkers[336] have suggested terminating the propofol infusion at least 30 minutes prior to diagnostic corticography. It is surprising to see that Samra and associates[337] were unable to demonstrate a significant change in epileptiform activity with sedative doses of propofol administered in patients suffering from partial complex epilepsy. These authors concluded that propofol sedation can be used for patients with epilepsy undergoing temporal lobectomy under local anesthesia. Furthermore, propofol has an advantage over two other short-acting agents, methohexital and alfentanil, as it does not produce any "false" spikes or electrographic seizures. In conclusion, the use of propofol is neither associated with cortical epileptic activity nor with the aggravation of seizures. Patients with known and controlled epilepsy may receive propofol anesthesia. Moreover, propofol may be used to treat convulsions unresponsive to conventional treatment. This agent seems particularly useful for the induction of coma therapy for controlling refractory epilepsy. Compared to barbiturates, burst suppression is more easily controlled, awakening is more rapid, and there are no hepatic side effects.[328]

Etomidate

Etomidate is an ultra-short-acting nonbarbiturate hypnotic agent with EEG changes similar to those of barbiturates.[338] In nonepileptic patients, epileptiform discharges are commonly observed, but no EEG abnormalities are apparent.[339] In epileptic patients, etomidate generates interictal spiking and at times initiates clinical seizures.[339-341] In patients with a history of seizures, it is therefore better to exercise great caution.[342] Etomidate has been used to induce epileptiform activity during diagnostic ECoG.[339,340] Using larger doses, Wauquier and coworkers[343] showed that etomidate has strong anticonvulsant properties, which could make it useful for treating refractory status epilepticus.[344]

Benzodiazepines

Benzodiazepines are potent beta activity activators. Occasionally high-voltage theta and delta activity occur, and burst suppression is not seen. Benzodiazepines are very efficacious anticonvulsants.[345] These drugs should not be used when diagnostic corticography is planned. For presurgical invasive investigations,

for example, implantations of depth electrodes, midazolam may be utilized as part of a continuous intravenous infusion technique.

Local Anesthetics

Local anesthetics have a biphasic effect on the EEG.[275,346] At low plasma concentrations, lidocaine has anticonvulsant action.[347] At high concentrations, local anesthetics have excitatory effects and may induce seizures.[348] High doses of local anesthetics during epilepsy surgery using ECoG should be avoided.[294] Larger than maximum recommended doses are frequently necessary for anesthetizing adequately the scalp and other sensitive structures. However, few reports of toxic reactions have been published.[349,350] Possible explanations include the concomitant use of epinephrine which slows down systemic absorption, the phenytoin-related increased detoxification process,[351] and too-low accepted plasma levels.[351] Low doses of propofol have been recommended for treating lidocaine toxicity.[353]

ANTIEMETICS—DROPERIDOL

Droperidol is frequently used in combination with fentanyl for providing neuroleptanalgesia during awake craniotomies. In small doses, it has a prolonged antiemetic effect.[354] Droperidol has no effect on the EEG[278] when given alone. At low doses, in combination with fentanyl, increased alpha activity is observed; high doses cause high-amplitude delta and beta activity.[355] In epileptic patients spike activity remains unchanged.[356] In combination with inhalation agents, neuroleptic agents appear to induce seizure activity.[296,297]

OPIOIDS

Various excitatory phenomena occasionally occur following the administration of opioids. These effects are dose-related and more apparent in the presence of high doses of potent opioids. Detailed studies using surface electrodes have failed to document any EEG evidence of seizure activity in humans after fentanyl, alfentanil, and sufentanil in high doses.[357-359] On the other hand, an increase in delta activity arises after the rapid infusion of very large doses of sufentanil, with a demonstrable ceiling effect.[360] The administration of fentanyl has resulted in a distinct seizure activity in deep temporal lobe structures of patients with complex partial seizure disorders; however, no cortical seizure activity or motor activity was observed.[361] Fentanyl, alfentanil, and sufentanil have been compared one with another and found to be very similar in their effects.[362-364]

During anesthesia opioids are utilized to produce analgesia and to reduce the demands for larger concentrations of inhalation or intravenous agents.[365-368] Patients chronically medicated with AEDs (antiepileptic drugs) develop an increased tolerance to opioids and a typical dose-effect relationship has been demonstrated for fentanyl.[369]

NEUROMUSCULAR BLOCKING AGENTS

Neuromuscular blocking agents (neuromuscular relaxants) have no effect on the electrical central activity. Great concern was expressed when EEG evidence of cerebral arousal was reported following the administration of large doses of atracurium.[370] The phenomenon was attributed to an increased concentration of laudanosine, the major end-product of the metabolism of atracurium. In anesthetized dogs, concentrations of laudanosine greater than 10 μg/ml induced electroencephalographic epileptic spiking.[371] In humans, no data substantiating a similar effect have been reported.[371-373]

Numerous studies have demonstrated major interactions between several AEDs and the muscle relaxants. Accelerated recovery has been observed with pancuronium,[374,376] doxacurium,[375] vecuronium,[377,378] pipericuronium,[379] and metocurine.[380,381] Atracurium appeared at first to be resistant to this action, but conflicting results have questioned the originally reported effect.[382,383] Succinylcholine has demonstrated opposite effects in patients on AEDs medication.[384]

Synergistic with the effect of AEDs on the activity of muscular relaxants is the action of steroids, which are frequently prescribed to epileptics in preparation for a surgical procedure. In the presence of betamethasone, resistance to the neuromuscular action of vecuronium was observed.[385]

ANESTHETIC MANAGEMENT

Based on the location and the structure of the epileptogenic abnormalities, a variety of surgical interventions are performed under local or general anesthesia. The main disadvantages using local anesthetics are the limitation in head fixation, the extra time involved, and the availability of an experienced neuroanesthesiologist. These restrictions aside, local anesthesia remains a useful technique when approaching an epileptogenic lesion in crucial zones such as the motor and speech areas.[386] When preoperative anatomic and electrophysiologic studies have clearly demarcated the epileptogenic zone in the noncrucial area, general anesthesia can be used quite satisfactorily. Most resections are performed nowadays under general anesthesia.

The importance of the team approach in the neurosurgical management of the epilepsy patient has already been stressed. Not unexpectedly, the neuroanesthesiologist comes late on stage and has limited time to establish a close relationship with the patient and family.[35] Although general anesthesia techniques and the extensive use during surgery of short-acting sedation agents have reduced the importance of communication between the anesthesiologist and the patient, a thorough preoperative assessment should be made.

PREANESTHETIC EVALUATION

The preanesthetic assessment is facilitated by the long and meticulous approach of the other participants, which precedes the decision to operate. In addition to the general medical evaluation of the systems, attention should be paid to some features particular to the epileptic patient.

Psychosocial Factors

Psychological and socioeconomic factors deeply affect the epileptic patient who lives with a constant sense of dread that another attack may supervene.[387] Epilepsy is frequently associated with stigmatizing dysmorphologies or neurologic impairments; these may reflect the original CNS abnormality or the side effects of previous surgical procedures or antiepileptic medication. Obtunded intellectual activity, facial or peripheral paresis, marks left by injuries, or even the social significance of a protective helmet are stigmatizing and may result in distorted mental processes and at times frankly psychotic attitudes.[388,389] The importance of the psychological approach is particularly evident in children.[388] Although many children with epilepsy learn and behave normally, a disproportionate number are learning-disabled and suffer minor behavioral disturbances. Children with epilepsy, particularly if they are brain-injured, are prone to a variety of behavioral disturbances that include impulsivity, temper tantrums, and attention deficit disorders with or without hyperactivity. By the second decade, some form of psychological dysfunction may be found in more than one-third of patients with epilepsy, with 11 percent of the group manifesting signs of overt psychotic thinking.

PHARMACOLOGIC FACTORS

Patients presenting for epilepsy surgery have all been treated for a variable period of time with one or many antiepileptic drugs (AEDs). Toxic reactions consequent to the use of AEDs, as well as side effects and interactions with anesthetics, are well documented and necessitate obtaining a full disclosure of all medications used in the past months. At the time of in-hospital preoperative assessment, antiepileptic medication may be acutely changed either to increase and optimize drug treatment, to evaluate the response of the seizure activity to new drugs, or to facilitate observation of vital and interictal activity consecutive to drug withdrawal.

A short review of the effects of AEDs on major systems can be seen below.

Most AEDs are metabolized by oxidative enzymes in the hepatocytes. Elevation of liver enzymes has been reported in 5 to 10 percent of patients, but these changes are rarely of clinical significance.[390,391] Carbamazepine, phenytoin, valproic acid, and phenobarbital are all effective in reducing the frequency of partial seizures.[392] Phenobarbital, however, is used as a second-line drug in most cases, since it tends to cause sedation and depression in adults and hyperactivity and aggression in children.

Carbamazepine is effective for the treatment of partial and generalized tonic-clonic seizures. The maintenance dose often depends on the extent to which CBZ induces its own metabolism. The drug can cause a range of idiosyncratic reactions, the most common being a morbilliform rash, which develops in about 10 percent of patients. Mild leukopenia is common, but blood dyscrasia and toxic hepatitis are rare. At high plasma concentrations, CBZ has an antidiuretic hormone-like action and the resulting hyponatremia is usually mild and asymptomatic. If however, the plasma sodium concentration falls below 125 mmol per liter, confusion and decreasing control of seizures may occur.

In addition to its ability to induce its own metabolism, CBZ can accelerate the hepatic oxidation and conjugation of other lipid-soluble drugs.[393] The metabolism of VPA, corticosteroids, anticoagulant and antipsychotic drugs, nondepolarizing muscle relaxants, and opioids is increased (see above). Paradoxically, whereas PHT induces the metabolism of CBZ, CBZ inhibits the metabolism of PHT. Thus, adding PHT decreases plasma carbamazepine concentration by about one-third, whereas adding CBZ increases plasma PHT concentrations by a similar amount. Drugs that inhibit the metabolism of CBZ sufficiently to cause toxic effects include cimetidine, propoxyphene, erythromycin, isoniazid, diltiazem, and verapamil. The substantial between-dose variation in plasma CBZ concentrations makes their interpretation problematic.

Phenytoin is effective for the treatment of partial and tonic clonic seizures. It is one of a handful of drugs for which the kinetic change from first order (in which the extent of metabolism is directly correlated with the amount of available drugs) to saturation occurs at therapeutic doses. Accordingly, a moderate increment in the dose can cause an unexpectedly large rise in the plasma concentration.

Phenytoin can cause a range of dose-related and idiosyncratic adverse effects. Reversible cosmetic changes (gum hypertrophy, acne, hirsutism, facial coarsening) although often mild, can be troublesome. Neurotoxic symptoms (drowsiness, dysarthria, tremor, ataxia, and cognitive difficulties) become increasingly likely when the plasma drug concentration exceeds 20 μg per ml.

Phenytoin can induce the oxidative metabolism of many lipid-soluble drugs, including VAP, anticoagu-

lant agents, corticosteroids, opioids, and cyclosporine. Theophylline half-life is reduced in the presence of PHT and patients may require an upward adjustment of their doses. It is a potent inducer of CBZ biotransformation, causing up to a 50 percent reduction in CBZ levels. A similar effect on VPA has been reported. Because its metabolism is saturable, inhibitory interactions are particularly likely to have neurotoxic effects. Drugs that inhibit the metabolism of PHT include amiodarone, cimetidine, impramine, and some sulfonamides (sulfadiazine, sulfamethiazole, sulfaphenazole). Phenytoin affects pituitary and adrenal functions by induction of P-450 hepatic enzyme, with resultant accentuation of endogenous hormone metabolism. Accelerated metabolism of exogenously administered steroid hormones may occur as well. Hypothalamic function can be affected with altered release of antidiuretic hormone.

Valproic acid is effective in patients with all types of seizures, especially in those with iodiopathic generalized epilepsy. Common side effects of VPA are dose-related tremor, weight gain due to appetite stimulation, thinning or loss of hair, and menstrual irregularities. The incidence of hepatotoxic effects is less than 1 in 20,000. Approximately 20 percent of all patients receiving the drug have hyperammonemia without hepatic damage.

Valproic acid is a potent inhibitor of hepatic metabolic processes, including oxidation, conjugation, and epoxidation and this may affect PHT, CBZ, PB, and LTG. Aspirin displaces VPA from its binding sites on plasma proteins and inhibits its metabolism. It has been suggested that VPA might increase surgical bleeding due to quantitative thrombocytopressive[394,395] and functional defects in platelet aggregation.[396] Valproic acid may also decrease plasma coagulation factors.[236] Postoperative hemorrhagic complications have been reported in patients who received VPA.[233,234] Consequently many epilepsy centers discontinue VPA preoperatively. A recent report by Ward and associates[397] has questioned this practice and does not recommend routinely discontinuing the treatment before craniotomy.

Phenobarbital abolishes partial and generalized toxic-clonic seizures. The drug can cause fatigue and listlessness in adults and insomnia, hyperactivity, and aggressivity in children. Memory, mood, and learning capacity may be impaired. Depression and arthritic changes have been reported.

Phenobarbital is among the best examples of an enzyme inducer and it will accelerate the metabolism of many lipid-soluble drugs, including PHT. The pharmacokinetic interactions with antiepileptic medication are important as many drugs demonstrate unexpected effects. Additional information concerning these drug interactions can be obtained from specialized sources.[398,399]

Laboratory Tests

In comparison with the many invasive and noninvasive diagnostic techniques used during the presurgical evaluation, the preanesthetic diagnostic tests are few. Unless indicated for medical problems unrelated to the epileptic condition, only the very basic laboratory tests will be required. These include a complete hematology count, liver function tests, and plasma drug levels for the AEDs. Coagulation studies are routinely performed prior to any major neurosurgical procedure, as is an electrocardiogram.

ANESTHESIA FOR INVASIVE DIAGNOSTIC PROCEDURES

The importance of intracranial recordings in the preoperative evaluation of epileptic patients has been discussed in a previous section. For these invasive procedures, general anesthesia is always used. The choice of agents is dictated by the local conditions and preferences of the neuroanesthesiologist. Proconvulsant agents such as enflurane are best avoided. Patients are monitored as is customary for routine neurosurgical procedures. A precordial Doppler monitor will be included because the patient's head may be placed higher than the level of the heart. The use of a central line for treatment of air embolism, however, is controversial. In our center a central line is not part of our routine.

After termination of the surgical procedure, the patient is returned to the postanesthetic recovery unit and closely observed until full return of consciousness is noted. Complications of these procedures include intracranial hemorrhage,[400] neurologic deficits, and infection.[401] Any delay in awakening or a slow recovery of neurologic function, particularly with evidence of lateralization, should alert the neurosurgical staff and demands immediate attention.

GENERAL ANESTHESIA FOR RESECTION OF EPILEPTOGENIC STRUCTURES

As a rule, patients arrive in the operating suite unpremedicated. If neither ECoG or cortical mapping is contemplated, the patient's usual antiepileptic medication is administered early in the morning prior to surgery, and anxiety is controlled with a short-acting benzodiazepine.[345] The intraoperative use of electrophysiological diagnostic techniques, including activation, precludes the administration of any sedative with anticonvulsant properties. With the exception of patients presenting with hyperactive epileptic features, who would be at risk otherwise, the AEDs are withdrawn for at least 48 h. Forty-eight hours prior to surgery

all patients are started on a corticosteroid regimen of hydrocortisone, prednisone, or dexamethasone to minimize brain swelling.

Epilepsy patients are likely to convulse at any time, particularly when they are off medication. It is therefore sound practice to keep ready at a convenient location (usually the anesthetic workstation) a potent antiepileptic agent that can be used at immediately to abort a toxic-clonic phenomenon in the short period preceding the induction of anesthesia. Methohexital is preferred by the author (D.T.), but sodium thiopental, propofol, or midazolam are acceptable alternatives. In the presence of a difficult venous access, a large enough intramuscular injection of midazolam may save the day.

Positioning requires breaking the table at various angles to improve comfort, and padding of exposed body parts, and attention to details (e.g., eye protection) are important, since long procedures tend to magnify any small shortcomings. It has been our practice to use straps and retainers to limit movements of free parts, should the patient awaken or develop a seizure during the procedure. An unobstructed view of the patient is essential if cortical stimulation of the motor area is contemplated. A bladder catheter is always inserted. A heating-cooling blanket is wrapped around the patient. Placement of a large-bore (gauge 16) intravenous catheter is performed in the unpremedicated awake patient, while the introduction of an intraarterial catheter is usually postponed until after induction.

The induction of anesthesia is achieved with an ultrashort-acting barbiturate or with propofol. Considering the many hours to come between the induction with sodium pentothal, methohexital, or propofol and the recording of the ECoG (if requested), there is little to be gained by using one agent in preference to another. Intubation is facilitated by the administration of a neuromuscular blocking drug. Variations of heart rate and blood pressure in response to intubation are prevented by the additional injection of intravenous lidocaine, an opioid, and/or esmolol. After endotracheal intubation, controlled ventilation is initiated in a conventional way with a nitrous oxide : oxygen mixture or, as preferred by the author (D.T.), with an air : oxygen mixture. Isoflurane is subsequently added to the breathing gases and delivered throughout the procedure at concentrations adequate to maintain hypnosis and amnesia. Concentrations below 0.5 MAC are known to interfere minimally with electrical brain activity.[93,94] When the time comes for the recording of interictal electrical activity and brain mapping, the concentrations can be rapidly reduced (see above).

From the outset, analgesia is provided using any one of the potent narcotic agents available. Fentanyl, alfentanil, and sufentanil have demonstrated similar activity and efficacy during the conduct of anesthesia,[362-364] and the choice is a matter of personal preference. Computer assisted continuous infusion (CACI) has the potential for maintaining analgesia at a constant level throughout the procedure and is thought[402,404] to optimize any total intravenous anesthesia technique. Intermittent administration of drugs on the contrary will result in variable plasma drug levels over time, with larger total doses utilized ultimately. With all its disadvantages, however, this approach corresponds better to the analgetic requirements during epilepsy surgery. Indeed, as observed during procedures under local anesthesia,[30,32] the largest part of the surgical procedure is painless, with painful episodes restricted to the incision of the extracranial tissues, the exposure of the brain, and the final sutures at the end of the procedure. Under these circumstances and in view of the wide variation in stimulation, a steady level of analgesia appears unnecessary. It has been our practice to use large amounts of sufentanil, in divided doses,[405-407] from the start to cancel out the stimulating effect of the pins and headholder and all the other painful maneuvers preceeding the exposure of the brain.[408]

For the first 30 min, the total sufentanil dose averages 5.0 to 7.5 μg/kg. Moderate hypotension and bradycardia are frequently observed and may be compensated by the rapid administration of intravenous fluids, vagolytic substances (atropine or glycopyrrolate), and vasopressors (ephedrine or phenylephrine). In most cases, no additional sufentanil will be required until the end of the procedure, about 6 h later. Respiratory depression, requiring narcotic reversal with small amounts of naloxone, has been observed in less than 30 percent of the cases. An alternative technique places reliance for maintaining an adequate level of anesthesia on continuous propofol administration with or without nitrous oxide.[409] Whatever the method that is elected, consideration should be given to the effect of all agents on the ECoG and the spontaneous or activated epileptic patterns. Mechanical ventilation is used in all patients. To facilitate control of respiration, nondepolarizing muscle relaxants are administered from the outset. Providing that mapping of the brain cortex is not planned, relaxation is maintained until the end of the procedure. However, if cortical stimulation and mapping are contemplated, only intermediate- or short-acting agents are used during the first part of the procedure and are deliberately withheld to allow for observation of the peripheral muscle responses. A return of better than 90 percent of the strength of the M. adductor pollicis, as estimated with a TOF technique, is generally required.

Intraoperatively, the prerolandic motor area is identified by direct stimulation of the nonparalyzed patient. Motor responses are usually crude and require large currents that prevent very fine spatial resolution. Somatosensory evoked potential localization of hand-related sensory cortex in patients under general anesthesia has been proposed by Woods and coworkers.[410] Some technical factors are important to achieve for successful mapping:

- The craniotomy must be large enough to permit access to the motor area
- The stimulator current must be sufficiently large to alter functions in the cortex, but not so large as to evoke a seizure
- All stimulations use a 60-Hz train of biphasic pulses, each phase 2 ms in duration, delivered from a constant current stimulator across 1 mm diameter carbon bipolar ball electrodes
- A small current, starting at 2 mA, between pulse peaks is applied for 4 s to cortex adjacent to a ECoG electrode. The stimulation is repeated at increasing currents until the patient reports a response or until afterdischarges are evoked. Larger than 7 mA currents are not indicated because a seizure is likely to occur. Some stimulators are calibrated in volts and have an inbuilt large impedance system, usually of the order of 1 kΩ. A 1 volt increment represents a 1 mA increase.

The absence of muscular paralysis, deemed necessary to optimize the motor response to cortical stimulation of the motor strip, combined with a very light level of anesthesia, to avoid interference with the ECoG, represents a state of inadequate anesthesia. As a result, patients often wake up and at times attempt to move. In some instances, verbal reassurance may succeed in controlling the patient, but it is often necessary to resort at once to pharmacologic means of control. A few patients may, as a response to stimulation, proceed with focal seizures that may progress to full tonic-clonic convulsions. The early administration of an appropriate dose of barbiturate (methohexital or pentothal) or propofol will help abort a full-fledged seizure.

As reported in detail in the first part of this section, nondepolarizing muscle relaxants have a shorter half-life in all patients chronically medicated with antiepileptic drugs. Other substances, such as steroids, frequently used at the time of neurosurgical procedures, will also shorten the duration of action of muscle relaxants.[385]

In keeping with modern trends, carbon dioxide levels are maintained at normal physiologic levels. This approach has always been privileged in epilepsy anesthesia because hyperventilation is well known to possess activation properties.[411] This feature is explained by the decrease in mesencephalic reticular function activity observed in the presence of hypocapnia.[412] Isert[413] has reviewed the nature of the arterial end-tidal CO_2 gradient and concluded that capnography alone cannot be used to confidently predict the true arterial P_{CO_2} value. Russell and coworkers support this view.[414] We feel that knowing the true state of ventilation is important in our patient management and believe that arterial P_{CO_2} should always be compared with end-tidal values.

Droperidol is used for its antiemetic properties.[354] In small amounts the drug has no effect on the ECoG, while the control of vomiting and nausea extends over many hours. Other antiemetic agents are not used, although ondansetron appears to be a valid alternative. Metoclopramide is contraindicated in epilepsies.[415]

The total amount of drugs administered is kept to a minimum in anesthesia for epilepsy surgery because all agents will affect the brain's electrical activity. Although the advantages obtained from infiltrating the scalp and adjacent tissues with a local anesthetic are less obvious in the asleep patient than in the awake one, the reduction in anesthetic drug requirements should not be ignored. As an additional benefit, the vasoconstriction resulting from infiltration with a 1:200,000 epinephrine solution limits the volume of blood loss at opening.

Craniotomies for epilepsy surgery are long procedures and require a large exposure of the brain and these factors should result in a higher than average incidence of bleeding. A cautious, unhurried approach throughout the procedure will minimize blood loss. In our experience we rarely infuse blood and satisfy ourselves with compensating fluid loss, blood and urine.

Monitoring during the procedure is kept simple as the majority of patients coming for surgery are healthy except for their neurologic dysfunction. In recent years, elevation of the head to improve acess to deep mesial structures has resulted in the utilization of a precordial Doppler monitor for observation of potential air embolisms.[416] After the complete removal of the epileptogenic tissue, the AED level is restored. Phenytoin, 15 mg/kg is administered intraoperatively.

The use of structural and functional neuroimaging to confirm location of noninvasive ictal EEG has eliminated the need for intracranial recording in all but a few patients.[417] However, there still exists a large enough cohort of epileptics with a surgically remediable syndrome in whom treatment should not be undertaken on the basis of structural imaging alone. For them, confirmation of focal epileptogenicity is necessary, and this usually requires ictal EEGs. Tailored excisions of epileptogenic structures are perfomed under general anesthesia, or, at times, local anesthesia.

The anesthetic management, in those instances where ECoG is an intrinsic part of the procedure, consists of two phases. The first extends from the beginning of the induction until the end of the resection, and includes the critical moments of recording of the ECoG, of mapping the motor area, and of activation of the epileptogenic foci. The second phase starts when the monitoring of the brain electrical activity is no longer required and ends with the return of the patient to the postanesthetic recovery unit (PARU).

The first phase has been covered in detail, although additional comments are warranted in view of the controversy regarding the effects of anesthetic agents on the different aspects of brain activity. The second phase is straightforward and follows the now well accepted methods of neuroanesthetic management of brain surgery.

Several aspects of general anesthesia for epilepsy surgery are controversial. There appears to be no agreement regarding the effects of anesthetic agents on the interictal electrocorticogram, on the validity of epileptic activity observed in these conditions, or on the accuracy of the activation techniques. With the exception of information obtained from chronic intracranial electrode recordings, intraoperative electrophysiologic identification of the epileptogenic zone depends only on interictal epileptiform activity. The localizing value of these tracings is quite controversial. Some reports have indicated that interictal activity and sites of onset may not always overlap.[418]

Part of the controversy may result from the different conditions for recording. Indeed, many general anesthetic agents, including propofol, alter the interictal activity.[292,333,335,337,419,420] To bring some light into the issue, the recommendation of Spencer to proceed with anesthetic standardization at the time of the ECoG should be followed.[421]

Even more confusing are the conflicting reports regarding the validity of changes on the ECoG observed after activation. Fundamental to the understanding of the activation process is the realization that inhibitory central nervous system structures are more sensitive to depression factors than are excitatory zones. Methohexital is a very potent activator of epileptic activity.[319–324] Several authors, however, have questioned the validity and the specificity of the observed ictal recording. Fiol and coworkers[422] observed that in patients undergoing temporal lobectomy for epilepsy, new spike foci were induced in 43 percent of the cases, both in the focal epileptic region and outside it. In a retrospective study of alfentanil activating property, Cascino and associates[423] also found evidence of false spread of activity. Etomidate,[340,341] enflurane,[279,293] and chlorpromazine[424] have been used as activating agents and may provide false information. Wyler[325] considers methohexital a specific agent that activates the epileptogenic zone essentially.

Postanesthetic Management

In the PARU vital signs and neurologic responses are closely monitored for the next 12 h (overnight). Hypotension is corrected with fluid administration and if indicated (hematocrit values below 25 percent) with blood replacement. Epinephrine or phenylephrine are rarely indicated. Bradycardia is managed with vagolytic agents. Severe hypertension and tachycardia are treated with a beta-blocker (esmolol) or a combined alpha- and beta-blocker (labetalol). Moderate hypertension is frequently related to agitation and sometimes to pain and appropriate measures should be considered for correction. At times, abnormal movements of a dystonic or myoclonic nature, unilateral or bilateral, as well as other abnormal neurologic symptoms (hypo- or hyperreflexia, disconjugated eye movements, tremor) or shivering may be confused with postsurgical seizure activity. In our experience small aliquots of propofol, large enough to provide sedation without interfering with spontaneous respiration, will remedy the situation. With doses as low as 25 μg/kg per min, patients remain alert and answer questions, they become sedated and side effects tend to decrease in number and importance.

As a rule, prophylactic antibiotics are not administered in our center, but other centers consider their use justified. Corticosteroid treatment initiated prior to surgery is pursued for a few days. Histamine H2 antagonists are commonly administered along with the steroids. Important variations in the level of AEDs, particularly phenytoin and carbamazepine, have been observed. As the occurrence of early postoperative seizures may be related to variations in the AEDs level, it appears wise to follow plasma levels closely during the first week.

LOCAL ANESTHESIA

"Regional anesthesia is necessary for best results in craniotomies for the radical treatment of focal epilepsy. The patient must be conscious and alert while electrical stimulation is being carried out . . . anesthetists desire to abolish all pain and anxiety, but it is not always wise".[30] This admonition by W. Penfield has haunted neurosurgeons and anesthesiologists alike for many years, who have had to deal with inadequate anesthetic agents and would not jeopardize the successful outcome of the surgery for the doubtful benefit of alleviating discomfort and fatigue. It can be viewed as ironic that general anesthesia is now used in the majority of epilepsy surgical procedures at a time when safe, conscious, analgesia techniques are available and adequately complement local anesthesia in the awake patient. So dominant in the field are anatomically uniform resections that one has to wonder if there is still a place for tailored operations based on information acutely collected from the exposed cortex at the time of surgery.[425]

Anatomically uniform operations are based on the assumption that the pathophysiology and location of eloquent areas have a relation to anatomic landmarks that is generally the same across all cases considered suitable for operation.[426] However, there is evidence that for temporal lobe epilepsy there is variability between cases in both the location of the focus within the temporal lobe and the location of language within the dominant temporal lobe.[427] The variability in the extent of the epileptogenic zone and the eloquent areas justifies a tailored approach with cortical mapping under local anesthesia for many authors.[428,429] Hermann and Wyler reviewed the results of dominant temporal lobectomies under general versus local anesthesia on language outcome and showed more naming deficits under general anesthesia.[428]

The original local anesthetic technique as reported by Pasquet[31] has been modified in subsequent years with the introduction of neuroleptanalgesia[35,349] and superseded by the use for sedation of propofol.[430] The effects of propofol sedation on seizures and intracranially recorded epileptiform activity in patients with partial epilepsy have been critically reviewed by Samra and coworkers.[337] Their report corroborated the experience of many centers and confirmed propofol to be the safest agent for sedation during interventions in awake patients for resection of epileptogenic foci. The time-honored technique based on neuroleptic agents[35,349,362] is still used, although the doses of droperidol have been drastically reduced.

Technical Aspects

The preanesthetic preparation has been considered earlier in the text. It is very important to obtain the confidence of the patient to assure the successful outcome of the procedure. It should be stressed that sleep and full alertness will alternate. The painful episodes, which are limited to the initial phase of the procedure, will be performed at a time sedation and analgesia are achieved with intravenous agents. The anesthesiologist's continuous presence at the bedside will assure that additional medication is administered if required.

On the day of surgery, only steroids are given prior to admission to the operating suite. Anxiety should be dealt with without use of pharmacologic means. All participants in the operating room should be fully aware that the procedure will take place in an awake patient. Unnecessary verbal comments and noise should be kept to a minimum. The temperature in the room should be comfortable for the patient. Anesthesia

TABLE 21-10
Sedation Scores

Grades	Degree of Sedation
1	Fully awake and oriented
2	Drowsy
3	Eyes closed but rousable to command
4	Eyes closed but rousable to mild physical stimulation
5	Eyes closed and unarousable to mild physical stimulation.

SOURCE: Wilson et al.,[436] with permission.

equipment and medication for the control of a seizure episode should be at hand.

After transfer to the table, an intravenous line is secured at once, and a saline infusion started at a low flow rate, which will be maintained throughout the procedure. Bladder catheterization is not part of our protocol because it will in most instances unnecessarily aggravate the patient. To limit the discomfort of a full bladder, the drip rate is adjusted to 1 ml/kg per h. The patient is positioned on the well-padded table in accordance with surgical demands. The lateral position is preferred because freedom of the airway is easier to maintain. However, the most judicious position for facilitating surgical approach will be chosen and is acceptable. A nasal cannula is affixed to the face, which permits concomitant delivery of oxygen and monitoring of exhaled CO_2. Although the reliability of the displayed values is questionable in absolute terms,[431] a breath-by-breath observation of respiration is obtained. Experience at our center[349] and by others[362,432] using a neuroleptic analgesia technique, has demonstrated that adequate ventilation could be maintained in such conditions. More recently Rosa and coworkers[433] and Silbergeld and associates[430] have reported similar views using propofol.

Sedation is initiated at this stage (Table 21-10). A bolus of propofol (300 μg/kg) is administered,[434] followed by a continuous infusion at 100 μg/kg per min. Small increments of fentanyl (1μg/kg) are injected at 3-min intervals. A minute amount of droperidol (.015 μg/kg) is administered for prevention of nausea and vomiting.[435] An appropriate level of sedation is achieved on the average within 10 min.[436] At grade 3 to 4, one can consider positioning the head. Using a foam headring is unfortunately no longer acceptable because stereotactic identification mandates a fixed relationship between instrumentation and physical landmarks so the patient's head must be secured firmly. A three-pin Mayfield head-holder is applied after infiltration of the sites of pin placement with local anesthesia. Not only are patients able to tolerate the head-

holder well, but the head remains secure even during a seizure. While the surgeon appropriately relates external physical features (ear, eye, nose) with landmarks on the computer image obtained from MRI investigations, a steady level of sedation and analgesia is established. The patient's arm and leg opposite the surgical site are padded and restrained for his/her own protection lest harm occurs during a seizure episode. Drapes must be placed in a way that allows access to the face and also allows the anesthesiologist to converse with the patient. Face and arm must be clearly visible and permit monitoring the peripheral response to cortical stimulation.

A fairly large craniotomy incision is usually required, extending down to the zygoma for maximum visualization of the tip of the temporal lobe and the inferior temporal circumvolution. Local anesthesia is achieved with a mixture of bupivacaine, 0.25 percent, and lidocaine, 1.0 percent, both with 1:200,000 epinephrine. Girvin[437] has claimed that this anesthetic formulation has lasted as long as 12 h, but this might be slightly exaggerated. As a tribute to the "Founder," nupercaine 1 : 1500 and 1 : 4000 is still used at the Montreal Neurological Institute and Hospital,[30] but the agent is no longer commercially available.

Optimal points of injection for scalp anesthesia include the origin of the greater and lesser occipital nerves below the superior nuchal line, the auriculotemporal nerve just in front of the ear, and the supraorbital nerve above the eyebrow. Finally, an injection made into the subcutaneous tissue of the anterior temporal region will join the zygomatic arch with the lateral part of the superior orbital ridge. The local injection not only controls pain but provides a marked degreee of hemostasis. To optimize the hemostasis the injections must be made into the subcutanuous tissue of the scalp and not exclusively into the subgaleal region. At least 10 to 15 ml of solution must be injected into the deep part of the temporalis muscle, extending from the supraorbital ridge through to the posterior part of the zygoma.

The total amount of local anesthetic agent is rather large. As mentioned earlier in this section, toxicity to local anesthetics is rare.[349] Sedation with propofol may have an additional protective effect.[354]

Intracranial structures that are painful to touch and traction include the dura and meningeal vessels. Once the dura is exposed, pain sensation is blocked by intradural injections of small quantities of local anesthetic on each side of the middle meningeal artery and its major branches.

The patients are usually awakened before opening the dura. The propofol infusion which was titrated down from its original rate so as to maintain a grade 3 to 4 sedation score is now set to 0. Patients wake up and within 5 to 10 min are able to speak and answer commands. As mentioned earlier, it is our practice to discontinue the propofol at least 30 min before ECoG, although some anesthesiologists will wait until the last few minutes. The patients usually awaken abruptly and demonstrate no lingering confusion. Spontaneous seizures occasionally have occurred in severe epileptics[332] asleep with propofol. Methohexital may be needed to control these seizures. Experience has shown that subsequent recording and stimulation may be possible, provided minimal amounts of the barbiturate are used (0.5 mg/kg).

With the patient awake and the brain exposed, direct cortical readings are performed. A post is placed on the skull at the edge of the craniotomy and array of 16 to 24 electrodes affixed to it. Details about the electrodes can be found in the text. The goal of ECoG recording is to delineate the full extent of interictal epileptiform activity. Following the recording of spontaneous electrical ativity, the exposed cortex is stimulated to map out important neurologic areas. Depending on the degree of surgical confidence and on the location of the planned resection, only topographic landmarks are used for identification of the central sulcus and the central area. Of course, if more clinical and functional data are needed, additional mapping with stimulation is performed. Stimulation of the motor cortex results in involuntary movements of the face and extremities. The area representing the face and mouth is at the inferior portion of the precentral gyrus (motor cortex), just above the temporal lobe. Although the patient is usually aware of the involuntary movements, direct observation is important. Stimulation of the postcentral gyrus (sensory cortex) may result in paresthesia, tingling, or prickly sensations in tongue, gums, face, and extremities. It is important to instruct the patient prior to the procedure to report any unusual feeling. The patient may also be asked to perform certain tasks during stimulation. Usually the effect of stimulation on speech is evaluated during counting or reciting such familiar concepts as days of the week or months of the year. Stimulation of the speech area is signaled by an abrupt interruption in speech, which will resume immediately upon cessation of the stimulation. If localization of the seizure focus is still in doubt after cortical recording, depth electrodes are positioned toward deeper structures in the vicinity of the amygdala and the hippocampus. Spontaneous activity is again recorded, followed by stimulation.

Stimulation mapping has been a useful technique for investigation of the human cortical organization, particularly for language and memory.[438] Some of these findings have implications for planning resections very close to eloquent areas. Avoiding cortical sites related by stimulation to recent verbal memory has been shown to be of value in decreasing the likelihood of a postoperative memory deficit.

Activation of epileptic activity is attempted at this stage. A 0.5 mg/kg of methohexital is administered and its effect on the ECoG is observed. Discussion about the validity of the procedure appears elsewhere in this text.

After the epileptogenic focus is identified and functional areas of the exposed brain have been mapped out, resection is initiated. The brain itself has no sensation, so pain is experienced only with traction or coagulation of blood vessels. To avoid an increase in sympathetic activity (tachycardia, hypertension, increased systemic vascular resistance) in anxiety and pain with unwanted side effects, for example, hemorrhage and movements, the propofol infusion is reinitiated and additional amounts of fentanyl administered. It may or may not be necessary to repeat the recording after the temporal resection has been completed. If postresection recording and testing of speech and motor ability is not necessary, sedation may be used more generously. For the remainder of the procedure the patient is allowed to doze off.

It is our contention that the continuous infusion of propofol during resection of an epileptogenic focus under local anesthesia has considerably facilitated the anesthetic management of the procedure.

Twenty-five years of experience with fentanyl and droperidol should not, however, be ignored. Neuroleptanalgesia has proved to be a safe technique[349] and represents a valid alternative in those parts of the world where propofol is not available or is considered too expensive. Time has demonstrated that large amounts of droperidol (0.15 to 0.50 μg/kg)[140] are not necessary since side effects of the agent are annoying. Extrapyramidal reactions to droperidol have been classified as dystonia with spasms of tongue, face, neck, and back, as parkinsonism with rigidity and tremor, and as akathesia or motor restlessness. These reactions are likely to occur at higher dosage, but even low doses have caused reactions.[439] Antiemetic effect is achieved with much smaller doses.[435]

Methohexital as part of the neuroleptanalgesia technique has played an important role in controlling uncooperative individuals. Bolus doses of 1 mg/kg methohexital can be repeated safely at regular intervals and respiration should be monitored continuously. Higher doses depress respiration, and in an extreme situation will force the anesthesiologist to resort to general anesthesia with "under the drapes" intubation.

Gignac and coworkers[362] have compared the three most commonly used narcotic agents in North American anesthesia and found no benefit of the newer agents over fentanyl. Appreciable savings will result from using fentanyl instead of the other agents.

Monitoring

Noninvasive monitoring is used as a rule for conscious sedation analgesia. Hemodynamic parameters are monitored with an ECG tracing displaced continuously on the video screen and heart rate is obtained from the ECG or the pulse oximeter. Noninvasive blood pressure measurements are displayed every 5 min. End-tidal CO_2 is continuously sampled at the nose, and the information is utilized essentially as a means to monitor respiratory rate. The oxygenation status of the patient is followed with a pulse oximeter attached to an extremity. We do not monitor temperature and tend to rely on the subjective report of the patient. Blood loss is estimated and corrected when it approaches 20 percent of circulating blood volume.

COMPLICATIONS OF EPILEPSY SURGERY

As with all intracranial surgical procedures, a certain number of complications are to be expected but they are not frequent. General complications include acute postoperative hemorrhage, infection, and hydrocephalus. Their occurrence is directly related to the surgical difficulties encountered at the time of the procedure and are independent of the anesthetic technique used. Specific complications may be subdivided in transient and permanent deficits, which relate directly to the nature of the original lesion, the location of the epileptogenic focus, and the extent of the surgical removal. However, as stated eloquently by Girvin,[440] the most frequent and prominent risk of epilepsy surgery is the failure to achieve the goal of the investigation and treatment.

THE PROBLEM OF STATUS EPILEPTICUS

Status epilepticus (SE) can be defined as a condition in which prolonged or recurrent seizures, or epileptic events, persist for more than 30 min. Repeated events associated with impaired consciousness should be considered to represent SE when the recurrence rate does not permit return of consciousness to be defined as status. Status epilepticus causes a wide spectrum of clinical symptoms, with a highly variable pathophysiologic, anatomic, and etiologic basis.[441] Status epilepticus is not merely the rapid repetition of seizures, but it incorporates different conditions that do not necessarily conform to a specific seizure type as defined in the classification of the ILAE.

Most types of epileptic seizures can manifest as SE; although there is no official ILAE classification of SE as yet, it could be classified, as suggested by Gastaut,[442] by type of seizure. A new classification scheme has been proposed by Shorvon[441] in which classification of

SE is based not only on seizure type, but on other features including age and cerebral maturity, and clinical characteristics such as etiology, EEG, anatomy, clinical pattern, and pathophysiologic mechanisms of the epilepsy. For a more detailed discussion, the reader is referred to the excellent monograph on status epilepticus by Shorvon.[441]

EPIDEMIOLOGY AND ETIOLOGY

Status epilepticus is a common emergency. It occurs more frequently in children and in the elderly, and in patients with structural cerebral pathology.[443] By far the most commonly reported form of SE is tonic-clonic (or convulsive status), which accounts for approximately 40 to 50 percent of the total. In the United States alone, convulsive status affects more than 50,000 people each year, and in a great proportion of patients the episode of status represents the initial manifestation of their epilepsy (~12 to 18 percent). The other forms of SE, while not as common, are well documented and are important in the differential diagnosis of acute confusional states. They include absence status (< 1 percent) and complex partial status (~6 to 8 percent). Finally, SE occurs relatively frequently during the neonatal period, often due to metabolic or infectious etiologies. It is also more common in mentally handicapped patients presumably because of diffuse cerebral abnormality. The annual incidence of SE in a general population is estimated to be approximately 450 to 650 cases per 1,000,000 persons in the United States and SE accounts for 1 to 5 percent of all hospital admissions for epilepsy.

The etiologies of SE vary, reflecting the referral bases of the institutions performing the investigations (adult versus pediatric centres, and status as the presenting symptom of epilepsy versus status as an intercurrent event or as a manifestation of well-established epilepsy). As already mentioned, the frequency of status is greatest in children, and most episodes occur before 5 years of age.[444,445] In the first year, 75 percent of episodes of SE were in the context of an acute illness, whereas this number falls to 28 percent in children over 3 years of age. In older children and adults, frequent causes of SE include poor antiepileptic drug compliance or drug withdrawal (~31 percent), ethanol-related status (~28 percent), drug toxicity or abuse and withdrawal (~9 percent), central nervous system infection (~8 percent), metabolic disorders (~14 percent), cerebrovascular diseases (~10 percent), cerebral tumors (~7 percent), trauma (~10 percent), febrile SE (~12 percent, almost exclusively found in children). The cause may also be multifactorial. No etiology is identified in approximately 20 percent of events resulting in a diagnosis of idiopathic or cryptogenic SE.

TABLE 21-11
Status Can Be Divided in Stages

Premonitory stage	Usually in patients with established epilepsy. May last several hours.
Early status (0–30 min)	This is the stage where physiologic mechanisms compensate for the greatly enhanced metabolic activity (adaptive or early compensated phase).
Established status (30–120 min)	Defined as status that has continued for 30 min in spite of early-stage treatment. Physiologic decompensation has begun (maladaptive or late decompensated phase).
Refractory status (> 120 min)	Seizures continue after initiation of therapy, prognosis is worse, and there is a high mortality and morbidity.

PHYSIOPATHOLOGY OF STATUS EPILEPTICUS

Status epilepticus has a distinct natural history that consists of a sequence of events evolving over a predictable course. The natural history of SE involves a gradual worsening through different stages (Table 21-11). It has been noted that during tonic-clonic SE particularly, motor seizures are frequently restricted in their distribution. In addition, focal or lateralized convulsive activity does not necessarily indicate that a localized structural lesion is responsible for the status. At later stages in the sequence of events, motor activity diminishes or even disappears. Therefore, the end-stage may consist of ongoing epileptiform discharges recorded by EEG without motor accompaniment, or a form of "electromechanical dissociation" between motor events and brain discharges.[446,447]

Status epilepticus, both convulsive and nonconvulsive, can lead to profound, life-threatening, systemic, metabolic, and physiologic disturbances. These factors usually account for the poor prognosis associated with this disorder. Status itself, however, independent of metabolic and physiologic disturbances, may lead to lasting brain dysfunction, and prolonged status may result in permanent neuronal damage.

Tonic-clonic status is often preceded by a premonitory stage during which seizure activity progressively increases from its habitual level, resulting in a clinical deterioration. In patients who have an acute symptomatic event, however, status often starts abruptly. Physiologic changes in tonic-clonic SE are usually divided into two phases[441,448,449] with an early compensated phase I, and a late decompensated phase II (Figure 21-9). The transition from early to late phase occurs after approximately 30 min, and it is for this reason that

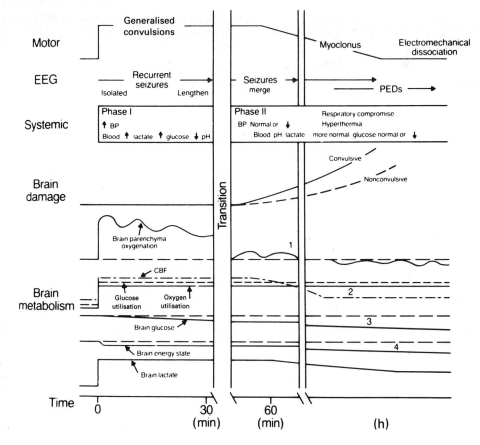

Figure 21-9 Summary of systemic alterations and brain metabolism in generalized convulsive status epilepticus (SE). Various events are aligned with respect to a time line (0 to 30 min, transition, 30 to 60 min, and hours of SE). (1) loss of reactivity of brain oxygen tension later in SE; (2) mismatch between the sustained increase in O₂ and glucose utilization and a fall in cerebral blood flow; (3) depletion of brain glucose (and glycogen); and (4) decline in the brain energy state. (From Lothman EW: The biochemical basis and pathophysiology of status epilepticus. *Neurology* 1990; 40(suppl 2);13, with permission.)

TABLE 21-12
Treatment Protocol for Tonic-clonic Generalized Status Epilepticus[a]

Stage	General Measures	AEDs	Usual Route of Administration
Premonitory stage	Continued neurologic observation, diagnose status epilepticus by observing continued seizure activity or one additional seizure.	Diazepam Lorazepam Midazolam Paraldehyde	10 mg iv bolus (max. 5 mg/min) 4 mg iv bolus (max. 2 mg/min) 5 mg iv bolus (max. 4 mg/min) 5–10 ml in 5–10 ml of water or oil by rectal bolus
Early status (0–30 mins)[b]	Ensure adequate cardiorespiratory function, iv line, administer O_2, initiate regular ECG and BP monitoring, draw blood for emergency investigations, intubation may be considered.	*First line* Diazepam Lorazepam *Second line* Midazolam Phenytoin Paraldehyde Lidocaine	 10–20 mg iv bolus 4–8 mg iv bolus 5–10 mg iv bolus 15–18 mg/kg iv loading dose (max. 50 mg/min) solution 4% in saline 50–100 ml/h iv infusion i.v. bolus and short infusion
Established status (30–120 min)	Set up second iv line (large veins), administer thiamine 100 mg iv and glucose D50W–50 ml iv, treat acidosis, establish etiology, admission to ICU, intubation has to be considered, EEG/ECG monitoring.	*First line* Phenytoin Phenobarbital *Second line* Diazepam Midazolam Paraldehyde	 repeat 7 mg/kg iv 10–20 mg/kg iv loading dose (< 100 mg/min) iv infusion[c] iv infusion[d] iv infusion
Refractory status (> 120 min)	Full anesthesia required, EEG/ECG monitoring, arterial line, initiate pressor therapy when required, monitoring of AED levels, intracranial pressure monitoring where appropiate.	*First line* Pentobarbital Propofol *Second line* Isoflurane	 iv bolus and infusion iv bolus and infusion inhalation

[a] This protocol is a guide only; it is by no means restrictive or exhaustive, and should be applied to adult patients.
[b] Time starts at seizure onset.
[c] Fresh solution, 10–20 mg in 250 ml 5% dextrose, infusion rate of 4–8 mg/h.
[d] Fresh solution,
NOTE: BP= blood pressure; iv = intravenous; EEG =electroencephalography; ECG = electrocardiography; ICU = intensive care unit; AED = antipiletic drug.
SOURCE: Adapted from Epilepsy Foundation of America's Working Group on Status Epilepticus[252] and Shorven,[441] with permission.

30 min is the time limit usually defined to represent SE. During the adaptive or early compensated phase, cerebral metabolism is greatly increased due to seizure activity, but physiologic mechanisms are sufficient to meet the metabolic demands, and cerebral tissue is protected from hypoxia or other metabolic damages. The major physiologic changes are related to the increased CBF and metabolism (hyperglycemia, lactic acidosis), autonomic activity, and cardiovascular changes (including hypertension, tachycardia, cardiac arrhythmia, hypersecretion and perspiration, hyperpyrexia, vomiting, and incontinence). Later, if not controlled, the status enters a phase of decompensation during which the increased cerebral metabolic demands cannot be fully met, resulting in hypoxia; altered cerebral function (failure of cerebral autoregulation, hypoglycemia, falling energy state, and cerebral edema resulting in rising intracranial pressure); altered systemic metabolic patterns (hypoglycemia, -natremia, -kalemia, hyperkalemia, metabolic and respiratory acidosis, multiorgan failure, consumptive coagulopathy, rhabdomyolysis, and myoglobulinuria); and progressively deteriorating cardiovascular functions (systemic hypoxia, hypotension, falling cardiac output, pulmonary edema, respiratory collapse, arrhythmia, pulmonary embolism, hyperpyrexia).

TREATMENT
Morbidity and mortality from SE are related to three factors: (1) the damage to the CNS caused by the acute insult precipitating the SE; (2) the systemic stress from repeated seizures; and (3) the injury from repetitive electrical discharges within the CNS. The most important clinical factors determining outcome are the etiology and the time from the onset of SE until treatment is initiated. The worst prognosis is found in those in whom status results from a serious intracranial process such as encephalitis, stroke, or cerebral hemorrage.

The best prognosis is seen in patients without structural lesions. The appropriate therapy initiated at the right time will limit the damage caused by the SE. A common error in the management of status is that AEDs are given in inadequate doses. For most drugs, serum concentration above the usually accepted therapeutic range for the management of chronic epilepsy are necessary in order to successfully terminate SE.

Although status is not technically considered to be present until the seizure activity has lasted for 30 min, it is recommended that emergency therapy not be delayed and that everyone who is still convulsing on admission to the emergency room should be treated aggressively. In addition, the management of SE is best carried out using a predetermined protocol (Table 21-12); continuous observation and skilled nursing care, adherence to a clear plan, prompt administration of effective drugs, and attention to adequate oxygen supply to the brain are critical. In addition, the AEDs selected should be administered intravenously, and maintenance AED therapy should be initiated as soon as possible.

Finally, in exceptional instances, one may consider a surgical approach in extremely severe and intractable status epilepticus. This may occur in a patient with focal cortical lesions with extreme epileptogenicity located in low-threshold cortical areas, such as the central cortex. We have described two patients who underwent surgical therapy for a life-threatening focal status epilepticus due to occult cortical dysplasia.[450]

References

1. Bruegel P: *The Pilgrimage of the Epileptics to the Church of St. John at Molenbeek (1569)*. Vienna, Graphische Sammlung Albertina.
2. Bruegel P: *The Extraction of the Stone of Madness (1556–1557)*. Brussels, Bibliothèque Royale Albert I.
3. Meador KJ, et al: History of epilepsy surgery. *Neurology* 1988; 38(suppl):383.
4. Dudley DW: Observations on injuries of the head. *Transylvania J Med* 1828; 1:9.
5. Smith S: The surgical treatment of epilepsy, with statistical tables, comprising all recorded cases of ligature of the carotid artery and also of trefining the cranium by American surgeons. *New York Med J* 1852; 1:220.
6. Billings JS: The surgical treatment of epilepsy. *Cincinnati Lancet and Observer* 1861; 4:334.
7. Jackson JH: *Selected Writings of John Hughlings Jackson*, vol 1, *On Epilepsy and Epileptiform Convulsions*. London, Hodder and Stoughton, 1931.
8. Macewen W: Tumour of the dura mater removed during life in a person affected with epilepsy. *Glas Med* 1879; 12:210.
9. Horsley V: Brain Surgery. *Br Med J* 1886; 2:670.
10. Taylor DC: One hundred years of epilepsy surgery: Sir Victor Horsley's contributions. In Engel J Jr (ed): *Surgical Treatment of the Epilepsies*. New York, Raven Press, 1987:11.
11. Krause F, Heyman F: *Lehrbuch der Chirurgischen Operationen*. Berlin, Wien, Urban & Schwarzenberg, 1914.
12. Sachs E: The subpial resection of the cortex in the treatment of Jacksonian epilepsy (Horsley operation) with observations on area 4 and 6. *Brain* 1935; 58:492.
13. Foerster O: Zur Pathogenese und Chirurgischen Behandlung der Epilepsie. *Zehrblatt fur Chirurgie* 1925; 52:531.
14. Foerster O, Penfield W: Der Narbenzug am und im gehirn bei traumatischer Epilepsie in seiner bedeutung fur das Zustandekommen der Anfalle, und fur der therapeutische Bekampfung derselben. *Z Neurol Psychiatry* 1930; 125:475.
15. Foerster O, Penfield W: The structural basis of traumatic epilepsy and results of radical operation. *Brain* 1930; 53:99.
16. Caton R: The electrical currents of the brain. *Br Med J* 1875; 2:278.
17. Berger H: Uber das Elektrenkephalogram des Menschen. *Arch Psychiatr Nervenkr* 1929; 87:527.
18. Foerster O, Altenburger H: Electrobiologische Vorgange an der menschilchen Hirninde. *Dtsch A Nervenheilk* 1935; 153:277.
19. Gibbs FA, et al: The electro-encephalogram in epilepsy and in conditions of impaired consciousness. *Arch Neurol Psychiatry* 1935; 34:1133.
20. Gibbs FA, et al: The electro-encephalogram in diagnosis and localization of epileptic seizures. *Arch Neurol Psychiatry* 1936; 36:1225.
21. Gibbs EL, Gibbs FA: Diagnostic and localizing value of electro-encephalographic studies in sleep. *Res Publ Assoc Res Nerv Ment Dis*, vol 26. Baltimore, Williams & Wilkins, 1947:366–376.
22. Jasper H: Electrocorticograms in man. *Electroencephalogr Clin Neurophysiol* 1949; 2(suppl):15.
23. Jasper H, et al: EEG and cortical electrograms in patients with temporal lobe seizures. *Arch Neurol Psychiatry* 1951; 65:272.
24. Penfield W, Steelman H: The treatment of focal epilepsy by cortical excision. *Ann Surg* 1947; 126:740.
25. Penfield W, Flanigin H: Surgical therapy of temporal lobe seizures. *Arch Neurol Psychiatry* 1950; 64:491.
26. Penfield W, Jasper H: *Epilepsy and Functional Anatomy of the Human Brain*. Boston, Little, Brown, 1954.
27. Talairach J, et al: Approche nouvelle de la neurochirurgie de l'épilepsie. *Neurochirurgie* 1974; 20(suppl).
28. Talairach J, Bancaud J: Stereotaxic exploration and therapy in epilepsy. In Vinken PJ, Bruyn GW (eds): *The Epilepsies Handbook of Clinical Neurology*. Amsterdam, North Holland, 1977:758–782.
29. Talairach J, Bancaud J: Stereotaxic approach to epilepsy. *Prog Neurol Surg* 1973; 5:297.
30. Penfield W: Combined regional and general anesthesia for craniotomy and cortical exploration. Part I. Neurosurgical considerations. *Curr Res Anesth Analg* 1954; 33:145.
31. Pasquet A: Combined regional and general anesthesia for craniotomy and cortical exploration. Part II. Anesthetic considerations. *Curr Res Anesth Analg* 1954; 33:156.
32. Gilbert RGB, Brindle GF: Anesthetic management for surgery of temporal lobe epilepsy. *Intern Anesth Clin* 1966; 4:842.
33. Trop D: Sedation during surgery of temporal lobe epilepsy. Proc Annual Meeting Canada Anesthesia Society, Montebello, Quebec, 1964.
34. Brindle GF: The use of neuroleptic agents in the neurosurgical unit. *Clin Neurosurg* 1969; 16:234.
35. Trop D: Conscious sedation analgesia during the neurosurgical treatment of epilepsies: Practice at the Montreal Neurological Institute. In Varkey G (ed): *Anesthetic Considerations for Craniotomy in Awake Patients*. Intern Anesthesiol Clin No 3. Boston, Little, Brown, 1986:175–184.
36. Ives JR, et al: The on-line computer detection and recording of spontaneous temporal lobe epileptic seizures from patients with implanted depth electrodes via a radiotelemetry link. *Electroencephalogr J* 1974; 37:199.

37. Gotman J: Automatic recognition of interictal epileptic activity in prolonged EEG recordings. *Electroencephalogr Clin Neurophysiol* 1979; 46:510.

38. Gloor P: Contributions of electroencephalography and electrocorticography to the neurosurgical treatment of epilepsies. *Adv Neurol* 1975; 8:59.

39. Ajmone-Marsan C: Depth electroencephalography and electrocorticography. In Aminoff MC (ed): *Electrodiagnosis in Clinical Neurology.* New York, Churchill-Livingstone, 1980:167–196.

40. Crandall PH, et al: Clinical application of studies on stereotactic implanted electrodes in temporal epilepsy. *J Neurosurg* 1963; 20:827.

41. Wyllie E, Lüders H: Classification of seizures. In Wyllie E (ed): *The Treatment of Epilepsy: Principles and Practices.* Pennsylvania, Lea & Febiger, 1993:359–361.

42. Commission on Classification and Terminology of the International League Against Epilepsy: Proposal for revised clinical and electroencephalographic classification of epileptic seizures. *Epilepsia* 1981; 22:489.

43. Commission on Classification and Terminology of the International League Against Epilepsy: Proposal for classification of epilepsies and epileptic syndromes. *Epilepsia* 1989; 30:389.

44. Wolf P: Epileptic seizures and syndromes: terms and concepts. In Wolf P (ed): *Epileptic Seizures and Syndromes.* London, John Libbey, 1994:3–7.

45. Gloor P: The EEG and differential diagnosis of epilepsy. In van Duijn H, et al (eds): *Current Concepts in Clinical Neurophysiology.* The Hague, NV Drukkerij Trio, 1977; 9–21.

46. Lüders H, et al: An expansion of the international classification of seizures to provide localization information. *Neurology* 1993; 43:1650.

47. Lüders H, et al: The international classification today: Disadvantages. In Wolf P (ed): *Epileptic Seizures and Syndromes.* London, John Libbey, 1994:15–20.

48. Theodore WH, et al: The secondarily generalized tonic-clonic seizure: A videotape analysis. *Neurology* 1994; 44:1403.

49. Engel J, Jr: *Seizures and Epilepsy.* Contemporary Neurology Series, vol 31. Philadelphia, FA Davis, 1989.

50. Wyllie E: *The Treatment of Epilepsy: Principles and Practices.* Philadelphia, Lea & Febiger, 1993.

51. Wolf P: *Epileptic Seizures and Syndromes.* London, John Libbey, 1994.

52. Hopkins A, et al: *Epilepsy.* London, Chapman & Hall Medical, 1995.

53. Anderson VE, Rich SS: Mapping epilepsy genes: A bridge between clinical and molecular studies. In Wolf P (ed): *Epileptic Seizures and Syndromes,* London, John Libbey, 1994:183–192.

54. Scheffer IE, et al: Autosomal dominant frontal lobe epilepsy: A new syndrome. *Epilepsia* 1993; 34(suppl. 6):30

55. Berkovic SF, et al: Familial temporal lobe epilepsy: A new syndrome with adolescent/adult onset and a benign course. In: Wolf P (ed): *Epileptic Seizures and Syndromes.* London, John Libbey, 1994:257–263.

56. Genton P, Guerrini R: Idiopathic localization-related epilepsies; the non-rolandic types. In Wolf P (ed): *Epileptic Seizures and Syndromes.* London, John Libbey, 1994:241–256.

57. Annegers JF: The epidemiology of epilepsy. In Wyllie E (ed): *The Treatment of Epilepsy: Principles and Practices.* Philadelphia, Lea & Febiger, 1993:157–164.

58. Hauser WA, et al: The prevalence of epilepsy in Rochester, Minnesota, 1940–1980. *Epilepsia* 1991; 32:429.

59. Hauser WA, Kurland LT: The epidemiology of epilepsy in Rochester, Minnesota, 1935 through 1967. *Epilepsia* 1975; 16:1.

60. Reynolds EH, et al: Why does epilepsy become intractable? Prevention of chronic epilepsy. *Lancet* 1983; 2:952.

61. Mattson RH, et al: Comparison of carbamazepine, phenobarbital, phenytoin and primidone in partial and secondary generalized tonic-clonic seizures. *N Engl J Med* 1985; 313:145.

62. Bourgeois BFD: General concepts of medical intractability. In: Lüders H (ed): *Epilepsy Surgery.* New York, Raven Press, 1991:77.

63. Schmidt D: Medical intractability in partial epilepsies. In Lüders H (ed): *Epilepsy Surgery.* New York, Raven Press, 1991:83–90.

64. Lüders H, Awad I: Conceptual considerations. In: Lüders H (ed): *Epilepsy Surgery,* New York, Raven Press, 1991:51–62.

65. Engel J, Jr: Update on surgical treatment of the epilepsies: Summary of the second international Palm Desert conference on the surgical treatment of the epilepsies (1992). *Neurology* 1993; 43:1612.

66. Powell GE: The new Maudsley series of temporal lobectomy. I: Short-term cognitive effects. *J Clin Psychol* 1985; 24:109.

67. Rausch R: Factors affecting neuropsychological and psychosocial outcome of epilepsy surgery. In Lüders H (ed): *Epilepsy Surgery.* New York, Raven Press, 1991:487–493.

68. Jackson GD: New techniques in MR. *Epilepsia* 1994; 35:S2.

69. Leppik IE, Schmidt D: Summary of the first international workshop on compliance in epilepsy. *Epilepsy Res* 1988; 1(suppl):179.

70. Rowan A, et al: The value of prolonged EEG/video monitoring as a routine diagnostic procedure in epilepsy. In: Canger R, et al (eds): *Advances in Epileptology. XIth Epilepsy Symposium.* New York, Raven Press, 1980:139–142.

71. Wilkus RJ, et al: Intensive EEG monitoring and psychological studies of patients with pseudoepileptic seizures. *Epilepsia* 1984; 25:100.

72. Fish DR, Marsden CD: Epilepsy masquerading as a movement disorder. In Marsden CD, Fahn S (eds): *Movement Disorders 3.* Oxford, Buterrworth-Heinemann, 1994:346–358.

73. So NK: The clinical neurophysiology of epilepsy surgery. In Hopkins A, et al (eds): *Epilepsy.* London, Chapman & Hall Medical, 1995:283–308.

74. Andermann F: Identification of candidates for surgical treatment of epilepsy. In Engel J, Jr (ed): *Surgical Treatment of the Epilepsies.* New York, Raven Press, 1987:51–70.

75. American Electroencephalographic Society. Guideline 13: Guidelines for standard electrode position nomenclature. *J Clin Neurophysiol* 1994; 11:111.

76. Rovit RL, et al: Sphenoidal electrodes in the electrographic study of patients with temporal lobe epilepsy. *J Neurosurgery* 1961; 18:151.

77. Sperling MR, et al: Mesial temporal spikes: A simultaneous comparison of sphenoidal, nasopharyngeal, and ear electrodes. *Epilepsia* 1986; 27:81. .

78. Binnie CD, et al: Distribution of temporal spikes in relation to the sphenoidal electrodes. *EEG Clin Neurophysiol* 1989; 73:403

79. Quesney LF, et al: Contribution of naso-ethmoidal electrode recording in the electrographic exploration of frontal and temporal lobe epilepsy. in Dam M, et al (eds): *Advances in Epileptology, XIIth Epilepsy International Symposium.* New York, Raven Press, 1981:293–304.

80. Quesney LF: Extracranial EEG evaluation. in Engel J Jr (ed): *Surgical Treatment of the Epilepsies.* New York, Raven Press, 1987:129.

81. Risinger MW: Electroencephalographic strategies for determining the epileptogenic zone. In Lüders H (ed): *Epilepsy Surgery.* New York, Raven Press, 1991:337–347.

82. Quesney LF, et al: Extracranial EEG evaluation. In Engel J Jr (ed): *Surgical Treatment of the Epilepsies.* New York, Raven Press, 1993:173–195.

83. Quesney LF, et al: Pre-operative extracranial and intracranial EEG investigation in patients with temporal lobe epilepsy:

Trends, results and review of pathophysiologic mechanisms. *Acta Neurol Scand* 1988; 117(suppl):52.

84. Cahan LD, et al: Review of the 20-year UCLA experience with surgery for epilepsy. *Clev Clin Q* 1984; 51:313.

85. Wieser HG, et al: Comparative value of spontaneous and chemically and electrically induced seizures in establishing the lateralization of temporal seizures. *Epilepsia* 1979; 20:47.

86. Williamson PD, et al: Complex partial seizures of frontal lobe origin. *Ann Neurol* 1985; 18:497.

87. Spencer SS, et al: Reliability and accuracy of localization by scalp ictal EEG. *Neurology* 1985; 35:1567.

88. Sammaritano M, et al: False lateralization by surface EEG of seizure onset in patients with temporal epilepsy and gross focal cerebral lesions. *Ann Neurol* 1987; 21:361.

89. Williamson PD, Spencer SS: Clinical and EEG features of complex partial seizures of extratemporal origin. *Epilepsia* 1986; 27(suppl 2):546.

90. Laxer KD, Garcia PA: Imaging criteria to identify the epileptic focus: Magnetic resonance imaging, magnetic resonance spectroscopy, positron tomography scanning, and singlephoton emission computed tomography. *Neurosurg Clin North Am* 1993:199.

91. Spencer SS: MRI, SPECT, and PET imaging in epilepsy: Their relative contributions. *Epilepsia* 1994; 35:S72.

92. Kuzniecky RI, Jackson GD: *Magnetic Resonance in Epilepsy.* New York, Raven Press, 1995.

93. Kuzniecky RI, et al: Magnetic resonance imaging in temporal lobe epilepsy: Pathological correlations. *Ann Neurol* 1987; 22:341.

94. Jack CR Jr, et al: Temporal lobe seizures: Lateralization with MR volume measurements of the hippocampal formation. *Radiology* 1990; 175:423.

95. Jackson GD, et al: Hippocampal sclerosis can be reliably detected by magnetic resonance imaging. *Neurology* 1990; 40:1869.

96. Berkovic SF, et al: Hippocampal sclerosis in temporal lobe epilepsy demonstrated by magnetic resonance imaging. *Ann Neurol* 1991; 29:175.

97. Cascino GD, et al: Magnetic resonance imaging-based volume studies in temporal lobe epilepsy: pathological correlations. *Ann Neurol* 1991; 30:31.

98. Cook MJ, et al: Hippocampal volumetric and morphometric studies in frontal and temporal lobe epilepsy. *Brain* 1992; 115:1001.

99. Cendes F, et al: Early chilhood prolonged febrile convulsions, atrophy and sclerosis of mesial structures, and temporal lobe epilepsy: MRI volumetric study. *Neurology* 1993; 43:1083.

100. Petroff OAC, et al: In vivo phosphorus nuclear magnetic resonance spectroscopy in status epilepticus. *Ann Neurol* 1984; 16:169.

101. Matthews PM, et al: A proton magnetic resonance spectroscopy study of focal epilepsy in humans. *Neurology* 1990; 40:985.

102. Kuzniecky RI, et al: In vivo 31P nuclear magnetic resonance spectroscopy of human temporal lobe epilepsy. *Neurology* 1992; 42:1586.

103. Laxer KD, et al: Increased pH and inorganic phosphate in temporal lobe seizure foci, demonstrated by (^{31}P) MRS. *Epilepsia* 1992; 33:618.

104. Jackson G, et al: Single volume proton MRS in patients with intractable temporal lobe epilepsy: A multicenter pilot study. *Epilepsia* 1993; 34(suppl 6):144.

105. Cendes F, et al: Proton MR spectroscopic imaging in temporal lobe epilepsy. *Ann Neurol* 1994; 35:211.

106. Gadian DG, et al: ^{1}H magnetic resonance spectroscopy in the investigation of intractable epilepsy. *Acta Neurol Scand* 1994; 152(suppl):116.

107. Arnold DL, et al: Proton magnetic specstroscopy imaging for metabolic characterization of demyelinating plaques. *Ann Neurol* 1992; 31:235.

108. Cendes F, et al: Imaging of axonal damage *in vivo* in Rasmussen's syndrome. *Brain* 1995; 118:753.

109. Cendes F, et al: Proton magnetic spectroscopic images and MRI volumetric studies for lateralization of temporal lobe epilepsy. *Magn Reson Imaging* 1995; 13:1187.

110. Garcia PA, et al: Proton magnetic resonance spectroscopic imaging in patients with frontal lobe epilepsy. *Ann Neurol* 1995; 37:279.

111. Youkin DP, et al: Cerebral metabolic effects of neonatal seizures measured with in vivo ^{31}P NMR spectroscopy. *Ann Neurol* 1986; 20:513.

112. Belliveau JW, et al: Functional mapping of the human visual cortex by magnetic resonance imaging. *Science* 1991; 254:716.

113. Connelly A, et al: Functional mapping of activated human primary cortex with a clinical MR imaging system. *Radiology* 1993; 188:125.

114. Cohen JD, et al: Activation of prefrontal cortex in a nonspatial working memory task with functional MRI. *Hum Brain Map* 1994; 1:293.

115. Morris GL, et al: Functional magnetic resonance imaging in partial epilepsy. *Epilepsia* 1994; 35:1194.

116. Rueckert L, et al: Magnetic resonance imaging functional activation of left frontal cortex during covert word production. *J Neuroimag* 1994; 4:67.

117. Jackson G, et al: Epilepsy and tumors near the motor cortex: preoperative identification of the motor strip using functional MRI. *Epilepsia* 1993; 34:120.

118. Penfield W: The evidence for a cerebral vascular mechanism in epilepsy. *Ann Intern Med* 1933; 7:303.

119. Engel J, Jr, et al: Patterns of human local cerebral glucose metabolism during epileptic seizures. *Science* 1982; 218:64.

120. Engel J, Jr, et al: Local cerebral metabolism during partial seizures. *Neurology* 1983; 33:400.

121. Editorial: PET and SPECT in epilepsy. *Lancet* 1989; 1:135.

122. Rowe CC, et al: Patterns of postictal cerebral blood flow in temporal lobe epilepsy: Qualitative and quantitative analysis. *Neurology* 1991; 41:1096.

123. Newton MR, et al: Postictal switch in blood flow distribution and temporal lobe seizures. *J Neurol Neurosurg Psychiatry* 1992; 55:891.

124. Henry TR, et al: Positron emission tomography. In Engel J Jr (ed): *Surgical Treatment of the Epilepsies,* 2d ed. New York, Raven Press, 1993:211–232.

125. Jackson GD, et al: Functional magnetic resonance imaging of focal seizure. *Neurology* 1994; 44:850.

126. Detre JA, et al: Localization of subclinical ictal activity by functional magnetic resonance imaging: correlation with invasive monitoring. *Ann Neurol* 1995; 38:618.

127. Berkovic SF, et al: Localization of epiletic foci using SPECT. In: Lüders H, (ed): *Epilepsy Surgery.* New York, Raven Press, 1991:251–256.

128. Harvey AS, et al: Frontal lobe epilepsy: Clinical seizure characteristics and localization with ictal ^{99m}Tc-HMPAO SPECT. *Neurology* 1993; 43:1966.

129. Ho SS, et al: Parietal lobe epilepsy: clinical features and seizure localization by ictal SPECT. *Neurology* 1994; 44:2277.

130. Theodore WH, et al: Neuroimaging in refractory partial seizures: Comparison of PET, CT and MRI. *Neurology* 1986; 36:750.

131. Abou-Khalil BW, et al: Positron emission tomography studies of cerebral glucose metabolism in chronic partial epilepsy. *Ann Neurol* 1987; 22:480.

132. Radtke RA, et al: Temporal lobe hypometabolism on PET:

predictor of seizure control after temporal lobectomy. *Neurology* 1993; 43:1088.

133. Henry TR, et al: Hippocampal neuronal loss and regional hypometabolism in temporal lobe epilepsy. *Ann Neurol* 1994; 36:925.

134. Rubin E, et al: Cerebral metabolic topography in unilateral temporal lobe epilepsy. *Neurology* 1995; 45:2212.

135. Abou-Khalil BW, Kessler R: Positron emission tomography in extratemporal epilepsy. *Neurology* 1991; 41(suppl 1):171.

136. Engel J, Jr., et al: PET in relation to intracranial electrode evaluations. *Epilepsy Res* 1992; 5(suppl):111.

137. Chugani HT, et al: Infantile spasms: I. PET identifies focal cortical dysgenesis in cryptogenic cases for surgical treatment. *Ann Neurol* 1990; 24:406.

138. Henry TR, et al: Decreased in vivo glucose metabolism and central benzodiazepine binding and mesial temporal lobe epilepsy. *Neurology* 1992; 32:245.

139. Savic I, et al: Comparison of [^{11}C]flumazenil and [^{18}F]FDG as PET markers of epileptic foci. *J Neurol Neurosurg Psychiatry* 1993; 56:615.

140. Savic I, et al: [^{11}C]flumazenil positron emission tomography visualizes frontal epileptogenic regions. *Epilepsia* 1995; 36:1225.

141. Bromfield EB, et al: Cerebral activation during speech discrimination in temporal lobe epilepsy. *Epilepsy Res* 1991; 9:49.

142. Bookheimer SY, et al: Multimodal functional imaging for language localization in epilepsy. *Neurology* 1993; 43:193.

143. Olivier A, et al: Stereotaxic seizure monitoring in patients with "bitemporal epilepsy": indications, technique and results. *Proc Am Assoc Neurol Surg*, No 14, Toronto, April 1977.

144. Olivier A, et al: The indications for and the role of depth electrode recording in epilepsy. *Appl Neurophsyiol* 1983; 46:33.

145. Olivier A, de Lotbinire A: Stereotactic techniques in epilepsy. *Neurosurgery State of the Art Reviews* 1987; 2:257.

146. Wyler AR, et al: Subdural strip electrodes for localizing epileptogenic foci. *J Neurosurg* 1984; 60:195.

147. Gloor P: Volume conductor principles: their application to the surface and depth electroencephalogram. In Wieser HG, Elger CE (eds): *Presurgical Evaluation of Epileptics*. Berlin, Springer-Verlag, 1987:59–68.

148. Barnett GH, et al.: Epidural peg electrodes for the presurgical evaluation of intractable epilepsy. *Neurosurgery* 1990; 27:113.

149. Wyllie E, Awad I: Intracranial EEG and localization studies. In Wyllie E (ed): *The Treatment of Epilepsy: Principles and Practices*. Philadelphia, Lea & Febiger, 1993:1023–1038.

150. Talairach J, et al: *L'Exploration Chirurgicale Stéréotaxique du Lobe Temporal dans l'Epilepsie Temporale. Repérage Anatomique Stéréotaxique et Technique Chirurgicale*. Paris, Masson, 1958.

151. Olivier A, et al: Stereotactic systems and procedures for depth electrodes placement: technical aspects. *Appl Neurophysiol* 1983; 46:37.

152. Goldring S, Gregorie M: Surgical management of epilepsy using epidural recording to localize the seizure focus. *J Neurosurg* 1984; 60:457.

153. Lüders H, et al: Chronic intracranial recording and stimulation with subdural electrodes. In Engel J (ed): *Surgical Treatment of the Epilepsies*. New York, Raven Press, 1987:297–321.

154. Olivier A, et al: Depth electrodes implantation at the Montreal Neurological Institute and Hospital. In Engel J (ed): *Surgical Treatment of the Epilepsies*. New York, Raven Press, 1987: 595–601.

155. Germano I, et al: Reoperation for recurrent temporal lobe epilepsy. *J Neurosurg* 1994; 81:31.

156. Olivier A, et al: Image guided surgery of epilepsy. *Neurosurg Clin North Am*, 1996; 7(2):229.

157. Branch C, et al: Intracarotid sodium amytal for the lateraliza-tion of cerebral speech dominance: Observations in 123 patients. *J Neurosurg* 1964; 21:399.

158. Wada J, Rasmussen T: Intracarotid injection of sodium amytal for the lateralization of cerebral speech dominance: Experimental and clinical observations. *J Neurosurg* 1960; 17:226.

159. Corkin S, et al: Somatosensory thresholds. Contrasting effects of post-central gyrus and posterior parietal-lobe excisions. *Arch Neurol* 1970; 22:41.

160. Jones-Gotman M, et al: Neuropsychological testing for localizing and lateralizing the epileptogenic region. In Engel J Jr (ed): *Surgical Treatment of the Epilepsies*, 2d ed, New York, Raven Press, 1993:245–262.

161. Jones-Gotman M, et al: Learning and retention of words and designs following excision from medial or lateral temporal-lobe structures. *Neuropsychologia* 1996 (in press).

162. Majdan A, et al: Performance of healthy subjects and patients with lesions of the temporal region on matched tests of verbal and visuospatial learning. *J Clin Exp Neuropsychol* 1996 (in press).

163. Penfield W, Milner B: Memory deficit produced by bilateral lesions in the hippocampal zone. *Arch Neurol Psychiat* 1958; 79:475.

164. Scoville W, Milner B: Loss of recent memory after bilateral hippocampal lesions. *J Neurol Neurosurg Psychiat* 1957; 20:11.

165. Press G, Amaral D, Squire L: Hippocampal abnormalities in amnesic patients revealed by high-resolution magnetic resonance imaging. *Nature* 1989; 341:54.

166. Düyckaerts C, et al: Bilateral and limited amygdalohippocampal lesions causing a pure amnesic syndrome. *Ann Neurol* 1985; 18:314.

167. Woods B, et al: Are hippocampal lesions sufficient to cause lasting amnesia? *J Neurol Neurosurg Psychiatry* 1982; 45:243.

168. Zola-Morgan S, et al: Human amnesia and the medial temporal region: Enduring memory impairment following a bilateral lesion limited to field CA1 of the hippocampus. *J Neurosci* 1986; 6:2950.

169. Jones-Gotman M: Commentary: Psychological evaluation—testing hippocampal function. In Engel J Jr (ed): *Surgical Treatment of the Epilepsies*. New York, Raven Press, 1987: 203–211.

170. Novelly RA, et al: Selective memory improvement and impairment in temporal lobectomy for epilepsy. *Ann Neurol* 1984; 15:64.

171. Ojemann G, Dodrill C: Verbal memory deficits after left temporal lobectomy for epilepsy. *J Neurosurg* 1985; 62:101.

172. Rausch R, Babb TL: Hippocampal neuron loss and memory scores before and after temporal lobe surgery for epilepsy. *Arch Neurol* 1993; 50:812.

173. Sass KJ, et al: Verbal memory impairment correlates with hippocampal pyramidal cell density. *Neurology* 1990; 40:1694.

174. Smith ML: Memory disorders associated with temporal-lobe lesions. In Boller F, Grafman J (eds): *Handbook of Neuropsychology*, vol 3. New York, Elsevier, 1989:91–106.

175. Fletcher JM: Memory for verbal and nonverbal stimuli in learning disability subgroups: analysis by selective reminding. *J Exp Child Psychol* 1985; 40:244.

176. Glosser G, et al: Assessing visual memory disorders. *J Cons Clin Psychol* 1989; 1:82.

177. Milner B, Petrides M: Behavioral effects of frontal-lobe lesions in man. *Trends Neurosci* 1984; 7:403.

178. Milner B, et al: Frontal lobes and the temporal organization of memory. *Human Neurobiol* 1985; 4:137.

179. Milner B, et al: Frontal-lobe contribution to recency judgment. *Neuropsychologia* 1991; 29:601.

180. Jones-Gotman M: Localization of lesions by psychological testing. *Epilepsia* 1991; 32:41.

181. Jones-Gotman M, Milner B: Design fluency: the invention of nonsense drawings after focal cortical lesions. *Neuropsychologia* 1977; 15:673.

182. Milner B: Psychological aspects of focal epilepsy and its neurosurgical management. In Purpura D, et al (eds): *Advances in Neurology.* New York, Raven Press, 1975:299–321.

183. Hermann B, et al: Pathological status of the mesial temporal lobe predicts memory outcome from left anterior temporal lobectomy. *Neurosurgery* 1992; 31:652.

184. Trenerry M, et al: MRI hippocampal volumes and memory function before and after temporal lobectomy. *Neurology* 1993; 43:1800.

185. Sperling M, et al: Predictors of outcome after anterior temporal lobectomy: The intracarotid amobarbital test. *Neurology* 1994; 44:2325.

186. Chelune GJ: Hippocampal adequacy versus functional reserve: predicting memory functions following temporal lobectomy. *Arch Clin Neuropsychol* 1995; 10:413.

187. Jones-Gotman M: Presurgical neuropsychological evaluation for localization and lateralization of seizure focus. In Luders H (ed.): *Epilepsy Surgery.* New York, Raven Press, 1991; 469–476.

188. Bouwer M, et al: Duration of sodium amytal effect: Behavioral and EEG measures. *Epilepsia* 1993; 34:61.

189. Ravdin L, et al: Serial recovery of language during the intracarotid amobarbital procedure. *Brain Cogn* 1996 (in press).

190. Loring D, et al: Amobarbital dose effects on Wada memory testing. *J Epilepsy* 1992; 5:171.

191. Loring D, Meador K, Lee G, et al: Wada memory performance predicts seizure outcome following anterior temporal lobectomy. *Neurology* 1994; 44:2322.

192. Fedio P, et al: Semantic, phonological and perceptual changes following left and right intracarotid injection (Wada) with a low Amytal dosage. *Brain Cogn* 1996 (in press).

193. Helmstaedter C, et al: Patterns of language dominance in focal left and right hemisphere epilepsies: Relation to MRI findings, EEG, sex and age at onset of epilepsy. *Brain Cogn* 1996 (in press).

194. Perria L, et al: Determination of side of cerebral dominance with amobarbital. *Arch Neurol* 1961; 4:173.

195. Serafetinides E, et al: EEG patterns induced by intracarotid injection of sodium amytal. *Electroenceph Clin Neurophysiol* 1965; 18:170.

196. Gotman J, et al: Intracranial EEG study of brain structures affected by internal carotid injection of amobarbital. *Neurology* 1992; 42:2136.

197. Ahern G, et al: Quantitative analysis of the EEG in the intracarotid amobarbital procedure. I. Amplitude analysis. *Electroenceph Clin Neurophysiol* 1994; 91:21.

198. Dade LA, Jones-Gotman M: Sodium amobarbital memory tests: What do they predict? *Brain Cogn* 1996 (in press).

199. Risse G, et al: A reconsideration of bilateral language representation based on the intracarotid amobarbital procedure. *Brain Cogn,* 1996 (in press).

200. Snyder P, et al: Mixed speech dominance in the intracarotid sodium amytal procedure: validity and criteria issues. *J Clin Exp Neuropsychol* 1990; 12:629.

201. Rausch R, et al: Intraarterial amobarbital procedures. In Engel J Jr (ed): *Surgical Treatment of the Epilepsies,* 2d ed. New York, Raven Press, 1993; 341–357.

202. Milner B, et al: Study of short-term memory after intracarotid injection of sodium amytal. *Trans Am Neurol Assoc* 1962; 87:224.

203. Jack CR, et al: Selective posterior cerebral artery amytal test for evaluation of memory function before surgery for temporal lobe seizures. *Neuroradiology* 1988; 168:787.

204. Wieser HG: Anterior cerebral artery amobarbital test. In Luders H (ed): *Epilepsy Surgery.* New York, Raven Press, 1991:515–523.

205. McMackin D, et al: Assessment of the functional effect of intracarotid sodium amobarbital procedure using co-registered MRI/HMPAO-SPECT and SEEG. *Brain Cogn* 1996 (in press).

206. Kneebone A, et al: Intracarotid amobarbital procedure as a predictor of material-specific memory change after anterior temporal lobectomy. *Epilepsia* 1995; 36:857.

207. Powell G, et al: Lateralization of memory functions in epileptic patients by use of the sodium amytal (Wada) technique. *J Neurol Neurosurg Psychiatry* 1987; 50:665.

208. Engel J Jr, et al: Correlation of criteria used for localizing epileptic foci in patients considered for surgical therapy of epilepsy. *Ann Neurol* 1981; 9:215.

209. Perrine K, et al: Wada memory disparities predict seizure laterality and postoperative seizure control. *Epilepsia* 1995; 36:851.

210. Wyllie E, et al: Intracarotid amobarbital procedure: II. Lateralizing value in evaluation for temporal lobectomy. *Epilepsia* 1991; 32:865.

211. Savard G, et al: Postictal psychosis after partial complex seizures: a multiple case study. *Epilepsia* 1991; 32:225.

212. Bruton CJ, et al: Epilepsy, psychosis, and schizophrenia: Clinical and neuropathological correlations. *Neurology* 1994; 44:34.

213. Mendez MF, et al: Schizophrenia in epilepsy: Seizure and psychosis variable. *Neurology* 1993; 43:1073.

214. Ketter TA, et al: Anticonvulsant withdrawal-emergent psychopathology. *Neurology* 1994; 44:55.

215. Gotman J, Marciani MG: Electroencephalographic spiking activity, drug levels and seizure occurrence in epileptic patients. *Ann Neurol* 1985; 17:597.

216. Marciani MG, et al: Patterns of seizure activation after withdrawal of antiepileptic medication. *Neurology* 1985; 35:1537.

217. Theodore WH, et al: Seizures during barbiturate withdrawal: Relation to blood level. *Ann Neurol* 1987; 22:644.

218. Bromfield EB, et al: Phenytoin withdrawal and seizure frequency. *Neurology* 1989; 39:905.

219. Duncan JS, et al: Discontinuation of phenytoin, carbamazepine, and valproate in patients with active epilepsy. *Epilepsia* 1990; 31:324.

220. So N, Gotman J: Changes in seizure activity following anticonvulsant drug withdrawal. *Neurology* 1990; 40:407.

221. Marks DA, et al: Clinical and electrographic effects of acute anticonvulsant withdrawal in epileptic patients. *Neurology* 1991; 41:508.

222. Malow BA, et al: Carbamazepine withdrawal: effects of taper rate on seizure frequency. *Neurology* 1993; 43:2280.

223. So NK: Effect of anticonvulsant withdrawal on spiking and seizure activity. In Luders H (ed): *Epilepsy Surgery.* New York, Raven Press, 1991:355–360.

224. Specht U, et al: Discontinuation of clonazepam after long-term treatment. *Epilepsia* 1989; 30:458.

225. Kalinowsky LB: Convulsions in nonepileptic patients on withdrawal of barbiturates, alcohol and other drugs. *Arch Neurol Psychiatry* 1942; 48:946.

226. Essig CF: Clinical and experimental aspects of barbiturate withdrawal convulsions. *Epilepsia* 1967; 8:21.

227. Theodore WH: Abrupt withdrawal of antiepileptic drugs for intensive video EEG monitoring. In Wyllie E (ed): *The Treatment of Epilepsy: Principles and Practices.* Philadelphia, Lea & Febiger, 1993:1009–1013.

228. Ludwig BI, Ajmone-Marsan CA: EEG changes after withdrawal of medication in epileptic patients. *EEG Clin Neurophysiol* 1975; 39:173.

229. Gotman J, Koffler DJ: Interictal spiking increases after seizures

but does not after decrease in medication. *EEG Clin Neurophysiol* 1989; 72:7.

230. Engel J, Jr, Crandall PH: Falsely localizing ictal onset with depth EEG telemetry during anticonvulsant withdrawal. *Epilepsia* 1983; 24:344.

231. Marciani MG, Gotman J: Effects of drug withdrawal on location of seizure onset. *Epilepsia* 1986; 27:423.

232. Spencer SS, et al: Ictal effects of anticonvulsant medication withdrawal in epileptic patients. *Epilepsia* 1981; 22:297.

233. Ranganathan C, et al: Valproate and epilepsy surgery. *J Epilepsy* 1993; 6:142.

234. Tetzlaff JE: Intraoperative defect in haemostasis in a child receiving valproic acid. *Can J Anaesth* 1991; 38:222.

235. Spencer SS, Packey DJ: Antiepileptic drug management before and after epilepsy surgery. In Levy RH, et al (eds): *Antiepileptic Drugs*. New York, Raven Press, 1995:189–200.

236. Loiseau P: Sodium valproate, platelet dysfunction and bleeding. *Epilepsia* 1981; 22:141.

237. Richardson SGN, et al: Sodium valproate and platelet function. *Br Med J* 1976; 1:221.

238. Dale BM, et al: Fibrinogen depletion with sodium valproate. *Lancet* 1978; 1:1316.

239. Kreuz W, et al: Valproate therapy induces von Willebrand disease type I. *Epilepsia* 1992; 33:178.

240. Cruz-Rodriguez RF, et al: Carbamazepine toxicity after epilepsy surgery. *Epilepsia* 1989; 30:640.

241. Penfield W, Jasper H: *Epilepsy and the Functional Anatomy of the Human Brain*. Boston, Little, Brown, 1954.

242. Penfield W, Roberts L: *Speech and Brain Mechanisms*. Princeton, Princeton University Press, 1959.

243. Ojemann GA, et al: Cortical Stimulation. In Engel J Jr (ed): *Surgical Treatment of the Epilepsies*, 2d ed. New York, Raven Press, 1993:399–414.

244. Perrine K: Future directions for functional mapping. *Epilepsia* 1994; 35(6).

245. Picard C, Olivier A: Sensory cortical tongue representation in man. *J Neurosurg* 1983; 59:781.

246. Spencer DD, et al: Access to the posterior medial structures in the surgical treatment of temporal lobe epilepsy. *Neurosurgery* 1984; 15:667.

247. Niemeyer P: The transventricular amygdalo-hippocampectomy in temporal lobe epilepsy. In Baldwin M, Bailey P (eds): *Temporal Lobe Epilepsy*. Springfield (IL), Charles C Thomas, 1958:461–482.

248. Wieser HG, Yasargil MG: Die "selectieve Amygdalohippokampektomie," Eine chirurgische Behandlungsmethode fur mediobasal-limbischen Epilepsie. *Neurochirurgia* 1982; 25:39.

249. Wieser HG: Selective amygdalohippocampectomy: Indications, investigative techniques and results. *Adv Techn Stand Neurosurg* 1986; 13:40.

250. Rasmussen T: Hemispherectomy for seizures revisited. *Can J Neurol Sci* 1983; 10:71.

251. Tinuper P, et al: Functional hemispherectomy for treatment of epilepsy associated with hemiplegia: Rationale, indications, results and comparison with callosotomy. *Ann Neurol* 1988; 24:27.

252. Villemure JG, Rasmussen T: Functional hemispherectomy-methodology. *J Epilepsy*, 1990; 3(suppl):177.

253. Morrel F, et al: Multiple subpial transsection: A new approach to the surgical treatment of focal epilepsy. *J Neurosurg* 1989; 70:231.

254. Van Wagenen W, Herren RY: Surgical division of commisural pathways in the corpus callosum. Relation to spread of an epileptic attack. *Arch Neurol Psychiatry* 1940; 44:740.

255. Bogen JE, Vogel PJ: Commissurotomy in man: Preliminary case report. *Bull LA Neurol Soc* 1962, 7:169.

256. Wilson DH, et al: Central commissurotomy for intractable generalized epilepsy: series 2. *Neurology* 1982; 32:687.

257. Spencer DD, et al: Corpus callosotomy for epilepsy. I. Seizure effects. *Neurology* 1988; 38:19.

258. Olivier A, et al: Anterior callosotomy in the treatment of intractable epilepsies. *Boll Lega It Epil* 1988; 64:81.

259. Oguni H, et al: Anterior callosotomy in the treatment of medically intractable epilepsies: A study of 43 patients with a mean follow-up of 39 months. *Ann Neurol* 1991; 30:357.

260. Alonso-Vanegas M, et al: Callosotomy for treatment of drop attacks. *J Neurosurg* 1996; 84:343A.

261. Falconer MA: Place of surgery for temporal lobe epilepsy during childhood. *Br Med J* 1972; 2:631.

262. Andermann F: Selection and investigation of candidates for surgical treatment of temporal lobe epilepsy in childhood and adolescence. In Blaw M, et al (eds): *Topics in Child Neurology*. Spectrum, Jamaica, 1977:167–171.

263. Rasmussen T: Cortical resection in children with focal epilepsy. In Parsonage M et al (eds): *Advances in Epileptology: XIVth Epilepsy International Symposium*, New York, Raven Press, 1983:249–254.

264. Shields WD, et al: Surgically remediable syndromes of infancy and early childhood. In Engel J Jr (ed): *Surgical Treatment of the Epilepsies*, 2d ed. New York, Raven Press, 1993:35–48.

265. Peacock WJ, et al: Special considerations for epilepsy surgery in childhood. In Engel J Jr (ed): *Surgical Treament of the Epilepsies*, 2d ed. New York, Raven Press, 1993:541–547.

266. Duchowny MS: Epilepsy surgery in children. *Current Op Neurol* 1995; 8:112.

267. Huttenlocher PR, Hapke RJ: A follow-up study of intractable seizures in childhood. *Ann Neurol* 1990; 28:699.

268. Sillanpä M: Remission of seizures and predictors of intractability in long-term follow-up. *Epilepsia* 1993; 34:930.

269. Grattan-Smith JD, et al: Hippocampal sclerosis in children with intractable temporal lobe epilepsy: Detection with MR imaging. *AJR* 1993; 161:1045.

270. Kuks JBM, et al: Hippocampal sclerosis in epilepsy and childhood febrile seizures. *Lancet* 1993; 342:1391.

271. Chugani HT, et al: Infantile spasms: II. Lenticular nuclei and brain stem activation on positron emission tomography. *Ann Neurol* 1992; 31:212.

272. Chugani HT: Infantile spasms. *Current Op Neurol* 1995; 8:139.

273. Vinters HV, et al: Neuropathological study of resected cerebral tissue from patients with infantile spasms. *Epilepsia* 1993; 34:772.

274. Kramer U, et al: Morbidity of depth and subdural electrodes: children and adolescents versus young adults. *J Epilepsy* 1994; 7:7.

275. Modica PA, et al: Pro- and anti-convulsant effects of anesthetics (part 2). *Anesth Analg* 1990; 70:433.

276. Modica PA, et al: Pro- and anti-convulsant effects of anesthetics (part 1). *Anesth Analg* 1990; 70:303.

277. Backman LE, et al: Electroencephalography in halothane anesthesia. *Acta Anaesthesiol Scand* 1964; 8:115.

278. Pichlmayr I, et al: Electroencephalographic patterns induced by various anesthetics and perioperative influences. In Pichlmayr I, et al (eds): *The Electroencephalogram in Anaesthesia*. Berlin, Springer-Verlag, 1984; 90–124.

279. Michenfelder JD: *Anesthesia and the Brain*. New York, Churchill-Livingstone, 1988.

280. Clark DL, et al: Neural effects of isoflurane in man. *Anesthesiology* 1973; 39:261.

281. Avramov MN, et al: Electroencephalographic changes during vital capacity breath induction with halothane. *Br J Anaesth* 1991; 66:211.

282. Neigh JL, et al: The electroencephalographic pattern during

anesthesia with ethrane: effects of the depth of anesthesia, Pa_{CO_2} and nitrous oxide. *Anesthesiology* 1971; 35:482.

283. Kavan EM, et al: Electrographic alterations induced in limbic and sensory systems during induction of anaesthesia with halothane, methoxyflurane, diethyl ether, and enflurane. *Br J Anaesth* 1972; 44:1234.

284. Lebowitz MH, et al: Enflurane induced central nervous system excitation and its relation to carbon dioxide tension. *Anesth Analg* 1972; 51:355.

285. Rosen I, Soderberg M: Electroencephalographic activation in children under enflurane anesthesia. *Acta Anaesthesiol Scand* 1975; 19:361.

286. Grant IS: Delayed convulsions following enflurane anaesthesia. *Anaesthesia* 1986; 41:1024.

287. Ohm WW, et al: Delayed seizure activity following enflurane anesthseia. *Anesthesiology* 1975; 42:367.

288. Allan NS: Convulsions after enflurane. *Anaesthesia* 1984; 39:605.

289. Burchiel KJ, et al: Relationship of pre and postanesthetic EEG abnormalities to enflurane-induced seizure activity. *Anesth Analg* 1977; 56:509.

290. Opitz A, et al: Enflurane anesthesia for epileptic patients. *Anaesthetist* 1977; 26:329.

291. Opitz A, Oberwetter WD: Enflurane or halothane anesthesia for patients with cerebral convulsive disorders? *Acta Anaesthesiol Scand* 1979; 71(suppl):43.

292. Ito BM, et al: The effect of isoflurane and enflurane on the electrocorticogram of epileptic patients. *Neurology* 1988; 38:924.

293. Flemming DC, et al: Diagnostic activation of epileptogenic foci by enflurane. *Anesthesiology* 1980; 52:431.

294. Kraemer DL, Spencer DD: Anesthesia in epilepsy surgery. In Engel J Jr (ed): *Surgical Treatment of the Epilepsies*. New York, Raven Press, 1993:527.

295. Darimont PC, Jenkins LC: The influence of intravenous anaesthetics on enflurane-induced central nervous system seizure activity. *Can Anaesth Soc J* 1977; 24:42.

296. Sprague DH, Wolf S: Enflurane seizures in patients taking amitriptyline. *Anesth Analg* 1982; 61:67.

297. Vohra SB: Convulsions after enflurane in a schizophrenic patient receiving neuroleptics. *Can J Anaesth* 1994; 41:420.

298. Newberg LA, et al: Systemic and cerebral effects of isoflurane at and above concentrations that suppress cortical activity. *Anesthesiology* 1983; 59:23.

299. Eger EI: Are seizures caused by isoflurane or nitrous oxide? *Anesthesiology* 1985; 62:698.

300. Hughes DR, et al: Control of epilepsia partialis continua and secondarily generalised status epilepticus with isoflurane (letter). *J Neurol Neurosurg Psychiatry* 1992; 55:739.

301. Sakaki T, et al: Isoflurane in the management of status epilepticus after surgery for lesions around the motor area. *Acta Neurochir* 1992; 116:38.

302. Dworacek B, DeVlieger M: Absence of electroencephalographic excitation pattern under isoflurane anesthesia. *Acta Anaesth Belg* 1984; 35:211.

303. Lüders H (ed): Protocols for surgery of epilepsy in different centers. In *Epilepsy*. New York, Raven Press, 1992:781–818.

304. Smith M: Anaesthesia for epilepsy and stereotactic surgery. In Walters JM, et al (eds): *Anaesthesia and Intensive Care for the Neurosurgical Patient*. Oxford, Blackwell 1994:318–344.

305. Hymes JA: Seizure activity during isoflurane anesthesia. *Anesth Analg* 1985; 64:367.

306. Poulton TJ, Ellingston RJ: Seizure associated with induction of anesthesia with isoflurane. *Anesthesiology* 1984; 61:471.

307. Rampil IJ, et al: The electroencephalographic effects of desflurane in humans. *Anesthesiology* 1991; 74:434.

308. Avramov MN, et al: Effects of different speeds of induction with sevoflurane on the EEG in man. *J Anesth* 1987; 1:1.

309. Scheller MS, et al:Cerebral effects of sevoflurane in the dog: comparison with isoflurane and enflurane. *Br J Anaesth* 1990; 65:388.

310. Faulconer A, et al: The influence of partial pressure of nitrous oxide on the depth of anesthesia and the electro-encephalogram in man. *Anesthesiology* 1994; 10:601.

311. Horbein TF, et al: The minimum alveolar concentration of nitrous oxide in man. *Anesth Analg* 1982; 61:533.

312. Matta BF, Lam AM: Nitrous oxide increases cerebral blood flow velocity during pharmacologically-induced EEG silence in humans. *J Neurosurg Anesthesiol* 1995; 7:79.

313. Gloor P: *Contributions of Electroencephalography and Electrocorticography to the Neurosurgical Treatment of the Epilepsies*. New York, Raven Press, 1975:59–105.

314. Stevens JE, et al: Effects of nitrous oxide on the epileptogenic property of enflurane in cats. *Br J Anaesth* 1983; 55:145.

315. Hoffman WE, et al: Nitrous oxide added to isoflurane increases brain artery blood flow and low frequency brain electrical activity. *J Neurosurg Anesthesiol* 1995; 7:82.

316. Stoica I: Rapid electroencephalographic activation by small doses of natriumevipan. *Epilepsia* 1965; 6:54.

317. Jewkes DA: The postoperative period—some important complication. *Clin Anesthesiol* 1987; 1:517.

318. Partinen M, et al: Status epilepticus treated by barbiturate anaesthesia with continuous monitoring of cerebral function. *Br Med J* 1981; 282:520.

319. Rockoff MA, Goudsouzian NC: Seizures induced by methohexital. *Anesthesiology* 1981; 54:333.

320. Musella L, et al: Electroencephalographic activation with intravenous methohexital in psychomotor epilepsy. *Neurology* 1971; 21:594.

321. Gumpert J, Paul R: Activation of the electroencephalogram with intravenous Brietal (methohexitone): The findings in 100 cases. *J Neurol Neurosurg Psychiatry* 1971; 34:646.

322. Paul R, Harris R: A comparison of methohexitone and thiopentone in electrocorticography. *J Neurol Neurosurg Psychiatry* 1970; 33:100.

323. Wilder B: Electroencephalogram activation in medically intractable epileptic patients. *Arch Neurol* 1971; 25:415.

324. Austin EJ, et al: Methohexital activation of epileptiform discharges in the human electrocorticogram. *Epilepsia* 1986; 27:624.

325. Wyler AR, et al: Methohexital activation of epileptogenic foci during acute electrocorticography. *Epilepsia* 1987; 28:490.

326. Aasly J, et al: Effects of amobarbital and methohexital on epileptic activity in mesial temporal structures in epileptic patients. An EEG study with depth electrodes. *Acta Neurol Scand* 1984; 70:423.

327. Smith I, et al: Propofol. An update on its clinical use. *Anesthesiology* 1994; 81:1005.

328. Borgeat A, et al: The nonhypnotic therapeutic applications of propofol. *Anesthesiology* 1994; 80:642.

329. Seifert HA, et al: Sedative doses of propofol increase beta activity of the processed electroencephalogram. *Anesth Analg* 1993; 76:976.

330. Mahla ME, et al: Prolonged anesthesia with propofol or isoflurane: intraoperative electroencephalographic patterns and postoperative recovery. *Semin Anesth* 1992; 11(suppl 1):31.

331. Van Hemelrijk J, et al: EEG-assisted titration of propofol infusion during neuroanesthesia. *J Neurosurg Anesth* 1992; 4:11.

332. Hodkinson BP, et al: Propofol and the electroencephalogram. *Lancet* 1987; 2:1518.

333. Ebrahim ZY, et al: The effect of propofol on the electroencephalogram of patients with epilepsy. *Anesth Analg* 1994; 78:275.

334. Drummond JC, et al: Masking of epileptiform activity by pro-pofol during seizure surgery. *Anesthesiology* 1992; 76:652.

335. Rampil IJ, et al: Propofol sedation may disrupt interictal epileptiform activity from a seizure focus. *Anesth Analg* 1993; 77:1071.

336. Smith SJM, et al: Propofol effects on the electroencephalogram during epilepsy surgery. *Epilepsia* 1993; 34(suppl 6):41.

337. Samra SK, et al: Effects of propofol sedation on seizures and intracranially recorded epileptiform activity in patients with partial epilepsy. *Anesthesiology* 1995; 82:843.

338. Doenicke A, et al: Plasma concentration and EEG after various regimens of etomidate. *Br J Anaesth* 1982; 54:393.

339. Ebrahim ZY, et al: Effect of etomidate on the electroencephalogram of patients with epilepsy. *Anesth Analg* 1986; 65:1004.

340. Gancher S, et al: Activation of epileptogenic activity by etomidate. *Anesthesiology* 1984; 61:616.

341. Koerner MK, et al: Etomidate for the activation of epileptiform abnormalities. *Epilepsia* 1986; 27:624.

342. Reddy RV, et al: Excitatory effects and electroencephalographic correlation of etomidate, thiopental, methohexital, and propofol. *Anesth Analg* 1993; 77:1008.

343. Wauquier A: Profile of etomidate, a hypnotic, anticonvulsant and brain protective compound. *Anaesthesia* 1983; 38(suppl):26.

344. Hoffman P, Schokenhoff B: Etomidate as an anticonvulsive agent. *Anaesthetist* 1984; 33:142.

345. Gotman J, et al: Correlations between EEG changes induced by diazepam and the localization of epileptic spikes and seizures. *Electroencephalogr Clin Neurophysiol* 1982; 54:614.

346. Tucker GT: Pharmacokinetics of local anaesthetics. *Br J Anaesth* 1986; 58:717.

347. Pascual J, et al: Role of lidocaine (lignocaine) in managing status epilepticus. *J Neurol Neurosurg Psychiatry* 1992; 55:49.

348. Wagman IH, et al: Effects of lidocaine upon spontaneous cortical and subcortical electric activity. *Arch Neurol* 1968; 18:277.

349. Archer DP, et al: Conscious-sedation analgesia during craniotomy for intractable epilepsy: A review of 354 consecutive cases. *Can J Anaesth* 1988; 35:338.

350. DeJong RH, Walts LF: Lidocaine-induced psychomotor seizures in man. *Acta Anaesthesiol Scand* 1966; 23(suppl):598.

351. Freund PR, et al: Caudal anesthesia with lidocaine or bupivacaine: Plasma local anesthetic concentration and extent of sensory spread in old and young patients. *Anesth Analg* 1984; 63:1017.

352. Bishop D, Johnstone RE: Lidocaine toxicity treated with low-dose propofol. *Anesthesiology* 1993; 78:788.

353. Palve H, et al: Maximum recommended doses of lignocaine are not toxic. *Br J Anaesth* 1995; 74:704.

354. Loeser EA, et al: Comparison of droperidol, haloperidol and prochlorperazine as postoperative anti-emetics. *Can J Anaesth* 1979; 26:125.

355. Nilsson E, Ingvar DH: EEG findings in neuroleptanalgesia. *Acta Anaesthesiol Scand* 1967; 11:121.

356. Opitz A, et al: General anesthesia in patients with epilepsy and status epilepticus. In Delgado Escueta AV, et al (eds): *Status Epilepticus: Mechanisms of Brain Damage and Treatment.* New York, Raven Press, 1983:43–47.

357. Smith NT, et al: EEGs during high-dose fentanyl-, sufentanil-, or morphine-oxygen anesthesia. *Anesth Analg* 1984; 63:386.

358. Sebel PS, et al: Effects of high dose fentanyl anesthesia on the electroencephalogram. *Anesthesiology* 1981; 55:203.

359. Benthuysen JL, et al: Physiology of alfentanil-induced rigidity. *Anesthesiology* 1986; 64:440.

360. Chi OZ, et al: Power spectral analysis of EEG during sufentanil infusion in humans. *Can J Anaesth* 1991, 38:275.

361. Tempelhoff R, et al: Fentanyl-induced electrocorticographic

362. Gignac E, et al: Comparison of fentanyl, sufentanil and alfentanil during awake craniotomy for epilepsy. *Can J Anaesth* 1993; 40:421.

363. From RP, et al: Anesthesia for craniotomy: A double-blind comparison of alfentanil, fentanyl, and sufentanil. *Anesthesiology* 1990; 73:896.

364. Mutch WAC, et al: Continuous opioid infusion for neurosurgical procedures: A double-blind comparison of alfentanil and fentanyl. *Can J Anaesth* 1991; 38:710.

365. Westmoreland CL, et al: Fentanyl or alfentanil decreases the minimum alveolar anesthetic concentration of isoflurane in surgical patients. *Anesth Analg* 1994; 78:23.

366. McEwan AI, et al: Isoflurane minimum alveolar concentration reduction by fentanyl. *Anesthesiology* 1993; 78:864.

367. Bailey PL, et al: Differences in magnitude and duration of opioid-induced respiratory depression and analgesia with fentanyl and sufentanil. *Anesth Analg* 1964; 70:8.

368. Vuyk J, et al: Pharmacodynamic interaction between propofol and alfentanil when given for induction of anesthesia. *Anesthesiology* 1996; 84:288.

369. Tempelhoff R, et al: Anticonvulsant therapy increases fentanyl requirements during anaesthesia for craniotomy. *Can J Anaesth* 1990; 37:327.

370. Lanier WL, et al: The cerebral effects of pancuronium and atracurium in halothane anethetized dogs. *Anesthesiology* 1985; 63:589.

371. Chapple DJ, et al: Cardiovascular and neurological effects of laudanosine. *Br J Anaesth* 1987; 59:218.

372. Yate PM, et al: Clinical experience and plasma laudanosine concentrations during infusion of atracurium in the ICU. *Br J Anaesth* 1987; 59:211.

373. Parker CJR, et al: Disposition of infusions of atracurium and its metabolite laudanosine, in patients in renal and respiratory failure. *Br J Anaesth* 1988; 61:531.

374. Hickey DR, et al: Phenytoin-induced resistance to pancuronium: Use of atracurium infusion in management of a neurosurgical patient. *Anaesthesia* 1988; 43:757.

375. Ornstein E, et al: Accelerated recovery from doxacurium-induced neuromuscular blockade in patients receiving chronic anticonvulsant therapy. *J Clin Anesth* 1991; 3:108.

376. Roth S, Ebrahim ZY: Resistance to pancuronium in patients receiving carbamazepine. *Anesthesiology* 1987; 66:691.

377. Whalley DG, Ebrahim ZY: Influence of carbamazepine on the dose-response relationship of vecuronium. *Br J Anaesth* 1994; 72:125.

378. Platt PR, Thackray NM: Phenytoin-induced resistance to vecuronium. *Anaesth Intensive Care* 1993; 21:185.

379. Jellish WS, et al: Accelerated recovery from pipecuronium in patients treated with chronic anticonvulsant therapy. *J Clin Anesth* 1993; 5:105.

380. Kim CS, et al: Decreased sensitivity to metocurine during long-term phenytoin therapy may be attributable to protein binding and acetylcholine receptor changes. *Anesthesiology* 1992; 77:500.

381. Ornstein E, et al: Resistance to metocurine-induced neuromuscular blockade in patients receiving phenytoin. *Anesthesiology* 1985; 63:294.

382. Ornstein E, et al: The effect of phenytoin on the magnitude and duration of neuromuscular block following atracurium or vecuronium. *Anesthesiology* 1987; 67:191.

383. Tempelhoff R, et al: Resistance to atracurium-induced neuromuscular blockade with intractable seizure disorders treated with anticonvulsants. *Anesth Analg* 1990; 71:665.

384. Melton AT, et al: Prolonged duration of succinylcholine in

patients receiving anticonvulsants: evidence for mild up-regulation of acetylcholine receptors? *Can J Anaesth* 1993; 40:939.

385. Parr SM, et al: Interaction between betamethasone and vecuronium. *Br J Anaesth* 1991; 67:447.

386. Rasmussen T: Surgical therapy of frontal lobe epilepsy. *Epilepsia* 1963; 4:181.

387. Thompson PJ, Oxley J: Socioeconomic accompaniments of severe epilepsy. *Epilepsia* 1988; 29 (suppl):59.

388. Pritchard PB, et al: Psychological complications of temporal lobe epilepsy. *Neurology* 1980; 30:227.

389. Lüders HO, et al: General principles. In: Engel J Jr (ed) *Surgical Treatment of the Epilepsies*, 2d ed. New York, Raven Press, 1993 .

390. Pellock JM: Carbamazepine side effects in children and adults. *Epilepsia* 1987; 28:S64.

391. Pellock JM, Willmore LJ: A rational guide to routine blood monitoring in patients receiving antiepileptic drugs. *Neurology* 1991; 41:961.

392. Brodie MJ, Dichter MA: Antiepileptic drugs. *N Engl J Med* 1996; 334:168.

393. Brodie MJ: Drug interactions in epilepsy. *Epilepsia* 1992; 33(suppl)1:S13.

394. Delgado MR, et al: Thrombocytopenia secondary to high valproate levels in children with epilepsy. *J Child Neurol* 1994; 9:311.

395. May RB, Sunder TR: Hematologic manifestations of long-term valproate therapy. *Epilepsia* 1993; 34:1098.

396. Gidal B, et al: Valproate-mediated disturbances of hemostasis: Relationship to dose and plasma concentration. *Neurology* 1994; 44:1418.

397. Ward MM, et al: Preoperative valproate administration does not increase blood loss during temporal lobectomy. *Epilepsia* 1996; 37:98.

398. Kutt H: Pharmacokinetic interactions with antiepileptic medication. In Wyllie E (ed). *The Treatment of Epilepsy: Principles and Practice*. Philadelphia, Lea & Febiger, 1993:775–784.

399. Leppik IE: Antiepileptic drug interactions: An overview. In: Faingold CL, Fromm GH (eds): *Drugs for Control of Epilepsy*. Boca Raton, CRC Press, 1991:390–399.

400. Spencer DD: Depth electrode implantation at Yale University. In: Engel J Jr (ed): *Surgical Treatment of the Epilepsies*. New York, Raven Press, 1987:603–607.

401. Pilcher WH, et al: Complications of epilepsy surgery. In: Engel J Jr (ed): *Surgical Treatment of the Epilepsies*. New York, Raven Press, 1993:565–581.

402. White PF: Use of continuous infusion versus intermittent bolus administration of fentanyl or ketamine during outpatient anesthesia. *Anesthesiology* 1983; 59:294.

403. Fragen RJ: Appendix. In: Fragen RJ (ed): *Drug Infusions in Anesthesiology*. New York, Raven Press, 1991:217–218.

404. White PF, et al: Comparison of alfentanil with fentanyl for outpatient anesthesia. *Anesthesiology* 1986; 64:99.

405. Tuman KLJ, et al: Sufentanil-midazolam anesthesia for coronary artery surgery. *J Cardiothor-Vasc Anesth* 1990; 4:308.

406. Phibin DM, et al: Fentanyl and sufentanil anesthesia revisited: How much is enough? *Anesthesiology* 1990; 73:5.

407. Glass PSA, et al: Plasma concentration of fentanyl with 70% nitroux oxide to prevent movement at skin incision. *Anesthesiology* 1993; 78:842.

408. Ausema ME, et al: Plasma concentrations of alfentanil required to supplement nitrous oxide anesthesia for general anesthesia. *Anesthesiology* 1986; 5:362.

409. Smith C, et al: The interaction of fentanyl on the Cp50 of propofol for loss of consciousness and skin incision. *Anesthesiology* 1994; 81:820.

410. Woods CC, et al: Localisation of human sensorimotor cortex during surgery by cortical surface recordings of somatosensory evoked potentials. *J Neurosurg* 1988; 68:99.

411. Bickford RG: Activation procedures and special electrodes. In: Klass DW, Daly DD (eds): *Current Practice of Clinical Electroencephalography*. New York, Raven Press, 1979:269–305.

412. Bonvallet M, Dell P: Reflections on the mechanisms of action of hyperventilation upon the EEG. *Electroencephalogr Clin Neurophysiol* 1956; 8:170.

413. Isert P: Control of carbon dioxide levels during neuroanesthesia: Current practice and an appraisal of our reliance upon capnography. *Anesth Intens Care* 1994; 22:435.

414. Russel GB, Graybeal JM: The arterial to end-tidal carbon dioxide difference in neurosurgical patients during craniotomy. *Anesth Analg* 1995; 81:806.

415. Albibi R, McCallum RW: Metoclopramide: Pharmacology and clinical application. *Ann Intern Med* 1983; 98:86.

416. Scuplak SM, et al: Case report: Air embolism during awake craniotomy. *Anesthesia* 1995; 50:338.

417. Engel J Jr: Surgery for seizures. *N Engl J Med* 1996; 334:647.

418. Awad IA, et al: Intractable epilepsy and structural lesions of the brain: mapping resection strategies, and seizure outcome. *Epilepsia* 1991; 32:179.

419. Artru A, et al: Nitrous oxide: Suppression of local epileptiform activity during inhalation and spreading of seizure activity following withdrawal. *J Neurosurg Anesthesiol* 1991; 2:189.

420. Yamamura T, et al: Fast oscillatory EEG activity induced by analgesic concentrations of nitrous oxide in man. *Anesth Analg* 1981; 60:283.

421. Spencer DD: Postscript: Technical controversies. In: Engel J Jr (ed): *Surgical Treatment of the Epilepsies*, 2d ed. New York, Raven Press, 1993:583–591.

422. Fiol M, et al: Methohexital (Brevital) effect on electrocorticogram may be misleading. *Epilepsia* 1990; 31:524.

423. Cascino GD, et al: Alfentanil induced epileptiform activity in patients with partial epilepsy. *J Clin Neurophysiol* 1993; 10:520.

424. Stewart LF: Chlorpromazine: Use to activate electroencephalographic seizure patterns. *Electroenceph Clin Neurophysiol* 1957; 9:427.

425. Ojemann GA: Awake operations with mapping in epilepsy. In: Schmidek HH, Sweet WH (eds): *Operative Neurosurgical Techniques*, 3d ed. Philadelphia, WB Saunders, 1995:1317–1322.

426. Ojemann GA: Awake operations in the treatment of epilepsy. In: Shorvon S et al (eds): *Treatment of Epilepsy*. London, Blackwell, 1996:752–758.

427. Rasmussen T: Localization aspects of epileptic seizure phenomena. In: Thompson R, Green J (eds): *New Perspectives in Cerebral Localization*. New York, Raven Press, 1982:177–203.

428. Hermann B, Wyler A: Comparative results of dominant temporal lobectomy under general or local anesthetic: Language outcome. *J Epilepsy* 1988; 1:127.

429. Hermann B, et al: Language function following anterior temporal lobectomy. *J Neurosurg* 1991; 74:560.

430. Silbergeld DL, et al: Use of propofol (Diprivan) for awake craniotomies: Technical note. *Surg Neurol* 1992; 38:271.

431. Waldan T, et al: Reliability of CO_2 measurements from the airway by a pharyngeal catheter in unintubated, spontaneously breathing subjects. *Acta Anesthesiol Scand* 1995; 39:637.

432. Manninen P, Contreras J: Anesthetic considerations for craniotomy in awake patients. *Int Anesthesiol Clin* 1986; 24:157.

433. Rosa G, et al: Effect of low-dose propofol administration on central respiratory drive, gas exchanges and respiratory pattern. *Acta Anaesthesiol Scand* 1992; 36:128.

434. Forrest FC, et al: Propofol infusion and the suppression of consciousness: The EEG and dose requirements. *Br J Anaesth* 1994; 72:35.

435. Gan TJ, et al: Double-blind comparison on ondansetron, dro-

peridol and saline in the prevention of postoperative nausea and vomiting. *Br J Anaesth* 1994; 72:544.

436. Wilson E, et al: Sedation during spinal anesthesia: Comparison of propofol and midazolam. *Br J Anaesth* 1990; 64:48.

437. Girvin J: Neurosurgical considerations and general methods for craniotomy under local anesthesia. *Int Anesthiol Clin* 1986; 24(3):89.

438. Ojemann G: Cortical organization of language. *J Neurosci* 1991; 11:2281.

439. Melnice BM: Extrapyramidal reactions to low-dose droperidol. *Anesthesiology* 1988; 69:424.

440. Girvin JP: Complications of epilepsy surgery. In: Lüders H (ed): *Epilepsy Surgery*. New York, Raven Press, 1991; 653–660.

441. Shorvon S: *Status Epilepticus*, Cambridge, University Press, 1994.

442. Gastaut H: Classification of status epilepticus. In: Delgado-Escueta AV, et al (eds): *Status Epilepticus. Advances in Neurology*, vol. 34. New York, Raven Press, 1987:34:15.

443. Hauser WA: Status epilepticus: Epidemiologic considerations. *Neurology* 1990; 40(suppl 2):9.

444. Aicardi J, Chevrie JJ: Convulsive status epilepticus in infants and children. *Epilepsia* 1970; 11:187.

445. Phillips SA, Shanahan RJ: Etiology and mortality of status epilepticus in children. *Arch Neurol* 1989; 46:74.

446. Aminoff MJ, Simon RP: Status epilepticus: Causes, clinical features and consequences in patients. *Am J Med* 1980; 69:657.

447. Treiman DM, et al: A progressive sequence of electroencephalographic changes during generalised convulsive status epilepticus. *Epilepsy Res* 1990; 5:49.

448. Lothman EW: The biochemical basis and pathophysiology of status epilepticus. *Neurology* 1990; 40(suppl 2):13.

449. Brown JK, Hussain IHMI: Status epilepticus. I. Pathogenesis. *Dev Med Child Neurol* 1991; 33:3–17.

450. Desbiens R, et al: Life-threatening focal status epilepticus due to occult cortical dysplasia. *Arch Neurol* 1993; 50:695.

451. Barry E, Hauser WA: Status epilepticus and antiepileptic medication levels. *Neurology* 1994; 44:47.

452. Epilepsy Foundation of Americas Working Group on Status Epilepticus: Treatment of convulsive status epilepticus. *JAMA* 1993; 270:854.

453. Lowenstein DH, Allredge BK: Status epilepticus in an urban public hospital in the 1980s. *Neurology* 1993; 43:483.

454. Heh CW, et al: Exacerbation of psychosis after discontinuance of carbamazepine treatment. *Am J Psychol* 1988; 45:878.

455. Sironi VA, et al: Interictal acute psychosis in temporal lobe epilepsy during withdrawal of anticonvulsant therapy. *J Neurol Neurosurg Psychiatry* 1979; 42:724

Chapter 22 _____

STEREOTACTIC SURGERY AND ABLATIVE PROCEDURES FOR PAIN

PHILLIP L. GILDENBERG

MARY B. NEAL

IGNATIUS DISTEFANO

FUNCTIONAL STEREOTACTIC SURGERY
   Procedure
ANESTHETIC CONSIDERATIONS
   Monitored Anesthesia Care
   Agents
   Craniotomy under Local Anesthesia
   Use of General Anesthesia
NONSTEREOTACTIC FUNCTIONAL NEURO-SURGERY

Stereotactic surgery is a technique to aim a probe, usually an electrode or biopsy cannula, with great accuracy to a target within the brain. The probe may also be an x-ray or proton beam, a surgical forceps or other instrument, or even the surgeon's eye view of a surgical field. Historically, stereotactic surgery concerns the use of a device that can be adjusted to point to the target, which is defined by a three-dimensional Cartesian coordinate system. The target may be visualized directly, or the position of the target may be defined by three coordinates that refer to landmarks in the skull or brain.

Stereotactic techniques have been used in the animal laboratory since 1908.[1] The coordinate system in animals is related to landmarks on the skull. However, it was not until 1947 when Spiegel and Wycis[2] used internal landmarks within the brain visualized by intraoperative x-ray that stereotactic techniques became accurate enough to use in patients. When computed tomography (CT) was introduced around 1974 and magnetic resonance (MR) imaging in 1985, techniques were developed to use those images to direct a probe at any target lesion seen in the imaging study.[3-7]

Functional Stereotactic Surgery

The first clinical stereotactic procedures involved *functional neurosurgery*, that is, techniques were used to change the function of a malfunctioning nervous system.[2,8-10] Such neurosurgery involves correction of movement disorders, alleviation of severe intractable pain, localization of epileptogenic foci, or modification of behavioral disorders. Functional neurosurgery is still an important and growing use of stereotaxis today. There are also many stereotactic techniques in functional neurosurgery. A few examples are cordotomy or spinal cord stimulation to treat cancer or chronic pain, or techniques to insert a needle into the gasserian ganglion under x-ray guidance to apply an electrical current or inject substances to partially deaden the trigeminal nerve to treat trigeminal neuralgia.

Study of the history of clinical stereotactic neurosurgery reveals how it has changed as technological advances in related fields have been incorporated into clinical techniques.[3] During the first three decades after its introduction in the late 1940s, clinical stereotactic surgery depended on intraoperative x-ray visualization of landmarks within the brain, ordinarily structures adjacent to the third ventricle.[9] The landmarks were demonstrated at first with pneumoencephalography and later with positive contrast ventriculography. An atlas, which represented the anatomy of a representative brain, was consulted to measure the relationship between the visualized landmarks, most commonly the anterior and posterior commissures, and the intended target, such as the ventral lateral nucleus of the thalamus or the medial globus pallidus, which could not be directly visualized on x-ray.[9,11,12] Because of variability of the size and shape of individual brains, such localization can be only approximate. Once an electrode was in the proper neighborhood, however, the area could be explored by stimulation and electronic recording to identify the target with great accuracy. Such neurophysiologic techniques remain the basis of stereotactic functional neurosurgery even today. After localization, the target is destroyed by making a small lesion to interrupt the neurons in and passing through the target. A high-frequency (radiofrequency) electrical current has been most commonly used, which heats the immediately surrounding tissue to a temperature that produces coagulation. Other techniques have involved the use of direct current, freezing, mechanical disruption, or even the use of radioisotopes.

Because of the requirement in functional neurosurgery for intraoperative physiologic testing to verify that the proper target had been hit or to assess the immediate effects of producing a lesion, it is usually necessary to operate under local anesthesia. Coordination between the neurosurgeon and the anesthesiologist is critical because many sedatives or anesthetic agents alter the neurologic activity that is important to verify a target.[13-15] The procedure may be long and stressful, so it is necessary to ensure the patient's comfort and safety, attain patient cooperation, and monitor the patient closely, all without compromising the necessary neurophysiologic observations. In the 1940s through the 1960s, few agents were available to accomplish these goals safely without compromising neurophysiologic target localization.

Functional stereotactic surgery was an important and widely used treatment for Parkinson's disease during the 1950s and most of the 1960s, with thousands of such operations being performed each year.[10,16–18] However, when L-dopa was introduced in 1968, stereotactic surgery for Parkinson's disease almost came to a halt. The field of stereotactic surgery was preserved at several academic institutions but was little used for the next decade.[3]

When CT scanning was introduced in 1972, it was only natural that it would become married to stereotactic surgery.[4] Both systems are organized in Cartesian space, both involve visualization of the internal anatomy of the brain, and both can localize a specific point within the brain in relation to other identifiable cerebral structures.

It was possible for the first time with CT to visualize directly an abnormal mass within the brain and to localize it in three dimensions with accuracy. Each slice of an axial scan provided information to localize any point within the head in two dimensions (anteroposterior and lateral). It was necessary to measure accurately the location of the slice in space to obtain the third dimension (vertical).[19,20] The most common way that is now accomplished is by attaching to a frame secured to the patient's head a series of straight and diagonal rods, each of which is intersected by each axial slice. The vertical coordinate is a reflection of the height of the slice above the frame and can be calculated by the position of the diagonal rods in relation to the vertical rods. Thus, the location of these fiducial rods makes it possible to calculate from information on a single two-dimensional slice the precise position of any point in three dimensions, providing all the information necessary to direct a probe to the target point with accuracy limited only by the thickness of the CT (or MR) slice.[21]

The ability to target directly any mass seen on CT or MR scanning opened up a new field, that of imaging-based stereotactic surgery. The position in space of a mass identified on imaging could be defined with great accuracy to insert a probe to any given point within the mass. It became possible to biopsy previously inaccessible masses, to aspirate abscesses or cysts, or to insert radioactive isotopes or cannulae into which such isotopes might be inserted to irradiate tumors from the inside out. It became feasible for a surgeon to direct a resection of a tumor volume defined by the edge of an enhancing mass on imaging by defining a point or a series of points stereotactically, each of which was identified on a two-dimensional image.[22]

The field of imaging-based stereotactic surgery advanced to an even more sophisticated level when three-dimensional computerized reconstruction of the head and its contents became possible. The data from a CT or MR scan is transferred by tape or Ethernet into a computer work station. By stacking the images of the head, each slice could be piled accurately on the other. By including a fiducial system on the scan, the position of each locus within the head could be accurately identified in stereotactic space. To define a mass lesion, the border of the target is outlined in each of the individual two-dimensional slices on which it appears. When all the slices are stacked in the computer, the edges of the mass are filled in, or interpolated, to form a three-dimensional volume. The position, size, shape, and orientation of the target mass are then used to direct the surgeon during tumor resection or other stereotactic treatment.[22–24]

Stereotactic radiosurgery can also use the same three-dimensional reconstruction to direct a specific high dose of radiation to a mass with minimal radiation to overlying cerebral structures. Radiation can be applied from an external source. There can be multiple radiation sources, as in the gamma knife,[24] or a linear accelerator x-ray beam can be successively directed from many angles,[25] as with linear accelerator-based stereotactic radiosurgery such as the XKnife. In *brachytherapy* or *interstitial radiation,* isotopes can be placed temporarily or permanently inside a tumor to radiate it from within, which is interstitial radiation or brachytherapy.[26]

Because the same landmarks used with ventriculography in functional neurosurgery can also be visualized on CT or MR, it has become possible to perform functional stereotactic surgery without the need for an invasive injection of contrast into the ventricle or intraoperative x-ray. For instance, the anterior and posterior commissures can be visualized on both sagittal and axial MR and used to target a variety of anatomic structures for electrode insertion.

Renewed activity in functional stereotactic neurosurgery for movement disorders has coincided with advances in image-based stereotaxis. Also, as it has become increasing apparent that L-dopa does not offer permanent control of parkinsonian disability, there has been a renewed interest in the use of stereotactic surgery to treat patients with Parkinson's disease. At the forefront of that revival is the production of lesions in the globus pallidus, stereotactic pallidotomy. Such surgery may alleviate some of the severe side effects of long-term L-dopa administration, such as dyskinesia, a repeated sudden fluctuation between severe dyskinesia, on the one hand, and severe rigidity and bradykinesia or freezing, the so-called on-off phenomenon.[27] Because the symptoms vary widely, depending on the response to the prior dose of medication, parkinsonian patients are particularly fragile and require close monitoring both during and after surgery.[28]

Other movement disorders treated with stereotactic surgery include hemiballism, dyskinesia, and tremors of other etiologies.[16] Regardless of the movement disorder, the target generally involves the same extrapyramidal loop within the basal ganglia. That reverberating pathway is essential for smooth motor control and regulation of muscle tone and extends from the secondary motor cortex to the putamen, then to the globus pallidus (pallidum), then by way of the ansa lenticularis and lenticular fasciculus to the ventrolateral and ventral intermediate area of the thalamus, from which it returns to the cortex. The best target for tremor, regardless of etiology, lies in the thalamus, in the ventral lateral nucleus, or the ventral intermediate nucleus (V. im), the target for a thalamotomy. It is presently held that the best target for bradykinesia, rigidity, and side effects of L-dopa lies in the ventral posterior pallidum, the target for stereotactic pallidotomy.

Certain types of pain are also managed by functional stereotactic surgery, particularly cancer pain, and especially that involving the head or neck, which is too high for a cordotomy, which involves interrupting the pain pathways in the spinal cord. That same spinothalamic pathway can be interrupted in the midbrain, however, so that the patient may have loss of pin stick pain sensation over the entire contralateral body, limbs, face, and head.[29] Even so, the patient may still complain of severe incapacitating cancer pain. In addition, if the multisynaptic pathway extending to the limbic system is also interrupted just medial to the spinothalamic tract, the patient may have relief of the suffering as well as the somatic pain, with a much more satisfactory clinical result.

Another common target for stereotactic treatment of cancer pain is in the thalamus, where the primary target is in the intralaminar area or centrum medianum, those areas involved with the limbic system.[30,31] Pain of neuropathic origin, such as infiltration of the brachial plexus with a Pancoast tumor, may also respond to such surgery.[32]

PROCEDURE

The general procedure of stereotactic surgery involves several discrete steps often in different locations. Depending on the individual hospital, the initial stage may occur in the operating room, the CT scanning room, or in an induction area adjacent to the MR or CT scanner. After appropriate monitoring is established, the head ring is applied to the patient's head by means of pins or rods that extend through the scalp and fix tightly to the skull. A fiducial localizing system, usually involving radiopaque rods or beads, is attached to the head ring or frame, and the appropriate imaging study is done. In most institutions, the patient is then transported to the operating room while the measurements and calculations are done on the scanner console or films. The patient is moved to the operating table. Many stereotactic head frames can also be used as head holders by attaching them to the operating table, often through an adjustable bracket. Depending on the procedure, all or only a small area may be shaved. Draping may be minimal, as for a biopsy or functional surgery, or elaborate, as for a stereotactic-directed craniotomy. After the surgery, the head ring is removed.

Anesthetic Considerations

The anesthetic management for all stereotactic surgical procedures begins outside the operating room. Some of the most challenging anesthetics to administer are those managed in a non-operating room location. The lack of the familiar operating room environment with available personnel who are familiar with the needs of the anesthesiologist can make routine procedures and techniques extremely difficult. In an emergency, the anesthesiologist must have all necessary equipment close at hand.

In many institutions, the patients must be transported long distances for all stereotactic cases, either in the middle or a multistep procedure or at the conclusion of the required neuroradiologic study. This frequently involves passage through long hospital corridors and can include several elevator rides to move from the CT scanner or the MR scanner or to return to the operating room and the postanesthesia care unit. The management of the anesthetized patient for all stereotactic cases must provide the ideal conditions for the necessary radiologic studies while maintaining the patient's safety at all times during the series of planned procedures.

The anesthesiologist must be thoroughly familiar with the neuroradiology suite and available equipment. The time required for setting up and checking equipment will be much greater than for even the most complex procedure in a standard operating room.

Whether the procedure requires general anesthesia or monitored anesthesia care, the requirements for a thorough preanesthesia evaluation are the same for patients scheduled for stereotactic surgery as those for any other surgical procedure. The evaluation must include a careful medical history, necessary consultations from subspecialists if indicated by the history, and all appropriate laboratory studies. If the stereotactic procedure is done with MR, a careful history must be obtained regarding implanted ferrous metals that are attracted to the magnet, for example, iron, cobalt, and nickel. Patients with pacemakers are not candidates for MR because the pacemaker may revert to an asynchronous mode or fail completely. Displacement of leads secondary to the magnetic torque has even been reported, and use of non-MR compatible leads can cause enough distortion in the magnetic field to introduce significant error in the stereotactic targeting, which requires a homogeneous magnetic field. Additional care must be taken to determine if any ferromagnetic materials have been used during previous surgical procedures. Metallic foreign bodies in vital areas (brain, eye, cardiac valve) are likely to cause damage as a result of torque and displacement secondary to attraction by the magnet.[33,34] Eye makeup using certain pigments may heat enough in the magnetic field to burn the eyelids.

In addition, the anesthesiologist and the neurosurgeon must discuss the anesthetic requirements for each patient. Few other surgical procedures require such continual modifications of the requirements for anesthesia or such close and active collaboration between the surgical and anesthesia teams.

The explanation to the patient of the requirements for anesthesia should address each step in the events of these complex procedures. The informed patient is far more cooperative.

It cannot be stressed enough that the patient becomes an active participant when the stereotactic procedure is conducted under local anesthesia. For much of the procedure, the anesthesiologist is the one in the most favorable position to communicate with the patient, for often the surgeon is standing behind the patient. Active, concerned, involved communication is the first and the most important agent to allay the patient's anxiety, lessen pain perception, and minimize the need for pharmacologic agents throughout the procedure. The patient is awake, so it is inexcusable for anyone in the operating room to carry on an unrelated conversation that indicates to the patient lack of concern or attention. Calm reassurance and explanation constitute an important part of anesthesia care.

During much of the procedure and associated sedation, the surgeon rather than the anesthesiologist is at the patient's head. Any surgeon should know the basics of maintaining the patient's airway by elevating the jaw and should be alert for and communicate with the anesthesiologist at the first sign of airway insufficiency.

When heavy sedation of intravenous anesthesia is required for head ring placement, the patient passes through a phase of uninhibited poor self-control while emerging from narcosis. Scanning, especially MR, may coincide with this phase and require that sedation be prolonged through the imaging procedure. If excessively deep sedation or long-acting agents can be minimized during the early stages, it may be possible to time the changing levels of sedation to avoid the need for deep sedation during the scan. (See also Chap. 21.)

MONITORED ANESTHESIA CARE

For many stereotactic procedures the only painful portion is the attachment of the head ring at the very beginning of the process. Monitored anesthesia care (MAC) is an ideal way to care for these patients. Heavy sedation can be administered in conjunction with local infiltration of the scalp at the site of pin placement. It is important, however, that if neurophysiologic monitoring is planned, no agent is used that would interfere with that monitoring later in the procedure. The actual placement of the head ring takes less than 5 min. The patient can then be allowed to awaken following the attachment of the ring and the radiologic procedure can be done without further sedation. The only requirement for a successful radiologic study is that the patient does not move during the scanning process. Because the procedure is not painful, most patients can handle this without difficulty.

General anesthesia presents particular problems with patients undergoing MR. The MR head ring for most systems obscures access to the patient's face, so intubation must be done before the head ring is applied. Some, but not all, CT head rings have adequate access to the patient's airway, so the intubation and extubation can be accomplished during the procedure.

If the airway were to become compromised during the procedure, the head ring may prevent adequate access to clear the airway or to intubate the patient. Consequently, *it is very important that the tools required to remove the head ring in an emergency remain with the patient throughout the entire procedure.* It would be disastrous to have an airway emergency as the patient arrives in the operating room and find that the wrench to remove the head ring was left behind in the radiology suite.

There are differences in the amount of sedation or anesthesia required, however, based on whether the patient must undergo CT scanning or MR. CT scans are generally of much shorter duration than MR studies and do not require complete immobilization for the duration of the scan. Less of the patient's body is surrounded by machinery in the CT scanner and there is less noise. Emotional distress during MR has been found to occur in about 9 percent of adult patients.[35] The level of distress was great enough in these patients to prevent adequate scanning. Patients who do not tolerate the confined space and the attendant noise are more common in the pediatric population and this approaches 100 percent at the age of 7 to 8 years. Transient claustrophobia has been reported to occur in 1 to 5 percent of the adult population undergoing MR scanning.[36] Some degree of sedation in all patients makes the experience of MR more pleasant. Patients who are being treated for movement disorders may require enough sedation to suppress the involuntary movements during the MR scan. For some patients heavy sedation or even general anesthesia may be best even through the procedure does not cause any physical pain. This may create a dilemma in functional surgery where the patient must be awake during the operative portion of the procedure. If even the greatest effort will not allow imaging to be done with safe sedation, it may not be possible to offer the patient the benefit of such surgery. It is generally *not* feasible to intubate the patient, apply the head ring, scan the patient, and then extubate the patient to do the remainder of the procedure under local monitored anesthesia.

Venous air embolism is a potential complication of stereotactic surgery under local anesthesia (MAC), which may not be immediately apparent. The clinical presentation is very much different than under general anesthesia. The episode may begin wtih a cough or perhaps a period of uncontrollable coughing. The patient may experience chest pain or tightness, along with a feeling of anxiety or apprehension, not unlike a myocardial infarction.[37] Vital signs are initially unchanged, but the pulse rate may then rise. It is only if the episode continues unrecognized or untreated that the patient may abruptly develop labored breathing and shock.[38] Management begins at the first recognizable cough, with the surgeon irrigating the incision to fill the subdural space with saline to replace the air that may enter along side the electrode or biopsy cannula. The entire opening in the bone is then occluded with wet gelfoam to prevent further introduction of air. The backrest of the operating table is lowered, or the entire table tilted in the Trendelenburg position. After the episode subsides, which may take 2 or 3 min, the procedure may usually be completed in safety, as long as the patient has returned to neurologic and physiologic baseline.

ADVANTAGES AND DISADVANTAGES OF MAC

Most functional stereotactic procedures require that the patient be awake during the later critical part of the surgery. Even when not required for neurophysiologic monitoring, however, there are more advantages of MAC for CT and MR stereotactic procedures than disadvantages. The neurosurgeon frequently needs to communicate with the patient during biopsy procedures, and good verbal communication is mandatory

during functional procedures. If bleeding or other complications were to occur, it would be apparent much sooner. For the anesthesiologist, the primary advantage is that the patients control their own airway, which brings an increased degree of safety during all periods of patient transport and positioning.[39]

The main disadvantage of MAC for stereotactic procedures is the rare occurrence of loss of airway requiring emergency management. If jaw thrust and airway opening in conjunction with stopping the sedating agents are not sufficient to restore adequate ventilation, the head ring may have to be removed for emergency intubation. This takes less than a minute, but the entire stereotactic procedure would have to be started over because the crucial positioning of the coordinates has been disrupted. Alternatively, the patient may be intubated with the head ring in place, which may require a flexible fiberoptic scope. In our practice, airway difficulties requiring removal of the head ring have occurred only once in almost 500 cases. However, in six cases, the patient was too agitated to proceed, even when the amount of sedation approached respiratory depression, so the procedure was aborted. All six patients returned within a few days and had the stereotactic biopsy performed successfully under general anesthesia. Newer CT head rings take this into account and are designed with sufficient access to the face to manage the airway without removing the ring.

MONITORING STANDARDS

Standards of monitoring have been set by the American Society of Anesthesiologists. These standards include (1) the required presence of qualified anesthesia personnel (remote monitoring, i.e., television, is occasionally required for personal safety, for instance, in the radiology suite); (2) monitoring of oxygenation, including oxygen analyzer, and a pulse oximeter; (3) monitoring of ventilation, ideally using capnography; (4) monitoring circulatory function, including electrocardiography (ECG), blood pressure, and auscultation of heart sounds or pulse plethysmography (oximetry); and (5) a readily available means to measure patient temperature continuously.[40]

It is necessary to follow these standards at all anesthetizing locations. Problems with monitoring in radiology suites have been well described.[41-46] MR creates unique and difficult requirements on equipment to be used for anesthesia and monitoring because of the powerful magnetic field. Virtually all anesthetic equipment contains ferromagnetic materials, which precludes its use in the MR. Modifications to standard equipment have been described,[44,47-49] and manufacturers now produce equipment specifically designed for use at the MR site.[42,43,45] It is extremely important for the anesthesiologist to be actively involved in the design and equipment purchases for the MR installation.

Monitoring equipment especially designed for the MR is available, and most of this equipment functions appropriately during the scanning procedure.[50] Difficulty does exist with the ECG interpretation because artifacts do occur.[50-52] The ECG is frequently distorted to the point that only the ventricular rate can be determined.

There have been multiple reports of cases of first-, second-, and third-degree burns that have occurred in the MR scanner,[53,54] primarily from the oscillating radiofrequency magnetic field.[53] Particular care must be used in the placement of all cables, leads, and wires (ECG leads and cable, pulse oximetry probe and cable). No potential conductor should be allowed to come in contact with the patient's skin at more than one location. Coils and loops must be removed from all cables, leads, and wires. Only equipment designated to be MR compatible should be used. An important concern is to use only MR-compatible oxygen or gas tanks on the anesthesia equipment. Fatal injury to the patient has been reported when an oxygen tank was violently pulled into the magnet with the patient in postiion for scanning.

One final practical consideration, the anesthesiologist must check his or her own personal equipment to make sure that it will not be attracted to the magnet or destroyed. Magnetically coded items (credit cards, bank cards, digital watches, audio or video tapes) may be altered or erased by the magnetic field. Pens, clipboards, scissors, and metal connectors on earpieces may be attracted by the magnet. A careful pocket check before entering the magnetic field will eliminate these difficulties.

AGENTS

Many different methods of anesthesia for MR and CT have been described.[42,55-62] These range from conscious sedation from oral medications, intramuscular injections, or intravenous administration to unconscious sedation and general anesthesia. Agents used have included cocktails of atropine-meperidine-promethazine, ketamine, secobarbital, thiopental, pentobarbital, chloral hydrate, diazepam, methohexital, midazolam, fentanyl, and propofol.

Good communication is required between the surgeon and the anesthesiologist to establish the anesthesia requirements before the case begins. If neurophysiologic monitoring is to be done, significant constraints are imposed on the amount and duration of sedation. Otherwise, patient comfort and safety are the primary considerations in selection of a sedative agent.

We now use propofol as the primary component of our anesthetic technique for most CT and MR procedures, including those that require general anesthesia.

Induction of anesthesia is carried out after all standard monitoring equipment is in place. For sedation and head ring placement we administer midazolam (0.01 to 0.06 mg/kg) at 0.5-mg intervals until the patient is relaxed but still readily communicates when asked questions. This is followed with intravenous lidocaine (0.5 mg/kg) prior to the slow administration of propofol (0.5 to 1.5 mg/kg) observing for onset of heavy sedation without loss of spontaneous ventilation. The scalp is infiltrated with 1% lidocaine with epinephrine 1:100,000 (2 to 3 ml) at each pin site. If the patient is uncomfortable during the pin placement from the sensation of squeezing of the skull, additional amounts of propofol (10 mg) are administered. Appropriate pediatric doses for propofol have been reported.[58,63] For children aged 1 to 10 years, induction doses of propofol 1.5 to 2 mg/kg followed by a constant infusion rate of 100 μg/kg per min are generally effective.

Management is similar for functional stereotactic surgery where intraoperative neurophysiologic or neurologic clinical monitoring is required, except to limit to a single initial dose of midazolam and to discontinue propofol and all other sedatives no later than the conclusion of scanning.

CRANIOTOMY UNDER LOCAL ANESTHESIA

Some functional neurosurgical procedures require open craniotomy under local anesthesia, particularly if mapping of functional cortical areas is necessary before tumor resection or if such functional areas and epileptogenic foci must be identified before resection for the treatment of epilepsy. Such procedures have been facilitated enormously by the introduction of pulse oximetry and propofol anesthesia. Oximetry allows deep sedation while ensuring adequate oxygenation. Propofol allows an anesthetic level of sedation without a long-lasting suppression of the electrocorticogram or depth electroencephalogram.

The patient is prepared as for any craniotomy, but long-lasting suppressive agents are avoided. The initial positioning and application of the head holder are performed under propofol anesthesia without intubation, which makes it possible to use a three-point head holder, such as the Mayfield, to hold the patient's head securely in position throughout the surgery. We have had patients remain solidly in position even with a grand mal seizure with the cranium opened and the head thus secured.[64] Local anesthesia (ordinarily Xylocaine 1% with epinepherine 1:100,000) is administered to block each of the nerves innervating the scalp (the supraorbital, occipital, and temporal nerves) and along the line of incision, as well as deep to the temporalis fascia to ensure good denervation of all tissues to be incised, including the temporalis muscle. The sites of penetration of the invasive points for the head holder are thoroughly infiltrated.

The patient may sleep under propofol anesthesia as the bone flap is fashioned. If the patient is asleep, either a hand drill and Gigli saw or a power burr hole and craniotome can be used, but if the patient is only sedated or only lightly anesthetized, it is better to avoid noisy power instruments. The dura has sensation that cannot be blocked until it is exposed by stripping it from the inner table, which is best done with the patient asleep. The dura can be anesthetized very rapidly on exposure to the local anesthetic, which can be used to irrigate the surface of the dura as it is uncovered. Once it is anesthetized, however, all sedation may be discontinued and priority given to neurophysiologic recording and the patient's conscious participation in the procedure, which may take from 1 to 6 h. The patient must remain calm and comfortable with a minimum of pharmacologic sedation throughout that time. Actively reassuring communication with the patient is important and can best be done by the anesthesiologist.

Once the tissue to be resected has been defined, sedation or anesthesia may be resumed. Because manipulation of blood vessels causes pain, and because it is not possible to provide sufficient local anesthesia before manipulation or coagulation of vessels, resumption of propofol anesthesia may be necessary. It must be kept in mind, however, that additional recording may be done after resection, so a mutually acceptable plan should be discussed between the surgeon and anesthesiologist. Once postresection recording has been completed, the patient may be allowed to sleep during the closure. The scalp is blocked by injecting the supraorbital, occipital, and temporal nerves as well.

USE OF GENERAL ANESTHESIA

If the stereotactic case will require general anesthesia in the operating room for an extensive surgical procedure after scanning, general anesthesia is most safely induced before the head ring is placed. The difficulties of transporting an intubated anesthetized patient must be carefully considered. Thoughtful preparation will make this difficult task safer for the patient and less anxiety producing for the anesthesiologist. If general anesthesia is planned, it is desirable to have a knowledgeable anesthesia assistant available to assist the anesthesiologist throughout the procedure and transportation. If an airway accessible CT head ring is available and if only a CT scan is required, there is the option of doing the imaging study under local anesthesia (MAC), transferring the patient to the operating room, and there intubating the patient under general anesthesia, in which case endoscopic intubation may be the best technique.

The induction of general anesthesia is carried out, in either case, after all standard monitoring equipment is in place. In the CT scanner this is often done on the operating room stretcher, which is immediately adjacent to the radiologic table. The area is small and the mobility is severely limited. The radiologic table is not equipped to provide the Trendelenburg position. If MR is required as the first radiologic study, anesthesia is induced in a separate induction area where a standard anesthesia machine and equipment can be safely used, and an MR-compatible ventilator or anesthesia machine must be available at the scanner.

Many different techniques have been reported for general anesthesia in the CT and MR scanner.[44,45,47,62,65–67] The range includes paralysis with pancuronium and ventilation in the critically ill patient, total intravenous techniques using thiopental, narcotics, propofol, or inhalation techniques using specially adapted circuits. We feel that total intravenous techniques offer the greatest safety for the patient, less interaction and interference with the scanning equipment, and significantly increased ease of transport.

Our standard induction technique begins with midazolam (0.01 to 0.06 mg/kg) at 0.5-mg intervals until the patient is relaxed but still readily communicates when asked questions. This is followed with lidocaine (0.5 mg/kg) and D-tubocurare (3 mg) prior to the slow administration of propofol (1 to 2.5 mg/kg). When the patient is unresponsive and has no lid reflex, succinylcholine (1.5 to 2 mg/kg) is administered. At laryngoscopy the vocal cords are further anesthetized with topical 4% lidocaine. Once intubated, the patient is allowed to recover from the succinylcholine. We maintain anesthesia with a propofol infusion of 75 to 150 μg/kg per min. If controlled ventilation is required we use the Bio-Med IC-2A or Omni-Ventilator Series DHBC ventilator in the MR scanner, although other MR compatible anesthesia machines are commercially available.

The head ring is applied while the patient is recovering from the relaxant and takes only a few minutes. For MR, the patient is then positioned on the moveable MR stretcher, which is used to transport the patient to the scanner inside the large shielded room. Care is taken to remove all ferromagnetic objects (laryngoscope) from the transport gantry. It is important to use only MR compatible ECG leads. With the patient spontaneously ventilating the patient is positioned in the MR scanner and the initial study completed under propofol anesthesia. Transportation to the operating room is accomplished with propofol anesthesia and appropriate monitors.

We do not use the laryngeal mask airway for stereotactic procedures that require general anesthesia because (1) the head position cannot be changed in the operating room once the surgical procedure is underway; (2) the anesthesiologist will have very limited access to the airway; (3) controlled ventilation will be required intraoperatively, and (4) the MR head ring interferes with proper positioning of the mask. Considerations for general anesthesia in the pediatric population are addressed in depth in pediatric textbooks.[66,67]

Nonstereotactic Functional Neurosurgery

The pain pathways may be interrupted at levels below the brain, which does not involve cerebral stereotactic techniques per se. The most established procedure involves interruption of pain pathways within the spinal cord, or anterolateral cordotomy. This procedure has been a staple of cancer pain management since its introduction at the turn of this century.[68] It involves interrupting the pain pathway in the lateral spinothalamic tract as it ascends in the anterolateral edge of the spinal cord, where it is separated from the nerves conducting touch and proprioception in the posterior columns and the motor fibers, which are more dorsal in the lateral funiculus. The original technique, which is still often done, involved a laminectomy, usually under general anesthesia, to expose the spinal cord and the section of the anterior outer quadrant with a sharp blade. Anesthesia is the same as for any other laminectomy, although the use of epidural anesthesia has been described, which allows sensory testing to control the incision in the spinal cord.

Percutaneous cervical cordotomy was introduced in the 1960s to insert an isotope[69] or a needle electrode under x-ray guidance at the C2[70] or lower cervical levels[71,72] to interrupt those same pathways with the heating effect of a radiofrequency current, providing equivalent pain relief without the necessity of a surgical exposure. The percutaneous procedure is done under local anesthesia, so the position of the electrode may be monitored by stimulation and the effect of the lesion as it is produced. These procedures are not truly stereotactic, in that they do not involve a three-dimensional Cartesian coordinate system, but rely on the visualization of the landmarks about the spinal canal in the vicinity of the target. MAC is important for this percutaneous technique because it is necessary to test for sensory loss after production of each increment of the lesion and to test for motor function to ensure safety. Midazolam may provide sufficient sedation to allay anxiety without interference with clinical testing during the cordotomy.

Such interruption of pain pathways is most appropriate for cancer pain, but other techniques are more appropriate for chronic pain of benign origin that involve spinal cord stimulation. Originally based on the Melzack-Wall gate control theory,[73] the observation

was made that stimulation of the large non-pain fibers that happen to be gathered in the dorsal columns might "close the gate" to inhibit pain signals entering the spinal cord by the small pain-transmitting C fibers.[74]

The implantation is done in two stages.[75] The first requires MAC. An electrode is introduced into the epidural space through a Tuohy needle under local anesthesia, so the position of the electrode may be readjusted until stimulation produces projection of sensation to the general area of the patient's pain. The patient must report the sensation as stimulation is applied to various pairs of the several contacts of the electrode, which had been inserted. Ordinarily a several day period of trial stimulation is then done to ensure that the patient has pain relief and tolerates the sensation of the stimulator. If the result is good, the electrode is attached at a separate surgery under general anesthesia to a stimulator inserted under the skin at a convenient site. Some stimulators contain a lithium battery, are totally implantable, and are controlled with an external computer that communicates through a radio signal. Other stimulators involve an implanted portion that does have a power supply incorporated; both the control and the energy for the stimulation impulse are transmitted through the skin by a radiofrequency signal from a battery-operated control unit the patient carries.

One other percutaneous pain procedure has particular challenges for the anesthesiologist, that of trigeminal rhizotomy.[76] Partial interruption or injection of the gasserian ganglion usually involves fluoroscopic visualization of the base of the skull to identify the landmarks allowing localization of the foramen ovale, through which the mandibular nerve, the third division of the trigeminal nerve, exits the skull. A needle inserted through this opening may be advanced along the anterior border of the petrous ridge to Meckel's cave, a folding of the dura housing the trigeminal gasserian ganglion. Injection of glycerol or other neurolytic substance is usually done into the ganglion itself. Interruption of nerve fibers by radiofrequency heating may selectively involve individual one or two divisions distal to the ganglion.

Injection procedures may require patient participation to identify when the ganglion is entered, but more often are based solely on radiologic targeting. Radiofrequency coagulation of individual divisions of the nerve, on the other hand, requires that the patient be able to report when low threshold electrical stimulation indicates that the electrode is in contact with the proper division, which presents a special anesthetic challenge. The patient, who is often elderly, must be calm enough to allow insertion of the needle-electrode through the cheek and allow probing of the base of the skull to find the foramen. Penetration of the dura at the foramen is particularly painful, but almost immediately thereafter the patient must be alert enough to cooperate with stimulation localization of the electrode. Threshold stimulation is applied and the patient reports where the sensation is felt. The patient must then be asleep for the application of the heating current for 30 to 60 s, which would be intolerably painful if the patient were awake. Local anesthetic cannot be used because it would cause a loss of indicators of nerve function. Immediately after lesion production, the patient must be alert enough to test for loss of sensation with a pin. If sensory loss is inadequate or if more than one division is involved, the procedure is repeated. The patient must be alert enough to help again with electrode stimulation for localization. The lesion may have to be repeated two or three times, each time with the patient asleep and immediately afterward awake for testing.

To add to the difficulty, the face is in the surgical field, and inaccessible to the anesthesiologist. The electrode insertion is so close to the nose that there is insufficient room to insert a nasal oxygen catheter, but oxygen may be allowed to flow over the face from tubing placed just below the patient's chin.

The neurosurgeon should prep the cheeks and also angles of jaw bilaterally, because it may be necessary for the surgeon to hold the jaw forward to maintain the airway when the patient is fully anesthetized, so the surgeon should be familiar with this maneuver. Excellent communication must be maintained between the neurosurgeon and anesthesiologist, and both must be thoroughly familiar with the anesthetic requirements.

The availability of propofol has significantly improved anesthesia management for radiofrequency trigeminal rhizotomy. Although sufficient midazolam may ensure that the patient is not too anxious to cooperate and to hold still, intermittent intravenous anesthesia is required. In addition, intravenous anesthesia may be required during penetration of the dura at the foramen ovale, depending on how difficult it is to find. Minimal doses of propofol are desirable because the patient must be awake immediately after penetration of the needle to report sensation produced by stimulation of the nerve. After the electrode is properly localized, deeper anesthesia without respiratory depression is required for the 60 s that the nerve is heated for lesion production. The patient must then awaken for sensory testing. If there is still inadequate sensory loss, the stimulation and lesion-making cycles may have to be repeated several times.

References

1. Horsley V, Clarke RH: The structure and functions of the cerebellum examined by a new method. *Brain* 1908; 31:45.
2. Spiegel EA, et al: Stereotaxic apparatus for operations on the human brain. *Science* 1947; 106:349.
3. Gildenberg PL: Whatever happened to stereotactic surgery? *Neurosurgery* 1987; 20:983.
4. Gildenberg PL: Computerized tomography and stereotactic surgery. In Spiegel EA (ed): *Guided Brain Operations*. Basel, Karger, 1982:24–34.
5. Heilbrun MP: *Stereotactic Neurosurgery. Concepts in Neurosurgery*, vol. 2. Baltimore, Williams & Wilkins, 1988.
6. Gildenberg PL, et al: Calculation of stereotactic coordinates from the computer tomographic scan. *Neurosurgery* 1982; 10:580.
7. Kelly PJ: Applications and methodology for contemporary stereotactic surgery. *Neurol Res* 1986; 8:2.
8. Spiegel EA, et al: Effect of thalamic and pallidal lesions upon involuntary movements in choreoathetosis. *Trans Am Neurol Assoc* 1950; 75:234.
9. Spiegel, EA, Wycis HT: *Stereoencephalotomy, Part I*. New York, Grune & Stratton, 1952.
10. Hassler R, Riechert T: Indikationen und Lokalisationsmethode der gezielten Hirnoperationen. *Nervenarzt* 1954; 25:441.
11. Talairach J, et al: Atlas d'anatomie stereotaxique, 1957.
12. Schaltenbrand G, Bailey P: *Introduction to Stereotaxis with an Atlas of the Human Brain*. Stuttgart, Thieme, 1959.
13. Gildenberg PL: Surgery for seizures. In Frost EAM (ed): *Clinical Anesthesia in Neurosurgery*. Boston, Butterworth, 1984:265–278.
14. Gildenberg PL: Stereotactic surgery. In Frost EAM (ed): *Clinical Anesthesia in Neurosurgery*, Boston, Butterworth, 1984:293–315.
15. Zukic A, Kelly PJ: Neuroleptic analgesia for stereotactic surgery. *Appl Neurophysiol* 1983; 46:167.
16. Gildenberg PL: Functional neurosurgery. In Schmidek HH, Sweet WH, (eds): *Operative Neurosurgical Techniques*, 2d ed. New York, 1988:1035–1068.
17. Cooper IS: Results of 1000 consecutive basal ganglia operations for parkinsonism. *Ann Intern Med* 1960; 52:483.
18. Spiegel EA, Wycis HT: *Stereoencephalotomy. Part II. Clinical and Physiological Applications*. New York, Grune & Stratton, 1962.
19. Kaufman HH, Gildenberg PL: New head-positioning system for use with computed tomographic scanning. *Neurosurgery* 1980; 7:147.
20. Gildenberg PL: General concepts of stereotactic surgery. In Lunsford LD, (ed): *Modern Stereotactic Neurosurgery*, Boston, Martinus Nijhoff, 1988:3–12.
21. Brown RA, et al: Stereotaxic frame and computer software for CT-directed neurosurgical localization. *Invest Radiol* 1980; 15:308.
22. Kelly PJ: Stereotactic technology in tumor surgery. *Clin Neurosurg* 1989; 35:215.
23. Kelly PJ, et al: Evolution of contemporary instrumentation for computer-assisted stereotactic surgery. *Surg Neurol* 1988; 30:204.
24. Lunsford LD, et al: Image-guided stereotactic surgery: A 10-year revolutionary experience. *Stereotact Funct Neurosurg* 1990; 54–55:375.
25. Kooy HM, et al: Treatment planning for stereotactic radiosurgery of intracranial lesions. *Int J Radiat Oncol Biol Phys* 1991; 21:683.
26. Gutin PH, et al: Brachytherapy of recurrent malignant brain tumors with removable high-activity iodine-125 sources. *J Neurosurg* 1984; 60:61.
27. Laitinen LV, Hariz MI: Leksell's posteroventral pallidotomy in the treatment of Parkinson's disease. *J Neurosurg* 1992; 76:53.
28. Parr-Day K: Postanesthesia care of the pallidotomy patient. *Journal of Post Anesthesia Nursing* 1994; 9(5):274.
29. Nashold BSJ: Extensive cephalic and oral pain relieved by midbrain tractotomy. *Conf Neurol* 1972; 34:382.
30. Tasker RR: Thalamotomy. *Neurosurg Clin North Am* 1990; 1:841.

31. Watkins ES: Stereotactic thalamotomy for intractable pain. Proceedings of the American Association of Neurological Surgeons Meeting, St. Louis, 1966 (abstr).

32. Spiegel EA, Wycis HT: Present status of stereoencephalotomies for pain relief. *Conf Neurol* 1966; 27:7.

33. Shellock FG, Crues JV: MRI: Safety considerations in magnetic resonance imaging. *Magn Reson Imaging Decisions* 1988; 2:25.

34. Kelly WM, et al: Ferromagnetism of intraocular foreign body causes unilateral blindness after MR study. *Am J Neuroradiol* 1986; 7:243.

35. Flaherty JA, Hoskinson K: Emotional distress during magnetic resonance imaging. *N Engl J Med* 1989; 320:467.

36. Fishbain DA, et al: Long-term claustrophobia following magnetic resonance imaging. *Am J Psychiatry* 1988; 145:1038.

37. Gildenberg PL, et al: The efficacy of Doppler monitoring for the detection of venous air embolism. *J Neurosurg* 1981; 54:75.

38. Adornato DC, et al: Pathophysiology of intravenous air embolism in dogs. *Anesthesiology* 1978; 49:120.

39. Gildenberg PL, Katz J: Stereotactic surgery. In Frost EAM (ed): *Clinical Anesthesia in Neurosurgery*, 2d ed. Boston, Butterworth-Heinemann, 1991:383–400.

40. Standards for basic intraoperative monitoring. 1986; ASA Newsletter No. 12.

41. Karlik SJ, et al: Patient anesthesia and monitoring at a 1.5-T MRI installation. *Magn Reson Med* 1988; 7:210.

42. Patterson SK, Chesney JT: Anesthetic management for magnetic resonance imaging: Problems and solutions. *Anesth Analg* 1992; 74:121.

43. Shellock FG: Monitoring sedated pediatric patients during MR imaging. *Radiology* 1990; 177:586.

44. Nixon C, et al: Nuclear magnetic resonance: Its implications for the anaesthetist. *Anaesthesia* 1986; 41:131.

45. McArdle CB, et al: Monitoring of the neonate undergoing MR imaging: Technical considerations. *Radiology* 1986; 159:223.

46. Roth JL, et al: Patient monitoring during magnetic resonance imaging. *Anesthesiology* 1985; 62:80.

47. Smith DS, et al: Anesthetic management of acutely ill patients during magnetic resonance imaging. *Anesthesiology* 1986; 65:710.

48. Rao CC, et al: Modification of an anesthesia machine for use during magnetic resonance imaging. *Anesthesiology* 1988; 68:640.

49. Ramsay JG, et al: A ventilator for use in nuclear magnetic resonance studies. *Br J Anaesth* 1986; 58:1181.

50. Jorgensen NH, et al: ASA monitoring standards and magnetic resonance imaging. *Anesth Analg* 1994; 79:1141.

51. Dimick RN, et al: Optimizing electrocardiograph electrode placement for cardiac-gated magnetic resonance imaging. *Invest Radiol* 1987; 22:17.

52. Wendt RE, et al: Electrocardiographic gating and monitoring in NMR imaging. *Magn Reson Imaging* 1988; 6:89.

53. Kanal E, Shellock FG: Burns associated with clinical MR examinations. *Radiology* 1990; 175:585.

54. Shellock FG, Slimp GL: Severe burn of the finger caused by using a pulse oximeter during MR imaging. *AJR Am J Roentgenol* 1989; 153:1105.

55. Kain ZN, et al: A first-pass cost analysis of propofol versus barbiturates for children undergoing magnetic resonance imaging. *Anesth Analg* 1994; 79:1102.

56. Bloomfield EL, et al: Intravenous sedation for MR imaging of the brain and spine in children: Pentobarbital versus propofol. *Radiology* 1993; 186:93.

57. Thompson JR, et al: The choice of sedation for computed tomography in children: A prospective evaluation. *Radiology* 1982; 143:475.

58. Valtonen M: Anaesthesia for computerised tomography of the brain in children: A comparison of propofol and thiopentone. *Acta Anaesth Scand* 1989; 33:170.

59. Hanigan WC, et al: Clinical utility of magnetic resonance imaging in pediatric neurosurgical patients. *J Pediatr* 1986; 108:522.

60. Packer RJ, et al: Magnetic resonance imaging of lesions of the posterior fossa and upper cervical cord in childhood. *Pediatrics* 1985; 76:84.

61. Geiger RS, Cascorbi HF: Anesthesia in an NMR scanner. *Anesth Analg* 1984; 63:622.

62. Boutros A., Pavlicek W: Anesthesia for magnetic resonance imaging. *Anesth Analog* 1987; 66:367.

63. Frankville DD, et al: The dose of propofol required to prevent children from moving during magnetic resonance imaging. *Anesthesiology* 1993; 79:953.

64. Gildenberg PL, Katz J: Surgery for seizures. In Frost EAM (ed): *Clinical Anesthesia in Neurosurgery*, 2d ed. Boston, Butterworth-Heinemann, 1991:335–345.

65. Barnett GH, et al: Physiological support and monitoring of critically ill patients during magnetic resonance imaging. *J Neurosurg* 1988; 68:246.

66. Cole CJ, et al: *A Practice of Anesthesia for Infants and Children*, 2d ed. Philadelphia, WB Saunders, 1993:401–415.

67. Rasch DK, Webster DE: *Clinical Manual of Pediatric Anesthesia*, New York, McGraw-Hill, 1994.

68. Spiller WG, Martin E: The treatment of persistent pain of organic origin in the lower part of the body by division of the anterolateral column of the spinal cord. *JAMA* 1912; 58:1489.

69. Mullan S, et al: Percutaneous interruption of spinal pain tracts by means of a strontium-90 needle. *J Neurosurg* 1963; 20:931.

70. Rosomoff HL, et al: Percutaneous radiofrequency cervical cordotomy: Technique. *J Neurosurg* 1965; 23:639.

71. Lin PM, et al: An anterior approach to percutaneous lower cervical cordotomy. *J Neurosurg* 1966; 25:553.

72. Gildenberg PL: Percutaneous cervical cordotomy. *Clin Neurosurg* 1973; 21:246.

73. Melzack R, Wall PD: Pain mechanisms: A new theory. *Science* 1965; 150:971.

74. Shealy CN, et al: Electrical inhibition of pain by stimulation of the dorsal columns. Preliminary clinical report. *Anesth Analg* 1967; 46:489.

75. Hosobuchi Y, et al: Preliminary percutaneous dorsal column stimulation prior to permanent implantation. Technical note. *J Neurosurg* 1972; 37:242.

76. Gybels JM, Sweet WH: *Neurosurgical Treatment of Persistent Pain. Pain and Headache*, vol. 11. Basel, Karger, 1989.

Chapter 23

ELECTROCONVULSIVE THERAPY

LOIS L. BREADY

DEBRA S. TYLER

Electroconvulsive therapy (ECT) uses electrically induced grand mal seizures in the treatment of severe psychiatric disorders. Described over 50 years ago, it is used most often as a treatment for major depression. A *somatic* therapy, it differs in many ways from pharmacotherapies that have grown and developed more recently. The principles of ECT involve the intentional production of a grand mal seizure, induced while the patient is rendered insensible through the administration of a short-acting general anesthetic. Anesthesiologists are involved in the pre-ECT evaluation, induction of anesthesia, airway management, monitoring, and recovery of the patient, all of which may occur in areas of the hospital distant from the operating room.

Electroconvulsive therapy has been the subject of over 1800 published research studies, articles, and letters in the past decade, the majority of which have supported its safety and efficacy.[1] There are a great many details of ECT implementation, many of which are discussed elsewhere in this chapter, and there are controversies about virtually every aspect of the therapy. Controlled studies have been performed to evaluate some of the questions, and, where available, will be described. The interested reader is encouraged to refer to cited sources for futher information.

History

Throughout recorded history, there have been observations that epilepsy and schizophrenia rarely occurred together. Paracelsus used camphor to produce seizures in the sixteenth century, as a treatment for psychosis and mania. Others used this technique in the late nineteenth century. In the 1930s, a number of therapies

TABLE 23-1
Development of Convulsive Therapies for Mental Illness

1930s
  Treatments for Mental Illness
    Continuous sleep
    Leucotomy
    Insulin shock
    Seizures: Camphor, Indoklon, Metrazole
1937
  Electroconvulsive Therapy

were introduced in attempts to treat patients with severe mental illness; continuous sleep, insulin coma, leucotomy, and various convulsive therapies were described (Table 23-1). Ladislas J. von Meduna, a Hungarian neuropsychiatrist and pathologist, observed that schizophrenic patients often showed clinical improvement after epileptic seizures. He produced camphor-induced seizures in schizophrenic patients and observed some improvement. Seeking a faster and more pleasant method than the intramuscular camphor in oil, he began using intravenous pentylenetetrazol (Cardiozol, or Metrazol) in 1934. He reported on the use of this technique, including, "The best evidence for the simplicity of the procedure is the fact that 60 to 80 patients can be treated in one morning with the aid of only one assisting physician and at most two or three nurses."[2]

Other investigators described production of seizures with other means, including the injection of "vasodilator substances" into the cisterna magna by suboccipital puncture.[3] Von Meduna and others found that seizures initiated with pharmacoconvulsants such as pentylenetetrazol, other convulsant agents, and insulin were difficult to control. Occasionally, cerebral hyperexcitability resulted in continuation of seizure activity beyond a desirable end point.

In 1937 in Italy, Ugo Cerletti and Luciano Bini induced seizures in animals with an electrical stimulus.[3] They observed that placement of the electrodes on the tongue and rectum caused the death of the animals, whereas bitemporal placement resulted in more predictable convulsions. In 1939, Lothar Kalinowski and others introduced ECT to the United States. Within 2 years, electrically induced seizure therapy would largely replace pharmacoconvulsive therapies and become the leading somatic therapy for major mental disorders.

In 1957, J. C. Krantz discovered that the inhalation of hexafluorodiethylether (Indoklon) produced convulsions. The drug enjoyed a brief period of use and apparently was as effective as ECT, but it was withdrawn from the market by the manufacturer because it was not profitable.

ANESTHESIA AND IMPROVEMENTS IN ECT

The use of curare in 1940 by Bennett was a major advancement in ECT.[4] The explorations of Richard C. Gill in the Amazon jungle led to the importation of crude curare to the United States, and its purification and standardization revolutionized many areas of medical practice, including ECT. The harmful side effects of convulsions, notably associated bone and teeth fractures, could thus be controlled (before the use of curare, vertebral compression fractures occurred in about 50 percent of patients treated with ECT[5]). Gallamine was introduced in 1948 by Hughenard and Bone; however, it was not until 1951, when succinylcholine was introduced, that the current drug of choice was applied to ECT.[6,7] The introduction of the short-acting barbiturate methohexital further improved the technique of ECT because it provided a smooth induction without adversely affecting the electroconvulsion. By the 1960s, ECT had been rendered much safer with the introduction of short-acting drugs, supplemental oxygen, and ventilatory support.[6,8]

CONTROVERSIES

The advent of psychopharmacologic agents in the late 1950s slowed ECT use, and it fell into some disfavor. The anti-ECT contingent cited the "brutal" nature of the therapy, compared with pharmacologic treatment. Compelling articles about memory disturbances, specifically amnesia, helped to mobilize opposition to the treatment. In 1975 in California, ECT was severely restricted.[8] Several other states adopted similar legislation and ECT use was limited.

With time, as drug-resistant patients failed to improve, and as the political and financial pressures on medicine for rapid, cost-effective therapies have increased, the pendulum of public support has swung again, and ECT has experienced a resurgence.[7,9–15] The majority of organized medicine now supports ECT when used appropriately. The psychiatric associations of the United States, Canada, and Great Britain call ECT an effective, relatively safe treatment for a small percentage of psychiatric patients. Approximately 100,000 ECTs are administered annually in the United States (compared with about twice that number per year in the United Kingdom).

How Does Electroconvulsive Therapy Work?

PROPOSED MECHANISMS

There are a number of current theories as to the mechanism(s) of action of ECT[16,17] (Table 23-2). One point of

TABLE 23-2
Current Theories of Mechanism of ECT

Neurophysiologic
    Regional changes in blood flow
    Changes in cerebral microcirculation
    Changes in neurometabolic activity

Neuroendocrinologic
    Acute endocrine discharge of corticotropin and prolactin
    Hypothalamic peptides—antidepressin

Neurochemical
    Changes in ion transport, neurotransmitter release, and bio-
        genic amines
    Stimulation of β-adrenergic receptors

view is that the patients and their families, in their interactions with psychiatrists who firmly believe in the merits of ECT, absorb a positive expectation of the treatment, indicating that there is a strong placebo effect.[18] Several double-blind studies refute this etiology, at least as a sole explanation for the beneficial effects of ECT. Patients in those studies were subjected to standard ECT or to anesthesia without ECT ("sham ECT"). Of six studies reported in the literature,[19–24] only one failed to demonstrate a superior antidepressant effect of the "real" ECT, and that one study used a technique of ECT later shown to have low efficacy.[23] Subsequent studies by Sackheim evaluated issues such as electrode positioning and intensity of stimulation, both of which play important roles in efficacy of ECT.[25,26] Thus, there appears to be little question remaining that ECT does, in fact, have bona fide efficacy in the treatment of depressive illness apart from a placebo effect.

What, then, are other theories? These may be roughly divided into neurophysiologic, neuroendocrinologic, and neurochemical theories. The theory most strongly favored at this time is the neuroendocrinologic, and much research is ongoing in the area.

Although there is some controversy about this (as with many other aspects of ECT!), the most firmly held tenet is that *the generalized seizure is the therapeutic process of ECT*. When seizures are not successfully stimulated by subtherapeutic levels of ECT, or are blocked by drugs that raise the seizure threshold, the antidepressant efficacy is greatly reduced.[27] Seizures are less likely to be therapeutic if the stimulus is not greater than the seizure threshold. This is especially important for unilateral ECT. The speed of response of unilateral and bilateral ECT is related to the degree to which the electrical dose exceeds the seizure threshold.[28]

Seizure threshold is influenced by many variables. Factors found by some investigators to *increase seizure threshold* include male gender, bilateral electrode placement, advancing age, and repeated courses of ECT.[29] Titration of the stimulus dose is sometimes necessary

to ensure the efficacy and safety for ECT.[30] Some practitioners have reported success in producing ECT seizures in patients whose seizure threshold was elevated, by prior administration of theophylline or caffeine, or by inducing hyperventilation. These modalities are described elsewhere in the chapter.

Determination of a patient's seizure threshold is performed before ECT using a "dose titration" technique. This technique consists of successive incremental stimuli, until a seizure is observed, and the threshold is then calculated as the arithmetic mean between the stimulus required for a seizure and the previous unsuccessful stimulus. Unnecessary cognitive side effects can be avoided in patients with low seizure thresholds.[28]

PROGNOSTIC FACTORS FOR EFFICACY

Psychiatrists have attempted to identify patients most likely to benefit from ECT. O'Leary and colleagues, in the Nottingham ECT trial, studied prospectively the power of delusions or agitation to predict response to ECT, using a simulated treatment control group. They found that neither delusions nor agitation predicted greater treatment response.[31] Other investigators have looked at a variety of other indicators (e.g., physical signs, neuroendocrine values), but no useful correlations have been identified to date.

Indications for ECT in 1996[6,12,30]

In 1990, the American Psychiatric Association (APA) published a task force report on ECT.[30] They reported data validating the efficacy of ECT for all subtypes of major depression and mania, as well as for psychotic schizophrenia exacerbations with catatonic or affective symptomatology (Tables 23-3 and 23-4). ECT may be

TABLE 23-3
Indications for ECT

Major depression

Need for faster onset of action
    Severe suicidal potential
    Catatonia
    Marked malnutrition and dehydration

Anticipated side effects less than drug therapy
    Elderly
    Heart block
    Pregnancy

Acute mania

Other disorders
    Catatonia
    Organic delirium
    Intractable epilepsy
    Endocrinopathies
    Parkinson's disease

SOURCE: Adapted from Coffey and Weiner.[6]

TABLE 23-4
Psychoses for Which ECT May be Effective[32]
(with DSM-IV Codes)

Major depression with psychotic features
    Single episode [296.24]
    Recurrent [296.34]
Bipolar major depression with psychotic features
    Depressed [296.54]
    Mixed [296.64]
    Not otherwise specified [296.74]
Mania (bipolar disorder)
    Mania [296.44]
    Mixed type [296.64]
    Not otherwise specified [296.74]
Atypical psychosis [298.94]
Schizophrenia
    Catatonia [295.2x]
    Schizophreniform [295.40]
    Schizoaffective [295.70]

SOURCE: Reproduced with permission from Fink.[32]

considered a first-line treatment for patients with severe melancholic states, patients exhibiting nihilistic or paranoid delusions, or patients who have responded to ECT in the past.[32]

DEPRESSION

The most common indication for ECT in current therapy is major depression. Patients with the diagnosis of depression account for up to 90 percent of ECT referrals in the United States, and for which the response rate is 80 percent or higher.[6] Several rating scales exist for standardized measurement of depression; one widely used is the Hamilton rating scale, a 17-item scale for depression.[33] It can be used to assess the severity of depression before and after a course of ECT, providing a relatively objective method of measuring change in mood.

In practice, ECT is prescribed only after a patient fails to respond to one or more courses of psychotropic medications. Patients who are unable to take antidepressant drugs, or who find the side effects intolerable (including many patients with cardiac disease), may be well treated with ECT.[29] In some particularly severe situations, however, use of ECT as a first-line treatment may be indicated. Such indications might include depression associated with severe malnutrition, catatonia, or active suicidal or homicidal activity. These are clinical scenarios in which the patient is at grave risk to himself or herself or to others.

MANIA

In the past decade the clinical indications for ECT have been expanded, and it has been used for most affective

disorders. ECT is effective in the treatment of acute mania.[34] Although lithium carbonate is the first-line therapy and is highly effective in the majority of manic patients (or those with bipolar disorder in the manic phase), ECT is associated with remission or marked clinical improvement in 80 percent of manic patients, including patients unresponsive to psychopharmacotherapy.[35] Manic patients may not need prolonged or multiple daily treatments. Electrode placement in patients with mania is a controversial issue and warrants further investigation and individual evaluation for each patient.

CATATONIA

Catatonia, or "lethal catatonia," is a common feature in patients with severe affective disorders and represents a real risk to the patient's well-being; catatonic patients become malnourished and are at greatly increased risk for deep-vein thrombosis and pulmonary emboli. Although the use of ECT in patients with schizophrenia is controversial, schizophrenia with catatonia is particularly responsive to ECT.[36]

PARKINSON'S DISEASE

Parkinson's disease can be treated successfully with ECT.[37–40] It is thought that dopamine may be released with ECT, which presumably plays a role in the mechanism of improvement for those patients.[41,42] Patients referred for ECT are those who are refractory to antiparkinson medications or those intolerant to drug side effects. Patients with severe disability such as bedridden patients or those with "on-off syndrome" (severe fluctuation of extrapyramidal symptoms ranging from dyskinetic movements to freezing immobility) are the usual candidates for this form of therapy.[40] Pharmacotherapy has not provided as much improvement in motor deficits as has ECT.[43]

OTHER INDICATIONS

Other conditions where ECT might be used are more controversial.[36] Organic deliria, epilepsy, hypopituitary states, and neuroleptic malignant syndrome are medical disorders with studies of ECT efficacy in progress. Reflex sympathetic dystrophy has been reportedly successfully treated with ECT.[44] The literature contains scores of individual case reports describing (usually) a positive response to ECT given to treat a great variety of disorders (after failure of conventional therapies) such as aggressive behavior after closed head injury, eating disorders, alcoholism, and others.

TABLE 23-5
Relative Contraindication

Increased intracranial pressure
  Intracerebral mass
  Increased ICP without mass
  Intracerebral bleeding, recent CVA

Recent myocardial infarction (within 1 month)

Unstable aneurysms, AV malformations

Retinal detachment

Pheochromocytoma

ASA physical status 4 or 5

SOURCE: Reproduced by permission from American Psychiatric Association Task Force for ECT.[30]

Contraindications

Of note is the fact that the APA Task Force cited *no absolute contraindications* to ECT, a departure from much of the literature published prior to that time and a position that may present some difficulties to the anesthesiologist, particularly regarding adequate care for the patient with multiple medical problems. Each patient must be reviewed individually and the level of risk measured against the severity of the psychiatric illness. Suicide rates can be as high as 10 to 15 percent in patients with major affective disorders, and thus ECT may be instituted in patients with relative contraindications[30] (Table 23-5).

A traditional contraindication to ECT, and one that still must be dealt with judiciously, is the presence of an *intracranial space-occupying lesion* such as a brain tumor. The pronounced increase in cerebral blood flow (CBF), together with alterations in membrane permeability, suggest the risk of herniation or worsening of neurologic dysfunction. A number of reports from the 1950s through 1970s did indeed recount neurologic deterioration when ECT was given to patients with brain tumors.[45-47] These ECTs, were, however, given without the "modification" of anesthesia and supplemental oxygenation. Maltbie and colleagues[48] reported results of ECT *with* anesthesia in a group of 35 patients with brain tumors, recording outcomes on behavioral, mental, and neurologic levels. In that report, 21 percent of patients had improvement in behavior without decrement of mental or neurologic function, and 13 percent had improved behavior *with* deterioration of mental and neurologic functions. Thus, only about one-third had any behavioral benefit. The remaining 66 percent had no improvement in behavior and either the same or worsened mental and neurologic functions.[48] When ECT is considered to be necessary for a patient with a known intracranial space-occupying lesion, it is prudent to administer steroids prophylactically to reduce the peritumor edema.[48]

TABLE 23-6
Commonly Prescribed Antidepressant Medications

Generic Names	Trade Names
Tricyclics	
Amitriptyline HCl	Elavil
Amoxapine	Asendin
Desipramine HCl	Norpramin, Pertofrane
Doxepin HCl	Adapin, Sinequan
Imipramine HCl	Janimine, Tofranil
Maprotiline HCl	Ludiomil
Nortriptyline HCl	Pamelor
Protriptyline HCl	Vivactil
Trimipramine HCl	Surmontil
Atypical	
Fluoxetine HCl	Prozac
Trazodone HCl	Desyrel
Monoamine oxidase inhibitors	
Isocarboxazid	Marplan
Phenelzine sulfate	Nardil
Tranylcypromine sulfate	Parnate
Tranylcypromine/ Trifluoperizine	Parstelin
Nialamide	Niamid
Pargyline	Eutonyl
Selegiline L-deprenyl	Eldepryl

Pharmacologic Alternatives to ECT

PSYCHOPHARMACOLOGIC MEDICATIONS

Medications commonly prescribed for the treatment of major psychiatric disorders include tricyclic antidepressants (TCAs), atypical antidepressants (fluoxetine and trazodone), monoamine oxidase inhibitors (MAOIs), neuroleptics, anxiolytics, valproate, carbamazepine, and lithium (Tables 23-6 and 23-7). Lithium

TABLE 23-7
Commonly Prescribed Neuroleptic Medications

Generic Names	Trade Names
Phenothiazines	
Chlorpromazine HCl	Thorazine
Triflupromazine HCl	Vesprin
Mesoridazine besylate	Serentil
Thioridazine HCl	Mellaril
Acetophenazine maleate	Tindal
Fluphenazine HCl	Prolixin
Perphenazine	Trilafon
Trifluoperazine HCl	Stelazine
Thioxanthenes	
Chlorprothixene	Taractan
Thiothixene HCl	Navane
Other heterocyclic compounds	
Haloperidol	Haldol
Loxapine succinate	Loxitane
Molindone HCl	Moban
Pimozide	Orap

is given to patients with bipolar disorder. Patients with major depression who are treated with available antidepressants can expect a response rate of about 65 to 70 percent. Efficacy of the various types of antidepressants is generally considered to be about equal; differentiation is thus made, and medications changed, based on side effect profiles.[49]

The majority of patients who present for ECT have been treated with one or more antidepressant medications, with less than complete success. ECT may be administered to patients in whom psychopharmaceutical agents are discontinued, or, on occasion, the drugs may be maintained. It is important to review these classes of medications briefly and to highlight potential interactions. (See also Chap. 12.)

TRICYCLIC ANTIDEPRESSANT DRUGS

The TCAs are commonly used in the treatment of depression. They are structurally related to the phenothiazines and are thought to work by blocking the uptake of norepinephrine into the presynaptic nerve terminals. Because the side effects are usually less troublesome, the secondary amine TCAs nortriptyline and desipramine are preferred over most of the other TCAs.[49] Important side effects are related to their nonspecific interaction with cholinergic, histaminergic, serotonergic, and dopaminergic receptors in the central nervous system (CNS). Anticholinergic effects include sedation and cardiac toxicity (tachycardia, conduction blocks). Enhanced response to epinephrine and norepinephrine occur with acute administration of TCAs, but this may not be as worrisome with chronic administration secondary to the down-regulation of receptors after long-term usage. In general, however, the elderly or patients with cardiac disease may be more sensitive to the cardiotoxic effects of these drugs.

ATYPICAL ANTIDEPRESSANT DRUGS

Atypical antidepressant drugs or selective serotonin reuptake inhibitors (SSRIs) include fluoxetine (Prozac), sertraline, and paroxetine. The SSRIs as a group are associated with headache, nausea, and sexual dysfunction. The SSRIs inhibit cytochrome P-450 isoenzymes, and all have been reported to increase plasma concentrations of concurrently administered TCAs.[49] Fluoxetine has been associated with provocation of grand mal seizures,[50] although it appears to have an anticonvulsant effect in epilepsy-prone rats.[51] Some practitioners have reported a prolongation of ECT-induced seizures, and thus prefer to discontinue the drug 14 days before ECT.[52]

MONOAMINE OXIDASE INHIBITORS

The MAOIs bind irreversibly to the enzyme monoamine oxidase and thereby increase intraneuronal levels of amine neurotransmitters. This is associated with

TABLE 23-8

Comparison between Neuroleptic Malignant Syndrome (NMS) and Malignant Hyperthermia (MH)

	NMS	MH
Similarities		
Elevated temperature		
Muscle rigidity		
Hypermetabolism		
Diaphoresis		
Rhabdomyolysis		
Elevated serum CK levels		
Respond to dantrolene		
Hyperkalemia after succinylcholine		
Differences		
Trigger	Neuroleptic agents	Inhalational agents, succinylcholine
Muscle rigidity	Neurogenic	Myogenic
Etiology of syndrome	?Antagonism of CNS dopaminergic receptors	MH susceptible skeletal muscle
Hyperthermia	Impaired thermoregulation	Hypermetabolism
	Decreased heat dissipation	

both antidepressant and antihypertensive effects, which last 2 to 3 weeks after the last dose. Severe hypertension may occur with ECT and with the use of indirect-acting sympathomimetic agents such as ephedrine. In addition, hyperpyrexic coma may occur with the use of narcotics, most notably meperidine.[53,54] Traditional recommendations are that MAOIs should be discontinued at least 2 weeks before ECT (or any other elective procedure) if possible. This is a highly controversial issue, and ECT has been given to patients receiving MAOIs without apparent morbidity.[55] Recent literature may show improved antidepressant response with ECT, and the co-administration of antidepressant medications.[56]

NEUROLEPTIC AGENTS

Neuroleptic agents are used in a variety of psychotic states. They are thought to act by blocking dopaminergic systems in the CNS. Common side effects include acute dystonia, akasthisia, parkinsonism, perioral tremor, tardive dyskinesia, and the most serious side effect, *neuroleptic malignant syndrome* (NMS), a clinical disorder characterized by muscle rigidity, hypermetabolism, fever, diaphoresis, rhabdomyolysis, and increased serum creatine kinase (CK).

NEUROLEPTIC MALIGNANT SYNDROME

The etiology of NMS is unknown, but it occurs only in patients receiving neuroleptic agents. Although it clinically resembles malignant hyperthermia (MH), and does respond to administration of dantrolene, other features differentiate the two entities (Table 23-8). Whether NMS and MH do in fact overlap is a subject of some controversy.[57] A recent report detailed the case of a 52-year-old schizophrenic man with a past history of NMS, who underwent general anesthesia for temporomandibular joint surgery. Postoperatively, he developed catatonia (so-called lethal catatonia) although he had a satisfactory outcome after ECT treatments.[58]

LITHIUM CARBONATE

Lithium carbonate is frequently used for the treatment of affective disorders. It has been associated with a variety of cardiac abnormalities such as T-wave flattening and sinus node dysfunction, and Kellner and colleagues report that "there is more literature about the potential toxic effect of the combination of lithium and ECT than any other psychotropic agent."[59] Lithium tends to act as an imperfect sodium ion and can interfere with the action of depolarizing and nondepolarizing agents. It has also been reported to prolong recovery from barbiturates. Traditional recommendations are that lithium should be discontinued for 3 days before ECT and should not be begun again until 2 or 3 days after the patient's last ECT. Delirium has been reported to be more common in patients receiving lithium while undergoing ECT. The mechanism is unclear, and it has been suggested that the disruption of the blood-brain barrier after ECT may lead to increased concentrations of lithium in the CNS. Several reports detail greater memory loss, confusion, and atypical neurologic findings after receiving ECT while being treated with lithium.[60-62] Other series report no difference in outcomes between patients who did or did not receive lithium.[63-65] This topic is another area of some controversy in the psychiatric community and is well discussed by Small and Milstein.[66] For the anesthesiologist presented with a patient receiving lithium, there is no consensus regarding management; the literature supports both sides of the issue, although hundreds of such patients are given ECT each year.

RESERPINE

Reserpine is prescribed for hypertension less frequently than in decades past and is very rarely used for its antipsychotic effects, but serious side effects have been reported when ECT is administered to patients receiving reserpine. It is recommended that they have a 2-week drug holiday before ECT. Serious complications such as hypotension, cardiac arrhythmias, and even death are attributed to the effects of intraneuronal catecholamine depletion caused by this drug.

OTHER DRUGS

Other drugs with potential for problematic interactions in the patient receiving ECT include theophylline, sedative hypnotics, and echothiophate eye drops. These should all be discontinued, when possible, before ECT treatment.[59]

DRUG BINDING AND INTERACTIONS

α_1-ACID GLYCOPROTEIN

α_1-Acid glycoprotein (AGP) is the major protein to which basic drugs bind in serum and is responsible for abnormalities in platelet serotonin uptake. In addition, this protein inhibits phagocytosis, neutrophil activation, and platelet aggregation. Alterations of AGP are potentially of concern in the psychiatric population because the TCAs are basic drugs that bind tightly to AGP. Elevations in the levels of this protein might effectively reduce the level of unbound drug and thereby limit its effectiveness, whereas decreases in AGP would lead to higher-than-desired blood levels. AGP levels are known to be elevated in depressed patients[67] and may be altered in epileptic patients. DeVane and colleagues reported mixed findings in a study of patients undergoing ECT, with considerable intrapatient variability in AGP levels from treatment to treatment.[68] At this time, it is not entirely clear whether or not concerns about alterations of AGP in patients undergoing ECT are founded.

PLASMA CHOLINESTERASE

Patients with plasma cholinesterase (pseudocholinesterase, PCE) deficiency or atypia may exhibit prolonged apnea after ECT in which succinylcholine is used. Jaksa and Palahniuk reported an attempted organophosphate suicide, in whom the antagonism of PCE resulted in prolonged effect after succinylcholine.[69] Some patients with Alzheimer's disease are treated with tacrine (tetrahydroaminoacridine), which is an anticholinesterase.[70] PCE would be expected to be inhibited, prolonging the effect of succinylcholine.

BURST-SUPPRESSION ISOFLURANE ANESTHESIA

Isoflurane reduces both the frequency and the number of spontaneous epileptiform bursts. It also increases the stimulus required to evoke epileptiform bursts. In 1993, Engelhardt and coworkers reported a study in which 12 patients who were severely depressed received either burst-suppression isoflurane anesthesia or ECT treatments or both. Three patients improved with isoflurane alone, and 9 patients required isoflurane and ECT to improve.[71]

In a more recent report, Langer and associates studied ECT versus isoflurane narcotherapy in drug-refractory depressed women. The antidepressant effects were comparable between the two groups and of note were the findings that the isoflurane group continued to improve *after* the term of treatment, whereas the ECT patients tended to relapse. Secondly, the isoflurane group improved in most psychometric variables, whereas the ECT patients demonstrated deterioration.

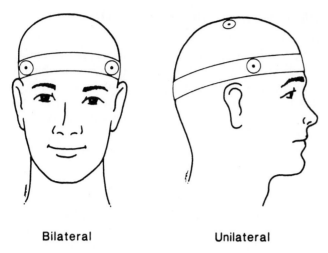

Bilateral   **Unilateral**

Figure 23-1 Electrode placement for ECT. (Reproduced by permission from Dubovsky.[35])

Finally, the electroencephalographic (EEG) patterns of the isoflurane patients remained normal or were improved, whereas the EEGs in ECT patients appeared more abnormal and developed theta/delta power.[72] Further studies of this modality are underway.

At the time of this writing, ECT is considered "standard therapy," is easier to administer, and continues to be the therapy of choice; however burst-suppression isoflurane anesthesia may be a coming alternative to patients who object to ECT.

Details of ECT[12,73,74]

GENERAL INFORMATION

Electroconvulsive therapy is a ritualized and labor-intensive therapy. The psychiatrist, various support personnel, the patient, and the anesthesiologist must all come together two or three times per week, generally in a location of limited familiarity to all, for the induction of a brief general anesthetic and induction of seizures. The skin is prepared at the electrode sites, electrode jelly is applied, and the electrodes are fixed to the scalp by means of a tight elastic headband (Fig. 23-1). The goal is to create a low-impedance pathway for stimulus current, without damaging the patient's skin, because the process is typically repeated for 6 to 12 sessions.

In general, a seizure should last *at least 20 s* (some authorities quote 30 s as the briefest acceptable seizure) but not longer than 2 min by visual inspection, and 3 min as judged by EEG monitoring. Treatments are usually given three times per week on alternate days for 6 to 12 treatments. Maletzky suggests that the aggregate duration of convulsive therapy should average between 210 and 1000 s,[75] although Sackeim vigorously

disputes this.[74] Mainstream thinking continues to adhere to the concept of a minimum acceptable seizure duration, however, and a great many studies include the concept in their design.

Each ECT session produces a generalized central seizure that spreads through the cortex and concludes with electical silence of up to 1.5 min (postictal suppression). This period is clinically associated with severe obtundation and loss of consciousness. After the postictal suppression, delta waves return, followed by theta waves, and EEG returns to pre-ECT baseline within 20 to 30 min. Immediate speed of recovery from the ECT postictal state is influenced by placement of electrodes (bilateral placement causes a longer recovery than unilateral placement), age of the patient (older patients take longer to recover), and the cumulative effect of a series of ECT can prolong recovery. With subsequent ECTs, the interictal EEG becomes slower and its amplitude becomes greater. Return to normal EEG develops over several months to a year after completion of ECT.

Administration of ECT has changed significantly in the past 50 years. In the United States, the typical patient receiving ECT is over 60 years of age, with a diagnosis of major depression. Relapse rates after treatment of affective disorders with either ECT or medications can be high (ranging from 50 to 95 percent). Older adults appear to be at greater risk for rehospitalization, especially in the first 18 months. Maintenance ECT has emerged as an alternative treatment for patients who relapse repeatedly or cannot tolerate psychotropic medications. Maintenance ECT appears to be safe, efficacious, and well tolerated by patient, and studies to date detail promising results. However, further controlled studies are needed to fully establish its role in psychiatric practice.

Following is an overview of many of the details of ECT, including the devices used.

SEIZURE MONITORING

Seizure monitoring is achieved by observation of the patient, EEG monitoring, and by the "isolated limb" or "cuff" technique.[76] Of these modalities, the EEG is the most accurate[77,78] and is described elsewhere in this chapter. The isolated limb may be an arm or a leg, to which is applied a noninvasive blood pressure cuff. The cuff is inflated to a pressure higher than the patient's systolic pressure before the administration of muscle relaxant. Thus, the motor manifestations of the seizure that ensue from the electrical stimulaton can be seen in the unparalyzed limb. Compared with EEG monitoring, the cuff method usually underestimates duration of the seizure.[79] Patients in whom a peripheral tourniquet is contraindicated include those with sickle cell disease and severe peripheral vascular disease (a

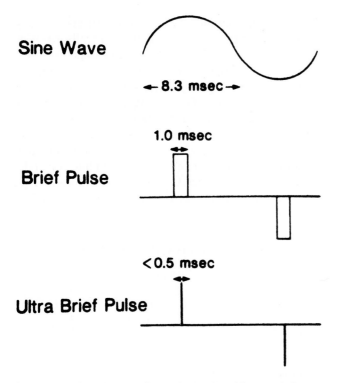

Figure 23-2 Stimulus waveforms. (Reproduced by permission from Dubovsky.[35])

relative contraindication). Patients requiring hemodialysis, in whom an indwelling arteriovenous fistula has been inserted, should not have that extremity occluded.

DEVICES

Instruments approved for use in ECT are classified based on the waveform they produce (Fig. 23-2). The variables that are altered for each patient are stimulus frequency, pulse width, and total stimulus duration.[80] The intricacies of stimulus parameters are discussed by Abrams.[81] The intensity of the current relative to the area of the brain through which it passes may be related to the neurobiologic effects of ECT. The type of electrical stimulus can strongly affect the minimal intensity of electrical stimulation required to produce seizures. Clinical facilities vary in the ECT devices they possess and use. The most commonly used wave form is the *brief-pulse stimulus,* an undulating alternating current of 60 cycles per s (in the United States), which rapidly reaches a peak current intensity and has a rapid offset.[74] The wave form for the brief-pulse stimulus is a *square wave.* The square wave requires less electrical energy and this is important because many sequelae are associated with higher doses of electrical energy.

Older machines produced stimulation that is slow to reach peak intensity and slow to decrease ("sine-wave stimulus") and is less efficient in eliciting seizures. Many of the undesirable sequelae of ECT (amnesia, confusion) are thought to be related to the use of higher doses of electrical energy, as is necessary with sine-wave units, and in general sine-wave devices are considered to be obsolete.

UNIPOLAR (UNILATERAL) VERSUS BIPOLAR (BILATERAL)

One of the important decisions in ECT is the use of unipolar or bipolar electrode placement, as illustrated in Fig. 23-1. Bilateral ECT is performed when an electrode is placed over each cerebral hemisphere; unilateral ECT involves the placement of both electrodes over one hemisphere. An advantage of *bipolar* lead placement is the institution of a more rapid response; however, this technique is associated with more cognitive impairment. *Unilateral* treatment delivered over the nondominant hemisphere requires careful determination of the threshold and may not be as rapid, effective, or enduring as bilateral treatment. Unilateral ECT is associated with less cognitive disruption, however.

There may be an additional difference between unipolar and bipolar ECT, which could be of clinical significance to the anesthesiologist. Swartz and colleagues reported a study of alternating unilateral ECT in 21 men with melancholia. The ECTs given to the right side of the head resulted in greater heart rate elevations than the ECTs given to the left side.[82] This is consistent with a right cerebral hemisphere dominance in heart rate control.

SINGLE VERSUS MODIFIED MONITORED MULTIPLE ECT

Modified monitored multiple ECT (MMMECT) is the method of eliciting multiple monitored ECTs in a single session, with the seizures occurring at 1- to 3-min intervals.[83] It offers the theoretical advantage of less exposure to anesthesia, shorter hospital stay, and less memory loss. Side effects include more drowsiness, disorientation, and confusion. Safety and efficacy studies are lacking, but concern has been expressed regarding the apparently increased risk of cognitive and cardiovascular sequelae and increased incidence of prolonged seizures.[84] For the anesthesiologist, the scheduling of a MMMECT represents a somewhat different procedure than the single ECT. The patient will need to be unconscious and paralyzed for a greater period of time; consider planned intubation of these patients. Succinylcholine's effect is likely to be too brief for the MMMECT, and a longer-acting nondepolarizing relaxant such as mivacurium might be preferable.[85]

TABLE 23-9
Indications for Maintenance ECT

Rapid relapse after course of ECT

Severe illness

Major depressive disorder with psychotic features

Parkinson's disease

Relapse despite adequate maintenance medication

Inability to tolerate maintenance medication

Noncompliance with medications

History of response to ECT better than response to medications

SERIES VERSUS MAINTENANCE

The patient with major depression is typically treated with a series of 6 to 12 ECTs, given on an inpatient basis. During the first year after successful ECT treatment of depression, the depression is likely to recur in many patients, and there may be a subset at even greater risk for recurrence. Investigators working with maintenance ECT report that patients treated with maintenance ECT after failing numerous trials of antidepressant medications experienced a 67 percent reduction of rehospitalization, suggesting that this very challenging subset of patients may be better managed with maintenance ECT.[86] Newer work supports intermittent single ECTs, usually administered to patients on an outpatient basis, once a month. As with many other aspects of ECT, the subject of maintenance ECT is one of some ongoing controversy.[87-89] Indications for maintenance ECT are listed in Table 23-9.

SCHEDULES—TWO VERSUS THREE TIMES WEEKLY

In a double-blind study, Lerer and coworkers[90] compared 52 consenting, medication-free patients with major depressive disorders. These subjects were randomly assigned to bilateral, brief-pulse, constant-current ECT administered over 4 weeks at rates of two or three times per week. The twice-weekly group had a sham ECT (induction of anesthesia and administration of muscle relaxant) performed each week, for a total of three "treatment" episodes. Both groups had significant improvement of the Hamilton depression scale scores, with a more rapid response occurring in the three-times-weekly group. However, the three-times-weekly group also had a greater incidence of cognitive effects. The authors recommended twice-weekly ECT for most patients, with use of three-times-weekly ECT reserved for patients in whom early onset of clinical effect is more important.[90]

LOCATION OF ECT

Electroconvulsive therapy can be performed on a psychiatric unit, in the operating room suite, adjacent to the operating room [e.g., in a postanesthesia care unit (PACU)], or in purpose-built facilities. Ideally, the location will be one with all the appropriate supplies, equipment (routine and emergency), and monitors available, with well-trained personnel present for the ECT and for the post-ECT emergence time. Areas that are quieter and appear less "clinical" than the average PACU find favor with the patients and the psychiatric personnel but may not be available in all health care facilities. In the two teaching hospitals of the University of Texas Health Science Center at San Antonio where ECT is performed, the location of choice is an isolation room of the PACU.

TECHNIQUES TO ENHANCE SEIZURES

On occasion, induction of a seizure is unsuccessful, and thus various techniques have been developed to induce or enhance seizure duration (Table 23-10). Following is a brief description of several of these interventions.

HYPERVENTILATION

Hyperventilation has long been recognized to contribute to prolongation of seizures with ECT. Bridenbaugh and colleagues reported that seizures induced in the presence of hypocapnia (end-tidal CO_2 of 2.5%) were of longer duration than those produced when the end-tidal CO_2 was 8.5%.[91] A more recent study reported by Pande and coworkers did *not* find hyperventilation to be of universal assistance in prolongation of seizures, however.[92]

THEOPHYLLINE

Theophylline lowers the seizure threshold in animals[93] and has been associated with seizures and status epilepticus in animals and humans.[94] When administered chronically to patients undergoing ECT, undesirably prolonged seizures have been reported.[95] Swartz and coworkers reported the use of oral theophylline to facilitate seizures in patients in mid-course ECT, who had developed an elevated seizure threshold.[96] Patients were given sustained-release theophylline 200 to 400 mg orally at 10 P.M., the evening preceding ECT.[96] Rasmussen and associates reported a study of seven patients given ECT while being treated with theophylline

TABLE 23-10
Techniques to Enhance Seizures

Hyperventilation

Theophylline

Caffeine

Delay between methohexital and ECT

for obstructive lung disease.[97] Of the 77 ECT seizures, only one was prolonged.

CAFFEINE

Caffeine facilitates seizures of greater duration in animals[98] and in humans,[99,100] and for that reason, some practitioners prescribe its use for patients whose seizures are considered too brief for therapeutic effect. Typical doses are 300 to 1000 mg orally, and 125 to 242 mg intravenously.[99] There have been some case reports of complications with its use, however, including the apparent precipitation of supraventricular tachycardia in a patient receiving clozapin and caffeine, who underwent ECT.[101] Its use is the subject of ongoing investigations. The anesthesiologist caring for an ECT patient might be requested to give caffeine intravenously after a failed or too-brief seizure and should be familiar with this indication.

DELAY BETWEEN METHOHEXITAL AND ECT

Past studies showed that methohexital given before ECT caused a reduction of seizure duration.[102] Collins and Scott hypothesized that, if the seizure-shortening property of methohexital is related to brain concentration, and if brain concentration falls rapidly (accounting for the rapid emergence after a single dose of methohexital), then the *time elapsed* between induction with methohexital and administration of ECT might influence the length of seizure. They described a small study in which this hypothesis was prospectively tested and found that *delaying the ECT* after methohexital injection (average 110 s, range 68 to 176 s) was associated with a lengthening of the seizure from 25.8 s to 33.2 s.[103] This technique, as well as some of those described elsewhere, may be of value in the management of the ECT-resistant patient.

Physiologic Responses to ECT

The physiologic effects of ECT are wide ranging, and are described in the following paragraphs (Table 23-11).

CARDIOVASCULAR RESPONSES

Seizure activity is thought to be the therapeutic aspect of ECT, and it is accompanied by significant physiologic responses. Concurrent with the shock, the parasympathetic system is stimulated, with reduced rhythmicity of the sinoatrial node, producing bradycardia, followed by asystole, with a dramatic fall in blood pressure. This phase lasts about 60 s. Immediately after the shock, cardiac rhythm returns, and there is a sympathetic surge. At that point the patient experiences hypertension and bradycardia, and then tachycardia,

TABLE 23-11
Physiologic Effects of Electroconvulsive Therapy

Cardiovascular effects
  Immediate
    Parasympathetic stimulation
      Bradycardia
      Hypotension
  Late (after 1 min)
    Sympathetic stimulation
      Tachycardia
      Hypertension
      Dysrhythmias
      Increased myocardial O_2 consumption
Cerebral effects
  Increased cerebral O_2 consumption
  Increased cerebral blood flow
  Increased intracranial pressure
Ophthalmologic effects
  Increased intraocular pressure
Gastrointestinal effects
  Increased intragastric pressure

SOURCE: Reproduced by permission from Gaines and Rees.[10]

increased cardiac output, and sometimes arrhythmias. These changes are well illustrated in Fig. 23-3, which shows the effects of ECT on a dog not given atropine.

The arrhythmias that occur with the sympathetic surge are likely to be sinus and ventricular tachycardias and premature ventricular contractions (PVCs), which may be multifocal and/or bigeminy or trigeminy. *This sympathetic discharge combined with electrical stimulation of convulsions increases the myocardial oxygen demand and may be a significant stress on patients with limited cardiac reserve.* Although the healthy patient usu-

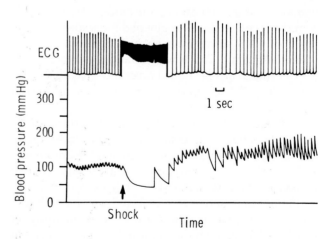

Figure 23-3 This figures shows the effects of ECT on a dog not given atropine. During the 5-s shock, the dog was asystolic, with a dramatic fall in blood pressure. Immediately following the shock, cardiac rhythm returned, the animal exhibited hypotension and bradycardia, followed then by tachycardia. (Reproduced by permission from Marks.[230])

ally has maximum hypertension by 60 s after the shock, the elderly patient, or others with slower circulation times, may not have a peak blood pressure as quickly. Partridge and colleagues reported that in normotensive patients undergoing ECT, systolic blood pressure increased 155 percent and heart rate increased 164 percent.[104]

The cardiovascular effects of ECT have been elucidated in animal models. The *parasympathetic response* is mediated via the vagus nerve, and the *sympathetic response* is a reflection of hippocampal activation and circulating catecholamines.[105]

ELECTROCARDIOGRAPHIC CHANGES

Electrocardiographic (ECG) changes associated with ECT have been described. Changes in T waves and in the QT intervals have been reported, as have other ECG abnormalities including altered QRS waves, nodal and ventricular paroxysmal tachycardias, extrasystoles, bigeminy, trigeminy, and atrioventricular dissociation. On occasion, the T-wave changes have been diagnosed initially as subendocardial infarction[106] and have been described in other patients undergoing ECT.[107,108] In a prospective study of 29 patients undergoing 85 ECTs, Dec and coworkers found that there were no *persistent* ECG changes or elevations in creatine phosphokinase or serum glutamic oxalaminase transaminase levels.[109] Twenty-four percent of the patients in that study had stable preexisting cardiovascular disease (conduction system disease, recent myocardial infarction, depressed ventricular function).

There are a variety of theories as to why ECT should be associated with ST-segment depression. If the ST-segment depression is a reflection of segmental myocardial ischemia, that would be consistent with observations in other clinical circumstances. Alternatively, some believe that the ST-segment depression is a direct effect of CNS stimulation on cardiac repolarization, without ischemia. This leaves the anesthesiologist with the question: *Does the patient experience myocardial ischemia with ECT?* A number of studies have addressed this issue.

In a recent study, using real-time recording of ST segments, Steiner and colleagues demonstrated myocardial injury in a patient undergoing ECT under general anesthesia.[110] A 79-year-old patient with known coronary artery disease and several previous myocardial infarctions underwent ECT and developed hypotension immediately afterward. The availability of real-time ST-segment data assisted in the subsequent management of refractory myocardial failure and myocardial infarction.[110]

Wells and Davies reported the use of *noninvasive electrical bioimpedance monitoring* in ECT.[111] As expected, induction of anesthesia was associated with a decrease in cardiac output and increase in heart rate. With the seizure, heart rate increased 20 percent, blood pressure increased 34 percent, and cardiac output increased 81 percent.[111]

Certainly, the hemodynamic changes associated with ECT may unmask previously unsuspected coronary insufficiency with ECT. Knos and coworkers reported such a case in a 64-year-old man without history of cardiac dysfunction, who developed ST depression with ECT and awoke complaining of chest pain. His course of ECT was interrupted by cardiac consultation, catheterization, and coronary artery bypass grafting, after which the ECT treatments resumed![112]

ECHOCARDIOGRAPHIC CHANGES

The echocardiogram may be affected by ECT.[113] Messina and coworkers, in a small clinical series, demonstrated a statistically significant correlation between ECG and echocardiographic changes during ECT. Eleven patients, all with normal baseline ECGs, underwent ECT with additional echocardiographic monitoring. Five of the patients developed hypokinesis of one or more contiguous myocardial segments.

How, then, do we answer the question posed earlier? *Do* patients experience myocardial ischemia with ECT? Strong evidence supports the diagnosis of myocardial ischemia associated with ST-segment changes, and appropriate management should be planned and implemented when this occurs, particularly in patients at risk for limited myocardial reserve. A variety of pharmacologic regimens have been developed to lessen the hemodynamic consequences of ECT, and they are described below.

PHARMACOLOGIC MODULATION

Pharmacologic modulation of the bradycardic, tachycardic, and hypertensive responses to ECT via pretreatment with anticholinergic drugs has been attempted by many groups over the years. Before further discussion of the management of the hemodynamic changes associated with ECT, it is important to note that hypertensive patients should have the institution of antihypertensive medications well before the start of ECT. We have observed that a solid foundation of antihypertensive therapy enables better control of the hemodynamics of the ECT period.

Prevention of Bradycardia

Patients pretreated with atropine have been reported to have vagally mediated arrhythmias at an incidence of 0 to 19 percent.[114,115] Without an anticholinergic before induction of anesthesia and ECT, the incidence is 30 to 70 percent.[5] Some studies have failed to show benefit with pretreatment, and, in fact, the anticholinergic activity of atropine may produce undesirable side effects such as tachycardia and delirium. Drug interactions with antidepressants such as TCAs is also a concern. Many practitioners prefer to give glycopyrrolate, which appears to offer the advantage of its quarternary structure and consequent inability to cross the normal blood-brain barrier.

Prevention of Tachycardia and Hypertension

Numerous agents have been used over the years, including sodium nitroprusside, clonidine, α- and β-adrenergic blockers, calcium channel antagonists, nitroglycerin, lidocaine, and other agents. These drugs are no longer given as frequently because the sympatholytic agents labetalol and esmolol are now available. They provide good control of hypertension and tachycardia, and their duration of action is better suited to the demands of the peri-ECT period. Further discussion of specific management follows elsewhere in this chapter.

"MYOCARDIAL STUNNING"

Myocardial stunning has been reported after ECT.[116] Myocardial stunning was described in 1982 and is defined as a prolonged but reversible myocardial contractile dysfunction.[117,118] The diagonosis is a clinical one. Zhu and coworkers[116] described data on a 77-year-old woman without cardiac history, who underwent ECT. After the ECT, the ECG revealed ST-segment elevation in six leads although she denied chest pain. An echocardiogram revealed an ejection fraction of 35 percent, but coronary angiography showed only mild coronary artery disease. Within 4 days, the ECG and echocardiographic changes had normalized and ejection fraction was 65 percent. Treatment with 15 mg labetalol before subsequent ECTs prevented recurrence.[116]

RESPIRATORY RESPONSES

During the tonic phase of ECT apneusis of approximately 12 s occurs, followed by a clonic phase of apnea of 30 to 50 s. In the days before preoxygenation and intentional positive-pressure ventilation prior to the ECT, patients developed hypoxemia frequently. This probably played a role in some post-ECT cognitive problems (amnesia, confusion).

NEUROLOGIC EFFECTS

There is no evidence that structural damage occurs to the nervous system with ECT, provided that hypoxemia is avoided, as described above. ECT affects CBF and intracranial pressure (ICP); causes EEG changes and some alterations in the magnetic resonance imaging (MRI); may affect the seizure threshold, at least in the peri-ECT period and perhaps longer; and has been related to causation of cognitive defects.

INTRACRANIAL PRESSURE AND CEREBRAL BLOOD FLOW

The ICP increases immediately after ECT secondary to an increase in CBF. This increased flow accompanies an increase in cerebral oxygen consumption and can be dramatic. The increased CBF may last for several hours after ECT. Saito and colleagues have recently reported their study of oxygenation of brain tissue using near-infrared spectrophotometry, and flow velocity at the middle cerebral artery (MCA) using transcranial Doppler ultrasonography, in depressed patients undergoing ECT.[119] They found that oxyhemoglobin fell during the seizure and then rebounded. MCA velocity of blood flow increased almost 240 percent (from about 45 cm/s to 106 cm/s). Within 10 min, velocity flow had returned to normal. They concluded that electrically induced seizures caused a temporary imbalance in energy consumption and supply, which normalized rapidly on cessation of the seizure.[119] This may indicate that autoregulation of CBF may be lost during the ECT-induced seizure.

ELECTROENCEPHALOGRAPHIC CHANGES

The EEG during ECT appears similar to spontaneous grand mal seizures. In the early phase, there is a gradual increase of rhythmic activity in the alpha and beta ranges. During the clonic phase, the EEG demonstrates repetitive polyphasic spikes and wave complexes, synchronous with the clonic movements of the patient. After the clonic phase, there occurs a period of EEG suppression, during which the patient is refractory to further seizure induction. Normalization of the EEG after ECT is rather variable; after the final treatment of an ECT series, the EEG trends toward an increase in alpha activity over days to weeks and has typically returned to normal by 3 months.[9]

MAGNETIC RESONANCE IMAGING

The MRI studies of ECT-treated patients fails to provide evidence of cerebral ischemia (i.e., lactate) but do indicate an increase in regional brain lipid, thought to be related to neurotransmitters.[120] Structural changes have been sought, but do not appear to occur.[121] Little is known about the effects of ECT on brain physiochemistry. Further study with serial MRI spectroscopy using quantitation of T1 and T2 relaxation times may provide insight into the cognitive deficits encountered after ECT treatments.[120,122]

PERSISTENT ELEVATION OF SEIZURE THRESHOLD

There is some suggestion that a given patient's seizure threshold may become persistently elevated by the use of ECT, although these findings have not been universally observed. Tomasson and coworkers noted increased frequency of failed and shortened seizures in men who had prior ECT treatment.[123] However, Krueger and associates did not find a persistent elevation of seizure threshold with ECT.[124]

Coffey and colleagues compared the seizure threshold at the first and sixth ECT treatments in 62 depressed patients. They reported that the seizure threshold increased by an average of 47 percent, but that *any* increase was experienced by only 56 percent of the patients. Patients who were likely to experience an increase in the seizure threshold were older and no other study factors played a role.[125,126] Thus, the apparent differences may stem from sample size and composition of the study groups. Further investigations are ongoing. The anesthesiologist caring for ECT patients would anticipate that after several ECTs, some patients might become more resistant to the ECT, and require a second shock of higher intensity. On occasion, one or more of the techniques outlined elsewhere in the chapter might become necessary.

ROLE OF PREEXISTING SEIZURE DISORDERS
Patients with preexisting seizure disorders have been reported to experience prolonged seizures with ECT.[127] In other cases, patients with epilepsy treated with anticonvulsants have had some difficulty achieving seizure with ECT.[128]

COGNITIVE DEFICITS
Multiple cognitive deficits are known to occur after ECT and have represented a substantial component of the public arguments against ECT. *Amnesia* is usually the predominant symptom and may appear within a few treatments. Other problems of cognitive impairment include disturbances in language, verbal fluency, naming abilities, and perceptual learning. There appears to be a linear relationship between the amount of electrical energy when using the sine-wave form of ECT and the severity of amnesia. With the advent of the brief-pulse stimuli, the severity and prevalence of ECT-induced amnesia has been falling, perhaps by as much as 50 percent.[25] Several mechanisms have been proposed as potential etiologies for these deficits. Increases in intracellular free acetylcholine, cholinergic dysfunction, and breakdown in the blood-brain barrier have been proposed,[129-131] and studies are ongoing.

NEUROENDOCRINE EFFECTS

HYPOTHALAMIC-PITUITARY-ADRENAL AXIS
The hypothalamic-pituitary-adrenal (HPA) axis is activated by ECT, resulting in a release of β-endorphin, corticotropin, cortisol, prolactin, and possibly growth hormone in humans.[132,133] Vasopressin, oxytocin, thyrotropin-releasing hormone (TRH), thyroid-stimulating hormone (TSH), and other peptides are also released. Repeated ECT treatment in animals increases the formation of corticotropin-releasing factor mRNA in the hypothalamic paraventricular nucleus. ECT resembles *chronic stress,* and the HPA axis responds to stress by increasing corticotropin-releasing factor (CRF)-mediated secretion of corticotropin and cortisol. In animals and in depressed humans, hypercortisolism is consistently found.[134,135] Thyroid-stimulating hormone and somatomedin A do not seem to be consistently affected by ECT. Thus, it appears that ECT produces a selective response from the HPA axis. Weinger and colleagues[136] demonstrated that pretreatment with esmolol 1 mg/kg significantly attenuated ECT-induced epinephrine secretion. Considerable efforts are being made to elucidate the role of hormonal changes and clinical response to ECT, with the hope being that identification of a peptide *antidepressin* will occur.

DOPAMINE
Another of the mechanisms by which ECT is thought to act is by enhancing dopamine function, although which of the many dopaminergic agonist-receptor complexes are involved is not yet clear. (Parkinson's disease is also considered to derive from dopamine deficiency; thus ECT is a logical modality to be studied, as described elsewhere in this chapter.)

γ-AMINOBUTYRIC ACID
Recently, Devanand and coworkers have examined the effects of ECT on plasma γ-aminobutyric acid (GABA) function in humans.[137] GABA is the principal inhibitory neurotransmitter in the brain and modulates other neurotransmitter and peptide systems. Several studies have suggested that patients with major depression have reduced levels of cerebrospinal fluid and plasma GABA.[138] Devanand and colleagues showed that, after ECT, free plasma GABA was significantly reduced for up to 1 h after the seizure.[137] Further studies are ongoing in this area.

GLUCOSE CONTROL
While ECT treatments are ongoing, regulation of glucose is often impaired.[139-142] A number of factors probably contribute to this phenomenon, including the elevations of circulating catecholamines and cortisol, elevated glucagon, and inhibition of glucose-mediated insulin secretion. The anesthesiologist caring for ECT patients should be aware of this potential lability, and evaluate blood glucose measurements in diabetic patients, lest potentially problematic hyperglycemia occur. Insulin-treated diabetics should be placed on sliding-scale insulin during the course of the ECTs.

TABLE 23-12
Intraocular Pressures (IOP) Associated With ECT

Event	Right Eye IOP	Left Eye IOP
Baseline	15.6 mmHg	15.4 mmHg
After thiopental, succinylcholine, during fasciculations	16.2	16.2
During seizure	32.9	32.4
After 5 min	21.6	21.1
After 10 min	17.0	16.6

SOURCE: Data adapted from and used with permission from Epstein et al.[143]

OPHTHALMOLOGIC EFFECTS

INTRAOCULAR PRESSURE

Intraocular pressure (IOP) increases with ECT.[143,144] Epstein and colleagues studied 20 patients without glaucoma who underwent ECT. The pressure in both eyes was measured and was consistently equal. IOP during the seizure was doubled and had essentially returned to baseline by 10 min later[143] (Table 23-12). Patients with glaucoma or retinal tears or detachment are potentially at risk for worsening of their visual function and should be carefully evaluated by an ophthalmologist before the ECT series begins. Ideally, the ophthalmologist will be familiar with the ECT protocol because some ophthalmic medications may present potential drug interactions with drugs used in ECT (e.g., echothiophate inhibits PCE, timolol may be absorbed and contribute to bradycardia, etc.)

IMMUNOLOGIC FUNCTION

Association between major depression and immunosuppression has long been observed. Fischler and coworkers studied immune changes induced by ECT and found a significant increase in the absolute number and percentage of activated lymphocytes (OKT10+ and IL2R1+) after ECT for depression.[145] Within 1 h after ECT, they noted an acute decrease in the absolute number of total lymphocytes, T8+ and Leu11+ cells. Clinical importance of these observations awaits further investigations.

MUSCULOSKELETAL RESPONSES

During a convulsion, the unparalyzed patient is at risk for severe muscle contractions, and bones may be fractured. Before the routine use of muscle relaxants in ECT, vertebral body fractures were common, as were broken teeth. The addition of skeletal muscle paralysis has thus made the process of ECT much safer. With the use of succinylcholine, myalgias may be manifest, but this is rarely a clinical problem of any magnitude.

Anesthetic Management

GOALS OF CARE

Recognition of the specific risks inherent in ECT, as outlined above, facilitates the safest management of the patient presenting for ECT.[146] The goals of anesthetic management are prevention of hypoxemia, avoidance of musculoskeletal injuries associated with the seizure, and modification of cardiovascular responses. The anesthetic technique selected should be smooth in onset and pleasant for the patient, provide autonomic stability, be safe to use repeatedly, and be compatible with rapid recovery. The sequence of the peri-ECT period is depicted in Fig. 23-4. Pharmacologic modification has virtually eliminated the vertebral fractures and broken teeth experienced in times past.

PREOPERATIVE EVALUATION

Preoperative evaluation includes a detailed medical history and physical examination before the first ECT of a series, and abbreviated evaluations before each subsequent treatment. Patients may not be able to communicate effectively, and fear and anxiety may be overwhelming, especially with the first treatment, and thus the history may not be complete. Those patients who are older, or in whom symptoms or signs suggest cardiac dysfunction, should be evaluated by a cardiologist before the beginning of a series of ECT treatments.[147]

Old anesthesia records from previous ECT treatments or surgeries provide important information about previous drugs used for induction, complications from those drugs, ease of airway management, adjuncts used, and so forth.

INFORMED CONSENT

It is important that the patient, or if necessary, the patient's guardian and family, be aware of associated risks of anesthesia for ECT. Informed consent is mandatory, but obtaining informed consent from a patient presenting for ECT can be challenging, particularly in patients with psychosis or other severe psychiatric dysfunction.

LABORATORY EVALUATIONS

Recommendations regarding minimum pre-ECT laboratory values to be obtained range from hemoglobin, hematocrit, B_{12} levels to rule out subacute combined degeneration, and ECG within 48 h of the treatment to a much more extensive list (Table 23-13). A chest x-ray may not be warranted if review of the history and physical examination is negative, but recall that poor communication on the part of the severely de-

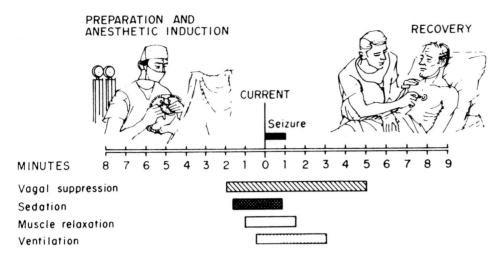

Figure 23-4 Diagram of the peri-ECT period. (Reproduced by permission from Rich and Smith.[231])

pressed patient may lead to underestimation of the abnormalities of the medical history.

PREMEDICATION

Preanesthetic medication with sedatives may depress seizure activity or prolong recovery time, and only rarely will a patient require any sedation. Pre-ECT use of anticholinergic agents is a controversial issue and must be individually considered, especially in patients with cardiovascular disease. If an anticholinergic drug is used, glycopyrrolate is preferable to atropine because of its reduced potential for causing tachycardia.

Patients with gastroesophageal reflux disease are given H_2 blockers and sodium citrate before each treatment, and thorough evaluation of airway management techniques must be made. Intubation of the trachea should be given careful consideration.

EQUIPMENT AND SUPPLIES

Prior to induction of general anesthesia for ECT, equipment and monitors are checked for availability and proper function (Table 23-14). A cardiac defibrillator

TABLE 23-13
Recommended Laboratory Investigations before ECT

Full blood count and B_{12}
Electrolytes, BUN, glucose
Thyroid function tests
Sickledex (where appropriate)
Urinalysis and urinary porphyrins
Chest x-ray
Electrocardiogram

SOURCE: Reproduced with permission from Marks.[230]

should be located near enough to the ECT location for prompt access. An intravenous catheter is inserted and monitors are applied. The ECT electrodes are applied to the scalp as described elsewhere in this chapter and depicted in Fig. 23-1. The electrolyte solution must not be allowed to drip and form a conduction path because the administered shock will pass through the gel rather than through the patient's head.

SELECTION OF ANESTHETIC AGENTS

Induction agents are selected according to the desired duration of action, affect on the seizure threshold, patient considerations, and length of recovery time.

METHOHEXITAL
Methohexital is an oxybarbiturate with a rapid onset and short duration of action. Methohexital does raise the seizure threshold, and decreases the duration of the seizures (compared with ECT without an induction agent).[148] The recommended dose of methohexital is 0.5 to 1.0 mg/kg. Depressed patients are more sensitive to induction agents and may require reduced drug dosages.[7]

Since the early endorsement by Pitts and coworkers, who praised the rapid recovery and lesser incidence of arrhythmias compared with other induction agents, methohexital became the most commonly used induction agent for ECT.[115] A more recent study by Mokriski and coworkers supported Pitts' enthusiasm; when compared in a randomized, double-blind study with thiopental and thiamylal, the methohexital group experienced longer seizures and fewer episodes of sinus bradycardia, premature atrial contractions, and PVCs.[149] When compared with thiopental in another study, methohexital-treated patients demonstrated a higher incidence of hiccup, muscle twitching, and salivation.[150]

TABLE 23-14
Customary Equipment and Monitors for ECT

Equipment	Monitors	Other Essentials	Readily Available
Oxygen	Noninvasive BP	ECT machine (with EEG)	Cardiac arrest cart, defibrillator
Ambu or anesthesia bag	Pulse oximeter		Dantrolene
Airway equipment	Precordial stethoscope		
Face masks, ETTs, LMA	ECG		
Laryngoscope	Tourniquet (isolated limb)		
Rubber mouth piece			
Anesthesia cart with drugs and supplies			
IV fluid, tubing, catheters			
Suction apparatus			

NOTE: BP, blood pressure; ETTs, endotracheal tubes; LMA, laryngeal mask airway

THIOPENTAL

Thiopental offers no apparent advantage over methohexital; and some studies have demonstrated a slower onset of anesthesia and a longer recovery time.[151] Thiopental may lead to greater hemodynamic instability than methohexital, particularly in patients with cardiovascular disease.[149]

BENZODIAZEPINES

Benzodiazepines must be used judiciously in the peri-ECT period, if at all. Diazepam and midazolam increase the seizure threshold and shorten seizure duration.[152] One study demonstrated more ECG abnormalities and patient recall.[153] Diazepam has been reported to delay both induction and recovery.[151] Loimer and colleagues studied midazolam as an induction agent for ECT and found that despite the appealing property of reversibility with flumazenil, the shortening of seizure duration (means decreased from 36 s to 20 s) was unacceptable.[154]

KETAMINE

Ketamine is reportedly a cerebral anticonvulsant in animals. However, it *increases the duration* of electrically induced seizures in both animals and humans.[148] Clinical experiences with ketamine for ECT were reported predominantly during the 1970s.[155,156] Some studies suggest that ketamine prolongs recovery and is associated with a greater incidence of nausea and ataxia,[157] and it is not used as a first-line induction agent for ECT by most practitioners.

ETOMIDATE

Etomidate in doses of 0.2 to 0.3 mg/kg intravenously has been used with ECT and has been shown to be acceptable; however, this was somewhat complicated by myoclonic jerking, increased muscle tone, and longer recovery time. Patients noted pain on injection, as well.[158,159] A retrospective study by Trzepacz and coworkers of ECT treatment of 28 depressed patients suggests that etomidate increases seizure duration during ECT, compared with thiopental.[160] Because of the retrospective nature of their study, comparison of patient outcomes was not possible. In a study of seizure duration in which etomidate and methohexital were compared, no difference in duration was found, however.[161]

PROPOFOL

Propofol significantly reduces the seizure activity duration, raising the concern that the ECT might be subtherapeutic.[162–166] A number of recent studies have addressed this issue and are discussed in the following paragraphs.

Fredman and associates reported that in three groups of ECT patients where propofol or methohexital were used as induction agents, dose-dependent decreases in the duration of motor and EEG seizure activity were found. Doses of propofol less than 1.5 mg/kg were associated with a clinically acceptable duration of EEG seizure activity.[167]

Comparing 13 adult outpatients undergoing ECT,[168] the same research team reported similar results. The use of propofol, 0.75 mg/kg, was associated with significantly shorter motor and EEG seizure durations compared with methohexital (34 s and 52 s versus 39 s and 61 s). Both groups had similar awakening times and hemodynamic stability and cognitive recovery were better after propofol. Thus, for *outpatients*, the slightly shorter (and thus, possibly somewhat less effective) ECT might be a consideration for the use of propofol.

Martensson and coworkers compared propofol with methohexital for induction of ECT patients and found a similar shortening of duration of propofol-induced seizures, without sacrificing efficacy.[169] Other groups who have reached similar conclusions include Malsch and colleagues[170] and Fear and coworkers.[171] Matters and associates compared methohexital and propofol and found no significant difference in psychometric recovery (measured by finger tap and digit symbol substitution tests) or duration of the seizure.[172] Thus, the rapid emergence customarily experienced after induction with propofol in other procedures may *not* be applicable in the setting of ECT.

Avramov and coworkers studied 10 outpatients being treated with maintenance ECT, in a total of 90 treatments.[173] They found that the durations of EEG and motor seizures were longest after induction with etomidate and shortest after induction with propofol, even in various doses. Awakening times were similar among the groups.

LIDOCAINE

Lidocaine raises the seizure threshold and has been reported to interfere with initiation of seizure activity.[60,174,175] Thus, its use before ECT-induced seizures is not recommended. *After* the seizure, however, if ventricular arrhythmias occur, lidocaine or procainamide may be indicated.[174]

NEUROMUSCULAR BLOCKADE

Several skeletal muscle relaxants are available that can be used with ECT; however, succinylcholine is the most widely used relaxant for single ECTs, principally because of the rapid onset and cessation of action.

SUCCINYLCHOLINE

Succinylcholine is administered in a dose of 0.5 to 1.0 mg/kg. The lower end of the dosing range is a lower dose than is cutomarily administered to facilitate intubation in an operating room setting and if the ECT patient has a normal airway and it can be managed by mask, intubation is not usually performed. Thus, the end point of the administration of succinylcholine is merely to blunt the impact of the muscle contractions secondary to the ECT, and a lower dose is sufficient.[176] If there is greater-than-normal need for complete muscle paralysis (e.g., need for tracheal intubation, myeloma, recent fracture, femoral head necrosis), a larger dose of succinylcholine is administered.

MIVACURIUM

Patients who have had prolonged periods of bed rest, patients with NMS, and those being treated with echothiophate eyedrops may not be good candidates for succinylcholine. Mivacurium has been used in situations in which there is concern about using succinylcholine (e.g., bedridden patients, those with history of MH, and patients with NMS due to neuroleptic agents). Kelly and Brull reported the successful repeated use of mivacurium in a patient who had developed a clinical syndrome presumed to be NMS (fever, rigidity, altered mental state, CF 1710 units/liter) after treatment with neuroleptic agents.[177] The neuroleptics were stopped, but emergency ECT was considered necessary. Anesthetic induction with thiopental and succinylcholine was uneventful, but the patient's temperature and CK rose later that day. Because the role of succinylcholine in the scenario was unclear, Kelly and Brull performed the remaining treatments with mivacurium (doses 0.12 to 0.16 mg/kg), using mask ventilation and reversal agents. Gitlin and colleagues reported their use of mivacurium for MMMECT, which requires somewhat longer anesthesia time than single ECT, typically 10 to 20 min, and for which their patients are intubated.[85] The dose used in that study was 0.25 mg/kg for normal patients and 0.15 mg/kg for a patient with myasthenia gravis.

ATRACURIUM

Atracurium has also been used in ECT with good success. Its duration of action is somewhat longer than that required for most single ECTs, and the reports of its use are predominantly before the clinical availability of mivacurium.[178]

MANAGEMENT OF THE AIRWAY

The patient undergoing ECT has increased requirement for oxygenation and ventilation during the course of the seizure, and maintenance of a patent airway is obviously required. The majority of ECT patients are managed with a regular anesthesia mask; after induction of anesthesia and injection of muscle relaxant, the patient is given positive-pressure ventilation for several breaths, the rubber oral bite block is inserted (Fig. 23-5), and the ECT is administered. (Although the rubber bite block appears to possess a nipple to which the airway tubing might be connected, the nipple does not provide a port through which significant ventilation, suction, and so forth can be provided. Thus, the rubber bite block is removed after the seizure, and other airway adjuncts are used.)

Swindells and Simpson showed that the degree of *desaturation* of patients undergoing ECT varied inversely with the number of breaths the patient received after muscle relaxation and before the shock.[179] Riley reported that failure to preoxygenate patients resulted in clinically significant desaturation after induction, which was of sufficient magnitude that they closed the study before its completion.[180] Thus, it would appear

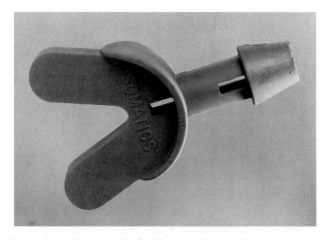

Figure 23-5 Photograph of rubber mouth piece (Somatics, Inc., Lake Bluff, IL). The molded mouthpiece allows firm apposition of patient's teeth without risk of dental fractures or injury to oral soft tissues. The nipple extends out from the patient's mouth but does not provide a port through which significant ventilation, suction, and so forth can be provided.

prudent both to *administer oxygen before induction of anesthesia*, and to *give positive-pressure ventilation* on the patient's loss of consciousness.

MASK

Patients with normal anatomy are managed satisfactorily with a standard anesthesia mask before and after the shock. On occasion, we have encountered significant difficulty with maintaining the airway, particularly in obese, edentulous patients. For routine anesthetics (i.e., not ECTs), insertion of a hard plastic oral airway often relieves the obstruction afforded by redundant tissues of the upper airway. The edentulous ECT patient, however, is at risk for laceration of oral soft tissues and gums if the shock is administered with a hard oral airway in place, and the rubber airway is used. Maintaining a patent airway after the seizure and during the time until spontaneous ventilation recurs can be very difficult in these patients. The ECT patient with teeth is at risk for breaking or avulsing incisors if the shock is administered with a hard oral airway in place, and one of us (LLB) has witnessed this occurrence.

LARYNGEAL MASK AIRWAY

We have been pleased to find that the largyngeal mask airway (LMA) is useful in the patient described above and can greatly facilitate adequate oxygenation during the postictal phase of the ECT. The construction of the LMA, with a 2.5- to 3-cm diameter tube protruding from the mouth, obviates its use *during* the shock, however, because of the risks of damage to teeth or the LMA.

TRACHEAL INTUBATION

Although not the routine airway management technique, intubation of the trachea with a cuffed endotracheal tube is necessary in several groups of patients as described elsewhere in this chapter. When an intubated patient is shocked, it is prudent to insert rolled gauze between the molars bilaterally, to enable the clenching of the masseters without risking damage to teeth, temporomandibular joints, or the endotracheal tube.

CONTROLLING HEART RATE AND BLOOD PRESSURE

The sympathetic response to ECT is manifested as hypertension and arrhythmias. These responses can be dramatic and life-threatening in patients with ischemic cardiovascular disease, hypertension, or vascular aneurysms.[181] Clonidine given orally 2 h before ECT, or nitroglycerin ointment 45 min prior to ECT reduces the hypertensive response.[182] Pretreatment with propranolol and lidocaine is considered ineffective.[151] Propranolol has also been implicated as a cause of asystole in several cases.[183–185] Nifedipine is another antihypertensive that can be used to treat hypertension.

ESMOLOL

The newer sympatholytic agents esmolol and labetalol have been reported to provide good control of hypertension and tachycardia in the dose range of 0.25 to 0.5 mg/kg intravenously, although several groups have reported good results with lower doses (Table 23-15). Some clinicians report concern about unopposed α-adrenergic stimulation with the use of β-blockers. Labetalol blocks both α and β receptors, but its longer duration of effect makes it somewhat less well suited to use for single ETCs.

Howie and coworkers described the use of *infusions of esmolol* (500 μg/kg per min before induction with methohexital and succinylcholine, 300 μg/kg per min after induction). They achieved significant reductions in mean and maximum heart rates and better blood pressure control. However, the duration of seizures decreased, as measured by clinical observation and by EEG.[186] In a follow-up study, they reported that reducing the second infusion rate from 300 μg/kg per min to 100 μg/kg per min resulted in seizures of normal duration.[187]

Kovac and colleagues combined bolus esmolol with infusion, at doses of 80-mg bolus followed by infusion of 24 mg/min.[188] This regimen achieved satisfactory control of blood pressure and heart rate. In a subsequent study, the group evaluated two esmolol bolus doses, 100 mg and 200 mg, on hemodynamic response to ECT.[189] Both doses produced satisfactory control of hemodynamics, but the 200-mg dose was associated

TABLE 23-15
Selected Esmolol Regimens for Controlling Tachycardia and Hypertension Associated With ECT

Regimen Number	Dose of Esmolol and Timing of Administration	Reference
1	100 mg IV 1 min preinduction	Kovac et al.[189]
2	2 mg/kg IV after induction, 2 min pre-ECT	O'Flaherty et al.[191]
3	1 mg/kg IV after induction	Weinger et al.[190]
4	1.3 or 4.4 mg/kg IV	Castelli et al.[192]

with a shorter duration of seizure. Thus, the group recommended the use of a 100-mg dose.

Weinger and colleagues[190] compared pretreatments of *bolus esmolol* (1.0 mg/kg), fentanyl, labetalol (0.3 mg/kg), lidocaine, and saline in a double-blind, randomized block-design study. The esmolol and labetalol patients had more pronounced attenuation of hemodynamic responses, with the esmolol arterial blood pressures somewhat less elevated than labetalol pressures. Retreatment for inadequate duration or failure of seizure production was necessary more frequently in the labetalol group. The authors recommended esmolol 1 mg/kg administered 1 min before induction of anesthesia.[190] O'Flaherty and coworkers[191] evaluated 10 patients undergoing 82 ECT treatments and compared esmolol 2 mg/kg, nitroglycerin 3 μg/kg, with placebo. The best clinical hemodynamics were obtained using esmolol, and in those cases, there was better control of heart rate and blood pressure.[191]

Castelli and associates[192] compared ECT patients pretreated with two different doses of esmolol, labetalol, or placebo. Placebo patients' peak increases in systolic blood pressure and heart rate were 55 mmHg and 37 beats per minute. Treatment with either dose of esmolol or labetalol caused reductions in peak systolic blood pressure and heart rate and with the esmolol, a return to normal values occurred more rapidly after ECT.[192] The doses of esmolol used were 1.3 or 4.4 mg/kg, and doses of labetalol were 0.13 or 0.44 mg/kg.

Administration of a bolus dose is generally more practical than that of an infusion, and the bolus esmolol techniques have become widely used.

LABETALOL
Labetalol has been studied apart from the use of esmolol. McCall and associates found that small doses of labetalol (5 and 10 mg per patient) attenuated the heart rate response to ECT without affecting blood pressure or seizure duration.[193] Stoudemire and colleagues administered labetalol, 2.5 to 5 mg per patient intravenously before ECT, and reported satisfactory outcomes in a predominantly elderly group (mean age 70 years).[194] Labetalol has been reported to be associated with asystole in the setting of ECT.[195] To quote Kauf-

man, "If beta blockers are utilized to control the haemodynamics of ECT, concomitant use of atropine or glycopyrrolate is suggested."[195]

Special Considerations

CHILDREN AND ADOLESCENTS

Use of ECT is rarely indicated for children less than 16 years of age. Indications for which ECT has been found to be effective include bipolar disorder and severe depression (e.g., suicide or starvation). Little information is available about efficacy for schizophrenia, delirium, and anorexia nervosa. ECT is considered *not* to be effective for treatment of autism or chronic organic brain syndromes.[196] Patients with NMS and with lethal catatonia have been treated with some success. In general, there is little information in the literature about use of ECT in children, and even less information in the form of controlled studies.

ELDERLY

The geriatric patient is at higher risk for concurrent disease, particularly cardiovascular and cerebrovascular disease.[197,198] In addition, these patients tend to be more sensitive to medications. A retrospective study by Philibert and coworkers[199] described comorbid illnesses in a group of 192 depressed patients aged 65 years and older and reviewed outcomes. The patients' comorbid illnesses are listed in Table 23-16 and are illustrative of the kinds of medical problems likely to be seen in the older ECT patients. They found that those patients treated with ECT had better outcomes.[199]

OSTEOPOROSIS

In the elderly female population, there is a high prevalence of osteoporosis, placing those patients at higher risk for fractures if they are not completely paralyzed for ECTs. Milstein and colleagues reviewed usefulness of pre-ECT radiographic screening of the skull and spine and recommended that older female patients be considered for spine films.[200]

TABLE 23-16
Comorbid Illnesses in 108 Geriatric Patients Treated with ECT

Disease	Number	Percent
Congestive heart failure	8	7.4
Myocardial infarction	10	9.3
Arrhythmia	78	72.2
Valvular disease	7	6.5
Other heart disease	2	1.9
COPD/Emphysema	6	5.6
Other lung disease	1	0.9
Hypertension	36	33.3
Diabetes	9	8.3
Organic brain disease	16	14.8
Cancer	8	7.4

NOTE: COPD, chronic obstructive pulmonary disease
SOURCE: Data adapted from and used with permission from Philibert et al.[199]

HEART DISEASE

Myocardial ischemia is a concern with ECT in the elderly because of the tachycardia and hypertension that occur with treatment. Patients with a history of myocardial infarction within the past 3 months are considered at high risk for ECT. Patients with prosthetic heart valves should have Coumadin continued.

Pacemaker patients require ready availability of a pacemaker magnet and knowledgeable assistance. Temporary conversion of the pacemaker from demand mode to a fixed (asynchronous) mode allows the ECT without inhibition of the pacer. After the ECT, the magnet is removed and the pacemaker is restored to a demand mode. Individual consultation with a patient's cardiologist is strongly recommended, lest the reprogramming be difficult.

There have been cases reported of ECT in patients with *automatic implantable cardiac defibrillators* (AICDs).[201] The AICD should be deactivated during the ECT, and it is suggested that a cardiologist be present in case the AICD is difficult to reprogram or if ventricular fibrillation occurs during ECT.

PREGNANCY

Special considerations also apply for pregnant patients. Behavior that is uncontrollable, combined with severe depression and poor nutritional intake, constitute clinical justification for ECT. Complications reported in this group include transient, benign fetal arrhythmias, mild vaginal bleeding, abdominal pain, and self-limited uterine contractions.[202] Sherer and colleagues reported recurrent mild abruptio placentae associated with ECT.[203] Patients with high-risk pregnancies, including twin pregnancy, have been managed with ECT, when it is indicated.[204,205] To reduce the risk of aspiration, it is recommended that ECT be performed under general anesthesia with endotracheal intubation. It is also recommended that an obstetrician be present and that fetal biophysical parameters be carefully monitored (uterine tocodynamometry) throughout the procedures.[202] The mother should be pretreated with glycopyrrolate rather than atropine (which crosses the placenta and interferes with fetal beat-to-beat variability), and left uterine displacement or frank lateral positioning should be implemented.

GASTROESOPHAGEAL REFLUX

With ECT, intragastric pressure increases dramatically,[206] almost certainly increasing the risk of regurgitation and aspiration in the patient with an incompetent lower esophageal sphincter. This is a common problem in the general population, and intubation of the trachea is indicated in patients with significant reflux disease. Pharmacologic modification of gastric contents is routinely used.

OTHER SPECIAL GROUPS

Case reports have been published which discuss management of ECT for patients with MH, heart transplant, and liver transplant.

MALIGNANT HYPERTHERMIA

Franks and colleagues described the management of a depressed patient for ECT, who had a prior history of masseter spasm after succinylcholine, elevated creatine phosphokinase, and scoliosis.[207] The patient was pretreated with dantrolene and heavily sedated because of her anxiety. Anesthesia for the ECTs consisted of thiamylal without a muscle relaxant and physical restraint of her limbs was provided by attendants. After nine ECT sessions she was markedly improved, and was eventually discharged on oral dantrolene, which relieved her anxiety. (It is noteworthy that the patient carried the diagnosis of MH based on a platelet bioassay, and data from subsequent platelet bioassays were used during the course of ECTs to manage her care. Because that assay is not now considered a valid test for MH, the importance of this case report is unclear.)

Lazarus and Rosenberg reported data on a 30-year-old man who underwent ECT for catatonia. He developed hyperthermia, muscle rigidity, tachycardia, and muscle soreness with ECTs (for which succinylcholine had been given). A caffeine-halothane contracture test was positive for MH susceptibility.[208]

If an ECT patient is known to be MH susceptible, a nontriggering anesthetic is administered, omitting succinylcholine and substituting a nondepolarizing agent. The barbiturates are considered protective against an MH crisis. Potent inhalational agents are not routinely administered during ECT. Routine prophylaxis of dantrolene is not recommended.

HEART TRANSPLANT

Jones[209] and Kellner and colleagues[210] described ECT in patients who had received cardiac transplants. The denervated heart responds differently to stimuli than the native heart does: lack of vagal innervation eliminates the risk of bradycardia with ECT, and response to stress and exercise is primarily by increased stroke volume, rather than by tachycardia. Hemodynamic responses to ECT in a patient who had received a heart transplant 5 years earlier were described by Pargger and coworkers.[211] In addition to having had a heart transplant, the patient suffered from insulin-dependent diabetes mellitus, hypertension, Parkinson's disease, chronic renal failure (treated with peritoneal dialysis), and had sustained a cerebral vascular accident. The patient was monitored noninvasively, with continuous ST-segment monitoring. Because of the concern that the transplanted heart might be supersensitive to catecholamines, he was given esmolol 100 mg before the first ECT. The esmolol was omitted in subsequent treatments, and hemodynamics were stable.[211]

LIVER TRANSPLANT

Showalter and colleagues described their management of a 63-year-old man who was suicidal 30 months after a liver transplant.[212] Special considerations in that case included supplementation of steroids, because of concern about adrenal suppression, and post-ECT fever spikes after two of the seven ECTs. The fevers were evaluated, but no cause was identified.

Complications

CARDIOVASCULAR

Complications common to ECT are most likely to be related to the cardiovascular system. This morbidity is estimated to be about 0.3 to 0.4 percent of patients treated with ECT.[213] Arrhythmias and myocardial ischemia occur most frequently in patients with a history of cardiac disease. Hypoxia, hypercapnia, respiratory acidosis, hypertension, and older age seem to be variables related to increased incidence of severe complications. Medications such as digitalis, diuretics, and antiarrhythmics can also be associated with more arrhythmias.[214] Of 40 patients with cardiac dysfunction (impaired left ventricular function, ventricular arrhythmias, or conduction defects) reported by Zielinski and coworkers, 38 were able to complete their courses of ECT, albeit with a significantly greater cardiac complication rate compared with ECT patients with normal hearts.[215] The major cardiac complications in that study were bundle branch blocks, PVCs, and intraventricular conduction defects. Zielinski emphasized that this group of patients had had prior difficulties with TCAs as well and that ECT was chosen only after serious consideration.

Rice and coworkers reviewed 1 year's ECT cases and found no cases of death or permanent cardiac morbidity during ECT.[216] Myocardial stunning has rarely been reported. Eitzman and coworkers described management of a 76-year-old woman who underwent ECT and developed ST-segment elevation and Q waves; echocardiogram revealed septal and apical akinesis. She was found to have coronary vasospasm by hyperventilation echocardiogram; she was successfully treated with nifedipine and had uneventful subsequent ECTs.[217]

NEUROLOGIC

Neurologic complications secondary to ECT are rare. There were reports in the early development of ECT that petechial hemorrhages, gliosis, and neuronal degeneration were evident after treatment. There is however, currently little evidence in humans that the electrically induced seizures produce cerebral damage.[121] CBF is increased from 100 to 400 percent over baseline, and this may be accompanied by *headache*.[218] Weisberg and colleagues reported an intracerebral hemorrhage after ECT in a 69-year-old patient.[219] Disorientation immediately after the electrically induced convulsion is noted in 12 percent of the elderly and 9 percent of younger patients. This disorientation has reportedly lasted close to 3 weeks after treatment in a few cases. The amount of electrical stimulation, type of wave form, and number of treatments directly affect the degree of cognitive defect.

Clinical and experimental studies indicate that when adequate oxygenation is provided, cerebral damage does not occur. Grand mal seizures in adequately oxygenated patients exhibit marked increases in lactate and carbon dioxide production.[5] Continuous seizure activity will cause a marked reduction of energy substrates, and with extreme neuronal hyperactivity that is not controlled, cell death will occur.

STATUS EPILEPTICUS

Status epilepticus is rarely precipitated by ECT.[79,220] Status epilepticus may not be obvious without an EEG because a patient may only appear to be more regressive, unresponsive, and mute. Crider and Hansen-Grant reported a case in which nonconvulsive status epilepticus appeared to be delayed emergence from anesthesia.[221] Diagnosis required EEG evaluation, and treatment is supportive.

COGNITIVE DEFICITS

The cognitive deficits mentioned elsewhere in this chapter have been addressed, at least in several groups' attempts to reduce the incidence and severity of amnesia.[222] Animal studies have suggested a role for L-triiodothyronine in ameliorating memory loss after ECT.[223] Khan and coworkers[130,131] reported a placebo controlled study in which depressed ECT patients were treated with low-dose TRH or placebo infusion. The TRH patients had an improved performance on a battery of neuropsychological tests.[130,131] Hofmann and coworkers reported a blunted TSH response at the end of ECT.[224] Further studies are ongoing in this field.

MUSCULOSKELETAL

Musculoskeletal complications are less common due to protection from paralytic agents. Before modified ECT, patients suffered from midthoracic vertebral compression fractures in up to 50 percent of cases.[5] Today, musculoskeletal injuries, damage to dentition, pulmonary aspiration, oral lacerations, and persistent myalgias occur rarely.

OTHER COMPLICATIONS

Other complications from ECT have been reported and descriptions follow.

Splenic rupture has been described in two patients with predisposing factors (a previous spontaneous splenic rupture that had been allowed to heal spontaneously and prior radiation therapy to the abdomen for Hodgkin's lymphoma).[225] Both patients presented with signs of hypotension in the post-ECT period, and thus demonstrated that the period immediately after ECT is a time of high risk.

Inadvertent shock of anesthesia personnel involved with the ECT has been reported.[226]

Recovery

Recovery from the ECT and from the anesthetic must be closely monitored by the anesthesiologist or other qualified staff, and emergency equipment must be readily available. In our experience, the psychiatrists usually prefer that patients *not* be sent back to the psychiatric unit with supplemental oxygen—the nasal prongs and tubing may present a risk to the suicide-prone individual.

The Future of ECT

A new technology, transcranial magnetic stimulation, has been developed.[227] This involves passage of current through a coil on the scalp, creating a magnetic field, which produces currents and depolarizes neurons in the cortex under the coil. With further refinements it may be possible to create an antidepressant effect by specific regional brain stimulation.[228]

Zyss[229] has described "deep magnetic brain stimulation." This technology, which allows more selective brain stimulation by time-varying magnetic field pulses, has fewer undesirable side effects and is painless.[229] Time will tell whether this newer technique will supplement or supplant the use of ECT.

Conclusions

Electroconvulsive therapy has evolved a great deal in the past 50 years, and with continued research, the mechanism of action will be more clearly defined. Patients range in physical status and should receive appropriate monitoring and care, according to the severity of their medical disorders. Teamwork among the anesthesiologist, psychiatrist, and PACU personnel can create a safe environment for the patient undergoing ECT.

References

1. Reid WH: Electroconvulsive therapy. *Texas Med* 1993; 89(5):58.
2. von Meduna L: General discussion of the Cardiozol therapy. *Am J Psychiatry* 1938; 94:40.
3. Bini L: Experimental research on epileptic attacks induced by the electrical current. *Am J Psychiatry* 1938; 94:172.
4. Bennett AE: Preventing traumatic complications in convulsive shock therapy by curare. *JAMA* 1940; 114:322.
5. Pitts FN: Medical physiology of ECT. In Abrams R, Essman WB (eds): *Electroconvulsive Therapy: Biological Foundations and Clinical Applications.* New York, Spectrum Publications, 1982:57–89.
6. Coffey ED, Weiner RD: Electroconvulsive therapy: An update. *Hosp Community Psychiatry* 41(5):515.
7. Gaines GY III, Rees DI: Anesthetic considerations of electroconvulsive therapy. *South Med J* 1992; 85:469.
8. Selvin BL: Electroconvulsive therapy—1987. *Anesthesiology* 1987; 67:367.
9. Kendell RE: The present status of electroconvulsive therapy. *Br J Psychiatry* 1981; 139:265.
10. Gaines GY III, Rees DI: Electroconvulsive therapy and anesthetic considerations. *Anesth Analg* 1986; 65:1345.
11. Scott AI: Contemporary practice of electroconvulsive therapy. *Br J Hosp Med* 1994; 51(7):334.
12. Weiner RD, Krystal AD: The present use of electroconvulsive therapy. *Annu Rev Med* 1994; 45:273.
13. Thompson JW, et al: Use of ECT in the United States in 1975, 1980, and 1986. *Am J Psychiatry* 1994; 151:1657.
14. Fink M: Optimizing ECT. *Encephale* 1994; 20(3):297.

15. Bready LL: Electroconvulsive therapy. In Bready LL, Smith RB (eds): *Decision Making in Anesthesiology,* 2nd ed. Philadelphia, Mosby-Year Book, 1992:346–347.

16. Fink M: How does convulsive therapy work? *Neuropsychopharmacology* 1990; 3(2):73.

17. Sackheim HA: Central issues regarding the mechanisms of action of electroconvulsive therapy: Directions for future research. *Psychopharmacol Bull* 1994; 30(3):281.

18. Crow TJ, Johnstone EC: Controlled trials of electroconvulsive therapy. *Ann N Y Acad Sci* 1986; 462:12.

19. Brandon S, et al: Electroconvulsive therapy: Results in depressive illness from the Leicestershire trial. *BMJ* 1984; 288:22.

20. Freeman CP, et al: Double-blind controlled trial of electroconvulsive therapy (E.C.T.) and simulated E.C.T. in depressive illness. *Lancet* 1978; 1:738.

21. Gregory S, et al: The Nottingham ECT study. A double-blind comparison of bilateral, unilateral and simulated ECT in depressive illness. *Br J Psychiatry* 1985; 146:520.

22. Johnstone EC, et al: The Northwick Park electroconvulsive therapy trial. *Lancet* 1980; 2:1317.

23. Lambourn J, Gill D: A controlled comparison of simulated and real ECT. *Br J Psychiatry* 1978; 133:514.

24. West ED: Electric convulsion therapy in depression: A double-blind controlled trial. *BMJ* 1981; 282:355.

25. Sackeim HA, et al: Effects of stimulus intensity and electrode placement on the efficacy and cognitive effects of electroconvulsive therapy. *N Engl J Med* 1993; 328:839.

26. Sackeim HA, et al: Physical properties and quantification of the ECT stimulus: I. Basic principles. *Convulsive Therapy* 1994; 10:93.

27. Ottosson JO: Seizure characteristics and therapeutic efficacy in electroconvulsive therapy. An analysis of the antidepressive efficiency of grand mal and lidocaine modified seizures. *J Nerve Ment Dis* 1962; 135:239.

28. Sackeim HA: Optimizing unilateral electroconvulsion therapy. *Convulsive Therapy* 1991; 7:201.

29. Sackeim HA, et al: Seizure threshold in electroconvulsive therapy. Effects of sex, age, electrode placement, and number of treatments. *Arch Gen Psychiatry* 1987; 44:355.

30. American Psychiatric Association Task Force for ECT: The practice of ECT: Recommendations for treatment, training, and privileging. *Convulsive Therapy* 1990; 2:85.

31. O'Leary D, et al: Which depressed patients respond to ECT? The Nottingham results. *J Affect Disord* 1995; 33(4):245.

32. Fink M: Indications for the use of ECT. *Psychopharmacol Bull* 1994; 30(3):269.

33. Strauss GD: Personality assessment of adults and children. In Kaplan HI, Sadock BJ (eds): *Comprehensive Textbook of Psychiatry VI,* 6th ed. Baltimore, Williams & Wilkins, 1995:521–635.

34. Mukherjee S, et al: Electroconvulsive therapy of acute manic episodes: A review of 50 years' experience. *Am J Psychiatry* 1994; 151:169.

35. Dubovsky SL: Electroconvulsive therapy: In Kaplan HI, Sadock BJ (eds): *Comprehensive Textbook of Psychiatry VI,* 6th ed. Baltimore, Williams & Wilkins, 1995:2129–2150.

36. Zwil AS, Pelchat RJ: ECT in the treatment of patients with neurological and somatic disease. *Int J Psychiatry Med* 1994; 24(1):1.

37. Zervas IM, Fink M: ECT for refractory Parkinson's disease. *Convulsive Therapy* 1991; 7:222.

38. Rasmussen K, Abrams R: Treatment of Parkinson's disease with electroconvulsive therapy. *Psychiatr Clin North Am* 1991; 14:925.

39. Faber R, Trimble MR: Electroconvulsive therapy in Parkinson's disease and other movement disorders. *Mov Disord* 1991; 6(4):293.

40. Kellner CH, et al: Electroconvulsive therapy and Parkinson's disease: The case for further study. *Psychopharmacol Bull* 1994; 30(3):495.

41. Fochtmann L: A mechanism for the efficacy of ECT in Parkinson's disease. *Convulsive Therapy* 1988; 4:321.

42. Kapur S, Mann JJ: Role of the dopaminergic system in depression. *Biol Psychiatry* 1992; 32:1.

43. Douyon R, et al: ECT and Parkinson's disease revisited: A naturalistic study. *Am J Psychiatry* 1989; 146:1451.

44. King JH, Nuss S: Reflex sympathetic dystrophy treated by electroconvulsive therapy: Intractable pain, depression, and bilateral electrode ECT. *Pain* 1993; 55:393.

45. Shapiro MF, Goldberg HH: Electroconvulsive therapy in patients with structural disease of the central nervous system. *Am J Med Sci* 1957; 233:186.

46. Dressler DM, Folk J: The treatment of depression with ECT in the presence of brain tumor. *Am J Psychiatry* 1975; 132:1320.

47. Gassell MM: Deterioration after electroconvulsive therapy in patients with intracranial meningioma. *Arch Gen Psychiatry* 1960; 3:504.

48. Maltbie AA, et al: Electroconvulsive therapy in the presence of brain tumor. Case reports and evaluation of risks. *J Nerv Ment Dis* 1980; 168:400.

49. Andrews JM, Nemeroff CB: Contemporary management of depression. *An J Med* 1994; 97(6A):24S.

50. Levine R, et al: Grand mal seizures associated with the use of fluoxetine. *J Clin Psychopharmacol* 1994; 14(2):145 (letter).

51. Yan QS, et al: Evidence that a serotonergic mechanism is involved in the anticonvulsant effect of fluoxetine in genetically epilepsy-prone rats. *Eur J Pharmacol* 1994; 252(1):105.

52. Gamage CA, Plant LD: Fluoxetine, electroconvulsive therapy, and prolonged seizures. Nursing assessment leads to patient safety. *J Psychosoc Nurs Ment Health Serv* 1995; 33(2):24.

53. Schwartz AJ, Wollman H: Anesthetic considerations for patients on chronic drug therapy: L-dopa, monoamine oxidase inhibitors, tricyclic antidepressants, and propranolol. *Anesthesiology* 1976; 44:98.

54. Roizen M: Monoamine oxidase inhibitors: Are we condemned to relive history, or is history no longer relevant? *J Clin Anesth* 1990; 2:293.

55. El-Ganzouri AR, et al: Monoamine oxidase inhibitors: Should they be discontinued preoperatively? *Anesth Analg* 1985; 64:592.

56. Sackheim HA: Continuation therapy following ECT: Directions for future research. *Psychopharmacol Bull* 1994; 30:501.

57. Caroff SN, et al: Malignant hyperthermia susceptibility in neuroleptic malignant syndrome. *Anesthesiology* 1987; 67:20.

58. Miller CE, et al: Lethal catatonia following temporomandibular joint surgery: A case report. *J Oral Maxillofac Surg* 1994; 52:510.

59. Kellner CH, et al: ECT-drug interactions: A review. *Psychopharmacol Bull* 1991; 27:595.

60. Hoenig J, Chaulk R: Delirium associated with lithium therapy in electroconvulsive therapy. *Can Med Assoc J* 1979; 116:837.

61. Remick RA: Acute brain syndrome associated with ECT and lithium. *Can Psychiatr Assoc J* 1978; 23:129.

62. Small JG, et al: Complications with electroconvulsive treatment combined with lithium. *Biol Psychiatry* 1980; 15:103.

63. Kirshna NR, et al: Response to lithium carbonate. *Biol Psychiatry* 1978; 13:601.

64. Perry P, Tsuang MT: Treatment of unipolar depression following electroconvulsive therapy. *J Affect Disord* 1979; 1:123.

65. Coppen A, et al: Lithium continuation therapy following electroconvulsive therapy. *Br J Psychiatry* 1981; 139:284.

66. Small JG, Milstein V: Lithium interactions: Lithium and electroconvulsive therapy. *J Clin Psychopharmacol* 1990; 10(5):346.

67. Healy D, et al: Alpha-1-acid glycoprotein in major depressive and eating disorders. *J Affective Dis* 1991; 22:13.

68. DeVane CL, et al: Effect of electroconvulsive therapy on serum concentration of alpha-1-acid glycoprotein. *Biol Psychiatry* 1991; 30:116.

69. Jaksa RJ, Palahniuk RJ: Attempted organophosphate suicide: A unique cause of prolonged paralysis during electroconvulsive therapy. *Anesth Analg* 1995; 80:832.

70. Chelliah J, et al: Inhibition of cholinesterase activity by tetrahydroaminoacridine and the hemisuccinate esters of tocopherol and cholesterol. *Biochim Biophys Acta* 1994; 1206:17.

71. Engelhardt W, et al: Intra-individual open comparison of burst-suppression-isoflurane-anesthesia versus electroconvulsive therapy in the treatment of severe depression. *Eur J Anaesthesiol* 1993; 10(2):113.

72. Langer G, et al: Isoflurane narcotherapy in depressive patients refractory to conventional antidepressant drug treatment. A double-blind comparison with electroconvulsive treatment. *Neuropsychobiology* 1995; 31(4):182.

73. Weiner RD: Back to the basics: Electricity and ECT. *Convulsive Rev* 1994; 10(2):135.

74. Sackeim HA, et al: Stimulus intensity, seizure threshold, and seizure duration: Impact on the efficacy and safety of electroconvulsive therapy. *Psychiatr Clin North Am* 1991; 14:803.

75. Maletzky BM: Seizure duration and clinical effect in electroconvulsive therapy. *Compr Psychiatry* 1978; 19:541.

76. Addersley DJ, Hamilton M: Use of succinylcholine in ECT. *BMJ* 1953; 1:195.

77. Fink M, Johnson L: Monitoring the duration of electroconvulsive therapy seizures: Cuff and EEG compared. *Arch Gen Psychiatry* 1982; 39:1189.

78. Lambert M, Petty F: EEG seizure duration monitoring of ECT. *Prog Neuropsychopharmacol Biol Psychiatry* 1994; 18(3):497.

79. Scott AIF, Riddle W: Status epilepticus after electroconvulsive therapy. *Br J Psychiatry* 1989; 155:119.

80. Weiner RD: ECT and seizure threshold. *Biol Psychiatry* 1980; 15:225.

81. Abrams R: Stimulus parameters and efficacy of ECT. *Convulsive Therapy* 1994; 10(2):124.

82. Swartz CM, et al: Heart rate differences between right and left unilateral electroconvulsive therapy. *J Neurol Neurosurg Psychiatry* 1994; 57(1):97.

83. Maletzky BM: Conventional and multiple-monitored electroconvulsive therapy. A comparison in major depressive episodes. *J Nerv Ment Dis* 1986; 174(5):257.

84. Weiner RD: Treatment optimization with ECT. *Psychopharmacol Bull* 1994; 30:313.

85. Gitlin MC, et al: Is mivacurium chloride effective in electroconvulsive therapy? A report of four cases, including a patient with myasthenia gravis. *Anesth Analg* 1993; 77:392.

86. Schwarz T, et al: Maintenance ECT: Indications and outcome. *Convulsive Therapy* 1995; 11(1):14.

87. Monroe RR: Maintenance electroconvulsive therapy. *Psychiatr Clin North Am* 1991; 14:947.

88. Kellner CH: Maintenance ECT, again. . . . *Convulsive Therapy* 1994; 10(3):187 (editorial).

89. Stiebel VG: Maintenance electroconvulsive therapy for chronic mentally ill patients: A case series. *Psychiatr Serv* 1995; 46(3):265.

90. Lerer B, et al: Antidepressant and cognitive effects of twice-versus three-times-weekly ECT. *Am J Psychiatry* 1995; 152:564.

91. Bridenbaugh RH, et al: Multiple monitored electroconvulsive treatment of schizophrenia. *Compr Psychiatry* 1972; 13:9.

92. Pande AC, et al: Effect of hyperventilation on seizure length during electroconvulsive therapy. *Biol Psychiatry* 1990; 27:799.

93. Walker J, et al: Effects of aminophylline on the electroencephalogram and seizure threshold of the rat. *Electroencephalogr Clin Peurophysiol* 1975; 38:553.

94. Zwillich CW, et al: Theophylline induced seizures in adults: Correllaton with serum concentrations. *Ann Intern Med* 1975; 82:784.

95. Devanand DP, et al: Status epilepticus following ECT in a patient receiving theophylline. *J Clin Psychopharmacol* 1988; 8:153.

96. Swartz CM, Lewis RK: Theophylline reversal of electroconvulsive therapy (ECT) seizure inhibition. *Psychosomatics* 1991; 32:47.

97. Rasmussen KG, Zorumski CF: Electroconvulsive therapy in patients taking theophylline. *J Clin Psychiatry* 1993; 54:11.

98. Francis A, Fochtmann L: Caffeine augmentation of electroconvulsive seizures. *Psychopharmacology (Berl)* 1994; 115(3):320.

99. McCall WV, et al: A reappraisal of the role of caffeine in ECT. *Am J Psychiatry* 1993; 150:1543.

100. Rosenquist PB, et al: Effects of caffeine pretreatment on measures of seizure impact. *Convulsive Therapy* 1994; 10(2):181.

101. Beale MD, et al: Supraventricular tachycardia in a patient receiving ECT, clozapine, and caffeine. *Convulsive Therapy* 1994; 10(3):228.

102. Ayd FJ: Methohexital (Brevital): A new anaesthetic for electroconvulsant therapy. *Diseases of the Nervous System* 1961; 22:388.

103. Collins IP, Scott IF: Anaesthetic technique in the practice of ECT. *Br J Psychiatry* 1995; 166(1)118 (letter).

104. Partridge BL, et al: Is the cardiovascular response to electroconvulsive therapy due to the electricity or the subsequent convulsion? *Anesth Analg* 1991; 72:706.

105. Welch CA, Drop L: Cardiovascular effects of ECT. *Convulsive Therapy* 1989; 5:35.

106. Gould L, et al: Electroconvulsive therapy-induced EKG changes simulating a myocardial infarction. *Arch Intern Med* 1983; 143:1786.

107. Graybar G, et al: Transient large upright T-wave on the electrocardiogram during multiple monitored electroconvulsive therapy. *Anesthesiology* 1983; 59:467.

108. Bennett BL, Bready LL; ECG changes with electroconvulsive therapy. *Anesth Analg* 1990; 70:338.

109. Dec GW Jr, et al: The effects of electroconvulsive therapy on serial electrocardiograms and serum cardiac enzyme values. A prospective study of depressed hospitalized inpatients. *JAMA* 1985; 253:2525.

110. Steiner LA, et al: Diagnosis of myocardial injury by real-time recording of ST segments of the electrocardiogram in a patient receiving general anesthesia for electroconvulsive therapy. *Anesthesiology* 1993; 79:383.

111. Wells DG, Davies GG: Hemodynamic changes associated with electroconvulsive therapy. *Anesth Analg* 1987; 66:1193.

112. Knos GB, et al: Electroconvulsive therapy-induced hemodynamic changes unmask unsuspected coronary artery disease. *J Clin Anesth* 1990; 2(1):37.

113. Messina AG, et al: Effect of electroconvulsive therapy on the electrocardiogram and echocardiogram. *Anesth Analg* 1992; 75:511.

114. Troup PJ, et al: Effect of electroconvulsive therapy on cardiac rhythm, conduction, and repolarization. *Pace* 1978; 1:172.

115. Pitts FN, et al: Induction of anesthesia with methohexital and thiopental in electroconvulsive therapy. *N Engl J Med* 1965; 273:353.

116. Zhu WX, et al: Myocardial stunning after electroconvulsive therapy. *Ann Intern Med* 1992; 117:914.

117. Braunwald E, Kloner RA: The stunned myocardium: Prolonged, post-ischemic ventricular dysfunction. *Circulation* 1982; 66:1146.

118. Bolli R: Mechanism of myocardial "stunning." *Circulation* 1990; 82:723.

119. Saito S, et al: The cerebral hemodynamic response to electrically induced seizures in man. *Brain Res* 1995; 673(1):93.

120. Woods BT, Chiu T-M: Induced and spontaneous seizures in man produce increases in regional brain lipid detected by in vivo proton magnetic resonance spectroscopy. In Bazan NG (ed): *Neurobiology of Essential Fatty Acids.* New York, Plenum Press, 1992:267–274.

121. Coffey CE, et al: Brain anatomic effects of electroconvulsive therapy. A prospective magnetic resonance imaging study. *Arch Gen Psychiatry* 1991; 48:1013.

122. Woods BT, Chiu T-M: In vivo 1H spectroscopy of the human brain following electroconvulsive therapy. *Ann Neurology* 1990; 28(6):745.

123. Tomasson K, et al: Failed and short seizures associated with prior electroconvulsive therapy. *Eur Arch Psychiatry Clin Neurosci* 1992; 241:307.

124. Krueger RB, et al: Does ECT permanently alter seizure threshold? *Biol Psychiatry* 1993; 33:272.

125. Coffey CE, et al: Seizure threshold in electroconvulsive therapy (ECT) I. Initial seizure threshold. *Biol Psychiatry* 1995; 37:713.

126. Coffey CE, et al: Seizure threshold in electroconvulsive therapy (ECT) II. The anticonvulsant effect of ECT. *Biol Psychiatry* 1995; 37:777.

127. Weiner RD: ECT-induced status epilepticus and further ECT: A case report. *Am J Psychiatry* 1981; 138:1237.

128. Hsiao JK, Evans DL: ECT in a depressed patient after craniotomy. *Am J Psychiatry* 1984; 141:442.

129. Khan A, et al: Electroconvulsive therapy. *Psychiatr Clin North Am* 1993; 16:497.

130. Khan A, et al: ECT and TRH: Cholinergic involvement in a cognitive deficit state. *Psychopharm Bull* 1993; 29:345.

131. Khan A, et al: Effects of low-dose TRH on cognitive deficits in the ECT postictal state. *Am J Psychiatry* 1994; 151:1694.

132. Kronfol A, et al: Effects of single and repeated electroconvulsive therapy sessions on plasma ACTH, prolactin, growth hormone and cortisol concentrations. *Psychoneuroendocrinology* 1991; 16:345.

133. Kamil R, Joffe RT: Neuroendocrine testing in electroconvulsive therapy. *Psychiatr Clin North Am* 1991; 14:961.

134. Dored G, et al: Corticotropin, cortisol and b-endorphin responses to the human corticotropin-releasing hormone during melancholia and after unilateral electroconvulsive therapy. *Acta Psychiatr Scand* 1990; 82:204.

135. Kling MA, et al: Effects of electroconvulsive therapy on the CRH-ACTH-cortisol system in melancholic depression: Preliminary findings. *Psychopharmacol Bull* 1994; 30:489.

136. Weinger MB, et al: Prevention of the cardiovascular and neuroendocrine response to electroconvulsive therapy: II. Effects of pretreatment regimens on catecholamines, ACTH, vasopressin, and cortisol. *Anesth Analg* 1991; 73:563.

137. Devanand DP, et al: Effects of electroconvulsive therapy on plasma GABA. *Convulsive Therapy* 1995; 11(1):3.

138. Petty F, et al: Plasma GABA in mood disorders. *Psychopharmacol Bull* 1990; 2:157.

139. Fakhri O, et al: Effect of electroconvulsive therapy on diabetes mellitus. *Lancet* 1980; 2:775.

140. Crammer J, Gillies C: Psychiatric aspects of diabetes mellitus: Diabetes and depression. *Br J Psychiatry* 1981; 139:171.

141. Finestone DH, Weiner RD: Effects on diabetes mellitus. *Acta Psychiatr Scand* 1984; 70:321.

142. Goldney R, et al: Depression, electroconvulsive therapy and diabetes mellitus. *Aust N Z J Psychiatry* 1983; 17:289.

143. Epstein HP, et al: Intraocular pressure changes during anesthesia for electroshock therapy. *Anesth Analg* 1975; 54:479.

144. Elliot DL, et al: Intraocular pressure changes during anesthesia for electroshock therapy. *Anesth Analg* 1975; 54:479.

145. Fischler B, et al: Immune changes induced by electroconvulsive therapy (ECT). *Ann N Y Acad Sci* 1992; 650:326.

146. Sedgwick JV, et al: Anesthesia and mental illness. *Int J Psychiatry Med* 1990; 20:209.

147. deSilva RA, Bachman WR: Cardiac consultation in patients with neuropsychiatric problems. *Cardiol Clin* 1995; 13:225.

148. Lunn RJ, et al: Anesthetics and electroconvulsive therapy seizure duration: Implications for therapy from a rat model. *Biol Psychiatry* 1981; 16:1163.

149. Mokriski BK, et al: Electroconvulsive therapy-induced cardiac arrhythmias during anesthesia with methohexital, thiamylal, or thiopental sodium. *J Clin Anesth* 1992; 4:208.

150. Greenan J, et al: Intravenous glycopyrrolate and atropine at induction of anesthesia: A comparison. *J Royal Soc Med* 1983; 76:369.

151. McCleave KJ, Blakemore WB: Anaesthesia for electroconvulsive therapy. *Anaesth Intensive Care* 1975; 3:250.

152. Stromgren LS, et al: Factors affecting seizure duration and number of seizures applied in unilateral electroconvulsive therapy anesthetics and benzodiazepines. *Acta Psychiatr Scand* 1980; 62:158.

153. Allen RE, Pitts FN Jr: Drug modification of ECT: Methohexital and diazepam. *Biol Psychiatry* 1979; 14:69.

154. Loimer N, et al: Midazolam shortens seizure duration following electronconvulsive therapy. *J Psychiatr Res* 1992; 26:97.

155. Brewer CL, et al: Ketamine ("Ketalar"): A safer anaesthetic for ECT. *Br J Psychiatry* 1972; 120(559):679.

156. Green CD: Ketamine as an anaesthetic for ECT. *Br J Psychiatry* 1973; 122(566):123.

157. McInnes EC, James NM: A comparison of ketamine and methohexital in electroconvulsive therapy. *Med J Aust* 1972; 1:1031.

158. O'Carroll TM, et al: Etomidate in electroconvulsive therapy. A within-patient comparison with alphaxalone/alphadalone. *Anaesthesia* 1977; 32:868.

159. Crispin A, Crommen AM: Progress in electroconvulsive therapy: The non-barbiturate anaesthetic drug etomidate. *Acta Psychatri Belg* 1977; 76:678.

160. Trzepacz PT, et al: Etomidate anesthesia increases seizure duration during ECT. A retrospective study. *Gen Hosp Psychiatry* 1993; 15(2):115.

161. Gran L, et al: Seizure duration in unilateral electroconvulsive therapy. A comparison of the anaesthetic agents etomidate and Althesin with methohexitone. *Acta Psychiatr Scand* 1984; 69:472.

162. Rouse EC: Propofol for electroconvulsive therapy. A comparison with methohexitone. Preliminary report. *Anaesthesia* 1988; 43(suppl):61.

163. Simpson KH, et al: Propofol reduces seizure duration in patients having anesthesia for electroconvulsive therapy. *Br J Anaesth* 1988; 61:343.

164. Dwyer R, et al: Comparison of propofol and methohexitone as anaesthetic agents for electronconvulsive therapy. *Anaesthesia* 1988; 43:459.

165. Boey WK, Lai FO: Comparison of propofol and thiopentone as anaesthetic agents for electroconvulsive therapy. *Anaesthesia* 1990; 45:623.

166. Rampton AJ, et al: Comparison of methohexital and propofol for electroconvulsive therapy: Effects on hemodynamic responses and seizure duration. *Anesthesiology* 1989; 70:412.

167. Fredman B, et al: Anaesthesia for electroconvulsive therapy: Use of propofol revisited. *Eur J Anaesthesiol* 1994; 11:423.

168. Fredman B, et al: Anesthesia for electroconvulsive therapy: Effects of propofol and methohexital on seizure activity and recovery. *Anesth Analg* 1994; 79:75.

169. Martensson B, et al: A comparison of propofol and methohexital as anesthetic agents for ECT: Effects on seizure duration, therapeutic outcome, and memory. *Biol Psychiatry* 1994; 35:179.

170. Malsch E, et al: Efficacy of electroconvulsive therapy after propofol and methohexital anesthesia. *Convulsive Therapy* 1994; 10:212.

171. Fear CF, et al: Propofol anaesthesia in electroconvulsive therapy. Reduced seizure duration may not be relevant. *Br J Psychiatry* 1994; 165:506.

172. Matters RM, et al: Recovery after electroconvulsive therapy: Comparison of propofol with methohexitone anaesthesia. *Br J Anaesth* 1995; 75:297.

173. Avramov MN, et al: The comparative effects of methohexital, propofol, and etomidate for electroconvulsive therapy. *Anesth Analg* 1995; 81:596.

174. Hood DD, Mecca RS: Failure to initiate electroconvulside seizures in a patient pretreated with lidocaine. *Anesthesiology* 1983; 58:379.

175. London SW, Glass DD: Prevention of electroconvulsive therapy-induced dysrhythmias with atropine and propranolol. *Anesthesiology* 1985; 62:819.

176. Pitts FN, et al: The drug modification of ECT II: Succinylcholine dosage. *Arch Gen Psychiatry* 1968; 19:595.

177. Kelly D, Brull SJ: Neuroleptic malignant syndrome and mivacurium: A safe alternative to succinylcholine? *Can J Anaesth* 1994; 41:845.

178. Messer GJ, et al: Electroconvulsive therapy and the chronic use of pseudocholinesterase-inhibitor (echotiophate iodide) eye drops for glaucoma. A case report. *Gen Hosp Psychiatry* 1992; 14:56.

179. Swindells SR, Simpson KH: Oxygen saturation during electroconvulsive therapy. *Br J Psychiatry* 1987; 150:695.

180. Riley R: Preoxygenation and electroconvulsive therapy. *Anesth Analg* 1987; 66:1057 (letter).

181. Jones RM, et al: Cardiovascular and catecholamine responses to ECT in untreated hypertensives compared with normotensives. *Anaesthesia* 1981; 36:795.

182. Lee JT, et al: Modification of electroconvulsive therapy induced hypertension and nitroglycerin ointment. *Anesthesiology* 1985; 62:793.

183. Wells DB, et al: ECT-induced asystole from a sub-convulsive shock. *Anaesth Intensive Care* 1988; 16:368.

184. Wulfson HD, et al: Propranolol prior to ECT associated with asystole. *Anesthesiology* 1984; 60:255.

185. Decina P, et al: Cardiac arrest during ECT modified by beta-adrenergic blockade. *Am J Psychiatry* 1984; 141:298.

186. Howie MB, et al: Esmolol reduces autonomic hypersensitivity and length of seizures induced by electroconvulsive therapy. *Anesth Analg* 1990; 71:384.

187. Howie MB, et al: Defining the dose range for esmolol used in electroconvulsive therapy hemodynamic attenuation. *Anesth Analg* 1992; 75:805.

188. Kovac AL, et al: Esmolol bolus and infusion attenuates increases in blood pressure and heart rate during electroconvulsive therapy. *Can J Anaesth* 1990; 37:58.

189. Kovac AL, et al: Comparison of two esmolol bolus doses on the haemodynamic response and seizure duration during electroconvulsive therapy. *Can J Anaesth* 1991; 38:204.

190. Weinger MB, et al: Prevention of the cardiovascular and neuroendocrine response to electronconvulsive therapy: I. Effectiveness of pretreatment regimens on hemodynamics. *Anesth Analg* 1991; 73:556.

191. O'Flaherty D, et al: Circulatory responses during electroconvulsive therapy. The comparative effects of placebo, esmolol and nitroglycerin. *Anaesthesia* 1992; 47:563.

192. Castelli I, et al: Comparative effects of esmolol and labetalol to attenuate hyperdynamic states after electroconvulsive therapy. *Anesth Analg* 1995; 80:557.

193. McCall WV, et al: Effects of labetalol on hemodynamics and seizure duration during ECT. *Convulsive Therapy* 1991; 7:5.

194. Stoudemire A, et al: Labetalol in the control of cardiovascular responses to electroconvulsive therapy in high-risk depressed medical patients. *J Clin Psychiatry* 1990; 51:508.

195. Kaufman KR: Asystole with electroconvulsive therapy. *J Intern Med* 1994; 235:275.

196. Bertagnoli MW, Borchardt CM: A review of ECT for children and adolescents. *J Am Acad Child Adolesc Psychiatry* 1990; 29:302.

197. Greenberg L, Fink M: The use of electroconvulsive therapy in geriatric pateints. *Clin Geriatric Med* 1992; 8:349.

198. Dubin WR, et al: The efficacy and safety of maintenance ECT in geriatric patients. *J Am Geriatric Soc* 1992; 40:706.

199. Philibert RA, et al: Effect of ECT on mortality and clinical outcome in geriatric unipolar depression. *J Clin Psychiatry* 1995; 56:390.

200. Milstein V, et al: Radiographic screening for ECT: Use and usefulness. *Convulsive Therapy* 1995; 11:38.

201. Goldberg RJ, Badger JM: Major depressive disorder in patients with the implantable cardioverter defibrillator. Two cases treated with ECT. *Psychosomatics* 1993; 34:273.

202. Miller LJ: Use of electroconvulsive therapy during pregnancy. *Hosp Community Psychiatry* 1994; 45:444.

203. Sherer DM, et al: Recurrent mild abruptio placentae occurring immediately after repeated electroconvulsive therapy in pregnancy. *Am J Obstet Gynecol* 1991; 165:652.

204. Livingston JC, et al: Electroconvulsive therapy in a twin pregnancy: A case report. *Am J Perinatol* 1994; 11:116.

205. Walker R, Swartz CM: Electroconvulsive therapy during high-risk pregnancy. *Gen Hosp Psychiatry* 1994; 16:348.

206. Hurwitz TD: Electroconvulsive therapy: A review. *Comp Psychiatry* 1974; 15:303.

207. Franks RD, et al: ECT use for a patient with malignant hyperthermia. *Am J Psychiatry* 1982; 139:1065.

208. Lazarus A, Rosenberg H: Malignant hyperthermia during ECT. *Am J Psychiatry* 1991; 148:541 (letter).

209. Jones ER Jr: Cardiac transplantation and depression. *Am J Psychiatry* 1991; 148:1271 (letter).

210. Kellner CH, et al: Electroconvulsive therapy in a patient with a heart transplant. *N Engl J Med* 1991; 325:663 (letter).

211. Pargger H, et al: Hemodynamic responses to electroconvulsive therapy in a patient 5 years after cardiac transplantation. *Anesthesiology* 1995; 83:625.

212. Showalter PE, et al: Electroconvulsive therapy for depression in a liver transplant patient. *Psychosomatics* 1993; 34:537 (letter).

213. Solomon JG: Electroconvulsive therapy: An overview. *VA Medicine* 1979; 106:180.

214. Weiner RD: The psychiatric use of electrically induced seizures. *Am J Psychiatry* 1979; 136:1507.

215. Zielinski RJ, et al: Cardiovascular complications of ECT in depressed patients with cardiac disease. *Am J Psychiatry* 1993; 150:6.

216. Rice EH, et al: Cardiovascular morbidity in high-risk patients during ECT. *Am J Psychiatry* 1994; 151:1637.

217. Eitzman DT, et al: Management of myocardial stunning associated with electroconvulsive therapy guided by hyperventilation echocardiography. *Ann Heart J* 1994; 127(4 Pt 1):928.

218. Weiner SJ: Headache and electroconvulsive therapy. *Headache* 1994; 34(3):155.

219. Weisberg LA, et al: Intracerebral hemorrhage following electroconvulsive therapy. *Neurology* 1991; 41:1849.

220. Grogan R, et al: Generalized nonconvulsive status epilepticus after electroconvulsive therapy. *Convulsive Therapy* 1995; 11:51.

221. Crider BA, Hansen-Grant S: Nonconvulsive status epilepticus as a cause for delayed emergence after electroconvulsive therapy. *Anesthesiology* 1995; 82:591.

222. Miller AL, et al: Factors affecting amnesia, seizure duration, and efficacy in ECT. *Am J Psychiatry* 1985; 142:692.

223. Stern RA, et al: Influence for L-triiodothyronine on memory following repeated electroconvulsive shock in rats: Implications for human electroconvulsive therapy: *Biol Psychiatry* 1995; 37(3):198.

224. Hofmann P, et al: TSH response to TRH and ECT. *J Affect Dis* 1994; 32:127.

225. Gitlin MC, et al: Splenic rupture after electroconvulsive therapy. *Anesth Analg* 1993; 76:1363.

226. Tammelleo AD: Doctor ''shocks'' nurse: $1.2 million verdict. *Nursing Law* 1993; 33(11):1.

227. Barker AT, et al: Non-invasive magnetic stimulation of the human motor cortex. *Lancet* 1985; 1:1106.

228. George MS, Wassermann EM: Rapid--rate transcranial magnetic stimulation and ECT. *Convulsive Therapy* 1994; 10:251.

229. Zyss T: Deep magnetic brain stimulation—The end of psychiatric electroshock therapy? *Med Hypotheses* 1994; 43:69.

230. Marks RJ: Electroconvulsive therapy: Physiological and anaesthetic considerations. *Can Anaesth Soc J* 1984; 31:541.

231. Rich CL, Smith NT: Anaesthesia for electroconvulsive therapy: A psychiatric viewpoint. *Can Anaesth Soc J* 1981; 28:153.

Chapter 24

NEURORADIOLOGY
Neuroradiologic Procedures

FERNANDO M. ZALDUONDO

E. RALPH HEINZ

The approach to detection and diagnosis of neurologic dysfunction has been revolutionized by modern neuroradiologic imaging, given its increasing ability to depict anatomic detail of normal and abnormal tissue. Exciting refinements in existing modalities such as computed tomography (CT), magnetic resonance imaging (MRI), magnetic resonance angiography (MRA), cervicocerebral vascular ultrasonography (US), positron emission tomography (PET) and single-photon emission computed tomography (SPECT), and the development of new modalities such as magnetic resonance spectroscopy (MRS) have widely expanded the neuroradiologist's diagnostic armamentarium. The result is significantly increased diagnostic sensitivity and specificity in defining not only the anatomic locus correlated with the clinical presentation but also the pathologic tissue's signature. This chapter provides an introduction to modern neuroradiologic imaging with examples of current applications of conventional imaging modalities. It is divided into the following sections: contrast media; the formation of an image by modality; comparison of MRI and CT; approach to neuroradiologic diagnosis; and an imaging review of neurologic disease.

Contrast Media

Conventional catheter angiography, angiography, and myelography require contrast material. Myelography employs an intrathecally administered contrast agent to outline the contents of the thecal sac and to depict intrinsic and extrinsic mass effect on the thecal sac. Catheter angiography relies on intraarterial injection of a contrast agent to define the arterial, capillary and venous anatomy of the craniospinal axis.

Computed tomography and magnetic resonance imaging, the most widely used neuroradiologic modalities, utilize intravenous contrast agents to improve diagnostic sensitivity. This is achieved by increasing lesional conspicuousness. Increased diagnostic specificity is achieved by characterization of enhancement patterns, including absence of enhancement. Nuclear medicine neuroradiologic studies rely on intravenous injectable radiopharmaceuticals for subsequent image formation. The concept of the blood-brain barrier is of paramount importance in understanding enhancement in pathologic lesions.[1]

BLOOD-BRAIN BARRIER

The term blood-brain barrier (BBB) was coined in 1921[2] following observations in the late 19th century that intravenous dye injections stained various organs but not the brain (choroid plexus stained). The BBB is instrumental in the maintenance of homeostasis of the brain's internal environment by means of specialized morphologic features of the capillary endothelium which has properties unique to the brain, retina, and inner ear. Continuous capillaries have a continuous or fused basement membrane.[1,3] Their endothelial cells have a narrow intercellular gap, are connected by a continuous belt of tight junctions, and are invested by a sheath of astrocytic foot processes.[1,3] Moreover, pinocytosis or vesicular transport is rarely present in the brain's capillary endothelium.[3] Capillaries in normal brain and areas of an intact BBB are impermeable to intravascular contrast media such that structures which are principally vascular exhibit enhancement. Minimal contrast enhancement is observed in normal brain parenchyma following contrast injection.

Fenestrated capillaries have a number of circular fenestrations or "pores," 30 to 100 nm in diameter, in the endothelial cells.[1] This type of capillary is present in areas where substantial exchange between blood and tissues takes place. In the brain, it is present in specialized areas named the circumventricular organs, thought to be involved in neurohumoral regulation of the circulation.[1] These areas include the pituitary and pineal glands, infundibulum, medial eminence of neurohypophysis, tuber cinereum, area postrema, choroid plexus, subfornical and subcommissural organs, organum vasculosum of the lamina terminalis, dura, and pia mater vessels.[1,3] Fenestrated capillaries exhibit pinocytotic activity accounting for the normally observed enhancement of these neural structures following intravenous contrast material administration.[3] On high-field strength magnetic resonance instruments, the normal meninges may enhance slightly, particularly where vascular structures reside.[4] Moreover, because the normal meninges lack a BBB, thin linear symmetric meningeal enhancement is a normal observation when not visualized on multiple contiguous sections.[4] This observation needs to be qualified as it applies only to short repetition time (TR) conventional spin echo pulse sequences. In the spine, for anatomic reasons, visualization of normal meningeal enhancement is much more unusual than in the brain.[4]

CONTRAST AGENTS

"Enhancement" refers to the increase in attenuation (in the case of computed tomography) and the increase in signal intensity (in the case of magnetic resonance imaging) as displayed on images. In the case of myelography, subarachnoid contrast agents outline both the contents of the thecal sac and any intrinsic and or extrinsic impressions on the thecal sac. In the case of conventional catheter angiography, contrast agents opacify the lumina of vessels, allowing for the study of the cervicocerebrospinal vasculature. Currently FDA-approved neuroradiologic contrast agents are divided into two categories: iodinated and paramagnetic.

Iodinated agents are used in catheter angiography, myelography, and computed tomography; paramagnetic agents are used in magnetic resonance imaging. The ideal contrast agent should be reproducibly efficacious in differentiating normal and abnormal anatomy by providing superb radiographic contrast, be tolerable and safe for the patient, and should be biologically inert and easily excretable. Dosages vary according to the patient's weight and age. Overall, children tend to have fewer adverse reactions to all types of contrast agents than do adults.[5]

IODINATED CONTRAST AGENTS

Important properties of water-soluble iodinated contrast agents utilized in computed tomography, myelography and catheter angiography include osmolality and hydrophilicity. These contrast agents are administered intravenously, intraarterially, and intrathecally.

Ionic monomers at concentrations ranging from 60 to 76 percent by weight are considered **high-osmolar contrast agents** (HOCA), possessing five to eight times the osmolality of human serum (290 mosm/kg). Nonionic monomers and dimers as well as ionic dimers are considered **low-osmolar contrast agents** (LOCA), having anywhere from two to three times the osmolality of human serum. Some LOCA are isoosmolar and slightly hypoosmolar relative to human serum.[6] All nonionic agents are LOCA, but not all ionic agents are HOCA. Specifically, ioxaglate (Hexabrix) is an ionic LOCA.

LOCA typically are of greater hydrophilicity, decreasing their protein and tissue-binding tendency and making LOCA more biologically inert.[6] The addition of hydroxyl groups to the contrast molecule increases its hydrophilicity at the expense of increases in overall molecule size and viscosity.

Currently, HOCA are extensively used for neuroangiographic procedures including interventional procedures. Advantages include low cost, low viscosity and anticoagulative properties. Disadvantages include higher osmolality and discomfort during intraarterial injection (especially during selective external carotid artery catheter angiography injection) and higher incidence of adverse reactions. LOCA are universally used at our institution for all neurodiagnostic procedures.

The incidence of mild, moderate, and severe reactions of both idiosyncratic (anaphylactoid) and nonidiosyncratic (chemotoxic, osmotoxic, direct organ toxicity and vasomotor) types is decreased with the use of LOCA.[6,7] The patient may experience pain, a warm sensation, and a metallic taste during contrast injection. This may increase anxiety, which in turn may contribute to contrast-related reactions.[5] During catheter angiography and enhanced computed tomography, a painful injection will increase the chance of patient motion during image acquisition, resulting in image degradation and possibly the need to repeat portions or even all of the study. This can also result in an increased total radiation exposure. In the case of catheter angiography, prolongation of the procedure and increased number of contrast injections is associated with increased morbidity and mortality.[8,9] It should be noted the intravenous route is associated with a higher rate of side effects than the intraarterial route. The current explanation for this observation is that in the intravenous route, large doses of contrast agents are delivered directly to the lung, resulting in histamine, serotonin, and other neurotransmitter release and providing greater stimulus for adverse reactions.[5] Although LOCA could result in a higher rate of thrombosis, particularly during arteriography,[10,11] this has not translated into clinically measurable adverse outcome when optimal technique is employed.[6] Warming the LOCA to 37°C will reduce its viscosity. Adequate heparinization of the angiographic saline flushing solution should resolve the potential problem of catheter tip clot formation when using LOCA.[5] Decreased incidence of adverse reactions seems to outweigh possible disadvantages of LOCA.

Iodinated contrast agents are nephrotoxic. A biphasic effect in the renal vasculature is noted. An initial mild vasodilatation is followed rapidly by a more prolonged vasoconstriction that rarely may lead to renal ischemia and breakdown of renal membrane basement junctions.[12] Patients with preexisting renal insufficiency, diabetes mellitus, and possibly congestive heart failure are at a higher risk (9 to 16 percent) for development of contrast agent-induced nephrotoxicity than is the general population (2 to 5 percent).[12] Although some studies have suggested that use of LOCA is associated with a reduction of contrast induced nephrotoxicity, this reduction has been at best subclinical and to date remains of questionable clinical significance.[12]

Dehydrated patients with multiple myeloma may be at a higher risk for contrast agent-induced renal insufficiency.[12] LOCA induce less sickling in vitro than do equivalent HOCA in patients with sickle cell disease (SS and SC).[12] Patients with pheochromocytoma are at risk for contrast-induced fatal hypertensive crisis. If use of a contrast agent is mandatory, an alpha-adrenergic blocker should be given.[12]

Although LOCA are safer and better tolerated than HOCA (overall adverse reaction incidence of 12.66 percent for HOCA and 3.13 percent for LOCA),[5,13] their significantly greater expense (10 to 25 times as much as an equivalent HOCA) has prevented their universal implementation.[12] Very young children must be given LOCA. Their lower osmolality lessens fluid shifts, and decreased pain during injection encourages much-needed compliance in these young patients.

Guidelines for treatment of contrast-induced reaction are continually being developed,[7,14] mandating continued education on the part of the radiologist who is usually the first line of defense clinically.

PARAMAGNETIC CONTRAST AGENTS

Gadolinium (III)-based contrast agents routinely utilized for MRI are considered to be safe and well tolerated, and are administered exclusively via the intravenous route. The overall incidence of adverse reactions for all MR agents ranges from 1 to 4 percent.[5] Few reports of severe or fatal reactions have been recorded.[15,16] Gadolinium is a paramagnetic metal containing seven unpaired outer shell electrons.

In contradistinction to the direct action of iodinated contrast agents, intravenous paramagnetic contrast agents used in MR imaging act indirectly by altering the T1 and T2 properties of neighboring protons adjacent to the site of contrast delivery.[17] Specifically, the T1 and T2 relaxation times are shortened translated to "enhancement" or signal intensity increment of structures with an altered blood-brain barrier permeability on T1-weighted images. Pathologic enhancement is typically produced by infection, inflammation, ischemia-infarction and/or neoplasm. Affected enhancing structures are displayed as brighter relative to neighboring unaffected structures, forming the basis of increased lesional conspicuousness.

The greatest worldwide experience with a paramagnetic agent has been with the ionic contrast agent gadopentetate dimeglumine or Magnevist (Berlex Laboratories, Wayne, NJ). Despite its excellent safety profile, paramagnetic contrast research and development has followed the trend of iodinated contrast agents inasmuch as nonionic agents were developed with hopes of further reducing the incidence of adverse reactions. The recently FDA-approved nonionic paramagnetic agents gadoteridol or ProHance (Squibb Diagnostics, Princeton, NJ) and gadodiamide or Omniscan (Nycomed, distributed by Winthrop) complete the currently available paramagnetic agents in neuroradiology in the United States.

Proposed guidelines for the selection of iodinated contrast agents (LOCA versus HOCA) and of gadolinium-based agents; for the development of premedication regimens in patients at increased risk for contrast-induced reactions; and for the development of standardized treatment algorithms for contrast-induced reactions have recently been formulated.[7,14]

The Formation of an Image: Basic Concepts by Modality

ULTRASONOGRAPHY

FORMATION OF AN IMAGE

Ultrasonography (US) utilizes sound waves of frequencies ranging between 1 and 30 MHz, much higher than frequencies detectable by the human ear. Electrically pulsed energy mechanically deforms and produces vibration of a crystal housed in a hand-held transducer or probe. A transducer-frequency specific sound wave is generated. This sound wave propagates through the patient's soft tissues and bounces off an acoustic interface, causing an echo. In turn, this bounced sound wave generates another vibration of the transducer crystal. The crystal generates an electrical voltage proportional to the magnitude of the returning echo. This signal is amplified and displayed in various formats interpretable as anatomic and physiologic information.

The time it takes for the emitted sound wave to return to the transducer is calculated and is assigned a depth. Visualization of adjacent tissues is improved when the difference between their acoustic textures is greatest. An example would be differentiating moving blood in the common carotid artery and internal jugular vein from the adjacent sternocleidomastoid musculature. This would be more apparent than differentiating liver from adjacent kidney,[18] given their smaller difference in echotexture. All US examples presented in this section are the result of high-resolution gray-scale imaging displayed as white on a black background.

As a general principle, the higher the frequency of the transducer, the higher the resolution of the image of superficial soft tissues, but the less the sound beam penetrates. Conversely, the lower the transducer's frequency, the deeper the sound beam penetrates. In the case of carotid ultrasound, a high-frequency transducer is optimal.

Ultrasound's attributes include its availability and relative low cost, documented safety and noninvasiveness. However, image quality depends on optimization of multiple scan parameters. This modality's sensitivity for lesion detection is operator-dependent; therefore, large modality-specific variability is not uncommon. Its main applications in diagnostic neuroradiology feature cervicocranial vascular disease, perinatal detection of cerebral and spinal structural abnormalities, and intraventricular and parenchymal hemorrhage.

CERVICOCRANIAL VASCULAR DISEASE

In the evaluation of cervicocranial atherosclerotic disease, the terms "gray scale," "spectral analysis," "duplex," and "color Doppler" abound. This section aims to present a succinct description of US terminology prior to a description of the role of US in the evaluation of carotid bifurcation.

The terms high-resolution gray scale or soft tissue imaging refer to the display of anatomy as bright spots on a black background. "Hyperechoic," "isoechoic," "hypoechoic" and "anechoic" are terms that characterize the echotexture of normal and abnormal anatomy. For example, simple cysts and moving blood are anechoic to hypoechoic and are displayed as "no echoes" or simply as black.

Spectral analysis provides physiologic information, namely flow in vessels, based on the Doppler principle. When a high-frequency sound wave emitted by the probe meets a moving interface such as red blood cells, the reflected sound wave has a different frequency. A frequency shift is produced akin to the change in frequency experienced by an observer (the ultrasound probe) when an ambulance siren moves toward or away from the observer (moving red blood cells). A higher returning frequency indicates that blood is moving toward the transducer. Conversely, a lower returning frequency indicates it is moving away. Pulsed Doppler utilizes the same transducer to emit and receive sound waves and analyzes the frequency shifts produced at a specified area generating arterial or venous spectral waveforms. Alternatively, in continuous wave Doppler, the sound wave is continuously generated by one transducer and continuously received by a second transducer housed in the same probe. Myriad scan parameters need to be optimized when imaging the carotid bifurcation to avoid inaccuracies in the determination of hemodynamically significant stenosis.

Arterial waveforms are displayed in a magnitude-over-time format, the so-called spectral analysis. In this format, directional information relative to the ultrasound probe conventionally is displayed as signal above or below an established baseline selected by the operator. Prototypical waveforms of a normal external carotid (ECA), internal carotid (ICA) and common carotid (CCA) are shown in Fig. 24-1A–C. The ECA waveform (Fig. 24-1A) is characterized by a sharp systolic upswing, a sharp systolic downswing and little or no end-diastolic flow, indicating a high-resistance arterial bed. The ICA waveform (Fig. 24-1B) is characterized by a less acute systolic downswing and a fairly large amount of persistent end-diastolic flow, indicating a low-resistance arterial bed. Spectral analysis includes determination of peak systolic velocity, end diastolic velocity, spectral broadening and flow volume. "Spectral broadening" refers to a higher number of frequencies present in the tracing indicative of turbulence.

"Duplex" ultrasound refers to the combined use of high-resolution gray scale imaging with physiologic information provided by spectral analysis, usually pulsed Doppler.[19] Although gray scale imaging and Doppler spectral analysis information usually correlate closely, occasionally there may be disagreement.[19]

"Color Doppler" allows display of blood flow and soft tissue over large anatomic areas, assigning color to flowing blood. By convention, red indicates flow toward the transducer and blue away from the transducer. The color represents the mean frequency shift produced by moving red blood cells in the sampled volume (Fig. 24-2). In this way, blood acts as a "natural" contrast agent, allowing detection of small channels of flow in narrowed vessels too small to resolve on conventional gray scale ultrasonography. This feature expedites examination time, promotes reproducibility

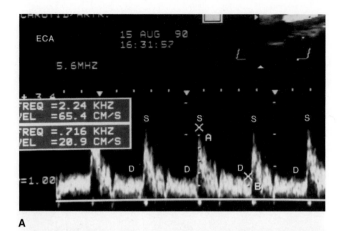

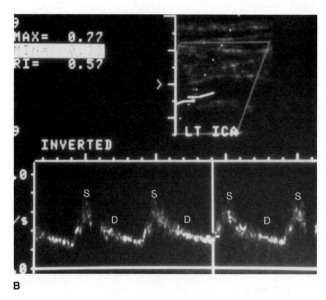

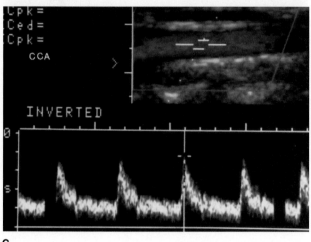

Figure 24-1 Carotid bifurcation ultrasound: Normal spectral waveforms. *A.* External carotid artery (ECA). *B.* Internal carotid artery (ICA). *C.* Common carotid artery (CCA). (Courtesy of BA Carroll, M.D., Duke University Medical Center.) *A.* The ECA waveform is characterized by a sharp systolic upstroke and downstroke (Ss) resulting in a narrow systolic peak. (Ds represent diastole.) *B.* The ICA waveform is characterized by a sharp systolic upstroke but a gentle downstroke resulting in a wider systolic peak (Ss) compared to the ECA (Fig. 24-1*A*). The diastolic component (Ds) is much higher than the ECA (Fig. 21-1*A*) given the low resistance of the internal circulation. Note the absence of spectral broadening indicative that frequencies are fairly homogeneous as flow is not disrupted by atherosclerotic plaque (compare to Fig. 24-3*B*). *C.* The CCA waveform essentially has a hybrid appearance.

of spectral information,[20] enhances diagnostic confidence, and helps clarify any possible source of disagreement between gray-scale and spectral analysis.[19] It is crucial for both the operator and the image interpreter to be aware of normal phenomena such as normal flow reversal along the posterior wall of the carotid bulb. This represents normal boundary layer separation (Fig. 24-2), a disturbance of normal laminar flow that occurs at all bifurcations.

The **N**orth **A**merican **S**ymptomatic **C**arotid **E**ndarterectomy **T**rial (NASCET) conducted at 50 medical centers in the United States and Canada established that patients with an ICA percentage diameter stenosis equal or greater than 70 percent but less than 100 percent would benefit from endarterectomy in the form of a decreased incidence of future cerebrovascular accidents.[21] Catheter angiography was used as the gold standard in establishing percentage diameter stenosis. This parameter is not directly measured by sonography, but rather indirectly as follows. Velocity of flow is proportional to frequency-induced shifts, a principle similar to that used by phase contrast magnetic resonance angiography (see MRA section later in this chapter). Tables of quantifiable parameters include several

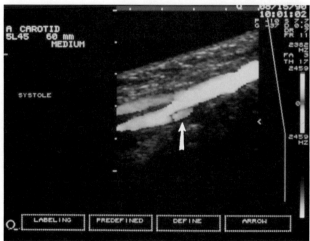

Figure 24-2 Carotid bifurcation: Normal ultrasound. (Courtesy of BA Carroll, M.D., Duke University Medical Center). Normal color Doppler sonography of the carotid bifurcation in the longitudinal plane demonstrates a normal area of flow reversal as laminar flow is disrupted at the carotid bifurcation. This is depicted by the change in tone as shown by the arrow along the dorsal aspect of the bulb at the origin of the internal carotid artery and is termed "boundary layer separation." This should not be misinterpreted as atherosclerotic plaquing.

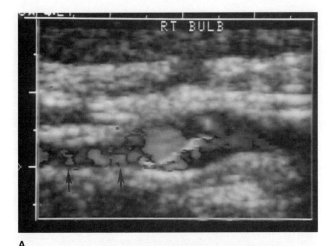

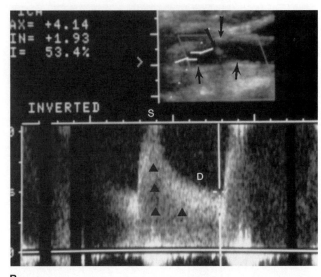

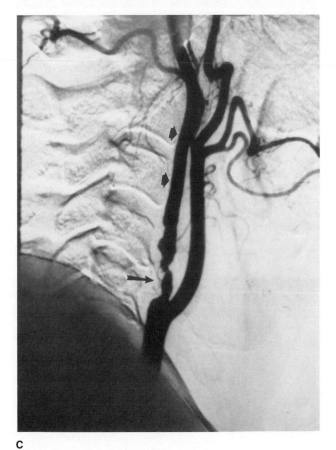

Figure 24-3 Carotid bifurcation: Severe hemodynamically significant stenosis. *A.* Color Doppler; *B.* Duplex ultrasound (Courtesy of BA Carroll, M.D., Duke University Medical Center) and *C.* Catheter angiogram. Carotid endarterectomy is indicated (NASCET criteria, see text). *A.* Color Doppler in the longitudinal plane demonstrates a post-stenotic jet displayed as a change in tone produced by severe atherosclerotic plaquing at the origin of the ICA (*arrows*). *B.* Duplex sonography displays a markedly increased peak systolic velocity and pronounced spectral broadening (*triangles*) indicative of disturbed laminar flow secondary to atherosclerotic plaquing (compare to the normal ICA waveform without spectral broadening, Fig. 24-1*B*). Arrows point to echogenic mural plaque. *C.* Lateral projection of a selective common carotid artery injection demonstrates irregular atherosclerotic plaquing of the proximal ICA resulting in greater than 70 percent luminal diameter stenosis (*arrow*) relative to the normal caliber ICA distally (*short arrows*).

ratios in the evaluation of cervical carotid arterial stenosis. The most commonly used ratio is peak systolic internal carotid artery velocity divided by peak systolic common carotid artery velocity. A study showed that peak ICA systolic velocity is the best single velocity parameter for quantification of luminal stenosis.[22] Stenosis is indirectly assessed by determining peak systolic velocities at the site of luminal narrowing. A post-

stenotic blood jet is faster than blood flow in a normal artery (Fig. 24-3*A*). Blood velocity increases with increasing stenosis up to a certain point, after which velocity drops. Flow reversal and turbulent nonlaminar flow is associated with a high-grade stenosis (Fig. 24-3*B*).

Characterization of atherosclerotic mural plaque and the presence of ulceration is clinically relevant.[23] Con-

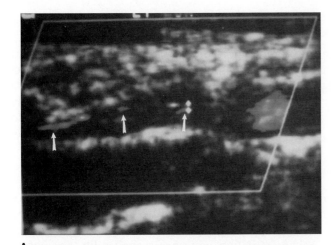

A

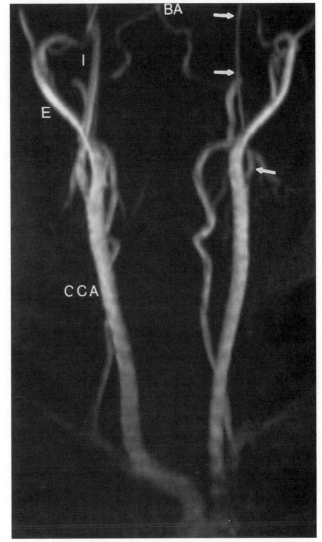

B

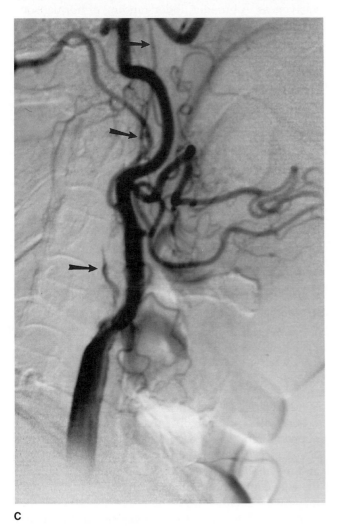

C

Figure 24-4   Carotid bifurcation: nearly occluded ICA: "string sign". *A.* Ultrasound (Courtesy of BA Carroll, M.D., Duke University Medical Center); *B.* MRA; *C.* Catheter angiogram. Carotid endarterectomy is indicated (NASCET criteria, see text). *A.* Color Doppler in the longitudinal plane demonstrates a string of flow (*arrows*) indicative of minimal residual patent lumen secondary to severe atherosclerotic plaquing. *B.* Maximum intensity projection MRA demonstrates a string-like left ICA (*arrows*). Note the normal caliber right ICA (I), right ECA (E), and right CCA (CCA). Basilar artery (BA). *C.* Lateral projection of a selective common carotid artery injection demonstrates a string-like ICA residual luminal opacification consistent with a preocclusive stage.

troversy abounds regarding the ability of any imaging modality to reproducibly and reliably establish the presence of ulceration. Limitations of US in evaluating carotid bifurcation disease feature calcification within a plaque (which may obscure the vessel lumen by the "shadowing" effect of calcium), tortuosity of the carotids, contralateral carotid disease, cardiac arrhythmia, and inability to measure other sites of stenosis, such as the origin of the great arteries in the aortic arch and the carotid siphon in the cavernous sinus.[18] As the

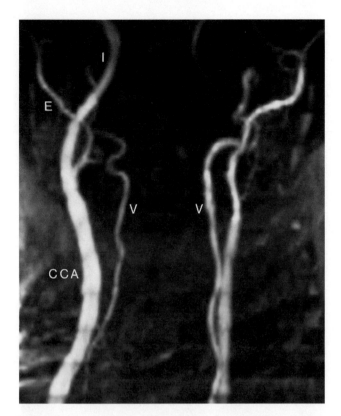

Figure 24-5 Carotid bifurcation: Occluded ICA. MRA. Carotid endarterectomy is not indicated (NASCET criteria, see text). No left ICA luminal signal is noted consistent with complete occlusion. This was confirmed on all source or "raw data" images (not shown). Compare to normal right ICA (I). ECA (E), CCA (CCA), Vs (vertebral arteries). Catheter angiogram (not shown) confirmed the finding.

severity of stenosis increases, the quality of sonographic imaging decreases along with the stenotic measurement accuracy.[19]

US is probably the best noninvasive modality for imaging *early* minimal atherosclerotic change. For carotid bifurcations with diameter stenosis of 50 percent of less, gray-scale imaging and color Doppler are most accurate. Spectral waveform analysis is best for diameter stenosis greater than 50 percent.[19] US tends to overestimate stenosis and occlusion, ultimately necessitating conventional catheter angiography for optimal quantitation. Nonetheless, US has the potential to distinguish between high-grade diameter stenosis and occlusion (Fig. 24-4), but it relies on optimal setting of physical parameters, which is operator-dependent. Establishment of internal carotid artery occlusion precludes carotid endarterectomy.[21]

US is excellent in establishing the directionality of blood flow in the vertebral arteries, noninvasively.[18] Transcranial Doppler offers inexpensive, portable, and rapid assessment of pediatric intracranial arterial circulation. However, up to 35 percent of studies of the adult intracranial anterior circulation are nondiagnostic because of insufficient sound beam penetration.[19] The combination of two-dimensional time-of-flight magnetic resonance angiography displayed as projection angiograms and duplex and color carotid US is a useful approach in helping detect and potentially grade the severity of ICA stenosis.[24] However, the gold standard to proceed to endarterectomy remains catheter angiography.

PEDIATRIC APPLICATIONS

Perinatal real-time US has become an essential component of the diagnostic armamentarium in studying pediatric patients, given its safety profile, absence of ionizing radiation, widespread availability, and noninvasiveness. A broader understanding of normal sonographic anatomy continues to be achieved. Pediatric applications in the brain include the diagnosis of hydrocephalus; hypoxic-ischemic diseases of prematurity, such as subependymal, intraventricular, and parenchymal hemorrhage; periventricular leukomalacia and periventricular cysts; periventricular hemorrhage venous infarction; TORCH (*Toxoplasma gondii*, rubella, cytomegalovirus, herpes) infections; vein of Galen arteriovenous fistula and dural sinus thrombosis; and evaluation of patients on extracorporeal membrane oxygenation.[18,25] Other important applications include the intrauterine evaluation of structural or developmental anomalies[25–27] such as encephalocele, anencephaly, myelomeningocele, and the Chiari II malformation, Dandy-Walker complex and simulators, agenesis of the corpus callosum, choroid plexus cyst, holoprosencephaly, hydranencephaly, schizencephaly, and, more recently, the antenatal diagnosis of diastematomyelia[28] and the tight filum terminale syndrome / tethered cord[29] (see Imaging Review of Neurologic Disease later in this chapter).

NUCLEAR MEDICINE

FORMATION OF AN IMAGE

Whereas the premier objective of most modalities in neuroradiology is to depict anatomy, nuclear medicine's objective is the study of physiology, function, and metabolism and low spatial resolution images are the rule compared to other modalities. Only recently, magnetic resonance applications such as spectroscopy, diffusion imaging, perfusion imaging, and functional imaging have begun to study function and metabolism.

Injectable and ingestable radiolabeled drugs (radiopharmaceuticals) consist of a radioactive label which provides a measurable signal and a ligand that determines organ-specific biodistribution. Radiopharmaceutical lipophilicity enables crossing of the intact blood-brain barrier. Efficient extraction from the blood

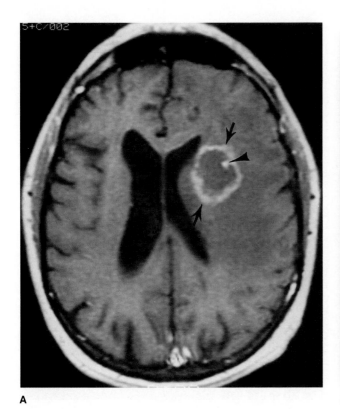

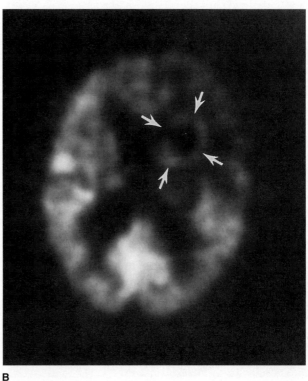

A   B

Figure 24-6   Primary cerebral lymphoma. *A.* MRI; *B.* PET scan (Courtesy of RE Coleman, M.D., Duke University Medical Center.) *A.* Axial enhanced T1 MRI of a 38-year-old man with AIDS demonstrates a large ring enhancing mass located in the periventricular white matter of the left frontal lobe (*black arrows*) with mass effect on the left lateral ventricle. In this clinical setting, main diagnostic considerations include primary CNS lymphoma, toxoplasmosis, and other infectious etiologies. Notice the focal nodular enhancement along the anterolateral margin of the ring (*arrowhead*). *B.* Corresponding axial PET scan demonstrates a ring-shaped areas of increased emission consistent with a metabolically active process. Biopsy proved to be a primary CNS B-cell lymphoma. Radiation therapy was promptly instituted. Absence of hypermetabolism would have favored an infectious process, most likely toxoplasmosis.

and intracellular incorporation allow the study of the tracer's distribution and accumulation over time in various body compartments.

Both x-rays and gamma rays are physically indistinguishable forms of electromagnetic radiation. In essense they are photons, differing only in their site of origin. X-rays are photons arising from orbital electrons rearrangements or from the deflection of electrons. Gamma rays are photons resulting from nuclear decay. While images in standard radiography, computed tomograpy, angiography, and myelography result from recording the passage of an external x-ray beam through the patient (transmission image), nuclear medicine images are produced when gamma rays resulting from nuclear decay within the patient are emitted and externally recorded (emission image).[30] This basic difference accounts for the need for specialized instrumentation for each modality.

Photons emitted by the patient following injection of a radiopharmaceutical are streamlined by a scattered radiation-reducing collimator attached to a gamma camera. The camera contains photon-sensitive scintillation crystals that can absorb the photons' energy and emit a light flash proportional to the absorbed photon's energy. In this way, the camera is able to measure not only the energy value but also the number of incident photons. The crystal is coupled to individual collimator holes and to specific photomultiplier tubes (PMT) that greatly amplify the crystal's light flashes by transducing them into electrons. In this way, PMT signal output quantitates incident photon energy. Following energy pulse discrimination by a pulse height analyzer, correction and electronic positioning circuitry, incident photons arising from the patient can be displayed as an image that accumulates information points over time.[30]

Image recording is performed with three major forms of equipment, resulting in a planar single-photon image, single-photon emission computed tomo-

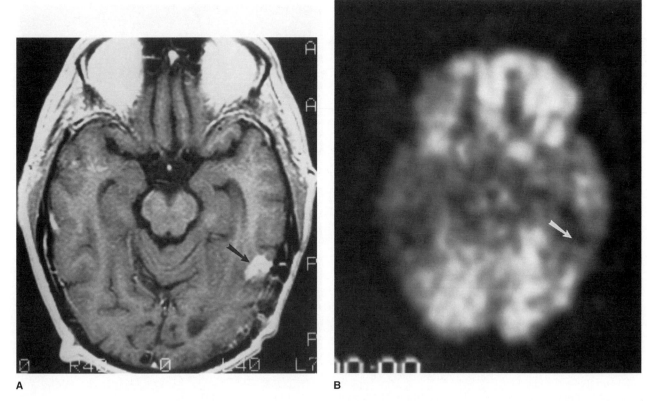

A   B

Figure 24-7   Radiation necrosis. *A.* MRI scan; *B.* PET scan (Courtesy of RE Coleman, M.D., Duke University Medical Center.) *A.* Axial contrast-enhanced MRI demonstrates a small nodular enhancement in the left posterior temporal lobe (*arrow*) of a 47-year-old man who underwent resection of a GBM followed by whole brain radiotherapy 4 months later. Main diagnostic considerations include recurrent tumor versus radiation necrosis. *B.* Axial FDG PET obtained the same day as the MRI demonstrates no signs of hypermetabolic activity (*arrow*) in the surgical bed indicative of radiation change. Based on imaging alone, a low-grade neoplasm cannot be entirely excluded. Stereotactic biopsy revealed radiation necrosis.

gram (SPECT), or positron emission tomogram (PET). The term "single-photon" refers to radionuclides which change to a more stable energy state by means of beta (−) decay, gamma decay, and electron capture with isotropic emission (uniform in all directions).[30] Each photon is independently recorded by an individual crystal. Radionuclides that decay by way of positron or beta (+) emission always release two high energy annihilation photons traveling 180 degrees from each other and require two physically opposed scintillation crystals or detector pairs arranged in a ring of detectors. This is known as coincidence detection.[30]

A planar single-photon image displays a one-to-one representation of radionuclide decay events distribution in the patient as recorded in the camera. A SPECT image is acquired by recording the patient's decay events distribution from different angles with a rotating gamma camera in much the same way as a CT scan is obtained. The main difference results in that this is a "nuclear emission computed tomogram"

rather than a "transmission computed tomogram." Multiple detector heads expedite the examination by recording more scintigraphic events for any given time. The information is reconstructed and displayed in any desired plane, allowing for multiplanar capability.[30]

Similarly, PET allows for multiplanar imaging capability. While PET has a significantly higher sensitivity and higher resolution compared to single-photon imaging, PET radiopharmaceuticals are short-lived, and almost all must be produced on site, usually from a cyclotron. The costs of installation and maintenance make these available mainly to a few large research institutions.[30] Currently, many of the applications initially utilized with PET imaging are being evaluated with SPECT, which is less costly and more widely available.[31–33]

Besides changes in regional blood flow measured by SPECT, PET defines regional utilization of glucose metabolism as well as oxygen and fatty acid metabolism, neurotransmitter receptor densities, and regional

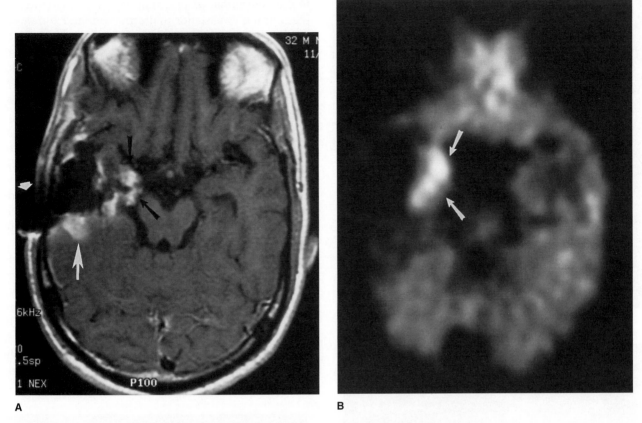

A

B

Figure 24-8   Recurrent glioblastoma multiforme (GBM). *A.* MRI; *B.* PET scan (Courtesy of RE Coleman, M.D., Duke University Medical Center.) *A.* Axial contrast-enhanced MRI of a 32-year-old man demonstrates a focal area of irregular peripheral enhancement along the medial margin of the right temporal lobe (*black arrows*), a new finding compared to prior MRI (not shown). The postsurgical cavity is evident in the right temporal region. Irregular enhancement along the posterior margin of the cavity had been stable for several months (*long white arrow*). Notice the signal dropout along the scalp soft tissues produced by an adjacent reservoir's magnetic susceptibility effect (*short white arrow*). *B.* Axial PET scan obtained the same day demonstrates increased emission (*white arrows*) corresponding to the new enhancement on the MRI consistent with recurrent tumor. There is no increased emission along the posterior margin of the postoperative cavity. Enhancement in this region on the MRI corresponds to stable radiation change.

pH. Although glucose is the brain's primary energy substrate and intuitively should be the imaging marker by excellence, it is metabolized and cleared at a rate faster than it can be imaged. PET employs a glucose analogue, 2-deoxyglucose (2-DG) labeled by a positron emitter such as ^{18}F or ^{11}C, resulting in fluorodeoxyglucose (FDG) injected intravenously. Like glucose, once it is transported to the brain, FDG is phosphorylated, becoming intracellular in the neuron without further breakdown given the substitution of H$^-$ for an OH$^-$ group. FDG resists degradation for a longer time than does glucose, allowing more time flexibility for imaging. Regional concentrations of 18 FDG reflect local cerebral metabolic rate for glucose[30] such that cerebral blood flow parallels glucose metabolism. Although FDG has traditionally been used with PET instruments,

more recently it has also proved diagnostic with SPECT instruments. Tracers commonly used with SPECT imaging include ^{123}I labeled *p*-iodo-*N*-isopropylamphetamine (IMP), ^{99m}Tc labeled agents like hexamethylpropyleneamine oxime (HMPAO), and ^{201}Th chloride (Th).

NEURORADIOLOGIC APPLICATIONS

Neuroradiologic applications include the evaluation of normal physiology, cerebral survival or brain death study;[34,35] cerebrospinal fluid (CSF) dynamics in the setting of normal pressure hydrocephalus, CSF rhinorrhea and otorrhea in the setting of fracture to the base of the skull, and ventricular shunt patency; differentiation of tumor from infection[31–33] (Fig. 24-6); differentiation of recurrent tumor from radiation necrosis[36–39] (Fig. 24-7 and 24-8); tumor grading; partial complex seizures

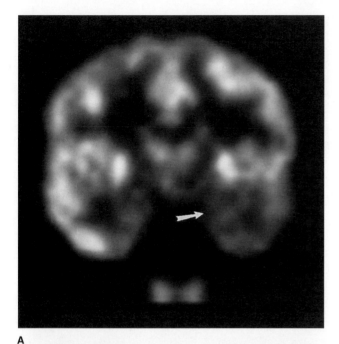

A

B

Figure 24-9 Mesial temporal sclerosis. *A.* PET scan; *B.* MRI (Courtesy of RE Coleman, M.D., Duke University Medical Center.) *A.* Coronal PET scan of a 26-year-old woman with partial complex seizures demonstrates focal decreased emission in the left hippocampus (*arrow*). *B.* Coronal oblique T2 MRI demonstrates a small left hippocampus of abnormal hyperintensity (*solid arrows*) relative to its counterpart (*open arrows*). The MRI and PET scan findings are consistent with mesial temporal sclerosis.

in the setting of mesial temporal sclerosis and localization of epileptogenic foci[40,41] (Fig. 24-9); neurodegenerative movement disorders and dementia (Fig. 24-10); and myriad psychiatric applications.[30] Applications of the conventional nuclear brain scan previously utilized

in the determination of cerebrovascular accidents, abscess, trauma, vascular malformation, and tumor are only of historical interest because the study has been replaced by computed tomography and magnetic resonance imaging, both of which provide higher resolution images.

In the setting of immunocompromise, including AIDS, patients on chemotherapy, and transplant recipients, differentiating toxoplasmosis from lymphoma has become an important clinical dilemma. An unwarranted trial of anti-toxoplasmosis medication can significantly delay the treatment of the radiosensitive CNS lymphoma. FDG PET (Fig. 24-6) and more recently Th SPECT[31,32] have been used successfully in establishing the correct diagnosis noninvasively, avoiding brain biopsy.

In glial tumor resection followed by whole brain and surgical bed radiotherapy, focal areas of enhancement in and around the tumor bed on CT or MRI studies cannot be accurately established as being tumor recurrence or tumor residual versus radiation change. FGD PET is consistently correlated with the brain MRI in determining whether the areas of enhancement on the MRI are hypermetabolic ("hot"), indicative of high-

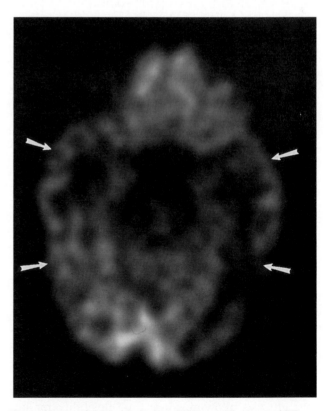

Figure 24-10 Alzheimer's disease. PET scan (Courtesy of RE Coleman, M.D., Duke University Medical Center.) Axial PET scan of a 56-year-old woman with progressive memory and cognitive deficits demonstrates symmetric bilateral focal decreased emission of the temporoparietal lobes diagnostic of Alzheimer's disease.

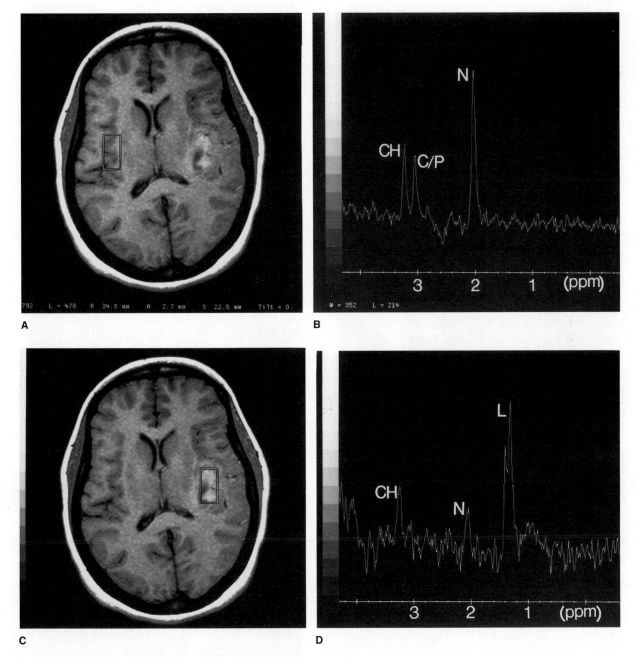

Figure 24-11 Magnetic resonance spectroscopy (General Electric 1.5T). *A–B.* Normal; *C–D.* Acute cerebrovascular accident. Tracings obtained from same patient during single examination (Courtesy of Robert D. Tien, M.D., Duke University Medical Center.) This 36-year-old woman with a history of intravenous drug abuse and endocarditis presented in the puerperium 3 weeks postpartum with acute onset of right body hemiparesis. *A.* Axial T1-weighted image through the insular cortex. A sampling volume is placed in the normal right insular cortex. *B.* Normal proton spectroscopy spectrum. Scale is in parts per million (ppm). Normal choline (CH), creatine/ phosphocreatine ratio (C/P), and *N*-acetylaspartate (N) spectral peaks. Note absence of a lactate peak. *C.* Same MR image as *A* with sampling volume placed in the swollen left insular cortex. *D.* Abnormal lactate peak (L) and decreased *N*-acetylaspartate peak (N) indicate acute infarction. Catheter angiogram (not shown) disclosed a mycotic aneurysm of an intrasylvian branch of the left middle cerebral artery in this location, responsible for the infarct.

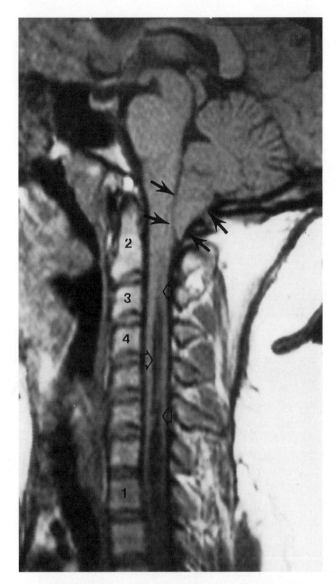

Figure 24-12   Chiari I malformation. MRI. Sagittal T1 MRI of an 8-year-old boy demonstrates cerebellar tonsillar ectopia protruding 12 mm below the foramen magnum (*long black arrows*) and a cervical cord syrinx (*short open arrows*) extending from C3 to T2, findings consistent with the Chiari I malformation. Note the dysplastic pointed appearance of the cerebellar tonsils.

grade neoplasm, (Fig. 24-8) or hypometabolic ("cold"), indicative of low-grade neoplasm or radiation change (Fig. 24-7). However, high-grade tumor such as anaplastic astrocytoma may exhibit hypometabolism,[39] making it indistinguishable from radiation change.[39]

FDG PET localization of a structural epileptogenic focus exhibiting decreased emission ("cold spot") in the interictal period became possible in 1982.[41] Recently, high-resolution MRI of the temporal lobes proved to have a higher sensitivity than PET in its ability to identify patients with partial complex seizures who would benefit from temporal lobectomy. When MRI and PET are used together, the predictive value for good postsurgical outcome is better than for either examination alone.[40] The ability to lateralize and further localize a seizure focus without placing depth electrodes represents a great advance in the surgical management of epilepsy.

CONVENTIONAL (CATHETER) ANGIOGRAPHY

The first cerebral arteriogram was performed by direct carotid artery puncture by Moniz in 1927, utilizing strontium bromide as contrast medium.[5] Angiography has come a long way since, with refinements in filming, contrast agent properties, arterial puncture site and technique, and catheter-guide wire manufacture, resulting in an easier, reproducible, and ultimately safer procedure.

High osmolar contrast agents (HOCA) utilized in selective carotid catheter angiography should contain only pure meglumine salts, since sodium ionic salts are associated with a higher incidence of seizures.[5] Iohexol, iopamidol, and ioversol are the most common low osmolar contrast agents (LOCA) used in the

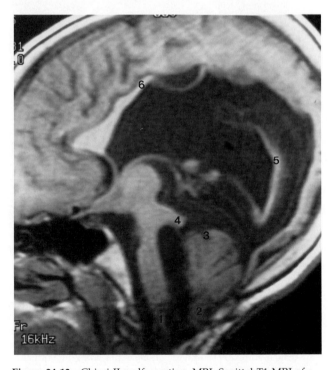

Figure 24-13   Chiari II malformation. MRI. Sagittal T1 MRI of a 10-year-old girl presenting with hydrocephalus and mental retardation demonstrates a small dysplastic posterior fossa and contents consistent with the Chiari II or Arnold-Chiari malformation. Cervicomedullary kinking (1), cerebellar tonsillar ectopia extending greater than 5 mm below the foramen magnum (2), towering cerebellum (3), and tectal beaking (4) are some of the features of this malformation. Colpocephaly (dilated occipital horns of the lateral ventricles) (5) and partial agenesis of the corpus callosum (6) are features that may be associated with this entity.

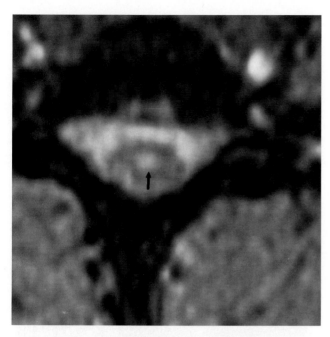

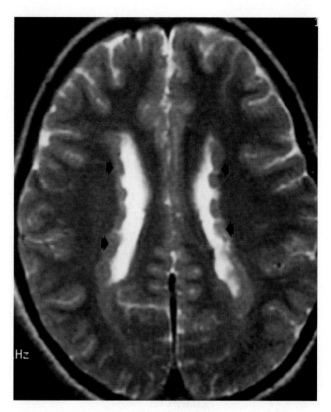

Figure 24-14   Syringohydromyelia. MRI. Axial gradient echo MRI at the C7 level of a 26-year-old woman with bilateral upper extremity shooting pains and muscle wasting following neck trauma, demonstrates a dilated central canal with ventral extension consistent with hydrosyringomyelia. No abnormal enhancements were demonstrated on the enhanced-T1 images to suggest underlying tumor (not shown).

Figure 24-16   Gray matter heterotopia. MRI. Axial T2 MRI of a 10-year-old girl presenting with seizures demonstrates an irregular lumpy-bumpy subependymal lateral ventricular surface (*arrows*) isointense to gray matter consistent with heterotopia of the subependymal type.

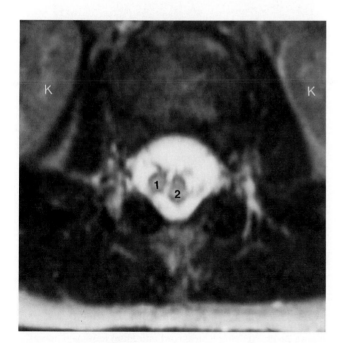

Figure 24-15   Diastematomyelia. MRI. Axial T2 MRI of an 8-year-old girl presenting with a hairy nevus in her midback demonstrates a "split" cord with a vertical cleft of CSF separating a right (1) and a left (2) hemicord at the midthoracic level. CT and plain films failed to disclose a bony or cartilaginous septum. A tethered cord, small syrinx, and Chiari II malformation were also present in this child (not shown). (K = kidney)

United States. Ioxaglate (Hexabrix), an ionic LOCA, also provides excellent delineation of intracranial and intraspinal vasculature and is believed to be as safe and efficient as the nonionic LOCA.

The safest and most widely used arterial access is the common femoral artery. With the introduction of the Seldinger technique,[42] transfemoral catheter techniques replaced direct carotid arterial puncture.[43] The introduction of digital substraction angiography (DSA) reduced the overall volume of intraarterial contrast and the overall duration of the procedure. Similar benefits derived from the introduction of biplane filming mode halving the number of contrast injections. Catheter-guide wire combinations are advanced into the aortic arch; subsequently the great arteries of the neck are selectively catheterized.

CERVICOCRANIAL ATHEROSCLEROTIC DISEASE
The North American Symptomatic Carotid Endarterectomy Trial (NASCET), a multi-institutional study, published in 1991, found an average 17 percent reduction in the incidence of stroke two years following carotid endarterectomy in symptomatic patients younger than age 80 who had internal carotid artery (ICA) diameter

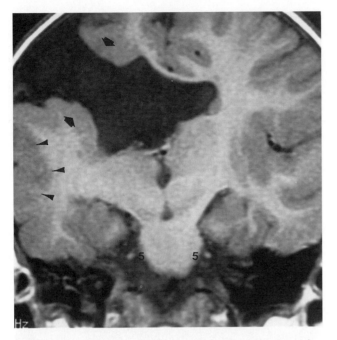

Figure 24-17 Unilateral open lip schizencephaly. MRI. Coronal T1 MRI of a 1-year-old boy presenting with left hemiparesis demonstrates a large CSF-containing cleft extending from the cortex of the frontoparietal convexity to the lateral ventricle. Gray matter (*arrows*) lines the large defect, diagnostic of schizencephaly. Note abnormally thick cortex representing pachygyria (*arrowheads*) contrasted with normal cortical thickness contralaterally. Note the normal appearance of the cisternal segment of the fifth nerves displayed in cross section ("5").

stenosis of 70 to 99 percent.[21] The European Carotid Surgery Trial (ECST) published in 1991 found an average 10 percent reduction of stroke incidence 3 years following surgery.[44] Patients with an occluded ICA did not benefit from surgery (Fig. 24-5). More recently, a prospective randomized multicenter trial was performed in patients in good general health with asymptomatic ICA diameter stenosis of 60 percent or greater the Asymptomatic Carotid Atherosclerosis Study (ACAS). Patients had a reduced 5-year risk of ipsilateral stroke if carotid endarterectomy was performed, with less than 3 percent perioperative morbidity and mortality added to aggressive management of modifiable risk factors.[45] The findings of this last study have not been widely applied clinically.

In the evaluation of carotid bifurcation atherosclerotic disease, selective common carotid arteriograms in at least two projections are obtained. The vessel responsible for the patient's neurologic deficit is studied first,[46] as determined by physical exam, duplex US with or without color Doppler, MRA, or computed tomography angiography (CTA). This way the most valuable information required in determining the need for carotid endarterectomy is obtained if circumstances preclude the completion of the examination. Catheter angiography provides information about the origin of

the great arteries from the aortic arch and of the carotid siphon, information that is factored in while determining the need to perform endarterectomy.

US, MRA,[24,27] and, more recently CTA,[48] represent alternatives to study the cervical carotid bifurcation noninvasively in an attempt to avoid catheter angiography and the potential complications inherent in such an invasive procedure. In a prospective study of 1002 angiograms,[49] the overall ischemic event rate between 0 and 24 h of the procedure was 1.3 percent; and it was 2.5 percent in patients studied for cerebrovascular disease. Only 0.1 percent of these events proved permanent. The ischemic event rate was 1.8 percent between 24 and 72 h following the procedure. Cerebral ischemic events occurred as a recurrence or worsening of a pre-existing condition twice as often as de novo ischemic events. All permanent deficits occurred as a worsening

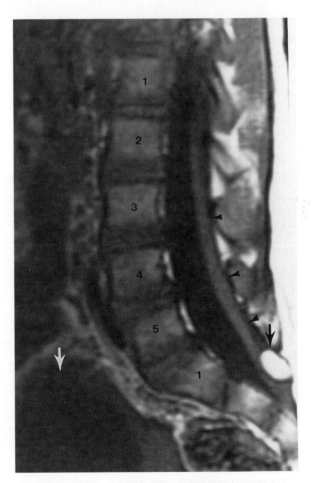

Figure 24-18 Tethered spinal cord and filum terminale lipoma. MRI. Sagittal T1 MRI of a 2-year-old boy presenting with urinary retention demonstrates a low lying conus medullaris which terminates at the sacral level. The cord is dorsally apposed in the caudal thecal sac (*arrowheads*), representing a tethered cord. A 1-cm oval-shaped homogeneous high signal mass (*black arrow*) is closely related to the dorsal margin of the lower cord, consistent with a lipoma to which the cord is tethered. The white arrow points to a dilated neurogenic bladder.

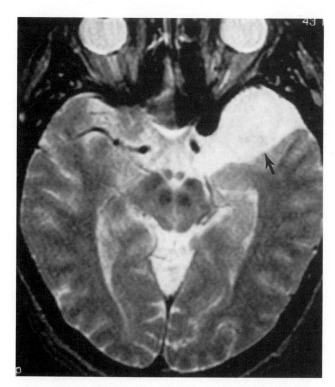

Figure 24-19   Arachnoid cyst. MRI. Axial T2 MRI of a 43-year-old man demonstrates a large extraaxial structure isointense to CSF occupying the anterior portion of the left middle cranial fossa (*arrow*), by far the most common location for an arachnoid cyst. Note evidence of temporal lobe dysgenesis. The patient presented for unrelated reasons.

of a preexisting deficit. A significant increase in the incidence of ischemic events in the first 24 h following angiography was established when the procedure lasted more than 1 h and when there was systolic hypertension. Trends toward higher incidence of ischemic events were recorded with large volumes of contrast agent, with increased serum creatinine, when stroke or transient ischemic attacks were the indications for the study, and when three or more catheters were used. In another prospective study of 1517 angiograms,[8] the incidence of all neurologic complications was 2.6 percent with an overall incidence of permanent deficit of 0.33 percent and of 0.63 percent in patients studied for cerebrovascular disease.

Other complications of catheter neuroangiography include transient global amnesia;[12,50–53] cortical blindness;[12,54] and multiple cholesterol emboli syndrome.[55] In an effort to study the carotid bifurcation noninvasively, US, MRA, and CTA continue to improve at a rapid pace, but catheter angiography remains the gold standard against which all other modalities are measured.

SUBARACHNOID HEMORRHAGE EVALUATION

In the evaluation of subarachnoid hemorrhage, it is critical to set a priority for injections to the vessel of

interest based on the findings of brain CT. If the CT scan is negative, a lumbar puncture with a persistently elevated number of red blood cells without signs of infection would exclude meningitis. The presence of a focal subarachnoid or parenchymal hematoma in a particular location on a CT scan will direct the angiographer to the first vessel to be injected.[46] If this finding is absent, injection of either carotid is acceptable as the anterior and the posterior communicating artery berry aneurysms are statistically the most common locations followed by middle cerebral artery trifurcation, basilar tip, and posterior inferior cerebellar artery. Finding the ruptured aneurysm does not complete the study because there is a 15 to 20 percent incidence of synchronous aneurysms[46,56] and coexistence of an arteriovenous malformation (AVM) should be excluded.

OTHER INDICATIONS

Other indications for catheter angiography include the evaluation of non-berry aneurysms (fusiform, my-

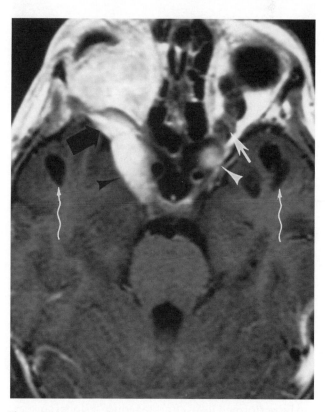

Figure 24-20   Neurofibromatosis type I: Optic nerve plexiform neurofibroma. MRI. Axial contrast-enhanced T1 MRI of an 18-year-old boy demonstrates a homogeneously enhancing right intraconal mass expanding the orbit and optic canal (*large black arrow*), resulting in exophthalmos. The epicenter of the mass is the right optic nerve, and it extends onto the prechiasmatic segment of the nerve (*black arrowhead*). Fusiform nonenhancing enlargement of the left optic nerve sheath (*white arrow*) and focal enhancement of the prechiasmatic segment of the left optic nerve (*white arrowhead*) are noted. Bilateral temporal lobe cystic structures of uncertain etiology are incidentally noted (*curved white arrows*).

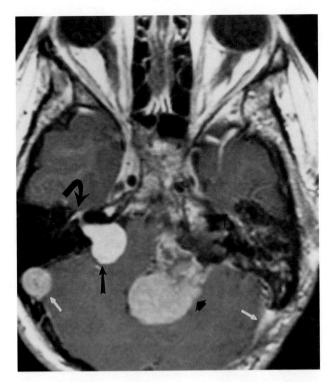

Figure 24-21 Neurofibromatosis type II: Bilateral vestibular schwanommas and multiple meningiomas. MRI. Axial contrast-enhanced T1 MRI of a 17-year-old girl with difficulty breathing demonstrates multiple enhancing masses in the posterior fossa compressing the brain stem. An inverted ice cream cone-shaped mass expands the right internal auditory canal and extends across the porus acusticus into the cerebellopontine angle cistern (*long black arrow*) consistent with an eighth nerve or vestibulocochlear schwannoma ("acoustic neuroma"). A smaller lesion involves the left eighth nerve (*black arrowhead*). More anteriorly, enhancement of the first genu and the tympanic segments of the right facial nerve represent a seventh nerve schwannoma (*curved black arrow*). A large mass expands the fourth ventricle and the left foramen of Luschka (*short black arrow*), representing an intraventricular meningioma. Last, en plaque/flat meningiomas abut the cerebellar hemispheres (*white arrows*).

cotic , giant, serpentine), arteriovenous malformations (Fig. 24-35) and other vascular lesions;[46] carotid cavernous fistula (Fig. 24-42) and other dural fistulae; arterial dissection (Fig. 24-41); vasculopathy, including fibromuscular dysplasia, various vasculitides (Fig. 24-31), and moya-moya; and tumoral vascular supply. Transcatheter embolization of AVM and tumor vasculature can be performed in an effort to reduce lesional surgical morbidity and mortality (see Chap. 25).

MYELOGRAPHY

The goal of myelography is to define the contents of the thecal sac and any intrinsic or extrinsic impressions on the thecal sac that could result in a complete or partial "block" (Fig. 24-89).[57] Contrast agents are infused intrathecally into the subarachnoid space, by-

passing the blood brain-barrier, diffusing through the CSF bathing the spinal cord and roots and the brain.

Earlier nonionic water-soluble contrast agents had to be mixed before the procedure (metrizamide: Amipaque). The newest myelographic contrast agents are low osmolar nonionic (LOCA), mix well with CSF, do not result in nerve root clumping, come already prepared, contain enough iodine to produce positive contrast, and are less neurotoxic than metrizamide. The only FDA-approved agents are iohexol and iopamidol, and current American College of Radiology guidelines specify the use of myelographic-specific iohexol and iopamidol indicated by the letter "M" following the contrast agent's name. Main complications related to myelography include headache, contrast-related complications, subdural or epidural contrast injection, spinal canal hematoma, meningitis, seizure, and various forms of neurologic deficit.[57]

Prior to the advent of noninvasive cross-sectional imaging (CT and MRI), myelography was the mainstay in the evaluation of spinal canal contents and adjacent structures. Disturbances in the contrast column contour are categorized as extradural and intradural. Intradural lesions can be further divided into extramed-

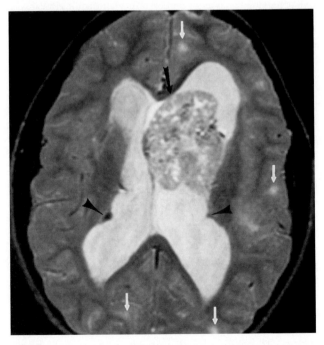

Figure 24-22 Tuberous sclerosis. MRI. Axial T2 MRI of a 9-year-old girl presenting with seizures, mental retardation, and adenoma sebaceum demonstrates a large intraventricular mass of heterogeneous signal at the left foramen of Monro (*black arrow*) responsible for obstructive hydrocephalus. This subependymal giant cell astrocytoma demonstrated homogeneous enhancement and dramatic growth over a 2-year period (*not shown*). Several hypointense subependymal nodules (*arrowheads*) and multifocal subcortical and cortical hyperintense nodules (*white arrows*) represent hamartomatous tubers.

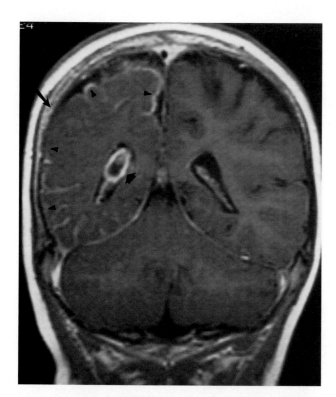

Figure 24-23 Sturge-Weber syndrome. MRI. Coronal contrast-enhanced T1 MRI through the posterior third of the brain of a 2-year-old boy with intractable seizures and a facial nevus along the distribution of V1. Right holohemispheric atrophy with ipsilateral calvarial thickening (*arrow*); diffuse leptomeningeal enhancing angiomatosis (*arrowheads*); and enlargement of the atrial choroid plexus (*short arrow*) are demonstrated.

ullary and intramedullary, where "medullary" refers to the spinal cord. Computed tomography following intrathecal administration of an iodinated contrast agent increased the specificity of myelography typically for delineation of extradural disease (Fig. 24-86), but the noninvasive and radiation-free spinal MRI (Fig. 24-87) may soon replace CT myelography except for certain indications. For further discussion on spinal lesions, refer to Approach to Neuroradiologic Diagnosis: General Principles later in this chapter (Fig. 24-77).

COMPUTED TOMOGRAPHY

FORMATION OF AN IMAGE

A computed tomogram represents reconstructed x-ray data obtained from multiple angles in the form of a "transmission scan," contrasted to nuclear medicine's "emission scan." With each revolution, an x-ray tube rotates around the patient. Multiple detectors record how much the x-ray beam is attenuated or absorbed along its path through the patient's soft tissues from the x-ray tube to the detector—hence the term "attenuation." Attenuation information from various angles is electronically integrated. A shade of gray is electroni-

cally assigned to the average attenuation value of each point in space expressed in Hounsfield units.

The intrinsic attenuation of a substance is directly related to its electron density,[58] hence the interchangeability of the terms "density" and "attenuation." Structures in the brain are said to be hypodense (of lower attenuation), isodense (of similar attenuation), or hyperdense (of higher attenuation) relative to brain parenchyma. The higher the electron density of the substance, the higher its attenuation value and the brighter its display on the CT image (Table 24-1). Iodinated contrast agents increase the attenuation of vascular structures, of the normal structures without a blood-brain barrier outlined earlier, and of lesions responsible for alteration of the BBB. Enhancement occurs as the iodine-containing contrast medium attenuates the x-ray beam, accentuating structural and lesional conspicuity.

By convention, computed tomography (CT) axial images are displayed with the patient's right to the reader's left and the patient's left to the reader's right (Fig. 24-25). This convention also applies to brain MRI and to brain PET and SPECT. Coronal sections can be acquired if the patient is able to hyperextend the neck when supine or prone. Quality computer reformatting into the sagittal and coronal planes can be performed from images acquired in the axial plane if high-resolution thin sections are obtained in a cooperative patient. Since inception of the technique CT scanning times have been dramatically reduced owing to technical advances.[59,60,61]

Given less stringent installation requirements and lower cost, CT instruments are more widely available than MRI. A CT examination is less costly and is ac-

TABLE 24-1
Computed Tomography Attenuation

High Attenuation
1. Metallic foreign object, aneurysm clip, ventricular catheter, etc.
2. Bone, calcification, ossification
3. Acute hemorrhage
4. Normally enhancing vascular structures
5. Highly proteinaceous lesions
6. High cellular to cytoplasmic ratio neoplasm

Intermediate Attenuation
1. Gray matter
2. White matter (slightly lower attenuation than gray matter)
3. Subacute hemorrhage (may be isodense to brain parenchyma)

Low attenuation
1. Air
2. Normal fat and fat containing substances and lesions
3. Cerebrospinal fluid
4. Chronic hemorrhage
5. Hyperacute hemorrhage: swirl sign (usually coexisting acute hemorrhage)
6. Edema, gliosis, demyelination, encephalomalacia, necrosis

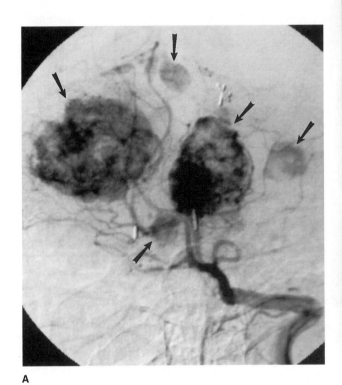

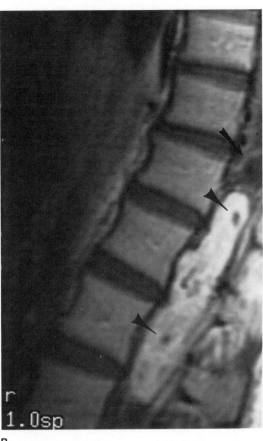

A   **B**

Figure 24-24   Von-Hippel-Lindau (VHL) syndrome. *A.* Angiogram; *B.* MRI. *A.* Left vertebral artery transfacial anteroposterior digital subtraction arteriogram (DSA) demonstrates myriad bilateral posterior fossa intense vascular blushes (*arrows*) corresponding to the highly vascular mural nodules of multiple hemangioblastomas in this 33-year-old woman with VHL syndrome. *B.* Sagittal contrast-enhanced T1 MRI of a 39-year-old woman with VHL syndrome demonstrates a sausage-shaped intramedullary enhancing thoracic spinal cord hemangioblastoma expanding the cord and the spinal canal. Notice the syrinx rostral to the mass (*arrow*). The mass spans the height of three lower thoracic vertebral bodies, which demonstrate posterior scalloping. Small foci of signal void (*arrowheads*) indicate vascular tumor nodules and/or dilated veins.

quired more quickly than an MRI examination. CT is study of choice for the detection of skull fractures and acute subarachnoid hemorrhage in the emergent setting, particularly given its availability and faster acquisition time, determination of calcification within a lesion, detection of salivary gland stone disease, and the study of the fine anatomy of the petromastoid temporal bone. However, a CT study delivers ionizing radiation to the patient and is relatively insensitive to posterior fossa pathology, given posterior fossa image degradation by beam hardening artifact produced by the interface of bone and parenchyma. CT's tissue contrast is limited compared with that achieved by MRI. Data acquisition is restricted to the axial and coronal planes and to a limited range of gantry angulation.

CT angiography (CTA), a recently developed technology, utilizes a spiral acquisition during the intravenous bolus administration of iodinated contrast media.

Spiral scanning is also referred to as helical or volume scanning because the traced path created by the movement of the x-ray beam during the acquisition resembles a helix. Unlike conventional CT scanning, a spiral acquisition is made while the patient is moved at a continuous constant speed through the scanning field while the x-ray tube rotates continuously. Advantages include faster imaging of larger anatomic regions during a breath-hold, thus minimizing motion artifact. Furthermore, one can perform noninvasive angiograms as peak arterial luminal opacification becomes possible over a larger region of interest. Recent studies have demonstrated a high degree of correlation of CTA and catheter angiography in the evaluation of cervical carotid atherosclerosis.[48] Refinements include the ability to obtain three-dimensional representation of information not achievable by catheter angiography or magnetic resonance angiography, such as plaque

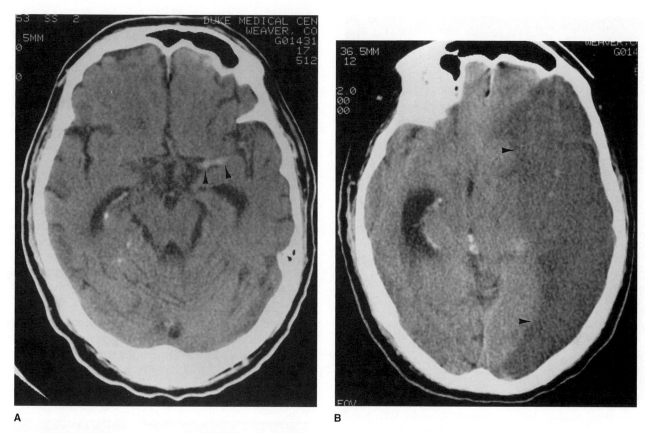

Figure 24-25   Hyperdense middle cerebral artery (MCA) sign. CT. *A.* Axial nonenhanced CT demonstrates focal asymmetric high density of the M1 segment of the left MCA (*arrowheads*) in a 65-year-old woman presenting with right hemiparesis. *B.* Axial nonenhanced CT obtained 48 hours later demonstrates interval development of a large nonhemorrhagic infarct along the distribution of the left MCA (*arrowheads*). Notice the cortical and subcortical low attenuation, sulcal effacement, and loss of differentiation between cortex and medulla as well as the subfalcial shift and entrapment of the right ventricular temporal horn.

calcification, ulceration, and size.[48] More recently, CTA has been used for the evaluation of cerebral aneurysms with promising results comparable to those obtained by 3-D time of flight and 3-D phase contrast magnetic resonance angiography.[61]

MAGNETIC RESONANCE IMAGING

Magnetic resonance imaging (MRI) has revolutionized neuroradiology over the last 15 years. The following discussion will touch on the basics of MRI and its logical developments, including magnetic resonance angiography (MRA) and magnetic resonance spectroscopy (MRS) among various recent developments. MRI has become the premier imaging modality in neuroradiology, with a rapidly enlarging set of indications. MRI has become the imaging modality of choice for myriad applications in neuroradiology[3,58,62–64] Given its intricate character, a basic understanding of the physics of image formation is imperative in order to interpret the many artifacts and mechanisms that lead to in-

creased or decreased image signal. Effective testing, image quality optimization, patient safety, and ultimately image interpretation hinge on such understanding.

FORMATION OF AN IMAGE

When the patient is placed in the MRI instrument, water protons are exposed to a strong and fairly homogeneous static external magnetic field (denoted **B**) measured in tesla (T) (1 tesla = 10,000 gauss). As a point of reference, the Earth's magnetic field is between 0.3 and 0.7 gauss. Clinical MRI instruments' magnetic field strength varies between 0.02 and 1.5 T. In the presence of a large static **B**, protons rearrange parallel or antiparallel relative to **B**, acquiring the most favorable possible energetic configuration. In doing so, protons precess or wobble about the long axis of **B** at a frequency proportional to **B** (resonant frequency). This phenomenon occurs because energy exchange takes places between **B** and the patient's protons.

The summation of parallel and antiparallel precess-

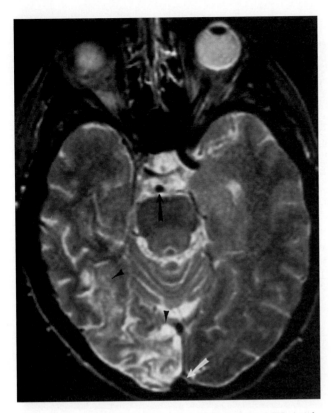

Figure 24-26   Posterior cerebral artery (PCA) infarct. MRI. Axial T2 MRI of a 73-year-old woman presenting with a left homonymous hemianopsia demonstrates abnormal hyperintensity involving the right PCA territory. The contrast-enhanced T1 sequence (not shown) demonstrated gyriform enhancement secondary to luxury perfusion indicative of a subacute infarction. A normal basilar artery flow void is demonstrated (*arrow*). Compare with Fig. 24-27, in which absence of basilar artery flow void indicates very slow flow or thrombosis. The white arrow points to the normal flow void of the superior sagittal sinus. Compare with the normal sagittal sinus luminal high signal on gradient echo sequences (Fig. 24-33*B*).

ing protons is logically termed Longitudinal Magnetization (LM) because it refers to the longitudinal arrangement of protons relative to **B**. However, LM of itself is not sufficient to create an image. To do so, energy in the form of a 90-degree radiofrequency (RF) pulse applied at the resonant frequency transforms LM into Transverse Magnetization (TM). This process is termed Resonance, during which protons shift from a low energy state to a high energy state.[65] When the RF pulse is turned off, protons now in a high energy state give off energy by progressively wobbling along **B**'s axis such that LM begins to be reestablished, a process known as Relaxation.[65] Energy is given off in two different and independent yet simultaneous ways, termed T1 or longitudinal relaxation time, and T2 or transverse relaxation time. T1 relaxation refers to the time it takes protons to *regain* their original LM following the application of an RF pulse. T2 relaxation refers to the time it takes a set of protons to *lose* their gained transverse

magnetization following the application of an RF pulse. In every image produced there are T1 and T2 effect contributions within certain time constraints.

Gradients are magnetic fields added to or subtracted from **B**, making it locally stronger or weaker. To achieve anatomic slice selection, spatial encoding and the representation of a three-dimensional set of information as a two-dimensional picture, gradients are applied in various directions within the desired imaging volume. By systematically varying the strength of gradients along a chosen direction and successively applying RF pulses and/or other gradients, electrical energy information emitted by the protons' varying states of energy is detected by an antenna-like coil. Differential T1 and T2 relaxation times of various protons within sampled tissues are translated into signal. Discrimination of signal intensity (SI) results in image formation, the cornerstone of MRI.

T1 and T2 relaxation times and proton density are intrinsic properties of the imaged protons within the sampled tissue. Imaging of hydrogen protons, in essence imaging of water, forms the basis of MRI. A high proton density or spin density refers to the number of

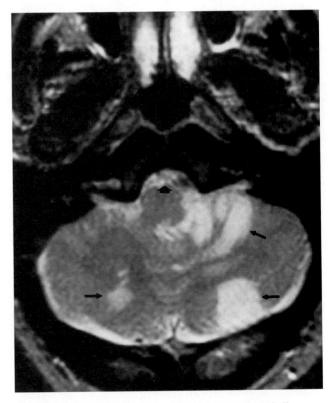

Figure 24-27   Basilar artery thrombosis and bland cerebellar embolic infarcts. MRI. Axial T2 MRI of a 65-year-old man demonstrates absence of the normally present basilar artery luminal flow void (*short arrow*) (Refer to Fig. 24-26 for a normal basilar artery flow void). Long arrows point to multiple small embolic cerebellar infarcts represented by multiple areas of abnormal high signal intensity in the cerebellar hemispheres.

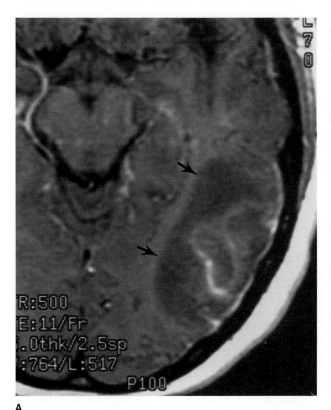

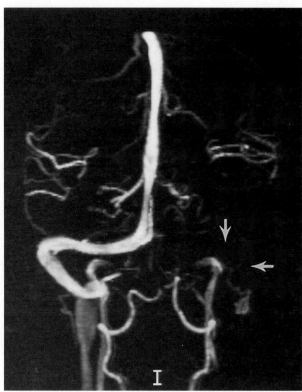

A

B

Figure 24-28   Venous infarct with hemorrhagic transformation secondary to dural sinus thrombosis. *A.* MRI; *B.* MRVenography. *A.* Detail of an axial contrast-enhanced T1 MRI of a 21-year-old, 12 weeks' pregnant woman demonstrates a cortical based area of heterogeneous high signal indicative of subacute hemorrhage in the left inferior posterior parietal region not conforming to an arterial territory (*arrows*). This represents a subacute hemorrhagic venous infarct. *B.* Coronal phase contrast magnetic resonance venography (velocity encoding of 20 cm/s) demonstrates absence of luminal signal in the expected course of the left transverse and sigmoid sinuses indicative of dural sinus thrombosis (*arrows*).

hydrogen protons available to emit a measurable signal used to create images.[66]

TR and TE are time parameters systematically varied by the operator to emphasize signal differences emitted by the sampled tissues. TR (time of repetition) refers to the time elapsed between two successive 90-degree RF pulses marking the beginning of a conventional spin echo (CSE) pulse sequence. TE (time to echo) refers to the time elapsed between the 90-degree pulse and time to sample the region studied during which formation of the echo (image) is produced. Use of a short TR and a short TE results in a T1-weighted image (T1W1) (Fig. 24-6A). Use of a long TR and a short TE yields a proton density or balanced image (PDI) (Fig. 24-54A). Use of a long TR and a long TE results in a T2-weighted image (T2WI) (Fig. 24-51). For a summary refer to Table 24-2.

Substances such as cerebrospinal fluid and edema have a long T2 relaxation time and are of high signal on T2-weighted images (vasogenic edema in Fig. 24-50 and Fig. 24-72B). Substances such as hemorrhagic

blood products (deoxyhemogobin and hemosiderin) have a short T2 relaxation time and are of low signal on T2-weighted images (Fig. 24-33). Substances such as fat (lipoma in Fig. 24-18), subacute hemorrhage (methemoglobin on subdural hematoma Fig. 24-40A) and pathologically enhancing lesions (epidural and marrow lymphoma in Fig. 24-90A) have a short T1 relaxation time and are of high signal T1-weighted images. Substances such as cerebrospinal fluid and edema have

TABLE 24-2
Relation of Repetition Time (TR) and Time to Echo (TE) to Image Weighing

T1-weighted image	Short[a]	Short[c]
Proton density image	Long[b]	Short
T2-weighted image	Long	Long[d]

[a] Less than 500 msec
[b] More than 1500 msec
[c] Less than 30 msec
[d] More than 80 msec

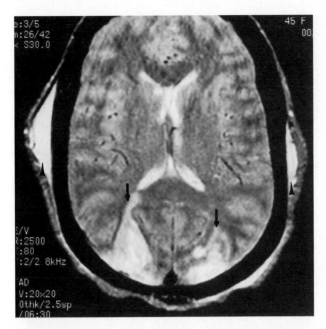

Figure 24-29 Supratentorial border zone (watershed) infarcts. MRI. Axial proton density MRI of a 45-year-old woman involved in a motor vehicle accident who presented with pronounced hypotension and paralysis demonstrates cortical and subcortical wedge-shaped areas of abnormal high signal with swollen gyri (*arrows*). They lie at the junction of the posterior and middle cerebral artery territories and represent watershed infarcts secondary to hypotension. Notice the high signal intensity scalp-deforming contusions (*arrowheads*).

a long T1 relaxation time and are of lower signal on T1-weighted images (CSF cleft in Fig. 24-17 and vasogenic edema in Fig. 24-72A). For a summary of characteristic signal intensity of normal and abnormal tissues, refer to Table 24-3.

SEQUENCES

Although strongly rivaled by faster sequences, conventional spin echo (CSE) imaging remains the most widespread, available, and simplest MRI sequence. A succinct description of the CSE sequence follows. The CSE sequence is composed of two different RF pulses. First, a RF pulse tilts protons 90 degrees, establishing transverse magnetization. As time elapses, protons begin to dephase. At a time midway between the 90-degree pulse and image sampling time or TE/2, a 180-degree RF pulse is applied to rephase protons. Rephasing dephasing protons allows for more signal to be detected, processed, and ultimately displayed as an image.

The demand to image patients who are unable to lie still for long periods of time; needed increased patient throughput; and the study of flowing blood has led to the development of imaging techniques faster than CSE. Patient populations who benefit from faster imaging feature the pediatric and at times the geriatric populations; uncooperative, debilitated, or disoriented patients; and patients with severe back pain and claustrophobia, among others. Gradient echo (GRE) sequences represent the most successful and widespread application to these needs (Figs. 24-14, 24-33B, 24-87).[3] More recently, fast spin echo, fast gradient echo, and echoplanar imaging have been developed, but discussion of these modalities is beyond the scope of this presentation.

SIGNAL INTENSITY

All MR sequences result in an image with differential signal intensity (SI). "Hyperintense," "isointense," and "hypointense" are terms referring to high, intermediate, and low signal of a tissue in question relative to

TABLE 24-3
Magnetic Resonance Imaging Signal Intensity (SI)

T1-weighted images
  Hyperintense or high SI
  1. Normal fat; fat-containing substances and lesions
  2. Proteinaceous lesions and fluid including mucin and melanin
  3. Early and late subacute hemorrhage: methemoglobin
  4. Slow blood flow
  5. Calcium (rarely)

  Intermediate SI
  1. Gray matter (slightly hypointense to white matter in adults)
  2. White matter
  3. Cerebrospinal fluid (hypointense to gray and white matter)
  4. Edema (hypointense to gray and white matter)

  Hypointense or low SI
  1. Air
  2. Cortical bone
  3. Normal arterial and fast venous blood flow
  4. Magnetic susceptibility artifact

T2-weighted images
  Hyperintense or high SI. Most pathology is hyperintense on T2-weighted images due to a higher concentration of water protons
  1. Cerebrospinal fluid
  2. Edema of all types
  3. Ischemia and infarction
  4. Demyelination
  5. Subacute hemorrhage in its extracellular stage: methemoglobin
  6. In fast spin echo, fat is relatively bright

  Hypointense or low SI
  1. Air
  2. Normal arterial and fast venous blood flow
  3. Acute hemorrhage: deoxyhemoglobin
  4. Subacute hemorrhage in its intracellular stage, methemoglobin
  5. Chronic hemorrhage: ferritin and hemosiderin
  6. Magnetic susceptibility artifact
  7. Fat (conventional spin echo)
  8. Cortical bone
  9. Calcium
  10. Melonin (not invariably)

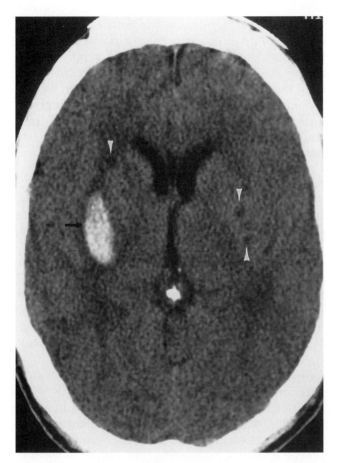

Figure 24-30 Hypertensive parenchymal hematoma. CT. Axial nonenhanced CT of a 42-year-old hypertensive man demonstrates a well-circumscribed lentiform shaped acute high attenuation putaminal hematoma (*arrow*) extending to the external capsular white matter, with surrounding edema, a typical location for a hypertensive hemorrhage. Note the small foci of low attenuation in the basal ganglia bilaterally, representing lacunar infarcts (*arrowheads*) typical of hypertensive patients.

the signal intensity of normal brain parenchyma. Signal intensity reflects tissue composition as represented by various image weightings.

A basic knowledge of the characteristics signal intensity of various substances is essential for effective interpretation of MR images, summarized in Table 24-3. Fat, protein (including hemorrhage in the subacute stage), slow flow, IV contrast enhancement of normal and pathologic tissue, and, rarely, calcium are displayed as bright on T1-weighted images. Adult gray and white matter, edema, and cerebrospinal fluid are of intermediate to low signal on T1-weighted images. Most pathologic processes are hyperintense on T2-weighted images due to a higher concentration of water protons. Cerebrospinal fluid, edema of various types, ischemia and infarction, demyelination (Fig. 24-52 to Fig. 24-55) and subacute hemorrhage in its extracellular stage (Fig. 24-41*B*) are displayed as bright on

T2-weighted images. Acute, early subacute and chronic hemorrhage are displayed as dark on T2-weighted images (Fig. 24-33). The combined interpretation of T1- and T2-weighted images at any given time allows for accurate determination of the age of a parenchymal hematoma (Fig. 24-72). Air, normal arterial blood flow (black arrow in Fig. 24-26), venous blood flow (white arrow in Fig. 24-26), cortical bone and magnetic susceptibility artifact from metal (white arrow in Fig. 24-8*A*) and air-brain interfaces are displayed as very dark on both T1- and T2-weighted images.

MAGNETIC RESONANCE ANGIOGRAPHY (MRA)
The two principal techniques utilized in MRA are Time-of-Flight (TOF) and Phase Contrast (PC).[67–70] This examination can be obtained at the same sitting during a conventional brain or spine MRI noninvasively without injecting contrast media and without the use of ionizing radiation. Other benefits over conventional catheter angiography include the capability to study multiple vessels simultaneously and, more recently, directional and velocity information.

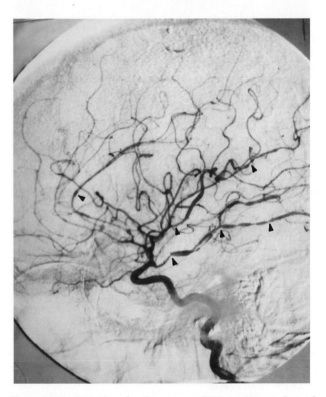

Figure 24-31 Vasculopathy: Lupus vasculitis. Angiogram. Lateral DSA of a selective right internal carotid artery injection of a 58-year-old woman with known systemic lupus erythomatosus demonstrates multiple areas of abnormal vessel narrowing and dilatation producing a beaded pattern involving the medium and small branches of the anterior, middle, and fetal origin posterior cerebral arteries (*arrowheads*). This is the angiographic hallmark of a vasculopathy.

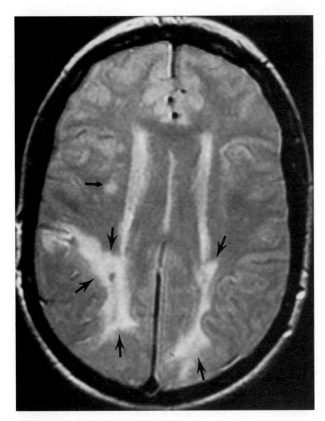

Figure 24-32 Vasculopathy: Cocaine abuse related vasculitis. MRI. Axial proton density MRI of a 35-year-old woman with a history of cocaine abuse demonstrates confluent (*large arrows*) and discrete (*small arrow*) supratentorial subcortical and periventricular white matter areas of hyperintensity corresponding to areas of cerebritis, ischemia, demyelination, or gliosis secondary to drug-related vasculitis.

Time-of-Flight (TOF)

MRA exploits flow-related enhancement of moving blood protons in a vessel relative to saturated stationary water protons. Even though this concept uses the word "enhancement," it does not refer to enhancement produced by intravenous contrast agent administration. Instead, flow-related enhancement refers to a process in which the signal intensity of moving blood protons is displayed as increased relative to the signal intensity of stationary protons.[68] The longitudinal magnetization of inflowing unsaturated blood protons is higher than that of saturated protons of stationary tissue because the blood does not experience saturation RF pulses. Conversely, protons from stationary tissue become saturated given repeated application of a "traveling" or "walking" saturation band. This RF pulse places a new saturation band next to each successive selected slice with a TR shorter than the T1 longitudinal relaxation time of stationary tissue.[69] This results in reduced longitudinal magnetization (signal) of stationary tissue, improving the conspicuousness of flowing blood.

Background suppression has been a relative deficiency of TOF techniques. Phase contrast MRA techniques achieve excellent background suppression at the expense of longer acquisition times. Recently developed magnetization transfer techniques when used in conjunction with TOF result in increased peripheral intracranial arterial definition approximating the excellent background suppression achieved by phase contrast MRA techniques.[71,72]

Phase Contrast (PC)

PC MRA detects changes in velocity-induced phase shifts of the transverse magnetization of moving blood protons along a set of gradients. Instead of relying on flow-related enhancement, PC MRA relies on moving protons' phase diffrences. PC MRA utilizes special gradients termed bipolar gradients of equal magnitude but opposite direction. These gradients are added, resulting in signal cancellation of stationary protons and differential display of moving protons. Compared with TOF MRA, PC MRA results in better stationary tissue suppression but takes longer to perform. Velocity information that includes speed and direction can be obtained with PC MRA, but not with TOF MRA. The operator can tailor a PC MRA examination by specifying the anticipated maximum blood velocity within the vessels to be studied, generally resulting in improved quality of the examination. Finally, substances with a short T1 relaxation time such as subacute hemorrhage within a thrombus can falsely simulate luminal blood flow signal in TOF MRA such that a diagnosis of dural sinus thrombosis or cervicocranial arterial dissection could potentially be dismissed as a normal study. This is not a potential pitfall for PC MRA. PC principles have been applied to the study of CSF dynamics.[73–75]

2D and 3D

Both TOF and PC MRA can be acquired in the two-dimensional (2D) or the three-dimensional (3D) mode. In the 2D acquisition mode, thin slices of tissue are excited sequentially and reconstructed by stacking them on top of each other. Therefore, the 2D mode has the disadvantage of being sensitive to patient motion such as swallowing while not being sensitive to blood flow along the plane of the slice, as seen with tortuous or looping vessels. In the 3D acquisition mode, repeated sampling of an entire thick slab or volume is performed, allowing display of slices thinner than possible with the 2D mode. However, the 3D mode is not as sensitive to slow blood flow as the 2D mode is. Signal from slow flowing blood may be lost toward the end of the excited volume. Because slow flowing blood remains for a longer time within the excited volume, it shows the saturation effect seen with station-

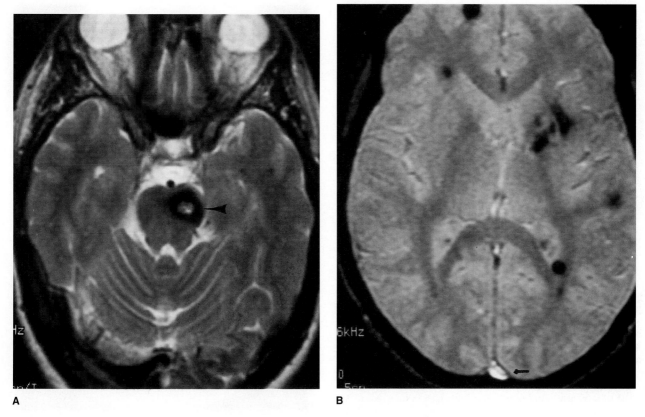

A   **B**

Figure 24-33   Cavernoma. *A.* Conventional spin echo MRI; *B.* Gradient echo MRI. *A.* Axial T2 MRI of a 45-year-old woman demonstrates a left pontine, round, well circumscribed area of central heterogeneous high and low signal representing subacute and acute blood products and a peripheral hypointense ring (*arrowhead*) representing chronic blood products. Notice the relative absence of mass effect given the size of the lesion. *B.* Axial 45-degree flip angle gradient echo MRI of a 19-year-old woman demonstrates multiple bilateral supratentorial hypointense foci without significant mass effect or edema consistent with multiple cavernous angiomas. The gradient echo sequence is exquisitely sensitive to the magnetic susceptibility effect produced by acute and chronic blood products such as deoxyhemoglobin, ferritin, and hemosiderin (see Tables 24-3 and 24-6). It displayed several lesions that were not visualized in the conventional spin echo sequence (not shown). Note that blood flow in the superior sagittal sinus (*arrow*) and arteries is normally of high signal on a gradient echo sequence, whereas it normally is of low signal on conventional spin echo sequences (*white arrow* in Fig. 24-26).

ary tissue. Saturation effects are more pronounced with 3D TOF than with 3D PC. However, 3D PC is slightly more sensitive to turbulence than is 3D TOF.

MOTSA

More recently, multiple overlapping thin slab acquisition (MOTSA) MRA was developed, combining the strengths of 2D and 3D imaging. With this technique, several volumes of tissue smaller than those typically used in 3D imaging but larger than the slices used in 2D imaging are stacked on top of each other to create an MR angiogram.[76]

MAXIMUM INTENSITY PROJECTION (MIP)

An MRA is displayed utilizing a technique known as maximum intensity projection (MIP) (Figs. 24-4*B* and

24-5). A MIP can be displayed as images rotated at 10 to 20 degree intervals to better assess the three-dimensional character of the vascular information. The data in the MIP projection can be cropped to include only the region of interest to eliminate extraneous superimposable background signal to improve delineation of flowing intravascular spins.

Clinical Applications

Besides the study of cervicocranial atherosclerotic disease, MRA has been utilized in the detection of aneurysms greater than 3 mm;[68,77,78] the preoperative assessment of the nidus, arterial feeders and venous drainage of an AVM; arterial dissection (Fig. 24-41, *C*);[79–81] intracranial venous anatomy, including evaluation of dural

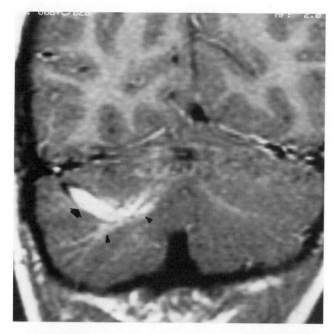

Figure 24-34 Developmental venous anomaly (DVA) or "venous angioma". MRI. Coronal contrast-enhanced T1 MRI through the posterior fossa of a 10-year-old boy presenting for unrelated causes demonstrates a typical DVA. Enlarged medullary or radial veins (Medusa head appearance) (*arrowheads*) drain to a dominant central transcortical collector vein (*arrow*), which in turn drains into the transverse sinus.

sinus thrombosis (Fig. 24-28B);[82] large vessel occlusion; and subclavian steal syndrome.[83] Current standard MRA methodology used at our institution is outlined on Table 24-4.

MAGNETIC RESONANCE SPECTROSCOPY

Magnetic resonance spectroscopy (MRS) combines the spatial information provided by conventional MRI and

TABLE 24-4
Dedicated MRA Technique for a Given Anatomic Region

Technique	Indication
2D TOF	Carotid bifurcation
	Dural sinuses
3D TOF	Circle of Willis
	Other intracranial vasculature
2D PC	Localizer MRA prior to 3D PC MRA
	Establishing velocity and flow direction
	Dural sinuses
3D PC	Intracranial vasculature
MOTSA	Carotid bifurcation
	Circle of Willis
	Other intracranial vasculature

NOTE: MRA, magnetic resonance angiography; TOF, time of flight; PC, phase contrast; 2D, two-dimensional; 3D, three-dimensional; MOTSA, multiple overlapping thin slab acquisition.

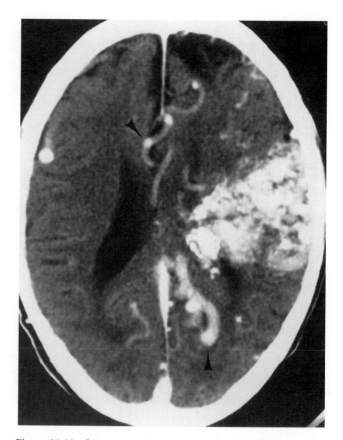

Figure 24-35 Supratentorial pial arteriovenous malformation (AVM). CT. Contrast-enhanced axial CT demonstrates an intensely enhancing tangle of dilated tortuous vessels in the left frontoparietal eloquent region. The base of the malformation abuts the cortical gray matter and its apex points to the lateral ventricle, its typical configuration. Notice the relative absence of mass effect given the large size of the lesion. Engorged tortuous draining veins (*arrowhead*) are easily discernible.

the chemical information provided by spectroscopy.[84,85] Spectroscopy was used long before MRI was developed. MRS is being used increasingly in conjunction with conventional MRI, allowing identification of chemical states of various elements without destruction of the sample. Chemical information in the form of metabolite maps provides functional information of the tissue under scrutiny.

MRS requires very high magnetic field strengths attainable only by MR instruments with superconducting magnets. Information is displayed as spectra, with peak areas being proportional to the amount of each chemical present in the sample (Fig. 24-11B, D). Most of the signal in conventional MRI arises from the water and fat present in concentrations four orders of magnitude higher than that of other metabolites. Therefore, MRI is at least 10,000 times more sensitive than MRS.[85] Because water and fat peaks overwhelm the much smaller metabolite peaks in a MRS spectrum, water and fat suppression techniques have been developed

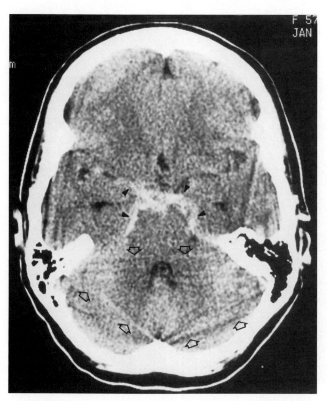

Figure 24-36   Subarachnoid hemorrhage. CT. Axial nonenhanced CT of a 57-year-old woman presenting with "sudden onset of the worst headache of her life." Abnormal high attenuation (*arrowheads*) fills the posterior portion of the suprasellar, interpeduncular, and ambient cisterns, indicating acute subarachnoid hemorrhage. Conventional angiography disclosed a ruptured posterior communicating artery aneurysm (not shown). Note the horizontally and diagonally oriented linear artifacts appearing to emanate from the internal occipital protuberance and cerebellar surfaces of the petromastoid temporal bone (*open arrows*). This is the x-ray beam hardening artifact CT is subject to that results in degradation of posterior fossa structure evaluation.

to increase sensitivity and specificity in the detection of other metabolites.[85] MRS is much more sensitive than MRI to small fluctuations in local magnetic field inhomogeneities because spectra reflect very small differences in the local magnetic field. Consequently, local magnetic field variations may broaden the peaks in spectra, decreasing its resolution and sensitivity.[85]

Among a growing number of clinical applications of MRS[85,86] are early detection of stroke[87] (Fig. 24-11); neonates born to HIV-infected mothers[88]; activity of multiple sclerosis plaques[89]; and the study of Alzheimer's disease.[90]

CT versus MRI

CT PREFERRED OVER MRI

CT instruments are more widely available than MRI, given their less stringent installation requirements and

lower cost. A CT examination is less costly and faster than an MRI examination. CT is the study of choice for the detection of skull fractures and acute subarachnoid hemorrhage (Fig. 24-36) in the emergent setting, particularly given its availability and faster acquisiton time. MRI is relatively insensitive in the detection of calcium, and CT remains the study of choice for finding and characterizing the matrix of calcification or ossification within a lesion, which may make possible specific identification of a lesion (Fig. 24-62), detection of salivary gland ductal stone disease, and study of the fine anatomy of the petromastoid temporal bone. However, a CT study delivers ionizing radiation to the patient; further, it is relatively insensitive to subtle but important pathology in the posterior fossa, given image degradation by beam-hardening artifact (Fig. 24-36), its tissue contrast is limited compared with that achievable with MRI, and acquisition is restricted to the axial and coronal planes and a limited range of gantry angulation.

For patients in whom MRI is contraindicated, CT is the study of choice. Extremely claustrophobic patients and patients with metallic implants, electromagnetic devices, pacemakers, foreign bodies, certain replaced cardiac valves, clips from recent surgery, and ferromagnetic cerebral aneurysm clips cannot undergo MRI examination.[95]

MRI PREFERRED OVER CT

MRI instruments, although not as widely available as CT, have dramatically increased in numbers in the last 5 years. MRI does not utilize ionizing radiation. Its multiplanar capability, with no need to reformat or change gantry angulation, and its ability to better characterize tissue water content are its strongest advantages.

MR is superior to CT in the evaluation of the posterior fossa (Fig. 24-27) as it is not subject to the highly degrading beam-hardening artifact of CT (Fig. 24-36). Other areas optimally imaged by MR but not by CT include the pineal gland region (Fig. 24-67); sellar and parasellar structures (Fig. 24-63–24-66); limbic system, including hippocampi (Fig. 24-9*B*); cranial nerves (Fig. 24-17, 24-65, 24-71); internal auditory canal and cerebellopontine angle (Fig. 24-68, 24-69); leptomeninges; appropriateness of myelination and neuronal migration abnormalities (Fig. 24-16, 24-17). Establishing the presence or absence of flow in arteries and dural sinuses (Fig. 24-27, 24-28*B*); arterial dissection (Fig. 24-41*B*, *C*); parenchymal lesion detection and detection of additional lesions; detection of diffuse axonal injury; detection of non-accidental trauma in children; and CSF flow studies are other clinical scenarios in which CT plays no diagnostic role. Other advantages of MRI

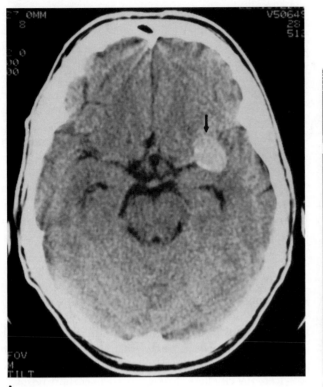

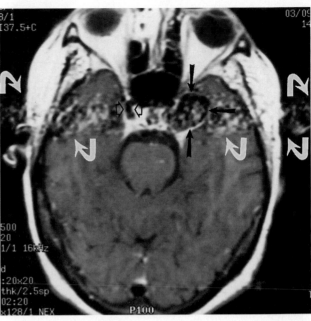

A   **B**

Figure 24-37 Middle cerebral artery (MCA) bifurcation aneurysm. *A.* CT *B.* MRI. *A.* Axial non-enhanced CT of a 67-year-old man presenting with headaches demonstrates an oval-shaped, well-circumscribed mass of homogeneous high attenuation and focal mural calcification in the cistern of the left MCA (*arrow*). *B.* Corresponding axial T1 contast-enhanced MRI obtained the same day demonstrates that the lesion is of heterogeneous signal (*three long black arrows*). The periodic artifactual signal extending beyond the confines of the skull along the phase-encoding direction (*curved white arrows*), a confirmatory sign of blood flow through the lesion, confirms the diagnosis of aneurysm. Notice the normal flow void of the cavernous segment of the right ICA (*short open black arrows*).

include its superior tissue contrast, its multiplanar capability without need to reformat (Fig. 24-13, 24-17), its superior ability to establish the intraaxial or extraaxial origin of a lesion (Fig. 24-65), and its ability to more accurately date a hematoma (Fig. 24-40*A*).

In the evaluation of spinal canal contents, MRI is clearly superior to CT, myelography, and postmyelographic CT, given its superb tissue contrast between spinal cord and CSF, obviating the instillation of intrathecal contrast medium with its concomitant potential complications. This is exemplified by the superior detection rate of disseminated CSF metastases following CNS and non-CNS malignant tumors (Fig. 24-78, 24-85)[96] and most intraspinal canal lesions (Fig. 24-83, 24-87, 24-88, and 24-90) as well as in the detection of acute cord injury and cord vascular malformations (Fig. 24-81, 24-82). CT myelogram remains useful when an osteophyte and a disc herniation cannot be clearly

differentiated by MRI, for detection of subtle cervical rootlet avulsion injury, and for the evaluation of the bony matrix of tumor.

Given the complexity of MRI physics, this modality is subject to myriad artifacts which will confound the inexperienced interpreter. However, the timely and appropriate recognition of the very same artifacts will often increase diagnostic specificity (Fig. 24-37*B*). At times artifacts will hinder evaluation of valuable anatomy (Fig. 24-8*A*), and may result in false-positive findings.

Approach to Neuroradiologic Diagnosis

GENERAL PRINCIPLES

COMPARTMENTS

Establishing the location or compartment of a lesion as intraaxial or extraaxial is crucial, given implications

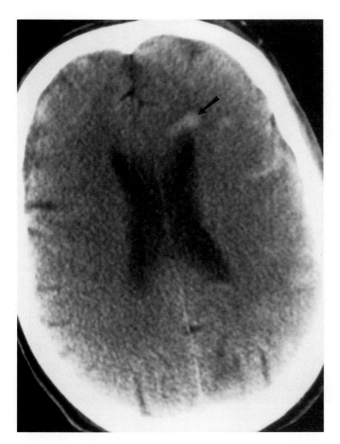

Figure 24-38   Diffuse axonal injury. CT. (Courtesy of JM Provenzale, MD; Duke University Medical Center). Axial non-enhanced CT of a 55-year-old man following a motor vehicle accident demonstrates a small irregular focus of high attenuation in the left corona radiata abutting the anterior margin of the body of the corpus callosum. Findings are consistent with hemorrhagic contusion as seen in diffuse axonal injury.

for prognosis and the formulation of a differential diagnosis. Extraaxial lesions are those arising extrinsic to the brain and spine, often from the meninges or superficial to the meninges. Intraaxial lesions are those arising from the central nervous system axis: the brain and spine. Although there are definite exceptions, a few general observations can be made about lesional location. In general, intraaxial lesions are more common and carry a poorer prognosis; they tend to be more aggressive and/or more often malignant than extraaxial lesions.

Ascribing a lesion to an intraaxial location is usually possible when brain parenchyma surrounds the lesion, when the gray-white matter junction or corticomedullary junction and cortical vessels are centrifugally (outwardly) displaced toward the inner table. The result is effacement of superficial sulci and subarachnoid spaces or of basal cisterns. Bone alterations are uncommon with intraaxial lesions. Typical examples of intraaxial lesions include primary CNS neoplasms such

as glioblastoma multiforme (Fig. 24-60), metastasis (Fig. 24-72), abscess (Fig. 24-46), infarction (Fig. 24-25B), inflammatory lesions (Fig. 24-52), parenchymal hematoma related (Fig. 24-72) or unrelated (Fig. 24-30) to tumor, and pial arteriovenous malformation (Fig. 24-35).

Ascribing a lesion to an extraaxial location is usually possible when brain parenchyma is centripetally (inwardly) displaced from the inner table with resultant widening of the subarachnoid space or cistern. The corticomedullary junction and subcortical white matter is said to "buckle." Bone alterations such as scalloping, hyperostosis, erosion, osteolysis, and fracture are common given the proximity or involvement of the dura with the inner table. Dural alterations such as thickening and tail-like enhancement often but not exclusively confirm the extraaxial character of a lesion. Typical extraaxial lesions include meningioma (Fig. 24-68); leptomeningeal carcinomatosis (Fig. 24-73); arachnoid cyst (Fig. 24-19); dermoid and epidermoid (Fig. 24-69); dural arteriovenous fistula (Fig. 24-42); calvarial and bony vertebral lesions (Figs. 24-89 and 24-90); epidural

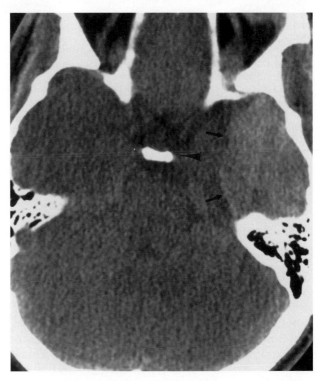

Figure 24-39   Epidural hematoma. CT. Axial nonenhanced CT of a 21-year-old man sustaining head trauma demonstrates a lentiform or biconvex acute high density hematoma in the left middle cranial fossa (*arrows*) compressing the temporal lobe producing uncal herniation. A nondepressed squamosal temporal bone fracture lacerated the middle meningeal artery resulting in the hematoma. The left uncus herniates into the suprasellar cistern (*arrowhead*).

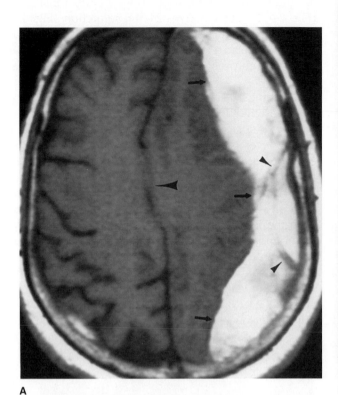

A

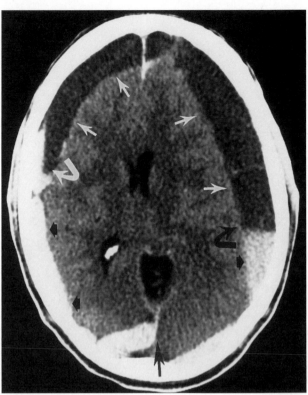

B

Figure 24-40 Subacute and mixed subdural hematomas. *A.* MRI; *B* CT. *A.* Axial nonenhanced T1 MRI of a 55-year-old woman with polycythemia and no history of trauma presenting with worsening mental status demonstrates an inwardly concave hemorrhagic fluid collection (*arrows*) at the left convexity with adjacent sulcal effacement. This represents a subacute (methemoglobin) subdural hematoma. Notice subfalcial shift (*large arrowhead*). Membrane formation is noted (*small arrowheads*). *B.* Axial nonenhanced CT of a 48-year-old alcoholic man with a history of frequent falls demonstrates a hematocrit effect within a left convexity subdural hematoma (*curved black arrow*). The high attenuation gravity-dependent component indicates acute blood (*short black arrows*) and the low attenuation non-dependent component indicates a preexisting chronic subdural hematoma (*white arrows*). A compartmentalizing fibrous membrane accounts for a vertically oriented sharp hematocrit effect within the right convexity subdural (*curved white arrow*). Note the inwardly displaced cerebral parenchyma outlined by all noncurved arrows and how the falx cerebri prevents the subdural from crossing the midline (*long black arrow*).

(Figs. 24-39 and 24-90) and subdural hematoma (Fig. 24-40) and empyema; and developmental spinal stenosis from varying contributions of disc herniation (Fig. 24-87), facet arthrosis, degenerative spondylosis (Fig. 24-84), and underlying congenital spinal canal stenosis.

At times, absolute determination of the intraaxial or extraaxial character of a lesion is not possible. This is more often the case with CT of the brain and spine. Multiplanar capability and superior tissue contrast of MRI of the brain and spine often but not infallibly will solve the dilemma. When its location remains indeterminate, the differential diagnosis of a lesion thus needs to be broadened to include both extraaxial and intraaxial entities.

In the head, intraaxial lesions can be further compartmentalized into parenchymal and intraventricular,

in either the supratentorial or the infratentorial compartment. In the spinal canal, intraaxial lesions are compartmentalized into intradural extramedullary and intradural intramedullary (Fig. 24-77). In the head, extraaxial lesions can be further compartmentalized into orbital, sellar, and parasellar, including cavernous sinus region, pineal region, and cerebellopontine angle region. In the spinal canal, extraaxial lesions are mainly extradural (Fig. 24-77) and include lesions in the epidural space and the bony structures defining the perimeter of the spinal canal. Accurate assignment of the origin of a mass to a particular compartment when evaluating cerebral or spinal imaging results in a compartment-specific differential diagnosis. This, in conjunction with the demographic information of the patient, including age, sex, past medical history and

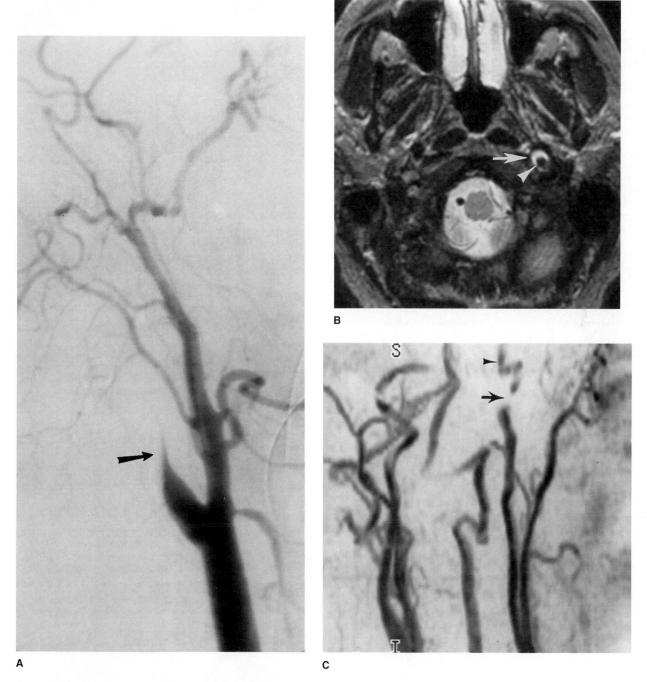

Figure 24-41   Internal carotid artery (ICA) dissection. *A.* Angiogram; *B.* MRI; *C.* MRA. *A.* Lateral digital subtraction angiogram of a right common carotid injection in a 41-year-old man involved in a motor vehicle accident demonstrates abrupt tapering of the opacified lumen of the proximal ICA (*arrow*) with a characteristic ''flame-shaped'' occlusion indicative of a mural hematoma from carotid dissection. *B.* Axial T2 MRI of a 48-year-old man presenting with a left Horner's syndrome and neckache demonstrates an eccentric crescentic hyperintense mural hematoma involving the vertical portion of the petrous segment of the left ICA (*arrow*). Total arterial diameter is increased compared to the normal right ICA given the intramural hematoma. The true lumen is narrowed but preserved (*arrowhead*), indicating patency. On catheter angiography, this artery would appear narrowed. *C.* Two-dimensional time-of-flight MRA of the same patient as Fig. 24-41*B* demonstrates focal absence of luminal signal of the corresponding segment of the left ICA (*arrow*). MRA overestimated the stenosis. Luminal signal a short distance distal to the signal defect and preservation of central luminal flow void in Fig. 21-41*B* indicate preservation of flow.

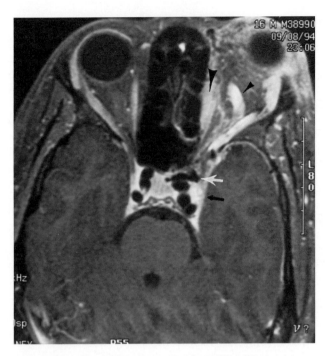

Figure 24-42 Carotid-Cavernous Fistula (CCF). MRI. Axial fat-suppressed enhanced T1 MRI through the orbits and cavernous sinus of a 16-year-old man who sustained a bicycle accident and facial fractures. The patient presented with 6 weeks of worsening exophthalmos, chemosis, and a periorbital bruit. The left cavernous sinus bulges outward (*black arrow*), an additional abnormal flow void separate from that of the cavernous internal carotid artery (*white arrow*), and a massively dilated superior ophthalmic vein (SOV) (*short arrowhead*) are consistent with arterialized flow through the cavernous sinus secondary to a fistulous communication between the cavernous segment of the ICA and the cavernous sinus. Retrograde filling of the SOV and venous congestion results in the diffusely enlarged extraocular muscles (*long arrowhead*) and exophthalmos.

clinical presentation, further tailors the list of differential possibilities to the particular clinical scenario.

MASS EFFECT AND HERNIATIONS

Given the static volume of the normal adult calvarium, space occupying processes will result in local alterations of the normal anatomic relationships of the intracranial contents. Extreme cases will manifest as local and distal alterations of normal anatomic relationships. This observation is also valid in the case of the dynamic normally growing pediatric calvarium. However, given the presence of fontanels and appositional growing sutures, the pediatric patient can afford greater room for intracranial content displacement. The same is true in the case of the diffusely or focally atrophied adult brain which can accommodate larger lesions before experiencing herniations.

The detection of positive mass effect is indicative of pathologic focally increased volume within the intracranial compartment increasing diagnostic sensitivity.

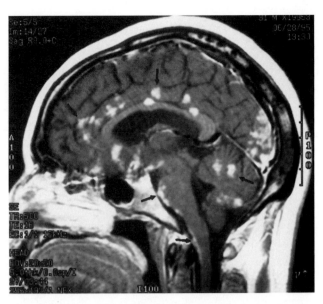

Figure 24-43 Neurosarcoidosis. MRI. Sagittal contrast-enhanced T1 MRI of a 31-year-old man demonstrates thick irregular nodular leptomeningeal enhancement along the subarachnoid cisterns coating cranial nerves, pons, medulla, and ventral upper cervical spine (*arrows*). This is a florid case of neurosarcoidosis. Differential considerations include infectious granulomatous disease such as tuberculosis and histoplasmosis.

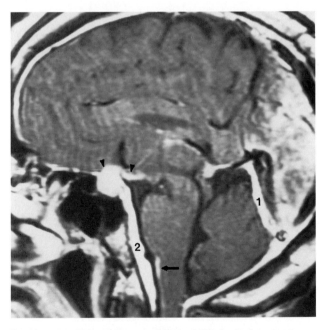

Figure 24-44 Tuberculous meningitis. MRI. Sagittal contrast-enhanced T1 MRI of a 60-year-old man with 4+ skin test (PPD) presenting with severe headaches and panhypopituitarism demonstrates diffuse intracranial dural enhancement. The dura is markedly thickened along the tentorium cerebelli (1) and the clivus (2). Abnormal pial enhancement of the medulla oblongata (*arrow*) is noted. Abnormal ehnahcement involves the suprasellar cistern and undersurface of the hypothalamus (*arrowheads*) with mass effect on the optic apparatus and pituitary infundibulum accounting for the endocrinologic deficit of this patient.

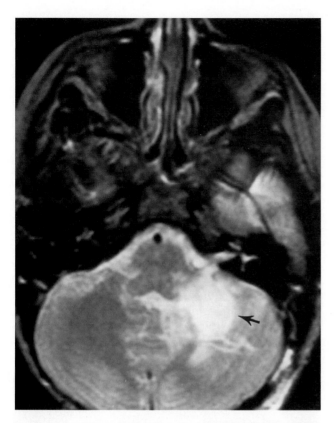

Figure 24-45 Listeria cerebritis. MRI. Axial T2 MRI through the posterior fossa of a 6-year-old girl demonstrates a poorly defined hyperintense mass centered in the left middle cerebellar peduncle (*arrow*) with extension onto the dorsal pons and medial cerebellar hemisphere. Mass effect on the fourth ventricle and minimal nodular enhancement was evident in other sections. Culture of biopsied material grew *Listeria monocytogenes.*

In conjunction with attenuation alterations in the case of CT and signal intensity alterations in the case of MRI, the detection of mass effect results in increased diagnostic specificity. A sufficiently large lesion usually is associated with a positive mass effect. This is evident by parenchymal "shifts" or herniations of the brain and spine relative to dural condensations (falx cerebri, tentorium cerebelli), bony foramina (foramen magnum), and wings of the sphenoid bone. Lesions with associated mass effect include intracranial hemorrhages in any compartment, acute and subacute infarctions, most infectious and inflammatory processes, and most neoplastic processes. Not uncommonly, a small lesion such as a metastatic deposit will exhibit disproportionately striking edema, resulting in significant mass effect and compression of vital structures.

The absence of mass effect in conjunction with attenuation and signal intensity alteration further contributes to diagnostic specificity. For example, progressive multifocal leukoencephalopathy results in parenchymal imaging characteristics alterations but typically lacks appreciable mass effect (Fig. 24-49). Low-grade

infiltrating neoplasm typified by gliomastosis cerebri results in localized gyral girth enlargement and signal intensity alteration (Fig. 24-61).

Negative mass effect is indicative of pathologic focally decreased volume also increasing diagnostic sensitivity and specificity. For example, following surgical resection of a tumor, the residual adjacent parenchyma will soften and show attenuation and signal alterations indicating encephalomalacia (Fig. 24-8A). This is apparent by attenuation or signal intensity changes in conjunction with dilatation of an adjacent subarachnoid cistern or ventricular horn, termed "ex vacuo" dilatation, a compensatory enlargement given adjacent parenchymal volume loss. Negative mass effect may occur following severe closed head injury, after a large cortical infarct, and more extensively following whole brain radiation and/or systemic chemotherapy (Fig. 24-74).

The severity and clinical significance of mass effect is further evaluated in terms of shifts of normal anatomic structures in the presence of a space occupying process.

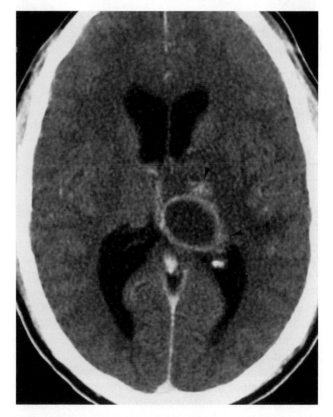

Figure 24-46 Bacterial brain abscess. CT. Axial enhanced CT of a non-immunocompromised 33-year-old man demonstrates a thin ring enhancing lesion with central low attenuation in the left thalamus consistent with an abscess. Culture of the biopsied tissue grew *S. pneumonia*. Note the satellite nodular enhancing lesions anterior and posterolateral to the dorminant abscess (*arrowheads*), which increase the specificity of the lesion. Note the midline shift experienced by the internal cerebral veins.

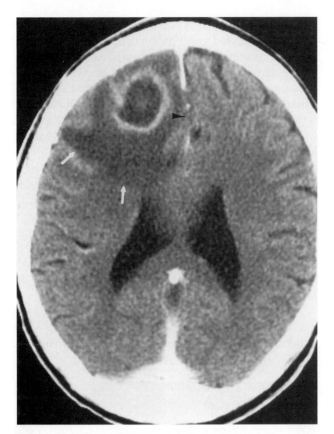

Figure 24-47 Toxoplasmosis. CT. Axial enhanced CT of a 30-year-old man with AIDS presenting with fever and change in mental status demonstrates a right subcortical white matter ring-enhancing mass with central low attenuation. Surrounding white matter vasogenic type low attenuation represents edema (*white arrows*) with associated mass effect and midline shift (*arrowhead*). The patient responded favorably to anti-toxoplasmosis drug regimen.

Shifts are divided into subfalcial, uncal, transalar, and transtentorial categories.

Subfalcial shift, also termed midline shift, refers to lateral displacement of midline structures such as the septum pellucidum and frontal horns, third ventricle, internal cerebral veins, vein of Galen, straight sinus, or pineal gland under the falx cerebri (Figs. 24-40, 24-46, and 24-57). Uncal herniation refers to medial displacement of the medial temporal lobe or uncus into the supraseller cistern (Fig. 24-39), with resultant compression of the upper brain stem. This results in torquing of the upper brain stem with consequent widening of the ipsilateral ambient cistern. Transalar herniation refers to anterior displacement of middle cranial fossa contents (temporal lobe) to the anterior cranial fossa or displacement of anterior cranial fossa contents (frontal lobe) to the middle cranial fossa over ala or wings of the sphenoid bone. Transtentorial herniation may be descending or ascending. Descending transtentorial herniation refers to downward displacement of cere-

bral parenchyma and brain stem through the tentorial incisura, typically pressing and/or stretching the posterior cerebral artery and sometimes resulting in inferior herniation of the cerebellar tonsils and medulla oblongata through the foramen magnum (Fig. 24-59). This typically occurs after other types of supratentorial shifts have developed. Ascending transtentorial herniation refers to superior displacement of the cerebellum and/or brain stem through the tentorial incisura, resulting in effacement of the quadrigeminal plate cistern (Fig. 24-73).

NUMBER OF LESIONS
AND LESIONAL DISTRIBUTION

Establishment of a lesion as solitary or as multiple has diagnostic implications beyond prognostic importance. This information is used in conjunction with the location of the lesion to improve diagnostic specificity. The following are useful guidelines, but are not without exceptions. Multiple lesions at the corticomedullary junction favor blood-borne processes such as met-

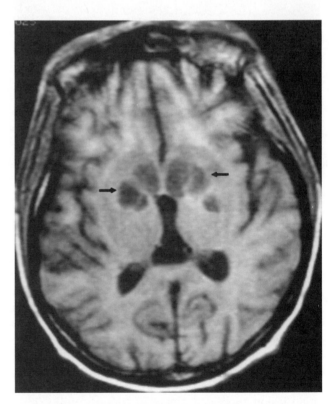

Figure 24-48 Cryptococcosis. MRI. Axial enhanced T1 MRI of a 28-year-old woman with AIDS presenting with fever and change in mental status demonstrates multifocal nonenhancing foci or low signal involving the inferior portions of the basal ganglia (*arrows*) along the distribution of perivascular spaces of Virchow-Robin. This is the typical appearance of the gelatinous pseudocysts packed with *Cryptococcus neoformans* seen in cryptococcal meningitis. Other forms of involvement including enhancing parenchymal cryptococcomas and enhancing leptomeningitis are less common forms of presentation.

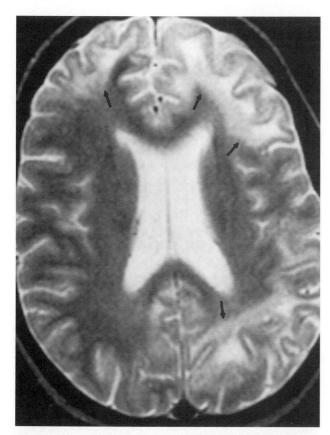

Figure 24-49 Progressive multifocal leukoencephalopathy (PML). MRI. Axial T2 MRI of a 26-year-old woman with AIDS presenting with change in personality demonstrates bilateral multifocal areas of hyperintensity involving the subcortical white matter (*arrows*) without appreciable mass effect. Enhanced images (not shown) revealed absence of enhancement. These two features are the hallmark of PML. The patient suffered a rapidly declining course.

astatic disease and septic emboli / abscesses. However, in closed head injury this distribution supports the diagnosis of diffuse axonal injury (Fig. 24-38) and contusions. Multiple small lesions following arterial territories strongly favor embolic infarcts. Synchronous primary CNS glial tumors are rare, but multifocal lymphoma is not infrequent in the immunocompromised population (Fig. 24-70).[69] Multiple lesions restricted to the periventricular white matter oriented perpendicular to the long axis of the lateral ventricles abutting the ependymal surface and lesions involving the corpus callosum and / or the middle cerebellar peduncles are highly suspicious for a demyelinating process such as multiple sclerosis (Fig. 24-54*A*). The presence of the not uncommon solitary lesion in itself is less specific than the presence of multiple lesions, and other critera need to be studied to arrive at a reasonable and manageable differential diagnosis.

EDEMA PATTERNS
Correct identification of one of any of four possible edema patterns will improve diagnostic specificity.

Edema is identified on CT by low attenuation relative to normal brain parenchyma. On MRI, it is identified by high signal intensity relative to normal brain parenchyma on T2-weighted images and slight hypointensity on T1-weighted images. Mass effect usually accompanies the edema surrounding a lesion. This tissue attenuation and signal intensity alterations are consistent in appearance, regardless of compartment. The four major edema patterns include vasogenic, ischemic, cytotoxic, and periventricular interstitial. Not uncommonly they overlap.

Vasogenic edema refers to white matter edema. Disruption of the blood-brain barrier results in fluid shifts from the systemic circulation to the neural extracellular space. The appearance is that of finger-like extensions of abnormal attenuation or signal to the subcortical white matter respecting the cortical gray matter. This edema pattern classically accompanies neoplasms (Fig. 24-72) and such infectious processes as cerebritis and abscess (Fig. 24-46, 24-47, 24-50).

Ischemic edema refers to gray *and* white matter edema. Disruption of the sodium-potassium pump re-

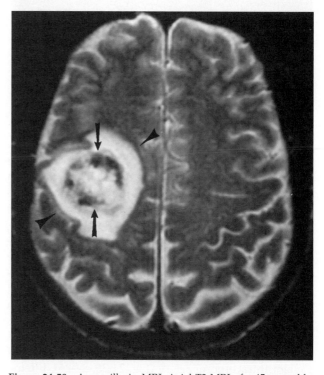

Figure 24-50 Aspergillosis. MRI. Axial T2 MRI of a 45-year-old man who had a renal transplant demonstrates a rounded mass of heterogeneous high and low signal (*arrow*) in the right posterior frontal centrum semiovale consistent with an aspergilloma (fungus ball). Surrounding white matter hyperintensity represents vasogenic edema (*arrowheads*). The lesion demonstrated ring enhancement (not shown). This presentation carries a favorable prognosis compared with the more aggressive meningoencephalitic presentation of *Aspergillus fumigatus*, which results in hemorrhagic infarction from vascular invasion.

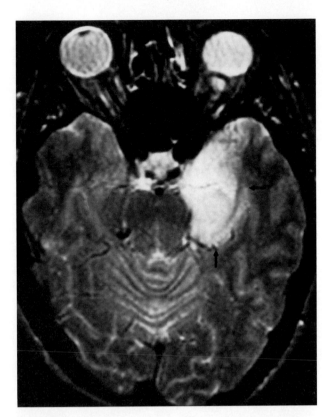

Figure 24-51 Herpes encephalitis. MRI. Axial T2 MRI of a 57-year-old woman presenting with a deteriorating mental status and stupor demonstrates inhomogeneous high signal intensity involving the medial left temporal lobe including the amygdala and hippocampus (*arrows*). Other sections revealed involvement of the insular region with sparing of the basal ganglia. The findings are classic for herpes simplex (type I) encephalitis.

sults in an intracellular influx of sodium cations with concomitant intracellular fluid shifts. This results in further shift of fluid from the intravascular compartment into both the extracellular and the intracellular neural compartments.[64] The result is massive swelling of the neural cells, with edema manifested as effacement of adjacent sulci and subarachnoid spaces. The cortical gray matter is not respected such that there is poor differentiation between cortex (gray matter) and medulla (subcortical white matter). This edema pattern is classically present during arterial and venous infarcts. The arterial infarct edema will tend to follow a territorial distribution corresponding to the supply of a major intracerebral artery (Fig. 24-25, 24-26). Edema in a venous infarct will tend not to follow a clear-cut arterial territorial distribution (Fig. 24-28A). The venous infarct will tend to be clinically silent if located in the temporal region and will tend to be hemorrhagic more often than will arterial infarcts (Fig. 24-28A). Thrombosis of a nearby dural sinus or deep vein will be detected if a dedicated contrast-enhanced CT or nonenhanced magnetic resonance venogram (MRV) is

performed (Fig. 24-28B). Coexistence of ischemic and vasogenic edema may limit their clear-cut differentiation at times at the expense of diagnostic specificity.

Cytotoxic edema is essentially similar to ischemic edema but is not limited to a single arterial or venous territory. Instead, it results from a global hypoxic-anoxic insult, usually secondary to diffuse cerebral hypoperfusion from transient or persistent hypotension.[63] Radiologically, diffuse supratentorial cortical gray matter becomes hypodense relative to white matter, the so-called "reversal sign"[97] as the normal attenuation relationship between gray and white matter is reversed (Table 24-1). This pattern is usually but not always associated with irreversible brain damage.[98] Border zone or watershed infarcts result in the setting of hypotension sufficiently profound to result in cytotoxic edema but sufficiently prolonged to result in global cerebral anoxia (Fig. 24-29).

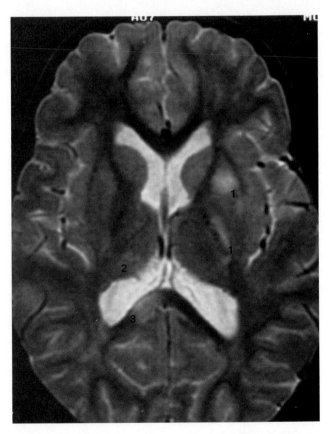

Figure 24-52 Acute disseminated encephalomyelitis (ADEM). MRI. Axial T2 MRI of a 3-year-old girl with an upper respiratory viral infection several weeks prior to the study presenting with acute lower extremity weakness and urinary retention. Multple poorly marginated areas of hyperintensity involve the left globus pallidus and putamen at various locations (1), the right thalamus (2), and the right side of the splenium of the corpus callosum (3). Other areas of involvement (*not shown*) included the upper brain stem, the middle cerebellar peduncles, and the cervical spine. The findings are typical for ADEM. The patient's symptoms subsided without intervention.

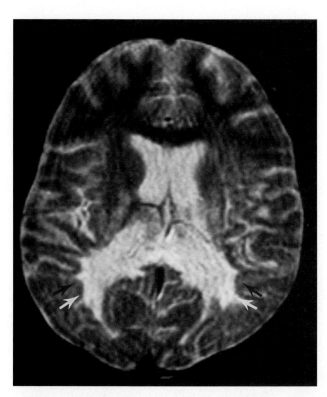

Figure 24-53   Adrenoleukodystrophy. MRI. Axial T2 MRI of a 6-year-old boy demonstrates bilaterally symmetric posterior periventricular white matter hyperintensity (*black* and *white arrows*). This process typically progresses from posterior to anterior. Contrast enhancement may be seen along the advancing leading edge, indicative of active demyelination (not shown). This image is degraded by motion artifact.

Periventricular interstitial edema results when the ventricular ependyma is unable to contain ventricular CSF within its confines in the setting of hydrocephalus. The ependymal lining stretches and/or tears,[64] and extracellular fluid accumulates in the periventricular white matter initially surrounding the frontal horns and later surrounding the bodies of the lateral ventricles. Radiologically, the ventricular-white matter interface becomes blurred, and a confluent band of periventricular white matter hypodensity develops on CT and hyperintensity develops on T2-weighted MRI images.

ENHANCEMENT PATTERNS
A variety of enhancement patterns has been described, including homogeneous, heterogeneous, ringlike, serpentine, gyriform, and intravascular. Similar to absence of mass effect, absence of enhancement can increase diagnostic specificity. Some lesions displaying homogeneous enhancement include meningioma (Figs. 24-68 and 24-21), low- and intermediate-grade glioma, and lymphoma in the non-immunocompromised patient. Some lesions displaying heterogeneous enhancement include high-grade glioma (Fig. 24-60),

infarction, and cerebritis. Some lesions displaying ring enhancement include high-grade glioma, lymphoma in the immunocompromised patient (Fig. 24-6*A*), metastasis (Fig. 24-72), abscess (Fig. 24-46, 24-47), resolving infarction, resolving hematoma, radiation necrosis, and active multiple sclerosis plaques. Some lesions displaying serpentine enhancement include arteriovenous malformation (Fig. 24-35), and developmental venous anomaly (Fig. 24-34). Some lesions displaying gyriform enhancement include subacute infarct and ischemic or injured tissue following trauma. Some lesions displaying no enhancement after intravenous contrast administration include low-grade noninfiltrative or infiltrative glioma (Fig. 24-61), arachnoid cyst (Fig. 24-19), dermoid and epidermoid cysts (Fig. 24-69), and viral infection, such as most cases of progressive multifocal leukoencephalopathy (Fig. 24-49).

Normally, the leptomeninges enhance (nonpathologic leptomeningeal enhancement is not apparent in contiguous images).[4] Linear and nodular enhancements are typical of infectious granulomatous (tuberculous) (Fig. 24-44) and noninfectious granulomatous (neurosarcoid) (Fig. 24-43) meningitis, nongranulomatous infectious meningitis, and meningeal carcinomatosis (Fig. 24-73, 24-85).

Finally, identification of flow voids (focal round or tubular areas of low signal on conventional spin echo imaging) within a lesion which may or may not exhibit enhancement after IV contrast are characteristic of certain highly vascular lesions (Fig. 24-24*B*).

Imaging Review of Neurologic Disease

The following short presentation offers some classic imaging examples of various cerebral and spinal conditions at the risk of obviating entities considered by authorities to be representative of the field of neuroradiology. This neuroradiologic imaging sampler provides examples in the following categories: developmental; vascular; trauma; infectious and inflammatory; demyelinating disease; neoplastic; neurodegenerative; hydrocephalus and increased intracranial pressure; and the three spinal compartments. The reader is referred to various recent modern outstanding neuroradiology textbooks for in-depth discussions and presentations of these and a myriad of other entities.[3,58,62–64, 98]

DEVELOPMENTAL

The Chiari malformations represent the congenital disorders of neural tube closure first described by Chiari in 1891.[62] Specifically, they refer to hindbrain anomalies in which cerebellar tissue descends into the cervical spinal canal in association with hydrocephalus.

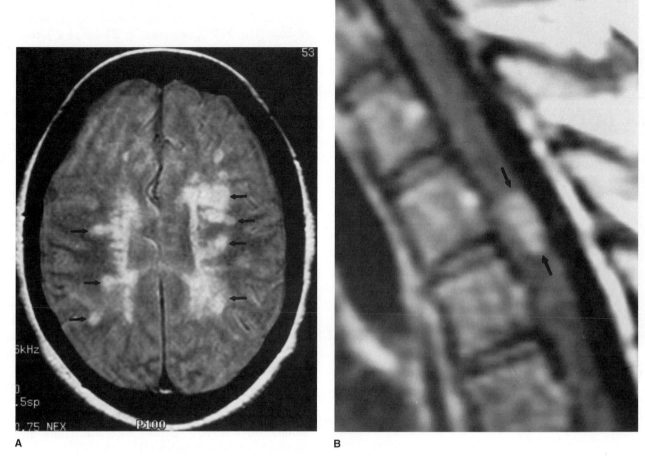

Figure 24-54   Multiple sclerosis (MS). MRI (*A.* Brain; *B.* Thoracic spine). *A.* Axial proton density MRI of a 45-year-old woman with a history of optic neuritis, abnormal visual evoked potentials, and oligoclonal bands on her CSF demonstrates multiple plaquelike lesions of abnormal hyperintensity relative to CSF in the centrum semiovale (*arrows*). The lesions are oriented perpendicular to the long axis of the lateral ventricles corresponding to demyelination along the perivenular spaces, typical of multiple sclerosis. Some plaques exhibited enhancement following contrast administration (not shown). *B.* Sagittal enhanced T1 MRI of the same patient demonstrates an enhancing intradural intramedullary MS plaque (*arrows*) principally involving the dorsal white matter of the lower cervical cord. The lesion spans the height of one vertebral body.

In the Chiari I malformation, sometimes termed congenital caudal cerebellar tonsillar ectopia,[62] the cerebellar tonsils are dysplastic, acquiring a peglike pointed configuration, and are inferiorly displaced across the foramen magnum. This is optimally demonstrated by MRI in the sagittal plane (Fig. 24-12). Tonsillar position differences normally occur with age, with expected normal tonsillar ascent occurring with increasing age. In the first decade of life, 6 mm or more is the criterion for tonsillar ectopia; 5 mm or more in the second and third decades; 4 mm or more in the fourth to eighth decades; and 3 mm or more afterwards.[58] In this condition there are usually no associated brain anomalies. Mild to moderate hydrocephalus is present in 25 percent of cases. Hydrosyringomyelia (Fig. 24-12) or any

pathologic CSF-containing cord cavity[58] that may or may not be continuous with the central canal is seen in 30 to 60 percent of all patients with the Chiari I malformation, usually involving the cervical region. One-quarter of patients will have bony abnormalities, mainly basilar invagination, atlantooccipital assimilation, and fused cervical vertebrae.

The Chiari II malformation, also termed Arnold-Chiari malformation, is a complex anomaly of unelucidated etiology involving skull and dura, cerebellar hemispheres, CSF spaces, spine and spinal cord.[58] Patients have a high incidence of associated supratentorial anomalies.[62] MRI elegantly displays many of the abnormalities of the Chiari II malformation, among which feature cervicomedullary kinking, towering cer-

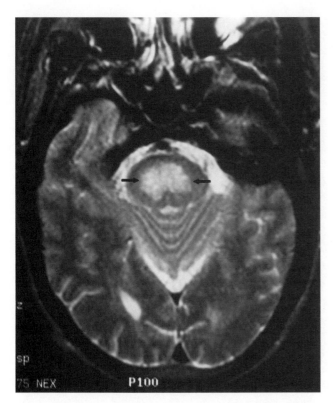

Figure 24-55 Central pontine myelinolysis. MRI. Axial T2 MRI of a 55-year-old man with a history of alcohol abuse presenting with pronounced hyponatremia demonstrates abnormal hyperintensity involving the central portion of the pons bilaterally (*black arrows*). Hyponatremia had been too rapidly corrected, resulting in osmotic myelinolysis of the pons.

ebellum, and tectal beaking (Fig. 24-13). Communicating hydrocephalus is present in 90 percent of cases.[58] There may be agenesis or dysgenesis of the corpus callosum with colpocephaly (disproportionately enlarged atria and occipital horns) (Fig. 24-13), gray matter heterotopias (Fig. 24-16), polymicrogyria, and stenogyria (contracted narrow gyri). Myelomeningocele is present at birth in virtually all cases, and following surgical closure nearly all patients develop hydrocephalus.[62] Syringohydromyelia (Fig. 24-14) is seen in 50 to 90 percent of cases, and diastematomyelia, sagittal clefting of the spinal cord (Fig. 24-15), is seen in 15 to 20 percent of cases.[58]

Gray matter heterotopia and schizencephaly represent disorders of cellular migration and sulcation that almost always present with a seizure disorder.[62] Gray matter heterotopias refer to collections of normal neurons situated ectopically in abnormal locations secondary to arrest of neuronal migration along the radial-glial fiber network.[62] Various types have been described, namely band (double cortex or laminar) and nodular. In turn, these may be focal, diffuse or subependymal (Fig. 24-16). MRI is much more sensitive

than CT in the detection of heterotopia.[62] On MRI, the heterotopia is isointense to gray matter on pulse sequences and displays no enhancement after contrast administration. Schizencephaly or split brain refers to a heterotopic gray matter-lined CSF-filled cleft extending from the pia to an ependymal surface. In the closed lip variety, the cleft walls are in apposition (Fig. 24-17); in the open lip variety, associated with a worse prognosis, the cleft walls are separated (not shown).[58] MRI optimally depicts the gray matter lined cleft. The main differential consideration is a porencephalic cyst which occurs after a localized insult to otherwise normal brain. In this condition, there is communication between the pia and an ependymal surface, but the cleft is not lined by heterotopic gray matter.

Early during embryogenesis, the caudal portion of the spinal cord extends to the caudal end of the spinal canal. With development, the vertebral bodies grow at a faster rate than the spinal cord and the caudal portion of the cord undergoes retrogressive differentiation.[62] Controversy remains, but by birth to 2 months of age the conus medullaris should normally terminate above the L2-L3 disc level 98 percent of the time.[62] Tethered cord and tight filum terminale syndrome are a common feature of most spinal malformations, and result from failure of involution of the terminal embryonic neural tube or from failure of normal nerve fiber lengthening.[58] Imaging findings feature a low-lying conus medullaris (Fig. 24-18), lateral or at times superior course of the exiting nerve roots and a thickened filum terminale (greater than 2.0 mm measured at L5-S1).[62] Spinal dysraphism typically accompanies this condition. Other abnormalities, namely lipoma (Fig. 24-18), diastematomyelia (Fig. 24-15), myelomeningocele, and scoliosis, are often associated with tethered cord.

Arachnoid (leptomeningeal) cyst is a benign congenital CSF-like fluid-filled extraaxial cyst within the arachnoid membrane that may result in parenchymal compression. When cysts are large enough and occur in their most common location, the middle cranial fossa, temporal lobe dysgenesis may be present (Fig. 24-19).[58] When uncomplicated, this nonenhancing lesion is isointense to CSF on all pulse sequences. Differential considerations include epidermoid (Fig. 24-69), open-lip schizencephaly (Fig. 24-17), loculated hygroma, and old infarct.[58]

The phakomatoses or neurocutaneous syndromes are disorders of histogenesis,[58] heterogeneously affecting the central nervous system with peculiar cutaneous manifestations. The main forms feature neurofibromatosis types I and II, tuberous sclerosis, Sturge-Weber syndrome, and Von Hippel-Lindau syndrome. Many other rare syndromes have been described but are beyond the scope of this presentation.

The Natural Institutes of Health has only defined

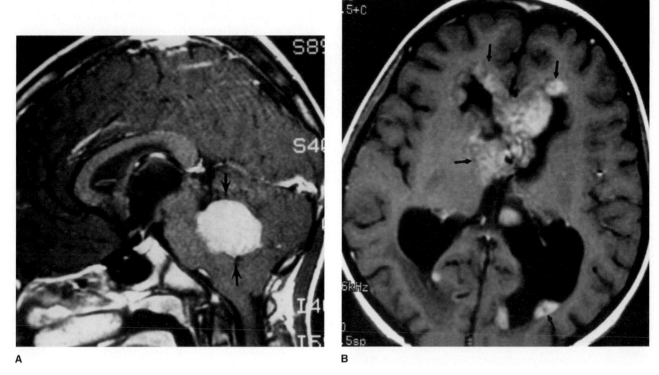

A   **B**

Figure 24-56 Primitive neuroectodermal tumor (PNET): Medulloblastoma. Intraventricular spread. MRI *A.* Sagittal enhanced T1 MRI of a 7-year-old boy, presenting with worsening headaches and vomiting, demonstrates a large homogeneously enhancing intraventricular mass massively distending the fourth ventricle (*arrows*). This is the typical appearance of a medulloblastoma, a form of primitive neuroectodermal tumor originating from the posterior medullary velum of the fourth ventricle. *B.* Axial enhanced T1 MRI of a 16-year-old girl who had a suboccipital craniectomy with resection of a posterior fossa medulloblastoma several years ago presenting with worsening headaches and vomiting. Multiple enhancing irregular masses coat the ependymal surfaces of the third and lateral ventricles (*arrows*), most pronounced along the frontal horns, representing metastatic disease.

two types of neurofibromatosis (NF), although NF is a group of heterogeneous diseases,[58] namely type 1 (NF-1) and type 2 (NF-2). NF-1 or von Recklinghausen disease is the most common of all phakomatoses, accounting for over 90 percent of all NF cases, and cutaneous manifestations are common. Lesions in NF-1 may include cerebral and spinal neoplasms, non-neoplastic "hamartomatous" lesions, skull and meningeal dysplasias, eye and orbital abnormalities, vascular abnormalities, visceral and endocrine tumors, and musculoskeletal lesions following a systemic mesodermal dysplasia. MRI best delineates the optic nerve and retroorbital segments of the optic nerves which is crucial in detection and follow-up of optic nerve gliomas and their posterior extensions (Fig. 24-20). While only 25 percent of all cases of optic nerve gliomas are associated with NF-1, this tumor occurs in 5 to 15 percent of cases of NF-1.[58] Plexiform neurofibromas are the hallmark of NF-1 and are diagnostic, found in one-third of all patients with this condition,[58] most commonly involving the first division of the trigeminal

nerve. Benign nonneoplastic hamartomatous lesions representing hyperplastic or dysplastic foci of glial proliferation are present in 80 percent of cases,[58] typically involve the basal ganglia, optic radiations, brain stem, cerebellar peduncles, and rarely the spinal cord[58] without associated mass effect and usually without enhancement after contrast administration.

Neurofibromatosis type 2 (NF-2) is much less common than NF-1, and cutaneous manifestations are rare. Bilateral eighth nerve schwannomas are diagnostic of NF-2 (Fig. 24-21). Multiple schwannomas involving other cranial nerves, multiple intracranial meningiomas (Fig. 24-21), multiple fusiform or dumbbell spinal schwannomas more common than meningiomas, and conus medullaris ependymomas are suggestive of NF-2.

Since the classic clinical triad of a papular facial nevus (adenoma sebaceum), seizures, and mental retardation is present in less than 50 percent of patients with tuberous sclerosis, the neuroradiologic findings of this condition can decisively establish the diagno-

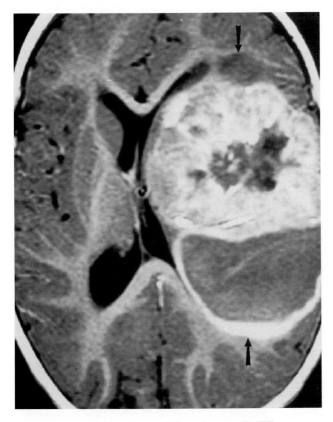

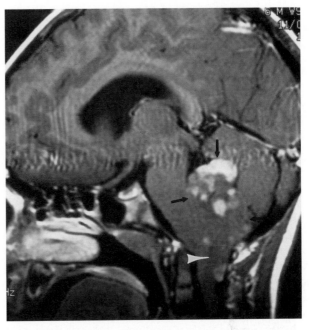

Figure 24-57 Primitive neuroectodermal tumor (PNET): Ependymoblastoma. MRI. Axial enhanced T1 MRI of a 6-month-old girl with macrocrania and progressive right hemiparesis demonstrates a very large heterogeneously enhancing mass of complex internal architecture (*arrows*) essentially replacing the left hemisphere. In this age group, main diagnostic considerations besides PNET must include glioblastoma multiforme and germ cell tumor.

Figure 24-59 Ependymoma. MRI. Sagittal enhanced T1 MRI of a 6-year-old boy presenting with headache and vomiting demonstrates a large heterogeneously nodular enhancing mass filling and expanding the fourth ventricle (*arrows*). Most of the mass is isointense to gray matter. It compresses the brain stem and insinuates along the midline foramen of Magendie (*arrowhead*) to the dorsal subarachnoid space of the upper cervical canal. Growth along the recesses of the fourth ventricle is typical of ependymoma but not of medulloblastoma.

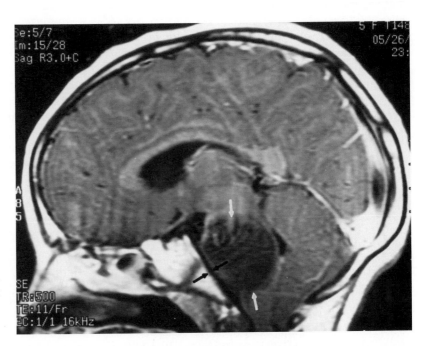

Figure 24-58 Pontine glioma. MRI. Sagittal enhanced T1 MRI of a 5-year-old girl demonstrates a large nonenhancing hypointense mass expanding the pons (*arrows*) obliterating the prepontine cistern (*opposing black arrows*). This is the typical appearance of a pontine glioma.

TABLE 24-5
Evolution of a Parenchymal Hematoma: Computed Tomography

	Timing	Attenuation
Hyperacute	Minutes to hours	Swirl sign (hypodense amidst hyperdense)
Acute	Hours to 1 week	Hyperdense
Subacute	1 to 6 weeks	Isodense
Chronic	Greater than 6 weeks	Hypodense

sis.[58] This condition is characterized by widespread hamartomas in multiple organ systems. CNS lesions consist of cortical tubers, white matter lesions, subependymal nodules (95 percent of cases), and giant cell astrocytomas typically at or near the foramen of Monro (15 percent of cases) (Fig. 24-22).[58] Recent studies attempt to correlate number of CNS lesions with seizure onset, infantile spasm, and mental impairment.[99]

In the Sturge-Weber syndrome (encephalotrigeminal angiomatosis), normal cortical venous drainage fails to develop in the presence of a leptomeningeal angioma, resulting in venous congestion, chronic cortical ischemia, cerebral atrophy, and secondary skull changes (Fig. 24-23). Dystrophic tram-track calcification paralleling gyri of the middle layers of the affected cerebral cortex develops as a result. An ipsilateral facial angioma develops, termed "port-wine stain" nevus flammeus, typically in the distribution of the first division of the trigeminal nerve. The pial angioma exhibits enhancement after contrast administration (Fig. 24-23). Gyriform cortical enhancement secondary to ischemic change, prominent medullary and subependymal veins, and an enlarged ipsilateral choroid plexus secondary to increased collateral deep venous drainage also may display striking enhancement (Fig. 24-23).[58] MRI and more recently MRA have proved to display the features of this entity to best advantage.[100,101]

Multiple CNS hemangioblastomas, one CNS hemangioblastoma in the presence of a visceral manifestation,

or one central or one visceral manifestation in a patient with an affected first-order family member constitute the Von-Hippel Lindau (VHL) syndrome.[58] VHL is a multiple organ system syndrome characterized by CNS and visceral angiomas, neoplasms, and cysts. Cerebellar hemangioblastomas represent 7 to 12 percent of all posterior fossa tumors and are found in up to two-thirds of patients with VHL.[58] The typical lesion exhibits an intensely dense prolonged vascular stain in catheter angiography (Fig. 24-24*A*) corresponding to a mural nodule on cross-sectional imaging. This enhancing tumor involves the spinal cord 15 percent of the time, is present in 10 to 30 percent of patients with VHL, and is often associated with a syrinx or a syrinx-like cyst with or without prominent flow voids representing afferent and efferent vessels feeding the lesion (Fig. 24-24*B*).[58]

VASCULAR

HEMORRHAGE

Detection of intracranial hemorrhage is one of the most common indications for emergent neuroradiologic cross-sectional imaging, given its typical clinical presentation of acute and/or progressive neurologic deterioration. Having a basic understanding of how CT (Table 24-5) and MRI (Table 24-6) portray hemorrhage in its various stages of evolution is of paramount importance in the management and prognostication of patients.

Etiologies

The differential diagnosis for parenchymal hemorrhage in the absence of trauma is vast and includes hypertensive bleed (Fig. 24-30); arterial or venous infarct with hemorrhagic transformation (Fig. 24-28); benign and malignant neoplasm including metastatic disease (Fig. 24-72); vascular malformation (Fig. 24-35); nonneoplastic hemorrhagic cyst (Rathke cleft cyst, complicated arachnoid cyst, complicated colloid cyst); amyloid angiopathy; infection such as herpes simplex

TABLE 24-6
Evolution of a Parenchymal Hematoma: Magnetic Resonance Imaging
(conventional spin echo, 1.5 Tesla instrument)

		Signal Intensity		Hemoglobin Blood Product
	Timing	T1WI	T2WI	
Acute	Hours to 1 week	Iso[a]	Lo[b]	Deoxyhemoglobin
Subacute	Weeks to months	Hi[c]	Lo then hi	Methemoglobin
Chronic	Months to years	Iso	Lo periphery	Hemosiderin, ferritin

[a] Iso, isointense to adult gray matter.
[b] Lo, hypointense to adult gray matter.
[c] Hi, hyperintense to adult gray matter.
NOTE: T1WI, T1-weighted image; T2WI, T2-weighted image.

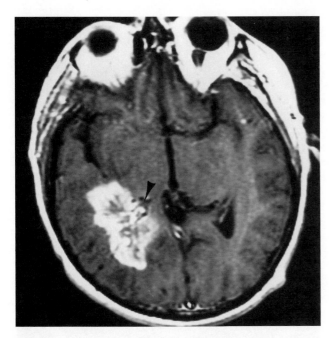

Figure 24-60   Glioblastoma multiforme (GBM). MRI. Axial enhanced T1 MRI of a 50-year-old man presenting with nausea, vomiting, and headaches demonstrates a heterogeneously peripherally enhancing mass in the right para-atrial white matter with subependymal and choroid plexus invasion (*arrowhead*). Its central low signal is suggestive of cystic necrosis. Pathology studies revealed GBM.

type II necrotizing encephalitis; inflammatory (rarely acute demyelinating encephalomyelitis and multiple sclerosis); angiogenic fungi such as *Aspergillus fumigatus* (Fig. 24-50); vasculitis as seen with sympathomimetic and recreational drug use such as amphetamine, phenylpropanolamine (PPA), phencyclidine (PCP), ephedrine, and cocaine (Fig. 24-32); blood dyscrasias; and coagulopathies. The most relevant clinical question is whether the etiology of a parenchymal hematoma is neoplastic or non-neoplastic. Finding the answers is extremely difficult because there is considerable radiologic imaging overlap and no absolute criteria.[58] Clinical presentation is probably the most reliable piece of information in making this distinction because tumors tend to have a protracted progressive course, whereas completed infarcts typically present with an acute neurologic deficit.

Certain generalizations are useful broad guidelines in differentiating tumoral hemorrhage from such non-tumor etiologies as infarct. The hematoma of an underlying tumor tends to be more heterogeneous and complex in attenuation and signal characteristics (blood intermixed with tumor); tends to have an incomplete hemosiderin rim on MRI[58]; and usually has nonhemorrhagic areas that enhance after IV contrast administration.[58] The pattern of enhancement of an infarct tends to be gyriform or linear, and occasionally fine adjacent

dural enhancement is evident.[94] Sometimes, infarcts display thin ring enhancement, whereas tumors commonly enhance as thick rings.[94] Changes in the imaging pattern over days to weeks favor infarct.[94] When sequential studies reveal persistent mass effect and edema as well as delayed and disordered evolution of the hematoma, tumor is favored.[58] Infarcts and tumors hemorrhage centrally, but infarcts frequently exhibit extravascular blood products at the periphery of the lesion.[94] Moreover, a lesion that involves more than one vascular territory is unlikely to be an infarct.[94]

Exclusion of trauma-related hemorrhage, contusion, edema, and mass effect represents one of the most common indications for a CT scan of the brain and a spinal MRI in the emergency room. A few examples include subarachnoid hemorrhage (Fig. 24-36), subdural (Fig. 24-40), epidural (Fig. 24-39), and deep white matter (Fig. 24-38) hematomas; and spinal cord contusion (Fig. 24-81).

Computed Tomography

A linear relationship exists between attenuation value and hematocrit[91] with the exception of hyperacute hemorrhage in which clot retraction has not taken place (Table 24-5). In the case of hyperacute hemorrhage,

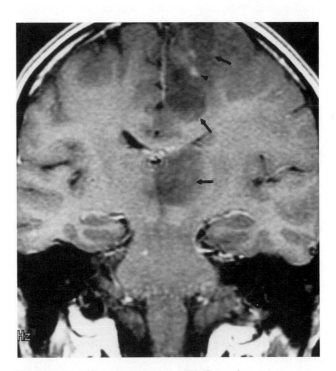

Figure 24-61   Gliomatosis cerebri. MRI. Coronal contrast enhanced T1 MRI of a 16-year-old boy presenting with headache and personality change demonstrates cortical enlargement involving the left paramedian convexity gray and subcortical white matter and the ipsilateral thalamus (*arrows*) with minimal enhancement (*arrowhead*). Biopsy of this diffusely infiltrating process disclosed the unusual diagnosis of gliomatosis cerebri.

irregular areas of intermediate to low attenuation also known as the "swirl sign"[92] are present amidst the hematoma. Because the diagnosis of acute cerebral hemorrhage depends on the ability to detect focal areas of high attenuation, no intravenous contrast is administered as it could impair the radiologist's ability to make the diagnosis. Normally enhancing structures may decrease the conspicuousness of the area of hemorrhage, particularly in the subarachnoid compartment. For example, enhancement of the arteries of the circle of Willis may hinder the detection of subarachnoid hemorrhage in the supresellar cistern.

The hematocrit of a fresh hematoma and the high mass density of the globin moiety of the hemoglobin molecule are responsible for the high attenuation of acute hemorrhage on CT (Fig. 24-30).[58] Over time, the hematocrit within a hematoma decreases and a corresponding decrease in attenuation value[92] and mass effect is observed unless re-hemorrhage ensues (Fig. 24-40B). Profoundly anemic patients (hemoglobin of 8 to 10 g/dl) do not necessarily follow this rule; acute hemorrhage in this setting may be isodense and therefore less conspicuous.[93]

Magnetic Resonance Imaging

Understanding hemorrhage as displayed by MRI is a challenging endeavor, not only because of its protean appearances but also because to date its pathophysiology has not been completely elucidated. Table 26-6 shows an abbreviated version of the evolution of a parenchymal hematoma in conventional spin echo imaging. Intrinsic factors that may influence the MR appearance of intracranial hemorrhage include macroscopic structure of the clot, hemoglobin molecule oxidation state, red blood cell morphology, protein concentration/clot hydration, size and location of the hematoma and surrounding edema.[58] Extrinsic confounding factors include the instrument's magnetic field strength and the choice of the appropriate pulse sequence.[58] Whereas at times the signal intensity of a hematoma decisively establishes its approximate age, as in the case of acute hemorrhage (Fig. 24-81) and subacute hemorrhage (Fig. 24-40A), a mixed pattern of signal intensity is a more common scenario (Fig. 24-33A, Fig. 24-72).

ATHEROSCLEROSIS

The clinical diagnosis of stroke is inaccurate in 13 percent of cases.[58] Neuroradiologic evaluation is performed to confirm the diagnosis of a cerebrovascular accident, to exclude a structural lesion such as tumor, AVM or subdural hematoma, and to exclude parenchymal hemorrhage, which dictates prognosis and management. While 60 percent of brain CTs are obtained shortly after symptoms are normal,[58] several findings

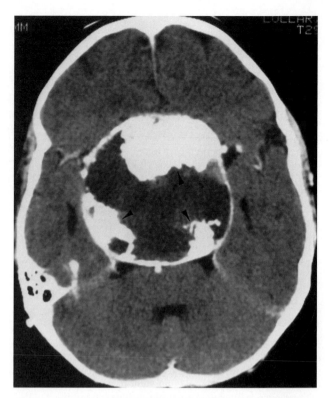

Figure 24-62 Craniopharyngioma. CT. Axial contrast-enhanced CT of a 19-year-old man presenting with headache and visual deficits demonstrates a huge rounded mass with large irregular mural calcification (*arrowheads*) and a larger central component of low attenuation. The epicenter of the lesion is the suprasellar cistern. The mass markedly compresses the brain stem, surrounding parenchyma, and ventricles.

may be present in early stroke. A hyperdense middle cerebral artery (Fig. 24-25A) has been reported in up to one-half of patients with MCA territory stroke[58] as a result of acute intraluminal thrombus. Other findings include loss of gray-white matter interface along the lateral insular ribbon or along the cortex, and obscuration of the lentiform nucleus. Low attenuation involving gray and white matter, sulcal effacement, edema and increasing mass effect are seen with completion of the infarct (Fig. 24-25B). MRI detects early infarcts more often and more accurately than does CT,[58] with a variety of findings. Besides sulcal effacement, gyral swelling, and loss of gray-white matter interface, MRI-specific findings include intravascular contrast enhancement, edema displayed as increased signal intensity on T2-weighted images (Fig. 24-26), and absence of normal arterial flow void (Fig. 24-27).

Whereas arterial infarcts conform to a typical vascular territory distribution, venous infarcts do not (Fig. 24-28A). Venous infarcts are not uncommonly underdiagnosed because clinical signs and symptoms are often nonspecific. They are more often hemorrhagic and are associated with dural sinus and/or cortical vein thrombosis. A high index of suspicion in the clinical setting of pregnancy/puerperium, infection, dehydration, oral contraceptive agents, coagulopathy, blood dyscrasias, adjacent tumor, and trauma (among others) is required to make the diagnosis. Both CT and MRI can detect venous thrombosis. MRI has the added benefit of multiplanar display, demonstrating luminal thrombus to greater advantage in various planes. MRA (sometimes termed MRV for magnetic resonance venography when parameters are adjusted to display dural sinus blood flow) noninvasively maps the flow defect to better advantage (Fig. 24-28*B*).

Peripheral border zones between the terminal capillary beds of major cerebral cortical and cerebellar arteries, usually near the junction of their supplied parenchyma, experience the greatest decrease in cerebral blood flow during generalized systemic hypotension of diverse etiologies. These areas, also termed watershed, differ in the fetus and premature infant stage when compared with term infants and adults. Most severely and frequently affected is the parietooccipital brain in the area where the middle, posterior, and anterior cerebral arteries converge (Fig. 24-29).[58]

Lacunar infarcts are deep cerebral infarcts up to 1 cm

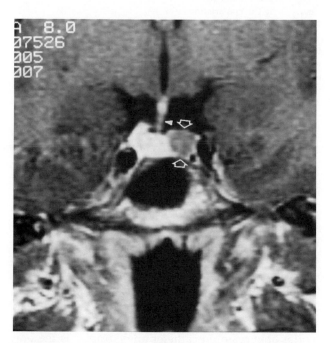

Figure 24-63 Pituitary microadenoma: prolactinoma. MRI. Coronal enhanced T1 MRI with special attention to the sella turcica of a 21-year-old woman presenting with galactorrhea, amenorrhea, and elevated serum prolactin demonstrates an 8-mm focal rounded mass in the left side of the pituitary gland (*short open white arrows*) enhancing to a lesser degree than normal gland tissue. The infundibulum is deviated to the right (*white arrowhead*) and the superior margin of the left side of the gland bulges in a convex fashion, adjunctive but nonspecific signs for an underlying microadenoma. This lesion was not detectable by CT (not shown).

that classically involve the deep gray matter structures, namely the thalamus and basal ganglia, accounting for up to 25 percent of all strokes,[58] along the lenticulostriate branch distribution (Fig. 24-30).

The most common nontraumatic etiology of adult intracranial hemorrhage is hypertension,[58] some cases resulting from ruptured Charcot-Bouchard microaneurysms of the lenticulostriate perforating arteries. Preferential involvement of the putamen, rest of the basal ganglia, external capsule (Fig. 24-30), pons, and dentate nuclei is the norm.

VASCULITIS

Multiple classifications have been proposed for vasculitides, a heterogeneous group of uncommon CNS disorders typified by necrosis and/or inflammation of the vessel wall.[58] The more traditional system groups them into bacterial, mycotic, necrotizing, and collagen-vascular etiologies.[58] Systemic lupus erythematosus may involve the peripheral and central nervous systems. SLE-related CNS vasculitis is uncommon, with a wide gamut of angiographic changes,[58] including a normal arteriogram, subtle small vessel changes, and large vessel changes with fusiform aneurysmal dilatation alternating with tandem stenosis and mural irregularity (Fig. 24-31). Drug-induced arteritis as a result from direct toxic injury to the vessel wall or from hypersensitivity from impurities within the preparation has become more prevalent. Over-the-counter, prescription, and illegal drugs have all been implicated (Fig. 24-32). A recent study concluded that a negative MRI excludes intracranial vasculitis more definitively than does a negative catheter angiogram.[102]

VASCULAR MALFORMATIONS

Cavernous hemangiomas or cavernomas represent 10 to 15 percent of all CNS vascular malformations.[103] Mulberry-like blood-filled lesions, in contrast with parenchymal arteriovenous malformations, venous angiomas, and capillary telangectasias, do *not* have intervening neural tissue. Most commonly they are incidental asymptomatic supratentorial lesions (80 percent),[58] occurring less frequently in the brain stem, cerebellum, and spinal cord. MRI is best for detection and diagnosis. The absence of mass effect and edema in a lesion of heterogeneous signal with a central subacute hemorrhagic focus and a peripheral chronic hemorrhagic hypointense rim are characteristic (Fig. 24-33*A*). The risk of lesional rupture is extremely low. Multiplicity occurs in 50 to 80 percent (Fig. 24-33*B*).[58] Seizures, headache, and focal neurologic deficits may be the presenting signs.

Developmental venous anomaly (DVA), also termed venous angioma, represents the most common intracranial vascular malformation[58] and does not have an

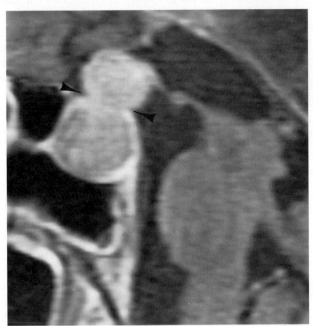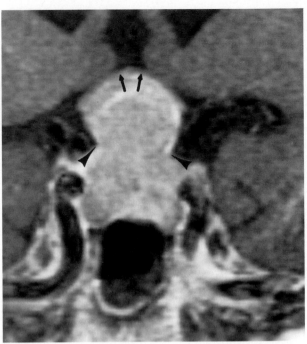

A

B

Figure 24-64   Pituitary macroadenoma. MRI. Sagittal (*A*) and coronal (*B*) enhanced T1 MRI of a 52-year-old man with bitemporal hemianopsia demonstrates a large homogeneously enhancing mass which expands the sella turcica and grows onto the suprasellar cistern. Note the constricting waist produced by the diaphragma sella (*arrowheads*) producing the "figure-of-eight" appearance. The symptoms are explained by compression and superior displacement of the optic chasm, which drapes over the mass (*arrows*). The flow voids of the cavernous segment of the ICAs flanking the mass are unremarkable. Compare to Fig. 24-63 in which the prolactinoma remains confined to the sella turcica and the suprasellar cistern and optic chasm remain undisturbed. Note extrinsic impression on the floor of the third ventricle.

arterial component. Surgical resection is contraindicated since DVA represents anomalous thin-walled veins draining normal brain parenchyma. These anomalies are most commonly adjacent to the frontal horn of the lateral ventricle, followed in frequency by the cerebellum. Up to one-third are associated with cavernomas.[58,104] Most commonly they are solitary and asymptomatic. The typical appearance is that of a tangle of dilated medullary veins (Medusa head) radially converging onto an enlarged transcortical collector vein that drains into a superficial dural sinus (70 percent[58] (Fig. 24-34) or into an ependymal surface. Unless the DVA is hemorrhagic, absence of mass effect and edema are the norm.

Parenchymal or pial arteriovenous malformation (AVM) is a congenital, usually solitary (98 percent)[58] vascular anomaly in which the capillary bed is absent and arterial blood is shunted to the venous system via a nidus. Most are supratentorial (85 percent).[58] Most AMVs declare themselves as hemorrhage and seizures. Intralesional aneurysms are more common than first thought.[105] Tight tangles of enlarged tortuous feeding and draining vessels is the typical appearance, which

can be displayed by CT (Fig. 24-35), MRI, MRA, and/or catheter angiography. Main relevant prognostic factors include the overall AVM size, size of the nidus, intranidal aneurysm, periventricular versus intraventricular location, venous drainage pattern, and eloquence.[106]

Subarachnoid hemorrhage is the most common presentation of an intracranial aneurysm[58] (Fig. 24-36). While catheter angiography remains the definitive diagnostic test in the diagnosis of intracranial aneurysm, in particular given the high rate of multiple lesions, CT (Fig. 24-37*A*) and MRI also can be diagnostic (Fig. 24-37*B*). When more than one aneurysm is found, visualization of contrast extravasation adjacent to the offender aneurysm on catheter angiography is the only pathognomonic sign.[58] Very helpful signs include surrounding clot as seen on CT or MRI, largest size, and irregular lobulated shape ("tit" sign).[58] Helpful signs include localized subarachnoid hemorrhage on CT and localized vasospasm on catheter angiography.[58]

TRAUMA

Diffuse axonal injury (DAI) or shearing injury occurs when sudden acceleration-deceleration or rotational

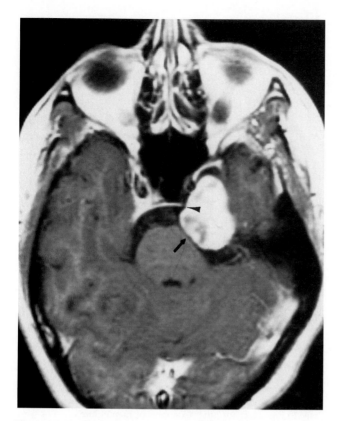

Figure 24-65   Trigeminal schwannoma. MRI. Axial enhanced T1 MRI of a 43-year-old woman demonstrates an inhomogeneously enhancing dumbbell shaped mass in the region of the left cavernous sinus and Meckel's cave representing a preganglionic, ganglionic, and postganglionic trigeminal nerve schwannoma. The focally constricting waist (*arrowhead*) reprsents the dural orifice of Meckel's cave, where the Gasserian ganglion normally resides, now enlarged by the mass. The posterior margin of the mass flattens of the left side of the belly of the pons (*arrow*) where the cisternal segment of the fifth nerve resides.

forces are exerted in the brain during closed head injury. These lesions occur most commonly at the supratentorial gray-white matter junction, the corpus callosum (Fig. 24-38), and dorsolateral upper brainstem and superior cerebellar peduncles.[58,107] Up to 20 percent of these injuries are hemorrhagic (Fig. 24-38).

Epidural hematomas represent 1 to 4 percent of patients imaged for trauma[58] and are the result of laceration of the middle meningeal artery, typically supratentorial. The hemorrhage typically assumes a biconvex configuration (Fig. 24-39) as it strips the dura away from the inner table. It may cross the midline and the tentorium, extending across dural attachments, but it does not cross sutures. Venous epidural hematomas are less common and usually involve laceration of the sphenoparietal sinus or the transverse sinus in association with fractures, resulting in anterior margin of the middle cranial fossa and posterolateral margin of the posterior cranial fossa hematomas.

Subdural hematomas account for 10 to 20 percent

of patients imaged for trauma[58] and are the result of stretching and tearing of bridging cortical veins where they traverse the subdural space en route to drain to a dural sinus. Like epidural hematomas, most are supratentorial. However, they tend to be more extensive and assume a lentiform configuration (Fig. 24-40). They may cross sutures but do not extend across dural attachments (Fig. 24-40B). Bilateral supratentorial, isolated interhemispheric, and posterior fossa subdural hematomas should raise the suspicion of nonaccidental trauma (child abuse).[58,62] Membrane formation (Fig. 24-40A) occurs over time as the collection becomes encapsulated, which may display enhancement after IV contrast. Chronic subdural hematomas are often loculated. Recurrent hemorrhage into a chronic subdural hematoma results in mixed density extraaxial collections that not uncommonly exhibit hematocrit effects (chronic hemorrhage-acute hemorrhage levels) (Fig. 24-40B).

Craniocervical arterial dissection, a common etiology of stroke in patients younger than 40, may be spontaneous or traumatic.[79-91] Most dissections involve

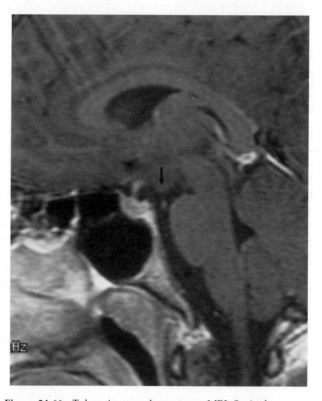

Figure 24-66   Tuber cinereum hamartoma. MRI. Sagittal enhanced T1 MRI of a 15-year-old mentally retarded boy presenting with gelastic seizures demonstrates a small nonenhancing mass in the tuber cinereum of the hypothalamus (*arrow*) between the pituitary infundibulum anteriorly and the mammillary bodies posteriorly. Compare to Fig. 24-64A to appreciate the normal appearance of the tuber cinereum. This lesion was not detectable by CT (not shown).

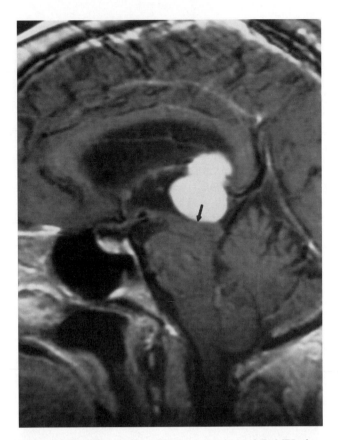

Figure 24-67 Pineocytoma. MRI. Sagittal enhanced T1 MRI of a 50-year-old woman presenting with ataxia and upward gaze paralysis (Parinaud's syndrome) demonstrates a large lobular homogeneously enhancing pineocytoma, a pineal cell origin tumor, compressing the quadrigeminal plate (*arrow*) and straddling onto the posterior recesses of the third ventricle resulting in obstructive hydrocephalus.

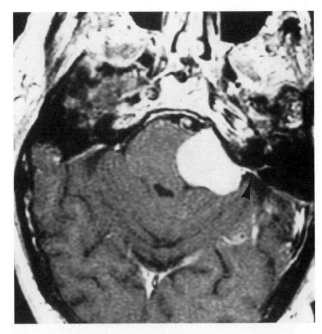

Figure 24-68 Cerebellopontine angle (CPA) meningioma. MRI. Axial enhanced T1 MRI of a 69-year-old man demonstrates a homogeneously enhancing mass widening the left CPA cistern and compressing the pons. Note the contiguous enhancing "dural tail" (*arrowhead*), suggestive but not specific for meningioma. Refer to Fig. 24-21 for other examples of meningioma.

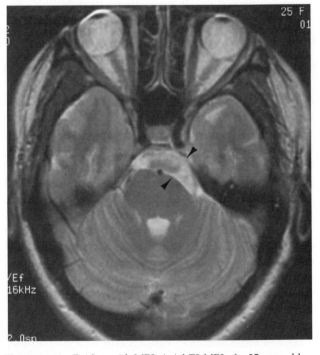

Figure 24-69 Epidermoid. MRI. Axial T2 MRI of a 25-year-old woman demonstrates an area of heterogeneous high signal slightly hypointense to CSF (*arrowheads*) widening the left cerebellopontine angle cistern and flattening the left belly of the pons, representing an epidermoid cyst. Epidermoids do not enhance and are isointense to CSF on T1-weighted images. Mass effect and intrinsic interstices usually allow for identification.

the internal carotid and the vertebral artery, typically at points of transition where the artery is fixed by dura or bone or other structure. Hemorrhage into the media secondary to an intimal tear may involve intracranial and extracranial vessels. Extracranial dissections could also result following rupture of the vasa vasorum.[81] Tapering irregular (and less commonly smooth) narrowing, sometimes to occlusion, is the typical appearance in catheter angiography (Fig. 24-41*A*) produced by the mass effect of the intramural hematoma on the contrast-opacified true lumen. Other findings include focal narrowing with an adjacent distal segment of dilatation, dissecting aneurysm, delayed runoff of contrast, and distal branch occlusion.[81] MRI and MRA represent effective noninvasive diagnostic tools (Fig. 24-41*B* and *C*). Conditions predisposing for spontaneous dissection include "trivial trauma," such as vigorous coughing and vomiting, and strenuous exercise, and chiropractic manipulation as well as fibromuscular dysplasia, cystic medial necrosis, type IV Ehlers-Danlos syndrome, and Marfan syndrome.[81] Patients

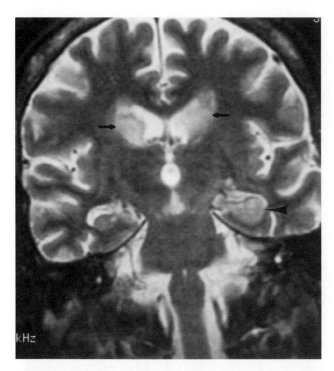

Figure 24-70 Primary cerebral lymphoma. MRI. Coronal T2 MRI of a 30-year-old man with AIDS demonstrates periventricular masses with subependymal invasion in the frontal horns (*arrows*), a spread pattern typical of primary CNS B-cell lymphoma. Note involvement of the left hippocampus (*arrowhead*). Diffuse parenchymal volume loss given the patient's age is consistent with HIV encephalopathy. These lesions demonstrated strong enhancement following contrast administration (not shown).

are at risk for occlusive infarction and for acute or nonacute embolic events. Close to 90 percent of patients completely recover or suffer minor neurologic disability.[81]

Carotid-cavernous fistula (CCF) is the most common traumatic dural arteriovenous fistula in which there is a single abnormal direct communication between the cavernous segment of the internal carotid artery and the cavernous sinus, resulting in reversed increased arterialized flow typically involving the superior ophthalmic vein (Fig. 24-42). Phase contrast MRA can display directional information in this setting. Venous hypertension results in chemosis, proptosis, bruit, and enlargement of extraocular muscles. A less common form, a spontaneous indirect CCF, typically occurs in middle-aged women in which multiple abnormal fistulous channels between the same vessels develop.[58]

INFECTIOUS AND INFLAMMATORY

Neurosarcoidosis occurs in 5 percent of patients with sarcoid, usually affecting the leptomeninges (basal more common than diffuse), pituitary gland and infundibulum, hypothalamus/floor of third ventricle, and

optic chiasm.[3,58] This is demonstrated on MRI as irregular nodular enhancement of the involved areas (Fig. 24-43). Less commonly, this entity may present as focal extraaxial or parenchymal masses mimicking a neoplastic process.[58]

Chronic tuberculous meningitis occurs more commonly in children than in adults.[3] Extensive basal and at times diffuse thick exudative enhancing meninges is typical. En plaque-enhancing thickened dural and at times heavily calcified basal meninges can be the sequelae of this condition (Fig. 24-44). Arterial structures coursing in the exudate-studded basal cisterns can become obliterated, resulting in spasm with consequent thrombosis and associated infarction.

Cerebritis is the earliest stage of abscess[58] occurring prior to development of a capsule. Cerebritis presents as a poorly marginated area of signal alteration on all MR pulse sequences (Fig. 24-45) or as an area of low attenuation on CT, which may or may not display subtle ill-defined enhancement.

Cerebral abscess develops after the stage of cerebritis. An abscess in an immunocompetent patient presents as a thin, smooth ring-enhancing lesion most commonly at the gray-white matter junction of the frontoparietal lobes, although abscesses may involve the deep structures (Fig. 24-46). Peripheral vasogenic edema and central liquefactive cystic necrosis are com-

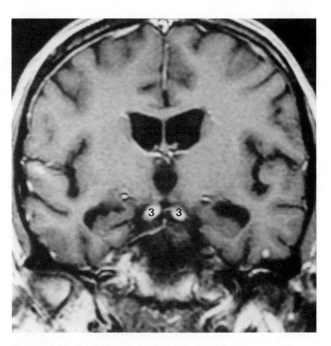

Figure 24-71 Lymphomatous leptomeningeal carcinomatosis. MRI. Coronal enhanced T1 MRI of a 39-year-old man with AIDS presenting with progressive bilateral third nerve palsies demonstrates bilateral abnormal circumferential leptomeningeal enhancement and enlargement of the third nerves (3) in the perimesencephalic and suprasellar cisterns. CSF cytology revealed lymphoma.

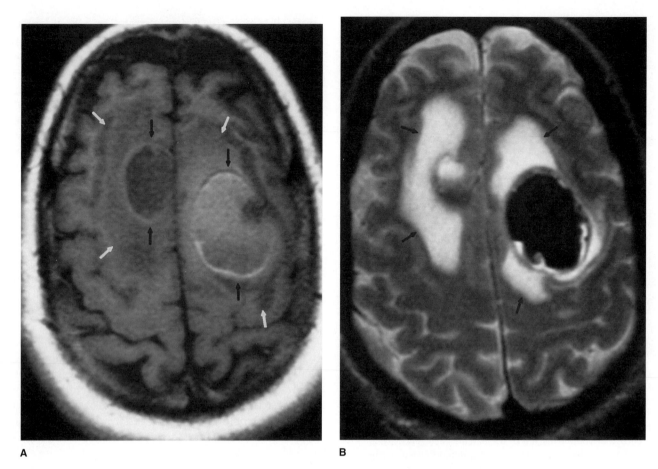

A

B

Figure 24-72 Parenchymal hemorrhagic metastatic melanoma. MRI. *A.* Axial enhanced T1 MRI and (*B.*) axial T2 MRI of a 44-year-old man with melanoma (original lesion in the nuchal region) presenting with progressive aphasia and right hemiparesis. The T1 image demonstrates bilateral oval-shaped peripheral rim enhancing heterogeneous signal intraaxial masses at the corticomedullary junction of the centrum semiovale (*black arrows*). The white arrows point to surrounding vasogenic edema, isointense to gray matter. Black arrows in the T2 image point to surrounding vasogenic type white matter edema. The right-sided lesion demonstrates signal characteristics of hyperacute hemorrhage. The left-sided lesion demonstrates signal characteristics of early subacute hemorrhage. Refer to Table 24-6 for details of signal intensity of evolving hematomas.

mon features. The presence of satellite or daughter abscesses (Fig. 24-46), asymmetric thickness of the lesional walls such that the medial wall is thinner than the more vascularized lateral wall, and a hypointense rim on T2-weighted images further suggest the diagnosis.

In immunocompromised patients, multiple lesions are more common, and the abscess wall is thicker and more irregular, making differentiation from neoplasm more difficult.[58] This is illustrated by CNS toxoplasmosis (Fig. 24-47), the second most common CNS pathogen in the setting of AIDS, which is often difficult to radiologically differentiate from lymphoma (Fig. 24-6). Subependymal involvement strongly favors lymphoma over toxoplasmosis.

CNS cryptococcal meningitis followed by cryptococcomas are the most common manifestation of the third most common pathogen affecting AIDS patients (5 percent),[58] the most common pathogen being the human immunodeficiency virus (HIV) itself.[58] Cryptococcal organisms fill the medullary perivascular spaces, forming gelatinous pseudocysts (Fig. 24-48).

Progressive multifocal leukoencephalopathy (PML) is produced by the papovavirus (Fig. 24-49). It affects immunocompromised patients and has a dismal prognosis. Lesions most commonly involve the parietooccipital subcortical white matter, exhibit minimal to no mass effect, and usually do not enhance following IV contrast. Cavitary change is a late manifestation.[58] In the clinical setting of immunosuppression, the other main diagnostic considerations include CMV and HIV encephalitis.

CNS aspergillosis usually occurs in the immunosuppressed patients, rarely inciting a granulomatous reaction in other settings. It may involve the CNS by direct extension from sinonasal infection or, more commonly, by hematogenous dissemination[3,58] (Fig. 24-50). This fungus is angiogenic and may result in hemorrhagic lesions secondary to vasculopathy with thrombosis and infarction of the anterior intracranial circulation.[3] When not attributable to hemorrhagic blood products, low signal on T2-weighted images more recently has been attributed to the high concentration of trace metals in these lesions.[108,109]

Herpes simplex virus type 1 (oral) constitutes the most common nonepidemic viral meningoencephalitis in the United States and Europe[58] resulting from reactivation of latent infection of the Gasserian ganglion. Prompt diagnosis is crucial given its high mortality rate (up to 70 percent) and significant long-term morbidity when untreated or when treatment is delayed. Acyclovir is an effective treatment. MRI is more sensitive than CT (Fig. 24-51), demonstrating signal alteration with a predilection for the limbic system, principally involving the medial temporal lobe. Sparing of the basal ganglia[62] may be a differentiating feature from neoplasm.

The most common parasitic CNS infection is cysticercosis (not shown) affecting the CNS in up to 90 percent of cases.[58]

DEMYELINATING DISEASE

Acute disseminated encephalomyelitis (ADEM) represents an autoimmune response to a recent viral infection or vaccination in which periventricular demyelinating foci develop, usually in children and young adults.[58,62,110] MR is more sensitive than CT for demonstrating signal alterations related to demyelination, which may be widely distributed (Fig. 24-52) and may rarely involve the spinal cord.

Childhood adrenoleukodystrophy is a recessive X-linked metabolic encephalopathy. Abnormal accumulation of saturated very long chain fatty acids results in demyelination in patients between the ages of 3 and 10 years, most commonly affecting the occipital white matter (Fig. 24-53).[111] The visual, auditory, and motor pathways are commonly involved.[111,112] Unlike the usual presentation of multiple sclerosis, adrenoleukodystrophy affects large areas of white matter, displaying a typical posterior-to-anterior progression.[58,111]

Multiple sclerosis (MS) is the most common demyelinating disease after vascular and age-related demyelination.[58] The sensitivity of MRI for detecting MS exceeds that of oligoclonal bands, evoked potentials, and CT.[58] Most lesions detected by MRI are clinically silent. Typical demyelinating lesions, termed plaques, develop along the perivenular spaces of the periventricular white matter oriented perpendicular to the long

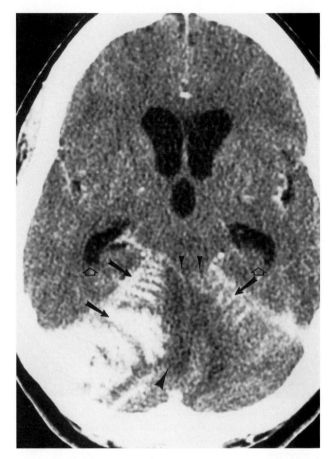

Figure 24-73   Metastatic breast carcinoma. CT. Axial enhanced CT through the posterior fossa of a 44-year-old woman with breast cancer presenting with worsening headache and ataxia demonstrates striking enhancement and widening of the cerebellar foliae (*long arrows*), representing metastatic leptomeningeal carcinomatosis. Abnormal low density in the cerebellum (*arrowhead*) represents parenchymal metastases and edema. The fourth ventricle is completely effaced, resulting in obstructive hydrocephalus evidenced by dilated temporal horns of the lateral ventricles (*short arrows*). Effacement of the quadrigeminal plate cistern (*small arrowheads*) indicates ascending transtentorial herniation.

axis of the lateral ventricles (Fig. 24-54*A*) with a predilection for the corpus callosum. The brain stem and middle cerebellar peduncles are the most common infratentorial locations. Lesions are typically multiple, but when solitary and large may mimic neoplasm. Enhancement is highly variable and transient, presumably correlated with demyelinating plaque activity.[58] Optic neuritis is the most common cranial neuropathy in MS. More recently, magnetic resonance spectroscopy[58] and magnetization transfer techniques have demonstrated that conventional MRI underestimates the true size of the plaque.[113] Spinal cord plaques may be found at any segment and have a nonspecific appearance (Fig. 24-54*B*), with a wide differential diagno-

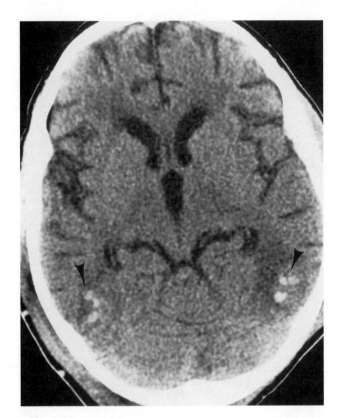

Figure 24-74 Mineralizing microangiopathy. CT. Axial non-enhanced CT of a 15-year-old girl with a resected posterior fossa medulloblastoma followed by high-dose chemotherapy and whole-brain radiotherapy. Multiple bilateral symmetric foci of smudgy high attenuation in the subcortical and periventricular white matter represent dystrophic calcification as a result of treatment. Surrounding low attenuation represent areas of demyelination. Also notice the generalized parenchymal volume loss markedly advanced for the patient's stated age.

sis discussed later in this chapter (Spine: Intramedullary Intradural).

Osmotic myelinolysis (myelin loss) classically occurs in chronic alcoholism, rapid correction of hyponatremia, and rarely with hypernatremia. The most common form is central pontine myelinolysis (Fig. 24-55), but extrapontine involvement, mainly basal ganglia, thalami, midbrain, and subcortical white matter have also been reported.[58] The transverse fibers are most affected, with relative sparing of the corticospinal tracts.[58]

NEOPLASTIC

According to Osborne,[58] no universally accepted pathologic classification of brain tumors has been proposed. The following is her modification of the 1993 World Health Organization and Russell and Rubinstein classifications, which includes glial tumors (gliomas), nonglial tumors, and metastatic tumors. Glial tumors are further subdivided into astrocytomas, oligodrogli-

omas, ependymal tumors, and choroid plexus tumors. Nonglial tumors are further subdivided into neuronal and mixed neuronal-glial tumors, meningiomas and mesenchymal tumors, pineal region tumors, embryonal tumors, cranial and spinal nerve tumors, hematopoietic neoplasms, pituitary tumors, local extension from regional tumors, and cysts and tumor-like lesions.

Glial tumors are vastly more common than neuronal tumors in adults by a ratio of 100 to 1.[58] Metastases account for one-third of all brain tumors in adults,[58] but are very rare in children.

The general term primitive neuroectodermal tumor (PNET) is used to describe undifferentiated tumors in children with partial neuronal, glial, and or mesenchymal differentiation.[58] This definition was later expanded to include other primitive tumors,[58] but the term remains controversial among neuropathologists.[3] The prototype of this tumor is the infratentorial or cerebellar medulloblastoma (Fig. 24-56*A*), comprising 25 percent of all intracranial tumors in children and second only to cerebellar astrocytoma.[3] Medulloblastoma displays a high rate of early CSF dissemination (up to 50 percent at the time of diagnosis) (Fig. 24-

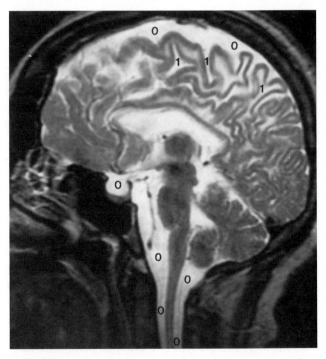

Figure 24-75 Olivopontocerebellar degeneration (OPCD). MRI. Sagittal T2 MRI of a 31-year-old woman with a family history of OPCD presenting with progressive ataxia and memory loss demonstrates pronounced diffuse volume loss involving brain parenchyma (deep wide sulci: 1s), brain stem, and cervical spinal cord demonstrated by an accommodating capacious subarachnoid space (0s). Note the decreased ventral pontine bulge. The cerebellum is not markedly involved. The patient's daughter was affected at an earlier age.

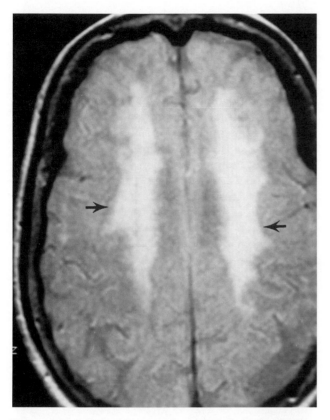

Figure 24-76   Subcortical arteriosclerotic encephalopathy (SAE). MRI. Axial proton density MRI on a 76-year-old hypertensive man demonstrates bilateral irregular supraventricular white matter hyperintensity (*arrows*) indicative of small vessel disease. Similar signal abnormalities were present in the periventricular white matter and the brain stem (not shown).

56*B*).[58] Characteristically, the tumor arises from the roof and posterior medullary velum of the fourth ventricle, bulging anteriorly into the fourth ventricle in the midline 75 percent of the time.[58] It is the most likely CNS tumor to metastasize outside the CNS.[3] Contrast-enhanced MR is superior to CT or CT myelography in the detection of subarachnoid dissemination and in the surveillance for therapy response.[58,96] Other tumors included in the category of PNET include ependymoblastoma (Fig. 24-57), cerebral neuroblastoma, pineoblastoma, medulloepithelioma, and melanotic vermian PNET of infancy.[3]

Brain stem glioma usually occurs in childhood and adolescence and has a dismal prognosis.[3] These are usually solid infiltrating tumors with variable enhancement, typically expanding the brain stem (Fig. 24-58) and sometimes encasing the basilar artery.[58] Involvement of the pons predominates, not uncommonly extending to the medulla oblongata and midbrain, at times displaying an exophytic component.

Intracranial ependymoma is another tumor of childhood and adolescence arising adjacent or close to an ependymal surface. When infratentorial, its most com-

mon location, it arises from the floor of the fourth ventricle. Typical finger-like tumor extensions along the fourth ventricle foramina downward into the dorsolateral subarachnoid space of the upper cervical spine (Fig. 24-59) have led the growth to be termed "plastic" ependymoma.[3] These tumors display calcification (45 percent) more often than any other posterior fossa tumor.[3]

Glioblastoma multiforme, the most common primary intracranial CNS tumor (up to 20 percent), is the most malignant of all glial tumors, with the worst prognosis given early, fast, and extensive dissemination.[58] While most common after age 50, it may present at any age, ranking high among primary brain tumors in newborns and children under 2 years.[58] The lesion, usually located in the cerebral hemispheric white matter, heterogeneously enhances with a central or eccentric area of cystic necrosis (Fig. 24-60) and exhibits striking vasogenic edema and mass effect.

Gliomatosis cerebri[114] is a diffusely infiltrating low-grade neoplasm involving at least two lobes of the brain (Fig. 24-61) which has microscopic findings distinct from the more common diffuse glioma. The most common presentation is behavioral changes, usually

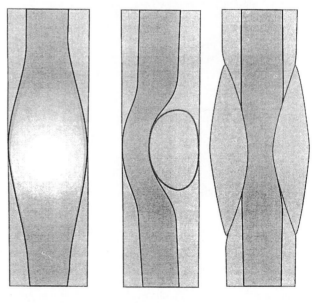

Intra-Medullary   **Extra-Medullary**   **Extra-Dural**
Intra-Dural

Figure 24-77   Diagrammatic representation of lesions on the three spinal compartments: intramedullary intradural, extramedullary intradural, and extradural. In this diagram, the spinal cord is depicted as the dark tubular structure surrounded by the lighter cerebrospinal fluid. The confines of the subarachnoid space represent the outer limits of the thecal sac. Note how the shape and caliber of the subarachnoid space and the spinal cord change for each example. Refer to the text for more specific descriptions.

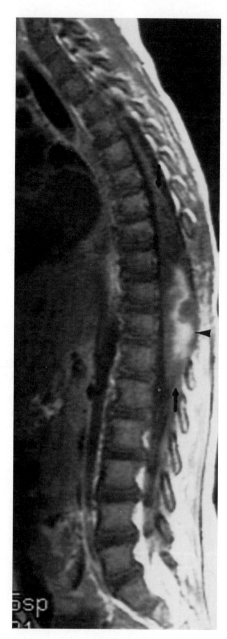

Figure 24-78 Spinal anaplastic astrocytoma. MRI. Sagittal enhanced T1 MRI of a 3-year-old boy demonstrates pronounced intramedullary cord expanding astrocytoma extending from the T7 to the L1 vertebral level involving the lower cord and conus medullaris (*arrows*). Inhomogeneous enhancement is demonstrated (*arrowhead*). Several rounded areas of intermediate to low signal represent cystic change. While the degree of tumor enhancement in the brain tends to correlate with tumor grading, enhancement of primary cord tumors does not.

derived from involvement of the temporal lobes and diencephalon.[114] The neurologic deficits are slight and out of proportion to the widespread extent of parenchymal involvement.

Craniopharyngioma arises from squamous rests along Rathke's cleft; it is the most common nonglial brain tumor in the pediatric population (with a second

incidence peak in adults) and typically has intrasellar and suprasellar components.[58] Characteristically these lesions are partially cystic and partially solid, with more than 90 percent exhibiting calcification (Fig. 24-62).

Pituitary adenomas are slow-growing neoplasms arising from the adenohypophysis or anterior lobe and are classified as microadenomas (Fig. 24-63) if under 10 mm and as macroadenomas (Fig. 24-64) if over 10 mm.[3] Not without exception, microadenomas tend to be hormonally active, whereas macroadenomas tend to present as a result of compression of the optic apparatus (Fig. 24-64*B*). Determination of cavernous sinus invasion can be difficult even by MRI.[3]

Schwannomas account for one-third of primary trigeminal nerve and Meckel's cave tumors.[58] Trigeminal schwannoma is the most common type to involve the

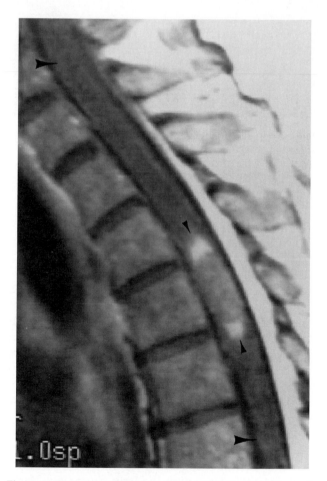

Figure 24-79 Intramedullary metastasis. MRI. Sagittal enhanced T1 MRI of a 46-year-old woman with squamous cell carcinoma of the cervix and a lung nodule presenting with thoracic sensory and motor deficits demonstrates a solitary mildly enhancing sausage-shaped intramedullary cord expanding metastatic deposit (*small arrowheads*) at T4. Abnormal hypointensity of the cord extends rostral to C7 and caudal to the conus (*large arrowheads*), representing adjacent and remote edema, not an uncommon finding with intramedullary metastatis.

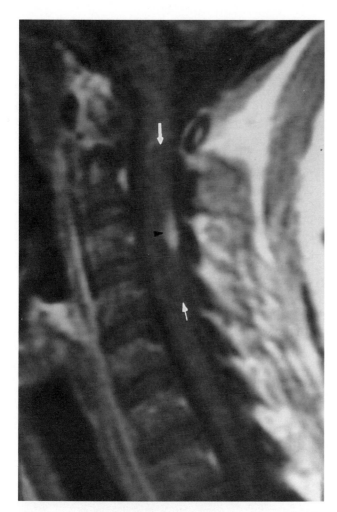

Figure 24-80 Lupus myelitis. MRI (Courtesy of JM Provenzale, M.D., Duke University Medical Center.) Sagittal contrast-enhanced T1 MRI of a 37-year-old woman with SLE demonstrates abnormal low signal of the cord extending from the C2 to the C4 vertebral levels (*arrows*). A small focal area of nodular enhancement involving the dorsal white matter at the C3 vertebral level is noted (*arrowhead*). Corresponding hyperintensity on proton density and T2 images (not shown) was apparent. The more extensive rostrocaudad involvement of the cord is typical of lupus myelitis (average of 3 to 4 vertebral bodies' height) compared with a typical multiple sclerosis plaque (Fig. 24-54*B*). Clinical and radiologic response was apparent following steroid therapy.

typically isointense to gray matter on T1-weighted images and slightly hyperintense on T2-weighted images.[58] It is best evaluated by MRI.

Pineal region tumors are divided into germ cell tumors (strong male predominance), pineal parenchymal cell tumors (Fig. 24-67), and others, such as meningioma, astrocytoma, and metastases. The complex anatomy of the pineal region is best depicted by the multiplanar capability of MRI (Fig. 24-67).

The most common cerebellopontine angle (CPA) cistern mass is the vestibulocochlear (acoustic) schwannoma (Fig. 24-21), followed by meningioma (Fig. 24-68) and epidermoid (Fig. 24-69). The acoustic schwannoma may be limited to the internal auditory

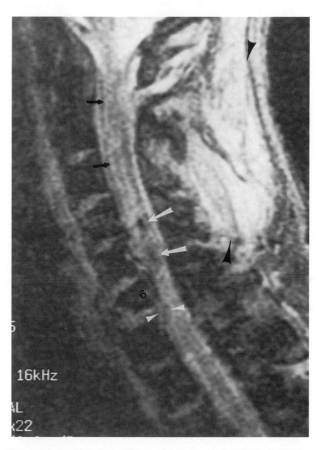

Figure 24-81 Spinal cord hemorrhagic contusion. MRI. Sagittal gradient echo MRI of a 32-year-old man sustaining a burst fracture of the C6 vertebra demonstrates abnormal focal low signal of the cord (*white arrows*) representing acute hemorrhagic contusion. Bony retropulsion of the posterior two-thirds of the vertebra is evident, focally obliterating the ventral subarachnoid space and compressing the cord. Traumatic posterior herniation of the adjacent C6–C7 disk (*white arrowheads*) further contributes to cord compression. Abnormal high signal and expansion of the spinal cord rostral to the fracture represents edema (*black arrows*). Note the abnormal high signal in the dorsal soft tissues of the craniocervical junction (*black arrowheads*) representing contusion. The wealth of information available in this study could not be obtained with CT, myelography, or postmyelographic CT.

central skull base. This extraaxial lesion is encapsulated, well-marginated, and is usually ovoid or lobulated morphologically. It enhances heterogeneously, given commonly present cystic and hemorrhagic components. Schwannomas involving the cisternal and Gasserian segments of the fifth nerve have a typical morphology (Fig. 24-65).

Hypothalamic (tuber cinereum) hamartoma is a pedunculated or sessile mass located between the pituitary infundibulum and the mammillary bodies (Fig. 24-66). It does not enhance after IV contrast and is

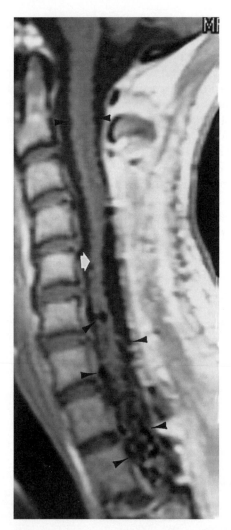

Figure 24-82   Spinal arteriovenous malformation (AVM). MRI. Sagittal enhanced T1 MRI of a 36-year-old woman demonstrates multiple abnormal dilated tortuous flow voids along the ventral and dorsal surfaces of the cord (*arrowheads*), representing an AVM. T2 images (not shown) demonstrated abnormal cord hyperintensity, representing ischemia/infarction from secondary to chronic blood steal and venous hypertension. The end stage is pronounced atrophy of the cord (*arrows*).

that increase diagnostic specificity,[116] and may make such invasive studies as a CT cisternogram unnecessary.

Primary cerebral lymphoma is typically of the B-cell, non-Hodgkin's variety, and occurs in younger patients in the setting of immunocompromise, particularly AIDS.[58] Most lesions abut the ependyma. Typical locations feature the basal ganglia, periventricular white matter (Fig. 24-6*B*) and corpus callosum (Fig. 24-70). Rarely, lymphomas may be diffusely infiltrating, termed lymphomatosis cerebri, in which case it may be difficult to differentiate from gliomatosis cerebri.[58] Metastatic lymphoma may present as dural or leptomeningeal enhancement, at times coating cranial nerves (Fig. 24-71). Subarachnoid dissemination is usually not detectable by CT[3] and requires IV contrast-enhanced MRI. Not uncommonly, repeated CSF cytologic analysis is required to establish subarachnoid dissemination when MRI is negative.

Metastatic disease to the brain has myriad manifestations. By far the most common parenchymal lesions classically occur at the corticomedullary or gray-white

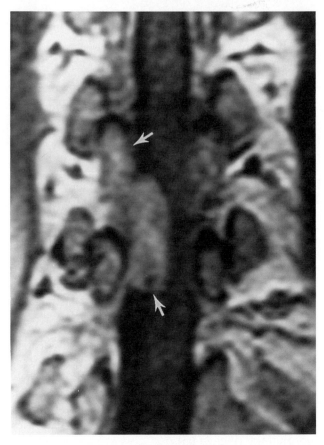

Figure 24-83   Spinal schwannoma. MRI. Coronal enhanced T1 MRI of a 22-year-old woman demonstrates an enhancing intradural extramedullary schwannoma extending across the right T9–T10 neural exit foramen assuming a dumbbell morphology (*arrows*).

canal (IAC), or it may extend across the porus acusticus into the CPA cistern. The CPA meningioma may rarely extend into the IAC, simulating an acoustic schwannoma. However, a dural tail and eccentricity relative to the porus acusticus favor meningioma (Fig. 24-68).[115] Whereas these two lesions enhance, an epidermoid does not. An epidermoid may be difficult to differentiate from arachnoid cyst (Fig. 24-19) and from CSF itself, given approximate signal characteristics on all conventional MRI pulse sequences. Similarly, the difficulty is also encountered in CT, given similar attenuation values. Indirect evidence of the presence of a mass may be the only sign of this lesion (Fig. 24-69). Recently, new pulse sequences have been developed

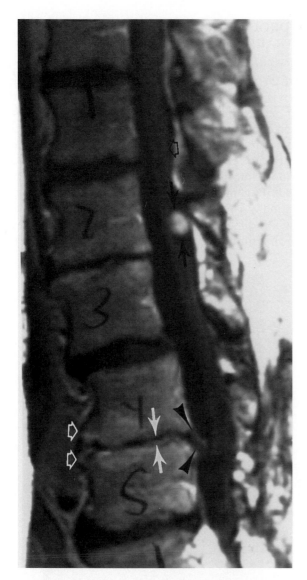

Figure 24-84   Cauda equina ependymoma. Degenerative disk disease and degenerative spondylosis. MRI. Sagittal enhanced T1 MRI of the lumbar spine of a 50-year-old man demonstrates a small well circumscribed oval-shaped enhancing intradural mass abutting the cauda equina (*long black arrows*) just below the conus medullaris (*open short black arrow*), representing an ependymoma. The L2–L3 and the L4–L5 (*white arrows*) disk heights are markedly reduced consistent with degenerative disk disease. Note the bridging anterior vertebral body osteophytes (*open short white arrows*) and posteriorly extruded disk material at L4–L5 (*arrowheads*). Note that there are vertebral body malalignments at L3–L4 and at L5–S1 secondary to degenerative ligamentous laxity.

matter junction (Fig. 24-72) as a result of hematogenous dissemination. The most common primary tumors to metastasize to brain include lung, breast, melanoma, gastrointestinal, and genitourinary, in descending order of frequency.[58] Leptomeningeal (Fig. 24-73) and skull metastases are not uncommon. Contiguous extension of sinonasal cavity or base-of-skull tumors is not

uncommon. Pachymeningeal and carcinomatous limbic encephalitis constitute rarer manifestations of CNS metastases.[58]

Mineralizing microangiopathy refers to perivascular dystrophic calcification as a result of cranial radiation and chemotherapy usually for systemic or CNS neoplastic disease. The basal ganglia and the gray-white matter junction are the most commonly affected sites (Fig. 24-74).

NEURODEGENERATIVE

Neurodegenerative disorders encompass a wide range of conditions in which various parts of the central nervous system gradually and progressively disintegrate.

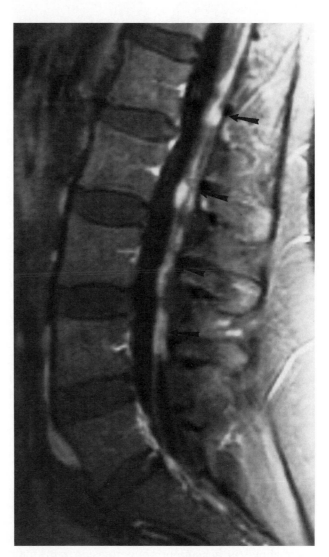

Figure 24-85   Intradural drop metastasis. MRI. Sagittal fat-suppressed enhanced T1 MRI of a 45-year-old woman with breast cancer demonstrates unsuspected abnormal irregular nodular enhancing lesions along the cauda equina (*arrows*) consistent with carcinomatosis.

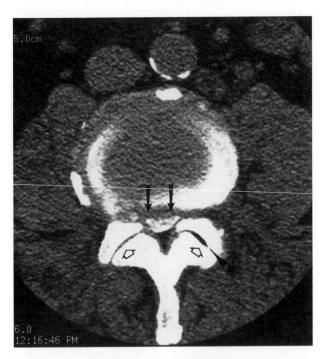

Figure 24-86 Spinal stenosis. Postmyelographic CT. Axial postmyelographic CT through L3–L4 intervertebral disk of a 72-year-old woman demonstrates bilateral facet joint hypertrophic change with exuberant ossification of the posterior longitudinal ligament resulting in severe central, lateral recess, and exit canal stenosis. A congenitally "tight" canal is evident, given the short sagittal dimension of the pedicles. Superimposed disk herniation would exacerbate spinal stenosis.

One scheme divides these disorders into dementias; degeneration of extrapyramidal nuclei; degeneration of the substantia nigra and related systems; degeneration of cerebellum, brain stem (Fig. 24-75) and spinal cord; and degeneration of motor system, primary or acquired. Alzheimer's disease is the most common disease in this category and is the most common etiology of dementia. Hippocampal formation atrophy has been implicated in Alzheimer's dementia.[3,58,117] Hippocampal atrophy coexisting with abnormal intrinsic T2 prolongation (hyperintensity) represents the hallmark of mesial temporal sclerosis (Fig. 24-9*B*) in the setting of partial complex seizures.

Subcortical arteriosclerotic encephalopathy (SAE), previously termed Binswanger disease, is a form of multi-infarct dementia.[118] Hypertension-related[3] changes of the long penetrating medullary arteries results in chronic ischemic changes, typically involving the supratentorial periventricular white matter, subcortical white matter (Fig. 24-76), and brain stem. Coexistence of lacunar infarcts (Fig. 24-30) with the changes noted above further supports hypertension as the main etiology of this common condition. Accompanying subcortical infarcts and diffuse cerebral volume loss manifested as deep and wide sulci and prominent ventricles complete the constellation of findings.

HYDROCEPHALUS AND INCREASED INTRACRANIAL PRESSURE

The ventricular system has an approximate volume of 20 to 25 ml of cerebrospinal fluid. Ventricular enlargement is not synonymous with hydrocephalus. Ventricular enlargement may indicate hydrocephalus, but when in conjunction with enlargement of the intracranial subarachnoid spaces it may indicate central and cortical atrophy. Hydrocephalus has classically been divided into intraventricular obstructive (noncommunicating) and extraventricular obstructive (communicating).[58] The former refers to obstruction from compression of the ventricular system (Fig. 24-64, 24-67, 24-73), within the ventricular system (Figs. 24-22 and

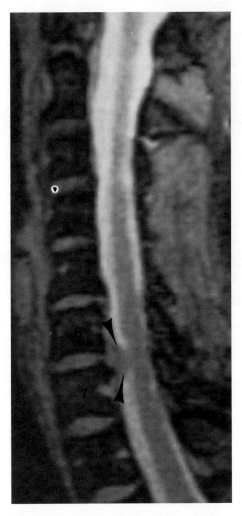

Figure 24-87 Cervical disk herniation. MRI. Sagittal gradient echo MRI of a 35-year-old woman presenting with a C7 radiculopathy demonstrates a large extradural mass isointense to and in direct contiguity with the C6–7 disk obliterating the ventral subarachnoid space, posteriorly displacing and invaginating the ventral surface of the cord (*arrowheads*). This is a large acute hydrated disk herniation with cord compression. Notice the similarity of the defect produced by the disk in this case to that of Fig. 24-89.

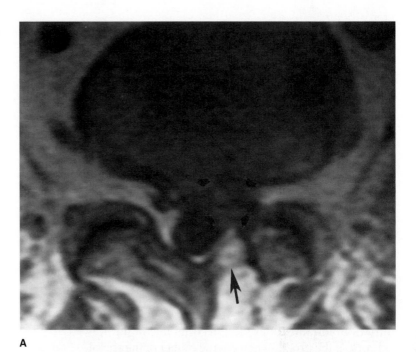

A

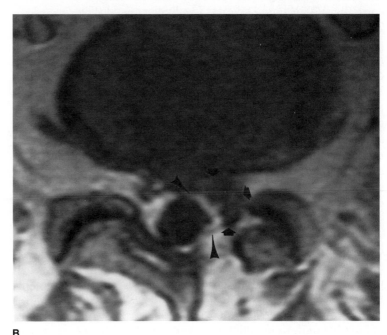

B

Figure 24-88   Recurrent lumbar disc herniation. MRI.
A. non-enhanced axial T1; *B.* IV contrast enhanced
axial T1 lumbar spine MRI through the L4–5 disk
level of a 53-year-old woman with recurrent left L5
radiculopathy. The nonenhanced image demonstrates
a posterior left paracentral rounded extradural mass
isointense to disc (*four short arrows*) focally exerting
mass effect on the thecal sac. It is difficult to
differentiate thecal sac from disk material from any
possible scar tissue. A laminectomy defect from prior
diskectomy is noted (*long arrow*). Following
gadolinium (*B*), a thin band of enhancement
(*arrowheads*) representing scar or granulation tissue
related to prior surgery is noted between the
recurrent non-enhancing recurrent herniated disk
(*three short arrows*) and the thecal sac medially.
Myelography and postmyelogram CT would not be
able to differentiate recurrent disk herniation from
scar.

24-56), including the fourth ventricular foramina
(Fig. 24-59), with resultant proximal ventricular system
dilatation. The latter refers to obstruction within the
subarachnoid spaces, the cisterns, or to decreased
arachnoid granulations CSF absorption. Alternatively,
communicating hydrocephalus may be the result of
overproduction of CSF by a choroid plexus tumor.[58]
Hydrocephalus may be the result of multifactorial
mechanisms. When one notes focal ventricular dilatation, the result of local parenchymal volume loss or
atrophy, this is called "ex-vacuo dilatation."

"Normal pressure" hydrocephalus is a poorly understood condition in which there is communicating
hydrocephalus but the CSF pressure measured by
lumbar puncture is less than 160 mm of water. The
ventricles, especially the temporal horns, are dilated,
but the sulci are not as apparent as would be expected
for the degree of ventricular dilatation. Timely diag-

nosis is essential because the patient may benefit from ventricular shunt decompression.

SPINE

MRI is the study of choice for imaging the spinal canal contents and adjacent structures. It has surpassed myelography, post-myelographic CT, and CT for the detection and diagnosis of most spinal pathology. A myelographic effect can be obtained using heavily T2-weighted gradient echo images with magnetization transfer.[119] Specific situations still demand the use of the other modalities, either in conjunction with or in lieu of MRI. The following portion of the neuroradiologic imaging sampler is logically divided into examples of intramedullary intradural, extramedullary intradural, and extradural entities.

INTRAMEDULLARY INTRADURAL

Intradural intramedullary lesions originate in the spinal cord. If the process enlarges the caliber of the spinal cord, the subarachnoid space is focally narrowed (Fig. 24-77). Most intramedullary entities are malignant neoplasms,[58] namely gliomas. Close to 95 percent of these are ependymomas and astrocytomas (Fig. 24-78).[58] Less common tumors include hemangioblastoma (Fig. 24-24B), metastatic disease (Fig. 24-79), lipoma, and nonneoplastic cysts.[58] Other intramedullary processes include acute transverse myelitis (ATM) (Fig. 24-54B, and 24-80), infection, granulomatous disease, vascular malformation (Fig. 24-82), and trauma (Fig. 24-81). Radiation, post-traumatic, and compressive myelopathy secondary to spondyloarthropathy, hydrosyringomyelia (Fig. 24-12, 24-14), and toxic and metabolic etiologies complete the list of intramedullary entities.

Acute transverse myelitis refers to the rapid onset of sensory, motor, and usually autonomic dysfunction referable to a spinal level in the absence of cord compression or prior neurologic disease.[120,121] Prior to the advent of MRI, this was a diagnosis of exclusion.[120] ATM is a general term that encompasses a vast array of possible underlying etiologies, featuring viral infection, post-vaccination,[120] acute demyelinating encephalomyelitis,[122] multiple sclerosis (Fig. 24-54B), systemic lupus erythematosus (Fig. 24-80), AIDS myelopathy, vascular insult, and vascular malformation (Fig. 24-82).[123]

EXTRAMEDULLARY INTRADURAL

Intradural extramedullary masses originate outside the spinal cord but within the dura. Ipsilateral to the mass, the subarachnoid space widens. The spinal cord is displaced and/or deformed away from the mass (Fig. 24-77). Nerve sheath tumors, namely schwannoma (Fig. 24-83) and neurofibroma, and meningioma account for up to 90 percent of intradural extramedullary lesions.[58]

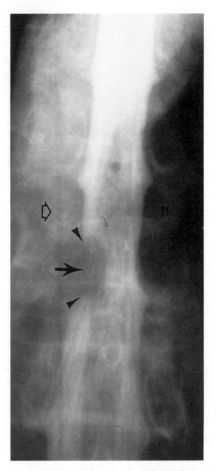

Figure 24-89 Vertebral bone marrow metastasis and epidural carcinomatosis. Myelogram. MRI. Frontal view of a myelogram of a 65-year-old man with prostate cancer demonstrates a focal extradural defect (*arrow*) narrowing the right subarachnoid gutter (*arrowheads*) of the contrast column at T11, representing epidural carcinomatosis. T11 demonstrates blastic transformation and absence of the pedicle ring (*outlined arrow*) consistent with adjacent bony metastases.

When large, these tumors result in smooth enlargement of the exit canals. Ependymoma (Fig. 24-84), paraganglioma, various cysts, and benign tumor-like masses are less common. A disk herniation can rarely become intradural.[3,58]

Common malignant tumors in this compartment include "drop" metastases from primary cerebral and spinal tumors and non-CNS tumors, featuring lung, breast, melanoma, lymphoma, and leukemia. Thick, nodular, irregular enhancing lesions coat the surface of the spinal cord and the cauda equina roots (Fig. 24-85). This appearance may also be produced by granulomatous disease.

EXTRADURAL

Extradural lesions originate outside the dura and include lesions of the bony skeleton, ligaments and disks, paraspinous soft tissues, and epidural space. Focal extrinsic compression of the thecal sac narrowing the

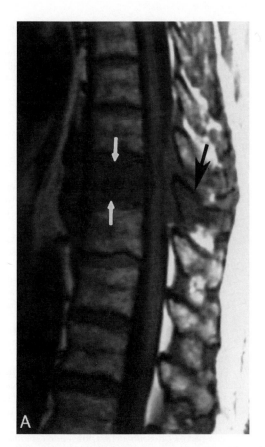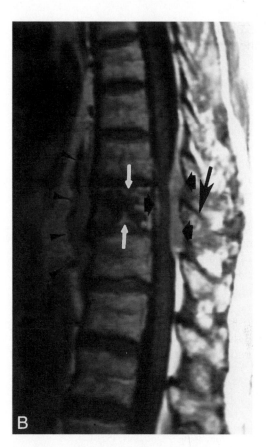

Figure 24-90   Vertebral marrow and epidural lymphoma resulting in cord compression. *A.* Sagittal T1 pre-IV contrast MRI of a 70-year-old man with lower back pain demonstrates abnormally low signal intensity of the marrow of an upper thoracic vertebral body (*white arrows*) and posterior element (*long black arrow*) with associated ventral and dorsal epidural impressions on the thecal sac which smoothly efface the subarachnoid space (refer to Fig. 24-77). *B.* Same patient following IV contrast. Note the heterogeneous enhancement of the involved marrow (*white arrows*), spinous process (*long black arrow*), and the more conspicuous enhancement of the epidural components of the mass (*short black arrows*). Also note the enhancement of a prevertebral soft tissue mass (*arrowheads*). Biopsy disclosed non-Hodgkin's lymphoma.

subarachnoid space is the hallmark of extradural lesions. A "myelographic block" may occur if the lesion is large enough to impede the CSF flow around it.

The most common benign extradural thecal sac impressions are the result of traumatic fracture and degenerative spondylosis. Bony and/or disk retropulsion into the spinal canal may compromise the neural structures (Fig. 24-81). Degenerative spondyloarthropathy features degenerative disk disease (Fig. 24-84), osteophytosis (Fig. 24-84), and posterior element arthrosis, which can compromise neural structures (Fig. 24-86), at times necessitating surgery (Fig. 24-87). A synovial cyst in the setting of facet arthropathy and even an intradural nerve sheath tumor may result in radiculopathy[58] mimicking disk herniation.

Postoperative back pain is routinely evaluated with IV contrast-enhanced MRI to differentiate nonenhancing recurrent disk herniation from enhancing granulation tissue (Fig. 24-88).[124] Spinal stenosis may be congenital or acquired. A congenitally narrow spinal canal is more susceptible to symptomatic compression of neural structures. Acquired spinal stenosis is typically the result of degenerative spondylosis and degenerative disk disease with or without accompanying disk herniation.

Nontraumatic fractures of pathologic bone may also result in an extradural lesion. Etiologies include osteopenia, primary benign or malignant bone tumor, and metastatic bone tumor (Fig. 24-90).[58] Neoplastic and non-neoplastic bone cysts may expand the vertebra, resulting in extradural compression. Osteomyelitis, diskitis, and paraspinous infectious, neoplastic, and vascular masses may result in extradural impression. Epidural lipomatosis and the rare angiolipomas complete the list of benign extradural lesions.

Metastases represent the most common malignant extradural neoplasm (Fig. 24-89, 24-90).[58] Not uncommonly, metastatic disease to the vertebral marrow has an accompanying epidural component, which may compromise the spinal cord (Fig. 24-89, 24-90). Primary malignant extradural extraskeletal tumors such as chordoma and lymphoma are uncommon.[58]

Conclusion

This has been a review of the rapidly expanding field of diagnostic neuroradiology, excluding head and neck imaging. Neuroradiology will continue to search for improved imaging techniques that will provide increased sensitivity and specificity in the evaluation of neurologic disease. Presentations included a discussion of contrast media, the formation of an image, comparison of MRI and CT, approach to neuroradiologic diagnosis, and an imaging review of neurologic diseases. The combination of a thorough knowledge of normal anatomy and pathology, familiarization with new technologies, and the capacity for clinical correlation makes the neuroradiologist an important partner in the diagnosis of neurologic disease. We hope this presentation will serve as a useful and compact neuroimaging reference for the neuroanesthesiologist.

References

1. Sage MR, Wilson AJ: The blood-brain barrier: An important concept in neuroimaging. *AJNR* 1994; 15:601.
2. Stern L, Gautier R: Rapports entre le liquide céphalo-rachidien et la circulation sanguine. *Arch Int Physiol Biochim* 1921; 17:138.
3. Atlas SW (ed): *Magnetic Resonance Imaging of the Brain and Spine*, 2d ed. Philadelphia, Raven-Lippincott, 1996.
4. Sze G: Anatomy and pathology of the meninges in the head and spine. In Huckman, MS (ed): *ARRS Neuroradiology Categorical Course Syllabus*. 1992:91–105.
5. Byrd SE, et al: Contrast agents in neuroimaging. *Neuroimaging Clin North Am* 1994; 4:9.
6. Amin MM, et al: Ionic and nonionic contrast media: Current status and controversies. *Appl Radiol* 1993:41.
7. *Manual on iodinated contrast media*. Reston, VA: American College of Radiology, 1991.
8. Earnest F, et al: Complications of cerebral angiography. *AJR* 1994; 142:247.
9. Mani RL, et al: Complications of catheter cerebral angiography: Analysis of 5,000 procedures. I. Criteria and incidence; II. Relation of complication rates to clinical and arteriographic diagnoses; III. Assessment of arteries injected, contrast medium used, duration of procedure, and age of patient. *AJR* 1978; 131:861.
10. Granger CB, et al: Fibrin modification by ionic and nonionic contrast media during cardiac catheterization. *Am J Cardiol* 1992; 69:821.
11. Kurisu Y, Tada S: The anticoagulant effect of ionic and nonionic low-osmolar contrast media in dogs. *Invest Radiol* 1992; 27:686.
12. Zagoria RJ: Iodinated contrast agents in neuroradiology. *Neuroimaging Clin North Am* 1994; 4:1.
13. Cohan RH, et al: Extravascular extravasation of radiographic contrast media: Effects of conventional and low-osmolar agents in the rat thigh. *Invest Radiol* 1990; 25:504.
14. Cohan RH, et al: Treatment of reactions to radiographic contrast material. *AJR* 1988; 151:263.
15. Jordan RM, Mintz RD: Fatal reaction to gadopentetate dimeglumine. *AJR* 1995; 164:743.
16. Goldstein HA, et al: Safety assessment of gadopentetate dimeglumine in U.S. clinical trials. *Radiology* 1990; 174:17.
17. Saini S, et al: Advances in contrast-enhanced MR imaging. *AJR* 1991; 156:235.
18. Sanders RC: *Clinical Sonography: A practical guide*, 2d ed. Boston, Little, Brown, 1991.
19. Carroll BA: Carotid sonography. *Radiology* 1991; 178:303.
20. Polak JF, et al: Internal carotid artery stenosis: Accuracy and reproducibility of color-Doppler-assisted duplex imaging. *Radiology* 1989; 173:793.
21. North American Symptomatic Carotid Endarterectomy Trial (NASCET) Collaborators: Beneficial effect of carotid endarterectomy in symptomatic patients with high grade carotid stenosis. *N Engl J Med* 1991; 325:445.
22. Hunink MGM, et al: Detection and quantification of carotid artery stenosis: Efficacy of various Doppler velocity parameters. *AJR* 1993; 160:619.
23. Imparato AM, et al: The importance of hemorrhage in the relationship between gross morphologic characteristics and cerebral symptoms in 376 carotid artery plaques. *Ann Surg* 1983; 197:195.
24. Polak JF, et al: Detection of internal carotid artery stenosis: Comparison of MR angiography, color Doppler sonography, and arteriography. *Radiology* 1992; 182:35.
25. Filly RA: Ultrasound evaluation of the fetal neural axis. In Callen PW (ed): *Ultrasonography in Obstetrics and Gynecology*, 3d ed. Philadelphia, WB Saunders, 1994:189–234.
26. Cohen HL, Haller JO: Advances in perinatal neurosonography. *AJR* 1994; 163:801.
27. Sherman NG, Rosenber HK: Ultrasound essentials for imaging neonatal brains. *Diagnostic Imaging* 1994; 164:108.
28. Anderson NG, et al: Diastematomyelia: Diagnosis by prenatal sonography. *AJR* 1994; 163:911.
29. Rowland CA, Gibson PJ: Ultrasound determination of the normal location of the conus medullaris in neonates. *AJNR* 1995; 16:469.
30. Palmer EL, et al: *Practical Nuclear Medicine*. Philadelphia, WB Saunders, 1992.
31. O'Malley JP, et al: Diagnosis of intracranial lymphoma in patients with AIDS: Value of 201Tl single-photon emission computed tomography. *AJR* 1994; 163:417.
32. Ruiz A, et al: Use of Thallium-201 brain SPECT to differentiate lymphoma from toxoplasma encephalitis in AIDS patients. *AJNR* 1994; 15:1885.
33. Hoffman JM, et al: FDG-PET in differentiating lymphoma from nonmalignant central nervous system lesions in patients with AIDS. *J Nucl Med* 1993; 34:567.
34. Larar GN, Nagel JS: Technetium-99m HMPAO cerebral perfusion scintigraphy: Considerations for timely brain death declaration. *J Nucl Med* 1992; 33:2209.
35. Idea RJ, Lewis DH: Diagnosis of brain death in an emergency trauma center. *AJR* 1994; 163:927.
36. Di Chiro G, Fulham MJ: Virchow's shackles: Can PET-FDG challenge tumor histology? *AJNR* 1993; 14:524.
37. Di Chiro G, et al: Cerebral necrosis after radiotherapy and/or intra-arterial chemotherapy for brain tumors: PET and neuropathologic studies. *AJNR* 1987; 8:1083.
38. Doyle WK, et al: Differentiation of cerebral radiation necrosis from tumor recurrence by ([18F]) FDG and 82Rb PET. *J Comput Assist Tomogr* 1987; 11:563.
39. Davis KW, et al: [18F]2-Fluoro-2-Deoxyglucose-Positron emission tomography correlation of gadolinium-enhanced MR imaging of central nervous system neoplasms. *AJNR* 1993; 14:515.
40. Heinz ER, et al: MR and positron emission tomography in

the diagnosis of surgically correctable temporal lobe epilepsy. *AJNR* 1994; 15:1341.

41. Engel J Jr, et al: Comparative localization of epileptic foci in partial epilepsy by PET and EEG. *Ann Neurol* 1982; 12:529.

42. Seldinger SI: Catheter replacement of needle in percutaneous arteriography. *Acta Radiol* 1953; 39(Suppl):368.

43. Chynn KY: Transfemoral carotid and vertebral angiography. *Acta Radiol* 1969; 9:244.

44. European Carotid Surgery Trialists' Collaborative Group. MRC European Carotid Surgery Trial: Interim results for symptomatic patients with severe (70–99%) or with mild (0–29%) carotid stenosis. *Lancet* 1991; 337:1235.

45. Executive Committee for the Asymptomatic Carotid Atherosclerosis Study: Endarterectomy for asymptomatic carotid artery stenosis. *JAMA* 1995; 273:1421.

46. Wolpert SM, Caplan LR: Current role of cerebral angiography in the diagnosis of cerebrovascular disease. *AJR* 1992; 159:191.

47. Bowen BC, et al: MR angiography of occlusive disease of the arteries in the head and neck: current concepts. *AJR* 1994; 162:9.

48. Cumming MJ, Morrow IM: Carotid artery stenosis: A prospective comparison of CT angiography and conventional angiography. *AJR* 1994; 163:517.

49. Dion JE, et al: Clinical events following neuroangiography: A prospective study. *Stroke* 1987; 18:997.

50. Fisher CM, Adams RD: Transient global amnesia. *Acta Neurol Scand* 1964; 40(suppl 9); 36:1.

51. Wales LR, Nov AA: Transient global amnesia: complication of cerebral angiography. *AJNR* 1981; 2:275.

52. Pexman JHW, Coates RK: Amnesia after femorocerebral angiography. *AJNR* 1983; 4:979.

53. Giang DW, Kido DK: Transient global amnesia associated with cerebral angiography performed with the use of iopamidol. *Radiology* 1989; 172:195.

54. Studdard WE, et al: Cortical blindness after cerebral angiography. *J Neurosurg* 1981; 54:240.

55. Rosansky SJ: Multiple cholesterol emboli syndrome after angiography. *Am J Med Sci* 1984; 288:45.

56. Lin JP, Kricheff II: Angiographic investigation of cerebral aneurysms. *Radiology* 1972; 105:69.

57. Shapiro R: *Myelography,* 4th ed. Chicago, Year Book, 1984.

58. Osborn AG: *Diagnostic Neuroradiology.* St. Louis, Mosby Year-Book, 1994.

59. Lee JT, et al: *Computed Body Tomography with MRI Correlation,* 2d ed. New York, Raven Press, 1989.

60. Zeman RK, et al: *Helical/Spiral CT: A Practical Approach.* New York, McGraw-Hill, 1995.

61. Schwartz RB, et al: Evaluation of cerebral aneurysms with helical CTA: Correlation with conventional angiography and MR angiography. *Radiology* 1994; 192:717.

62. Barkovitch JA: *Pediatric Neuroimaging.* 2d ed. New York, Raven Press, 1995.

63. Latchaw RE: *MR and CT Imaging of the Head, Neck, and Spine,* 2d ed. St. Louis, Mosby Year-Book, 1991.

64. Woodruff WW: *Fundamentals of Neuroimaging.* Philadelphia, WB Saunders, 1993.

65. Prorok RJ, Sawyer AM: *Signa Advantage applications guide,* vol IV: *Fast package/Signa release.* General Electric Company, 1992.

66. Schild HH: *MRI Made Easy (. . . Well Almost).* Berlin, Bergkamen, 1990.

67. Bowen BC, et al: MR angiography of occlusive disease of the arteries of the head and neck: current concepts. *AJR* 1994; 162:9.

68. Atlas SW: MR angiography in neurologic disease. *Radiology* 1994; 193:1.

69. Turski P et al: *Vascular Magnetic Resonance Imaging,* vol III. General Electric Medical Systems, 1990.

70. Huston III J, Ehman RL: Comparison of time-of-flight and phase-contrast MR neuroangiographic techniques. *Radiographics* 1993; 13:5.

71. Elster AD, et al: Improved detection of gadolinium enhancement using magnetization transfer imaging. *Neuroimaging Clin North Am* 1994; 4:185.

72. Elster AD, Mathews VP: Magnetization transfer amplifies tissue contrast. *Diagnostic Imaging* 1995; 73:53.

73. Atlas SW, et al: Aqueductal stenosis: Evaluation with gradient-echo rapid MR imaging. *Radiology* 1988; 169:449.

74. Enzmann DR, Pek NJ: Normal flow of intracranial and intraspinal CSF defined with phase-contrast cine MR imaging. *Radiology* 1991; 178:467.

75. Bhadelia RA, et al: Analysis of cerebrospinal fluid flow waveforms with gated phase-contrast MR velocity measurements. *AJNR* 1995; 16:389.

76. Blatter DD, et al: Cerebral MR angiography with multiple overlapping thin slab acquisition. Part II. Early clinical experience. *Radiology,* 1992; 183:379.

77. Huston III J, et al: Blinded prospective evaluation of sensitivity of MR angiography to known intracranial aneurysms: Importance of aneurysm size. *AJNR* 1994; 15:1607.

78. Araki Y, et al: A pitfall in detection of intracranial unruptured aneurysms on three-dimensional phase-contrast MR angiography. *AJNR* 1994; 15:1618.

79. Gelbert F, et al: MRI in spontaneous dissection of vertebral and carotid arteries. *Neuroradiology* 1990; 33:111.

80. Klufas RA, et al: Dissection of the carotid and vertebral arteries: Imaging with MR angiography. *AJR* 1995; 164:673.

81. Provenzale JM: Dissection of the craniocervical arteries. In Taveras JM, Ferrucci JT (eds): *Radiology: Diagnosis-Imaging-Intervention.* Philadelphia, JB Lippincott, 1995.

82. Vogl TJ, et al: Dural sinus thrombosis: Value of venous MR angiography for diagnosis and follow-up. *AJR* 1994; 162:1191.

83. Drutman J, et al: Evaluation of subclavian steal with two-dimensional phase-contrast and two-dimensional time-of-flight MR angiography. *AJNR* 1994; 15:1642.

84. Kohler: *Signa Advantage PROBE/SV: Single-Voxel Proton Brain Exam Applications Guide,* vol V. General Electric Medical Systems, 1993.

85. Young I, Charles HC (eds): *MR Spectroscopy.* London, Martin Dunitz, 1995.

86. Henriksen O: Review article: MR spectroscopy in clinical research. *Acta Radiol* 1994; 35:96.

87. Barker PB, et al: Acute stroke: Evaluation with serial proton MR spectroscopic imaging. *Radiology* 1994; 192:723.

88. Cortey A, et al: Proton MR spectroscopy of brain abnormalities in neonates born to HIV-positive mothers. *AJNR* 1994; 15:1853.

89. Grossman RI, et al: MR proton spectroscopy in multiple sclerosis. *AJNR* 1992; 13:1535.

90. Meyerhoff DJ, et al: Effects of normal aging and Alzheimer's disease on cerebral 1H metabolites. Abstract, p. 1931. *Soc Magn Reson Med,* Berlin, 1992.

91. Scott WR, et al: Computerized axial tomography of intracerebral and intraventricular hemorrhage. *Radiology* 1974; 112:73.

92. Cohen WA, Wayman LA: Computed tomography of intracranial hemorrhage. *Neuroimaging Clin North Am* 1992; 2:75.

93. Boyko OB, et al: Contrast-enhanced CT of acute isodense subdural hematoma. *AJNR* 1991; 12:341.

94. Kricheff II: Strategies for the evaluation of supratentorial brain neoplasms. In: Huckman MS (ed): *ARRS Neuroradiology Categorical Course Syllabus.* 1992, 9.

95. Shellock FG: *Pocket Guide to MR Procedures and Metallic Objects: Update 1994.* New York, Raven Press, 1995.

96. Heinz ER, et al: Detection of cerebrospinal fluid metastasis: CT myelography or MR? *AJNR* 1995; 16:1147.

97. Han BK, et al: Reversal sign on CT: Effects of anoxic/ischemic cerebral injury in children. *AJNR* 1989; 10:1191.

98. Grossman RI, Yousem DM: *Neuroradiology.* St. Louis, Mosby-Year Book, 1994.

99. Shepherd CW, et al: MR findings in tuberous sclerosis complex and correlation with seizure development and mental impairment. *AJNR* 1995; 16:149.

100. Benedikt RA, et al: Sturge-Weber syndrome: Cranial MR imaging with Gd-DTPA. *AJNR* 1993; 14:409.

101. Vogl ThJ, et al: MR and MR angiography of Sturge-Weber syndrome. *AJNR* 1993; 14:417.

102. Harris KG, et al: Diagnosing intracranial vasculitis: The roles of MR and angiography. *AJNR* 1994; 15:317.

103. Martin N, Vinters H: Pathology and grading of intracranial vascular malformations. In Barrow DL (ed): *Intracranial Vascular Malformations.* Park Ridge IL, American Association of Neurological Surgeons, 1990:1.

104. Wilms G, et al: Simultaneous occurrence of developmental venous anomalies and cavernous angiomas. *AJNR* 1994; 15:1247.

105. Turjman F, et al: Aneurysms related to cerebral arteriovenous malformations: superselective angiographic assessment in 58 patients. *AJNR* 1994; 15:1601.

106. Golfinos JG, et al: The management of unruptured intracranial vascular malformation. *Barrow Neurological Institute Quarterly.* 1992; 8:2.

107. Mittl Jr RL, et al: Prevalence of MR evidence of diffuse axonal injury in patients with mild head injury and normal head CT findings. *AJNR* 1994; 15:1583.

108. Ashdown BC, et al: Aspergillosis of the brain and paranasal sinuses in immunocompromised patients. *AJR* 1994; 162:155.

109. Miaux Y, et al: MR of cerebral aspergillosis in patients who have had bone marrow transplantation. *AJNR* 1995; 16:555.

110. Baum PA, et al: Deep gray matter involvement in children with acute disseminated encephalomyelitis. *AJNR* 1994; 15:1275.

111. Jensen ME, et al: MR imaging appearance of childhood adrenoleukodystrophy with auditory, visual, and motor pathway involvement. *Radiographics* 1990; 10:53.

112. Loes DJ, et al: Childhood cerebral form of adrenoleukodystrophy: Short-term effects of bone marrow transplantation on brain MR observations. *AJNR* 1994; 15:1767.

113. Hiehle Jr JF, et al: Magnetization transfer effects in MR-detected multiple sclerosis lesions: comparison of gadolinium-enhanced spin-echo images and nonenhanced T1-weighted images. *AJNR* 1995; 16:69.

114. Felsberg GJ, et al: Radiologic-pathologic correlation: gliomatosis cerebri. *AJNR* 1994; 15:1745.

115. Harnsberger HR: *Handbook of Head and Neck Imaging,* 2d ed. St. Louis, Mosby Year-Book, 1995.

116. Tien RD, et al: Variable bandwidth steady-state free-precession MR imaging: A technique for improving characterization of epidermoid tumor and arachnoid cyst. *AJR* 1995; 164:689.

117. Drayer BP: Degenerative disorders of the central nervous system: An integrated approach to the differential diagnosis. *Neuroimaging Clin North Am* 1995; 1:135.

118. Golomb J, et al: Nonspecific leukoencephalopathy associated with aging. *Neuroimaging Clin North Am* 1995; 5:33.

119. Finelli DA, et al: Use of magnetization transfer for improved contrast on gradient-echo MR images of the cervical spine. *Radiology* 1994; 193:165.

120. Provenzale JM, et al: Lupus-related myelitis: Serial MR findings. *AJNR* 1994; 15:1911.

121. Campi A, et al: Acute transverse myelopathy: Spinal and cranial MR study with clinical follow-up. *AJNR* 1995; 16:115.

122. Tartaglino LM, et al: MR imaging in a case of postvaccination myelitis. *AJNR* 1995; 16:581.

123. Friedman DP, et al: Vascular neoplasms and malformations, ischemia, and hemorrhage affecting the spinal cord: MR imaging findings. *AJR* 1994; 162:685.

124. Dina TS, et al: Lumbar spine after surgery for herniated disk: Imaging findings in the early postoperative period. *AJR* 1995; 164:665.

Anesthesia and Neuroradiologic Procedures

CECIL O. BOREL

PREPARATION FOR THE PROCEDURE
 Nausea and Vomiting
 Allergic Reaction Prophylaxis
 Anxiolysis
CHOICE OF ANESTHETIC TECHNIQUE
 Monitored Anesthesia Care
 General Anesthesia
INDUCTION AND MAINTENANCE OF ANESTHESIA
EMERGENCE AND POSTANESTHETIC CARE
ANESTHESIA FOR SPECIAL PROCEDURES
 CT-Guided Stereotactic Surgery
 CT Scans/CT Myelogram
 Magnetic Resonance Imaging
CONCLUSION

Anesthesia for radiologic studies is fundamentally similar to other anesthetics where basic principles apply, but complicated when alterations in technique are required to perform an adequate radiologic study or procedure.[1] The goals of anesthetic management are patient safety and comfort in the radiologic suite; as in any other location, these are the responsibility of the anesthetist. Usually, radiologic procedures that require anesthetics are not performed in the operating room, and the anesthetist will be away from extra supplies, emergency drugs, or familiar equipment and back-up help. The size or location of radiologic equipment limits access to the patients and their airways during the procedure. Frequent changes in position, movement in and out of scanners, or the movement of contrast agents may be an integral part of the study, and should be anticipated in the anesthesia plan. The radiologist may also require ideal "operating" conditions so that the study or intervention can be performed optimally. Many radiologic procedures are not particularly painful but require that the patient be absolutely still for a long period of time; deep levels of general anesthesia may not be necessary for successful completion of these procedures. When performed skillfully, anesthetic management during radiologic studies receives enthusiastic support from radiologists and gratitude from patients.

Preparation for the Procedure

NAUSEA AND VOMITING

Preparing the patient to undergo a radiologic study or procedure involves minimizing or anticipating adverse occurrences unique to the procedure. As in other procedures, there are risks of nausea, vomiting, and aspiration, and these may be exacerbated by the studies. There is a particular risk in procedures where the patient is positioned with the stomach higher than the head, or where embolizing material is likely to induce nausea and vomiting. An empty stomach is required for patients undergoing elective procedures. Where anxiety contributes to nausea, or nausea is a likely complaint, administration of an antiemetic is appropriate. Neutralization of gastric acid secretion is also an important preventive measure. Histamine receptor blockers may be doubly helpful in decreasing gastric acid secretion and providing histamine receptor blockade in the event of an allergic reaction.[2] When the patient is likely to be positioned so that the stomach is higher than the head, the addition of metoclopramide is useful, promoting gastric motility to empty the stomach. Metoclopramide may be administered orally, intramuscularly, or intravenously, but should be given at least 2 h before the procedure to allow adequate emptying to occur.

ALLERGIC REACTION PROPHYLAXIS

The risk of allergic reaction to contrast media or therapeutic agent is a consideration in preparing patients for these studies or procedures. A review of previous reaction to contrast agents, seafood allergy, or penicillin will help identify a patient at risk.[2] The use of beta-blockers may increase the risk of suffering a severe anaphylactoid reaction in patients with high risk of allergic reaction.[3] Pretreatment for prevention of allergic reactions appears to reduce the risk and severity of subsequent allergic reactions.[4] Two protocols for preventive regimens are shown in Table 24-1.

ANXIOLYSIS

The compassionate control of anxiety or pain of a procedure is a suitable role for the anesthetist. A patient

TABLE 24B-1
Pretreatment Protocols to Prevent Anaphylactoid Reactions to Radiocontrast Media

Marshall and Lieberman[4]
   Prednisone 50 mg orally at 13, 7, and 1 h before procedure
   Diphenhydramine 50 mg IM 1 h before procedure
   Cimetidine 300 mg orally 1 h before procedure
   Ephedrine 25 mg orally 1 h before procedure (not for hypertensive patients)
Wittbrodt and Spinler[2]
   Prednisone 50 mg orally at 13, 7, and 1 h before procedure
   Diphenhydramine 50 mg IM 1 h before procedure (discontinue beta-blockers)

may request very heavy sedation for the procedure because of a previously painful procedure or untoward reaction. Most radiologic procedures are not painful, but many appear frightening. Intravenous administration of short-acting benzodiazepenes supplemented with narcotics is useful for mild-to-moderately painful procedures. Most patients will have a satisfactory experience when a minor tranquilizer is administered orally 2 h before the procedure and supplemental sedation is given intravenously when necessary during the procedure. In patients in whom intracranial pressures may be elevated, neither narcotics or sedatives are safe because of the risk of raising P_{CO_2} and increasing intracranial pressure.

Choice of Anesthetic Technique

MONITORED ANESTHESIA CARE

Local anesthesia is appropriate for adult patients who are coherent and cooperative, especially when the procedure will be short, insertion of catheters will be the only stimulation, or neurologic examination will be necessary during the investigation. Local anesthesia is also ideal for the comatose or critically ill patient unlikely to move during investigation. The role of the anesthetist is to monitor airway status and vital signs during the procedure. The anesthetist should be available for emergency airway management or resuscitation in the event of an untoward reaction, and thus should provide airway equipment, IV access, suitable monitoring modalities, and emergency drugs for this eventuality.

Local anesthesia supplemented with intravenous sedation is indicated for adult, awake patients when the procedure is likely to be prolonged or uncomfortable, but not frankly painful. Using mild sedation it is possible to maintain enough patient interaction and participation to allow neurologic evaluation. Since the airway will not be controlled during the procedure, access to the airway should be maintained so that it is relatively easy to establish airway control in the event of an emergency. The use of a precordial stethoscope with transmitter, ECG monitoring, end-tidal CO_2 and respiration monitor, pulse oximeter, and automatic blood pressure cuff enhance the ability to monitor the patient when the anesthetist must be away from the airway or must resuscitate the patient in an emergency situation. Measures to ensure comfort during the procedure such as bladder catheterization, egg-crate mattress padding of the table, and padding of extremities seem to make long procedures more tolerable.

GENERAL ANESTHESIA

Though local/sedation techniques are ideal for many radiologic procedures, there are situations in which this anesthetic approach would be quite difficult. In patients who have raised intracranial pressure, sedation techniques may cause CO_2 retention, increasing intracranial pressure. These patients need airway control and controlled ventilation if sedation is required. Combative, disoriented patients are likely to become worse with light sedation, and may suffer airway compromise with further sedation. Since such compromise may occur at a time when it is difficult to reach the airway, intubation and general anesthesia are usually more appropriate for these patients. For very long procedures in which absolute control of patient movement will be important, sedatives are unlikely to be adequate for the duration. Some embolization procedures are painful at sites remote from the catheter insertion. Sedation/narcotic combinations may not be sufficient for control of visceral or vascular pain. Young children who are likely to be frightened, uncomfortable, or uncooperative often benefit from a general anesthetic rather than a poor attempt at sedation and local anesthesia.[5]

General anesthesia, by contrast, is indicated if the following is likely: a long difficult procedure; an uncooperative patient where ideal investigational conditions are necessary; a procedure where airway compromise or access will be limited or a large part of the procedure; or hyperventilation procedures. A "light" general anesthetic, endotracheal intubation, and moderate relaxation is sufficient for pain management and prevention of movement to optimize imaging. Techniques that do not increase cerebral blood flow are desirable if intracranial pressure is elevated. Nitrous oxide must be avoided if air is injected into a closed space to provide air contrast. The anesthetic should be easily and quickly reversible so that neurologic sequelae can be evaluated in the radiologic suite, allowing further diagnostic studies or interventions to be performed immediately when necessary.

Induction and Maintenance of Anesthesia

All the standard equipment for administering an anesthetic safely should be available prior to the induction of anesthesia. Because anesthetic administration is not routine in many radiologic suites, extra effort is necessary to ascertain the location and availability of anesthetic equipment before induction: suction; oxygen supply; airway equipment; drugs for anesthesia and resuscitation; and monitoring equipment. Oversights in set-up are greatly magnified by the difficulty of getting emergency or extra equipment from a store room located near the operating rooms several floors away.[1]

Special equipment is necessary for anesthetizing patients in radiology suites or scanners. Extra long airway tubing, IV tubing with extensions, and long monitoring probe connectors are essential for the patient to slide in and out of the scanning apparatus. Since the patient's position relative to the radiologic equipment is usually predetermined, it may be necessary to position the anesthesia machine and equipment in unusual locations, such as at the left side of the patient. Monitoring equipment with electronic display must remain visible during filming, when the anesthetist will be standing in a protected environment. When in doubt, reviewing equipment location and changes in patient positioining with the radiologist prior to induction of anesthesia avoids the difficulty of correcting problems once the anesthetic is underway.

Induction of anesthesia usually can be carried out with the patient already positioned on the x-ray table. This avoids difficult movement onto the table once the patient is anesthetized. If a problem occurs during the procedure, the patient can be immediately returned to the position prior to induction so that emergency airway management and resuscitation can take place; if the patient was induced on a stretcher and positioned on the table after induction, the stretcher should remain immediately available in the event emergency management is necessary.

Anesthesia should be maintained at a depth sufficient for the rapid completion of investigational and interventional procedures. Judicious use of muscle relaxants eliminates movement artifact in the anesthetized patient, and allows for a rapid emergence and reversal for neurologic assessment after the procedure. Inhalation, infusion, and N_2O-narcotic have all been used successfully in this situation when general anesthesia is required.

Emergence and Postanesthetic Care

There is no better place to assess poor emergence due to intracerebral hemorrhage or occlusion of cerebral vasculature than in the area where the studies have been performed. Patients who receive general anesthesia or deep sedation should be observed in a postanesthesia recovery room following emergence to monitor airway and cardiovascular status. Those patients at risk for neurologic or cerebrovascular compromise in the hours following embolization procedures are candidates for overnight monitoring in an intensive care unit where skilled services are immediately available.

Anesthesia for Special Procedures

CT-GUIDED STEREOTACTIC SURGERY

Using CT scanning techniques, stereotactic procedures offer an alternative to traditional craniotomy for diagnosis and treatment of tumor, abscess, and other intracranial lesions.[6] Stereotaxis can also be used therapeutically to treat movement disorders and central pain syndromes. Damage to adjacent structures can be minimal, which is especially important when working in deep structures within the brain.

The lesion is located relative to an external reference frame applied with compression pins fitted tightly to the skull. This external frame fits inside the scanner and is included in the scan of the lesion, permitting calculation of the precise trajectory of the biopsy probe. The Leksell frame and the Brown-Roberts-Wells (BRW) frame are both used for CT-guided stereotactic procedures. The Leksell is a square frame that allows access to the patient's head and airway. The BRW frame is cylindrical and fits completely around the head, giving little access to the airway once it is in place. Both frames are held with four pins in the skull placed under local anesthesia. The head must remain immobile with reference to the frame because the trajectory of the biopsy probe is calculated by referencing external markers on the frame to the lesion visualized by CT. Airway management becomes difficult once the procedure is underway because of the position of the patient's head and body in the gantry.

Several factors are important to consider when selecting anesthetic techniques in this situation. Since the biopsy is usually performed on mass lesions, patients undergoing this procedure are considered to have raised intracranial pressure, or brain which may be very intolerant of changes in intracranial volume. Techniques that increase P_{CO_2} are not safe in this context. Patients will have the frame placed around the head, and the head will be within the body of the scanner for much of the time, making access to the airway and usual airway management difficult. The procedure itself will involve creation of the burr hole and fixation of pins; painful procedures often well tolerated with local anesthesia. Once the scanning and passage of the

biopsy probe begin, there must be no change in relation of the patient to the frame, a situation facilitated by absolute stillness of the patient as well as head fixation in the frame.

Cooperative patients tolerate the procedure well under local anesthesia. The benefit of this approach is the continuous assessment of neurologic function as the biopsy probe follows the planned trajectory to the lesion. This approach is necessary to avoid damage to the speech center when biopsying lesions in the left temporal lobe, or assessing the response of movement or pain to external stimulation. Unfortunately, sedation muddles the neurologic evaluation, and may place the airway at risk, so it must be used judiciously, if at all, for these procedures.

General anesthesia is usually necessary with children or uncooperative adults. The airway can be easily controlled with endotracheal intubation, and hyperventilation can be used in the event of raised intracranial pressure. General anesthesia provides excellent analgesia for the burr hole and pin fixation, and will provide absolute patient immobility at crucial periods of the procedure.

Postoperatively, there is a small but significant risk of epidural, subdural, or intracerebral bleeding. The patient should recover in a place where frequent neurologic examination can be carried out.

CT SCANS/CT MYELOGRAM

CT procedures on small children will frequently require participation of an anesthetist. For a good quality study the patient must be completely motionless. In the child older than 12 to 18 months, oral sedation may not be sufficient to keep the child still. Multiple unsuccessful attempts at deepening levels of sedation are not as safe as a light general anesthetic with endotracheal intubation. The child will be at less risk of hypoventilation and hypoxia from the general anesthetics than the additive and longer-duration effects of the drugs used for sedation. This is especially true for children with brain tumors or hydrocephalus where intracranial compliance is poor.

Patients having CT scans for extracranial lesions can be managed with intramuscular or intravenous ketamine mixed with a small amount of midazolam and atropine. This produces a quiet child capable of being scanned easily after the head is positioned and taped in place. Since ketamine does not depress ventilation as greatly as other intravenous anesthetics, less airway support is required during the scan when the anesthetist must be away from the patient's airway.

Children undergoing myelography usually start in the lateral position for the lumbar puncture, and are then turned supine and from side to side with the legs elevated to facilitate movement of the dye through the subarachnoid space. During this maneuver the patient's head is kept flexed to prevent movement of dye through the foramen magnum. Absolute control of the airway must be maintained during this process so that the endotracheal tube does not become dislodged and the child extubated. For the actual scan, the child is supine and the airway is easily secured.

MAGNETIC RESONANCE IMAGING

As MRI becomes increasingly common and useful, more acutely ill and uncooperative patients will become candidates for MRI studies. Anesthesia and monitoring in the MRI scanner presents several problems.[7] Ferromagnetic equipment must be excluded from the magnetic field. There is limited access to the patient and decreased visibility in the magnet. Monitoring equipment malfunctions because of electromagnetic interference produced by changing magnetic field gradients and rapidly switching radiofrequency currents. The MR image is degraded by stray radiofrequency currents produced by monitoring equipment and leads.

The principal decision to be made by the anesthesiologist is the location of the anesthesia machine, ventilator, and monitoring equipment in relation to the magnet.[8] Equipment may be either inside or outside the magnetic field. If the equipment is kept outside the field, all anesthesia equipment must be kept outside the Gauss line at which attraction of ferromagnetic items is likely, usually between 30 and 50 Gauss lines.[7] This often results in having the ventilator, anesthesia machine, and monitoring equipment 10 to 20 feet from the face of the magnet. Very long ventilatory tubing will be required to reach the patient, which results in a large compressible volume of gas in the circuit. Long intravenous and pressure monitoring tubing will be necessary to maintain infusion delivery and invasive monitoring during the study. If the equipment will be close to the magnet, it must be composed of non-ferromagnetic components or must be permanently attached.[9] Monitoring equipment powered by unfiltered electrical current may produce interference when placed close to the magnet. Battery-powered monitors must be permanently fixed, since batteries are highly attracted to magnetic fields.

The airway should be maintained with an endotracheal tube in unconscious patients or in patients receiving general anesthesia, because the head and airway are invisible and inaccessible during the scanning procedure. Standard laryngoscopes are metallic but not ferromagnetic, and will undergo a degree of torque if used in proximity to the magnet. The batteries are also highly magnetic. A plastic laryngoscope with a paper-covered battery can be used in close proximity to the magnet. In most situations anesthesia can be induced and the patient intubated outside the 50 Gauss line so that standard equipment can be used. The use of a RAE tube is helpful in routing the ventilator tubing and providing clearance while the head is in the magnet.[10]

Positive pressure ventilation can be maintained by a variety of techniques and devices. In situations where airway and ventilatory management are uncommon occurrences in the scanner, a simple arrangement of plastic disposable Mapleson D circuitry with extension tubing to about 30 feet will permit manual ventilation with oxygen and air mixtures from piped gas supplies. Several nonferromagnetic, gas-powered ventilators have been specifically developed for use in the scanner and appear capable of ventilating critically ill patients requiring PEEP. The 225 SIMV (Monaghan Medical Corp) and the Narco Airsheild VC 20-1 are functional in a 1.5 T field.[9,11] Siemens-Elema 900C ventilators have been used successfully in a 1.5 T magnet when located at least 1.2 m away from the magnet.[12] Alternatively, the ventilator on the anesthesia machine may be used temporarily to ventilate unanesthetized critically ill patients. Pressurized oxygen can be supplied by wall outlets or by aluminum cylinders to power the machines.

A patient placed in the bore of the magnet will be hidden from view, and will therefore require monitoring of vital functions. Ferromagnetic equipment within the bore of the magnet must be avoided, and loops of wire, (even nonferromagnetic wire) within the bore can significantly degrade image detection.[7] All direct electrical connections between equipment within the magnet and outside may introduce radiofrequency interference. Voltage induced in the wire leads may pose a burn and electrical shock hazard to the patient.[13] ECG leads V_5 and V_6 maximize QRS detection and minimize artifact.[14] ECG monitoring can also be improved by twisting the cable, keeping electrodes close together, positioning electrodes near the center of the scanner, and maintaining the plane of any loop of cable parallel to the magnetic field lines.[15] Blood pressure is usually monitored noninvasively with an automatic cuff, outfitted with extended tubing and located as far from the magnet as possible.[13] Pulse oximetry has proved particularly useful in monitoring patients during scanning. Pulse oximeters are susceptible to interference from the changing magnetic field, and will occasionally be deactivated by radiofrequency pulses. Oximeter monitors may be placed within 2 m of the magnet, but greater distances provide longer periods of uninterrupted monitoring.[13] The probe should be placed on a distal extremity as far from the scan site as possible because severe burns to the finger have been caused by a loop of wire from a pulse oximeter probe.[16] End-tidal CO_2 monitoring provides a good index of breathing rate, airway patency, circuit integrity, and gas exchange. An aspirating-type of CO_2-monitor is better than a direct-reading type, because the direct-reading CO_2 windows will be within the bore of the magnet and may introduce artifact or injury. Long extension tubing is necessary to collect gas samples because the CO_2 analyzer must be located at a distance from the patient. The long extension tubing introduces a delay in CO_2 measurements by several breaths. Blood pressure and arterial oxygenation may be monitored invasively if the pressure transducers are connected to long extension tubing and remain outside the magnet.[7]

Anesthetic techniques for MR scanning follow the principles stated earlier in the chapter. For patients requiring general anesthesia, the induction is carried out on an MRI rolling gurney at a safe distance from the magnet. The patient is then rolled into the magnet and reconnected to airway and monitoring equipment. Most "light" general anesthetic techniques have proved satisfactory for MR scans.

As MR scanning becomes increasingly popular and useful, its use in critically ill and other patients requiring general anesthesia will undoubtedly increase. There seems to be no contrain dication for considering most patients as candidates for MRI anesthesia whenever they are suitable candidates for MRI.

Conclusion

Although managing an anesthetic in a radiographic suite makes many anesthetists uncomfortable, the rewards of helping a patient through a difficult and frightening procedure far outweigh the difficulties of providing safe anesthetic care. Recently, many strategies have evolved to allow full monitoring, deliver anesthetics, and maintain mechanical ventilation in the radiographic suite. Imaging techniques are rapidly developing, and the operative use of magnetic resonance imaging and CT-guided stereotactic imaging is likely to increase. Anesthesiologists must continue to develop safe and effective approaches to patient care in these areas.

References

1. Manninen PH: Anaesthesia outside the operating room. *Can J Anaesth* 1991; 38:126.
2. Wittbrodt ET, Spinler SA: Prevention of anaphylactoid reactions in high-risk patients receiving radiographic contrast media. *Ann Pharmacother* 1994; 28:236.
3. Lang DM, et al: Increased risk for anaphylactoid reaction from contrast media in patients on beta-adrenergic blockers or with asthma. *Ann Intern Med* 1991; 115:270.
4. Marshall GD, Lieberman PL: Comparison of three pretreatment protocols to prevent anaphylactoid reactions to radiocontrast media. *Ann Allergy* 1991; 67:70.
5. Schulman SR: Anesthesia for external-beam radiotherapy. In Halperin EC, et al (eds): *Pediatric Radiation Oncology*, 2d ed. New York, Raven Press, 1994:576–587.
6. Gatenby RA, et al: CT-guided biopsy for the detection and staging of tumors of the head and neck. *AJNR* 1984; 5:287.
7. Peden CJ, et al: Magnetic resonance for the anesthetist. Part I: Physical principles, applications, and safety aspects. *AJR* 1992; 47:240.
8. Peden CJ, et al: Magnetic resonance for the anaesthetist. Part II: Anaesthesia and monitoring in MR units. *AJR* 1992; 47:508.
9. Rao CC, et al: Modification of an anesthesia machine for use during magnetic resonance imaging [letter]. *Anesthesiology* 1988; 68:640.
10. Nixon C, et al: Nuclear magnetic resonance. Its implications for the anaesthetist. *AJR* 1986; 41:131.
11. Smith DS, et al: Anesthetic management of acutely ill patients during magnetic resonance imaging [letter]. *Anesthesiology* 1986; 65:710.
12. Mirvis SE, et al: MR imaging of ventilator-dependent patients, preliminary experience. *AJR* 1987; 149:845.
13. Patteson SK, Chesney JT: Anesthetic management for magnetic resonance imaging: Problems and solutions. *Anesth Analg* 1992; 74:121.
14. Dimick RN, et al: Optimizing electrocardiograph electrode placement for cardiac-gated magnetic resonance imaging. *Invest Radiol* 1987; 22:17.
15. Wendt RE, et al: Electrocardiographic gating and monitoring in NMR imaging. *Magn Reson Imaging* 1988; 6:89.
16. Shellock FG, Slimp GL: Severe burn of the finger caused by using a pulse oximeter during MR imaging. *AJR* 1989; 153:1105.

INTERVENTIONAL NEURORADIOLOGY

WILLIAM L. YOUNG

JOHN PILE-SPELLMAN

The enormous progress in neuroanesthesia care over the past five decades has made possible simultaneous advances in neurosurgical science. *Interventional neuroradiology* (INR) is a hybrid of traditional neurosurgery and neuroradiology. INR may be broadly defined as treatment of central nervous system (CNS) disease by endovascular access for the purpose of delivering therapeutic agents, including both drugs and devices.[1-7] Development of novel materials and techniques has allowed unprecedented access into the distal cerebral and spinal cord vasculature, opened new therapeutic avenues, and offered means to understanding CNS pathophysiology.

In this rapidly developing field, anesthesiologists have much to offer in the prevention of morbidity and mortality during INR procedures. The various types of INR procedures[6,8] and primary areas of anesthetic care interaction are shown in Table 25-1. This chapter reviews basic concepts in treating the various disease processes and emphasizes the synergistic interaction between anesthesiologist and interventionalist. Briefly, the three primary functions of the anesthesiologist in the interventional suite are (1) provision of a physiologically stable and immobile patient, (2) manipulation of the systemic blood pressure as dictated by the needs of the procedure, and (3) emergent care of catastrophic complications.

Rapid development in this discipline has raised controversy as to what it should be called (endovascular therapy, surgical neuroangiography, endovascular neurosurgery, interventional neuroradiology, etc.). This reflects the interest of both neuroradiologists and neurosurgeons.[9,10] Formal guidelines for training and certification are being considered by the concerned professional societies. Local practices worldwide vary considerably.[6,8] At some institutions, the INR service is separate and autonomous from the division of neuroradiology. Many INR services have separate ward and admitting privileges and designated intensive care unit (ICU) space, and patients are cared for by the INR service from admission to discharge.

As the frontiers of INR expand, care of these patients will demand more of the anesthesiologist's participation. Many of the risks encountered in this newer arena are the same as during traditional operative neurosurgery (e.g., aneurysmal rupture or cerebral ischemia from vascular occlusion) and the anesthesiologist's manipulation of systemic and cerebral hemodynamics (e.g., deliberate hypotension or hypertension) is also the same. Although many of the risks and responses are for the most part conceptually the same, there are many important differences in the working environment.

Historically, the pioneers in INR provided light intravenous sedation with rudimentary monitoring for their adult patients. Anesthesia coverage appears to be becoming the standard of care. One recent survey estimated that 75 percent of INR services have the "anesthesia service monitor procedures in radiology suite or operation room."[6] Some centers have employed anesthesiologists in an "on call" fashion.[11] As the complexity of procedures and breadth of patient populations expands, the distinction between the interventional angiography suite and the operating room will blur. The need for sophisticated sedation techniques, monitoring, and physiologic manipulation will increase.

We emphasize that many of the techniques described are the result of the continuing evolution of the authors' clinical experience. In some instances recommendations are based on clinical intuition, and many

TABLE 25-1
Interventional Neuroradiologic Procedures and Primary Anesthetic Considerations

Procedure	Major Anesthetic Considerations
Special Diagnostic Procedures	
• Superselective angiography and functional testing	Cerebral ischemia ICH
• Test occlusion	Cerebral ischemia ICH Blood pressure control[a]
Therapeutic Procedures	
• Therapeutic embolization of vascular malformation	Cerebral ischemia ICH Pulmonary embolism
Intracranial arteriovenous malformations	Deliberate hypotension Postprocedure NPPB
Dural arteriovenous fistulae	Deliberate hypercapnia
Extracranial AVM	Deliberate hypercapnia
Carotid cavernous fistula	Deliberate hypercapnia Postprocedure NPPB
Cerebral aneurysms	Aneurysmal rupture Blood pressure control[a]
• Sclerotherapy of venous angiomas	Airway swelling Hypoxia Hypoglycemia Intoxication from ethanol
• Balloon angioplasty of occlusive cerebrovascular disease	Cerebral ischemia ICH Deliberate hypertension Concomitant coronary artery disease
• Balloon angioplasty of cerebral vasospasm secondary to aneurysmal subarachnoid hemorrhage	Cerebral ischemia ICH Blood pressure control[a]
• Therapeutic carotid occlusion for giant aneurysms and skull base tumors	Cerebral ischemia ICH Blood pressure control[a]
• Thrombolysis of acute thromboembolic stroke	ICH Concomitant coronary artery disease Blood pressure control[a]
• Intra-arterial chemotherapy of head and neck tumors	Airway swelling Intracranial hypertension
• Embolization for epistaxis	Airway control

[a] Blood pressure control refers to deliberate hypo- or hypertension.

NOTE: ICH, intracranial hemorrhage; NPPB, normal perfusion pressure breakthrough

remain to be scientifically validated in future clinical trials or studies.

INR Considerations Pertinent to Anesthetic Care

GENERAL COMMENTS ON INR PROCEDURES

Diagnostic neuroradiology has advanced tremendously in recent years; cerebral angiography was a surgical procedure in the 1950s.[12] Even standard *diagnostic* cerebral angiography has a low but significant morbidity associated with it. Large studies estimate the permanent neurologic morbidity at about 0.3 percent.[13,14]

Interventional neuroradiology is a complex endovascular intervention carried out on a vessel with proven pathology. The procedures performed in INR practice are inherently more dangerous than diagnostic studies. In a recent review of our series,[15] the total 30-

day rate of complications was 33 of 243 procedures (14 percent). Although the total for death and major complications was only 3 of 243 (1.2 percent),[15] it is probably more reasonable to expect catastrophic outcomes for major cerebrovascular treatments to be closer to 5 percent, similar to operative neurovascular series. For example, Purdy and colleagues reported in 1991 an incidence of intracranial hemorrhage (ICH) during arteriovenous malformation (AVM) embolization of 11 percent (7 of 63), with a poor outcome of 5 percent (3 of 63), even in experienced hands.[16] A primary goal of anesthesia coverage is immediate intervention in the event of catastrophe such as ICH or acute vascular insufficiency.

THERAPEUTIC GOALS

Because INR therapy is relatively new, precise indications and efficacy of many of the treatment modalities require further definition. For a detailed discussion of indications and experience, the reader is referred elsewhere.[1-8,17-23] However, a basic grasp of the terms, general concepts, and methodology is desirable for optimal anesthesia care and further development of the field.

The goals of INR therapy, as in any surgical or invasive therapy, must be well defined. In general, goals fall into three classes of treatment: (1) *definitive*, such as certain dural and spinal fistulae; (2) *adjunctive* therapy for surgery or radiotherapy, for example, preoperative embolization of AVM feeding arteries that will be difficult to control during craniotomy; or (3) *palliative*, for example, intraarterial chemotherapy for a malignant and inoperable brain tumor.

Many of the considerations described below are also applicable to certain complex neuroradiologic diagnostic procedures. *Superselective angiography* can define complex angioarchitecture not visualized on routine angiography. Proximal carotid or vertebral artery *test occlusion* may be used. Finally *provocative testing* with deliberate hypotension during test occlusions or superselective anesthesia functional examination (SAFE), such as intraarterial amobarbital administration into vascular territories at risk, fall into this category.

ENDOVASCULAR ACCESS AND METHODS

The INR procedures typically involve placing special catheters into the arterial circulation of the head, neck, or spinal cord. The transfemoral approach is used in most cases although direct carotid or brachial puncture may be used in special circumstances. The umbilical artery may be used in neonates.

Catheters are usually measured as "French" (F), which equals the circumference in millimeters

TABLE 25-2
Approximate Sizes

French	Millimeter	Mils	Gauge
1	0.33	13	29
1.5	0.5	20	25
2	0.66	26	
2.7	0.9	35	
2.9	0.96	38	
3	1	40	19.5
3.7	1.25	49	18
4	1.35	52	
4	1.67	66	16
6	2	78	14.5
7	2.3	92	

(3 F is about 1 mm diameter); wires are measured in "Mils," which is diameter in thousandths of an inch (040 Mils = 1 mm or 3 F). Gauge, used for needles, is the number of items laid side-to-side that are required to make an inch (14 g = about 6.3 F = about 083 mm). Table 25-2 shows sizes for comparisons (see Rüfenacht and Latchaw[24] for a detailed discussion of this topic).

As illustrated in Fig. 25-1, transfemoral access is accomplished by the placement of a large introducer sheath into the femoral artery, usually 7.5 F. The transfemoral puncture site may be infiltrated with a local anesthetic, such as 0.25% bupivicaine. Because of the proximity of the femoral nerve, inadvertent femoral nerve block may result in a motor and sensory deficit that must be differentiated from CNS damage. Through this introducer a 7.0 *coaxial* catheter is then positioned by fluoroscopic control into the carotid or vertebral arteries. Finally, a 1.5 to 2.7 F *superselective* microcatheter is then introduced into the cerebral circulation. There are both wired-guided and flow-directed microcatheters. The superselective catheter may be used to deliver drugs, embolic agents, or balloons to the desired location.

Transfemoral *venous* access can be used to reach the dural sinuses and, in some cases, the arterial side of the AVMs as well. Direct percutaneous puncture is used for access to superficial venous malformations.

THERAPEUTIC MATERIALS

The nature of the disease, purpose of the embolization, size and penetration of emboli and vessels, and permanency of occlusion are among the factors taken into consideration for agent selection. The ideal choice and combination of agents is controversial.[22,25,26] Table 25-3 summarizes the various materials in current use.

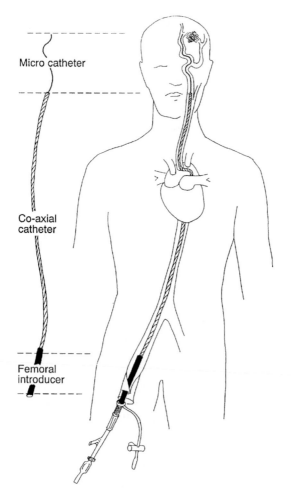

Figure 25-1 Catheter placement. Representation of a typical arrangement of the transfemoral coaxial catheter system showing the femoral introducer, the coaxial catheter, and the microcatheter (superselective catheter). (Adapted from Young WL: *Clinical Neuroscience Lectures.* Cathenart Publishing, Munster, IN, 1995, with permission.)

Glues are of particular usefulness in our experience, the newest being *N*-butyl cyanoacrylate (NBCA). It is a low viscosity liquid monomer that polymerizes to a solid form on contact with ionic solutions, including blood and saline, but remains liquid in a 5% dextrose in water solution. It is blended with radiopaque tantalum powder and an oil-based agent such as ethiodized oil (a contrast agent used for lymphography and hysterosalpingography). Depending on the clinical situation, the radiologist may adjust how fast the glue solidifies once it is injected into the circulation by adjusting the polymerization time. Increasing the amount of oil can vary polymerization time from a few milliseconds to over 5 s.

No vascular stents are available at present; however, the early results of using stents designed for other purposes are promising.[27]

IMAGING TECHNOLOGY

Necessary radiologic imaging methods include high-resolution fluoroscopy and high-speed digital subtraction angiography (DSA). High-speed DSA can provide up to 30 images per second. To remove bone shadows and other nonvascular structures from the images, a "scout" film is taken before each run, as shown in Fig. 25-2. This scout film serves as a "mask." The mask is subtracted by computer from all subsequent images in the run so that only vessels opacified with contrast are visualized.

Injection of contrast through distally placed superselective catheters yields a level of specificity to delineate vascular anatomy and the pathologic nature of the diseases in detail not obtainable with the proximal—internal carotid—injection used for conventional angiography. This is particularly pertinent for certain complex AVMs and aneurysms.

To facilitate placement of superselective catheters into the distal circulation, a technique called "roadmapping" is used. To make a "roadmap," a bolus of contrast is injected into the circulation from the proximal coaxial catheter (e.g., the internal carotid or vertebral artery) to obtain an image that demonstrates the vascular anatomy. The computer then superimposes this image on the live fluoroscopy image so that the radiologists can see the progress of the radiopaque

TABLE 25-3
Materials Used in Interventional Neuroradiology Procedures[a]

Balloons	Detachable
	Nondetachable
Solid agents	Polyvinyl alcohol particles
	Oxidized cotton
	Suture material
	Coils
	Simple coils
	Detachable coils
	Silastic pellets
Liquid agents	Cyanoacrylates (NBCA)
	USP grade 95% ethanol
Thrombolytic agents	Urokinase
	Streptokinase
	Tissue plasminogen activator
Chemotherapeutic agents for tumors	

[a] This list is not meant to be all inclusive and is for illustrative purposes only.

NOTE: NBCA, *N*-butyl cyanoacrylate.

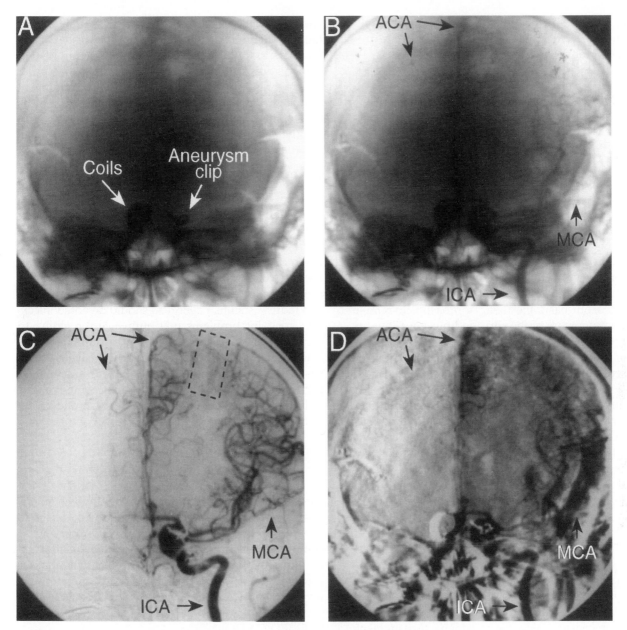

Figure 25-2 Digital subtraction angiography and image degradation. *A.* A scout antero-posterior skull film. This patient had two paraclinoid carotid aneurysms; one was treated with endovascular coils and the other by surgical clipping. *B.* The same view with contrast injected through the internal carotid artery. *C.* The contrast injection with background subtraction. The subtraction process makes vessel identification much clearer. Further, this digital subtracted vascular image (or "map") may be used as a backdrop during live fluoroscopy to serve as a "roadmap" for the passage of microcatheters into the distal circulation. Note the smaller vessels are only visualized well with background subtraction. The rectangular dotted-line box represents the "watershed" cortical zone between the anterior cerebral artery (ACA) and middle cerebral artery (MDA). (See also Figs. 25-4 and 25-12.) *D.* An example of how patient motion profoundly degrades the image. (Adapted from Young WL: *Clinical Neuroscience Lectures.* Cathenart Publishing, Munster, IN, 1995, with permission.)

catheter (especially the tip) against the "roadmap." Any motion during this stage of the procedure profoundly degrades the image.

Anesthetic Considerations

CHOICE OF ANESTHETIC MANAGEMENT: INTRAVENOUS SEDATION VERSUS GENERAL ANESTHESIA

The choice of primary anesthetic technique must be governed by two major considerations: (1) the dictates of the procedure and (2) the experience and expectations of the surgical and anesthetic team. Our bias is to perform procedures that can benefit from functional evaluation of the treated area (e.g., glue embolization of cerebral AVMs) during intravenous sedation. Our remarks, therefore, are made with this bias in mind.

In adults, our basic anesthetic approach is to render the patient unaware of the surroundings yet allow for rapid return to consciousness for intermittent assessment of neurologic function during manipulation of the vasculature. This goal is, at the present time, most easily achieved using deep intravenous sedation and allowing the patient to breathe spontaneously with an unprotected airway. There is no good nomenclature for such an anesthetic state so we will, for the sake of simplicity, refer to it as intravenous sedation in the following discussion. In earlier reviews we have used the term "conscious sedation." However, this term can be misleading in that it does not adequately communicate the concerns of the anesthesiologist regarding airway management to the rest of the operative team. Small children and uncooperative adult patients will require more traditional general anesthesia with endotracheal intubation. General anesthesia is also routinely used for certain procedures, as described in following sections.

A major consideration for anesthetic management during INR is that, while the patients receive intravenous sedative drugs, the routine and potential emergency management of these cases is much more interactive than a typical "monitored anesthesia care" (MAC) case due to frequent changes in level of consciousness and manipulation of systemic arterial blood pressure. In addition, the nature of many of the potential complications requires immediate intervention of the anesthesiologist.

Although MAC is appropriate for a diagnostic procedure or a minor surgical procedure that is performed primarily with local anesthesia supplemented by minimal sedation, active manipulation of hemodynamics and sensorium render a description more akin to "dynamic akinetic sedation with controlled hemodynamics" (DASCH). *Dynamic* refers to repeated lightening and deepening of sedation, *akinetic* stresses the importance of an immobile patient, and *controlled hemodynamics* refers to the physiologic trespass by manipulation of blood pressure. Acronyms aside, a challenging problem in orienting new staff to the INR environment is that the anesthetic care of these patients may be potentially much more involved than in other, superficially similar, settings.

PREPROCEDURE CONSIDERATIONS

HISTORY

In addition to the usual preanesthetic evaluation of the neurosurgical patient, previous experience with angiography, history of prior anticoagulation or coagulation disorders, protamine allergy (including insulin use, fish allergy, and prior vasectomy), recent steroid use, and contrast reactions (including general atopy and iodine/shellfish allergies) should be noted. Neck, back, or joint problems may influence the ability to secure the airway or tolerance to lying supine for several hours. In the population with occlusive cerebrovascular disease, control of preprocedure essential hypertension is critical for perioperative hemodynamic stability.[28] Pregnancy in female patients should be determined.

PHYSICAL EXAMINATION

Intravenous sedation may predispose certain patients to airway obstruction; checking the patency of the nares will let the anesthesiologist know which side is less likely to present a problem if the need arises to place a nasal cannula intraoperatively. Of special concern is the patient with a tumor or venous malformation that involves the upper airway. The potential for postprocedure swelling that might compromise the airway should be carefully discussed with the INR team.

PREMEDICATION

An anxiolytic may be given, if appropriate to the patient's sensorium. In patients in whom oral secretions are foreseen to be or have previously been a problem, atropine or glycopyrrolate can be administered intravenously in the angiography suite.

Prophylaxis for cerebral ischemia is in a state of development. Nimodipine may be useful in the treatment of cerebral ischemia in the setting of ischemic stroke[29] and subarachnoid hemorrhage (SAH).[30-32] Because of the lack of impressive side effects,[33,34] we use oral nimodipine as a premedication in patients with an appreciable risk of cerebral ischemia. This calcium channel blocker is also felt to lessen the incidence of traumatic vessel spasm during catheter passage; nifedipine is used by some for this purpose.[35] The above notwithstanding, efficacy of calcium channel blockers

TABLE 25-4
Anesthesia Setup: Drugs and Equipment Recommended
for Typical Intravenous Sedation Interventional
Neuroradiology Cases

Equipment	Routine Drugs	Emergency Drugs
Infusion pumps	Midazolam	Protamine
Portable monitor for transport	Fentanyl	Thiopental
	Droperidol	Succinylcholine
O₂ tank for transport	Propofol for bolus and infusion	Nondepolarizing muscle relaxant
Laryngoscopy and airway supplies	Heparin	Atropine
Source of suction	Phenylephrine for bolus and infusion	Lidocaine
Anesthesia machine with ventilator	Esmolol for infusion	Ephedrine
		Mannitol
	Labetolol	

for such prophylactic purposes has not been documented to be effective by randomized, controlled studies.

Other authors have described additional considerations for premedication, including corticosteroids, anticonvulsants, aspirin, and antibiotics.[20]

ROOM PREPARATION

Ideally, the INR suite should be equipped for anesthetic care exactly as is a standard operating room. Suction, gas evacuation, oxygen, and nitrous oxide should be available from wall outlets. Dedicated 20-ampere power lines, including emergency circuits, should be available. A dedicated telephone line for the anesthesia team for laboratory communication and management of neurologic catastrophes is essential. A refrigerator for drugs should be in the room or immediately accessible. Emergency equipment for cardiopulmonary resuscitation, including defibrillator and materials for surgical airway access, should be immediately available. The anesthesia machine should ideally have the ability to provide CO₂ gas (discussed in the section on induced hypercapnia). Adequate spotlighting should be available to maintain the anesthesia record and observe monitors because the room lights are often dimmed for viewing of the fluoroscopy screens. Long or extension tubing from the anesthesia gas circuit is desirable.

Many angiography suites have doors that automatically switch off fluoroscopy when they are opened. This can be detrimental in the event of emergencies (i.e., if someone enters the room during a critical manipulation of the intracerebral catheters). An entry "maze" is preferable that allows room access at all times but still provides radiation protection to those outside of the room.

Routine equipment and drugs to have at hand are listed in Table 25-4. Because the risk of intracranial hemorrhage or vascular occlusion is ever present, airway, intubation, and induction materials and vasoactive drugs must be prepared for immediate use and remain near the head of the table.

CONDUCT OF ANESTHESIA

PATIENT POSITIONING

Because the procedures may take many hours, having the patient as comfortable as possible before beginning sedation is essential. No amount of intravenous sedation can substitute for careful patient positioning. A comfortable air or foam mattress and some type of device for good head and neck positioning are needed. After the femoral introducer sheath has been placed, a pillow may be placed under the knees to obtain a modest amount of flexion, which may improve patient tolerance to prolonged periods of lying supine. Because patients may return for multiple treatments, continued patient acceptance is important. Head position needs to be maintained constant, so a headrest that discourages movement or paper tape across the patient's forehead is used as a "reminder." Use of rigid fixation should be avoided because it might increase the likelihood of aspiration if emesis occurs.

INTRAVENOUS VASCULAR ACCESS

To maximize the distance between the fluoroscopy unit and the anesthesiologist, extension tubing in the intravenous lines is recommended. In one line, a stopcock or infusion port near the patient can be used for continuous drug infusions. A second line may be used for bolus injections through a port furthest from the image intensifier during fluoroscopy, to minimize staff radiation exposure. When the patient is draped with arms restrained and advanced toward the image intensifier, access to intravenous sites is difficult. Therefore, anesthetics and vasoactive drugs should be in-line and ready to infuse before the patient is moved into final position, and all lines should be clearly labeled.

ARTERIAL PRESSURE MONITORING

We use direct transduction of arterial pressure in any intracranial or spinal cord procedure; it is certainly indicated whenever the likelihood exists for manipulation of systemic pressure with vasoactive agents, in procedures involving the posterior fossa or upper cervical cord, or when mitigating medical considerations exist. There is little, if any, additional risk to the patient, because the arterial system is cannulated as part of the treatment. For the typical intracranial procedure, three arterial pressures are easily monitored. Pressure transducers and access stopcocks for blood withdrawal and zeroing are mounted either on the sterile field or toward the anesthesia team. The advantage of having the stopcocks and transducers on the field is that the radiology team assumes the care of the various connections as part of their setup and the likelihood of inadvertently flushing or injecting the wrong catheter is greatly reduced. The disadvantage is that the anesthesia team cannot draw blood samples and zero the transducers. We opt for the former.

Although some institutions also perform radial artery catheterizations, the femoral artery introducer sheath is easily used as the real-time monitor of arterial pressure. A disadvantage is that it consistently underestimates the systolic and overestimates the diastolic pressure, due to the coaxial catheter passing through it. However, the mean pressures are reliable and may be used to safely monitor the induction of either hyper- or hypotension. The femoral catheter is continually flushed with an intraflow device at 3 ml/h of heparinized saline, which does not appreciably influence the mean pressure recording.

The second pressure is transduced from the coaxial catheter (or a balloon catheter to give a "stump" pressure) in the carotid or the vertebral artery. The reasons for monitoring this pressure are several. Thrombus formation and vascular spasm at the catheter tip or migration of the catheter may be diagnosed by damping of the waveform. Also, leads in the introducer collar for the superselective catheter will appear as a loss of pressure in the coaxial tracing. A high volume (100 ml/h) continuous heparinized flush is passed through the coaxial tip to discourage thrombus formation (this infusion characteristically results in an approximate 20 mmHg increase in the coaxial pressure and should be turned off for quantitative readings). A flush system malfunction can be suggested by a change in or loss of the waveform.

Finally, the pressure at the tip of a superselective catheter may be monitored. This is useful during intracranial AVM embolization. The use of microcatheters for mean pressure measurements has been validated by Duckweiler and colleagues.[36]

OTHER SYSTEMIC MONITORING

Other monitors should include a 5-lead electrocardiogram (ECG) (ideally with automated ST-segment trending) and automatic blood pressure cuff (Table 25-5). In patients at risk for myocardial ischemia, a baseline recording of the ECG may be helpful for later comparisons during hemodynamic manipulation. A pulse oximeter probe is placed on the great toe of the leg that will receive the femoral catheters. This can give an early warning of femoral artery obstruction or distal thromboembolism. It is also useful when the femoral sheath must be removed and the site compressed for hemostasis, particularly in smaller children where overvigorous compression can lead to permanent occlusion of the vessel.

TABLE 25-5
Common Monitoring for Intravenous Sedation and Blood Pressure Manipulation

Systemic Monitoring
5-lead ECG (ideally with automated ST-segment trending)
Pulse oximeter (on limb receiving catheter)
Pet_{CO_2} (or at least measurement of respiratory rate)
Temperature probe (axillary or bladder catheter)
Bladder catheter
Direct arterial pressure measurement

CNS Monitoring Options
Neurologic examination
EEG
Somatosensory and motor-evoked potentials
Transcranial Doppler ultrasound (TCD)
^{133}Xe cerebral blood flow (CBF)
Tomographic CBF (stable Xe or SPECT)

NOTE: Pet_{CO_2}, partial pressure of end-tidal CO_2; CNS, central nervous system; EEG, electroencephalogram; SPECT, single photo emission computed tomography

Oxygen (2 to 4 liter/min) is given by nasal cannula with a system to sample and monitor partial pressure of end-tidal CO_2 (Pet_{CO_2}). Low flows and humidification of the O_2 may improve patient tolerance. For the patient spontaneously breathing O_2, an indicator of respiratory rate is recommended if Pet_{CO_2} is not available and may be useful for detecting abnormal respiratory patterns that may be encountered during procedures involving the posterior fossa.

Temperature may be monitored in a number of ways, such as an axillary probe or bladder catheter thermistor. Shivering is a troublesome problem because it results in patient motion and image degradation, and every effort should be made to keep the patient's temperature near normal (except in the case of a neurologic catastrophe).

All patients undergoing transfemoral procedures receive bladder catheters to assist in fluid management as well as for patient comfort. A significant volume of heparinized flush solution may be necessary over the course of the procedure and radiographic contrast is an osmotic diuretic. Administration of other diuretics such as mannitol or furosemide may also be required for fluid management or in the event of a catastrophe. Condom-type catheters are not recommended.

When the patient's condition warrants placement of a central venous or pulmonary artery catheter, central catheters may be positioned using fluoroscopy. Similarly, the endotracheal tube position for general anesthesia cases is easily verified by fluoroscopy of the chest during passage of the coaxial catheters.

CNS MONITORING

During many procedures the neurologic examination provides adequate monitoring of CNS integrity, as the INR team will follow the neurologic examination as an index of distal ischemia. Adjuncts, especially useful during general anesthesia or planned proximal occlusions, include EEG,[37,38] somatosensory[37] and motor-evoked potentials, transcranial Doppler ultrasound (TCD),[39] and ^{133}Xe cerebral blood flow (CBF) monitoring.[19]

Other methods of determining the cerebral hemodynamic effect of proximal carotid or vertebral occlusion that may be used during the period of anesthesia care include CBF measurement with stable ^{133}Xe computed tomography (CT) scanning or single photon emission computed tomography (SPECT).[40–43] There is still debate as to which of the physiologic imaging procedures yields the most appropriate information for a given clinical setting.[44]

ANESTHETIC TECHNIQUES

Intravenous Sedation

Primary goals of anesthetic choice for sedation include alleviating pain or discomfort, providing anxiolysis and patient immobility, but at the same time allowing for a rapid decrease in the level of sedation when neurologic testing is required.

The procedures, in general, are not painful, exceptions being sclerotherapy and chemotherapy. An element of pain may be associated with injection of contrast into the cerebral arteries (burning) and with distension or traction on them (headache). Discomfort, however, from long periods of lying still is the rule. Insertion of the bladder catheter and, to a lesser extent, the initial groin puncture for the femoral cannulation are two notable points of discomfort.

The procedure is also psychologically stressful. A risk of serious stroke or death is present. This may be particularly important in a patient who has already suffered a preoperative hemorrhage or stroke.

Movement by the patient will decrease the usefulness of the roadmapping techniques and could potentially result in a complication. For example, a guidewire or catheter could penetrate a vessel wall and still appear to reside within the lumen.

Anesthetic agents are selected to meet the above goals. Our primary approach to intravenous sedation is to establish a base of neurolept anesthesia by titration (per 70 kg) of 100 to 150 μg/kg of fentanyl, 2 to 4 mg of droperidol, and 3 to 5 mg of midazolam after intravenous access and O$_2$ administration has been started. The goal of this initial drug titration is to render the patient immobile and generally unaware of the surroundings, but still arousable with adequate spontaneous ventilation. A small bolus of propofol may be useful as the bladder catheter is passed.

When the patient is in final position and draping begins, a propofol infusion is started at low levels (10 to 20 μg/kg per min) and then titrated slowly to result in an unconscious patient with a patent airway. The use of propofol gives the anesthesiologist some degree of control when a rapid return to consciousness is needed for neurologic assessment.

All patients should receive supplemental O$_2$ during intravenous sedation techniques. Placement of nasopharyngeal airways may cause troublesome bleeding in anticoagulated patients and is generally avoided. If the need for a nasopharyngeal airway is expected, it is prudent to place it before anticoagulation and to observe meticulous hemostasis.

Droperidol may be useful in a neurolept technique because of its antiemetic effect, α-adrenergic blockade, and our impression that it renders a calmer, more motionless patient than do benzodiazepines alone. Postprocedure dysphoria is a theoretical concern and dopadrenergic blockade can result in extrapyramidal symptoms in normal patients as well as in those with Parkinson's disease.[45]

Other sedation regimens and variations are possible[2,35,46–48] and must be based on the experience of the practitioner and the goals of anesthetic management for a particular procedure. In our experience and in that of others, chloral hydrate and ketamine-based techniques have little to offer.[47] A predominantly propofol-based technique is possible. Our enthusiasm for this method, however, quickly waned because of an unacceptably high incidence of upper airway obstruction, which led to nasopharyngeal airway placement in an anticoagulated patient and enough epistaxis to complicate airway control. In addition, troublesome behavioral disinhibition occurred frequently.

Laryngeal mask airways may have a place in the management of deep intravenous sedation in these cases.* If they are used, care must be taken to ensure that there is not excessive motion during the period when the depth of anesthesia is decreased to remove the airway. Coughing or bucking with the large, stiff introducer catheters in the neck vessels may result in vascular injury.

General Anesthesia with Endotracheal Intubation

Small children and uncooperative adult patients require general anesthesia with endotracheal intubation. General anesthesia is also routinely used for certain procedures such as aneurysm ablation, sclerotherapy, and certain cases of chemotherapy. Children from 12 to 15 years old will usually tolerate intravenous seda-

---

* Irene Osborn, MD; David J. Stone, MD: Personal communication.

tion if the procedure is carefully explained to them and their parents preoperatively and if they are well coached on what to expect during treatment.

No evidence suggests that general anesthesia with endotracheal intubation should differ in the INR suite from its usual intraoperative application, be it for adult or pediatric cases. Anesthetic choice and cerebral protection during neurosurgical procedures is extensively reviewed elsewhere.[49] A theoretical argument could be made for eschewing the use of N_2O because of the possibility of introducing air emboli into the cerebral circulation, but no data support this.

When general anesthesia is used, it is frequently to obtain a motionless patient to improve the quality of the images. This is especially pertinent to INR treatment of spinal pathology, where sometimes exhaustive multilevel angiography must be performed. Because chest excursion during positive-pressure ventilation may interfere with roadmapping, radiologists frequently request apnea for DSA in spinal procedures. An effective alternative to apnea is to adjust the ventilator to a relatively rapid rate and small tidal volume. Adequate gas exchange can be maintained during brief periods without degrading the image quality by excessive chest excursion. If available, this may be an ideal application for high-frequency jet ventilation.

An additional anesthetic technique is a "hybrid" of traditional general anesthesia and intravenous sedation and is usually applied for intraoperative "wake up" to assess spinal cord function. However, it may also be used for intracranial procedures in patients who have difficulty maintaining an acceptable airway with intravenous sedation but need to be functionally evaluated during the course of embolization. Our method is to use nasotracheal intubation and maintain anesthesia using a nitrous-narcotic technique. Before neurologic testing is needed, 4% lidocaine is instilled around the cuff of the endotracheal tube. The N_2O is then discontinued and the narcotic infusion titrated downward until the patient is able to follow commands but tolerate the presence of the endotracheal tube.

ANTICOAGULATION
Careful management of coagulation is required to prevent thromboembolic complications during and after the procedures, although algorithms for anticoagulation remain controversial.[2,16,17] It is certainly indicated whenever permanent or test occlusion is performed. Distal thromboembolism or clot propagation can be a major source of complications after major vascular occlusion.

Whether heparinization should be used for *every* case of intracranial catheterization is not clear. Some would argue that anticoagulation increases the risk of intracranial hemorrhage. We feel that heparinization should be routinely performed during *any* superselective cath-

eterization. In addition to thrombus formation from foreign bodies in the circulation, a considerable amount of thrombogenic endothelial damage may be done by the passage of the superselective catheter.

After placement of the femoral introducer catheter, a baseline activated clotting time (ACT) is obtained. Heparin, 5000 units/70 kg, is given and another ACT is checked to verify a target prolongation of at least two to three times baseline. ACT is monitored at least every hour. If an ACT is not drawn on schedule because of some extenuating circumstance, 2000 units heparin is given empirically every hour. The risk of overdosing the patient on heparin in this fashion is minimal compared to the risk of inadvertent thrombus formation. Heparin dose and ACT may be entered in a graphic manner on the anesthesia record so that it is easier to follow trends at a glance.

In our practice, heparin is continued through the first postprocedure night. The rationale for postprocedure anticoagulation is both to protect against the thrombogenic effects of endothelial trauma and the inherently thrombogenic nature of the materials instilled, such as glue or coils, which can cause retrograde thrombosis in embolized vessels. A period of 24 h is felt to be sufficient for a "pseudoendothelial" layer to form and prevent either retrograde or antegrade thrombus formation that may propagate along the arterial tree (and the venous system in AVMs) with potentially disastrous results. The heparin effect is then allowed to wane on the first postprocedure day. Because the patient is heparinized, the large introducer sheath in the groin is left in place the first postprocedure night and removed before discharge to the floor on the following morning.

Sometimes the procedure may be aborted before any foreign material is deposited or significant endothelial trauma has occurred. For example, superselective angiography or provocative testing may reveal that a lesion is not amenable to treatment. In this event, heparin may be electively reversed with protamine at the conclusion of the procedure and the femoral catheter removed in the angiography suite. However, our practice is evolving in this respect. Because of the endothelial damage that occurs with intracranial navigation of microcatheters, an argument can be made for continuing heparin therapy for the first night postoperatively, even when no embolic materials have been placed.

An occasional patient may be refractory to attempts to obtain adequate anticoagulation. Switching from bovine to porcine heparin or vice versa may be of use. If antithrombin III deficiency is suspected, administration of fresh frozen plasma may be necessary.

OTHER LABORATORY TESTS TO MONITOR
A baseline arterial blood gas (ABG) at the time of the first ACT is useful to determine a baseline Pa_{O_2} to

Sa_{O_2} gradient as well as the Pa_{CO_2} to Pet_{CO_2} gradient. Although the correlation between Pa_{CO_2} and Pet_{CO_2} is usually good during general anesthesia,[50] monitoring Pet_{CO_2} through the nasal cannula is less precise and the discrepancy between end-tidal and arterial values is greater. In 33 patients anesthetized with the neurolept/propofol technique described above, mean ± SD Pet_{CO_2} was 32 ± 9 mmHg when Pa_{CO_2} was 46 ± 7 mmHg, with an average gradient of 14 ± 9 mmHg.[15]

The patients receive large quantities of fluid and contrast media and may diurese considerably and a baseline hematocrit determination is helpful. The issue of optimal hematocrit in the brain-injured patient is controversial.[51,52] Based on available evidence, both extremes of hemodilution and hemoconcentration should be avoided. Because intravenous ethanol administration may result in hypoglycemia,[53] monitoring blood glucose may be considered in sclerotherapy patients who might be prone to hypoglycemia.

SUPERSELECTIVE ANESTHESIA FUNCTIONAL EXAMINATION (SAFE)

Before therapeutic embolization, SAFE is performed to determine if the tip of the catheter has been inadvertently placed proximal to the origin of nutritive vessels to eloquent regions, either in the brain or spinal cord.[11,38,54] Such testing is an extension of the Wada and Rasmussen test[55] in which amobarbital is injected into the internal carotid artery (ICA) to determine hemispheric dominance and language function. Its primary application is in the setting of AVM treatment, but it may also be used for tumor or other vascular malformation work.

An additional setting for the use of SAFE is in the preoperative evaluation of the patient being considered for surgical treatment of epilepsy. Confident identification of the laterality of memory is essential before temporal resection. Not infrequently, however, intracarotid artery injection of amytal will fill both the anterior and the middle cerebral artery territories and cause inattention that makes memory examination unreliable. This can be alleviated by superselective amytal injection of the vesels feeding the territory planned for surgical resection.

Before testing, the level of sedation should be decreased, for example, by stopping the propofol infusion. In rare instances, it may be necessary to use naloxone or flumazenil to antagonize other intravenous agents, but this should be avoided by not oversedating the patient with fixed agents. A baseline, focused neurologic examination under residual light sedation is performed by the INR team. Sodium amobarbital (30 mg) or lidocaine (30 mg), mixed with contrast, is then given via the superselective catheter and an angiogram obtained of the distribution of the drug/contrast mixture. The doses and volume (0.5 to 3 ml) of agent may be altered to fit the clinical situation. Sodium amobarbital is used for investigating gray matter areas. Lidocaine may be used for evaluating the integrity of white matter tracts, especially in the spinal cord.[56,57] Injection of lidocaine may result in seizures when used in the brain, particularly in areas such as motor strip. Besides being disquieting to the patient and increasing the risk of aspiration, seizure activity can result in a transient focal neurologic deficit. A postictal paralysis, for example, can confuse interpretation of the test. For this reason, the barbiturate is usually given first, followed by lidocaine. If the amobarbital is negative, it may protect against cortical seizure but not significantly interfere with assessment of lidocaine's effect on white matter tracts. Not all authors agree on the use of lidocaine for intracerebral testing.[38]

After drug injection, the neurologic examination is repeated. Attention is directed to areas at risk as well as "quiet areas" where a deficit might be missed if only a motor or sensory examination is performed, such as dominant parietal lobe.

Generally, SAFE is reliable, but false-positive tests can occur with overinjection and reflux into normal vessels. Underinjection, or a "sump" effect from an AVM, may lead to false-negative results.[3] Systemic recirculation of the anesthetic may, in some cases, result in generalized sedation. Rauch and colleagues described the use of electroencephalographic (EEG) monitoring, coupled with a clinical examination, to enhance the sensitivity of SAFE.[38]

It has been argued that knowledge of neuroanatomy and angioarchitecture can replace functional testing for the purpose of AVM embolization. The problem with this approach is at least twofold. First, there is considerable variation in the normal localization of function and, second, cerebral pathology may cause neurologic function to shift from its native location to another. Functional relocalization (transference) is a poorly understood phenomena but appears to be operative in several disease states, including ischemic stroke.[58,59] For example, Chollet and coworkers studied finger movement on a previously plegic hand after unilateral stroke. They found significant regional CBF changes after activation in both the contralateral and ipsilateral primary sensorimotor cortex and in both cerebellar hemispheres.[58,59] The mechanisms for this functional transference are unknown. Diaschisis may be involved in the transference or recovery of function.[60] After the inhibition of a distant site, an active repair process may ensue.

Our surgical experience indicates that resection in eloquent regions is more frequently associated with new deficits, suggesting that transfer should be relatively rare. Others have also proposed that AVMs, as opposed to tumors, do not displace cerebral function from adjacent tissues.[61] However, a recent large pro-

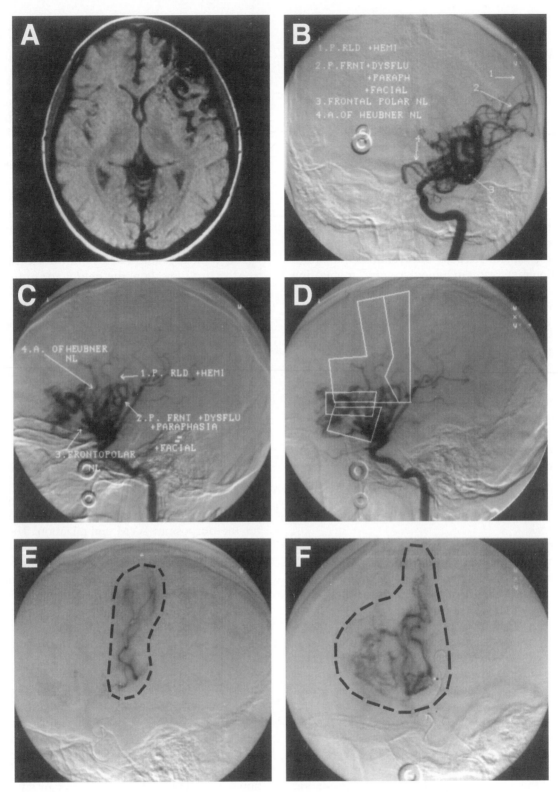

Figure 25-3 Selective anesthetic testing to local cerebral function. This case is a 34-year-old female who presented with headache from intracranial hemorrhage but was neurologically intact. *A*. T1 axial MRI that shows the left frontal AVM. Four pedicles were tested for eloquence. These vessels are shown in *B* (anteroposterior carotid injection) and *C* (lateral carotid injection). Corresponding territories are shown in *D*. The following results were obtained: No anesthetic-induced deficits were encountered after anesthetic injection of the *artery of Heubner* (66 mmHg at a systemic mean of 86), the *orbital frontal artery* (54 mmHg at a systemic mean of 87 mmHg) or the *fronto-polar*

spective surgical series did not find eloquence of the operative site to be related to outcome.[62] Therefore, functional localization in patients with AVMs remains a controversial topic.

An example of how language function was found in an unexpected location is shown in Fig. 25-3. Whether localization was a result of the AVM itself or from a spontaneous intracerebral hemorrhage is an open question.

DELIBERATE HYPOTENSION

The two primary indications for elective deliberate hypotension are (1) to slow flow in an AVM-feeding artery before injection of glue, termed *flow arrest*, and (2) to test cerebrovascular reserve in patients undergoing carotid occlusion. In most cases, the level of sedation is decreased so that neurologic examinations can be followed during the period of deliberate hypotension. In awake patients, nausea and vomiting can be a problem. It is for this reason that droperidol is an attractive choice as part of the sedative regime. An additional dose of droperidol (1.25 mg) may be given for anti-emesis just before starting hypotension (which usually begins at least 2 h after the initial dose). If nausea is known to be a problem from prior experience, ondansetron may be considered. Some practitioners expectantly give ondansetron in procedures that involve induced hypotension. Before beginning hypotension, one should confirm that the patient is fully oxygenated and the airway unobstructed.

Most of the AVM patients treated are relatively young and fit. Most importantly, they are not under general anesthesia and the adjunctive hypotensive effect of general anesthesia is absent during intravenous sedation. Therefore, it may be considerably more challenging to induce hypotension in this setting; sometimes surprisingly large doses of hypotensive agents may be necessary.

Our first-line agent is usually esmolol, given as a 1 mg/kg bolus and titrated to target systemic blood pressure at an infusion rate beginning at 0.5 mg/kg per min. High levels of infusion are often needed and boluses of labetolol (50 to 100 mg) are useful as an adjunct. Adrenergic blockers have the advantage of

not directly affecting CBF[63] and have the theoretical advantage of shifting the autoregulatory curve to the left.[64] Trimethaphan probably also shares such an effect.[65] Disadvantages of trimethaphan include tachyphylaxis and the large doses needed for awake patients. Use of large doses may result in pupillary dilation, which may confound the neurologic examination, and inhibition of plasma pseudocholinesterase.

Sodium nitroprusside (SNP) and nitroglycerin are standard hypotensive agents and may be used in INR.[35] A relative disadvantage of both drugs is that it is easy to overshoot and render the patient momentarily severely hypotensive. Although this can be treated without incident in the patient under general anesthesia with endotracheal intubation, the onset of hypotension-induced emesis and nausea in an awake patient can be disastrous in the INR setting from several standpoints. It can decrease the total amount of time available to the team for the procedure because of continued discomfort and interfere with angiographic visualization because of motion artifact. The nausea may be confused with acute intracranial hypertension from vascular perforation. Retching can cause migration of the intracranial catheters from the desired location, cause further endothelial damage, or produce vessel perforation. Additional theoretical considerations for cerebral vasodilators, including dihydralazine, is the potential for interfering with collateral perfusion to an ischemic region and the possibility of increasing cerebral blood volume in a patient with decreased intracranial compliance.

The above considerations regarding SNP notwithstanding, the drug may have some beneficial effects in the setting of cerebral ischemia as it is a nitric oxide (NO) donor. Zhang and colleagues showed that high-dose intracarotid SNP improved CBF and decreased infarct size.[66] Accumulating evidence indicates that manipulation of vascular tone in borderzone areas adjacent to a regional or focal ischemic process can be manipulated. Several independent lines of evidence suggest NO is beneficial in the initial stages of cerebral ischemia. L-Arginine, the precursor of NO, increases CBF to ischemic territories and attenuates focal ischemic damage.[67] Stimulation of the fastigial nucleus, a

Figure 25-3 (*Continued*)   branch (no pressures available). Anesthetic injection into the *peri-Rolandic branch* (*E*) resulted in contralateral paresis. Anesthetic injection into the *pre-frontal branch* (*F*) resulted in a facial weakness, dysfluency and paraphasic errors. The pressure in the pre-frontal branch was 46 mmHg at a systemic mean of 85 mmHg. Thus, this case is an example of a patient with decreased pressure in normal tissue adjacent to an AVM; language function has shifted anteriorly from the area where it is traditionally believed to reside. The influence of the prior hemorrhage is indeterminate in this case. Further studies are needed to document the relationship of functional shifts to local arterial pressure reductions and the influence of prior hemorrhage. (Adapted from Young WL: *Clinical Neuroscience Lectures.* Cathenart Publishing, Munster, IN, 1995, with permission.)

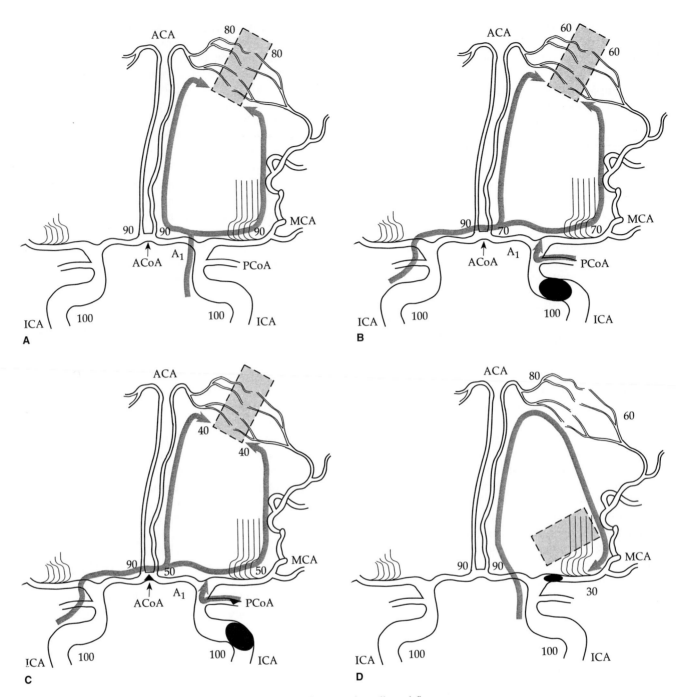

Figure 25-4 Depiction of collateral pathways. The basic considerations for collateral flow disturbances are presented in the following series of panels. The principle collateral conduits are the anterior communicating artery (ACoA), which connects to the contralateral carotid circulation, and the posterior communicating artery (PCoA), which connects to the vertebrobasilar circulation. The *shaded boxes* refer to the "watershed" areas between the territories of the anterior cerebral artery (ACA) and middle cerebral artery (MCA) circulations. This is the "equal pressure boundary" between multiple sources of arterial input pressure and may shift according to changes in vascular anatomy. The *small black triangles* represent regions of hemodynamically significant stenosis in collateral pathways. The *thick gray lines* represent the general sources and direction of arterial flow. The *numbers* represent hypothetical mean arterial pressure (in mmHg) that might be encountered in each scenario. The *black ovals* represent an obstruction to arterial flow; these might be balloon-tipped catheters or an arterial embolus. The arterial pressure values are illustrative only and other potential collateral pathways exist; the purpose of this illustration is to set forth the basic considerations of cerebral collateral flow. The lenticulostriate arteries which arise from the first portion of the MCA are seen as multiple thin curved lines. *A.* Normal: Flow supplies the ACA

procedure that increases neocortical CBF by local release of NO, improves CBF in ischemic regions and decreases infarct size.[68] Some investigators, but not all, reported NO synthase inhibitors enlarge infarct size.[66] These NO-related considerations remain to be placed in clinical perspective.

The most important factor in choosing a hypotensive agent is the ability to safely and expeditiously achieve the desired reduction in blood pressure while maintaining the patient physiologically stable. These goals can be achieved with a number of different agents and the experience of the clinician with a given agent is an important factor.

BLOOD PRESSURE AUGMENTATION (DELIBERATE HYPERTENSION)

Frequently a situation will arise in which the patient will experience cerebral ischemia from either a planned or inadvertent vascular occlusion. As reviewed by Young and Cole, the systemic blood pressure should be increased to drive adequate flow via collaterals to the area of ischemia as a temporizing measure.[69] The primary routes of collateral circulation are the willisian channels (anterior communicating artery, posterior communicating artery, and the ophthalmic via the external carotid artery).

The second main recourse for collateral flow in the hemispheres are the surface connections between pial arteries that bridge major arterial territories between anterior (ACA), middle (MCA), and posterior (PCA) cerebral arteries. These connections are called by various names. *Pial-to-pial anastomoses* or *collaterals* seem to be the most logical, but they are also called *leptomeningeal pathways*[70] (Fig. 25-4). These pathways may protect the so-called border zones or watershed areas between vascular territories. There is considerable confusion with this terminology.[71] Physiologically, a

more precise term might be "equal pressure boundary,"[72] where, under normal circumstances, pial flow does not cross collateral pathways into an adjacent territory because the pressure on either side of this distal territorial boundary is equal. There is considerable variation in the anatomic location of these boundaries. Examples would be large proximal vessel occlusions (carotid occlusion or moyamoya disease) or high-flow AVMs. Border zones may shift during the course of treatment if the vascular architecture is altered.

Collateral pathways are most efficacious during chronic ischemia, when they may gradually enlarge over time. Acutely, it is frequently necessary to augment blood pressure to effectively drive flow across them. Absence of adequate collateral pathways, especially in the circle of Willis, is a normal anatomic variant, so deliberate hypertension is not guaranteed to succeed. Deliberate hypertension can be used to treat acute cerebral ischemia by improving pial-to-pial collateral flow across a "watershed," as shown in Fig. 25-4.

Our first-line agent is a phenylephrine bolus (about 1 μg/kg) followed by titrated infusion to increase the pressure up to levels that reverse the neurologic deficit, empirically, 30 to 40 percent above baseline. The ECG and ST-segment monitor should be carefully inspected for signs of myocardial ischemia. Blood pressure goals must be tempered by the patient's preexisting medical status. Based on the best available evidence, deliberate hypertension in the face of symptomatic cerebral ischemia from vascular occlusion during AVM embolization should not be avoided because of fear of rupturing the malformation.[73]

If the heart rate is very low to start, for example, due to preoperative β-blockade or sinus node disease, an alternate choice would be dopamine, with or without phenylephrine. In our experience, use of dopamine

---

Figure 25-4 (*Continued*)   and MCA via the ipsilateral carotid artery. Although they are both patent, no appreciable flow is delivered through the ACoA or PCoA. *B.* Occluded internal carotid with normal collateral pathways. With an occlusion of the ICA, pressure decreases in the distal territory and flow now is recruited from the ACoA and PCoA conduits. The distal "watershed" remains in the same location but pressure is reduced significantly. *C.* Occluded internal carotid with poor collateral pathways. In this case, there is stenosis of both the ACoA and PCoA conduits. Therefore, the distal "watershed" is now severely hypotensive and at risk for infarction. Although not shown in the Figure, augmentation of systemic mean arterial pressure would improve the distal cerebral pressure by compensating for the pressure drop across the stenotic conduit pathways. *D.* Occluded first portion of the MCA: watershed shift. In this case, the occluded vessel is the first part of the MCA (M_1), which is distal to the conduit pathways of the circle of Willis. The only available collateral pathway is for flow to cross the pial-to-pial surface connections of the normal "watershed" (seen in *A* through *C*) and retrogradely fill the proximal portion of the MCA. The "watershed" has shifted now to the territory supplied by the lenticulostriate arteries; this circulation is the farthest from the arterial pressure input and is an "end-arterial" territory; the hypotension here is severe. (Adapted from Young WL: *Clinical Neuroscience Lectures.* Cathenart Publishing, Munster, IN, 1995, with permission.)

alone to induce hypertension frequently results in unacceptable tachycardia.

DELIBERATE HYPERCAPNIA

Venous malformations of the face or dural fistulas have the potential to drain into intracerebral veins or sinuses. During general anesthesia, hypercapnia is desirable for circumstances where agents are injected into the venous circulation. By increasing the Pa_{CO_2} to 50 to 60 mmHg, cerebral venous outflow will greatly exceed extracranial venous outflow and the pressure gradient will favor movement of either a sclerosing agent, chemotherapeutic agent, or glue away from critical intracranial drainage pathways. Although actual pressure gradients have never been studied, increased intracranial outflow is readily demonstrable in clinical practice with angiography. Addition of CO_2 gas to the inspired gas mixture is the easiest and safest way to achieve hypercapnia. Airway collapse and atelectasis are prevented by maintaining adequate tidal volume. However, hypoventilation may be used if CO_2 gas is not available; in this case, addition of positive endexpiratory pressure may be useful to maintain oxygenation.

TRANSPORT AND POSTPROCEDURE CONSIDERATIONS

After intracranial or intraspinal procedures, patients spend the first postprocedure night in the ICU. Complicated cases may go first to CT or SPECT scan; only rarely is an emergent craniotomy indicated. Blood pressure control, either modest hypotension in the case of AVM embolization or deliberate hypertension in the patient with occlusive or vasospastic cerebrovascular disease, should be continued during transport.

Postprocedure nausea and vomiting can be due to anesthetic agents or the large volumes of contrast agent. This general topic is reviewed elsewhere.[74] For procedures in the posterior fossa, small degrees of ischemia and swelling from contrast not infrequently result in symptomatic local brain swelling in the postprocedure period. In the more capacious supratentorial compartment, such minor swelling is rarely symptomatic. In the posterior fossa, this may present as delayed deficits or decreased sensorium during the course of the first evening after the procedure, particularly if cerebrospinal fluid (CSF) pathways become obstructed. This eventuality should be factored into decisions regarding airway management.

COMPLICATIONS AND SPECIAL CONSIDERATIONS

NEUROLOGIC CATASTROPHES

Complications during instrumentation of the cerebral vasculature can be rapid and dramatic and require

TABLE 25-6
Management of Neurologic Catastrophes[a]

Initial Resuscitation
Communicate with radiologists
Call for assistance
Secure the airway and hyperventilate with 100% O_2
Determine if problem is hemorrhagic or occlusive
Hemorrhagic: immediate heparin reversal (1 mg protamine for each 100 units of heparin activity) and low normal pressure
Occlusive: deliberate hypertension, titrated to neurologic examination, angiography or physiologic imaging studies (i.e., TCD, CBF, etc.)

Further Resuscitation
Head up 15° in neutral position
Titrate ventilation to a Pa_{CO_2} of 26–28 mmHg
Mannitol 0.5 g/kg, rapid IV infusion
Anticonvulsants—Dilantin (give slowly: 50 mg/min) and phenobarbitol
Titrate thiopental infusion to EEG burst suppression
Allow body temperature to fall as quickly as possible to 33°–34°C
Consider dexamethasone 10 mg if clinically appropriate

[a] These are only general recommendations and drug doses, which must be adapted to specific clinical situations and in accordance with a patient's preexisting medical condition. In some cases of asymptomatic or minor vessel puncture or occlusion, less aggressive management may be appropriate.

NOTE: TCD, transcranial Doppler; CBF, cerebral blood flow

a multidisciplinary collaboration.[16] Having a well thought out plan for dealing with intracranial catastrophes may make the difference between an uneventful outcome and death. A catastrophe plan outline is shown in Table 25-6, based on currently recommended approaches to the treatment of acute cerebral injury.[49,75]

If a neurologic catastrophe occurs, rapid and effective communication between the anesthesia and radiology teams is critical. The appropriate neurology and neurosurgical consultants should be contacted as soon as possible. The anesthesiologist should know enough about the nature and extent of the problem to effectively treat it. The primary responsibility of the anesthesia team is to preserve gas exchange and, if indicated, secure the airway. If endotracheal intubation is necessary, a thiopental and relaxant induction should not be avoided because of the possibility of a transient decrease in perfusion pressure.

Simultaneous with airway maintenance, the first branch in the decision-making algorithm is for the anesthesiologist to communicate with the INR team and determine whether the problem is hemorrhagic or occlusive.

In the setting of vascular occlusion, a method to

increase distal perfusion by blood pressure augmentation is the primary strategy and may be combined, if applicable, with thrombolysis. Note that thiopental will probably provide some degree of protection even after an occlusion.[76] Deliberate hypertension may be used in the setting of acute hemispheric ischemia from large vessel occlusion distal to the circle of Willis to improve collateral perfusion, as shown in Fig. 25-4.

If the problem is hemorrhagic, *immediate* reversal of heparin is indicated. Protamine is given as rapidly as possible to reverse heparin without undue regard for the systemic blood pressure. The cardiac output need only be as high as is necessary to achieve reversal of heparin (due to experience with cardiopulmonary bypass, there is a reflexive reluctance for most anesthesiologists to administer protamine rapidly enough). The dispatch with which heparin is reversed may very well be the critical step between a good and a poor outcome from the bleed.

As an emergency reversal dose, 1 mg protamine can be given for each 100 units "heparin effect." In other words, whatever was the initial dose required to increase the ACT to its maintenance level should be the target for emergency reversal. For example, if 5000 units heparin initially resulted in an ACT of 250 s, then 50 mg would be a reasonable reversal dose at any time during the case with an ACT of 250 s. The ACT can then be used to fine-tune the final protamine dose. Blood pressure control requires second-to-second communication with the radiologist. While bleeding is in process and during reversal of heparin, the blood pressure should be kept as low as possible. These recommendations are based on clinical experience and intuition. Ideally, some index of cerebral perfusion would be used to optimize both cerebral perfusion pressure (CPP) and CBF (see Eng[77]).

In concert with securing the airway, thiopental should be considered as a first-line method of lowering blood pressure; it will also prevent seizure activity from acute SAH. Once the bleeding has been controlled, especially if by temporary vascular occlusion, blood pressure should be kept as high as clinically appropriate after consulting with the INR team.

Bleeding catastrophes are usually heralded by headache, nausea, vomiting, and vascular pain related to the area of perforation. The radiologist can often see the contrast extravasating seconds before the patient becomes symptomatic. In cases of vessel puncture, heparin reversal *before* withdrawing the offending wire or catheter back into the lumen of the vessel may keep the perforation partially blocked until hemostatic function is restored. Rupture or perforation of vessels is often treatable with glue, coils, or balloons.

If an episode of suspected contrast extravasation or vessel puncture turns out not to be a bleed, the patient can be re-heparinized. If significant mass effect is present, the decision to intervene operatively can be undertaken after consultation with the other specialists involved.

Sudden loss of consciousness is not always due to ICH. Seizures, as a result of contrast or temporary ischemia, and the resulting postictal state can also result in an obtunded patient.

CONTRAST REACTIONS

This subject is dealt with extensively in the literature, especially for the older ionic contrast agents.[78] Most important for modern INR is the use of low osmolality non-ionic contrast agents such as iohexol, which in its usual application for INR is an iodine-salt concentration of 300 mg/ml. This corresponds to an osmolality of 672 mosm/kg, as opposed to the older ionic agents with a osmolality of some 2000 mosm/kg.[79] Although fatal reactions probably occur at the same frequency as with ionic agents (on the order of 1 : 100,000 exposures), non-ionic agents have a lower incidence of mild and moderate reactions.[79-82]

Despite a controversy over the general use of non-ionic agents and cost effectiveness for radiologic imaging, for INR purposes the lower osmotic activity allows for relatively generous use in single cerebral vessels. A single vascular pedicle may receive in the vicinity of 100 to 200 ml contrast during the course of a procedure. This could not be accomplished with older ionic agents.

For patients having a history of reactions, pretreatment with steroids and antihistamines is recommended.[78] Prednisone 50 mg, the evening before and the morning of the procedure, and diphenhydramine, 50 mg intravenously before starting the procedure, is our current regimen.

To prevent renal complications, intraoperative fluid management should be aimed at maintaining euvolemia to offset the diuretic effect of the injected contrast. Maintaining an isotonic or slightly hypertonic state for neurosurgical patients[83] is generally not a problem because contrast-induced diuresis usually encourages a hypertonic state. However, patients who have undergone diagnostic procedures in the previous week before an INR procedure are frequently volume depleted and can be hemodynamically unstable.

RADIATION SAFETY

As a potential risk to anesthesia personnel,[84] three sources of radiation exposure are typically encountered from the imaging equipment: *direct* (from the x-ray tube), *leakage* (through the collimators' protective shielding), and *scattered* (reflected from the patient and the area surrounding the body part being imaged). A fundamental knowledge of radiation safety is essential for staff working in an environment such as the angiography suite. All personnel should wear lead aprons and thyroid shields and have exposure badges. Movable lead glass shields are positioned for the anesthesia team to stand or sit behind. Note that DSA delivers considerably more radiation than routine fluoroscopy and personnel should either leave the room or stand behind lead barriers during DSA. A common error made by new staff is to turn their back (which is usually unshielded) toward the x-ray source during anesthetic care of the patient.

Because the amount of exposure drops off proportionally to the square of the distance from the source of radiation (inverse square law), activity near the head of the patient should be kept at a minimum during fluoroscopy. For example, a person standing near the head of the table (and the radiation source) may receive a hundredfold greater radiation exposure than one at the foot of the table. There must be effective communication between anesthesia and radiology teams to take optimal care of the anesthetized or sedated patient and minimize staff exposure to ionizing radiation.

The annual recommended limit for occupational whole-body exposure is 5000 mrems.[85] With proper precautions the anesthesia team should be exposed to less than 0.1 mrem/h.

Specific Procedures

THE VASCULAR MALFORMATIONS

THERAPEUTIC EMBOLIZATION
OF INTRACRANIAL AVMs

Background

AVMs are a complex tangle of abnormal vessels joined by multiple fistulae and thought to arise as an embryologic failure in the otherwise normal differentiation of primordial vascular channels into mature arteries, capillary bed, and veins. AVMs are a treatable cause of neurologic morbidity, usually found in young adults.[86] The primary goal of treatment is to decrease the risk of spontaneous bleeding and this is best accomplished by total surgical obliteration. The risk of bleeding from an AVM is in the range of 2 to 4 percent a year. Approximately one-third of these patients will die from the bleed, one-third will have a significant stroke, and one-third will escape unscathed. These figures depend greatly on the series reported. Risk for bleeding is higher in the smaller, higher pressure AVMs with aneurysms or in venous occlusive disease.[87]

The anesthesiologist should be aware of several important differences between aneurysms and AVMs. Approximately 10 percent of patients with AVMs also harbor intracranial aneurysms. Some of these aneu-

rysms are "flow-related" and felt to be formed by the high shear stresses imposed by high flows through the parent artery supplying the fistula. Our general approach is to treat the symptomatic lesion first,[88] but this is controversial and treatment is probably best individualized for a particular case. Note that the converse is not true; the incidence of AVMs in aneurysm patients is probably much closer to the incidence of AVMs in the general population. Intracerebral hemorrhage from aneurysms is usually associated with *subarachnoid hemorrhage*, whereas AVMs more commonly bleed into the ventricle or into parenchyma. This explains why the occurrence of *vasospasm* is distinctly uncommon in AVM cases. Spontaneous hemorrhage during the perioperative period as a result of variations in systemic blood pressure are probably less likely as well,[73] due to a "buffering" capacity of the fistula on changes in systemic pressure.[89]

There are three modes for treatment of AVMs: endovascular embolization, radiosurgery, and surgical excision. Treatment strategies, especially for complex lesions, frequently involve more than one modality. Typically, patients who present for embolization have large, complex AVMs made up of several discrete fistulas with multiple feeding arteries. The goal of the therapeutic embolization is to obliterate as many of the fistulas and their respective feeding arteries as possible. Although in rare cases INR treatment is aimed at total obliteration, embolization is usually used as an adjunct in preparation for surgery or radiotherapy.[90] Radiosurgery of AVMs remains a controversial issue.[91]

As a presurgical adjunct, embolization is thought to facilitate operative removal, with less bleeding and better outcome than if the lesion was untreated. Obliteration of deep feeders, in particular, can make surgery easier[10,92] and thereby should reduce the surgical risk. Therefore, preoperative embolization has been suggested to make the surgical risk for a given lesion better.[93,94] There are other potential benefits. Staging obliteration of arteriovenous shunts theoretically allows the surrounding brain to accommodate to the alteration of hemodynamics and may prevent "normal perfusion pressure breakthrough" (NPPB).[95,96] Obliteration of high-flow feeders may be of benefit in patients with progressive neurologic deficits or intractable seizures, ostensibly by diminishing steal,[1] but more likely by decreasing mass effect from expanding vascular structures.[97] Because intranidal aneurysms appear to increase risk of spontaneous hemorrhage from AVMs,[98] obliteration of intranidal aneurysm during the initial embolization may decrease the rate of intercurrent hemorrhage during the course of treatment. However, embolization may increase intranidal pressure and could theoretically increase this intercurrent ICH risk.[87] This area needs further study.

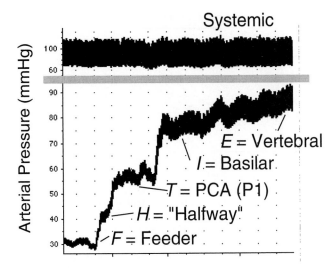

Figure 25-5 Recording made of vascular pressures in a patient with an occipital AVM fed by the posterior cerebral artery. Data taken from ———.[109] Vascular zones (E, I, T, H and F) are described in Fig. 25-6. The catheter was positioned in the feeding artery (*zone F*) and slowly pulled back through *zone H*, the P_1 segment (*zone T*), basilar artery (*zone I*) and finally into the extracranial vertebral artery (*zone E*). As the catheter was withdrawn slowly from the distal feeding artery adjacent to the fistula, the pressure can be seen to increase, with step increases at branch points. The simultaneously recorded systemic arterial pressure is also shown. Note that the pressure in the proximal portion of the posterior cerebral artery (PCA), which irrigates a large area of normal, eloquent tissue, is modestly hypotensive in this asymptomatic patient. (Adapted from Young WL: *Clinical Neuroscience Lectures.* Cathenart Publishing, Munster, IN, 1995, with permission.)

Changes in Cerebral Arterial and Venous Pressures from AVMs

Ample evidence indicates that AVMs induce arterial hypotension and venous hypertension in the input and outflow conduits to the fistula.[36,87,89,96,99–107]

Unfortunately, the extent of transmission of such pressure changes to neighboring vascular territories and the consequences of altering them with treatment has been the subject of more speculation than experimental observation. Arterial pressure appears to decrease gradually as one proceeds distally out along the vascular tree, although the pressure changes are exaggerated at major branch points.[108] This is shown in Figs. 25-5 and 25-6. These observations have significant bearing on any presumed effects of decreased perfusion pressure on autoregulatory function. The important point is that *relatively large arterial distributions* (i.e., PCA territory in Fig. 25-5) are subjected to relative hypotension.

It is now clear that distal cerebral hypotension is the exception rather than the rule. For example, in a study of 41 patients undergoing surgery or embolization, distal feeding artery pressure (mean ± SE) was 38 ± 2 at a systemic pressure of 77 ± 2 mmHg: 56 percent had

a distal pressure of 40 mmHg or less, 36 percent had a distal pressure between 40 and 60 mmHg and 8 percent had greater than 60 mmHg.[109]

Less is known about how AVMs affect the venous circulation, primarily because the veins are more difficult to study. Changes in central venous pressure and systemic arterial pressure affect draining vein pressure (DVP) more as a venous than as an arterial structure, implying that the fistula possesses some internal resistance.[89] Note that it is often assumed that the largest AVMs have the lowest feeding pressure and highest draining vein pressure.[110] Although deep venous drainage has not been systemically studied, *superficial* DVP and feeding arterial pressure appear to have a parallel relationship; that is, higher arterial pressure is associated with higher venous pressure.[89] However, the net transnidal pressure gradient (feeding artery-DVP), appears to be lower in larger AVMs.

Perfusion Changes Due to AVMs

Arteriovenous malformations may exert a deleterious effect on brain function by several mechanisms, including mass effects (e.g., hematoma, edema, or gradually expanding abnormal vascular structures such as ve-

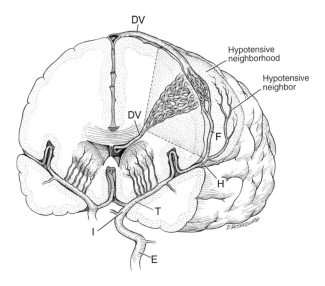

Figure 25-6 Regional cerebral hypotension induced by AVMs. Coronal-oblique view of intracranial circulation to AVM demonstrating anatomic vascular zones and surrounding functional area subject to chronic hypotension ("hypotensive neighborhood"). One vessel perfusing the hypotensive neighborhood, labeled the "hypotensive neighbor," is illustrated. E = extracranial, I = intracranial, T = transcranial Doppler (TCD) insonation site, H = pressure measured at half the distance from T to F, supplying functional tissue and shunt, and F = feeder. Draining veins (DV) are also indicated. NOTE: There is also a hypotensive neighborhood, perfused by hypotensive neighbors, in the volume of brain which has bene cut away for illustrative purposes. (Adapted from Young WL: *Clinical Neuroscience Lectures.* Cathenart Publishing, Munster, IN, 1995, with permission.)

nous aneurysms), metabolic depression (diaschisis), and seizure activity. However, a largely unproven but conceptually attractive paradigm is often discussed to explain many instances of pretreatment defects—ascribed to "cerebral steal"—and certain catastrophic posttreatment complications of brain swelling and ICH. This has been termed *normal perfusion pressure breakthrough* (NPPB)[95] or "circulatory breakthrough." These models propose the following:

1. Perfusion pressure is reduced to the lower limit of autoregulation by both arterial hypotension and venous hypertension in neighboring vascular territories.
2. Arteriolar resistance in these adjacent territories is at or near a state of maximal vasodilation. If perfusion pressure decreases, "steal" ensues.
3. Chronic hypotension results in "vasomotor paralysis" and deranged autoregulatory capability.
4. Reversal of arterial hypotension after treatment is not matched by a corresponding increase in cerebrovascular resistance and results in hyperemia and, in its worst case, swelling or ICH.

Such a model implies that it is not the AVM itself but, rather, decreased perfusion pressure in adjacent functional tissue, which is responsible for both pretreatment ischemic and posttreatment hyperemic symptoms. In principle, this model assumes mechanisms encountered in other conditions of reduced perfusion pressure, for example, occlusive atherosclerotic disease.[111]

The intraoperative appearance of diffuse bleeding from the operative site or brain swelling and the postoperative occurrence of hemorrhage or swelling have been attributed to NPPB or "hyperemic" complications. A difficulty in studying the problem arises in the heterogeneous set of criteria used by different authors in defining exactly what a "hyperemic" complication is. Although the incidence of postoperative "hyperemic complications" has been estimated to be as high as 25 to 50 percent, it is probably lower than 5 percent.[112]

Despite much discussion of NPPB, there is little direct experimental evidence that it exists. In human studies, chronic hypotension does not necessarily result in vasoparalysis in the arteriolar resistance bed. Autoregulation to increases in perfusion is generally maintained in cerebral tissue adjacent to AVMs preoperatively and postsurgery. More importantly, the lower limit of pressure autoregulation appears to be shifted to the left[105] (Fig. 25-7). This adaptive shift to the left places the lower limit at a level considerably lower than what is considered the normal lower limit of pressure autoregulation (50 or 60 mmHg).[95,113] This

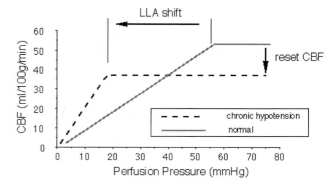

Figure 25-7 Schematic depiction of adaptation of cerebral autoregulation during chronic hypotension. Cerebral blood flow is shown as a function of cerebral perfusion pressure. It appears that the lower limit of autoregulation is reset to a lower point in chronically hypotensive vascular territories adjacent to AVMs (adaptive autoregulatory displacement) and that there is a minimal, nonischemic reduction in CBF in such territories. (Adapted from Young WL: *Clinical Neuroscience Lectures*. Cathenart Publishing, Munster, IN, 1995, with permission.)

shift to the left may also be associated with a mild decrease in resting CBF, which is well above the ischemic range.[114] These mild decreases in CBF may be attributable to a phenomena similar to diaschisis[115,116] or perhaps a down-sizing of the local neuronal population. Although CO_2 reactivity may be impaired in brain regions surrounding AVMs,[100] there is generally a preserved responsiveness to CO_2 pre- and postsurgical resection, which lends further support to the notion of intact autoregulatory capacity.[105]

Cerebral steal is felt by many authors to explain focal neurologic deficits in AVM patients; steal is attributed to local hypotension. The definition of steal is far from uniform and includes recurrent reversible and stable nonprogressive focal deficits. Even seizures have been interpreted by some as being steal induced,[117] although this is exceedingly rare in occlusive cerebrovascular disease. The incidence of patients presenting with focal deficits *possibly* attributable to steal ranges from less than about 8 percent in our experience to as high as 25 to 50 percent.[99,118,119] There are numerous reports of neurologic deficits or CBF reductions that have either partially or completely resolved with AVM obliteration.[120–128] Further, Batjer and colleagues concluded that local hypoperfusion by SPECT imaging, which they defined as steal, *was present in every one of their patients.*[129] Although the concept of steal has been proposed to explain such observations, none of the studies to date have related alterations in CBF to specific vascular patterns *and* actual measurement or estimation of vascular pressures.

As we have recently described,[97] focal deficits are a rare presentation (<10 percent) and not necessarily associated with localized cerebral hypotension. It is highly likely that local mass effects are more important than local "hemodynamic failure" to account for symptomatic focal neurologic deficit unrelated to intracerebral hemorrhage.

Therefore, the diagnoses of steal and NPPB are, if they exist, exceedingly rare. As regards intraoperative management, the diagnosis of NPPB should be a diagnosis of exclusion after all other correctable causes for malignant brain swelling or bleeding have been excluded. Our empirical bias is that autonomic or adrenergic blockade may be of use, in addition to other supportive and resuscitative measures, in preventing and treating this syndrome. This has indirect support from reports of both sympathetic activation after AVM resection[130] and the potential activation of perivascular autonomic innervation to the cerebral vasculature after treatment.[131] An alternative approach to explain hemorrhage and swelling after AVM treatment has been termed "venous overload"[132] or "occlusive hyperemia,"[133] emphasizing that iatrogenic venous outflow obstruction can also result in complications.

Endovascular Treatment of AVMs

The primary agent in our practice is NBCA. Polyvinyl alcohol particles (PVA), coils, or silk thread are recanalized in days to weeks and used only as an adjunct for surgery planned within that period. Proximal occlusion with coils or sutures is not useful for long-term management[22,134] because it appears to only temporarily decrease flow through the fistula; it leaves the low resistance arteriovenous connection intact and therefore capable of recruiting flow from other channels.[135] The most deleterious type of recruitment is from deep perforating arteries, which make surgical resection especially difficult.[92]

Depending on the tortuosity of the vascular pathway and other technical considerations, it may either be very difficult or extremely easy for the INR team to place the catheter tip exactly where they want it. The ease of passing the superselective catheter will determine, in part, how many pedicles can be embolized on a given day. The patients, despite best efforts, usually will not tolerate more than 4 to 5 h of intravenous sedation and remain still enough to allow satisfactory performance of the neuroimaging procedures.

As the superselective catheter is passed distally, pressure measurements may be made at the tip of the catheter. The pressure will typically decrease in a stepwise fashion as it is advanced distally.[36,109] When the catheter has been placed in position for potential glue injection, the level of sedation is decreased and a baseline neurologic examination is performed. Functional anesthetic testing (SAFE) is then performed. If this test is positive, that is, a focal neurologic deficit is encountered, then the catheter is repositioned or

embolization of that pedicle may be aborted. If negative, the glue or embolic material can be injected.

Choice of Anesthetic Technique

Choice of anesthetic technique is a controversial area; there are generally two schools of thought on how to manage the patient undergoing embolization of an AVM. One is to rely on the knowledge of neuroanatomy and vascular architecture to ascertain the likelihood of neurologic damage after deposition of glue. The "anatomy" school, therefore, will prefer to embolize under general anesthesia. Arguments for this approach include improved visualization of structures with the absence of patient movement, especially if temporary apnea is used. Further, it is argued that if the glue is placed "intranidal," by definition no normal brain is threatened.

The other school, which we might call the "physiologic" school, trades off the potential for patient movement for the increased knowledge of the true functional anatomy of a given patient. As shown in Fig. 25-3, localization of cerebral function may not always follow textbook descriptions, as described in the section above on SAFE. Furthermore, the AVM nidus or a previous hemorrhage may result in a shift or relocalization of function. The "physiologic" approach demands, at the present, deep intravenous sedation and waking the patient for SAFE before injection of embolic material. This is our preferred approach.

Flow Arrest

Once the superselective catheter is in optimal position, profound but tolerable systemic hypotension is induced while the radiologists prepare the glue for injection. Hypotension slows the flow through the fistula and provides for a more controlled deposition of embolic material, the glues in particular. Deliberate hypotension is used to achieve *flow arrest*. Ideally, there would be zero flow through the AVM at the time of glue injection so that the distribution of glue would be totally controlled by the radiologist. (Complications of glue injection are described at the end of this section.)

Flow arrest, therefore, is only partial. Adequate flow arrest occurs at a different systemic pressure for each patient. In fact, it seems that flow through the fistula remains relatively constant until a certain pressure is reached, when it drops off sharply. As the pressure is lowered, the radiologist will perform several contrast injections with fluoroscopy and visually determine the optimal systemic pressure to slow the flow through the fistula. Typically, we will reduce systemic mean arterial pressure (MAP) to about 50 mmHg, but greater or lesser degrees depend on the speed of the contrast transit through the fistula.

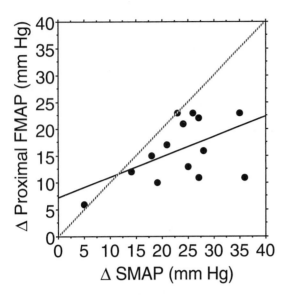

Figure 25-8 Correlation between systemic, arterial and AVM feeding pressures. There is a disparity between changes in the mean arterial pressure measured in an AVM feeding artery (FMAP) and changes in the systemic mean arterial pressure (SMAP). This data was taken from Young WL, et al,[105] and was a study of 14 patients during 15 embolization procedures. SMAP was increased with a phenylephrine infusion. The SMAP and FMAP were recorded simultaneously at the beginning and end of the phenylephrine challenge. The ΔFMAP is shown as a function of ΔSMAP with the line of identity indicated. Since the microcatheter placement in this series was rather proximal (to measure normal cortical regions using ^{133}Xe washout), the disparity between *distal* FMAP and SMAP may be even more pronounced than this study indicates. (From Young WL, et al: Columbia University AVM Study Project. *Neurosurgery* 1994; 35:389–396, with permission.)

This subject has not been rigorously studied, and it is not clear whether systemic hypotension decreases shunt flow solely on the basis of a reduction in pressure or by limiting total (and in the case of an AVM, increasing) flow to the brain or by some combination of both factors. In any event, in the presence of a cerebral fistula, reducing systemic pressure does not affect downstream feeding artery pressure to the same degree, and different patients may require different degrees of hypotension to adequately slow flow through the fistula for glue deposition. The converse is true as well. Increasing systemic pressure is not uniformly transmitted to the AVM nidus (Fig. 25-8); there appears to be a "buffering" of changes in systemic pressure at the level of the nidus.

Another technique used to achieve flow arrest is to place a balloon catheter via the other femoral artery. The balloon is positioned proximal to the superselective catheter to be used for gluing. Prior to glue injection, the balloon may be inflated to either slow or completely arrest distal flow. But this technique necessitates passage of another intracranial catheter from the contralateral femoral artery and the attendant risks of vessel rupture from balloon overinflation.

Postprocedure Complications

Measurement of immediate postembolization pressures has been suggested as a means of following the course of hemodynamic changes[36,104] and predicting postprocedure complications,[103] as large increases in feeding artery pressure appear to be associated with ICH. Additional studies are needed to further define the clinical utility of such measurements. At the present time, unfortunately, immediate postembolization pressure measurements are only practical with thread, coils, or PVA. Available superselective catheters must be withdrawn immediately after glue injection (so that they are not cemented into place). It is possible to "chase" glue from the microcatheter with non-ionic solutions, but this reduces the operator control over glue deposition.

As discussed above, the pressures in the proximal feeding artery are quite low, that is, 40 to 60 percent of MAP. Near the entry to a high-flow AVM nidus the pressure may be as low as 15 to 25 percent of MAP. Because AVM feeding arteries supply variable amounts of normal brain, abrupt restoration of normal systemic pressure to a chronically hypotensive vascular bed may overwhelm autoregulatory capacity and result in hemorrhage or swelling (NPPB). It is, in part, for this reason that the target range for posttreatment blood pressure is maintenance of 10 to 20 percent below the patient's normal ward blood pressure. As discussed above, the exact pathophysiology of hemodynamic complications after treatment of AVMs remains controversial.[136]

Although any injected embolic material can occlude normal vessels, injection of the glue is fraught with particular hazards. Injection of glue is a critical moment (not unlike the moment when a surgeon closes the clip on the neck of an aneurysm). The catheter may become glued to the vessel. If the catheter cannot be removed by intermittent firm, gentle traction, it may be necessary to leave the catheter intravascularly, where it will eventually endothelialize.

Similarly, the catheter, as it is withdrawn, may drag a piece of glue into the proximal part of the artery and occlude it. In this event, territories fed by nutrient vessels distal to the occlusion may become ischemic. Glue that is carried out into the draining vein can cause venous outflow obstruction and result in ICH.

Glue may also pass into the pulmonary circulation. Small amounts (<0.5 ml) may not be clinically significant. Larger amounts, however, may result in a syndrome similar to acute idiopathic pulmonary embolism; flow arrest techniques probably decrease the incidence of such occurrences.[137] Since the glue is extremely thrombogenic, it may pick up thrombus en route and form more clot once lodged in the pulmonary vasculature. This is of particular concern in small children. At the time of gluing, the anesthesiologist must be ready to intervene immediately in the event of catastrophe.

OTHER CNS VASCULAR MALFORMATIONS
Dural Fistulae

Dural arteriovenous fistulae (DAVF), initially thought to be a congenital disorder, is currently considered an acquired lesion resulting from venous dural sinus stenosis or occlusion, opening of potential arteriovenous shunts, and subsequent recanalization. The use of the term *fistula*, rather than *malformation*, is preferable because it stresses the concept that they are fed by branches of the external carotid artery and the pathophysiology includes some degree of venous hypertension. Although there is no true intracerebral arterial supply, DAVF drain through intracerebral structures (e.g., cortical veins) and patients may present with focal neurologic deficits, seizure, or hemorrhage.[138] Other presentations include chemosis, proptosis, and bruits.

Dural arteriovenous fistulae may be treated by multistaged embolization.[139] SAFE may be performed as in cases of intracranial AVMs. NBCA is usually used as an embolic agent. Both transarterial and transvenous approaches can be used to access the dural sinuses.

Carotid Cavernous and Vertebral Fistulae

Carotid cavernous fistulae (CCF) are direct fistulae usually caused by trauma to the cavernous carotid artery leading to communication with the cavernous sinus.[1] They are usually associated with basal skull fracture but can result from penetrating injuries, collagendeficiency diseases, ruptured aneurysms, arterial dissection, or fibromuscular dysplasia. The detachable balloon has nearly totally replaced the surgical treatment of CCF.[140]

Vertebral artery fistulae are connections to surrounding paravertebral veins, usually as a result of penetrating trauma, but may be congenital, result from blunt trauma, or be associated with neurofibromatosis. In addition to cerebral involvement, spinal cord function may also be impaired.

Both CCF and vertebral fistulae may induce arterial hypotension and venous hypertension in neighboring circulatory regions, analogous to true cerebral AVMs. NPPB has rarely been described after fistula interruption,[141] so attention to postprocedure blood pressure control is warranted.

Vein of Galen Malformations

These are relatively uncommon but complicated lesions that present in infants and require a multidisciplinary approach. The patients may have intractable congestive heart failure, intractable seizures, hydrocephalus, and mental retardation.[7] Several approaches have been attempted, including transarterial and transvenous.[142] Morbidity and mortality are high in these cases. Anesthetic considerations for INR therapy are the same as for surgical treatment.[143]

In infants with high output failure, preexisting right-to-left shunts, and pulmonary hypertension, a relatively small pulmonary glue embolism can be fatal.

Craniofacial Venous Malformations

Craniofacial venous malformations (or angiomas) are congenital disorders and, in addition to causing significant cosmetic deformities, may impinge on the upper airway and interfere with swallowing. Many of these lesions are resistant to conventional surgery, cryosurgery, or laser surgery. In our practice, USP grade 95% ethanol opacified with contrast is injected percutaneously into the lesion under fluoroscopic guidance, resulting in a chemical burn to the lesion, eventually shrinking it (100% ethanol may be contaminated with benzene). Sclerotherapy alone may be adequate treatment or it may be combined with surgery.[144]

Venous angiomas may occur anywhere in the body and are usually treated at multiple sessions. The procedures are short (30 to 60 min) but painful and general anesthesia with endotracheal intubation is used. Complex airway involvement may require endotracheal intubation with fiberoptic techniques[145] or elective preprocedure tracheostomy. Because *marked* swelling occurs immediately after ethanol injection, the ability of the patient to maintain a patent airway must be carefully considered in discussion with the radiologist. An example of acute swelling is shown in Fig. 25-9. More graphic examples of venous malformations impinging on the airway are available elsewhere.[144]

Ethanol has several noteworthy side effects. First, on injection it can cause changes in the pulmonary vasculature and create a short-lived shunt or a ventilation perfusion mismatch. Desaturation on the pulse oximeter is frequently noted after injection; in our experience at least a 2 to 3 percent drop in O_2 saturation is noted in about 25 percent of cases; more significant decreases are rare. There have been unpublished anecdotal reports of cardiac arrest during ethanol sclerotherapy, as well as hypoglycemia. The systemic effects of ethanol in this setting need further study.

Placing the patient on 100% O_2 during ethanol injection is a possible consideration. The predictable intoxication and other side effects of ethanol may be evident after emergence from anesthesia, particularly post-emergence agitation in children.

Sodium tetradecyl sulfate (Sotradecol) has also been used as a sclerosing agent to treat venous malforma-

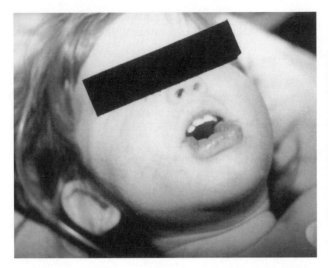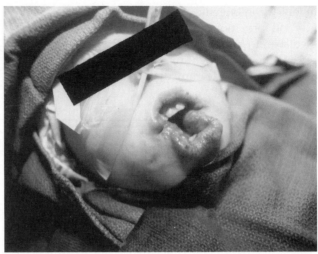

Figure 25-9   Soft tissue swelling after ethanol sclerotherapy. Example of marked soft tissue swelling after 95% ethanol sclerotherapy. The first panel shows a five-year-old girl with a venous malformation of the lower lip. In the second panel, the patient has just undergone ethanol injection, and the dramatic degree of swelling can be readily appreciated. (From Young WL, Pile-Spellman J: *Anesthesiology* 1994; 80:448, with permission.)

tions. Although it is relatively painless on injection, in our experience it is not as efficacious as ethanol.

TEST AND THERAPEUTIC CAROTID AND VERTEBRAL ARTERY OCCLUSION

BACKGROUND

Carotid occlusion, both permanent and temporary, may be used in several circumstances.[146–148] Skull base tumors frequently involve the intracranial or petrous portion of the carotid artery or its proximal willisian branches. Large or otherwise unclippable aneurysms may be partly or completely treated by proximal vessel occlusion. To assess the consequences of carotid occlusion in anticipation of surgery, the patient may be scheduled for a test occlusion. Cerebrovascular reserve is evaluated by a multimodal combination of angiographic, clinical, and physiologic tests. Such testing is used to arrive at the safest course of action for a given patient's clinical circumstances.

The vertebral artery may also be occluded in a similar fashion. The following discussion is directed at carotid occlusions, but the same general principles apply.

Because each ICA provides one-third of the brain's blood supply, acute occlusion must result in dramatic CBF redistribution if neuronal function is to be maintained. Many tests have been introduced to assess this capability.[43,149–173] Cross-compression angiography was one of the earliest tests to assess cerebrovascular reserves preoperatively.[159] Unfortunately, it was found unreliable because angiographic vessel opacification

is a poor physiologic indicator of CBF. Subsequently developed techniques include the measurement of intraoperative ICA-occluded stump pressure,[151,160,161] angiographic catheter back pressure,[162,163] and retinal artery pressure.[164,165] More recent techniques include transcranial Doppler,[166] dynamic CT scanning,[167] ^{133}Xe CBF,[148,158,159] SPECT,[43,168,169] stable xenon CT CBF,[170–172] and positron emission tomography (PET).[173]

Despite these sophisticated methods, patients may still develop cerebral infarction after permanent ICA occlusion.[174] The causes are multifactorial and include technical factors and development of thrombosis and embolism in the immediate postoperative period. Direct testing of cerebrovascular reserve is discussed below and refinements of such "stress tests" will hopefully lower the incidence of delayed post-occlusion stroke.

CONDUCT OF PROCEDURE

The following is a synopsis of our current protocol for management of carotid test occlusion. First, after routine carotid and vertebral angiograms, the anatomic integrity of the circle of Willis is assessed, that is, the ability of blood to cross the two posterior communicating arteries and the anterior communicating artery. The radiologists will compress the ipsilateral carotid during contrast injection into the contralateral carotid to assess the cross-filling from the other hemisphere via the anterior communicating artery. Ipsilateral carotid compression followed by vertebral injection of contrast will demonstrate posterior communicating artery patency.

A catheter with both a lumen and a balloon is placed in the carotid artery. The balloon is long enough so that distal ICA branches that may serve as a source of collateral circulation are blocked. A baseline neurologic examination is performed, TCD velocity of the MCA is recorded, and CBF is measured by intracarotid ^{133}Xe injection. Baseline femoral and carotid pressures are noted.

The balloon is then inflated; the stump pressure in the carotid distal to the balloon is recorded. Stump pressure is a useful adjunct to CBF measurement. By itself, a normal stump pressure does not guarantee normal CBF, but very low stump pressure appears to be reliably associated with low CBF.[175] There appears to be a good correlation between stump pressures and other indices of CBF.[176,177] This is especially pertinent where one can determine that there is no angiographic evidence of stenotic disease between the ICA and distal vasculature. It is our clinical impression that the blood pressure often increases 10 to 15 percent with inflation of the balloon. The anesthesiologist must also be prepared to treat hemodynamically significant bradycardia during inflation of the balloon.

The neurologic examination is repeated. As in the case with SAFE, attention is directed to areas at risk, such as watershed regions, as well as "quiet areas." After a few minutes of equilibration, ^{133}Xe CBF and TCD values are measured.

Immediately thereafter, a SPECT tracer can be given. At the present time Ceretec is used, which is ^{99M}technetium-labeled hexamethylpropylamineoxime (HMPAO). Ceretec is a tracer that rapidly crosses the blood-brain barrier and binds to cerebral tissues and takes a "snapshot" of the blood flow distribution (not quantitative CBF levels) to the brain at that instant; the relatively long half-life of Ceretec (about 6 h) allows for the patient to go to the nuclear medicine department after the procedure to have the "snapshot" developed by placement in the SPECT scanner.

To more completely assess the extent of cerebrovascular reserve, deliberate hypotension is begun after 15 min of observation of the patient at spontaneous postocclusion MAP. The *lack* of cerebral ischemic symptoms at relative normotension does not yield information on the status of cerebrovascular reserve. During subsequent craniotomy, the blood pressure may be considerably lower, especially with rapid blood loss. Also, the postoperative surgical patient is notoriously prone to sags in arterial blood pressure. Finally, superimposition of an embolic event, either perioperatively or at some later time, will require some degree of cerebrovascular reserve to prevent infarction.

For these reasons, the blood pressure is lowered gradually to determine at what point the patient begins to show evidence of cerebral ischemia.[19] We usually

TABLE 25-7
Criteria for Failing Balloon Test Occlusion

The major criteria for failure of the balloon test occlusion are:

1. The occurrence of a neurologic deficit in the territory that is tested.

   Usually this starts as a difficulty to focus, then sleepiness, immediately followed by a facial palsy and weakness of the upper extremity (pronator drift) and the lower extremity.

   On the dominant hemisphere, speech difficulty is observed, with aphasia, dysphasia, or a comprehension deficit.

   On the nondominant hemisphere, a dense contralateral hemineglect may be noted.

2. Other criteria include, usually in association with a neurologic deficit:
   CBF values <20 ml/100 g per min

3. Stump pressure measurements <35 mmHg

4. TCD MCA velocities <30 cm/s with a pulsatility index (PI) <0.50

5. A major attention deficit assessed by specialized neuropsychological testing

6. A minor attention deficit associated with upper extremity weakness and absence of angiographic evidence of collaterals

NOTE: TCD, transcranial Doppler; MCA, middle cerebral artery

begin with esmolol (and consider adding nitroglycerin in a patient with coronary artery disease) and slowly bring the pressure down as the radiologist continually assesses neurologic function. One must proceed cautiously with blood pressure reduction to rationally interpret the neurologic examination. Frequently, the first sign of impending cerebral ischemia is yawning. If the radiologist feels that the patient is becoming symptomatic, the balloon is deflated and the hypotensive agent(s) discontinued. Depending on the clinical circumstances, phenylephrine (or another clinically appropriate agent) can be used to bring the blood pressure back toward normal levels.

The patient's hematocrit, Pa_{CO_2}, and blood pressure at the time when the test occlusion is considered "passed" or "failed" should be noted. Our criteria are shown in Table 25-7. The lowest systemic pressure obtained before symptoms, if any, and the results of the other imaging modalities are considered in formulating a treatment plan regarding INR occlusion or the advisability of vascular sacrifice during surgical resection. Although uniform guidelines have yet to be formulated, significant asymmetry on SPECT[43] (or stable ^{133}Xe CT) or significant decrease in ^{133}Xe CBF or TCD velocities[19] after test occlusion may be useful in selecting patients for extracranial-to-intracranial bypass procedures if the carotid artery must be sacrificed.[178] Limitations of SPECT scanning in this setting are discussed elsewhere.[163]

INTRACRANIAL ANEURYSMS

TREATMENT OF CEREBRAL ANEURYSMS

Modern neurosurgical and neuroanesthetic techniques, coupled with improved postoperative management, have improved the care of the patient with intracerebral aneurysms.[179] Most lesions can be safely obliterated surgically with preservation of the parent vessel. However, difficulties in the management of certain types of aneurysms remain, such as giant or fusiform aneurysms.[180] In addition, patients with medical risks or poor neurologic grade may not be surgical candidates. The two basic approaches for INR therapy are occlusion of proximal parent arteries and obliteration of the aneurysmal sac.

For some giant aneurysms, cervical carotid balloon ligation may be performed with or without subsequent extracranial-to-intracranial bypass.[178] The test occlusion protocol described above with physiologic monitoring may be useful in predicting which patients have borderline cerebrovascular reserve.[181]

The aneurysmal sac may be obliterated by use of coils and/or balloons. The newest form of treatment for aneurysms is the Guglielmi detachable coil (GDC).[182,183] This is a curlicue type of platinum coil that is attached to a stainless steel guidewire. The coil is passed through a superselective catheter into the aneurysmal sac and then detached by passing an electric current through the guidewire, which causes the stainless steel portion to detach from the platinum coil by electrolysis, leaving the coil curled up in the sac. Small aneurysms may only need one coil; larger sacs may take several. Because these procedures can be quite long (especially for large lesions requiring multiple GDC coils) and the lesser need to follow the neurologic examination, these cases are most often done under general anesthesia with endotracheal intubation.

Endovascular obliteration of the aneurysmal sac while sparing the parent vessel is still challenging.[184] Manipulation of the sac may cause distal thromboembolism and rupture. Incomplete obliteration may result in recurrence and hemorrhage. An example is shown in Fig. 25-10. This case also illustrates a current drawback to packing the dome; that is, packing of the coils leaves the neck of the aneurysm exposed to the blood column and therefore further growth.

Some aneurysms are treated with a combination of parent vessel sacrifice and obliteration of the sac with coils. Therefore, it is important for the anesthesiologist to fully understand what the tactics of any given session are going to be to optimally manage the patient.

An attractive strategy is that of taking a "hot" aneurysm (just ruptured) and transforming it into a "cold" aneurysm by packing the dome with coils. Therefore, *acute* rebleed may be prevented, allowing a delayed lower risk treatment of the remaining aneurysm. This strategy is, in part, based on the assumption that it is generally the dome that bleeds, whereas aneurysms grow at the neck.[185] However, in a significant number of cases the bleeding site may not be the dome of the aneurysm. Further, in some cases packing the neck with coils clearly makes surgical clipping more difficult.

The anesthesiologist should be prepared for aneurysmal rupture and acute SAH at all times in any treatment scenario, either from spontaneous rupture of a leaky sac or direct violation of the aneurysm wall by vascular manipulation. At the present time there is not the same degree of certainty that the lesion has been completely removed from the circulation after coil ablation of the aneurysm as there is with application of a surgical clip. There may be areas of the dome that are still in contact with the arterial blood column. Therefore, careful attention to postprocedure blood pressure control is warranted.

TREATMENT OF CEREBRAL VASOSPASM FROM ANEURYSMAL SAH

Angioplasty for Vasospasm

In cases of symptomatic vasospasm refractory to deliberate hypertension and intravascular volume expansion, angiography can be performed to assess the contribution of large proximal conductance vessels (usually internal carotid, MCA, or ACA).[186] Angioplasty is usually reserved for patients who have already had the symptomatic lesion surgically clipped (for fear of re-rupture) and is done early in the course of symptomatic ischemia to prevent transformation of a bland infarct into a hemorrhagic one. A balloon catheter is guided under fluoroscopy into the spastic segment and inflated to mechanically distend the constricted area.

There is a correlation between the extent of SAH and resultant reductions in both CBF[187] and the cerebral metabolic rate of O_2.[188] However, a vasospastic segment functions in a fashion analogous to an atherosclerotic stenosis and induces a pressure drop across its length.[189] The microvasculature distal to the spastic segments is probably maximally vasodilated.[190] Dilating the spastic arterial segment alleviates the pressure drop and improves distal perfusion. As in the case of occlusive carotid disease reported by Schroeder,[189] angiographic evidence of a narrowed vessel does not necessarily correlate with an actual hemodynamic impairment. More importantly, a good angiographic result does not guarantee patient improvement, which occurs in only about half the cases.

These procedures are commonly performed in patients who are *in extremis* and are therefore frequently intubated, on vasopressor agents, and have either ven-

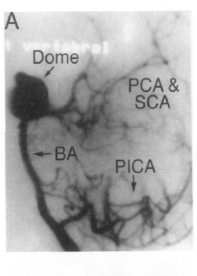

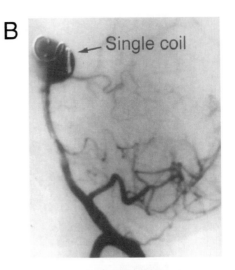

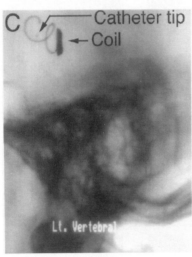

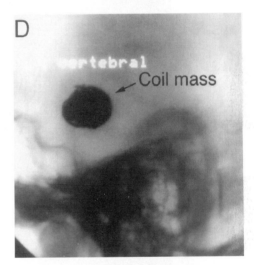

Figure 25-10   Endovascular treatment of a basilar aneurysm with coils. *A.* Lateral subtracted vertebral injection showing a giant basilar aneurysm (the dome is indicated). PCA = posterior cerebral artery; SCA = superior cerebellar artery; BA = basilar artery; PICA = posterior inferior cerebellar artery. *B.* Lateral subtracted vertebral injection showing a single coil placed within the dome. *C.* Lateral scout film showing the single coil. Note also the opaque tip of the microcatheter. *D.* Lateral scout film showing the mass of coils after procedure. *E.* Immediate post-procedure angiogram. *F.* One year post-procedure angiogram. Note how the coils have been packed into the dome, leaving the base of the aneurysm exposed to the arterial blood column. (Adapted from Young WL: *Clinical Neuroscience Lectures.* Cathenart Publishing, Munster, IN, 1995, with permission.)

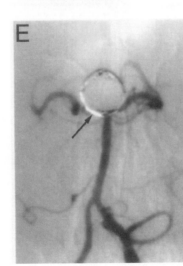

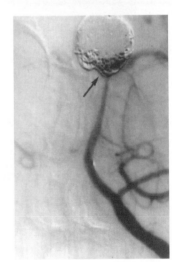

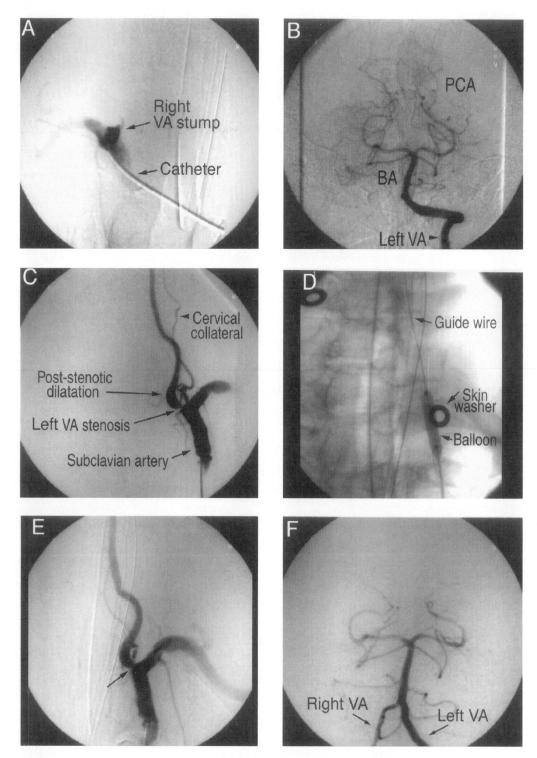

Figure 25-11 Angioplasty of occlusive vascular disease. This case is an elderly man who presented with a brainstem stroke referable to the right distal vertebral artery territory in the distribution of the posterior inferior cerebellar artery (PICA). This case illustrates the importance of collateral flow evaluation in the treatment of stenotic lesions. *A*. The catheter is in the right subclavian artery in the chest. Contrast injection reveals the stump of the right vertebral artery (VA) and is completely occluded. *B*. Antero-posterior view of the distal left vertebral artery (injection of contrast is into the left subclavian artery which is below the field of view). Note that the right vertebral does not fill. Other angiographic studies demonstrated that collateral pathways from the anterior (carotid) circulation were not present (posterior communicating arteries). BA = basilar artery; PCA = posterior cerebral artery; VA = vertebral artery. *C*. Injection of contrast into

tricular drainage or other intracranial pressure (ICP) monitoring equipment in place. Blood pressure management after angioplasty must take into consideration the presence and age of any existing cerebral ischemia or cerebral infarction. If deliberate hypertension was being used to ameliorate a focal neurologic deficit before angioplasty, blood pressure should probably be managed in the normal range after angiographic demonstration of a significantly widened spastic segment.

Papaverine

Another approach to vasospasm is to use a pharmacologic means to dilate the vasospastic segment. Superselective intra-arterial papaverine has had success.[191-196] Papaverine is a nonspecific vasodilator of the alkaloid class. Its direct action on smooth muscle is thought to be primarily related to inhibition of cyclic adenosine monophosphate phosphodiesterases, with some effect on cyclic guanosine monophosphate phosphodiesterases as well.[197] There are, however, probably other actions that include calcium channel blockade,[198] adenosine blockade,[199] or an effect on protein kinase C.[200] The drug is a potent cerebral vasodilator.[201] Therefore, acute increases in ICP are possible. There are sometimes inexplicable focal neurologic deficits attributable to papaverine, which may or may not be related to a direct effect on ICP.[202] It is also interesting to note that in the animal models of MCA occlusion, papaverine improved local blood flow but did not affect ultimate infarct size,[66] which may represent a time-dependent effect. For example, it is possible that when low arterial concentrations are reached during systemic elimination of papaverine, a vasoconstrictor effect may become evident.[200]

MANAGEMENT OF OCCLUSIVE CEREBROVASCULAR DISEASE

ANGIOPLASTY OF CEREBRAL CONDUCTANCE VESSELS

Angioplasty for atherosclerosis has been tried in cervical and intracranial arteries with favorable results.[203,204] Indications, and efficacy, in relation to surgical endar-terectomy are controversial and remain to be worked out. This is especially true for extracranial carotid disease. Vertebral angioplasty is less controversial because many symptomatic vertebral lesions are relatively inaccessible by surgery.

At present, patients offered carotid angioplasty are poor surgical candidates because of advanced age or concomitant medical disease. Encouraging initial results, coupled with clearer indications for revascularization from the North American Symptomatic Carotid Endarterectomy Trial,[205-207] will speed the development and application of this form of angioplasty.

Risk of distal thromboembolism and long-term restenosis are the major issues to be resolved regarding this procedure. There are several approaches to reduce distal thromboembolism. One tactic is to perfuse blood distally during angioplasty and to aspirate distally during deflation of the balloon to retrieve embolic material. The second is to perform angioplasty under proximal flow arrest and to aspirate possible debris before flow is reestablished. The third tactic is to do angioplasty under distal flow arrest and to aspirate possible emboli before the distal balloon is deflated.[208] Finally, use of stents[27] may offer some protection against embolic events. Stents additionally offer the promise that restenosis will be prevented.

Anesthetic considerations for this procedure include those discussed in the section concerning deliberate hypertension and the general considerations pertinent to the care of the carotid endarterectomy patient. An example is shown in Fig. 25-11 to illustrate the issue of blood pressure control during angioplasty. During the period the balloon is being passed across the stenotic area and then inflated there is a potential for distal hypotension. Therefore, induced hypertension is indicated. When the balloon is deflated, however, there will be areas of brain exposed to a suddenly normalized perfusion pressure and there is the potential for brain swelling or hemorrhage, so maintenance of a lower than normal MAP is indicated in the period immediately following balloon deflation.

Figure 25-11 (*Continued*)   the left subclavian artery reveals a tight stenosis of the ostium of the left vertebral artery. Note the post-stenotic dilation. The smaller vessel running parallel with the vertebral artery represents deep cervical collateral flow. The pressure drop secondary to the proximal vertebral stenosis causes enlargement of anastomotic muscular branches emanating from the subclavian artery to feed the distal vertebral and partial compensate for proximal stenosis. *D.* Using a washer to mark the site of the stenosis, a balloon catheter is placed over a wire. The balloon straddles the stenosis and is then inflated with contrast. *E.* Note the alleviation of the tight stenosis, alleviation of post-stenotic dilation, and an apparent decrease in the deep cervical collateral flow. *F.* Injection of the left subclavian now fills the right vertebral in a retrograde fashion and there is a general improvement in vertebrobasilar opacification. (Adapted from Young WL: *Clinical Neuroscience Lectures.* Cathenart Publishing, Munster, IN, 1995, with permission.)

THROMBOLYSIS OF ACUTE THROMBOEMBOLIC STROKE

In acute occlusive stroke, it is possible to recanalize the occluded vessel by superselective intraarterial thrombolytic therapy.[209,210] Thrombolytic agents can be delivered in high concentration by a microcatheter navigated close to the clot. Neurologic deficits may be reversed without additional risk of secondary hemorrhage if treatment is completed within 6 h from the onset of carotid territory ischemia and within 24 h in vertebrobasilar territory. More time is available for treatment of posterior circulation lesions because the local collateral circulation may be better (that is, there is a shorter distance between collateral territories) and the patients probably present sooner than for most anterior circulation thromboembolic events. Randomized trials of safety and efficacy are in progress. An example is shown in Fig. 25-12.

Dissolution of thrombus is mediated by fibrinolysis within the thrombus (thrombolysis). Degradation of fibrin is catalyzed by plasmin activated from plasminogen. Formation of plasmin is promoted by appearance of plasminogen activator. Exogenous plasminogen activators, such as urokinase (UK), streptokinase (SK), or acylated plasminogen-streptokinase activator complex (APSAC), have been used in thrombolytic therapy. UK, which is a serine protease produced from human urine of fetal renal cell culture, directly activates plasminogen.

In contrast, SK, derived from culture of β-hemolytic streptococcus, has no direct effect on plasminogen. SK combines with plasminogen to form a plasminogen-streptokinase complex, which activates circulating plasminogen to plasmin. Free plasmin in the circulating blood activated by these agents degrades fibrin and fibrinogen, causing fibrinolysis. These exogenous agents also inactivate prothrombin (II) factors V and VIII, thereby inhibiting systemic coagulation. Also, fibrin degradation products (FDP) act as a potent anticoagulant. Thus, large doses of these agents could cause a prolonged systemic anticoagulant state. SK is less expensive than UK, and mass production is easy. However, the half-life of SK is longer (18 to 83 min) than that of UK (11 to 18 min), and it has more side effects than UK, such as fever or allergy, because of its immunogenic properties. Activity may be unstable in patients with previous streptococcus infection. APSAC has been considered to be more fibrin specific in ongoing studies.

In contrast to these exogeneous plasminogen activators that act nonspecifically on circulating plasminogen, tissue plasminogen activator (tPA) and single chain urokinase plasminogen activator (scuPA) are endogenous plasminogen activators with high fibrin specificity. tPA is a serine protease with a short half-

life (5 to 8 min) produced initially from melanoma cell culture and recently by recombinant DNA technique. Although associated with fibrin, tPA is activated in the thrombus and converts plasminogen to plasmin, which is protected from the neutralizing effect of α_2-antiplasmin by fibrin, as described above. Although scuPA has no direct activity to plasminogen, it is activated and converted to UK by plasmin in the thrombus, which causes the localized fibrinolysis. Endogenous plasminogen activators have been considered to have few anticoagulant effects. High doses of tPA, however, may produce systemic fibrinolysis and plasminogen destruction through inactivation of clotting factors. The indications, contraindications, and optimal doses are unknown for thrombolysis. Excellent reviews are available.[210–213]

One of the impediments in development in this area has been the fear of increasing the risk of hemorrhagic transformation in the acute infarction patient. But recent and accumulating evidence suggests that this paradigm (based on early autopsy series) may no longer be tenable.[214] The incidence of postthrombolysis hemorrhage may be at least equal to, if not lower than, the incidence of spontaneous hemorrhage transformation.

Anesthetic considerations for these patients include the usual concerns for elderly patients with symptomatic and most probably widespread atherosclerotic disease. Blood pressure management is a particularly important consideration. Patients with acute thromboembolic stroke are commonly spontaneously hypertensive, and, in the face of a nonhemorrhagic focal neurologic deficit, should not have their blood pressure aggressively treated. After clot lysis, blood pressure should probably be maintained in the normal range and ideally titrated to some index of CBF to prevent hyperperfusion injury. Although the pathogenesis of hemorrhagic transformation may be related to collateral blood flow to ischemic regions, acting in concert with systemic hypertension,[214] studies in the clinical setting are lacking concerning both blood pressure management and the use of other cerebral protective techniques.

As INR methods develop, this area could evolve into one very interactive with anesthesia care because of the high incidence of systemic disease present in these patients, coupled with the high morbidity associated with acute thromboembolic stroke.

SPINAL CORD LESIONS

Embolization may be used for intramedullary spinal AVM, dural fistulas, or tumors invading the spinal canal.[21,215] The experience of the anesthesiologist and INR team will determine the optimal choice of anesthetic technique for a given patient. For cases done

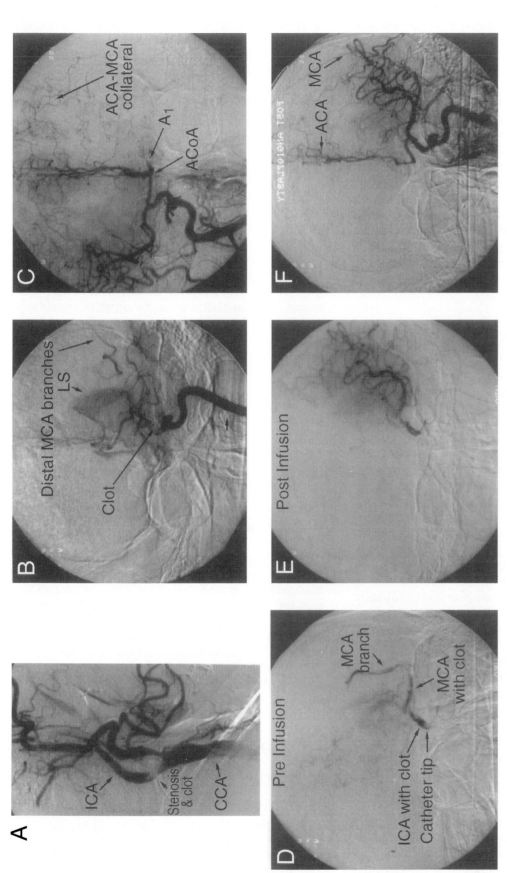

Figure 25-12 This case is an elderly man who presented with left face and arm weakness and was immediately referred for evaluation. A CT scan was normal. *A.* This lateral carotid angiogram over the neck shows severe stenosis of the right proximal internal carotid artery and the suggestion of clot in the arterial lumen. (ICA = internal carotid artery; CCA = common carotid artery). *B.* Intracranial AP view of injection of contrast into the right internal carotid artery. Note the contrast hangs up near the bifurcation of the ICA into the MCA and ACA. There is poor ACA filling and spotty filling of the MCA, suggesting that a large amount of clot is present in the proximal MCA. The lenticulostriate arteries can be seen to fill and drain into the internal cerebral vein, compared with the profound decrease in filling seen in the rest of the MCA territory. LS = lenticulostriate. *C.* AP view of the contralateral ICA injection. Note how blood flow crosses the anterior communicating artery to supply the contralateral ACA territory. It fails to fill the first portion of the ACA (A₁) and hence MCA because of clot (see below). However, the ACA does partially fill, in a retrograde fashion, the MCA territory via tenuous pial-to-pial surface anastomoses down towards the MCA stem (compare with Figs. 25-2 and 25-4). *D.* Superselective angiogram with the catheter tip in the distal ICA just before the bifurcation of the ACA and MCA. An infusion of 1,200,000 units of urokinase was begun 3 h after onset of symptoms and continued for one hour. Note the irregular contrast pattern in the vessel lumens, which represents clot. *E.* Superselective angiogram with the catheter tip in the proximal MCA. At the end of the infusion, the MCA vessels are now completely visualized. *F.* This AP view is injection of contrast into the right internal carotid artery after both thrombolysis, as shown in Panels *D* and *E,* and balloon angioplasty of the proximal stenosis, shown in *A.* The MCA and ACA appear to fill normally with no further evidence of intravascular clot. The patient did well and sustained a small MCA territory infarct with a minor residual deficit. (Adapted from Young WL: *Clinical Neuroscience Lectures.* Cathenart Publishing, Munster, IN, 1995, with permission.)

with general anesthesia with endotracheal intubation, an intraoperative wake-up test may be requested. It is useful to review the wake-up procedure with the patient before the case begins. Patients requiring general anesthesia who are scheduled for intraoperative wake-up and neurologic testing generally receive a N_2O/narcotic regimen. Neuromuscular blockade, if used, should be readily reversible for the wake-up test.

For selected lesions, somatosensory and motor-evoked responses may be helpful in both anesthetized and sedated patients. When using motor-evoked potential monitoring during general anesthesia, we titrate neuromuscular blockade to a reduction of single twitch height to about 40 to 50 percent of baseline. Optimal anesthetic regimens for use of intraoperative motor-evoked potentials are being developed.[216] Pressure measurements from balloon catheters placed in the rectum may be of occasional use in assessing sacral root function.

INTRAARTERIAL CHEMOTHERAPY AND EMBOLIZATION OF TUMORS

Preoperative embolization may be performed for many hypervascular tumors in intracranial, craniofacial, and spinal territories.[217,218] Superselective intraarterial administration of chemotherapeutic agents may be used for neoplasms refractory to conventional treatments or as a primary adjunct. SAFE may be used to assess the safety of vessel occlusion, or in some cases, eventual surgical sacrifice. Chemotherapy followed by vascular obliteration is a commonly used combination. Devascularizing the tumor bed prevents tumor swelling.

Hypervascular tumors can swell if there is venous occlusion, hemorrhage into the tumor bed, or significant tissue necrosis. These conditions are most likely to be seen when there is incomplete embolization of feeding arteries. Patients may present with an already compromised airway and treatment may result in further compromise. Systemic effects of chemotherapeutic agents are minimal because, even though standard intravenous doses are used, the drugs appear to become trapped in tissue being embolized.

Paragangliomas present the possibility for catecholamine release from the tumor during the course of embolization,[219] and the means to treat a hypertensive crisis should be at hand. In addition, swelling of carotid body tumors after embolization may result in symptomatic bradycardia.

EPISTAXIS

Hypertension, arteriosclerosis, coagulopathies, trauma, or vascular dysgenesis can cause intractable epistaxis uncontrolled by usual surgical maneuvers, such as intranasal packing. Numerous tortuous vessels, fed by branches of the external carotid artery, are usually visualized in nasal mucosa by angiography. PVA particles and oxidized cotton pledgets are used in obliterating these arteries.[218] Packing can be removed immediately after the embolization. Maintenance of an unobstructed airway and adequate gas exchange with minimal sedation is the primary goal of anesthetic management in these cases.

Conclusions

Interventional neuroradiology is a rapidly expanding field in the treatment of CNS disease. The selection of patients for operative neurosurgery will be profoundly influenced by the development of this specialty. The use of general anesthesia in the treatment of neurosurgical disease will probably decline as operative techniques, both in INR and in the areas of stereotactic and functional neurosurgery, progress. The traditional concepts of "conscious sedation," "monitored anesthesia care," and "general anesthesia" will have to be modified and techniques developed to allow rapid changes in sensorium in patients with unsecured airways and at the same time to provide manipulation of systemic arterial pressure and other physiologic functions.

Acknowledgments

The authors are indebted to Lotfi Hacein-Bey, MD, Huang Dong, MD, Kristy Z. Baker, MD, Patricia Fogarty-Mack, MD, and Shailendra Joshi, MD, for their comments and suggestions; the Neuroanesthesia Section of the Department of Anesthesiology and the Technologist and Nursing staff of the Neuroradiology Division for their part in patient care and development of protocols; to Joyce Ouchi for expert assistance in preparation of the manuscript; and to Bennett M. Stein, MD, J. P. Mohr, MD, and the other members of the Columbia University AVM project for their continued support. Portions of this work were supported by PHS RO1 NS27713 and RO1 NS34949.

References

1. Halbach VV, et al: Interventional neuroradiology. *Am J Roentgenol* 1989; 153:467 (review article).
2. Eskridge JM: Interventional neuroradiology. *Radiology* 1989; 172:991.
3. Barnwell SL: Interventional neuroradiology. *West J Med* 1993; 158:162 (review).
4. Brown MM: Surgery, angioplasty, and interventional neuroradiology. *Curr Opin Neurol Neurosurg* 1993; 6:66.

5. Bryan RN: Remarks on interventional neuroradiology (Commentary on Duckwiler GR et al, pp 621–623 and on Luessenhop AJ, pp 625–629). *AJNR: Am J Neuroradiol* 1990; 11:630.

6. Luessenhop AJ: Interventional neuroradiology: A neurosurgeon's perspective (see Commentary by Bryan RN, pp 630–632). *AJNR: Am J Neuroradiol* 1990; 11:625.

7. Setton A, Berenstein A: Interventional neuroradiology. *Curr Opin Neurol Neurosurg* 1992; 5:870.

8. Duckwiler GR, et al: A survey of vascular interventional procedures in neuroradiology (see Commentary by Bryan RN, pp 630–632). *AJNR: Am J Neuroradiol* 1990; 11:621.

9. Taveras JM: Training in interventional neuroradiology. *Am J Neuroradiol* 1989; 10:909 (editorial).

10. Martin NA: Neurosurgery and interventional neuroradiology. In Vinuela F, et al (eds): *Interventional Neuroradiology: Endovascular Therapy of the Central Nervous System*. New York, Raven Press, 1992:193.

11. Purdy PD, et al: Intraarterial sodium amytal administration to guide preoperative embolization of cerebral arteriovenous malformations. *J Neurosurg Anesth* 1991; 3:103.

12. Dyken ML: Controversies in stroke: Past and present (The Willis Lecture). *Stroke* 1993; 24:1251.

13. Earnest F 4th, et al: Complications of cerebral angiography: Prospective assessment of risk. *Am J Roentgenol* 1984; 142:247.

14. Dion JE, et al: Clinical events following neuroangiography: A prospective study. *Stroke* 1987; 18:997.

15. Young WL, Pile-Spellman J: Anesthetic considerations for interventional neuroradiology. *Anesthesiology* 1994; 80:427 (review).

16. Purdy PD, et al: Management of hemorrhagic complications from preoperative embolization of arteriovenous malformations. *J Neurosurg* 1991; 74:205.

17. Vinuela F, et al: *Inteventional Neuroradiology: Endovascular Therapy of the Central Nervous System*. New York, Raven Press, 1992.

18. Vinuela F, et al: Interventional neuroradiology. *Neuroimaging Clinics of North America: Interventional Neuroradiology* 1992; 2:1.

19. Anon VV, et al: Balloon occlusion of the internal carotid artery in 40 cases of giant intracavernous aneurysm: Technical aspects, cerebral monitoring, and results. *Neuroradiology* 1992; 34:245.

20. Berenstein A, Kricheff II: Catheter and material selection for transarterial embolization. Technical considerations. *Radiology* 1979; 132:619.

21. Anson JA, Spetzler RF: Interventional neuroradiology for spinal pathology. *Clin Neurosurg* 1992; 39:388.

22. Purdy PD, et al: Arteriovenous malformations of the brain: Choosing embolic materials to enhance safety and ease of excision. *J Neurosurg* 1992; 77:217.

23. Cross DT III: Interventional neuroradiology. *Curr Opin Neurol* 1993; 6:891 (review).

24. Rüfenacht DA, Latchaw RE: Principles and methodology of intracranial endovascular access. *Neuroimaging Clinics of North America: Interventional Neuroradiology* 1992; 2:251.

25. Germano IM, et al: Histopathological follow-up study of 66 cerebral arteriovenous malformations after therapeutic embolization with polyvinyl alcohol. *J Neurosurg* 1992; 76:607.

26. Vinuela F, et al: Progressive thrombosis of brain arteriovenous malformations after embolization with isobutyl 2-cyanoacrylate. *Am J Neuroradiol* 1983; 4:1233.

27. Vitek JJ, et al: Angioplasty and stenting in atherosclerotic stenosis on the bifurcation of the carotid artery and the neck portion of the vertebral artery. Presented at the April 23–27 American Society of Neuroradiology meeting in Chicago. Scientific Paper 163:1995.

28. Gelb AW, Herrick IA: Preoperative hypertension does predict post-carotid endarterectomy hypertension (Letter to the Editor) [Comment (with response) on Shuaib A, Hunter M, Anderson MA: Multiple intracranial hemorrhages after carotid endarterectomy, *Can J Neurol Sci* 1989; 16:345–347]. *Can J Neurol Sci* 1990; 17:95.

29. Gelmers HJ, et al: A controlled trial of nimodipine in acute ischemic stroke. *N Engl J Med* 1988; 318:203.

30. Ohman J, Heiskanen O: Effect of nimodipine on the outcome of patients after aneurysmal subarachnoid hemorrhage and surgery. *J Neurosurg* 1988; 69:683.

31. Pickard JD, et al: Effect of oral nimodipine on cerebral infarction and outcome after subarachnoid haemorrhage: British aneurysm nimodipine trial. *BMJ* 1989; 298:636.

32. Mee E, et al: Controlled study of nimodipine in aneurysm patients treated early after subarachnoid hemorrhage. *Neurosurgery* 1988; 22:484.

33. Warner DS, et al: Nicardipine HCl: Clinical experience in patients undergoing anaesthesia for intracranial aneurysm clipping. *Can J Anaesth* 1989; 36:219.

34. Stullken EH, et al: Implications of nimodipine prophylaxis of cerebral vasospasm on anesthetic management during intracranial aneurysm clipping. *J Neurosurg* 1985; 62:200.

35. O'Mahony BJ, Bolsin SNC: Anaesthesia for closed embolisation of cerebral arteriovenous malformations. *Anaesth Intens Care* 1988; 16:318.

36. Duckwiler G, et al: Intravascular microcatheter pressure monitoring: Experimental results and early clinical evaluation. *Am J Neuroradiol* 1990; 11:169.

37. Berenstein A, et al: Somatosensory evoked potentials during spinal angiography and therapeutic transvascular embolization. *J Neurosurg* 1984; 60:777.

38. Rauch RA, et al: Preembolization functional evaluation in brain arteriovenous malformations: The ability of superselective amytal test to predict neurologic dysfunction before embolization. *Am J Neuroradiol* 1992; 13:309.

39. Giller CA, et al: Prediction of tolerance to carotid artery occlusion using transcranial Doppler ultrasound. *J Neurosurg* 1993; 78:366 (abstr).

40. Yudd AP, Van Heertum RL, Masdeu JC: Interventions and functional brain imaging. *Semin Nucl Med* 1991; 21:153.

41. Eckard DA, Purdy PD, Bonte FJ: Temporary balloon occlusion of the carotid artery combined with brain blood flow imaging as a test to predict tolerance prior to permanent carotid sacrifice. *Am J Neuroradiol* 1992; 13:1565.

42. Nakano S, et al: Critical cerebral blood flow thresholds studied by SPECT using xenon-133 and iodine-123 iodoamphetamine. *J Nucl Med* 1989; 30:337.

43. Moody EB, et al: ^{99m}Tc-HMPAO SPECT imaging in interventional neuroradiology: Validation of balloon test occlusion. *Am J Neuroradiol* 1991; 12:1043.

44. Purdy PD: Imaging cerebral blood flow in interventional neuroradiology: Choice of technique and indications. *Am J Neuroradiol* 1991; 12:424 (commentary).

45. Patton CM Jr: Rapid induction of acute dyskinesia by droperidol. *Anesthesiology* 1975; 43:126.

46. Glauber DT, Audenaert SM: Anesthesia for children undergoing craniospinal radiotherapy. *Anesthesiology* 1987; 67:801.

47. Ferrer-Brechner T, Winter J: Anesthetic considerations for cerebral computer tomography. *Anesth Analg* 1977; 56:344.

48. Brann CA, Janik DJ: Anesthesia in the radiology suite. *Problems in Anesthesia* 1992; 6:413.

49. Drummond JC: Cerebral ischemia: State of the art management. *Anesth Analg* 1992 (suppl to vol. 74):1992 Review Course Lectures: 120.

50. Young WL, et al: Cerebral blood flow reactivity to changes in carbon dioxide calculated using end-tidal *versus* arterial tensions. *J Cereb Blood Flow Metab* 1991; 11:1031.

51. Todd MM, Weeks JB, Warner DS: Cerebral blood flow, blood volume, and brain tissue hematocrit during isovolemic hemodilution with hetastarch in rats. *Am J Physiol* 1992; 263:H75.

52. Korosue K, Heros RC: Mechanism of cerebral blood flow augmentation by hemodilution in rabbits. *Stroke* 1992; 23:1487.

53. Service FJ: Hypoglycemic disorders. In Wyngaarden JB, Smith LH Jr (ed): *Cecil Textbook of Medicine.* Philadelphia, WB Saunders, 1985; 1341.

54. Peters KR, et al: Intraarterial use of sodium methohexital for provocative testing during brain embolotherapy. *Am J Neuroradiol* 1993; 14:171.

55. Wada J, Rassmussen T: Intracarotid injection of sodium amytal for the lateralization of cerebral speech dominance: Experimental and clinical observations. *J Neurosurg* 1960; 17:266.

56. Doppman JL, et al: Spinal Wada test. *Radiology* 1986; 161:319.

57. Horton JA, et al: Embolization of intramedullary arteriovenous malformations of the spinal cord. *Am J Neuroradiol* 1986; 7:113.

58. Chollet F, et al: The functional anatomy of motor recovery after stroke in humans: A study with positron emission tomography. *Ann Neurol* 1991; 29:63.

59. Weiller C, et al: Functional reorganization of the brain in recovery from striatocapsular infarction in man. *Ann Neurol* 1992; 31:463.

60. Feeney DM, Baron J-C: Diaschisis. *Stroke* 1986; 17:817.

61. Sass KJ, et al: Neocortically based, congenital vascular malformations: III. Intrahemispheric localization of language functions. *J Clin Exp Neuropsychol* 1988; 10:86.

62. Hamilton MG, Spetzler RF: The prospective application of a grading system for arteriovenous malformations. *Neurosurgery* 1994; 34:2.

63. Schroeder T, et al: Effect of labetalol on cerebral blood flow and middle cerebral arterial flow velocity in healthy volunteers. *Neurol Res* 1991; 13:10.

64. Fitch W, et al: Autoregulation of cerebral blood flow during controlled hypotension in baboons. *J Neurol Neurosurg Psychiatry* 1976; 39:1014.

65. Werner C, et al: Ganglionic blockade improves neurologic outcome from incomplete ischemia in rats: Partial reversal by exogenous catecholamines. *Anesthesiology* 1990; 73:923.

66. Zhang F: Nitric oxide donors increase blood flow and reduce brain damage in focal ischemia: Evidence that nitric oxide is beneficial in the early stages of cerebral ischemia. *J Cereb Blood Flow Metab* 1994; 14:217.

67. Morikawa E, et al: L-Arginine decreases infarct size caused by middle cerebral arterial occlusion in SHR. *Am J Physiol* 1992; 263:H1632.

68. Zhang F, Iadecola C: Fastigial stimulation increases ischemic blood flow and reduces brain damage after focal ischemia. *J Cereb Blood Flow Metab* 1993; 13:1013.

69. Young WL, Cole DJ: Deliberate hypertension: Rationale and application for augmenting cerebral blood flow. *Problems in Anesthesia* 1993; 7:140.

70. Day AL: Arterial distributions and variants. In Wood JH (ed): *Cerebral Blood Flow: Physiologic and Clinical Aspects.* New York, McGraw-Hill, 1987:19.

71. Bladin CF, et al: Confusing stroke terminology: Watershed or borderzone infarction. [Comment on (with response by) van der Zwan A, Hillen B: Review of the variability of the territories of the major cerebral arteries. *Stroke* 1991; 22:1078–1084.] *Stroke* 1993; 24:477 (letter).

72. Van der Zwan A, et al: Variability of the territories of the major cerebral arteries. *J Neurosurg* 1992; 77:927.

73. Szabo MD, et al: Hypertension does not cause spontaneous hemorrhage of intracranial arteriovenous malformations. *Anesthesiology* 1989; 70:761.

74. Watcha MF, White PF: Postoperative nausea and vomiting: Its etiology, treatment, and prevention. *Anesthesiology* 1992; 77:162.

75. Young WL, McCormick PC: Perioperative management of intracranial catastrophes. *Crit Care Clin* 1989; 5:821.

76. Selman WR, et al: Barbiturate-induced coma therapy for focal cerebral ischemia: Effect after temporary and permanent MCA occlusion. *J Neurosurg* 1981; 55:220.

77. Eng CC, et al: The diagnosis and management of a perianesthetic cerebral aneurysmal rupture aided with transcranial Doppler ultrasonography. *Anesthesiology* 1993; 78:191.

78. Goldberg M: Systemic reactions to intravascular contrast media: A guide for the anesthesiologist. *Anesthesiology* 1984; 60:46 (review article).

79. Hirshfeld JW Jr: Low-osmolality contrast agents—who needs them? (Editorial comment on Steinberg EP, Moore RD, Powe NR, Gopalan R, Davidoff AJ: Safety and cost effectiveness of high-osmolality as compared with low-osmolality contrast material in patients undergoing cardiac angiography, pp. 425–430). *N Engl J Med* 1992; 326:482.

80. Caro JJ, et al: The risks of death and of severe nonfatal reactions with high- vs low-osmolality contrast media: A meta-analysis. *Am J Roentgenol* 1991; 56:825.

81. Caro JJ, et al: The cost-effectiveness of replacing high-osmolality with low-osmolality contrast media. *Am J Roentgenol* 1992; 159:869.

82. Steinberg EP, et al: Safety and cost effectiveness of high-osmolality as compared with low-osmolality contrast material in patients undergoing cardiac angiography (see comment by Hirshfeld JW Jr: Low-osmolality contrast agents—who needs them? pp 482–484). *N Engl J Med* 1992; 326:425.

83. Todd MM, Warner DS: Perioperative fluid management in neurosurgery. *Curr Opin Anaesthesiol* 1989; 2:599.

84. Aidinis SJ, et al: Anesthesia for brain computer tomography. *Anesthesiology* 1976; 44:420.

85. Sorenson JA, Phelps ME: *Physics in Nuclear Medicine*, 2d ed. Philadelphia, WB Saunders/Harcourt Brace Jovanovich, 1987:552.

86. Stein BM, Wolpert SM: Arteriovenous malformations of the brain: I. Current concepts and treatment. *Arch Neurol* 1980; 37:1.

87. Kader A, et al: The influence of hemodynamic and anatomic factors on hemorrhage from cerebral arteriovenous malformations. *Neurosurgery* 1994; 34:801.

88. Cunha e Sa MJ, et al: The treatment of associated intracranial aneurysms and arteriovenous malformations. *J Neurosurg* 1992; 77:853.

89. Young WL, et al: Arteriovenous malformation draining vein physiology and determinants of transnidal pressure gradients. *Neurosurgery* 1994; 35:389.

90. Vinuela F, et al: Combined endovascular embolization and surgery in the management of cerebral arteriovenous malformations: Experience with 101 cases. *J Neurosurg* 1991; 75:856.

91. Sisti MB, et al: Microsurgery for 67 intracranial arteriovenous malformations less than 3 cm in diameter. *J Neurosurg* 1993; 79:653.

92. Stein BM: General techniques for the surgical removal of arteriovenous malformations. In Wilson CB, Stein BM (ed): *Intracranial Arteriovenous Malformations.* Baltimore, Williams & Wilkens, 1984:143.

93. Jafar JJ, et al: The effect of embolization with N-butyl cyanoacrylate prior to surgical resection of cerebral arteriovenous malformations. *J Neurosurg* 1993; 78:60.

94. DeMeritt JS, et al: Outcome analysis of preoperative embolization with N-butyl cyanoacrylate in the treatment of cerebral arteriovenous malformations. *Am J Neuroradiol* 1995; 16:1801.

95. Spetzler RF, et al: Normal perfusion pressure breakthrough theory. *Clin Neurosurg* 1978; 25:651.

96. Spetzler RF, et al: Surgical management of large AVM's by staged embolization and operative excision. *J Neurosurg* 1987; 67:17.

97. Mast H, et al: "Steal" is an unestablished mechanism for the clinical presentation of cerebral arteriovenous malformations. *Stroke* 1995; 26:1215.

98. Norbash AM, et al: Correlation of pressure measurements with angiographic characteristics predisposing to hemorrhage and steal in cerebral arteriovenous malformations. *Am J Neuroradiol* 1994; 15:809.

99. Spetzler RF, et al: Relationship of perfusion pressure and size to risk of hemorrhage from arteriovenous malformations. *J Neurosurg* 1992; 76:918.

100. Barnett GH, et al: Cerebral circulation during arteriovenous malformation operation. *Neurosurgery* 1987; 20:836.

101. Hassler W, Steinmetz H: Cerebral hemodynamics in angioma patients: An intraoperative study. *J Neurosurg* 1987; 67:822.

102. Marks MP, et al: Vascular characteristics predictive of hemorrhage in cerebral AVM's. *J Neurosurg* 1993; 78:346 (abstr).

103. Ahuja A, et al: Pedicle pressure changes in cerebral arteriovenous malformations during therapeutic embolization: Relationship to delayed hemorrhage. *Stroke* 1993; 24:185 (abstr).

104. Jungreis CA, et al: Blood pressure changes in feeders to cerebral arteriovenous malformations during therapeutic embolization. *Am J Neuroradiol* 1989; 10:575.

105. Young WL, et al: Evidence for adaptive autoregulatory displacement in hypotensive cortical territories adjacent to arteriovenous malformations. *Neurosurgery* 1994; 34:601.

106. Miyasaka Y, et al: Correlation between intravascular pressure and risk of hemorrhage due to arteriovenous malformations. *Surg Neurol* 1993; 39:370.

107. Miyasaka Y, et al: Draining vein pressure increases and hemorrhage in patients with arteriovenous malformation (case report). *Stroke* 1994; 25:504.

108. Fogarty-Mack P, et al: The effect of arteriovenous malformations on the distribution of intracerebral arterial pressures. *Am J Neuroradiol* in press, 1996.

109. Fleischer LH, et al: Relationship of transcranial Doppler flow velocities and arteriovenous malformation feeding artery pressures. *Stroke* 1993; 24:1897.

110. Spetzler RF: Comment on Young WL, Prohovnik I, Ornstein E, Ostapkovich N, Sisti MB, Solomon A, Stein BM: The effect of arteriovenous malformation resection on cerebrovascular reactivity to carbon dioxide, pp 257–266. *Neurosurgery* 1990; 27:266.

111. Powers WJ: Cerebral hemodynamics in ischemic cerebrovascular disease. *Ann Neurol* 1991; 29:231.

112. Young WL, et al: Cerebral hyperemia after resection is related to "break-through" complications but not to feeding artery pressure. *Neurosurgery* 1996; 38:1085.

113. Nornes H, Grip A: Hemodynamic aspects of cerebral arteriovenous malformations. *J Neurosurg* 1980; 53:456.

114. Prohovnik I, et al: Rapid intra-cerebral ¹¹³Xe injections. *Stroke* 1994; 25:753 (abstr).

115. Fink GR: Effects of cerebral angiomas on perifocal and remote tissue: A multivariate position emission tomography study. *Stroke* 1992; 23:1099.

116. Hacein-Bey L, et al: Adaptive changes in autoregulation to chronic cerebral hypotension with arteriovenous malformations: An acetazolamide-enhanced single-photon emission CT study. *Am J Neuroradiol* 1995; 16:1865.

117. Luessenhop AJ: Natural history of cerebral arteriovenous malformations. In Wilson CB, Stein BM (eds): *Intracranial Arteriovenous Malformations.* Baltimore, Williams & Wilkins, 1984:12.

118. Batjer HH, Devous MD Sr: The use of acetazolamide-enhanced regional cerebral blood flow measurement to predict risk to arteriovenous malformation patients. *Neurosurgery* 1992; 31:213.

119. Manchola IF, et al: Arteriovenous malformation hemodynamics: A transcranial Doppler study. *Neurosurgery* 1993; 33:556.

120. Wade JPH, Hachinski VC: Cerebral steal: Robbery or maldistribution? In Wood JH (ed): *Cerebral Blood Flow: Physiologic and Clinical Aspects.* New York, McGraw-Hill, 1987:467.

121. Homan RW, et al: Quantification of intracerebral steal in patients with arteriovenous malformation. *Arch Neurol* 1986; 43:779.

122. Tyler JL, et al: Hemodynamic and metabolic effects of cerebral arteriovenous malformations studied by positron emission tomography. *Stroke* 1989; 20:890.

123. Sugita M, et al: Improvement of cerebral blood flow and clinical symptoms associated with embolization of a large arteriovenous malformation: Case report. *Neurosurgery* 1993; 33:748.

124. De Reuck J, et al: Positron emission tomography studies of changes in cerebral blood flow and oxygen metabolism in arteriovenous malformation of the brain. *Eur Neurol* 1989; 29:294.

125. Prosenz P, et al: Contribution to the hemodynamics of arterial venous malformations. *Stroke* 1971; 2:279.

126. Marks MP, et al: Cerebral blood flow evaluation of arteriovenous malformations with stable xenon CT. *Am J Neuroradiol* 1988; 9:1169.

127. Tarr RW, et al: Use of acetazolamide-challenge xenon CT in the assessment of cerebral blood flow dynamics in patients with arteriovenous malformations. *Am J Neuroradiol* 1990; 11:441.

128. Hachinski V, et al: Symptomatic intracranial steal. *Arch Neurol* 1977; 34:149.

129. Batjer HH, et al: Intracranial arteriovenous malformation: Relationships between clinical and radiographic factors and ipsilateral steal severity. *Neurosurgery* 1988; 23:322.

130. Porembka D, et al: The postoperative hyperdynamic cardiovascular response following intracranial excision of arterial venous malformation (AVM). *Anesthesiology* 1991; 75:A215 (abstr).

131. Macfarlane R, et al: The role of neuroeffector mechanisms in cerebral hyperfusion syndromes. *J Neurosurg* 1991; 75:845 (review article).

132. Wilson CB, Hieshima G: Occlusive hyperemia: A new way to think about an old problem. *J Neurosurg* 1993; 78:165 (editorial).

133. Al-Rodhan NRF, et al: Occlusive hyperemia: A theory for the hemodynamic complications following resection of intracerebral arteriovenous malformations. *J Neurosurg* 1993; 78:167.

134. Drake CG: Cerebral arteriovenous malformations: Considerations for and experience with surgical treatment in 166 cases. *Clin Neurosurg* 1979; 26:145.

135. Kader A, et al: Transcranial Doppler changes during staged surgical resection of cerebral arteriovenous malformations: A report of three cases. *Surg Neurol* 1993; 39:392.

136. Young WL, et al: Pressure autoregulation is intact after arteriovenous malformation resection. *Neurosurgery* 1993; 32:491.

137. Pelz DM, et al: Symptomatic pulmonary complications from liquid acrylate embolization of brain arteriovenous malformations. *Am J Neuroradiol* 1995; 16:19.

138. Berenstein A: Comment on Sugita M, Takahashi A, Ogawa A, Yoshimoto T: Improvement of cerebral blood flow and clinical symptoms associated with embolization of a large arteriovenous malformation: Case report, pp 748–751. *Neurosurgery* 1993; 33:752.

139. Halbach VV, et al: Dural fistulas involving the transverse and

sigmoid sinuses: Results of treatment in 28 patients. *Radiology* 1987; 163:443.

140. Debrun GM, et al: Indications for treatment and classification of 132 carotid-cavernous fistulas. *Neurosurgery* 1988; 22:285.

141. Halbach V, et al: Normal perfusion pressure breakthrough occurring during treatment of carotid and vertebral fistulas. *Am J Neuroradiol* 1987; 8:751.

142. Lylyk P, et al: Therapeutic alternatives for vein of Galen vascular malformations. *J Neurosurg* 1993; 78:438.

143. McLeod ME, et al: Anaesthetic management of arteriovenous malformations of the vein of Galen. *Can Anaesth Soc J* 1982; 29:307.

144. Lasjaunias P, Berenstein A: Endovascular treatment of the craniofacial lesions. In Lasjaunias P, Berenstein A (eds): *Surgical Neuroangiography*, vol 2. Heidelberg, Springer-Verlag, 1987:389.

145. Roberts JT, et al: A patient with massive oral-facial venous malformation. *J Clin Anesth* 1991; 3:76.

146. Andrews JC, et al: Management of the internal carotid artery in surgery of the skull base. *Laryngoscope* 1989; 99:1224.

147. Berenstein A, et al: Transvascular treatment of giant aneurysms of the cavernous carotid and vertebral arteries. *Surg Neurol* 1984; 21:3.

148. Debrun G, et al: Giant unclippable aneurysms: Treatment with detachable balloons. *Am J Neuroradiol* 1981; 2:167.

149. Leech PJ, et al: Cerebral blood flow, internal carotid artery pressure, and the EEG as a guide to the safety of carotid ligation. *J Neurol Neurosurg Psychiatry* 1974; 37:854.

150. Beatty RA, Richardson AE: Predicting intolerance to common artery ligation by carotid angiography. *J Neurosurg* 1968; 28:9.

151. Ehrenfeld WK, et al: Relation of carotid stump pressure to safety of carotid ligation. *Surgery* 1983; 93:299.

152. Gurdjian ES, et al: Carotid compression in the neck—Results and significance in carotid ligation. *JAMA* 1957; 163:1030.

153. Hacke W, et al: Monitoring of hemispheric or brainstem functions with neurophysiologic methods during interventional neuroradiology. *Am J Neuroradiol* 1983; 4:382.

154. Kwaan JHM, Peterson GJ, Connolly JE: Stump pressure. An unreliable guide for shunting during carotid endarterectomy. *Arch Surg* 1985; 115:1083.

155. Matas R: Testing the efficiency of the collateral circulation as a preliminary to occlusion of the great surgical arteries: Further observations, with special reference to the author's methods, including a review of other tests thus far suggested. *JAMA* 1914; 63:1441.

156. Meinig G, et al: Reduced risk of internal carotid artery ligation after balloon occlusion test. *Neurosurg Rev* 1982; 5:95.

157. Morioka M, et al: Balloon test occlusion of the internal carotid artery with monitoring of compressed spectral arrays (CSAs) of electroencephalogram. *Acta Neurochir (Wien)* 1989; 101:29.

158. Sundt TM, et al: Cerebral blood flow measurements and electroencephalograms during carotid endarterectomy. *J Neurosurg* 1974; 41:310.

159. Wilkinson HA, et al: Correlation of reduction in pressure and angiographic cross-filling with tolerance of carotid artery occlusion. *J Neurosurg* 1965; 22:241.

160. Miller JD, et al: Safety of carotid ligation and its role in the management of intracranial aneurysms. *J Neurol Neurosurg Psychiatry* 1977; 40:64.

161. Sweet WH, et al: A clinical method for recording internal carotid pressure. Significance of changes during carotid occlusion. *Surg Gynecol Obstet* 1950; 90:327.

162. Enzmann DR, et al: Carotid back pressures in conjunction with cerebral angiography. *Radiology* 1980; 134:415.

163. Steed DL, et al: Clinical observations on the effect of carotid artery occlusion on cerebral blood flow mapped by xenon computed tomography and its correlation with carotid artery back pressure. *J Vasc Surg* 1990; 11:38.

164. Heyman A, et al: Measurement of retinal artery and intracarotid pressures following carotid artery occlusion with the Crutchfield clamp. *J Neurosurg* 1960; 17:297.

165. Wylie EJ: Mini symposium: Unusual problems in carotid surgery—Overview. *Surgery* 1983; 93:297.

166. Powers AD, et al: Transcranial Doppler monitoring of cerebral blood flow velocities during surgical occlusion of the carotid artery. *Neurosurgery* 1989; 25:383.

167. Terada T, et al: Assessment of risk of carotid occlusion with balloon Matas testing and dynamic computed tomography. *Neurol Med Chir (Tokyo)* 1988; 28:142.

168. Monsein LH, et al: Assessing adequacy of collateral circulation during balloon test occlusion of the internal carotid artery with ^{99m}Tc-HMPAO SPECT. *Am J Neuroradiol* 1991; 12:1043.

169. Peterman SB, et al: Improved detection of cerebral hypoperfusion with internal carotid balloon test occlusion and ^{99m}Tc-HMPAO cerebral perfusion SPECT imaging. *Am J Neuroradiol* 1991; 12:1035.

170. de Vries EJ, et al: A new method to predict safe resection of the internal carotid artery. *Laryngoscope* 1990; 100:85.

171. Erba SM, et al: Balloon test occlusion of the internal carotid artery with stable xenon/CT cerebral blood flow imaging. *Am J Neuroradiol* 1988; 9:533.

172. Johnson DW, et al: Stable xenon CT cerebral blood flow imaging: Rationale for and role in clinical decision making. *Am J Neuroradiol* 1991; 12:201.

173. Powers WJ, et al: Regional cerebral blood flow and metabolism in reversible ischemia due to vasospasm: Determination by positron emission tomography. *J Neurosurg* 1985; 62:539.

174. Linskey ME, et al: Stroke risk after abrupt internal carotid artery sacrifice: Accuracy of preoperative assessment with balloon test occlusion and stable xenon-enhanced CT. *Am J Neuroradiol* 1994; 15:829.

175. McKay RD, et al: Internal carotid artery stump pressure and cerebral blood flow during carotid endarterectomy: Modification by halothane, enflurane, and innovar. *Anesthesiology* 1976; 45:390.

176. Kofke WA, et al: Comparison of 3-D Xe CBF, transcranial Doppler, and carotid stump pressure during carotid balloon test occlusion in humans. *J Neurosurg Anesth* 1991; 3:207 (abstr).

177. Jorgensen LG, Schroeder TV: Transcranial Doppler for detection of cerebral ischaemia during carotid endarterectomy. *Eur J Vasc Surg* 1992; 6:142.

178. Onesti ST, et al: Cerebral revascularization: A review. *Neurosurgery* 1989; 25:618.

179. Solomon RA, et al: Early aneurysm surgery and prophylactic hypervolemic hypertensive therapy for the treatment of aneurysmal subarachnoid hemorrhage. *Neurosurgery* 1988; 23:699.

180. Solomon RA, et al: Deep hypothermic circulatory arrest for the management of complex anterior and posterior circulation aneurysms. *Neurosurgery* 1991; 29:732.

181. Fox AJ, et al: Use of detachable balloons for proximal artery occlusion in the treatment of unclippable cerebral aneurysms. *J Neurosurg* 1987; 66:40.

182. Guglielmi G, et al: Endovascular treatment of posterior circulation aneurysms by electrothrombosis using electrically detachable coils. *J Neurosurg* 1992; 77:515.

183. Guglielmi G, et al: Electrothrombosis of saccular aneurysms via endovascular approach. *J Neurosurg* 1991; 75:8.

184. Higashida RT, et al: Intracranial aneurysms: Interventional neurovascular treatment with detachable balloons—results in 215 cases. *Radiology* 1991; 178:663.

185. Crompton MR: Mechanism of growth and rupture in cerebral berry aneurysms. *BMJ* 1966; 1:1138.

186. Newell DW, et al: Angioplasty for the treatment of symptomatic vasospasm following subarachnoid hemorrhage. *J Neurosurg* 1989; 71:654.

187. Ishii R: Regional cerebral blood flow in patients with ruptured intracranial aneurysms. *J Neurosurg* 1979; 50:587.

188. Carpenter DA, et al: Cerebral oxygen metabolism after aneurysmal subarachnoid hemorrhage. *J Cereb Blood Flow Metab* 1991; 11:837.

189. Schroeder T: Hemodynamic significance of internal carotid artery disease. *Acta Neurol Scand* 1988; 77:353 (review article).

190. Grubb RL, et al: Effects of subarachnoid hemorrhage on cerebral blood volume, blood flow, and oxygen utilization in humans. *J Neurosurg* 1977; 46:446.

191. Clouston JE, et al: Intraarterial papaverine infusion for cerebral vasospasm after subarachnoid hemorrhage. *Am J Neuroradiol* 1995; 16:27.

192. Kaku Y, et al: Superselective intra-arterial infusion of papaverine for the treatment of cerebral vasospasm after subarachnoid hemorrhage. *J Neurosurg* 1992; 77:842.

193. Kassell NF, et al: Treatment of cerebral vasospasm with intra-arterial papaverine. *J Neurosurg* 1992; 77:848.

194. Livingston K, Hopkins LN: Intraarterial papaverine as an adjunct to transluminal angioplasty for vasospasm induced by subarachnoid hemorrhage. *Am J Neuroradiol* 1993; 14:346.

195. Marks MP, Steinberg GK, Lane B: Intraarterial papaverine for the treatment of vasospasm. *Am J Neuroradiol* 1993; 14:822.

196. Morgan MK, et al: The use of intraarterial papaverine in the management of vasospasm complicating arteriovenous malformation resection. *J Neurosurg* 1995; 82:296.

197. Aoki H, et al: Relationship between cytosolic calcium concentration and force in the papaverine-induced relaxation of medial strips of pig coronary artery. *Br J Pharmacol* 1994; 111:489.

198. Iguchi M, et al: On the mechanism of papaverine inhibition of the voltage-dependent Ca^{++} current in isolated smooth muscle cells from the guinea pig trachea. *J Pharmacol Exp Ther* 1992; 263:194.

199. Phillis JW, et al: Effects of anoxia on cerebral blood flow in the rat brain: Evidence for a role of adenosine in autoregulation. *J Cereb Blood Flow Metab* 1984; 4:586.

200. Jin Y, et al: The effects of papaverine on phorbol dibutyrate-induced vasoconstriction in brain slice microvessels. *J Neurosurg* 1994; 81:574.

201. Fogarty-Mack P, et al: Superselective intra-arterial papaverine: Effect on regional cerebral blood flow in patients with arteriovenous malformations. *J Neurosurg* in press, 1996.

202. Mathis JM, et al: Transient neurologic events associated with intraarterial papaverine infusion for subarachnoid hemorrhage-induced vasospasm. *Am J Neuroradiol* 1994; 15:1671.

203. Tsai FY, et al: Percutaneous transluminal angioplasty of the carotid artery. *Am J Neuroradiol* 1986; 7:349.

204. Higashida RT, et al: Transluminal angioplasty for atherosclerotic disease of the vertebral and basilar arteries. *J Neurosurg* 1993; 78:192.

205. North American Symptomatic Carotid Endarterectomy Trial Collaborators: Beneficial effect of carotid endarterectomy in symptomatic patients with high-grade carotid stenosis. *N Engl J Med* 1991; 325:445.

206. North American Symptomatic Carotid Endarterectomy Trial (NASCET) Steering Committee: North American Symptomatic Carotid Endarterectomy Trial: Methods, patient characteristics, and progress. *Stroke* 1991; 22:711.

207. North American Symptomatic Carotid Endarterectomy Trial (NASCET) Investigators: Clinical alert: Benefit of carotid endarterectomy for patients with high-grade stenosis of the internal carotid artery (Special Report)—National Institute of Neurological Disorders and Stroke: Stroke and Trauma Division. *Stroke* 1991; 22:816.

208. Theron J, et al: New triple coaxial catheter system for carotid angioplasty with cerebral protection [followed with Commentary by Ferguson R: Getting it right the first time, pp 875–877]. *Am J Neuroradiol* 1990; 11:869.

209. del Zoppo GJ, et al: Local intra-arterial fibrinolytic therapy in acute carotid territory stroke: A pilot study. *Stroke* 1988; 19:307.

210. Brott T: Thrombolytic therapy for stroke. *Cerebrovasc Brain Metab Rev* 1991; 3:91.

211. Wardlaw JM, Warlow CP: Thrombolysis in acute ischemic stroke: Does it work? *Stroke* 1992; 23:1826.

212. Zeumer H: Fibrinolysis in cerebrovascular diseases of the central nervous system. In Vinuela F, et al (eds): *Interventional Neuroradiology: Endovascular Therapy of the Central Nervous System.* New York, Raven Press, 1992:141.

213. Zeumer H: et al: Intravascular thrombolysis in central nervous system cerebrovascular disease. *Interventional Neuroradiology* 1992; 2:359.

214. Lyden PD, Zivin JA: Hemorrhagic transformation after cerebral ischemia: Mechanisms and incidence. *Cerebrovasc Brain Metab Rev* 1993; 5:1.

215. Theron J, et al: Spinal arteriovenous malformations: Advances in therapeutic embolization. *Radiology* 1986; 158:163.

216. Kalkman CJ, et al: Effects of propofol, etomidate, midazolam, and fentanyl on motor evoked responses to transcranial electrical or magnetic stimulation in humans. *Anesthesiology* 1992; 76:502.

217. Manelfe C, et al: Preoperative embolization of intracranial meningiomas. *Am J Neuroradiol* 1986; 7:963.

218. Davis KR: Embolization of epistaxis and juvenile nasopharyngeal angiofibromas. *Am J Roentgenol* 1984; 148:209.

219. LaMuraglia GM, et al: The current surgical management of carotid body paragangliomas. *J Vasc Surg* 1992; 15:1038.

Chapter 26

INTRACRANIAL ANEURISMS AND A-V MALFORMATIONS

Surgical Considerations

BRYCE K. WEIR

Aneurysms

EPIDEMIOLOGY

INCIDENCE OF SUBARACHNOID HEMORRHAGE FROM ANEURYSMS

About 1 in 100 adults may harbor an intracranial aneurysm. In over half of such cases, rupture of this lesion causes death. The annual incidence of aneurysmal subarachnoid hemorrhage (SAH) is approximately 10/100,000.[1-3] Almost every racial group appears to be affected by aneurysms, but certain countries such as Finland and Japan seem to have particularly high rates. Contrary to what used to be taught, aneurysms are not congenital lesions, and their incidence in the first few decades of life is extremely low. They are degenerative, acquired structures that become progressively more common with aging.[2,3] Because of the population mix of society, the most common age at presentation is in the sixth decade. Smoking is probably a risk factor for the development and rupture of aneurysms; hypertension also may have a causal relationship, but the data are less clear than for smoking.[1,3] Aneurysmal subarachnoid hemorrhage accounts for about one-tenth of all cerebrovascular accidents.[4] Males outnumber females until about age 50; females progressively predominate thereafter.

NATURAL HISTORY AFTER RUPTURE

About 1 patient in 6 with a ruptured aneurysm will die within minutes and will not be admitted to the hospital.[3] Aneurysms are therefore an important group in forensic pathology series. Of patients who survive to be admitted to the hospital, about one-quarter will still die, and only just over one-half will recover completely. The natural history is seldom seen now that therapeutic intervention is commonly undertaken. From early population studies it was known that for every five cases of untreated ruptured aneurysms, there would be one death after the first day, two deaths by the end of the first week, three deaths by the end of the first six months, and four deaths after 20 years.[3]

PROGNOSTIC FACTORS FOR OUTCOME

The rate and volume of bleeding are probably the fundamental determinants of outcome. This determines the neurologic condition of the patient on presentation at the hospital. Patients who have only a severe headache and who never lost consciousness fare much better than patients who arrive comatose. Sicker patients do worse.[5] Old age and poor general health play an important adverse role. A large number of these patients will give a history of hypertension. The presence of significant clots within the substance of the brain or the ventricles is also prognostic for a poor outcome. Patients who have a repeat hemorrhage are much less likely to survive than those who have only one. Without treatment, at least one-half of cases with ruptured aneurysms will re-rupture within six months and thereafter at a rate of approximately 3 percent per year. The risk of rupture of multiple aneurysms or incidentally discovered aneurysms is not known with as much certainty, but it probably approaches a 1 to 3 percent risk of rupture per year.[1,3,4]

TIMING OF SURGERY; POSTOPERATIVE AND MANAGEMENT MORTALITY

Most neurosurgeons now try to operate early to definitively clip a ruptured aneurysm, since the greatest risk to the patient's life following hospital admission is rebleeding. Until fairly recently a substantial number of neurosurgeons held the opinion that patients would do better overall if they were allowed to recover from the initial insult before having the superimposed trauma of an operation. Nowadays, there are ways of preventing and treating the cerebral vasospasm that used to be a powerful disincentive to early surgery. Since the death rate from the initial effects of the hemorrhage diminishes with the passage of time, as does the chance for rebleeding, it follows that, if surgery is delayed for two or three weeks, it will be performed on survivors, so that the postoperative mortality rate will be less than for all patients operated upon early.

However, it is likely that the overall management mortality (deaths while waiting for operation versus postoperative deaths) for all cases will be reduced by early surgery. It also seems reasonable that neurologic outcome will be correspondingly improved by earlier surgery.[3,5] Delaying surgery may still be justified in cases of overwhelming medical contraindications, or extreme technical difficulty due to the adverse size and location of an aneurysm. The red, angry, swollen brain that discouraged earlier generations of aneurysm surgeons can to a large extent be ameliorated by techniques that reduce intracranial pressure, such as draining spinal fluid, osmotic diuretics, and neuroanesthetic control of blood gases and other parameters.

GENETICS OF ANEURYSMS AND ASSOCIATED DISEASE STATES

FAMILIAL ANEURYSMS
Between 1 in 20 and 1 in 10 patients with ruptured aneurysms will have one or more first-order relatives who also had a ruptured aneurysm. Such a history should be sought in all cases, and it is our current practice to offer siblings of such patients the opportunity of having magnetic resonance angiography carried out. Those found to have unruptured asymptomatic aneurysms are offered prophylactic surgery in most cases. The exact mechanism of transmission of the tendency to develop aneurysms is unknown, but it is probably a dominant method of transmission with variable penetrance.[3,6]

ADULT POLYCYSTIC KIDNEY DISEASE
Almost one in twenty cases in most large series of aneurysms has suffered from polycystic kidney disease.[2,3,6] Such patients usually give a family or personal history of this disease and will show albuminuria, azotemia, and hypertension in almost all cases. The severe coexisting kidney disease is an adverse factor in patients who have ruptured aneurysms. Careful management of blood pressure and the electrolyte / fluid status

in such patients has greatly improved the outlook. It seems reasonable to offer magnetic resonance angiography since as many as one-third of patients with polycystic kidney disease are found to have aneurysms at autopsy. The chance of these lesions having ruptured is about 1 in 10.

COARCTATION OF THE AORTA
Almost 1.0 percent of patients with aneurysms reported in the neurologic literature have been found to have coarctation of the aorta.[2] It is estimated that 1 patient in 20 with aortic coarctation will develop an aneurysm. In all reported cases the patients have been hypertensive. Coarctation is somewhat more common in young males. Untreated, these lesions can lead to aortic rupture, bacterial endocarditis, and congestive heart failure, as well as rupture of intracranial aneurysms. All patients with aneurysms should be checked for upper body hypertension, particularly younger patients.[3]

SICKLE CELL DISEASE
Almost any neurologic sign or symptom can result in this hereditary form of chronic hemolytic anemia. About one patient in five with sickle cell disease will have neurologic complications. Thrombosis is more common than hemorrhage, and hemorrhage from an aneurysm is quite rare. Other manifestations include chronic hemolytic anemia, hyperbilirubinemia, recurrent painful crises, multiple infarctions, and shortened life expectancy. Patients presenting with subarachnoid hemorrhage from ruptured aneurysms who suffer from sickle cell disease should be adequately hydrated, the electrolyte imbalance should be corrected, and any underlying infection treated.[1,4] Adequate oxygenation is imperative, and acidosis and hypothermia should be studiously avoided. Partial exchange transfusions are considered an effective way of breaking the vicious cycle of sickling. Some authorities have advocated partial exchange transfusions to reduce the amount of hemoglobin S to less than 30 or 40 percent prior to angiography and surgery.

DRUG ABUSE
It is estimated that there may be more than five million cocaine abusers in North America currently. This drug produces intense generalized vasoconstriction with resultant hypertension. It appears to be associated with the rupture of intracranial aneurysms at an earlier age than would otherwise be expected. In addition, the history of cocaine abuse has been associated with a very high management mortality. Knowledge of the patient's addiction may be useful in the acute medical management and perhaps more importantly in the rehabilitation of such patients.[4]

OTHER DISEASES

It is not established with certainty whether essential hypertension increases the risk of developing an aneurysm, but it is very likely. There is conflicting evidence. It has also been suggested that patients are more likely to develop multiple aneurysms if they are hypertensive. About 30 to 40 percent of ruptured aneurysm patients have preexisting significant hypertension.[1-5]

Other relatively rare conditions that have been associated with the occurrence of intracranial aneurysms include fibromuscular dysplasia, Marfan's syndrome, tuberous sclerosis, Ehlers-Danlos syndrome, hereditary hemorrhagic telangiectasia, moyamoya disease, and pseudoxanthoma elasticum.[2,3]

SYMPTOMS AND SIGNS OF SUBARACHNOID HEMORRHAGE FROM ANEURYSMS

SYMPTOMS

Headache

The rupture of an intracranial aneurysm usually leads to the very *sudden* onset of the *worst* headache in the patient's life. Despite its very dramatic and severe symptomatology, it is amazing that the diagnosis is so frequently missed by the patients and their families and even more so by their initial medical attendants. Common misdiagnoses include influenza, meningitis, cervical disc disease, migraine headaches, heart attacks, and malingering. Since migraine and other chronic headache syndromes are so common in the general population, it is to be expected that many patients with ruptured aneurysms will give such a history. Usually, however, the patient will say that the headache of ruptured aneurysm is clearly different and more severe than the previous migraine headaches. Occasionally the entity of benign orgasmic headache can lead to diagnostic confusion, since such headaches are often instantaneous and very severe. Since true aneurysms can also rupture during the hypertensive challenge induced by sexual orgasm, it is important to investigate such headaches thoroughly. Usually in the benign nonaneurysmal headaches, there is a history of multiple similar headaches under similar circumstances.[2,3]

Malaise

Most patients following an aneurysmal rupture feel ill and may be irritable, uncooperative, and combative. This occasionally leads to misdiagnosis, particularly if the patient were drinking or taking drugs at the time of the rupture.

SIGNS

Impaired Consciousness

Consciousness may be impaired to any degree, including deep coma, although some patients will have re-covered completely by the time of medical presentation. Then the correct diagnosis depends on a high index of suspicion based on the history of a sudden onset of the worst headache of the patient's life.

Neck Stiffness

This finding is given considerable importance in most textbooks, but it may be absent in the early hours after hemorrhage and may not be evident in a patient who is in deep coma.

Ophthalmologic Signs

The presence of hemorrhages on ophthalmologic examination is important confirmatory evidence of the recent occurrence of subarachnoid hemorrhage and is prognostic for a poorer outcome.[8]

Focal Neurologic Deficits

Aphasia or hemiplegia is relatively unusual at the onset of subarachnoid hemorrhage. Their likelihood increases with the occurrence of intracerebral hemorrhage. This type of bleeding becomes more common after subsequent episodes of aneurysmal rupture. In the interval between 4 and 14 days after the subarachnoid hemorrhage, the possibility of delayed cerebral infarction from severe, angiographically demonstrable vasospasm becomes a likely cause of focal deficits. It is critical during this time to avoid volume depletion and hypotension and to ameliorate any electrolyte abnormality, particularly hyponatremia.[1,6]

Fever

Subarachnoid blood is a potent stimulus to temperature elevation. Patients with larger volume subarachnoid clots are more likely to get high fever and also delayed cerebral ischemia. There is a convincing body of experimental work demonstrating that modest temperature reductions are efficacious in reducing infarct size to a variety of insults. It makes sense to combat abnormal temperature elevations in patients, particularly in the period of maximal risk of delayed infarction from vasospasm.[3]

Biochemical and Hematologic Changes

The most common abnormality after subarachnoid hemorrhage is hyponatremia, which usually progresses after a few days and will be maximal a week or two following the bleeding. Opinion varies widely as to the optimal hematocrit for a patient after a subarachnoid hemorrhage. Some authorities deliberately recommend hemodilution and a hematocrit around 30 percent to increase cerebral blood flow. The author favors maintaining a hematocrit normal for a particular patient. Oxygen delivery to the brain is a more important parameter than absolute level of cerebral blood flow, which increases with hemodilution.[3]

REBLEEDING

PROGNOSTIC FACTORS

The larger the hole in the aneurysm at the initial rupture, the larger the volume of blood likely to be deposited in the subarachnoid space. This, in turn, produces a worsened neurologic state. It makes sense, therefore, that a bad prognostic factor for rebleeding is impaired neurologic status. The shorter the interval from hemorrhage, the higher the rebleeding rate will be. Females have a rebleeding rate about twice that of males, and patients in poor general medical condition are also more prone to early rebleeding. High levels of hypertension are also associated with an increased risk. Older patients rebleed more commonly than younger ones. About one patient in five will rebleed in two weeks, and about one in three will rebleed at two months if definitive clipping is not undertaken. Rebleeding rates are about halved in the initial two weeks if antifibrinolytic agents are used. Unfortunately, their use is associated with doubling of the mortality rates from delayed ischemia, so that there is no net gain from the use of antifibrinolytics. Therefore, most neurosurgeons have abandoned their use and opted instead for early surgery with definitive clipping of the bleeding point.[3]

METHODS FOR REDUCING REBLEEDING RATES

In the early period immediately following aneurysmal rupture it is important to lower the patient's blood pressure if possible. This can be done with analgesics and antihypertensive agents such as sodium nitroprusside. After the first few days following subarachnoid hemorrhage, the risk of lowering the blood pressure increases, since the patient is then into the time interval of vasospasm and delayed ischemia. At that point it is probably best to let the patient's blood pressure go where it will. Rebleeding may be stimulated by lumbar puncture or rapid ventricular drainage when the aneurysm is still unsecured. Lowering the intracranial pressure may be done as a calculated risk if cerebral perfusion is already compromised by intracranial hypertension.[3]

It is conceivable that endovascular techniques may be used to secure an aneurysm at the time of initial angiography; if this prevents early rebleeding, then surgery could be performed under optimal conditions on a delayed basis. The role of endovascular techniques is currently undergoing intensive investigation, but at the time of this writing application of an aneurysm clip across the neck of the lesion represents the gold standard of therapy.[4]

MEDICAL COMPLICATIONS

Given that the average patient age is just over 50, it is not surprising that those with SAH from aneurysms suffer from many preceding diseases. The most common probably is hypertension, which is present in between one and two of every five patients. It is a poor risk factor and is prognostic for cerebral infarction as well as death. The most common postoperative medical complications in one large series were hypertension, pneumonia, anemia, gastrointestinal bleeding, cardiac arrhythmias, electrolyte disorders, hypotension, atelectasis, diabetes, adult respiratory distress syndrome, and cardiac failure.[5,7] Each of these affected more than 2 percent of the series. Less common, but often more lethal, were pulmonary embolisms (at 0.8 percent) and myocardial infarction (at 0.7 percent).

Most patients who die from ruptured aneurysms in the first day or two will show pathologic evidence of pulmonary edema. Neurogenic pulmonary edema is of extremely rapid onset. This is a life-threatening early complication in patients who are initially deeply comatose. There may be a history of vomiting and pink foam pouring from the airways, and patients are cyanotic and show abnormal respiratory patterns. The skin may be moist and cool, and hypoxia and hypocapnia occur. Treatment consists of intubation, vigorous suctioning, and oxygenation. Lasix and dobutamine have been reported to be therapeutic in neurogenic pulmonary edema.

About one-third of patients will show ECG abnormalities, which can be of any type. They are a reflection of subendocardial ischemia, hemorrhage, or myocardial necrosis. Changes are more likely to occur if the patient is hypokalemic and they spontaneously reduce in frequency and severity in the 10 days following SAH.[3]

Risk factors for pulmonary embolism include a previous occurrence, advanced age, obesity, paresis, cardiac failure, and lower limb trauma. Compression stockings are routinely used, and many neurosurgeons are employing low-dose heparin prophylactically.

It used to be thought that hyponatremia resulted from inappropriate secretion of antidiuretic hormone, but recently there has been persuasive evidence that it is more likely due to cerebral salt wasting. This has practical consequences in that the treatment for inappropriate antidiuretic hormone secretion is fluid restriction, and this in itself can be dangerous in the setting of potential delayed cerebral ischemia from vasospasm. Cerebral salt wasting can be treated with saline replacement. The clinical and laboratory differentiation of these syndromes is sometimes difficult and usually hinges on the fact that patients with cerebral salt wasting are volume-depleted in comparison to those with inappropriate antidiuretic hormone secretion.[3] Leukocytosis is common in response to subarachnoid blood.[3]

Almost 5 percent of patients will suffer from some

degree of gastrointestinal bleeding. This can be sudden and life-threatening and should be thought of in any unexpected episode of hypotension and tachycardia.[3]

Seizures can be expected to develop in almost one patient in ten.[2-4] They are more likely in patients who have intracerebral hemorrhage or infarction. There is no convincing evidence that prophylactic anticonvulsant therapy is beneficial in the acute phase after SAH, although giving them is a common practice. The generalized seizure-like activity occurring at the time of SAH is not prognostic for the subsequent development of seizures. The mean time of onset of seizures after SAH is 20 months, and more than 90 percent of cases will have had their first seizure by three years.

TYPES OF ANEURYSMS

SACCULAR
The great majority of aneurysms are less than one inch in maximum diameter. The surgical results of treating ruptured aneurysms are to some extent a function of their size, with poor results being associated with larger and therefore technically more difficult aneurysms. They result from disintegration of the elastic layer of the artery at the flow separator region in response to the ceaseless pounding of the arterial pulse wave.[3]

GIANT
These lesions make up about 5 percent of all aneurysms.[2,3] They can range in size up to 10 cm or so. Larger aneurysms tend more frequently to be partially filled with onion-like layers of laminated thrombus than do smaller aneurysms. The necks of these giant aneurysms are often thick and brittle; with the growth of such aneurysms, important arteries may be incorporated into the wall so that simple neck clipping is much less likely to be an option than with smaller aneurysms. Removal of thrombus may be necessary before the neck can be accurately clipped. Large size is no insurance against rupture. There is sometimes a need for innovative and complex surgical approaches, including bypassing of the affected arterial segments or direct surgery under induced cardiac arrest and hypothermia. Sometimes in a very old patient, or when there are minor or no symptoms, giant aneurysms are best left alone.

SPECIAL
Fusiform aneurysms are elongate, cigar-shaped arterial enlargements commonly associated with severe atherosclerosis, but may result from certain degenerative processes in childhood. Dissecting aneurysms result from a tear in the luminal endothelial layer that permits the blood column to dissect in between the endothe-

lium and the media. Blood may actually tear through the media and produce an SAH. In the vertebral and basilar arteries these are sometimes associated with trauma. Treatment may consist of trapping the dissected segment if there has been frank rupture.[3]

Aneurysms may develop when the vessel wall is weakened by small emboli of infectious or neoplastic material. Drug addicts and patients with infective endocarditis are prone to these bacterial aneurysms. The two relatively common types of tumors associated with multiple peripheral cerebral aneurysms are choriocarcinoma and cardiac myxomas.[2,3]

Aneurysms can also be traumatic in origin. In some cases there may be sharp contact between the falx or the sphenoid ridge and the pericallosal or middle cerebral arteries which can traumatize the vessel wall, leading to the development of a traumatic aneurysm over two or three weeks. The occurrence of SAH in this time frame after a severe head injury should lead to the consideration of a traumatic aneurysm.[2,3]

PATHOLOGY

PATHOLOGIC CHANGES AFTER RUPTURE
Since saccular aneurysms are by far the most common aneurysms, and since they are usually located at vessel bifurcations in the subarachnoid space, it follows that most hematomas following rupture are located in the subarachnoid space. However, with the resultant fibrosis that takes place, subsequent episodes of bleeding are more likely to direct the pathologic stream of blood into the brain or into the ventricles via the brain. In most clinical series, about one in five patients will be found to have an intracerebral hemorrhage and about the same number to have some amount of intraventricular blood.[3,5,7] These are ominous developments and commonly cause death, so that in pathologic series the incidence of bleeding in the brain or ventricles is at least double that of clinical series. Infarction of the brain can result from hematomas with direct brain destruction or shifts and vascular compromise. An additional important cause of delayed brain infarction is cerebral vasospasm.

HYDROCEPHALUS
Acute
The sudden deposition of a large jelly-like clot throughout the subarachnoid space can block spinal fluid passage through the basal subarachnoid cisterns. Between one in ten to fifteen patients will show acute ventricular dilatation in the first few hours following aneurysmal rupture. This condition of spinal fluid blockage can lead to a spuriously poor neurologic grade. It is usually necessary to institute ventricular drainage to normalize intracranial pressure. One of the advantages of early

clipping of an aneurysm is that ventricular drainage can be instituted at surgery without the usual concern that excessive lowering of intracranial pressure will cause an increase in transmural aneurysmal pressure that increases the tendency of unclipped aneurysms to rupture.[3]

Chronic

Between one in ten to fifteen patients will develop an insidious ventriculomegaly in the weeks following subarachnoid hemorrhage. This is an important cause of (1) failure to improve in the patient who is initially comatose; or (2) a secondary slow decline in patients who were initially in good condition. Virtually every patient with a ruptured aneurysm should have a CT scan about a month after the bleed to ensure that no chronic hydrocephalus is developing. The symptoms usually include impairment of consciousness, dementia, gait disturbance, and incontinence.[3]

PHYSIOLOGY

INTRACRANIAL PRESSURE

At the time of aneurysmal rupture the intracranial pressure can equal that of mean blood pressure and result in global impairment of blood flow to the brain. That this is not always the case is indicated by the fact that a majority of patients do not actually lose consciousness. It is reasonable to place a ventricular catheter to record intracranial pressure in patients who are obtunded or comatose, especially grade 4 or 5 patients, if there is doubt as to whether the patient should be subjected to craniotomy. Once the aneurysm is clipped, maintenance of the intracranial pressure below 20 mmHg is reasonable. There has been some evidence that excessive drainage of spinal fluid may predispose to the subsequent onset of clinical hydrocephalus.[3]

CEREBRAL BLOOD FLOW

Normal blood flow is approximately 50 ml/100 g per min. The larger the volume of subarachnoid blood and the greater the intracranial pressure, the more likely it is that neurologic grade will be poor and that the cerebral blood flow will be reduced. Once severe diffuse vasospasm exists, there is almost always a regional reduction in blood flow. Subarachnoid hemorrhage is a common cause for the loss of autoregulation, which is the ability of the brain to maintain normal steady flow in the face of a changing systemic blood pressure between a mean arterial blood pressure of 50 and 150 mmHg. Under physiologic circumstances, the cerebral blood flow is linearly responsive to the Pa_{CO_2} between 20 and 100 mmHg; and an increase in Pa_{CO_2} of 1 mmHg

is associated with an increase in cerebral blood flow of 2 ml/100 g per min.[3,6]

CEREBRAL OXYGEN METABOLISM AND DELIVERY

There is a significant reduction in cerebral metabolic rate for oxygen after subarachnoid hemorrhage. This can occur even when the cerebral blood flow and oxygen extraction fraction values are normal. Cerebral metabolic rate for oxygen is dependent on the cerebral blood flow, the total arterial oxygen content, and the oxygen extraction fraction. The total arterial oxygen content in turn depends on the hemoglobin concentration and the arterial oxygen saturation. It is important in the post-subarachnoid hemorrhage state to attempt to optimize oxygen delivery to the brain. This is *the* critical parameter, not the cerebral blood flow itself. Under some circumstances hemodilution can increase the cerebral blood flow, yet actually reduce the oxygen delivery. Maintaining hemoglobin concentration at a normal range is probably a reasonable policy.[3]

ANATOMY

COMMON LOCATIONS OF ANEURYSMS

About nine out of ten aneurysms are on the anterior circulation and about one in ten on the posterior.[2,3] There are three common sites in the anterior circulation: internal carotid–posterior communicating, anterior communicating, and middle cerebral artery bifurcation. There are three relatively uncommon sites: internal carotid–ophthalmic, internal carotid artery bifurcation, and distal anterior cerebral artery. The remaining anterior circulation sites are rare. The most common site in the posterior circulation is the basilar apex, with the remaining sites all being uncommon. About one patient in five with an aneurysm will have more than one. In females, the proximal internal carotid circulation is more commonly involved; in males, the anterior communicating artery region is favored. The internal carotid artery bifurcation is a relatively common location in childhood.

POSITIONING AT SURGERY BY LOCATION OF ANEURYSM

The supine position with a slight hyperextension of the neck and medial tilt is most commonly employed for supratentorial aneurysms. The true lateral position is used for patients where the basilar apex is being approached from the subtemporal route. Posterior circulation aneurysms from the vertebral artery to the upper basilar trunk are usually approached with the patient in the semilateral position. The sitting position is rarely if ever employed.[3]

SPECIAL CONSIDERATIONS

PEDIATRIC PATIENTS

Fewer than one in twenty patients with ruptured aneurysm will be under the age of 20 years. Most children with aneurysms present with typical subarachnoid hemorrhage. About one-half of children with subarachnoid hemorrhage will have aneurysms, and about one-quarter will have arteriovenous malformations.[2,3] Children are much more resistant to the effects of vasospasm than are adults. Because of their unique potential for neurologic recovery, heroic therapeutic measures are indicated, even in those with poor initial neurologic grade.

ANEURYSMS DURING PREGNANCY

Subarachnoid hemorrhage causes about one in twenty-five deaths in pregnancy. The rate of rupture from aneurysms increases progressively during pregnancy and is highest on the day of delivery. Most patients who die from subarachnoid hemorrhage have had previous pregnancies without rupture. Ruptured aneurysms in patients who are pregnant should be treated as if the patient were not pregnant. Whether or not a cesarean section should be performed would depend on the individual circumstances of the case. For instance, if a patient is suffering from delayed cerebral ischemia several days after aneurysmal rupture and aneurysm clipping, a C-section might be preferable to normal vaginal delivery. In many other circumstances this would not be the case despite a recent subarachnoid hemorrhage.[2-4]

ANEURYSMS AND ARTERIOVENOUS MALFORMATIONS

About 1.0 percent of patients with an aneurysm will also have coincidental arteriovenous malformations (AVMs).[2-4] On the other hand, about one in fifteen patients with an AVM will be found to have an aneurysm. The high flow through some arteriovenous malformations probably is an inciting factor to the development of aneurysms on proximal arteries feeding the malformation. Occasionally after removal of the AVMs proximal aneurysms will decrease in size or totally regress. In patients with both aneurysms and arteriovenous malformations, the chance of one or the other being the source of a hemorrhage is about equal. The pattern of bleeding is important in making the correct diagnosis. Subarachnoid hemorrhage is much more common with a ruptured aneurysm, and intraparenchymal bleeding in relationship to the AVM suggests that this is the more likely site of rupture. Both lesions should be treated, if this is feasible, when doubt remains as to the source of the hemorrhage. If the aneurysm is considered to be the cause of the subarachnoid hemorrhage, an associated arteriovenous malformation may be left until later if surgery is indicated for the AVM at all.

TECHNIQUES OF MANAGING ANEURYSMS

CLIPPING

The microsurgical placement of an aneurysm clip flush with the aneurysm-bearing artery is the gold standard of treatment.[8] Late clip failure is virtually unknown with the modern generation of clips. Late rebleeding from a clipped aneurysm is such an unusual event that routine angiographic assessment is not indicated. The common most problems in clip application are incomplete occlusion of the neck with residual aneurysmal filling or the continued existence of an aneurysmal pathologic wall proximal to the clip that can subsequently balloon and rupture. The clip may also inadvertently occlude nearby normal vessels. The employment of intraoperative angiography reduces these hazards.

PROXIMAL LIGATION

Occasionally the location of an aneurysm, such as the cavernous carotid, makes direct operative approach and clipping hazardous. Other factors related to the size or morphology of the aneurysm may also make direct clipping hazardous or impossible. In such circumstances the occlusion of the common or internal carotid artery in the neck produces a high likelihood of total thrombosis of the aneurysm, particularly when located more proximally on the internal carotid. The hazards of carotid occlusion are immediate hemodynamic ischemia due to failure of collateral circulatory pathways, thrombosis within the carotid distal to the clamp with extension or embolization to cause ischemic infarction, and late hemodynamic symptoms when the effects of aging may make previously adequate compensatory mechanisms fail. Carotid ligation, however, particularly for unruptured aneurysms, has a very low acute mortality and morbidity. The alternatives such as cardiac standstill and deep hypothermia usually entail higher risk.[4]

COILING

The placement of thrombogenic material into aneurysms has been performed for many decades. Recently, however, with the development of endovascular techniques, this has become a much more attractive treatment option.[1] The placement of thrombogenic coils is becoming a more widely employed technique, but at the time of writing is still not an approved standard therapy. It will be some years before we know the long term failure rate. It appears that normal endothelial formation over the coiled wires may not take place or may do so only partially. It is also possible that many of the coiled aneurysms that are not 100 percent occluded may show late growth.

OTHER

Occasionally, aneurysms can be satisfactorily treated by placing a clip on a proximal intracranial vessel. This procedure is clearly hazardous with respect to the distal circulation and not entirely satisfactory in that it provides incomplete security from aneurysmal rupture.

It is likely that in the near future endovascular stents will become an attractive option for some types of aneurysms. The placement of intraaneurysmal polymerizing materials may also become a standard treatment at some point in the future.

VASOSPASM

DEFINITION

Vasospasm is the prolonged, intense constriction of the larger conducting arteries in the subarachnoid space which are initially surrounded by subarachnoid clot. The narrowing of the vessels is best demonstrated by cerebral angiography. It is likely that spasmogens are released from the breakdown of red blood cells trapped by a fibrin mesh in the abnormal environment of the subarachnoid space. Significant narrowing develops gradually over the first few days after aneurysmal rupture, and the vessel narrowing usually is not severe enough to cause ischemic symptoms for four days or so. The spasm is usually maximal about a week after the hemorrhage. Symptoms from infarction are also most common at around this time. The chance of the patients' beginning to develop symptomatic infarction after two weeks on the basis of vasospasm is extraordinarily low.

For patients in all neurologic grades the chance is about 50-50 that significant angiographic vasospasm will develop. Between one-quarter and one-fifth of patients will get symptoms of delayed ischemia, and in between one-third and one-half there will be CT evidence of infarction due to vasospasm. Vasospastic infarction severe enough to cause death will occur in between one in twenty and one in six patients. Vasospasm is one of the leading causes of death after aneurysmal rupture along with the effects of the initial hemorrhage and later rebleeding.[3]

The more severe the initial hemorrhage and the larger the volume of subarachnoid clot, the more likely it is that severe diffuse vasospasm will develop. For infarction to develop, there usually has to be an extreme degree of narrowing over a long segment and a failure of collateral flow. Many other factors are important, however, including the circulating blood volume, cardiac output, blood pressure, intracranial pressure, and the age of the brain.

TIME COURSE

Vasospasm is almost never observed angiographically in the first three days following aneurysmal rupture. If it is seen on the first angiogram it probably indicates that the patient had a previously unsuspected bleeding episode prior to the one that brought the patient to medical attention. The vasospasm is maximal around seven to eight days following the rupture and has usually subsided by two or three weeks.[3]

DIAGNOSIS
Clinical

Progressive impairment in level of consciousness or increase in focal neurologic deficit occurring more than four days after the bleeding episode should raise the suspicion of vasospasm. If operation has been conducted early the differential diagnosis includes postoperative bleeding or swelling, electrolyte abnormality—particularly hyponatremia, hypoxia from respiratory complications, developing hydrocephalus, or sepsis. It is important not to use vasospasm as a catch-all explanation for any late deterioration.[3,4]

Transcranial Doppler and Angiography

As the caliber of the major conducting arteries is reduced, the velocity of blood going through them generally increases. A progressive increase in this velocity may be a harbinger of problems due to vasospasm. Patients who develop clinical evidence of ischemia from vasospasm often have mean velocities in the middle cerebral arteries of over 200 cm/s.[1,4] Occasionally, the existence of intracranial hypertension will cause a spuriously low mean middle cerebral velocity. There are many exceptions to the linkage between increased velocities and ischemia, so that close clinical correlation is required and angiographic confirmation of severe diffuse vasospasm remains the gold standard.

Flow Studies: Xe-CT, PET, Isotopes

Several technologies currently are available for obtaining regional cerebral blood flow estimates. The xenon-CT scan and positron emission tomography (PET) scan provide excellent quantitative data but are not generally available. Single photon emission tomography is generally more common, but the data are not quantitative.[4]

TREATMENT
Prophylaxis

Early surgery permits the mechanical removal of fresh blood clot by suction and irrigation.[3] Once the offending aneurysm has been secured by a clip it is possible to place tissue plasminogen activator within the subarachnoid space, either at the time of surgery or subsequently through catheters, to facilitate the early fibrinolysis of the clot, thus reducing the amount of decaying blood pressing against the arteries. This appears to be an effective way of preventing vasospasm. These fibrinolytic agents have a potential to cause bleeding by dissolving normal clot, so only patients at high risk of developing vasospasm should be chosen for this type of prophylaxis.

Calcium Antagonists

The one drug currently approved for use after subarachnoid hemorrhage in North America is the calcium antagonist nimodipine. Its use was associated with a reduced tendency toward postaneurysmal cerebral infarction. Its clinical effectiveness was not based on its ability to prevent or reverse angiographically demonstrable vasospasm.[3,7]

Endothelin Antagonists

Endothelin is the most potent naturally occurring vasoconstrictor. It can be produced by vascular endothelium and smooth muscle cells. In animal models, endothelin antagonists have been associated with a reduced incidence of chronic vasospasm following clot placement. Such compounds have not yet gone to clinical trials.

Induced Hypertension

While this therapeutic modality has never been subjected to prospective clinical trial, it is nevertheless widely employed in the setting of delayed ischemia after aneurysmal rupture.[1,4,7] All experienced neurosurgeons have seen instances of dramatic reversal of focal neurologic deficits by induction of arterial hypertension. This is usually done in association with normalization of the circulating blood volume with fluid administration or transfusion. Very close clinical observation is indicated when patients are receiving agents such as dopamine or dobutamine in this setting. Xenon blood flow studies have demonstrated that in certain patients induced hypertension is associated with a reduction in regional cerebral blood flow. While such patients are undoubtedly exceptional, this is an important caveat.

Hypervolemia

The avoidance of hypovolemia is perhaps more important than the institution of hypervolemia. The old days of intentional dehydration are gone forever. The optimal hematocrit varies from patient to patient, but it is probably reasonable to maintain it within the normal range. Crystalloid solutions are given to meet normal daily requirements. Glucose solutions are avoided. Human serum albumin is commonly used as a volume expander in doses of 1 g/kg per day divided in 4 to 6 doses/day, each administered over 30 to 60 min.

In critically ill patients or in those with compromised pulmonary function, a Swan-Ganz catheter should be in place and appropriate monitoring used to avoid circulatory overload and pulmonary edema, as well as to ensure the optimization of cardiac output.[1,2,6]

Angioplasty

If the patient is in imminent danger from severe diffuse vasospasm refractory to hypertension and hypervolemia, these spastic arterial segments may be forcibly dilated by means of small, sausage-shaped balloons placed through intraarterial catheters. In expert hands, this is associated with the permanent reversal of vasospasm and clinical improvement in one-half to two-thirds of patients. There is a serious risk of arterial rupture, however, so the procedure should be restricted to experienced interventional neuroradiologists on the advice of experienced clinicians.[1,4]

Intraarterial Papavarine

The proximal segment of the anterior cerebral artery, the posterior cerebral arteries, and distal middle cerebral arteries are not amenable to balloon dilatation because of size or angle of take-off. The instillation over several hours of high concentrations of intra-arterial papavarine has been associated with reversal of spasm in some cases.[4] There has been a tendency for spasm to recur, and the infusion may have to be repeated, but it is sometimes associated with clinical improvement. Again, this is not a therapy to be undertaken lightly or before the failure of more conventional means.

Arteriovenous Malformations (AVMs)

EPIDEMIOLOGY

AVMs are between one-seventh and one-tenth as prevalent as aneurysms. They have been found in about .05 percent of some general autopsy series.[4,9,10] AVMs represent between one-tenth and one-twentieth of all non-aneurysmal cerebrovascular malformations. Other types are capillary telangiectasia, venous malformations, and cavernous malformations. Patients may show one or two of these malformation types in contiguity.

The yearly mortality from an untreated AVM is 1 to 1.5 percent, and this rate is not dependent on the mode of presentation. In addition, there is an approximate 1 percent annual risk of serious morbidity. The anticipated mortality rate from a hemorrhage is 10 to 15 percent, and the chance of permanent morbidity is double that. Mortality rate is higher for infratentorial AVMs.[4]

In one of the largest series in which patients were followed untreated for an average of 12 years, one-fifth remained well, one-tenth were in fair condition, one-fifth were disabled, and one-quarter died. There was a one in six mortality from the AVM itself. One-quarter of patients had been lost to follow-up, so conceivably as many as one-half of the patients could have died from the AVM. The estimated yearly morbidity was 3.5 percent, and mortality was 1 to 2 percent annually. Once an AVM has hemorrhaged, there is a 6 percent chance of repeat bleed in the next year and 2 percent per year thereafter. In addition to the 10 percent mortality resulting from rupture, the 30 percent chance of permanent morbidity must be considered.

GENETICS AND ASSOCIATED DISEASES

FAMILIAL AVMS

Reports exist but are extraordinarily rare, much more so than with aneurysms. Familial clusters could conceivably be due to chance.

INHERITED SYNDROMES WITH AVMS

The *Wyburn-Mason syndrome* is characterized by intracranial AVM with associated extracranial and retinal malformations. There can be AVMs in the skin, retina, brain, mandible, and maxilla. Presenting symptoms are usually visual loss, proptosis, chemosis, and cutaneous telangiectasia. Hemorrhage may occur either inside or outside the brain.[4,9]

Hereditary hemorrhagic telangiectasia (or Rendu-Osler-Weber syndrome) is a genetic disorder characterized by widely scattered AVMs of the skin and viscera. Major AVMs can occur in the lung. Patients frequently present with epistaxis, hemoptysis, or gastrointestinal hemorrhage. The pulmonary vascular abnormalities can result in septic emboli to the brain with abscess formation. The patients may be polycythemic because of chronic hypoxia. Brain AVMs occur in about 1 percent of cases, which is higher than would be expected in the general population.[4,9]

The *Sturge-Weber syndrome* is characterized by encephalotrigeminal angiomatosis. There is diffuse gross reddening of the brain surface, most commonly in the posterior aspect of the brain, caused by a diffuse network of thin vessels on the pial surface. There is linear calcification in the cortex.[4,9]

SYMPTOMS AND SIGNS

Symptoms and signs can result from compression of normal neurologic structures; hydrocephalus; hemorrhage into the brain, subarachnoid space, or ventricles; seizures from ischemic neuronal or hemorrhagic damage; bruit; neurologic dysfunction from mass effect; ischemia; increased intracranial pressure from increased venous pressure; or impaired neurologic function from vascular steal.

BLEEDING AND REBLEEDING

About one-half of AVMs present with hemorrhage. The rebleeding rate in the first year after hemorrhage from an AVM is about 6 percent, and 2 percent per annum thereafter.[4,9,10] There is some suggestion that bleeding rates are higher with smaller AVMs, and in those associated with the temporal lobe, presenting with neurologic deficits, in females, and with an increased number of hemorrhages. AVMs that drain through deep veins may be slightly more likely to bleed. There may also be an increased tendency to bleed if draining veins have stenotic portions. If a patient gives a history of more than two bleeding episodes from an AVM, there is one chance in four of yet another hemorrhage within one year. The risk of rebleeding from AVMs that have already bled once was studied in six series of 639 patients who averaged 15 years of follow-up. The average rate of rebleeding in the first year was 8 percent, and thereafter was 3 percent. In comparison, the risk of bleeding from unruptured AVMs in seven series totalling 543 patients who were followed for an average of 14 years was 2.2 percent. The range of bleeding rates for unruptured AVMs was 1.5 to 4 percent, and for rebleeds from ruptured AVMs the annual rebleeding rate was 2 to 6 percent.

The apparent observation that small AVMs are more likely to rebleed than large ones may only reflect the fact that they would not be diagnosed unless they bled, and large ones may be relatively more prone to seizures or progressive neurologic deficits. Some have suggested that bleeding is more likely for AVMs with an arterial aneurysm within the nidus. Low-flow lesions, as judged angiographically, may have a higher tendency to rebleed than do high-flow lesions. Direct arteriovenous fistulas are an unusual cause of hemorrhage.

AVMs should be sought vigorously in young patients with normal blood pressure who have no bleeding disorder when they present with intracerebral hemorrhage. Most cerebellar hemorrhages in patients under the age of 40 are from AVMs.

Fatal rebleeding within the first two weeks after a hemorrhage from an AVM occurs in fewer than 1 percent of cases.[4] The mortality from an AVM rupture is 10 to 15 percent, and the morbidity is 30 percent.

With few exceptions the treatment of hemorrhage from an AVM does not require an immediate operation. Exceptions may occur when the hematoma is very large or when it occurs in the posterior fossa. AVMs in the cerebellum with hematomas larger than 3 cm in diameter generally require urgent evacuation. Most neurosurgeons wait at least several weeks after a hemorrhage from an AVM so that significant neurologic recovery will already have taken place spontaneously and patients will be in optimal medical condition. Even when intracerebral hematomas are removed in a delayed fashion there can be an accelerated neurologic recovery after clot removal.[4,9]

In one series about one patient in four presenting with epilepsy developed a hemorrhage within the next 15 years. It is not known whether the risk of bleeding in a previously unruptured AVM increases or decreases with increasing age. There is no large body of convincing data.[4]

SEIZURES

One-fifth to two-thirds of patients will present with seizures. More than half of patients with AVMs will have at least one seizure by age 30. More than two-thirds of patients with AVMs will have seizures at some point. The average age of patients at the time of first seizure is 25 years, which is later than the mean for onset of bleeding. The nature of the seizure is related to the location of the AVM.[4]

When AVMs are in the medial temporal lobe, seizures are relatively more common. When they occur in the cerebellum, seizures are absent. Similarly, deep supratentorial AVMs involving the basal ganglia and ventricles do not usually present with seizures, but hemorrhage and other symptoms are common. More than two-thirds of AVMs present by age 40.[9]

On the basis of 11 series with 746 cases, AVMs under 2 cm were associated with epilepsy in 11 percent of cases, and AVMs over 4 cm were associated with epilepsy in 37 percent of cases. Patients with smaller AVMs were eight times more likely to present with hemorrhage than seizures. In patients with larger AVMs, the chance of presenting with hemorrhage was just under two times that for seizures.[4] When patients are treated with excision and/or embolization, about one-third are free of seizures postoperatively, based on the results of 319 epileptic patients with AVMs drawn from eight series. In 440 treated patients who did not have seizures preoperatively, between 4 and 30 percent developed their first seizure after the treatment. Approximately one-third of patients with AVMs will present with seizures, and about one-third will be cured of seizures by having their AVMs excised.

Up to 117 patients were observed over 20 years without specific treatment. One in five developed epilepsy after hemorrhage from their AVMs. The chance of developing seizures was much lower if the patient had no history of hemorrhage. The mechanism of epileptogenesis may be either ischemia from blood flow steal or irritation by the breakdown products of the hematoma. In four series of 41 AVMs operated for seizures and treated by excision of the AVM alone, 56 percent were seizure-free at follow-up, which was only a few years at most. In three series of 44 patients operated for epilepsy who were treated with AVM excision plus excision of epileptogenic cortex, the success rate was somewhat higher, with 75 percent being seizure-free postoperatively. In seven surgical series of AVMs, seizures presented for the first time postoperatively in 7 percent of patients. There is probably a more persuasive rationale for the routine use of anticonvulsants in AVM than in aneurysm surgery.[4]

OTHER PRESENTATIONS

About one-quarter present with headache, bruit, or progressive neurologic deficit.[4, 9, 10] Fewer than one-tenth of AVMs are symptomatic by the end of the first decade, and the most common decade in which they become symptomatic is the third. They do tend to present at an earlier age than aneurysms. Symptoms most commonly develop in the mid-decades of life; with advancing age it becomes rare for an arteriovenous malformation not to cause any symptoms.

Headache can be in any location and may have variable characteristics of duration and severity. The AVM can cause chronic, recurrent, and progressive incapacitating headache. It may be in any location. These headaches can mimic migraine headaches. AVMs situated in the occipital lobe tend to present with severe headache, and associated visual disturbances are common. Headaches may or may not resolve after the AMV is excised.

Hydrocephalus is a relatively common complication if the patient has intraventricular hemorrhages.

Between one-tenth and one-twentieth of patients with AVMs present with progressive neurologic deficit. This is considered to be due to the AVMs stealing blood from the adjacent normal brain because of the low resistance in the malformation and the preferential flow through it.[4,9]

Posterior fossa AVMs usually present with an intracerebral hemorrhage. Epilepsy is not a feature. There may be fluctuating neurologic symptoms resulting from intrinsic AVMs of the brain stem. The majority of brain stem AVMs will rupture, and there is a high chance of fatality. The usual presenting signs are ataxia, dysarthria, nystagmus, and those related to hydrocephalus. A very rare symptom is trigeminal neuralgia.[4,9]

MEDICAL COMPLICATIONS

These are much the same as those that occur with aneurysmal rupture, although neurogenic pulmonary edema is more rare in our experience.

PATHOLOGY

By the seventh week of gestation the circle of Willis is complete in fetal development. Capillary precursors are beginning to penetrate the hemispheres. By week eight the deep venous galenic system appears. Internal vascularization of the brain is essentially complete by week twelve.[4]

An arteriovenous malformation is a developmental anomaly due to the failure of normal evolution of embryonic vascular networks. The usual malformation has fewer and larger vessels between the arterial input and the venous outflow than would exist in normal brain. As a result, this is a low-resistance lesion, and early venous filling on angiography is a fairly constant feature. There is great variation in the size of the vessels comprising the nidus of the malformation. There is generally gliosis in and around the nidus. Almost all AVMs show some hemosiderin-laden macrophages. About one-third of cases operated upon for epilepsy with no history of hemorrhage will show some evidence of remote blood staining. About one-tenth of AVMs will show some mineralization of the vessel walls or intervening parenchyma. Some vessels associated with the AVM may undergo spontaneous thrombosis, and this can incite reactive inflammatory changes. There is usually some thickening of the overlying leptomeninges. Normal patterns of venous drainage are frequently absent in association with AVMs, perhaps congenitally absent, but the normal draining pattern may become evident after they are excised.[9]

AVMs are usually characterized by grossly dilated, serpentine afferent and efferent vessels. There may be a racemose tangle of pathologic vessels and rapid circulation time with arteriovenous shunting. Usually, the supplying arteries are dilated and elongated. Tortuosity involves both the proximal and terminal arterial tangles. The intrinsic vascularity consists of closely packed pathologic vessels. Brain tissue in the interstices becomes progressively uncommon toward the center of the nidus. Draining veins may become enormous. The differential diagnosis is angioblastic meningioma, hemangioblastoma, or vascular metastases. The vascular channels may show fibromuscular hyperplasia or thinning of the walls. The luminal surface of feeding arteries may show plaque-like mounds of disorganized smooth muscle cells, fibroblasts and connective tissue. The elastica may be fragmented and patchy.

AVMs are highly variable in shape, but the most common is probably conical, with the apex extending toward the ventricular system. All sizes up to hemispheric can occur, and all regions of the central nervous system may be affected. These are congenital lesions. Multiple lesions are extremely uncommon. It is also uncommon for them to be associated with types of vascular malformations other than aneurysms, but such associations are well documented. Flow rate can be extremely high or only mildly elevated.[9]

The feeding arteries may terminate entirely within the AVM nidus or, in certain cases, may communicate directly with draining veins, in which case the AVM is termed an *AV fistula*. Other arteries may partially drain into the AVM, but can bypass it to supply normal brain. Finally, arteries can be contiguous with the AVM without supplying any blood to it.[9]

PHYSIOLOGY

Since AVMs are congenital lesions and can undergo expansion during life, normal brain functions may be displaced in the brain from their usual locations.

AVMs sometimes increase in size, and sometimes stay the same after the patient comes for observation. They very rarely spontaneously regress or disappear. In three series comprised of 49 cases followed for an average of about five years, one-half were larger, one-third were the same, and about one-twentieth were either smaller or had disappeared.[4]

Representative pressures based on operative recordings from patients suggest that a mean systemic arterial blood pressure of 110 mmHg can be associated with a mean arterial blood pressure just proximal to the AVM of 60 mmHg, a venous blood pressure post-AVM of 18 mmHg, and an immediate increase in the arterial blood pressure immediately proximal to an excised AVM of 10 to 20 mmHg.[4] Pressures in feeding arteries are therefore low and may be only half that of systemic arteries. The venous pressure on the other hand is relatively high.

Normal perfusion pressure breakthrough is a theory based on the assumption that vessels in the ischemic brain surrounding an AVM are maximally dilated and lose their ability to contract. Once the AVM is acutely excised, adjacent small vessels may rupture.[4,9,10] Traumatic swelling and hemorrhage from multiple sites during or just following the one-stage excision of a large AVM is called normal perfusion pressure breakthrough. This is a dramatic if uncommon event. The original article naming this phenomenon was based on a single case report, and two additional case reports were mentioned from the literature. It is extremely rare, but it has become popular for neurosurgeons to attribute intraoperative and immediate postoperative swelling and hemorrhage to this phenomenon. It has been suggested that it can be prevented by keeping the blood pressure low postoperatively and by achieving a graded reduction in the flow of very large AVMs prior to excision. It is associated with large AVMs that have long and big feeding arteries. Generally, in the preoperative angiogram, there is a lack of filling of adjacent normal brain and high, fast flow through the malformation. Following excision there may be a marked increase in the pressure within the feeding artery. It has been suggested that the likelihood of this development can be reduced by staged occlusion of feeding vessels through embolization and by maintenance of low blood pressure in the intraoperative and postoperative period. Intraoperative angiography is useful in identifying residual portions of AVMs that are prone to cause deep hemorrhage and swelling.

In nine series reported between 1979 and 1990 comprising 1318 patients, only 1.2 percent were considered to have developed normal perfusion pressure breakthrough.[4]

Delayed postoperative swelling and hemorrhagic venous infarction are due to spreading thrombosis in arteries proximal to the removed bed and veins distal to it. The deterioration can be delayed, since it takes time for the thrombus to grow back to the point in an artery where it occludes circulation to distal normal brain or, in the case of venous thrombosis, for the thrombus to extend distally to the point where it occludes venous drainage from normal brain structures. If severe swelling and multiple hemorrhages have occurred from brain adjacent to the bed of a high-flow AVM, consideration should be given to prolonged sedation postoperatively and maintenance of a low blood pressure. Retrograde arterial thrombosis occurred in 7 percent of one series of 76 operations.[4]

Careful monitoring is required after excision of an AVM. The intracranial pressure should be monitored and controlled, as should the arterial pressure if the AVM has been large and its removal difficult.

The most common cause of severe acute intraoperative brain swelling and hemorrhage from multiple points is deep intraparenchymal or intraventricular hemorrhage from friable retracted deep arteries, or from a retained deep portion of the nidus which is transected. Acute venous occlusion prior to the total arrest of arterial input may also contribute. Controlled hypotension may be useful, as well as such general measures as hypocapnia, osmotic diuretics, and barbiturates. All of these measures, if employed too vigorously or for too long, may paradoxically increase the tendency to ischemic infarction of adjacent brain.

ANATOMY

In one large series of parenchymal AVMs, approximately one-third were fed from one vascular territory, approximately one-third had only one feeder, and about one-third drained into the deep venous system. Almost two-thirds drained into the superficial venous system, and approximately one-half were served by the middle cerebral artery, two-fifths by the posterior cerebral artery, and one-third by the anterior cerebral artery. The venous drainage of an AVM is classified as being superficial, deep, or combined. The draining veins should be counted. Stenosis of draining veins should be sought. This feature may be associated with an increased risk of bleeding. Rarely, AVMs are angiographically occult.[9]

One-tenth to one-sixth of all AVMs occur in the posterior fossa. About two-thirds are in the cerebellum, and the remainder in the brain stem. Rarely do they occur in the cerebellar pontine angle or on the surface of the brain stem and cerebellum.[4,9]

TECHNIQUES OF MANAGEMENT

SURGICAL EXCISION

The ideal treatment is one-stage total surgical excision of an uncomplicated AVM with no damage to the surrounding brain. This is not always possible. Some large inaccessible AVMs involving vital areas are best left alone. Many factors come to bear on the decision to operate. The degree of technical difficulty is increased by size, the presence of ill-defined margins, deep location, deep arterial supply, and deep venous drainage. Extensively arterialized cortical draining veins can be a problem. The surgical approach makes use of dissection within fissures and gives preference to transcortical dissection.

Since more than two-thirds of patients will make a complete recovery from the effects of an initial hemorrhage, it is the practice of most experienced surgeons to wait a month or two before undertaking a major surgical excision that could involve long periods of induced hypotension and retraction.[4,9,10]

INTRAOPERATIVE TECHNIQUE

The level of the AVM should be maintained as high as possible in relation to the heart to reduce venous congestion. Intraoperative hypertension should be avoided, and means of lowering blood pressure pharmacologically should be available.

RESULTS OF SURGERY

Major surgical series of AVMs include Olivecrona's 81 excisions by 1954, with only a 9 percent mortality, and Yasargil's 414 supratentorial AVM excisions with a mortality rate of only 2.4 percent and a major morbidity of 2.9 percent.[4,9]

In Heros' series of 250 excisions, 61 percent had excellent results, 19 percent good, 11 percent fair, 9 percent poor, and 0.8 percent died. Most surgical series report an overall mortality rate of under 5 percent and a serious morbidity rate of under 10 percent. In Stein's series of 180 superficial AVMs, the following complications were encountered: eight hemi-motor or sensory deficits, 16 hemianopias, 2 postoperative aphasias, and

1 akinetic mute state. In five cases the removal was incomplete. There was only minimal resolution of stable preoperative neurologic deficits. Postoperative bleeding requiring reoperation occurred in 3 percent of cases. In the UCLA series of 100 cases, minor new deficits occurred in 13 percent, major new deficits in 4 percent, and mortality in 1 percent of cases. [4,10]

Posterior fossa AVMs are a great technical challenge. They are usually not amenable to embolization. They can be approached from the transtentorial route underneath the temporal lobe, but more commonly using a suboccipital or far lateral suboccipital approach. The sitting position may be employed in some cases, or the modified lateral position. In Drake's series of posterior fossa AVMs, four out of five proved amenable to excision. Seventy-three percent of 86 posterior fossa AVMs had excellent to good results. The mortality rate was 12 percent. There was a 12 percent incidence of postoperative hemorrhage, and half of these patients died. To a large extent the surgical results depended on the preoperative neurologic state and the size of the AVM. In one series of 16 cases, one patient was disabled preoperatively and remained so, two patients underwent significant neurologic deterioration, and two died. In addition, two cases did not have any significant removal accomplished. In about three patients out of five complete removal can be achieved. [4]

The most commonly used classification for AVMs currently is that of Spetzler and Martin, who utilized six grades. [4] Three points are given in relation to size, one in relation to the "eloquence" of adjacent brain, and one according to whether or not there is a deep vascular component (arterial or venous). A lesion larger than 6 cm in the dominant Broca's area with lenticulostriate feeders and drainage into the internal cerebral venous system would be classified as a grade 6, which by their definition is inoperable. The higher the grade the more difficult is the surgical removal and the higher will be the anticipated mortality and permanent morbidity. The Spetzler-Martin grading system does not take into account the presence or absence of intracerebral hemorrhage, the neurologic grade of the patient, or the age of the patient and the general medical status. All of these factors are obviously also important in determining surgical outcome.

EMBOLIZATION

In order to make some very large AVMs operable, a variety of materials including particles, glue, and metallic coils can be embolized into the feeding vessels or nidus of the malformation. [4] Although relatively infrequent, there can be total angiographic cure of an AVM in this fashion. It is important to use nonabsorbable materials to ensure permanence of effect. Preoperative embolization of deep penetrating vessels is ex-

tremely helpful, but unfortunately it is usually easier to embolize large surface arteries, which are the ones most easily sealed by the surgeon. If the larger surface arteries are closed off too far in advance of the surgery, the deep penetrating ones undergo compensatory hypertrophy and this makes the operation more difficult and dangerous. Arteriovenous malformations are removed in a stepwise fashion, with occlusion of the feeding vessels as close to the nidus as possible and development of a plane of dissection abutting the nidus. Draining veins are maintained intact until the final stage of the removal.

For certain unusual types of AVMs, such as some of the "vein of Galen" varieties, embolization is the procedure of choice. [4] Preoperative embolization is an important adjunct in the preparation of the patient for surgical excision of posterior fossa AVMs. In one series of 79 posterior fossa AVMs, management mortality was 7 percent, and morbidity was 8 percent. Selective preoperative embolization was performed in over 50 percent of cases and has become progressively more utilized. Half the patients had presented with hemorrhage, half had headaches, just under half had neurologic deficits, and about one-quarter had seizures. Almost half had improvement in their neurologic deficits postoperatively, and one-fifth were unchanged. About one-third of patients had worsening of their neurologic status with surgery. There were no deaths in this series, and only a 6 percent incidence (two cases) of disabling morbidity.

Even very experienced interventional neuroradiologists have experienced fatalities from embolizing procedures. Mortality rates have been reported in the range of 1 to 2 percent. Residual portions of AVMs following embolization can be treated either surgically or occasionally, if they are under 3 cm in diameter, by stereotactic radiosurgery. Acute hemorrhage may be induced, and the surgical team should be prepared to intervene under certain circumstances.

RADIOTHERAPY

Focused radiation or radiosurgery has become a more popular technique for smaller AVMs. The nidus has to be under 3 cm in maximum diameter for best results. With the gamma knife, 50 Gy of radiation in a single dose obliterates 85 percent of AVMs within two years. A single dose of 10 Gy is equivalent to 40 Gy by fractionation. Permanent radiation-related complications are around 3 percent for the gamma knife. Such therapy is increasingly employed to take care of residual fragments of the nidus after surgery or embolization. [4]

SPECIAL CONSIDERATIONS

PEDIATRIC AVMS

Intracerebral hemorrhage accounts for most admissions of children with AVMs (excluding the so-called vein of Galen types). The mortality rate for first hemorrhages ranges between 7 and 13 percent, and this rises to 25 to 41 percent for a second hemorrhage. Neurologic deficits are often severe immediately after the bleeding episode, but children can make remarkable improvements over time.[4]

AVMS AND PREGNANCY

The physiologic changes occurring with pregnancy may predispose arteriovenous malformations to hemorrhage. The risk of repeat bleeding during pregnancy from a ruptured AVM appears to be high and three of eleven cases did so in one series. In another series of ten cases, three rebled during the pregnancy. This suggests that a somewhat more aggressive approach to rupture should be taken during pregnancy than at other times.[10] During surgery, it seems reasonable to avoid the straight supine position in favor of the semilateral. Fetal monitoring should be used. Extreme hypotension should be avoided and careful consideration given to the use of osmotic diuretics, since there have been reports of induced fetal electrolyte abnormalities. Phenobarbital is probably a safer drug than Dilantin during pregnancy. In a large series of AVMs in pregnant females, hemorrhages tended to cluster toward the last trimester of pregnancy and immediately postpartum, although none were reported to have occurred during labor.[4]

RADIOLOGY

The CT scan may show serpiginous calcifications; after augmentation there may be marked contrast enhancement. On the MRI, the anatomy is usually better delineated, with flow voids being evident and evidence of previous hemorrhages showing up as hyperintensities. Angiography is the gold standard study and classically shows enlarged tortuous feeding arteries, a compact nidus, and early visualization of draining veins.[4]

References

1. Awad IA (ed): Current management of cerebral aneurysms. *Neurosurgical Topics,* AANS, 1993:327.
2. Fox JL: *Intracranial Aneurysms.* New York, Springer-Verlag, 1983:1462.
3. Weir B: *Aneurysms Affecting the Nervous System.* Baltimore, Williams & Wilkins, 1987:671.
4. Carter LP et al (eds): *Neurovascular Surgery.* New York, McGraw-Hill, 1994:1446.
5. Kassell NF et al: The International Cooperative Study on the Timing of Aneurysm Surgery. Part I. Overall management results. *J Neurosurg* 1990; 73:18.
6. Ratcheson RA, Wirth FP (eds): *Ruptured Cerebral Aneurysms,* Vol 6: *Concepts in Neurosurgery.* Baltimore, Williams & Wilkins, 1994:208.
7. Haley EC et al: A randomized trial of two doses of nicardipine in aneurysmal subarachnoid hemorrhage. A report of the Cooperative Aneurysm Study. *J Neurosurg* 1994; 80.
8. Samson DS, Batjer HH: *Intracranial Aneurysm Surgery Techniques.* Mount Kisko NY, Futura Publishing, 1990:248.
9. Yasargil MG: *Microneurosurgery.* New York, Thieme Medical, 1984–1988.
10. Wilson CB, Stein BM (eds): *Intracranial Arteriovenous Malformations.* Baltimore, Williams & Wilkins, 1984:342.

Anesthetic Management

PHILIPPA NEWFIELD

RUKAIYA K. A. HAMID

ARTHUR M. LAM

INTRAOPERATIVE ANEURYSMAL RUPTURE
HYPOTHERMIC CIRCULATORY ARREST FOR
GIANT ANEURYSMS AND COMPLEX VERTE-
BROBASILAR ANEURYSMS
    Brain Protection During Circulatory Arrest
    Anesthetic Considerations
SUBARACHNOID HEMORRHAGE AND PREG-
NANCY
    Pathophysiology of Cerebrovascular Accidents
      During Pregnancy
    Physiologic Changes During Pregnancy
    Diagnosis
    Management of Patients After SAH

The goal of anesthetic management in the surgical treatment of intracranial aneurysms (Table 26-1) is to facilitate the operation and the patient's recovery while minimizing the risk of aneurysmal rupture, cerebral ischemia, neurologic deficit, and associated systemic morbidity. The functional survival after aneurysmal rupture has been so low that efforts are directed at improving the case management as well as the operative mortality (Table 26-2).

Grading of Aneurysms

Because the systemic and neurologic effects of aneurysmal rupture and subarachnoid hemorrhage (SAH) are protean and affect every organ system (Table 26-3), the anesthesiologist's evaluation includes assessment of the patient's physical status, both systemic and neurologic. A system for the grading of patients after SAH was introduced by Botterell[1] in 1956 to facilitate the assessment of surgical risk, the prediction of outcome, and the evaluation of the patient's condition as it evolved from the post-hemorrhage period to that immediately preceding operation. The five grades describe the patient's level of consciousness and degree of neurologic impairment as I to V, each grade representing increased severity (Table 26-4).

Botterell's system was modified by Hunt and Hess[2] to include descriptions of the accompanying headache and neurologic deficits and a provision for the effect of serious systemic illness (e.g., hypertension, diabetes, chronic pulmonary disease, vasospasm) that would move the patient into the next, less favorable category (Table 26-5). The World Federation of Neurological

TABLE 26-1
Cerebral Aneurysms: Localized Dilatations
of Intracranial Arteries

Berry	Traumatic	Neoplastic
Mycotic	Fusiform	Atherosclerotic

TABLE 26-2
Cerebral Aneurysms in North America: Epidemiology

SAH patients/year	28,000
Died immediately	10,000
Admitted to hospital	18,000
Died/disabled	9,000
Rebleeding	3,000
Vasospasm	3,000
Medical complications	1,000
Surgical complications	2,000
Functional survival	9,000

NOTE: SAH = subarachnoid hemorrhage.

Surgeons subsequently developed a grading scale based on the Glasgow Coma Scale[3] (Table 26-6) in which the preoperative level of consciousness was found to correlate most directly with outcome.[4] The patients who are in good condition immediately before surgery (Grades I and II) are likely to do well, whereas patients who are moribund preoperatively have a high mortality and morbidity (Table 26-7).

The severity of the associated cerebral and systemic pathology also correlates with the clinical grade. Poor-grade patients are more likely to have impairment of cerebral autoregulation[5-8] and the cerebrovascular response to hypocapnia,[7,8] intracranial hypertension,[9] and vasospasm,[10] as well as fluid and electrolyte imbalance,[11-13] myocardial dysfunction,[14] cardiac arrhythmias,[15] and respiratory impairment (Table 26-8). In one series,[16] the incidence of at least one severe, life-threatening medical complication after SAH was 40 percent; the proportion of deaths from medical complications was 23 percent. The deaths attributed to the direct effects of the initial hemorrhage (19 percent), rebleeding (22 percent), and vasospasm (23 percent) were of comparable proportion.

Fluid and Electrolyte Balance

Fully one-third to all of patients demonstrate a diminution in intravascular volume after SAH that correlates

TABLE 26-3
Effects of Aneurysmal Rupture

↑ ICP secondary to hematoma
Disturbance of CSF flow → hydrocephalus
Direct brain destruction
Cerebral infarction secondary to vasospasm
Systemic fluid and electrolyte imbalance
Cardiac irregularities
Respiratory impairment

NOTE: ICP = intracranial pressure; CSF = cerebrospinal fluid.

TABLE 26-4
Botterell Clinical Grade

Grade	Criteria
I	Consciousness with or without meningeal signs
II	Drowsy without significant neurologic deficit
III	Drowsy with neurologic deficit and probable cerebral clot
IV	Major neurologic deficits present
V	Moribund with failing vital centers and extensor rigidity

SOURCE: From Botterell EH et al. *J Neurosurg* 1956; 13:1, with permission.

with the clinical grade.[13,16–20] In keeping with this association, patients who have evidence of intracranial hypertension on computed tomographic (CT) scan are more likely to be hypovolemic.[13] Such hypovolemia may in turn increase the degree of vasospasm and lead to cerebral ischemia and infarction.[13,19,21] Maroon and Nelson[22] have identified bed rest, negative nitrogen balance, supine diuresis, decreased erythropoiesis, and iatrogenic blood loss as factors contributing to the hypovolemia.

The hyponatremia that accompanies the hypovolemia, noted in 30 percent of patients who have vasospasm,[23] was originally thought to be due to the development of a syndrome of inappropriate[24,25] and then "appropriate" secretion of antidiuretic hormone in response to the hypovolemia. Now, however, investigators believe that distension of the ventricles, as with post-SAH hydrocephalus, causes the release of atrial natriuretic factor from the hypothalamus.[26–28] If this is the case, rather than fluid restriction, patients should be treated with normal or hypertonic (3 percent) saline, which is in keeping with the use of hypertensive hyper-

TABLE 26-5
Clinical Grading After Subarachnoid Hemorrhage: Hunt and Hess Modification

Grade 0	Unruptured aneurysm
Grade 1	Asymptomatic or minimal headache and slight nuchal rigidity
Grade 2	Moderate to severe headache, nuchal rigidity, no neurologic deficit other than cranial nerve palsy
Grade 3	Drowsiness, confusion or mild focal deficit
Grade 4	Stupor, moderate to severe hemiparesis, possible early decerebrate rigidity, vegetative disturbances
Grade 5	Deep coma, decerebrate rigidity, moribund appearance

NOTE: Serious systemic diseases (hypertension, atherosclerotic heart disease, diabetes, chronic pulmonary disease, severe vasospasm seen on angiography) cause placement of the patient into the next less favorable category.
(SOURCE: From Hunt WE, Hess RM. *J Neurosurg* 1968; 28:14, with permission.)

TABLE 26-6
World Federation of Neurological Surgeons' Grading Scale

WFNS Grade	GCS Score	Motor Deficit
I	15	Absent
II	14–13	Absent
III	14–13	Present
IV	12–7	Present or absent
V	6–3	Present or absent

NOTE: WFNS = World Federation of Neurological Surgeons; GCS = Glasgow Coma Scale
SOURCE: From Drake CG. *J Neurosurg* 1988; 68:985, with permission.

volemia to improve cerebral perfusion in the presence of vasospasm.[22]

Half to three-quarters of patients also develop hypokalemia, commonly in association with the use of diuretics, and hypocalcemia after SAH,[29] and require appropriate replacement. Hyperkalemia and hypernatremia occur as well, but less frequently. The electrolyte imbalance was not noted to correlate with the use of corticosteroids, saline, or potassium chloride.[16]

Cardiac Sequelae

Electrocardiographic (ECG) abnormalities occur in 50 to 100 percent of patients after SAH,[30–36] particularly during the perioperative period. The most common ECG abnormalities are inversion of the T-wave and depression of the ST segment. Other morphologic changes include the appearance of U-waves, prolongation of the Q-T interval, and, rarely, the appearance of Q-waves.

Disturbances of rhythm are seen in 30 to 80 percent of patients after SAH.[16] Although premature ventricular complexes are most common, sinus bradycardia, sinus tachycardia, atrioventricular dissociation, atrial extrasystole, atrial fibrillation, bradycardia-tachycardia, and ventricular tachycardia and fibrillation occur, as well.[37] These may be life-threatening in 5 percent of patients in the first 48 hours after SAH.[16,38] In one series, 15 percent of patients had prolongation of the Q-T interval

TABLE 26-7
Predictors of Mortality after Subarachnoid Hemorrhage

Decreased level of consciousness
Increased age
Thickness of subarachnoid clot on CT scan
Elevated blood pressure
Preexisting medical illness
Basilar aneurysm

TABLE 26-8
Signs and Symptoms of Subarachnoid Hemorrhage from Intracranial Aneurysmal Rupture

---

Meningeal irritation
  Excruciating headache
  Meningismus
  Photophobia
  Confusion, dysphasia

Focal neurologic signs

Depressed level of consciousness

Coma

Cranial nerve palsies

Seizures

Nausea and vomiting

Elevated temperature

Electrocardiographic abnormalities

Increased sympathetic activity, hypertension

Hypovolemia

Hyponatremia, electrolyte imbalance

Clotting abnormalities

Leukocytosis

Proteinuria, glycosuria

---

associated with at least one episode of moderate or severe arrhythmia.[16]

The onset of arrhythmia is most frequently within the first seven days after SAH; the peak occurrence is between days 2 and 3. The duration of the changes may vary. The ECG may return to normal in 10 days,[39] or the abnormalities may persist for up to six weeks.[40] The abnormalities may also change from one day to the next,[15] and may occur intraoperatively and postoperatively.[41,42]

The exact etiology of these ECG abnormalities is unknown. They have been attributed to post-SAH injury to the posterior hypothalamus with release of norepinephrine from the adrenal medulla and sympathetic cardiac efferents and resultant ischemic subendocardial changes.[33,43–47] This relation to hypothalamic injury is supported by the coexistence of high levels of urinary catecholamines, ECG changes (T-wave inversion, Q-waves, Q-T prolongation),[46] hypertension, and hypothalamic and cardiac lesions,[48,49] including subendocardial hemorrhages and myocytolysis.

Electrolyte disturbances may also play a role in the genesis of the ECG changes after SAH. Hypokalemia has been reported to depress the ST segment, decrease the amplitude of the T-wave, increase the amplitude of the U-wave, prolong the Q-T interval, and cause arrhythmias.[29] More recently, however, the presence of hypokalemia did not correlate significantly with cardiac arrhythmias.[16]

Specific types of ECG changes have been associated with poor outcomes.[50–52] The extent of myocardial dysfunction has correlated with the severity of neurologic injury.[53] Echocardiographic studies have failed, however, to establish a relationship between ECG abnormalities and myocardial dysfunction.[14] While the incidence of ECG abnormalities was statistically greater in patients who had an increased amount of intracranial blood or an intracerebral clot on CT scan after SAH, neither the amount of blood seen on CT scan nor the incidence of ECG abnormalities was useful in predicting patient outcome.[54] Other series have demonstrated a higher incidence of ECG abnormalities in patients whose neurologic status is poor,[34,52] and a correlation between the amount and distribution of subarachnoid blood on CT scan and the development of cerebral vasospasm.[55]

The ECG changes and myocardial damage associated with SAH are frequently suggestive of the kind of ischemia associated with coronary atherosclerosis or thrombosis.[56] Plasma creatine kinase (CK) and its cardiac-specific isoenzyme, CK-MB, increase in 50 percent of patients after SAH.[57] The total CK and the ratio of CK-MB to total CK, however, are rarely consistent with transmural infarction. The ventricular wall dysfunction noted in 27 to 33 percent of patients after SAH[14,53] has been associated with increased morbidity, including pulmonary edema, formation of intra-atrial thrombus, and embolic stroke.

The prophylactic administration of beta-adrenergic blocking drugs or autonomic antagonists has improved cardiac outcome in some patients after SAH,[58–60] but not in others.[33,61] A small prospective study of prophylactic adrenergic blockade demonstrated a strong trend toward less neurologic deficit and fewer deaths at one year.[62]

Most of the ECG abnormalities are neurogenic rather than cardiogenic in origin,[29] although some patients do have myocardial infarctions after SAH.[63] Since it is important to minimize rebleeding by proceeding with surgical therapy in a timely fashion, the concern exists regarding how to determine whether the patient's cardiac status is precarious enough to mandate delaying surgery.[64] The measurement of serial cardiac enzymes and the assessment of ventricular function by echocardiography may provide information about the degree of ischemia. An increase in total creatine kinase, however, was not statistically associated with an increased frequency of cardiac arrhythmias.[16]

Although the vast majority of total arrhythmias in one series[16] were considered mild (66 percent) or moderate (29 percent), there was a 5 percent incidence of severe arrhythmia. The presence of a severe arrhythmia or significant cardiogenic pulmonary edema might necessitate the postponement of surgery until treatment is instituted. The use of a pulmonary artery catheter to monitor pulmonary capillary wedge pressure and cardiac output may facilitate management of both the patient's cardiac dysfunction and the response to hypertensive hypervolemic hemodilution (see below), should that be indicated for the treatment of delayed ischemic deficit or vasospasm.

Respiratory System

Pulmonary complications, including cardiogenic and neurogenic pulmonary edema[65-67] and pneumonia, increase the morbidity and mortality of SAH. Solenski[16] studied the medical complications in the placebo limb of a large, randomized controlled trial of the calcium antagonist nicardipine after SAH[68] and noted that 23 percent of deaths were from medical complications. Pulmonary complications were the most common non-neurologic cause of death in patients after SAH and, as such, were responsible for 50 percent of all deaths from medical complications at three months. Pneumonia and adult respiratory distress syndrome (28 percent) and pulmonary emboli (16 percent) led the list of fatal pulmonary complications.

As a percentage of the total medical complications, Solenski[16] noted that pulmonary edema and pneumonia occurred in 23 percent and 22 percent of patients, respectively. The majority (60 percent) of patients who developed pulmonary edema did so between days 0 and 7 after SAH; the highest number of cases occurred on day 3. The frequency of pulmonary edema increased in patients older than 30 years. Previous lung or heart disease (myocardial infarctions, arrhythmias, angina, congestive heart failure) and prophylactic and therapeutic hypertensive hypervolemic therapy were not associated with an increased risk of pulmonary edema.

Hepatic dysfunction was frequently observed in patients who developed pulmonary edema ($p < .001$). Poor clinical grade at the time of admission also correlated with a higher frequency of respiratory dysfunction, suggesting neurogenic influences (e.g., sympathetic discharge after initial hemorrhage).[35] An increase in the frequency of pulmonary edema was also associated with the day of surgery or the day after surgery ($p < .05$). The significance of Solenski's study is that it substantiates the need to prevent, recognize, and treat potential medical complications of SAH, especially pulmonary problems, to reduce the overall mortality rate.

Other Medical Complications

Hepatic dysfunction including hepatic failure and hepatitis[64,69] numbers among the medical complications

TABLE 26-9
Neurologic Deterioration after Subarachnoid Hemorrhage

Rebleeding
Hydrocephalus
Vasospasm
Delayed ischemic deficit
Cerebral infarction

after SAH. A total of 24 percent of 455 patients in Solenski's series[16] had hepatic dysfunction, either at the time of admission or during the first 14 days after SAH. Severe dysfunction occurred in 4 percent. Only 2 percent of patients had a clinical history of preexisting hepatic disease. No association existed between hepatic dysfunction and age, use of alcohol 24 h before admission, or use of nonsteroidal anti-inflammatory drugs, anticonvulsant drugs, or histamine-2 receptor blocking drugs. Poor clinical grade, on the other hand, correlated positively such that patients who had hepatic dysfunction were judged to have a poor clinical grade at the time of admission twice as frequently as patients who had normal liver function. Almost half the patients with hepatic dysfunction also had pulmonary edema, suggesting a role for passive congestion.

Almost 8 percent of patients develop renal dysfunction after SAH, and 15 percent of those have severe dysfunction.[16] The highest frequency is reported in the patients receiving antibiotic therapy. Nearly 20 percent of the renal failure patients had sepsis, but increasing age did not increase the risk of renal dysfunction.

During the first 14 days after SAH, 4 percent of patients were reported to develop thrombocytopenia.[16] Sepsis was associated with 35 percent of the thrombocytopenic patients. Over half had more severe neurologic deficits by clinical grade. Antibiotic use, with or without sepsis, also correlated with an increased incidence of thrombocytopenia. Neither age nor the use of minidose heparin or anticonvulsant drugs was significantly correlated. Other reported hematologic disorders include disseminated intravascular coagulation[70] and leukocytosis.[71]

Medical Treatment of Subarachnoid Hemorrhage and Vasospasm

In the effort to reduce the total case management mortality for craniotomy for the securing of intracranial aneurysms, pharmacologic and mechanical therapies have been developed to enhance the cerebral circulation and mitigate against the devastating sequelae of rebleeding and vasospasm (Table 26-9). Such treatments have implications for the conduct of anesthesia for both emergent and elective surgery.

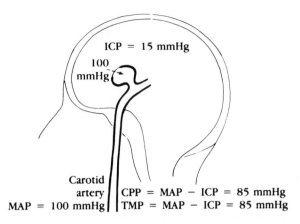

Figure 26-1 The transmural pressure (TMP) of the aneurysm. TMP is equal to the difference between the mean arterial pressure (MAP) and the intracranial pressure (ICP).[162] (From Newfield P and Cottrell J: *Neuroanesthesia*: *Handbook of Clinical and Physiologic Essentials*, 2d ed. Little, Brown, Boston, 1991.)

Rebleeding after the initial SAH, as indicated by data from the International Cooperative Study on the Timing of Aneurysm Surgery, is highest, at 4 percent, during the first 24 h after SAH and then decreases subsequently to 1.5 percent per day.[72] The cumulative risk of rebleeding is 19 percent at 2 weeks and 50 percent at 6 months.[73] After this, the risk of rebleeding decreases to 3 percent per year. The overall incidence of rebleeding is 11 percent,[74] which represents 8 percent of the mortality and morbidity.[4] The administration of the antifibrinolytic drugs epsilon aminocaproic acid and tranexamic acid decreases the probability of rebleeding[75] by preventing dissolution of the clot sealing the rent in the aneurysm. Although the use of epsilon aminocaproic acid has reduced the incidence of rebleeding from 23 to 13 percent, there is an associated increase in the occurrence of vasospasm and hydrocephalus,[76] resulting in no improvement in overall outcome.[77,78]

While the obliteration of the aneurysm is the only definitive means of preventing rebleeding, treatment while the patient awaits operation includes prevention of hypertensive episodes and the concomitant increases in transmural pressure [mean arterial pressure minus intracranial pressure (ICP) Fig. 26-1]. Systolic blood pressures in excess of 160 mmHg have been associated with an increase in the incidence of rebleeding.[79] To this end, narcotic analgesics and sedatives will reduce pain and anxiety. Short-acting hypotensive drugs (nitroprusside, esmolol, labetalol) are used for control of labile hypertension or transient episodes induced by therapeutic interventions. On the other hand, the maintenance of the patient's ward pressure as the lower limit of acceptable blood pressure is essential to avoid initiation or exacerbation of vasospasm through an undue decrease in cerebral perfusion pressure [mean arterial pressure minus intracranial pressure

(ICP)]. Early surgery has diminished but not eliminated the risk of rebleeding.

A host of pharmacologic attempts at inducing vasodilatation of spastic vessels in the treatment of vasospasm has been ineffective[80,81] because vasospasm involves a structural alteration in the vessel wall, rather than just a spastic contracture or failure of relaxation of the smooth muscle in the media of the vessels. Calcium channel blocking drugs, including nicardipine[82] and nimodipine, are currently in wide use for the prevention of delayed ischemic deficit after SAH (Table 26-10). Nimodipine diminishes the myoplasmic calcium in smooth muscle cells and impedes the entry of extracellular calcium necessary for the contraction of the smooth muscle.

The administration of nimodipine to all patients within 96 h of SAH has reduced the incidence of poor outcome by 40 to 70 percent.[83–88] In all the nimodipine studies, the incidence, severity, and distribution of angiographically detected vasospasm was not significantly different in the nimodipine and placebo groups. It is speculated, therefore, that nimodipine decreases the severity of vasospasm-induced neurologic deficit by: (1) modification of microcirculatory blood flow (i.e., dilatation of pial conducting vessels or decreased platelet aggregation) not apparent on conventional angiography; or (2) a direct neuronal effect.[89] The use of the experimental calcium antagonist fausidil was recently associated with an improvement in angiographic vasospasm.[90]

Since calcium antagonists tend to reduce patients' blood pressure, patients may require hydration immediately before induction of anesthesia and careful attention to fluid balance intra- and postoperatively.

HYPERTENSIVE HYPERVOLEMIC HEMODILUTION

The mechanical treatment of vasospasm is predicated on the augmentation of cerebral perfusion pressure in ischemic areas of the brain that have impaired autoreg-

TABLE 26-10
Treatment of Vasospasm

Maintenance of cerebral perfusion

Augmentation of blood pressure and cardiac output

Inotropes (dopamine, dobutamine)

Calcium-channel blockers (nimodipine, nifedipine)

Intravascular volume expansion

Relative hemodilution (hematocrit 32 percent)

Correction of hyponatremia

Transluminal angioplasty

Recombinant tissue plasminogen activator

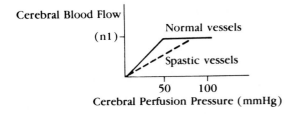

Figure 26-2 Cerebral blood flow response to changes in cerebral perfusion pressure in the presence of normal autoregulation and impaired autoregulation due to cerebral vasospasm.[162] (From Newfield P, Cottrell J: *Neuroanesthesia: Handbook of Clinical and Physiologic Essentials*, 2d ed. Little Brown, Boston, 1991, with permission.)

ulation (Fig. 26-2). Since perfusion pressure depends in part on the intravascular volume and mean arterial pressure, this boosting of cerebral blood flow (CBF) is accomplished by "Triple H therapy," or hypertensive hypervolemic hemodilution: the augmentation of blood pressure and cardiac output, the expansion of intravascular volume, the preservation of relative hemodilution (hematocrit of 32 percent to promote blood flow through the cerebral microvasculature), and the avoidance of hyponatremia.[10,22,23,91–95]

The key to the successful use of Triple H therapy is its early application before mild ischemia evolves to infarction. Because the risk of rebleeding can be as high as 19 percent,[47] however, both hypertension and hypervolemia are induced with caution in the period preceding surgical securing of the aneurysm by clip ligation, wrapping, gluing, or balloon occlusion. With early operation, the likelihood of rebleeding from Triple H therapy is diminished.[92–94] Other adverse intracerebral sequelae of Triple H therapy include hemorrhage into areas of infarction, exacerbation of cerebral edema, and a rise in ICP. The systemic complications include myocardial infarction (2 percent), pulmonary edema (7 to 17 percent), coagulopathy (3 percent), and dilutional hyponatremia (3 to 35 percent).[10,23,91,92]

For the anesthesiologist, it is crucial to maintain the blood pressure and intravascular volume in the normal range during surgery and to augment both as the aneurysm is being secured. Serial measurement of the hematocrit intraoperatively and during the recovery period will facilitate achievement of the appropriate degree of hemodilution through the administration of crystalloid and blood as necessary. Hetastarch and dextran solutions are relatively contraindicated because of their potential for interference with coagulation.[96,97] Five percent albumin may be used in addition to crystalloid.

Previous reports on the management of hypervolemic hemodilution after SAH equated the optimal volume expansion to a central venous pressure (CVP) of 10 mmHg and a pulmonary capillary wedge pressure (PCWP) of 12 to 20 mmHg.[91–94,98] Levy and Gianotta[98] studied nine patients after SAH and determined that, while increasing the PCWP from 8 to 14 mmHg significantly increased the stroke volume index, left ventricular stroke work index, and cardiac index, further expansion of the intravascular volume to raise the PCWP above 14 mmHg actually caused a decline in cardiac index. They noted no correlation between changes in the CVP and the PCWP during augmentation of the intravascular volume and recommend following the PCWP rather than the CVP.

The administration of intravenous fluids alone may not effect an adequate degree of hypervolemia because of the resultant vagal response and diuresis. This may necessitate the use of atropine, 1 mg IM every 3 to 4 h, to increase the heart rate and aqueous vasopressin (Pitressin), 5 units IM, to reduce the urine output to less than 200 ml per h.

Vasopressor drugs, including dopamine, dobutamine, and phenylephrine may also be required to raise the blood pressure to reverse the signs and symptoms of the ischemic deficit. It the patient's aneurysm has not been clipped, the systolic blood pressure is increased to 120 to 150 mmHg. Once the aneurysm has been secured, systolic blood pressures in the range of 160 to 200 mmHg may be maintained. The resultant change in CBF may be indicated with the use of the transcranial Doppler (TCD) monitor, and improvement in vasospasm is signalled by a decrease in flow velocity. This is a useful monitor because of the correlation between elevated middle cerebral artery erythrocyte velocities and delayed ischemia after SAH.[99] Vasospasm and hypoperfusion coexist in patients who demonstrate lateralizing neurologic deficits.

TRANSLUMINAL ANGIOPLASTY

Transluminal angioplasty, the mechanical dilation of a cerebral vessel at a segment of spastic narrowing by the use of an inflatable intravascular balloon, caused improvement in the patients' level of consciousness and regression of focal ischemic deficits.[100] The factor crucial to the success of this technique is early intervention at the point at which the chance of reversing the neurologic deficit is greatest. The vessels are also more responsive to dilation in the earlier stages of spasm, presumably because collagen deposition and fibrosis in the vessel wall increase with time. The salutary effects of such localized angioplasty have persisted over time and the complication rate has been low. One series reported the reversal of deficits within 12 to 48 h in 75 percent of patients treated.[101]

OTHER PHARMACOLOGIC INTERVENTIONS

The intrathecal administration of recombinant tissue plasminogen activator (rtPA) has been shown to dissolve subarachnoid clots, thereby preventing vasospasm in primates[102] and humans.[103] The use of rtPA in human trials reduced the severity of angiographic vasospasm and improved the clinical neurologic grade of the patients.[104]

Alternatively, the super-selective intra-arterial infusion of papaverine (2 mg over 10 s) has been shown to be effective in dilating spastic distal vessels not accessible to angioplasty techniques.[105]

CNS Complications

The central nervous system (CNS) is affected directly by the initial trauma and subsequent sequelae of aneurysmal rupture and SAH. The resultant vascular disruption, hematoma, and hydrocephalus lead to cerebral ischemia and infarction, impaired cerebral autoregulation, disordered cerebrovascular response to changes in carbon dioxide tension (Pa_{CO_2}), cerebral edema, and intracranial hypertension. The presence of a giant aneurysm may additionally impair intracranial compliance and exacerbate the difficulty of anesthetizing these patients.

AUTOREGULATION

Cerebral autoregulation refers to both the hemodynamic response of CBF to changes in cerebral perfusion pressure and the ability of the cerebral vasculature to dilate in response to tissue hypoxia. The CNS damage attendant upon SAH interferes with autoregulation and the extent of the impairment correlates directly with the clinical grade of the patient.[5-8] Patients demonstrate a decrease in CBF and cerebral metabolic rate, as well.[106-109] The impairment in autoregulation is also closely related to the degree of vasospasm (Fig. 26-2).[8]

For this reason, the treatment for a neurologic deficit of new onset after SAH is to augment the cerebral perfusion through an increase in the systemic blood pressure with vasopressor drugs and expansion of the intravascular volume.[91] This is especially crucial when the deficit is correlated with a decrease in the systemic pressure to a level below the patient's previous blood pressure. The patient's "ward" pressure in the immediate post-admission period thus becomes the lower limit of acceptable blood pressure in the perioperative management. Furthermore, disease states such as hypertension and the use of vasodilating drugs that affect the conductance or resistance vessels in the brain (hydralazine, sodium nitroprusside, nitroglycerine, calcium channel blocking drugs which patients may receive after SAH) can influence autoregulation as well. Their effects thus need to be factored into the preservation of the patient's "normal" blood pressure.[110]

CARBON DIOXIDE RESPONSE

Carbon dioxide (CO_2) influences cerebrovascular resistance and has a direct effect on CBF. CO_2 diffuses rapidly across the blood-brain barrier (BBB), influences the pH of the extracellular fluid, and affects arteriolar resistance. The CSF does have the capacity to buffer itself against these alterations in pH by active exchange of bicarbonate (HCO_3) such that CO_2-induced cerebral vasoconstriction dissipates over 6 to 10 h.[111] In this buffered system, CBF changes 2 to 4 percent in a linear fashion for each mmHg change in Pa_{CO_2} from 20 to 80 mmHg at normotension. Although the linearity of the response diminishes at the extremes of the range, doubling the Pa_{CO_2} from 40 to 80 mmHg doubles the CBF, and decreasing the Pa_{CO_2} from 40 to 20 mmHg decreases the CBF by half.

The effect of the Pa_{CO_2} on CBF is in turn modified by the systemic arterial blood pressure. The ability of the cerebral circulation to respond to changes in Pa_{CO_2} is diminished by moderate hypotension.[112] The Pa_{CO_2} also influences the autoregulatory mechanism such that hypocapneic conditions facilitate the maintenance of the stability of the CBF over a wider range of blood pressures than does hypercapnia.[110] Consequently, a decrease in cerebrovascular reactivity to CO_2 may reflect a local decrease in cerebral perfusion pressure distal to a spastic vessel or the structural damage attendant upon ischemic cerebrovascular disease,[113] head injury,[114] or SAH.[115,116] The cerebrovascular response to hyperventilation is preserved, however, after SAH.[5,7,8] A decline in CO_2 reactivity, unlike the SAH-induced impairment in autoregulation, usually does not occur in the absence of extensive disruption of cerebral homeostasis.[7]

INTRACRANIAL HYPERTENSION

The very presence of intracranial aneurysms, particularly giant aneurysms, and SAH and the resultant hematoma, edema, and hydrocephalus all have the potential for causing intracranial hypertension. The increase in intracranial pressure (ICP) immediately after SAH can approach the systemic blood pressure. Teleologically, this may serve to limit the volume of blood able to leak through the rent in the wall of the aneurysm.[117] For this reason, a rapid reduction of ICP is liable to lead to further hemorrhage by increasing the transmural pressure (MAP-ICP) gradient across the wall of the aneurysm.

The clot itself from the initial rupture or rebleeding can cause a mass effect, with a shift of the intracranial contents and impairment of local cerebral perfusion.[4] Cerebral edema may also develop, as can acute hydrocephalus secondary to obstruction of the CSF drainage pathways by intraventricular or intraparenchymal clots. Blood in the subarachnoid space also causes hydrocephalus through the formation of arachnoidal adhesions that prevent reabsorption of CSF.[118] The incidence of hydrocephalus is reported to be about 15 percent. Since the clinical features of hydrocephalus, including progressive obtundation and small, nonreactive pupils, are present in only about half the cases, a CT scan is necessary to distinguish hydrocephalus from other causes of neurologic deterioration[119] including rebleeding, edema, and infarction.

It is best to treat hydrocephalus after the aneurysm has been secured, because reducing the ICP before this point increases the risk of rebleeding by increasing the transmural pressure gradient across the wall of the aneurysm. Severe intracranial hypertension may be relieved, however, by a preoperative ventriculostomy, which may serve during the induction of anesthesia as a monitor of ICP and during surgery as a method for the drainage of CSF to enhance brain relaxation and improve access to the aneurysm. Only in rare cases is a permanent shunt required for the treatment of the hydrocephalus.

Vasospasm can also cause an elevation in ICP. The decrease in CBF secondary to the vasoconstriction induces vasodilatation in the distal vessels with an accompanying increase in cerebral blood volume[107,109] and ICP. Hypovolemia in the face of intracranial hypertension may lead to cerebral ischemia and infarction because of impaired perfusion.

After SAH, the ICP is reflected in the patients' clinical grade. Patients judged to be Grade I or II generally have normal ICP (but not necessarily normal intracranial elastance), whereas Grade IV and V patients generally have intracranial hypertension.[9] Patients whose ICP is elevated immediately before operation require the same anesthetic precautions as all patients who have intracranial hypertension including hyperventilation and the use of cerebrovasoconstricting drugs to reduce cerebral blood volume.

Surgical Intervention

TIMING OF SURGERY

The timing of surgery for aneurysmal clip-ligation has been a subject of recent scrutiny and reevaluation by neurosurgeons.[120] Because the outcome after operative intervention was correlated with the patients' clinical condition at the time of surgery, neurosurgeons had previously delayed the procedure to enable patients to recover from the acute effects of SAH and the ischemic complications of vasospasm. Operations performed 7 to 10 days after SAH usually disclosed a slack, easily manipulable brain and a firmer, tougher aneurysmal sac that was less likely to rupture during dissection.

There were also problems associated with the postponement of surgery, however. Mortality increased to as high as 40 percent in patients who rebled during this waiting period.[73] It was also hazardous to use hypertensive hypervolemic hemodilution to treat delayed ischemia from vasospasm before the aneurysm had been secured. The case management mortality after SAH therefore continued to be high, despite good operative results.

The proponents of early surgery in the first 24 to 48 h after SAH cite the advantages of the prevention of rebleeding, the reduction in the incidence of vasospasm by the removal of blood from the subarachnoid space,[121] and the ability to use volume expansion and deliberate hypertension with relative safety to treat vasospasm once the aneurysm has been clipped.[93] Other considerations favoring early operative intervention include the reduction in medical complications (pneumonia, deep-vein thrombosis, pulmonary embolus, electrolyte imbalance, gastric ulcer), anxiety on the part of the patients and their families, and the cost of prolonged hospitalization.

The International Cooperative Study on the Timing of Aneurysm Surgery, a nonrandomized, prospective study,[4,122] tabulated the results of contemporary surgical and medical management of 3521 aneurysm patients in 68 neurosurgical centers around the world. At the time of admission, 75 percent of the patients were in good condition. Surgery was performed in 83 percent of the patients. Vasospasm, rebleeding, and the effects of the initial hemorrhage were the leading causes of death. At the end of the first 6 months, 58 percent of the patients had made a complete recovery and 26 percent were dead. Predictors for mortality included a decreased level of consciousness, increased age, thickness of the subarachnoid clot on CT scan, elevated blood pressure, preexisting medical illness, and basilar aneurysms.

The neurosurgeons participating in the study noted a 50 percent incidence of brain swelling or "tightness" when patients were operated on day 0 or 1 after SAH, as opposed to a 20 percent incidence when surgery was performed on day 10 or later. Despite this, dissection of the aneurysm was judged to be no more difficult during the early operations than the late; and there was no difference in the incidence of intraoperative aneurysmal rupture between early and late surgery.

The International Cooperative Study reported a 6 percent incidence of rebleeding in patients operated on within the first three days after SAH, as opposed to a 14 percent incidence for those operated 7 to 11 days after SAH. Despite this reduction in the rate of rebleeding, the overall management results indicated a mortality of 20 percent and good outcome in 60 percent of patients whether they had early (0 to 3 days after

TABLE 26-11
Diagnosis of Subarachnoid Hemorrhage

Clinical history	Lumbar puncture	Magnetic resonance scan
Physical examination	Computed tomographic scan	Angiography

SAH) or late (11 to 14 days) surgery. This similarity of overall morbidity and mortality was attributed primarily to the development of vasospasm. The outcome was least favorable and the mortality was highest when surgery was performed 7 to 10 days after SAH, which coincided with the peaking of vasospasm. In alert patients, timing was not a factor at all. In the subset of North American patients, however, results were best in patients operated on 0 to 3 days after SAH.[74]

These data from the International Cooperative Study indicate that early operation may have an advantage because of the reduction in rebleeding, especially when combined with clinically proven methods for treating vasospasm. It must be borne in mind, however, that the outcomes reported in this study represent the collective results of institutions that have considerable experience in the management of aneurysm patients, and therefore may not be applicable to other centers. Of note is the fact that the outcomes reflected considerable variability among the participating centers, related to case mix and patient management.

PREOPERATIVE EVALUATION

Because the sequelae of SAH involve every organ system, the preoperative evaluation of the patient scheduled for operation to secure an intracranial aneurysm includes a review of the neurosurgical diagnostic studies (Table 26-11), a neurologic examination, a notation of ward blood pressures and any association between a decrease in blood pressure and neurologic deterioration, and attention to fluid and electrolyte balance and hematocrit. The patient's cardiac history and ECG are reviewed, as 60 percent of patients will have electrocardiographic abnormalities (ST or T-wave changes, U-waves, Q-T prolongation, arrhythmia) after SAH from increased vagal and sympathetic neural output (see above). Since the extent of myocardial impairment is related to the patient's degree of neurologic dysfunction, poorer-grade patients and those who have a history of ischemic heart disease, arrhythmia, or cardiomyopathy may warrant further investigation including cardiology consultation, echocardiogram (although echocardiographic abnormalities do not always correlate well with ECG abnormalities after SAH), determination of serum myoglobin and CK isoenzymes, myocardial nuclear scanning, and perioperative cardiovascular monitoring.

Patients who receive nimodipine or nicardipine, the calcium-channel blocking drugs given prophylactically (see above) to reduce the neurologic complications of vasospasm after SAH, have been noted to become hypotensive in the preoperative period secondary to systemic vasodilatation.[82,87,123] These patients also had lower blood pressures intraoperatively,[123–125] and required smaller doses of hypotensive drugs to induce hypotension.[125] Because of the vasodilatation, patients treated with nimodipine or nicardipine require careful monitoring of intravascular volume (CVP or PCWP) and blood pressure in the perioperative period.

PREMEDICATION

When considering premedication, it is important to note that patients should continue to receive their calcium-channel blocking drugs (nimodipine or nicardipine), anticonvulsant drugs (phenytoin), and steroids (dexamethasone) up to the time of operation. Drugs that reduce gastric acidity (cimetidine, ranitidine) and volume and hasten gastric emptying (metoclopramide) may also be given before induction of anesthesia. Sedative, hypnotic, and anxiolytic drugs and narcotics are used sparingly in the immediate preoperative period to avoid respiratory depression, with its attendant increase in CBF, cerebral blood volume, and, potentially, ICP, and the masking of deterioration in the patient's neurologic condition. In addition to the reassurance offered by the anesthesiologist during the preoperative visit, small doses of intravenous narcotic (morphine, 1 to 4 mg, or fentanyl, 25 to 50 μg) and benzodiazepine (midazolam, 1 to 2 mg) may be administered by the anesthesiologist to good-grade patients, in order to prevent rebleeding from anxiety-induced surges in blood pressure. Poor-grade patients who already have depressed levels of consciousness are not candidates for preoperative sedation unless an endotracheal tube is in place and they are mechanically ventilated. In this case, they may even require muscle relaxation during transport to the operating room.

MONITORING

The patient undergoing craniotomy for aneurysmal clip-ligation requires close monitoring to ensure neurologic, cardiovascular, and pulmonary well-being and to optimize the status of each organ system. To facilitate this and the diagnosis and treatment of physiologic perturbations, the following modalities are monitored during anesthesia (Table 26-12):

1. Cardiac rate and rhythm using the V5 lead of the ECG for detection of ischemia
2. Direct intraarterial blood pressure

TABLE 26-12
Intraoperative Monitoring

Cardiac rate and rhythm
  Electrocardiogram with V5 lead

Direct intra-arterial blood pressure

Central venous pressure or pulmonary capillary wedge pressure

End-tidal CO_2, oxygen saturation

Intermittent blood gases, serum electrolytes, glucose, osmolarity

Brain temperature
  Nasopharyngeal, esophageal thermistor

Urinary output
  Indwelling catheter

Neuromuscular blockade
  Peripheral nerve stimulator

Electrophysiologic monitors
  Electroencephalogram
  Somatosensory evoked potentials

Transcranial Doppler ultrasonography

Jugular bulb oxygen saturation

Noninvasive cerebral oximetry

3. Degree of neuromuscular blockade

4. Central venous pressure (CVP) via the antecubital, subclavian, or jugular route as a guide to intra- and postoperative volume expansion

5. Pulmonary artery wedge pressure and cardiac output for patients who have cardiac compromise or severe vasospasm

6. End-tidal CO_2, oxygen saturation via pulse oximetry

7. Intermittent arterial blood gases, glucose, electrolytes, osmolarity, and hematocrit

8. Brain temperature using a tympanic or nasopharyngeal thermistor

9. Urinary output via an indwelling catheter

10. Electrophysiologic monitors: EEG, evoked potentials

11. Cerebral blood flow velocity via transcranial Doppler ultrasonography

12. Jugular bulb venous oxygen saturation

Adequate intravenous access is as essential as adequate monitoring. One or two large-bore intravenous catheters should be inserted peripherally, in addition to the CVP or PA catheter. Intravenous cannulation and monitoring should be accomplished before positioning for surgery, which may limit access to arteries and veins, and before interventions that will affect blood pressure, ICP, transmural pressure, and CBF. Once the patient is positioned for the operation, the arterial pressure transducer is secured at the level of the brain to reflect cerebral perfusion, and moved accordingly if the patient's position is changed.

In addition to the beat-to-beat monitoring of the pa-

tient's blood pressure, an arterial catheter will facilitate sampling for measurement of arterial blood gases and serum electrolytes, glucose, hematocrit, and osmolarity. Potassium may be depleted by the administration of mannitol and furosemide. Further, mannitol will increase serum osmolarity while decreasing brain water. No further brain relaxation is achieved by additional doses of mannitol, however, if the serum osmolarity exceeds 320 mosm, making this an important parameter to measure if the brain is "tight."[126] Serum glucose should also be maintained in the normal range (less than 200 mg/dl) to avoid the hyperglycemic exacerbation of ischemic injury to the CNS.

The measurement of CVP is mandatory for patients undergoing craniotomy for the securing of an intracranial aneurysm. In patients known to be hypovolemic preoperatively, the CVP is a guide to volume repletion in the setting of fluid shifts from osmotic and loop diuresis and the potential for considerable blood loss. For this reason, four to six units of blood should be typed, cross-matched, and readily available when the operation begins.

Since CVP and left ventricular end-diastolic pressure correlate poorly in SAH,[68] pulmonary artery catheterization may be necessary when patients have severe, symptomatic vasospasm and require hypervolemic hypertension, are in poor condition and at greater risk for developing complications from the treatment of postoperative vasospasm, or have coronary artery disease or ventricular dysfunction and may need prophylactic hypertensive hypervolemic hemodilution. Whatever the intraoperative scenario, the postoperative management of all patients relies heavily on the CVP and pulmonary capillary wedge pressure as indicators of intravascular volume. The insertion of a CVP catheter should therefore include a large-bore sheath introducer to facilitate conversion to a pulmonary artery catheter.

Central venous cannulation may be accomplished after induction of anesthesia and before positioning by way of the internal jugular, subclavian, or brachial (medial antecubital) vein. Because patients may have intracranial hypertension or a decrease in intracranial compliance, access to the internal jugular vein is accomplished with no or at most 5 to 10 degrees of head-down tilt. The central venous catheter itself will not cause venous obstruction, although the creation of a hematoma may interfere with cerebral drainage. When the possibility exists that the carotid artery may be occluded at the level of the neck on the side ipsilateral to the aneurysm, the internal jugular vein on the contralateral side may be cannulated. Alternatively, the subclavian approach brings with it the risk of pneumothorax, and the antecubital approach has less chance of central cannulation. Radiologic guidance with a flotation-tipped catheter or the use of the change in P-wave configuration on ECG may improve the probability of appropriate placement.[127]

The temperature of the brain is most closely reflected in the tympanic and nasopharyngeal temperatures. After the cranial flap is turned, a thermistor may be placed on the surface of the brain to measure the temperature of the brain directly.

ELECTROPHYSIOLOGIC MONITORING

Electrophysiologic monitoring may allow intraoperative detection of cerebral ischemia and possibly alteration of surgical technique. However, this is not routinely used because the changes are not always specific and the recording sites not always accessible.

ELECTROENCEPHALOGRAM (EEG)

This modality has been used to determine the lowest blood pressure tolerable during induced hypotension, but the results are not consistent.[128,129] This is not surprising as significant deterioration in EEG can be compatible with normal neurologic recovery. Tempelhoff and coworkers described the use of intraoperative bihemispheric computer-processed EEG and found changes correspond to postoperative outcome.[130] However, the series is too small to draw any conclusions. In contrast, EEG monitoring may be indicated when temporary occlusion is planned, either to determine the duration of tolerance or for titration of anesthetic agents when pharmacologic metabolic suppression is desired. Direct cortical EEG recording has also been described.[131] The value of electrophysiologic monitoring during cerebral aneurysm surgery has been reviewed by Emerson and Turner.[132]

EVOKED POTENTIALS

Somatosensory evoked potential (SSEP) monitoring has been investigated for use during procedures on both anterior and posterior circulation aneurysms while brain stem auditory evoked potential (BAEP) monitoring has been primarily investigated for use during procedures on vertebobasilar aneurysms.[133-147] Both monitors are probably most useful when temporary or permanent occlusion is planned. Evoked potentials can be recorded during barbiturate coma and are therefore the only electrophysiologic monitor available when maximal pharmacologic metabolic suppression is used. Common to all electrophysiologic monitoring, even during temporary occlusion, SSEP monitoring lacks specificity and a significant false-positive rate can be expected. For aneurysms in the vertebrobasilar system, BAEP monitoring complements the use of spontaneous breathing as a monitor of brain stem function.[133-135] The simultaneous use of SSEP and BAEP monitoring during temporary or permanent occlusion provides additional enhancement in sensitivity and specificity.[135] A summary of the literature on use of SSEP during temporary arterial occlusion is shown in Table 26-13.

JUGULAR BULB OXYGEN SATURATION

Cerebral metabolic rate (CMR_{O_2}) is the product of cerebral blood flow (CBF) and arteriovenous oxygen content difference (AVD_{O_2}) derived from blood samples obtained from arterial blood and jugular bulb blood. Thus AVD_{O_2} reflects the balance between metabolic demand and blood supply. When hemoglobin concentration stays relatively constant and arterial oxygen saturation is 100 percent, then AVD_{O_2} is reflected by $(1 - Sjv_{O_2})$, where Sjv_{O_2} is the jugular bulb oxygen saturation. Thus, when blood flow is higher than what is needed, Sjv_{O_2} will increase; conversely, when CBF is inadequate, Sjv_{O_2} will decrease.

Although jugular venous oximetry has found wide acceptance in the intensive care management of the injured brain, there are relatively few data on its potential use in cerebral aneurysm surgery. As hyperventilation is frequently employed during cerebral aneurysm surgery to improve surgical conditions, and because excessive hyperventilation can cause cerebral ischemia, intermittent or continuous jugular bulb oxygen saturation measurement may be useful in determination of the optimal level of hyperventilation.

Matta and coworkers have demonstrated the feasibility and safety of intermittent jugular venous saturation monitoring in a series of neurosurgical patients, including patients undergoing aneurysm clipping.[148] The most common cause of desaturation (<50 percent) is hyperventilation; and this occurred in about 60 percent of the patients studied. Severe desaturation (Sjv_{O_2} < 45 percent) was observed in 10 percent of the patients studied, with many of these episodes occurring despite a Pa_{CO_2} > 25 mmHg. Inadequate CBF due to a low systemic blood pressure can also lead to jugular venous desaturation, although the effects are less dramatic than those seen with hyperventilation. The potential utility of continuous jugular venous oximetry for optimal intraoperative blood pressure management in patients with cerebral aneurysms was shown by Moss and coworkers.[149]

TRANSCRANIAL DOPPLER ULTRASONOGRAPHY

Although transcranial Doppler (TCD) as a diagnostic tool is well established in the fields of neurology and neurosurgery, study of its potential application as a monitor of intracerebral hemodynamics during anesthesia and surgery has only just begun. Despite the

TABLE 26-13
SSEP Monitoring During Temporary Arterial Occlusion for Cerebral Aneurysm Surgery

	No. of Patients	Temporary Occlusion	False-Positive (%)	False-Negative (%)	Year
Manninen et al.[136]	70	52	11	47	1993
Mizoi and Yoshimoto[137]	124	97	57	25	1993
Schramm et al.[138]	113	34	40	34	1990
Manninen et al.[141]	157	97	43	14	1990
Mooij et al.[142]	5	5	?	0	1987
Momma et al.[143]	40	40	60	5	1987
Kidooka et al.[144]	31	15	38	22	1987
Symon et al.[145]	34	15	40	7	1984

presence of many theoretical and practical limitations, TCD represents the first step toward achieving the goal of noninvasive continuous CBF monitoring during anesthesia.

Intraoperative use of TCD is generally limited to the middle cerebral artery (MCA) via the transtemporal route. As the MCA carries about 75 to 80 percent of the ipsilateral carotid artery blood flow, a change in MCA flow (Vmca) is representative of the change in hemispheric blood flow. However, the Vmca is proportional to cerebral blood flow only when the diameter of the vessel insonated remains constant. As the basal cerebral arteries are conductance vessels, generally they do not dilate or constrict as the vascular resistance changes. Carbon dioxide tension,[150] systemic blood pressure,[151] and inhaled anesthetics[152] have all been shown to have negligible effects on the diameter of the MCA, although the effects of the latter are still in dispute.[153] However, the occurrence of vasospasm renders this relationship invalid. Indeed, the increase in flow velocity with constriction of the basal cerebral artery (as in vasospasm) represents one of the most important and established uses of the TCD.[154] Moreover, TCD measurements can only give relative indexes of CBF. Although correlation between absolute flow velocity and CBF in any given population is poor, good correlation between relative changes in flow velocity and CBF has been demonstrated.[155,156]

Both flow velocity and waveform changes may be useful during cerebral aneurysm surgery. The former may be useful during induced hypotension to assess the ability of the patient to autoregulate, and the latter can be used to diagnose or confirm perioperative aneurysm rupture prior to opening of dura. One of the reasons for the decline in the use of induced hypotension during clipping of cerebral aneurysms is the unpredictable cerebrovascular response to induced hypotension in patients with subarachnoid hemorrhage.

Continuous monitoring with TCD allows the anesthesiologist to determine the patient's ability to tolerate induced hypotension, as well as the effect of hyperventilation on CBF during this vulnerable period. The validity of TCD for determination of the lower limit of autoregulation has been confirmed.[157]

Although the incidence of aneurysmal rupture during induction of anesthesia with modern techniques is low (<1 percent), the diagnosis may not be readily apparent until the time of dural incision, resulting in difficult operating conditions with a swollen congested brain. TCD has been used intraoperatively to confirm the diagnosis and facilitate management in a patient whose aneurysm ruptured shortly after induction of anesthesia.[158] Although access and fixation remain significant limitations, the development of specially designed frames has made intraoperative monitoring feasible in many situations.[159]

Anesthesia

INDUCTION

The induction of anesthesia is a critical juncture for the patient who has an unsecured intracranial aneurysm, because rupture at this time can be fatal. The incidence of aneurysmal rupture during the induction of anesthesia ranges from less than 1 to 2 percent in reported series;[160] the attendant mortality approaches 75 percent. The smooth induction of anesthesia therefore requires mitigation against the sympathetically-mediated hypertensive response to maneuvers such as laryngoscopy and intubation and the attendant increase in transmural pressure (Fig. 26-1), obliteration of coughing and straining once the endotracheal tube is in place, and maintenance of adequate cerebral perfusion pressure in a patient who may already have vasospasm and an impairment of autoregulation.[161]

The relationship between the transmural pressure across the wall of the aneurysm and the wall tension of the aneurysm is linear. Either an increase in the mean arterial pressure (as during sympathetic stimulation in the face of light anesthesia) or a decrease in the ICP (as by hyperventilation, administration of mannitol, CSF drainage, or opening of the cranial vault at a time when the blood pressure is elevated) will raise the transmural pressure and enhance the possibility of aneurysmal rupture.[162] The goal, therefore, is to minimize the transmural pressure while maintaining the cerebral perfusion pressure during the induction of anesthesia. This necessitates a compromise between the risk of cerebral ischemia from a decrease in cerebral perfusion pressure (by way of a decrease in mean arterial pressure) and the benefit of reducing the chance of rupture of the aneurysm through a reduction in the transmural pressure (also by way of a decrease in mean arterial pressure).

The extent to which the blood pressue is intentionally reduced during the induction of anesthesia depends on the clinical grade of the patient. The ICP of good-grade patients (Grades O, I, II) is usually normal[9] (see above) so that a decrease in blood pressure to 30 to 35 percent below ward values (or a systolic blood pressure of 100 mmHg) is not detrimental in the absence of evidence of cerebral ischemia. Poor-grade patients (IV, V), in contrast, already have intracranial hypertension and a reduction in cerebral perfusion pressure, the combination of which may cause ischemia. A decrease in the blood pressure of these patients may exacerbate the potential for cerebral ischemia. While the blood pressure in poor-grade patients should be reduced less than in good-grade patients, and for a shorter time, measures should still be taken to blunt the sympathetic response to laryngoscopy and endotracheal intubation.

Good-grade patients do not require hyperventilation during the induction of anesthesia, since they generally do not have a decrease in intracranial compliance. In the absence of intracranial hypertension, the reduction in CBF caused by hyperventilation will reduce the ICP and increase the transmural pressure (when the mean arterial pressure remains constant or rises), risking rupture of the aneurysm. Poorer-grade patients, conversely, may have an increase in ICP, and will benefit from moderate hyperventilation to enhance cerebral perfusion.

The intravenous induction of anesthesia is designed to confer loss of consciousness while maintaining cardiovascular and intracerebral homeostasis in the face of catechol-stimulating maneuvers (Table 26-14). Anesthesia is induced by the intravenous administration of thiopental (3 to 5 mg/kg) or etomidate (0.1 to 0.3 mg/kg). Propofol also achieves rapid loss of consciousness,

TABLE 26-14
Induction of Anesthesia: Aneurysmal Clip-Ligation

Optimal head position	
Deep level of anesthesia	
Sufentanil	0.5–1.0 μg/kg
Fentanyl	3.0–5.0 mg/kg
Thiopental	3.0–5.0 mg/kg
Propofol	1.0–2.0 mg/kg
Vecuronium	0.1 mg/kg
Low-dose isoflurane	
Controlled ventilation	100% O_2
Normal CO_2 (35–40 mmHg)	
Before laryngoscopy	
Lidocaine	1.5 mg/kg
Thiopental	2.0–3.0 mg/kg
Propofol	0.5 mg/kg
Brief, gentle laryngoscopy	
Intubation	

reduction in CBF, ICP, and cerebral metabolic oxygen requirement, maintenance of cerebral autoregulation and cerebrovascular CO_2 responsiveness, cerebral protection, and reasonable cardiovascular stability.[163] Slow incremental administration of smaller doses (1.0 to 1.5 mg/kg) will mitigate against systemic hypotension and the possibility of attendant compromise of cerebral perfusion. Propofol has the added advantages of prompt awakening and a decrease in the incidence of postoperative nausea, and is appropriate for inclusion in the pharmacopeia of neuroanesthesia provided cerebral perfusion is maintained through the prevention or prompt treatment of any reduction in blood pressure.

The addition of a narcotic (fentanyl, 3 to 7 μg/kg,[164] or sufentanil, 0.5 to 1.0 μg/kg), lidocaine, 1.5 mg/kg,[165] and a benzodiazepine (midazolam, 0.1 to 0.2 mg/kg) during the induction of anesthesia will further blunt the patient's response to sympathetic stimulation as from laryngoscopy, intubation, and the application of three-point skull-fixation devices. The prior infiltration of the scalp and periosteum with local anesthetic may also avoid the hypertensive response to the insertion of pins into the outer table of the skull.[166]

If the patient does not have an increase in intracranial elastance, isoflurane may be introduced before laryngoscopy to augment the depth of anesthesia. Ventilation is controlled with 100 percent oxygen to achieve an arterial Pa$_{CO_2}$ of 35 to 40 mmHg when the intracranial elastance is normal, and 25 to 30 mmHg when intracranial elastance is impaired.

MUSCLE RELAXANTS

For muscle relaxation, the major advantage of vecuronium[167,168] and atracurium,[169,170] nondepolarizing muscle relaxants of intermediate duration, is that they do not increase ICP in the presence of a reduction in intracranial compliance. Pipecuronium, a long-acting nondepolarizing muscle relaxant which combines prolonged duration of action with cardiovascular stability, did not affect ICP or cerebral perfusion pressure in patients who had intracranial tumors but no intracranial hypertension at the time of the drug's administration.[171]

Succinylcholine (SCH) has been demonstrated to raise ICP in animals[172] and humans,[173, 174] owing to an increase in muscle spindle afferent activity. While pretreatment with a small dose of pancuronium blocked neither the afferent muscle activity nor the increase in CBF in dogs,[175] administration of a defasciculating dose of a nondepolarizing muscle relaxant to patients either prevented or diminished the increase in ICP,[173,174] regardless of the presence or absence of an intracranial space-occupying lesion. Deepening the level of anesthesia also mitigates against the rise in ICP.[176]

The administration of SCH has also been associated with ventricular fibrillation in patients after SAH, possibly secondary to an acute increase in serum potassium. Manninen demonstrated, however, that the elevation in serum potassium was not detrimental when patients received SCH within four days of their SAH.[177] Nonetheless, susceptible patients include those who are comatose but nonparetic, have flaccid paralysis, spasticity, or clonus secondary to head injury, or move their extremities in response to pain but not to command.

Consequently, neuroanesthesiologists had limited their use of SCH to rapid-sequence induction for emergency operation on unprepared patients. Alternatively, intubation may be accomplished by pretreatment of the patient with a "priming" dose of nondepolarizing relaxant (atracurium, 0.1 mg/kg, or vecuronium, 0.015 mg/kg) during preoxygenation. This small dose is then followed by a larger dose (atracurium, 0.7 mg/kg, or vecuronium, 0.15 mg/kg) given immediately after the sleep-inducing dose of thiopental or propofol. Intubating conditions are obtained in 60 to 90 s.[178]

To the options for the achievement of muscle relaxation during rapid-sequence induction is now added the short-acting, nondepolarizing muscle relaxant, rocuronium. Although the half-life is about 20 min, relaxation sufficient to facilitate tracheal intubation occurs in 30 to 60 s after administration in infants, children, and adults. Rocuronium also does not adversely affect either CBF or ICP, and offers a true alternative to SCH. Its short duration of action may necessitate the use of a longer-acting muscle relaxant after endotracheal intubation.

After the patient is asleep and relaxed, further pharmacologic intervention is necessary before laryngoscopy and endotracheal intubation to prevent the sympathetically-mediated rise in blood pressure. Both anesthetic and cardioactive drugs may be used. Fentanyl, 1.5 to 10 μg/kg,[164] or sufentanil, 0.5 to 1.0 μg/kg, is effective, especially for poor-grade patients or those who have a decrease in intracranial compliance. The use of a higher concentration of an inhalational anesthetic is appropriate only for patients who have normal intracranial dynamics.

Alternatively, additional thiopental, 1 to 2 mg/kg,[179] or intravenous lidocaine, 1.5 to 2.0 mg/kg, may be administered 1 to 2 min before laryngoscopy to preserve hemodynamic stability. Lidocaine in lower doses also confers sedation and produces a dose-related decrease in CBF and cerebral metabolic rate for oxygen;[180] higher concentrations may induce seizures, however.

CARDIOACTIVE DRUGS

Cardioactive drugs also counteract the hypertensive response to laryngoscopy and intubation. The beta-adrenergic antagonists propranolol,[181] 1 to 2 mg, and esmolol, 0.5 mg/kg,[182–184] will block the chronotropic and inotropic effects of sympathetic stimulation. Esmolol has no significant effect on CBF or ICP.[185] Labetalol, a combined alpha- and beta-adrenergic antagonist, has been used to treat hypertension in a dose of 5 to 20 mg IV and to induce hypotension. Besides the absence of toxicity, tachyphylaxis, and rebound hypertension, labetalol does not affect CBF, even when given in doses sufficient to reduce the mean arterial pressure by 45 percent.[186] Further, labetalol caused no significant changes in ICP in a canine model, with and without intracranial hypertension, despite a reduction in mean arterial pressure of 27 to 38 percent.[187]

When esmolol and labetalol were compared in terms of their ability to control hypertension during emergence from anesthesia for intracranial surgery, both drugs were effective, but labetalol was associated with a higher incidence of bradycardia in the immediate postoperative period.[184] Esmolol may thus be the preferred drug for control of hypertension at the conclusion of surgery and, by extrapolation, in the immediate preintubation period, which is generally followed by little stimulation and an ensuing fall in blood pressure.

Sodium nitroprusside (SNP), 100 μg, has been recommended for administration before laryngoscopy and intubation to prevent hypertension. SNP, a potent, direct-acting cerebral vasodilator, can increase cerebral blood volume and ICP[188,189] secondary to the dilation of capacitance vessels. Although SNP is valuable for immediate control of hypertension because of its rapid onset and brief duration, it may be detrimental in patients who have a reduction in intracranial compliance. For these patients, the prior use of hyperventilation and intravascular cerebral vasoconstricting drugs such as barbiturates may mitigate against the increase in ICP from cerebral vasodilatation.

Nitroglycerin (TNG) also causes an increase in cerebral blood volume from the dilation of capacitance vessels and a concomitant increase in CSF pressure,[190,191] which may be greater than that induced by SNP. In addition, the brain-surface oxygen tension in cats was not maintained as well with TNG as with SNP.[192] SNP therefore remains the better choice for rapid control of blood pressure during neurosurgical procedures.

An alternative is offered by the calcium-channel blocking drugs nicardipine and diltiazem, for the rapid control of intraoperative hypertension during cerebral aneurysm surgery.[193] Nicardipine increases local cerebral blood flow and internal carotid artery blood flow velocity, while diltiazem changes neither. The recommended doses are nicardipine, 0.01 to 0.02 mg/kg, and diltiazem, 0.2 mg/kg (or 10 mg). Both drugs are useful and safe in that they do not decrease local CBF or blood flow velocity.

When the patient is scheduled for emergency surgery and preoperative fasting is not an option, the patient is treated as if he/she has a full stomach. While the induction of anesthesia in this situation is designed to prevent regurgitation and aspiration, the problem of hypertension from sympathetic stimulation becomes especially significant because of the attendant risk of rerupture of the aneurysm, which would be particularly deleterious at this juncture. A rapid-sequence induction with preoxygenation and cricoid pressure is indicated with the addition of fentanyl, 10 μg/kg, sufentanil, 0.1 μg/kg, esmolol, 0.5 mg/kg, or labetalol, 0.2 to 0.4 mg/kg, to a supranormal induction dose of thiopental to reduce the risk of hypertension from laryngoscopy and intubation. Propofol is not recommended because of the possibility of systemic hypotension. Muscle relaxation may be conferred by SCH after a dose of curare or metocurine to prevent fasciculation (and a rise in ICP),[174] vecuronium, 0.15 to 0.20 mg/kg, or rocuronium, 0.6 mg/kg.

Although ventilation with cricoid pressure after the induction of anesthesia is offered as an alternative technique to rapid-sequence induction to avoid systemic hypertension by permitting titration of dose to response for the hypnotic and narcotics, the risk of regurgitation and aspiration is considerable enough to render first securing the airway of paramount importance. The use of a "priming" dose of nondepolarizing muscle relaxant in this setting has been associated with regurgitation and aspiration, so that this technique is less than optimal.[194]

Whatever the choice of technique for anesthesia and muscle relaxation in the unprepared patient, the crucial objective is to prevent the hypertensive response to laryngoscopy and intubation. If the blood pressure does rise in response to airway manipulation, the stimulus is discontinued, the patient is ventilated by mask with cricoid pressure, the depth of anesthesia is augmented, and sympatholytic drugs are administered before the laryngoscopy is repeated.

INTUBATION

Fiberoptic intubation is the most effective technique for securing the difficult airway before the induction of anesthesia. The challenge in this instance, known to increase the risk of aneurysmal rupture, is to prevent hypertension and coughing in response to manipulation of the airway while avoiding respiratory depression and obtundation from sedation. Topical anesthesia for fiberoptic intubation is achieved in 20 to 30 min by the patient's inhalation of nebulized 4 percent lidocaine.

The combination of fentanyl and midazolam in small incremental doses of 25 μg and 0.5 mg, respectively, will confer sedation in those patients who have normal intracranial compliance. The sedation will also diminish the coughing elicited by the translaryngeal injection of 2.5 ml of 4 percent lidocaine through the cricothyroid membrane, an alternative or adjunct to nebulized anesthesia. Alternatively, or in addition to nebulization and translaryngeal injection, bilateral superior laryngeal nerve blocks may be performed by the injection of 0.50 to 0.75 ml of 2 percent lidocaine on both sides of the arch of the hyoid bone.

In the situation in which tracheal intubation is impossible but ventilation is adequate, the patient's trachea may be intubated fiberoptically through an intubating mask. It is essential during this period of airway manipulation to maintain oxygenation and ensure adequate anesthesia with intravenous or—if the intracranial dynamics are normal—inhalational drugs, monitoring the blood pressure all the while. Use of the light wand and retrograde intubation over a translaryngeal guide wire are alternative techniques when oxygenation is assured. If ventilation as well as intubation are impossible, transtracheal jet ventilation is a temporizing measure while fiberoptic intubation is performed. Failing success fiberoptically, the patient may require cricothyroidotomy or tracheotomy.

MAINTENANCE OF ANESTHESIA

The selection of drugs for the maintenance of anesthesia is predicated on the need to optimize cerebral perfusion, protect against cerebral ischemia and edema, minimize brain retractor pressure by providing cerebral relaxation (i.e., reduction in brain volume through a reduction in CBF, cerebral blood volume, and CSF), manipulate blood pressure to decrease the transmural pressure during dissection and clipping of the aneurysm, and facilitate rapid emergence. In the absence of intraoperative complications, patients deemed to be in good condition preoperatively (Grades I, II, and III) should be awakened at the conclusion of the operative procedure. Their tracheas are extubated promptly to permit timely assessment of their neurologic status. Intravenous and inhalational drugs may be used alone or in combination to achieve these goals and prevent aneurysmal rupture.

INHALATIONAL ANESTHETICS

As cerebral vasodilators, all the inhalational anesthetics have the potential for increasing ICP. With the exception of nitrous oxide (N_2O), they also depress cerebral metabolism. The vasodilator and metabolism-enhancing properties of N_2O[195] are augmented when N_2O is combined with an inhalational anesthetic.[176,196–200] Intravenous anesthetics, on the other hand, attenuate the tendency of N_2O to increase CBF and CMR_{O_2}.[195,201,202] In humans, N_2O decreased the cerebral metabolic rate for oxygen[203] and caused cerebral vasodilatation[204] and an increase in ICP.[205] This increase in ICP could be limited by the prior administration of morphine[206] or the creation of hypocapneic conditions. In some animal studies, however, hypocapnia failed to prevent the increase in CBF and ICP.[207]

It is advisable, therefore, to avoid N_2O, especially during the induction of anesthesia, in patients who have a decrease in intracranial compliance, and to introduce N_2O only after intravenous vasoconstricting drugs have been given and hypocapnia has been established. The discontinuation of N_2O should be considered when cerebral relaxation is difficult to achieve. N_2O may also increase ICP by diffusing into an intracranial air space more quickly than the nitrogen in the air diffuses out, necessitating prompt diagnosis of pneumocephalus by computed tomographic scan and evacuation to relieve the resultant compression.

Isoflurane produces a minimal increase in CBF[208,209] and a decrease in cerebral metabolism.[210,211] The increase in ICP associated with the administration of isoflurane can be prevented or partially blocked by hypocapnia or the administration of barbiturates.[212–214] Since isoflurane has been reported to increase ICP despite hypocapnia in patients who have space-occupying lesions,[215] it is prudent to use isoflurane as an adjuvant anesthetic in low concentrations or to avoid it altogether in patients known to have a decrease in intracranial compliance. Isoflurane may also confer a degree of cerebral protection, at least in the early phase of ischemic insult, because of its metabolic depressive effect.[216,217]

The cerebrovascular effects of desflurane (4 to 6 per-

cent), similar to those of isoflurane,[218] include dose-dependent cerebral vasodilatation and a decrease in the cerebral metabolic rate with no significant effect on ICP.[219] Cerebrovascular reactivity to changes in Pa_{CO_2} is preserved.[220] The low blood-gas solubility may permit rapid awakening, an advantage for facilitating prompt postoperative neurologic evaluation.

INTRAVENOUS ANESTHETICS

The preponderance of the evidence regarding the effect of narcotics on CBF and ICP indicates that they are safe for intraoperative administration in the presence of hyperventilation and vasoconstricting drugs. On the one hand, sufentanil increased CSF pressure significantly and decreased cerebral perfusion pressure during elective resection of supratentorial tumors.[221] Both fentanyl and sufentanil were associated with elevation of the ICP in patients who had head trauma,[222,223] despite hyperventilation; and sufentanil increased CBF velocity.[224] On the other hand, fentanyl, sufentanil, and alfentanil improved cerebral relaxation[225] and did not alter brain retractor pressure[226] during craniotomy in patients anesthetized with isoflurane and hyperventilated. Sufentanil also failed to increase CBF in healthy human volunteers[227,228] (in the absence of cerebral vasoconstricting drugs). While doses of narcotics in the clinical range have modest depressive effects on CBF and the cerebral metabolic rate for oxygen, narcotic-induced seizures are associated with a marked increase in CBF, the cerebral metabolic rate for oxygen, and the cerebral metabolic rate for glucose.[229]

In combination with the inhalational anesthetics or as an alternative, narcotics may be administered intermittently or by infusion. Either fentanyl (25 to 50 μg IV as a bolus and 1 to 2 μg/kg per h as an infusion) or sufentanil (10 to 20 μg as a bolus and 0.1 to 0.2 μg/kg per h as an infusion) may be combined with isoflurane (0.5 to 1 percent) or administered with an infusion of pentothal or propofol (40 to 60 μg/kg per min) for the maintenance of anesthesia.

While high-dose fentanyl (50 to 100 μg/kg) and sufentanil (5 to 10 μg/kg) will definitely interfere with prompt awakening and neurologic assessment,[230] a total dose of 10 μg/kg of fentanyl or 2 μg/kg of sufentanil will not prolong recovery at the end of the operation. With regard to the issue of rapid emergence, there is no clinically significant difference between fentanyl and alfentanil.[231] Propofol may be most effective for short-term extension of the duration of the anesthetic as the operation nears conclusion. There was also no difference demonstrated, for that matter, regarding intraoperative hypertension, rapidity of emergence, or postoperative hypertension among patients anesthetized with thiopental/sufentanil, thiopental/fentanyl, or isoflurane when these drugs were used with nitrous oxide and vecuronium.[232] To a certain extent, how drugs are used is more important than the choice of the agents.

The use of long-acting intravenous drugs as the primary anesthetic technique is appropriate when there is no plan to extubate the patient's trachea at the end of the operation, either because of poor preoperative status or a catastrophic intraoperative event (e.g., aneurysmal rupture necessitating ligation of a feeding vessel, brain swelling). These patients probably will require continued intubation and postoperative ventilatory support.

Good-grade patients may be awakened in the operating room and their tracheas extubated at the end of the operation. The avoidance of coughing, straining, hypercarbia, and hypertension is essential. Propofol or lidocaine may be used to reduce the laryngotracheal and hemodynamic responses to emergence and extubation. Patients whose aneurysms have been wrapped or who have multiple aneurysms should have their blood pressure maintained within 20 percent of their normal range (120 to 160 mmHg) during emergence. Although the residual depressant effects of narcotics may be reversed with naloxone, 0.05 $\mu g/kg$, larger doses of naloxone can be hazardous because they may cause sudden, violent awakening of the patient and marked increases in systemic blood pressure.

If the patient fails to demonstrate the preoperative neurologic status or, worse, fails to awaken at the conclusion of the operation, the residual anesthetic effects of sedatives, narcotics, and inhalational and muscle relaxant drugs should be dissipated or reversed, and the Pa_{CO_2} normalized. Other causes of residual depression of the patient's level of consciousness include hypoxia and hyponatremia, and these should be treated or ruled out. The persistence of diminished responsiveness or a new neurologic deficit for two hours after surgery has ended mandates a CT scan to diagnose the presence of intracranial or subdural hematoma, hydrocephalus, pneumocephalus, infarction, or edema. A magnetic resonance angiogram or an intra-arterial angiogram may demonstrate the existence of vascular occlusion.

FLUID ADMINISTRATION

The intraoperative administration of fluid is guided by the patient's maintenance fluid requirement, blood loss, urine output, and CVP or PCWP. After SAH, patients have a decrease in circulating blood volume.[22] This hypovolemia has been associated with cerebral ischemia and perioperative neurologic deficits, especially in the presence of vasospasm. To prevent a hypotensive response to the induction of anesthesia, the intravascular volume is expanded acutely before the

induction, and also in anticipation of aneurysmal clipping and the use of controlled hypotension, since hypovolemic hypotension adversely affects organ perfusion.

Full restoration of the intravascular volume to a state of modest hypervolemia occurs during the securing of the aneurysm to optimize CBF and militate against the possibility of postoperative vasospasm.[94] Most of the fluid is administered as glucose-free crystalloid, because both focal and global cerebral ischemia are exacerbated by elevated serum glucose levels.[233–236] Plasmalyte, normal saline, and Normo-Sol are superior to Ringer's lactate. Since Ringer's lactate is hyposmolar to plasma, this may contribute to the formation of cerebral edema when the blood-brain barrier is disrupted. The resultant hyponatremia has also been associated with an increase in the incidence of delayed ischemic deficit.[21]

The use of blood and blood products is indicated to maintain the hematocrit in the low normal range of 30 to 35 percent, as hemodilution enhances cerebral perfusion in humans. Five percent albumin may confer some rheologic advantages by making red blood cells more "slippery." Hetastarch in amounts exceeding 500 ml is relatively contraindicated, however, because of the possibility of interference with hemostasis and resultant intracranial bleeding.[96,97]

Cerebral Volume Reduction

To facilitate the surgical approach to the aneurysm, the volume of the intracranial contents may be reduced and brain relaxation improved after the opening of the dura. All maneuvers are timed to prevent aneurysmal rupture secondary to the increase in transmural pressure from the decrease in ICP induced by hyperventilation, administration of mannitol, or drainage of CSF. The carbon dioxide tension is moderately reduced to the range of 30 to 35 mmHg until the dura is incised—in the absence of a preoperative increase in intracranial elastance—and then hyperventilation to a Pa_{CO_2} of 25 to 30 mmHg is instituted to decrease CBF, cerebral blood volume, and brain bulk. Higher levels of CO_2 tension are appropriate in patients who have vasospasm to avoid exacerbation of the ischemic injury and during the period of induced hypotension.

Mannitol, an osmotic diuretic, is given in a dose of 0.25 to 1.0 g/kg to decrease brain water through creation of an osmotic gradient. Although the peak reduction in cerebral volume occurs at 60 to 90 min after administration, the onset of action is within 10 to 15 min. Giving the mannitol should therefore be timed to avoid any marked decrease in cerebral blood volume and ICP—with an attendant rise in transmural pres-

TABLE 26-15
Aneurysmal Manipulation

Systemic hypotension	Local hypotension	Modifiers
Isoflurane	Temporary clips	Captopril
Nitroprusside	(with normal BP)	Saralasin
Adenosine	Carotid compression	Clonidine

sure and the possibility of aneurysmal rupture—before the dura is opened.[237] Since the rapid administration of mannitol can cause both systemic hypotension and an acute increase in intravascular volume detrimental to patients who have compromise of their cardiac function, furosemide is added to potentiate the action of mannitol and diminish the dose.[238,239] Although the combination of mannitol and furosemide confers relative potassium-sparing, fluid and electrolyte balance is monitored closely after their administration.

The drainage of CSF facilitates surgical exposure. The surgeon may put in a ventricular catheter or drain the basal cisterns intraoperatively. Alternatively, a lumbar subarachnoid catheter is inserted after induction of anesthesia and before positioning for surgery. While the cranium is still closed, the avoidance of leakage of CSF is essential to prevent a decrease in ICP and the concomitant rise in transmural pressure. If the ICP is elevated preoperatively, the subarachnoid puncture and escape of CSF may also lead to tonsilar herniation.

Controlled Hypotension

For surgical clip-ligation of intracranial aneurysms, patients require precise intraoperative control of blood pressure to prevent rebleeding, facilitate clip placement, and counteract vasospasm (Table 26-15). Lowering of the blood pressure during microscopic dissection of the aneurysm has been advocated to reduce the risk of rupture by decreasing aneurysmal wall tension and augmenting the malleability of the neck of the aneurysm. The maneuver is effective because the wall of the aneurysmal sac thins as the aneurysm increases in size. The likelihood of rupture increases, since less pressure is required to enlarge it to the bursting point.[240] Therefore, the lower the pressure, the better. Hypotension also facilitates visualization of the aneurysmal neck and adjacent vessels by diminishing bleeding.

Patients who have normal brains will tolerate a reduction of the mean arterial pressure to 50 mmHg. The limits of autoregulation in chronically hypertensive patients are higher than for normotensive patients so that the hypertensive patient's blood pressure should be reduced to no more than 50 mmHg less than the normal

pressure.[241] Even more modest reductions in blood pressure of no more than 20 to 30 mmHg are advisable in patients who have anemia, fever, cerebral hematoma, occlusive cerebrovascular disease, and the probability of prolonged retractor pressure.[242] Harp and Wollman also pointed out long ago that the concomitant use of hyperventilation and hypotension may decrease CBF sufficiently to increase the risk of focal ischemia significantly.[243] Consequently, patients should be normocarbic during the period of induced hypotension.[244]

Sodium nitroprusside (SNP) and isoflurane are the drugs most commonly used for the intraoperative reduction of blood pressure.[245] SNP decreases peripheral vascular resistance by metabolic or spontaneous reduction to nitric oxide.[246] Pharmacologically, SNP is notable for its rapid onset, short half-life, dilatation of resistance vessels, and neutral effect on cardiac output. The deleterious effects of SNP include cyanide and thiocyanate toxicity, intracranial hypertension, rebound hypertension, abnormalities of coagulation, increased pulmonary shunting, hypothyroidism, mitochondrial damage, and decreases in myocardial, liver, and skeletal muscle oxygen reserves.

Cyanide is a metabolite of SNP. Toxic blood levels of greater than 100 μg/dl develop when more than 1 mg/kg of SNP is administered within 2.5 h or when more than 0.5 mg/kg per h is administered within 24 h.[247] Treatment of cyanide toxicity includes the intravenous administration of thiosulfate. In the presence of abnormal renal function, hydroxocobalamin is substituted. The dose of SNP itself may be reduced by the concomitant use of captopril.[248]

SNP may increase the ICP of patients who have a decrease in intracranial compliance because of its dilation of capacitance and resistance vessels.[249,250] Patients who have space-occupying lesions are at even greater risk since venous return could be impeded by the mass with a resultant increase in cerebral blood volume and ICP[251] and a compromise in regional cerebral perfusion. Even after the cranium is opened and the ICP equals atmospheric pressure, the SNP-induced cerebral vasodilation may cause cerebral swelling and a disturbance in perfusion in areas under retraction.[252]

The dose for inducing hypotension with SNP is 0.5 to 10 mg/kg per min and is increased slowly. The infusion is discontinued if the target mean arterial pressure is not achieved with 10 mg/kg per min within the first 10 to 15 min to preclude the possibility of cyanide toxicity.

Isoflurane lowers the blood pressure through peripheral vasodilatation. When compared with SNP, isoflurane attenuates the "stress response" to induced hypotension.[253] Although the use of isoflurane has been associated with exacerbation of ST-segment changes and the shunting of blood from regions of the myocardium dependent on collateral circulation,[254] there is no increase in pulmonary shunting or dead space with isoflurane-induced hypotension.

Isoflurane reduces the cerebral metabolic rate and maintains CBF, but at clinical doses isoflurane confers less protection than thiopental in an in vitro hippocampal slice model.[255] When primates underwent middle cerebral artery occlusion, Gelb demonstrated no difference in lesion size or neurologic score between groups in which either isoflurane or SNP was used to induce hypotension.[256] Even in the presence of mild hypothermia, isoflurane did not offer greater cerebral protection than halothane in a rat model of focal ischemia.[257]

Since isoflurane's interference with cardiac output[247] and autoregulation[258] is dose-related, combining isoflurane with either labetalol,[259] an alpha- and beta-blocking drug, or enalapril,[260] an angiotensin-converting enzyme inhibitor, will facilitate the achievement of adequate levels of hypotension with less than 1 percent isoflurane. Both labetalol and esmolol, a beta-adrenergic blocking drug with a half-life of 9 min, are indeed useful by themselves[261,262] or as adjuncts for induced hypotension because they do not cause cerebral vasodilatation, tachycardia, or rebound hypertension.[187]

Temporary Occlusion

While controlled hypotension decreases aneurysmal wall tension and bleeding and facilitates clip application, lowering the blood pressure can also compromise regional CBF. SAH impairs cerebral autoregulation and perfusion[5-8] and interferes with the cerebrovascular response to induced hypotension.[161] Because patients in whom cerebral autoregulation and perfusion are abnormal have a higher incidence of ischemia, infarction, and postoperative neurologic deficit,[263] neurosurgeons avoid the use of induced hypotension, especially where there is angiographic evidence of vasospasm.[264] Instead, they now routinely use temporary proximal occlusion of the parent vessel to reduce the risk of aneurysmal rupture during manipulation of the aneurysm.[265-267]

Application of temporary clips produces "local hypotension" and reduction of transmural pressure without the problems attendant upon systemic hypotension. The risks of focal cerebral ischemia and infarction distal to the temporary occlusion, cerebral edema, and damage to the parent vessel do exist, however, and are directly related to the duration of the temporary occlusion and the integrity of the collateral circulation. The chance of developing a new neurologic deficit after temporary proximal occlusion is exacerbated by advanced age (greater than 61 years of age), poor preoperative neurologic status, and aneurysms involving the distributions of the perforating arteries of the distal basilar and horizontal segment of the middle cerebral artery.[268]

To optimize collateral circulation during the period of temporary proximal occlusion, the patient's blood pressure is maintained in the high-normal range.[269] Boosting the systemic blood pressure will improve CBF and cerebral perfusion pressure and may militate against ischemia in a threatened vascular territory by improving collateral circulation.[270]

The blood pressure may be raised at the time of temporary occlusion by the administration of dopamine, norepinephrine, or phenylephrine.[271] The pure alpha-agonist phenylephrine does not cause direct vasoconstriction of the cerebral vessels and augments CBF because of the rise in systemic blood pressure. Because cardiac afterload is increased when the blood pressure is raised pharmacologically, patients who have coronary artery disease are at risk for the development of cardiac ischemia. Hemodynamic monitoring, including a pulmonary artery catheter, is therefore critical when induced hypertension is planned in this patient population.

Temporary proximal occlusion is the quintessential example of a situation fraught with the hazard of focal cerebral ischemia. Vascular occlusion of short duration with prompt reperfusion usually presents no problem. Although Samson[268] concluded that 15 to 20 min of temporary occlusion is a critical threshold for the development of postoperative cerebral infarction, the reduction of CBF to less than 5 to 10 ml/100 g per min for more than 10 min has led to cell death.[272] Drugs administered to extend the duration of occlusion have demonstrated a reduction in ischemic damage in humans and in animal models. Such protection may be conferred by a decrease in the neuronal electrical activity and consequently in the metabolic demand. The drugs that act as cerebral vasoconstrictors may also redistribute blood from normal to ischemic areas and reduce the damage attendant upon focal ischemia.[273]

Cerebral Protection

Other mechanisms of pharmacologic cerebral protection include prevention of the intracellular entry of calcium,[274] prevention of the sequestration of calcium by the mitochondria,[275] and alteration of free fatty acid metabolism and the arachidonic acid cascade.[276] The antagonism of the N-methyl D-aspartate (NMDA) receptor, which inhibits the action of glutamate and other excitatory amino acid neurotransmitters, confers a cerebroprotective effect, since glutamate can become neurotoxic under conditions of cerebral ischemia.[277,278] The increased concentrations of extracellular glutamate released during ischemia activate the NMDA receptor to open the membrane channels, allowing an influx of sodium. Membrane depolarization occurs subsequently, as well as a secondary passive influx of chloride and water, which causes cellular swelling.[279] This eventually leads to lysis of the cell membrane and cell death. The NMDA antagonists have their greatest potential effect in the penumbra of mild to moderate focal ischemia, where their ability to block receptor-activated calcium influx may prevent lethal injury.

With reperfusion of ischemic tissue, a later effect of uncontrolled calcium influx is the release of oxygen free radicals because of the availability of oxygen once again in previously ischemic tissue.[280] The superoxide radical is formed by the conversion of hypoxanthine to xanthine. This reaction is catalyzed by xanthine oxidase, which is formed when the uncontrolled rise of intracellular calcium leads to the proteolytic conversion of xanthine dehydrogenase. The free radical component of injury assumes importance when the duration of ischemia is prolonged and affects the microvasculature most adversely. Damage to the microvascular endothelium causes thrombosis and permanent occlusion, with conversion of selective neuronal necrosis to pan-necrosis and infarction.

Natural free-radical scavengers include vitamin C, vitamin E, catalase, glutathione peroxidase, and superoxide dismutase. Techniques have been designed to prevent ischemic damage by free radicals: anoxic reperfusion to deliver free radical scavenging drugs; free-iron chelation; and inhibition of xanthine oxidase. Most anesthetics are relatively poor free-radical scavengers, so their protective role may be limited during the reperfusion phase.

In view of the complexity of the sequelae of ischemic injury to the CNS, it is not surprising that reduction of the cerebral metabolic rate for oxygen alone does not offer adequate cerebral protection. Furthermore, since the efficacy of many anesthetic drugs in decreasing the cerebral metabolic rate depends on a reduction in cerebral electrical activity, barbiturates and other metabolic rate depressants are beneficial only in circumstances in which some electrical activity is present. There is no further reduction in metabolic rate once the electroencephalogram (EEG) becomes isoelectric. Accordingly, barbiturates have improved outcome after focal ischemic insult,[230,281-284] but not after global ischemic insult when the EEG is attenuated or isoelectric.[285-287] In an animal model of hypothermic circulatory arrest, thiopental prevented the increase in the cerebral energy state normally observed with hypothermia and caused a decrease in the energy state of the brain during hypothermic circulatory arrest and

subsequent reperfusion.[288] These results suggest that thiopental administration before a period of hypothermic circulatory arrest may be detrimental to the preservation of the energy state of the brain.

In contrast to the barbiturates, the inhalational anesthetic isoflurane offers no benefit during focal ischemia (see above).[256,281,283,289] Isoflurane does provide better protection than other volatile anesthetics from incomplete regional ischemia in humans,[290] as evidenced by the significantly lower incidence of encephalographic ischemic changes during carotid endarterectomy with isoflurane anesthesia (18 percent) than with either halothane (25 percent) or enflurane (26 percent). A recent account of six aneurysm patients who underwent craniotomy for clip ligation under isoflurane anesthesia reported good outcomes. EEG burst suppression was easily induced, and the patients awakened quickly after surgery.[291]

Although there have been no controlled human studies of the protective effects of intravenous drugs during aneurysm surgery, the ability to institute protective measures prophylactically, before the onset of ischemia, offers beguiling possibilities. A number of drugs and combinations of drugs have been administered to extend the duration of vascular occlusion. Giving high-dose mannitol (2 g/kg) before temporary occlusion has been advocated because it enhances the microcirculation and increases regional CBF in areas of ischemia.[292,293] Samson and Batjer[257] saw neurologic recovery in their patients after 32 to 60 min of occlusion using the protocol of normotension, normovolemia, mannitol administration, and burst-suppression-inducing doses of etomidate or barbiturates. Yoshimoto and Suzuki[294] reported temporary occlusion of up to 80 min without adverse neurologic sequelae with the administration of mannitol. In view of the fact that the production of free radicals may contribute to neuronal damage from ischemia, Suzuki has added vitamin E (500 mg) and dexamethasone (50 mg) to mannitol (100 g), the "Sendai cocktail."[295]

Patients have received barbiturates before temporary vascular occlusion in an uncontrolled fashion to facilitate aneurysmal clip ligation. McDermott and coworkers reported good results in 36 patients who received barbiturates, but had no control group.[296] Batjer and colleagues[297] also failed to include a control group in their study of 14 patients who received sufficient etomidate to produce burst suppression on the EEG before the securing of large and giant cerebral aneurysms. Although the outcome was determined to be good in 10 of the 14 patients, the absence of a control group makes it impossible to attribute these results to the use of etomidate. The inclusion of hypothermia in the treatment of basilar artery aneurysms also obscured whatever protective effect barbiturates may have had in the report by Spetzler and associates.[298]

When considering the use of barbiturates, it is important to bear in mind that the recommended dose of thiopental, 5 to 6 mg/kg, will decrease the blood pressure, and the time to awakening and extubation will be prolonged. If the hypotension associated with the use of barbiturates is not corrected, greater ischemic damage might result than if barbiturates had not been given and normotension had been maintained. Etomidate, 0.4 to 0.5 mg/kg, produces a smaller decrease in blood pressure and less delay in extubation. Ravussin and Tribolet[299] demonstrated that the administration of propofol to the point of EEG burst suppression, with a presumed protective effect, will still permit extubation of the patient's trachea in the operating room.

The monitoring of EEG activity permits the use of a dose of barbiturate sufficient to induce burst suppression of EEG activity just before temporary vascular occlusion. This is a helpful end-point since no further metabolic benefits are derived from doses greater than those needed to produce burst suppression or electrical silence.[300,301] Additional doses of barbiturate may be given as indicated by the EEG. If collateral circulation is reduced to the point of interfering with delivery of the drug, however, further administration may be ineffective. The relative advantage of such poor collateral flow is that any drug that has already accumulated in the ischemic area would remain there because of the diminished washout.

Electrophysiologic monitoring is also useful as an indicator of neuronal well-being. The continued presence of a normal EEG or evoked potential pattern is an indication that the brain is tolerating the proximal occlusion and that the surgeon may proceed with the dissection. Conversely, any deterioration of the electrophysiologic pattern signals the need for a brief period of reperfusion. Both the EEG and evoked potentials may be used in conjunction with mannitol as the cerebroprotective drug, but only the evoked potentials remain unaffected by the anesthetic drugs that are used for pharmacologic protection. Regardless of the monitoring parameters, maintenance of the blood pressure in the normal to slightly above normal range during the period of temporary occlusion will optimize collateral blood flow.

Even mild hypothermia has been shown to be cerebroprotective by virtue of decreasing the release of excitatory neurotransmitters (e.g., glutamate) and increasing the release of inhibitory neurotransmitters (e.g., gamma-aminobutyric acid).[302–306] Hypothermia also reduces cerebral oxygen demand by 7 to 8 percent per 1°C, and this effect continues after the EEG becomes isoelectric. It is thus salutary to maintain the patient's body temperature in the range of 33 to 35°C while the

TABLE 26-16
If the Aneurysm Ruptures

Before the skull is opened	During dissection
Suspect if ↑ BP	Hypotension
Realize ICP also ↑	Carotid compression
Thiopental, BP control	Intracranial occlusion
	Barbiturates
	Blood product replacement

NOTE: BP = blood pressure; ICP = intracranial pressure.

patient is at risk for cerebral ischemia and to reduce any increase in body temperature above normal. Since the patient's body temperature does drift 2 to 3°C during the course of an operation, this mild degree of hypothermia may be maintained intraoperatively without active attempts at cooling the patient. Complete rewarming may be difficult with conventional methods (convective heaters, circulating water blankets, etc.).[307]

Moderate hypothermia (28 to 32°C) has been used to extend the duration of vascular occlusion.[295] The potential complications of myocardial depression, cardiac arrhythmias and ischemia, coagulopathy, increased blood viscosity, prolonged drug clearance, increased rates of infection, and increased oxygen consumption from postoperative shivering may militate against its routine use.[308]

Intraoperative Aneurysmal Rupture

Rupture of the aneurysm (Table 26-16) during induction of anesthesia or during the operation can be catastrophic; mortality and morbidity are increased. The incidence of intraoperative rupture is 19 percent:[122] aneurysmal leak occurs in 6 percent and rupture in the other 13 percent of cases.

The occurrence of aneurysmal rupture varies with the stage of the operation and the location and size of the aneurysm itself. Batjer and Samson[309] reported that 7 percent of the ruptures occurred before dissection of the aneurysm, 48 percent during dissection, and 45 percent during clip application.

An abrupt increase in blood pressure during or after induction, with or without bradycaria, may indicate that the aneurysm has bled and the ICP may increase as well. At this juncture, aneurysmal rupture may be diagnosed by the use of transcranial Doppler ultrasound,[158] and the efficacy of management monitored thereafter. Therapy is directed toward the maintenance of cerebral perfusion, control of intracranial hypertension, and reduction of the transmural pressure of the aneurysm. Thiopental or SNP will decrease the blood pressure, although hypotension can be detrimental.

While postponement of the operation will afford an opportunity for cerebral recovery from the events of the acute rupture, "rescue clipping" of the aneurysm after rupture during induction has been successful.[160]

Intraoperative rupture of the aneurysm calls for rapid achievement of surgical control. The mean arterial pressure may be reduced to 40 to 50 mmHg to facilitate clip-ligation of the neck of the aneurysm or temporary proximal and distal occlusion of the parent vessel. When the parent vessel is occluded, blood pressure is increased to normal during the period of temporary occlusion to enhance collateral perfusion. This may be preferable to the use of hypotension after rupture.[310] Alternatively, the ipsilateral carotid artery may be manually compressed for up to three min to produce a bloodless field. If the bleeding is sufficient to cause acute hypovolemia, induced hypotension may not be an option. In this case, the blood that is lost is replaced immediately with whole blood, blood products, or colloid to maintain intravascular volume.

Although barbiturates and etomidate have been advocated for protection against focal ischemia, their efficacy has not been demonstrated in this clinical situation, and their effects can be detrimental in hypovolemic patients. Stable patients may receive thiopental or etomidate before temporary occlusion.

Hypothermic Circulatory Arrest for Giant Aneurysms and Complex Vertebrobasilar Aneurysms

Giant cerebral aneurysms are defined as being greater than 2.5 cm in diameter and represent a subset of cerebral aneurysms that may present technical difficulty due to their size or lack of an anatomic neck. They often have perforating vessels originating in the wall of the neck, as well as a high likelihood of changes. The incidence of giant aneurysms is 2 percent of all patients in the Cooperative Study.[4] Most giant aneurysms present with symptoms of a mass lesion, such as headache, visual disturbance, and/or cranial nerve palsies.

Surgical treatment of these aneurysms is associated with significant perioperative morbidity and mortality. Drake and coworkers reported that, in their series of 174 patients with giant aneurysms who underwent standard surgical treatment, 71.5 percent had good outcomes, 13 percent were severely disabled, and 15.5 percent died.[311] The series of 174 included 73 patients with giant basilar aneurysms which were associated with a greater complication rate of nearly 50 percent (23 percent had poor outcome, and 25 percent died).

Surgery for giant aneurysms remains a formidable challenge, and some neurosurgeons advise their patients against operative intervention unless immediate life-threatening risks are documented.[312] Two surgical techniques are used for the management of giant aneurysms considered otherwise inoperable: the use of proximal and distal temporary occlusion to collapse the aneurysm, or the use of circulatory arrest under profound hypothermia (Table 26-17 Protocol 1). Although the former approach has been advocated by some surgeons,[309,313] it is not considered uniformly applicable. The latter approach had been used as a general approach for all cerebral aneurysms, but fell into disfavor as improvement in microsurgical technique and neuroanesthesia allowed conventional approaches to achieve superior results. Similarly, many complex aneurysms of the vertebrobasilar system are considered inoperable because of difficulty of access and visualization. With improvement in cardiopulmonary bypass technology, there is revived interest in using this technique for giant aneurysms and complex vertebrobasilar aneurysms, with several series reporting good results, mortality ranging from 0 to 25 percent.[312,314–322]

The main advantages of hypothermic circulatory arrest for giant aneurysms include: (1) decompression of the aneurysmal sac; (2) better visualization of the anatomy; (3) a totally bloodless field; and (4) easy manipulation and placement of the clip. Circulatory arrest can be performed using closed-chest femoral vein-femoral artery bypass or open chest with median sternotomy and ventricular venting. The closed-chest method is associated with lower morbidity and is generally preferred. The most devastating complication from this technique is postoperative intracranial hemorrhage.

The major issues concern brain protection and complications of cardiopulmonary bypass. For details on physiology and management of cardiopulmonary bypass, the readers should consult a standard textbook on cardiovascular anesthesia.

BRAIN PROTECTION DURING CIRCULATORY ARREST

Cerebral hypoxia and ischemia are the factors that limit the duration of the circulatory arrest. The metabolic oxygen consumption of the brain may be divided into an "active component," which can be regarded as any neuronal activity, and a "basal component," which is related to maintenance of cellular integrity. Pharmacologic and nonpharmacologic methods that decrease the metabolic oxygen consumption will increase the duration of arrest tolerated. At the present time, these include the use of barbiturates and profound hypothermia. A number of investigators have reported good results with giant aneurysms utilizing the combination of barbiturate therapy and profound hypothermia dur-

TABLE 26-17
Protocol 1: Protocol for Circulatory Arrest

1. Placement of arterial line and large-bore intravenous catheters prior to induction. The usual precautions with induction of patients with cerebral aneurysm apply.

2. Once anesthesia is induced and the trachea intubated, place the following: either a central venous line or pulmonary artery catheter, a second arterial line to allow phlebotomy, lumbar subarachnoid drain, and electrophysiologic monitors (EEG and/or SSEP/BAEP). Nasopharyngeal/esophageal/tympanic temperature probes should be used to estimate brain temperature, whereas rectal/bladder temperature probe should be placed to monitor core temperature. Anticipate periods of stimulation as during intubation, head pinning, and periosteal retraction which can cause a hypertensive response.

3. Begin surface cooling by lowering room temperature and using a cooling blanket. Cold (refrigerated) intravenous fluids will facilitate cooling. The rate of decrease should proceed at approximately 0.2°C/min.

4. If barbiturates are to be used, administer 3 to 5 mg/kg bolus of thiopental to induce a burst suppression pattern of 1:5 ratio on EEG or isoelectric EEG. This can be followed with a continuous infusion of thiopental at 0.1 to 0.5 mg/kg per min. Once cooling begins, the infusion is continued at this rate for the entire period on cardiopulmonary bypass.

5. Hemodilute to a hematocrit of 28 to 30 percent by collecting blood into an anticoagulant solution kept at room temperature. Maintain intravascular volume with up to 4 liters of cold intravenous saline containing 4 to 6 meq/liter of KCl.

6. After the aneurysm is dissected and hemostasis obtained, extracorporeal circulation via femoral artery-femoral vein bypass is begun when the patient's temperature reaches 32 to 34°C. Occasionally two venous cannulas are required for adequate venous return. Just prior to initiating bypass, ensure surgical hemostasis, then heparinize with 300 to 400 IU/kg to maintain ACT of 450 to 500 s. Hetastarch should not be used to replenish intravascular volume.

7. The patient is cooled to 15 to 18°C nasopharyngeal temperature. Rectal or bladder temperature will lag behind by 5 to 7°C. Be aware of ECG changes; at 28°C, the myocardium is extremely irritable and may fibrillate continuously. Fibrillation should be stopped with 40 to 80 meq of KCl, and if persistent, defibrillate with 100 to 250 watts/s and administer additional doses of KCl, if necessary.

8. Circulatory arrest occurs at 15 to 18°C and should be limited to the period of clip application. EEG should be isoelectric before arrest. If barbiturates were not used earlier, they may be added at this point to achieve a silent EEG. Elevate the patient's head slightly to facilitate venous drainage, keeping in mind that too much exsanguination carries the potential risk of air embolism and a no-reflow phenomenon in small vessels.

9. The circulatory arrest time should be limited to less than 60 min for optimal results. During arrest it is critically important to keep the ambient temperature low to prevent the brain from warming up. Some surgeons advocate surgical dissection under low perfusion pressure on bypass to minimize the circulatory arrest time.

10. Once the aneurysm is clipped, bypass is reestablished and patient rewarmed at a rate of 0.2 to 0.5°C/min. Too rapid rewarming can cause tissue acidosis and hypoxia. Sodium nitroprusside may be used to allow a more homogeneous rewarming. Check ACT frequently during rewarming. Additional heparin may be necessary.

11. With rewarming, the heart will fibrillate. Cardioversion with 200 to 400 joules through external defibrillating pads and antiarrhythmic agents may be required to restore a normal sinus rhythm. In addition, the patient may require inotropic support.

12. Extracorporeal circulation is discontinued when the patient's temperature is 35 to 36°C and the heart can maintain a normal cardiac output and sinus rhythm. Allow an extra 20 min of rewarming before discontinuation of bypass to minimize the after-drop in temperature from heat redistribution. Supplement with warmed intraveneous solutions and surface forced-air rewarming.

13. The ACT is corrected with protamine sulfate to 100 to 150 s. The autologous blood containing platelet-rich plasma is transfused as well as other blood products necessary to restore hemostasis. Full coagulation profile is determined. Two to four units of fresh frozen plasma and 6 to 12 units of platelet concentrate usually are needed.

ing circulatory arrest.[312,314,315,317,319,323] However, similar results have also been obtained with profound hypothermia alone.[4,316]

BARBITURATES

Barbiturates reduce the cerebral metabolic rate (CMR_{O_2}) attributed to the active component to a maximum of 50 percent. Additional administration beyond that required to cause electrical silence in the EEG will not decrease the metabolic rate further.[300] However, barbiturates also may have other actions including free-radical scavenging and membrane stabilization.[317] Therefore, barbiturates may provide additional cerebral protection even during profound hypothermia, but this remains controversial. Barbiturate therapy is most effective in preventing cerebral injury secondary to temporary focal ischemia. It is less well established in the situation of temporary global ischemia.

Two modes of administering barbiturates (primarily sodium thiopental) prior to cooling and arrest are used: a single bolus or a continuous infusion. Where a single dose of thiopental was given, the amount ranged from 30 to 40 mg/kg as a bolus administered over 30 min.[319,320,323] In most of the reported series, however, EEG monitoring was not utilized to determine the endpoint. Monitoring of EEG allows the anesthesiologist to titrate the loading dose as well as the maintenance infusion to achieve EEG burst suppression throughout the procedure.[281,317] A simple bihemispheric two-channel EEG device will suffice. Burst suppression may be

TABLE 26-18
Relationship of Temperature, % Δ in Cerebral Metabolic Rate, and Time Period of Tolerated Circulatory Arrest

Temperature in °C	% of Cerebral Metabolic Rate	Period of Tolerated Circulatory Arrest (min)
38	100	4 to 5
30	50	8 to 10
25	25	16 to 20
20	15	32 to 40
10	10	64 to 80

accomplished with an initial loading dose of 3 to 5 mg/kg followed by a continuous infusion varying from 0.1 to 0.5 mg/kg per min for the entire period on cardiopulmonary bypass. With profound hypothermia at temperatures below 18°C, EEG is rendered isoelectric even without pharmacologic suppression. (In contrast, evoked responses are abolished between 15 to 18°C). It is recommended that the infusion rate previously established be maintained during circulatory arrest.[312]

HYPOTHERMIA

Hypothermia is a nonpharmacologic method of reducing the CMR_{O_2} and is different from barbiturates in that it not only reduces the active component but also the basal component of the CMR_{O_2}. Hypothermia causes a significant reduction in cerebral oxygen consumption and has been demonstrated to protect the brain during anoxic conditions.[324] The period of circulatory arrest tolerated at normothermia is only 4 to 5 min, but doubles for every 8°C temperature reduction.[325] Thus, the CMR_{O_2} decreases to 50 percent of normal with hypothermia to 30°C, 25 percent of normal at 25°C, 15 percent of normal at 20°C, and 10 percent of normal at 15°C.[326] At 15°C continuous circulatory arrest can therefore be theoretically tolerated for 32 to 40 min. The maximum time of deep hypothermic arrest has not been definitively established, but in clinical practice it has been safely used for up to 60 min (Table 26-18).[316]

As substantial gradients in temperature can develop between the brain and the periphery during cooling and rewarming, it is important to monitor the brain temperature accurately before circulatory arrest. Williams and coworkers reported close correlation of brain temperature measured with esophageal, tympanic membrane, and nasopharyngeal sensors.[316] In contrast, rectal and bladder temperatures are unreliable. Direct brain temperature monitoring has also been advocated.[312] To improve safety, at least two temperature monitoring sites should be used.

The depth of hypothermia and duration of circulatory arrest reported in various series for treatment of

giant aneurysms are summarized in Table 26-19. Note that the amount of time necessary for the clipping is usually less than the tolerable safe limit at the respective temperature. The results also suggested that temperature should be decreased to 15 to 18°C as the series with the highest mortality (25 percent) was associated with circulatory arrest at 25°C.

Cardiovascular Effects of Hypothermia

Hypothermia induces characteristic cardiovascular changes.[317,325] As temperature decreases, systemic vascular resistance increases while cardiac output decreases. To allow high pump flow to facilitate rapid cooling and subsequent rewarming, use of vasodilators such as sodium nitroprusside may be necessary. Progressive bradycardia occurs as temperature approaches 30°C, and the atria frequently begin to flutter or fibrillate below 30°C. The ventricles usually fibrillate below 28°C. As continuous ventricular fibrillation may cause ischemic injury to the heart, electrical activity should be terminated with administration of 40 to 80 meq of KCl to the pump, or with cardioversion using 100 to 250 watts/s.

Hematologic Effects of Hypothermia

The coagulation system is severely perturbed by hypothermia and the problem is compounded by inadequate surgical hemostasis or incomplete reversal of heparin with protamine.[316,317,319,331] Hypothermia-induced coagulopathy is caused by a multitude of factors: (1) hypothermia affects the platelet count by inducing thrombocytopenia, probably from splenic sequestration; (2) it causes a reversible platelet dysfunction; (3) hypothermia slows down the enzyme-mediated steps in the coagulation cascade as well as the metabolism of heparin. The dilutional effect of priming solutions with cardiopulmonary bypass on factors I, II, V, VII, and XIII also contributes to difficulty with hemostasis. Because of the significant risk of coagulation abnormality following bypass, and the usually fatal consequence of intracranial hemorrhage, hetastarch should not be used in these procedures.

Hypothermia also causes an increase in viscosity leading to sludging of the red blood cells. However, this can be effectively treated by deliberately lowering the hematocrit with phlebotomy and simultaneously replacing the blood volume with crystalloids. The phlebotomy not only decreases the hematocrit, but also preserves platelet-rich autologous blood for subsequent transfusion during the rewarming phase. The decreased hematocrit reduces oxygen carrying capacity, but is partially compensated by the increased amount of dissolved oxygen due to the increased solubility during hypothermia. The hemoglobin-oxygen dissociation curve, however, is also shifted to the left,

TABLE 26-19
Circulatory Arrest for Treatment of Giant and Complex Vertebrobasilar Aneurysms

Authors and Years	No. of Cases	Body Temp (°C)	DURATION OF ARREST Median (min)	DURATION OF ARREST Range (min)	Major Morbidity (%)	Mortality (%)
Woodhall et al, 1960[318]	1[a]	12	30	—	100	0
Patterson and Ray, 1962[327]	7	14–17	25	9–43	0	30
Michenfelder et al, 1964[328]	15	13–16	17	0–39	40	20
Drake et al, 1964[322]	10	13–17	14	2–18	40	30
Sundt et al, 1972[329]	1	13	30	—	100	0
McMurtry et al, 1974[321]	12[e]	28–29	9	1–28	50	8
Baumgartner et al, 1983[319b]	15[d]	16–21.5	19	0–51	20	0
Gonski et al, 1986[330]	40	25	10	0–35	23	25
Spetzler et al, 1988[317b]	7	17.5–21	11	7–53	29	14
Thomas et al, 1990[323b]	1	15.4	35	—	0	0
Solomon et al, 1991[312b]	14	15–22.5	22	8–51	50	0
Williams et al, 1991[316]	10[c]	8.4–13.7	25	1.25–60	20	10
Ausman et al, 1993[315b]	9	17–18	20	12–37	22	33
Greene et al, 1994[314b]	2	15–18	40–70	40–70	0	0

[a] Patient with metastatic bronchogenic carcinoma.

[b] Barbiturate therapy was also used.

[c] Only 4 out of 10 are giant aneurysms. The patient who died had an AVM; the patients with morbidity included 1 with AVM and 1 with aneurysm.

[d] 2 of 15 are patients with medullary hemangioblastoma.

[e] 1 of 12 with AVM.

and may reduce unloading of oxygen in ischemic tissue.

Hyperglycemia

Hypothermia prevents proper utilization and metabolism of glucose and may cause hyperglycemia. Hyperglycemia may exacerbate neuronal damage during ischemia[235,236] and therefore should be treated with insulin. Frequent monitoring of serum glucose and electrolytes in addition to acid-base balance is therefore absolutely essential.

ANESTHETIC CONSIDERATIONS

In addition to the normal evaluation of the patient with SAH, preoperative consideration of patients scheduled for hypothermic circulatory arrest must include special emphasis on coexisting cardiac, pulmonary, hematologic, or neurologic disorders that could modify or exclude the patient from the therapy. For example, patients with aortic valve insufficiency may require the open-chest method to prevent ventricular distension.

Although induction of anesthesia is similar to what has been covered previously regarding monitors, blood pressure control, and intubation, there are several additional monitors that should be considered.

These include electroencephalography (EEG), somatosensory evoked potentials (SSEP), brain stem auditory evoked potentials (BAEP), and transesophageal echocardiography. The EEG monitors cortical activity and is necessary as an end-point for barbiturate-induced burst suppression when barbiturates are used for added protection. SSEP, on the other hand, is a measure of the sensory conduction to the cortex and can be recorded even during barbiturate-induced silent EEG. BAEP reflects the function of the auditory pathway through the brain stem and may be useful during procedures on vertebrobasilar aneurysms.[317] However, during profound hypothermia at 15 to 18°C, all electrophysiologic activity is abolished. Nevertheless, SSEP monitoring may allow assessment of neurologic function during cooling as well as rewarming and may have prognostic value. Transesophageal echocardiography allows visualization of the cardiac chambers and assessment of ventricular function and is useful in management of patients with cardiac disease.[312] In addition, TCD has also been used during these procedures,[312] presumably to monitor blood flow and emboli, although its value has not been established.

The overall management necessitates a team effort requiring effective communication among all participants. To administer anesthesia safely for hypothermic circulatory arrest, a thorough understanding of the cardiovascular and hematologic pertubations in response to hypothermia must be appreciated. The technique also demands a knowledge of the use of the various electrophysiologic monitors to guide and to maintain cerebral protection. Although the actual practice varies among different centers, a suggested protocol is appended.

The major and most feared postoperative complication associated with hypothermic cardiac arrest for aneurysm surgery is coagulopathy leading to cerebral hemorrhage. A small leak at the operative site can be disastrous. To reduce this risk, the surgeon should complete the dissection of the aneurysm and verify absolute hemostasis prior to initiating hypothermic circulatory arrest. Heparinization should be evaluated and followed with the activated clotting time (ACT), and maintained within 400 to 450 s. Once rewarming has occurred and the patient no longer requires bypass, protamine sulfate is titrated to reverse the effect of heparin until the ACT is between 100 and 150 s. The phlebotomized blood removed earlier is retransfused, and additional blood products such as fresh frozen plasma, cryoprecipitate, and platelets are often required. Meticulous surgical hemostasis is again necessary before dural closure begins.

The anesthesiologist must also watch for the expected cardiovascular complications associated with cardiopulmonary bypass and correct any rhythm abnormalities during the cooling or rewarming phase. The patient may also require inotropic support during the warming and immediate postoperative course. With or without additional barbiturate protection, the patient is generally transferred directly to the intensive care unit for continued care. Extubation of the trachea and assessment of neurologic function usually can be accomplished within 12 to 24 h. In some cases a CT scan may be required in the interim.

In summary, with careful selection of patients and combined efforts of the anesthesia and surgery team, many patients with giant cerebral aneurysms previously considered inoperable can now be treated surgically under profound hypothermia and circulatory arrest.

Subarachnoid Hemorrhage and Pregnancy

The intense desire for maternal welfare along with optimal fetal outcome presents an important anesthetic challenge in itself. This task may become substantive for the anesthesiologist when compounded by a neurologic insult that jointly endangers the mother and her unborn baby.

Intracranial hemorrhage (ICH) can cause catastrophic complications during pregnancy and is considered an important nonobstetric cause of maternal morbidity and mortality. The etiologies of ICH are diverse and warrant a thorough understanding by the anesthesiologist to facilitate optimal perioperative management. Anesthesiologists must therefore be fully aware of the diagnosis, possible neurovascular complications, and timely management of these life-threatening events in the perioperative period. The complexity of management increases because the medical and neurologic problems are superimposed on the gravid state of the patient.

Cerebrovascular accidents (CVA) can cause a hemorrhagic or an ischemic insult. Intracranial hemorrhage can either be subarachnoid (SAH) or intraparenchymal. Generally, SAH results from cerebral aneurysmal rupture, or bleeding from an arteriovenous malformation (AVM). SAH has been reported to be the third leading cause of nonobstetric maternal morbidity.[332] Intraparenchymal (intracerebral) hemorrhage is associated with AVMs, hypertensive disorders, and eclampsia. The incidence of ICH varies from 0.01 to 0.05 percent of all pregnancies[333,334] or 1 in 10,000 pregnancies.[335] Aneurysms are responsible in 77 percent and AVMs in 23 percent of cases. ICH occurs antepartum in 92 percent and postpartum in 8 percent of patients.[336]

The morbidity and mortality from ICH during pregnancy are significant. Mortality rates range as high as 73 to 83 percent[332] and account for 5 to 12 percent of all maternal deaths during pregnancy.[332,334,337] The fetal mortality is 17 percent.[336] As with the nongravid population, women who have angiomatous hemorrhage are younger than those who have aneurysmal hemorrhage.[332,334,336,338] About 50 percent of the patients who present with SAH during pregnancy have a ruptured AVM, as compared with 10 percent in the nonpregnant group.[334,338,339] In the nonpregnant patient, SAH is more commonly caused by the rupture of an intracerebral aneurysm than by an AVM. In pregnancy, these occur with equal frequency.[334,338] SAH from an aneurysm during pregnancy usually occurs in multiparous women between 25 to 35 years of age,[340] whereas bleeding from an AVM occurs in patients between 18 to 25 years of age and parity is not a factor.[341]

The risk of rebleeding after a hemorrhage during the same pregnancy is 27 percent.[339] AVMs tend to rupture at any stage of pregnancy,[338] but most commonly between 20 weeks of gestation and 6 weeks postpartum. The relationship of aneurysmal hemorrhage to stage of pregnancy has been reported as follows: first trimester, 6 percent; second trimester, 31 percent; third trimester, 55 percent; and postpartum, 86 percent.[337] The tendency to rupture may be related to hemodynamic, hormonal, and coagulation changes that occur during the third trimester,[342] including the increase in blood volume.

PATHOPHYSIOLOGY OF CEREBROVASCULAR ACCIDENTS DURING PREGNANCY

Cerebral aneurysms represent a structural abnormality of the intracranial arteries and usually arise at the branch points of major vessels. Involvement of the vessels derived from the internal carotid artery is much more common than posterior circulation involvement.[343] Approximately 85 percent of aneurysms occur in the anterior circulation on the anterior communicating, internal carotid, and middle cerebral arteries. Aneurysms in the posterior circulation occur at the apex of the basilar artery and at the origin of the posterior-inferior cerebellar artery.[344] The wall of the aneurysm is thin, and there is degeneration of the muscularis. The pressure across the wall is equal to the difference between the mean arterial pressure and the intracranial pressure. The probability of rupture is related to the size of the aneurysm.[345] Approximately 1 percent of reproductive-age women harbor cerebral aneurysms, and one-fourth of patients with aneurysms have multiple lesions.[346]

Arterial aneurysms are the most common cause of nontraumatic SAH, and the spontaneous rupture of an aneurysm has been temporally related to the use of "crack" cocaine.[347] Eclampsia is also a common cause of ICH during pregnancy.[332] Amias[348] reported a relationship between pregnancy-associated hypertension and ruptured cerebral aneurysm. An aggressive regimen of antihypertensives is indicated when blood pressure rises above 160/110 mmHg as chronic hypertensives are at increased risk of rupture of intracranial aneurysms. Robinson[338] reported a ruptured aneurysm in association with severe preeclampsia. The onset of aneurysmal bleeding has also occurred during an elective cesarean section.[333]

Vasospasm is a frequent complication of SAH.[340] There are two possible mechanisms. Vasoconstrictive substances are released by activated platelets, cerebral tissue, or red blood cells. The decomposing products of hemolyzing blood, including protein and hemoglobin catabolites, may also be vasoactive.[344] Vascular compression and/or vasospasm may produce ischemia and infarction in 5 to 7 days after the initial SAH and cause delayed neurologic deficits.[345,349]

AVMs are congenital lesions. While sometimes detected in infancy, they are most commonly diagnosed in the third or fourth decade of life.[345,350] Intracranial AVMs present with intracerebral hemorrhage in 50 percent of cases. Ten percent of patients die after the first hemorrhage, and roughly 14 percent are disabled.[344] AVMs are a network of thin-walled vessels in which the arterial blood passes directly to the draining veins because there are no intervening capillaries. AVMs commonly extend from the surface of the brain into the parenchyma and can occur in the spinal cord.[349] Ten percent of all intracranial hemorrhages are caused by AVMs. This represents the third most common cause of intracranial bleeding after saccular aneurysms and spontaneous intraparenchymal hemorrhage.[344]

A sudden, albeit transient, increase in blood pressure leads to distension and rupture of the vascular malformation. The likely predisposing factor for this increase in blood pressure is coughing, straining, intercourse, or emotional distress. It is estimated that about 10 percent of the bleeding episodes will be fatal.[351] There is a well-known association between AVMs and aneurysms, which usually occur on a major feeding artery to the AVM. When bleeding occurs in this setting, it is usually from rupture of the aneurysm.[344]

Neurologic signs and symptoms result from the intracranial hypertension attendant upon leakage and dispersion of the blood. Patients may have severe explosive headache, nausea, nuchal rigidity from meningeal irritation, drowsiness, irritability, seizures, coma, or death, depending on the severity of the hemorrhage.[344] Irritation of the brain parenchyma may cause autonomic disturbances, with consequent hypertension, cardiac dysrhythmias, or pulmonary edema.

PHYSIOLOGIC CHANGES DURING PREGNANCY

Although no specific correlation has been established between SAH and pregnancy, there are numerous reports of rupture of aneurysms and AVMs during pregnancy, labor, delivery, and during the postpartum period.[332–339,342] No single factor has been directly implicated, but the physiologic changes (Table 26-20) that occur during pregnancy may be responsible for the catastrophe. Pregnancy has a stimulating effect on aneurysmal growth,[352,353] especially during the third trimester. There is an increased incidence of rupture during this period.[337]

The hemodynamic stress of increased blood volume, increased heart rate, increased cardiac output and stroke volume, pregnancy-induced hypertension in the third trimester, and hormonal alterations of pregnancy which cause changes in the walls of the arteries and veins may all contribute to the increased risk of rupture of intracerebral lesions during pregnancy.[354,355] The hemodynamic alterations of pregnancy do not, however, alter CBF or the cerebral metabolic rate for oxygen.[356]

The blood flow to the uterus is directly proportional to the mean perfusion pressure and inversely proportional to the uterine vascular resistance. As such, any factors that reduce perfusion pressure or increase vas-

TABLE 26-20
Physiologic Changes of Pregnancy: Implications for Anesthetic Management

Physiologic Changes	Anesthetic Management
1. Increase in CO	Careful monitoring of intravascular volume
2. Increase in uterine size	Aortocaval compression in supine position: maintain left lateral uterine displacement perioperatively
3. Reduced FRC, increased O_2 consumption	Preoxygenation, higher FiO_2
4. Increase in minute ventilation, decrease in Pa_{CO_2}, left shift of oxyhemoglobin dissociation curve, reduced release of oxygen to the fetus	Monitor changes in Pa_{CO_2} closely, prevent hyperventilation; avoid decrease in CO, uterine blood flow, O_2 supply to the fetus
5. Decrease in gastric emptying, gastroesophageal reflux	Aspiration prophylaxis, rapid-sequence induction
6. Maternal hyperventilation, reduced Pa_{CO_2}, cerebral vasospasm, cerebral ischemia/infarction	Monitor ET_{CO_2}; maintain adequate cerebral perfusion pressure
7. Reduced MAC for inhalation anesthetics	Avoid overdose and cardiovascular depression
8. Decreased epidural and subarachnoid space	Decreased local anesthetic requirement for regional anesthesia
9. Uterine blood flow is not autoregulated and is proportional to mean perfusion pressure	Avoid hypotension and consequent decrease in uterine blood flow with reduced O_2 delivery to the fetus
10. Decrease in serum cholinesterase	Monitor neuromuscular blockade after succinylcholine use

NOTE: FRC = Functional residual capacity; MAC = Minimal alveolar concentration; CO = Cardiac output.

cular resistance will adversely affect placental perfusion, with consequent ill-effects on the fetus. Maternal hypotension should be avoided during operation.

Pregnancy itself causes a progressive increase in minute ventilation and a decrease in functional residual capacity. Changes in minute ventilation, the mechanical effect of positive pressure ventilation, and a decrease in the partial pressure of CO_2 may reduce placental blood flow to the fetus. Respiratory alkalosis shifts the oxygen-hemoglobin dissociation curve to the left and increases the affinity of maternal hemoglobin for oxygen, thereby reducing fetal oxygen supply. Hypocapnia also reduces uterine blood flow with attendant fetal hypoxia and acidosis.[357] Maternal Pa_{CO_2} should therefore be maintained at about 30 mmHg.

DIAGNOSIS

The diagnosis of SAH is established by the following: (1) history; (2) physical examination and neurologic assessment; and (3) laboratory tests, including CBC, electrolytes, glucose, BUN, creatinine, and coagulation profile, electrocardiogram (ECG), CT scan, angiography, lumbar puncture (LP), and magnetic resonance imaging (MRI).

HISTORY
Although it may not be possible to elicit a complete history at the time of first examination owing to the emergent nature of the situation, every attempt should be made to document the nature and onset of symptoms, any associated conditions (bleeding disorder, myocardiopathy, seizure disorder, moyamoya disease,

sickle-cell hemoglobinopathy), and a history of drug and alcohol abuse. Both cocaine and alcohol abuse have been linked to intracerebral hemorrhage.[347,358] Studies indicate that 2 to 9 percent of pregnant women are heavy drinkers,[359] and about 8 to 17 percent of pregnant women abuse cocaine.[360]

NEUROLOGIC ASSESSMENT

The clinical features of cerebrovascular accidents in pregnant women are not any different than in the general population.[336] The initial investigation needs to be prompt and thorough in order to differentiate cerebrovascular accidents from other disorders presenting with severe headaches associated with neurologic signs. The differential diagnosis includes preeclampsia, chronic hypertension, seizure disorder, intracranial tumors, abscesses and other space-occupying lesions, sagittal sinus thrombosis,[361] meningitis, encephalitis, demyelinating disease, cerebral arterial occlusive disease,[362,363] and moyamoya disease,[364] all of which may worsen during pregnancy and are associated with intracerebral hemorrhage.[364-367] Pituitary apoplexy,[336] abuse of cocaine[347] and alcohol,[358] disseminated intravascular coagulation, ectopic endometriosis, subacute bacterial endocarditis, and choriocarcinoma[368] may also produce symptom complexes that are indistinguishable from ICH and should be included in the differential diagnosis.

Aneurysmal rupture causes a sudden rise in intracranial pressure (ICP) and a consequent decrease in cerebral perfusion pressure. The resultant signs and symptoms depend on the extent of the hemorrhage

TABLE 26-21
Complications of Subarachnoid Hemorrhage: Hematoma, Intracranial Hypertension, Hydrocephalus, Vasospasm, Infarction, Bleeding

Early Complications (Hematoma/increased ICP)	Late Complications (Vasospasm/hydrocephalus/rebleed)
1. Nerve palsy, hemiparesis, decreased LOC	1. Permanent hemiparesis
2. Cardiac dysrhythmias	2. Myocardial infarction
3. Transient systemic hypertension	3. Persistent hypertension
4. Impaired vision	4. Vitreous hge/blindness
5. Fluid, electrolyte disturbances	5. Neurologic deterioration/death

NOTE: LOC = Level of consciousness; hge = Hemorrhage.

(Table 26-21). It has been suggested that 50 to 60 percent of these patients may have a "warning leak" and experience a less severe headache from a less severe episode of bleeding in the weeks or months prior to the acute event.[369,370] The clinical examination after SAH may reveal fever, nuchal rigidity, and high blood pressure. There may be focal neurologic deficits caused by hematoma, hydrocephalus, ischemia, or recurrent bleeding, including aphasia, hemiparesis, and hemianopsia. Seizures may be the presenting symptom in some cases of SAH from AVM. Hypothalamic irritation from the subarachnoid bleeding may cause a variety of systemic abnormalities. Contraction of intravascular volume or secretion of atrial natriuretic hormone may lead to electrolyte disturbances.[344] SAH may also mimic eclampsia, especially as severe hypertension and proteinuria may develop after SAH.[332,371]

EVALUATION
An aggressive work-up to delineate the etiology of intracranial hemorrhage in the pregnant patient is vital in the cause-specific perioperative management designed to contain subsequent morbidity and avoid mortality.

Routine Blood Tests
Coagulation profile: prothrombin time, partial thromboplastin time, platelet count, and fibrinogen; electrolytes; osmolarity; glucose; BUN; creatinine.

Electrocardiogram
Patients will need a 12-lead ECG and possibly a cardiology consultation if there are severe ECG abnormalities or cardiac dysfunction.

Electroencephalogram
Essential in patients who have seizures, for characterization of the discharge focus and also for follow-up during medical therapy.

Computed Tomographic Scan (CT Scan)
This is noninvasive, immediate, and often diagnostic, showing a hematoma within the brain, an intracerebral bleed, or blood around the brain surface after SAH. The location, form, and distribution of hemorrhage, together with direct enhancement of the aneurysm, permit accurate diagnosis. Moreover, early visualization of the extent of the clot in the subarachnoid cisterns is a reliable way of predicting the subsequent development of vasospasm. Cerebral AVMs may be demonstrated in unenhanced and more commonly in enhanced scans.[344]

Lumbar Puncture (LP)
Because of the possibility of precipitating a rerupture of the aneurysm or transtentorial herniation, LP is indicated after SAH only in patients who have a normal CT scan or when CT is not available.[344] This will show blood, xanthochromia, or a combination of both in the spinal fluid.

Angiography
This is used to demonstrate the aneurysmal neck and sac and their relation to parent arteries, or any other source of bleeding such as an AVM. Reactive narrowing of the cerebral arterial tree after SAH occurs in approximately 30 percent of patients and is identifiable angiographically. Vasospasm is associated with neurologic deterioration in 50 percent of these patients.[340] Four-vessel angiography will also identify multiple lesions. The reported incidence of multiple intracranial aneurysms is approximately 15 percent. In patients who have aneurysms, 1.1 percent are reported to have intracranial AVMs as well.[344] Abdominal shielding to avoid exposure of the infant is recommended for all radiographic procedures.[343] Iodinated contrast drugs do not cross the placenta, but may cause fetal dehydration from their osmotic effect.

Magnetic Resonance Imaging (MRI)
Magnetic resonance angiography permits visualization of aneurysms larger than 2 mm in diameter. As such, MRI is excellent for screening family members of patients who have documented aneurysms and for periodic visualization of people who have small, asymptomatic aneurysms.

MANAGEMENT OF THE PATIENT AFTER SAH

Subarachnoid hemorrhage from rupture of an aneurysm or AVM is a medical emergency with a high maternal and fetal mortality.[336] Consequently, diagnosis and neurosurgical treatment must be pursued in a vigorous and timely fashion.[361]

TABLE 26-22
Management of Subarachnoid Hemorrhage in Pregnancy

Lesion	Pregnancy	Management
1. Incidental aneurysm	Before 26 weeks	Risk of SAH regardless of the mode of delivery → surgical treatment of aneurysm reduces risk for both mother and baby[377]
2. Incidental aneurysm	34–36 weeks	C-section → Aneurysm clipping under same anesthetic.[377] The "take-home" rate is same as full-term infants
3. Corrected aneurysm	Any stage	Negligible risk of bleeding, needs normal obstetric management[343]
4. Ruptured aneurysm	Before 26 weeks	Aneurysm surgery and then vaginal delivery at term according to obstetric indications[397]
5. Ruptured aneurysm	Beyond 26 weeks	Moribund patient → C-section → to save the infant. Perinatal morbidity and mortality > 60%, due to pulmonary immaturity, intraventricular hemorrhage and infection
6. Ruptured aneurysm, unstable patient	Beyond 34 weeks	Neuroresuscitation to stabilize pt. CT/angiogram → C-section and aneurysm surgery; maintain uterine tone during lengthy surgery[381,377]
7. Ruptured aneurysm	In utero death	Aneurysm surgery and then vaginal delivery
8. Unruptured AVM	Term pregnancy	No C-section, when no adverse circumstances prevail[375]
9. Ruptured AVM	Before 26 weeks	Conservative management (risk of rebleed less than aneurysm)
10. Ruptured AVM, unstable	Term pregnancy	Neuroresuscitation → CT/angiogram → C-section → surgery and excision of AVM[380]

MEDICAL MANAGEMENT

The general management of pregnant patients after SAH is no different than in the nonpregnant population.[339,372] The basic needs are to provide an atmosphere of calm and comfort in order to prevent recurrent hemorrhage (Table 26-22). The patient should receive supportive therapy such as analgesics, sedatives, and anticonvulsants as needed. The goal is to maintain normal cerebral perfusion while minimizing the chance of exceeding the bursting pressure of the aneurysm.

SURGICAL MANAGEMENT

Surgery is the treatment of choice for aneurysms, offering better results for the mother (11 percent versus 63 percent) and the fetus (5 percent versus 27 percent)[332,373] than conservative management. The one-year mortality rate in the general population without surgery is 50 percent.[374] Conservative management during pregnancy is associated with a high risk of maternal mortality from rebleeding.[352] The most important step in the management of rebleeding is the prompt control of ICP with hyperventilation and mannitol. The risk of further hemorrhage is increased after recurrent hemorrhage from aneurysms. A second bleed in the preoperative period is an indication for immediate surgery. Without surgery, 5 to 7 percent of patients will bleed again within the first year, and perhaps 2 to 3 percent per year thereafter.[351]

According to Forster,[375] the absence of prior bleeding from an AVM is not a useful guide to the safety of undertaking pregnancy. Women of child-bearing age who harbor a cerebral AVM run a 5 percent risk of hemorrhage. This risk is significantly higher in the third trimester compared with the first and second trimesters. Convulsive disorder is a common presentation for AVM, and sometimes may be difficult to control medically. Unless operation is required for life-threatening hematoma, surgery for AVM usually can wait until recovery from the effects of the intracerebral bleed. Unlike aneurysms, the risk of rehemorrhage is small with AVMs.

The decision to operate needs to be individualized (Table 26-22) depending on the type and number of lesions, the neurologic deficit, the progression of signs and symptoms, the tendency to rebleed (aneurysm or AVM), any coexisting condition (such as sickle-cell anemia, moyamoya disease, or bleeding disorder), site, size, and surgical accessibility of the lesion, and the need for special techniques such as profound hypotension with adverse effects on the fetus. In this situation, a cesarean section is performed before craniotomy for clipping of the aneurysm if the fetus is at or near term. The risk of bleeding during vaginal delivery, however, is not significantly different from that during cesarean birth. Further, no significant differences exist in maternal and fetal mortality between vaginal and cesarean delivery in untreated aneurysms.[336]

PERIOPERATIVE MANAGEMENT

Management of SAH during pregnancy is similar to that in nonpregnant patients and depends on the neurologic condition of the mother and the stage of the pregnancy. Craniotomy for aneurysm is performed under neurosurgical criteria, while cesarean section is done for obstetric indications.

TABLE 26-23
Protocol 2. Perioperative Anesthetic Management of Combined Procedure for C-section and Craniotomy for Cerebral Vascular Surgery

1. Preoperative assessment of patient/fetus/medical management/investigations, any complications. Assess patient's airway and peripheral IV, central venous, arterial monitoring access.

2. Develop understanding, gain confidence by clear yet carefully worded explanation of risks of anesthesia and special techniques (epidural block/hypotensives) to both patient and family.

3. Prepare patient for acid aspiration prophylaxis: nonparticulate antacid, anticholinergic, metoclopramide, ranitidine, famotidine.

4. Prepare OR: check anesthesia machine, suction device. Have extra laryngoscope and difficult airway management equipment available.

5. While patient is on the OR bed, provide for left lateral displacement of the uterus to prevent supine hypotensive syndrome and aorto-caval compression.

6. Patient to breathe 100% O_2 while monitors placed: ECG, BP, pulse oximetry, continuous fetal monitoring.

7. Prepare and drape patient. Identify cricoid cartilage. Have assistant stand on the side to apply Sellick's maneuver.
   - Recheck suction, drugs, intubation equipment. Continue PreO$_2$.
   - IV bolus lidocaine 1.5–2 mg/kg over 2–3 min to attenuate hypertensive response to laryngoscopy, and also for its cerebral vasoconstrictor effect.
   - Rapid sequence induction with Sellick's maneuver.
   - Thiopental IV 3–4 mg/kg and succinylcholine.
   - Brief intubation.
   - Monitor pulse oximetry/fetal heart rate continuously; continue 100% until delivery.

8. Neonatologist in attendance to resuscitate infant if necessary.

9. Maintain anesthesia during C-section with inhalational agent (if ICP is normal—otherwise narcotic, propofol) and 100% O_2 until the delivery of the baby. Then narcotic and oxytocin are added, while continuously monitoring the blood pressure, ET_{CO_2} and maintaining minimal hyperventilation.

10. Reduce Pa_{CO_2} after dura is opened to relax the brain.

11. Diuresis to relax brain and improve operating conditions with furosemide rather than mannitol as this can cause fetal dehydration in high doses.

12. Maintain anesthesia during craniotomy with nitrous oxide, oxygen, isoflurane, narcotic, and muscle relaxant.

13. Blood pressure is controlled to facilitate dissection and clipping of the aneurysm by hypotension or by temporary proximal occlusion with super-normal blood pressure.

14. Maintain oxytocin infusion throughout the operation to ensure uterine contraction in the postpartum period.

15. Extubate trachea when patient is responsive after reversal of relaxant if clinical conditions permit.

The perioperative management depends on the neurologic evaluation, viability of the fetus, effect of anesthetic techniques and drugs on intracranial pressure, utero-placental transfer of the drugs and their teratogenicity, and effect on uterine relaxation. In general, the timing and method of operative correction should be decided on neurosurgical grounds, without regard to the status of the pregnancy.[343,376,377] Support exists for the performance of both procedures—a primary cesarean section and then craniotomy for clipping of the cerebral aneurysm under general anesthesia—in a situation of term pregnancy.[378–380] Clipping of the cerebral aneurysm under general anesthesia without ill-effects on the uterine tone has also been reported.[381] A cesarean section is indicated when the mother is moribund after SAH to preserve a fetus deemed mature enough for delivery.[336]

Patients who have AVMs are more likely to suffer intracranial hemorrhage during labor than are those who have aneurysms.[339] If an AVM is amenable to surgical treatment, there is no need to delay this treatment because of pregnancy,[343] although a case of successful management of pregnancy to term followed by delivery without incident has been reported.

The basic requisites of intraoperative management are the maintenance of adequate cerebral perfusion and a favorable operative field. Maintaining fetal homeostasis and uterine relaxation, preventing fetal depression, and monitoring fetal heart rate and uterine contraction are paramount (Table 26-23 Protocol 2).

The basic management consists of:

1. Smooth *induction*. Avoid rebleeding from rise in blood pressure and cerebral ischemia from hypotension and hypovolemia. Positioning the patient first to ensure left lateral tilt avoids the supine hypotensive syndrome.

2. Controlled *laryngoscopy*. Avoid both rise in blood pressure[382] and rise in ICP.[383]

3. Prevent *aspiration* of gastric contents. As with any other cesarean section, it is imperative to prevent regurgitation and aspiration of stomach contents. Metoclopramide,[384] ranitidine,[385] anticholinergics,[386] and famotidine[387] have been used preoperatively to

reduce both gastric volume and acidity in pregnant women.[384] Oral sodium citrate given immediately before induction has also been shown to increase the pH of stomach contents.[388,389] A rapid-sequence induction with thiopental, succinylcholine or rocuronium, IV lidocaine, fentanyl, and propranolol or SNP and cricoid pressure[390] have been used with good results.[357,379,391]

4. Avoid *fetal depression.* Discontinue long-acting drugs such as diazepam and phenobarbital and use drugs that do not depress the infant.

5. Prevent *uterine relaxation.* Avoidance of inhalational drugs like halothane is important to prevent uterine relaxation with consequent hemorrhage in the postpartum period. Isoflurane to 1 percent has been used in such situations[379] with good outcome, as it has been shown to reduce awareness and blood loss during cesarean section.[392]

6. Control of *BP.* Systemic hypertension increases the CBF, cerebral blood volume, and ICP and may induce rebleeding.[393] Controlled hypotension[261,394] or temporary proximal occlusion meets surgical requirements. The use of SNP in obstetrics is still controversial owing to the potential for fetal toxicity from cyanide and fetal hypoxia from the hypotension-induced reduction in placental perfusion. With judicious use of SNP, however, fetal compromise may be kept at bay.[395–397]

7. Control of *ICP.* Mannitol, an osmotic diuretic, may have adverse effects on the fetus, including dehydration and bradycardia.[333,398]

8. Management of *ruptured aneurysm intraoperatively.* Aggressive restoration of the acute blood loss, hypotension (anesthesia, SNP, or ipsilateral carotid compression), avoidance of excessive ventilation, and a relaxed brain.

9. Maintain *uterine tone.* Oxytocin has been safely infused after combined neuroresuscitation and cesarean section and continued throughout the subsequent angiogram and six-hour craniotomy for clipping of a saccular aneurysm of the middle cerebral artery with hippocampal herniation and evacuation of a large hematoma in the left temporoparietal region.[381] The hypertension caused by methylergonovine maleate and prostaglandins for treatment of uterine atony may be detrimental before the aneurysm is secured.

10. *Ventilation* during anesthesia has to be carefully matched to the needs of the patient with due consideration for the unborn baby. Hyperventilation may aggravate preexisting cerebral vasospasm and will also cause utero-placental insufficiency due to vasoconstriction with attendant fetal hypoxia and acidosis.[399]

11. Continuous *BP monitoring.* This is essential when hypotensive drugs are employed. Monitoring arterial blood gases in the perioperative period will confirm adequate oxygenation, effective CO_2 elimination, and metabolic homeostasis. An unexplained metabolic acidosis may indicate the early occurrence of cyanide toxicity.

12. *Urinary output.* Good urine output is an indication of the adequacy of intravascular volume and organ perfusion and the effectiveness of diuresis.

13. *Fluids, electrolytes,* glucose, and osmolarity must be monitored closely to detect and treat contracted intravascular volume and disordered sodium and potassium balance.

Acknowledgments

The authors would like to acknowledge the invaluable assistance of Judy Fletcher and Phillip Gordon, M.D. in the critical appraisal and preparation of the manuscript.

References

1. Botterrell EH et al: Hypothermia and interruption of the carotid or carotid and vertebral circulation in the surgical management in intracranial aneurisms. *J Neurosurg* 1956; 13:1.

2. Hunt WE, Hess RM: Surgical risk as related to time of intervention in the repair of intracranial aneurisms. *J Neurosurg* 1968; 28:14.

3. Drake CG: Report of World Federation of Neurological Surgeons Committee on a universal subarachnoid hemorrhage grading scale. *J Neurosurg* 1988; 68:985.

4. Kassell NF et al: The International Cooperative Study on the Timing of Aneurysm Surgery. Part I: Overall management results. *J Neurosurg* 1990; 73:18.

5. Dernbach PD et al: Altered cerebral autoregulation and CO_2 reactivity after aneurysmal subarachnoid hemorrhage. *Neurosurgery* 1988; 22:822.

6. Ishii R: Regional cerebral blood flow in patients with ruptured intracranial aneurisms. *J Neurosurg* 1979; 50:587.

7. Tenjiu H et al: Dysautoregulation in patients with ruptured aneurysms: Cerebral blood flow measurement obtained during surgery by a temperature-controlled thermoelectrical method. *Neurosurgery* 1988; 23:705.

8. Voldby B et al: Cerebrovascular reactivity in patients with ruptured intracranial aneurisms. *J Neurosurg* 1985; 62:59.

9. Voldby B, Enevoldsen EM: Intracranial pressure changes following aneurysm rupture. I: Clinical and angiographic correlations. *J Neurosurg* 1982; 56:186.

10. Awad IA et al: Clinical vasospasm after subarachnoid hemorrhage: Response to hypervolemic hemodilution and arterial hypertension. *Stroke* 1987; 18:365.

11. Diringer MN et al: Plasma atrial natriuretic factor and subarachnoid hemorrhage. *Stroke* 1988; 19:1119.

12. Diringer MN et al: Suprasellar and intraventricular blood predict elevated plasma atrial natriuretic factor in subarachnoid hemorrhage. *Stroke* 1991; 22:577.

13. Nelson RJ et al: Association of hypovolemia after subarachnoid hemorrhage with computed tomographic scan evidence of raised intracranial pressure. *Neurosurgery* 1991; 29:178.

14. Davies KR et al: Cardiac function in aneurysmal subarachnoid

haemorrhage: A study of electrocardiographic and echocardiographic abnormalities. *Br J Anaesth* 1991; 67:58.

15. Stober T et al: Cardiac arrhythmias in subarachnoid hemorrhage. *Acta Neurochir (Wien)* 1988; 93:37.

16. Solenski NJ et al: Medical complications of aneurysmal subarachnoid hemorrhage: A report of the multicenter cooperative aneurysm study. *Crit Care Med* 1995; 23:1007.

17. Landolt AM et al: Disturbances of the serum electrolytes after surgery of intracranial arterial aneurysms. *J Neurosurg* 1972; 37:210.

18. Solomon RA et al: Depression of circulating blood volume in patients after subarachnoid hemorrhage: Implications for the management of symptomatic vasospasm. *Neurosurgery* 1984; 15:354.

19. Wijdicks EFM et al: Hyponatremia and cerebral infarction in patients with ruptured intracranial aneurysms: Is fluid restriction harmful? *Ann Neurol* 1985; 17:137.

20. Wijdicks EFM et al: Volume depletion and natriuresis in patients with a ruptured intracranial aneurysm. *Ann Neurol* 1985; 18:211.

21. Hasan D et al: Hyponatremia is associated with cerebral ischemia in patients with aneurysmal subarachnoid hemorrhage. *Ann Neurol* 1990; 27:106.

22. Maroon JC, Nelson PB: Hypovolemia in patients with subarachnoid hemorrhage: Therapeutic implicaitons. *Neurosurgery* 1979; 4:223.

23. Hasan D et al: Effect of fluid intake and antihypertensive treatment on cerebral ischemia after subarachnoid hemorrhage. *Stroke* 1989; 20:1511.

24. Fox JL et al: Neurosurgical hyponatremia: The role of inappropriate antidiuresis. *J. Neurosurg* 1971; 34:506.

25. Wise BL: Syndrome of inappropriate antidiuretic hormone secretion after spontaneous subarachnoid hemorrhage: A reversible cause of clinical deterioration. *Neurosurgery* 1978; 3:412.

26. Diringer MN et al: Cerebrospinal fluid atrial natriuretic factor in intracranial disease. *Stroke* 1991; 21:1550.

27. Doczi T et al: Increased concentration of atrial natriuretic factor in the cerebrospinal fluid of patients with aneurysmal subarachnoid hemorrhage and raised intracranial pressure. *Neurosurgery* 1988; 23:16.

28. Rosenfeld JV et al: The effect of subarachnoid hemorrhage on blood and CSF atrial natriuretic factor. *J Neurosurg* 1989; 71:32.

29. Rudehill A et al: A study of ECG abnormalities and myocardial specific enzymes in patients with subarachnoid haemorrhage. *Acta Anaesth Scand* 1982; 26:344.

30. Burch GE et al: A new electrocardiographic pattern observed in cerebrovascular accidents. *Circulation* 1954; 9:719.

31. Kreus KE et al: Electrocardiographic changes in cerebrovascular accidents. *Acta Med Scand* 1969; 185:327.

32. Stober T, Kunze K: Electrocardiographic alterations in subarachnoid hemorrhage. *J Neurol* 1982; 227:99.

33. Marion DW et al: Subarachnoid hemorrhage and the heart. *Neurosurgery* 1986; 18:101.

34. Manninen PH et al: Perioperative monitoring of the electrocardiogram during cerebral aneurysm surgery. *J Neurosurg Anesthesiol* 1990; 2:16.

35. Weintraub BM, McHenry LC: Cardiac abnormalities in subarachnoid hemorrhage: A resume. *Stroke* 1974; 5:384.

36. Brouwers PJAM et al: Serial electrocardiographic recording in aneurysmal subarachnoid hemorrhage. *Stroke* 1989; 20:1162.

37. Di Pasquale G et al: Holter detection of cardiac arrhythmias in intracranial subarachnoid hemorrhage. *Am J Cardiol* 1987; 59:596.

38. Andreoli A et al: Subarachnoid hemorrhage: Frequency and severity of cardiac arrhythmias. A survey of 70 cases studied in the acute phase. *Stroke* 1987; 18:558.

39. Vidal B et al: Cardiac arrhythmias associated with subarachnoid hemorrhage: Prospective study. *Neurosurgery* 1979; 5:675.

40. Harries AD: Subarachnoid haemorrhage and the electrocardiogram: A review. *Postgrad Med J* 1981; 57:294.

41. Manninen PH et al: Perioperative monitoring of the electrocardiogram during cerebral aneurysm surgery. *J Neurosurg Anesth* 1990; 2:16.

42. Manninen PH et al: Electrocardiographic changes during and after isoflurane-induced hypotension for neurovascular surgery. *Can J Anaesth* 1987; 34:549.

43. Cruickshank JM et al: Possible role of catecholamines, corticosteroids, and potassium in the production of electrocardiographic abnormalities associated with subarachnoid haemorrhage. *Br Heart J* 1974; 36:697.

44. Weidler DJ: Myocardial damage and cardiac arrhythmias after intracranial hemorrhage. A critical review. *Stroke* 1974; 5:759.

45. Hunt D, Gore I: Myocardial lesions following experimental intracranial hemorrhage: Prevention with propranolol. *Am Heart J* 1972; 83:232.

46. Harrison MJG: Influence of haematocrit on the cerebral circulation. *Cerebrovasc Brain Metab Rev* 1989; 1:55.

47. Greenhoot JH, Reichenbach DD: Cardiac injury and subarachnoid hemorrhage. A clinical, pathological, and physiological correlation. *J Neurosurg* 1969; 30:521.

48. Doshi R, Neil-Dwyer G: A clinicopathologic study of patients following a subarachnoid hemorrhage. *J Neurosurg* 1980; 52:295.

49. Doshi R, Neil-Dwyer G: Hypothalamic and myocardial lesions after subarachnoid hemorrhage. *J Neurol Neurosurg Psychiatry* 1977; 40:821.

50. Cruickshank JM et al: Electrocardiographic changes and their prognostic significance in subarachnoid hemorrhage. *J Neurol Neurosurg Psychiatry* 1974; 37:775.

51. Rudehill A et al: ECG abnormalities in patients with subarachnoid hemorrhage and intracranial tumors. *J Neurol Neurosurg Psychiatry* 1987; 50:1375.

52. Galloon S et al: Prospective study of electrocardiographic changes associated with subarachnoid haemorrhage. *Br J Anaesth* 1972; 44:511.

53. Pollick C et al: Left ventricular wall motion abnormalities in subarachnoid hemorrhage: An echocardiographic study. *J Am Coll Cardiol* 1988; 12:600.

54. Manninen PH et al: Association between electrocardiographic abnormalities and intracranial blood in patients following acute subarachnoid hemorrhage. *J Neurosurg Anesthesiol* 1995; 7:12.

55. Fisher CM et al: Relation of cerebral vasospasm to subarachnoid hemorrhage visualized by computerized tomographic scanning. *Neurosurgery* 1980; 6:1.

56. White JC et al: Preanesthetic evaluation of a patient with pathological Q waves following subarachnoid hemorrhage. *Anesthesiology* 1985; 62:351.

57. Kaste M et al: Heart type creatinine kinase isoenzyme (CKMB) in acute cerebral disorders. *Br Heart J* 1978; 40:802.

58. Neil-Dwyer G et al: Beta-blockage benefits patients following a subarachnoid hemorrhage. *Eur J Clin Pharmacol* 1984; 28 (suppl):25.

59. Neil-Dwyer G et al: Beta-blockers, plasma total creatinine kinase and creatinine kinase myocardial isoenzymes and prognosis in subarachnoid hemorrhage. *Surg Neurol* 1986; 25:163.

60. Cruickshank JM et al: Reduction of stress catecholamine-induced cardiac necrosis by beta-selective blockage. *Lancet* 1987; 2:585.

61. Grad A et al: Effect of elevated plasma norepinephrine on

electrocardiographic changes in subarachnoid hemorrhage. *Stroke* 1991; 22:746.

62. Walter P et al: Beneficial effects of adrenergic blockade in patients with subarachnoid haemorrhage. *Br Med J* 1982; 284:1661.

63. Koselko P et al: Subendocardial haemorrhage and ECG changes in intracranial bleeding. *Br Med J* 1964; 1:1479.

64. Samra SK, Kroll DA: Subarachnoid hemorrhage and intraoperative electrocardiographic changes simulating myocardial ischemia: Anesthesiologist's dilemma. *Anesth Analg* 1985; 64:86.

65. Ciongolia K, Poser CM: Pulmonary edema secondary to subarachnoid hemorrhage. *Neurology* 1972; 22:867.

66. Weir B: Pulmonary edema following fatal aneurysm rupture. *J Neurosurg* 1978; 49:502.

67. Schell AR et al: Pulmonary edema associated with subarachnoid hemorrhage. *Arch Intern Med* 1987; 147:591.

68. Haley EC et al: A randomized controlled trial of high-dose intravenous nicardipine in aneurysmal subarachnoid hemorrhage. A report of the Cooperative Aneurysm Study. *J Neurosurg* 1993; 78:537.

69. Weir B: Medical, neurologic, and ophthalmologic aspects of aneurysms. In: *Aneurysms Affecting the Nervous System*. Baltimore, Williams & Wilkins, 1987:54–119.

70. Spallone A et al: Disseminated intravascular coagulation as a complication of ruptured intracranial aneurysm. Report of two cases. *J Neurosurg* 1983; 59:142.

71. Parkinson D, Stephensen S: Leukocytosis and subarachnoid hemorrhage. *Surg Neurol* 1984; 21:132.

72. Kassell NF, Torner JC: Aneurysmal rebleeding: A preliminary report from the Cooperative Aneurysm Study. *Neurosurgery* 1983; 13:479.

73. Jane JA et al: The natural history of intracrannial aneurysms. Rebleeding rates during the acute and long-term period and implications for surgical management. *Clin Neurosurg* 1979; 24:176.

74. Haley Jr EC et al: The International Cooperative Study on Timing of Aneurysm Surgery: The North American experience. *Stroke* 1992; 23:205.

75. Kassell NF et al: Antifibrinolytic therapy in the treatment of subarachnoid hemorrhage. *Clin Neurosurg* 1986; 33:137.

76. Kassell NF et al: Antifibrinolytic therapy in the acute period following aneurysmal subarachnoid hemorrhage. *J Neurosurg* 1984; 61:225.

77. Fodstad H et al: Antifibrinolysis with tranexamic acid in aneurysmal subarachnoid hemorrhage: A consecutive controlled clinical trial. *Neurosurgery* 1981; 28:21.

78. Pinna G et al: Rebleeding, ischaemia and hydrocephalus following antifibrinolytic treatment for ruptured cerebral aneurysms: A retrospective clinical study. *Acta Neurochir* 1988; 93:77.

79. Brown MF, Benzel EC: Morbidity and mortality associated with rapid control of systemic hypertension in patients with intracranial hemorrhage. *J Neurosurg* 1990; 75:53.

80. Cook DA: The pharmacology of cerebral vasospasm. *Pharmacology* 1984; 29:1.

81. Wilkins RH: Attempted prevention or treatment of intracranial arterial spasm: An update. *Neurosurgery* 1986; 18:808.

82. Flamm ES et al: Dose-escalation study of intravenous nicardipine in patients with aneurysmal subarachnoid hemorrhage. *J Neurosurg* 1988; 68:393.

83. Allen GS et al: Cerebral arterial spasm: A controlled trial of nimodipine in patients with subarachnoid hemorrhage. *N Engl J Med* 1983; 308:619.

84. Mee E et al: Controlled study of nimodipine in aneurysm

85. Neil-Dwyer G et al: Early intervention with nimodipine in subarachnoid hemorrhage. *Eur Heart J* 1988; 88:41.

86. Pickard JD et al: Effect of oral nimodipine on cerebral infarction and outcome after subarachnoid haemorrhage: British Aneurysm Nimodipine Trial. *Br Med J* 1989; 298:636.

87. Tettenborn D, Dycka J: Prevention and treatment of delayed ischemic dysfunction in patients with aneurysmal subarachnoid hemorrhage. *Stroke* 1990; 21 (suppl IV):85.

88. Petruk KC et al: Nimodipine treatment in poor-grade aneurysm patients: Results of a multicenter double-blind placebo-controlled trial. *J Neurosurg* 1988; 68:505.

89. Meyer FB: Calcium antagonists and vasospasm. *Neurosurg Clin North Am* 1990; 1:367.

90. Shibuya M et al: Effect of AT 877 on cerebral vasospasm after aneurysmal subarachnoid hemorrhage: Results of a prospective placebo-controlled double-blind trial. *J Neurosurg* 1992; 76:571.

91. Kassell NF et al: Treatment of ischemic deficits from vasospasm with intravascular volume expansion and induced arterial hypertension. *Neurosurgery* 1982; 11:337.

92. Buckland MR et al: Anesthesia for cerebral aneurysm surgery: Use of induced hypertension in patients with symptomatic vasospasm. *Anesthesiology* 1988; 69:116.

93. Solomon RA et al: Early aneurysm surgery and prophylactic hypervolemic hypertensive therapy for the treatment of aneurysmal subarachnoid hemorrhage. *Neurosurgery* 1988; 23:699.

94. Levy M et al: Cardiac performance enhancement from dobutamine in patients refractory to hypervolemic therapy for cerebral vasospasm. *J Neurosurg* 1993; 19:494.

95. Wood JM, Kee DB: Hemorrheology of the cerebral circulation in stroke. *Stroke* 1985; 16:765.

96. Cully MD et al: Hetastarch coagulopathy in a neurosurgical patient. *Anesthesiology* 1987; 66:706.

97. Damon L et al: Intracranial bleeding during treatment with hydroxyethyl starch. *N Engl J Med* 1987; 317:964.

98. Levy ML, Giannotta SL: Cardiac performance indices during hypervolemic therapy for cerebral vasospasm. *J Neurosurg* 1991; 75:27.

99. David SM et al: Correlation between cerebral arterial velocities, blood flow, and delayed ischemia after subarachnoid hemorrhage. *Stroke* 1992; 23:492.

100. Zubkov TN et al: Balloon catheter technique for dilatation of constricted cerebral arteries after aneurysmal SAH. *Acta Neurochir (Wien)* 1984; 70:65.

101. Newell DE et al: Angioplasty for the treatment of symptomatic vasospasm following subarachnoid hemorrhage. *Neurosurgery* 1989; 71:654.

102. Findlay JM et al: Effect of intrathecal thrombolytic therapy on subarachnoid clot and chronic vasospasm in a primate model of SAH. *J Neurosurg* 1988; 69:723.

103. Zabramski JM et al: Phase I trial of tissue plasminogen activator for the prevention of vasospasm in patients with aneurysmal subarachnoid hemorrhage. *J Neurosurg* 1991; 75:189.

104. Ohman J et al: Effect of intrathecal fibrinolytic therapy on clot lysis and vasospasm in patients with aneurysmal subarachnoid hemorrhage. *J Neurosurg* 1991; 75:197.

105. Kaku Y et al: Superselective intraarterial infusion of papavarine for the treatment of cerebral vasospasm after subarachnoid hemorrhage. *J Neurosurg* 1992; 77:842.

106. Carpenter DA et al: Cerebral oxygen metabolism after aneurysmal subarachnoid hemorrhage. *J Cereb Blood Flow Metab* 1991; 11:837.

107. Grubb RL et al: Effects of subarachnoid hemorrhage on cere-

patients treated early after subarachnoid hemorrhage. *Neurosurgery* 1988; 22:484.

bral blood volume, blood flow, and oxygen utilization in humans. *J Neurosurg* 1977; 46:446.

108. Jakobsen M et al: Cerebral blood flow and metabolism following subarachnoid hemorrhage: Cerebral oxygen uptake and global blood flow during the acute period in patients with SAH. *Acta Neurol Scand* 1990; 82:174.

109. Martin WRW et al: Cerebral blood volume, blood flow, and oxygen metabolism in cerebral ischaemia and subarachnoid haemorrhage: An in-vivo study using positron emission tomography. *Acta Neurochir* 1984; 70:3.

110. Paulson OB et al: Cerebral autoregulation. *Cerebrovasc Brain Metab Rev* 1990; 2:161.

111. Raichle ME et al: Cerebral blood flow during and after hyperventilation. *Arch Neurol* 1970; 23:394.

112. Harper AM: Autoregulation of cerebral blood flow: Influence of the arterial blood pressure on the blood flow through the cerebral cortex. *J Neurol Neurosurg Psychiatry* 1966; 29:398.

113. Bullock R et al: Cerebral blood flow and CO_2 responsiveness as an indicator of collateral reserve capacity in patients with carotid arterial disease. *Br J Surg* 1985; 72:348.

114. Enevoldsen EM, Jensen FT: Autoregulation and CO_2 responses of cerebral blood flow in patients with acute severe head injury. *J Neurosurg* 1978; 48:689.

115. Nelson RJ et al: Transcranial Doppler ultrasound studies of cerebral autoregulation and SAH in the rabbit. *J Neurosurg* 1990; 73:601.

116. Shinoda J et al: Acetazolamide reactivity on cerebral blood flow in patients with subarachnoid haemorrhage. *Acta Neurochir (Wien)* 1991; 109:102.

117. Nornes H: The role of intracranial pressure in the arrest of hemorrhage in patients with ruptured intracranial aneurysm. *J Neurosurg* 1973; 39:226.

118. Borgmann R: Natural course of intracranial pressure and drainage of CSF after recovery from subarachnoid hemorrhage. *Acta Neurol Scand* 1990; 81:300.

119. Van Gijn J et al: Acute hydrocephalus after aneurysmal hemorrhage. *J Neurosurg* 1985; 63:355.

120. Ohman J, Heiskanen O: Timing of operation for ruptured supratentorial aneurysm: A prospective randomized study. *J Neurosurg* 1989; 70:55.

121. Taneda M: Effect of early operation for ruptured aneurysms on prevention of delayed ischemic symptoms. *J Neurosurg* 1982; 57:622.

122. Kassell NF et al: The International Cooperative Study on the Timing of Aneurysm Surgery. Part II: Surgical results. *J Neurosurg* 1990; 73:37.

123. Stulken EH et al: Implications of nimodipine prophylaxis of cerebral vasospasm on anesthetic management during intracranial aneurysm clipping. *J Neurosurg* 1985; 62:200.

124. Stulken EH et al: The hemodynamic effects of nimodipine in patients anesthetized for cerebral aneurysm clipping. *Anesthesiology* 1985; 62:346.

125. Warner DS et al: Nicardipine HCl: Clinical experience in patients undergoing anesthesia for intracranial aneurysm clipping. *Can J Anaesth* 1989; 36:219.

126. Eng CC, Lam AM: Cerebral aneurysms: Anesthetic considerations. In: Cottrell JE, Smith DS (eds): *Anesthesia and Neurosurgery*, 3d ed. St Louis, CV Mosby, 1994:376–405.

127. Colley PS, Artru AA: ECG-guided placement of Sorenson CVP catheter via arm veins. *Anesth Analg* 1984; 63:953.

128. Blume WT: Monitoring the safe levels of hypotension: III. The role of electroencephalography. *Int Anesthesiol Clin* 1982; 20:125.

129. Jones TH et al: EEG monitoring for induced hypotension for surgery of intracranial aneurysms. *Stroke* 1979; 10:292.

130. Tempelhoff R et al: Use of computerized electroencephalographic monitoring during aneurysm surgery. *J Surg* 1989; 71:24.

131. Young WL et al: Direct cortical EEG monitoring during temporary vascular occlusion for cerebral aneurysm surgery. *Anesthesiology* 1989; 71:794.

132. Emerson RG, Turner CA: Monitoring during supratentorial surgery. *J Clin Neurophysiol* 1993; 10:404.

133. Lam AM et al: Brainstem auditory evoked potential monitoring during vertebrobasilar occlusion therapy for posterior fossa aneurysms. *Anesthesiology* 1984; 61:A347.

134. Lam AM et al: Monitoring of brainstem auditory evoked potentials during basilar artery occlusion in man. *Br J Anaesth* 1985; 57:924.

135. Manninen PH et al: Monitoring of brainstem function during vertebral basilar aneurysm surgery. *Anesthesiology* 1992; 77:681.

136. Manninen PH et al: Evoked potential monitoring during posterior fossa aneurysm surgery: A comparison of two modalities. *Can J Anaesth* 1993; 41:92.

137. Mizoi K, Yoshimoto T: Permissible temporary occlusion time in aneurysm surgery as evaluated by evoked potential monitoring. *Neurosurgery* 1993; 33:434.

138. Schramm J et al: Surgical and electrophysiological observations during clipping of 134 aneurysms with evoked potential monitoring. *Neurosurgery* 1990; 26:61.

139. Friedman WA et al: Monitoring of somatosensory evoked potentials during surgery for middle cerebral artery aneurysms. *Neurosurgery* 1991; 29:83.

140. Friedman WA et al: Evoked potential monitoring during aneurysm operation: Observations after fifty cases. *Neurosurgery* 1987; 20:678.

141. Manninen PH et al: Monitoring of somatosensory evoked potentials during temporary arterial occlusion in aneurysm surgery. *J Neurosurg Anesthesiol* 1990; 2:97.

142. Mooij JJ et al. Somatosensory evoked potential monitoring of temporary middle cerebral artery occlusion during aneurysm operation. *Neurosurgery* 1987; 21:492.

143. Momma F et al: Effects of temporary arterial occlusion on somatosensory evoked responses in aneurysm surgery. *Surg Neurol* 1987; 27:343.

144. Kidooka M et al: Monitoring of somatosensory-evoked potentials during aneurysm surgery. *Surg Neurol* 1987; 27:69.

145. Symon L et al: Perioperative use of somatosensory evoked responses in aneurysm surgery. *J Neurosurg* 1984; 60:269.

146. Landi A et al: Intraoperative monitoring by means of somatosensory evoked potentials during cerebral aneurysm surgery. *Agressologie* 1990; 31:363.

147. Little JR et al: Electrophysiological monitoring during basilar aneurysm operation. *Neurosurgery* 1987; 20:421.

148. Matta BF et al: A critique of the intraoperative use of jugular venous bulb catheters during neurosurgical procedures. *Anesth Analg* 1994; 79:745.

149. Moss E et al: Effects of changes in mean arterial pressure on SjO_2 during cerebral aneurysm surgery. *Br J Anaesth* 1995; 75:527.

150. Huber P, Handa J: Effect of contrast material, hypercapnia, hyperventilation, hypertonic glucose and papaverine on the diameter of the cerebral arteries—angiographic determination in man. *Invest Radiol* 1967; 2:17.

151. Giller CA et al: Cerebral arterial diameters during changes in blood pressure and carbon dioxide during craniotomy. *Neurosurgery* 1993; 32:737.

152. Lam AM, Matta BF: Isoflurane and desflurane do not dilate the middle cerebral artery appreciably. *Anesth Analg* 1995; 80:S262.

153. Schregel W et al: The effect of halothane, alfentanil and propofol on blood flow velocity, blood vessel cross section and

blood volume flow in the middle cerebral artery. *Anaesthetist* 1992; 41:21.

154. Aaslid R et al: Evaluation of cerebrovascular spasm with transcranial Doppler ultrasound. *J Neurosurg* 1984; 60:37.

155. Bishop CCR et al: Transcranial Doppler measurement of the middle cerebral flow velocity: A validation study. *Stroke* 1986; 17:913.

156. Dahl A et al: A comparison of regional cerebral blood flow and middle cerebral artery blood flow velocities: Simultaneous measurements in healthy subjects. *J Cereb Blood Flow Metab* 1992; 12:1049.

157. Larsen FS et al: Transcranial Doppler is valid for determination of the lower limit of cerebral blood flow autoregulation. *Stroke* 1994; 25:1985.

158. Eng CC et al: The diagnosis and management of a perianesthetic cerebral aneurysmal rupture aided with transcranial Doppler ultrasonography. *Anesthesiology* 1993; 78:191.

159. Lam AM: Intraoperative transcranial Doppler monitoring (letter). *Anesthesiology* 1995; 82:1536.

160. Tsementzis SA, Hitchcock ER: Outcome from rescue clipping of ruptured intracranial aneurysms during induction of anesthesia and endotracheal intubation. *J Neurol Neurosurg Psychiatry* 1985; 48:160.

161. Farrar JK et al: Effects of profound hypotension on cerebral blood flow during surgery for intracranial aneurysms. *J Neurosurg* 1981; 55:857.

162. Colley PS: Intracranial aneurysms: Anesthetic management. In: Newfield P, Cottrell JE (eds): *Neuroanesthesia: Handbook of Clinical and Physiologic Essentials.* 2d ed. Boston, Little, Brown, 1991:194–214.

163. Ravussin P et al: Propofol v. thiopental-isoflurane for neurosurgical anesthesia: Comparison of hemodynamics, CSF pressure, and recovery. *J Neurosurg Anesthesiol* 1991; 3:85.

164. Kautto UM: Attenuation of the circulatory response to larynoscopy and intubation by fentanyl. *Acta Anaesth Scand* 1982; 26:217.

165. Hamill JF et al: Lidocaine before endotracheal intubation: Intravenous or laryngeal? *Anesthesiology* 1981; 55:578.

166. Colley PS, Dunn R: Prevention of the blood pressure response to skull pin head-holder by local anesthesia. *Anesth Analg* 1979; 58:241.

167. Stirt JA et al: Vecuronium: Effect on intracranial pressure and hemodynamics in neurosurgical patients. *Anesthesiology* 1987; 67:570.

168. Rosa G et al: Effects of vecuronium bromide on intracranial pressure and cerebral perfusion pressure. *Br J Anaesth* 1986; 58:437.

169. Minton MD et al: Intracranial pressure after atracurium in neurosurgical patients. *Anesth Analg* 1985; 64:113.

170. Rosa G et al: The effects of atracurium besylate (Tracrium) on intracranial pressure and cerebral perfusion pressure. *Anesth Analg* 1986; 65:381.

171. Rosa G et al: The effects of pipecuronium bromide on intracranial pressure and cerebral perfusion pressure. *J Neurosurg Anesthesiol* 1991; 3:253.

172. Lanier WL et al: Cerebral stimulation following succinylcholine in dogs. *Anesthesiology* 1986; 64:551.

173. Minton MD et al: Increase in intracranial pressure from succinylcholine. Prevention by prior nondepolarizing blockade. *Anesthesiology* 1986; 65:165.

174. Stirt JA et al: Defasciculation with metocurine prevents succinylcholine-induced increases in intracranial pressure. *Anesthesiology* 1987; 67:50.

175. Lanier WL et al: Cerebral function and muscle afferent activity following intravenous succinylcholine in dogs anesthetized with halothane: The effects of pretreatment with a defasciculating dose of pancuronium. *Anesthesiology* 1989; 71:87.

176. Lam AM et al: Nitrous oxide-isoflurane anesthesia causes more cerebral vasodilation than an equipotent dose of isoflurane in humans. *Anesth Analg* 1994; 78:462.

177. Manninen PH et al: The effect of succinylcholine on serum potassium in patients with acutely ruptured cerebral aneurysms. *Anesth Analg* 1989; 68:S180.

178. Mehta MP et al: Facilitation of rapid endotracheal intubation with divided doses of neuromuscular blocking drugs. *Anesthesiology* 1985; 62:392.

179. Unni VKN et al: Prevention of intracranial hypertension during laryngoscopy and endotracheal intubation: Use of a second dose of thiopentone. *Br J Anaesth* 1984; 56:1219.

180. Sakabe T et al: The effects of lidocaine on canine metabolism and circulation related to the electroencephalogram. *Anesthesiology* 1974; 40:433.

181. Safwat AM et al: Use of propranolol to control rate-pressure product during cardiac anesthesia. *Anesth Analg* 1981; 60:732.

182. Cucchiara RF et al: Evaluation of esmolol in controlling increases in heart rate and blood pressure during endotracheal intubation in patients undergoing carotid endarterectomy. *Anesthesiology* 1986; 65:528.

183. Parnass SM et al: A single bolus dose of esmolol in the prevention of intubation-induced tachycardia and hypertension in an ambulatory surgery unit. *J Clin Anesth* 1990; 2:215.

184. Muzzi DA et al: Labetalol and esmolol in the control of hypertension after intracranial surgery. *Anesth Analg* 1990; 70:68.

185. Bunegin L et al: Effect of esmolol on cerebral blood flow during intracranial hypertension and hemorrhagic hypovolemia. *Anesthesiology* 1987; 67:A424.

186. Gustafson C et al: Haemodynamic effects of labetalol-induced hypotension in the anaesthetized dog. *Br J Anaesth* 1981; 53:585.

187. Van Aken H et al: Effect of labetalol on intracranial pressure in dogs with and without intracranial hypertension. *Acta Anaesth Scand* 1982; 26:615.

188. Griswold WR et al: Nitroprusside induced intracranial hypertension. *JAMA* 1981; 246:2679.

189. Marsh ML, et al: Changes in neurologic status and intracranial pressure associated with sodium nitroprusside administration. *Anesthesiology* 1979; 51:336.

190. Dohi S et al: The effects of nitroglycerin on cerebrospinal fluid pressure in awake and anesthetized humans. *Anesthesiology* 1981; 54:511.

191. Cottrell JE et al: Intracranial pressure during nitroglycerin-induced hypotension. *J Neurosurg* 1980; 53:309.

192. Maekawa T et al: Brain-surface oxygen tension and cerebral cortical blood flow during hemorrhagic and drug-induced hypotension in the cat. *Anesthesiology* 1979; 51:313.

193. Abe K et al: Effect of nicardipine and diltiazem on internal carotid artery blood flow velocity and local cerebral blood flow during cerebral aneurysm surgery for subarachnoid hemorrhage. *J Clin Anesth* 1994; 6:99.

194. Musich J, Walts LF: Pulmonary aspiration after a priming dose of vecuronium. *Anesthesiology* 1986; 64:517.

195. Sakabe T et al: Cerebral effects of nitrous oxide in the dog. *Anesth* 1978; 48:195.

196. Algotsson L et al: Effects of nitrous oxide on cerebral haemodynamics and metabolism during isoflurane anaesthesia in man. *Acta Anaesth Scand* 1992; 36:46.

197. Hoffman WE et al: Nitrous oxide added to isoflurane increases brain artery blood flow and low frequency brain electrical activity. *J Neurosurg Anesthesiol* 1995; 7:82.

198. Roald OK et al: Cerebral effects of nitrous oxide when added to low and high concentrations of isoflurane in the dog. *Anesth Analg* 1991; 72:75.

199. Drummond JC et al: The effect of nitrous oxide on cortical blood flow during anesthesia with halothane and isoflurane, with and without morphine, in the rabbit. *Anesth Analg* 1987; 66:1083.

200. Seyde WC et al: The addition of nitrous oxide to halothane decreases renal and splanchnic flow and increases cerebral blood flow in rats. *Br J Anaesth* 1986; 58:63.

201. Artru AA et al: Electroencephalogram, cerebral metabolic, and vascular responses to propofol anesthesia in dogs. *J Neurosurg Anesthesiol* 1992; 4:99.

202. Phirman JR, Shapiro HM: Modification of nitrous oxide induced intracranial hypertension by prior induction of anesthesia. *Anesthesiology* 1977; 46:150.

203. Smith AL, Wollman H: Cerebral blood flow and metabolism: Effects of anesthetic drugs and techniques. *Anesthesiology* 1972; 36:378.

204. Sakabe T et al: Cerebral responses to the addition of nitrous oxide to halothane in man. *Br J Anaesth* 1976; 48:957.

205. Moss E, McDowall DG: ICP increases with 50% nitrous oxide in oxygen in severe head injuries during controlled ventilation. *Br J Anaesth* 1979; 51:757.

206. Phirman JR, Shapiro HM: Modification of nitrous oxide-induced intracranial hypertension by prior induction of anesthesia. *Anesthesiology* 1977; 46:150.

207. Todd MM: The effects of Pa_{CO_2} on the cerebrovascular response to nitrous oxide in the halothane-anesthetized rabbit. *Anesth Analg* 1987; 66:1090.

208. Algotsson L et al: Cerebral blood flow and oxygen consumption during isoflurane and halothane anaesthesia in man. *Acta Anaesth Scand* 1988; 32:15.

209. Madsen JB et al: The effect of isoflurane on cerebral blood flow and metabolism in humans during craniotomy for small supratentorial tumors. *Anesthesiology* 1987; 66:332.

210. Madsen JB et al: Cerebral blood flow and metabolism during isoflurane-induced hypotension in patients subjected to surgery for cerebral aneurysms. *Br J Anaesth* 1987; 59:1204.

211. Newman B et al: The effect of isoflurane-induced hypotension on cerebral blood flow and cerebral metabolic rate for oxygen in humans. *Anesthesiology* 1986; 64:307.

212. Adams RW et al: Isoflurane and cerebrospinal fluid pressure in neurosurgical patients. *Anesthesiology* 1981; 54:97.

213. Campkin TV: Isoflurane and cranial extradural pressure, a study in neurosurgical patients. *Br J Anaesth* 1984; 56:1083.

214. Gordon E et al: The effect of isoflurane on cerebrospinal fluid pressure in patients undergoing neurosurgery. *Acta Anaesth Scand* 1988; 32:108.

215. Grosslight K et al: Isoflurane for neuroanesthesia: Risk factors for increases in intracranial pressure. *Anesthesiology* 1985; 63:533.

216. Messick JM et al: Correlation of regional cerebral blood flow (rCBF) with EEG changes during isoflurane anesthesia for carotid endarterectomy: Critical rCBF. *Anesthesiology* 1987; 66:344.

217. Lam AM: Isoflurane and brain protection: Lack of clear-cut evidence is not clear-cut evidence of lack. *J Neurosurg Anesthesiol* 1990; 2:315.

218. Ornstein E et al: Desflurane and isoflurane have similar effect on cerebral blood flow in patients with intracranial mass lesions. *Anesthesiology* 1993; 79:498.

219. Lutz LJ et al: The cerebral, functional, metabolic and hemodynamic effects of desflurane in dogs. *Anesthesiology* 1990; 73:125.

220. Lutz LJ et al: The response of the canine cerebral circulation to hyperventilation during anesthesia with desflurane. *Anesthesiology* 1991; 74:504.

221. Marx W et al: Sufentanil, alfentanil, and fentanyl: Impact on cerebrospinal fluid pressure in patients with brain tumors. *J Neurosurg Anesthesiol* 1989; 1:3.

222. Albanese J et al: Sufentanil increases intracranial pressure in patients with head trauma. *Anesthesiology* 1993; 79:493.

223. Sperry RJ et al: Fentanyl and sufentanil increase intracranial pressure in head trauma patients. *Anesthesiology* 1992; 77:416.

224. Trindle MR et al: Effects of fentanyl versus sufentanil in equi-anesthetic doses on middle cerebral artery blood flow velocity. *Anesthesiology* 1993; 78:454.

225. Bristow A et al: Low-dose synthetic narcotic infusions for cerebral relaxation during craniotomies. *Anesth Analg* 1987; 66:413.

226. Herrick IA et al: Effects of fentanyl, sufentanil, and alfentanil on brain retractor pressure. *Anesth Analg* 1991; 72:359.

227. Mayer N et al: Sufentanil does not increase cerebral blood flow in healthy human volunteers. *Anesthesiology* 1990; 73:240.

228. Weinstable C et al: Effect of sufentanil on intracranial pressure in neurosurgical patients. *Anaesthesia* 1991; 46:837.

229. Keykhah MM et al: Influence of sufentanil on cerebral metabolism and circulation in the rat. *Anesthesiology* 1985; 63:274.

230. Shupak RC, Harp JR: Comparison between high-dose sufentanil-oxygen and high-dose fentanyl-oxygen for neuroanaesthesia. *Br J Anaesth* 1985; 57:375.

231. Mutch WA et al: Continuous opioid infusion for neurosurgical procedures. A double-blind comparison of alfentanil and fentanyl. *Can J Anaesth* 1991; 38:710.

232. Grundy BL et al: Three balanced anesthetic techniques for neuroanesthesia: Infusion of thiopental sodium with sufentanil or fentanyl compared with inhalation of isoflurane. *J Clin Anesth* 1992; 4:372.

233. Pulsinelli WA et al: Increased damage after ischemic stroke in patients with hyperglycemia with or without diabetes mellitus. *Am J Med* 1983; 74:540.

234. Sieber FE et al: Glucose: A reevaluation of its intraoperative use. *Anesthesiology* 1987; 67:72.

235. Lam AM et al: Hyperglycemia and neurologic outcome in patients with head injury. *J Neurosurg* 1991; 75:545.

236. Lanier W et al: The effects of dextrose infusion and head position on neurologic outcome after complete cerebral ischemia in primates: Examination of a model. *Anesthesiology* 1987; 66:39.

237. Rosenorn J et al: Mannitol induced rebleeding from intracranial aneurysm. *J Neurosurg* 1983; 59:529.

238. Pollay M et al: Effect of mannitol and furosemide on blood-brain osmotic gradient and intracranial pressure. *J Neurosurg* 1983; 59:445.

239. Cottrell JE et al: Furosemide and mannitol-induced changes in intracranial pressure and serum osmolality and electrolytes. *Anesthesiology* 1977; 47:28.

240. Ferguson GG: The rationale for controlled hypertension. In: Varkey GP (ed): *Anesthetic Considerations in the Surgical Repair of Intracranial Aneurysms*. Boston, Little, Brown, 1992.

241. Miller ED Jr: Deliberate hypotension. In: Miller RD (ed). *Anesthesia*, 3d ed. New York, Churchill-Livingstone, 1990:1347–1367.

242. Lownie S et al: Brain retractor edema during induced hypotension. The effect of the rate of return of blood pressure. *Neurosurgery* 1990; 27:901.

243. Harp JR, Wollman H: Cerebral metabolic effects of hyperventilation and deliberate hypotension. *Br J Anaesth* 1973; 45:256.

244. Sullivan HG et al: The critical importance of Pa_{CO_2} during intracranial aneurysm surgery. *J Neurosurg* 1980; 52:426.

245. Lagerkranser M: Controlled hypotension in neurosurgery. *Pro J Neurosurg Anesthesiol* 1991; 3:150.

246. Johns RA: Endothelium-derived relaxing factor. Basic review and clinical applications. *J Cardiothorac Vasc Anesth* 1991; 5:69.

247. Cottrell JE, Hartung J: Induced hypotension In: Cottrell JE, Smith DS (eds): *Anesthesia and Neurosurgery*, 3d ed. St Louis, CV Mosby, 1994:425–434.

248. Thomsen LJ et al: Cerebral blood flow and metabolism during hypotension induced with sodium nitroprusside and captopril. *Can J Anaesth* 1989; 36:392.

249. Michenfelder JD, Milde JH: The interaction of sodium nitroprusside, hypotension and isoflurane in determining cerebral vasculature effects. *Anesthesiology* 1988; 69:870.

250. Morris PJ et al: Changes in canine intracranial pressure in response to infusions of sodium nitroprusside and trinitroglycerin. *Br J Anaesth* 1982; 54:991.

251. Cottrell JE et al: Intracranial pressure changes induced by sodium nitroprusside in patients with intracranial mass lesions. *J Neurosurg* 1978; 488:329.

252. Pinaud M et al: Cerebral blood flow and cerebral oxygen consumption during nitroprusside-induced hypotension to less than 50 mmHg. *Anesthesiology* 1989; 70:255.

253. Mcnab MSP et al: The stress response to induced hypotension for cerebral aneurysm surgery: A comparison of two hypotensive techniques. *Can Anaesth Soc J* 1988; 35:111.

254. Reiz S et al: Coronary hemodynamic effects of general anesthesia and surgery. *Regional Anesth* 1982; 7 (suppl): S8.

255. Bendo AA et al: Comparison of the protective effect of thiopental and isoflurane against damage in the rat hippocampal slice. *Brain Res* 1987; 403:136.

256. Gelb A et al: Primate brain tolerance to temporary focal cerebral ischemia during isoflurane or sodium nitroprusside-induced hypotension. *Anesthesiology* 1989; 70:678.

257. Sano T et al: A comparison of the cerebral protective effects of isoflurane and mild hypothermia in a model of incomplete forebrain ischemia in the rat. *Anesthesiology* 1992; 76:221.

258. Van Aken H et al: Cardiovascular and cerebrovascular effects of isoflurane-induced hypotension in the baboon. *Anesth Analg* 1986; 65:565.

259. Toivonen J et al: Labetalol attenuates the negative effects of deliberate hypotension induced by isoflurane. *Acta Anaesth Scand* 1992; 36:84.

260. Van Aken H et al: Influence of converting enzyme inhibition on isoflurane induced hypotension for cerebral aneurysm surgery. *Anaesthesia* 1992; 47:261.

261. Ornstein E et al: Deliberate hypotension in patients with intracranial arteriovenous malformations: Esmolol compared with isoflurane and sodium nitroprusside. *Anesth Analg* 1991; 72:639.

262. Goldberg ME et al: A comparison of labetalol and nitroprusside for inducing hypotension during major surgery. *Anesth Analg* 1990; 70:537.

263. Kelly PJ et al: Cerebral perfusion, vascular spasm, and outcome in patients with ruptured intracranial aneurysms. *J Neurosurg* 1977; 47:44.

264. Ruta TS, Mutch WAC: Controlled hypotension for cerebral aneurysm surgery: Are the risks worth the benefits? *J Neurosurg Anesthesiol* 1991; 3:153.

265. Charbel FT et al: Temporary clipping in aneurysm surgery: Techniques and results. *Surg Neurol* 1991; 36:83.

266. Jabre A, Symon L: Temporary vascular occlusion during aneurysm surgery. *Surg Neurol* 1987; 27:47.

267. Pool JL: Aneurysms of the anterior communicating artery, bifrontal craniotomy, and routine use of temporary clips. *J Neurosurg* 1961; 18:98.

268. Samson DS et al: A clinical study of the parameters and effects of temporary arterial occlusion in the management of intracranial aneurysms. *Neurosurgery* 1994; 34:22.

269. Wasnick JD, Conlay LA: Induced hypertension for cerebral

270. Young WL, Cole DJ: Deliberate hypertension: Rationale and application for augmenting cerebral blood flow. *Probl Anesth* 1993; 7:140.

271. Cole DJ et al: The effect of hypervolemic hemodilution with and without hypertension on cerebral blood flow following middle cerebral artery occlusion in rats. *Anesthesiology* 1989; 71:580.

272. Jones TH et al: Thresholds of focal cerebral ischemia in awake monkeys. *J Neurosurg* 1981; 54:773.

273. Schell RM, Cole DJ: Cerebral protection and neuroanesthesia. *Anesthesiol Clin North Am* 1992; 10:453.

274. Vanhoutte PM: Calcium entry blockers and vascular smooth muscle. *Circulation* 1982; 65 (suppl):11.

275. Siesjo BK: Cerebral circulation and metabolism. *J Neurosurg* 1984; 60:883.

276. Siesjo BK: Pathophysiology and treatment of focal cerebral ischemia. Part II. Mechanisms of damage and treatment. *J Neurosurg* 1992; 77:337.

277. Choi DW, Rothman SM: The role of glutamate neurotoxicity in hypoxic-ischemic neuronal death. *Ann Rev Neurosci* 1990; 13:171.

278. Albers GW: Potential therapeutic uses of N-Methyl-D-aspartate antagonists in cerebral ischemia. *Clin Neuropharmacol* 1990; 13:177.

279. Choi DW et al: Pharmacology of glutamate neurotoxicity in cortical cell culture: Attenuation by NMDA antagonists. *J Neurosci* 1988; 88:185.

280. Ikeda Y, Long DM: The molecular basis of brain injury and brain edema: The role of oxygen-free radicals. *Neurosurgery* 1990; 27:1.

281. Nussmeier N et al: Neuropsychiatric complications after cardiopulmonary bypass: Cerebral protection by a barbiturate. *Anesthesiology* 1986; 64:165.

282. Spetzler RF et al: Barbiturate therapy for brain protection during temporary vascular occlusion. In: Weinstein PR, Faden AI (eds): *Protection of the Brain from Ischemia*. Baltimore, Williams & Wilkins, 1990:253–258.

283. Spetzler RF, Hadley MN: Protection against cerebral ischemia: The role of barbiturates. *Cerebrovasc Brain Metab Rev* 1989; 1:212.

284. Smith A et al: Barbiturate protection in acute focal cerebral ischemia. *Stroke* 1974; 5:1.

285. Abramson N et al: Randomized clinical study of thiopental loading in comatose survivors of cardiac arrest. *N Engl J Med* 1986; 314:397.

286. Gisvold S et al: Thiopental treatment after global brain ischemia in pigtailed monkeys. *Anesthesiology* 1984; 60:888.

287. Steen P et al: No barbiturate protection in a dog model of complete cerebral ischemia. *Ann Neurol* 1979; 5:343.

288. Siegmann MG et al: Barbiturates impair cerebral metabolism during hypothermic circulatory arrest. *Ann Thorac Surg* 1992; 54:1131.

289. Warner D et al: Reversible focal ischemia in the rat: Effects of halothane, isoflurane and methohexital anesthesia. *J Cereb Blood Flow Metab* 1991; 11:794.

290. Michenfelder JD: Isoflurane when compared to enflurane and halothane decreases the frequency of cerebral ishemia during carotid endarterectomy. *Anesthesiology* 1987; 67:336.

291. Meyer FB, Muzzi DA: Cerebral protection during aneurysm surgery with isoflurane anesthesia. *J Neurosurg* 1992; 76:541.

292. Little JR: Modification of acute focal ischemia by treatment with mannitol. *Stroke* 1978; 9:4.

293. Yoshimoto T et al: Experimental cerebral infarction. III. Protec-

tive effect of mannitol in thalamic infarction in dogs. *Stroke* 1978; 9:217.

294. Yoshimoto T, Suzuki J: Intracranial definitive aneurysm surgery under normothermia and normotension utilizing temporary occlusion of brain artery and preoperative mannitol administration. *Neurol Surg* 1976; 4:775.

295. Suzuki J: Temporary occlusion of trunk arteries of the brain during surgery. In: Suzuki J (ed): *Treatment of Cerebral Infarction: Experimental and Clinical Study.* New York, Springer-Verlag, 1987.

296. McDermott MW et al: Temporary vessel occlusion and barbiturate protection in cerebral aneurysm surgery. *Neurosurgery* 1989; 25:54.

297. Batjer H et al: Use of etomidate, temporary arterial occlusion, and intraoperative angiography in surgical treatment of large and giant cerebral aneurysms. *J Neurosurg* 1988; 68:234.

298. Spetzler RF et al: Aneurysms of the basilar artery treated with circulatory arrest, hypothermia, and barbiturate cerebral protection. *J Neurosurg* 1988; 68:868.

299. Ravussin P et al: Total intravenous anesthesia with propofol for burst suppression in cerebral aneurysm surgery. Preliminary report of 42 patients. *Neurosurgery* 1993; 32:236.

300. Michenfelder JD: The interdependency of cerebral functional and metabolic effects following massive doses of thiopental in the dog. *Anesthesiology* 1974; 41:231.

301. Muizelaar JP: The use of electroencephalography and brain protection during operation for basilar aneurysms. *Neurosurgery* 1989; 25:899.

302. Busto R et al: The importance of brain temperature in cerebral ischemic injury. *Stroke* 1989; 20:1113.

303. Busto R, et al: Effect of mild hypothermia on ischemia-induced release of neurotransmitters and free fatty acids in rat brain. *Stroke* 1989; 20:904.

304. Minamisawa H et al: The influence of mild body and brain hypothermia on ischemic brain damage. *J Cereb Blood Flow Metab* 1990; 10:365.

305. Minamisawa H et al: The effect of mild hyperthermia and hypothermia on brain damage following 5, 10 and 15 minutes of forebrain ischemia. *Ann Neurol* 1990; 28:26.

306. Baker C et al: Reduction by delayed hypothermia of cerebral infarction following middle cerebral artery occlusion in the rat: A time-course study. *J Neurosurg* 1992; 77:438.

307. Baker C et al: Deliberate mild intraoperative hypothermia for craniotomy. *Anesthesiology* 1994; 81:361.

308. Bissonette B: Body temperature and anesthesia. *Anesthesiol Clin North Am* 1991; 19:849.

309. Batjer H, Samson D: Intraoperative aneurysmal rupture: Incidence, outcome and suggestions for surgical management. *Neurosurgery* 1986; 18:701.

310. Gianotta SL et al: Management of intraoperative rupture of aneurysms without hypotension. *Neurosurgery* 1991; 28:531.

311. Drake CG: Giant intracranial aneurysms: Experience with surgical treatment in 174 patients. *Clin Neurosurg* 1979; 26:12.

312. Solomon RA et al: Deep hypothermic circulatory arrest for the management of complex anterior and posterior circulation aneurysms. *Neurosurgery* 1991; 29:732.

313. Symon L, Vajda J: Surgical experiences with giant intracranial aneurysms. *J Neurosurg* 1984; 61:1009.

314. Greene KA et al: Cardiopulmonary bypass, hypothermic circulatory arrest and barbiturate cerebral protection for the treatment of giant vertebrobasilar aneurysms in children. *Pediatr Neurosurg* 1994; 21:124.

315. Ausman JI et al: Hypothermic circulatory arrest and the management of giant and large cerebral aneurysms. *Surg Neurol* 1993; 40:289.

316. Williams MD et al: Cardiopulmonary bypass, profound hypothermia, and circulatory arrest for neurosurgery. *Ann Thorac Surg* 1991; 52:1063.

317. Spetzler RF et al: Aneurysms of the basilar artery treated with circulatory arrest, hypothermia, and barbiturate cerebral protection. *J Neurosurg* 1988; 68:868.

318. Woodhall B et al: Craniotomy under conditions of quinidine-protected cardioplegia and profound hypothermia. *Ann Surg* 1960; 152:37.

319. Baumgartner WA et al: Reappraisal of cardiopulmonary bypass with deep hypothermia and circulatory arrest for complex neurosurgical operations. *Surgery* 1983; 94:242.

320. Silverberg G et al: Hypothermia and cardiac arrest in the treatment of giant aneurysms of the cerebral circulation and hemangioblastoma of the medulla. *J Neurosurg* 1981; 55:337.

321. McMurtry JG et al: Surgical treatment of basilar artery aneurysms: Elective circulatory arrest with thoracotomy in 12 cases. *J Neurosurg* 1974; 40:486.

322. Drake CG et al: The use of extracorporeal circulation and profound hypothermia in the treatment of ruptured intracranial aneurysm. *J Neurosurg* 1964; 21:575.

323. Thomas AN et al: Anaesthesia for the treatment of a giant cerebral aneurysm under hypothermic circulatory arrest. Case report. *Anaesthesia* 1990; 45:383.

324. Steen PA, Michenfelder JD: Barbiturate protection in tolerant and nontolerant hypoxic mice: Comparison with hypothermic protection. *Anesthesiology* 1979; 50:404.

325. Michenfelder JD et al: Induced hypothermia: Physiologic effects, indications and techniques. *Surg Clin North Am* 1965; 45:889.

326. Pierce EC II: In: *Extracorporeal Circulation for Open-Heart Surgery.* Springfield IL, Charles C Thomas, 1969.

327. Patterson RH, Ray BS: Profound hypothermia for intracranial surgery: Laboratory and clinical experience with extracorporeal circulation by peripheral cannulation. *Ann Surg* 1962; 156:377.

328. Michenfelder JD et al: Clinical experience with a closed-chest method of producing profound hypothermia and total circulatory arrest in neurosurgery. *Ann Surg* 1964; 159:125.

329. Sundt TM et al: Excision of giant basilar aneurysms under profound hypothermia. Report of a case. *Mayo Clin Proc* 1972; 47:631.

330. Gonski A et al: Profound hypothermia in the treatment of intracranial aneurysms. *Aust NZ J Surg* 1986; 56:639.

331. Cohen JA et al: Plasma heparin activity and antagonism during cardiopulmonary bypass with hypothermia. *Anesth Analg* 1977; 56:564.

332. Barno A, Freeman DW: Maternal deaths due to spontaneous subarachnoid hemorrhage. *Am J Obstet Gynecol* 1976; 125:384.

333. Daane TA, Tandy RW: Rupture of congenital intracranial aneurysms in pregnancy. *Obstet Gynecol* 1960; 15:305.

334. Miller HJ, Hinckley CM: Berry aneurysms in pregnancy: A 10 year report. *South Med J* 1970; 63:279.

335. Graham JG: Neurologic complications of pregnancy and anaesthesia. *Clin Obstet Gynecol* 1982; 29:333.

336. Dias MS, Sekhar LN: Intracranial hemorrhage from aneurysms and arteriovenous malformation during pregnancy and the puerperium. *Neurosurgery* 1990; 27:855.

337. Barrett JM et al: Pregnancy related rupture of arterial aneurysms. *Obstet Gynecol* 1976; 125:384.

338. Robinson JL et al: Subarachnoid hemorrhage in pregnancy. *J Neurosurg* 1972; 36:27.

339. Robinson JL et al: Arteriovenous malformation, aneurysms and pregnancy. *J Neurosurg* 1974; 41:63.

340. Fisher CM et al: Cerebral vasospasm with ruptured saccular aneurysm: The clinical manifestations. *Neurosurgery* 1977; 1:245.

341. Maymon R, Fejgin M: Intracranial hemorrhage during pregnancy and puerperium. *Obstet Gynecol Survey* 1990; 45:157.

342. Sadasivan B et al: Vascular malformations and pregnancy. *Surg Neurol* 1990; 33:305.

343. Holcomb WL Jr, Petrie RH: Cerebrovascular emergencies in pregnancy. *Clin Obstet Gynecol* 1990; 33:467.

344. Crowell RM: Aneurysms and arteriovenous malformations. *Neurol Clin* 1985; 3:291.

345. Wiebers DO et al: The natural history of unruptured intracranial aneurysms. *N Engl J Med* 1981; 304:696.

346. Stehbens WE: Aneurysms and anatomical variation of cerebral arteries. *Arch Pathol* 1963; 7:45.

347. Henderson CE, Torbey M: Rupture of intracranial aneurysm associated with cocaine use during pregnancy. *Am J Perinatol* 1988; 5:142.

348. Amias AG: Cerebral vascular disease in pregnancy. 1: Haemorrhage. *J Obstet Gynecol Br Common W* 1970; 77:100.

349. Rosen MA: Cerebrovascular lesions and tumors in the pregnant patient. In: Newfield P, Cottrell JE (eds): *Neuroanesthesia: Handbook of Clinical and Physiological Essentials*, 2d ed. Boston, Little, Brown, 1991:230–248.

350. Drake CG: Cerebral arteriovenous malformations. *Clin Neurosurg* 1979; 26:145.

351. Itoyama Y et al: Natural course of unoperated intracranial arteriovenous malformations: Study of 50 cases. *J Neurosurg* 1989; 71:805.

352. Pool JL: Treatment of intracranial aneurysms during pregnancy. *JAMA* 1965; 192:109.

353. Weir BK, Drake G: Rapid growth of residual aneurysm neck during pregnancy. *J Neurosurg* 1991; 75:780.

354. Barrett JM et al: Pregnancy related rupture of arterial aneurysms. *Obstet Gynecol Surv* 1982; 37:557.

355. de la Monte SM et al: Risk factors for the development and rupture of intracranial berry aneurysms. *Am J Med* 1985; 78:957.

356. Chesley LC: Cardiovascular changes in pregnancy. *Obstet Gynecol Annu* 1975; 4:71.

357. Lennon RL et al: Combined cesarean section and clipping of the intracerebral aneurysm. *Anesthesiology* 1984; 60:240.

358. Hillbom M, Kaste M: Alcohol intoxication: A risk factor for primary subarachnoid hemorrhage. *Neurology* 1982; 32:706.

359. Valiant GE: *Alcoholism and Drug Dependence*. Cambridge, Harvard University Press, 1983.

360. Evans A, Gillogley K: Drug use in pregnancy: Obstetric perspectives. *Clin Perinatol* 1991; 18:23.

361. Simolke GA et al: Cerebrovascular accidents complicating pregnancy and the puerperium. *Obstet Gynecol* 1991; 78:37.

362. Grossett DG: Stroke in pregnancy and the puerperium: What magnitude of risk? Editorial. *J Neurol Neurosurg Psychiatry* 1995; 58:129.

363. Jennett WB, Cross JN: Influence of pregnancy and oral contraception on the incidence of stroke in women of childbearing age. *Lancet* 1967; 1:1019.

364. Amin-Hanjani S et al: Moyamoya disease in pregnancy: A case report. *Am J Obstet Gynecol* 1993; 69:395.

365. Bingham WF et al: Moyamoya disease in pregnancy. *Wis Med J* 1980; 79:21.

366. Enomoto H, Goto H: Moyamoya disease presenting as intracerebral hemorrhage during pregnancy: Case report and review of literature. *Neurosurgery* 1987; 20:33.

367. Hashimoto K et al: Occlusive cerebrovascular disease with moyamoya vessels and intracranial hemorrhage during pregnancy: Case report and review of literature. *Neurol Med Chir (Tokyo)* 1988; 28:588.

368. Wilterdink JL, Feldmann E: Cerebral hemorrhage. In: Devinsky O et al (eds): *Neurological Complications of Pregnancy*. New York, Raven Press, 1994:13–23.

369. Okawara SH: Warning signs prior to rupture of an intracranial aneurysm. *J Neurosurg* 1973; 38:575.

370. King RB, Saba MI: Forewarnings of major subarachnoid hemorrhage due to congenital berry aneurysm. *NY State J Med* 1974; 74:638.

371. Tuttleman R, Gleicher N: Central nervous system hemorrhage complicating pregnancy. *Obstet Gynecol* 1981; 58:651.

372. Donaldson JO: *Neurology of Pregnancy*. Philadelphia, WB Saunders, 1978:115–156.

373. Minielly R et al: Subarachnoid hemorrhage secondary to ruptured cerebral aneurysm in pregnancy. *Obstet Gynecol* 1979; 53:64.

374. Locksley HB: Natural history of subarachnoid hemorrhage, intracranial aneurisms and arteriovenous malformations. *J Neurosurg* 1966; 25:321.

375. Forster DMC et al: Risk of cerebral bleeding from arteriovenous malformations. *Sterotact Funct Neurosurg* 1993; 61:20.

376. Hunt HB et al: Ruptured berry aneurysms and pregnancy. *Obstet Gynecol* 1974; 43:827.

377. Reichman OH, Karlman RL: Berry aneurysm surgery in the pregnant patient. *Surg Clin North Am* 1995; 75:115.

378. Conklin KA et al: Anaesthesia for caesarean section and cerebral aneurysm clipping. *Can Anaesth Soc J* 1984; 31:451.

379. Whitburn RH et al: Anaesthesia for simultaneous caeserean section and clipping of intracerebal aneurysm. *Br J Anaesth* 1990; 64:642.

380. Buckley TA et al: Caesarean section and ablation of cerebral arterio-venous malformation. *Anaesth Int Care* 1990; 18:248.

381. Kofke WA et al: Cesarean section following ruptured cerebral aneurysm and neuroresuscitation. *Anesthesiology* 1984; 60:242.

382. Stoelting RK: Attenuation of blood pressure response to laryngoscopy and tracheal intubation with sodium nitroprusside. *Anesth Analg* 1979; 58:116.

383. Kepes ER et al: Conduct of anesthesia for delivery with grossly raised cerebrospinal fluid pressure. *NY State J Med* 1972; 72:1155.

384. O'Sullivan GM et al: The effects of magnesium trisilicate mixture, metoclopramide and ranitidine on gastric pH, volume and serum gastrin. *Anaesthesia* 1985; 40:246.

385. Gillett GB et al: Ranitidine and single-dose antacid therapy as prophylaxis against acid aspiration syndrome in obstetric practice. *Anaesthesia* 1984; 39:638.

386. Dewan DM et al: Antacid anticholinergic premedication in the parturient. *Anesthesiology* 1980; 53:S308.

387. Boulay K et al: Effects of oral ranitidine, famotidine and omeprazole on gastric volume and pH at induction and recovery from general anaesthesia. *Br J Anaesth* 1994; 73:475.

388. May AE: The confidential enquiry into maternal deaths 1988–1990. *Br J Anaesth* 1994; 73:129.

389. Gomber S et al: Preanaesthetic oral ranitidine, omeprazole and metoclopramide for modifying gastric fluid volume and pH. *Can J Anaesth* 1994; 7:879.

390. Sellick BA: Cricoid pressure to control regurgitation of stomach contents during induction of anaesthesia. *Lancet* 1961; 2:404.

391. Stoelting RK: Circulatory change during direct laryngoscopy and tracheal intubation: Influence of duration of laryngoscopy with or without prior lidocaine. *Anaesthesia* 1977; 47:381.

392. Warren TM et al: Comparison of the maternal and neonatal effects of halothane, enflurane and isoflurane for Cesarean delivery. *Anesth Analg* 1983; 62:516.

393. Fox EJ et al: Complications related to pressor response to endotracheal intubation. *Anesthesiology* 1977; 47:524.

394. Turner JM, Powell K: Intracranial pressure changes in neurosurgical patients during hypotension induced with sodium nitroprusside or trimetaphan. *Br J Anaesth* 1977; 49:419.

395. Donchin Y et al: Sodium nitroprusside for aneurysm surgery in pregnancy. Report of a case. *Br J Anaesth* 1978; 50:849.

396. Rigg D, McDonough A: Use of sodium nitroprusside for deliberate hypotension during pregnancy. *Br J Anaesth* 1981; 53:985.

397. Willoughby JS: Sodium nitroprusside, pregnancy and multiple intracranial aneurysms. *Anaesth Int Care* 1984; 12:358.

398. Bruns PD et al: The placental transfer of water from fetus to mother following the intravenous infusion of hyperosmotic mannitol to the maternal rabbit. *Am J Obstet Gynecol* 1963; 86:160.

399. Levinson G et al: Effects of maternal hyperventilation on uterine blood flow and fetal oxygenation and acid-base balance. *Anaesthesia* 1974; 40:340.

Chapter 27

CAROTID ARTERY DISEASE
Surgical Management
H. D. ROOT

HISTORY OF CAROTID DISEASE AND ENDAR-TERECTOMY
EXTRACRANIAL CAROTID VASCULAR DISEASE
    Symptoms
    Pathophysiology
    Natural History
    Medical Management
INDICATIONS FOR SURGICAL INTERVENTION
    Symptomatic Group
    Asymptomatic Group
SURGICAL TECHNIQUE
COMPLICATIONS
OUTCOME
ALTERNATE THERAPIES
    Extracranial-Intracranial (EC-IC) Bypass
    Angioplasty
VERTEBRAL ARTERY DISEASE

History of Carotid Disease and Endarterectomy

Overall, stroke or cerebrovascular accident, is the third leading cause of death in the United States and the second leading cause of death due to cardiovascular disease.[1] The true incidence is difficult to verify, but is estimated to be approximately 160 patients per 100,000 population per year. Because approximately 20 percent of these patients will die as a result of their first stroke, we consider here the remaining 80 percent, of whom 60 percent will regain much or most of their function through rehabilitative efforts and healing of the brain tissue and reorientation of neurologic function. The remaining 40 percent represent varying degrees of disability ranging from a vegetative state requiring assistance in carrying out daily bodily activities to minor impairment. This is a severe psychologic and socioeconomic burden on the patient, as well as on the patient's family.

In 1875, a patient with right hemiplegia and blindness in the left eye was found to have an occlusion of the left carotid artery in the neck.[2] Other correlations by

Drake in 1968[3] and Hollenhorst in 1966[4] linked carotid arterial disease with amaurosis fugax. It is the latter author whose name is applied to the cholesterol crystals and plaques noted in the retinal vasculature of patients who are complaining of amaurosis fugax.

Association was made repeatedly between severe stenosis and/or ulceration of the carotid artery and the syndrome of transient ischemic attacks affecting the opposite arm and/or leg along with evidence of fibrin and platelet emboli in the retinal arteries (Fig. 27-1). Finally, in 1953, the English surgeons Eastcott, Pickering, and Rob proposed relieving the obstruction in the extracranial internal carotid artery of a woman in England.[5] They successfully resected the diseased segment and reanastomosed the internal carotid to the common carotid artery and the patient remained free of symptoms for over 15 years. Later, DeBakey[6] and Carrea and coworkers[7] cited carotid artery procedures they had performed prior to the English Surgeons Report, but their findings were published later.

These landmark carotid artery procedures were ushered in by the development of vascular surgery, begun in 1949 by Jean Kunlin,[8] who performed the first femoral-popliteal bypass with reversed saphenous vein. Repairing damaged arteries and veins during the Korean conflict gave added courage to potential vascular surgeons in becoming more aggressive with these problems. Simultaneously, open heart surgery was rapidly developing in the early 1950s, again adding reassurance that operating on arteries was an acceptable and rewarding adventure.

Since Eastcott's report,[5] the literature has burgeoned on indications/conraindications for carotid endarterectomy, expected morbidity and mortality outcome, and, most recently, better delineation of the natural history of the diseased carotid arteries and symptomatic and asymptomatic patients.

Extracranial Carotid Vascular Disease

SYMPTOMS

In patients with extracranial carotid artery disease, the pattern of development of the atheromatous plaque follows those found elsewhere; at points of bifurcation of major vessels and, in this case, at the point where the common carotid bifurcates into the external and internal carotid arteries. There is great variation in the amount of plaque development in the common carotid artery, but, characteristically, the internal carotid artery and the bulb are severely involved for approximately the first 3 cm (Fig. 27-2). The external carotid artery may also be involved for a distance of approximately 2 cm. Variations on this pattern are notable; for example, the common carotid arteries may have stenoses at

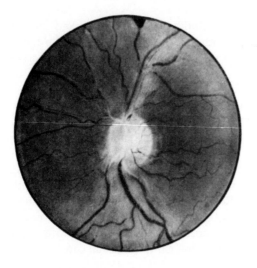
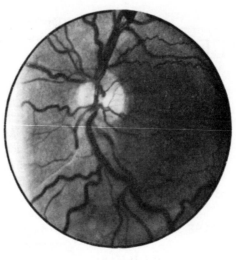

Figure 27-1 *Left* Platelet emboli entering the retinal arteries of a man aged fifty-one, who had transient blindness of that eye in recurrent attacks lasting up to 5 min. *Right* Four and a half minutes later: the emboli have almost passed. Fourteen days after his last attack a left carotid arteriogram showed complete occlusion, and symptoms ceased.

their origins either from the innominate artery or from the aortic arch. There are variations in the amount of plaque formation and obstruction in the common carotid artery between points of origin and bifurcation. There may also be simultaneous atherosclerotic obstruction at the origins of the vertebral arteries.

The symptoms associated with the extracranial disease basically follow three patterns:

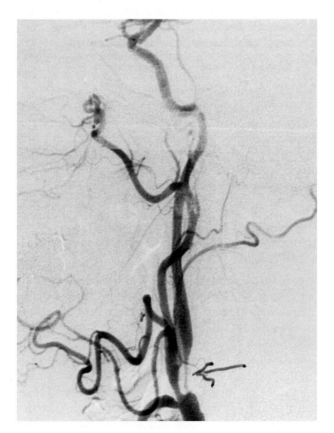

Figure 27-2 High-grade stenosis in internal carotid artery (*arrow*), narrowing of external carotid and common carotid arteries.

1. Intermittent symptoms of complete blindness appear, such as amaurosis fugax, lasting for several seconds upwards to several minutes; or symptoms of partial retinal ischemia, such as a closing down of the visual field likened to a shade being pulled over the eye, limiting the upward gaze and, sometimes, the lower gaze. Multiple scotomata may appear because showering of atheromatous emboli is probably occurring. Eastcott has shown platelet emboli entering retinal arteries with such symptoms, which were cleared a few minutes later.[5] Complete occlusion of the retinal artery with thrombosis, resulting in unilateral blindness, occurs in approximately 2 percent of patients with severe symptoms.

2. Events of brain ischemia, transient ischemic attacks (TIA), typically occur in the distribution of the middle cerebral artery in which sensory and/or motor function is temporarily interrupted in those somatic areas served by the ischemic portions of the brain. Such brief events may be noted as tingling and/or numbness, or loss of motor function for up to 24 h, with complete recovery noted by the patient between such events. Hemiplegic symptoms in all of the above are typically contralateral to the diseased carotid artery. However, TIAs may occur on the ipsilateral side of the brain where, of the two diseased internal carotid arteries, the more severe appearing disease is demonstrated by arteriogram. Facial weakness has been noted in approximately 10 percent of the patients.[1] Debate continues on whether the TIAs lasting 24 h or longer may actually be completed strokes, or the term "reversible ischemic neurologic deficit" (RIND) may be appropriate. Allow 72 h at maximum for complete clearing of symptoms of a RIND; thereafter, the term "stroke" is applied which becomes an important issue in deciding the timing of a carotid endarterectomy.

3. Less well defined and more easily confused with

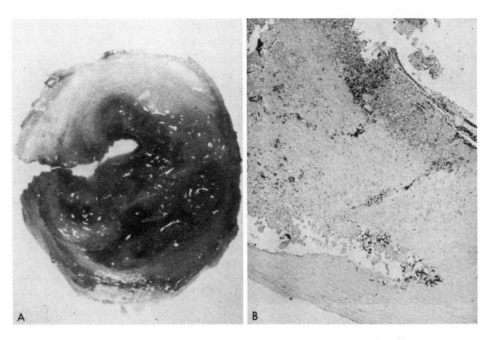

Figure 27-3 *A.* Cross section through a proliferative arteriosclerotic plaque taken at the bifurcation of the common carotid artery. Note the tiny lumen that remains. The material is glistening and consists primarily of cholesterol and necrotic atheromatous debris. *B.* Microscopic section, ×10. The atheromatous portion of the diseased intima is at the upper part of the photograph. The small spaces or clefts distributed throughout the initial lesion represent cholesterol crystals. [From Moore WS: Pathology of extracranial cerebrovascular disease. In Rutherford RB (ed): *Vascular Surgery,* 2d ed, 1984. Reproduced by permission of W. B. Saunders.]

other types of deranged physiology, are episodes of dizziness or exaggerated orthostatic symptoms. Grouped with this constellation can be signs of global ischemia, for example, changes in personality, dulling of sensorium, and apathy developing in patients who may have bilateral disease and collaterals through vertebral flow inadequate to maintain minimum cerebrovascular needs. It is now realized that those patients with symptoms have at least double the risk of developing a stroke (2 percent per year) versus those patients who may have high grade stenosis of the extracranial carotid system but without symptoms.[9]

PATHOPHYSIOLOGY

These areas of narrowing and obstruction typically are composed of atheromatous deposits with cavitation of some of the degenerating plaques, partially or completely filled with thrombus in various degrees of degeneration (Fig. 27-3). The atheromatous plaques extend throughout the media and smooth muscle of the arterial wall so that, on removal of the plaque, a few elastic fibers and adventitia are the only elements remaining in the wall of the diseased artery (Fig. 27-4). The basic mechanisms of deposition of the atherosclerosis are unknown, but the association of greater disease attack rates in those patients who smoke cigarettes or who have sustained hypertension over long periods of time has been noted.[1] The relationship with serum cholesterol levels and high density lipoprotein or low density lipoprotein has not been clearly established at this point. Carotid artery atherosclerosis with narrowing does occur in patients who have never smoked cigarettes, but in patients who are presented in the literature and in Moore's personal experience,[1] at least 95 percent of the patients have been heavy cigarette smokers at some time in their lifetime. These carotid lesions may be associated with severe coronary artery disease and lower extremity arterial disease. The association is clear enough to warrant careful evaluation of the patient's coronary artery system when contemplating operative procedures, for example, carotid endarterectomy.[10]

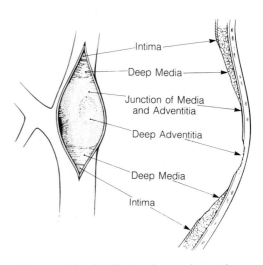

Figure 27-4 Arterial wall following the usual carotid endarterectomy. The deepest plane extending into the adventitia is found at the site of the most heavily concentrated disease (posterolateral bulb) and is usually no more than 1 cm² in size. [From Clagett GP: Vein patch graft closure for carotid endarterectomy. In Ernst CB, Stanley JC (eds): *Current Therapy in Vascular Surgery,* 2d ed, 1991. Reproduced by permission of B. C. Decker.]

Varying degrees of fibrosis and scarring occur in the walls of the artery and, simultaneously, around the artery, giving evidence of an inflammatory process that may produce scarring and attachment to contiguous tissues, such as jugular vein, hypoglossal nerve, or cervical strap muscles. The same type of inflammatory-scarring association is seen in other sites of atherosclerotic deposits, such as the aorta, the iliacs, and femoral arterial system. The issue of genetic susceptibility and P53 gene presence has not been fully explored but, obviously, there are clusters of patients whose family members have manifestations of vascular disease in much higher associated rates than in other families, even with a similar history of chronic cigarette smoking.[7] Fibromuscular dysplasia with characteristic "beading" of the carotid artery is an uncommon cause of carotid artery obstruction.

NATURAL HISTORY

One of the more difficult and yet extremely important aspects of this disease is the attempt to describe the natural history in order to predict the rate of progress and the eventual outcome of atherosclerotic deposits in the carotid and vertebral arteries. Through ultrasound studies and arteriograms of the carotid arteries in many study groups, slow progression of narrowing of the arteries has been described and, in other groups, rapid progression has been recognized as rapid change from initial TIAs through complete thrombosis and major stroke.[11] Thus, in attempting to plan therapy appropriate to each patient, this natural history must be recognized as extremely variable. Prospective randomized studies are mandatory.[11]

In the general population at age 70 years, the predicted stroke rate is 0.6 percent per year.[11] In patients with asymptomatic carotid stenosis on one side, the stroke rate is 1.5 percent per year.[12] These are identified by duplex ultrasound scans. Those patients with a history of a prior myocardial infarction (MI) also have a stroke rate of 1.5 percent per year. In patients with symptomatic stenosis of one internal carotid artery of over 60 percent, the stroke rate was 2 percent per year. In patients with transient ischemic attacks, the stroke rate was 6 percent per year, and those with prior strokes, 10 percent per year. In patients with atrial fibrillation unrelated to carotid disease, the stroke rate is 5 percent per year. Further information from the North American Surgical Carotid Endarterectomy Trial (NASCET) study,[13] regarding the natural history of carotid artery/atherosclerotic disease showed that if patients were symptomatic from their carotid stenosis, the risk of ipsilateral stroke at two years was 26 percent if the patients were treated medically, in other words, with anti-platelet therapy.

In the asymptomatic patients, 30 percent of people over 50 years of age have some evidence of carotid artery atherosclerotic disease. The incidence of carotid stenosis of more than 50 percent has been estimated, on the basis of ultrasonography, to be 4 percent among middle-aged and older people.[14] According to data from Bornstein,[15] less than 1 percent of people in these age groups have stenosis of 80 percent or more. In a 12-year German study of 500 patients with at least 80 percent carotid artery stenosis, the annual rate of ipsilateral stroke was 2.4 percent.[16] For patients with less than 75 percent stenosis, the annual rate of stroke was 1 percent in both the German study and a Canadian study.[16] The risk of fatal coronary artery disease increases with the degree of carotid stenosis. In the Canadian studies,[17,18] the annual rate of death, mostly from myocardial infarction, was 6.5 percent. In a recently reported asymptomatic carotid atherosclerosis study (ACAS),[19] in which 1662 patients were followed for an average of 2.7 years, the 5-year risk of stroke was 10.6 percent in the medically treated group. Thus, it is apparent that for patients with physical findings of bruits in the region of the common carotid artery bifurcation, which can be separated from bruits of cardiac origin, ultrasound duplex scanning should be employed for monitoring these lesions. Any patient with symptoms suggestive of TIAs, RINDS, amaurosis fugax, or global ischemia should initially undergo ultrasound evaluation of the carotid and vertebral arteries. A patient who has symptoms of TIAs or amaurosis fugax should undergo carotid angiography if the patient is to be considered a candidate for endarterectomy.

MEDICAL MANAGEMENT

Medical management of patients with asymptomatic carotid occlusive disease secondary to atherosclerosis consists primarily of careful cardiac evaluation to rule out nonvalvular or valvular-based atrial fibrillation, which in itself would be a major consideration for anticoagulant therapy to prevent cerebral embolic events. Careful management of the patient's hypertension, smoking, diabetes, cardiac symptoms from coronary artery narrowing, and cholesterol levels are all a part of adequate medical therapy.

Consideration of the optimum antiplatelet therapy remains in evolution. The patient, of course, must be convinced of the extreme importance of giving up cigarette smoking because of the profound negative influence it has by creating disease in susceptible areas, such as carotid artery bifurcation.

In those patients who have evidence of both asymptomatic atrial fibrillation and carotid artery stenosis, it appears that warfarin is of benefit, as noted in a number of studies.[20-25] Thus, the overall reduction of ischemic-CNS events and the relative risk of patients who are treated with warfarin, as compared to placebo, was 64 percent with a *p*-value of less than .001.[21] Data from trials in case control studies indicate that patients with nonvalvular atrial fibrillation, who are less than 60 years old and have no other risk factors, do not have an increased risk of stroke, as compared with normal subjects.[26,27] With advancing age, the complications of warfarin therapy, such as hemorrhagic events, reduces the measurable effectiveness of the anticoagulation, especially in patients who are not dependable in terms of following their medication schedules and monitoring their prothrombin times.

In patients who have TIAs, it is still not clear that warfarin will be of any value in reducing the stroke rate due to disease of the major cerebral arteries or lacunar disease. There have been no good studies of patients with TIAs or minor strokes who have received a randomized placebo or warfarin clinical trial. At present, there are large trials underway examining the benefit of a combination of warfarin and heparin in patients with acute or progressing stroke.

As of now, the major emphasis on managing patients with asymptomatic carotid disease is through the use of platelet inhibitors. Sulfinpyrazone, aspirin, and dipyridamole all inhibit platelet aggregation in vitro.[28] On the basis of studies that have demonstrated the presence of white platelet-fibrin thrombi in the retinal arteries in patients with amaurosis fugax, these drugs were given to patients with recurrent transient monocular blindness and found to be beneficial.[29,30] White platelet-fibrin material has also been observed in the cortical artery exposed for EC-IC bypass surgery.

In the Canadian cooperative clinical trial of aspirin, sulfinpyrazone, and placebo, the combined incidence of stroke and death was reduced by 31 percent among patients who took 1300 mg aspirin per day alone or with sulfinpyrazone, as compared to the placebo group.[31]

Sulfinpyrazone alone was ineffective. A subgroup analysis showed a statistically significant reduction of 48 percent in relative risk of stroke or death among the men, but no significant reduction in these relative risks of outcomes among women. Although over 14,000 patients with TIAs or minor strokes of noncardiac origin have been studied in 15 different randomized trials evaluating five platelet-inhibiting drugs, aspirin seems to be the major drug that shows effectiveness in reducing the stroke rate. These studies have some flaws in terms of their lack of evaluation of the probable causes of the cerebral ischemia.[31-33] Concern over the potential problems of simultaneously inhibiting the production of platelet thromboxane A_2 and the production of endothelial prostacyclin[34,35] has led to trials of lower doses of aspirin; for example, 75 to 300 mg daily. Although low doses of aspirin have proved effective in reducing the incidence of recurrent myocardial infarction and stroke among patients with unstable angina or acute MI, the benefit of low doses of aspirin is less certain in patients with TIAs or minor strokes of arterial origin.[36,37] Currently, there is a randomized trial underway to compare the effectiveness of a low-dose aspirin (125 mg) or a high-dose aspirin (1300 mg) schedule in reducing recurrent TIAs or strokes.

Ticlopidine is the only other platelet-inhibiting drug that has been beneficial in clinical trials. It inhibits platelet aggregation induced by adenosine diphosphate and other agonists, apparently by interfering with a membrane-fibrinogen interaction, thereby blocking the platelet glycoprotein (II.b./III.a. receptor).[38,39] The onset of maximum effect on the platelets is delayed 24 to 48 h, as compared to the maximum benefit in 20 min for aspirin on the cyclooxygenase system. In large studies, ticlopidine seems not to be any more effective than aspirin in patients with minor stroke or TIAs. The side effects include suppression of bone marrow, diarrhea, rash, and bleeding during surgery.

On the basis of the imperfect data cited above, aspirin is the drug of first choice for patients with transient cerebral ischemia, presumably not due to cardiac origin. Aspirin, in combination with warfarin, may have some additional benefit, but in the NASCET study, a daily dose of 650 mg or more was superior to a daily dose of 325 mg or less in preventing stroke during the first 30 days after surgery.[13] The chief complication of aspirin therapy, GI bleeding, is not dose related and, therefore, in patients with high-grade stenosis of internal carotid arteries, 650 mg of aspirin daily seems to be a reasonable dose.

Indications for Surgical Intervention

SYMPTOMATIC GROUP

HISTORY OF MANAGEMENT

With the growing acceptance of surgical carotid endarterectomy, beginning with the first report by Eastcott[5] of resection and reanastomosis of the diseased internal carotid artery, and with the development of increasing numbers of surgeons trained in vascular surgery techniques, the number of carotid endarterectomies skyrocketed to a peak of 110,000 procedures known to

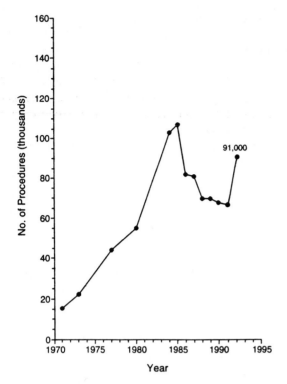

Figure 27-5 Number of carotid endarterectomies performed in the United States from 1971 to 1992. (From Barnett HJM: Drugs and surgery in the prevention of ischemic stroke. *N Engl J Med*, January 26, 1995. Reproduced by permission.)

have been performed in 1985. These included both symptomatic and asymptomatic groups of patients with narrowing of their carotid arteries secondary to atherosclerosis. In Winslow's study of carotid endarterectomy,[40] 44 percent of patients were asymptomatic in these earlier series. This bandwagon effect "enhanced the popularity of the procedure," but unexpected developments then intervened and the number of procedures declined (Fig. 27-5)[41] to approximately 70,000 in 1991 and 1992. Now, however, in 1994, the number of procedures has gone back up to approximately 91,000. The low levels of perioperative complications reported by the experienced vascular surgeons in their studies were not matched by the experience in most other hospitals in the United States. Data from the National Hospital Discharge Survey and other sources revealed that the average rate of stroke and death in the perioperative period was about 10 percent.[37] Thus, it was suddenly realized that, although the operation of endarterectomy appears relatively simple, the morbidity and mortality were alarming. Several reports from various private hospitals with morbidity/mortality combinations of 22 percent caused a revulsion among many neurologists and surgeons and required careful reassessment, so that when the international clinical trials were begun, institutions were

chosen to participate only if the morbidity/mortality of carotid endarterectomy in the institution was less than 5 percent.[13] The National Outcome Studies from many centers have been using this as a standard for acceptance of proper carotid endarterectomy outcomes.

NASCET STUDY RESULTS

The above-mentioned North American Surgical Carotid Endarterectomy Trial (NASCET), which began enrolling patients in 1987 with an interim report in 1991,[13] was the first international study to compare in a randomized manner all symptomatic patients considered candidates for carotid endarterectomy with 30 percent or greater degrees of diameter narrowing; they were enrolled under the direction of Dr. Barnett at the University of Western Ontario, London, Ontario, Canada. This study group is currently still enrolling patients in its study, but the early report in 1991 indicated that, for symptomatic patients with a diameter stenosis of 70 percent or greater of the internal carotid, medical care alone was inferior to carotid endarterectomy at 2 and 3 years respectively.[13,42] Similarly, the European Carotid Surgery Trial (ECST)[43] confirmed the benefit of carotid endarterectomy in a similar group of patients with high-grade stenosis. The absolute difference between the risk of stroke among patients receiving medical care alone and among those undergoing surgery was unequivocal. In the NASCET study, the risk of ipsilateral stroke in 2 years was 26 percent for patients treated medically and 9 percent for those treated surgically. The benefit was slightly smaller in the ECST: At 3 years, the absolute difference was 14 percent, as compared with 17 percent at two years in NASCET.

The third study, conducted within the U.S. Department of Veterans Affairs (V.A.), was stopped when the benefit of surgery for patients with severe stenosis in NASCET and ECST became evident. In this V.A. study, 189 patients with carotid stenosis of at least 50 percent revealed no benefit of surgery, unless TIAs during or after treatment were considered along with stroke in the analysis of outcome events.[44] At present, surgery has not been demonstrated to be superior to medical management in patients with less than 70 percent carotid stenosis, but both trials continue to enroll symptomatic patients, with a goal of studying approximately 2000 patients each and then following them for a minimum of 5 years. For their follow-up surveillance, these patients have annual ultrasonography of their carotids. Ultrasonography, in the hands of most technologists, is not as accurate as arteriography and, for that reason, arteriography is the basis for determining the degree of stenosis in NASCET. They report that ultrasonography has a sensitivity of only 67 percent and a specificity of 78 percent for detecting severe stenosis. Strandness,[45] with his ultrasonography techniques, however, has refuted this disparity and feels strongly that ultrasonography should be fully depended on for following these symptomatic patients.[46,47] If endarterectomy is to be recommended, however, the rate of perioperative morbidity and mortality must be no greater than 5 percent, as required in the NASCET study. Otherwise, the benefits of carotid endarterectomy over medical therapy are diminished. The discrimination of predictable stroke rate between patients with 70, 80, or 90 percent degrees of stenosis has not yet been detectable in the NASCET study.

Subgroup analysis of NASCET data provides additional information. Gasecki[48] concluded that carotid endarterectomy can be performed safely within 30 days of a nondisabling stroke and that waiting longer exposes the patient to increased risk of recurrent stroke.

INDICATIONS FOR CAROTID ENDARTERECTOMY

Currently, patients with transient ischemic attacks as described above, or monocular temporary blindness with or without evidence of retinal Hollenhorst plaques in conjunction with detectable extracranial carotid artery disease, are candidates for carotid endarterectomy, if the degree of carotid stenosis is at least 70 percent. These data may be modified as the final evaluation of the NASCET study is released. All surgical consideration should be based on a very low morbidity and mortality from carotid endarterectomy, if the benefits of endarterectomy in patients with 30 to 70 percent degrees of stenosis are to be identified. In addition, Eliasziw showed that, if treated medically, the presence of ulceration in the plaque as evidenced by angiogram increased the incidence of stroke threefold.[49]

ASYMPTOMATIC GROUP

HISTORY OF MANAGEMENT
The history of management is that of multiple trials comparing aspirin and other platelet-inhibiting drugs, controlled as outlined above. The asymptomatic patients with varying degrees of stenosis initially suspected because of bruits detected at routine physical examination, should be followed with ultrasonography to detect progressive and advancing degrees of stenosis in the carotids.

MULTI-INSTITUTIONAL STUDY RESULTS
The role of carotid endarterectomy in patients with asymptomatic disease is not demonstrated so clearly as in the symptomatic group. At present, it is known that the incidence of asymptomatic carotid stenosis increases with age.[13] It has been estimated that 30 percent of people over 50 years of age have some evidence of carotid artery disease. The incidence of carotid stenosis of more than 50 percent has been estimated, on the basis of ultrasonography, to be 4 percent among people middle-aged and older; less than 1 percent of people in these age groups have stenosis of 80 percent or more.[50] Patients in two large studies who underwent carotid ultrasonography are reported below.[51,52] In an 8-year Canadian study of 696 patients, the annual rate of ipsilateral stroke was 2.5 percent among patients with at least 75 percent stenosis of one carotid artery. In a 12-year German study[52] of 500 patients with at least 80 percent stenosis, the annual rate of ipsilateral stroke was 2.4 percent. For patients with less than 75 percent stenosis, the annual rate of stroke was 1 percent in both studies. The risk of fatal coronary artery disease increases with the degree of carotid stenosis. In fact, the Canadian study showed that the annual rate of death from MI was 6.5 percent.[53]

The results of three randomized trials of endarterectomy in patients with asymptomatic carotid disease have been published. In the asymptomatic patients with carotid artery stenosis (CASANOVA) trial, patients with stenosis of more than 90 percent were excluded, and those with bilateral disease were randomly assigned to medical treatment or underwent endarterectomy for the more severely affected carotid artery.[53] Only 25 percent of the 440 patients in the trial received medical treatment alone. No benefit was found for carotid endarterectomy. After 71 patients had been enrolled, the Mayo Asymptomatic Carotid Endarterectomy (MACE)[54] study was discontinued because myocardial infarction and several ischemic events had occurred in eight and three patients, respectively, in the endarterectomy group, as compared with none in the aspirin group. The third trial with negative results was the Department of Veterans Affairs study with 444 patients.[55] The 30-day rate of postoperative stroke or death in the 203 patients who underwent endarterectomy was 4.4 percent. The stroke-free survival curves with the medical and surgical groups overlapped, both during the early weeks of follow-up and thereafter. The incidence of TIAs, especially amaurosis fugax, was reduced in the surgical group; however, there was no reduction in the number of strokes. A much larger study, the Asymptomatic Carotid Atherosclerosis Study (ACAS) found a benefit from endarterectomy, as compared with medical treatment, in 1162 patients followed for an average of 2.7 years. This was in patients with 60 percent diameter stenosis or greater. The 5-year risk of stroke was 10.6 percent in the medical group and 4.8 percent in the surgical group.[14] This reflects a 5.8 percent absolute risk reduction in 5 years, which is just above 1 percent per year. A number of these patients were followed with ultrasonography alone. Most of the patients, however, were entered for having been operated on, if they had over 60 percent of stenosis shown by angiogram. The 30-day rate of stroke or death was 2.3 percent, half of which were due to complications of the angiogram. The ipsilateral stroke rate was reduced by 1 percent per year; but a 16 percent reduction occurred in females. This study was begun in 1987 and supported by the National Institutes of Health.

CURRENT INDICATIONS FOR CEA

At present, in the asymptomatic group of patients, the indication for carotid endarterectomy would include those patients with 60 percent or greater degree of diameter stenosis of a carotid artery. This would have to be confirmed by arteriogram. The patients should be selected very carefully, and significant cardiac disease should be evaluated for preliminary improvement, either by medical therapy or coronary bypass. These endarterectomies should not be undertaken by a surgeon whose results do not meet the national standards of no more than 5 percent combined morbidity and mortality of the carotid endarterectomy.

Further data from the ACAS study are eagerly awaited. Undoubtedly, modification of our patient management will occur, but it should be based on good data.

Surgical Technique

We prefer to do carotid endarterectomy with the patients under general anesthesia because of ease of surgical dissection, good relaxation of the patient, and better exposure of the high-lying carotid bifurcation. The choices of anesthetic agents and the methods of management are covered in the following section. At the present time, it appears desirable to maintain the patient's blood pressure at least equal to the preoperative pressure. There is the impression that sustaining mild hypertension (i.e., 20 to 40 mm above the preoperative blood pressure levels) during carotid endarterectomy, may be of some benefit in reducing the incidence of ischemic stroke, but there is little data to support this. It is important that the patients come to the operating room while on aspirin therapy to diminish the likelihood of the white fibrin platelet clots so well described by Eastcott 40 years ago.[5]

The patient is positioned supine with a roll between the scapulae, the head rotated to the contralateral side for good visibility and easy access by the surgeon and his assistant. If the procedure is to be performed under cervical nerve block and local anesthetic supplement,

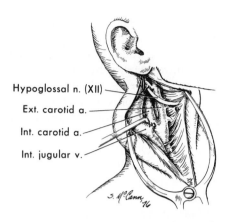

Figure 27-6   Exposure of the common carotid in its distal 5.0 cm and the internal-external carotid with their relationships to adjacent structures. [From Moore WS: Operative technique. In Rutherford RB (ed): *Vascular Surgery*, 2d ed, 1984. Reproduced by permission.]

then provision for airway management must be included with the positioning and draping of the patient.

We give one dose of broad spectrum antibiotics such as ticarcillin and clavulanate 1 h before the incision is made. This has not been proven to be of benefit because the incidence of infection in cervical incisions is extremely low. While a randomized study has not been carried out to demonstrate this, it is in keeping with the antibiotic management in patients undergoing other open surgical procedures.

In a patient with elastic, nonwrinkled skin where cosmesis may be an extremely important issue, for example, in women, a collar incision just below the level of the thyroid cartilage with extension along the plane of the sternocleidomastoid aiming toward the ipsilateral mastoid process may be employed. In the more typical male of seventh or eighth decade with flabby skin of the neck, an incision is made along the anterior border of the sternocleidomastoid in a plane from the suprasternal notch to the mastoid bone. Oozing from skin edges in a patient dosed with aspirin is to be expected, but it is a reasonable price to pay for the benefit of the protection from platelet thrombi. Exposure of the common carotid in its distal 5 cm and the internal carotid/external carotid is accomplished with a standard method (Fig. 27-6). Encircling umbilical tape is applied around the common carotid artery for control early in the procedure. Minimal handling by dissection or motion of the carotid bulb is important in case unrecognized friable thrombi are present in the atherosclerotic plaque of the carotid bulb. Careful exposure of the distal internal carotid artery, with careful deference to the hypoglossal, the vagus, and the spinal accessory nerves, is mandatory. Encirclement of the internal carotid artery, at least 2 cm distal to the obvious plaque of the internal carotid, is desirable. An elastic rubber vascular loop is easily utilized. Similarly, the external carotid artery is encircled with an elastic vessel loop and removable clips may be applied to the superior thyroid artery or the ascending pharyngeal if its point of origin requires it. These are removed after completion of the endarterectomy.

Patient monitoring is intense and will basically include the EEG, arterial blood pressure from an indwelling radial artery catheter, and venous pressure from a central line. In the patient who is at severe cardiac risk, a triple lumen catheter is often inserted so that cardiac outputs, mixed venuos saturations, and chamber pressures can be monitored. There should be close communication between anesthesiologist and surgeon in the event that ischemic events take place, and the need for an intralumenal shunt can be assessed.[56,57] This area will be covered in detail below.

Intravenous administration of heparin is then instituted, unless the patient has been brought to the operating room under heparin therapy because of crescendo TIAs. After waiting an appropriate time period for the heparin to become effective and while in close coordination with the anesthesiologist, the common carotid, internal carotid, and external carotid vessels are occluded. An arteriotomy anteriorly located is quickly made. The common carotid and internal carotid arteries are opened with a distal end of the arteriotomy going past the point of the termination of the evident plaque.

At this point, an intraluminal shunt may be placed (Fig. 27-7). The classic indications are: ICA stump pressure less than 50 mmHg, or EEG evidence of ischemia. It depends on the surgeon whether one is used for other reasons. In our teaching institution, with vascular fellows and chief residents, we utilize a shunt routinely to eliminate the question of need and to familiarize them with the technique, thus minimizing the complications from its use. The shunt is inserted into the internal carotid initially with free back bleeding from the internal carotid to eliminate air and debris. With free bleeding from the shunt, the end is inserted into the common carotid artery which is then reoccluded by an occluding tape. This should consume no more than 2 or 3 min. The alternative is to measure carotid stump pressure and, if in the safe range of at least 50 mmHg with occlusion of the external and common carotid arteries, the shunt may be omitted. Choice of shunt is dependent on the experience of the surgeon. With most vascular surgeons, usually, if a patient has had a prior stroke the stump pressure is ignored and a shunt is used.

The plaque is then dissected free from its cleavage plane (Fig. 27-7), which is usually quite evident on the yellowish cholesterol plaque. This is removed in a technique that allows thinning out or removal of just

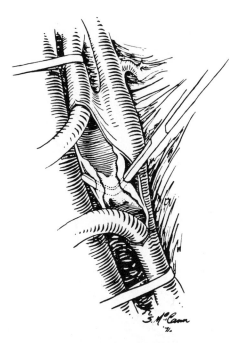

Figure 27-7   Technique of completing circumferential mobilization of the atheromatous lesion by utilizing the closed jaws of a right-angle clamp. [From Moore WS: Operative technique. In Rutherford RB (ed): *Vascular Surgery*, 2d ed, 1984. Reproduced by permission of W. B. Saunders.]

the plaque in the internal carotid artery and, if it "feathers" appropriately, no further therapy is necessary at that end. If the removal of the plaque does not leave a smooth surface at the cranial end, then tacking sutures are applied to the transected end of the internal carotid artery plaque where the dissection has stopped. The plaque is dissected from the external carotid and taken down the common carotid until all significant narrowing obstructive disease is removed. Tacking sutures may be used on the common carotid end of the endarterectomy, if a blunt end of the transected plaque is remaining. After thorough irrigation and debridement of the operative site, closure is begun with a 7-0 monofilament polyester suture at the internal carotid arteriotomy end. Very carefully placed sutures to minimize circumferential narrowing are continued to the bulb where a 6-0 suture is begun (Fig. 27-8). The closure is pursued from either end of the endarterectomy and, before final closure, the shunt is removed with good back bleeding allowed from the internal carotid to eliminate all possible bubbles and clots. This should consume no more than 2 or 3 min of time after the shunt is removed.

Selective or routine patching of the endarterectomy closure is again an option of the individual surgeon (Fig. 27-8). It is fairly standard to use a vein patch or synthetic graft patch for small internal carotid arteries, such as are typically found in the female, or in someone

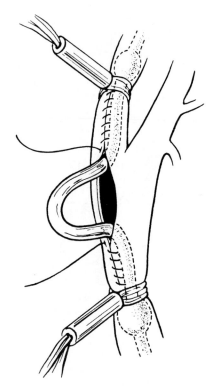

Figure 27-8   Partial closure of the arteriotomy with a suture beginning at each end. The arteriotomy is closed as far as the emergence of the internal shunt will permit. [From Moore WS: Operative technique. In Rutherford RB (ed): *Vascular Surgery,* 2d ed, 1984. Reproduced by permission of W. B. Saunders.]

with recurrent carotid artery stenosis. The results, whether complications or long-term outcome, seem to be equivalent between the patched and nonpatched closure of the arteriotomy.[58]

Hemostasis is carefully achieved and the cervical incision closed with approximation of the deep fascial layer, and then a subcutaneous suture is applied so that the skin lies easily approximated. Skin tapes are then applied and the patient recovered from anesthesia. Careful monitoring of postoperative blood pressure, with support for either hypotension or hypertension, is carefully done in conjunction with the anesthesiologist. These variant blood pressures occur in about 50 percent of the patients and usually last no more than 24 h postoperatively.[59] Monitoring in the intensive care unit–recovery room is important for evidence of cranial nerve injury or evidence of postoperative stroke.

Complications

The usual complications in the immediate postoperative period are severe hypotension or severe hypertension, which must be controlled carefully. The dreaded major surgical complication is a fresh stroke involving the ipsilateral brain. If this occurs, the patient should be promptly returned to the operating room. The arteriotomy is examined by Doppler flow study of the vessel in the operating room, looking for evidence of thrombus. The vessel should be reopened and the thrombus cleared from the artery with reinstitution of flow. On occasion, these episodes of postoperative stroke may occur in a delayed manner, perhaps 12 to 24 h later, which is suggestive of a thrombus build-up, typically a white platelet thrombus in a patient who had not been on preoperative aspirin.

The patient is examined neurologically for evidence of damage to the cranial nerves, including evidence of paresis of the ipsilateral vocal cord. Evidence of damage to the ramus mandibularis branch of the facial nerve is sought; such damage is usually due to pressure from an unwisely applied retractor over the edge of the mandible during the procedure. Barring neurologic complications, the patient is monitored in the ICU for 24 h, or until hemodynamically stable, and the patient is able to swallow without difficulty. Discharge from the hospital is typical within 3 days.

Outcome

The morbidity and mortality associated with extracranial carotid arterial surgery has been evaluated carefully with the development of the aforementioned national and international controlled studies of the benefits of carotid endarterectomy. At present, the accepted combined morbidity and mortality rate of less than 5 percent is the national norm. It is not unusual now to find series with 0.6 to 0.8 percent mortality and 2 to 3 percent morbidity, mainly that of neurologic deficit, either brief or permanent. A smaller percentage of patients may have temporary paresis of the hypoglossal nerve or, uncommonly, a fixed injury of that nerve. Less commonly injured are the vagus, the spinal accessory, or the glossopharyngeal nerves. Wound hematomas requiring evacuation postoperatively occur in approximately 5 percent of the patients.[60] Careful attention to hemostasis in patients who come to the operating room while on aspirin therapy will minimize this wound complication.

The postoperative control of blood pressure is extremely important to prevent CNS damage from severe and malignant hypertension, which also can increase the likelihood of wound hematoma secondary to bleeding through the suture line. Blood pressure variations are usually easily controllable with pharmacologic means and are self-limiting with the patient's blood pressure returning to the preoperative norm within 48 h.

In spite of careful preoperative screening of patients for cardiac disease, the surgical mortality of approximately 1 percent is largely associated with acute MIs, typically at 48 to 72 h postoperatively.

Patients who have been followed for 5 or more years after carotid endarterectomy have demonstrated that approximately 80 to 85 percent will have no further attacks of TIAs. In most series, the mortality rate over five years is around 30 to 35 percent, half of which is due to cardiac events and only about 4 percent may be due to strokes. For a series studying the long-term outcome of asymptomatic patients who had carotid endarterectomy, Thompson and colleagues[61] showed that 91 percent remained asymptomatic over a mean period of 55 months. Four and one-half percent developed TIAs, with almost all of these on the contralateral side. In the series of Lees and Hertzer,[60] after a mean follow-up of 8.6 years and after 390 carotid endarterectomies in 335 patients, 17 percent suffered late strokes, 7 percent of which were ipsilateral to the carotid endarterectomy. Of these patients, 25 percent developed contralateral asymptomatic stenosis. Of the entire series of 335 patients, approximately 90 percent were asymptomatic on the ipsilateral hemisphere after a mean follow-up of 8.6 years. In general, the long-term outcome of these patients depends somewhat on the preoperative indications for the operation. Asymptomatic patients have a lower incidence of developing TIAs or strokes in the late follow-up, whereas those patients operated on because of TIAs developed new symptoms in about 15 to 20 percent of cases, and approximately 5 percent developed stroke. All of these older data will probably be modified as we obtain information from the NASCET study. These patients are to be followed by duplex ultrasound examination annually, which may reveal developing stenosis or asymptomatic occlusion of the carotid artery that was operated on. These events do occur and the patients may suffer no symptoms. In the old literature, these patients were not studied. Suffice it to say that these patients need to undergo reexamination, at least on an annual basis, by duplex scan, plus a search for symptoms. It is to be anticipated that their advancing vascular disease will become manifest through cardiac events, as well as lower-extremity ischemic events.

Alternate Therapies

EXTRACRANIAL-INTRACRANIAL (EC-IC) BYPASS

If stenosis or occlusions of the carotid and vertebral arteries are not correctable (for example, with intracranial obstructions) and patients have compelling, crescendo TIAs, attempts at revascularization by utilizing the superficial temporal artery connected to one of the meningeal or middle cerebral arteries have been developed by the neurosurgeons.[62] The technique is demanding and the mortality and morbidity are such that a controlled study was conducted on the benefits of EC-IC and reported several years ago. The study is thought to be controversial, mainly because of patient selection and probable omission of groups of patients from the study in many institutions. Nevertheless, the conclusion from this study was that there seemed to be no therapeutic benefit from EC-IC for the usual indications, as stated.[64] The technique is important and special circumstances may require its application; but at present, it has no apparent role in patients who have cerebral ischemic events.[9,61,63]

ANGIOPLASTY

The development of angioplasty techniques is rapidly advancing, both in Europe and the United States. A trial in Europe is comparing balloon angioplasty with carotid endarterectomy in patients with symptomatic extracranial carotid disease.[65] Concern seems appropriate regarding the possibility of dislodging emboli that could lodge in the brain or retina. More data are needed to assess the role of angioplasty in patients with carotid artery disease.

Vertebral Artery Disease

Symptoms specific to vertebral artery stenosis are those involving the posterior brain. Bilateral intermittent visual changes, such as exaggerated orthostatic dizziness, are often subtle and difficult to evaluate as are the other symptoms of vertebral arterial insufficiency. Because of the great potential for collateral flow from the anterior circulation (e.g., carotid, via the circle of Willis) as well as through the posterior circulation, it is highly likely that severe stenoses of the vertebral, osteal, and/or main vertebral artery, occur in the absence of symptoms. In the presence of combined internal carotid artery stenoses and vertebral artery stenoses with symptoms suggestive of posterior brain ischemia and/or global ischemia, management is usually approached by correcting the carotid artery stenoses first, with relief of symptoms to be expected, if the circle of Willis is complete and collateral potential is present. However, it is appropriate to correct both the vertebral stenosis and the internal carotid stenosis at the same time. Transposition of the origin of the vertebral artery into the side of the common carotid artery is the usual technique, since access to the vertebral artery for an endarterectomy is more difficult (Fig.

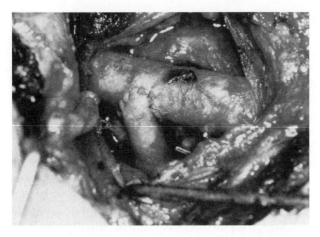

Figure 27-9 Completion of the anastomosis. [From Edwards WH: Direct vertebral artery reconstruction for vertebral basilar insufficiency. In Ernst CB, Stanley JC (eds): *Current Therapy in Vascular Surgery,* 2d ed, 1991. Reproduced by permission.]

27-9). Flow through the common carotid artery easily supports both anteroposterior circulation, so long as arch aortogram shows no stenosis at the origin of the common carotid arteries. The vertebral artery disease is the neglected sister of the four-vessel blood supply to the brain. It is now becoming more widely recognized as a source of vague symptoms and is more aggressively treated than in the past.

Subclavian steal is a clinical syndrome in which the patient notes weakness of the hand and/or arm on usage, with induction of vertigo and, occasionally, global ischemic symptoms. These symptoms are secondary to the retrograde flow that occurs from the brain down the vertebral in order to meet the blood supply needs of the arm when the subclavian artery origin is stenotic. This anatomic situation is present much more commonly than previously realized and most patients seem to be asymptomatic, even though retrograde flow from the brain to the arm is occurring. The brain can withstand the burden of supplying collateral flow to the arm, provided that the anterior circulation is unimpeded and the circle of Willis complete enough to allow perfusion of the entire brain.

When symptoms as noted above do develop, corrective measures can be applied. A short graft from the side of the common carotid artery to the side of the subclavian artery, utilizing a 6-mm Dacron or polytetrafluorethylene graft, is a popular choice. Occasionally, a saphenous vein graft is also utilized. If the patient has no symptoms related to the arm with the retrograde flow through the vertebral, another option is transposing the vertebral artery to the side of the common carotid to supply the brain and prevent retrograde steal. The anatomic opportunities and the probability of arm ischemia will dictate the surgical choices in the above situation. The long-term results are satis-

factory in about 90 percent of patients. Development of restenoses or advancing carotid artery atherosclerotic disease may require subsequent consideration.

Bibliography

1. Moore WS: Pathology of extracranial cerebrovascular disease. In Rutherford R (ed): *Vascular Surgery,* 2d ed. Philadelphia, WB Saunders, 1984:1202.
2. Gowers WR: On a case of simultaneous embolism of central retinal and middle cerebral arteries. *Lancet* 1875; 2:794.
3. Drake WE, Drake MAL: Clinical and angiographic correlates of cerebrovascular insufficiency. *Am J Med* 1968; 45:253.
4. Hollenhorst RW: Vascular status of patients who have cholesterol emboli in the retina. *Am J Ophthalmol* 1966; 61:1159.
5. Eastcott HHG, et al: Reconstruction of internal carotid artery in a patient with intermittent attacks of hemiplegia. *Lancet* 1954; 2:994.
6. DeBakey ME: Successful carotid endarterectomy for cerebrovascular insufficiency. Nineteen-year follow-up. *JAMA* 1975; 233:1083.
7. Carrea R, et al: Surgical treatment of spontaneous thrombosis of the internal carotid artery in the neck. Carotid-carotid anastomosis: Report of a case. *Acta Neurol Lat Am* 1955; 1:71.
8. Kunlin J: Le traitment de l'artérite obliterante par la greffe veineuse. *Arch Malad Coeur et Vaiss* 1949; 42:371.
9. Sergeant PT, et al: Carotid endarterectomy for cerebrovascular insufficiency: Long term follow-up of 141 patients followed up to 16 years. *Acta Chirurgica Belgica* 1980; 79(8):309.
10. Salasidis GC, et al: Carotid artery duplex scanning in preoperative assessment for coronary artery revascularization: The association between peripheral vascular disease, carotid artery stenosis and stroke. *J Vasc Surg* 1995; 21:154.
11. Johnson BF, et al: Clinical outcome in patients with mild and moderate carotid artery stenosis. *J Vasc Surg* 1995; 21:120.
12. Hart R: Personal communication.
13. North American Symptomatic Carotid Endarterectomy Trial Collaborators: Beneficial effect of carotid endarterectomy in symptomatic patients with high-grade carotid stenosis. *N Engl J Med* 1991; 325:445.
14. Clinical Advisory: Carotid endarterectomy for patients with asymptomatic internal carotid artery stenosis. Press release of the National Institute of Neurological Disorders and Stroke, National Institutes of Health. Bethesda MD, 1994.
15. Bornstein NM, et al: Significance of plaque ulceration in symptomatic patients with high-grade carotid stenosis. *Stroke* 1994; 25:304.
16. Barnett HJM, et al: Drugs and surgery in the prevention of ischemic stroke. *N Engl J Med* 1995; 332:238.
17. Norris JW, et al: Vascular risks of asymptomatic carotid stenosis. *Stroke* 1991; 22:1485.
18. Hennerici M, et al: Natural history of asymptomatic extracranial arterial disease: Results of a long-term prospective study. *Brain* 1987; 110:777.
19. The Asymptomatic Carotid Atherosclerosis Study Group: Study design of randomized prospective trial of carotid endarterectomy for asymptomatic atherosclerosis. *Stroke* 1989; 20:844.
20. Petersen P, et al: Placebo-controlled, randomized trial of warfarin and aspirin for prevention of thromboembolic complications in chronic atrial fibrillation: The Copenhagen AFASAK Study. *Lancet* 1989; 1:175.
21. The Boston Area Anticoagulation Trial for Atrial Fibrillation Investigators: The effect for low-dose warfarin on the risk of

stroke in patients with nonrheumatic atrial fibrillation. *N Engl J Med* 1990; 323:1505.

22. Connolly SJ, et al: Canadian Atrial Fibrillation Anticoagulation (CAFA) Study. *J Am Coll Cardiol* 1991; 18:349.

23. Stroke Prevention in Atrial Fibrillation Investigators: Stroke Prevention in Atrial Fibrillation Study: Final results. *Circulation* 1991; 84:527.

24. Ezekowitz MD, et al: Warfarin in the prevention of stroke associated with nonrheumatic atrial fibrillation. *N Engl J Med* 1992; 327:1406. [Erratum, *N Engl J Med* 1993; 328:148].

25. EAFT (European Atrial Fibrillatin Trial) Study Group: Secondary prevention in non-rheumatic atrial fibrillation after transient ischaemic attack or minor stroke. *Lancet* 1993; 342:1255.

26. The Stroke Prevention in Atrial Fibrillation Investigators: Predictors of thromboembolism in atrial fibrillation. I. Clinical features of patients at risk. *Ann Intern Med* 1992; 116:1.

27. Moulton AW, et al: Risk factors for stroke in patients with nonrheumatic atrial fibrillation: A case-control study. *Am J Med* 1991; 91:156.

28. Mustard JF, et al: The effect of sulfinpyrazone on platelet economy and thrombus formation in rabbits. *Blood* 1967; 29:859.

29. Harrison MJG, et al: Effect of aspirin in amaurosis fugax. *Lancet* 1971; 2:743.

30. Mundall J, et al: Transient monocular blindness and increased platelet aggregability treated with aspirin. *Neurology* 1972; 22:280.

31. The Canadian Cooperative Study Group: A randomized trial of aspirin and sulfinpyrazone in threatened stroke. *N Engl J Med* 1978; 299:53.

32. Acheson J, et al: Controlled trial of dipyridamole in cerebral vascular disease. *BMJ* 1969; 1:614.

33. Gent M, et al: A secondary prevention, randomized trial of suloctidil in patients with a recent history of thromboembolic stroke. *Stroke* 1985; 16:416.

34. Burch JW, et al: Sensitivity of fatty acid cyclocygenase from human aorta to acetylation by aspirin. *Proc Natl Acad Sci USA* 1978; 75:5181.

35. Moncada S, Vane JR: Prostacyclin: Its biosynthesis, actions and clinical potential. *Philos Trans R Soc Lond Biol* 1981; 294:305.

36. Bornstein NM, et al: Failure of aspirin treatment after stroke. *Stroke* 1994; 25:275.

37. Dyken ML: Controversies in stroke: past and present: The Willis Lecture. *Stroke* 1993; 24:1251.

38. DiMinno G, et al: Functionally thrombasthenic state in normal platelets following the administration of ticlopidine. *J Clin Invest* 1985; 75:328.

39. Saltiel E, Ward A: Ticlopidine: A review of its pharmacodynamic and pharmacokinetic properties, and therapeutic efficacy in platelet-dependent disease states. *Drugs* 1987; 34:222.

40. Winslow CM, et al: The appropriateness of carotid endarterectomy. *N Engl J Med* 1988; 319:124.

41. Barnett HJM, et al: Drugs and surgery in the prevention of ischemic stroke. *N Engl J Med* 1995; 322:244.

42. Dyken ML: Controversies in stroke: Past and present. The Willis Lecture. *Stroke* 1993; 24:1251.

43. European Carotid Surgery Trialists' Collaborative Group: MRC European Carotid Surgery Trial: Interim results for symptomatic patients with severe (70–99%) or with mild (0–29%) carotid stenosis. *Lancet* 1991; 337:1235.

44. Mayberg MR, et al: Carotid endarterectomy and prevention of cerebral ischemia in symptomatic carotid stenosis. *JAMA* 1991; 266:3289.

45. Dawson DL, et al: The role of duplex scanning and arteriography before carotid endarterectomy: A prospective study. *J Vasc Surg* 1993; 18:673.

46. Howard G, et al: A multicenter validation study of Doppler ultrasound versus angiography. *J Stroke Cerebrovasc Dis* 1991; 1:166.

47. Moneta GL, et al: Correlation of North American Symptomatic Carotid Endarterectomy Trial (NASCET) angiographic definition of 70% to 99% internal carotid artery stenosis with duplex scanning. *J Vasc Surg* 1993; 17:152.

48. Gasecki AP, et al: Early endarterectomy for severe carotid artery stenosis after a nondisabling stroke: Results from the North American Symptomatic Carotid Endarterectomy Trial. *J Vasc Surg* 1994; 20:288.

49. Eliasziw M, et al: Significance of plaque ulceration in symptomatic patients with high-grade carotid stenosis. North American Symptomatic Carotid Endarterectomy Trial. *Stroke* 1994; 24:304.

50. Bornstein NM, Norris JW: Management of patients with asymptomatic neck bruits and carotid stenosis. *Neurol Clin* 1992; 10:269.

51. Norris JW, et al: Vascular risks of asymptomatic carotid stenosis. *Stroke* 1991; 22:1485.

52. Hennerici M, et al: Natural history of asymptomatic extracranial arterial disease: Results of a long-term prospective study. *Brain* 1987; 110:777.

53. The CASANOVA Study Group: Carotid surgery versus medical therapy in asymptomatic carotid stenosis. *Stroke* 1991; 22:1229.

54. Mayo Asymptomatic Carotid Endarterectomy Study Group: Effectiveness of carotid endarterectomy for asymptomatic-carotid stenosis. *Mayo Clin Proc* 1989; 64:897.

55. Hobson RW II, et al: Efficacy of carotid endarterectomy for asymptomatic carotid stenosis. *N Engl J Med* 1993; 328:221.

56. Gewertz BL, McCafferty M: Intraoperative monitoring during carotid endarterectomy. *Curr Probl Surg* 1987; 24:475.

57. Ivanovic LV, et al: Spectral analysis of EEG during carotid endarterectomy. *Ann Vasc Surg* 1986; 1:112.

58. Claggett GP, et al: Vein patch versus primary closure for carotid endarterectomy. *J Vasc Surg* 1989; 9:213.

59. Pearce W: Perioperative care in major vascular operations. In Rutherford R (ed): *Vascular Surgery*, 2d ed. Philadelphia, WB Saunders, 1984:428.

60. Lees C, Hertzer N: Postoperative stroke after carotid endarterectomy. *Arch Surg* 1981; 116:1561.

61. Thompson JB, et al: Asymptomatic carotid bruit long term outcome after CEA. *Ann Surg* 1978; 188:308.

62. Yasargil MG, et al: Microneurosurgical arterial reconstruction. *Surgery* 1970; 67:221.

63. The EC/IC Bypass Study Group: Failure of EC-IC bypass to reduce the risk of ischemic stroke. *N Engl J Med* 1985; 313:1191.

64. Brown MM: Balloon angioplasty for cerebral vascular disease. *Neurol Res Suppl* 1992; 14:159.

CAROTID ARTERY DISEASE
Neuroanesthetic Management
ROSEMARY HICKEY

PREOPERATIVE ASSESSMENT AND PREPARATION
Cerebrovascular and Cardiovascular Disease
Carotid Endarterectomy and Coronary Artery Bypass Surgery

The mortality from stroke has declined in the United States since the 1970s; this has been attributed to improved diagnosis and treatment of risk factors. Despite this favorable trend, however, stroke remains a major health problem in the United States, representing both the third leading cause of death and a major cause of disability. Ischemic stroke syndromes most commonly result from arterial narrowing or occlusion and are classified according to the nature and time course of cerebral ischemic symptoms. These syndromes [transient ischemic attack (TIA), reversible ischemic neurologic deficit (RIND), stroke syndromes] are described in Chap. 27A. Surgical procedures such as carotid endarterectomy and extracranial-intracranial (EC-IC) bypass have been used as preventative treatments in certain of these ischemic stroke syndromes. Since the recent confirmation of the long-term benefits of carotid endarterectomy in patients with symptomatic internal carotid stenosis of 70 percent or greater,[1] the frequency of this procedure has increased dramatically. EC-IC procedures, on the other hand are now infrequently performed because of lack of documentation of their efficacy (see "Extracranial-Intracranial Bypass" below). This portion of the chapter will focus on anesthetic management of patients with ischemic cerebrovascular disease undergoing carotid endarterectomy and EC-IC bypass procedures. Preoperative evaluation, monitoring techniques, anesthetic choice, and postoperative complications will be reviewed.

Preoperative Assessment and Preparation

CEREBROVASCULAR AND CARDIOVASCULAR DISEASE

Preoperative assessment should focus on evaluation of the manifestations of arteriosclerosis, particularly in the cerebrovascular and cardiovascular systems. Evaluation of the cerebrovascular system should include careful documentation of the presence of transient or permanent neurologic deficits. This is essential in order to follow neurologic progress in the perioperative period, as well as helping to identify the patient's perioperative risk. Neurologic risk factors for carotid endarterectomy, as defined by Sundt and coworkers, include a progressive neurologic deficit, a deficit of less than 24 h duration, frequent daily TIAs, and multiple neurologic deficits secondary to cerebral infarctions.[2] Sundt and colleagues reported that patients with these unstable or progressing neurologic findings were at the highest risk (10 percent) for developing new postoperative neurologic deficits.[2] Other risk factors have also been identified. McCrory and colleagues recently evaluated 1160 patients retrospectively to determine the extent to which clinically significant adverse events could be predicted from preoperative clinical data.[3] They noted that significant predictors of adverse events were age (75 years or greater), symptom status (ipsilateral symptoms versus asymptomatic or nonipsilateral symptoms), severe hypertension (preoperative diastolic blood pressure of greater than 110 mmHg), carotid endarterectomy performed in preparation for coronary artery bypass surgery, history of angina, evidence of internal carotid artery thrombus, and internal carotid artery stenosis near the carotid siphon.[3] The presence of two or more of these risk factors was associated with a nearly two-fold increase in risk of an adverse event.[3] Because these authors found that patients with ipsilateral hemispheric symptoms were at greater risk of carotid endarterectomy complications compared to those who were asymptomatic or had nonipsilateral symptoms (8.5 percent had either stroke or myocardial infarction or died during the postoperative period), they further examined preoperative risk factors in these patients.[4] They found that the overall frequency of adverse outcomes was higher in the patients with complete ipsilateral carotid occlusions, ipsilateral intraluminal thrombus, or ipsilateral carotid siphon stenosis.[4] Those patients over age 75 had a greater risk of myocardial infarction but not of stroke or death.[4]

Cerebrovascular evaluation should also include notation of results of noninvasive tests (e.g., carotid duplex scan, transcranial doppler studies) as well as angiographic demonstration of vascular insufficiency. Cerebral angiography is the most reliable method of assessing the cerebral vascular system and demonstrating the location of the responsible lesion and the extent of arteriosclerotic narrowing of the vessel lumen. The adequacy of collateral circulation around the circle of Willis, as well as the presence of bilateral carotid disease, should be evident from angiography. Computed tomography (CT) or magnetic resonance imaging (MRI) may also have been performed to study the extent and location of infarcted brain tissue, as well as to rule out other lesions that mimic cerebral vascular occlusive disease.

In evaluating the cardiovascular system, it should be kept in mind that hypertension and coronary artery disease are frequently present. Hypertension, present in approximately 80 percent of the patients, should be medically controlled preoperatively. Asiddao and coworkers have demonstrated that postoperative hypertension and transient neurologic deficits are more frequent in patients with poor preoperative blood pressure (BP) control (BP > 170/95) than in those with adequate control or normotension.[5] Excessive lowering of the blood pressure should be avoided, however, because of the risk of developing symptomatic focal ischemia. Coronary artery disease (CAD) is frequently present in patients presenting for carotid endarterectomy, and is known to be the major cause of death in patients with cerebrovascular disease. Hertzer and coworkers reported the results of coronary angiography in 506 patients with extracranial cerebrovascular disease.[6] They noted that only 7 percent of these patients had normal coronary arteries.[6] Severe, surgically correctable CAD was documented in 28 percent of this series, and 7 percent of these patients had severe CAD that already was inoperable.[6] Chimowitz and colleagues recently examined the cardiac outcome of patients with asymptomatic carotid stenosis presenting for carotid endarterectomy.[7] They noted that 45 percent of patients had a history of CAD (history of CABG, angina, symptomatic MI, or evidence of an asymptomatic MI by ECG). During the study (follow-up average of 47.9 months), 43 percent of patients with CAD and 33 percent of patients without a history of CAD had cardiac ischemic events.[7] In patients without a history of CAD, factors that were independently associated with cardiac events included diabetes, intracranial occlusive disease, and peripheral vascular disease.[7] Thus, patients with these co-existing diseases, even in the absence of known CAD, should be considered high risk for adverse cardiac events.

Urbinati and coworkers assessed the prevalence and prognostic role of silent CAD in patients who were undergoing carotid endarterectomy for symptomatic high-grade carotid stenosis.[8] These patients underwent exercise ECG testing and thallium-201 myocardial scintigraphy.[8] They noted that silent CAD, as defined by abnormal testing in patients with no history, symptoms or ECG signs of CAD, was found in 25 percent of patients.[8] Although silent CAD did not affect the perioperative outcome in these patients, it did strongly influence the long-term prognosis.[8] During a 5.4-year follow up, cardiac ischemic events occurred in 29 percent of patients with silent CAD but only 1.2 percent of patients without CAD.[8] These results stress the importance of silent CAD in patients with severe carotid stenosis.

The strong association between carotid and cardiac disease as well as the increased risk posed by cardiac disease thus warrants careful preoperative assessment. Evidence of heart disease should be sought by historical data, particularly noting the presence of stable or unstable angina, previous myocardial infarction, or congestive heart failure. Signs of cardiac enlargement or failure should be sought on physical examination and chest radiograph. The electrocardiogram should be examined for abnormalities of cardiac rhythm or evidence of ischemia/infarction. Further cardiac diagnostic workup is individualized and coordinated with the cardiologist. This may include exercise ECGs and exercise thallium imaging,[9] dipyridamole thallium imaging, echocardiography, MUGA and coronary angiography. Fleisher and Beattie reported the results of a survey of cardiovascular anesthesiologists to determine the practice of preoperative cardiac evaluation of patients undergoing major vascular surgery.[10] They noted that in patients undergoing carotid endarterectomy, 59 percent of patients underwent preoperative cardiovascular testing.[10] This compared to 73 percent of patients undergoing aortic surgery and 54 percent of patients undergoing lower extremity revascularization.[10] There was no significant difference between university and private practices in the percentage of patients in whom testing was performed.[10] Dipyridamole or exercise thallium imaging was the most common test used, and Holter monitoring was the least common.[10] Testing was thought to modify perioperative monitoring in 80 percent of university institutions and 89 percent of private institutions.[10]

CAROTID ENDARTERECTOMY AND CORONARY ARTERY BYPASS SURGERY

Combined carotid endarterectomy and coronary artery bypass surgery has been advocated by some centers.[11-14] The basis for this recommendation has been the recognition of two patient groups: the first group includes those patients with known coronary artery disease who are found to have advanced carotid artery lesions preceding elective myocardial revascularization. The second group of patients are those that are scheduled for carotid endarterectomy who are found to have severe, surgically correctable coronary artery disease. The possibility of cerebral infarction after coronary artery bypass grafting (CABG) in the former group of patients and the high incidence of myocardial infarction after carotid endarterectomy in the latter group, has motivated interest in a combined surgical approach. Since 1972, when combined carotid and coronary artery surgery in patients with co-existing ischemic heart disease and cerebrovascular disease was proposed by Bernhard and colleagues,[15] numerous articles have been published about this issue. However, despite growing experience, the controversy in management and timing of surgical intervention in these two patient groups has not been totally resolved and in many instances depends on the specific referral pattern prevalent at the time and place the patient initially presents. Potential difficulties with a combined procedure include the necessity for heparinization that makes bleeding from the neck wound more likely and the delayed ability to detect new neurologic deficits postoperatively because of slow awakening from the cardiac anesthetic. The specific cause of a new neurologic deficit may also be difficult to ascertain because both procedures have associated neurologic risks.

OTHER DISEASES

Other diseases that are frequently present and require preoperative assessment includes diabetes mellitus and chronic obstructive pulmonary disease (COPD). Diabetes mellitus is present in approximately 20 percent of patients presenting for cerebral vascularization techniques,[6] and frequently requires insulin therapy. As noted by Chimowitz, patients with carotid stenosis and no history of CAD but who have diabetes have a risk of cardiac events similar to that of patients with a history of CAD.[7] Severe, inoperable coronary artery disease is also especially common among diabetics (14 percent incidence reported by Hertzer and coworkers in patients under evaluation for extracranial reconstruction[6]). The adequacy of blood glucose control should be ascertained preoperatively and the absence of ketoacidosis confirmed. Manifestations of common complications of diabetes mellitus should be sought, including renal failure, sensory and autonomic neuropathy (delayed gastric emptying, sick-sinus syndrome), coronary and peripheral atherosclerosis (silent MIs), and retinal/vitreous hemorrhage and blindness.[16]

Cigarette smoking has a number of undesirable effects in the perioperative period including an increase in airway irritability and secretions and a decrease in mucociliary transport. It also decreases forced vital capacity (FVC) and mid maximal expiratory flow rate (MMEF), and increases the incidence of postoperative pulmonary complications. Patients with chronic obstructive pulmonary disease should be given optimal medical treatment preoperatively, most often including aerosol therapy with bronchodilators. Corticosteroids may be required if there is a history of their recent prolonged use. To lower the likelihood of perioperative respiratory complications, cigarette smoking should be stopped for eight weeks preoperatively. There is also a significant reduction in carboxyhemoglobin levels in the first few days following cessation of smoking which is beneficial.

DRUG THERAPY

The patient's current drug therapy should be reviewed preoperatively. These patients are usually receiving several drugs on a long term basis. Frequent medications include antihypertensives, anticoagulant and antiplatelet therapy and cardiac medications. Insulin, antacids, and histamine (H_2) antagonists are also commonly administered. It is particularly important to continue all significant cardiovascular medications up to and including the morning of surgery, as perioperative discontinuation of these therapies may lead to perioperative ischemia.

PREMEDICATION

Premedication should be individualized but generally is given in small doses to avoid obscuring the development of new neurologic deficits. We commonly use a benzodiazepine (midazolam) and/or narcotic (fentanyl), titrating to effect when the patient arrives in the operating room. An antacid is also given preoperatively (sodium citrate) and in patients at higher risk of reflux (such as the diabetic or obese patient), metoclopramide and ranitidine are also given.

Choice of Anesthesia

Anesthesia for the patient undergoing carotid endarterectomy may be accomplished with either a regional or general anesthetic. Proponents of regional anesthesia point out that awake neurologic assessment is the ultimate test for the presence of cerebral ischemia. The time of onset of neurologic deficit is also apparent in the awake patient. This may enable the specific cause of the deficit (temporary cerebral ischemia during carotid occlusion, emboli, reperfusion injury, or carotid artery thrombosis) to be more easily determined[17] and in some instances corrected. Regional anesthesia has been used to allow selective placement of intraarterial bypass shunts during carotid cross clamping.[17-22] Changes in

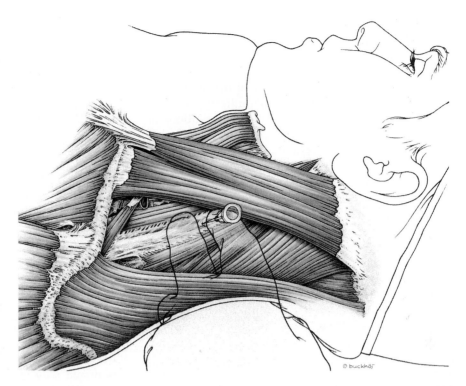

Figure 27-10   The single injection interscalene technique is performed by locating the interscalene groove between the anterior and middle scalene muscles. The needle is inserted between the palpating fingers in a direction that is perpendicular to the skin in all planes with a slight caudad direction. (Reprinted with permission from Winnie AP: Interscalene perivascular technique of brachial plexus block. In: *Plexus Anesthesia*. Philadelphia, W. B. Saunders, 1983:176.)

consciousness, hemiparesis, aphasia, visual disturbances, and inappropriate restlessness may all indicate cerebral ischemia in the awake patient.[18,20] If the patient tolerates the trial occlusion without developing any change in neurologic status, the procedure may proceed without a shunt being placed. If signs of cerebral ischemia develop, a shunt is placed to restore carotid flow. Based on this process of selective shunting by following neurologic status in patients receiving local anesthesia, 20 percent or less of patients may require shunt placement.[17-22] The proposed advantage of this approach is that the benefit of shunting is given to those who specifically need it to maintain cerebral blood flow and the complications of shunting are avoided in those with adequate collateral flow.

REGIONAL ANESTHESIA

A regional anesthetic for carotid endarterectomy is accomplished by a deep cervical plexus block. This may be performed by either a multiple injection technique or perhaps more simply by a single injection interscalene technique.[23] The single injection interscalene technique (Fig. 27-10) relies on the premise that the cervical plexus, like the brachial plexus, lies in the space between the anterior and middle scalene muscles and is enveloped by a fascial sheath that is continuous from the transverse processes of the cervical vertebrae to beyond the axilla. The cervical plexus is blocked by a single injection of local anesthetic within this fascial

sheath. The procedure is performed as follows: the patient is placed supine with the head turned opposite to the side being blocked. The lateral margin of the clavicular head of the sternocleidomastoid muscle is identified at the level of C4 (determined by noting the superior margin of the thyroid cartilage). The index and middle finger of the anesthesiologist's palpating hand are then rolled laterally across the anterior scalene muscle until the interscalene groove, between the anterior and middle scalene muscles, is palpated. A regional block needle (short bevel) is then inserted between the palpating fingers in a direction perpendicular to the skin in all planes with a slight caudad direction. The needle is then advanced and when a paresthesia is obtained, 10 to 15 ml of anesthetic solution is injected. The slight caudad direction is critical because if a nerve is not encountered by the advancing needle, the transverse process of the cervical vertebrae will provide a shield to deter further needle advancement into the epidural or subarachnoid spaces. An immobile needle technique[24] may be used in which a small bore intravenous extension tubing is placed between the needle and the syringe containing the anesthetic solution to provide stabilization of the needle during injection. Because the deep cervical block anesthetizes the cervical nerve roots themselves, it is not necessary to also perform a superficial cervical plexus block. In order to facilitate patient comfort when the head is turned to the side during the operative procedure, an additional injection to block the accessory nerve is beneficial. This is done by infiltrating the substance of the sternocleidomastoid muscle with 5 ml of local anesthetic below its attachment to the mastoid process.[25] If the upper end of the incision overlaps the area innervated by the trigeminal nerve or if the midline is crossed, additional local infiltration may be performed by the surgeon. Possible complications of deep cervical plexus block include unintentional subarachnoid, epidural, or vertebral artery injection. The risk of these complications is minimized by maintaining a slight caudad needle direction and by careful aspiration prior to injection. Other possible complications include block of the phrenic nerve leading to a paralyzed diaphragm, block of the recurrent laryngeal nerve leading to hoarseness, and block of the cervical sympathetic chain leading to Horner's syndrome. Castresana and coworkers recently evaluated the incidence of hemidiaphragmatic paresis in patients undergoing carotid endarterectomy with cervical plexus block anesthesia.[26] They noted that by fluoroscopy, 61 percent of patients had abnormal diaphragmatic motion.[26] There was a mean increase in Pa_{CO_2} of 4 mmHg, and in one patient with COPD, Pa_{CO_2} increased from 42 to 52 mmHg.[26] Thus, the authors recommended that cervical plexus block should be used with caution in patients with severe COPD. Also, if preexisting diaphragmatic paresis is already present, this should also be considered.

Spread to the lower roots of the brachial plexus can be minimized by maintaining digital pressure distal to the injection and by limiting the dose of local anesthetic. Fifteen milliliters or less is usually sufficient to provide anesthesia of the dermatomes necessary for carotid endarterectomy (C2-C4). The specific local anesthetic used often is dependent on the anticipated duration of the surgical procedure. One percent mepivacaine and 0.5% bupivacaine as well as a mixture of 1% mepivacaine and 0.2% tetracaine (made by dissolving 40 mg of tetracaine crystals in 20 ml of 1% mepivacaine) can all be used successfully. Epinephrine in a concentration to 1:200,000 is added to the local anesthetic solution, unless patient factors contraindicate its use.

REGIONAL VERSUS GENERAL

The choice of regional versus general anesthesia often depends on the preference and experience of both the surgeon and the anesthesiologist. Because of the ability to provide direct monitoring of cerebral function in the conscious patient, regional anesthesia may be particularly beneficial in settings where electrophysiologic monitoring is not available. Intraoperative neurologic changes have been correlated with postoperative neurologic outcome. Davies and coworkers reported a series of 389 patients undergoing carotid endarterectomy under cervical plexus block and noted that intraoperative neurologic changes predicted a high risk of postoperative stroke.[27] They noted that trial carotid artery cross clamping resulted in neurologic changes in 24 percent of patients, and these changes usually responded to declamping and shunt insertion.[27] However, patients who developed an intraoperative neurologic change had a significantly greater incidence of developing either temporary (11 percent) or permanent (6.6 percent) neurologic complications, compared to patients who did not develop intraoperative neurologic changes, where the incidence of temporary or permanent neurologic changes were 5 percent and 1.1 percent, respectively.[27]

It is important to keep in mind that the trachea will not be anesthetized by the regional block so it is possible that the patient may cough during the procedure. Constant communication should be maintained with the patient throughout the surgery because even though neurologic function may appear adequate at the time of carotid artery clamping, signs of cerebral ischemia may be delayed and occur at a time when surgical attention is directed elsewhere.[28] Proper patient selection is necessary to minimize the possibility of having to convert to general anesthesia midway through the procedure. Excessively anxious patients may not be able to lie still for the duration of the procedure or may experience claustrophobia due to the close proximity of the drapes. Also, if uncontrolled hemorrhage develops, the necessity to convert to general anesthesia with rapid intubation may become necessary.

One benefit of the regional block technique may be in the control of postoperative hypertension. Corson and colleagues reported that perioperative blood pressure was unstable for a significantly longer period of time after general anesthesia (mean, 24.6 h) than regional cervical block anesthesia (mean, 2.1 h) and that vasoactive drugs were required for significantly longer periods of time following general anesthesia.[29] The patients receiving regional anesthesia in this study were able to either return directly to the ward, or if they did go to the intensive care unit, it was for a significantly shorter period of time than the group receiving general anesthesia.[29] Likewise, Allen and coworkers noted that the use of cervical block anesthesia was associated with fewer perioperative cardiopulmonary complications and a shorter postoperative hospitalization when compared with general anesthesia.[21] Regional anesthesia was also associated with a significantly shorter operative time in this study, probably related to the fact that fewer patients in the regional group (19.2 percent) required use of a carotid artery shunt compared to those receiving a general anesthetic (42.1 percent).[21]

Monitors

CARDIOVASCULAR, GENERAL MONITORS

Whether the patient receives regional or general anesthesia, monitoring is primarily directed toward detecting any changes that develop in the cardiovascular and cerebrovascular systems. Electrocardiographic (ECG) monitoring is done with a five-lead system, with four electrodes on the extremities and a fifth electrode in the V_5 position (anterior axillary line in the fifth intercostal space). Leads II and V_5 are then displayed simultaneously, to detect arrhythmias as well as myocardial ischemia. ST segment analysis is also displayed. Other cardiovascular monitors should include an arterial line and in select instances a central venous line or pulmonary artery catheter. An arterial line is useful for continuous recording of blood pressure, which is often labile in these patients, and for intermittent determination of arterial blood gases. It is particularly beneficial during the period of carotid cross clamping, when maintenance of cerebral perfusion pressure is critical. A central venous catheter is useful for infusion of vasoactive drugs and, if placed, it is usually from an antecubital or subclavian approach. A pulmonary artery catheter is reserved for those patients with limited myocardial reserve associated with poor ventricular function or severe, uncorrected coronary artery disease. If available, two dimensional transesophageal echocardiography (2D-TEE) is a sensitive monitor of myocardial ischemia as detected from acute segmental wall motion abnormalities.[30]

MONITORING THE ADEQUACY OF CEREBRAL PERFUSION

Monitoring of the cerebrovascular system is directed toward assessing the adequacy of cerebral perfusion during the period of carotid cross clamping. Various modalities have been used for this, including jugular venous oxygen saturation, internal carotid artery occlusion pressure, regional cerebral blood flow, raw and processed electroencephalography (EEG), somatosensory evoked potentials, and the transcranial Doppler.

Jugular venous oxygen saturation (Sv_{O_2}) values of 50 percent or higher at the time of carotid artery cross clamping were originally felt to indicate adequate cerebral perfusion.[31] However, it was noted by Larson and coworkers that no reliable relationship could be established between Sv_{O_2} and cerebral function during trial carotid occlusion under local anesthesia.[32] The technique has now been largely abandoned for carotid surgery, with the realization that it is more a reflection of global hemispheric perfusion than focal cerebral ischemia.

Internal carotid artery occlusion pressure (stump pressure) is the pressure measured in the distal internal carotid artery when the common carotid artery is clamped. It represents the back pressure resulting from collateral circulation via the contralateral carotid artery and vertebrobasilar systems. It has the advantage of being easy and inexpensive to perform and has been widely used in the past. Unfortunately, however, it has not proven to be a reliable indicator of cerebral perfusion. The suggested minimally acceptable stump pressure of 50 to 55 mmHg[33] has been shown to be only a crude index of flow. McKay and coworkers demonstrated that only 58 percent of patients undergoing carotid endarterectomy demonstrated a positive correlation between regional cerebral blood flow (rCBF) and stump pressure (i.e., when both were either above or below their critical values of 18 to 24 ml/100g per min and 50 torr, respectively).[34] A poor correlation between stump pressure and EEG evidence of ischemia has been demonstrated[35] and neurologic changes have been seen in awake patients with presumably adequate stump pressure.[36] Stump pressure has been shown to vary when measured serially during normocapnic anesthesia.[37] McKay and colleagues also demonstrated that the relationship between stump pressure and rCBF is influenced by the anesthetic technique.[34] In the absence of transient ischemia during occlusion (rCBF > 18 ml/100g per min), halothane and enflurane anesthesia were associated with higher rCBFs and lower stump pressures than neuroleptanesthesia.[34] Besides the anesthetic, other factors such as Pa_{CO_2} may alter the relationship between stump pressure and flow by causing changes in cerebrovascular resistance. Manipulation of these variables may result in either cerebral vasodilation or cerebral vasoconstriction, both of which may alter the relationship between pressure and flow. Additional difficulties may arise in interpreting stump pressures. A stenotic or occlusive vascular lesion may exist between the measurement site and the area of brain at risk, making the stump pressure unreliable in predicting flow to that region. Also, the brief period that is used to measure stump pressure may not indicate changes that occur during the more prolonged period necessary for the endarterectomy.

Regional cerebral blood flow has been used to assess the adequacy of cerebral perfusion during carotid cross clamping. Sundt and coworkers have used a technique in which 200 to 300 μCi of xenon-133 diluted with saline to a total volume of 0.2 to 0.3 ml is injected into the common carotid artery (with the external carotid artery temporarily occluded).[38] A scintillation probe placed over the motor strip on the ipsilateral side is then used to calculate clearance curves, and from the initial slope of the curves, rCBF is determined. Blood flows are obtained prior to carotid occlusion, during occlusion, and after restoration of flow and if a shunt is in place additional measurements are taken. Using the technique, Sundt was able to correlate rCBF measurements with continuous EEG monitoring. He reported that reductions in flow with carotid occlusion below a critical range created changes in the EEG. Although this critical range varied according to the anesthetic used, occlusion flows of less than 10 ml/100g per min always produced rapid EEG changes, and flows of less than 15 ml/100g per min usually caused EEG changes. Other investigators have reported similar correlations between rCBF and EEG monitoring.[39,40] The complex nature and expense of this technique, however, has limited its use to only a few institutions.

The standard or unprocessed EEG has long been recognized as a sensitive indicator of the adequacy of cerebral perfusion. A 16-channel system is generally used and recordings are made continuously throughout the operative procedure. Intraoperative neurologic complications have correlated well with EEG changes indicative of ischemia. Sundt and coworkers reported that in a series of 1145 carotid endarterectomies, no patient had a prolonged or fixed neurologic deficit without an associated EEG abnormality.[38] McFarland and colleagues, in his series of 392 carotid endarterectomies, also reported that the EEG was predictive of neurologic deficits occurring during surgery, and all of his patients with no significant EEG changes during surgery awoke without apparent neurologic deficit.[41] Both of these investigators used EEG monitoring as the basis for selective shunt placement. Redekop and Ferguson correlated intraoperative EEG changes with the risk of stroke during 293 carotid endarterectomies performed without the use of a shunt.[42] They noted that the risk of postoperative neurologic deficit was significantly higher in patients developing major EEG changes (4 of 22, 18.2 percent) than in those without such changes (5 of 271, 1.8 percent).[42] Ipsilateral attenuation of amplitude/slowing are the most commonly seen changes during carotid cross clamping.[41] Despite the benefits of raw EEG monitoring and its use for carotid endarterectomy in many major institutions,[43] its use has been limited by a number of factors, mostly technical in nature. An experienced EEG technician often in combination with a neurologist is necessary to set up the cumbersome equipment and interpret the large amount of data that is generated. To improve the practicality of monitoring, some institutions rely primarily on a well-trained EEG technician with a physician electroencephalographer available for backup and consultation.[44] To alleviate the problem of displaying meaningful EEG data to the anesthesiologist in a short period of time, various processed methods of EEG analysis have been devised, including the compressed spectral array and density spectral array.

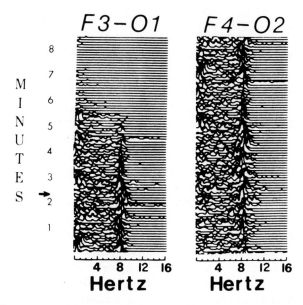

Figure 27-11 Intraoperative CSA recording during test clamping of the left carotid artery. After clamping (at the arrow) the 8 Hz activity in the left fronto-occipital channel (F3-O1) continued to be symmetrical for 1 min, and then progressively deteriorated. (Reprinted with permission from Myers RR, et al: Monitoring of cerebral perfusion during anesthesia by time compressed fourier analysis of the electroencephalogram. *Stroke* 8:331, 1977.)

The compressed spectral array (CSA) presents a power spectrum analysis of the EEG in the form of a plot of amplitude versus frequency for each period of time known as an epoch (usually 2 to 16 s). By shifting the origin of the plot vertically with time, a three dimensional graph is created in which there appears to be hills at those frequencies making large contributions to the EEG, and valleys at frequencies that contain less power.[45] The spectral edge (SE), which is the frequency below which most (95 to 99 percent) of the EEG in the current spectrum lies, is also displayed on the CSA monitor. The benefit of the CSA in demonstrating cerebral ischemia has been shown by Myers and coworkers[46] (Fig. 27-11) and Chiappa and colleagues.[47] A disadvantage of the CSA is that time and amplitude are both compressed onto the same axis, which makes determination of the temporal relationship of events somewhat difficult.[48] Also, the hills created by high amplitude activity may obscure subsequent low amplitude activity at the same frequency.

Density spectral analysis (DSA) allows display of the power spectrum analysis without loss of data hidden behind the hills of the CSA. The display is a density-modulated gray scale in which each epoch of the spectral analysis is displayed as a line of varying density or a series of dots of various sizes.[45] The areas of maximum intensity (or largest dots) correspond to the frequencies that make the largest contribution to the EEG spectrum.[45] Using DSA for detection of cerebral ischemia during carotid endarterectomy, Kearse and co-workers noted that the DSA was not as reliable in detecting mild 16-channel analog EEG ischemic pattern changes, as it was in detecting severe changes.[49] However, in many institutions 16-channel EEG monitoring is not available, and therefore CSA/DSA monitoring appears appropriate. The equipment displaying the CSA/DSA may also include a display of the raw EEG for a limited number of channels (usually two to four channels). This allows for correlation of the CSA/DSA with raw EEG activity.

Somatosensory evoked potentials (SSEPs) may also be useful during carotid endarterectomy. Branston and colleagues found a threshold relationship between cortical cerebral blood flow and cortical SSEPs.[50] If the local cortical cerebral blood flow was greater than 16 ml/100g per min, the SSEP was not affected; however at flows less than approximately 12 ml/100g per min, the evoked potential was abolished.[50] Complete loss of certain components of the SSEP has been associated with a worsening of neuropsychological abilities and in some instances with subsequent strokes.[51] Changes in the SSEP that have been reversed with shunt insertion or raising the arterial blood pressure have also been demonstrated.[52] In terms of reliability, Horsch and coworkers reported a sensitivity of intraoperative SSEP monitoring in predicting neurologic outcome of 60 percent with a specificity of 100 percent.[53] Lam and coworkers compared the use of conventional electroencephalogram and somatosensory evoked potentials for detecting postoperative neurologic deficits and reported a sensitivity and specificity of 50 percent and 92 percent for EEG and 100 percent and 94 percent for SSEP, respectively, differences that were not statistically significant.[54] Two of 64 patients in this series had transient neurologic deficits postoperatively, with both having SSEP changes, whereas one had EEG changes.[54] It was also noted that amplitude reduction greater than 50 percent was a better indicator of postoperative neurologic deficit than latency increase (increase in central conduction time greater than 1 ms), because of the lack of sensitivity of latency changes.[54] It is also important to note that the use of the N_{20} component (the primary short-latency component) for analysis of amplitude is more appropriate than the later components, because the later components are more susceptible to anesthetic influence which may interfere with interpretation.[54] Shunts were not used in this study, regardless of changes in the EEG or SSEP, providing a unique opportunity to correlate monitoring changes with postoperative neurologic deficits. Other authors have used SSEP changes to determine the need for shunt insertion (Fig. 27-12).[55,56] Fiori and Parenti recently reported results of two channel computerized EEG and SSEP monitoring during 255 ca-

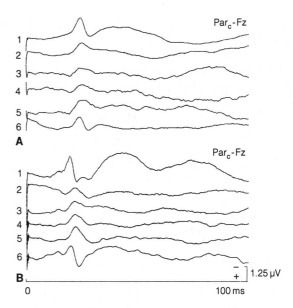

Figure 27-12   Intraoperative SEPs in two patients with SEP changes within 2 min after clamping: *A.* Trace 1: preclamping; Trace 2: 2 min after clamping; Traces 3, 4: 5 and 30 min after shunt application; Traces 5, 6: late improvement after awakening. *B.* Trace 1: preclamping; Trace 2, 3: 1 and 2 min after clamping; Trace 4: 30 min after shunt application; Trace 5, 6: late improvement before awakening. (Reprinted with permission from Amantini A, et al: Monitoring of somatosensory evoked potentials during carotid endarterectomy. *J Neurol* 1992; 239:241.)

rotid endarterectomies.[57] They used CSA (onset of clear asymmetry between the two channels with the lost of fast frequencies ipsilateral to the cross clamp) and SSEP (complete loss of the cortical wave) changes to determine the need for shunting.[57] Other SSEP changes (central conduction time increase > 1 ms or N_{20} amplitude reduction > 50 percent) were treated with increasing the systolic arterial pressure.[57] They noted no false negatives (patients that did not have loss of the cortical SSEP wave and EEG changes never developed clinical symptoms) with the monitoring combination, and their one case with persisting EEG asymmetry showed an irreversible postoperative deficit.[57]

Recently, transcranial Doppler ultrasonography (TCD) has evolved as a means of monitoring blood flow velocity in the middle cerebral artery of patients undergoing carotid endarterectomy. This technique has the potential to detect hemodynamic changes as well as embolic phenomenon. McDowell examined the stroke rate in patients classified as having no (velocity > 41 percent of baseline), mild (velocity 16 to 40 percent of baseline), or severe (velocity 0–15 percent of baseline) ischemia at the time of carotid cross clamping.[58] They noted that for patients with no ischemia by TCD, stroke rate was significantly lower without the use of a shunt. For patients with severe ischemia by TCD, strokes were less frequent with a shunt.[58] For mild ischemia by TCD, shunting did not significantly affect the stroke rate.[58] These authors, therefore, concluded that shunting is not necessary for most carotid surgery, but is recommended when severe TCD ischemia is present (approximately 10 percent of patients in their series). They also noted that neurologic morbidity was usually, but not always, preceded by both EEG and TCD evidence of ischemia. They suggested that the reason that in some cases one of these techniques may show ischemia when the other does not, may be related to the fact that the EEG is a good indicator of cerebral cortical activity, and the TCD is a better test of deeper portions of the hemisphere such as the basal ganglia and internal capsule.[58]

Jansen and coworkers have noted that the TCD provides direct feedback about thromboembolism that is not detected by EEG alone.[59] They noted that the immediate acoustic feedback from the TCD may have a direct influence on the surgical technique, alerting the surgeon of embolic phenomenon.[59] In a comparison of preoperative and postoperative CT scans or MRIs of the brain, Jansen and colleagues noted that there was a significant relation between the number of embolic signals during the surgical dissection of the carotid artery and the occurrence of intraoperative infarcts as detected by new lesions on CT or MRI (although four of five infarcts were clinically silent).[60] The TCD has also been used for assessing the effect of carotid endarterectomy in removing the suspected source of cerebral microemboli.[61] Preoperative TCD evaluation with determination of the number of high-intensity transient signals per hour indicating microemboli can be compared with postoperative TCD studies.[61] Van Zuilen and coworkers noted that carotid endarterectomy resulted in a significant reduction in the number of high-intensity transient signals per hour seven days and three months after surgery.[61] They suggest that ongoing microemboli to the brain at that time may prompt reevaluation of the operated carotid artery or a search for other sources of microemboli. A case report of incipient carotid artery thrombosis diagnosed by TCD has been reported (Fig. 27-13).[62] In this case report, it was noted on closure of the neck that MCA velocity began to fall and intermittent signals consistent with microembolism were detected.[62] As these continued to worsen, it was decided to reexplore the operative site and a thrombotic stenosis in the internal carotid artery was noted.[62] With removal of the thrombosis, the MCA velocity increased and no further microembolization was detected.[62]

In summary, many techniques have been suggested to determine the adequacy of cerebral perfusion during carotid endarterectomy. Sv_{O_2} and stump pressure are of limited benefit. The unprocessed 16-channel EEG and measurement of rCBF are valuable, but lack of

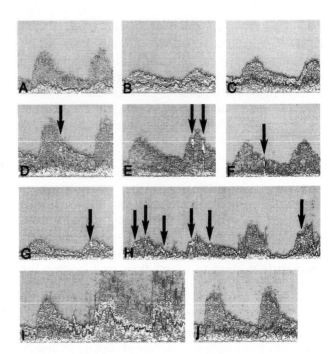

Figure 27-13   TCD printouts showing MCA velocity changes and detection of emboli (emboli are indicated by arrows). *A.* Start of operation. Average velocity = 48 cm/s. *B.* Carotid artery clamped. Average velocity decreases to 24 cm/s. *C.* Shunt opened. Average velocity = 42 cm/s. *D.* Flow restored through carotid artery. Average velocity = 68 cm/s. First embolus noticed. *E.* and *F.* MCA velocity falling. More emboli noted. *G.* Artery is nearly occluded. Emboli are still occuring. *H.* Reopening neck. Handling ICA results in numerous emboli followed by velocity increase from 26 to 40 cm/s. *I.* Injection of contrast during on-table arteriography results in flow disturbance. *J.* End of operation. Average velocity = 57 cm/s, maintained after the procedure. (Reprinted with permission from Gaunt ME, et al: On-table diagnosis of incipient carotid artery thrombosis during carotid endarterectomy by transcranial doppler scanning. *J Vasc Surg* 1994; 20:104.)

technical support and equipment availability may preclude their use. SSEPs are useful to those that are experienced in their application. Processed EEG techniques such as the CSA and the DSA are beneficial to the anesthesiologist because of the ease of their use for the amount of information that is obtained. The transcranial Doppler is a recent addition to monitoring techniques and appears useful to provide both hemodynamic and embolic information relating to perfusion of the jeopardized brain territory.

Anesthetic Technique

ANESTHETIC INDUCTION AND MAINTENANCE

The goal of anesthetic induction is to maintain stable cardiovascular parameters such that cerebral and myocardial blood flows are maintained. These patients are often hypertensive, with a depleted volume status, and careful fluid replacement prior to and during induction is beneficial in minimizing blood pressure liability. Esmolol is beneficial in blunting the increases in heart rate and arterial blood pressure associated with endotracheal intubation.[63] Because its duration of action is so brief, its effects will not linger to the time of carotid cross clamping when beta blockade is undesirable. A variety of anesthetic agents may be chosen for induction. The combination that we have found most successful includes narcotics (usually fentanyl), thiopental or etomidate, lidocaine, and a nondepolarizing muscle relaxant (usually vecuronium or rocuronium). Laryngoscopy is of short duration with care provided to avoid rough airway manipulation. After confirmation of tracheal tube placement by bilateral breath sounds and end-tidal CO_2 recordings, the tracheal tube is carefully and securely taped, keeping in mind that once the drapes are placed, access to the airway is usually limited. Ventilation is then controlled to maintain normocarbia.

Like the induction agent, various anesthetic agents may all be used successfully for anesthetic maintenance. We prefer to use a base of narcotics (usually fentanyl) with or without nitrous oxide with the addition of isoflurane. Although a difference in neurologic outcome following carotid endarterectomy has not been shown among the different inhalational agents, isoflurane relative to halothane and enflurane offers an advantage. Michenfelder and coworkers found that the critical cerebral blood flow (CBF), below which the majority of patients developed ischemic changes within 3 min of carotid occlusion, was lower for isoflurane than halothane or enflurane.[64] We maintain muscle relaxation throughout the case, usually with vecuronium or rocuronium. These muscle relaxants have the advantage of lacking significant cardiovascular effects that may be associated with adverse alterations in myocardial oxygen supply and demand. Their intermediate duration of action necessitates frequent monitoring of neuromuscular status and frequent dosing to maintain paralysis. Reversal of its effects at the end of the case is rarely a problem.

Arterial blood gases are checked shortly after induction and then intermittently as necessary to assess the adequacy of oxygenation and to make sure that arterial carbon dioxide (Pa_{CO_2}) is maintained within a normal range. At one time it was recommended that hypercarbia should be maintained in an attempt to increase CBF. However, blood vessels to ischemic brain may be maximally dilated. Raising Pa_{CO_2} would then dilate only the normal vessels so that flow would actually be diverted from diseased to normal areas (intracranial steal). Conversely, hypocapnia would constrict the normal vessels so that flow would increase to the ischemic area (Robin Hood effect). The response to CO_2 in any given patient, however, may be variable. Waltz

and colleagues found that a normal response (an increase in CBF with an increase in Pa_{CO_2}), an attenuated response (only a slight increase in CBF with an increase in Pa_{CO_2}), and a paradoxical response (a decrease in CBF with an increase in Pa_{CO_2}) could all be seen in patients undergoing carotid endarterectomy.[65] The effects of Pa_{CO_2} manipulation cannot be totally predicted in these patients and maintenance at their level of normocapnia is now felt to be the safest approach. Thiel and coworkers recently looked at preoperative cerebrovascular reactivity to carbon dioxide inhalation in an attempt to predict intraoperative SEP changes with carotid clamping.[66] They wanted to determine if patients with poor intracerebral collaterization, as reflected by impaired cerebrovascular reactivity to CO_2 inhalation on preoperative TCD testing, would have an increased risk of cerebral ischemia during carotid surgery. They found, however, that the incidence of critical SEP changes was not significantly different between patients showing impaired carbon dioxide reactivity and the remaining patients.[66]

The maintenance of adequate oxygenation is also of utmost importance in these patients. Cerebral oxygen delivery is dependent upon both the CBF and the oxygen content of the arterial blood. It is not only necessary to assure that CBF remains adequate, but also that the oxygenation of the blood that reaches the brain is not compromised. Unless necessary to avoid hypoglycemia, the intraoperative use of glucose containing solutions should be avoided. Even modest elevations in brain glucose may augment post-ischemic cerebral injury.

Arterial blood pressure should be maintained within a range that is normal for that patient and during the period of carotid cross clamping at or slightly above this level. Knowledge of the patient's preoperative blood pressure recordings in relation to neurologic status is most helpful in determining that range. Cerebral autoregulation, which maintains CBF relatively constant within a mean arterial pressure range of approximately 50 to 150 mmHg may be impaired in these patients. They are often hypertensive, which shifts the upper and lower limits of autoregulation to higher levels. Autoregulation may also be lost in areas of cerebral ischemia. Therefore, maintenance of mean arterial blood pressure (MAP) will be a critical factor in the maintenance of CBF. When excessive reductions in MAP occur, particularly during the time of carotid cross clamping, cerebral perfusion pressure (CPP) and the adequacy of CBF via collateral circulation will be compromised. If MAP falls below an acceptable range for that patient, a reduction in concentration of the volatile anesthetic agent, which in our instance is usually isoflurane, is first attempted. This usually is effective in restoring MAP to acceptable levels. In those instances in which it is not effective, vasopressors such as phenylephrine may be added. While MAP should not be allowed to decrease, it is also important to avoid marked increases in blood pressure that may be associated with factors such as light anesthesia or overtreatment with vasopressors. These patients, as mentioned earlier, often have significant cardiovascular disease. Increases in blood pressure and heart rate increase myocardial oxygen requirements which may lead to myocardial ischemia. There is evidence to suggest that the intraoperative use of vasopressors in patients with heart disease undergoing carotid endarterectomy may increase the risk of cardiac complications. Riles and coworkers reported that the risk of myocardial infarction increased from 2.9 percent to 8.1 percent with the intraoperative use of metaraminol in patients with a history of heart disease.[67] Smith and colleagues implicated phenylephrine in the development of intraoperative myocardial ischemia.[68] In this study of 60 patients undergoing carotid endarterectomy, blood pressure was kept within 20 percent of each patient's average ward systolic pressure by halothane or isoflurane (with N_2O) either at a low concentration alone or at a higher concentration with phenylephrine added to support blood pressure.[68] Myocardial ischemia was measured intraoperatively by left ventricular end-systolic wall stress and rate-corrected velocity of fiber shortening, as determined by echocardiography.[68] The incidence of myocardial ischemia was higher in those patients who received phenylephrine than those patients who had light anesthesia to maintain similar systolic pressures.[68] Although no patient in this study developed a perioperative MI, the differences in echocardiograms suggested that maintenance of blood pressure may be better achieved by lowering the concentration of inhalational agent than adding phenylephrine. These issues gain particular importance when one considers that myocardial infarction is the leading cause of both perioperative and late death following carotid endarterectomy.

Surgical manipulation in the area of the carotid sinus during carotid mobilization may cause marked alterations in heart rate and blood pressure. Stretch of the afferent nerve fibers may produce reflex bradycardia/hypotension. The reflex can be modified by the local infiltration of lidocaine, which is done routinely by some surgeons. Temporarily halting surgical manipulation, and, if necessary, the intravenous administration of atropine, are effective methods of treatment. Perkins and coworkers reported the effects of lidocaine accidently injected into the carotid artery during intraoperative attempts to block carotid sinus nerve activity.[69] They reported two cases in which transient EEG alterations consistent with severe cerebral dysfunction were observed during carotid endarterectomy. The proximity in time of the EEG changes to the carotid

sinus injection, the appearance of bisynchronous spikes, and the transient nature of the changes suggested that they were secondary to CNS lidocaine toxicity rather than ischemia. Although this complication is probably uncommon, it should be kept in mind as a possibility when EEG changes develop shortly after carotid sinus infiltration. Bishop and Johnstone reported a case in which signs of CNS toxicity of lidocaine developed in a patient receiving local injection of lidocaine into the wound and around the carotid artery during carotid endarterectomy.[70] These symptoms were successfully treated with small boluses of propofol followed by a low dose infusion.[70]

USE OF A SHUNT TO MAINTAIN CEREBRAL PERFUSION

During the period of carotid cross clamping, attempts are made to detect signs indicative of inadequate cerebral perfusion. The various monitoring devices that may be used for this purpose have already been discussed. Some surgeons will routinely employ a shunt as a means of cerebral protection, some use one selectively based on an assessment of collateral circulation, and others rarely if ever use a shunt. Proponents of routine shunting note that it allows an unhurried pace for the endarterectomy, enhances the technical facility with which it is inserted, and avoids the hazards of a rushed insertion at a critical stage during the endarterectomy.[71] They also point out that if meticulous surgical technique is used, many of the potential complications of a shunt may be avoided.[72] Others use methods to assess the cerebral circulation in an attempt to limit the use of intraoperative shunts to those instances in which evidence of cerebral ischemia is present. Sundt and coworkers used selective shunting based on a correlation between EEG changes and a fall in CBF below the critical level required for adequate perfusion during the period of carotid occlusion.[73] This series of 1935 patients was retrospectively analyzed and divided into four risk categories for surgery based on medical and neurologic risks and angiographic findings.[73] They found that shunts were required in 30 percent of the low risk group and 56 percent of the high risk group.[73] Based on the severity of reductions of CBF during the period of carotid occlusion (CBF $\leq$10 ml/100g per min), they concluded that 12 percent of all patients would have sustained a major deficit without shunting.[73] The risk of shunting, determined by EEG abnormalities during placement or use of the shunt and in some instances documented by visualization of atherosclerotic material traversing the shunt, was 0.5 percent in his series.[73] Although this incidence was low, it was felt that the risk was significant enough not to routinely employ a shunt. As an alternative to selective shunting, some surgeons perform carotid endarterectomy routinely without a shunt. They have advocated that the risk of temporary carotid clamping has been exaggerated and that most intraoperative stroke is the result of embolization, the risk of which is increased by the use of a shunt. They also report that equally good or superior results may be achieved without the use of a shunt.[74] Another potential complication of shunting is improper placement of the shunt, such as subintimal insertion.

A prospective, randomized study by Gumerlock and Neuwelt suggested that the use of a shunt in their neurosurgical practice (residency training program) was associated with fewer postoperative neurologic deficits.[75] In their study of 118 patients undergoing carotid endarterectomy without cerebral monitoring techniques, there were no cerebral infarctions in the shunted group and six in the unshunted group, a difference which was statistically significant.[75] Halsey reported a retrospective study of 1495 carotid endarterectomies monitored with transcranial Doppler, and each group was subdivided according to shunt use.[76] He noted that in patients with severe ischemia by transcranial Doppler that persisted, the rate of severe stroke was very high when no shunt was used (46 percent).[76] If ischemia did not occur with transcranial Doppler monitoring, the stroke rate was higher with shunting (4.4 percent), than when no shunt was used (0.7 percent).[76]

ANESTHETIC EMERGENCE

The concentration of inhaled anesthetic is gradually tapered toward the end of the procedure. Lidocaine 1 mg/kg may be given to help prevent excessive coughing during emergence. Neuromuscular blockade is allowed to partially recover but is not fully reversed until the anesthesiologist has adequate access to the airway. The N_2O or air is then discontinued and the patient is allowed to breathe 100% oxygen. Confirmation of recovery from neuromuscular blockade and maintenance of adequate arterial oxygenation is necessary prior to extubation. A prompt and smooth emergence with extubation in the operating room is ideal. This allows immediate assessment of neurologic function and evaluation of any abnormalities present. If the patient does not awaken promptly or if ventilation is inadequate, the patient may be transferred to the recovery room with the endotracheal tube in place. ECG and direct arterial pressure monitoring should be continued in the recovery room as blood pressure is often labile during this period. Treatment of hypertension during emergence from anesthesia and in the immediate postoperative period is often necessary. We have found that this is usually best accomplished with esmolol and/or labetelol.

Postoperative Complications

ABNORMALITIES OF SYSTEMIC BLOOD PRESSURE

Hypertension is a common complication following carotid endarterectomy, occurring in approximately 60 percent of patients. Blood pressure elevation is often greatest in the first 2 to 3 h following surgery but may remain elevated for 24 or more hours.[77,78] Preoperative hypertension, particularly uncontrolled, is a major determinant for the development of postoperative hypertension.[4,79] Patients who develop postoperative hypertension have an increased risk of neurologic deficit.[78,79] Hans and Glover reported the relationship of cardiac and neurologic complications to blood pressure changes in 330 patients undergoing carotid endarterectomy.[78] They noted that of the four patients developing perioperative myocardial infarction, none had postoperative hypertension.[78] However of the 11 patients (3.3 percent) that developed new neurologic deficits, 10 of these patients had experienced postoperative hypertension.[78] Control of postoperative hypertension is also important to minimize the risk of postoperative intracerebral hemorrhage, which is most commonly related to a post-endarterectomy hyperperfusion syndrome. This syndrome is typically seen in patients with a high-grade stenotic lesion who develop a major increase in CBF after completion of the endarterectomy.[38]

Carotid baroreceptors have been postulated to be involved in the etiology of postoperative hypertension and hypotension. They are present in the adventitial tissue at the carotid bifurcation and are innervated by the carotid sinus nerve. Efferent impulses from the carotid sinus travel to the vasomotor center in the medulla. Carotid sinus stimulation inhibits central nervous system sympathetic activity resulting in a reduction of heart rate and blood pressure, while carotid sinus inactivation causes the reverse effect.[77] Surgical techniques during carotid endarterectomy may entail dissection/division of the carotid sinus nerve. The decrease of carotid baroreceptor impulses secondary to carotid sinus nerve trauma may play a role in the development of postoperative hypertension. Post-endarterectomy hypotension may also reflect abnormal carotid sinus nerve activity.[77,80] Baroreceptor function diminishes with age and in the presence of cerebrovascular disease. It is hypothesized that atheromatous plaques dampen the pressure wave reaching the carotid sinus baroreceptors.[80] With endarterectomy, removal of the plaque results in increased stimulation of the baroreceptors, producing bradycardia and hypotension.[80] This response, which may be exaggerated in the presence of hypovolemia, is usually short-lived, as the baroreceptors theoretically reset to a new level of stimulation.[80] Local anesthetic injected into the carotid sinus region may help prevent this complication.[81-83]

MYOCARDIAL INFARCTION

The incidence of myocardial infarction varies according to the series reported but is approximately 2 percent, and is the most frequent cause of perioperative mortality. Riles and coworkers reported an overall incidence of myocardial infarction following carotid endarterectomy of 2.3 percent, increasing from 0.5 percent for patients without heart disease to 4.9 percent for patients with known preexisting heart disease.[67] Patients over the age of 75 also have a greater risk of perioperative myocardial infarction.[3] Musser and coworkers retrospectively examined death and adverse cardiac events according to the Goldman Index.[84] They noted that the incidence of myocardial infarction, fatal myocardial infarction, and death from all causes increased with increasing Goldman class assignment. For the Goldman classes I, II, and III, the rates of myocardial infarction were 0.9 percent, 2.7 percent, and 15.4 percent respectively. Thus the strong association between cardiac disease and carotid disease is again emphasized.

NEUROLOGIC COMPLICATIONS

Neurologic deficits following carotid endarterectomy may result from a variety of factors. Riles and coworkers recently examined the cause of perioperative stroke in 3062 carotid endarterectomies performed from 1965 through 1991.[85] Patients receiving local anesthesia were shunted if they demonstrated signs of ischemia with test clamping and patients receiving general anesthesia had an intraarterial shunt placed.[85] More than 20 different mechanisms of perioperative stroke were identified, but could be grouped into five major categories.[85] These included postoperative thrombosis and embolism ($n = 25$), intracerebral hemorrhage ($n = 12$), ischemia during carotid artery clamping ($n = 10$), strokes from other mechanisms associated with the surgery ($n = 8$), and stroke unrelated to the reconstructed artery ($n = 8$).[85] Dividing the operative experience into time periods, they noted a recent decrease in perioperative stroke caused by ischemia during clamping and intracerebral hemorrhage, with postoperative thrombosis and embolism remaining the major cause of neurologic complications.[85] They also noted that most perioperative strokes (65 percent) could be traced back to technical mishaps occurring during placement of a shunt, endarterectomy or carotid artery reconstruction.[85] Peer and coworkers examined the records of patients (27 of 920 endarterectomies) requiring early reoperation during a 10-year period with respect to operative findings and clinical outcome.[86] They noted that early reexploration was required in 3 percent of patients, for either expanding hematoma (6 patients) or suspected thrombosis associated with a new neurologic deficit (21 patients).[86] In the patients with a new neurologic deficit, thrombosis was confirmed in 19 of the 21 cases (91 percent), more often due to arterial narrowing than to an intimal defect.[86] Prompt repair resulted in improvement in clinical status in 50 percent of patients, with severe contralateral disease more common among patients with residual deficits. Thus, postoperative thrombosis is a serious complication whose consequences may be improved by emergent reexploration.

HEMORRHAGE

Postoperative hemorrhage at the wound site may result from disruption or bleeding at the arteriotomy site or from surrounding tissues. Bleeding into the neck may rapidly lead to airway compromise. This necessitates reintubation and surgical evacuation of the hematoma. Prompt exploration can be lifesaving in these instances.[86]

CRANIAL NERVE INJURIES

Cranial nerve injuries may also be identified in the postoperative period. The incidence of clinically recognized nerve deficits is approximately 3 percent[87-89] but may be higher if more aggressive diagnostic tests and specialist evaluations are performed.[88] The hypoglossal is the nerve most exposed to injury during carotid endarterectomy, but fortunately is usually easily identified and thus rarely severed.[87] Temporary injury due to traction or pressure is more common.[87] The recurrent laryngeal nerve and mandibular branch of the facial nerve are the other nerves most commonly injured. Damage to the recurrent laryngeal nerve may result in hoarseness due to vocal cord paralysis. Hypoglossal nerve injury may lead to inarticulate speech and difficulty chewing food, and injury to the mandibular branch of the facial nerve results in drooping of the corner of the mouth.[87] The possibility of serious airway problems secondary to bilateral cranial nerve injuries mandates careful preoperative evaluation to detect residual cranial nerve deficits prior to sequential carotid endarterectomies.

LOSS OF CAROTID BODY FUNCTION

Bilateral carotid endarterectomy results in loss of carotid-body function, with loss of the usual compensatory circulatory or respiratory responses to hypoxia.[90] A persistent elevation in Pa_{CO_2} may occur.[90] The potential for exaggeration of respiratory depressant effects with premedicant drugs such as morphine should be kept in mind, particularly in those patients with coexisting chronic obstructive pulmonary disease.[91]

Extracranial-Intracranial Bypass

The number of extracranial-intracranial (EC-IC) bypass procedures performed has been dramatically reduced as a result of an international randomized trial published in the mid-1980s. The study included 1377 patients with symptomatic atherosclerosis of the internal carotid or middle cerebral artery who were randomized to receive either medical care alone or EC-IC bypass with medical care.[92,93] The results did not support the use of surgical therapy because non-fatal and fatal stroke occurred more frequently and earlier in the patients who had surgery.[92] There was also no subgroup of patients with different angiographic lesions that could be identified to benefit from surgery,[92] and there was no significant difference in the long term functional status between the surgical and nonsurgical groups.[93]

ANESTHETIC MANAGEMENT

Anesthetic management of patients undergoing EC-IC bypass is similar in many aspects to that for carotid endarterectomy. Careful preoperative assessment of associated diseases, particularly those of the cardiovascular system, is mandatory. Although the role of the procedure has dramatically declined, the major previous indication was to increase collateral blood flow in patients with cerebrovascular insufficiency from atheromatous disease related to an inaccessible internal carotid or middle cerebral artery stenosis or occlusion. The procedure is still sometimes used to increase intracranial blood flow prior to carotid occlusion in the treatment of otherwise inoperable intracranial aneurysms.[94] The surgical procedure involves the construction of an anastomosis between the extracranial superficial temporal artery and a cortical branch of the middle cerebral artery. Posterior circulation procedures are performed in the sitting position and necessitate precautions for risks associated with this position such as air embolism and cardiovascular instability. Procedures involving the anterior circulation are performed in the supine position with the head turned laterally. Care should be taken to avoid severe rotation of the cervical spine and preoperatively the patient should be assessed to determine the effect of head positioning on neurologic function.

A major goal of the anesthetic technique for EC-IC bypass procedures is the maintenance of adequate cerebral perfusion. Systemic arterial pressure is monitored continuously with an arterial line and blood pressure is kept within a normal range for that patient. Arterial blood gases are followed to ensure adequate oxygenation and the maintenance of Pa_{CO_2} within a normal range. The procedure is performed at high magnification through a narrow exposure, and respiratory variations may cause a distracting brain bounce. Smaller inspiratory volumes and lower airway pressures (with increased respiratory rate) along with adequate muscle relaxation help to minimize brain surface movement. High frequency ventilation (HFV) has the advantage of reducing ventilator-synchronous brain movement.[96] A major disadvantage of HFV, however, is that it is seldom or never used by most anesthesiologists and therefore lacks the familiarity associated with traditional ventilatory techniques.

Routine monitors are similar to those used for carotid endarterectomy. Besides the intraarterial catheter, they include ECG, esophageal stethoscope, temperature monitor, urinary catheter, anesthetic gas and CO_2 monitoring, and pulse oximetry. In posterior circulation bypass procedures performed in the sitting position a central venous line is inserted, and in patients with severe cardiac risks, a pulmonary artery catheter may be inserted. Induction is accomplished with a combination of agents, usually including thiopental, narcotics, lidocaine and a nondepolarizing muscle relaxant. Other combinations of drugs may also be used successfully as long as care is provided to maintain stable cardiovascular parameters. Anesthetic maintenance may be achieved with a variety of agents, usually narcotics with or without nitrous oxide, and isoflurane. Muscle relaxation is maintained throughout the procedure and a peripheral nerve stimulator is used to assess muscle paralysis. A cortical branch of the middle cerebral artery (such as the angular artery) is clamped during the period of the anastomosis[97] and this clamp time is considerably longer than that necessary to perform carotid endarterectomy. Regional CBF may be significantly increased after the anastomosis, although this may not bring the flow into the normal range.[98] The anesthetic should be tailored such that prompt awakening is possible. This is usually not a problem because the majority of the procedure is minimally stimulating and requires only small doses of anesthetics.

POSTOPERATIVE COURSE

Postoperatively, arterial blood pressure is maintained at normotensive levels to optimize flow through the newly anastomosed vessel and low molecular weight dextran may be infused.[97] The mortality and morbidity associated with the procedure varies on the basis of the patient's preoperative neurologic condition, and was 1 percent and 4 percent, respectively, in a group of 415 superficial temporal to middle cerebral artery bypass procedures reported by Sundt and coworkers.[99] The 30-day surgical mortality and major stroke morbidity in the ECIC study was also similar, reported as 0.6 percent and 2.5 percent, respectively.[92] Technical complications may include occlusion of the superficial temporal arterial pedicle or damage to the cortical vessels.[99] Although major cerebral infarction is infrequent, minor ischemic strokes and transient deficits are more common.[99] Postoperative intracerebral hemorrhage may also be a risk, particularly in patients who have had a recent stroke and had a period of marked postoperative elevation of blood pressure.[100] Other local complications include wound infections and scalp necrosis. Serious systemic complications, particularly cardiac, account for a majority of postoperative deaths.[99]

References

1. Easton JD, Wilterdink JL: Carotid endarterectomy: trials and tribulations. *Ann Neurol* 1994; 35:5-17.
2. Sundt TM, et al: Carotid endarterectomy. Complications and preoperative assessment of risk. *Mayo Clin Proc* 1975; 50:301.
3. McCrory DC, et al: Predicting complications of carotid endarterectomy. *Stroke* 1993; 24:1285.
4. Goldstein LB, et al: Multicenter review of preoperative risk factors for carotid endarterectomy in patients with ipsilateral symptoms. *Stroke* 1994; 25:1116.
5. Asiddao CB, et al: Factors associated with perioperative complications during carotid endarterectomy. *Anesth Analg* 1982; 61:631.
6. Hertzer NR, et al: Coronary angiography in 506 patients with extracranial cerebrovascular disease. *Arch Intern Med* 1985; 145:849.
7. Chimowitz MI, et al: Cardiac prognosis of patients with carotid stenosis and no history of coronary artery disease. *Stroke* 1994; 25:759.
8. Urbinati S, et al: Frequency and prognostic significance of silent coronary artery disease in patients with cerebral ischemia undergoing carotid endarterectomy. *Am J Cardiol* 1992; 69:1166.
9. Urbinati S, et al: Preoperative noninvasive coronary risk stratification in candidates for carotid endarterectomy. *Stroke* 1994; 25:2022.
10. Fleisher LA, Beattie C: Current practice in the preoperative evaluation of patients undergoing major vascular surgery: a survey of cardiovascular anesthesiologists. *J Cardiothorac Vasc Anesth* 1993; 7:650.
11. Rizzo RJ, et al: Combined carotid and coronary revascularization: the preferred approach to the severe vasculopath. *Ann Thorac Surg* 1992; 54:1099.
12. Chang BB, et al: Carotid endarterectomy can be safely performed with acceptable mortality and morbidity in patients requiring coronary artery bypass grafts. *Am J Surg* 1994; 168:94.
13. Vassilidze TV, et al: Simultaneous coronary artery bypass and carotid endarterectomy. Determinants of outcome. *Texas Heart Institute Journal* 1994; 21:119.
14. Halpin DP, et al: Management of coexistent carotid and coronary artery disease. *Southern Med Journal* 1994; 87:187.
15. Bernhard VM, et al: Carotid artery stenosis: association with surgery for coronary artery disease. *Arch Surg* 1972; 105:837.
16. Bready LL: Diabetes mellitus. In Bready LL, Smith RB (eds): *Decision Making in Anesthesiology.* Toronto, B.C. Decker, 1987:180.
17. Steed DL, et al: Causes of stroke in carotid endarterectomy. *Surgery* 1982; 92:634.
18. Bosiljevac JE, Farha SJ: Carotid endarterectomy: Results using regional anesthesia. *Am Surg* 1980; 46:403.
19. Donato AT, Hill SL: Carotid arterial surgery using local anesthesia: A private practice retrospective study. *Am Surg* 1992; 58:446.
20. Shah DM, et al: Carotid endarterectomy in awake patients: Its safety, acceptability, and outcome. *J Vasc Surg* 1994; 19:1015.
21. Allen BT, et al: The influence of anesthetic technique on perioperative complications after carotid endarterectomy. *J Vasc Surg* 1994; 19:834.
22. Benjamen ME, et al: Awake patient monitoring to determine the need for shunting during carotid endarterectomy. *Surgery* 1993; 114:673.
23. Winnie AP, et al: Interscalene cervical plexus block: A single injection technic. *Anesth Analg* 1975; 54:370.
24. Winnie AP: An "immobile needle" for nerve blocks. *Anesthesiology* 1969; 31:577.
25. Ramamurthy S, et al: A simple technic for block of the spinal accessory nerve. *Anesth Anal* 1978; 57:591.
26. Castresana MR, et al: Incidence and clinical significance of hemidiaphragmatic paresis in patients undergoing carotid endarterectomy during cervical plexus block anesthesia. *J Neurosurg Anesth* 1994; 6:21.
27. Davies MJ, et al: Neurologic changes during carotid endarterectomy under cervical block predict a high risk of postoperative stroke. *Anesthesiology* 1993; 78:829.
28. Frost EAM: Some inquiries in neuroanesthesia and neurological supportive care. *J Neurosurg* 1984; 60:673.
29. Corson JD, et al: The influence of anesthetic choice on carotid endarterectomy outcome. *Arch Surg* 1987; 122:807.
30. Smith JS, et al: Intraoperative detection of myocardial ischemia in high-risk patients: Electrocardiography versus two-dimensional transesophageal echocardiography. *Circulation* 1985; 72:1015.
31. Lyons C, et al: Cerebral venous oxygen content during carotid thrombintimectomy. *Ann Surg* 1964; 160:561.
32. Larson CP, et al: Jugular venous oxygen saturation as an index of adequacy of cerebral oxygenation. *Surgery* 1967; 62:31.
33. Boysen G, et al: On the critical lower level of cerebral blood flow in man with particular reference to carotid surgery. *Circulation* 1974; 49:1023.
34. McKay RD, et al: Internal carotid artery stump pressure and cerebral blood flow during carotid endarterectomy. *Anesthesiology* 1976; 45:390.
35. Kelly JJ, et al: Failure of carotid stump pressures. Its incidence as a predictor for a temporary shunt during carotid endarterectomy. *Arch Surg* 1979; 114:1361.
36. Kwaan JHM, et al: Stump pressure. An unreliable guide for shunting during carotid endarterectomy. *Arch Surg* 1980; 115:1083.
37. Beebe HG, et al: Carotid artery stump pressure: Its variability when measured serially. *J Cardiovasc Surg* 1989; 30:419.
38. Sundt TM, et al: Correlation of cerebral blood flow and electroencephalographic changes during carotid endarterectomy. *Mayo Clin Proc* 1981; 56:533.
39. Halsey JH, et al: Blood velocity in the middle cerebral artery

and regional cerebral blood flow during carotid endarterectomy. *Stroke* 1989; 20:53.

40. Messick JM, et al: Correlation of regional cerebral blood flow (rCBF) with EEG changes during isoflurane anesthesia for carotid endarterectomy: Critical rCBF. *Anesthesiology* 1987; 66:344.

41. McFarland HR, et al: Continuous electroencephalographic monitoring during carotid endarterectomy. *J Cardiovasc Surg* 1988; 29:12.

42. Redekop G, Ferguson G: Correlation of contralateral stenosis and intraoperative electroencephalogram change with risk of stroke during carotid endarterectomy. *Neurosurgery* 1992; 30:191.

43. Chemtob G, Kearse LA: The use of electroencephalography in carotid endarterectomy. *Int Anesthesiol Clin* 1990; 28:143.

44. Borresen TE, et al: EEG monitoring during carotid surgery: Who should do the monitoring? *Clin Electroencephalogr* 1993; 24:70.

45. Levy WJ, et al: Automated EEG processing for intraoperative monitoring: A comparison of techniques. *Anesthesiology* 1980; 53:223.

46. Myers RR, et al: Monitoring of cerebral perfusion during anesthesia by time compressed fourier analysis of the electroencephalogram. *Stroke* 1977; 8:331.

47. Chiappa KH, et al: Results of electroencephalographic monitoring during 367 carotid endarterectomies: Use of a dedicated minicomputer. *Stroke* 1979; 10:381.

48. Levy WJ, et al: Monitoring the electroencephalogram and evoked potentials during anesthesia. In Saidman LJ, Smith NT (eds): *Monitoring in Anesthesia.* Stoneham, Butterworth, 1984: 227.

49. Kearse LA, et al: Computer derived density spectral array in detection of mild analog electroencephalographic ischemic changes during carotid endarterectomy. *J Neurosurg* 1993; 78:884.

50. Branston NM, et al: Relationship between the cortical evoked potential and local cortical blood flow following acute middle cerebral artery occlusion in the baboon. *Exp Neurol* 1974; 45:195.

51. Brinkman SD, et al: Neuropsychological performance one week after carotid endarterectomy reflects intraoperative ischemia. *Stroke* 1984; 15:497.

52. Markland ON, et al: Monitoring of somatosensory evoked responses during carotid endarterectomy. *Arch Neurol* 1984; 41:375.

53. Horsch S, et al: Intraoperative assessment of cerebral ischemia during carotid surgery. *J Cardiovasc Surg* 1990; 31:599.

54. Lam AM, et al: Monitoring electrophysiologic function during carotid endarterectomy: A comparison of somatosensory evoked potentials and conventional electroencephalogram. *Anesthesiology* 1991; 75:15.

55. Amantini A, et al: Monitoring of somatosensory evoked potentials during carotid endarterectomy. *J Neurol* 1992; 239:241.

56. Fava E, et al: Role of SEP in identifying patients requiring temporary shunt during carotid endarterectomy. *Electroencephalogr Clinical Neurophysiol* 1992; 84:426.

57. Fiori L, Parenti G: Electrophysiological monitoring for selective shunting during carotid endarterectomy. *J Neurosurg Anesthesiol* 1995; 7:168.

58. McDowell HA, et al: Carotid endarterectomy monitored with transcranial doppler. *Ann Surg* 1992; 215:514.

59. Jansen C, et al: Carotid endarterectomy with transcranial doppler and electroencephalographic monitoring. A prospective study in 130 operations. *Stroke* 1993; 24:665.

60. Jansen C, et al: Impact of microembolism and hemodynamic changes in the brain during carotid endarterectomy. *Stroke* 1994; 25:992.

61. Van Zuilen EV, et al: Detection of cerebral microemboli by means of transcranial doppler monitoring before and after carotid endarterectomy. *Stroke* 1995; 26:210.

62. Gaunt ME, et al: On-table diagnosis of incipient carotid artery thrombosis during carotid endarterectomy by transcranial doppler scanning. *J Vasc Surg* 1994; 20:104.

63. Cucchiara RF, et al: Evaluation of esmolol in controlling increases in heart rate and blood pressure during endotracheal intubation in patients undergoing carotid endarterectomy. *Anesthesiology* 1986; 65:528.

64. Michenfelder JD, et al: Isoflurane when compared to enflurane and halothane decreases the frequency of cerebral ischemia during carotid endarterectomy. *Anesthesiology* 1987; 67:336.

65. Waltz AG, et al: Cerebral blood flow during carotid endarterectomy. *Circulation* 1972; 45:1091.

66. Thiel A, et al: Cerebrovascular carbon dioxide reactivity in carotid artery disease. Relation to intraoperative cerebral monitoring results in 100 carotid endarterectomies. *Anesthesiology* 1995; 82:655.

67. Riles TS, et al: Myocardial infarction following carotid endarterectomy: A review of 683 operations. *Surgery* 1979; 85:249.

68. Smith JS, et al: Does anesthetic technique make a difference? Augmentation of systolic blood pressure during carotid endarterectomy: Effects of phenylephrine versus light anesthesia and of isoflurane versus halothane on the incidence of myocardial ischemia. *Anesthesiology* 1988; 69:846.

69. Perkins WJ, et al: Cerebral and hemodynamic effects of lidocaine accidently injected into the carotid arteries of patients having carotid endarterectomy. *Anesthesiology* 1988; 69:78.

70. Bishop D, Johnstone RE: Lidocaine toxicity treated with low-dose propofol. *Anesthesiology* 1993; 78:788.

71. Whittemore AD: Carotid endarterectomy. An alternative approach. *Arch Surg* 1980; 115:940.

72. Schiro J, et al: Routine use of a shunt for carotid endarterectomy. *Am J Surg* 1981; 142:735.

73. Sundt TM, et al: The risk-benefit ratio of intraoperative shunting during carotid endarterectomy. Relevancy to operative and postoperative results and complications. *Ann Surg* 1986; 203:196.

74. Ott DA, et al: Carotid endarterectomy without temporary intraluminal shunt. *Ann Surg* 1980; 191:708.

75. Gumerlock MK, Neuwelt EA: Carotid endarterectomy: To shunt or not to shunt. *Stroke* 1988; 19:1485.

76. Halsey JH: Risks and benefits of shunting in carotid endarterectomy. *Stroke* 1992; 23:1583.

77. Bove EL, et al: Hypotension and hypertension as consequences of baroreceptor dysfunction following carotid endarterectomy. *Surgery* 1979; 85:633.

78. Hans SS, Glover JL: The relationship of cardiac and neurological complications to blood pressure changes following carotid endarterectomy. *Am Surg* 1995; 61:356.

79. Towne JB, Bernhard VM: The relationship of post operative hypertension to complications following carotid endarterectomy. *Surgery* 1980; 88:575.

80. Tarlov E, et al: Reflex hypotension following carotid endarterectomy: Mechanism and management. *J Neurosurg* 1973; 39:323.

81. Cafferata HT, et al: Avoidance of postcarotid endarterectomy hypertension. *Ann Surg* 1982; 196:465.

82. Pine R, et al: Control of postcarotid endarterectomy hypotension with baroreceptor blockade. *Am J Surg* 1984; 147:763.

83. Angell-James JE, Lumley JSP: The effects of carotid endarterectomy on the mechanical properties of the carotid sinus and

carotid sinus nerve activity in atherosclerotic patients. *Br J Surg* 1974; 61:805.

84. Musser DJ, et al: Death and adverse cardiac events after carotid endarterectomy. *J Vasc Surg* 1994; 19:615.

85. Riles TS, et al: The cause of perioperative stroke after carotid endarterectomy. *J Vasc Surg* 1994; 19:206.

86. Peer PM, et al: Carotid exploration for acute postoperative thrombosis. *Am J Surg* 1994; 168:168.

87. Rogers W, Root HD: Cranial nerve injuries after carotid artery endarterectomy. *South Med J* 1988; 81:1006.

88. De Bord JR, et al: Carotid endarterectomy in a community hospital surgical practice. *Am Surg* 1991; 57:627.

89. Hobson RW, et al: Efficacy of carotid endarterectomy for asymptomatic carotid stenosis. *N Engl J Med* 1993; 328:221.

90. Wade JG, et al: Effect of carotid endarterectomy on carotid chemoreceptor and baroreceptor function in man. *N Engl J Med* 1970; 282:823.

91. Lee JK, et al: Morphine-induced respiratory depression following bilateral carotid endarterectomy. *Anesth Analg* 1981; 60:64.

92. EC/IC Bypass Study Group: Failure of extracranial-intracranial arterial bypass to reduce the risk of ischemic stroke. *N Engl J Med* 1985; 313:1191.

93. Haynes RB, et al; for the EC/IC Bypass Study Group: Functional status changes following medical or surgical treatment for cerebral ischemia. Results of the extracranial-intracranial bypass study. *JAMA* 1987; 257:2043.

94. Barnett DW, et al: Combined extracranial-intracranial bypass and intraoperative balloon occlusion for the treatment of intracavernous and proximal carotid artery aneurysms. *Neurosurgery* 1994; 35:92.

95. Sundt TM, Piepgras DG: Occipital to posterior inferior cerebellar artery bypass surgery. *J Neurosurg* 1978; 48:916.

96. Todd MM, et al: The effects of high-frequency positive pressure ventilation on intracranial pressure and brain surface movements in cats. *Anesthesiology* 1981; 54:496.

97. Fein JM: Extracranial to intracranial bypass grafting: Anterior circulation. In Wilkins RH, Rengachary SS (eds): *Neurosurgery.* New York, McGraw-Hill, 1985:1272.

98. Carter LP, et al: Cortical blood flow during extracranial-intracranial bypass surgery. *Stroke* 1984; 15:836.

99. Sundt TM, et al: Results, complications, and follow-up of 415 bypass operations for occlusive disease of the carotid system. *Mayo Clin Proc* 1985; 60:230.

100. Heros RC, Nelson PB: Intracerebral hemorrhage after microsurgical cerebral revascularization. *Neurosurgery* 1980; 6:371.

Chapter 28

SUPRATENTORIAL AND PITUITARY SURGERY

Supratentorial Neurosurgery

VISWANATHAN RAJARAMAN

CARSWELL H. JACKSON

CHARLES L. BRANCH, JR.

PATRICIA H. PETROZZA

Diagnosis Of Raised Intracranial Pressure[1-9] (Table 28-1)

A clear understanding of the signs and symptoms of raised ICP from focal brain abnormalities is vital for timely intervention in situations of intracranial hypertension. The urgency of severe elevations in ICP may not permit an orderly investigation of the underlying causes. Appropriate emergent measures, operative and otherwise, may successfully relieve a dangerous degree of intracranial hypertension and save the patient's life (Fig. 28-1).

HEADACHE

Headache is the most common symptom of raised ICP. While headache is a very nonspecific, common symptom, the headache from intracranial hypertension has certain characteristics. It often awakens the patient from sleep. It may be temporal, frontal, or involve the whole head. It is an unreliable indicator of the side

TABLE 28-1
Mechanisms of Raised Intracranial Pressure

1.	Mass Lesions	Hematoma, tumor, abscess
2.	CSF Accumulations	Hydrocephalus
		a. Impaired absorption—meningitis, subarachnoid hemorrhage, etc.
		b. Obstructive—congenital, due to tumors and other masses
		c. Increased production—choroid plexus Papilloma
3.	Cerebral Edema	Increased brain water content
		a. Vasogenic—vessel damage (tumor, abscess, contusion)
		b. Cytotoxic—cell membrane pump failure (hypoxia, ischemia, toxins)
		c. Hydrostatic—high transmural pressure (dysautoregulation, postdecompression)
		d. Interstitial—high CSF pressure—e.g., hydrocephalus
4.	Congestive (vascular) brain swelling	Increased cerebral blood volume
		a. Arterial vasodilatation
		b. Venous obstruction

or site of lesion. It is often described as bursting or throbbing, and at its greatest intensity may be associated with scalp tenderness. Patients may complain of neck pain and stiffness, which should not be mistaken for meningitis, since a lumbar puncture in such a situation could lead to fatal brain herniation. The pain is often aggravated by change of posture, coughing, and straining. The severity gradually increases, and the

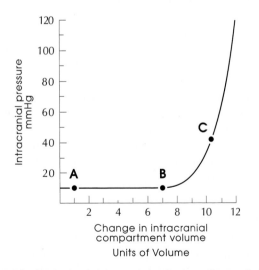

Figure 28-1 Intracranial pressure–volume curve. There is little elevation of pressure from points A to B—the compensatory phase. Small changes in volume result in large increases in pressure between B and C.

recognition of progression is important in distinguishing intracranial hypertension from headache of other causes. When the headache is severe, as in later stages of intracranial hypertension, there may be clouding of consciousness with mental confusion, lack of attention or alertness, and transient signs of neurologic dysfunction.

VOMITING

Vomiting occurs in later stages and is observed more often in children than in adults. In lesions of the posterior cranial fossa, however, especially those arising in the region of the fourth ventricle, vomiting may be an early and only symptom. This may result from direct irritation of the vomiting center of the medulla as well as a rise in ICP. Vomiting with raised ICP is classically described as "projectile" because it is not preceded by nausea. Vomiting may or may not be related to the headache, but when present with it, may result in some relief of the headache, possibly due to associated hyperventilation.

VISUAL SYMPTOMS

A variety of visual symptoms occur with intracranial hypertension. Severe headache may be accompanied by transient total loss of vision or by hemianopia. Such attacks may be related to sudden change of posture and must be regarded as a warning that the intracranial hypertension requires urgent management. More commonly, blurring or mistiness of vision, transient at first and later continuous, progresses to impairment of visual acuity. This is usually associated with papilledema. Significant loss of acuity is a late feature. Diplopia, or double vision, is intermittent at first and commonly results from abducens paresis. It is usually, but not always, unilateral. The site of paresis is not an indication of the site of the lesion responsible for raised ICP and is therefore often spoken of as a "false localizing sign." Other cranial nerves are rarely involved, although numbness from fifth cranial nerve involvement and facial weakness from seventh nerve involvement have been described in cases of idiopathic intracranial hypertension.

ALTERATION IN CONSCIOUSNESS

Disturbance of consciousness occurs in the late stages of raised ICP. The patient is at first apathetic and disinterested and seemingly lacks awareness of the surroundings, appearing lethargic and drowsy. As drowsiness deepens, coma supervenes, and there is no longer a purposeful response to verbal and then to painful stimuli. In the recording of such changes in the level of consciousness, terms such as stupor, semi-coma, and

TABLE 28-2
Glasgow Coma Scale

Eyes	Open	Spontaneously	4
		To verbal command	3
		To pain	2
	No response		1
Best motor response	To verbal command: Obeys		6
	To painful stimulus: Localizes pain		5
		Flexion-withdrawal	4
		Flexion-abnormal	3
		Extension	2
		No response	1
Best verbal response		Oriented and converses	5
		Disoriented and converses	4
		Inappropriate words	3
		Incomprehensible sounds	2
		No response	1
Total			3–15

obtundation should be avoided in favor of simple objective statements of the patient's response to standard stimuli. These observations are formalized in the Glasgow Coma Scale (GCS)[10] which records the patient's eye opening, motor and verbal responses (Table 28-2). Coma is defined as the state in which there is no eye opening even to painful stimuli, failure to obey simple commands, and failure to utter recognizable words—corresponding to a GCS sum score of less than 8. Progressive impairment of consciousness indicates a dangerous degree of intracranial hypertension, and the speed with which consciousness is lost bears some relation to the rate at which the mass is developing. In a patient with a slowly growing tumor, drowsiness and lethargy may be present for several days before coma ensues. In cases of intracranial hemorrhage, an alert patient complaining of severe headache may lapse into coma within hours. Loss of consciousness depends on two factors, diminution in cerebral blood flow to a critical level and interruption of brain stem function. The relative share of these two factors will vary with the nature of the causative lesion, its location, and its speed of evolution. In a slowly evolving benign supratentorial lesion, severe displacement of the brain stem can take place without consciousness being disturbed. On the other hand, in a more rapidly evolving situation, such as a chronic subdural hematoma, consciousness may be impaired to a greater degree with a similar degree of brain stem displacement. However, at operation the ICP frequently is not very high. The degree of accommodation to conditions that impede cerebral blood flow and distort the brain stem depends, therefore, on the rate of a lesion's development. Disturbance of consciousness may not always be progressive; periods of confusion can alternate with lucidity. In other instances, a period of delirium and intense rest-lessness may occur before the patient slips into coma. It is important to recognize these symptom complexes, because inappropriate use of sedation for a patient's confusion associated with increased ICP can have serious consequences.

PAPILLEDEMA

A characteristic sign of raised ICP is papilledema. The appearance of the optic disc on funduscopic examination in well-developed papilledema is unmistakable. This is the result of a block to the axoplasmic transport in the optic nerve coupled with impaired venous return. While its presence is a reliable indicator of raised ICP, the converse is not true. With the increasing use of modern neuroimaging techniques, brain pathologies that permit the development of papilledema are being detected at an earlier stage. In other cases, absence of papilledema may be related to anatomic variations and the extent to which the subarachnoid space extends along the optic nerve. In still others, the eyes may be affected to a dissimilar degree.

Brain Shifts and Herniation Syndromes

It is well recognized that raised ICP in the absence of a mass lesion is well tolerated. The best examples in clinical practice are patients with idiopathic intracranial hypertension. These patients have normal cerebral function despite persistent elevation of ICP. The displacement of cerebral tissue and distortion of the brain stem or its vascular supply cause the devastating effects of intracranial hypertension. The compartmentalization of the cranial cavity into right and left halves and supra- and infratentorial regions leads to minor

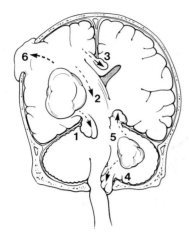

Figure 28-2   Types of brain herniations. 1. Transtentorial herniation. 2. Central transtentorial herniation. 3. Subfalcine herniation. 4. Tonsillar herniation. 5. Upward transtentorial herniation. 6. Extracalvarial herniation.

pressure differentials between parts of the brain. While a focal lesion in one part of the brain may cause certain signs and symptoms, the brain herniation that results from mass effect can produce so-called false-localizing signs, which appear incompatible with the suspected locale of the tumor. It is important to recognize these syndromes of brain shifts, not only to distinguish them from the underlying focal pathology, but also to be alert to possible impending catastrophe if remedial measures are not undertaken promptly (Fig. 28-2).

TRANSTENTORIAL HERNIATION

Unilateral mass lesions, especially when low in the brain or involving the temporal lobe, cause medial displacement of the uncus and the hippocampal gyrus over the sharp free edge of the tentorium. This manifests clinically with progressive enlargement of the ipsilateral pupil, which loses reaction to light whether stimulated directly or consensually. The exact mechanism underlying the development of third nerve palsy is not fully understood. At least three different mechanisms have been proposed: the direct impingement of the uncus over the ventral surface of the nerve; the counter pressure against the petroclinoid ligament; and, in yet other instances, dorsal compression by the posterior cerebral artery, which is dragged downwards by the transtentorial caudal shift of the brain stem. The early development of pupillary dilatation is due to the damage to the pupillo-constrictor fibers on the superior / dorsal surface of the third nerve. The medial displacement of the temporal lobe also causes pressure on the lower part of the internal capsule, and the medial margin of the hippocampus compresses the crus cerebri. Either or both of these give rise to contralateral

extremity weakness, which progresses to spastic hemiplegia. In later stages, the limbs adopt an abnormal flexion or extensor posture sometimes termed decorticate and decerebrate, respectively. The decorticate abnormality signifies predominant internal capsule damage, whereas the decerebrate posture points to predominant midbrain involvement. As the herniation worsens, the signs become bilateral, with both pupils dilated and nonreactive and all four limbs spastic and paralyzed in a symmetrical state of extensor rigidity. Associated with the early pupillary changes, the patient's level of consciousness deteriorates; by the time hemiplegia is evident, the patient is deeply unconscious. Without appropriate treatment, heart rate and blood pressure changes, including the Cushing response of hypertension and bradycardia, may become evident. Respirations deepen, later becoming periodic before death occurs from respiratory arrest.

The speed at which these events develop varies considerably. If the lesion is an extradural hematoma, the patient may slip into deep coma, with extensor rigidity and pupillary abnormalities within hours of the accident. In cases of a rapidly growing tumor, the symptoms and signs may develop over days. However, edema, necrosis, and hemorrhage may cause more rapid deterioration. Therefore, the clinical signs of tentorial herniation always indicate a clinical situation of grave urgency.

Minor variations in the clinical presentation of transtentorial herniation have been described. Some authors have divided transtentorial herniation into three types: anterior, posterior, and central. The foregoing discussion relates primarily to anterior tentorial herniation with medial displacement of the uncus as the predominant feature. When the mass lesion is located posteriorly, as in an occipital lobe tumor, the posterior parts of the hippocampal gyrus are more involved and produce a herniation through the posterior part of the tentorial hiatus. In this situation and in cases of bilateral supratentorial mass lesions, such as bilateral subdural hematoma, the dorsal aspect of the mid-brain, including the tectal plate, suffers the brunt of the compression, and bilateral ptosis, defective upward gaze, and bilateral fixed pupils occur before consciousness is lost. In rare situations, a slowly progressive mass lesion may cause such a severe lateral shift that the contralateral crus cerebri is pressed against the sharp edge of the tentorium on the opposite side. This leads to an ipsilateral paralysis of the limbs, yet another instance of a false localizing sign. Such a presentation has often been called the Kernohan phenomenon.

Autopsy studies have documented the extensive pathologic changes that accompany transtentorial herniation. Often a deep groove in the uncus and the hippocampal gyrus is readily identifiable post-mortem. Necrosis and swelling of the prolapsed brain may lead to incarceration in the hiatus, and the wedged tissue between the free margin of the tentorium on the side of the brain stem may persist even after the causative mass has been removed. Indentation, stretching, and kinking of the third nerve by the uncus, the petroclinoid ligament, and the posterior cerebral artery are often obvious. The downward displacement of the brain stem produces stretching and narrowing of the midline perforating vessels arising from the basilar artery. This may lead to ischemic necrosis and/or hemorrhage of the brain stem. These mid-brain and pontine hemorrhages may be petechial, linear, or irregular and may even extend as high as the internal capsule. Ischemic and hemorrhagic infarction of the calcarine cortex is not uncommon after massive transtentorial herniation. This condition is directly related to the stretching and kinking of the posterior cerebral arteries. Cortical infarctions elsewhere in the brain have also been described, especially in the arterial boundary zones between the anterior and middle and the middle and posterior cerebral arteries. These infarctions are thought to arise from persistent raised ICP and falling cerebral perfusion pressure leading to widespread areas of ischemia.

SUBFALCINE HERNIATION

In more superiorly positioned tumors with predominantly lateral displacements, the medial surface of the hemisphere bulges under the falx. This process is called subfalcine or cingulate herniation. It is more marked with lesions of the anterior part of the hemisphere where the falx is narrow. The pericallosal and callosomarginal arteries may be compressed, leading to infarctions in the region of the distal anterior cerebral artery. The third ventricle is compressed from side to side and is shifted across the midline, and is easily detected by CT or MRI. In most instances, subfalcine herniation is not associated with any specific symptoms or signs, though unilateral or bilateral leg weakness has been documented.

TONSILLAR HERNIATION

Masses in the posterior cranial fossa classically displace the lower cerebellum, especially the tonsils, down through the foramen magnum. This causes compression of the medulla and stretching of the upper cervical nerve roots. The neck stiffness of cerebellar herniation may be mistaken for meningism, and patients may be mistakenly subjected to lumbar puncture, with disastrous herniation resulting. The direct pressure of the cerebellar tonsils upon the posterior columns of the upper cervical cord and the counterpressure on the ventral medulla from the foramen magnum may produce a combined loss of postural sensibility and spasticity with extensor plantar response. Sudden death is particularly common with cerebellar herniation and is usually due to respiratory arrest or, less frequently, from vomiting and aspiration with medullary irritation. The lack of pupillary abnormalities may contribute to delayed detection.

UPWARD TRANSTENTORIAL HERNIATION

Upward herniation of the cerebellum through the tentorial hiatus is an uncommon herniation syndrome. It may be observed after overenthusiastic ventricular drainage in cases of obstructive hydrocephalus and, less commonly, in posterior fossa mass lesions. The clinical signs and symptoms of such brain shift are often subtle. The pupils are often small but still reactive, with possible impairment of upward gaze. There may be attacks of extensor rigidity, often referred to as "cerebellar fits" in the older literature. This is due to the wedging of the herniating cerebellar tissue between the free edge of the tentorium and the midbrain. The pons and the medulla are also compressed against the clivus. It must be recognized that infratentorial mass lesions are likely to distort and compress the fourth ventricle and/or the aqueduct early in the course of their development. This can cause enormous increases in ICP due to obstructive hydrocephalus.

The signs and symptoms of raised ICP must be distinguished from those of the causative lesion and the ones due to brain herniation and shift. Finally, accurate assessment of the speed with which these three symptom complexes evolve is needed to guide the urgency with which investigative and management measures must be carried out.

General Presentation of Neurosurgical Lesions

The clinical presentation of neurosurgical disorders is due to one of three mechanisms: signs and symptoms resulting from the focal lesion; those from raised ICP; and finally those due to brain herniation and shift. The latter have been discussed in detail in the beginning of the chapter. In the majority of situations, focal lesions of the brain manifest themselves as focal cerebral dysfunction with almost mathematical accuracy. Broadly speaking, these can be divided into signs and symptoms due to irritation or abnormal electrical activity of the part of the brain affected and those due to impaired function.

SEIZURES

Seizures are one of the common manifestations of a supratentorial lesion. In nearly half the patients with supratentorial tumors they are the initial presenting symptom.[11] They are likely to occur whether the tumor is extracerebral or intracerebral, but are more likely to complicate a frontal temporal lesion than an occipital one. They may be focal, which suggests development of the abnormal electrical activity in one area of the cerebral cortex, or nonfocal (generalized). Loss of consciousness is the primary event in generalized epilepsy, and convulsions may follow that affect all four limbs. Occasionally there may be little or no convulsive activity. Generalized epilepsy may be the result of lesions anywhere in the supratentorial compartment, but is more frequently seen with frontal and parietal lesions.

Focal epilepsy on the other hand has localizing significance. It may take different forms depending on the part of the brain affected. Focal motor convulsions with twitching of the tongue, face, or an extremity are seen in lesions involving the precentral gyrus of the frontal lobe. Following the convulsion, the area affected may be paralyzed for a variable period (Todd's paralysis), and this further adds to the localizing value. Deviation of head and eyes toward the opposite side, called adversive seizures, is due to lesions in and around Broadman area eight, the frontal eye-field. Perisylvian lesions may present with speech arrest and/or dysphasia and are commonly followed by facial motor or sensory phenomena.

Seizures originating in the parietal lobe, especially the postcentral gyri, may present with sensory epilepsy with feelings of numbness, tingling, or loss of postural sensibility in the limbs which are paroxysmal and at times followed by twitching or abnormal movement in the same distribution. Focal epilepsy originating in the occipital lobe presents as hallucinations of light and colors not recognizable as objects in the opposite visual field. In contrast, posterior temporal lobe epilepsy can present as visual hallucination of formed objects. Focal temporal lobe epilepsy is the most common form of epilepsy and can take on a variety of forms. The first of three main varieties consists of momentary absences, pure lapses of consciousness during which there is loss of contact with reality, and in which the flow of speech is broken but the patient does not lose consciousness. Such episodes often pass unnoticed by onlookers. Psychic phenomena such as olfactory and visual hallucination and déjà vu are another mode of presentation. Auditory hallucinations almost always point to an underlying psychosis rather than epilepsy. The third kind of presentation includes a variety of automatisms comprised of complex, well coordinated, but mostly purposeless activity. Attacks may be brief, such as smacking of lips, facial grimacing, clasping of hands, or sometimes more elaborate gestures.

IMPAIRED FUNCTION

Impaired function of focal areas of the brain clinically manifest as recognizable syndromes and aid in the clinical diagnosis of a supratentorial lesion. It must be admitted, however, that with advances in neuroimaging techniques and ready availability of CT and MRI scans, this aspect of clinical neurology is rapidly losing its significance. Presently, its value lies in optimal counseling of patients and family regarding progression, recovery, and rehabilitation. The signs and symptoms produced by the involvement of different parts of the brain are briefly summarized below.

FRONTAL LOBE

Lesions of the posterior frontal lobe cause hemiplegia when they involve projection fibers transversing the white matter to the corona radiata and the internal capsule. More localized weakness, such as a lower extremity weakness, occurs when the superior and medial part of the lobe, the paracentral lobule, is involved. Posterior inferior frontal cortical lesions on the dominant side may cause expressive dysphasia and/or facial weakness. Lesions of the anterior and basal portion of the frontal lobe give rise to few or no symptoms until they become large. Extensive dysfunction of the frontal lobe leads to the triad of apathy, lack of initiative, and social indifference. Impairment of memory in the early stages is often mild, but with progression frank dementia finally supervenes.

PARIETAL LOBE

Anterior parietal lobar lesions interfere with discriminative sensibility, including joint position sense, tactile localization, two-point discrimination, and stereognosis. Severe loss of these modalities of sensation can significantly impair normal coordinated movement. Subcortical lesions may manifest with sensory and visual inattention, whereas a more posterior and inferior lesion may involve the optic radiation, producing a lower quadrantic hemianopia. Lesions of the posterior inferior dominant parietal lobe abutting the temporal lobe can lead to disturbance of language function, which may manifest as dysphasia, dyslexia, and/or dysgraphia. Gerstmann's syndrome due to a lesion in the left angular gyrus consists of dysgraphia, dyscalculia finger agnosia, and right-left disorientation. Lesions affecting the parietal temporal occipital junction can produce more complex disturbances such as agnosia, a disorder of awareness or appreciation in the presence of normal sensory, motor, and visual sensibilities, or apraxia, a disorder of performance of coordinated activity in the absence of any motor or sensory loss.

OCCIPITAL LOBE

Hemianopia, loss of one-half field of vision, is a characteristic sign of occipital lobe involvement. Such a deficit may go unnoticed by the patient except that he or she complains of a tendency to collide with objects in the affected half field. More rarely, a left homonymous hemianopia may cause difficulty in reading because the word beginning each line cannot be easily identified as the eyes scan the printed page.

TEMPORAL LOBE

Lesions of the temporal lobe may remain silent until the patient presents with features of raised ICP. Posteriorly placed lesions may present with receptive dysphasia, and tumors in a deeper location may involve the sweeping fibers of the optic radiation (Meyer's loop) and cause a contralateral superior quadrantic hemianopia. Lesions of the medial temporal lobe may cause severe loss of memory for recent events, and the patient may confabulate and present the syndrome of Korsakov's psychosis. More often lesions in this region present with temporal lobe epilepsy with visual, olfactory, or gustatory hallucinations. Still others may present with déjà vu, dreamy states, automatic movements such as smacking of lips, chewing and swallowing, or with emotional instability with an inclination to bad temper and/or paranoia.

CORPUS CALLOSUM

Lesions in this region have a particular tendency to spread along the commissural pathways, thereby involving both hemispheres. Anterior callosal lesions spreading into the two frontal lobes presents as a characteristic butterfly-shaped mass and tend to reach a large size before greatly disturbing ICP. These lesions are commonly malignant, infiltrative gliomas in elderly subjects, and progressive dementia and personality change may be the only clue to their presence. When the middle third of the corpus callosum is affected, bilateral signs of motor and sensory disturbance may develop. Lesions of the posterior third commonly present with disorders of occular movement, particularly upward gaze, because of the downward pressure on the superior colliculi.

BASAL GANGLION AND THALAMUS

Lesions in these regions directly involve the fibers of the internal capsule with consequent contralateral motor, sensory, and hemianopic defects. Tremor and other complex involuntary movements are rarely caused by tumors in this region. Similarly, the thalamic pain syndrome of Dejerine and Roussy is more common after infarction or hemorrhage rather than a neoplasm.

LATERAL VENTRICLES

Lesions arising in and predominantly confined to the lateral ventricles tend to attain large sizes, molding themselves to the ventricular cavity. CSF tends to pass around the surfaces of such tumors, and hydrocephalus and raised ICP may not develop until late. Patients present with features of generalized raised ICP with no localizing signs. Occasionally, a mild motor or sensory or hemianopic defect may be produced with involvement of the structures adjacent to the walls of the ventricle.

THIRD VENTRICLE AND HYPOTHALAMUS

The most common lesion in this location is a glioma, and it tends to occupy the posterior parts of the cavity. Other lesions in this region include colloid cyst and craniopharyngioma, which arise in the anterior part, and less common lesions including choroid plexus papilloma, epidermoid cyst, and teratoma. Tumors arising in the pineal region tend to involve the posterior third ventricle. However, germ cell tumors, the commonest lesion in this location, are known to spread along the floor of the third ventricle to involve the anterior hypothalamus and the optic apparatus. Hydrocephalus and features of intracranial hypertension predominate; rarely, the characteristic symptom of sudden and transient loss of tone in the limbs may be encountered. Anteriorly placed lesions in this region may present a variety of endocrine abnormalities including diabetes insipidus, obesity, hypogonadism, or precocious puberty. Optic chiasmal involvement may lead to bitemporal hemianopia, which characteristically begins with inferior quadrant anopsia due to compression from above.

OPTIC NERVE AND CHIASM

Tumors restricted to the optic nerve usually arise within the orbit and give rise to progressive failure of visual acuity and proptosis. Proximal spread of the tumor to involve the optic chiasm leads to bilateral symptoms. Such a progression may not take place for several years, but precludes any successful surgical treatment of the lesion or correction of visual loss once it has occurred.

Neoplasms

Intracranial neoplasms comprise a significant proportion of the workload of a neurosurgical service. While

TABLE 28-3
Types and Incidence of Intracranial Tumors

	%
Gliomas	45–50
a. Astrocytoma (25%)	
b. Oligodendroglioma (5%)	
c. Anaplastic glioma of glioblastoma (50%)	
Metastatic tumors	20–30
Meningioma	15
Medulloblastoma	6
Schwannomas	6
Pituitary adenoma	5
Craniopharyngioma	3
CNS lymphoma	
Neurocytoma	
Ganglioglioma	
Hemangioblastoma	

metastasis from systemic cancer is the most common type of intracranial tumor, gliomas constitute the single largest group of neoplasms encountered in a general neurosurgical practice. The relative incidence of the different types of tumors requiring surgical intervention is presented in Table 28-3. To this list must be added congenital tumors, such as teratomas, epidermoids and dermoids, which account for about 1 to 2 percent of all intracranial tumors, primary CNS lymphoma, which has registered increasing frequency in recent years, and tumors involving the scalp and skull. The diagnosis of intracranial tumors is based on clinical presentation and radiologic characteristics. Manifestations of lesions at different sites and the signs and symptoms of raised ICP have been discussed earlier in the chapter. While a definitive diagnosis should await histopathologic confirmation, advances in neuroradiologic techniques have enabled a more confident presumptive preoperative diagnosis, thereby facilitating early management strategies. Another important advance has been the development of computer-guided stereotactic systems, which enable biopsy confirmation of ambiguous lesions with very low morbidity.

The distinction between benign and malignant tumors is less clear-cut in the brain than elsewhere in the body, as primary CNS tumors rarely metastasize outside the brain. Malignancy depends on other aspects of tumor behavior, such as rate of growth, tendency to infiltrate diffusely, and spread along CSF pathways. Another important consideration in the management of intracranial tumors is the location of the lesion, whatever its nature: involvement of vital centers may threaten life directly or limit surgical ac-

cessibility. A surgeon's natural reaction to a tumor is to remove the whole of it. Such a straightforward solution may not always be possible in the brain, where loss of function of adjacent essential areas of the brain may result. Success of a neurosurgical operation depends not only on the length of survival but on the quality as well. Therefore, different forms of radiotherapy may be used alone or in conjunction with surgery for the control of symptoms, prolongation of life, and in rare instances even to effect cure. Chemotherapy and immunotherapy have been tried extensively and can be useful palliative measures in specific instances. The general principles of tumor surgery, radiotherapy, and chemotherapy are outlined below, followed by a brief discussion of some of the common neoplasms.

GENERAL SURGICAL PRINCIPLES

Surgical intervention is aimed at complete removal of such benign lesions as meningiomas, congenital cysts, and other tumor-like conditions when they are readily accessible and resectable without compromise of neurologic function. Even if a tumor is resectable, a particular patient's interest may not always be best served by total resection, taking into account its rate of growth and the patient's natural expectation of life. Satisfactory control of symptoms may be obtained by partial resection with much less risk to adjacent neurologic structures than a radical operation. In other instances, relief of raised ICP and/or the establishment of tissue diagnosis are the primary considerations. CSF diversionary procedures to relieve CSF pathway obstruction and debulking of aggressive tumors play an important role in the control of the symptoms and signs of raised pressure and improve the quality of survival. Recovery of focal neurologic deficits following surgical resection of tumors is less straightforward. It is dependent on several variables, including the location of the lesion, the duration of symptoms, the preoperative Karnofsky performance score (Table 28-4), and the type of deficit. Visual acuity recovers well when chiasmal compression is relieved, unless marked optic atrophy is already established. Hemiplegia is at least partly improved after evacuation of a tumor cyst, but may be aggravated, albeit temporarily, following excision of a solid tumor close to the motor cortex. Epilepsy may undergo a temporary or permanent remission following surgery. Cognitive functions are less predictable, although the increased alertness following relief of ICP, in general, improves the level of functioning.

RADIOTHERAPY

The susceptibility of the normal brain tissue to irradiation limits the value of this treatment mode. However,

TABLE 28-4
Karnofsky Performance Status

Definition	Percent	Criteria
Able to carry on normal activity and to work. No special care is needed.	100	Normal; no complaints; no evidence of disease
	90	Able to carry on normal activity; minor signs or symptoms of disease
Unable to work. Able to live at home, care for most personal needs. A varying amount of assistance is needed.	80	Normal activity with effort; some signs or symptoms of disease
	70	Care for self. Unable to carry on normal activity or to do active work
Unable to care for self. Requires equivalent of institutional or hospital care. Disease may be progressing rapidly.	60	Requires occasional assistance, but is able to care for most of his or her needs
	50	Requires considerable assistance and frequent medical care
	40	Disabled; requires special care and assistance
	30	Severely disabled, hospitalization is indicated although death is not imminent
	20	Very sick; hospitalization necessary; active supportive treatment necessary
	10	Moribund; fatal processes progressing rapidly
	0	Dead

SOURCE: Karnofsky D, et al: Triethylene melamine in the treatment of neoplastic disease. *Arch Intern Med* 87:477–516, 1951, with permission.

for lesions located in eloquent areas of the brain and those situated deep, which cannot be surgically removed without prohibitive loss of function, various forms of radiotherapy offer the best palliation. Conventionally, external beam radiation is administered in fractions of 15 to 18 mgy (150 to 180 rads) per treatment to a cumulative dose of 450 to 600 mgy (4500 to 6000 rads) depending on the site of the lesion. Often, in addition to this whole brain radiation, focal boost to the center of the lesion is also added. In other instances, cytoreductive surgery is followed by radiation therapy to control residual tumor and/or to prevent recurrences. Stereotactic biopsy followed by external radiation is a far better option than either surgery or no treatment at all.

Stereotactic radiosurgery, a term used to describe a variety of techniques involving focused radiation for the treatment of cerebral lesions, is a new modality for the treatment of several intracranial neoplasms and is gaining popularity. Presently, radiosurgery utilizes three techniques: the proton beam; the Gamma knife; and the linear accelerator. Using a variety of stereotactic guidance systems and treatment planning using sophisticated computerized reconstructions, precise radiation in very high doses is delivered to the target area without damaging the surrounding healthy brain tissue.[12] The application of this technique is well established for the management of small (<3 cm) metastases and in the control of growth of certain benign intracranial tumors.[13]

Another radiotherapeutic maneuver showing promise is the intratumoral/intracystic placement of radioactive seeds (interstitial brachytherapy).[14]

Cranial irradiation does not usually cause any systemic disturbances, but temporary or permanent epilation may occur. Some degree of cerebral swelling is not uncommon during the early stages of treatment, and this can be adequately controlled with small doses of steroids. Much more significant is the delayed development (usually 9 months to 3 years) of recurrence of the original symptoms or of raised ICP due to the development of radionecrosis. The exact mechanism underlying this is not completely understood but is related to ischemia due to fibrinoid necrosis in the small vessels surrounding the lesion. It is associated with significant vasogenic edema and its distinction from tumor recurrence can often be difficult.

CHEMOTHERAPY

In contrast to malignancies elsewhere in the body, primary intracranial exoplasms have only shown minimal to modest response to a variety of antineoplastic drugs. The best results have been registered with the use of the nitrosureas (BCNU, CCNU).[15] Randomized, controlled trials of combination chemotherapy regimens have shown little benefit.[16] A variety of newer techniques, including intra-arterial and intratumoral delivery of chemotherapeutic agents, are being attempted.[17] Another approach involves alteration of the blood-brain barrier with intra-arterial mannitol in conjunction with a variety of chemotherapeutic agents.[18]

GLIOMAS

Gliomas are the most common intracranial neoplasm and range in their malignant potential from benign to most malignant. They can involve any part of the brain or the spinal cord and show great histologic variation even within an individual tumor. Their biologic behavior is determined by the most anaplastic component of its cell population.

ASTROCYTOMA

This is by far the most common of the gliomas, comprising 10 to 15 percent of intracranial neoplasms. They may be composed of well differentiated cells similar to the different types of astrocytes (fibrillary, protoplasmic, gemistocytic) or of poorly differentiated cells as in anaplastic tumors. Diffuseness without any definite edge or margin to the tumor is the chief characteristic of low-grade astrocytoma. Nearly 90 percent of patients harboring these lesions present with seizures, and a minority have neurologic deficits at presentation. The tumors appear as ill-defined, low-density lesions on CT scan, showing no contrast enhancement. MR scans, in general, demonstrate a larger area of involvement, but there is only minimal or no associated edema. Histologically, the pilocytic variety of astrocytoma is the most benign and can be removed without recurrence. Tumors located in the medial or anterior temporal or frontal lobes may be completely removed by lobectomy with excellent long-term results. Such complete excisions may not be possible in other cerebral locations, but still the long-term outcome is quite favorable, especially in young patients.[19] Postoperative radiation therapy is not routine. Recurrent tumors are managed by reoperation and/or radiotherapy.

OLIGODENDROGLIOMA

These comprise 2 to 5 percent of all gliomas. Histologically, they are composed of uniform, small, round cells with clear cytoplasm; they usually grow slowly. Over half of these tumors show some degree of calcification, an important point in radiologic diagnosis. They are more common in the cerebral hemispheres and appear as lesions of heterogeneous density with areas of calcification on the CT scan. Treatment is aimed at total removal, followed by radiotherapy if histologic features of malignancy are present. Chemotherapy is also particularly effective in the management of certain anaplastic oligodendrogliomas.[20]

EPENDYMOMA

These tumors are derived from the ependymal cells lining the ventricular walls and the central canal of the spinal cord. About 40 percent of these arise in the supratentorial compartment. Although the majority are related to some part of the lateral ventricle and are often lobulated with some cystic components, tumors occasionally may arise in the substance of the brain from ependymal cell rests. The solid components are firm and calcification is not uncommon. Histologically, they are characterized by solid clusters of cells with rosette formation. They appear as heterogeneous lesions on the CT scan with variable enhancement. With early diagnosis, supratentorial ependymomas are often amenable to gross total resection; with postoperative radiotherapy, long-term survival up to 20 years has been reported.[21]

MALIGNANT GLIOMAS

These include the Grade III gliomas, also known as anaplastic gliomas in certain classification schemes, and the most malignant of all brain tumors, the glioblastoma multiforme. These tumors are characterized by a fast rate of growth and by rapid progression of symptoms. Radiologically, anaplastic tumors are more radiodense than the surrounding brain tissue, are irregular and are associated with significant surrounding edema. The more malignant lesions may appear circumscribed with central areas of radiolucent necrosis. Glioblastomas arising in the frontal lobe may extend from one side to the other via the corpus callosum, producing the characteristic butterfly-shaped lesions on the CT scan. Irregular areas of enhancement representing viable tumor are the rule. MR scan is more sensitive in defining the solid portion of the tumor and the extent of vasogenic edema (Fig. 28-3).

Histologically, the distinction between anaplastic gliomas and glioblastoma multiforme is based on the presence or absence of necrosis, endothelial proliferation, and features of anaplasia. These tumors are highly cellular with nuclear pleomorphism and frequent mitoses. These may arise de novo or from pre-existing lower grade gliomas of different types.

While the management of these two tumors is similar, a definitive histologic diagnosis is vital, for even with the best available treatment, the median survival for glioblastoma multiforme is 32 weeks and that for anaplastic astrocytoma 63 weeks.[22] The prognostic factors influencing survival in the order of decreasing importance are (1) the age of the patient; (2) the preoperative Karnofsky status; and (3) the extent of tumor resection. Patients less than 40 years of age and in good neurologic condition have a median survival of nearly two years, compared to a survival time of less than six months for patients over 65 years. While there is still debate about the effect of cytoreductive surgery in glioblastomas, there is evidence to support gross total

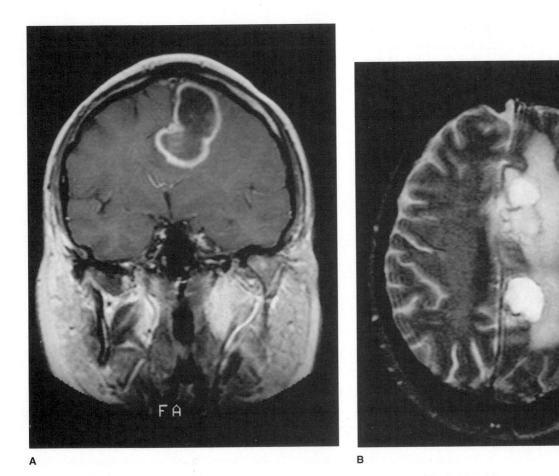

Figure 28-3   Glioblastoma multiforme. *A.* Coronal T1-weighted MRI after gadolinium contrast enhancement. Note the tumor crosses the midline and has solid enhancing parts and a non-enhancing necrotic area. *B.* Axial T2-weighted image in the same patient shows extensive vasogenic edema in the white matter.

resection whenever the tumor involves non-eloquent areas of the brain, especially if the patient is young and in good neurologic condition.[23] Tumors crossing the midline usually have a poorer prognosis. Postoperative radiotherapy and, in the younger patient, chemotherapy in carefully selected patients may provide a few additional months of life.

PRIMARY CNS LYMPHOMA

These tumors have shown an increased incidence in the last two decades not only in patients who have acquired or therapeutically induced immunodeficiency but also among immunocompetent people. Radiologically, they are paraventricular in location, being iso- or hyperdense, with strong contrast enhancement on CT scan. Spread along the ventricular pathways and diffuse involvement of the leptomeninges is not uncommon. MRI scans are more sensitive and can yield a confident presumptive diagnosis. Histologically, most of these are B-cell lymphomas with high-grade

malignant charactersitics. Treatment consists of establishing a tissue diagnosis, either by stereotactic biopsy or excision, followed by a combination of steroids, radiotherapy, and chemotherapy. These tumors respond to the above combination, often with complete radiologic resolution of the lesions. The overall prognosis, however, is dismal, with the median survival of six months in the immunocompromised patient and 13 months in others.[24]

MENINGIOMAS

Meningiomas arise from arachnoidal cap cells, and while the majority are in relation to the coverings of the brain, intraosseous and intraventricular tumors are not unknown. They account for about 15 to 20 percent of all intracranial tumors and may occur at any age, with a peak incidence around 45 years. Most of these tumors are located in the cerebral convexity or the parasagittal area. Those arising from the skull base are most commonly located in the region of the olfactory groove and the sphenoid wing. Other less common sites of involvement include the tentorium, the foramen magnum, the petrous ridge, and the orbit. Macroscopically, these tumors have a broad base of attachment, appear globular with a smooth or nodular surface, and often produce hyperostosis of the adjacent bone. Microscopically, most of these lesions are benign, with uniform cell types arranged in whorls and other interlacing patterns with a rich fibrovascular network. While cellular pleomorphism and frequent mitoses may be seen in certain types of meningiomas, truly malignant meningiomas are uncommon.

Clinically, these are slow-growing lesions with a long history of symptoms and signs. Rapid deterioration may be related to the progression of the surrounding vasogenic edema, brain shifts and obstruction of CSF pathways, tumor degenerations such as cyst formation and hemorrhage, or simply exhaustion of intracranial compensatory mechanisms. Definitive preoperative diagnosis is often possible based on their location, shape, and characteristic radiologic findings. They appear as iso- or hyperdense dural based lesions that show uniform contrast enhancement on the CT scan (Fig. 28-4). While most meningiomas are associated with surrounding edema, certain histologic varietes such as the hemangioblastic and the hemangiopericytic types may exhibit extensive, often holohemispheric edema. Changes in the adjacent bone are also well demonstrated on scans displayed on bone windows. MR scans are useful in displaying the tumor and its relationships in the coronal and sagittal planes. Angiography and preoperative embolization may be useful in certain highly vascular tumors.

Surgery for meningiomas aims at total removal of the tumor and the involved dura. When bone is infiltrated, the affected part of the skull also should be removed and reconstructed by cranioplasty. Complete removal of the tumor and the affected dura results in long-term cure, with a recurrence rate of only 9 percent. This increases to 19 percent when the dura is only cauterized and not totally removed.[25] While convexity meningiomas may be amenable to such radical removal, tumors involving the skull base and those partly invading the dural venous sinuses may not allow complete dural excision. Advances in microneurosurgical techniques and surgical approaches to the skull base over the last two decades have made possible a more complete excision of these lesions. Treatment of recurrent tumors in reoperation whenever feasible. Conventional external beam radiation, interstitial radiation (brachytherapy), and stereotactic radiosurgery have all been used in the management of residual tumors in inaccessible locations to prolong the interval before recurrence. It must be remembered, however, that some of these tumors may be extremely slow

growing, and ones not causing any significant symptoms or found in otherwise medically compromised patients can be followed periodically until surgery is needed.

While surgical excision of a relatively less vascular convexity meningioma may be a fairly straightforward operation, significant blood loss and hemodynamic instability is to be expected in a large vascular meningioma related to the major venous sinuses. Further, intraoperative complications such as air embolism due to opening of a major venous sinus, catastrophic brain swelling due to occlusion of major venous channels, and interference with vital functions, especially in skull-base tumors in close proximity to the brain stem, can make intraoperative management by the anesthesiologist quite challenging.

PHAKOMATOSIS

The phakomatoses comprise a group of familial or hereditary disorders characterized by a triad of central-peripheral nervous system tumors, skin lesions, and abnormalities involving the viscera.

Tuberous sclerosis is an autosomally dominant hereditary disorder presenting with epilepsy, low intelligence, and angiofibromas of the skin (adenoma sebaceum). A variety of other skin lesions and hamartomous lesions affecting abdominal organs and phakomas of the eyes are also known to occur. The intracranial lesions of neurosurgical importance are "the tubers," hamartomous, subependymal nodules often with calcification and at times interfering with CSF circulation. Others may present with subependymal giant cell astrocytomas which characteristically enhance with contrast administration on the CT scan.

Neurofibromatosis has been classified into several types, but type 1 (von Recklinghausen's disease) and type 2 (bilateral acoustic neuromas) are the ones of neurosurgical importance. Both these conditions are inherited as autosomal dominant disorders, and the underlying genetic abnormality has been traced to chromosome 17 in NF-1 and to chromosome 22 in NF-2. These two disorders are clinically distinct, with Type 1 presenting multiple cutaneous and subcutaneous neurofibromas, café-au-lait skin lesions, intracranial meningiomas, and gliomas. Surgical intervention is directed at those lesions which are symptomatic and progressive. NF-2 patients present with auditory symptoms, and because of the bilaterality of the tumors, their management is a neurosurgical challenge. Surgical treatment aims at complete removal of larger or symptomatic lesions while preserving hearing at least on one side. Nondisabling lesions are often closely monitored with frequent MR scans.

Von Hippel-Lindau disease or familial hemangi-

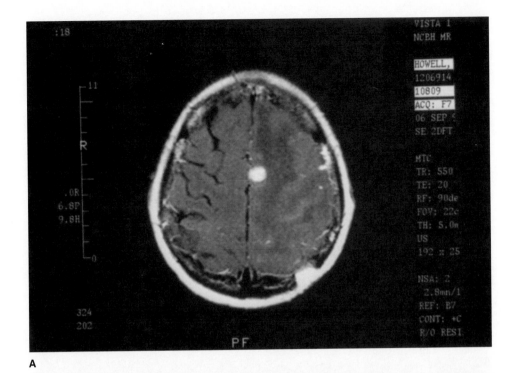

A

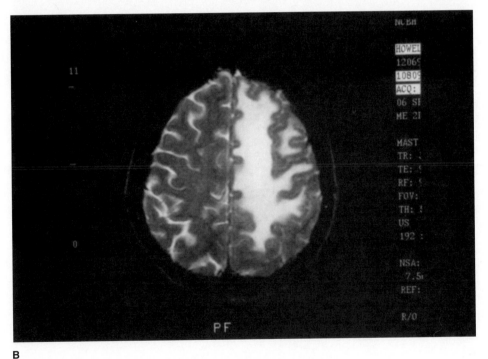

B

Figure 28-4 Meningioma. *A.* CT scan of a 36-year-old woman with a two-month history of mild headache and one-day history of left focal seizures. The mass is hyperdense, globular, arising from the convexity and causes significant brain shift. *B.* The tumor enhances uniformly after IV contrast administration.

oblastoma is also an autosomal dominant disorder characterized by hemangiomas of the retina, hemangioblastomas in the central nervous system (especially the cerebellum), and cysts of the pancreas, liver, and kidneys.

Sturge-Weber syndrome is characterized by a facial port-wine nevus, epilepsy, cerebral hemangioendo-

theliomatosus, and a variety of ocular lesions. The diagnosis often can be made at birth, and, in children, MR scans may demonstrate intracranial lesions before the characteristic railroad pattern of calcification becomes apparent. Neurosurgical treatment involves lobectomy or hemispherectomy to control intractable seizures.

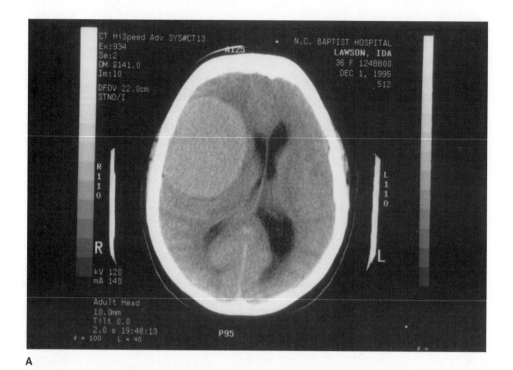

A

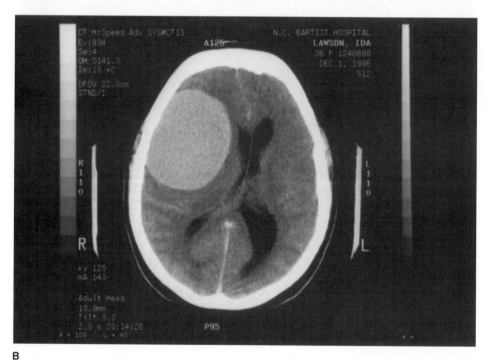

B

Figure 28-5 Cerebral metastasis. Solitary left parietal metastasis from a primary in the colon. *A.* T1-weighted post-contrast MRI. Note the fullness of the left hemisphere with obliteration of sulci. *B.* T2-weighted MRI in the same patient demonstrates extensive edema.

CEREBRAL METASTASES

Cerebral metastases from systemic cancer are the most common intracranial neoplasm. Only 50 percent of these patients are of adequate overall medical condition with a favorable systemic prognosis, so they can tolerate a surgical intervention. Nearly half harbor multiple lesions. Metastatic lesions are often associated with extensive vasogenic edema (Fig. 28-5). While surgical excision of solitary cerebral metastasis has been practiced for several years, it was not until 1990 when Patchell and co-workers[26] published the results of a prospective randomized study, demonstrating a median survival of 40 weeks and functional independent survival of 38 weeks in the surgical group versus 15 and 8 weeks, respectively, in the nonsurgical group, that such a management strategy came to be universally accepted. The most common metastatic lesions of the brain are those from lung, breast, melanoma, colon, and kidney. More recent studies from the M. D. Anderson Cancer Center, Houston TX, have demonstrated the value of reoperation for recurrent metastatic brain tumors[27] as well as surgical treatment for easily accessible multiple brain metastasis[28] in selected groups of patients. Stereotactic radiosurgery is also particularly suited for the treatment of multiple brain metastasis, as these lesions are usually small, spherical, and often deep-seated. Early results have been very promising.[13] In most patients with cerebral metastases, however, whole-brain radiation is still the appropriate palliative measure, allowing 3 to 6 months of quality survival.

PINEAL REGION TUMORS

Tumors arising from the pineal gland and others in the region of the posterior third ventricle present with certain characteristic ocular signs, hydrocephalus, and, in some cases, hypothalamic disturbance. Nearly 80 percent of the tumors at this site are malignant and are of germ cell origin. Suspected malignant lesions at this site can often be confirmed by stereotactic biopsy and treated with external beam radiation. Until recently, direct surgical excision carried high rates of morbidity and mortality because of the deep location within the cranium. With advancements in microneurosurgical techniques, total surgical excision, especially of the benign lesions, has become the goal. A variety of surgical approaches have been employed, and in addition to the tedious and often lengthy nature of these operations, they may be associated with increased complications of hemorrhage, due to the close relationship of several deep venous structures. Many of these operations also employ unique positioning of the patient at surgery and may be accompanied by a complicated postoperative course. The most common malignant lesion at this site is the germinoma, and this tumor not uncommonly spreads along the floor of the third ventricle to involve the hypothalamus and the chiasmal region, producing a variety of hypothalamic, endocrine, and visual disturbances. The benign lesions in this region include the meningioma, epidermoid and dermoid.

LATERAL VENTRICULAR TUMORS

The most common lateral ventricular tumors include meningiomas and the choroid plexus papilloma. The latter is often associated with significant hydrocephalus caused by a combination of increased CSF production and CSF pathway obstruction secondary to micro- or macrohemorrhages. These lesions are irregular, lobulated and demonstrate significant calcification, producing a characteristic radiologic appearance on both CT and MR scans. Surgical excision, whether by a transcortical or a transcallosal approach or endoscopically through a ventriculoscope, is the treatment of choice. Postoperative CSF diversionary procedures are often required.

Infections

Microorganisms reach and colonize the CNS via the blood stream and/or by direct extension of infection from the paranasal sinuses and middle ear. Infections of the CNS may be generalized as in meningitis or localized as in abscess. Meningitis, whether bacterial, fungal, or viral in origin, rarely requires any neurosurgical intervention. Postmeningitis hydrocephalus may require CSF diversionary measures such as a VP shunt.

BACTERIAL INFECTIONS

Extracerebral infections, such as subgaleal abscess and osteomyelitis of the skull bone, usually develop secondary to trauma or neurosurgical procedure. Like abscesses elsewhere in the body, their treatment involves aspiration, debridement of the bone, and drainage of purulent material along with administration of appropriate antibiotics.

Epidural abscesses also follow trauma or, more commonly, craniotomy and require removal of the overlying bone flap, drainage of the pus, and use of appropriate antibiotics. In contrast, subdural empyema is a more serious disorder with a high mortality rate. Infection at this location causes thrombosis of the major cortical draining veins and can lead to frank meningitis, intraparenchymal abscess formation, and venous infarctions of the brain. They are, therefore, associated with a disproportionate amount of cerebral edema, high incidence of seizures, focal neurologic deficits, and, if not treated early, rapid mental deterioration leading to coma and even death. Their management often requires large craniotomy flaps for the adequate drainage of often thick purulent material, in addition to antibiotics.

Brain abscesses occur either from direct spread of infection from the mastoid or paranasal sinuses, or they may develop secondary to infection in the lungs, heart, or kidneys. Children with congenital heart disease and patients with AIDS are especially susceptible. In the early stage of cerebritis, they can often be managed with antibiotics. With the liquefaction of the infected and dead brain tissue, a firm wall develops around this region when the host is able to contain the infection. They appear as ring enhancing lesions on the CT scan with significant vasogenic edema and mass effect (Fig. 28-6). Deep-seated and multiple brain abscesses are treated by a combination of antibiotics and repeated stereotactic aspirations. Larger abscesses and

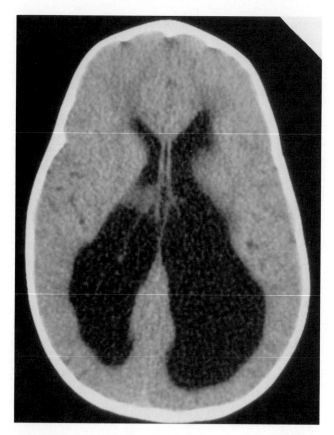

Figure 28-6 Hydrocephalus. CT scan of a 11-month-old child with enlarged head. Asymmetrical enlargement of the different parts of the ventricular system is not uncommon, especially if hydrocephalus follows intraventricular hemorrhage.

those which are multiloculated or have very thick walls require surgical excision. The high morbidity associated with cerebral abscess formation is to a large extent related to the extensive cerebral edema that often accompanies abscess formation. Concurrent management of the source of sepsis is also very important.

VIRAL INFECTIONS

Relative to the incidence of viral infections in the general population, CNS infections and more specifically those requiring neurosurgical intervention are extremely rare. The common viruses that come to neurosurgical attention are HIV and herpes simplex. HIV infection can present in a variety of ways, including AIDS dementia complex, meningoencephalitis, myelopathy, and peripheral neuropathies. Most of these conditions are diagnosed on the basis of CSF studies, CT/MRI scans, PNCV and EMG studies, and occasionally muscle and nerve biopsies. Intracranial neurosurgical intervention is seldom, if ever, required. Herpes simplex on the other hand, can cause an acute necrotiz-

ing encephalitis preferentially affecting the temporal lobes and subfrontal regions with significant mass effect. A disease of adults with no gender preference, it may present insidiously or in a fulminating manner, with personality and behavior changes, fever, and headache. Neurosurgical intervention may involve craniotomy for biopsy and, in fulminant cases, excision of the necrotic temporal lobe to relieve mass effect.

FUNGAL AND PARASITIC INFECTIONS

The incidence of fungal and parasitic infections of the brain is increasing in the United States with the greater prevalence of AIDS and patients undergoing immunosuppressive therapy. Pathogenic fungal infections are caused by histoplasma, coccidioides, and blastomyces. More common are the opportunistic infections, which include candida, aspergillus, cryptococcus, and mucormycosis. Neurosurgical intervention is aimed primarily at stereotactic biopsy diagnosis of nonresolving granulomas caused by aspergillus, cryptococcus, and the mucor family of fungi.

Toxoplasmosis is the most common cause for enhancing mass lesions in AIDS patients. Diagnosis is often established based on serum and CSF antibody titers. In those few patients with unresponsive lesions despite anti-toxoplasma treatment, confirmation by stereotactic biopsy is indicated. The other common parasitic infection encountered especially in the southern and western parts of the United States is cysticercosis. This disease, caused by pork tapeworm (*Taenia solium*), is acquired by consuming poorly washed/cooked fresh vegetables that have been contaminated by tapeworm larvae. CNS lesions include multiple cysts, which lodge in the parenchyma, basilar cisterns, and ventricular system. Clinical presentation is due to epilepsy, focal neurologic deficit, or symptoms of hydrocephalus. VP shunt for the relief of hydrocephalus and, rarely, excision of the cyst may be required.

Hydrocephalus and Arachnoid Cyst

Hydrocephalus refers to an excessive accumulation of CSF within the ventricular system of the brain. It is caused either by an increased rate of CSF formation, obstruction to its normal circulation, or by defective absorption. Based on its etiology, it may be classified as congenital, when it is due to a CNS malformation, or acquired, secondary to infection, trauma, or tumor.

CONGENITAL HYDROCEPHALUS

Most cases of congenital hydrocephalus are noncommunicating and are caused by aqueductal stenosis and fourth ventricular outflow obstruction. While some of these are inherited as X-linked disorders, others may be associated with myelomeningocele and Dandy-Walker syndrome. Hydrocephalus develops in nearly 95 percent of children with myelomeningocele and in nearly 50 percent of children with Arnold-Chiari malformation and occipital encephaloceles. Dandy-Walker syndrome is characterized by a large posterior fossa cyst thought to be due to the congenital atresia of the foramina of Luschka and the foramen of Magendie. If recognized early and treated appropriately, many of these children can lead a near-normal life in the absence of other complicating congenital malformations.

ACQUIRED HYDROCEPHALUS

Postnatal complications such as intraventricular hemorrhage, especially in pre-term infants, can lead to the development of communicating hydrocephalus because of interference with CSF absorption. Similarly, among adults, any event leading to intraventricular or subarachnoid hemorrhage such as head trauma, tumors, and aneurysm/AVM rupture can lead to the development of communicating hydrocephalus. Bacterial and tuberculous meningitis, because of the intense inflammatory response that these conditions elicit in the basal subarachnoid space and around the CSF absorptive surfaces, can cause both communicating and noncommunicating hydrocephalus. Tumors, especially those involving the posterior fossa, can cause obstruction to CSF circulation at the aqueduct of Sylvius and/or the fourth ventricle, leading to the development of noncommunicating hydrocephalus. Supratentorial neoplasms, by causing mass effect, may distort the ventricular system and cause obstruction at the foramen of Monro, the aqueduct of Sylvius, or the third ventricle. Another condition now being increasingly recognized, especially in the elderly population, is the syndrome of normal pressure hydrocephalus. This communicating type of ventricular dilatation is thought to be related to defective CSF absorption and in some cases may be related to a remote history of meningitis or subarachnoid hemorrhage.

Clinical manifestations of hydrocephalus include features of raised ICP and those due to the underlying cause. Diagnosis is made by the demonstration of progressive enlargement of the head or by ultrasonography in neonates and infants. In older children and adults, demonstration of ventriculomegaly by CT scan of the brain coupled with clinical features of raised pressure is diagnostic (Fig. 28-6). The syndrome of normal pressure hydrocephalus in its classic form includes the triad of gait ataxia, incontinence, and dementia.

Some of the cases of acquired hydrocephalus can be effectively treated by adequately managing the under-lying cause; for example, complete excision of fourth ventricular and lateral ventricular tumors. In all other instances, some form of CSF diversionary procedure must be performed. The most common of these is the placement of a Silastic catheter from the lateral ventricle to the peritoneum (VP shunt). Most of these systems include a valve assembly and a flushing chamber to regulate the rate of CSF drainage. Shunting may also be performed to other body cavities, including the right atrium, the pleural space, and so on. Communicating hydrocephalus, especially in adults, can also be effectively treated by the placement of a shunt from the lumbar subarachnoid space to the peritoneum (LP shunt).

Complications following CSF shunts include infection, malfunction, hemorrhage, and over- or under-drainage. Revision and replacement of the shunt system are therefore not uncommon in these patients, and control of shunt infection often requires complete removal of the system and temporary external drainage of CSF. Excessive reduction of ICP should be avoided preoperatively since that might promote the development of subdural hematoma. Further, the number and movement of personnel within the operating room should be kept to the minimum to help prevent shunt infection.

ARACHNOID CYSTS

These are uncommon congenital lesions that occur in the subarachnoid space and have their own wall consisting of a semitransparent membrane similar to the normal arachnoid. The cyst contents are clear and watery, resembling normal cerebrospinal fluid. The surrounding brain is almost always normal except for the indentation and impression caused by the longstanding cyst. While these cysts may occur anywhere in the brain, the common sites include the sylvian fissure, the suprachiasmatic region, cerebral convexity, the cerebellopontine angle, and the cisterna magna. Many of these lesions are found incidentally and require no specific treatment. Symptomatic cysts often present with features of raised ICP and/or focal neurologic symptoms. Treatment in such cases includes excision of the cyst wall or marsupialization and, in rare instances, the placement of a catheter from the cyst to the normal subarachnoid space.

Other Conditions

PNEUMOCEPHALUS

Air may enter the cranium through a dural defect and collect in the subdural, subarachnoid space or in the ventricles. If the defect is in close proximity to a brain laceration, the collection may occur within the substance of the brain. This condition develops in fractures involving the paranasal sinuses, the roof of the nose, or mastoid air cells. In rare instances, it may be the result of erosion of the cranial base by a tumor, commonly a fronto-ethmoidal osteoma or from a mucocele of the frontal or sphenoid sinus. Tension pneumocephalus leading to cerebral compression may occur, especially if the defects are small and the mucosal surfaces or the dural tears act as a one-way valve, trapping air within the cranium with straining, coughing, or sneezing. In rare instances, it may follow lumbar CSF drainage. While small collections of air without associated active CSF leak may heal spontaneously with time, larger collections and tension pneumocephalus require burr hole evacuation and/or repair of the site of leak. It is important to remember that a certain degree of air collects in the subdural space after every craniotomy and most of it is absorbed in the immediate postoperative period.

RADIATION NECROSIS

The normal brain tissue surrounding a tumor is susceptible to damage from the effects of radiation therapy, but this does not become clinically apparent until long after treatment (at least 9 months and usually about 3 years). Clinical manifestations of postradiation necrosis include localizing neurologic signs, dementia, and papilledema. The affected tissue becomes ischemic due to fibrinoid necrosis of small vessels, but the reason for the long latent period is still not known. Radiologically, these lesions are often indistinguishable from the original tumor and are often associated with significant edema. Positron emission tomography may be useful in distinguishing this condition by demonstrating a relative lack of metabolic activity. Management of this condition includes prevention by careful planning of radiation portals and dosimetry, use of steroids, often in high doses, to mitigate the effects of edema, and, in certain conditions, surgical excision of the necrotic area.

Supratentorial Neurosurgery— Patient Positioning

Optimal positioning of the patient is vital to any neurosurgical procedure. Most supratentorial lesions can be adequately operated upon in one of the three standard positions: supine, lateral, and prone. Proper positioning of the patient in the operating room requires advance planning and can be quite challenging. Both surgical and anesthetic teams will require access to the patient. In most institutions, the anesthesiologist and

anesthetic equipment are positioned to the left of the patient regardless of the side being operated upon, as this allows unimpeded surgical access to the scrub nurse, especially for a right-handed surgeon. Alternatively, the head-end of the operating table can be reversed 180 degrees to approach right- and left-sided lesions, with the anesthesiologist and his/her equipment on the side opposite from the operation. In either case, advanced communication between surgical and anesthetic teams allows efficient use of time and space in the operating room.

SUPINE POSITION

The supine position is the most versatile in neurosurgery. Frontal, temporal, and parietal craniotomy approaches are most commonly performed with the patient in this position. The head and neck are positioned just above the level of the heart to ensure adequate venous drainage without increasing the risk of venous air embolism. For midline and subfrontal lesions, the head is kept straight but extended at the neck to allow the frontal lobes to fall away from the base of the skull with gravity. For a right- or left-sided lesion, a soft roll is placed under the ipsilateral shoulder so that the head may be turned to the opposite side without much neck rotation. In general, optimal positioning aims to bring the site of the lesion uppermost and parallel to the floor. The head is secured to the operating table using a three-point head holding device such as the Mayfield three-pin headrest. The pins of the holding device should be positioned so that they remain well away from the craniotomy site with its axis at or below the equatorial plane to prevent accidental slipping during the course of the operation. More posterior and paramedian lesions may require the head to be flexed at the neck.

LATERAL POSITION

This position is preferred for posterior parietal and occipital lesions and in patients in whom neck rotation is either restricted or not desirable. Again, the three-point headrest is used to fix the skull. The patient is then turned to the lateral position with the surgeon controlling the head in synchronous movement with the rest of the body, maintaining a neural head-neck position. A well padded, soft roll is placed under the dependent axilla to protect the brachial plexus, and the head frame is then secured to the operating table. All pressure points are securely padded. The hips and knees are flexed anatomically. The dependent upper extremity is allowed to rest on an arm board, and the superior upper extremity is secured anatomically over several layers of sheets and padding.

PRONE POSITION

Midline and paramedian occipital lobe lesions are best dealt with in a prone patient. Again, the three-point headrest is applied, and the patient is then turned prone onto the operating table, resting on chest rolls. All pressure points, especially the elbow, wrist, and ankle are adequately padded. The arms are tucked by the sides. The hips and knees are flexed slightly. The head and neck are kept neutral with respect to the rest of the body.

SITTING POSITION

This position is sometimes used in the management of pineal region tumors. Anesthetic and operative considerations of this position are discussed in the chapter on posterior fossa surgery.

The position of the patient during the procedure should permit adequate access so that the surgical team can operate in comfort throughout. The patient should be adequately secured to the table, as changes in table height and tilt may be needed intraoperatively. All anatomic pressure areas and traction points require padding to prevent ischemic injury. The final position of the patient on the table should be such that an awake patient would be comfortable, without hemodynamic or neurologic compromise. Achieving this can be time-consuming and may provide quite variable stimulation to the patient. Intense periods of stimulation, such as during induction with laryngoscopy and application of the three-point head frame, are interspersed with varying times of minimal stimulation. Maintaining stable hemodynamics to assure cerebral perfusion requires vigilance and skill.

Supratentorial Neurosurgery— Anesthetic Considerations

Optimal anesthetic care of the patient with a supratentorial mass begins preoperatively. It is only through an integrated assessment of the exact location of the supratentorial lesion, the apparent degree of CNS compromise, surgical and positioning considerations, and the patient's pre-existing medical condition that an effective anesthetic technique can be planned. Examination of the patient's neuroradiologic studies will reveal the size and location of the lesion. Peritumoral edema, distortion of the ventricular system, and the presence of midline shift on CT and/or MRI indicate that ICP elevations are likely, and anesthetic techniques are focused on maximizing surgical exposure and preventing cerebral ischemia. While superficial lesions may compromise intracranial volume, such tumors often are relatively easy to remove. Adjunctive techniques such as hyperventilation to decrease intracranial volume may be required only briefly. Lesions deep within the brain, regardless of size, or tumors in proximity to vital structures, such as the intracerebral arteries, may require specialized intraoperative monitoring and maximal efforts to facilitate surgical exposure.

Most patients are extremely anxious about the craniotomy, and may express concern about anesthetic care. The neuroanesthesiologist establishes rapport with the patient by discussing this issue along with the patient's general medical condition. Preexisting medical conditions, such as cardiac disease, influence the selection of anesthetic agents and monitoring techniques. A history of endocrine dysfunction, often associated with pituitary lesions, should be elicited. In addition, the evaluation focuses on signs and symptoms of elevated ICP.

Headaches, central nervous system depression, nausea and vomiting, as well as visual disturbances and papilledema are all indicative of increased ICP. Most often patients with brain tumors who exhibit these symptoms, will be treated preoperatively with the corticosteroid, dexamethasone. Dexamethasone decreases peritumoral edema, possibly through inhibition of the Na^+-K^+ ATPase pump and promotion of a decrease in vascular permeability. By the time the neuroanesthesiologist encounters the patient, signs and symptoms from a tumor may no longer be present.[29]

The presence of preoperative neurologic deficits should be documented. Neuroimaging studies may hint at likely postoperative deficits, depending on the location of the lesion. Following the operation, an attentive neuroanesthesiologist, in concert with the surgeon, can differentiate anticipated transient deficits from those which are unexpected and necessitate immediate re-exploration of the operative site. Preexisting motor deficits influence the choice of neuromuscular relaxants as well as the site of blockade monitoring. Many patients with supratentorial lesions present with seizures. While the seizures are usually controlled preoperatively with anticonvulsant therapy, the anesthesiologist must continue therapy perioperatively to prevent waning of therapeutic blood levels. Patients on chronic anticonvulsant therapy often require more frequent dosing of relaxants to maintain the desired level of neuromuscular blockade.[30]

Preoperative laboratory studies for the patient undergoing craniotomy for a supratentorial mass should include hematocrit, blood chemistry (particularly glucose and creatinine) as well as a type and screen for blood products. Cross-matched blood should be available for a patient with a large meningioma, hemangioblastoma, or other tumor type demonstrating increased vascularity on neuroimaging studies.

Dexamethasone can elevate blood glucose. Since the detrimental effects of an elevation in glucose on wound healing and on outcome from a cerebral ischemic event are well known,[31] glucose should be controlled to levels less than 250 mg/dl during neurosurgical procedures. Creatinine is an important indicator of renal function in patients requiring diuretic therapy to facilitate intracranial exposure.

Patients undergoing craniotomy for supratentorial lesions require standard perioperative monitoring including ECG, noninvasive blood pressure, pulse oximetry, temperature, and capnography. Direct, intra-arterial pressure monitoring offers the convenience of sampling capability for frequent blood gas, electrolyte, and hematocrit determinations, and provides a continual assessment of mean arterial pressure. Transducing the arterial blood pressure at the level of the patient's foramen magnum will allow one to maintain and monitor an adequate cerebral perfusion [cerebral perfusion pressure (CPP) = MAP − ICP] at >60 torr if an ICP monitor is employed prior to craniotomy. Once the dura is opened, ICP equals atmospheric pressure, and CPP is solely dependent upon MAP. Continual assessment of MAP allows titration of vasoactive infusions to maintain CPP.

In many patients a steady relationship exists between ET_{CO_2} and Pa_{CO_2}. This may not be the case in patients with pre-existing pulmonary diseases, including those related to cigarette smoking.[32] In such instances, frequent blood gas tension determinations serve to guide hyperventilation therapy.

If the potential exists for significant intraoperative hemorrhage, or a lengthy surgical procedure is anticipated, central venous pressure monitoring is useful to guide fluid therapy and blood replacement. A multiorificed central venous catheter should be placed to treat a possible embolism (VAE) if the patient's head is elevated 30° above the heart level.[33] A precordial Doppler for early detection of VAE is required as well.[34]

Since much intracranial surgery is performed by microscopic techniques, motionless conditions must be assured. Additionally, many patients are usually fixed in a three-point headrest, secured with pins anchored into the cranium itself. Forceful movements can cause scalp lacerations or even neck injury. Neuromuscular blockade monitoring is advantageous.

Special caution must be taken in the patient presenting with hemiparesis. Disuse atrophy allows for an increase in the density of acetylcholine receptors at the neuromuscular junction.[35] Monitoring of neuromuscular blockade in an extremity where there is an increase in receptors may lead to an underestima-

tion of the degree of neuromuscular relaxation and a relative overdose of relaxant. Blockade may be prolonged at a time when rapid neurologic assessment of the patient is required. Care must be taken to assure placement of the monitor on a neurologically intact extremity.

In a patient with a supratentorial mass, anesthesiologists focus on controlling intracranial volume and maximizing surgical exposure. During induction one must assure that the patient's head is elevated and positioned without embarrassment to jugular venous drainage.[36,37] Adequate oxygenation must be assured. Arterial oxygen tensions <50 mmHg cause marked increases in cerebral vasodilatation and blood flow.[38]

Diuretic therapy is commonly employed to facilitate intracranial exposure. Mannitol, an osmotic diuretic of high molecular weight, causes water to be drawn into the intravascular space across an intact blood-brain barrier along an osmotic gradient.[39] Hematocrit, blood viscosity, and cerebrovascular resistance are lowered. Cerebral blood flow may actually increase, and oxygen delivery to brain tissue may improve. In patients with an elevated ICP, prompt reductions in ICP follow mannitol therapy.[40] A common dose is 0.5 to 1.0 g/kg administered by infusion at the beginning of the craniotomy. Caution must be exercised in using osmotic diuretics in patients with congestive heart failure because of the transient increase in blood volume. Mannitol may also afford cerebral protection, possibly through improvements in the cerebral microcirculation.[41]

The loop diuretic furosemide inhibits the Na^+-K^+ ATPase pump to allow free water excretion via the kidney. This yields an overall reduction in plasma volume, and presumably in cerebral blood volume. Furosemide may also mildly depress cerebrospinal fluid formation.[42] A dose of 0.5 mg/kg is common. Electrolyte losses must be closely monitored if furosemide is administered in addition to mannitol.

Cerebrospinal fluid drainage is occasionally employed to increase intracranial access to supratentorial lesions. The neurosurgeon can locate the lateral ventricle intraoperatively and allow cerebrospinal fluid drainage by gravity. Care must be taken to maintain the CSF drain height to prevent overly vigorous drainage. More commonly, a lumbar CSF drain may be placed following anesthetic induction. Opening the drain before the dura is open and vigorous CSF drainage causing hypertension must be avoided.[43]

Hyperventilation can be very effective in reducing intracranial volume. Carbon dioxide freely diffuses across the blood-brain barrier, affecting cerebral arteriolar resistance through changes in pH.[44] Carbon dioxide tension and cerebral blood flow are linearly related between 20 and 80 mmHg. Hyperventilation below Pa_{CO_2} 25 is not recommended, as blood flow is severely compromised, shifting the oxyhemoglobin dissociation curve to the left. Cerebral ischemia may result with anaerobic metabolism and the production of lactic acidosis.[45]

In a patient with signs and symptoms of increased ICP, preoperative sedation should be administered only in the presence of the anesthesiologist. Sedative agents may prevent an accurate preoperative neurologic examination, and narcotic agents may cause the patient to hypoventilate allowing a rise in Pa_{CO_2}. Bearing this in mind, however, patients presenting for craniotomy are frequently apprehensive. Sympathetic stimulation can cause an increase in mean arterial pressure and possibly exacerbate intracranial hypertension. Carefully titrated amounts of benzodiazepine can be used with caution. Likewise, local anesthesia to blunt sympathetic responses should be used for potentially painful procedures, such as attaining arterial and intravascular access.

The selection of anesthetic agents is probably less important than a *very carefully conducted* anesthetic, with particular attention to hemodynamic and ICP control. The effects of individual anesthetic agents on cerebral blood volume and ICP should be considered as well as requirements for intraoperative monitoring and rapid postoperative neurologic assessment.

The ideal intravenous induction agent for the patient undergoing supratentorial craniotomy should maintain cerebral perfusion pressure, prevent extreme changes in mean arterial pressure, and preferably decrease, but certainly not increase, ICP. Thiopental has a successful history of use during induction. This agent depresses cerebral metabolic function (CMR_{O_2}) and reduces cerebral blood flow concomitantly.[46,47] ICP is lowered, but myocardial depression and peripheral vasodilatation can be profound. The resulting decline in mean arterial pressure may compromise cerebral perfusion. Combining a reduced dosage of thiopental with modest doses of narcotics during induction often makes cardiac depression clinically insignificant in patients with good myocardial function.

Midazolam, a benzodiazepine, offers an acceptable alternative because the effects on cerebral metabolic rate and cerebral blood flow are similar to thiopental, and myocardial depression from an induction dose is modest.[48] Etomidate tends to maintain cardiovascular stability on induction and renders a dose-dependent decrease in CBF and the cerebral metabolic rate of oxygen consumption, while preserving CO_2 reactivity.[49] Use is not widespread because of associated myoclonus, which resembles seizure activity in appearance, and suppression of adrenal function. Often the neurosurgical patient is managed with corticosteroids, however, and adrenal suppression associated with an induction dose is short-term. Etomidate offers an advantage in a patient with cardiovascular compromise.

Propofol depresses cerebral blood flow and ICP; however, systemic vasodilatation may reduce mean arterial pressure to such a degree as to compromise cerebral perfusion.[50] Ketamine has been shown to increase ICP, probably via cerebrovasodilatation as well as sympathomimetic effects on mean arterial pressure.[51] The effect on ICP may be blunted by hyperventilation, but ketamine nonetheless is generally avoided in the patient with a supratentorial lesion.

A common induction sequence for a patient for a supratentorial tumor involves the use of thiopental 3 to 5 mg/kg, 5 μg/kg of fentanyl, 100 mg of lidocaine and small doses of esmolol or additional thiopental to blunt the cardiovascular responses to laryngoscopy. Hyperventilation is instituted following loss of consciousness and a nondepolarizing neurovascular relaxant is administered once an adequate mask airway is assured.

Hemodynamic responses to a muscle relaxant may prompt its selection since, in general, these agents exhibit no effect on cerebral blood flow or ICP. Pancuronium is a sympathomimetic and may increase mean arterial pressure. D-Tubocurarine, metocurine, and atracurium may cause vasodilatation due to histamine release, which may be a factor in a patient with severely reduced intracranial compliance.[52–54] Laudanosine, a metabolite of atracurium, may cause seizures in dogs, but this phenomenon has not been reported in humans.[55] Vecuronium and rocuronium render very stable hemodynamics.[56]

The effects of the depolarizing relaxant, succinylcholine, on ICP are more controversial. Succinylcholine has been shown in some animal and human studies to cause an increase in ICP. This most likely results from fasciculations and an increase in muscle spindle activity, which in turn increases cerebral blood flow.[57] This increase is probably attenuated by prevention of muscle spindle activity. Pretreatment with a nondepolarizing muscle relaxant has been shown to prevent the increase in ICP seen with succinylcholine.[58]

Historically, the use of volatile anesthetics in the neurosurgical patient with a supratentorial lesion has enjoyed a long record of safety. This seems surprising when one considers the effects of these agents on the cerebral vasculature, ICP, and systemic vascular resistance. Halothane, for example, causes cerebrovascular dilatation, increases cerebral blood flow, and increases cerebral blood volume.[59] In the patient with a mass lesion, ICP may rise. Simultaneously, halothane causes myocardial depression and decreases MAP. As a result, CPP declines, potentially into the ischemic range. Enflurane and, less so, isoflurane also cause cerebrovasodilatation and increased cerebral blood flow.[60,61] Enflurane in concentrations of 1.5 to 2.0 MAC when combined with hyperventilation can induce seizure activity on electroencephalographic recordings.[62]

The success of inhalational agents historically in neurosurgical anesthesia has probably occurred because the effects of low doses of these agents on cerebral blood flow and intracranial pressure are attenuated by hyperventilation and adjuvant methods of reducing brain bulk.[63] In most cases, halothane or isoflurane may be used without deleterious effects on ICP as components of a carefully conducted anesthetic, with the usual practices of hyperventilation and diuresis.

The newer volatile agents, desflurane and sevoflurane, behave similarly to isoflurane. Cerebrovascular dilatation and a coupled decrease in cerebral metabolic rate occur in a dose-dependent fashion.[64,65] Responsivity to carbon dioxide is maintained, so the effect of increased cerebral blood flow is very much attenuated by hyperventilation. These agents appear safe in the patient presenting with a supratentorial lesion, and may even be advantageous because their insolubility allows rapid elimination of the volatile anesthetic on emergence.

Nitrous oxide, an agent with a long history of use in neuroanesthesia, can increase ICP in man. Cerebral blood flow increases through vasodilatation.[66] Often deleterious effects on ICP are blocked by common neuroanesthetic techniques of hyperventilation, narcotic, and barbiturate administration.[67] However, in circumstances where surgical exposure is extremely limited, cerebral relaxation techniques often include the discontinuation of nitrous oxide.

Nitrous oxide is 30 times more soluble than nitrogen, and freely diffuses into an air-filled space.[68] A tension pneumocephalus may result if the dura is closed over a large intracranial pocket in the presence of nitrous oxide. Clinically, the patient manifests a decreased sensorium, neurologic deficit and/or seizures in the PACU.[69]

Narcotics are often the foundation of maintenance anesthesia for craniotomy. The ability to provide hemodynamic stability, without deleterious effects on ICP, and allow for rapid emergence at the conclusion of the case make narcotics invaluable adjuncts. Carbon dioxide reactivity is preserved.[70] However, controversy remains over the effect of narcotics upon cerebral blood flow. Sufentanil has been reported to cause a marked increase in ICP through cerebral vasodilatation.[71] Alfentanil also has been shown, in some studies, to increase ICP.[72] If one examines the effects of fentanyl, sufentanil, alfetanil, and most recently remifentanil on ICP, cerebral blood flow, and CPP in subjects who are

hyperventilated and receive adequate anesthesia, in general the effects of narcotics are minimal.[73,74]

Careful titration of narcotics is required to avoid respiratory depression and delays in emergence postoperatively. While these effects can be antagonized, naloxone has been shown to increase mean arterial pressure, cerebral blood flow, and ICP.[75] Remifentanil, with its rapid clearance by an esterase metabolism, may provide a very clear emergence from general anesthesia, thus enabling one to quickly assess the patient neurologically with almost complete elimination of anesthetic agents that can alter mental status.[76]

Fluid management of the neurosurgical patient has received much attention. Hyperglycemia exacerbates ischemic brain injury, so dextrose-containing solutions should be avoided.[31] Additionally, many patients experience alterations in glucose tolerance secondary to exogenous steroids. The risk of cerebral ischemia is certainly present in the patient with a supratentorial lesion, as cerebral perfusion may become compromised with changes in mean arterial pressure or ICP. Intraoperative brain retraction generating pressures in excess of 20 mmHg can also cause disruptions in blood flow, causing ischemia.[77]

Osmotic gradients are primarily responsible for movement of water between the vasculature and the brain's extracellular space.[78] Of the non-glucose-containing solutions, few data support the use of one isotonic solution over another. Theoretically, normal saline, with its slight hypertonicity, may help to reduce cerebral edema, given an intact blood-brain barrier.

The use of hydroxyethyl starch deserves discussion. This colloid provides intravascular expansion with little effect on brain edema, but its use is limited in the patient undergoing craniotomy. In volumes greater than 1000 ml, hydroxyethyl starch may prolong PTT and actually promote fibrinolysis. This results in part from a decrease in factor VIII and von Willebrand activity.[79] Obviously, a decline in coagulability in the patient having craniotomy can lead to catastrophic hematoma formation and cerebral compromise.

Occasionally, intraoperative surgical exposure is compromised in the anesthetized patient. Initial steps include determination of an arterial blood gas to assure adequate oxygenation and hyperventilation to a Pa_{CO_2} of 25 mmHg. Reassessment of the patient's position to assure modest head elevation and unobstructed jugular venous drainage should also occur. An additional dose of furosemide or mannitol may be helpful, with careful attention given to serum osmolality and electrolyte concentrations. If conditions improve with small doses of thiopental, inhalational anesthetics are often discontinued and a total intravenous technique initiated.

In most cases, neurosurgeons want an adequate neurologic assessment as soon as possible after craniectomy. Special care must be taken to facilitate a smooth and rapid anesthetic emergence. Coughing allows a tremendous increase in intrathoracic pressure that impairs jugular drainage and elevates ICP. It is best avoided and often can be minimized through the use of lidocaine, 50 to 100 mg, during closure of the skin incision. Likewise, elevations in mean arterial pressure can cause hematoma formation at the surgical site. Labetalol, a mixed α or β antagonist, allows careful control of blood pressure and heart rate without deleterious effects on cerebral vasculature.

Immediately postoperatively, the anesthesiologist aims to eliminate residual anesthetics that could complicate evaluation of the craniotomy patient. Obviously, respiratory depression from narcotic overdosage and resulting hypercarbia are to be avoided. Persistence of an unanticipated neurologic deficit requires immediate attention, as brain tissue may be compromised in a life-threatening fashion. Neuroradiologic studies and/or surgical re-exploration must be considered, and emergency therapy for intracranial hypertension may be required.

General Complications Following Supratentorial Surgery

Despite careful preoperative planning and meticulous intraoperative technique, adverse postoperative events occur. Anticipation of such complications and diligent postoperative care are essential to a successful outcome. Some of the common and often avoidable complications following supratentorial neurosurgery are discussed below.

WOUND BREAKDOWN AND INFECTION

Scalp wound breakdown after elective surgery is extremely uncommon because of the excellent vascularity of the scalp. It more often complicates surgery following trauma and in situations where there has been loss of tissue. Postcraniotomy infections are most often superficial and restricted to the scalp and the subgaleal space. The scalp is usually closed in two layers to achieve hemostasis and prevent the formation of a subgaleal hematoma, a potential focus for infection. A delay in the clearance of the normal postoperative subgaleal fluid collection, the appearance of the cardinal signs of infection, namely, swelling, tenderness, and redness (often not very obvious) and/or persistent discharge from the wound should alert one to the possibility of scalp infection. Early detection allows

rapid control of infection, if necessary by open drainage and irrigation along with appropriate antibiotics. Every effort should be made to detect osteomyelitis of the underlying bone flap, for its involvement necessitates bone plate removal in most cases.

In cases of infections beyond the galea, removal of the bone plate and irrigation of the epidural space almost always results in good infection control. In such instances, cranioplasty to cover the resulting defect should be delayed at least 6 to 12 months. Subdural empyema as a complication of elective supratentorial surgery is extremely rare. It may follow operations in which the paranasal or mastoid air sinuses have been violated or in instances where a subdural drain has been left in place, for example, following evacuation of a subdural hematoma. The clinical manifestations may include fever, seizures, and wound drainage. CT and/or MR scans may show fluid collections in subdural space with enhancement of its margins. Treatment of such accumulations include not only complete drainage and irrigation of the subdural cavity but also removal of the bone plate and prolonged course of antibiotic therapy.

Postoperative meningitis and intracerebral abscess formation are exceedingly rare. Blood in the CSF space may produce meningism and pyrexia at an early stage after supratentorial craniotomy. The persistence of such symptoms with associated leukocytosis should raise one's suspicion of meningitis, prompting an early analysis of the CSF. While a mild degree of pleocytosis is not uncommon after a craniotomy, leukocyte counts in excess of 100 indicate infection. The operative cavity is occasionally the site of a late intracranial abscess after weeks or months. The use of a foreign body at the time of operation, ventricular catheters or drains, and violation of potentially infected sinuses during the craniotomy all predispose to infection at this site. Early diagnosis even with CT and MR scanning can often be difficult, but infection should be suspected whenever the edema, mass effect, and enhancement of the resection cavity is beyond that expected. When infection is suspected, diagnosis and treatment may include needle aspiration and possible re-exploration along with appropriate antibiotics. Such intracranial infections are rarely if ever associated with concomitant scalp infection.

HEMORRHAGE

Postoperative hemorrhage is the most serious complication of neurosurgery and can have a devastating effect on outcome if not detected early. Careful hemostasis during opening and subsequent closure of the scalp wound in two layers will help prevent most subgaleal hematomas. In a recent 5-year survey of operated postoperative hematoma following 6668 neurosurgical procedures, Palmer and co-workers reported an overall rate of 1.1 percent.[80] Forty-three percent of these were intraparenchymal, 35 percent extradural, 12 percent subdural, and 10 percent involved the subgaleal space. A small collection of epidural blood following every craniotomy is not uncommon. Significant collections, especially after large craniotomy flaps, can be avoided by placing epidural tack-up sutures around the bone edges and using Gelfoam or Surgicel packing between the bone-dura interface.

Subdural and intracerebral hematomas are more common following emergency craniotomies and surgery for benign neoplasms such as meningiomas than after removal of intrinsic brain tumors. In one series, postoperative hematomas complicated 6.2 percent of cases following meningioma surgery compared with a 2.2 percent rate following surgery for intrinsic supratentorial tumors.[81] With every intracranial operation, the surgeon should meticulously achieve hemostasis under normotensive conditions prior to dural closure. Routine use of the Valsalva maneuver by the anesthesiologist can help demonstrate potential sites of venous bleeding. The operative site should be thoroughly irrigated with saline until the returns are completely clear. Hemostatic agents such as Gelfoam or Surgicel can only help control minor capillary ooze in the presence of normal host hemostatic mechanisms. Avoidance of increased blood pressure and violent coughing upon emergence and at extubation is a must.

Observation of the patient in the immediate postoperative period is directed primarily at detecting clot formation. To facilitate early diagnosis, the anesthesiologist must have the patient awake, answering simple questions, and moving limbs to command before they leave the operating room. Any subsequent deterioration in the level of consciousness, strength, or size of the pupils should raise a strong suspicion of an intracranial hematoma. A clot may form within hours of leaving the OR, and a patient who is allowed to "sleep off" the operation with either long-acting anesthetic agents or postoperative sedation may never wake up. Discomfort after craniotomy is seldom great and can be alleviated without masking changes in the conscious level by judicious use of analgesics. In a recent study of the timing of postoperative hematoma, 90 percent[81] of hematomas requiring reoperation occurred within 6 h of surgery. Further, nearly two-thirds of patients requiring reoperation had preoperatively identifiable risk factors for a preoperative bleeding disorder, with use of antiplatelet agents being the most common risk factor.[80]

SEIZURES

Every supratentorial operation carries some risk of epilepsy, the risk depending on pre-existing seizures, the underlying pathologic lesion, and on cortical damage caused by the surgery. Surgery in and around the sensory motor cortex carries a much higher risk than in the occipital region. An early postoperative seizure may herald or precipitate postoperative complications. It is imperative, therefore, that every patient undergoing supratentorial surgery be pretreated with adequate amounts of anticonvulsants to maintain sufficient therapeutic levels in the postoperative period.

CSF OBSTRUCTION AND LEAK

Spillage of blood into the subarachnoid space and ventricular system can interfere with free CSF circulation and its absorption at the arachnoidal villi, leading to the development of hydrocephalus. Clinically significant hydrocephalus, however, is more commonly observed following surgery for benign, longstanding lesions that have already caused interference with normal CSF circulation. It is also associated with operations for such conditions as craniopharyngioma, epidermoids, and dermoids, where the release of the cyst contents into the subarachnoid space elicits a strong chemical meningitic reaction.

Another manifestation of impaired CSF circulation is the formation of pseudomeningocele. Every attempt should be made to close the dura in a watertight fashion following craniotomy. However, in the absence of an preoperative CSF circulation abnormality, postoperative CSF leak and pseudomeningocele are rare. With the normalization of pressures within the cranial cavity, a pseudo-dura forms with time. There is, however, a greater likelihood of scar formation and adherence of the cerebral cortex, which can potentially make reoperation more difficult. Treatment of CSF leak and pseudomeningocele requires reoperation and closure of the leak and attention to underlying hydrocephalus and CSF outflow obstruction.

CSF leaks from the scalp wound also reflect an underlying problem of raised pressure and/or impaired circulation. Minor leaks may be contained by simple oversewing of the wound. They are much more common when the ventricular system has been entered during surgery. CSF otorrhea and rhinorrhea are likely to complicate procedures when paranasal sinuses and mastoid air cells have been entered during the operation. Whatever the source or site of leak, this problem requires immediate attention because of the potential development of meningitis. Continuous lumbar CSF drainage in the postoperative period is effective in most instances. More persistent leaks demand exclusion of underlying raised pressure or hydrocephalus and may require reoperation and direct closure of the site of leak.

ISCHEMIA

Focal ischemia following supratentorial craniotomy is most often due to excessive or prolonged retraction of the brain during surgery. Widespread disruption of the blood-brain barrier and subsequent development of edema in the region of retraction have been demonstrated in both experimental and clinical studies involving retraction pressure measurements. Intentional and inadvertent occlusion of vessels also may contribute. Venous infarction and extensive brain swelling may follow occlusion of major draining veins, for example, during surgeries in and around the venous sinuses. Management of ischemic complications is essentially preventive, for there is no effective treatment once infarction has occurred. Hyperglycemia should be avoided to prevent extension of the ischemic area. Interventions with barbiturates, etomidate, hypothermia, hypertension, and hypervolemia may be needed to retrieve some function in the region of ischemic penumbra.

RAISED ICP

Many of the above-mentioned complications can lead to raised ICP which can further compromise neurologic function. Other more readily correctable causes in the immediate postoperative period include carbon dioxide retention due to inadequate ventilation, effects of drugs and anesthetics, and raised body temperature. Hypoventilation, whether due to impaired brain stem function or excessive sedation from narcotics, can significantly impair recovery from the operation and even cause permanent neurologic deterioration by causing severe vasodilatation and raised ICP. Fever and raised body temperature can cause significant elevation of cerebral metabolism and blood flow, leading to raised ICP. Anesthetic agents and other drugs may rarely induce hyperthermia, and its effect on ICP may persist for several hours after the operation. Other agents such as volatile anesthetics and vasoactive drugs may raise ICP by causing cerebral vasodilatation.

SYSTEMIC COMPLICATIONS

Intracranial operations must be regarded as major surgical procedures and are subject to systemic complications like surgery elsewhere in the body. The frequency and severity of such complications is to a large extent determined by the preoperative medical condition of the patient. Optimal control of blood pressure helps prevent worsening of vasogenic edema that follows manipulation of brain tissue. Atelectasis remains the most common pulmonary complication, especially following lengthy intracranial procedures and those performed in the lateral decubitus position. The use of high-dose steroids in patients undergoing supratentorial craniotomy predisposes them to an increased risk of stress ulcers and gastrointestinal bleeding. Urinary tract infections due to indwelling catheters and impairment of renal function by the variety of antibiotics, anticonvulsants, steroids, and diuretic agents used in the management of the neurosurgical patient should be anticipated and appropriate preventive measures instituted. Prolonged bed rest and immobilization of limbs due to paralysis significantly increase the incidence of venous thromboembolism. Routine use of pneumatic compression boots in the intra- and perioperative period is therefore highly desirable. Though some studies have demonstrated the safety of perioperative use of low-dose heparin,[82] it has not gained universal acceptance for intracranial procedures. Endocrine and other electrolyte disturbances such as SIADH and diabetes insipidus are particularly prone to occur following surgeries in and around the hypothalamus and the pituitary gland.

Conclusions

Supratentorial neurosurgery involves the management of a variety of disorders, and this chapter has attempted to provide a broad overview of some of the common conditions. A more detailed discussion of the conditions presented in this chapter may be found in the referenced journal articles. For details regarding the more rare supratentorial lesions, the interested reader should consult a standard neurosurgical text.

References

1. Miller JD, Dearden M: Measurement, analysis and the management of raised ICP. In Teasdale GM, Miller JD (eds): *Current Neurosurgery*. Edinburgh, Churchill-Livingstone, 1992:119–156.
2. Langfitt TW: Increased intracranial pressure. *Clin Neurosurg* 1969; 16:436.
3. Pollay M: Formation of cerebrospinal fluid. Relation of studies of isolated choroid plexus to the standing gradient hypothesis. *J Neurosurg* 1975; 42:665.
4. McComb JG: Recent research into the nature of cerebrospinal fluid formation and absorption. *J Neurosurg* 1983; 59:369.
5. Pickard JD, et al: Steps towards cost-benefit analysis of regional neurosurgical care. *Br Med J* 1990; 301:629.
6. Minns RA: *Problems of Intracranial Pressure in Childhood. Clinics in Developmental Medicine 113/114*. London, Mackeith Press, 1991.
7. Klatzo I: Neuropathological aspects of brain edema. *J Neuropathol Exp Neurol* 1967; 26:1.

8. Schulta HS, et al: Brain swelling produced by injury and aggravated by arterial hypertension. A light and electron microscopic study. *Brain* 1968; 91:281.

9. Fishman RA: Brain edema. *N Engl J Med* 1975; 293:706.

10. Teasdale G, Tennett B: Assessment of coma and impaired consciousness. A practical scale. *Lancet* 1974; 2:81.

11. Ettinger AB: Structural causes of epilepsy: tumors, cysts, stroke and vascular malformations. *Neurol Clin* 1994; 12:41.

12. Davey P, et al: Clinical indications for the radiosurgical treatment of brain tumors. *Can J Oncol* 1994; 4:273.

13. Phillips MH, et al: Stereotactic radiosurgery: A review and comparison of methods. *J Clin Oncol* 1994; 12:1085.

14. Sneed PK, et al: Brachytherapy of brain tumors. *Stereotact Funct Neurosurg* 1992; 59:157.

15. Obbens EA, Shapiro WR: Brain tumor chemotherapy. *Cancer Chemother Biol Response Modif* 1994; 16:628.

16. Shapiro WR, et al: Randomized trial of three chemotherapy regimens and two radiotherapy regimens in postoperative treatment of malignant glioma. Brain Tumor Cooperative Group Trial 8001. *J Neurosurg* 1989; 71:1.

17. Grossman SA, et al: The intracerebral distribution of BCNU delivered by surgically implanted biodegradable polymers. *J Neurosurg* 1992; 76:640.

18. Neuwelt EA, et al: Therapeutic efficacy of multiagent chemotherapy with drug delivery enhancement by blood brain barrier modification in glioblastoma. *Neurosurgery* 1986; 19:573.

19. Pollack IF, et al: Low grade gliomas of the cerebral hemispheres in children: an analysis of 71 cases. *J Neurosurg* 1995; 82:536.

20. Cairncross JA, et al: Aggressive oligodendroglioma: A chemosensitive tumor. *Neurosurgery* 1992; 31:78.

21. Healey EA, et al: The prognostic significance of postoperative residual tumor in ependymoma. *Neurosurgery* 1991; 28:666.

22. Nazzaro JM, Neuwelt EA: The role of surgery in the management of supratentorial intermediate and high grade astrocytomas in adults. *J Neurosurg* 1990; 73:331.

23. Winger MJ, et al: Supratentorial anaplastic gliomas in adults. The prognostic importance of extent of resection and prior low grade glioma. *J Neurosurg* 1989; 71:487.

24. Hockberg FH, Miller DC: Primary CNS lymphoma. *J Neurosurg* 1988; 68:835.

25. Simpson D: The recurrence of intracranial meningiomas after surgical treatment. *J Neurol Neurosurg Psychiatry* 1957; 20:22.

26. Patchell RA, et al: A randomized trial of surgery in the treatment of single metastasis to the brain. *N Engl J Med* 1990; 322:494.

27. Bindal RK, et al: Reoperation for recurrent metastatic brain tumors. *J Neurosurg* 1995; 83:600.

28. Bindal RK, et al: Surgical treatment of multiple brain metastasis. *J Neurosurg* 1993; 79:210.

29. Leenders KL, et al: Dexamethasone treatment of brain tumor patients: Effects on regional cerebral blood flow, blood volume and oxygen utilization. *Neurology* 1985; 35:1610.

30. Ornstein E, et al: Resistance to metocurine-induced neuromuscular blockade in patients receiving phenytoin. *Anesthesiology* 1985; 63:294.

31. Lanier WL, et al: The effects of dextrose infusion and head position on neurologic outcome after complete cerebral ischemia in primates: Examination of a model. *Anesthesiology* 1987; 66:39.

32. Fairley HB: Respiratory monitoring. In Blitt CD (ed): *Monitoring in Anesthesia and Critical Care Medicine*. New York, Churchill-Livingstone, 1985:229.

33. Bunegin L, et al: Positioning the right atrial catheter—a model for reappraisal. *Anesthesiology* 1981; 55:343.

34. Maroon JC, Albin MS: Air embolism diagnosed by doppler ultrasound. *Anesth Analg* 1974; 53:399.

35. Gronert GA, et al: Canine gastrocnemius disuse atrophy: Resistance to paralysis by dimethyl tubocurarine. *J Appl Physiol* 1984; 57:1502.

36. Feldman Z, et al: Effect of head elevation on intracranial pressure, cerebral perfusion pressure, and cerebral blood flow in head-injured patients. *J Neurosurg* 1992; 76:207.

37. Lipe HP, Mitchell PH: Positioning the patient with intracranial hypertension: How turning and head rotation affect the internal jugular vein. *Heart Lung* 1980; 9:1031.

38. Brown MM, et al: Fundamental importance of arterial oxygen content in the regulation of cerebral blood flow in man. *Brain* 1985; 108:81.

39. Rudehill A, et al: Pharmacokinetics and effects of mannitol on hemodynamics, blood and cerebrospinal fluid electrolytes, and osmolality during intracranial surgery. *J Neurosurg Anesthesiol* 1993; 5:4.

40. Ravussion P, et al: Changes in CSF pressure after mannitol in patients with and without elevated CSF pressure. *J Neurosurg* 1988; 69:869.

41. Little JR: Morphological changes in acute focal ischemia. Response to osmotherapy. *Adv Neurol* 1980; 28:443.

42. Melby JM, et al: Effect of acetazolamide and furosemide on the production and composition of cerebrospinal fluid from the cat choroid plexus. *Can J Physiol Pharmacol* 1982; 60:405.

43. Barker J: An anaesthetic technique for intracranial aneurysms. *Anaesthesia* 1982; 30:557.

44. Koehler RC, Traystman RJ: Bicarbonate ion modulation of cerebral blood flow during hypoxia and hypercapnia. *Am J Physiol* 1982; 243:H33.

45. Paulson OB, Sharbrough FW: Physiologic and pathophysiologic relationship between the electroencephalogram and the regional blood flow. *Acta Neurol Scand* 1974; 50:194.

46. Michenfelder JD: The interdependency of cerebral functional and metabolic effects following massive doses of thiopental in the dog. *Anesthesiology* 1974; 41:231.

47. Pierce EC Jr, et al: Cerebral circulation and metabolism during thiopental anesthesia and hyperventilation in man. *J Clin Invest* 1962; 41:1664.

48. Griffin JP, et al: Intracranial pressure, mean arterial pressure, and heart rate following midazolam or thiopental in humans with brain tumors. *Anesthesiology* 1984; 60:491.

49. Renou AM, et al: Cerebral blood flow and metabolism during etomidate anaesthesia in man. *Br J Anaesth* 1978; 50:1047.

50. Pinaud M, et al: Effects of propofol on cerebral hemodynamics and metabolism in patients with brain trauma. *Anesthesiology* 1990; 73:404.

51. Takeshita H, et al: The effects of ketamine on cerebral circulation and metabolism in man. *Anesthesiology* 1972; 36:69.

52. Stoelting RK: The hemodynamic effects of pancuronium and d-tubocurarine in anesthetized patients. *Anesthesiology* 1972; 36:612.

53. Savarese JJ: Histamine, d-tubocurarine, and CSF pressure. *Anesthesiology* 1975; 42:369.

54. Basta SJ, et al: Histamine-releasing potencies of atracurium, dimethyl tubocurarine and tubocurarine. *Br J Anaesth* 1983; 55:105S.

55. Lanier WL, et al: The cerebral effects of pancuronium and atracurium in halothane-anesthetized dogs. *Anesthesiology* 1985; 63:589.

56. Stirt JA, et al: Vecuronium: Effect on intracranial pressure and hemodynamics in neurosurgical patients. *Anesthesiology* 1987; 67:5870.

57. Marsh ML, et al: Succinylcholine-intracranial pressure effects in neurosurgical patients. *Anesth Analg* 1980; 59:550.

58. Minton MD, et al: Increases in intracranial pressure from succinylcholine: prevention by prior nondepolarizing blockade. *Anesthesiology* 1986; 65:165.

59. Jennett WB, et al: Effect of anaesthesia on intracranial pressure in patients with space-occupying lesions. *Lancet* 1969; 1:61.

60. Adams RW, et al: Isoflurane and cerebrospinal fluid pressure in neurosurgical patients. *Anesthesiology* 1981; 54:97.

61. Eintrei C, et al: Local application of [133]Xenon for measurement of regional cerebral blood flow (rCBF) during halothane, enflurane, and isoflurane anesthesia in humans. *Anesthesiology* 1985; 63:391.

62. Wollman H, et al: Cerebral blood flow and oxygen consumption in man during electroencephalographic seizure patterns induced by anesthesia with ethrane. *Fed Proc* 1969; 28:356.

63. Adams RW, et al: Halothane, hypocapnia, and cerebrospinal fluid pressure in neurosurgery. *Anesthesiology* 1972; 37:510.

64. Lutz LJ, et al: The cerebral functional, metabolic, and hemodynamic effects of desflurane in dogs. *Anesthesiology* 1990; 73:125.

65. Kitaguchi K, et al: Effects of sevoflurane on cerebral circulation and metabolism in patients with ischemic cerebrovascular disease. *Anesthesiology* 1993; 79:704.

66. Sakabe T, et al: Cerebral responses to the addition of nitrous oxide to halothane in man. *Br J Anaesth* 1976; 48:957.

67. Henriksen HT, Jorgensen PB: The effect of nitrous oxide on intracranial pressure in patients with intracranial disorders. *Br J Anaesth* 1973; 45:486.

68. Artru AA: Nitrous oxide plays a direct role in the development of tension pneumocephalus intraoperatively. *Anesthesiology* 1982; 57:59.

69. Raggio JF, et al: Expanding pneumocephalus due to nitrous oxide anesthesia. *Neurosurgery* 1979; 4:261.

70. Michenfelder JD, Theye RA: Effects of fentanyl, droperidol, and innovar or canine cerebral metabolism and blood flow. *Br J Anaesth* 1971; 43:630.

71. Marx W et al: Sufentanil, alfentanil, and fentanyl: Impact on cerebrospinal fluid pressure in patients with brain tumors. *J Neurosurg Anesthesiol* 1989; 1:3.

72. Jung R, et al: Cerebrospinal fluid pressure in patients with brain tumors: Impact of fentanyl versus alfentanil during nitrous oxide-oxygen anesthesia. *Anesth Analg* 1990; 71:419.

73. Cuillerier DJ, et al: Alfentanil sufentanil and fentanyl: Effect on cerebral perfusion pressure. *Anesth Analg* 1990; 70:S75.

74. Werner C, et al: Effects of sufentnail on cerebral hemodynamics and intracranial pressure in patients with brain injury. *Anesthesiology* 1995; 83:721.

75. Turner DM, et al: Cerebral and systemic vascular effects of naloxone in pentobarbital-anesthetized normal dogs. *Neurosurgery* 1984; 14:276.

76. Hoffman WE, et al: Effects of remifentanil, a new short-acting opioid, on cerebral blood flow, brain electrical activity, and intracranial pressure in dogs anesthetized with isoflurane and nitrous oxide. *Anesthesiology* 1993; 79:107.

77. Albin MS, et al: Brain retraction pressure during intracranial procedures. *Surg Forum* 1975; 26:499.

78. Zornow MH, et al: The acute cerebral effects of changes in plasma osmolality and oncotic pressure. *Anesthesiology* 1987; 67:936.

79. Stump DC, et al: Effects of hydroxyethyl starch on blood coagulation, particularly factor VIII. *Transfusion* 1985; 25:349.

80. Palmer JD, et al: Postoperative hematoma: A 5 year survey and identification of avoidable risk factors. *Neurosurgery* 1994; 35:1061.

81. Taylor WAS, et al: Timing of postoperative intracranial hematoma development and implications for the best use of neurosurgical intensive care. *J Neurosurg* 1995; 82:48.

82. Powers SK, Edwards MSB: Prophylaxis of thromboembolism in the neurosurgical patients. A review. *Neurosurgery* 1982; 10:509.

Pituitary Surgery

SAMUEL ROBERT BOWEN

DAVID L. KELLY, JR.

PATRICIA H. PETROZZA

CLINICAL PRESENTATION OF PITUITARY ADENOMAS
  Signs and Symptoms Secondary to Mass Effect
  Signs and Symptoms of Hypersecretory Pituitary Adenomas
  Diagnostic Endocrine Evaluation
  Diagnosing Endocrinopathies
  Radiologic Evaluation
TREATMENT
  Introduction
  Medical Therapy
  Radiation Therapy
  Surgical Therapy
  Postoperative Complications with the Transsphenoidal Approach
  Intracranial Complications
ANESTHETIC MANAGEMENT
  Preoperative Preparation
  Intraoperative Management

The list of differential diagnoses of a sellar or suprasellar mass is very extensive (Table 28-5). For the scope of this chapter, we will concentrate on the diagnosis and treatment of pituitary adenomas, since they are the most common tumors in that area. However, the other tumors on the list must be considered when the diagnosis is not clear. Detailed descriptions of these lesions can be found in other neurosurgical texts.[1]

Clinical Presentation of Pituitary Adenomas

Signs and symptoms can be grouped in two broad categories: (1) those due to mass effect in that region; and (2) those secondary to endocrine hypersecretion syndromes.

SIGNS AND SYMPTOMS SECONDARY TO MASS EFFECT

With mass effect, the most common objective findings at presentation are visual. Bitemporal hemianopsia or any other visual field defect are the most frequent visual deficits. Usually, with bitemporal hemianopsia,

TABLE 28-5
Differential Diagnosis of Sellar Mass

Abscesses	Lymphomas
Aneurysms	Melanomas
Chordomas	Meningiomas
Craniopharyngiomas	Olfactory neuroblastomas
Dermoid and epidermoid cysts	Paragangliomas
Gangliocytomas	Pituitary adenomas or carcinomas
Germinomas	Rathke's cleft cyst
Hemangioblastoma	Sarcoidosis
Histiocytosis	Sarcomas
Hypothalmic and optic gliomas	Skeletal tumors
Lipomas	Teratomas

the superior temporal quadrants are affected first, then the inferior quadrants are affected. Unilateral central scotoma with a contralateral superior temporal quadrantanopsia also can be seen and is usually due to compression of the optic nerve at the chiasm. Fibers from the opposite optic nerve, known as von Willebrand's knee, come across the chiasm and bend anteriorly into the central anterior optic nerve prior to traveling down the optic tract. Marcus Gunn pupil is seen occasionally due to compression at the optic nerve. Patients may present with extraocular muscle dysfunction, or facial numbness from cranial nerve compression, but these signs are seen only with invasion of the cavernous sinus, and thus are uncommon with most pituitary adenomas. With extension of the tumor into the frontal lobes, personality changes are often seen. If the tumor extends into the temporal lobe, seizures may be the presenting symptom.[2]

Hypothalamic and pituitary dysfunction are caused by local tumor mass effect. Compression on the infundibulum causes varying degrees of hypopituitarism. Pituitary hypofunction is rarely seen with pituitary microadenomas, but with large null cell macroadenomas pituitary hypofunction is present in approximately 35 percent of patients at presentation. Diabetes insipidus can be seen with compression of the infundibulum or posterior pituitary, although it is rarely seen with a pituitary adenoma. When present, it should alert the diagnostician to other possibilities. Hypogonadism is another symptom of pituitary hypofunction characterized by loss of libido and decreased beard growth in males; in females there is decrease in axillary and pubic hair, amenorrhea, uterine and vaginal atrophy, decrease in vaginal secretions, and dyspareunia. Hypothyroidism from hypopituitarism causes decreased energy, lethargy, cold intolerance, dry skin, and myxedema, just as primary hypothyroidism does. Decreased adrenal function is seen with decreased production of ACTH from the pituitary gland. Nausea and vomiting, postural hypotension, hyperthermia, and general fatigue are some of the more common symptoms caused by this relative lack of cortisol.

Prolactin levels often increase slightly secondary to compression of the infundibular stalk and loss of dopamine inhibition of prolactin release. This phenomenon is known as the stalk effect. Prolactin levels, although elevated, are rarely greater than 150 units from the stalk effect alone. If prolactin levels are >150, it is likely that the patient has a prolactin secreting tumor.[2]

Headaches are a common symptom caused by local tumor mass effect. These headaches may result from compression on the diaphragma sellae. With large tumors, headaches may actually be a symptom of hydrocephalus caused by obstruction of the foramen of Monro. The other signs of hydrocephalus, such as papilledema, lethargy, or coma, should be carefully sought in these patients with significant headaches.

Pituitary apoplexy is a rare but well-known condition. It is caused by hemorrhage into, or infarction of, a pituitary neoplasm. Severe headache, acute visual impairment, and altered mental status are some of the symptoms commonly associated with this disorder. Subarachnoid hemorrhage, electrolyte abnormalities, and acute adrenal insufficiency are also sometimes seen with pituitary apoplexy and can cause severe illness in these patients.[2]

SIGNS AND SYMPTOMS OF HYPERSECRETORY PITUITARY ADENOMAS

Prolactin-secreting adenomas are the most common hyperfunctional pituitary tumors. In women, galactorrhea, infertility, amenorrhea, or oligomenorrhea are the most common symptoms. In men, prolactinomas tend to be larger at the time of diagnosis, and presenting signs and symptoms are more likely to be from direct mass effect of the tumor. This is because the common endocrine symptoms of hyperprolactinemia, such as decreased libido, impotence, and oligospermia are much less apparent than the amenorrhea or galactorrhea women have at presentation. Galactorrhea in men is an obvious finding, but occurs much less often than it does in women.[2,3]

Growth hormone-secreting tumors produce different syndromes, depending on the age of the patient. Acromegaly occurs only in adults whose epiphyses have fused. Enlargement of the extremities in adults causes changes in shoe size and ring size. These changes in ring size and shoe size are the most common symptoms at presentation. Frontal bossing, enlargement of the mandible, and increasing hat size are the common face and head changes. These patients also have systemic disturbances, including hypertension, diabetes, cardiomegaly, congestive heart failure, osteoarthritis, and respiratory disease, which can cause serious morbidity.[1]

Growth hormone-secreting tumors in children cause gigantism. Gigantism is different from acromegaly in that, with the former, the increase in the size of the body parts tends to be more proportional. Gigantism is caused by increased growth hormone levels prior to fusion of the long bone epiphyses. This allows the bones to grow in both length and width.

Cushing's disease is caused by an overproduction of ACTH from a pituitary tumor. The pituitary adenoma produces ACTH, which stimulates the adrenals to produce more cortisol, which then produces the end-organ changes. Centripetal obesity, hirsutism, striae, infections, poor wound healing, muscle wasting, acne, buffalo hump, and amenorrhea or oligomenorrhea are some of the many symptoms of Cushing's disease or syndrome. The overproduction of cortisol also has associated medical conditions which include hypertension, osteoporosis, impaired glucose tolerance, and erythrocytosis.[1,4,5]

TSH-secreting adenomas are a rare type of pituitary adenoma, the symptoms of which are manifested as weight loss, tachycardia, nervousness, and other signs and symptoms seen with hyperthyroidism. Because of the rarity of TSH-secreting adenomas, primary hyperthyroidism must be carefully ruled out in order to prove that the pituitary gland is the cause of increased serum T4 levels. To prove that hyperthyroidism has been caused by a TSH-secreting adenoma, the patient must have: (1) increased serum T4; (2) increased or abnormally high TSH; and (3) evidence of a pituitary tumor on imaging studies.[6]

Gonadotropin hypersecretion from pituitary adenomas is extremely rare. When present, these tumors usually overproduce FSH. Despite increased production of these gonadotropins, hypogonadism is the most common presenting symptom. This is because of the loss of the normal balance and cycle of hormones needed to produce gonadal growth and function. Although hypogonadism is the most common presenting symptom, not all FSH-secreting adenomas will necessarily be associated with this. Some patients can still have fairly normal gonadal function even with an FSH-secreting tumor. The TSH, LH, and FSH glycoprotein hormones all consist of both an α and β subunit. The α subunit is identical for all three hormones. Some null-cell tumors have been found to secrete the α subunit alone without any β subunit secretion.[7] Hypersecretion of the α subunit by itself is not associated with any clinical signs or symptoms, but can be used as a marker of the efficacy of treatment if the tumor has been found to secrete the α subunit.[2,8]

DIAGNOSTIC ENDOCRINE EVALUATION

Endocrine studies should be obtained for all patients suspected of having pituitary tumor for two main reasons: (1) to assess pituitary hormone reserve; and (2) to diagnose a hypersecretory adenoma.

First we shall discuss assessment of pituitary hormone reserve, starting with the adrenal axis.

A normal serum plasma cortisol is indicative of an intact hypothalamic-pituitary-adrenal axis. To test pituitary gland reserve, a cosyntropin (an ACTH analogue) stimulation test should be done. To perform this test, a baseline serum cortisol value is obtained; then 250 μg of cosyntropin is given IV or IM, with a repeat cortisol measurement being obtained 30 min later. The normal response is a rise of 7 μg/dl and a peak of >20 μg/dl. This same test can be performed using corticotropin-releasing factor to stimulate corticol production as well.[2]

In assessing the thyroid axis, it can be assumed that the axis is normal if the serum free T4 is normal. If serum T4 is low, then a thyrotropin-releasing hormone (TRH) stimulation test can be used to assess pituitary function. For this test, baseline TSH is measured, 500 μg of TRH is given intravenously, and TSH is measured 30 and 60 min later. A TSH level twice baseline at 30 min indicates normal function; a peak at 60 min indicates hypothalamic dysfunction.[2]

In assessing the gonadal axis, baseline values of FSH, LH, and estradiol in women, testosterone in men, are helpful. The main reason to assess these is to help guide replacement therapy.

Baseline prolactin levels should be obtained on anyone suspected of having a pituitary tumor, and will often be elevated due to the phenomenon called the "stalk effect." The stalk effect is seen with compression of the infundibular stalk and inhibition of dopamine transfer from the hypothalamus to the pituitary gland. Dopamine normally inhibits prolactin release in the pituitary; with impaired transmission of dopamine from the hypothalamus to the pituitary, there will be a subsequent rise in the prolactin released from the pituitary and serum prolactin levels. Although the stalk effect does increase serum prolactin, it rarely causes levels >150 μg/ml.

Studies of baseline growth hormone levels are not necessary in asymptomatic adults, but children should be evaluated to assess the need for possible replacement.

Posterior pituitary dysfunction is usually diagnosed clinically. These patients have polyuria and polydipsia from impaired release of antidiuretic hormone, the syndrome of which is called diabetes insipidus. If the diagnosis of diabetes insipidus is equivocal, then a water-deprivation test can be performed by withholding water and recording serum sodium and urine output. If the urine output remains high and the serum sodium increases, then the patient has impaired release of antidiuretic hormone.

DIAGNOSING ENDOCRINOPATHIES

Prolactin-secreting adenomas are the most common hypersecretory tumors, but positive diagnosis can sometimes be difficult. Two fasting morning prolactin levels of >150 nanograms/ml are very suggestive of a prolactinoma. Hypothyroidism, renal failure, phenothiazines, tricyclic antidepressants, and central-acting antihypertensives can all increase prolactin levels, although usually they will not cause them to increase more than 150 μg. TSH should be measured to rule out primary hypothyroidism in all patients with a moderately elevated prolactin level. Prolactin may also be elevated due to compression of the pituitary stalk and loss of dopamine inhibition. MRI may or may not show a lesion, so the diagnosis of a prolactinoma has to be made clinically on the basis of finding elevated prolactin and ruling out other causes.[2]

To rule out growth hormone adenomas, three tests are done, along with obtaining baseline levels. Basal growth hormone (GH) levels are increased in 90 percent of patients with active acromegaly. For these, blood is drawn in the morning in the fasting patient. These levels may be falsely elevated by exercise, stress, and hypoglycemia.

The GH-glucose-suppression test is helpful in differentiating between physiologic elevation of GH and elevation due to a GH adenoma. A glucose load suppresses GH secretion in normal individuals, even when GH is physiologically elevated. In patients with GH adenomas, a glucose load will not suppress the level of GH.

Somatomedins are proteins that mediate the effect of GH on peripheral tissue. They are always elevated in patients with acromegaly. Their measurement is useful when GH levels are low and for following a patient's response to treatment.

Thyrotropin-releasing hormone (TRH) stimulation is another test used for GH-secreting tumors. TRH induces release of GH in patients who have GH-secreting tumors, but not in normal patients. The response to this test is variable, though, and the test is expensive, so it is not used routinely.[2]

Gonadotropin-releasing-factor assays are important in certain instances. Ectopic gonadotropin-releasing factor has been shown to be a rare cause of acromegaly. This should be considered if a patient with acromegaly does not appear to have a pituitary source of increased growth hormone. This test is rarely needed, so it is done only in a few research centers.

The first step in diagnosing an adrenocorticotropin (ACTH) producing pituitary adenoma is to make the diagnosis of peripheral hypercortisolism or Cushing's syndrome.

Twenty-four-hour urinary free cortisol is an easy value to obtain, and when the level is twice normal, it is highly suggestive of hypercortisolism or Cushing's syndrome. Because it is an easy test to perform and is relatively inexpensive, it is a good initial screening test.

The overnight dexamethasone-suppression test is also useful for screening. One mg of dexamethasone is given at bedtime, and plasma cortisol is measured in the morning. If the level is 75 μg/dl or greater, then Cushing's *syndrome* is likely. This test is also good for screening and can be done as an outpatient procedure. These two tests are used to diagnose Cushing's syndrome, which is the clinical entity of hypercortisolism from any cause. Cushing's disease, on the other hand, is the clinical entity of hypercortisolism caused specifically by an ACTH-producing pituitary tumor. Cushing's *disease* is the cause of non-iatrogenic hypercortisolism in 60 to 80 percent of cases; adrenal tumors are the cause of 15 to 25 percent; and ectopic ACTH production is the cause in 5 to 15 percent.

Ectopic sources of ACTH production can be small-cell carcinomas of the lung, carcinoids, thymomas, pancreatic islet cell tumors, medullary carcinomas of the thyroid, or pheochromocytomas. Rarely, there can be ectopic production of corticotropin-releasing hormone by one of these tumors. Also of note is the fact that the most common cause of Cushing's syndrome is iatrogenic from exogenous steroids. Iatrogenic Cushing's syndrome should be diagnosed easily from a proper history.

Diagnosing Cushing's disease is the second step after the diagnosis of Cushing's syndrome has been made.

The dexamethasone-suppression test should be done first. Twenty-four-hour urinary excretion of 17-hydroxycorticosteroids is measured in response to dexamethasone administration. The standard six-day test consists of two days of basal samples, then two days of the patient taking 0.5 mg dexamethasone every 6 h (low-dose), and finally, two days of the patient taking 2.0 mg dexamethasone every 6 h (high-dose). Values are corrected to creatinine excretion. Basal values greater than 7 μg/g creatinine over 24 h are elevated. In normal patients, the basal level will decrease 50 percent or more during a low-dose test. Patients with Cushing's disease will now show suppression during a low-dose test, but will show suppression of up to 50 percent of basal levels on the second day of high-dose dexamethasone. Patients with ectopic ACTH production will not show suppression from either low- or high-dose dexamethasone.[2]

ACTH levels alone are not specific for pituitary versus ectopic ACTH, and are normal in approximately half of patients with ACTH-producing adenomas. To overcome this problem, ACTH levels are drawn from both petrosal sinuses, which contain blood from the pituitary gland. If ACTH is elevated, this usually is diagnostic of a pituitary source. This test can also help lateralize the tumor, and aiding the operating surgeon by indicating the side of the gland that contains the tumor. Corticotropin-releasing factor can also be given prior to petrosal sampling to further increase the specificity of the test.[9]

A metyrapone test also can be performed. This is done by testing basal secretion of 17-hydroxycorticosteroids in the urine, and then giving 750 mg of metyrapone every 4 h for 24 h, and then rechecking the urinary secretion of 17-hydroxycorticosteroids. Metyrapone blocks the final conversion of 11-deoxycortisol to cortisol, which causes a build-up of precursor steroids and an increased secretion of corticotropin-releasing factor. In patients with Cushing's disease, there will be at least a twofold rise in urine 17-hydroxycorticosteroids. Typically, in patients with an ectopic source of ACTH, there will be no rise in urine 17-hydroxycorticosteroids.[2]

It is important in diagnosing Cushing's disease or other hypersecretory pituitary tumors to remember that imaging studies may not always reveal a pituitary source. Hyperfunctioning adenomas can be too small for conventional studies to detect and yet still may produce clinical signs and symptoms. Also, patients may have a small pituitary tumor on imaging studies, but that tumor is not responsible for their clinical state. Therefore, it is of the utmost importance to rely primarily on the clinical studies for diagnosis and to use radiologic imaging as a diagnostic adjunct.

RADIOLOGIC EVALUATION

Increasingly improved technology and its indiscriminate use have led to more and more pituitary tumors being detected on imaging studies. These advances in radiology have helped both with diagnosis and with surgical treatment of pituitary adenomas.

Skull x-rays can be helpful, but are not required preoperatively. They can provide information about the size of the sella, the thickness of the floor of the sella, the site and configuration of the sphenoid sinus, and any abnormal calcification.

CT scans done with contrast material can detect most pituitary macroadenomas. Coronal sections are better for viewing the pituitary gland, whereas axial images may be better for viewing suprasellar masses. For smaller pituitary lesions, though, CT will often miss what might be seen on MRI.

MRI is the study of choice when looking for pituitary tumors. It is very good at differentiating soft tissue densities in the sellar region. Its limitation, though, is that it is poor in visualizing bony changes. Pituitary adenomas are seen as hypointense on T1 and hyperintense on T2. The normal pituitary gland enhances with gadolinium more so than do adenomas, so adenomas usually appear as hypointense lesions on contrast-enhanced MRI. Although with delayed contrast images, the reverse is usually true, and the tumor will enhance more than the surrounding gland.

MRI is helpful in showing tumor invasion into the cavernous sinus. Now, with the addition of MRA, aneurysms can be excluded from the differential diagnosis in a noninvasive manner.

Of special note, with the advent of MRI is the fact that many (11 to 23 percent) normal patients have been found to have pituitary microadenomas.[10] Thus, the diagnosis of a functioning adenoma cannot be made on the basis of radiographic data alone. Also, when a patient's symptoms are vague, the clinician has to be careful in assuring that a small pituitary tumor is the cause of those symptoms.[2]

Angiography is not done routinely today, but it can show invasion of the carotid artery or the cavernous sinus. It can also be helpful in ruling out an aneurysm when the diagnosis is not certain. Another form of angiography is petrosal sinus sampling. This is used mainly to help with the diagnosis of Cushing's disease, and the lateralization of an ACTH-secreting adenoma.

For cavernous sinus venography with petrosal sinus sampling, a catheter is placed into the inferior petrosal sinus to measure different hormone levels. High levels of ACTH in the sinus can confirm Cushing's disease, and if the level is higher on one side, it may help to localize a microadenoma. Cavernous sinus venography may show cavernous invasion, but other less invasive studies can also show such invasion, and cavernous sinus venography is not done routinely for this purpose alone.

Treatment

INTRODUCTION

Many decisions must be made before therapy is initiated. There are many different treatment options, including medication, radiation, and surgery. The patient's age and medical condition are always important, as is the type of tumor present and the symptoms and signs caused by the tumor. For example, asymptomatic patients with nonfunctioning adenomas less than 1.0 cm can be followed and may not need surgery unless the tumor reaches a size greater than 1.2 to 1.5 cm. At that point, the risk of future problems in young patients probably warrants surgery. In very old or medically impaired patients, it may be safer to follow larger tumors because of the increased risk of anesthetic and postoperative complications.

MEDICAL THERAPY

There is no medical cure for a pituitary adenoma. The available therapy acts by decreasing the level of hormone secretion and reducing tumor size, or by preventing some of the end-organ effects of the hormone. It does not ever obliterate the adenoma.

PROLACTIN-SECRETING ADENOMAS

The standard medical treatment is with bromocriptine, a dopamine agonist. The advent of this treatment has greatly reduced the amount of surgery needed for prolactinomas. Bromocriptine is probably not tumoricidal—it most likely works by reducing cell size and the amount of prolactin released by the tumor cells, but does not lyse the tumor cells. The side effects of bromocriptine are minimal, and long-term use has not shown any serious complications. In symptomatic patients, bromocriptine usually causes cessation of galactorrhea, return of menses, and possibly return of fertility. However, with removal of the drug, symptoms usually return promptly. Therefore, patients being treated with bromocriptine must take it for the rest of their lives.[11]

Bromocriptine may also lower the success rate of a surgical approach by causing fibrosis within the gland, making total tumor removal slightly more difficult. This is controversial, though, and should be considered a contraindication of treatment in young patients, although surgery prior to bromocriptine therapy is often the recommended treatment. These patients then do not have to take bromocriptine for the rest of their lives, and the chance of a surgical cure may be higher. CSF leak after bromocriptine therapy has been reported. It is probably the result of tumor shrinkage, exposing a pre-existing defect in the dura. This compli-

cation is rare, but it should be thought of when rhinorrhea is seen after bromocriptine therapy.[12]

Medical treatment for growth hormone-secreting adenomas has not been nearly as effective as with prolactinomas. Bromocriptine has been shown to reduce GH levels in up to 75 percent of patients with GH-secreting adenomas; however, only 20 percent had reduction to a normal level.[13] Some tumors secrete both GH and prolactin, and some of these tumors will shrink with bromocriptine. The dose of bromocriptine required for GH-secreting adenomas is also much higher than that required for prolactinomas. Because of the poor response to medical therapy, surgery is usually the recommended first-line treatment.[14,15]

With ACTH-secreting adenomas, several different drugs have been tried with very limited success. Mitotane, an adrenal toxin, is one such drug, but the success rate with its use has been poor.[16] Metyrapone, which inhibits the last step in steroid synthesis, has been used as an adjunct to surgical or radiation therapy. It helps reduce some of the end-organ symptoms.[17] Serotonin antagonists, such as metergline, have also been shown to decrease corticosteroid production and lead to symptomatic improvement.[18] Their use, though, is still not a cure and only minimally improves symptoms, making surgery the mainstay of therapy for patients with Cushing's disease.

RADIATION THERAPY

Radiation therapy may be used as an adjunct or as the primary treatment for pituitary adenomas. Radiation therapy is not without significant side effects and it probably should not be used without a tissue diagnosis. The efficacy of radiation therapy varies, depending on the tumor type. Owing to the popularity of transsphenoidal operations, the use of radiation therapy has appropriately diminished somewhat, although it is still beneficial in certain cases as an adjunct to surgical treatment.

With bromocriptine and the transsphenoidal operation, radiation therapy has become almost obsolete for use with prolactinomas. The response of prolactinomas to radiation therapy in the past has been unimpressive. Because of this, radiation should not be used as the primary treatment modality for these tumors.[19,20]

Radiation therapy has been used for GH-secreting tumors, even prior to assays of the hormone in the past. The results have been good for most of these patients. A study by Eastman and coworkers showed levels to be less than 10 ng/ml in 81 percent of patients at 10-year follow-up.[21] Almost all patients had symptomatic improvement as well. The problem Eastman found was not with continued acromegaly as much as with postradiation hypopituitarism, since 9 of 19

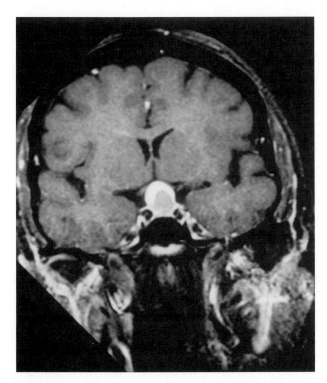

Figure 28-7 This T1 weighted MRI with gadolinium enhancement shows a 1.5 to 2.0 cm pituitary tumor. Notice how the normal surrounding gland enhances more than the adenoma.

developed significant hypopituitarism at 10-year follow-up. These patients had a total of 40 to 50 Gy (4000 to 5000 rads) of conventional radiation therapy.[21]

Cushing's disease is another pituitary adenoma in which the results of radiation therapy in the past have been favorable, with 50 to 80 percent of patients requiring no further therapy. Although the number of patients in these studies has been small, it may indeed be that radiation therapy is of value in Cushing's disease when surgery has failed to be curative. These patients also are at risk of developing postradiation hypopituitarism.

The exact efficacy of radiation therapy on nonfunctional adenomas has not been determined.

SURGICAL THERAPY

Surgical therapy is the primary treatment for most symptomatic adenomas. There are several surgical approaches to pituitary masses, but the majority can be removed adequately via the transsphenoidal approach. Some of the larger tumors though with significant growth outside the sella are best treated with a craniotomy. The most important decision in choosing the approach should be whether the tumor extends superiorly and laterally outside the sella. If the tumor extends superiorly yet stays in the midline, different techniques can be used to raise the intracranial pressure and cause

the tumor to be pushed down into the sellar region where it can be safely removed. If the tumor has obvious extension into the frontal or temporal lobes, then a craniotomy is the safest approach for adequate tumor removal. Examples are shown of both a tumor best treated via the transsphenoidal approach and one best treated with a craniotomy (Figs. 28-7 and 28-8).

The large majority of pituitary tumors can be removed via the transsphenoidal approach. There are small differences in the way different surgeons perform this surgery, but the basic technique should be the same. We will describe the operation as it is currently done at our institution. The patient is positioned on the operating table supine in the three-point headrest, with the head tilted approximately 15 degrees toward the left shoulder. It is important to keep the vertical plane in the perpendicular position because that position helps the surgeon stay in the midline during the approach. The nasal-oral area is prepared and draped with sterile towels. The abdomen is prepared and draped for harvesting adipose tissue. Before starting the procedure the oropharynx is packed to prevent significant drainage of surgical debris into the pharynx. The nasal mucosa is injected with local anesthetic mixed with epinephrine to help with hemostasis and dissection of the mucosa off of the nasal septum. The assistant usually harvests the fat graft while the surgeon starts the transsphenoidal approach.

The upper lip is retracted superiorly and an incision

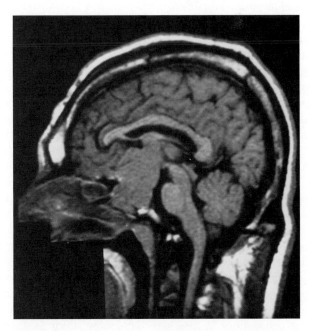

Figure 28-8 A sagittal T1-weighted MRI showing a large pituitary adenoma extending superiorly into the hypothalamus, third ventricle, and inferior frontal lobe. Because of the significant extrasellar extension of tumor, this patient was treated with a craniotomy.

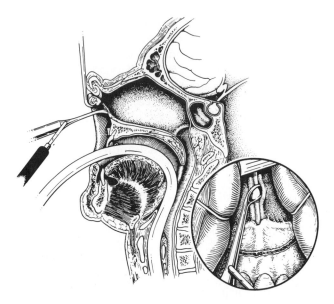

Figure 28-9 This shows the initial subchondral dissection.

is made horizontally in the gingival mucosa. The incisions should be so placed that enough tissue is left above the teeth for closure of the gingiva at the end of the procedure. The maxilla is exposed and then the soft tissue is dissected superiorly to expose the piriform aperture and the floor of the nares. Then, the cartilaginous septum is identified and an incision is made superiorly in the septum just slightly to one side. This facilitates a subchondral separation of the mucosa from the nasal septum (Fig. 28-9).

The mucosa is separated down to the nasal spine and then separated from it. The nasal septum is then fractured and moved to one side. The mucosa is then separated posteriorly down to the bony septum made up of the superior portion of the vomer and the inferior parts of the perpendicular plate of the ethmoid. The speculum is opened to fracture this septum and to bring the sphenoid sinus into view. There will remain a small bony remnant of the bony septum in the middle of the anterior wall of the sphenoid sinus (Fig. 28-10).

The sinus is then opened and the anterior wall is removed. The speculum should not be opened within the sinus for fear of fracturing the sphenoid bone. The mucosa of the sinus is removed using suction and cautery. The sellar floor is then usually easily identified. If the floor is not easily seen, a lateral skull x-ray can be obtained to verify its location. The degree of pneumatization of the sphenoid sinus is variable, and occasionally bone must be drilled posteriorly before the sellar floor is reached. The sellar floor is then opened and enlarged, with care being taken not to enter the cavernous sinus or circular sinus (the latter being a connection between the two cavernous sinuses). A stellate incision is then made in the dura

using an arachnoid knife. Again, care must be taken at this point to avoid entering the cavernous sinus or even injuring the carotid arteries (Fig. 28-11).

If any bleeding is encountered at this point, it is usually from the circular sinus. This bleeding may appear brisk, but usually can be controlled with simple packing with Gelfoam or other similar material. Occasionally, a patient may have an ectatic internal carotid artery, which can be injured if the dissection is carried too far laterally. If uncontrollable bleeding is encountered from any of these sources, the procedure may have to be aborted. However, this is very rare, and even with some moderate bleeding the case usually can be finished.

After the dura has been opened, the pituitary tumor usually can be easily seen. Most often, the tumor appears different from the normal gland (Fig. 28-12). It usually is soft and is easily removed using ring curettes, enucleators, suckers, or pituitary forceps. The diaphragma sellae is present just superior to the gland and comes into the field only as the tumor is removed and ICP raised. Care should be taken not to puncture this membrane in order to minimize a postoperative CSF leak.

With large tumors, only a small portion of normal gland may be left. This remaining gland is usually found posteriorly and superiorly. Care should be taken to preserve it if at all possible. When there is suprasellar extension of the tumor, a small cuff of tumor can be used to pull the suprasellar portion down into the sella for ease of removal.

Microadenomas 5 mm or less often are not easily seen initially. The next step then is to look laterally in

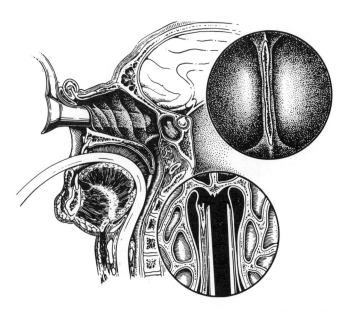

Figure 28-10 The remnant of the bony septum is being fractured by opening the speculum.

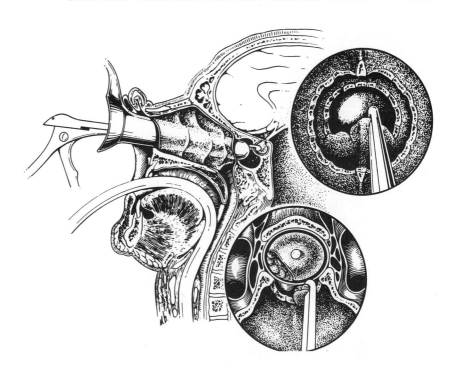

Figure 28-11 The removal of the sellar floor
and exposure of the pituitary.

the gutters, where they are often found. If still no tumor
material is apparent, then the gland can be incised.
Prolactinomas and growth hormone-secreting adenomas tend to be located laterally in the gland, so a
vertical incision placed laterally should be used.
ACTH-secreting tumors tend to be closer to the midline, and the incision should be started on the midline
when looking for these tumors.[2]

Once the tumor has been removed, hemostasis is
obtained. The intrasellar tumor bed and the sphenoid
sinus are then packed with the abdominal adipose tissue obtained earlier. The speculum is removed and

the midline structures are returned to their original
positions. The gingival mucosa is then closed with
absorbable sutures. Both nares are packed with sterile
gauze, which helps to reapproximate the nasal mucosa
as well as to effect hemostasis. The patient is then
extubated and taken to the recovery room.

Once the patient's condition has stabilized, he or she
is taken to the ICU and is kept NPO until the next day.
Postoperatively, strict hourly records are kept of the
oral and intravenous intake as well as urinary output.
Also, it is important in patients who have hypopituitarism to give them adequate hormonal replacement. If
the patient is doing well, he or she is transferred to
the floor after 24 h, and oral intake is liberalized. Intravenous antibiotics are continued until the nasal packs
are removed on postoperative day 5. Humidified air
is given to keep the nasal packs moist as long as they
are in place. On postoperative day 5, if everything
has gone well, the packs are removed, the intravenous
infusions are discontinued, and the patient is discharged to home.

CRANIOTOMY APPROACH

The two most common intracranial approaches are the
frontotemporal pterional and the subfrontal. Occasionally, if the tumor extends far posteriorly, a subtemporal
approach may be best.

Craniotomies for pituitary tumors are done as any
craniotomy would be for lesions in the same region.
A detailed discussion of craniotomies can be found in
the chapter concerning supratentorial surgery. Special
care must be taken to avoid damage to the important
vascular and neural structures in this region. Although

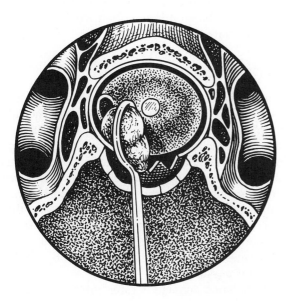

Figure 28-12 The extirpation of an adenoma using ring curets.

the morbidity and mortality may be slightly higher with a craniotomy, there are certain cases in which the intracranial approach is necessary for adequate and safe removal of the tumor and decompression of optic nerves and chiasm.

POSTOPERATIVE COMPLICATIONS WITH THE TRANSSPHENOIDAL APPROACH

CSF rhinorrhea has been reported in as high as 9 percent of cases, but in most studies is about 3 percent.[22-24] Untreated CSF rhinorrhea is a dangerous condition that can lead to meningitis or tension pneumocephalus. Certain factors increase the risk of postoperative CSF rhinorrhea: large tumor size; prior surgical or radiation therapy; presence of a preoperative leak; and occurrence of an intraoperative leak. CSF rhinorrhea occurs when the diaphragma sellae has been torn or when a large tumor has eroded through the sellae and its removal exposes a defect. Thus, to prevent postoperative leaks, care must be taken intraoperatively to protect the diaphragma sellae. Packing the sinus with autologous fat and trying to reconstruct the sella floor are also useful. If a leak occurs intraoperatively, a lumbar drain can be placed postoperatively in the hope of diverting the leak until the diaphragma sellae has healed. Occasionally, a leak may not be apparent until the nasal packing has been removed. The treatment in these cases is bed rest and placement of a lumbar drain. Once there has been no leakage for 24 to 48 h, then the lumbar drain can be removed. If lumbar drainage does not work, either the sinus can be repacked or the leak can be repaired from above through a craniotomy. Most can be treated without reoperation, as shown by Spazowilte and co-workers, who claim that only 2 percent of their patients with a postoperative CSF leak required operative repair.[25]

Hypopituitarism is another potentially serious postoperative complication. In a study by Faria and Tindall, permanent damage to one endocrine axis occurred in 4 percent of patients undergoing surgical removal of a pituitary tumor. The most common endocrine dysfunction postoperatively is diabetes insipidus, which occurs transiently in about 60 percent of patients, but permanently in fewer than 3 percent.[26] Because the great majority of patients will improve within six weeks, not all need to be treated initially. Of course, this is only possible in an awake patient who has an intact thirst mechanism and is able to keep up with his or her urinary loss. If patients continue to have diabetes insipidus, then treatment is usually initiated for both the patient's convenience and to prevent the renal pelvis from losing its concentrating abilities. If a patient presents with hypopituitarism or diabetes insipidus, they will probably have it postoperatively.

The best way to prevent postoperative hypopituitarism is with careful intraoperative preservation of normal gland tissue.

Cranial nerve injury is rarely seen following transsphenoidal surgery. It is usually transient and self-limited. Direct injury from instrumentation laterally and overpacking the sella are the two most common causes. The incidence of cranial nerve injury from the transsphenoidal approach has ranged from 0.4 to 6.0 percent in different studies. The 3d and 4th nerves are most frequently involved. Visual worsening or loss is a rare but devastating complication seen almost exclusively with large tumors with significant suprasellar extension.[27]

Nasal complications are rare, the most common being sinusitis from mucosal edema and obstruction of sinus drainage. This usually is self-limiting and is easily treated with appropriate antibiotics and decongestants. Mucoceles can occur as well, but can be prevented intraoperatively by adequate exenteration of the sinus mucosa. If excessive cartilage is removed for packing the sella, nasal deformities may occur, and it is the policy at our institution never to use nasal cartilage for packing the sella. Septal perforations can be annoying and have been reported in as many as 8 percent of patients.[24,28] They are related to operative or infectious damage to the mucoperichondrium. Packing of the nares will help reapproximate the mucosa, and usually prevents these perforations.

A rare but potentially dangerous complication is the formation of a carotid-cavernous (c-c) fistula. This is seen when a connection occurs directly between the carotid artery and the cavernous sinus from direct injury at the time of surgery. These can be very difficult to treat, as are carotid cavernous fistulas from any other cause. The workup and treatment in these iatrogenic fistulas should be no different than what is done with routine non-iatrogenic c-c fistulas.

INTRACRANIAL COMPLICATIONS

Although hemorrhage is a rare complication, it is one of the most common causes of operative mortality. Hemorrhage is much more commonly seen with craniotomies, but also has been reported with the transsphenoidal route. The bleeding may be intraparenchymal, subarachnoid, subdural, or even epidural. Intrasellar hemorrhage may be a cause of early postoperative visual worsening,[29] and should be thought of if this is seen. Treatment of hemorrhages after pituitary surgery is the same as that of other postoperative intracranial hemorrhages. Symptomatic accessible clots should be removed if possible.

Hypothalamic damage is rare, but potentially serious. Usually it is seen with tumors having significant suprasellar extension. Surgical trauma, ischemia, or secondary trauma from a hematoma are the most common causes of hypothalamic injury. Suprasellar tumors should be resected only under direct vision to help prevent hypothalamic damage.[30]

In summary, the advances made with microsurgical techniques and imaging have made pituitary surgery a very safe treatment option. The large majority can be well treated with good long-term results. The most common complications can usually be treated without causing serious morbidity. Careful surgical techniques during the procedure do help prevent some of the postoperative complications, and it is important to be extremely careful with large tumors extending outside the sella. Also, it is important to give appropriate follow-up for these patients, which includes reassessment of their pituitary reserve and the need for replacement therapy. In patients with known residual tumor, follow-up MRIs and visual field teting are important in assessing regrowth. Also, in those with functioning adenomas preoperatively, hormone levels must be followed postoperatively to assess the adequacy of surgical resection.

If a patient is found to have tumor regrowth or is not cured from the previous surgery, several options should be considered. In most instances, a second surgery can and should be undertaken if possible. Then, radiation therapy may be used as an adjunct or the primary treatment for tumor recurrence. Medical therapy can also be helpful in treating the symptoms of tumor recurrence, although in tumors other than prolactinomas, its long-lasting benefit is limited.

Anesthetic Management

Anesthesiologists should be knowledgeable about the surgical challenges posed by the position of the pituitary gland at the base of the brain. Within the sphenoid bone, the pituitary gland is surrounded by the osseous sella turcica (Fig. 28-13). The pituitary gland and its arachnoid covering pierce the roof of the sella, which is formed by the diaphragma sella. The anterior and posterior clinoid processes project from the sella laterally, while the true lateral wall of the sella is composed of the medial borders of each cavernous sinus. Each cavernous sinus contains the intracavernous portion of the internal carotid artery as well as the oculomotor, trochlear, abducens, and portions of the trigeminal cranial nerves.[31]

The optic nerves meet at the optic chiasm above the diaphragma sella. Variations exist in the true location of the chiasm relative to the tuberculum or anterior walls of the sella. In a transfrontal surgical approach, this distance may limit access to the pituitary gland.

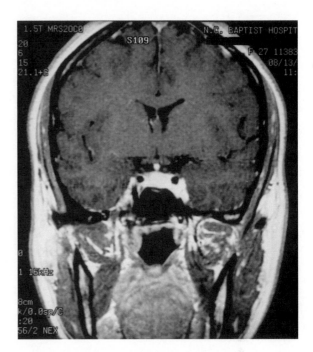

Figure 28-13 MRI scan: Coronal view with contrast demonstrating cavernous sinus surrounding the sella.

Anatomic variations have also been found in the distance between the cavernous portions of the right and left carotid arteries. The arteries may bulge to within millimeters of the midline.[32]

PREOPERATIVE PREPARATION

Patients for pituitary surgery are best managed when the results of imaging studies and a full endocrinologic work-up are available to the anesthesiologist. Rarely, pituitary surgery is emergent due to pituitary apoplexy. This acute clinical syndrome results from pituitary hemorrhage or infarction and is characterized by a patient symptom complex of headache, vomiting, ocular paresis and reductions in visual fields or acuity.[33] Often, urgent surgery is recommended to relieve compression on the optic chiasm and to decrease intracranial pressure. Significant visual recovery is possible if surgery is performed within a week of the apoplectic episode.[34] In most cases, replacement corticosteroids are indicated, and a large mass may require maneuvers such as the use of mannitol or hyperventilation to improve surgeons' access.[35]

Surgical approaches to tumors in the pituitary region include stereotactic, transsphenoidal, and subfrontal. Most often, the size of the initial lesion identified on imaging studies as well as the possibility of suprasellar or cavernous sinus extension dictate the surgical approach. To date, no neuroradiographic imaging technique can flawlessly predict parasellar extension of

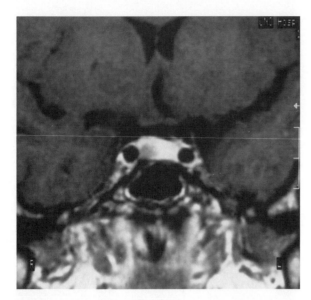

Figure 28-14 MRI scan: Coronal view with contrast from a patient with a pituitary adenoma. Note flow-void created by intracavernous portion of carotid artery.

tumors; however, refinements of MRI angiography and contrast hold promise (Fig. 28-14).[36]

In addition to the usual focused preanesthetic assessment for a neurosurgical patient, patients scheduled for pituitary surgery should have an assessment made of visual function, signs and symptoms of increased intracranial pressure, and a review of endocrinologic studies including growth hormone, cortisol, thyroid studies, and reproductive hormones. In patients with Cushing's syndrome, anesthetic considerations related to the presence of obesity and hypertension necessitate evaluation of the patient for gastroesophageal reflux, hypertension, hyperglycemia, sleep disorders, and cardiovascular dysfunction.[37] Hyperglycemia in patients with Cushing's syndrome is characterized by both reduced insulin sensitivity and non-insulin-mediated glucose disposal in the presence of enhanced insulin secretion.[38] Additionally, easy bruisibility and skin fragility may make intravascular access difficult.

A recent study of patients with Cushing's disease demonstrated that one-third of the subjects had sleep apnea characterized by nine or more episodes of oxygen desaturation an hour. Often these patients complained of excessive daytime drowsiness and snoring.[39] Since nasal packing is employed postoperatively following transsphenoidal surgery, a prior history of sleep apnea may complicate the postoperative course.

Left ventricular hypertrophy is frequently seen in Cushing's syndrome and is thought to be due to hypertension. Recent echocardiographic evidence indicates that left ventricular hypertrophy may be accompanied by asymmetric septal hypertrophy which resolves following adequate treatment of the illness.[40]

Patients with acromegaly will have hypertrophy of the facial bones as well as the mucosa, soft tissues around the larynx, and vocal cords.[41,42] Hypertension and cardiomyopathy as well as diabetes mellitus may be present.[43] The cardiomyopathy is thought to relate primarily to diastolic dysfunction and is not related to the presence of hypertension alone.[44] Myocardial hypertrophy and interstitial fibrosis are common in acromegalic hearts and, occasionally, this entity may progress to frank cardiac failure.

A significant number of patients with acromegaly have sleep apnea. This may be due to anatomic factors (peripheral sleep apnea) or central factors.[45,46] Overgrowth of facial bones, laryngeal structures and soft tissues of the hypopharynx may induce changes in a patient's voice and cause difficulties with mask ventilation and/or laryngoscopy. Adequate preoperative assessment of a particular patient's airway anatomy and careful planning for management for oral tracheal induction are crucial steps. Changes in vocal cord frequencies induced by excessive growth hormone begin to resolve within 10 days following pituitary resection.[47]

While prolactinomas are often characterized by symptoms related to the reproductive system in women, they tend to present later in men and may be associated with a significant intracranial mass.[48] Patients should be screened for the development of panhypopituitarism, particularly if they have undergone a rapid increase in symptomatology.

INTRAOPERATIVE MANAGEMENT

Anesthetic management of the patient for transsphenoidal pituitary surgery is directed toward achieving the goals of good surgical exposure, careful hemodynamic control to facilitate hemostasis, and facilitation of gross motor, visual, and extraocular muscle function examination early in the postoperative period. Careful tailoring of the anesthetic to a particular team's operative time is crucial, as a nasal packing requires a patient to breathe only through the mouth at the end of the procedure.

In most cases, a nitrous oxide/narcotic technique with the addition of inhalational agents as needed provides a smooth intraoperative course and early postoperative assessment. Some surgeons inject nitrous oxide into a subarachnoid catheter to better enhance the anatomy of the gland intraoperatively. If this is necessary, nitrous oxide must be eliminated from the anesthetic technique during and after this maneuver.[49] Most often, however, adequate visualization of the gland is obtained through the use of C-arm fluoroscopy with the addition of a Valsalva maneuver when requested.

Most patients are positioned on the operating table

with the back slightly elevated, and the head turned slightly away from midline. This facilitates placing of a speculum by the otolaryngologist who in many instances will perform the initial sublabial incision and bony approach to the sella. If cavernous sinus invasion is strongly suspected, or the patient's head is positioned significantly above 15 degrees from supine, adequate monitoring for venous air embolism should be employed.[50] Such monitoring would include use of end-tidal carbon dioxide and end-tidal nitrogen measurement, a precordial Doppler, and a central venous pressure catheter.

Often during the initial approach, the otolaryngologist will infiltrate the patient's mucosa with lidocaine with epinephrine or cocaine. If the cribriform plate and arachnoid are injected with local anesthetics, a total spinal anesthetic may occur.[51] In those patients who have been placed on preoperative beta-blockers, significant arterial hypertension may result from the unopposed alpha adrenergic effect of the cocaine.

Adjustments in the anesthetic depth utilizing inhalational anesthetic agents or cerebrovasodilators such as nitroglycerin or nitroprusside for short periods may be necessary as the actual sella is approached. In general, the neurosurgeon confines the resection to within the sella; however, bleeding related to branches of the carotid artery or to injury to the cavernous sinus may occur and can be difficult to control. After removal of the tumor, the neurosurgeon will inspect the site for hemorrhage and often close the defect utilizing a piece of fat taken from the patients abdomen. Complications related to the use of this fat have been reported and have been demonstrated postoperatively initially by difficulties with visual assessment and patient alertness. Symptomatic "overfilling" of the sella with fat is a reason for emergent reexploration.[52]

Upon closing, the otolaryngologist may insert stents into the nasal passages and then pack the nose with material such as iodoform gauze. A small pad will be placed over the nose, and the patient will be permitted to awaken. Often a smooth emergence can be facilitated by placing the patient in a semiseated position and assuring that commands are followed before extubation.

Very rarely, intraoperative diabetes insipidus has occurred during transsphenoidal resection.[53] This entity is often managed by careful urine electrolyte evaluation and fluid replacement as well as intermittent doses of subcutaneous aqueous vasopressin (10 U). Often surgeons prefer subcutaneous vasopressin with the short acting time of 4 to 6 h as apposed to intranasal desmopressin (DDAVP) as initial management. Monitoring in an intensive care unit is warranted in the patient who has developed diabetes insipidus. Additionally, a significant number of patients who have undergone transsphenoidal pituitary resection may develop hyponatremia. Typically, this syndrome appears approximately 6 or 7 days postoperatively and may be related to inappropriate secretion of antidiuretic hormones.[54] It is recommended that patients undergo an electrolyte determination approximately one week following surgery.

The provision of an early neurologic examination following transphenoidal surgery allows the surgeons and anesthesiologists to assess extraocular muscle function as well as the level of consciousness. Severe sequelae including carotid artery thrombosis and injury to the nerves traversing the cavernous sinus may be demonstrated by hemiplegia in the first case and difficulties with extraocular muscle function in the latter.[55,56]

Ninety-five percent of pituitary tumors are now resected through the transsphenoidal approach.[57] Careful individual assessment of the tumor location, endocrinologic abnormalities, and physical challenges of each patient is necessary for optimal outcome.

References

1. Tindall GT, Barrow DL: *Disorders of the Pituitary.* St. Louis, Mosby Year Book, 1986.
2. Tindall GT, Barrow DL: Tumors at the sellar and parasellar area in adults. In Youmans (ed): *Neurological Surgery,* 3d ed. Philadelphia, WB Saunders, 1990:3447–3498.
3. Coogan K, et al: Rarity and pituitary adenoma risk. *J Nat Cancer Instit* 1995; 8:1410.
4. Cost WS: A mineralocorticoid excess syndrome presumably due to excessive secretions of corticosterone. *Lancet* 1963; 1:362.
5. Krakoff L, et al: Pathogenesis of hypertension in Cushing's syndrome. *Am J Med* 1975; 58:216.
6. Tolis G, et al: Pituitary hyperthyroidism: Case report and review of the literature. *Am J Med* 1978; 64:177.
7. Ridgeway EC, et al: Pure alpha-secreting pituitary adenomas. *N Engl J Med* 1981; 304:1254.
8. Peterson RE, et al: Luteinizing hormone—and α-subunit-secreting pituitary tumor: Positive feedback of estrogen. *J Clin Endocrinol Metab* 1981; 52:692.
9. Manni A, et al: Simultaneous bilateral venous sampling for adenocorticotropin in pituitary dependent Cushing's disease: Evidence for lateralization of pituitary venous drainage. *J Clin Endocrinol Metab* 1983; 57:1070.
10. Herman-Bonert V, Fagen JA: Molecular pathogenesis of pituitary tumors. *Baillieres Clinical Endocrinology and Metabolism* 1995; 9:203.
11. Barrow DL, et al: Clinical and pathological effects of bromocriptine on prolactin-secreting and other pituitary tumors. *J Neurosurg* 1984; 60:1.
12. Landolt AM, Osterwalder V: Perivascular fibrosis in prolactinomas: Is it increased by bromocriptine? *J Clin Endocrinol Metab* 1984; 58:1179.
13. Besser GM, et al: Bromocriptine in the medical management of acromegaly. *Adv Biochem Psychopharmacol* 1980; 23:191.
14. Oppizzi G, et al: Dopaminergic treatment of acromegaly: Different effects on hormone secretion and tumor size. *J Clin Endocrinol Metab* 1984; 58:988.

15. Wass JAH, et al: Reduction of pituitary-tumour size in patients with prolactinomas and acromegaly treated with bromocriptine with or without radiotherapy. *Lancet* 1979; 2:66.

16. Luton JP, et al: Treatment of Cushing's disease by O,p'-DDD: Survey of 62 cases. *N Engl J Med* 1979; 300:459.

17. Jeffcoate WJ, et al: Metyrapone in long-term management of Cushing's disease. *Br Med J* 1977; 2:215.

18. Krieger DT, et al: Cyproheptadine-induced remission of Cushing's disease. *N Engl J Med* 1975; 293:893.

19. Antunes JL, et al: Prolactin-secreting pituitary tumors. *Ann Neurol* 1977; 2:148.

20. Kleinberg DL, et al: Galactorrhea: A study of 235 cases, including 48 with pituitary tumors. *N Engl J Med* 1977; 296:589.

21. Eastman RC, et al: Conventional supervoltage irradiation is an effective treatment for acromegaly. *J Clin Endocrinol Metab* 1979; 48:931.

22. Black PMcL, et al: Incidence and management of complications of transsphenoidal operation for pituitary adenomas. *Neurosurgery* 1987; 20:920.

23. Ciric I, et al: Transsphenoidal microsurgery of pituitary macroadenomas with long-term follow-up results. *J Neurosurg* 1983; 59:395.

24. Sherwen PJ, et al: Transseptal, transsphenoidal surgery: A subjective and objective analysis of results. *J Otolaryngol* 1986; 15:155.

25. Spaziante R, et al: Techniques of reconstruction of the sella and related structures. In Schmidek HH, Sweet WH (eds): *Operative Neurosurgical Techniques: Indications, Methods, and Results.* Orlando, Grune & Stratton, 1988:321.

26. Faria MA, Tindall GT: Transsphenoidal microsurgery for prolactin-secreting pituitary adenomas: Results in 100 women with the amenorrhea-galactorrhea syndrome. *J Neurosurg* 1982; 56:33.

27. Nelson AT, et al: Residual anterior pituitary function following transsphenoidal resection of pituitary macroadenomas. *J Neurosurg* 1984; 61:577.

28. Kennedy DW, et al: Transsphenoidal approach to the sella: The Johns Hopkins experience. *Laryngoscope* 1984; 94:1066.

29. Barrow DL, Tindall GT: Loss of vision after trans-sphenoidal surgery. *Neurosurgery* 1990; 27:60.

30. Laws ER Jr., Kern EB: Complications of transsphenoidal surgery. *Clin Neurosurg* 1976; 23:401.

31. Pearson BW, Laws ER Jr: Anatomical aspects of the transsphenoidal approach to the pituitary. In Laws ER Jr et al (eds): *Management of Pituitary Adenomas and Related Lesions with Emphasis on Transsphenoidal Microsurgery.* New York, Appleton-Century-Crofts, 1982:65–80.

32. Rhoton AL Jr, et al: Microsurgical anatomy of the sellor region and cavernous sinus. *Clin Neurosurg* 1977; 24:54.

33. Bonicki W, et al: Pituitary apoplexy: Endocrine, surgical and oncological emergency. Incidence, clinical course and treatment with reference to 799 cases of pituitary adenomas. *Acta Neurochir (Wien)* 1993; 120:118.

34. Bills DC, et al: A retrospective analysis of pituitary apoplexy. *Neurosurgery* 1993; 33:602.

35. Gaillard RC: Pituitary gland emergencies. *Baillieres Clin Endocrinol Metab* 1992; 6:57.

36. Knosp E, et al: Parasellar classification of pituitary adenomas. *Neurosurgery* 1993; 33:610.

37. Fallo F, et al: Left ventricular structural characteristics in Cushing's syndrome. *J Hum Hypertens* 1994; 8:509.

38. Page R, et al: Insulin secretion, insulin sensitivity and glucose-mediated glucose disposal in Cushing's disease: A minimal model analysis. *Clin Endocrinol* 1991; 35:509.

39. Shipley JE, et al: Sleep architecture and sleep apnea in patients with Cushing's disease. *Sleep* 1992; 15:514.

40. Sugihara N, et al: Cardiac characteristics and postoperative courses in Cushing's syndrome. *Am J Cardiol* 1992; 69:1475.

41. Bhatia ML, et al: Laryngeal manifestations in acromegaly. *J Laryngol Otol* 1966; 80:412.

42. Kitahata LM: Airway difficulties associated with anaesthesia in acromegaly. Three case reports. *Br J Anaesth* 1971; 43:1187.

43. Lie JT, Grossman SJ: Pathology of the heart in acromegaly: anatomic findings in 27 autopsied patients. *Am Heart J* 1980; 100:41.

44. Rossi E, et al: Acromegalic cardiomyopathy. Left ventricular filling and hypertrophy in active and surgically treated disease. *Chest* 1992; 102:1204.

45. Piper JG, et al: Perioperative management and surgical outcome of the acromegalic patient with sleep apnea. *Neurosurgery* 1995; 36:70.

46. Grunstein RR, et al: Central sleep apnea is associated with increased ventilatory response to carbon dioxide and hypersecretion of growth hormone in patients with acromegaly. *Am J Respir Crit Care Med* 1994; 150:496.

47. Williams RG, et al: Voice changes in acromegaly. *Laryngoscope* 1994; 104:484.

48. Wright RL, et al: Hemorrhage into pituitary adenoma. *Arch Neurol* 1965; 12:326.

49. Messick JM, et al: Anesthesia for transphenoidal surgery of the hypophyseal region. *Anesth Analg* 1978; 57:206.

50. Newfield P, et al: Air embolism during trans-sphenoidal pituitary operations. *Neurosurgery* 1978; 2:39.

51. Hill JN, et al: Total spinal blockade during local anesthesia of the nasal passages. *Anesthesiology* 1983; 59:144.

52. Slavin ML, et al: Chiasmal compression from fat packing after transsphenoidal resection of intrasellar tumor in two patients. *Am J Ophthalmol* 1993; 115:368.

53. Messick JM, et al: Anesthesia for transsphenoidal microsurgery. In Laws ER Jr, et al (eds): *Management of Pituitary Adenomas and Related Lesions with Emphasis on Transsphenoidal Microsurgery.* New York, Appleton-Century-Crofts, 1982:253–261.

54. Kelly DF, et al: Delayed hyponatremia after transsphenoidal surgery for pituitary adenoma. Report of nine cases. *J Neurosurg* 1995; 83:363.

55. Wilkins RH: Hypothalamic dysfunction and intracranial arterial spasm. *Surg Neurol* 1975; 4:472.

56. Laws ER Jr., Kern EB: Complications of transsphenoidal surgery. In Laws ER Jr et al (eds): *Management of Pituitary Adenomas and Related Lesions with Emphasis on Transsphenoidal Microsurgery.* New York, Appleton-Century-Crofts, 1982:329–346.

57. Wilson CB: Endocrine-inactive pituitary adenomas. *Neurosurgical Operative Atlas* 1992; 2:455.

Chapter 29

SURGERY AND ANESTHESIA OF THE POSTERIOR FOSSA

SUSAN S. PORTER

ABHAY SANAN

SETTI S. RENGACHARY

Surgery of the posterior fossa presents a unique set of circumstances that must be carefully considered by the operative neurosurgeon and anesthesiologist. Understanding the complex anatomy of the region is fundamental in planning approaches and preventing complications. Nowhere else in the body is there as dense a collection of critical neurovascular structures passing through such a rigidly confined space. Because of this combination of factors, the posterior fossa contents tolerate distortion poorly and produce symptoms that can progress rapidly. A wide variety of developmental, neoplastic, and vascular lesions in the posterior fossa can require neurosurgical intervention. Surgery of the posterior fossa is challenging because of its small space and little forgiveness in allowing retraction. Choosing the proper position and selecting the appropriate surgical approach are critical in obtaining proper exposure of the offending pathology. These decisions have important implications for anesthetic management, choice of monitoring techniques, deciding on the need for special techniques, and in assessing the risk of specific complications such as venous air embolism. The preparation for any surgical procedure involving the posterior fossa should always include communication among surgeon, patient, anesthesiologist, and nursing personnel to best anticipate and prepare for intraoperative needs and to properly educate and care for the patient throughout the perioperative period.

Historical Perspectives

In the early neurosurgical era (before the 1950s), most patients with a posterior fossa mass came to surgery in a miserable state. Already blind from papilledema, cachectic from vomiting, and drowsy from hydrocephalus, these patients faced the grim prospect of a difficult surgical procedure and an often bleak prognosis for successful treatment. Without imaging techniques other than air ventriculography, posterior fossa operations were, in truth, blind explorations. The already high pressure in the posterior fossa was further elevated by induction of anesthesia, a process often involving slow inhalation induction with concomitant respiratory depression, breath-holding, coughing, and risk of hypotension. On opening the dura, the swollen cerebellum often herniated and further exposure might require considerable retraction for the surgeon to see the lesion with the unaided eye. Death or devastating neurologic compromise was often the result.

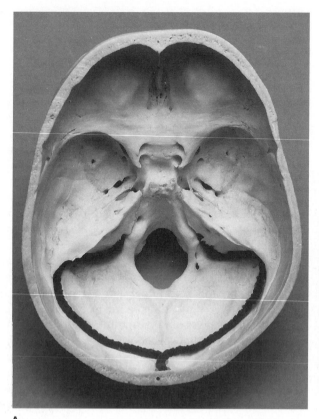

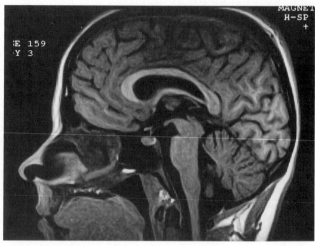

A   **B**

Figure 29-1   *A.* The bony confines of the posterior fossa. The paths of the transverse and sigmoid sinuses are marked in black. *B.* MRI (T1 weighted, sagittal section) shows the boundaries and contents of the posterior fossa.

At that time, local anesthesia was the anesthetic most commonly used for intracranial operations. The use of general anesthesia was uncommon, there being no easy means to manage the patient's airway. Inadequate ventilation contributed to further elevation of already precariously high intracranial pressure, risking intraoperative herniation and death. Intraoperative monitoring of blood loss, respiratory gas (particularly CO_2) monitoring, and detection of venous air embolism (VAE) were not possible. It was mandatory to operate expeditiously because prolonged surgery and anesthesia were dangerous and many factors were uncontrollable. Surgical delicacy and careful dissection were nearly unknown luxuries. Because posterior fossa surgery implied operation in an already small space of limited accessibility and the structures contained within were so vulnerable to injury by dissection and retraction, many lesions of the posterior fossa were deemed inoperable.

Today, anesthesia is a much safer process and there is little need to limit operative time due to excessive risk. Computed tomography (CT) and magnetic resonance imaging (MRI) can identify posterior fossa lesions early, before extensive destructive changes have

altered the anatomy or precipitated serious symptoms. Microsurgical techniques have reduced the need for retraction. The precordial Doppler and continuous respiratory gas monitoring have allowed early detection of venous air embolism and the use of bipolar coagulation has allowed blood loss to become controllable. Most cases of posterior fossa surgery can now be performed with minimal perioperative morbidity.

Anatomic Considerations

The posterior fossa is the largest of the cranial fossae (Fig. 29-1). Although the posterior cranial fossa refers strictly to bony boundaries, it is convenient to use the infratentorial compartment as a synonym. It is rigidly bounded by the clivus anteriorly, the occipital bone posteriorly, and the temporal bones laterally. The floor is formed by the occipital bone. The foramen magnum, through which the medulla oblongata becomes continuous with the spinal cord, is found on the floor of the posterior fossa. The roof of the posterior fossa is formed by the tentorium cerebelli, which contains a hiatus through which the midbrain becomes continuous with the diencephalon. Confined within this posterior fossa cavity are neural structures, cerebrospinal fluid (CSF) spaces, arterial and venous vessels, and venous sinuses.

The neural contents include the cerebellum, brain stem, and cranial nerves. Disturbance of the normal function of these structures accounts for the majority of symptoms produced by a posterior fossa mass. It is noteworthy that the posterior fossa contains every efferent pathway of the brain. Because of the combination of critical structures packed into this small area, elevated intracranial pressure (ICP) within the infratentorial space is tolerated even more poorly than the supratentorial space. The pathway of outflow of CSF through the aqueduct of Sylvius to the fourth ventricle and then through the foramen of Magendie and Lushka into the basal cisterns is located entirely within the posterior fossa. Pathologic conditions located here that result in edema or structural dislocation can obstruct CSF flow and produce secondary hydrocephalus.

The infratentorial space has a blood supply distinct from the supratentorial space. The paired vertebral arteries join anterior to the brain stem and form the basilar artery. Unlike the carotid arteries, a vertebral artery can become occluded during excessive turning of the head. Perhaps the most important anatomic feature of the cerebellum with regard to intraoperative risk and management is the presence of large venous sinuses throughout the infratentorial compartment. The torcula, superior petrosal sinuses, transverse sinus, and the sigmoid sinus are located within the dural folds of the tentorium (Fig. 29-2). The use of the sitting position during some posterior fossa procedures and the potential for these large sinuses to entrain air has focused a great deal of attention on the prevention and treatment of VAE.

Surgical Diseases

TUMORS

Tumors are the most common posterior fossa lesions requiring surgical intervention. The spectrum of disease varies markedly with age (Table 29-1). In childhood, primary central nervous system (CNS) tumors are second only to leukemia in incidence. Two-thirds of brain tumors occurring in this age group arise in the posterior fossa. Tumors can broadly be categorized into those arising from the neuraxis (intra-axial) and those arising from surrounding tissue (extra-axial). Each of these can be further subdivided into tumors arising from a specific location (Table 29-2). The pathology of the tumor can often be predicted from the age of the patient and the location of the tumor. A summary of the salient features of the major tumor types is presented in Table 29-3.

GENERAL CLINICAL PRESENTATION

The presence of so many eloquent neural structures within the posterior fossa implies that a mass lesion may produce a wide variety of signs and symptoms. This fact notwithstanding, the clinical presentation of a posterior fossa mass lesion can vary from nonspecific symptoms to lateralizing signs to symptoms that are the result of secondary hydrocephalus. Localizing signs and symptoms either indicate lesions that involve the neural structures very early, or are late signs indicative of growth into adjacent structures or mass effect. Nonspecific complaints such as fatigue, vomiting, anorexia, headache, and personality change may precede more localizing symptoms such as cerebellar ataxia and cranial nerve palsy. The classic triad of symptoms referable to a mass in the posterior fossa is headache, vomiting, and ataxia.

ELEVATED INTRACRANIAL PRESSURE

Elevated ICP from hydrocephalus is suggested by early morning headache, nuchal pain, vomiting, diplopia, unsteadiness of gait, urinary incontinence, and drowsiness. Hydrocephalus is common with intraaxial tumors of the fourth ventricle and other midline tumors. Early signs include a bulging fontanel in the infant and an enlarging blind spot in the adult. Papilledema is often present. Downward pressure on the brainstem may stretch the sixth (VI) cranial nerve along its long course and produce the well-recognized false localizing sign of unilateral or bilateral abducens (VI) nerve palsy.

Expansion of a midline tumor may produce a sufficient increase in ICP to cause tonsillar herniation, which is associated with meningismus, head tilt, downbeat nystagmus, and opisthotonus. Pressure on the pyramidal tracts may produce posturing that is mistaken for seizures ("cerebellar fits").[1] Coughing can produce further impaction of the tonsils against the medulla and precipitate clinical deterioration including loss of consciousness and respiratory arrest. Tonsillar herniation is more common in children because adults are able to articulate their symptoms much earlier.

Very high ICP produces hypertension and bradycardia, a phenomenon classically called the "Cushing response," Cushing being the first to systematically study the relationship between ICP and cardiorespiratory function.[2] Acute dynamic distortion of the vasomotor region of the medulla engenders reflex hypertension in an attempt to preserve flow to the critical regions of the brainstem. The bradycardia is mediated peripherally via the carotid sinus as a reflex response to

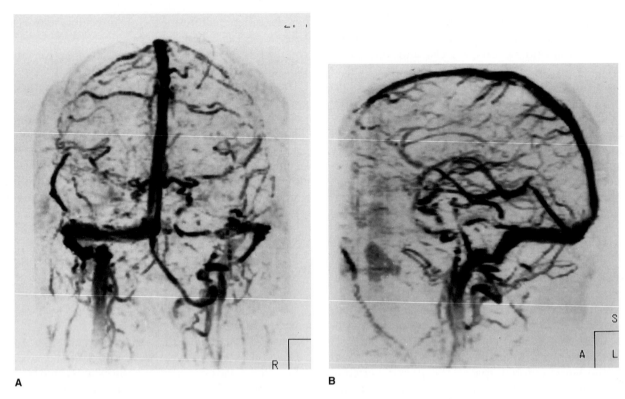

A   **B**

Figure 29-2   Magnetic resonance image venogram (anteroposterior view, *A*; lateral view, *B*) shows the large venous structures that may be encountered during surgical procedures in the posterior fossa.

systemic hypertension. Unfortunately, Cushing's triad often heralds imminent herniation and death.

SPECIFIC CLINICAL SYNDROMES

MIDLINE CEREBELLAR SYNDROME   Midline lesions of the cerebellum and fourth ventricular lesions tend to produce disturbances in equilibrium and an unsteady, wide-based gait that resembles inebriation. Nystagmus is common and hydrocephalus and papilledema occur early. Larger midline lesions push on the brain stem and can produce a facial or other cranial nerve palsy. This presentation is typical of the ependymoma and medulloblastoma.

LATERAL CEREBELLAR SYNDROME   Lateral cerebellar hemispheric lesions such as astrocytomas and hemangioblastomas can be expected to produce ataxia, dysmetria, asynergia, dysarthria, gaze paresis, dysdiadochokinesia, intention tremor, hypotonia, scanning speech, and an inability to discriminate weight. These signs are present ipsilateral to the lesion. Hydrocephalus and brain stem compression are less frequent and occur very late.

CEREBELLOPONTINE ANGLE SYNDROME   Expansion of a lesion into the cerebellopontine angle produces a clinical syndrome characterized by dysfunction of the facial (VII) and vestibulocochlear (VIII) cranial nerves. As the tumor enlarges, cerebellar dysfunction and hydrocephalus usually develop. This course is typical of the acoustic (VII) nerve schwannoma but can be mimicked by a meningioma.

BRAIN STEM SYNDROMES   Processes primarily involving the brain stem produce a combination of cranial nerve palsies and long tract signs such as spasticity. Ipsilateral cranial nerve palsy and contralateral motor and sensory deficits are characteristic. Further growth produces life-threatening respiratory dysfunction, bradycardia, hypertension, and hyperthermia. Signs isolated to the brain stem suggest the diagnosis of a glioma in the child and of clival chordoma in the adult.

MEDULLOBLASTOMA

Medulloblastoma arises from embryonal medulloblastic cells located in the anterior or posterior medullary velum (Fig. 29-3). They are regarded by many pathologists as a type of primitive neuroectodermal tumor (PNET). Eighty percent of cases occur before the age of 16 and this tumor is much more common in males. Roughly one-fifth of all pediatric brain tumors are me-

TABLE 29-1
Posterior Fossa Tumor Distribution by Age

Tumor Type	Percent of All Brain Tumors (within age group)	Percent of Infratentorial Tumors (within age group)
0–20 years		
Astrocytoma	20	36
Medulloblastoma	20	36
Brain stem glioma	10	18
Ependymoma	5	9
Total	55	99
20–60 Years		
Metastases	5	55
Vestibular schwannoma	3	33
Meningioma	1	11
Total	9	99
>60 Years		
Acoustic schwannoma	20	66
Metastases	5	16
Meningioma	5	16
Total	30	99

SOURCE: Adapted with permission from Butler AB, et al: Classification and biology of brain tumors. In Youmans JR (ed): *Neurological Surgery.* Philadelphia, WB Saunders, 1982:2685.

dulloblastomas.[3] Unlike most brain tumors, medulloblastomas frequently metastasize to extracranial sites or spread throughout the leptomeninges to produce spinal cord or nerve root syndromes. The tumor usu-

TABLE 29-2
Location of Tumors of the Posterior Fossa

	Intraaxial Tumors	
Cerebellum	Fourth Ventricle and Pons	Brainstem
Astrocytoma	Medulloblastoma	Glioma
Hemangioblastoma	Ependymoma	Hemangioblastoma
Metastasis	Choroid plexus papilloma Hemangioblastoma	
	Extraaxial Tumors	
Cerebellopontine Angle	Skull Base	
Vestibular schwannoma	Metastasis	
Meningioma	Chordoma	
Arachnoid cyst	Chondrosarcoma	
Epidermoid tumor		

ally presents with a brief history of rapidly evolving midline cerebellar signs but can distort the brain stem and produce brain stem syndromes. Obstructive hydrocephalus is common. A midline suboccipital approach is used to debulk the tumor and surgery is then followed by radiation therapy and chemotherapy. A 5-year survival of more than 70 percent can now be expected in patients who have undergone gross total resection of tumor. A plane usually exists between the tumor and the brain stem.

CEREBELLAR ASTROCYTOMA

Cerebellar astrocytomas are distinct from supratentorial astrocytomas in that they present in the first two decades of life and follow a much more benign course.[4] The tumor is usually a slow-growing, cystic mass confined to one cerebellar hemisphere. Therefore, these patients present with lateralizing ipsilateral cerebellar dysfunction (ataxia) and signs of elevated ICP are late. Gross total removal through a suboccipital approach is curative.

EPENDYMOMA

Ependymomas arise from the ependymal lining of the floor of the fourth ventricle. They usually also present in the first decade of life. By virtue of their location, ependymomas tend to invade the underlying brain stem. They also have a tendency to follow the CSF spaces and quickly obstruct the foramen of Magendie and Luschka. Like the medulloblastoma, ependymomas present with midline cerebellar signs but produce brain stem signs and hydrocephalus earlier. Like the medulloblastoma, a midline approach is used for attempts at resection. The 5-year survival rate is approximately 60 percent if a gross total resection is achieved.[5] Because they are firmly attached to the underlying brain any tug on the tumor causes distortion of the brain stem. This may result in cardiovascular instability during tumor dissection. The use of the ultrasonic aspirator (CUSA) reduces this problem by removing tissue without traction or retraction on surrounding structures.

BRAIN STEM GLIOMA

The majority of these lesions are diffusely infiltrating malignant lesions arising in the pons. An occasional lesion is found in the medulla and these are regarded as histologically benign but biologically malignant because of their location. Almost all patients are affected in childhood, and symptoms are often variable and insidious in onset and progression.[6–8] Ipsilateral palsy of the abducens (VI) and facial (VII) nerves combined with long tract signs of hemiparesis or ataxia is the classic presentation. Obstruction of CSF pathways is a very late problem and hydrocephalus places the diag-

TABLE 29-3
Salient Features of Major Tumor Types

Tumor Histology	Age of Presentation	Clinical Syndrome	Standard Approach	Anesthetic Concerns
Medullobastoma	Childhood	Midline cerebellar syndrome	Midline sub-occipital	Hemodynamic instability, ICP
Ependymoma	Childhood	Midline cerebellar syndrome	Midline sub-occipital	Hemodynamic instability, ICP
Cerebellar astrocytoma	Childhood	Lateral cerebellar syndrome	Lateral sub-occipital	
Brainstem glioma	Childhood	Brainstem syndrome	Midline or lateral suboccipital[a]	Hemodynamic instability, cranial nerve palsy, ?Leave intubated?
Pineal region	Young adulthood	Hydrocephalus Parinaud's syndrome	Supracerebellar infratentorial	Sitting position often used
Hemangioblastoma	Adulthood	Cerebellar or brainstem syndrome	Lateral sub-occipital	Polycythemia Occult pheochromocytoma, hypertension
Metastases	Adulthood	Lateral cerebellar syndrome	Lateral sub-occipital	ICP
Vestibular schwannoma	Late adulthood	Cerebellopontine angle syndrome	Lateral sub-occipital	
Meningiomas	Late adulthood	Variable	Variable	

[a] Surgery is rarely undertaken for pontine gliomas unless the tumor is exophytic.
NOTE: ICP, intracranial pressure.

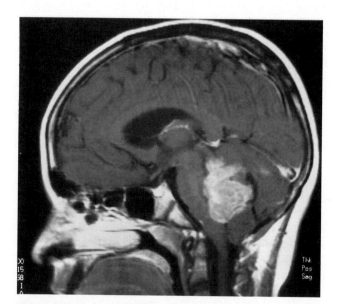

Figure 29-3 MRI (T1 weighted, gadolinium enhanced, sagittal section) shows a medulloblastoma. The tumor arises from the cerebellum and fills the fourth ventricle. A plane usually exists between the tumor and the brain stem.

nosis of a brain stem glioma in question. Surgical removal is not undertaken unless there is an exophytic portion that is amenable to excision. The surgical approach varies with the location of the mass. The postoperative course of these patients may be rocky. Extubation should not be considered for several days because clinical deterioration commonly occurs on postoperative day 2 or 3. The usual course of action is to obtain a closed or open biopsy and administer radiation therapy. Despite treatment, the prognosis is dismal. Most patients die within a few years, earlier if there is malignant transformation to glioblastoma.

VESTIBULAR SCHWANNOMA

These tumors, also called acoustic neurilemmoma, are benign tumors arising from the covering of the vestibular division of the vestibulocochlear (VIII) nerve. They occur in later adulthood with an equal sex distribution. The majority of these tumors are solitary but bilateral tumors can be found associated with type II neurofibromatosis. This is the classic tumor of the cerebellopontine angle and has a stereotypic presentation. The tumor arises inside the internal auditory canal and grows outward into the posterior fossa, where it can

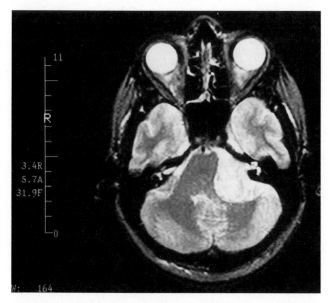

Figure 29-4 MRI (T2 weighted, axial section) shows a vestibular schwannoma. The tumor has enlarged the internal auditory canal and is growing in the cerebellopontine angle.

affect the cerebellum, cranial nerves (particularly the facial (VI) nerve), and the brain stem (Fig. 29-4). Tinnitus is an early symptom but is often ascribed to other causes. Vertigo, nausea, and vomiting may be misdiagnosed as middle ear dysfunction. Hearing loss can progress so gradually as to go unnoticed. Further tumor growth causes cerebellar compression and distortion of the trigeminal (V) nerve, which produces unilateral limb ataxia and facial anesthesia or pain, respectively. Hydrocephalus and lower cranial nerve dysfunction can develop as the tumor grows larger. The facial (VII) nerve is peculiarly insensitive to distortion by tumor (i.e., facial weakness is not a common preoperative finding) yet the nerve remains sensitive to operative manipulation. The patient may be operated in the sitting, lateral, or supine position. Depending on the preoperative hearing status and the anatomy of the tumor, a suboccipital or transtemporal approach may be selected. Intraoperative facial nerve monitoring and monitoring of brain stem auditory evoked responses (BAER) may be used. Total removal is curative. Postoperatively, the two most frequent complications are CSF leak and facial nerve palsy. The CSF leak responds well to spinal drainage. The danger of facial nerve paresis is that the eyelid cannot shut and secondary corneal ulceration may occur. In the immediate postoperative period, protective lubricants should be applied frequently; later a gold weight may be implanted into the eyelid to allow for passive closure.

MENINGIOMA

Meningiomas are derived from arachnoidal cap cells and a tenth of these lesions are found in the posterior fossa. They usually present in late adulthood and are more common in women. The mode of presentation varies with the tumor location. Most produce hemispheric cerebellar deficits, but those of the cerebellopontine angle can mimic vestibular schwannomas and those of the clivus can mimic chordomas. Meningiomas of the tentorium may grow into the middle and posterior fossae; a combined supratentorial and infratentorial approach is then needed for complete removal. Meningiomas of the foramen magnum have an unusual presentation in that they present with occipital or neck pain, hand atrophy, gait ataxia, cough, headache, and hypoglossal palsy. Cerebellar symptoms are uncommon. Meningiomas are histologically benign and surgical extirpation is curative. Postoperatively, one-third of patients may be expected to have permanent deficits of at least one cranial nerve.[9]

HEMANGIOBLASTOMA

Hemangioblastomas are the most common primary cerebellar tumor of adulthood. The tumor is highly vascular and usually exists within a cystic cavity as a mural nodule. As expected, cerebellar hemispheric disturbance is common. In as many as 50 percent of cases, the tumor secretes erythropoietin and produces a secondary polycythemia,[10] and this should not be misinterpreted as dehydration. Cerebellar hemangioblastomas may be associated with von Hippel-Lindau syndrome, an autosomal dominant condition in which retinal angiomatosis is present in addition to the cerebellar lesions.[11] These patients may have cysts in the pancreas, liver, or kidney. Occult renal cell carcinoma or pheochromocytoma may also complicate the condition. Sudden uncontrollable hypertension during anesthesia should prompt the anesthesiologist to consider the diagnosis of catecholamine storm secondary to undetected pheochromocytoma.

CHOROID PLEXUS PAPILLOMA

Posterior fossa choroid plexus papillomas occur in the fourth ventricle during the first decade of life. They usually present as hydrocephalus, either from obstruction of CSF pathways or excessive production of CSF. Complete surgical removal may be curative.

CHORDOMA

Chordomas are thought to arise from rests of primitive notochordal tissue in the clivus. They destroy the bone and present with cranial nerve and brain stem dysfunction. Approaches to the clivus are frequently complex and require a detailed understanding of skull base anatomy. Most of these tumors cannot be completely removed, and many may be considered inoperable. Removal is often associated with a temporary paresis of the lower cranial nerves so extubation should be performed only after recovery of the nerves has been demonstrated.

EPIDERMOID AND DERMOID TUMORS

Epidermoid and dermoid tumors are uncommon benign tumors that account for fewer than 1 percent of all posterior fossa tumors. Both are thought to be a result of aberrant dorsal neural tube closure. Epidermoid tumors are typically found in a lateral location (cerebellopontine angle, petrous apex), whereas dermoid tumors more often occur in the midline (fourth ventricle). These tumors present with headache, cerebellar findings, and cranial nerve involvement. Occasionally, the tumors release irritating fluid and cause repeated episodes of aseptic meningitis. Operative removal is curative.

METASTATIC LESIONS

Metastases may implant in the cerebellum and produce symptoms of a mass lesion. Lung and breast cancer are the most frequent tumors to metastasize to the posterior fossa. These tumors are highly vasogenic and the ICP is typically high. Surgery is undertaken for solitary lesions or lesions that threaten life.

PINEAL TUMORS

Pineal tumors are not located in the posterior fossa per se, but surgical access to these tumors is usually performed by traversing the posterior fossa, so a brief discussion of these lesions is pertinent. Tumors in this region may be of amazingly diverse histologic types including germ cell tumors, pineal tissue tumors, and glial tumors. Most tumors are of germ cell origin and occur in young adults. The pineal is located adjacent to the aqueduct of Sylvius and the superior colliculus and compression results in hydrocephalus and Parinaud's syndrome, respectively. Further enlargement causes cerebellar and hypothalamic disturbance. There is considerable controversy about the treatment of patients with pineal tumors. Some surgeons favor stereotactic biopsy and radiation therapy; others favor operative removal. Surgical access to the pineal gland is commonly attempted through a supracerebellar infratentorial approach with the patient in the sitting position. Hyperextension of the neck and trunk ("sea lion" position) with a biooccipital craniotomy has been recommended for patients who cannot tolerate the sitting position.[12]

VASCULAR LESIONS

The same vascular diseases that affect the supratentorial space also affect the posterior fossa, namely, arteriovenous malformations, aneurysms, infarctions, and hemorrhages; however, the tight confines of the posterior fossa impart a higher degree of urgency to many of these conditions.

ARTERIOVENOUS MALFORMATIONS

Arteriovenous malformations (AVMs) of the posterior fossa can involve either the parenchymal vessels or the transverse-sigmoid sinus complex. Those of the parenchymal vessels are thought to be congenital in origin and present with hemorrhage, headache, mass effect, or hydrocephalus. Operative removal requires a wide midline craniectomy so the arterial supply will always remain in control. Blood loss in these cases can be sudden and massive. The ability to maintain controlled hypotension and the capability to administer large volumes of blood are important anesthetic considerations.

Dural AVMs involving the lateral or sigmoid sinuses are probably acquired lesions resulting from aberrant recanalization of a previously thrombosed sinus. Pulsatile tinnitus with headache are the classic complaints. Increased ICP or focal neurologic deficit is unusual. Operative removal is usually preceded by arterial embolization, which helps to prevent excessive bleeding during surgery. A combined supratentorial-infratentorial approach is usually required to fully access the involved sinus.

Vein of Galen malformations are better thought of as arteriovenous fistulas. The symptoms on presentation depend on the degree of shunting and fall into three clinical patterns that can be grouped by age. Infants most commonly present with congestive heart failure and have a very high-flow fistula. On occasion as much as 80 percent of the cardiac output may be shunted from the arterial to the venous circulation. Not surprisingly, seizures and hydrocephalus are common. A holocranial bruit can be heard with a stethoscope. Intraoperatively, dramatic hemodynamic changes can occur suddenly. There is potential for massive blood loss and hypotension as the fistula is dissected. Sudden heart failure with acute pulmonary edema can occur when the feeding artery is ligated. Blood replacement can exceed several blood volumes. The challenge of intraoperative management is the maintenance of cardiovascular stability in the face of a rapidly changing blood volume.[13] Some centers use controlled hypotension to prevent circulatory overload when the fistula is obliterated. Other centers use hypothermia with circulatory arrest. Yet others use a combination of inotropic agents and pharmacologic afterload reduction. The reported operative mortality is over 50 percent. Recently, endovascular techniques have been used to attempt obliteration of the fistula by injection of coils into the fistula through a transtorcular puncture. Older children present with hydrocephalus from compression of the aqueduct of Sylvius. A cranial bruit can be heard but frank congestive heart failure is usually not a feature. Cardiomegaly, however, is common. Adults usually present with headaches. A cranial bruit and cardio-megaly are absent.

Cavernous malformations are commonly seen in the posterior fossa. They can cause neurologic deficit from repeated bleeding. Surgical risk (of serious postoperative neurologic deficit or death) depends on the location. Angiomas deep in the brain stem carry the worst risk and are largely considered inoperable. Those presenting at the surface of the brain stem are of intermediate risk to approach surgically, whereas those located in the cerebellar hemispheres are the least threatening.

ANEURYSMS

Fifteen percent of all intracranial aneurysms are found in the posterior fossa circulation. Approximately one-half of these are at the basilar tip and require an approach through the supratentorial space. Midbasilar aneurysms remain a challenge and can be approached anteriorly through the clivus or laterally through a subtemporal transtentorial approach. Aneurysms of the vertebral artery can be approached through a unilateral suboccipital craniectomy. The inability to retract brain in the posterior fossa renders some large aneurysms particularly difficult to treat. To produce a completely avascular field, some centers use deep hypothermia with cardiac standstill during the time the aneurysm is dissected and clipped. With a core temperature of between 15° and 20°C, circulatory arrest can be maintained for about 60 min. This technique requires expertise in both cardiovascular and neurosurgical anesthetic management.

SPONTANEOUS HEMORRHAGE

Spontaneous hypertensive hemorrhage may occur in the cerebellum or in the brain stem. Twenty percent of all hypertensive bleeding occurs in structures in the posterior fossa.[14] Patients with cerebellar bleeding may be treated surgically, but patients with brain stem hemorrhage are not good candidates for surgical intervention because of the uniformly poor prognosis. The rapid expansion of a hematoma may produce life-threatening tonsillar herniation. In response to increasing pressure in the posterior fossa compartment, the cerebellar tonsils bulge through the foramen magnum and in doing so compress the medulla against the bony rim of the foramen magnum. The clinical presentation of vomiting, unilateral ataxia, and unilateral facial palsy requires immediate attention. In contrast to the syndrome of transtentorial herniation, third nerve palsy and hemiparesis are absent. The patient may be alert and suddenly suffer a fatal respiratory arrest. Once diagnosed, surgical evacuation is both lifesaving and gratifying.

Traumatic epidural and subdural hemorrhages are much less common in the posterior fossa compared to those occurring in the supratentorial compartment. Only 5 to 10 percent of all extradural hematomas are found in the posterior fossa.[15] The mode of presentation is similar to a cerebellar hemorrhage. Evacuation is generally through a lateral suboccipital craniectomy. Unlike those that occur in the supratentorial space, the bleeding is usually venous in origin.

CEREBELLAR INFARCTION

Most cerebellar infarctions are due to embolic disease from atherosclerosis although infarctions in young patients are often due to a vertebral artery dissection. The most common distribution is that of the posterior inferior cerebellar artery. Initially, the patient presents with nausea, nystagmus, and ataxia. As the infarcted cerebellum swells, the brain stem is compressed and a gaze palsy followed by a facial palsy appears. If surgical resection of infarcted tissue is not performed, coma and death can ensue. A CT scan of the brain may be normal in appearance in the early stages. This condition, like cerebellar hemorrhage, is a neurosurgical emergency and rapid surgical extirpation is crucial. The operation of choice is a suboccipital decompression down to the level of the foramen magnum and resection of the infarcted cerebellar tissue that oozes out like toothpaste on opening the dura. Results after prompt resection of infarcted tissue are good. Because the supratentorial compartment does not suffer any intrinsic damage, full cognitive function can return even in a patient who was comatose preoperatively.

DEVELOPMENTAL DISORDERS

DANDY-WALKER COMPLEX

The Dandy-Walker complex refers to a collection of three related conditions: the Dandy-Walker malformation, the Dandy-Walker variant, and the mega cisterna magna. The Dandy-Walker malformation is defined by a triad of anatomic findings: (1) agenesis of the cerebellar vermis, (2) dilatation of the fourth ventricle, and (3) enlarged posterior fossa with upward displacement of the torcula.[16] These patients usually have hydrocephalus and require early shunting. The Dandy-Walker variant is similar to the Dandy-Walker malformation except that the posterior fossa is not enlarged. Mega cisterna magna refers to a retrocerebellar cyst that is unaccompanied by vermian hypoplasia.

CHIARI MALFORMATIONS

Most Chiari malformations can be grouped into two types based on anatomic features. The Chiari I malformation is characterized by descent of the cerebellar tonsils into the cervical spinal canal. This is thought to be secondary to a small posterior fossa volume.[17] Symptoms do not usually appear until adolescence or

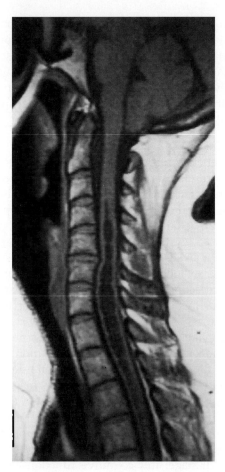

Figure 29-5 MRI (T1 weighted, sagittal section) shows a Chiari I malformation. The cerebellar tonsils are below the level of the foramen magnum and a syrinx is present in the cervical spinal cord.

young adulthood and consist of cough-induced headache, nuchal pain, downbeat nystagmus, and lower cranial nerve dysfunction. Syringomyelia often accompanies Chiari I malformations and may produce dissociated sensory loss and atrophy of the hands (Fig. 29-5). The Chiari I malformation is an isolated abnormality and is not usually accompanied by spina bifida, hydrocephalus, or other cranial abnormalities.

The Chiari II malformation is a more complex abnormality. Here not only does the inferior vermis herniate through the foramen magnum but other infratentorial abnormalities are also present as well, including a small bony posterior fossa, "beaking" of the quadrigeminal plate, and medullary kinking. Spina bifida, hydrocephalus, and syringomyelia are inevitably present. This malformation becomes symptomatic in 5 to 10 percent of neonates born with this condition. Lower cranial nerve dysfunction may produce stridor and respiratory compromise. Spasticity and quadriparesis will be progressive in untreated cases. Even with aggressive therapy, up to 30 percent of symptomatic infants die of respiratory complications.

The surgical therapy for Chiari I and II is similar. A suboccipital craniectomy and upper cervical laminectomy is the treatment of choice. Any adhering arachnoidal bands are sectioned and a generous duroplasty is performed. Treatment of hydrocephalus or an associated syrinx may require a ventriculoperitoneal or cystoperitoneal shunting. Some surgeons resect herniated cerebellar tissue or place a muscle plug in the obex, although both procedures have lost favor. Postoperatively, a sleep apnea-like syndrome may appear in the Chiari II patient, prompting emergency reintubation.

ARACHNOID CYSTS
Arachnoid cysts are CSF collections that are enclosed within the layers of the piaarachnoid. Most are asymptomatic but some are large enough to cause compression of the cerebellum and aqueduct of Sylvius. Marsupialization and cystoperitoneal shunting are performed for symptomatic cysts.

CRANIOCERVICAL DISORDERS
Both developmental and acquired disorders can affect the craniovertebral junction. These include Hurler's syndrome, Klippel-Feil syndrome, basilar invagination, inflammatory (mostly rheumatoid) disease, Down syndrome, and dwarfism. Problems range from small foramen magnum to atlanto-occipital instability to atlantoaxial dislocation. Symptoms are those of lower cranial nerve compression and brain stem or cervical cord compression. Surgical treatment includes realignment of the craniocervical axis and stabilization along with posterior fossa decompression. This may be approached posteriorly or sometimes via an anterior transoral route. These patients are often in dynamic or static traction preoperatively and this is continued postoperatively.

CRANIAL NERVE DYSFUNCTION
MICROVASCULAR DECOMPRESSION
Although Dandy[18] first proposed nearly a century ago that compression of a cranial nerve at its point of entry into the brain stem was a cause of cranial neuralgia, real examination of the utility of vascular decompression has been within the last 20 years in response to the work of Janetta.[19] Small vessels can often be found impinging on the root entry zone of cranial nerves, but the exact mechanism by which this may cause hyperactive nerve irritation is not clear. Surgical decompression of the cranial nerves has a fairly good success rate—over two-thirds of patients with trigeminal neuralgia or hemifacial spasm can expect relief.[20] The procedure involves a small retromastoid craniectomy through which the cerebellum is retracted medially to allow visualization of the root entry zones. The

operating microscope will usually reveal an offending arterial vessel loop but on occasion veins, tumors, or vascular malformations have also been identified. Removing the offending tumor or placing a cushion (shredded Teflon) between the artery and root entry zone offers relief in most cases. In general, monitoring of the affected cranial nerve is performed to establish the adequacy of decompression and avoid inadvertent neural injury.[21]

TRIGEMINAL NEURALGIA

Trigeminal neuralgia or tic douloureux is the most common and most clinically representative of the root entry zone compression syndromes. Patients describe paroxysmal episodes of excruciating and lancinating pain over the ipsilateral trigeminal distribution. The pain is usually in the cheek or gums. Particular trigger points may be identified that elicit the pain when touched and, on occasion, these patients will present with severe dehydration because of their reluctance to eat or drink. Patients who are refractory to medical treatment and are in good medical health are good candidates for microvascular decompression. The superior cerebellar artery is the most frequent offender. No special intraoperative electrophysiologic monitoring is usually performed because fifth nerve monitoring is not available. The pain relief can be immediate after surgery, but it may be several weeks before response is noted. Roughly 15 to 30 percent of patients will have a major recurrence within 5 years,[22] with the variability in incidence secondary to the stringency of diagnostic criteria applied. Atypical facial pain syndromes do not respond well to microvascular decompression.

Older patients and patients who cannot tolerate open craniotomy may be appropriate for neurodestructive procedures. A needle introduced percutaneously through the foramen ovale can give access to the trigeminal (gasserian) ganglion. Using injection of a neurolytic agent such as alcohol or using a radiofrequency probe, all or a portion of the ganglion can be destroyed. This procedure, percutaneous trigeminal rhizolysis (PTR) is performed under local anesthesia with sedation during the periods when the needle is passed intracranially. Periods of communication with the patient are essential during this procedure to allow the patient to provide feedback about the distribution of sensory deficit produced by rhizolysis. Although offering some chance at pain relief, this procedure is plagued with a high recurrence rate and is associated with the development of "anesthesia dolorosa" in the area of prior pain. This syndrome, which is literally translated as "painful numbness," is refractory to most attempts at therapy and is probably secondary to overzealous destruction of the trigeminal ganglion.

HEMIFACIAL SPASM

Hemifacial spasm is thought to be caused by pulsatile vascular irritation at the root entry zone of the seventh cranial nerve. The patient suffers from painful paroxysmal bouts of facial contraction. The offending vessel may include the vertebral, posterior inferior cerebellar, or anterior inferior cerebellar artery. Intraoperative monitoring of BAERs, electromyographic recording of facial nerve function, and recording of compound potentials directly from the eighth nerve are frequently used to try to avoid deafness from inadvertent manipulation of the cochlear nerve and to ensure that the facial nerve demonstrates a reduction in irritability after decompression. In expert hands, the success rate is near 90 percent.[19,23]

VESTIBULAR NERVE DYSFUNCTION

Disabling vertigo that cannot be referred to a specific process such as benign positional vertigo, vestibular neuritis, or Meniere's disease has been treated with microvascular decompression, or by sectioning the vestibular division of the vestibulocochlear nerve. The success rate has been reported at over 80 percent in well-selected patients.[24] The vertebral artery is the usual offender. BAERs are monitored intraoperatively to detect inadvertent cochlear nerve injury.

GLOSSOPHARYNGEAL NEURALGIA

This is a rare disorder that presents with paroxysms of pain in the posterior pharynx. These symptoms may be relieved with topical anesthesia. Some patients also manifest syncope.[25] The posterior inferior cerebellar artery is the usual culprit. Decompression has a reported long-term success rate of 80 percent.[26] Intraoperative cardiovascular instability may occur during nerve manipulation or decompression and transient lower cranial nerve palsy has been reported postoperatively.

Surgical Approaches

Surgical approaches to the posterior fossa may be grouped into those that enter the compartment directly (suboccipital, supracerebellar infratentorial, transtemporal, transoral) and those that enter through the supratentorial compartment (combined supratentorial infratentorial, occipital transtentorial, temporal transtentorial). These approaches are schematically depicted in Fig. 29-6.

SUBOCCIPITAL APPROACH

This is the most common approach to the posterior fossa (Fig. 29-7) and allows exposure of the vermis and cerebellar hemispheres with a midline incision or exposure of the cerebellar hemispheres and pontocerebellar angle with a lateral incision. The vertebral artery

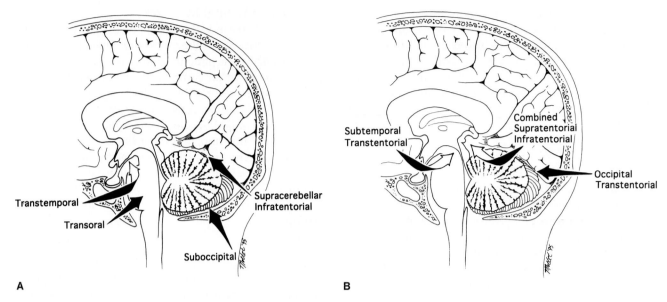

A   **B**

Figure 29-6 *A.* Surgical approaches that enter the posterior fossa directly include the suboccipital, supracerebellar infratentorial, transtemporal, and transoral. *B.* Surgical approaches that approach the posterior fossa through the supratentorial compartment include the combined supratentorial infratentorial, occipital transtentorial, and temporal transtentorial.

and the lower basilar artery can also be accessed. The incision is made from the level of the inion to the level of C3. The skin and muscle are retracted and the occipital bone is removed by either craniotomy or craniectomy.

SUPRACEREBELLAR INFRATENTORIAL APPROACH

This approach is suited for access to the pineal gland and surrounding structures and is perhaps the only

approach in which the sitting position is fully justifiable. Access to the pineal region through other approaches such as the occipital transtentorial or transcallosal approach requires considerable retraction and possible injury to the large surrounding venous channels. By going superior to the cerebellum, large veins are avoided. The sitting position allows the cerebellum to sag and improves the exposure. Gravity carries blood and CSF away from the pineal region and relieves the surgeon from repeatedly suctioning down a small hole with poor visibility.

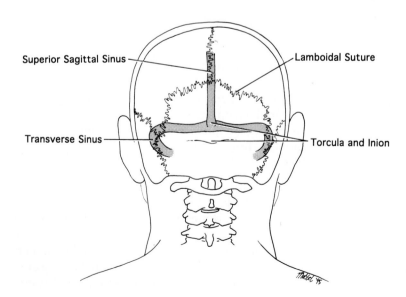

Figure 29-7 The suboccipital craniotomy is the most widely used surgical approach to the posterior fossa. The significant landmarks are indicated: the transverse sinus, superior sagittal sinus, lambdoidal suture, and the inion.

TRANSTEMPORAL APPROACH

Approaches through the temporal bone have been used to gain access to the cerebellopontine angle. They are usually performed in conjunction with a neuro-otologist and include the translabrynthine, retrolabrynthine, and middle fossa approaches.

TRANSORAL APPROACH

The transoral approach is used for access to the lower clivus and exposes the anterior brain stem and basilar artery. Special armored endotracheal tubes should be used for intubation. Alternatively, a tracheostomy should be performed if cranial nerve dysfunction is anticipated postoperatively. The intravenous administration of steroids before and after surgery may help minimize swelling of the tongue and secondary airway obstruction. The major complications using the transoral approach are continuing CSF leakage and meningitis.

COMBINED SUPRATENTORIAL INFRATENTORIAL APPROACH

This approach may be necessary to remove lesions that have a component both above and below the tentorial hiatus such as meningioma, vestibular schwannoma, and epidermoid cyst. A curvilinear incision is used that starts at the zygoma and curves around the ear to end below the mastoid tip. Sacrifice of the sigmoid sinus and sectioning of the tentorium may be performed to obtain better exposure.

OCCIPITAL TRANSTENTORIAL APPROACH

Lesions of the superior surface of the cerebellum can be difficult to approach through a standard posterior fossa approach because the lesion is parallel to the surgeon's line of sight. The suboccipital transtentorial approach involves making a supratentorial craniotomy and then by lifting the occipital lobes and dividing the tentorium, one can visualize the superior surface of the cerebellum. Lesions in the region of the pineal may also be approached this way.

SUBTEMPORAL TRANSTENTORIAL APPROACH

A subtemporal transtentorial approach affords access to the upper clivus, basilar artery, cerebellopontine angle, and the cerebellar peduncles. The temporal lobe is lifted and the tentorium divided parallel to the petrous ridge. Spinal drainage and mannitol are used to allow for adequate temporal lobe retraction. The fourth (IV) cranial nerve skirts the free edge of the tentorium and is susceptible to injury using this approach. Care

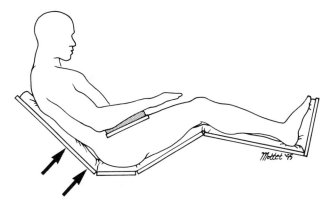

Figure 29-8 The lounging position is the term that best describes the position commonly called the "sitting" position. The back is elevated at 60° with the hips and knees flexed. The neck is flexed but space remains between the chin and chest. The arms are supported and well padded. Attaching the head-holder device to the operating table between the two heavy arrows ensures that the head and trunk will move as a single unit on adjustment of the operating table.

must be taken to avoid manipulation or interference with the draining veins of the temporal lobe to avoid postoperative infarction.

Positioning for Posterior Fossa Surgery

Positioning is an important part of the operative procedure and should be decided on by both the neurosurgeon and anesthesiologist. Adequate access to the patient including intravenous lines, the airway, and any additional monitors being used is critical, and the anesthesiologist must ensure this. All possible points of pressure or traction should be checked. Prior to draping, the anesthesiologist should be convinced that the patient would be comfortable in that position were the patient awake, and should be able to access all monitoring equipment with a minimum of disturbance to the operative field.

SITTING POSITION

The sitting position (Fig. 29-8) is perhaps the most controversial position in neurosurgery. The position was introduced to neurosurgery in 1913 by DeMartel and popularized in the United States in 1928 by Frazier. Its advocates feel that CSF and venous blood drainage are facilitated by gravity and that the cerebellar hemispheres also are displaced inferiorly by gravity. Therefore, optimal visualization of the surgical field is obtained without the use of suction or retraction. Its critics feel that the sitting position exposes the patient to unnecessary risks because other positions can provide similar operative conditions. Possible risks and bene-

TABLE 29-4
Risks and Benefits of the Sitting Position

	Benefits	Risks
Surgical	Improved access to tentorial hiatus	Intracranial hemorrhage
	Decreased blood loss	Quadriplegia
	Improved visibility	Pneumocephalus
	Preservation of cranial nerve function	
Anesthetic	Improved access to patient	Air embolism
	Improved ventilation	Hypotension
		Positional injuries

fits from both a surgical and anesthetic perspective are summarized in Table 29-4. The sitting position has been used most successfully to allow access to the cerebellopontine angle, the cerebellar hemispheres, the fourth ventricle, and the pineal gland.

Despite the well-entrenched term "sitting position," it should be noted that practically no neurosurgeon uses the classically described historic position any more and the patient is better described as "lounging." The back is elevated at approximately 60° with the thighs flexed at the hip and the legs flexed at the knee. The head-holder device should be attached to the table in such a manner that the head and trunk always move as a single unit. This will prevent injury or delay in an emergency situation that would require rapid repositioning. Before surgery begins, the operating team should familiarize themselves with the head-holder and operating table position. This will allow smooth and rapid change to and from the supine position if it is necessary.

Neuropathies of the brachial plexus, ulnar, common peroneal, and sciatic nerves have all been reported and should be guarded against. The arms should be supported and placed across the chest. Neither the elbows nor the lateral aspect of the knees should touch the metal frame required for the head-holder. The weight should be evenly distributed over the lower back, buttocks, and thighs. Extreme flexion at the hips exposes the sciatic nerve to excessive pressure and foot drop has been reported.[27,28]

The head is typically flexed but there should be at least a 1-in. space between the chin and chest to preserve airway patency and to allow venous drainage from the face and tongue. Massive swelling of the head, neck,[29] and tongue[30] have been reported following cases in which extreme flexion or a large oral airway were used. The position of the endotracheal tube should be rechecked after the final position is achieved to prevent endobronchial migration after neck flexion.[31]

Compression stockings or pneumatic boots should be used to prevent blood from pooling in the lower limbs. The pin sites used for head fixation should have a petrolatum-based antibiotic ointment placed around them because these can be a site of air entry.[32-34]

The response of the mean arterial pressure (MAP) and cerebral blood flow (CBF) to the sitting position is controversial. Experiments in dogs demonstrate a reduction in CBF in the sitting position only when the ICP is elevated.[35] Similar studies in humans have revealed conflicting results.[36-38] However, modern investigations convincingly argue that the sitting position does not seem to alter the MAP or the CBF in the vast majority of patients.[36,37]

There are some relative contraindications to the sitting position (Table 29-5). Known right-to-left shunts such as intracardiac defects or pulmonary arteriovenous fistula increase the risk that VAE will cross and be disseminated systemically. Severe hydrocephalus increases the risk of pneumocephalus and subdural hemorrhage. Severe hypovolemia or cardiovascular disease increases the risk of hypotension and stroke. A ventriculoatrial shunt may allow air to enter the venous system through the ventricles of the brain.

In addition to the risk of air embolism, there are several other reasons for decreasing use of the sitting position. One is that postoperative quadriplegia is a rare but known complication of the sitting position, most likely in the elderly, spondylotic spine.[39,40] Excessive flexion combined with low spinal cord perfusion pressure is thought to produce the vascular insult to the cervical spinal cord. Another less common complication of the sitting position is supratentorial hemorrhage.[41,42] The cause is not clear but thought to be secondary to altered ICP dynamics and venous disruption. Drainage of CSF is unchecked in the sitting position and subdural pneumocephalus can occur particularly in patients with preexisting CSF shunts.[43] Finally, the position induces a great deal of fatigue on the surgeon. Despite better exposure, the height and angle of the surgical approach can create discomfort

TABLE 29-5
Relative Contraindications to the Use of the Sitting Position

Intracardiac defect with right-to-left shunt

Pulmonary arteriovenous fistula

Severe hydrocephalus

Functioning ventriculoatrial shunt

Significant hypovolemia

Myocardial dysfunction

for the surgeon, who must work with his neck craned toward the ceiling and with his arms extended.

A study by Black and coworkers[36] retrospectively examined the relationship between perioperative complications and the position used (horizontal or sitting) in a single institution over a 4-year period (1981–1984). The risk of hypotension (defined as a 20 percent drop in MAP from awake baseline) in the sitting position was found to be overestimated. In fact, no difference in the incidence of hypotension was found between patients assuming the horizontal or sitting position. The clinical impression that blood loss was reduced in the sitting position was supported by the results: patients in the seated position required 2 units or more of packed red cells 3 percent of the time, whereas patients operated in the horizontal position had similar requirements 13 percent of the time. Cranial nerve function was better preserved in the sitting group by a significant margin. No morbidity could be attributed to venous air embolism. Despite these results, the authors admitted to an increasing preference for use of the horizontal position for posterior fossa surgery. At the beginning of the study period, the sitting position was used three times more frequently than the horizontal position. By 1984, the ratio had nearly reversed. A survey of British anesthesiologists revealed a similar result: In 1981, 53 percent of British centers always used the sitting position for posterior fossa cases but by 1991, the number had dropped to 20 percent.[44]

Many neurosurgeons feel that the supracerebellar infratentorial approach to the pineal region is the only indication remaining for the sitting position in posterior fossa neurosurgery. The sitting position provides excellent exposure and drainage of this region and lessens the risk of retraction injury. Most neurosurgeons feel that all other posterior fossa operations can be performed adequately in horizontal positions.

Currently, it is clear that the sitting position has potential risks that are much more substantial than the horizontal position. However, several studies have failed to demonstrate an excessive number of serious complications or a significantly increased risk of death or morbidity from the sitting position. Experienced practitioners argue that very few complications are unique to the sitting position and that meticulous attention to positioning and monitoring for air embolism can avoid most problems.[45–48] Nevertheless, the existence of horizontal positions that eliminate the potential risks associated with the sitting position without adversely affecting the surgical result is a strong argument for restricting the use of this position unless it demonstrates an obvious advantage in an individual case. The important point is that the location of the lesion and the medical condition of the patient should

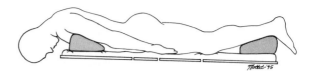

Figure 29-9 The head is distracted and flexed in the prone position. Chest rolls should be used to minimize pressure on the thorax and abdomen and allow free respiratory movement.

dictate the surgical approach. However, if needed, the current literature argues that given appropriate precautions and patient selection, the sitting position can be used safely.

PRONE POSITION

The prone position (Fig. 29-9) avoids most of the problems of air embolism that may occur with the sitting position. The prone position is ideally suited for midline lesions of the cerebellum and for exposure of the fourth ventricle. In adults, three-point fixation of the skull should be used because a horseshoe rest is too unstable, and the head may shift over time, causing pressure on the orbits, cheeks, or bridge of the nose. Furthermore, the weight of the adult head, when resting on a horseshoe, is great enough to create pressure necrosis of the forehead and blindness from retinal artery thrombosis. However, a horseshoe head rest with thick padding is suitable for a child's lighter head. A mild degree of facial and conjunctival edema is expected from this position. Chest rolls should be placed from the clavicles to the pelvis so that the thorax and abdomen are not mechanically compressed.

A modification of the prone position called the "sea lion" position has been described for approaching the pineal region in patients who cannot tolerate the sitting position.[12] After intubation, the neck and trunk are extended so that the orbitomeatal line is nearly parallel to the floor. The pineal region can then be approached through an occipital craniotomy with an interhemispheric approach. This position mandates the use of monitoring for venous air embolism because the head is significantly above heart level.

A head-prone position ("bunny crouch") has been described for posterior fossa surgery in infants with severe hydrocephalus in whom the sitting position is contraindicated because of the risk of subdural hematoma following rapid decompression. Access to the apex of the fourth ventricle may be achieved with this approach.[49] The infant is turned 180° so that the rump is at the head of the operating room table. The infant is then placed in a kneeling position with moderate flexion of the neck. By lowering the head of the bed,

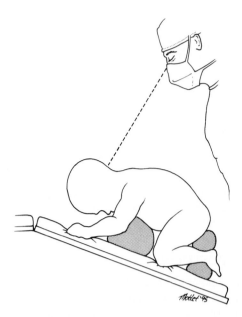

Figure 29-10 The "bunny crouch" position can be used in infants to allow access to the apex of the fourth ventricle.

the surgeon can achieve a direct line of sight to the apex of the fourth ventricle (Fig. 29-10). This position is only useful in infants with a crown-rump length less than 50 cm (about 1 year of age).

LATERAL POSITION

The lateral position (Fig. 29-11) is suited for lesions of the cerebellopontine angle and lesions of the clivus or foramen magnum. The lateral position has an advantage over the prone position for the anesthesiologist because there is direct access to the face, chest, and airway. It is a good position to use in patients who are obese or have a severe kyphotic deformity because ventilation is more efficient and ventilatory compliance is better in this position. Air embolism is rare. An axillary roll is mandatory to avoid neurovascular injury to the dependent arm. Padding should be placed between the legs and under the dependent knee to prevent compression of the common peroneal nerve. The lower leg is kept straight and the upper leg is

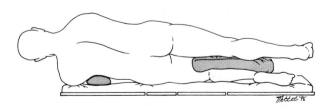

Figure 29-11 The use of the lateral position mandates an axillary roll and padding between the legs.

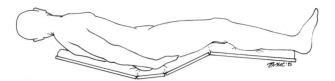

Figure 29-12 In the supine position, the head is rotated, extended, and flexed.

flexed slightly. The upper arm can either be placed adjacent to the head or in the larger person can be placed on an arm rest or bedside stand on the side of the table. The major disadvantage is that visualization may be compromised by the patient's superior shoulder. In this case, the shoulder may be forcibly depressed and held in place with wide adhesive tape.

SUPINE POSITION

The supine position (Fig. 29-12) can be used in the younger patient whose neck will tolerate a maximal degree of lateral rotation and flexion. A roll is placed under the ipsilateral shoulder to relieve tension on the neck. This position allows for excellent access to the cerebellopontine angle for tumors or microvascular decompression. The shoulder does not obstruct the view as in the lateral position and the risk for pressure-induced peripheral neuropathies is low. The only precaution is that this position may not be possible in the elderly patient due to limitation of neck mobility. In addition, excessive neck rotation may impair venous drainage and promote cerebellar congestion.

PARK-BENCH (SEMIPRONE) POSITION

The park-bench or semiprone position (Fig. 29-13) is useful in gaining rapid access to the cerebellar hemispheres. It is named "park-bench" because the patient's final position resembles an inebriate sleeping on a public park bench. The head should be turned about 30° and the neck should be maximally flexed. Because the patient can rapidly be placed in this posi-

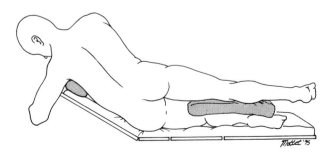

Figure 29-13 The park-bench position is used for emergency access to the cerebellar hemispheres.

TABLE 29-6
Position-related Complications of Posterior Fossa Surgery

Complication	Sitting	Prone	Lateral/3/4 Prone	Park-Bench
Nervous System				
Cerebral ischemia	++	+	—	+
Cervical cord ischemia	++	+	—	+
Cranial nerve palsy	+	++	++	++
Peripheral nerve injuries	+ (br. plexus, sciatic, peroneal)	+ (ulnar)	++ (br. plexus)	++ (br. plexus)
Tension pneumocephalus	++	++	+	—
Airway				
Facial/tongue edema	++	++	+	—
ET tube migration	++	++	+	+
Respiratory				
V/Q mismatch	+	+	++	+
Increased airway pressures	—	++	+	+
Cardiovascular				
Hypotension	++	++	—	—
Arrhythmias	++	++	±	++
Blood loss	+	++	±	+
Miscellaneous				
Orbital compression	—	+++	++	+
VAE	+++	—	++	—
PAE	++	+	?	?

NOTE: ET, endotracheal; PAE, paradoxical air embolism; VAE, venous air embolism.
SOURCE: Adapted with permission from Young ML: Posterior fossa: Anesthetic considerations. In Cottrell JE, Smith DS (eds): *Anesthesia and Neurosurgery*. St. Louis, Mosby-Year Book, 1994:345.

tion, it is frequently used in emergency evacuation of hematomas or resection of infarctions. The head-holder is not always used. Care must be taken not to twist the neck too much relative to the neck or venous obstruction can occur, exacerbating intracranial hypertension. Padding must be applied as in the lateral position. The position can sometimes be disorienting to the surgeon because the head is not in a standard surgical plane. Young and colleagues have reviewed and summarized the common complications of positioning patients for posterior fossa surgery (Table 29-6).

Special Conditions

VENOUS AIR EMBOLISM

Certain conditions can conspire to produce a risk of entrainment of air into the veins—venous air embolism

(VAE). The venous pressure at the operative site must be below atmospheric pressure and the vein noncollapsible. These two conditions are commonly met during posterior fossa surgery in the sitting position. The head is positioned well above the level of the heart, and many of the large veins exposed during posterior fossa surgery are tethered open by bony or dural attachments. Air embolism, however, is not unique to the sitting position or to intracranial surgery. Lumbar, peripheral limb, and intra-abdominal (particularly gynecologic or cesarean section) procedures also carry a risk of intraoperative air entrainment. This phenomenon was first described in the late 1600s[50] and continued to be identified in the medical literature until the etiology was finally pinned down in the mid-1800s.[51]

The reported incidence of VAE varies markedly in published reports.[48,52] The more sensitive the monitoring method, the higher the incidence of detected VAE.

TABLE 29-7
Incidence and Mortality of Venous Air Embolism (VAE)

Author, Year	No. of Patients	VAE (%)	VAE Mortality (%)
Michenfelder, 1969[54]	751	5	0
Michenfelder, 1972[55]	69	47	0
Albin, 1976[56]	180	25	0
Voorhies, 1983[57]	81	50	0
Standefer, 1984[45]	488	6	0
Matjasko, 1985[46]	554	23.5	0
Young, 1986[47]	255	30	0
Black, 1988[36]	333	45	0
von Gosseln, 1991[58]	704	7	0

After the introduction of the precordial Doppler probe by Maroon in 1968,[53] the reported incidence increased as the detection methodology became more sensitive. Despite detection of air embolism in nearly a third of all sitting patients, the actual risk of morbidity is very low (Table 29-7),[36,45–47,54–58] documenting the relative safety of the sitting position. This implies that the serious consequences of air embolism can be avoided with early recognition and appropriate therapy.

PATHOPHYSIOLOGY
The ability of entrained air to produce clinical sequelae depends on three factors: the amount of air entrained, the rate of air entry, and the presence or absence of a patent foramen ovale. The mechanism of injury and the final determinant of end-organ dysfunction depend primarily on the rate of air entry. Continuous entrainment of low volumes of air produces gradual dispersion of air bubbles, which have been mechanically broken up by the contractile action of the right atrium and ventricle, into the pulmonary circulation. Here the effect is an elevation of pulmonary vascular pressure secondary to both reflex pulmonary vasoconstriction and mechanical obstruction by air bubbles. The microvascular bubbles potentiate the injury by initiating the release of endothelial mediators that trigger free radical generation, complement activation, and an inflammatory response. This leads to progressive pulmonary hypertension, impaired gas exchange, and can lead to hypoxemia and CO_2 retention. The mechanical obstruction of the pulmonary capillaries and increased intrapulmonary shunting produce an increase in dead space manifest by a reduction in end-tital CO_2 (ETCO$_2$). Bronchoconstriction may also result, further complicating gas exchange. Further air entrainment leads to progressive decreases in cardiac output, hypotension, arrhythmias, and myocardial ischemia or failure.[59,60] Studies on the natural history of low-volume air embolism, however, tend to confirm the clinical experience that

the pathophysiologic effects are short-lived if air entrainment does not continue. A 60-cc bolus of air in sheep causes a 10-min reduction in cardiac output.[61] Ventilation/perfusion scan mismatch after minor air embolism in dogs returns to normal after 30 min.[62] Microbubbles in the lung vasculature of dogs, viewed through a glass window, undergo spontaneous resorption after 1 to 3 min.[63] Obviously, if air continues to enter the venous system, these short-lived effects will become more severe and result in more permanent damage. Low-volume air embolus is less well tolerated in small or pediatric patients and leads to significant clinical sequelae much earlier.[64]

The clinical response is somewhat different if there is sudden entry of a large bolus of air into the right heart, resulting in an "airlock" phenomenon that blocks the right ventricular outflow tract and leads to sudden cardiac arrest or cardiovascular collapse.[61,65,66] Studies in a dog model of air embolism have revealed that massive air embolism causes an air lock in the pulmonary outflow tract and extreme elevations in right ventricular pressure.[67] Dogs can tolerate 1000 cc of air given over 1 to 2 h but succumb to a 100-cc bolus injection.[65] Based on intraoperative experiences of air aspiration from atrial catheters, it is estimated that at least 50 cc of air must be entrained before clinical signs such as hypotension appear.[68] In man, the rapid entrainment of 300 to 500 cc of air is likely to be fatal if untreated.

PARADOXICAL AIR EMBOLISM
Pathophysiology
Anatomic patency of the foramen ovale (PFO) is reported at 27 percent[69] and functional patency, as assessed by a Valsalva maneuver during echocardiography, is estimated at 25 percent.[70] Therefore, the theoretical risk of paradoxical air embolism (PAE) is about 5 to 10 percent in the sitting position. Fortunately, the actual occurrence of PAE resulting in systemic air embolization appears to be much less than this. The most likely mechanism for PAE is through right-to-left shunting at the atrial level, but PAE has been reported in its absence,[71,72] and Lynch reported an 18 percent incidence of right-to-left shunt during Valsalva echocardiography in normal subjects.[73] High right-sided cardiac pressures may increase the risk of PAE because air may be shunted through a PFO, disseminating air into the systemic circulation. Air may enter the coronary circulation, causing myocardial ischemia or arrhythmias.[74,75] Air entering the cerebral circulation may cause cerebral infarction or multiple small microinfarcts visible on CT scanning.[76,77] In addition to passage through intracardiac defects such as ventricular septal defect (VSD) or PFO, transpulmonary passage of air has been noted on transesophageal

echocardiography (TEE).[71,78,79] Several factors may predispose a patient toward PAE during sitting craniotomy. Hypovolemia is thought to facilitate the occurrence of VAE and thus PAE.[80] Assumption of the sitting position facilitates a reduction in central venous and arterial blood pressure, more likely in elderly patients.[81,81] Perkins-Pearson noted that up to 50 percent of patients developed a right-to-left pressure gradient after an hour in the sitting position,[83] theoretically increasing their vulnerability to PAE. Some have advocated fluid loading prior to assumption of the sitting position to offset this risk as well as to treat the hemodynamic consequences of the position itself.[84] Once an episode of VAE is apparent, further VAE may promote PAE by secondary elevation of right heart pressures.[85] Some anesthetic techniques have been found to facilitate transpulmonary passage of air, whether through pulmonary vasodilating effects or other unknown mechanisms.[57,86] Although VAE is associated with a low mortality, clinical sequelae may have a variable impact depending on the amount of air disseminated. The same holds true for arterial embolism, but systemic air embolism remains very dangerous, and carries a mortality rate of around 70 percent if significant air is transferred.[46,87] The extreme danger of massive arterial air embolism is offset only by its exceptionally rare occurrence.

DETECTION OF AIR EMBOLISM

The detection of VAE has improved with the introduction of more sensitive monitoring. Using clinical criteria alone, Hunter[88] reported an 8 percent incidence of VAE in the sitting position. With the introduction of the esophageal stethoscope in the 1960s, the reported incidence nearly doubled.[89] Using precordial Doppler monitoring further increased the detection rate.[54]

Detection using clinical criteria alone (hypotension, hypoxemia, gasping respirations, arrhythmias) is too unreliable and occurs too late for the implementation of effective treatment. The classic finding of a "mill-wheel" murmur is rarely noted today, being one of the latest signs of VAE and associated with near-fatal doses of entrained air. Sloan and Kimovec[90] have reported that elevation of airway pressure resulting from reactive bronchoconstriction may be an additional sign of air embolism; however, this clinical sign is not specific for VAE.

The precordial Doppler probe is a sensitive device for detecting intracardiac air and has become the standard monitor used in cases where air embolism may occur. A 2.5-MHz continuous ultrasonic signal is emitted by the Doppler probe and the reflection is electronically converted to an audible sound. Air is an excellent acoustic reflector and produces a distinct change in the frequency of the emitted sound. The probe is typically placed along the right parasternal border at the fourth intercostal space to obtain right-sided heart sound (Fig. 29-14). Proper positioning can be confirmed by rapidly injecting a few milliliters of saline through a central venous catheter.[91,92] The probe can detect as little as 0.05 ml/kg of air.[93] The probe is ideally suited for thin patients because the signal is considerably degraded in the obese or in those with pulmonary disease significant enough to increase anteroposterior diameter of the chest. However, with persistence the Doppler can usually be positioned to allow detection of right-sided intracardiac sounds. False-positive signals from the precordial Doppler are uncommon, with the exception of injection of mannitol crystals.[94] Current investigations focusing on spectral analysis of the precordial Doppler signal may allow some degree of quantitation of the volume of entrained air in the future.[95]

Change in ET_{CO_2} tension is a useful monitor for the detection of VAE, occurring after Doppler detection but preceding any hemodynamic clinical signs. Air embolization into the pulmonary vasculature increases alveolar dead space, abruptly decreasing ET_{CO_2}. Nitrogen contained in the entrapped air diffuses into the alveolar air spaces, increasing the expired nitrogen content (ET_{N_2}). This can be detected if respiratory gas monitoring in use has the ability to detect nitrogen. Changes in ET_{N_2} are often small, however, and monitoring changes in ET_{N_2} may be no more sensitive than ET_{CO_2} in detecting VAE.[96] Unfortunately, neither changes in ET_{CO_2} and ET_{N_2} are specific for VAE because reduction in cardiac output or pulmonary perfusion can affect both measures, as can other conditions that increase alveolar-arterial CO_2 gradient (chronic obstructive pulmonary disease [COPD], bronchospasm, etc.). However, continuous ET_{CO_2} monitoring gives important information about adequacy of ventilation, disconnects, and estimates the arterial Pa_{CO_2} continuously. End-tidal nitrogen analysis is specific for detection of intravascular air, but is not as sensitive as the precordial Doppler for detection of subclinical VAE.[97]

The current studies suggest that the precordial transthoracic Doppler probe can safely and inexpensively detect clinically silent amounts of intracardiac air; therefore, the Doppler probe is recommended standard monitoring for those at risk of VAE. Some advocate placement of the Doppler in all cases of posterior fossa surgery regardless of position, but the risk of VAE is clearly related to the degree of head-up tilt, and the rates of detection and retrieval are higher in head-up positions. If a risk of PAE is suspected, the TEE should be used to allow detection of air crossing into the systemic circulation. Other monitoring that can be useful in validating the detection of VAE includes pulmonary artery pressure monitoring and use of continuous arterial oxygen and carbon dioxide content measurement.

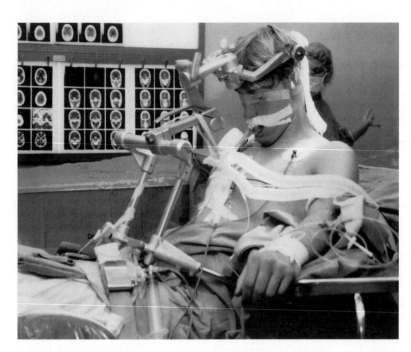

Figure 29-14 The precordial Doppler is positioned at the left sternal border and secured in position in a patient undergoing sitting craniotomy for resection of a cerebellar hemangioblastoma. (Adapted with permission from Cucchiara RF, et al: Anesthesia for intracranial procedures. In Barash PG, et al (eds): *Clinical Anesthesia*. London, JB Lippincott, 1989:860.)

Pulmonary artery catheter placement allows for the simultaneous detection of the increases in pulmonary arterial and central venous pressures and decreases in pulmonary capillary wedge pressure (PCWP) that accompany VAE. Matjasko and others have shown that the changes in PCWP following an episode of VAE occur later and are of less magnitude than changes in ET_{CO_2}, and that the additional risk of pulmonary artery catheterization is probably not justified unless otherwise mandated by the patient's condition.[46] The pulmonary artery catheter does allow detection of a potential gradient between left and right atrial pressure that may predispose to PAE,[98] but positioning the pulmonary artery catheter to allow simultaneous measurement of PCWP and air aspiration from the right atrial port is difficult. Air aspiration through the smaller-lumen pulmonary artery catheter is also inadequate compared to a multiorifice catheter.[99] Likewise, the use of continuous fiberoptic measurement of arterial O_2 and CO_2 content, or transcutaneous O_2 and CO_2 is no more sensitive and does not allow earlier detection than the use of pulse oximetry and ET_{CO_2}.[100,101] Figure 29-15 illustrates a clinical scenario in which the sequential changes in Doppler, ET_{CO_2}, and pulmonary, central venous, and arterial blood pressures are demonstrated. The standard use of ET_{CO_2} monitoring and a precordial Doppler probe offers sensitive detection of VAE at negligible risk. The use of both of these devices in cases at risk for VAE should allow detection of air emboli before they become clinically relevant.

Transesophageal echocardiography remains the most sensitive method of detecting intracardiac air. The probe is in widespread use during cardiac surgery and allows two-dimensional visualization of the car-

diac chambers in real-time using a 3.5 to 5.0 Hz intraesophageal probe inserted to lie behind the heart. When compared with the precordial probe, it is a more sensitive detector of intracardiac air. The TEE detection

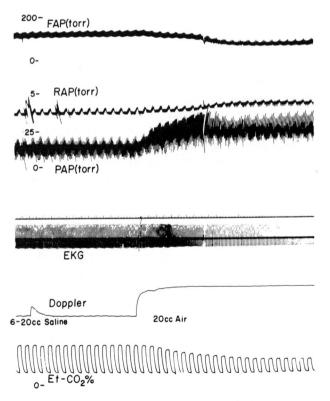

Figure 29-15 Sequential effect of an episode of VAE on precordial Doppler sounds, ET_{CO_2}, PA pressure, central venous pressure, and arterial blood pressure. (Adapted with permission from Chang JL, Albin MS, et al. *Neurosurgery* 7:135, 1980.)

threshold is approximately 0.02 ml/kg,[102] and it has the ability to visualize microbubbles in all chambers.[103] It is the only device that can detect ventricular or atrial septal defects preoperatively or visualize interatrial shunting intraoperatively,[104–106] and therefore the only device that is useful for the detection of PAE (Fig. 29-16). TEE can be added in patients who are suspected to be at risk of PAE (i.e., those with known intracardiac shunts). It can be used simultaneously with the precordial Doppler, although the technique is unwieldy, by directing the TEE toward the right ventricular outflow tract and left atrium.[107] Its general use is limited by the expense of the device and its large size, as well as the need for trained personnel to be available continuously for interpretation. The size of the probe implies some potential for injury to the esophagus or larynx if not inserted by an experienced technician or practitioner. Another consideration is that the use of TEE for early detection of VAE has not yet been proven to improve outcome when compared to the precordial Doppler, probably because the device is a qualitative measure, not quantitative. However, if air is detected in the left heart or aorta, aggressive measures can be taken to prevent further air entrainment and initiate treatment. The sensitivity of various monitoring methods in the detection of VAE is summarized in Table 29-8.

PREVENTION AND TREATMENT OF VAE

Most episodes of VAE can be prevented by the surgeon's attention to detail. Hemostasis should be rapid and complete. Bone wax should be liberally applied to all raw bone surfaces. Proper placement of a central venous catheter is an absolute necessity in the patient at risk for VAE to allow both confirmation of the diagnosis and to allow some degree of therapeutic intervention. When VAE occurs, the intracardiac air tends to temporarily accumulate near the junction of the superior vena cava and the right atrium. It then either passes on through into the right ventricle and pulmonary vasculature or collects in the auricle of the right atrium (Fig. 29-17). Attempts should be made to place the aspiration area of the central venous pressure catheter just above the superior vena cava-right atrial (SVC-RA) junction because, in the experimental model, over 80 percent of injected air can be aspirated from this area.[108] Moving the catheter tip into the right atrium reduces the fraction of injected air recovered substantially. Factors that affect the efficiency of air retrieval include catheter length and diameter, degree of inclination of the right atrium, number and size of orifices, and distance between orifices. Use of a multiorifice catheter[68,108] increases the recovered fraction most because it expands the zone of aspiration to include the SVC-RA junction and the atrium itself if the tip of the multiorifice catheter is placed 1 to 3 cm below the SVC-RA junction. Multiorifice catheters also develop

intraluminal clots less frequently, are able to aspirate at a faster rate, and rarely adhere to the atrial wall during suction.[68,109] Balloon-tipped catheters, while theoretically offering better positioning at the air-fluid interface,[110] have on further study been found to offer no additional advantage and are apparently less effective at air aspiration than multiorifice catheters.[111] Pulmonary artery catheters, angiography catheters (with or without balloon tip), and single- or multiorifice pulmonary artery catheter sheaths have all been studied to compare success in treatment of VAE.[112–114]

The right atrial catheter can be placed via any of multiple routes—through antecubital veins, the subclavian veins, or the external or internal jugular veins. Each site has advantages and disadvantages depending on the complications unique to the site of vascular cannulation, the position of the patient, and access to the catheter intraoperatively. Usually the catheter can be placed without difficulty independent of the site of insertion, but some feel that the antecubital fossa is the site of choice due to the lack of complication from that site and the accessibility.[115,116] Catheter position should be verified after the final surgical position is assumed because the catheter can move up to 4 to 5 cm with arm movement alone if an antecubital site is used.[117] Use of the subclavian vein allows best patient comfort postoperatively, but insertion site complications include pneumothorax and arterial puncture. Use of the internal jugular vein is limited by problems with access after positioning and with the fact that placement of a large-bore catheter in this vein may interfere with intracranial venous drainage and potentially affect intracranial compliance. However, multiorifice catheters are available both in long and short lengths, appropriate for either peripheral or central insertion sites.[119] Whatever the site, the puncture site should be dressed with a sterile transparent occlusive dressing to minimize the chance that air will be entrained from the puncture wound.[120] In clinical practice, correct catheter position can be confirmed by chest radiograph after the patient is positioned, or by using the catheter as an intravascular electrocardiographic (ECG) lead. Lead V from the ECG monitor is attached to the catheter, allowing continuous monitoring of the ECG morphology as the catheter is advanced. This can be done by using an alligator clip onto a metal catheter or stopcock hub or clipped to the wire guide, or by using a modified snap-button hub attachment that allows the lead to be snapped on to the catheter directly. Ideally, the catheter should be flushed with electrically conductive solution such as $NaHCO_3$ or saline.[118] When using a single-orifice catheter, the presence of a large P wave oriented negatively (downgoing) indicates a position above the sinoatrial (SA) node. When below the SA node, the P wave component will be positive (upright). (Alternatively, lead II can be used as the exploring

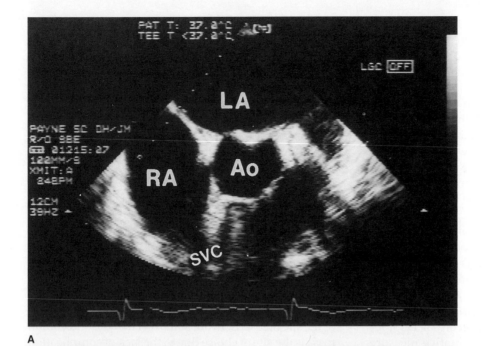

A

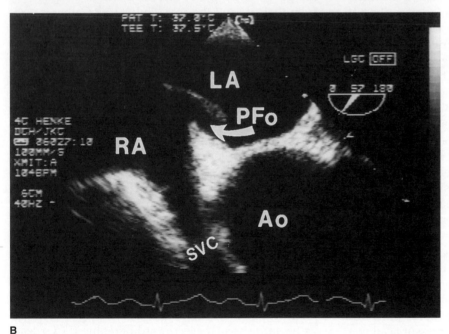

B

Figure 29-16 Venous air embolism and paradoxical air embolism can be visualized with transesophageal echocardiography. *A*. Normal sagittal image of both atria. *B*. Patent foramen ovale appearing as a defect in the interatrial septum. *C*. Air (white speckling) in the right atrium. *D*. Air crossing from the right atrium to the left atrium through a patent foramen ovale. RA, right atrium; LA, left atrium; SVC, superior vena cava; Ao, aorta; PFO, patent foramen ovale. (Echocardiographic images are courtesy of Dr. David C. Homans, Department of Internal Medicine, University of Minnesota Hospital and Clinics.)

electrode, in which case the P wave orientation will be in the opposite direction).[121] The SA node is found at or slightly below the level of the SVC-RA junction, and at this point the P wave component of the intravascular ECG is biphasic. The catheter should then be withdrawn about 2 to 3 cm to position the tip for most efficient air retrieval. When using a multiorifice catheter, the intravascular ECG waveform is thought to originate from the most proximal holes.[122,123] Hence, an intravascular ECG waveform suggesting a position above the SA node (large negative P wave on lead

V) should indicate that the catheter is appropriately positioned (Fig. 29-18). There have been suggestions that pressure monitoring alone can be used for verification of right atrial catheter position,[124] but since confirmation of position so largely influences efficacy, whatever method is chosen should be one that ensures all participating parties that the catheter is in optimal position.

Preoperative echocardiographic testing has been suggested to allow early detection of PFO or right-to-left shunts and thus allow identification of patients

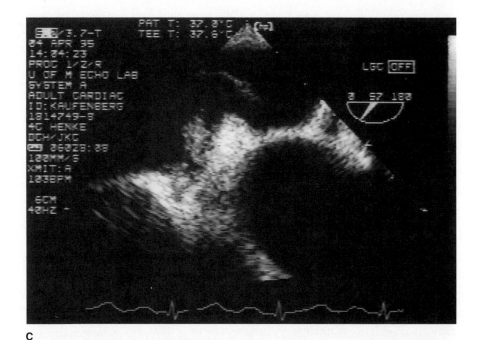

C

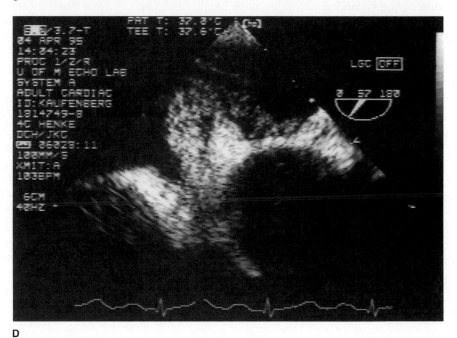

Figure 29-16   *(Continued)*   D

who should not be placed in surgical positions that facilitate VAE.[105,125] However, paradoxical systemic air embolization can occur in the absence of identified shunt and even in those with negative preoperative echocardiography.[72,126,127] Therefore, the absence of demonstrable intracardiac shunting on preoperative testing does not guarantee the lack of potential for PAE.

In the absence of other findings, changes in the Doppler signal alone should not provoke great alarm. The surgeon should be alerted and the application of a wet sponge will usually halt any ongoing air entrain-

ment. Aspiration from a right atrial catheter should be attempted, both to confirm the suspicion of VAE and to allow removal of some of the intracardiac air. Immediate aspiration of air from a right atrial catheter offers the quickest and most effective means of reducing clinical sequelae.[54,66,67] If Doppler sounds of air continue or there is significant reduction in ET_{CO_2} (>2 to 5 mmHg without other apparent cause) despite these measures and the site cannot be rapidly identified, either a Valsalva maneuver or jugular compression may increase venous bleeding to the point that the source of air

TABLE 29-8
Sensitivity of Monitoring for Venous Air Embolism

Monitor	Threshold (ml/kg air)	Reference
Transesophageal echo-cardiogram	0.01–0.19	101, 102, 103
Precordial Doppler	0.02–0.24	101, 102
Pulmonary artery pressure	0.5	208
End-tidal CO$_2$	0.5	208
Pulse oximetry	0.7–1.5	101, 208
Esophageal stethoscope	0.75	208
Arterial blood pressure	>1.0	208
"Mill-wheel" murmur	>2.0	208

entrainment can be located.[128–130] However, jugular compression, especially if bilateral, can cause intracranial venous hypertension and increase brain swelling, reducing cerebral perfusion. Neck compression may also result in carotid artery compression or activation of the carotid sinus reflex with resultant bradyarrhythmias. If air entrainment continues, or if an episode of massive air embolism occurs, the anesthesiologist should immediately notify the surgeon, who can then flood the operative field with saline and apply a wet laparotomy sponge to the wound. Attempts to withdraw air from the central venous catheter should continue, help should be solicited, and the head of the bed should be promptly lowered. Hypotension and hypoxia should be treated with supportive measures

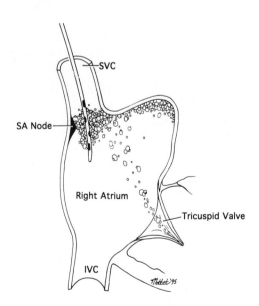

Figure 29-17 Air from venous air embolism first collects at the superior vena cava-right atrial junction and then is funneled into the right atrium or through the tricuspid valve into the lungs. [Adapted, with permission from Black S, Cucchiara RF: Tumor surgery. In Cucchiara RF, Michenfelder JD (eds): *Clinical Neuroanesthesia*. New York, Churchill-Livingstone, 1990:297.]

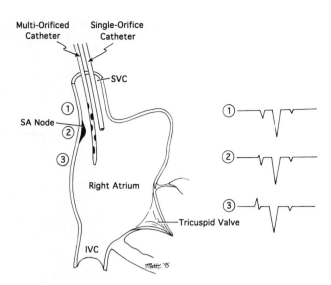

Figure 29-18 Use of intravascular ECG (IVECG). When using single-orifice catheters, tracing 2 indicates appropriate position of the catheter tip. When a multiorifice catheter is used, tracing 1 is more indicative of appropriate placement because the ECG recording site is felt to be located at the most proximal orifice. [Adapted, with permission from Black S, Cucchiara RF: Tumor surgery. In Cucchiara RF, Michenfelder JD (eds). *Clinical Neuroanesthesia*. New York, Churchill-Livingstone, 1990:297.]

(intravenous fluids, vasopressors, inotropes, antiarrhythmics) if needed. If N$_2$O is being used, it should be discontinued due to the risk of significantly increasing the size of intravascular air bubbles (N$_2$O is less soluble in plasma than in air and will rapidly diffuse into air-containing spaces exposed to blood flow). Although some advocate use of N$_2$O as a means of aiding diagnosis[131] of VAE and others have found no evidence of danger when N$_2$O is used in low concentrations,[132] use of N$_2$O in the face of continuing VAE could potentially convert a clinically insignificant air embolus into one that produces hypotension, hypoxia, and arrhythmias.[133] If the patient is severely hypotensive or hypoxic, placing the patient in Durant's position (head-down, left lateral decubitus, with Trendelenburg) should limit further entry of air into the pulmonary vasculature. The ideal position for placing the patient after massive VAE is undergoing reexamination. The value of the left lateral decubitus position was championed by Durant in the 1950s,[65] who demonstrated an improved survival of dogs placed in the left lateral decubitus position after massive VAE. He postulated that air buoyancy caused air to "float" out of the pulmonary outflow tract and into the atrium. Recently, Mehlhorn and coworkers have revisited this issue,[134] demonstrating that hemodynamics were not affected by body position in dogs subjected to massive air embolism. This result notwithstanding, it seems prudent to recommend the left lateral decubitus position as a

TABLE 29-9
Treatment of Venous Air Embolism (VAE)

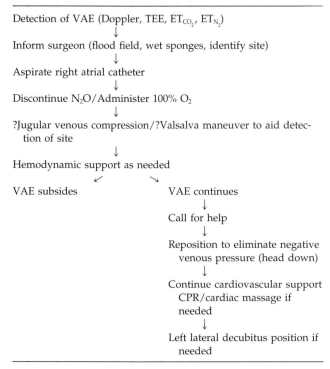

NOTE: CPR, cardiopulmonary resuscitation; ET_{CO_2}, end-tidal carbon dioxide; ET_{N_2}, end-tidal nitrogen; TEE, transesophageal echocardiography.

treatment adjunct for severe air embolism until further studies are performed. If cardiac arrest occurs, cardiopulmonary resuscitation should begin—open cardiac massage may be necessary. External cardiac massage alone may be effective in disrupting a large air bolus filling the right heart.[135] Table 29-9 reviews the suggested treatment regimen for an episode of VAE.

The application of positive end-expiratory pressure (PEEP) to prevent or treat VAE (by the indirect effect of increasing right atrial and therefore central venous pressure) is controversial. There are fears that elevation of right atrial pressure may increase the potential for transfer of intravenous air across a PFO and increase the incidence of paradoxical systemic air embolism.[136] Indeed, Perkins demonstrated that the left atrial pressure-right atrial pressure gradient was positive in the sitting position without PEEP, and reversed when 10 cm PEEP was applied to the respiratory circuit, potentiating conditions for PAE. Furthermore, addition of 10 cm of PEEP elevated right atrial pressure by only 5 cmH2O, a value unlikely to affect venous pressure in the cranial vault, which is some 20 cm above the heart. Their conclusions were that PEEP was insufficient to prevent VAE but was sufficient to potentiate PAE in susceptible individuals.[137] Other animal studies have failed to find any effect of PEEP on the left atrial-

right atrial gradient except at the time that PEEP was discontinued. At this time a "surge" of air was seen to cross a surgically created atrial septal defect.[99]

Proponents of PEEP argue that it raises intracranial venous pressure and prevents air entrainment.[57] However, little experimental evidence supports this. Superior saggital sinus pressure and transverse sinus pressure do not appear to increase after the application of either 10 or 15 cmH2O PEEP.[129,138,139] PEEP is contraindicated in patients with intracardiac defects due to enhanced risk of PAE. The application of PEEP to patients in the sitting position for neurosurgery should be restricted to those situations where it is necessary to support oxygenation.

Military antishock trousers (MAST) have been suggested as a means to prevent VAE in children.[140] Inflation to pressures between 30 and 40 mmHg raised jugular venous pressure to above atmospheric. There were no episodes of VAE in the MAST-treated group, whereas 26 percent untreated controls demonstrated episodes of VAE by Doppler. Because MAST appears to raise both right atrial and left atrial pressures equally, the authors argue that the risk of PAE was not increased. Application of such an antigravity suit to the lower body may provide some benefit in reducing venous pooling and may help attenuate the hypotension that accompanies the sitting position in the anesthetized patient.[141,142] However, the MAST suit is not consistently effective in maintaining initial elevations of central venous pressure for longer than about 30 min, and there appears to be little benefit to using it clinically.[143,144]

PREVENTION AND TREATMENT OF PAE

If cerebral air embolism is suspected, hyperbaric oxygen therapy may improve neurologic outcome. This is based largely on multiple case reports following PAE[145-147] and on the proven efficacy of hyperbaric therapy in the treatment of decompression sickness. Hyperbaric oxygen therapy may improve the sequelae of PAE in several ways: (1) high atmospheric pressure (6 atmospheres) reduces the physical size of the bubbles by up to 45 percent, and may help open blocked arterioles, restoring perfusion; (2) the higher alveolar Pa_{O_2} favors a nitrogen "washout" from the bubble to the alveoli as the nitrogen follows its concentration gradient; (3) the high arterial oxygen tension may salvage some ischemic tissue. Despite strong anecdotal evidence, the role of hyperbaric oxygen for cerebral air embolism has been criticized due to the lack of scientific evidence of its benefit.[148]

ELECTROPHYSIOLOGIC MONITORING

Multiple electrophysiologic modalities can be used intraoperatively and perioperatively to give information about the well-being of the nervous system. Such techniques are indicated in specific circumstances as dictated by the procedure and the area of nervous system at risk. Information about the integrity and function of the spinal cord, brain stem, cranial nerves, and cortex can all be obtained to assist in detecting intraoperative compromise or predict postoperative function. Electroencephalography, somatosensory evoked potentials (SSEP), motor evoked potentials (MEP), BAER, and cranial nerve monitoring can be used singly or in combination to achieve these goals.[149]

SOMATOSENSORY EVOKED POTENTIALS

Monitoring of SSEP allows assessment of the integrity of the electrical pathway involved in transmitting a sensory stimulus from a peripheral receptor to the somatosensory cortex. Potentials can be recorded at any point along this pathway, from peripheral nerve to plexus to spinal cord to subcortical brain structures to sensory cortex. The information gained can be useful in posterior fossa surgery for detection of cervical cord ischemia or stretch injury in patients in the sitting position[39] or in those undergoing procedures involving the upper cervical cord. Monitoring short-latency subcortical SSEP has been investigated as a measure of function of subcortical sensory pathways in cervical cord and posterior fossa surgery.[150] Cortical SSEP can be used to gauge the depth of anesthesia or to assess the presence of brain ischemia because cortical SSEP reflect information similar to the cortical EEG. However, it is important to realize that SSEP primarily reflect the integrity of the sensory pathways and may miss damage occurring in posterior descending motor tracts or in other areas of brain, specifically the brain stem, motor strip, pyramidal tracts, and cranial nerves.[151] The latency and amplitude of cortical components can vary significantly and may be affected by volatile anesthetics, physiologic changes, N_2O, and temperature.[152] This places limitations on the anesthetic choices and makes interpretation somewhat problematic.

BRAIN STEM AUDITORY EVOKED POTENTIALS

Brain stem auditory evoked responses are electrical signals generated by depolarizations in structures along the conductive pathway from the ear to the auditory cortex following stimulation (auditory click) of the eighth cranial nerve. All of the structures reflected by the waveform of the BAER are contained within the brain stem. These signals are robust and are very resistant to the depressant effects of anesthetics. Monitoring BAER, therefore, provides a means of assessing the intraoperative function of both the eighth (acoustic) cranial nerve and the brain stem.[153] This type of monitoring is used extensively during resection of acoustic nerve tumors,[154–157] microvascular decompression of the cranial nerves,[19,23] and other lesions of the medulla or brain stem.[158,159] Bilateral changes in BAER are indicative of brain stem compromise and can be of prognostic help in patients with postoperative neurologic deficit following brain stem tumor or hematoma decompression or in those with continuing coma.[160]

MOTOR EVOKED POTENTIALS

Motor evoked potentials can be recorded from muscle after stimulation of either the anterior spinal cord[161] or the motor cortex with electrical or magnetic stimuli.[162,163] These potentials allow assessment of the function of the motor pathways from stimulation site to periphery. Cortical MEP have been used clinically to monitor patients with cervical cord lesions, Chiari malformation, and medullary tumors to guide intraoperative decompression and to predict postoperative function, with fairly good results.[163,164] MEP are of somewhat limited utility due to the lack of generally available equipment and technical support, and by their sensitivity to depression by most anesthetic agents and muscle relaxants. MEP have been successfully recorded in patients undergoing open posterior fossa craniotomy under etomidate infusion.[164]

FACIAL NERVE POTENTIALS

Many investigators have reported success in preservation of facial nerve function after posterior fossa surgery, particularly after resection of acoustic nerve tumors or tumors involving the cerebellopontine angle. Spontaneous audio and visual recordings can be elicted from the facial muscles from needle electrodes placed subdermally. Facial MEP occur when the facial nerve is subjected to stretch, compression, or percussion. These evoked responses can guide the surgical resection of a tumor that envelops the nerve, especially when combined with direct stimulation recordings. This modality allows the surgeon to electrically stimulate areas of tumor near the nerve using a small sterile hand-held electrical probe, aiding in identifying the anatomic course of the facial nerve. Use of muscle relaxants must be limited during procedures in which this technique is used because paralysis will obliterate the electromyographic-evoked response.[165] Use of facial nerve monitoring has contributed to a 60 to 90 percent rate of at least partial facial nerve preservation in patients undergoing resection of tumors of the cerebello-pontine angle.[166] Direct seventh and eighth nerve recordings have also been used intraoperatively during microvascular decompression.[23]

Preoperative Evaluation

GENERAL MEDICAL CONDITION

Evaluation of the patient's preoperative status has important influence on the selection of surgical approach and surgical position. Unlike the relatively straightforward positioning needed during supratentorial surgery, positioning a patient to allow adequate access to posterior fossa structures may be difficult and challenging. The risks and benefits of surgical needs should be evaluated and discussed preoperatively. What may seem to be an ideal surgical position may be associated with unacceptable anesthetic risk. In a more practical vein, mobility and risk of neurologic compromise also must be considered. It is good practice to ask the patient, while awake, to assume the proposed operative position including any head flexion or rotation. If the position cannot be assumed in the awake cooperative patient, or if it is associated with exacerbation or new onset of neurologic deficit, it should not be used under anesthesia.

A thorough review of cardiovascular condition, pulmonary status, intravascular volume, airway anatomy, and some assessment of required vascular access should be made preoperatively. Cardiovascular status, including a history of hypertension, cardiac disease, or carotid disease is important in identifying patients at risk for hypotension, impaired cerebral perfusion, or abnormal cerebral autoregulation.[167,168] The sitting position may be additionally hazardous in these patients because of the risk of systemic hypotension under anesthesia in this position, resulting in significant reduction of cerebral and myocardial blood flow.[81,82,169–171] Although more horizontal positioning could theoretically help preserve cerebral and myocardial blood flow, no extensive comparative data document an increased risk of stroke or myocardial infarction in elderly or sick patients in the sitting position. In fact, Black found no difference in the incidence of perioperative hypotension related to position in 85 patients with cardiac disease operated in the horizontal or sitting position.[36]

Patients with intracranial hypertension may be hypovolemic related to vomiting, treatment with diuretics, or poor oral intake. Hypotension after induction of anesthesia or after positioning is more likely in these patients. Use of preloading with intravenous fluids (crystalloid or colloid), placement of thigh-high compression stockings, and close monitoring of arterial pressure during induction and positioning can limit the degree of hypotension. It should be remembered that hemangioblastomas can produce a polycythemia and this should not be misinterpreted as a sign of fluid depletion.

Patients with known intracardiac septal defects should not be placed in the sitting position because of the risk of paradoxical arterial cerebral air embolism. Improvements in noninvasive echocardiographic technology may make preoperative echocardiography a routine preoperative screening test for patients to be operated on in the sitting position even though results are currently nonpredictive.[125,126] At the present time, the most prudent course of action is to order echocardiography, including a contrast study, on any patient with a suspicious heart murmur.

The presence of pulmonary disease or obesity may make the sitting position attractive because of improved intraoperative ventilatory function, and in fact there may be less risk of hypoxemia due to intrapulmonary shunting in the sitting position than in the lateral or prone position.[172] Patients with significant pulmonary dysfunction may require higher inspired oxygen concentrations or the application of PEEP in the lateral or prone positions to counter the associated decrease in functional reserve capacity and restriction in chest wall expansion. Patients should be asked about a prior history of sleep apnea, dysphagia, recurrent or aspiration pneumonia, or disturbance with phonation. The airway should be carefully assessed for ease of intubation. If fiberoptic intubation appears necessary because of airway anatomy or the presence of cervical symptomatology, the procedure must be reviewed with the patient preoperatively to help allay anxiety. Oversedation should be avoided in patients with depressed level of consciousness or in those with elevated ICP to avoid hypoxemia and hypercarbia, and some thought should be given to prevention of the hypertensive response to airway manipulation and intubation in the awake patient. Any preexisting cranial nerve dysfunction or brain stem symptomatology may be exacerbated after surgical manipulation within the posterior fossa and such patients should be carefully evaluated before extubation to ensure they are awake, have adequate strength and airway reflexes present, and can maintain patency of the airway. Checking the patient's level of consciousness, ability to swallow, grimace, protrude the tongue, and breathe around the deflated cuff of the endotracheal tube will usually identify any problems. Any preexisting neurologic deficits or paresthesias should be well documented preoperatively. The operating team should pay particular attention to cervical range of motion in patients with craniocervical disorders and note if there is exacerbation or new onset of symptoms with the head position required for surgery or intubation.[173] The patient and family should be informed if there is a possibility of postoperative intubation due to a prolonged procedure, postoperative brain swelling, cranial nerve dysfunction, or respiratory insufficiency.

All cases performed in the sitting position will require a right atrial catheter and the best site for this should be determined preoperatively. This may require preoperative insertion of the central venous pressure catheter if the patient is obese or has limited venous access, but usually the right atrial catheter can be

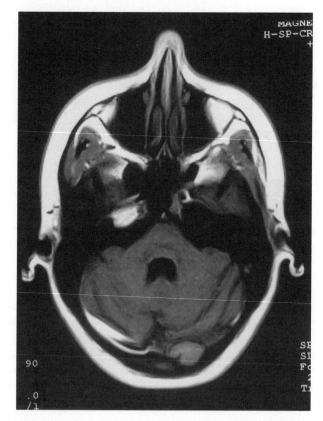

Figure 29-19 Axial MRI of the posterior fossa show the pons, cerebellar hemispheres, and the fourth ventricle. MRI offers superior resolution of the neural structures.

inserted after induction of anesthesia. The venodilation produced by general anesthesia will aid insertion, especially if an antecubital site is anticipated.

IMAGING

Magnetic resonance imaging is the best imaging modality currently available for anatomic delineation of the posterior fossa lesions (Fig. 29-19). In elective cases, the MRI is the study of choice because it is not affected by bony artifact, gives superior anatomic resolution, and is able to image in multiple planes. Occasionally, the CT scan will also be obtained if delineation of bony anatomy is necessary for planning an approach or if there is concern about the presence of intracranial calcification or bony invasion (Fig. 29-20). The bony confines of the infratentorial space can produce streak artifacts on the CT scan but because it is able to be performed more rapidly, it is a more appropriate scan to use in emergent situations.

Intraoperative Anesthetic Management

ANESTHETIC GOALS

The goals of anesthetic management for surgery of the posterior fossa include maintenance of cerebral perfu-

sion pressure and oxygenation, facilitating brain relaxation, ensuring hemodynamic stability, planning for appropriate hemodynamic monitoring or monitoring for air embolism, planning for rapid emergence to allow early neurologic evaluation, and using a technique that is compatible with any electrophysiologic monitoring that may be needed.

MONITORING

ROUTINE

Routine monitoring for posterior fossa surgery is the same as is indicated for all anesthetic procedures and includes noninvasive blood pressure, ECG, oxygen saturation, temperature, ET_{CO_2} and other respiratory gas monitoring if available, urinary output, and monitoring of neuromuscular blockade. An intraarterial catheter can be justified in nearly all cases of posterior fossa surgery due to the need for close monitoring of cerebral perfusion pressure and the length of time needed for surgery. Also, many patients undergoing posterior fossa surgery will be relatively inaccessible during the procedure, and real-time continuous monitoring of blood pressure and the ability to draw arterial blood for laboratory examinations make an arterial line desirable. More invasive monitoring (central venous or pulmonary artery pressure monitoring) should be dictated by the patient's preoperative condition, the presence of associated cardiorespiratory disease, the patient's expected responses to positioning or surgical manipulation, and the expected degree of blood loss. If con-

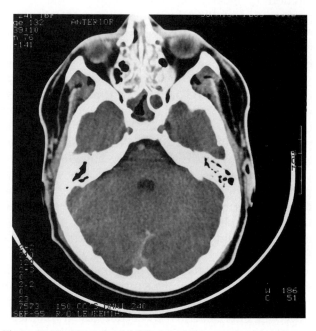

Figure 29-20 Normal axial CT scan of the posterior fossa. Bony structures are better defined on CT.

TABLE 29-10
Monitoring for Posterior Fossa Surgery

Type	Monitor	Indication
Routine	Noninvasive blood pressure Electrocardiogram Sa_{O_2} ET_{CO_2} Fi_{O_2} Inspired/expired agent Temperature Urinary output Neuromuscular blockade	
Invasive	Intraarterial catheter	Intracranial surgery Intracranial hypertension Inaccessible patient Cardiovascular respiratory disease Repetitive laboratory tests needed Controlled hypotension
	Central venous pressure	Cardiovascular/respiratory disease (if indicated) Excessive blood loss anticipated
	Pulmonary artery catheter/cardiac output	Cardiovascular/respiratory disease (if indicated)
Special	Multiorifice right atrial catheter	Risk of VAE
	Precordial Doppler	Risk of VAE
	End-tidal N_2	Risk of VAE
	Transesophageal echo	Risk of PAE
	Transcranial Doppler	Risk of PAE
	SSEP	Cervicomedullary surgery Sitting position ($\pm$) Controlled hypotension ($\pm$)
	MEP	Cervicomedullary surgery
	BAER	CP angle surgery, microvascular decompression Surgery involving brainstem or acoustic nerve
	VII nerve monitoring	CP angle surgery, microvascular decompression

NOTE: BAER, brainstem auditory evoked response; CP, cerebellopontine; MEP, motor evoked potential; PAE, paradoxical air embolism; SSEP, somatosensory provoked potential; VAE, venous air embolism.

trolled hypotension is needed for access to an aneurysm or AVM, arterial pressure and central venous or pulmonary artery pressure monitoring are mandatory.

SPECIAL

Special monitoring techniques are indicated if the procedure is associated with particular risks (i.e., spinal cord ischemia, positioning injury, brain stem or cranial nerve injury, VAE) or if special anesthetic techniques are to be used (i.e., controlled hypotension in a position that may potentiate cerebral or cord ischemia). Table 29-10 summarizes the types and indications for most monitoring techniques in posterior fossa surgery.[174]

INDUCTION AND MAINTENANCE OF ANESTHESIA

The goals of anesthetic induction, maintenance, and emergence should be to provide adequate depth of anesthesia for intubation (particularly in patients with poor intracranial compliance) and the procedure while avoiding hemodynamic instability and untoward movement; to optimize conditions for neurophysiologic monitoring; to help minimize bleeding; to allow smooth emergence, early awakening, and early neurologic assessment; and to prevent excessive postoperative pain.

No one particular technique is indicated to achieve

these ends. The choice of induction agents is best dictated by the patient's age and clinical condition. Use of higher doses of volatile anesthetics promotes greater degrees of hypotension in elderly patients or in those patients in the sitting position and can interfere with the interpretation of cortical EEG or cortical SSEP. Nitrous oxide may be best to avoid in three situations—if there is risk of VAE, when a patient with pulmonary disease is in the lateral or prone position due to the possible need for higher inspired Fi_{O_2}, and if deliberate hypotension is needed, when optimal Fi_{O_2} and oxygen-carrying capacity are important. The use of muscle relaxants is often necessary because paralysis facilitates ventilation (especially in the prone or lateral positions), prevents unwanted movement during periods of light anesthesia, and optimizes brain relaxation and visibility during microscopic surgery. Some authors have recently promoted the use of spontaneous ventilation to monitor brain stem function during posterior fossa procedures, relying on the changes in respiratory pattern to indicate the presence of brain stem compression or ischemia.[175,176] The potential disadvantages of spontaneous ventilation are several, however. Mechanical control of ventilation is necessary if hyperventilation is needed to facilitate brain relaxation, and the depressant effects of inhaled anesthetics and narcotics on respiratory control imply that a potentially significant degree of hypercarbia will be present for spontaneous ventilation to occur under general anesthesia. There may be associated problems with hypoxia and atelectasis if ventilation under anesthesia is not controlled. These problems are only exacerbated the longer the procedure lasts. Although the "gasp" response has been described in awake patients during an episode of VAE, spontaneous (i.e., negative-pressure) ventilation facilitates further air entry by increasing the pressure gradient favoring air entrainment during inspiration.[177] Therefore, spontaneous ventilation is best avoided in patients at risk for VAE.

If there appears to be a risk of intraoperative cerebral ischemia (i.e., temporary occlusion of a feeding vessel to an aneurysm or AVM, significant retraction pressure anticipated, etc.), glucose-containing solutions are best avoided because of the possibility of enhanced neuronal vulnerability to ischemia.[178] A moderate degree of intraoperative hypothermia (34°C) may be considered to allow some degree of cerebral protection should an ischemic insult occur, or if deliberate hypotension is contemplated as part of the anesthetic plan.[179]

SPECIAL TECHNIQUES

DELIBERATE HYPOTENSION

The use of some degree of induced hypotension may be desirable when approaching an intracranial aneu-

rysm or AVM, when a tumor is known to be quite vascular, or when microsurgical techniques are needed. Deliberate hypotension also reduces blood loss and lessens the risk of homologous blood transfusion. Reduction in MAPs to a level of 60 to 70 mmHg should have little effect on cerebral perfusion in normal areas of brain due to the presence of cerebral autoregulation of blood flow. Hypertensive patients are "right-shifted," requiring higher perfusion pressures to maintain the same level of cerebral perfusion,[167] and areas of brain involved with tumor or surrounding a mass lesion are generally thought not to exhibit normal autoregulatory responses.[180] Deliberate hypotension is therefore relatively contraindicated in patients with coronary or cerebrovascular disease, those with renal or hepatic insufficiency, those with severe pulmonary disease, or those with poor intracranial compliance (i.e., intracranial mass lesion). Lower cerebral perfusion pressure will also increase the susceptibility of brain to retractor-pressure ischemia. However, in those patients with isolated vascular lesions who have otherwise no contraindication, and with appropriate monitoring of intraarterial blood pressure, urinary output, and ECG, this technique can be used safely for minutes to hours intraoperatively. Either the volatile anesthetic agents or a rapid-acting vasodilator such as sodium nitroprusside, nitroglycerin, or trimethaphan can be used to reduce blood pressure. Isoflurane offers the advantage of preservation of cardiac output and mild vasodilatation, short duration of action, and some reduction in cerebral and spinal ischemic insult. The use of nitroprusside allows rapid titration and preservation of tissue blood flow but often is complicated by reflex tachycardia, rebound hypertension, the risk of toxicity, and activation of the renin-angiotensin system. This can be attenuated by pretreatment with converting-enzyme inhibitors or β blockers, which also reduce the needed dose of nitroprusside.[181] Nitroglycerin avoids these problems but may be frustrating to use due to lack of potency. Trimethaphan is easy to use and effective but produces pupillary dilation that may complicate postoperative neurologic assessment. The β_2-agonist esmolol is effective and of short duration (9 min) but suffers from lack of potency and is expensive. Often a combination of agents will allow the needed level of hypotension to be reached while avoiding large doses of any particular agent, thus reducing side effects and expense.

ELECTROPHYSIOLOGIC MONITORING

Inspired concentrations of volatile anesthetics greater than 1 MAC should not be used if SSEP monitoring is to be used.[152] Nitrous oxide may also enhance the depressant effect of volatile agents on SSEP morphology and significantly affects the amplitude of peripherally recorded motor evoked responses.[182,183] Complete neuromuscular block eliminates the electromyographic artifact that can contaminate SSEP waveforms, but the use of muscle relaxants will obliterate intramuscular recording of MEPs or evoked facial nerve recordings.[184] Somatosensory potentials are usually best recorded under conditions of complete neuromuscular blockade and nitrous oxide-narcotic-benzodiazepine anesthesia, or with techniques involving total intravenous anesthesia (propofol infusion).[152] MEP have been recorded successfully in patients undergoing intracranial surgery with continuous infusion of etomidate as the primary anesthetic.[163] The need for partial or for no muscle relaxation may be addressed by communicating with the surgeon and monitoring personnel in advance and is often solved by using an infusion of a relatively intermediate-acting neuromuscular blocking agent such as vecuronium along with an intravenous anesthetic technique with or without nitrous oxide. This allows titration of the infusion to the desired level of neuromuscular blockade and also allows rapid reversal at the end of the procedure. It is important to maintain a steady depth of anesthesia without sudden changes in anesthetic administration at times that are critical for interpretation of the electrophysiologic waveform.

Complications

CARDIOVASCULAR

HYPOTENSION
Placing the patient in the sitting position often results in postural hypotension related to a reduction in preload as blood pools in the lower extremities. This effect is enhanced by the autonomic blockade that results to some degree from general anesthesia. The reduction in blood pressure can be minimized by assuming the sitting position slowly, and by administration of intravenous fluids before sitting (1000 to 2000 ml crystalloid, 500 to 1000 ml colloid in the adult patient). This should be monitored by following central venous or pulmonary artery pressure during fluid loading. Compression stockings should be placed on the lower extremities to reduce venous pooling prior to induction. Despite these measures, some patients will still require treatment with vasopressors to maintain blood pressure at acceptable levels. Elderly patients, chronically hypertensive patients, and patients with poor myocardial function are those most at risk for refractory hypotension in the sitting position. These patients should be monitored more aggressively (intraarterial blood pressure, central venous pressure, pulmonary artery catheter) if use of the sitting position is contemplated.

ARRHYTHMIAS
Cardiac arrhythmias (both bradyarrhythmias and tachyarrhythmias) are frequently observed during surgical procedures around the cranial nerves or brain stem. Removal of brain stem lesions such as ependymomas, medulloblastoma, and brain stem gliomas are the most frequent offenders. Bradycardia, ventricular escape rhythms, junctional bradycardia, sinus arrest, and ventricular tachycardia are possible. Manipulation or cauterization near a cranial nerve entry zone or ganglion may be associated with severe hypertension, tachyarrhythmias, ventricular tachycardia, and ST depression. Often, cessation of the stimulus will abort the arrhythmia, but if necessary, appropriate treatment with atropine, vasopressors, vasodilators, or electroshock should be instituted. In the patient with coronary disease or myocardial dysfunction, this degree of hypertension or the presence of an arrhythmia may lead to significant myocardial ischemia or infarction or may lead to intraoperative cardiac failure and pulmonary edema. These problems should be anticipated, the patient aggressively monitored for such situations (pulmonary artery catheter, two-lead ECG), and the appropriate antiarrhythmics, inotropes, vasodilators, or vasopressors should be readily available. A pacing Swan-Ganz catheter may be desirable.

RESPIRATORY

RESPIRATORY FAILURE
Pulmonary edema or adult respiratory distress syndrome can be the result of massive VAE.[185,186] Mechanical obstruction of the pulmonary arterioles provokes intense pulmonary vasoconstriction, promoting acute transcapillary leak or myocardial dysfunction.[187] Furthermore, air bubbles may interact with capillary endothelium, initiating platelet, fibrin, and red cell deposition.[188] Secondary neutrophil infiltration of the endothelial surface follows, disrupting the underlying basal lamina.[189,190] The combination of pulmonary hypertension and elevated microvascular permeability promotes leakage of proteinaceous exudate into the lung parenchyma. Therapy includes mechanical ventilatory support, supplemental oxygen, PEEP, and administration of diuretics and antibiotics. Methylprednisolone[191] and superoxide dismutase[192] ameliorate the microvascular lung injury of air embolism in the sheep model. If venous air embolism has occurred, ventilation/perfusion pulmonary scans will remain abnormal into the postoperative period due to perfusion defects that are indistinguishable from thromboemboli.

AIRWAY
Airway obstruction may become a problem after posterior fossa surgery. If the patient has been operated in

the prone or excessively head-flexed position, the face and tongue may develop edema to such a degree that extubation is impossible.[29,30] This can be treated with continuing intubation and recovery in the head-up position until the edema resolves sufficiently to allow extubation. Airway obstruction may also occur because of persistent neuromuscular weakness due to hypothermia, oversedation, inadequate reversal of neuromuscular blocking agents, or cranial nerve dysfunction. These problems are more likely in patients with abnormal or difficult airway access identified preoperatively (e.g., morbid obesity), but may also occur in the previously healthy patient. Procedures around the brain stem or those involving the area of brain stem near the origins of cranial nerves VII through X are most likely to be associated with postoperative cranial nerve dysfunction resulting in obtundation of normal airway reflexes, inability to phonate or swallow, or airway obstruction. If there is concern, patients should be allowed to awaken completely, follow all commands, be able to protrude the tongue, swallow, and suction themselves before extubation. If these criteria cannot be met before extubation and removal of the endotracheal tube is desirable, deflating the cuff of the endotracheal tube and observing the ability of the patient to breathe around the occluded tube and phonate may help assess the function of the vocal cords and the degree of airway edema present. Assessment of gag reflex and swallowing ability should indicate the degree of susceptibility to aspiration following extubation.

ALTERATIONS IN INTRACRANIAL PRESSURE

The ICP of the posterior fossa may differ considerably from the supratentorial space. Standard techniques such as hyperventilation and mannitol are also effective in lowering elevated ICP from a posterior fossa lesion. CSF drainage by the lumbar route is contraindicated due to the risk of tonsillar herniation. Even ventricular drainage is not without risk—upward herniation of the cerebellum through the tentorial hiatus has been reported. This upward shift results in compression of the deep venous channels (veins of Galen and Rosenthal) and deformation of mesencephalon and posterior third ventricle. Clinical symptoms include autonomic dysfunction, loss of upward gaze, and progressive obtundation. The incidence of upward herniation after ventricular drainage is low (about 5 percent).[193,194] Nevertheless, precraniotomy ventricular drainage should be performed only if necessary. The correct therapy for hydrocephalus associated with a posterior fossa mass should be the prompt operative decompression or removal of the mass.

If a ventriculostomy is present, it is important that the drainage of CSF be monitored closely during surgery. This is particularly true in the sitting position where the careless placement of the drainage chamber (e.g., at the level of the operating table) can precipitate subdural bleeding from aggressive drainage of CSF and withdrawal of the brain surface from the cranial vault. If a preexisting shunt is in place, the surgeon should consider temporarily occluding it before placing the patient in the sitting position.

The ICP can be elevated by inattention during positioning. If the head is flexed excessively, the endotracheal tube may kink and produce sudden elevation of airway pressure, which is then transmitted to the venous circulation. Flexion may also cause the endotracheal tube to migrate into the right mainstem bronchus, promoting hypercarbia or hypoxia.[195] A distance of two finger breadths should remain between the chest and chin after the final position is achieved. Hyperflexion or excessive lateral rotation can also interfere with jugular venous drainage, elevating intracranial venous pressure and exacerbating intracranial hypertension.[196]

WOUND COMPLICATIONS

Even with meticulous attention to wound closure, a pseudomeningocele can develop postoperatively. Management depends on whether there is an associated CSF leak and whether hydrocephalus is present. Any degree of hydrocephalus should be treated first because this may spontaneously resolve the pseudomeningocele. A pseudomeningocele without hydrocephalus or CSF leak warrants only close observation because these often resolve. The presence of a CSF leak without hydrocephalus implies a local dural disruption. Initially, this can be treated with head elevation, wound aspiration, pressure dressing application, and perhaps lumbar CSF drainage. Failure of these more conservative measures implies that surgical reexploration and dural closure are needed.

PNEUMOCEPHALUS

The combination of hyperventilation, mannitol, and CSF drainage often dehydrates the brain significantly. Particularly in the sitting position, as the brain settles and CSF drains during the surgical procedure, air can enter the cranial vault. This is often referred to as the "inverted pop-bottle" syndrome—the soda drains out of an inverted pop bottle to be replaced by air.[197] After the dura is closed, this air becomes trapped subdurally, usually in the frontal regions, and can mimic a mass lesion (Fig. 29-21). Although a small amount of pneumocephalus occurs in virtually every craniotomy where the head is elevated to any degree and the dura is opened, symptomatic pneumocephalus occurs in

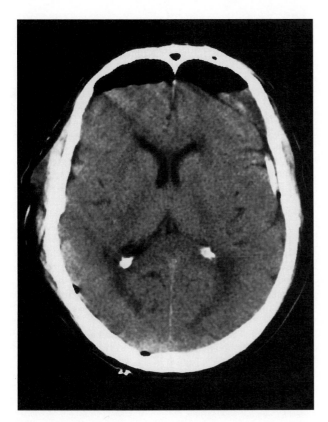

Figure 29-21 Some degree of pneumocephalus is common after sitting craniotomy. On occasion, tension pneumocephalus can develop (see text). This CT image shows subdural air collections in the frontal region.

only a small percentage.[45,198] Pneumocephalus is placed under tension when rehydration and normalization of Pa_{CO_2} result in reexpansion of brain. Moreover, the air mass may increase in size after dural closure if nitrous oxide is administered.[199,200] For this reason alone, nitrous oxide may be best avoided in patients in the sitting position.

Tension pneumocephalus typically presents as continuing lethargy or delayed emergence from anesthesia and less commonly as delayed neurologic deterioration in the immediate postoperative period. The diagnosis can be confirmed by either plain skull x-rays or CT scan. Placing the patient supine and on 100% oxygen to facilitate resorption is usually sufficient, but in exceptional cases, needle aspiration may be needed as a lifesaving maneuver. An attempt can be made to prevent pneumocephalus by irrigating the subdural space with saline before dural closure and by discontinuing hyperventilation during dural closure.

NEUROLOGIC COMPLICATIONS

Several noteworthy neurologic complications are associated with posterior fossa surgery. Midcervical quadriplegia following operations in the sitting position has

been reported, although it is rare. The precipitating insult is unclear but may be related to prolonged cervical flexion producing a stretch injury of the cord substance, resulting in an ischemic myelopathy.[39] Elderly, spondylotic patients may be particularly susceptible to this. There may also be a role played by hypoperfusion of the cervical cord if episodes of hypotension are not aggressively treated or if the acceptable level of mean arterial pressure is not maintained. Hypertensive patients demonstrate altered autoregulatory responses in the spinal cord that are similar to those in the brain.[201] Perfusion pressures needed to maintain normal cerebral and spinal cord blood flow are higher, and the lower limit of autoregulation is often a mean arterial pressure of 70 to 80 mmHg.

Supratentorial hemorrhage after posterior fossa surgery occurs in less than 1 percent of cases.[41,45] This complication is seen almost exclusively in the sitting position. The combination of iatrogenic dehydration and gravity settling of brain tissue can disrupt cortical bridging veins and result in an acute subdural hematoma. Rarely, hemorrhage is intraparenchymal, for which the mechanism is uncertain.[42,202]

Mutism following posterior fossa surgery (cerebellar mutism) is a recently described syndrome typically found in children who have undergone operations that require entry into the cerebellum, particularly the inferior vermis. The mutism is usually transient, occurring a few days postoperatively and resolving within 6 months. The cause is unclear but it may be related to dysfunction of the deep cerebellar nuclei, with loss of language coordination.[203]

Cranial nerve dysfunction secondary to operative manipulation may be obvious in the postoperative period. The facial nerve (VII) may be injured when tumors of the cerebellopontine angle are removed. In these patients, the cornea needs to be protected because the eyelids cannot oppose. Suspected intraoperative injury to the lower cranial nerves should prompt laryngoscopy prior to extubation to check the function of the larynx. A nasogastric tube should be placed at the end of the procedure and connected to low intermittent suction postoperatively to minimize risks of aspiration. If there is impairment of the swallowing mechanism, enteral alimentation may be necessary indefinitely or until swallowing function improves.

Aseptic meningitis occasionally occurs postoperatively due to meningeal irritation from blood in the CSF space. Spiking fevers and nuchal rigidity may appear as the patient is being weaned from steroid therapy. CSF analysis may reveal hypoglycorrhachia and pleocytosis that are indistinguishable from bacterial infection. The patient is treated with antibiotics pending CSF culture results. If there is no evidence of infection, antibiotics can be discontinued. The symptoms are often self-limiting but can be improved with reinstitution of small doses of corticosteroids for a short period of time.

Paradoxical air embolism with cerebral air embolism should be considered as the possible cause of any unexplained delay in awakening after surgery, especially after sitting craniotomy. A CT scan may reveal air in the cerebral vasculature. The transcranial Doppler may reveal a signal consistent with air in the middle cerebral artery and has been used intraoperatively for detection of cerebral arterial air bubbles.[204] Hyperbaric oxygen therapy is currently the only therapeutic intervention available to treat cerebral air embolism. Promptness of therapy is directly associated with the likelihood of successful outcome.[205-207]

Conclusions

The patient undergoing surgery of the posterior fossa can range from the infant with craniocervical dysplasia to the elderly patient with a metastatic tumor of the cerebellum. The surgical and anesthetic implications are complex and dictated by factors that involve the patients' underlying medical condition, their neurosurgical disease, the needs of the surgical procedure, and the limitations of monitoring and anesthetic choice. Many complications are unique to the posterior fossa, related both to the involved anatomy and to the surgical position. The synthesis of all of these factors implies that each case be thoughtfully considered, that adequate preoperative communication occur between all parties, and that the patient and family be fully informed. Posterior fossa surgery can be performed safely and successfully in nearly every case, and we are fortunate to have many anesthetic and monitoring choices to apply to each individual situation. Further progress in monitoring technology and development of new surgical equipment and anesthetic drugs can only make our management of such patients more completely tailored toward maximally reducing morbidity and optimizing outcome.

References

1. Haines SJ: Decerebrate posturing misinterpreted as seizure activity. *Am J Emerg Med* 1988; 6:173.
2. Cushing H: Some experimental and clinical observations concerning states of increased intracranial tension. *Ann J Med Sci* 1902; 124:375.
3. Park TS, et al: Medulloblastoma: Clinical presentation and management. Experience at the Hospital for Sick Children, Toronto, 1950–1980. *J Neurosurg* 1983; 58:543.
4. Hojer C, et al: Pilocytic astrocytomas of the posterior fossa. A followup study in 33 patients. *Acta Neurochir (Wien)* 1994; 129:131.
5. Ferrante L, et al: Fourth ventricle ependymomas. A study of 20 cases with survival analysis. *Acta Neurochir (Wien)* 1994; 131:67.
6. Epstein R, Wisoff J: Brainstem tumors in childhood: Surgical indications. In McLaurin R, et al (eds): *Pediatric Neurosurgery.* Philadelphia, WB Saunders, 1989:357.
7. Wen DY, Haines SJ: Posterior fossa: Surgical considerations. In Cottrell JE, Smith DS (eds): *Anesthesia and Neurosurgery,* 3d ed. St. Louis, Mosby-Year Book, 1994:326.
8. Panitch M, Berg B: Brainstem tumors of childhood and adolescence. *Am J Dis Child* 1970; 119:465.
9. Symon L, et al: Surgical management of posterior cranial fossa meningiomas. *Br J Neurosurg* 1993; 7:599.
10. Julow J, et al: Posterior fossa hemangioblastomas. *Acta Neurochir (Wien)* 1994; 128:109.
11. Rengachary SS, Blount JP: Hemangioblastoma. In Wilkins RH, Rengachary SS (eds): *Neurosurgery,* 2d ed. New York, McGraw-Hill, 1995:1205.
12. Iwabuchi T, et al: Biparieto-occipital craniotomy with hyperextended neck—"Sea-lion" position. *Acta Neurochir (Wien)* 1979; 51:113.
13. McLeod ME, et al: Anaesthetic management of arteriovenous malformations of the vein of Galen. *Can Anaesth Soc J* 1982; 29:307.
14. Freytag E: Fatal hypertensive intracerebral hematomas: A survey of the pathological anatomy of 393 cases. *J Neurol Neurosurg Psychiatr* 1968; 31:616.
15. Roda JM, et al: Posterior fossa epidural hematomas: A review and synthesis. *Surg Neurol* 1983; 19:419.
16. Altman NR, et al: Posterior fossa malformations. *AJNR Am J Neuroradiol* 1992; 13:69.
17. Badie B, et al: Posterior fossa volume and response to suboccipital decompression in patients with Chiari I malformation. *Neurosurgery* 1995; 37:214.
18. Dandy W: Concerning the cause of trigeminal neuralgia. *Am J Surg* 1934; 24:447.
19. Janetta PJ: Cranial rhizopathies. In Youmans JR (ed): *Neurological Surgery.* Philadelphia, WB Saunders, 1982:4169.
20. Haines S, et al: Microvascular relations of the trigeminal nerve. An anatomical study with clinical correlation. *J Neurosurg* 1980; 52:381.
21. Harner SG, et al: Improved preservation of facial nerve function with use of electrical monitoring during removal of acoustic neuromas. *Mayo Clin Proc* 1987; 62:92.
22. Mendoza N, Illingworth RD: Trigeminal neuralgia treated by microvascular decompression: A long-term followup study. *Br J Neurosurg* 1995; 9:13.
23. Moeller A, Janetta P: Microvascular decompression in hemifacial spasm. Intraoperative electrophysiological observations. *Neurosurgery* 1985; 16:612.
24. Moeller M, et al: Diagnosis and surgical treatment of disabling positional vertigo. *J Neurosurg* 1986; 64:21.
25. Ferrante L, et al: Glossopharyngeal neuralgia with cardiac syncope. *Neurosurgery* 1995; 36:58.
26. Resnick DK, et al: Microvascular decompression for glossopharyngeal neuralgia. *Neurosurgery* 1995; 36:64.
27. Keykhah MM, Rosenberg H: Bilateral footdrop after craniotomy in the sitting position. *Anesthesiology* 1979; 51:163.
28. Gozal Y, Pomeranz S: Sciatic nerve palsy as a complication after acoustic neurinoma resection in the sitting position. *J Neurosurg Anesth* 1994; 6:40.
29. Ellis SC, et al: Massive swelling of the head and neck. *Anesthesiology* 1975; 42:102.
30. McAllister RG: Macroglossia—A positional complication. *Anesthesiology* 1974; 40:199.
31. Toung TJK, et al: Movement of the distal end of the endotra-

cheal tube during flexion and extension of the neck. *Anesth Analg* 1985; 64:1029.

32. Cabezudo JM, et al: Air embolism from wounds from a pin-type head-holder as a complication of posterior fossa surgery in the sitting position. Case report. *J Neurosurg* 1981; 55:147.

33. Wilkins RH, Albin MS: An unusual entrance site of venous air embolism during operations in the sitting position. *Surg Neurol* 1977; 7:71.

34. Grinberg F, et al: Probable venous air embolism associated with removal of the Mayfield skull clamp. *Anesth Analg* 1995; 80:1049.

35. Ernst PS, et al: Intracranial and spinal cord hemodynamics in the sitting position in dogs in the presence and absence of increased intracranial pressure. *Anesth Analg* 1990; 70:147.

36. Black S, et al: Outcome following posterior fossa craniectomy in patients in the sitting or horizontal positions. *Anesthesiology* 1988; 69:49.

37. Nelson RJ, et al: Changes in blood flow during anaesthesia and surgery in the sitting position. *J Neurol Neurosurg Psychiat* 1987; 50:971.

38. Tindall GT, et al: Effects of the sitting position of blood flow in the internal carotid artery of man during general anesthesia. *J Neurosurg* 1966; 26:383.

39. Wilder BL: Hypothesis: The etiology of midcervical quadroplegia after operation with the patient in the sitting position. *Neurosurgery* 1982; 11:530.

40. Hitselberger WE, House WF: A warning regarding the sitting position for acoustic tumor surgery. *Arch Otolaryngol* 1980; 106:69.

41. Seiler RW, Zurbrugg HR: Supratentorial intracerebral hemorrhage after posterior fossa operation. *Neurosurgery* 1986; 18:472.

42. Haines SJ, et al: Supratentorial intracerebral hemorrhage following posterior fossa surgery. *J Neurosurg* 1978; 49:881.

43. Grundy BL, Spetzler RF: Subdural pneumocephalus resulting from drainage of cerebrospinal fluid during craniotomy. *Anesthesiology* 1980; 52:269.

44. Elton RJ, Howell RSC: The sitting position in neurosurgical anaesthesia: A survey of British practice in 1991. *Br J Anaesth* 1994; 73:247.

45. Standefer M, et al: The sitting position in neurosurgery: A retrospective analysis of 488 cases. *Neurosurgery* 1984; 14:649.

46. Matjasko J, et al: Anesthesia and surgery in the seated position: Analysis of 554 cases. *Neurosurgery* 1985; 17:695.

47. Young ML, et al: Comparison of surgical and anesthetic complications in neurosurgical patients experiencing venous air embolism in the sitting position. *Neurosurgery* 1986; 18:157.

48. Cucchiara RF: Safety of the sitting position. *Anesthesiology* 1984; 61:790.

49. Rayport M, Martin JT: New head-prone position for posterior fossa surgery in infants with severe hydrocephalus. *Childs Nerv Syst* 1992; 8:419.

50. Bedford RF: Venous air embolism: A historical perspective. *Semin Anesth* 1983; 2:169.

51. Young ML: Posterior fossa: Anesthetic considerations. In Cottrell JE, Smith DS (eds): *Anesthesia and Neurosurgery*, 3d ed. St. Louis, Mosby-Year Book, 1994:348.

52. Young ML: Posterior fossa: Anesthetic considerations. In Cottrell JE, Smith DS (eds): *Anesthesia and Neurosurgery*, 3d ed. St. Louis, Mosby-Year Book, 1994:349.

53. Maroon JC, et al: Detection of minute venous air emboli with ultrasound. *Surg Gynecol Obstet* 1968; 127:1236.

54. Michenfelder JD, et al: Air embolism during neurosurgery. An evaluation of right-atrial catheters for diagnosis and treatment. *JAMA* 1969; 208:1353.

55. Michenfelder JD, et al: Evaluation of an ultrasonic device

56. Albin MS, et al: Anesthetic management of posterior fossa surgery in the sitting position. *Acta Anaesth Scand* 1976; 20:117.

57. Voorhies RM, et al: Prevention of air embolism with positive end-expiratory pressure. *Neurosurgery* 1983; 12:503.

58. von Gosseln HH, et al: The lounging position for posterior fossa surgery: Anesthesiologist considerations regarding air embolism. *Childs Nerv Syst* 1991; 7:368.

59. Pfitzner J, et al: Hypoxaemia following sustained low-volume venous air embolism in sheep. *Anaesth Intens Care* 1988; 16:164.

60. Moosavi H, et al: Lung ultrastructure in noncardiogenic pulmonary edema induced by air embolization in dogs. *Lab Invest* 1981; 45:456.

61. Deal CW, et al: Hemodynamic effects of pulmonary air embolism. *J Surg Res* 1971; 11:533.

62. Hlastala MP, et al: Gas exchange abnormalities produced by venous gas emboli. *Respiration Physiology* 1979; 36:1.

63. Presson RG, et al: Fate of air emboli in the pulmonary circulation. *J Appl Physiol* 1989; 67:1898.

64. Cucchiara RF, Bowers B: Air embolism in children undergoing suboccipital craniotomy. *Anesthesiology* 1982; 57:338.

65. Durant TM, et al: Pulmonary (venous) air embolism. *Am Heart J* 1947; 33:269.

66. Adornato DC, et al: Pathophysiology of intravenous air embolism in dogs. *Anesthesiology* 1978; 49:120.

67. Alvaran SB, et al: Venous air embolism: Comparative merits of external cardiac massage, intracardiac aspiration, and left lateral decubitus position. *Anesth Analg* 1978; 57:166.

68. Albin MS, et al: Clinical considerations concerning detection of venous air embolism. *Neurosurgery* 1978; 3:380.

69. Hagen PT, et al: Incidence and size of patent foramen ovale during the first 10 decades of life: An autopsy study of 965 normal hearts. *Mayo Clin Proc* 1984; 59:17.

70. Gross CM, et al: Valsalva maneuver contrast echocardiography, a new technique for improved detection of right to left shunting in patients with systemic embolism. *Am J Cardiol* 1982; 49:995.

71. Black M, et al: Paradoxic air embolism in the absence of an intracardiac defect. *Chest* 1991; 99:754.

72. Marquez J, et al: Paradoxical cerebral air embolism without an intracardiac septal defect. *J Neurosurg* 1981; 55:997.

73. Lynch JJ, et al: Prevalence of right-to-left atrial shunting in a healthy population: Detection by Valsalva maneuver contrast echocardiography. *Am J Cardiol* 1984; 53:1478.

74. Gottdeiner JS, et al: Incidence and cardiac effects of systemic venous air embolism. Echocardiographic evidence of arterial embolization via noncardiac shunt. *Arch Intern Med* 1988; 148:795.

75. Durant TM, et al: Arterial air embolism. *Am Heart J* 1949; 38:481.

76. Hwang T, et al: Confirmation of cerebral air embolism with computerized tomography. *Ann Neurol* 1983; 13:214.

77. Hirabuki N, et al: Changes of cerebral air embolism shown by computed tomography. *Br J Radiol* 1988; 61:252.

78. Suriani RJ: Echocardiographic identification of paradoxical air embolism. *Anesthesiology* 1994; 81:1548.

79. Bedell EA, et al: Paradoxic air embolism during venous air embolism: Transesophageal echocardiographic evidence of transpulmonary air passage. *Anesthesiology* 1994; 80:947.

80. Pfitzner J, McLean AG: Venous air embolism and active lung inflation at high and low CVP: A study in upright anesthetized sheep. *Anesth Analg* 1987; 66:1127.

81. Coonan TJ, Hope CE: Cardiorespiratory effects of change of body position. *Can Anaesth Soc J* 1983; 30:424.

(Doppler) for the diagnosis of venous air embolism. *Anesthesiology* 1972; 36:164.

82. Darymple DG, et al: Cardiorespiratory effects of the sitting position in neurosurgery. *Br J Anaesth* 1979; 15:1079.

83. Perkins-Pearson NAK, et al: Atrial pressures in the seated position: Implications for paradoxical air embolism. *Anesthesiology* 1982; 57:493.

84. Colohan ART, et al: Intravenous fluid loading as prophylaxis for paradoxical air embolism. *J Neurosurg* 1985; 62:839.

85. Butler DB, Hills BA: Transpulmonary passage of venous air emboli. *J Appl Physiol* 1985; 59:543.

86. Yahagi N, et al: Effect of halothane, fentanyl, and ketamine on the threshold for transpulmonary passage of venous air emboli in dogs. *Anesth Analg* 1992; 75:720.

87. Bedford RF: Perioperative venous air embolism. *Semin Anesth* 1987; 6:163.

88. Hunter AR: Air embolism in the sitting position. *Anesthesia* 1962; 17:467.

89. Marshall BM: Air embolus in neurosurgical anaesthesia, its diagnosis and treatment. *Can Anaesthes Soc J* 1965; 12:255.

90. Sloan TB, Kimovec MA: Detection of venous air embolism by airway pressure monitoring. *Anesthesiology* 1986; 64:645.

91. Tinker JH, et al: Detection of air embolism. A test for positioning of right atrial catheter and Doppler probe. *Anesthesiology* 1975; 43:104.

92. Colley PS, et al: Assessment of a saline injection test for location of a right atrial catheter. *Anesthesiology* 1979; 50:258.

93. Edmund-Seal J, Maroon JC: Air embolism diagnosed with ultrasound. *Anaesthesia* 1969; 24:438.

94. Losasso TJ, et al: Doppler detection of intravenous mannitol crystals mimics venous air embolism. *Anesth Analg* 1990; 71:568.

95. Lui PW, et al: Spectral characteristics of embolic heart sounds detected by precordial Doppler ultrasound during venous air embolism in dogs. *Br J Anaesth* 1993; 71:689.

96. Drummond JC, et al: A comparison of pulmonary artery pressure, end-tidal carbon dioxide, and end-tidal nitrogen in the detection of venous air embolism in the dog. *Anesth Analg* 1985; 64:688.

97. Matjasko J, et al: Sensitivity of end-tidal nitrogen in venous air embolism detection in dogs. *Anesthesiology* 1985; 63:418.

98. Black S, et al: Parameters affecting occurrence of paradoxical air embolism. *Anesthesiology* 1989; 71:235.

99. Bedford RF, et al: Cardiac catheters for diagnosis and treatment of venous air embolism. A prospective study in man. *J Neurosurgery* 1981; 55:610.

100. Greenblatt G, et al: Detection of venous air embolism by continuous intra-arterial oxygen monitoring. *J Clin Monitoring* 1990; 6:53.

101. Gelnski JA, et al: Transesophageal echocardiography and transcutaneous O_2 and CO_2 monitoring for detection of venous air embolism. *Anesthesiology* 1986; 64:541.

102. Furuya H, et al: Detection of air embolism by transesophageal echocardiography. *Anesthesiology* 1983; 58:124.

103. Muzzi DA, et al: Comparison of a transesophageal and precordial ultrasonic Doppler sensor in the detection of venous air embolism. *Anesth Analg* 1990; 70:103.

104. Kondstadt SN, et al: Intraoperative detection of patent foramen ovale by transesophageal echocardiography. *Anesthesiology* 1991; 74:212.

105. Guggiari M, et al: Early detection of patent foramen ovale by two-dimensional contrast echocardiography for prevention of paradoxical air embolism during sitting position. *Anesth Analg* 1988; 67:192.

106. Sato S, et al: Echocardiographic detection and treatment of intraoperative air embolism. *J Neurosurg* 1986; 64:440.

107. Young ML: Posterior fossa: Anesthetic considerations. In Cot-trell JE, Smith DS (eds): *Anesthesia and Neurosurgery*, 3d ed. St. Louis, Mosby-Year Book, 1994:353.

108. Bunegin L, et al: Positioning the right atrial catheter: A model for reappraisal. *Anesthesiology* 1981; 55:343.

109. Colley PS, Artru AA: Bunegin-Albin catheter improves air retrieval and resuscitation from lethal venous air embolism in dogs. *Anesth Analg* 1987; 66:991.

110. Bunegin L, Albin MS: Balloon catheter increases air capture. *Anesthesiology* 1982; 57:66.

111. Diaz PM: Balloon catheter should increase recovery of embolized air. *Anesthesiology* 1982; 57:66.

112. Hanna PG, et al: In vitro comparison of central venous catheters for aspiration of venous air embolism: Effect of catheter type, catheter tip position, and cardiac inclination. *J Clin Anesth* 1991; 3:290.

113. Bowdle TA, Artru AA: Treatment of air embolism with a special pulmonary artery catheter introducer sheath in sitting dogs. *Anesthesiology* 1988; 68:107.

114. Hicks HC, Hummel JC: A new catheter for detection and treatment of venous air embolism. *J Neurosurg* 1980; 52:595.

115. Smith SL, et al: CVP catheter placement from the antecubital veins using a j-wire catheter guide. *Anesthesiology* 1984; 3:238.

116. Cucchiara RF, et al: Time required and success rate of percutaneous right atrial catheterization: Description of a technique. *Can Anaesth Soc J* 1980; 27:572.

117. Lee DS, et al: Migration of tips of central venous catheters in seated patients. *Anesth Analg* 1984; 63:949.

118. Young ML: Posterior fossa: Anesthetic considerations. In Cot-trell JE, Smith DS (eds): *Anesthesia and Neurosurgery*, 3d ed. St. Louis, Mosby-Year Book, 1994:352.

119. Kloosterboer TB, et al: Subclavian vein catheter as a source of air emboli in the sitting position. *Anesthesiology* 1986; 64:411.

120. Colley PS, Artru AA: ECG-guided placement of Sorenson CVP catheters via arm veins. *Anesth Analg* 1984; 63:953.

121. Young ML: Posterior fossa: Anesthetic considerations. In Cot-trell JE, Smith DS (eds): *Anesthesia and Neurosurgery*, 3d ed. St. Louis, Mosby-Year Book, 1994:353.

122. Warner DO, Cucchiara RF: Position of proximal orifice determines electrocardiogram recorded from multiorificed catheter. *Anesthesiology* 1986; 65:235.

123. Johans TG: Arrow brachial CVP air aspirating catheter placement with the IVECG technique. *Anesthesiology* 1988; 69:140.

124. Mongan P, et al: Pressure monitoring can accurately position catheters for air embolism aspiration. *J Clin Monit* 1992; 8:121.

125. Black S, et al: Preoperative and intraoperative echocardiography to detect right-to-left shunt in patients undergoing neurosurgical procedures in the sitting position. *Anesthesiology* 1990; 72:436.

126. Cucchiara RF, et al: Failure of preoperative echo testing to prevent paradoxical air embolism: Report of two cases. *Anesthesiology* 1989; 71:604.

127. Kronik G, Mosslacher H: Positive contrast echocardiography in patients with patent foramen ovale and normal right heart hemodynamics. *Am J Cardiol* 1982; 49:1806.

128. Iwabuchi T, et al: Dural sinus pressure as related to neurosurgical position. *Neurosurgery* 1986; 12:203.

129. Toung TJK, et al: Comparison of the effects of positive end-expiratory pressure and jugular venous compression on canine cerebral venous pressure. *Anesthesiology* 1984; 61:169.

130. Sharma K, Tripathi M: Detection of site of air entry in venous air embolism: Role of Valsalva maneuver. *J Neurosurg Anesthesiol* 1994; 6:209.

131. Shapiro HM, et al: Nitrous oxide challenge for detection of intravascular pulmonary gas following venous air embolism. *Anesth Analg* 1982; 61:304.

132. Losasso TJ, et al: Fifty percent nitrous oxide does not increase

the risk of venous air embolism in neurosurgical patients operated upon in the sitting position. *Anesthesiology* 1992; 77:21.

133. Munson ES, Merrick HC: Effects of nitrous oxide on venous air embolism. *Anesthesiology* 1986; 27:783.

134. Mehlhorn U, et al: Body position does not affect the hemodynamic response to venous air embolism in dogs. *Anesth Analg* 1994; 79:734.

135. Ericsson JA, et al: Closed-chest cardiac massage in the treatment of venous air embolism. *N Engl J Med* 1964; 270:1353.

136. Cucchiara RF, et al: Identification of patent foramen ovale during sitting position craniotomy by transesophageal echocardiography with positive airway pressure. *Anesthesiology* 1985; 63:107.

137. Perkins NAK, Bedford RF: Hemodynamic consequences of PEEP in seated neurological patients—Implications for paradoxical air embolism. *Anesth Analg* 1984; 63:429.

138. Zentner J, et al: Prevention of an air embolism by moderate hypoventilation during surgery in the sitting position. *Neurosurgery* 1991; 28:705.

139. Grady MS, et al: Changes in superior sagittal sinus pressure in children with head elevation, jugular venous compression, and PEEP. *J Neurosurg* 1986; 65:199.

140. Meyer PG, et al: Prevention of venous air embolism in paediatric neurosurgical procedures performed in the sitting position by combined use of MAST suit and PEEP. *Br J Anaesth* 1994; 73:795.

141. Gardner WJ, Dohn DF: The antigravity suit (G-suit) in surgery: Control of blood pressure in the sitting position and in hypotensive anesthesia. *JAMA* 1956; 162:274.

142. Marshall WK, et al: Cardiovascular responses in the seated position—Impact of four anesthetic techniques. *Anesth Analg* 1983; 62:648.

143. Martin JT: Neuroanesthetic adjuncts for surgery in the sitting position. II. The antigravity suit. *Anesth Analg* 1970; 49:588.

144. Tinker JH, Vandam LD: How effective is the G suit in neurosurgical operations? *Anesthesiology* 1972; 36:609.

145. Catron PW, et al: Cerebral air embolism treated by pressure and hyperbaric oxygen. *Neurology* 1991; 41:314.

146. Armon C, et al: Hyperbaric treatment of cerebral air embolism sustained during an open-heart surgical procedure. *Mayo Clin Proc* 1991; 66:565.

147. Bitterman H, Melamed Y: Delayed hyperbaric treatment of cerebral air embolism. *Isr J Med Sci* 1993; 29:22.

148. Layon AJ: Hyperbaric oxygen treatment for cerebral air embolism—Where are the data? *Mayo Clin Proc* 1991; 66:641.

149. Schramm J, et al: Neurophysiologic monitoring in posterior fossa surgery. I. Technical principles, applicability, and limitations. *Acta Neurochir (Wien)* 1989; 98:9.

150. Urasaki E, et al: Monitoring of short-latency evoked somatosensory evoked potentials during surgery for cervical cord and posterior fossa lesions—Changes in subcortical components. *Neurol Med Chir* 1988; 28:546.

151. York DH, et al: Utilization of somatosensory evoked cortical potentials in spinal cord injury—Prognostic limitations. *Spine* 1983; 8:832.

152. Grundy BL: Intraoperative monitoring of sensory-evoked potentials. *Anesthesiology* 1983; 58:72.

153. Radtke RA, et al: Intraoperative brainstem auditory evoked potentials: Significant decrease in postoperative morbidity. *Neurology* 1989; 39:187.

154. Clemis JD, Mitchell C: Electrocochleography and brain stem responses used in the diagnosis of acoustic tumors. *J Otolaryngol* 1977; 6:447.

155. Eggermont JJ, Con M, Brackmann DE: Electrocochleography and auditory brainstem electric responses in patients with pontine angle tumors. *Ann Otol Rhinol Laryngol* 1980; 89(Supp)75:1.

156. Linden RD, et al: Electrophysiological monitoring during acoustic neuroma and other posterior fossa surgery. *Can J Neurol Sci* 1988; 15:73.

157. Kalmanchey R, et al: The use of brainstem auditory evoked potentials during posterior fossa surgery as a monitor of brainstem function. *Acta Neurochir* 1986; 82:128.

158. Weilaard R, Kemp RB: Auditory brainstem evoked responses in brainstem compression due to posterior fossa tumors. *Clin Neurol Neurosurg* 1979; 81:185.

159. Schwartz D, et al: Intraoperative monitoring of auditory brainstem responses following emergency evaluation of a cerebellar AVM. *J Clin Monit* 1988; 5:116.

160. Lutsch J, et al: Brainstem auditory evoked potentials and early somatosensory evoked potentials in neurointensively treated comatose children. *Am J Dis Child* 1983; 137:421.

161. Levy WJ, York DH: Evoked potentials from the motor tracts in humans. *Neurosurgery* 1983; 12:422.

162. Levy WJ, et al: Motor evoked potentials from transcranial stimulation of the motor cortex in humans. *Neurosurgery* 1984; 15:287.

163. Lee WY, et al: Intraoperative monitoring of motor function by magnetic motor evoked potentials. *Neurosurgery* 1995; 36:493.

164. Welna JO, et al: Effect of partial neuromuscular blockade on intraoperative electromyography in patients undergoing resection of acoustic neuroma. *Anesth Rev* 1988; 15:75.

165. Schaller B, et al: Preoperative and postoperative auditory and facial nerve function in cerebellopontine angle meningiomas. *Otolaryngol Head Neck Surg* 1995; 112:228.

166. Lalwani AK, et al: Facial nerve outcome after acoustic neuroma surgery: A study from the era of cranial nerve monitoring. *Otolaryngol Head Neck Surg* 1994; 111:561.

167. Standgaard S, et al: Autoregulation of brain circulation in severe arterial hypertension. *Br Med J* 1973; 1:507.

168. Young ML: Posterior fossa: Anesthetic considerations. In Cottrell JE, Smith DS (eds): *Anesthesia and Neurosurgery*, 3d ed. St. Louis, Mosby-Year Book, 994:340.

169. Calliauw L, et al: The position of the patient during neurosurgical procedures on the posterior fossa. *Acta Neurochir (Wien)* 1987; 85:154.

170. Enderby GEH: Postural ischaemia and blood pressure. *Lancet* 1954; 1:185.

171. Toole JF: Effects of change on head, limb, and body position on cephalic circulation. *N Engl J Med* 1968; 279:307.

172. Lawson NA: The lateral decubitus position. In Martin JT (ed): *Positioning in Anesthesia and Surgery*. Philadelphia, WB Saunders, 1987:174.

173. Petrozza PH: Anesthesia for posterior fossa procedures. In Porter S (ed): *Problems in Anesthesia: Neuroanesthesia*. Philadelphia, JB Lippincott, 1990:124.

174. Awasthi D, et al: Intrinsic lesions of the spinal cord: Surgical and anesthetic management. In Porter SS (ed): *Anesthesia for Surgery of the Spine*. New York, McGraw-Hill, 1995:127.

175. Manninen PH, et al: Monitoring of brainstem function during vertebral basilar aneurysm surgery: The use of spontaneous ventilation. *Anesthesiology* 1992; 77:681.

176. Manninen PH: Spontaneous ventilation is a useful monitor of brain stem function during posterior fossa surgery. *J Neurosurg Anesthesiol* 1995; 7:63.

177. Scuplak SM, et al: Air embolism during awake craniotomy. *Anaesthesia* 1995; 50:338.

178. Sieber FE, et al: Glucose: A reevaluation of its intraoperative use. *Anesthesiology* 1987; 67:72.

179. Milde LN: Clinical use of mild hypothermia for brain protection: A dream revisited. *J Neurosurg Anesthesiol* 1992; 4:211.

180. Bedford RF, Colley PS: Intracranial tumors: Supratentorial and infratentorial. In: Matjasko J, Katz J (eds): *Clinical Controversies In Neuroanesthesia and Neurosurgery.* Orlando, FL: Grune & Stratton, 1986:135.

181. Porter SS, et al: Intravenous nitroglycerine versus nitroprusside/captopril for deliberate hypotension during posterior spine fusion in adults. *J Clin Anesth* 1989; 1(2):87.

182. Zentner J, Abner A: Nitrous oxide suppresses the electromyographic response evoked by electrical stimulation of the motor cortex. *Neurosurgery* 1989; 24:60.

183. Sebel PS, et al: Evoked potentials during isoflurane anesthesia. *Br J Anaesth* 1986; 58:580.

184. Tung H, et al: The effects of anesthestic and sedative agents on magnetic motor evoked potentials. *Anesthesiology* 1988; 69(Suppl 3A):A313.

185. Lam KK, et al: Severe pulmonary oedema after venous air embolism. *Can J Anaesth* 1993; 40:964.

186. Still JA, et al: Pulmonary edema following air embolism. *Anesthesiology* 1974; 40:194.

187. Perschau RA, et al: Pulmonary interstitial edema after multiple venous air emboli. *Anesthesiology* 1976; 45:364.

188. O'Quin RJ, Lakshminarayan S: Venous air embolism. *Arch Intern Med* 1982; 142:2173.

189. Albertine KH, et al: Quantification of damage by air emboli to lung microvessels in anesthetized sheep. *J Appl Physiol* 1984; 57:1360.

190. Flick MR, et al: Leukocytes are required for increased lung microvascular permeability after microembolization in sheep. *Circ Res* 1981; 48:344.

191. Jerome EH, et al: Timing of corticosteroid therapy. Effect on lung lymph dynamics in air embolism lung injury in awake sheep. *Am Rev Respir Dis* 1990; 142:872.

192. Flick MR, et al: Superoxide dismutase with heparin prevents increased lung vascular permeability during air emboli in unanesthetised sheep. *J Appl Physiol* 1983; 55:1284.

193. Hoffman HJ, et al: Metastasis via ventriculoperitoneal shunt in patients with medulloblastoma. *J Neurosurg* 1976; 44:562.

194. Raimondi AJ, Tomita T: Hydrocephalus and infratentorial tumors. Incidence, clinical picture, and treatment. *J Neurosurg* 1981; 55:174.

195. Lingenfelter AL, et al: Displacement of right atrial and endotracheal catheters with neck flexion. *Anesth Analg* 1978; 57:371.

196. Stone DJ, Harris MM: Anesthesia for increased intracranial pressure in adults. In Porter SS (ed): *Problems in Anesthesia: Neuroanesthesia.* Philadelphia, JB Lippincott, 1990:62.

197. Lunsford LD, et al: Subdural tension pneumocephalus. Report of two cases. *J Neurosurg* 1979; 50:525.

198. Di Lorenzo N, et al: Pneumocephalus and tension pneumocephalus after posterior fossa surgery in the sitting position: A prospective study. *Acta Neurochir (Wien)* 1986; 83:112.

199. Artru AA: Nitrous oxide plays a direct role in the development of tension pneumocephalus intraoperatively. 1982; 57:59.

200. Pandit UA, et al: Pneumocephalus after posterior fossa exploration in the sitting position. *Anaesthesia* 1982; 37:996.

201. Hickey R, et al: Autoregulation of spinal cord and cerebral blood flow: Is the spinal cord a microcosm of the brain? *Stroke* 1987; 17:1183.

202. Bucciero A, et al: Supratentorial intracerebral hemorrhage after posterior fossa surgery. *J Neurosurg Sci* 1991; 35:221.

203. Dailey AT, et al: The pathophysiology of oral pharyngeal apraxia and mutism following posterior fossa tumor resection in children. *J Neurosurg* 1995; 83:467.

204. Spencer MP, et al: Detection of middle cerebral artery emboli during carotid endarterectomy using transcranial Doppler ultrasonography. *Stroke* 1990; 21:415.

205. NHLBI workshop summary. Hyperbaric oxygen therapy. *Am Rev Respir Dis* 1991; 144:1414.

206. Dutka AJ: A review of the pathophysiology and potential application of experimental therapies for cerebral ischemia to the treatment of cerebral arterial gas embolism. *Undersea Biomed Res* 1985; 12:403.

207. Dutka AJ: Air of gas embolism. In Camporesi EM, Barker AC (eds): *Hyperbaric Oxygen Therapy: A critical review.* Bethesda, MD, Undersea and Hyperbaric Medical Society, 1991:1.

208. English JB, et al: Comparison of venous air embolism monitoring methods in supine dogs. *Anesthesiology* 1978; 48:425.

Chapter 30
AIR EMBOLISM
MAURICE S. ALBIN

"The timely removal of the air is the only rational treatment in all cases where simpler measures have proved inadequate in preventing a fatal outcome."
Nicholas Senn, 1885[1]

History[2–13]

The idea that venous air embolism (VAE) occurs exclusively during neurosurgical procedures in the sitting position appears to have dominated our thinking during the past two decades. In many ways, this false sense of security is contradicted by the development of our knowledge of this dangerous and sometimes fatal clinical entity, and therefore it is important to reacquaint ourselves with history. It is interesting that as early as 1667, Francisco Redi noted that animals (dogs, hares, foxes) died rapidly when a vein was opened and air blown into it. A brief survey of the understanding of VAE up to the end of the nineteenth century can be seen in Table 30-1. It must be remembered that ether and chloroform were not used for surgical procedures until 1846 and 1847, respectively, and hence, surgery before these dates had to be, of necessity, extraordinarily rapid, often resulting in the cutting or tearing of veins and sinuses. Because most

of these head, neck, and chest procedures were carried out in a chair or with the patient reclining, a large gravitational gradient between the incisional area and the right heart usually existed, thus promoting the entrainment of air. By the twentieth century, literally hundreds of clinical cases of VAE had already been described in the literature. Similarly, many hundreds of experiments had been carried out in a variety of animals to delineate the physiopathology of VAE. The depth of information on VAE gathered during the nineteenth century is appreciated in the work of Jean Zulema Amussat[5] and Nicholas Senn.[1] Amussat was the author of a 255-page book published in 1839 and dedicated solely to the problems posed by VAE (Figs. 30-1 and 30-2). Senn, a professor of Surgery at Rush Medical College and the University of Chicago, also had been a colonel in the US Army Medical Corps and published a 115-page dissertation on VAE in 1885 (Fig. 30-3). Between them, they collected and reviewed more than 250 clinical case reports, described hundreds of animal experiments performed to elucidate the pathophysiology of VAE, and described treatment modes, including cannulation of the right side of the heart. Amussat and Senn completely described the changes in heart tones that we now call the mill-wheel murmur and characterized the cyanosis, gasping respiration, and cardiovascular collapse that are the major clinical signs of severe VAE. They described the air lock due to air bubble accumulation that causes overdistension of the right side of the heart and to the consequent asphyxia from obstruction to the pulmonary circulation that produces acute cerebral ischemia. Amussat and Senn documented the finding that the development of gradients, described by Senn as "the force of gravitation," between the right side of the heart and the incisional area is a critical factor in air entrainment.

Although Amussat was mainly concerned about air entrainment during surgical procedures in the head and neck (he called this area the *région dangereuse*), he dedicated the last chapter of his book to VAE during parturition. As early as 1829, the surgeon Legallois stated that his father (an obstetrician) ". . . a vu trois fois l'air pénétrer dans le systèm sanguin par les veines utérines et occasioner instantanément la mort des femelles" (on three occasions he saw air penetrate into the blood of the uterine veins and instantly occasion the death of these women).[5,10] Many others described VAE in the nineteenth century related to hemorrhage during and after delivery and during attempts at abortion. Sir James Young Simpson (Fig. 30-4), who first used chloroform in deliveries, worked in Cormack's laboratory assisting in animal experiments concerning the relationship between the volume of air aspirated, the speed of aspiration, and the diameter of the vessel into which the air was introduced.[7] Karl Joseph von

TABLE 30-1
Early History of Venous Air Embolism

1667	Francisco Redi—Animals died when air was blown into the veins.
1683	Anton de Heyde—Air insufflation caused dilatation of the right heart in animals.
1681	Herder—Reported the hissing sound noted with the entrance of air into a vein in the human.
1686	Camerarius—Death occurred quickly after rapid air insufflation and more slowly after slow insufflation.
1811	Nysten—Animals tolerated small volumes of air, death due to distension of right ventricle.
1818	Bauchene—First human death during tumor excision in the right shoulder, reported by Magendie in 1821.
1821	Magendie—Elucidated physiopathology, advocated air aspiration via a cannula in the right atrium, described millwheel murmur.
1822	Dupuytren—Death during dissection of a neck tumor following a prolonged hissing noise. Right atrium distended and air found in the great vessels.
1823	Wattmann—Compressed torn vein digitally, then developed surgical technique to ligate and repair it. Wrote a 188-page book on air embolism that was published in 1843.
1829	Legallois—Death from VAE during parturition.
1830	Barlow—Death during surgery on neck tumor, with a hissing-gurgling noise present.
1832	J.C. Warren (Professor of Anatomy and Surgery, Harvard)—Two cases of VAE with one death at Massachusetts General Hospital.
1837	Cormack—Thesis for degree of Doctor of Medicine, "On the Presence of Air in the Organs of Circulation," 56 pages. Described heart sounds, pathology.
1839	Amussat—"Researches on the Accidental Introduction of Air into the Veins," 255 pages. Described therapy, heart sounds, physiopathology, treatment.
1844	Ericksen—"On the Proximate Cause of Death After Spontaneous Introduction of Air into the Veins, with Some Remarks on the Treatment of the Accident," 24 pages. Described heart sounds, pathophysiology, treatment.
1885	Senn—"An Experimental Study of Air-Embolism," 116 pages. Described pathophysiology, heart sounds, treatment.

Wattmann was the Professor of Surgery at Innsbruck, Austria and then Professor at the University of Vienna.[13] In 1843, he published a book on the problem of VAE and how to manage the surgical aspect of air entering a vein and developed a special forceps for hemostasis (Figs. 30-5, 30-6, and 30-7).

These early authors identified VAE in cases involving numerous vascular structures, including the internal and external jugular, facial, axillary, anterior thoracic, superficial cervical, femoral, internal saphenous, uterine, pulmonary, and diploic veins as well as the superior longitudinal and uterine sinuses. Equally important, they were therapeutic positivists advocating the prophylactic approach of hemostasis by compression, flooding the operative field, and vein ligation. In experimental studies, they showed that air in the right side of the heart could be evacuated by needle aspiration or by the introduction of a catheter or cannula into the jugular vein and subsequent aspiration.[2,5]

No organ system is immune from VAE,[3] and cases have been reported during head and neck, obstetric, gynecologic, organ biopsy, craniofacial, otorhinolaryngologic, neurosurgical, abdominal, urologic, cardiothoracic, orthopedic, oral surgical, and endoscopic procedures. VAE has also occurred after liver transplantation, after trauma, during medical procedures such as placement of peripheral or central venous lines, after diagnostic and therapeutic air injections, and following insertion of epidural catheters. The use of hydrogen peroxide for wound or cavity irrigation has

given rise to a number of reports of VAE and similarly, pulsed saline irrigation can be a source of embolic air entering the circulation. Orogenital sexual contact has also been reported as a cause of VAE.

This chapter deals primarily with VAE in the surgical environment and touches on the problem of arterial air embolism only in terms of the paradoxical movement of air to the left side of the heart through a patent foramen ovale (PFO) or into the brain during cardiac surgery when cardiopulmonary bypass (CPB) is used.

Physiopathology

Air can enter the venous circulation wherever a sufficient gradient exists between the right atrium and the upper area of the incision or point of entrance of air. Albin and coworkers have reported that a 5.0-cm gravitational gradient was sufficient to entrain air in a neurosurgical case.[14] Entry of 100 ml air into circulation has been fatal,[1,4,14] and it has been calculated that this amount of air can pass through a 14-gauge needle in 1 s with a gradient of 5.0 cm H_2O.[15] Increasing the elevation between an open vein in the skull and the right atrium by placing the patient in the sitting position or even by merely raising the head tends to increase this gradient and thus the risk of VAE.

Factors modifying air entrainment include the *body position, depth of ventilation, volume of air entering the vessel, rate of gaseous entry,* and *central venous pressure* tracted blood volume, with hemorrhagic hypovolemia, when a negative pressure is used during the expiratory phase of mechanical ventilation, and when a frame (Hasting's or four-poster) that favors a decreased intrathoracic pressure (up to −6 cmH$_2$O) by freeing the abdomen is used in the prone position.[21-23]

In terms of cardiovascular response, there is a marked difference between a constant infusion of gas and a single, large bolus injection of gas into the venous circulation. Deal and collaborators[24] showed that 60 ml air introduced into the right side of the sheep's heart produced an immediate drop in cardiac output and an increase in right ventricular pressure accompanied by a marked decrease in Pa$_{O_2}$ to anoxic levels. Both cardiac output and right heart pressure returned to normal gradually as a large amount of air dissipated into the pulmonary circulation.

Verstappen and coworkers,[25-28] in a series of seminal papers, experimented in dogs using air, O$_2$, N$_2$, and He. They found that after an intravenous gas injection, there was an acute obstruction of many branches of the pulmonary artery. Pulmonary artery pressure (PAP) rose to a maximum within 30 to 60 s and then

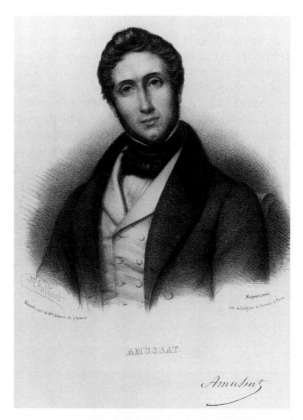

Figure 30-1   Jean Zulema Amussat (1844–1908). Surgeon during the Napoleonic Wars, physiologist, urologist, and inventor of a double-valved nasal ether inhaler. His book on venous air embolism (255 pages) published in *1839*, still remains a landmark as the most comprehensive exposition of the pathophysiology, diagnosis, and treatment of this problem.

(CVP). Because spontaneous inspiration reduces intrathoracic pressure, the gradient tends to increase with the tidal volume. A threshold exists for the transpulmonary passage of venous air emboli; this occurs at an infusion rate of 0.30 ml/kg per min in dogs and at 0.10 ml/kg per min in pigs.[16-18] The "spillover" increased as the pressure gradient across the pulmonary bed was augmented.[19] Hence, the volume of air moving through the portal of entry as well as the rate of entrainment may be critical in overwhelming the capacity of the lung to dissipate the air, or in the production of an air lock in the right side of the heart due to bubble coalescence and filming that increases surface tension. In 1981, Marquez and colleagues reported a death from VAE during a posterior fossa sitting-position procedure in a patient without an intracardiac septal defect.[20] Similarly, in 1991, Albin and coworkers reported a death during a lumbar laminectomy in the prone position where there was no septal defect[21]; large volumes of air were found in the brain, cardiac chambers, pulmonary vessels, and mesenteric vessels. Decreasing the CVP also helps to increase the pressure gradient, enhancing VAE; this may occur in the face of a con-

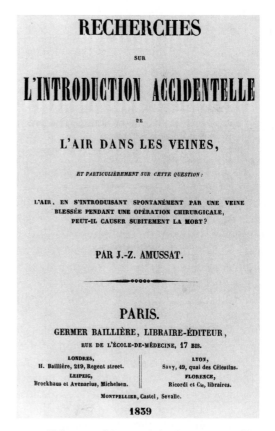

Figure 30-2   Title page of Amussat's book concerning "Research on the Accidental Introduction of Air Into the Veins." As a subtitle Amussat asks the question "If air is introduced spontaneously through a torn vein during a surgical operation can it cause sudden death?"

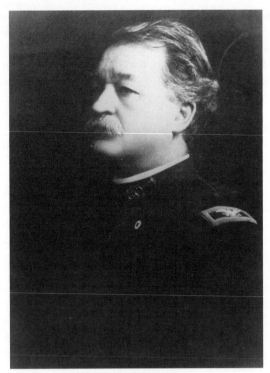

Nicholas Senn, M.D.
1844 - 1908

Figure 30-3 Nicholas Senn (1844–1908), Spanish-American War military surgeon, Professor of Surgery at the University of Chicago and Rush Medical College, author of *Principles of Surgery*, one of the first modern American books on surgical techniques and treatment (1890). His seminal paper on air embolism in 1885 ranks with Amussat's in its broad overview of this problem.

dropped to the original baseline value. The volume of gas determined the degree of obstruction; this was unrelated, however, to the type of gas used, with the exception of CO_2. The rate of disappearance of VAE depends on the diffusive property of the gas. Arterial oxygen tension falls dramatically after air embolization, and the degree of decrease in Pa_{O_2} is related to the volume of air in the right side of the heart. The decrease in end-tidal CO_2 ($ETCO_2$) tension and arterial oxygen tension is related to the amount but not to the type of gas injected, with the exception of CO_2, which, because of its very high blood solubility, produces a smaller effect from a given volume.

During venous gas infusion, PAP increases slowly, reaches a plateau, and, after termination of the infusion, returns to control levels. The rate of PAP increase depends on the rate of infusion and physical properties of the gas. The degree of embolization compatible with an efficient circulation is determined by the performance of the right ventricle. Decreases in alveolar CO_2 and in arterial oxygen tensions are observed. These are related to the increase in PAP, an index of elevated pulmonary vascular resistance.[25–28]

Adornato and coworkers[29] reported the cardiopulmonary effects of slow infusion versus a bolus injection of air into the external jugular veins of dogs. With slow infusion, there was a progressive increase in CVP, an abrupt increase in PAP to a plateau, a decrease in peripheral vascular resistance, and a compensatory increase in cardiac output. Blood pressure decreased moderately until decompensation occurred, at which point it dropped very sharply. The echocardiographic (ECG) changes consisted first of peaked P waves followed by ST-segment depression. Changes in heart sounds occurred only after significant cardiovascular decompensation and consisted first of a "drumlike" sound followed later by the classic mill-wheel murmur. A reflex gasp also occurred in animals breathing spontaneously, which appeared to be mediated by pulmonary receptors. During the gasp, a sudden decrease in CVP was seen, which potentially could draw additional air into the open vein. With injection of a large bolus of air, systolic PAP decreased, diastolic PAP and

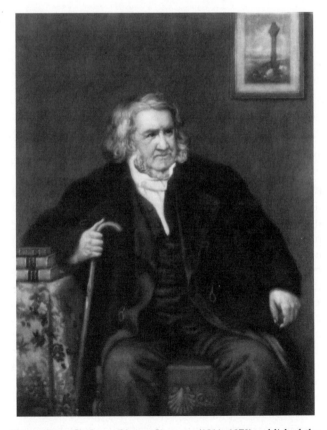

Figure 30-4 Sir James Young Simpson (1811–1870) published the first clinical papers on the use of chloroform as an anesthetic agent for surgery and obstetrics (1847). In earlier years he performed animal experiments on VAE working in the laboratory of John Rose Cormack in Edinburgh, Scotland. Cormack was a great contributor to our knowledge of the pathophysiology of venous air embolism, writing an important thesis "On the Presence of Air in the Organs of Circulation," in 1837.

pulmonary gas embolism. Berglund and Josephson[30] and Josephson and Ovenfors[31] demonstrated an increase in pulmonary air flow resistance and a decrease in dynamic lung compliance. These changes are similar to those observed after autologous thromboembolism, and Kahn and coworkers[32] showed that they can be blocked by the administration of heparin, producing thrombocytopenia, or by using serotonin antagonists. The proposed mechanism of airway constriction was related to thrombin-induced serotonin release from platelets.

As seen in the work of Verstappen and colleagues,[28] the more soluble the gas, the more diffusable it is in the blood; thus, embolization with CO_2 produces only minimal physiological disturbances compared with air. On the other hand, the differences in relative blood solubilities of the gases involved implies that some gases may diffuse more rapidly into than out of the bubbles, producing an increase in volume and augmenting the resulting physiologic dysfunction. Munson and Merrick[33] described a reduction of the quantity of gas required to produce physiologic alteration in the rabbit when N_2O was added to an inhaled halothane

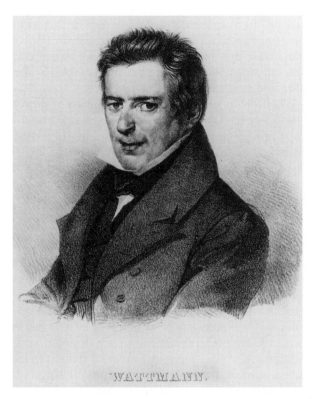

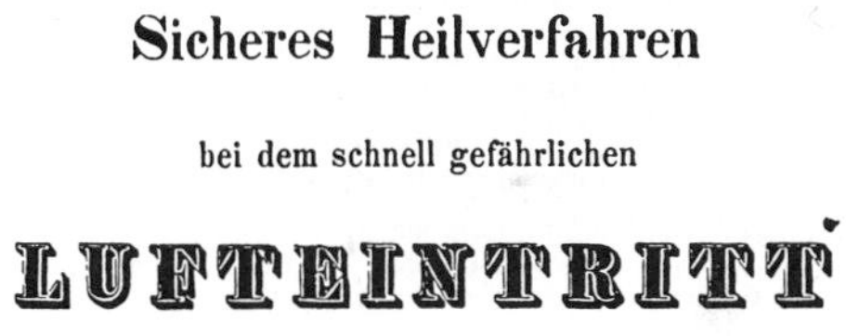

Figure 30-5   Karl Joseph von Wattmann (1789–1866), Professor of Surgery at the University of Innsbruck, Austria and then at the University of Vienna. His 188-page book on venous air embolism in 1843, "Certain Treatments for the Rapid and Dangerous Entrance of Air into the Veins" helped to pinpoint the surgical approach to dealing with a torn vein. He developed special hemostats to deal with this problem.

CVP increased, and systemic blood pressure fell dramatically. Postmortem studies demonstrated air in the right side of the heart. The authors concluded that cardiovascular collapse secondary to a slow infusion of air resulted from impairment of blood flow distal to the pulmonary artery because of air in the lungs, whereas decompensation following a bolus of air was caused by an air lock in the right heart that prevented effective cardiac output. Both mechanisms may be operative when VAE occurs in the operating room.

The effect of gas emoblism on respiration was also evaluated by Verstappen and collaborators.[26] During spontaneous ventilation, gas embolism produced a compensatory increase in minute volume depending on the degree of embolization. During controlled ventilation, pulmonary gas exchange was affected in relation to the extent of embolization; there was a decrease in end tidal O_2, a decrease in Pa_{O_2}, and an increase in Pa_{CO_2}. Increasing artificial ventilation improved the washout of CO_2 but did not affect the uptake of oxygen.

Pulmonary mechanics are also severely altered by

Sicheres Heilverfahren

bei dem schnell gefährlichen

LUFTEINTRITT

in die Venen

und dessen gerichtsärztliche Wichtigkeit.

———◆◆◆———

Von

Dr. Ch. Jos. Edl. v. Wattmann,

k. k. n. ö. Regierungsrathe, Leibchirurg, o. ö. Professor
der praktischen Chirurgie und der ersten chirurgischen
Klinik, Vorsteher des Operations-Institutes an der k. k.
Universität in Wien, und Mitgliede mehrerer
gelehrten Gesellschaften.

Mit einer chlographischen Tafel.

Wien, 1843.

Bei Braumüller und Seidel.
Graben, Sparkassegebäude.

Figure 30-6   Title page of Wattmann's book on air embolism published in 1843.

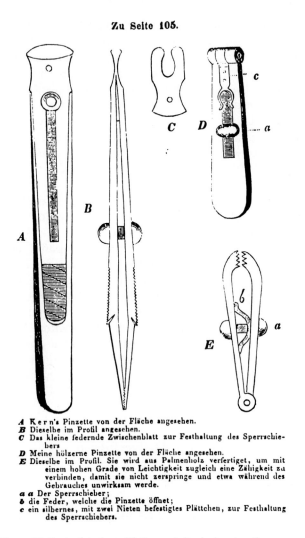

Zu Seite 105.

A Kern's Pinzette von der Fläche angesehen.
B Dieselbe im Profil angesehen.
C Das kleine federnde Zwischenblatt zur Festhaltung des Sperrschiebers
D Meine hölzerne Pinzette von der Fläche angesehen.
E Dieselbe im Profil. Sie wird aus Palmenholz verfertiget, um mit einem hohen Grade von Leichtigkeit zugleich eine Zähigkeit zu verbinden, damit sie nicht zerspringe und etwa während des Gebrauches unwirksam werde.
a a Der Sperrschieber;
b die Feder, welche die Pinzette öffnet;
c ein silbernes, mit zwei Nieten befestigtes Plättchen, zur Festhaltung des Sperrschiebers.

Figure 30-7 A plate from Wattmann's book showing the different hemostats used to clamp a torn vein. *D* shows a frontal view of the clamp and *E* illustrates a profile of Wattmann's instrument.

mixture. This was due to the differences in solubility between N_2O and O_2 in blood; because N_2O is nearly 35 times more soluble than N_2, the bubble volume increased owing to the large partial pressure gradient. At 50% inspired concentration of N_2O and O_2, air entering the circulation doubles in volume. Along the same lines, Presson and coworkers[34] reported an increase in bubble size when He or N_2O was added to the ventilating gases during air injection.

Similar physiologic consequences of VAE have been noted by other workers. Black and coworkers[35] noted that with venous air infusion in pigs, increases were seen in right atrial pressure (RAP), systolic and diastolic PAP, and pulmonary capillary wedge pressure (PCWP). Changes in left atrial pressure (LAP) varied; the rate of change of this parameter was significantly less than that of the PCWP. These animals also had

surgically created atrial septal defects to investigate the occurrence of paradoxical air embolism (PAE); it was noted that mean systemic arterial pressure was generally unchanged during VAE unless PAE occurred and produced myocardial ischemia.

When air in the pulmonary circulation, a decrease in alveolar P_{CO_2} and an increase in alveolar P_{N_2} occurs.[36] Impaired gas exchange due to ventilation/perfusion mismatch leads to a decrease in Pa_{O_2} and an increase in Pa_{CO_2}; pulmonary edema may also be seen.[37–40] If small amounts of air are infused, they may be eliminated by the lungs. The air bubbles lodge in pulmonary arterioles and diffuse across the arteriolar wall into the alveolar spaces.[41]

Large volumes of air may cross from the venous to the arterial system through known cardiac defects (such as an atrial septal defect) or through a probe patent foramen ovale (PFO) in patients without known cardiac disease.[42,43] The overall incidence of PFO in autopsy specimens has been noted to be 27.3 percent; thus, a fairly high percentage of the population is at risk for PAE.[43] The mean diameter of the PFO across all age groups was noted in the study of Hagen and coworkers to be approximately 5 mm.[43] Contrast echocardiography has been used to identify the presence of PFO.[44–48] Preoperative precordial echocardiography may be used as a screening method to determine which patients are at risk for PAE through a PFO. In a series of 101 neurosurgical patients, Black and colleagues[44] noted that the incidence of PFO on preoperative echocardiography was less than expected in the general population. In addition, an episode of PAE occurred in one patient, although no evidence of PFO was noted on preoperative testing. The authors concluded that the usefulness of preoperative echocardiography as a screening test may be limited. However, if a PFO is found on preoperative testing, this provides valuable information for patient management. Intraoperatively, transesophageal echocardiography is useful in determining the presence of right-to-left shunting in patients with PFO, and if a VAE occurs, it can establish the diagnosis of PAE.[45] A transcranial Doppler probe over the middle cerebral artery can image any microemboli liberated during contrast injection into the right atrium.[49] Concomitant use of echocardiography can determine the presence of PFO.

Another factor to be considered in the pathophysiology of PAE is the gradient between the right and left atria. There has been concern that factors that increase RAP relative to LAP increase the likelihood of PAE once VAE occurs.[50] In some patients, placement in the sitting position has been shown to result in an RAP greater than PCWP.[50,51] Application of positive end-expiratory pressure (PEEP) may also elevate RAP enough to exceed PCWP.[50] PEEP had previously been

TABLE 30-2
Incidence of Venous Air Embolism in the Sitting Position

Author	Year	No. of Patients	Percent Air
Michenfelder et al.[115]	1972	69	31.8
Tateishi[128]	1972	36	22.2
Millar[127]	1972	110	2.0
Albin et al.[14,96]	1976	400	25.0
Buckland and Manners[129]	1976	36	33.0
Davis et al.[149]	1977	156	60.0
Bedford et al.[104]	1981	100	35.0
Voorhies et al.[53]	1983	81	50.0
Standefer et al.[57]	1984	332	7.0
Matjasko et al.[55]	1985	554	22.0
Young et al.[58]	1986	255	30.0
Guggiari et al.[111]	1988	189	19.0

advocated as a means of prevention and acute treatment of VAE.[52,53] Its effectiveness was thought to be related to an increase in CVP so that air is less likely to be entrained. However, it has been demonstrated that PEEP may not be an effective method of increasing CVP.[54] Also, Black and associates[35] demonstrated in an animal model that although the application of PEEP is not associated with an increased incidence of PAE compared with other modes of ventilation, the release of PEEP frequently results in an increase in the amount of PAE or in new PAE. In view of the concerns about the effectiveness of PEEP in preventing or treating VAE and the possible increased risk of PAE, the use of PEEP is generally not recommended. If PAE does occur, it may result in serious coronary and cerebral ischemic complications. Arrhythmias, S-T segment changes, wallmotion abnormalities, and other evidence of myocardial ischemia may be seen with PAE in the coronary circulation.[35] Cerebral arterial air embolism may present clinically when air bubbles are visualized in the cerebral arterial tree, when electroencephalographic changes are noted intraoperatively, or when unexplained postoperative neurologic deficits occur.

Incidence

There are no reliable data on the overall incidence of VAE. The general exception to this statement is the large number of studies of VAE during neurosurgical procedures in the sitting position, indicating an overall incidence of about 24 percent (Table 30-2).[55-58] The past 20 years have brought an increasing awareness that VAE can occur in procedures other than neurosurgery.[3] This is especially true in obstetrics, where the exteri-

orized uterus may provide the gravitational gradient for air entrainment during cesarean sections.[59] In three studies, air was detected with the precordial Doppler in 10 to 47 percent of patients.[60-62]

Venous air embolism has been reported during hip procedures and other orthopedic surgery[21,63-66]; hysterectomy[67]; orogenital sex play during pregnancy[69]; urologic procedures including transvesical and retrograde radical prostatectomy[69-74]; transurethral resections, retrograde pyelography, and percutaneous nephrolithotomy; abdominal procedures[75,76]; trauma[77,78]; craniofacial and head and neck procedures[79,80]; catheterization, shunting, and endoscopy[81-85]; transfusion and fluid infusion[15]; otologic procedures[86,87]; pulmonary vascular embolism in the newborn[88]; and liver transplantation.[89,90] Even in neurosurgery, Albin and coworkers have reported that VAE may occur in the supine, prone, and lateral positions with gravitational gradients as small as 5.0 cm (Table 30-3).[14] Additionally, reports have surfaced of VAE after the use of H_2O_2 for wound irrigation and pulsed saline pressure-powered irrigation.[91-94]

Signs and Symptoms

The signs and symptoms of VAE may include gasping respiration in spontaneously breathing patients, increased CVP and PAP, arrhythmias, ECG changes, hypotension, abnormal heart sounds, alteration of heart rate (both tachycardia and bradycardia), decreased peripheral resistance, a change in cardiac output, and cyanosis. Figure 30-8 indicates the thresholds for the earliest changes in the parameters monitored in terms of milliliters per kilogram^{-1} per minute^{-1} of air infused

TABLE 30-3
Incidence of Venous Air Embolism in the Sitting, Lateral, Supine, and Prone Positions

Position	No. Patients	DETECTABLE AIR EMBOLISM No. cases	DETECTABLE AIR EMBOLISM Percent	Amount of Air Aspirated (ml)	Gradient (cm)
Sitting	400	100	25.0	2–500	20–65
Lateral	60	5[a]	8.3	3–200	5–18
Supine	48	7[b]	14.6	2–150	5–18
Prone	10	1[c]	10.0	45	7.5
Totals	518	113			

[a] Two cases, tic douloureux; two cases, hemifacial spasm; one case, tumor.

[b] Three cases, transsphenoidal hypophysectomy; three cases, intracranial tumor; and one case, tic douloureux (air was detected after reapplication of the pin head holder with the patient in the supine position before the patient was put in the sitting position).

[c] Ependymoma of the spinal cord.

SOURCE: Reproduced by permission from Albin and coworkers.[14]

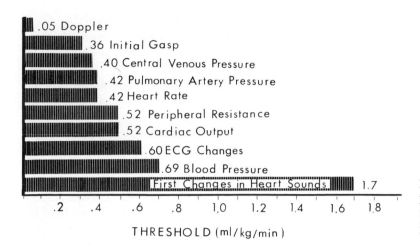

.05 Doppler
.36 Initial Gasp
.40 Central Venous Pressure
.42 Pulmonary Artery Pressure
.42 Heart Rate
.52 Peripheral Resistance
.52 Cardiac Output
.60 ECG Changes
.69 Blood Pressure
First Changes in Heart Sounds   1.7

THRESHOLD (ml/kg/min)

Figure 30-8 Thresholds for detection of various physiologic responses after air injection in animals. (Reproduced by permission from Frost E: Anesthesia for neurosurgical procedures in the sitting position. Lesson 4:1, 1977; *Weekly Anesthesia Update.*)

in the dog. It is important to note that the most *insensitive* parameter was the earliest change in heart sounds, indicating that this is a poor warning sign. The millwheel murmur was described quite accurately by the early pioneers of VAE treatment (see Table 30-1). It is caused by agitation of blood and air in the right ventricle and it is often not heard at all or is audible for only a short period of time. The entrance of air into the pulmonary vasculature produces severe pulmonary perfusion deficits in humans, as noted by Albin and coworkers using technetium-macroaggregated albumin scans[14] (Fig. 30-9).

Monitoring and Diagnosis

PRECORDIAL DOPPLER (Figure 30-10)

The ultrasonic Doppler technique has opened a new era in rapid, sensitive monitoring for air and air vol-

umes as small as 0.10 ml may be detected passing the sensor and we all owe a debt for Maroon and Edmonds-Seal for their pioneering effort in developing this modality.[95-103] The performance of the Doppler is generally related to correct placement of the transducer, usually over the third to sixth intercostal space to the right of the sternum. The Doppler signal caused by air entrainment is qualitative and does not indicate the quantity of air passing the beam. Although false-positive rates have been described, the more important false-negative rate has been shown to be 3 percent.[104]

The excellent reliability of the precordial Doppler in the detection of air bubbles was also noted by Fong and coworkers, who monitored patients undergoing cesarean section in the horizontal position using two-dimensional echocardiography and a precordial Doppler.[105] They found a perfect correlation between the precordial Doppler and echocardiography (k value = 1) in the 49 patients in the study, with an incidence of

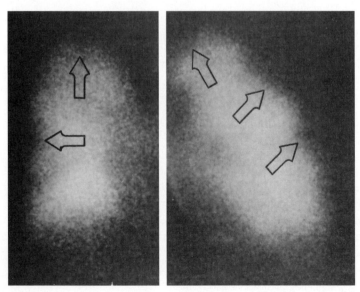

A   B

Figure 30-9 Technetium-macroaggregated albumin lung scans after the rapid entry (over a 30-min period) of a moderate amount of air (150 ml was aspirated through the central line) from the venous system during a neurosurgical procedure. Right (*A*) and left (*B*) lung scans taken 5 h after termination of surgery. The arrows indicate areas of scalloping along the lateral and medial aspects of both lungs fields. The lesions are segmental and multiple. (Reproduced by permission from Albin and coworkers.[14])

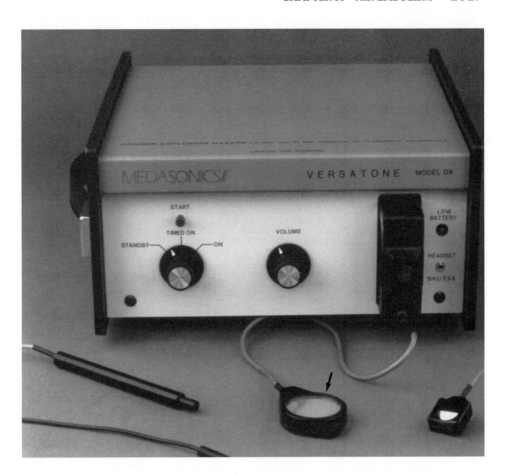

Figure 30-10 The Medasonic's Versatone® Doppler with various ultrasonic probes. The round precordial transducer is identified with the arrow. (Reproduced by permission from Medasonics, Fremont, CA)

VAE of 29 percent (14 of 49). Equally important, the emboli detected by the precordial Doppler were air bubbles and not signals characteristic of amniotic fluid or thromboemboli. Gibby has noted that the sensitivity of the precordial Doppler for air bubble detection lies in the same range as that of the transesophageal echocardiograph.[106] Although the precordial Doppler has excellent sensitivity and reliability, there is a time lag between the moment of Doppler activation with an auditory signal and manual aspiration of the central line. Thus, small volumes of air may pass the tip of the central line and enter the right atrium before aspiration is performed. Using a computerized pattern-recognition technique, Gibby developed an automated unit that gave a signal alarm in the presence of air, allowing the anesthesiologist to concentrate on other aspects of patient management without often losing or missing the elusive "chirp" characteristic of air.[107]

It is important for the beam pattern of the Doppler transducer to cover the right atrium completely with a depth of field that compensates for positional changes. One must ensure the presence of efficient radio frequency filtering, so that the signal is not lost while the electrocautery is being used. We have found the Versatone® unit to be highly effective (see Fig. 30-10)

(Medasonics, Fremont, CA). Figure 30-11 indicates the sensitivity of the precordial Doppler compared with other monitoring modalities.

TRANSESOPHAGEAL DOPPLER

Martin and Colley[108] developed a transesophageal Doppler probe containing a 360° transducer that was tested in animals. Their probe had good sensitivity with an ultrasonic output safe for biologic tissues. With this type of probe it would be possible to avoid the chest configuration problems that may affect the precordial Doppler, and by placing another probe at the appropriate location, it would also be possible to monitor the right and left sides of the heart simultaneously with a relatively inexpensive device.

END-EXPIRATORY CO₂

End-expiratory CO_2 is an effective and practical method of detecting VAE and the detectors have virtually eliminated the problem of interference by moisture buildup.[97,98,104,109] There is a decrease in ET_{CO_2} as air enters the circulatory system. Routine, continuous ET_{CO_2} monitoring, either with a dedicated device or as part of a

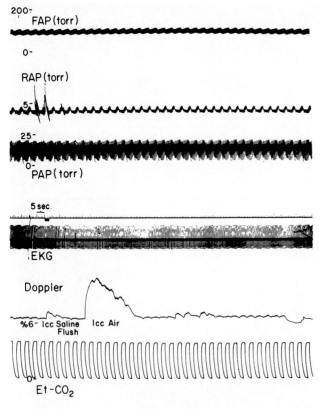

Figure 30-11 Comparison of sensitivity of monitoring techniques after injection of 1.0 ml saline and 1.0 ml air. Only the Doppler responds; the other parameters are unchanged. Et-CO$_2$, end-tidal P$_{CO_2}$; FAP, femoral artery pressure; PAP, pulmonary artery pressure; RAP, right atrial pressure. (Reproduced by permission from Chang JL and coworkers.[98])

mass spectroscopic unit, has become part of the standard of care during general anesthesia in the United States. It may permit detection of air embolism even in unexpected situations, such as when small gravitational gradients are present.

PULMONARY ARTERY PRESSURE

Munson and coworkers first reported the use of a pulmonary artery catheter for VAE detection in 1975, when they noted an increase in PAP accompanied by a decrease in ET$_{CO_2}$.[56] Marshall and Bedford found PAP increases to be sensitive to the presence of air but noted that precordial Doppler was superior in sensitivity.[110] In 1981, Bedford and coworkers noted that the PAP sensitivity to VAE was no greater than that of the ET$_{CO_2}$.[104] The small lumen of the pulmonary artery catheter at its atrial port, and the invasive character of this modality, makes its usefulness limited. Of interest was the finding by Chang and colleagues that propranolol could block the rise in PAP seen with the injection of a 20.0 ml bolus of air in dogs[98] (Fig. 30-12).

TRANSESOPHAGEAL ECHOCARDIOGRAPHY

Transesophageal echocardiography can be a useful tool for evaluating the presence of a PFO and visualizing air in the heart chambers.[111] It has been validated in both animal and human studies.[112,113] The limitations of transesophageal echocardiography lie in the need for an experienced interpreter and its costliness.

CENTRAL VENOUS PRESSURE

The CVP increases with air entry into the pulmonary circulation and the increased pulmonary vascular resistance resulting from release of vasoactive substances.[32,98] When large volumes of air enter the right atrium, an air lock that impedes venous return to the heart may be produced that causes an increase in CVP.

CENTRAL VENOUS CATHETER

Absolute verification of VAE depends on the ability to aspirate air from a previously injected central line. The use of a catheter in the right atrium for air aspiration and detection was first introduced by Michenfelder and coworkers in 1966.[114,115]

An effective design that allows for maximal air aspiration was achieved with the development of the multiorificed catheter, the effectiveness of which was verified in animal studies. Using a cast of a human right atrium to mimic some of the in vivo right atrial hemodynamic characteristics, Bunegin and coworkers compared the air aspiration characteristics of a 16-gauge multiorificed catheter at atrial inclinations of 60°, 80°, and 90° from the horizontal.[116] Optimal air aspiration occurred with the multiorificed tip positioned approxi-

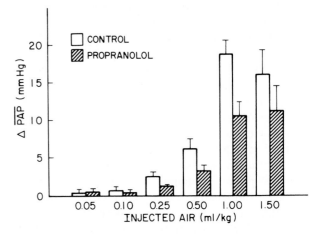

Figure 30-12 Net changes in PAP after venous air embolism in animals with and without β-adrenergic receptor blockade (propranolol). The PAP of the propranolol-treated group is significantly lower than that of the control group at levels of 0.25, 0.5, and 1.0 ml air/kg ($p = <.05$). (Reproduced by permission from Chang and coworkers.[98])

mately 2 cm below the junction of the superior vena cava and the atrium at an inclination of 80°, and as much as 80 percent of the incoming air could be aspirated. In animal studies, Colley and Artru showed that the multiorificed air aspiration catheter[116] had superior air aspiration qualities when compared to the single-orifice catheter.[118] To attenuate clot development the multiorificed catheter developed by Bunegin and coworkers has been heparin bonded. Using a 7 F single-orifice flow-directed catheter in the right atrial model, Bunegin and Albin were able to aspirate greater than 90 percent of the air at 80° inclination when the balloon was inflated but only 27 percent with the balloon down.[117] The multiorificed catheter is generally inserted from the antecubital fossa, preferably through the basilic (medial) vein, which is associated with a higher incidence of success than is the cephalic vein in passing to the superior vena cava.

The ECG trace may be used to assist in the proper positioning of the catheter by attaching it to an ECG lead. Leaving the wire in place or filling the catheter with sodium bicarbonate solution generally improves the quality of the trace. Characteristic P-wave changes may be seen as the catheter is advanced. As described by Cucchiara and associates, when the lead V is used, the P wave will initially be small with a negative deflection.[119] As the catheter tip approaches the right atrium, the P wave becomes progressively more negative until the right atrium is entered, at which point a small positive deflection is seen. When the catheter is in the midatrium, the P wave is large and biphasic. The catheter is then withdrawn so that an all-negative P wave is again seen, indicating that the catheter tip is again within the superior vena cava.[120,121] The optimal location for air aspiration has been demonstrated by Bunegin and colleagues in an in vitro model of the human right atrium.[116] They noted that the maximal yield resulted when the end of a single-orificed catheter was just above the junction of the superior vena cava and right atrium and when the distal tip of the multiorificed catheter was just below this level. A chest radiograph may be used to confirm the location of the catheter or the ECG trace may be used as described above. It should be kept in mind that the ECG trace from a multiorificed catheter may originate proximal to the distal tip (2.5 ± 0.6 cm) for the Bunegin-Albin air aspiration kit (Cook Inc, Bloomington, IN).[122] The central line has a tendency to migrate into the atrium when the patient is placed in the sitting position and this may necessitate a slight withdrawal of the catheter after positioning.[123] Because of the problem of catheter migration, one should consider taking a chest radiograph in the supine position and then with the patient sitting up after catheter insertion. The catheter position can also be checked by attaching the line to a strain gauge and an elevated pressure trace (15 to 30 mmHg) indicates the catheter has migrated to the right ventricle.[123] Positioning the catheter using the Doppler activation as an indication of proper atrial placement (the Tinker test)[124] can lead to false-positive results because Doppler activation can occur with the catheter tip placed high up in the superior vena cava.

There is a fairly high incidence of success in placing CVP catheters from the antecubital fossa. Smith and coworkers reported a 91 percent success rate in the placement of a catheter system equipped with a J-wire guide (Cook Bunegin-Albin air aspiration kit).[125] When the antecubital route is not successful, however, other methods of central access are used. These methods include cannulation of the subclavian, internal, and external jugular veins and the femoral vein in selected pediatric patients.

In a recent report, Albin and coworkers presented three cases of VAE during lumbar laminectomy in the prone position.[21] In one patient, the precordial Doppler indicated air bubbles passing the probe that could not be readily aspirated with the multiorificed catheter. Although the lag time between Doppler air bubble detection and catheter aspiration can be a factor in explaining this failure, it is possible that the volume of air obtained by catheter aspiration may be decreased in the prone position because of layering of air above the level of the catheter tip. Bunegin and Albin have carried out bench experiments (unreported) with the right atrial model in the horizontal (supine) plane, which suggest that a reduction in aspiration efficiency occurs in both the single and multiorificed catheters. This appears primarily to be due to the sinking of the higher density (relative to blood) catheters, whereas buoyancy keeps the air emboli floating near the upper surface of both the superior vena cava and the right atrium. Some improvement in aspirating air in this position was observed when a balloon-tipped single-orifice catheter was used. After balloon inflation with 0.75 to 1 ml air, the catheter floated to the upper surface, positioning itself among the air bubbles and permitting better aspiration. Artru demonstrated the difficulty in obtaining air aspiration in the prone position in animals when air entered via the inferior vena cava.[126] It is possible though that the presence of an aspirating atrial catheter may be able to prevent an air lock from developing.

In addition to the fact that routine monitoring for VAE is not carried out during spine surgery, our lack of knowledge of the actual incidence of VAE has been exacerbated by the malpractice crisis. In general, outcomes involving serious morbidity or death that are in the process of litigation are *now rarely reported in the medical literature even when the legal process has been terminated for a considerable period of time.* In talks and telephone conversations with anesthesiologists in many parts of the United States subsequent to the publication of this paper, it was astounding to find that the problem of VAE during spine surgery was encountered by many of our colleagues during the past decade and *never* reported. It is important that this problem be addressed because we are being lulled into a false sense of security, resulting in a skewed incidence rate of this complication.

ELECTROCARDIOGRAM

Electrocardiographic changes can occur with VAE, especially when large volumes of air are involved. These changes may include bradycardia, premature ventricular contractions, ST-T wave depression, variability of the P wave, and heart block.[96,127,128] ECG changes were shown to occur in 40 percent of the cases in which VAE was accompanied by Doppler signals.[129]

AIRWAY PRESSURE

The development of airway constriction after VAE is followed by a decrease in ventilatory compliance. Sloan and Kimovec reported a case of VAE[130] with the patient in the sitting position. Coincident with Doppler activation, a decrease in ET_{CO_2}, peak airway pressure increased from a stable baseline of 19.0 to a maximum of 25.0 mmHg. VAE was confirmed by the aspiration of 27 ml air from a central catheter. It has been described in animal studies that airway pressure, lung compliance and airway resistance are affected by VAE at volumes of 0.2 cc/kg,[32] which is similar for changes induced by VAE for ET_{CO_2}.

ARTERIAL BLOOD PRESSURE

Systemic arterial hypotension is a relatively late sign after VAE and in itself does not have the sensitivity necessary for early, rapid detection of VAE.[98]

TRANSCRANIAL DOPPLER (Fig. 30-13)

This monitoring modality has been used to access the velocity of flow in both intracranial and extracranial blood vessels. Recent experimental work has also demonstrated the ability of the transcranial Doppler both to detect and to differentiate small quantities of air (<0.8 μl) from particulate matter circulating in the middle cerebral artery of the rhesus monkey.[49] In the human, the transcranial Doppler has been able to detect air coursing through the middle cerebral artery during CPB procedures. The transcranial Doppler may serve as an ancillary monitor in detecting PAE through the pulmonary circulation or a PFO.

In general, it appears that the keystone to reliable,

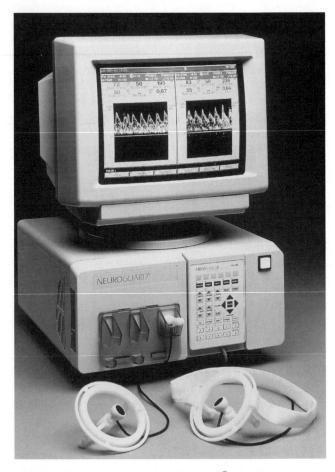

Figure 30-13 The Medasonic's Neuroguard® transcranial Doppler. This unit is equipped with bilateral probes which lie inside the probe holders that can be seen in front of the unit. (Reproduced by permission from Medasonics, Fremont, CA)

sensitive, and practical detection of VAE lies in the use of the precordial Doppler and ET_{CO_2} monitors combined with a previously inserted multiorificed catheter of which the tip lies in the superior vena cava just distal to its entrance into the right atrium. The use of end-tidal N_2 (ET_{N_2}) monitoring necessitates low total gas flows, an ET_{N_2} scale range of 2% or less, and very frequent gas sampling.[131] Transcutaneous CO_2 and O_2, Pa_{O_2} and Pa_{CO_2}, and changes in respiratory patterns all appear to indicate relatively late developments after air entrainment.[99,104,113] Finally, the detection of aberrant sounds with esophageal stethoscope (e.g., mill-wheel murmur) during an episode of VAE is a very late phenomenon and indicates that a considerable amount of air has entered the circulation[1,5,29] (see Fig. 30-8).

Treatment

The hallmark for treatment of VAE lies in early detection, rapid aspiration from the central line, and whenever possible, sealing off the source of air entry.[104] Air aspiration through a multiorificed catheter can help in the presence of an air lock caused by large volumes of air and will also decrease the amount of air entering the pulmonary circulation. This author well remembers aspirating more than 200 ml of air foam over a period of 3 min in a patient having a posterior fossa exploration in the lateral position with a 5.0-cm gradient.[14]

When large volumes of air have been entrained, it is sometimes necessary to aspirate several hundred milliliters of blood to capture the air, and this act may certainly produce blood volume depletion. It is our practice to use large syringes for aspiration, each one containing 3 or 4 ml heparinized saline. In the event that the deaerated blood is returned to the patient, the heparinized saline will avoid activation of clotting factors.

When VAE is apparent, in addition to central line aspiration, the surgeon should be notified, N_2O turned off, and the patient placed on 100% O_2. At a 50% concentration of O_2–N_2O, the volume of the entrained air is doubled.[33] It is our practice not to use N_2O at all in the sitting-position cases or during procedures in which a significant gravitational gradient exists. In the presence of continued VAE, the use of very brief bilateral internal jugular compression will allow the surgeon to find the open veins or sinuses.[114,132] The inflation of a previously applied neck tourniquet has been advocated by Sale as a method of visualizing the site of air entrance.[133] This technique may be hazardous in a patient with significant preexisting intracranial hypertension. Controversy has arisen as to whether decreasing the gradient by using PEEP to raise the CVP is effective in stopping air entrainment. This rise in CVP may decrease the gravitational gradient but may also increase the chance of PAE developing, as the RAP may become higher than LAP, permitting a shunt to develop in the presence of a probe PFO.[51]

Pneumocephalus occurs frequently during procedures in the posterior fossa, and the cortex may be partially displaced by the air bubble. The air can often be readily identified over the frontal lobes by skull radiography with the patient supine. Cases of tension pneumocephalus have been reported in which release of the pressure resulted in immediate improvement.[134–137] Whether or not N_2O should be used when pneumocephalus formation is a possibility remains a controversial issue.[138–140] This author has not used N_2O during neuroanesthetic procedures for many years.

Symptomatic treatment of VAE should be initiated as needed, including volume expanders and vasopressors for persistent hypotension. It was thought that the use of the left lateral decubitus position as described by Durant and colleagues[141] would improve cardiac output and venous return because the heart is dependent, thus decreasing the possibility of air moving through a PFO. Unfortunately, the work of Mehlhorn and coworkers[142] indicates that this position has minimal effect on outcome after VAE.

The diagnosis of cerebral air embolism after PAE or VAE overflowing the pulmonary circulation may not be easy to make. In patients undergoing a surgical procedure during which the possibility of VAE is present or where VAE has been diagnosed, one must suspect cerebral air embolism in the event the patient remains comatose past the expected time of emergence from anesthesia or awakens with a neurologic deficit. Under these conditions, a magnetic resonance imaging scan should be performed to detect whether intraaxial air is present. If cerebral air embolism is considered likely, the patient should be taken to a hyperbaric chamber and treatment started using the U.S. Navy Dive Table.[143] Cerebral air embolism has been reported as a complication of CPB in 0.12 to 0.14 percent of cases. Hyperbaric oxygenation appears to be the treatment of choice for cerebral air embolism, with the best outcome resulting from early recognition and early treatment.[143–148]

Summary

Air embolism is a subtle and ever-possible scourge during medical and surgical procedures and can result in severe morbidity and even mortality. Gravitational gradients as small as 5 cm may cause the entrainment of air from an open vein or sinus into the dependent heart. The adage "out of sight, out of mind" appears to be applicable to this problem because our perceptions are blinded, as anesthesiologists generally associate air embolism *only* with neurosurgical cases carried out in the *sitting position*. We are also blinded by our lack of a knowledge of history, because before the twentieth century, literally hundreds of cases of VAE in nonneurosurgical procedures were described in the medical literature.

The entrance of air into the venous circulation can start a process in which small volumes may coalesce in the right side of the heart owing to surface tension, break up because of the pumping action of the heart, and then vent through the lungs out of the body. When the entrained volume is large, an air lock may develop, impede venous return, and either pass directly through the pulmonary circulation and out through the lungs or, if there is a probe PFO, move into the left atrium and from there into the coronary sinuses, brain, and arterial circulation. Air may also move across the pulmonary bed into the left side of the heart when the filtering ability of the lungs is overwhelmed.

Signs of VAE include, in the order of increasing

severity, a change in the Doppler heart tones; a decrease in ET_{CO_2}; increases in CVP and PAP; hypotension, tachycardia or bradycardia; alterations in peripheral resistance, cardiac output, and the ECG; and the development of a mill-wheel murmur. This latter sign occurs last and indicates that a substantial quantity of air has entered the heart chambers. The key to the treatment of VAE lies in the ability to recognize it before hemodynamic problems occur and the precordial Doppler air bubble detector appears to have the greatest sensitivity, followed by ET_{CO_2} monitoring. A multiorificed central venous catheter of which the tip is 1 cm past the superior vena cava-atrial junction provides the best opportunity to aspirate air and thus to prevent or break up an air lock. If VAE is suspected, N_2O should be discontinued and the patient put on 100 percent O_2. At an O_2/N_2O ratio of 1 : 1, the volume of the embolus doubles as N_2O replaces the N_2 in the air bubble. If a patient suspected of having had a VAE remains comatose after a surgical procedure or awakens with a neurologic dysfunction, the possibility of cerebral air embolism must be considered, resulting from either PAE or passage of air through the pulmonary circulation to the left side of the heart. Under these circumstances, the central nervous system should be examined by computed tomography or magnetic resonance imaging for intraaxial brain or spinal cord air. The finding of intraaxial air may then necessitate treatment with hyperbaric oxygenation.

The key, though, in handling the problem of VAE can best be described in two Latin words *Praemonitus, Praemunitus,* "Forewarned is Forearmed."

References

1. Senn N: An experimental and clinical study of air embolism. *Surg Ann* 1885; 2:197.
2. Albin MS: The sights and sounds of air. *Anesthesiology* 1983; 58:113 (editorial).
3. Albin MS, et al: Venous air embolism is not restricted to neurosurgery! *Anesthesiology* 1983; 59:151 (letter).
4. Albin MS, Robinson D: Amussat (1796–1856) and Senn (1844–1908): The holy duo of venous air embolism. In Atkinson RS, Boulton RB (eds): *The History of Anaesthesia.* London, Royal Society Medical Services, 1989:539.
5. Amussat JZ: *Recherches sur l'Introduction Accidentelle de l'Air Dans les Veines.* Paris, Germer Bailliere, 1839:255.
6. Barlow M: An attempt to remove a tumor on the neck: Entrance of air in vein. Sudden death. *Med Chir Trans* 1930; 16:28.
7. Cormack JR: *On the Presence of Air in the Organs of Circulation* (thesis). Edinburg, John Carfrae and Son, 1837:56.
8. Cormack JR: The entrance of air by the open mouths of the uterine veins, considered as a cause of danger and death after parturition. *London Med J* 1850; 2:928.
9. Erichsen JE: On the proximate cause of death after spontaneous introduction of air into the veins, with some remarks on the treatment of the accident. *Edinburgh Med Surg J* 1944; 61:1.
10. Legallois E: Des maladies occasionees par la resorbtion de pus. *J Hebdomonaire Med* 1829; 3:166.
11. Lesky E: Notes on the history of air embolism. *Ger Med Monthly* 1961; 6:159.
12. Warren JC: Two cases of accidents, from admission of air into the veins during surgical operations. *J Med Sci* 1852; 20:545.
13. Wattmann CS: *Sicheres Heilverfahren bei dem Schnell Gefahrlichen Lufteintritt in die Venen und Dessen Gerichtsarztliche Wichtigkeit.* Vienna, Braumuller und Seidel, 1843:188.
14. Albin MS, et al: Clinical considerations concerning detection of venous air embolism. *Neurosurgery* 1978; 3:380.
15. Yeakel AE: Lethal air embolism from plastic storage container. *JAMA* 1968; 204:267.
16. Butler BD, Hills BA: The lung as a filter for microbubbles. *J Appl Physiol* 1979; 47:537.
17. Butler BD, Hills BA: Transpulmonary passage of venous air emboli. *J Appl Physiol* 1985; 59:543.
18. Vik A, et al: Venous air embolism in swine; transport of gas bubbles through the pulmonary circulation. *J Appl Physiol* 1990; 69:237.
19. Butler BD, Katz J: Vascular pressures and passage of gas emboli through the pulmonary circulation. *Undersea Biomed Res* 1988; 15:203.
20. Marquez J, et al: Paradoxical cerebral air embolism without an intracardiac septal defect. *J Neurosurg* 1981; 55:997.
21. Albin MS, et al: Venous air embolism during lumbar laminectomy in the prone position: Report of three cases. *Anesth Analg* 1991; 73:346.
22. DiStefano VJ, et al: Intraoperative analysis of the effects of position and body habitus on surgery of the low back. *Clin Orthop* 1974; 99:51.
23. Shenkin HN, Goldfedder P: Air embolism from exposure of posterior cranial fossa in prone position. *JAMA* 1969; 210:726.
24. Deal CW, et al: Hemodynamic effects of pulmonary air embolism. *J Surg Res* 1971; 11:533.
25. Verstappen FT, et al: Effects of pulmonary gas embolism on circulation and respiration in the dog. 1. Effects on circulation. *Pflugers Arch* 1977; 368:89.
26. Verstappen FT, et al: Effects of pulmonary gas embolism on circulation and respiration in the dog. 2. Effects on respiration. *Pflugers Arch* 1977; 368:97.
27. Verstappen FT, et al: Excretion of venous gas bubbles by the lung. *Pflugers Arch* 1977; 370:67.
28. Verstappen FT, et al: Origin of arterial hypoxemia during pulmonary gas embolism. *Pflugers Arch* 1977; 370:71.
29. Adornato DC, et al: Pathophysiology of intravenous air embolism in dogs. *Anesthesiology* 1978; 49:120.
30. Berglund E, Josephson S: Pulmonary air embolism: Physiological aspects. *Thorax* 1969; 24:509.
31. Josephson S, Ovenfors CO: Pulmonary air embolism: Radiological changes. *Thorax* 1969; 24:509.
32. Kahn MA, et al: Acute changes in lung mechanics following emboli of various gases in dogs. *J Appl Physiol* 1972; 33:774.
33. Munson ES, et al: Effect of nitrous oxide on venous air embolism. *Anesthesiology* 1966; 27:783.
34. Presson RG Jr, et al: The effect of ventilation with soluble and diffusable gases on the size of air emboli. *J Appl Physiol* 1991; 70:1064.
35. Black S, et al: Parameters affecting occurrence of paradoxical air embolism. *Anesthesiology* 1989; 71:235.
36. Brechner VL, et al: Pathological physiology of air embolism. *Anesthesiology* 1967; 28:240.
37. Chandler WF et al: Acute pulmonary edema following venous air embolism during a neurosurgical procedure. *J Neurosurg* 1974; 40:400.
38. Kuhn M, et al: Acute pulmonary edema caused by venous

air embolism after removal of a subclavian catheter. *Chest* 1987; 92:364.

39. Perschau RA, et al: Pulmonary interstitial edema after multiple venous air emboli. *Anesthesiology* 1983; 45:364.

40. Still JA, et al: Pulmonary edema following air embolism. *Anesthesiology* 1974; 10:194.

41. Presson RG Jr, et al: Fate of air embolism in the pulmonary circulation. *J Appl Physiol* 1989; 67:1898.

42. Gronert GA, et al: Paradoxical air embolism from a patent foramen ovale. *Anesthesiology* 1979; 50:548.

43. Hagen PT, et al: Incidence and size of patent foramen ovale during the first decades of life: An autopsy study of 965 normal hearts. *Mayo Clin Proc* 1984; 59:17.

44. Black S, et al: Preoperative and intraoperative echocardiography to detect right-to-left shunt in patients undergoing neurosurgical procedures in the sitting position. *Anesthesiology* 1990; 72:436.

45. Cucchiara RF, et al: Identification of patent foramen ovale during sitting position craniotomy by transesophageal echocardiography with positive airway pressure. *Anesthesiology* 1985; 63:107.

46. Fischler M, et al: Patent foramen ovale and sitting position. *Anesthesiology* 1984; 60:83.

47. Kronick G, Mosslacher H: Positive contrast echocardiography in patients with patent foramen ovale and normal right heart dynamics. *Am J Cardiol* 1982; 49:1806.

48. Lynch JJ, et al: Prevalence of right-to-left atrial shunting in a health population: Detection by Valsalva maneuver contrast echocardiography. *Am J Cardiol* 1984; 53:1478.

49. Albin MS, et al: The transcranial Doppler can image microaggregates of intracranial air and particulate matter. *J Neurosurg Anesth* 1989; 1:134.

50. Perkins-Pearson NAK, et al: Atrial pressure in the seated position. *Anesthesiology* 1982; 57:493.

51. Perkins-Pearson NAK, Bedford RF: Hemodynamic consequences of PEEP in seated neurological patients: Implications for paradoxical air embolism. *Anesth Analg* 1984; 63:429.

52. Muravchick S, et al: The use of PEEP to identify the source of cardiopulmonry air embolism. *Anesthesiology* 1978; 49:294.

53. Voorhies RM, et al: Prevention of air embolism with positive and expiratory pressure. *Neurosurgery* 1983; 12:503.

54. Toung T, et al: Comparison of the effects of positive end-expiratory pressure and jugular venous compression on canine cerebral venous pressure. *Anesthesiology* 1984; 61:169.

55. Matjasko, J, et al: Anesthesia and surgery in the seated position: Analysis of 554 cases. *Neurosurgery* 1983; 17:695.

56. Munson ES, et al: Early detection of venous air embolism using a Swan-Ganz catheter. *Anesthesiology* 1975; 42:223.

57. Standefer M, et al: The sitting position in neurosurgery: A retrospective analysis of 488 cases. *Neurosurgery* 1984; 14:649.

58. Young ML, et al: Comparison of surgical and anesthetic complications in neurosurgical patients experiencing venous air embolism in the sitting position. *Neurosurgery* 1986; 18:157.

59. Younker D, et al: Massive air embolism during cesarean section. *Anesthesiology* 1986; 65:77.

60. Handler JS, Bromage PR: Venous air embolism during cesarean delivery. *Reg Anaesth* 1990; 15:170.

61. Karupathy VR, et al: Incidence of venous air embolism during cesarean section is unchanged by the use of a 5° to 10° head-up tilt. *Anesth Analg* 1989; 69:620.

62. Malinow AM, et al: Precordial ultrasonic monitoring during cesarean delivery. *Anesthesiology* 1987; 66:816.

63. Frankel AH, Holzman RS: Air embolism during posterior spinal fusion. *Can Anaesth Soc J* 1988; 35:511.

64. Lang SA, et al: Fatal air embolism in an adolescent with Duchenne muscular dystrophy during Harrington instrumentation. *Anesth Analg* 1989; 69:132.

65. Michel R: Air embolism in hip surgery. *Anaesthesia* 1980; 35:858.

66. Ngai SH, Stinchfield EE: Air embolism during hip arthroplasties. *BMJ* 1974; 3:460.

67. Naulty SJ, et al: Air embolism during radical hysterectomy. *Anesthesiology* 1982; 57:420.

68. Fatteh A, et al: Fatal air embolism in pregnancy resulting from orogenital sex play. *Forensic Sci* 1973; 2:247.

69. Albin MS, et al: Venous air embolism during radical retropubic prostatectomy. *Anesth Analg* 1992; 74:151.

70. Hofsess DW: Fatal air embolism during transurethral resection. *J Urol* 1984; 131:355.

71. Miller RA, et al: Air embolism, a new complication of percutaneous nephrolithotomy. *J Urol* 1984; 90:337.

72. Pyron CL, Segal AJ: Air embolism: A potential complication of retrograde pyelography. *J Urol* 1983; 130:125.

73. Sale M: Fatal air embolism during transvesical prostatectomy. *Ann Clin Gynaecol Fenn* 1971; 60:151.

74. Vacanti CA, Lodhia KL: Fatal massive air embolism during transurethral resection of the prostate. *Anesthesiology* 1991; 74:186.

75. Befeler D, et al: Preventing air-embolism after abdominal injury. *Lancet* 1968; 2:1395.

76. Rich RE: Fatal pulmonary air embolism following lysis of adhesions. *Surgery* 1952; 32:126.

77. Adams VI, Hirsch CS: Venous air embolism from head and neck wounds. *Arch Pathol Lab Med* 1989; 113:498.

78. Crone KR, et al: Superior sagittal sinus air after penetrating craniocerebral trauma. *Surg Neurol* 1986; 25:276.

79. Hybels RL: Venous air embolism in head and neck surgery. *Laryngoscope* 1980; 90:946.

80. Phillips RJL, Mulliken JB: Venous air embolism during a craniofacial procedure. *Plast Reconstr Surg* 1988; 82:155.

81. Ahmat KP, et al: Fatal air embolism following anesthesia for insertions of peritoneal-venous shunt. *Anesthesiology* 1989; 70:702.

82. Baggish MS, Daniel JF: Death caused by air embolism associated with neodymium-ytrrium-aluminum-garnet laser surgery and artificial sapphire tips. *Am J Obstet Gynecol* 1989; 161:877.

83. Lowdon JD, Tidmore TL Jr: Fatal air embolism after gastrointestinal endoscopy. *Anesthesiology* 1988; 69:622.

84. Seidelin PH, et al: Central venous catheterization and fatal air embolism. *Br J Hosp Med* 1987; 38:438.

85. Wadhwa RK, et al: Gas embolism during laparoscopy. *Anesthesiology* 1978; 48:74.

86. Fairman HD, et al: Air embolism as a complication of inflation of the tympanum through the external auditory meatus: A clinicopathological study of a fatal case. *Acta Otolaryngol (Stockh)* 1968; 66:65.

87. Finsnes KA: Lethal intracranial complication following air insufflation with a pneumatic otoscope. *Acta Otolaryngol (Stockh)* 1973; 75:436.

88. Lee SK, Tanswell AK: Pulmonary vascular air embolism in the newborn. *Arch Dis Child* 1989; 64:507.

89. Bohrer H, Luz M: Bypass associated air embolism during liver transplantation. *Anaesth Intensive Care* 1990; 18:265.

90. Praser MC, et al: Massive venous air embolism during orthotopic liver transplantation. *Anesthesiology* 1990; 72:198.

91. Bassan MM, et al: Near fatal systemic oxygen embolism due to wound irrigation with hydrogen peroxide. *Postgrad Med J* 1982; 58:448.

92. Shah J, et al: Hydrogen peroxide may cause venous oxygen embolism. *Anesthesiology* 1984; 61:531 (letter).

93. Tsai SK, et al: Gas embolism produced by hydrogen peroxide irrigation of an anal fistula during anesthesia. *Anesthesiology* 1985; 63:316.

94. Brunicardi FC, et al: Air embolism during pulsed saline irrigation of an open pelvic fracture: Case report. *J Trauma* 1989; 29:700.

95. Tucker WS Jr: Symptoms and signs of syndromes associated with mill wheel murmurs. *N C Med J* 1988; 49:569.

96. Albin MS, et al: Anesthetic management of posterior fossa surgery in the sitting position. *Acta Anaesthesiol Scand* 1976; 20:117.

97. Brechner VL, Bethune RWM: Recent advances in monitoring pulmonary air embolism. *Anesth Analg* 1971; 50:255.

98. Chang JL, et al: Analysis and comparison of venous air embolism detection methods. *Neurosurgery* 1980; 7:135.

99. Edmonds-Seal J, et al: Air embolism: A comparison of various methods of detection. *Anaesthesia* 1971; 26:202.

100. English JB, et al: Comparison of venous air embolism monitoring methods in supine dogs. *Anesthesiology* 1978; 48:425.

101. Gildenberg L, et al: The efficacy of Doppler monitoring for the detection of venous air embolism. *J Neurosurg* 1981; 54:75.

102. Maroon JC, et al: Detection of minute venous air emboli with ultrasound. *Surg Gynecol Obstet* 1968; 127:1236.

103. Michenfelder JD, et al: Evaluation of an ultrsonic device (Doppler) for the diagnosis of venous air embolism. *Anesthesiology* 1972; 36:164.

104. Bedford RF, et al: Cardiac catheters for diagnosis and treatment of venous air embolism. *J Neurosurg* 1981; 55:610.

105. Fong J, et al: Are Doppler-detected venous emboli during cesarean section air emboli? *Anesth Analg* 1990; 71:254.

106. Gibby GL: Precordial Doppler is not obsolete for venous air embolism monitoring. *Anesthesiology* 1988; 68:829.

107. Gibby GL: Unattended, real-time monitoring for venous air emboli by a computerized Doppler system. *Anesthesiology* 1988; 69:A732.

108. Martin RW, Colley PS: Evaluation of transesophageal Doppler detection of air embolism in dogs. *Anesthesiology* 1983; 58:117.

109. Pattion WJ: End-tidal carbon dioxide levels in the early detection of air embolism. *Anaesth Intensive Care* 1975; 3:58.

110. Marshall JC, Bedford RF: Use of a pulmonary-artery catheter for detection and treatment of venous air embolism: A prospective study in man. *Anesthesiology* 1980; 52:131.

111. Guggiari M, et al: Early detection of patent foramen ovale by two-dimensional contrast echocardiography for prevention of paradoxical air embolism during sitting position. *Anesth Analg* 1988; 67:192.

112. Cucchiara RF, et al: Detection of air in upright neurosurgical patients by 2-D transesophageal echocardiography. *Anesthesiology* 1984; 60:353.

113. Glenski JA, et al: Transesophageal echocardiography and transcutaneous O_2 and CO_2 monitoring for detection of venous air embolism. *Anesthesiology* 1986; 65:541.

114. Michenfelder JD, et al: Air embolism during neurosurgery: An evaluation of right-atrial catheter for diagnosis and treatment. *JAMA* 1969; 208:1353.

115. Michenfelder JD, et al: Air embolism during neurosurgery: A new method of treatment. *Anesth Analg* 1966; 45:390.

116. Bunegin L, et al: Positioning the right atrial catheter: A model for reappraisal. *Anesthesiology* 1981; 55:343.

117. Bunegin L, Albin MS: Balloon catheter increases air capture. *Anesthesiology* 1982; 57:66.

118. Colley PS, Artru AA: Bunegin-Albin catheter improves air retrieval and resuscitation from lethal air embolism in dogs. *Anesth Analg* 1987; 66:991.

119. Cucchiara RK, et al: Time required and success rate of percuta-

neous right atrial catheterization: Description of a technique. *Can Anaesth Soc J* 1980; 27:572.

120. Martin JT: Neuroanesthetic adjuncts for surgery in the sitting position. III. Intravascular electrocardiography. *Anesth Analg* 1970; 49:793.

121. Rorie DK: Monitoring during cardiovascular surgery. In Torban S (ed): *Cardiovascular Surgery and Postoperative Care.* Chicago. Year Book, 1982:55.

122. Artru AA: The site of origin of the intravascular electrocardiogram recorded from multiorificed intravascular catheters. *Anesthesiology* 1988; 69:44.

123. Wolf S, et al: Spontaneous migration of a central venous catheter and its repositioning: Technical note. *Neurosurgery* 1980; 6:652.

124. Tinker JH, et al: Detection of air embolism, a test for positioning of right atrial catheter and Doppler probe. *Anesthesiology* 1975; 43:104.

125. Smith SL, et al: CVP placement from the antecubital vein using a J-wire catheter guide. *Anesthesiology* 1984; 60:238.

126. Artru AA: Placement of a multiorificed catheter in the inferior portion of the right atrium: Percentage of gas retrieved and success rate of resuscitation after venous air embolism in prone dogs with the abdomen hanging freely. *Anesth Analg* 1994; 70:740.

127. Miller RA: Neuroanaesthesia in the sitting position. *Br J Anaesth* 1972; 44:495.

128. Tateishi H: Prospective study of air embolism. *Br J Anaesth* 1972; 44:1306.

129. Buckland RW, Manners JM: Venous air embolism during neurosurgery. *Anaesthesia* 1976; 31:633.

130. Sloan TB, Kimovec MA: Detection of venous air embolism by airway pressure monitoring. *Anesthesiology* 1986; 64:645.

131. Matjasko J, et al: Sensitivity of end-tidal nitrogen in venous air embolism in dogs. *Anesthesiology* 1985; 63:418.

132. Tausk HC, Miller R: Anesthesia for posterior fossa surgery in the sitting position. *Bull N Y Acad Sci* 1983; 59:771.

133. Sale JP: Prevention of air embolism during sitting neurosurgery (the use of an inflatable neck tourniquet). *Anaesthesia* 1984; 39:795.

134. Leunda G, et al: Subdural tension pneumocephalus after posterior fossa operation: Is the inverted bottle phenomenon the only causative factor? *Surg Neurol* 1981; 15:303.

135. Lunsford LD, et al: Subdural tension pneumocephalus: Report of 2 cases. *J Neurosurg* 1979; 50:525.

136. Pandit UA, et al: Pneumocephalus after posterior fossa exploration in the sitting position. *Anaesthesia* 1982; 37:996.

137. Artru AA: Nitrous oxide plays a direct role in the development of tension pneumocephalus intraoperatively. *Anesthesiology* 1982; 57:59.

138. Friedman GA, et al: Discontinuance of nitrous oxide does not prevent tension pneumocephalus. *Anesth Analg* 1981; 60:57.

139. Saidman LJ, Eger EL II: Change in cerebrospinal fluid pressure during pneumoencephalography under nitrous oxide anesthesia. *Anesthesiology* 1965; 26:67.

140. Skahen S, et al: Nitrous oxide withdrawal reduces intracranial pressure in the presence of pneumocephalus. *Anesthesiology* 1986; 65:192.

141. Durant TM, et al: Pulmonary (venous) air embolism. *Am Heart J* 1947; 33:269.

142. Mehlhorn U, et al: Body position does not affect the hemodynamic response to venous air embolism in dogs. *Anesth Analg* 1994; 79:734.

143. *US Navy Diving Manual* (NAVSEA 0994-LP-001-9010), Vol. 1: Air Diving Revision 1. Washington, DC, US Government Printing Office, June 1985:8–37.

144. Armon C, et al: Hyperbaric treatment of cerebral air embolism

sustained during an open-heart surgical procedure. *Mayo Clin Proc* 1991; 66:565.

145. Fishman NH, et al: The importance of the pulmonary veins in systemic air embolism following open-heart surgery. *Surgery* 1969; 66:655.

146. Stoney WS, et al: Air embolism and other accidents using pump oxygenators. *Ann Thorac Surg* 1980; 29:336.

147. Calverley RK, et al: Hyperbaric treatment of cerebral air embolism: A report of a case following cardiac catheterization. *Can Anaesth Soc J* 1971; 18:665.

148. Winter PM, et al: Hyperbaric treatment of cerebral air embolism during cardiopulmonary bypass. *JAMA* 1971; 215:1786.

149. Davis RM, et al: Control of spasticity and involuntary movements. *Neurosurgery* 1977; 1:205.

Chapter 31

FUNCTIONAL ORGANIZATION AND PHYSIOLOGY OF THE SPINAL CORD

ROSEMARY HICKEY

TOD B. SLOAN

JAMES N. ROGERS

Spinal Cord Functional Organization

Knowledge of the functional anatomic features of the spinal cord is important in the management of spinal cord disorders. Since the functional organization of the spinal cord is too extensive a topic to be covered fully in the limited space, the reader is referred to major neuroanatomy textbooks for more detailed information.[1-4] This discussion is provided to present an overview of the salient organizational features.

The patterns of gray and white matter in the spinal cord vary according to the vertebral level. The cervical and lumbar enlargements have the largest cross section, owing to the large number of incoming and outgoing peripheral nerve fibers at these levels. The cervical enlargement extends from C3 to T1 and the lumbar enlargement from L1 to S2. At these points, the dorsal and ventral horns are particularly well developed. The thoracic cord can be distinguished by the characteristic lateral horn containing the autonomic preganglionic motor neurons. A cross section of the spinal cord shows the characteristic centrally placed gray matter and the surrounding white matter. The white matter is formed by ascending and descending tracts as well as intraspinal pathways.

Gray Matter

The gray matter (Fig. 31-1) consists of a large number of neurons and their processes, as well as an even greater number of neuroglial cells. The gray matter on cross section can be divided by cytoarchitectonic features such as the 10 laminae described by Rexed or subdivided into nuclei that really are cell columns that extend throughout the length of the spinal cord.

The majority of neurons in the gray matter are interneurons that serve important integrative functions. The interneurons have short and medium-length axons that remain in the same segment (intrasegmental interneurons), project to neighboring segments (intersegmental interneurons), or proceed to the opposite side of the spinal cord (commissural interneurons). The interneurons far outnumber the motor neurons and long-axoned ascending pathway neurons. They are involved in various reflex loops and serve as intermediaries between descending pathways and motor and sensory mechanisms and between peripheral afferent fibers and spinal cord neurons giving rise to ascending pathways. The interneuronal net is largely responsible for the readiness and flexibility of the body to various stimuli.

The nucleus posteromarginalis (Rexed lamina I) consists of a thin layer of cells that caps the tip of the dorsal horns. Axons of many cells contained in this nucleus join the spinothalamic pathway.

The substantia gelatinosa (Rexed laminae II, III) makes up much of the apex of the dorsal horn. The substantia gelatinosa is thought to act as a gating mechanism for the control of afferent input to the spinothalamic neurons ("gate control theory of pain"). Activity in the small unmyelinated C fibers keeps the gate "open" while activation of the large myelinated A fibers "closes" the gate. Activation of the A fibers excites small substantia gelatinosa cells that project to the spinothalamic neurons. This is thought to produce pre-

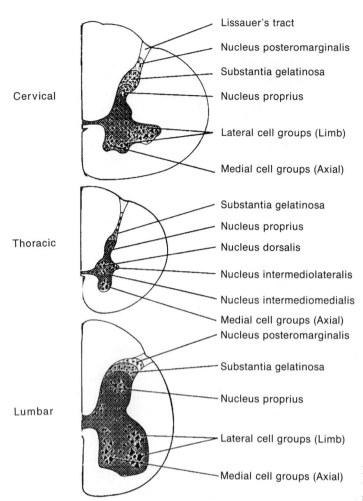

Cervical

- Lissauer's tract
- Nucleus posteromarginalis
- Substantia gelatinosa
- Nucleus proprius
- Lateral cell groups (Limb)
- Medial cell groups (Axial)

Thoracic

- Substantia gelatinosa
- Nucleus proprius
- Nucleus dorsalis
- Nucleus intermediolateralis
- Nucleus intermediomedialis
- Medial cell groups (Axial)
- Nucleus posteromarginalis
- Substantia gelatinosa

Lumbar

- Nucleus proprius
- Lateral cell groups (Limb)
- Medial cell groups (Axial)

Figure 31-1 In this cross section of the spinal cord, note that the relative amount of gray and white matter differs between spinal cord levels.

synaptic inhibition of the afferent input to the spino-thalamic neurons, preventing the pain impulses, which travel along the small fibers, from reaching the brain.

The middle portion of the gray matter is a heterogeneous region containing the intermediolateral and intermediomedial cell columns from T1 to L2. The intermediolateral cell column is responsible for forming the lateral horn. These columns contain the preganglionic visceral motor neurons of the sympathetic nervous system.

The motor cell columns are present in the ventral horn (Rexed lamina IX). The medial cell columns innervate the trunk and neck muscles. The lateral columns are present only in the cervical and lumbar enlargements and supply the limb muscles. Within the lateral columns there is somatotopic localization in the sense that the neurons supplying the distal musculature are dorsal to those supplying the proximal limb muscles.

White Matter

The white matter (Fig. 31-2) is divided into dorsal, lateral, and ventral funiculi that are arranged function-ally into ascending and descending pathways. The names of these pathways imply their origin and point of termination.

Ascending Sensory Pathways

The ascending sensory pathways can be divided into three groups: (1) pathways for pain and temperature, (2) pathways for tactile information and vibration and position sense, and (3) pathways for somatosensory impulses to the cerebellum.

Pathways for pain and temperature include the spinothalamic, spinoreticular, and spinotectal tracts. The cell bodies of most nociceptors and thermoreceptors lie in the dorsal root ganglion with axonal projections to the dorsal horn, specifically to Rexed laminae I, II, III, and V. Many of the fibers involved in pain and temperature transmission take part in various reflexes.

The spinothalamic tract is the main spinal cord pathway for pain and temperature impulse transmission. Its cells of origin are primarily located in Rexed laminae I, IV, and V. Most of the axons cross in the white

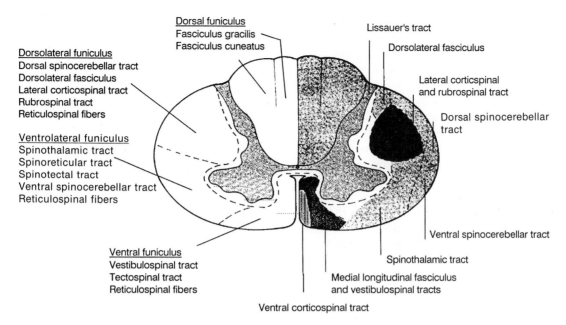

Figure 31-2   Spinal cord white matter is divided into funiculi that are comprised of ascending and descending pathways.

commissure in the same or adjacent segment and ascend in the anterolateral funiculus on the opposite side of the cord. As the fibers ascend, the more rostral levels will occupy increasingly deeper parts of the tract.

The spinoreticular tracts accompany the spinothalamic fibers and are both crossed and uncrossed. The spinoreticular fibers are involved in various reflex adjustments. The axons terminate in the reticular formation in the medial portion of the brain. This is the first link in the spinoreticulothalamic pathway responsible for activation of widespread areas of the cerebral cortex.

The spinotectal tract terminates in the tectum and the periaqueductal gray areas of the midbrain. The spinotectal tract establishes synaptic relationships with a "pain-inhibiting system" within the periaqueductal gray and midbrain raphe nuclei.

Pathways for tactile information and vibration and position sense include the dorsal column–medial lemniscus pathway and the spinocervicothalamic pathway. The dorsal column–medial lemniscus pathway is responsible for carrying tactile sensitivity and vibration and position sense to the ventral posterolateral nucleus (VPL) in the thalamus. The spinocervicothalamic pathway also carries tactile sensitivity to the VPL.

Descending Supraspinal Pathways

The motor pathways are located in Rexed's lamina IX according to a general somatotopic pattern. The axial musculature neurons are located medially, whereas the limb musculature neurons are located in the lateral portion of the ventral horn. In addition, the motor neurons related to the distal musculature are located more caudal and dorsal than neurons innervating the proximal musculature.

Descending supraspinal pathways are often referred to only as motor tracts. It is important to remember they also control activity in the sensory pathways and in spinal reflexes. The corticospinal and rubrospinal tracts make up the lateral group and terminate on laterally placed interneurons in the intermediate gray matter. These interneurons are related to the dorsolateral part of the ventral horn, involving the distal motor neurons important for skilled movements. Fibers contained in the corticospinal tract originate in the motor cortex and the premotor cortex. After passing through the internal capsule, the fibers cross to the opposite side at the level of the pyramidal decussation.

The rubrospinal tract is related closely to the corticospinal tract, both anatomically and physiologically. It descends through the spinal cord with the corticospinal tract and terminates at almost the same regions within the lateral aspect of the intermediate gray matter (Rexed laminae IV to VII). Both the corticospinal and rubrospinal tracts regulate activity in the distal and proximal musculature.

The vestibulospinal tracts originate from the lateral vestibular nucleus. The fibers terminate in the medial aspects of the ventral horn where they synapse with interneurons and motor neurons related to both trunk and limb muscles. The vestibulospinal tract acts as an important mediator of cerebellar influence on the lower motor neurons. It is also closely associated with the vestibular apparatus and the vestibular and spinal portions of the cerebellum and the control of postural reflexes.

The reticulospinal tracts are involved in many functions related to somatomotor and visceromotor functions such as cardiovascular and respiratory control. It is thought that the reticulospinal tract is involved with the vestibulospinal tract in the control of postural reflexes.

The descending pathways not only provide motor functions but also control the afferent input to the spinal cord, cerebellum, and forebrain and influence reflex transmission. These functions are the result of termination of the axons in Rexed laminae IV and V where they are in a position to control incoming impulses from muscles, joints, and skin.

Spinal Cord Reflexes

A reflex is a preprogrammed reaction that occurs in response to a stimulus. It consists of five elements: (1) a "receptor" receiving a stimulus, (2) an "afferent fiber" for input to the CNS, (3) a "reflex center" in the CNS, (4) an "efferent fiber" carrying the reflex impulse, and (5) the "effector organ."

Common stretch reflexes tested during a neurologic examination include:

1. Biceps reflex (C5-C6)
2. Brachioradialis reflex (C5-C6)
3. Triceps reflex (C7-C8)
4. Quadriceps (patellar) reflex (L3-L4)
5. Achilles reflex (S1)

These stretch reflexes are especially prominent in the antigravity muscles responsible for posture. Flexor and crossed extensor reflexes serve as an important protective mechanism such as achieving a rapid withdrawal of a limb in response to a painful stimulus.

Spinal Cord Blood Flow

Most studies of spinal cord blood flow (SCBF) suggest that the gray and white matter of the spinal cord are physiologically similar to their counterparts in the cerebral cortex. Several techniques have been utilized to measure SCBF including autoradiography, particle distribution (e.g., radioactive albumin or microspheres), and clearance of heat, ^{133}Xe, or hydrogen. The hydrogen clearance method has been used extensively and rests on its ability to measure the concentration of H_2 by the oxidation of molecular H_2 at the surface of a positively referenced platinum electrode.[5] Blood flow is directly

TABLE 31-1
Rat Spinal Cord Blood Flow by Hydrogen Clearance

	SCBF, ml/min per 100 g
Gray matter	
Rexed's laminae	
I	39.6
II	49.4
III (dorsal horn)	53.8
IV	50.1
V	52.3
VII, X (intermediate gray)	79.4
VIII	69.8
IX (ventral horn)	56.2
Mean gray matter	64.5
White matter	
Dorsal funiculus	21.0
Lateral funiculus	18.6
Ventral funiculus	23.3
Mean white matter	20.4

SOURCE: Adapted from Hayashi et al.[6]

proportional to the H_2 concentration. By using microelectrodes carefully placed in the spinal cord, regional flow can be determined. Shown in Table 31-1 are values obtained using this technique.[6] In general, mean gray and white matter blood flow is 64.5 and 20.4 ml/min per 100 g, respectively. Table 31-2 summarizes values obtained from different measurement techniques.

Regional variations in blood flow appear to relate to local anatomy. As shown in Table 31-1, small differences have been seen between different spinal cord regions; however, the major differences are between gray and white matter. As illustrated in Table 31-3, representative gray and white matter values appear independent of spinal level. Since the relative percentage of gray matter is higher in cervical and lumbar regions than in the thoracic region, the average blood flow for the cord as a whole will vary among cervical, thoracic, and lumbar regions.

Spinal Cord Oxygen Tension and Metabolism

Local oxygen tension can be measured within the spinal cord and local metabolism calculated by the Fick

TABLE 31-2
Spinal Cord Blood Flow

Technique	MEAN SCBF, ML/MIN PER 100 G	
	Gray Matter	White Matter
Hydrogen clearance[6]	64.5	20.4
^{14}C-antipyrine[7]	61.4	15.2
Autoradiography[7-10]	48.4–57.6	

TABLE 31-3
Spinal Cord Blood Flow, Tissue Oxygen Tension, and Oxygen Metabolism at Various Levels in the Spinal Cord

	Cervical	Thoracic	Lumbar
SCBF, ml/min per 100 g			
Gray matter	63	62	64
White matter	20	19	20
Tissue oxygen tension, mmHg			
Gray matter	17	19	16
White matter	15	16	15
Tissue oxygen consumption, ml/min per 100 g			
Gray matter	3.5	3.4	3.6
White matter	1.1	1.0	1.1

SOURCE: Reproduced with permission from Hayashi et al.[6]

principle. As noted in Table 31-3, oxygen tensions (17 mmHg in gray matter, 15 mmHg in white matter) and oxygen consumption (3.5 ml O_2/min per 100 g in gray matter and 1.1 ml O_2/min per 100 g in white matter) also appear to be relatively independent of spinal level.

The spinal cord tissue oxygen tension is thought to be directly proportional to the oxygen supply of the tissue and depends on the spinal cord's oxygen affinity and the diffusion coefficient for oxygen in the blood and spinal cord. Local tissue oxygen tension also decreases in proportion to spinal cord tissue oxygen consumption in a fashion similar to that reported in the brain.[11] Therefore, spinal cord oxygen tension is altered by the balance of supply and consumption. These values in the spinal cord are similar to values reported for the brain (5 to 30 torr).[12–14]

Control of Local Spinal Blood Flow

Similar to the brain, the spinal cord appears to regulate blood flow at a microvascular level in relation to local metabolic demands. Local blood supply is maintained by bidirectional flow between adjacent radicular arteries (protecting the cord from a reduction in perfusion of an individual radicular artery) and by capillary anastomoses within the spinal cord.

The relationship of oxygen consumption to blood flow appears to be maintained at a consistent ratio. The increased flow in the gray matter is matched by an increased density of the vascular bed. This vascular density is higher in the gray matter and in the ventral half of the spinal cord.[15] Within the gray matter, the highest blood flow appears to be in internuncial regions[16] and around catecholaminergic nerve terminals.[17] These regional variations probably match variations in metabolism and are similar to the vascular

density in the hypothalamus, where increased flow also is seen around catecholaminergic concentrations.

Spinal cord blood flow appears to follow changes in physiologic parameters similar to the brain. In studies where flows of the spinal cord and cerebral cortex were examined simultaneously, the response to various physiologic parameters suggests that the spinal cord mimics the cortex.[17–19] One difference between the spinal cord and cerebral cortex is that the spinal cord differs in the volume and arrangement of the gray matter and white matter. Because of the small size of the spinal cord, study of SCBF has been difficult. However, animal studies suggest a parallel between cerebral blood flow (CBF) and SCBF. Figure 31-3 summarizes the relationship of changes in blood pressure, oxygenation, and carbon dioxide on SCBF. These data have been garnered from several studies and suggest that the effects of these variables on SCBF mimic their effect on blood flow in the cerebral cortex.

Response to Blood Pressure

Autoregulation of SCBF has been demonstrated consistently in multiple studies.[18,19,21–28] Similar to the brain, mean arterial pressures (MAP) between 50 and 125 mmHg are associated with a plateau in SCBF. MAP values below 50 to 60 mmHg are associated with reductions in SCBF, and values above 125 mmHg are associated with increases in SCBF (Fig. 31-3A). In a manner similar to the cerebral cortex, the adjustment

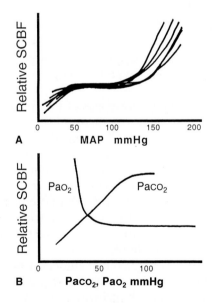

Figure 31-3 Alterations of spinal cord blood flow (SCBF) to physiologic changes as measured in studies in animals. The top panel (*A*) shows SCBF (relative scale) vs. mean arterial pressure (MAP) as redrawn from several studies.[23,25,26,28] The bottom panel (*B*) shows relative SCBF as a function of Pa_{CO_2}[21] or Pa_{O_2}.[20]

TABLE 31-4
Spinal Cord Blood Flow Autoregulation Studies

Model	Anesthesia	Manipulation	SCBF Determination Method	Autoregulatory Range, mmHg	Reference
Rat	Pentobarbital	Trimethaphan, neosynephrine	Microspheres	60–120	28
Cat	Nembutal	Hypovolemia, hypervolemia	^{131}I albumin	60–160	21
Dog	N$_2$O/O$_2$-halothane or pentobarbital	Graded hemorrhage	^{133}Xe	60–150	25
Rhesus	N$_2$O/O$_2$	Angiotension, norepinephrine	H$_2$ clearance	50–135	24
Rhesus	N$_2$O/O$_2$, pentobarbital	Hemorrhage, angiotension	H$_2$ clearance	50–125	23
Rhesus	N$_2$O/O$_2$	Hemorrhage, norepinephrine	H$_2$ clearance	50–125 50–135	26

of SCBF in response to changes in blood pressure is rapid but not instantaneous; transient rises in SCBF may occur with sudden hypertension within the autoregulatory range.[18,19] Studies demonstrating autoregulation of SCBF have been conducted in a variety of animal models with differing forms of anesthesia, and varying techniques of blood flow measurement. It should be recognized that many of these studies measure total or surface blood flow (white matter). Studies where the autoregulatory plateau range was reported are given in Table 31-4.

Several studies indicate that within the plateau range, the vascular resistance progressively increases as MAP increases,[21-23] suggesting that autoregulation is mediated via changes in vascular tone. The mechanism underlying these changes in vascular tone has not been clarified. It is unknown if an endothelium-relaxing factor (e.g., nitric oxide) acts as a mediator of vessel tone in the spinal cord, as has been suggested in cerebral vasculature.[29] With chronic hypertension, it is known that the cerebral autoregulatory curve is shifted to the right. Alteration in the spinal cord autoregulatory response with chronic hypertension, however, has not been examined.

The autoregulatory response of the spinal cord appears to be lost under conditions of hypoxia (Pa$_{O_2}$ between 30 and 45 mmHg),[25] hypercarbia[21,25] (Pa$_{CO_2}$ 85 to 100 mmHg),[25] and with spinal cord injury.[10,30] In these conditions the SCBF bears a linear relationship to MAP, although occasional autoregulation above MAP values of 90 to 100 mmHg has been demonstrated.[25] In studies where both SCBF and cortical flow were measured simultaneously, the two flows appeared to mimic each other within similar limits.[27,28]

Early reports suggested that autoregulation was dependent on a brain stem center that regulated the SCBF via neural (autonomic) pathways.[31] However, studies demonstrating preserved autoregulation after high cord transection have documented that autoregulation is more likely a local phenomenon, not dependent on brainstem regulation.[18,23,26]

Response to Hypoxia

Similar to the effect of hypoxia on CBF, hypoxia is also associated with increases in SCBF.[20–22,25] Studies examining graded ischemia show that the SCBF begins to rise when the Pa$_{O_2}$ falls 55 mmHg,[21] or an arterial oxygen saturation of 60 percent[32] (see Fig. 31-3B). One study suggested that the effect of hypoxia may be accentuated and the break point increased (70 mmHg) under conditions of hypercarbia.[21] Studies where white and gray matter SCBFs were measured separately suggest that hypoxia has a similar effect on both tissue types.[22] It is thought that the effect of hypoxia is mediated via vasodilation[25] and that this may explain the loss of autoregulation. Studies with spinal cord injury[25,33] suggest that hypoxia hyperemia may be abolished during the acute hypoperfusion phase following mechanical impact injury to the spinal cord.

Response to Changes in Pa$_{CO_2}$

Again similar to studies of cerebral blood flow, SCBF appears to be linearly related to alterations in Pa$_{CO_2}$, with plateau effects at high and low values of Pa$_{CO_2}$[19,21,22,25–27] (see Fig. 31-3B). When the response to varying Pa$_{CO_2}$ was studied in dogs, SCBF appeared to be directly related to Pa$_{CO_2}$ between 20 and 70 mmHg,[20] while above 70 mmHg there is no further increase in SCBF. This effect was similar in the gray matter, white matter, dorsal horn, and junction of the gray and white matter. The change in blood flow with Pa$_{CO_2}$ is similar to that of the cerebral cortex. One study in primates differed from the results in dogs. Kobrine reported that SCBF was linearly related to Pa$_{CO_2}$ between 50 and 90 mmHg with constant SCBF beyond these limits.[26] It is unclear why these results differ; however, if SCBF mimics cerebral blood flow, the lower and upper plateau regions of this curve may be below 20 and above 90 mmHg Pa$_{CO_2}$. When cortical blood flow and SCBF responses were studied simultaneously, the time profile (prompt change with changes in Pa_{CO_2}) and amount of change appeared similar.[18-20] This effect appears to be mediated by changes in vascular resistance with a decrease in resistance as Pa_{CO_2} rises above 20 to 30 mmHg and an increase in resistance below this value.[34] This change in vascular resistance appears to be responsible for a shift in the percentage of cardiac output (CO) to the spinal cord at various CO_2 values (0.42 percent CO at 21.1 mmHg Pa_{CO_2}, 0.68 percent at 28.2, 1.24 percent at 47.3).[34]

When rhesus monkeys were chronically exposed to hypercarbia (45.6 mmHg),[34] SCBF was shown to normalize, as did cerebral spinal fluid pH. This suggests that the effect of CO_2 on SCBF may be mediated via mechanisms also thought to be active in the cerebral cortex. Autoregulation of SCBF was also not demonstrable in this study, suggesting that a decrease in perivascular pH may mediate the loss of autoregulation seen under conditions of hypercarbia.

Similar to autoregulation, the CO_2 responsiveness of SCBF is also preserved with cord transection, which suggests that brainstem centers do not mediate the change in SCBF with alterations in Pa_{CO_2}.[18,19] Also similar to autoregulation, the responsiveness of SCBF to CO_2 may be abolished after impact spinal cord injury, during which time SCBF is reduced.[33,34] In the latter studies, a "steal" phenomena was observed during hypercarbia. It was thought this was due to vasodilation in adjacent uninjured areas of the cord where CO_2 reactivity was preserved.

Response to Autonomic Stimulation of the Spinal Cord Vasculature

In order to determine the effect of baroreceptor-mediated changes in SCBF via autonomic mechanisms, Marcus and coworkers utilized intravenous nicotine bitartrate or altered the perfusion pressure of an isolated carotid sinus.[22] Appropriate changes in bowel and muscle blood flow, blood pressure, and pulse indicated that the desired baroreceptor stimulation had been achieved. Despite these changes, and the demonstrably high concentrations of norepinephrine in spinal cord blood vessels (suggesting sympathetic innervation), SCBF did not change. This suggests that autonomic innervation of the spinal cord probably contributes minimally to regulation of SCBF. These responses are similar to those demonstrated in the cerebral cortex.[35,36]

Response to Regional Metabolic Stimulation

Marcus and colleagues also examined the effect of metabolic stimulation of spinal cord tissue.[22] Electrical stimulation of the sciatic and femoral nerves was performed in lambs above motor threshold for 10 min. This was associated with a bilateral increase (50 percent) in lumbosacral gray matter blood flow. Adjacent lumbar white matter as well as thoracic and cortical gray matter blood flow did not change. Since this stimulation paradigm has been associated with an increase in gray matter glucose metabolism,[37] the authors interpret these results to suggest coupling of regional SCBF and metabolism. This mimics the cerebral cortex where vasodilation is associated with increases in regional metabolic activity.[37-39] The relationship of blood flow to metabolism probably explains the relatively higher SCBF in gray matter compared with white matter because of the higher metabolic demand of gray matter.[37] This may also explain the higher overall blood flow in the cervical and lumbar cord where the percentage of gray matter is higher.

Response to Spinal Cord Trauma

Studies of SCBF during several forms of spinal cord injury (SCI) present conflicting patterns of SCBF alteration. Although studies uniformly demonstrate an altered response to hypoxia, Pa_{CO_2}, and autoregulation (see above), the actual values of SCBF have been shown to both increase and decrease following trauma.

The majority of studies suggest a prolonged decrease in SCBF to a degree that parallels the degree of injury. Studies using an extradural compression cuff demonstrate a profound reduction in SCBF that remains for 24 h.[30,40] Both white and gray matter SCBF were reduced (white matter SCBF was affected more than gray matter, but white matter flows recovered more rapidly). Similarly, extradural clip SCI produced a long-lasting (24 h) reduction in gray and white matter SCBF.[41] Other studies[33,34] utilizing an impact injury method have demonstrated a decrease in flow that was maximal in the gray matter, intermediate in the central white matter, and minimal in peripheral white matter.[34] The surface white matter may have different SCBF characteristics because of pial arteries present in the subarachnoid space that are known to behave differently than blood vessels in the cord.[20]

A few studies demonstrate an increase in SCBF following SCI. Studies with severe weight drop injury demonstrated a fourfold increase in lateral funiculus blood flow that returned to normal by 8 h and an associated decline in gray matter flow over the first 4 h.[30,42] This white matter hyperemia may be mediated by histamine release.[40]

These studies demonstrate alterations in SCBF both cephalad and caudad to the site of injury. The differences in flow (increase or decrease) are not easily ex-

plained by examining the various models utilized. However, it appears that various regions of the cord behave differently after SCI. Gray matter appears to be more sensitive to injury than white matter. As such, the decrease in gray matter SCBF and known higher metabolic rate suggest that the gray matter may be more vulnerable than the white matter following SCI.

Effects of Anesthetic Agents

Although extensive literature is available concerning the cerebral metabolic and vascular effects of anesthetic agents, fewer studies have addressed the effects of anesthetic agents on spinal cord physiology. In addition, noninvasive methods of measuring aspects of spinal cord physiology in the human are not available, so most data are derived from animal studies. It has been assumed by many investigators that the effects of anesthetic agents on the spinal cord mimic their effects in the brain, and this is likely to be qualitatively correct. To make true comparisons, however, investigators must examine brain and spinal cord parameters simultaneously, which has not been done in most cases. Besides the spinal cord vascular effects of agents administered systemically, there are also pertinent effects of agents administered in the subarachnoid or epidural spaces. In this section, we review the effects of both locally and systemically administered anesthetic agents on spinal cord physiology and review the important clinical implications of these effects.

LOCAL ANESTHETICS

There are varying results (Table 31-5) from studies that have determined the effects of subarachnoid local anesthetics on SCBF. In an animal model using microspheres to measure SCBF, Porter and coworkers noted no change in segmental SCBF with subarachnoid lidocaine, mepivacaine, or tetracaine.[43] Somatosensory cortical evoked responses were used to confirm the intrathecal anesthetic effects, with pentobarbital used as a baseline anesthetic in this study. Dohl and colleagues, in an animal model using hydrogen clearance to measure blood flow, also noted that the subarachnoid administration of lidocaine solutions (1, 2, 3, and 5%) failed to produce statistically significant changes in CBF or SCBF in halothane anesthetized animals.[44] Using a similar model, Dohi and coworkers also found no significant effect of subarachnoid tetracaine on SCBF or CBF.[45] Other authors, however, have noted changes in SCBF following subarachnoid local anesthetics. Crosby and colleagues, using a chronically implanted lumbar subarachnoid catheter in conscious rats, found by autoradiographic techniques that bupivacaine decreased

SCBF.[46] Using radioactive microspheres in pentobarbitone anesthetized animals, Kozody and coworkers also noted that subarachnoid bupivacaine significantly decreased SCBF to the cervical, thoracic, and lumbosacral cord.[47] Subarachnoid tetracaine, on the other hand, was found in a similar model by Kozody and coworkers to produce a regional spinal cord (lumbosacral) hyperemia (approximate doubling of SCBF) and generalized dural hyperemia.[48] Following subarachnoid lidocaine, Kozody and colleagues also noted regional spinal cord (lumbosacral) hyperemia, accompanied by a more rapid regional dural hyperemic response.[49]

From these studies, it is difficult to draw conclusions regarding the effects of various local anesthetic agents on SCBF. Varying effects have been seen in different studies using different models, with no consistent definable pattern.

The effects of local anesthetics on spinal metabolic activity have been examined by Crosby.[46] He noted that the subarachnoid administration of bupivacaine produced a reduction in spinal glucose utilization, as measured by the 2-[C] deoxyglucose utilization in conscious rats.[46] A reduction in spinal glucose utilization has also been noted by Cole and coworkers to occur with subarachnoid tetracaine.[50] These authors noted that the administration of spinal tetracaine prevented the increase in metabolism associated with somatosensory stimulation, and produced a decrease in spinal cord metabolism at the site of drug administration.[50] Thus the administration of a spinal anesthetic may block nociceptive neural traffic and its accompanying increase in metabolic activity.[50]

VASOCONSTRICTIVE AGENTS

Subarachnoid epinephrine does not appear to decrease SCBF below control values. Dohi and coworkers noted that the subarachnoid administration of 100, 300, and 500 μg of epinephrine did not significantly change SCBF.[45] Likewise, Kozody and coworkers[51] and Porter and colleagues[43] also noted that subarachnoid epinephrine did not significantly affect SCBF. When combined with a local anesthetic, however, epinephrine has been shown to prevent local anesthetic-induced vasodilation. Kozody and coworkers noted that the addition of epinephrine (200 μg) prevented the regional spinal cord hyperemia seen following subarachnoid tetracaine[48] or subarachnoid lidocaine.[49] Conflicting data exist concerning the effects of subarachnoid phenylephrine on SCBF. Kozody and coworkers noted that the administration of phenylephrine (5 mg) did not significantly alter SCBF.[51] When phenylephrine (0.1, 0.2, 0.3, and 0.5%), 1 ml, was injected into the subarachnoid space there were significant decreases in SCBF at concentrations of phenylephrine greater than 0.2%.[44]

TABLE 31-5
Local Anesthetics and Spinal Cord Blood Flow

Author	Species	Technique	Baseline Anesthetic	LA[a]	SCBF[b]
Porter et al.[43]	Cats	Microspheres	Pentobarbital	Lidocaine Mepivacaine Tetracaine	No change No change No change
Dohi et al.[44]	Dogs	Hydrogen clearance	Halothane	Lidocaine (1, 2, 3, 5%)	No change (lumbar)
Dohi et al.[44]	Dogs	Hydrogen clearance	Halothane	Tetracaine	No change (lumbar)
Crosby et al.[46]	Rats	Autoradiography	Conscious	Bupivacaine (0.75%)	↓ SCBF (27–34%) (lumbar)
Kozody et al.[47]	Dogs	Microspheres	Pentobarbitone	Bupivacaine	↓ SCBF (cervical, thoracic, lumbosacral)
Kozody et al.[48]	Dogs	Microspheres	Pentobarbitone	Tetracaine	↑ SCBF (lumbosacral) ↑ dural blood flow (cervical, thoracic, lumbosacral)
Kozody et al.[49]	Dogs	Microspheres	Pentobarbitone	Lidocaine	↑ SCBF (lumbosacral) ↑ dural blood flow (lumbosacral)

[a] LA, local anesthesia.
[b] SCBF, spinal cord blood flow.

These same authors also noted that when phenylephrine was added to lidocaine, there was a significant decrease in SCBF that was not seen when lidocaine alone was administered.[44]

OPIOIDS

Although it has long been recognized that local anesthetic agents administered along the spinal canal provide effective analgesia, the demonstration that opioids also provide effective analgesia by this route has led to a tremendous clinical interest in the subarachnoid and epidural administration of narcotics. Animal and human studies suggest that presynaptic and postsynaptic receptors in the substantia gelatinosa of the dorsal horn of the spinal cord are a major site of action of spinally administered opioids.[52] The narcotics result in a highly selective depressant action on nociceptive pathways in the dorsal horn, thus resulting in a block of pain conduction without a change in sympathetic tone or motor function.[53] Local anesthetics, on the other hand, act by axonal membrane blockade, predominantly in the spinal nerve roots,[52] and may be associated with sympathetic block and loss of motor function. Binding studies with opioid agonists have demonstrated the presence of multiple binding sites in the dorsal horn, which correspond to receptor populations found in guinea pig ileum (mu), mouse vas deferens (delta), and rat vas deferens (epsilon), as well as kappa and sigma receptors (spinal dog).[52] It appears that substance P may play a role in neuromodulation by spinally administered opioids. Substance P is found primarily in the terminals of small-diameter unmyelinated (C) and thinly myelinated (A-δ) sensor fibers, many of which subserve nociception.[54] It has been shown that in the spinal cord, presynaptic inhibition of evoked substance P release is mediated by opioid receptors (μ, κ, and δ).[54] Activation of these receptors and the inhibition of substance P release may be a major mechanism by which opioids exert their spinal analgesic action.[54] It is important to note that a major factor influencing the action of intraspinal narcotics is the lipid solubility of the drug. The more lipid-soluble agents (sufentanil, fentanyl) diffuse to the opiate receptors more quickly and produce more rapid onset than do the less-lipid-soluble agents such as morphine, which stay longer in solution in the CSF. The potential for delayed respiratory depression is also less with the more-lipid-soluble agents, as a result of shorter duration of action and less potential for rostral spread to supraspinal areas of the CNS (i.e., medullary respiratory centers).

Despite the widespread use of intrathecal and epidural narcotics, few data exist on the effects of these agents on SCBF and metabolism. Matsumiya and Dohi measured CBF and SCBF simultaneously following the intravenous or subarachnoid administration of morphine in dogs anesthetized with halothane.[55] They found that morphine hydrochloride, 1 mg/kg given intravenously, significantly reduced CBF and SCBF (to approximately 73 percent of control values).[55] Prior administration of the narcotic antagonist naloxone blocked this effect. The administration of subarachnoid morphine (0.2 mg), on the other hand, did not affect

CBF or SCBF.[55] These authors concluded that the effects of intravenous morphine on CBF and SCBF were via opiate receptors at supraspinal sites.[55] In terms of metabolism, it has been shown that subarachnoid morphine does not affect cerebral metabolic rates for oxygen (CMR_{O_2}) and glucose (CMR gluocse).[55] In addition, local glucose utilization in the spinal cord has been shown to be unaffected by the administration of epidural morphine.[56]

ALPHA₂ AGONISTS

An antinoceptive effect has been demonstrated in animal studies following the intrathecal administration of the α-2 adrenoreceptor agonist clonidine.[57] This effect is not reversed by the administration of naloxone, indicating a mechanism of action independent of opiate receptors. Activation of the postsynaptic α-2-adrenoreceptors in the substantia gelatinosa in the spinal cord is considered to be the mechanism of action of intrathecal and epidural analgesia with clonidine.[58] The ultimate usefulness of intraaxially administered clonidine is still being defined, although it may offer unique advantages in certain pain syndromes such as deafferentation pain and pain states that are resistant to opioids. The addition of clonidine to epidural narcotics for postoperative pain relief has been shown to enhance the analgesic effect of the epidural narcotic.[59] Side effects associated with the use of epidural clonidine include sedation and a decrease in blood pressure and heart rate.[60] Effects of epidural clonidine on CBF and SCBF have been examined in an animal model by Gordh and coworkers using a microsphere technique.[58] These authors noted that the lowest dose of epidural clonidine (3 μg/kg) did not affect regional blood flow to the spinal cord or to any other organ.[58] Higher doses, however, did result in alterations in SCBF, with the 10 μg/kg dose producing a significant reduction in both lumbar and thoracic SCBF. CBF was not significantly altered by epidural clonidine.[58] Although Eisenach and Grice could not confirm the reduction in SCBF seen with epidural clonidine in a conscious sheep model,[61] Crosby and coworkers noted a significant reduction in both SCBF and glucose utilization when subarachnoid clonidine was administered to conscious rats.[62] The significance of the redution in SCBF with clonidine is not clear. It may help explain clonidine's ability to prolong spinal anesthesia but does not appear to produce a flow-metabolism imbalance that leads to ischemia. The neurotoxic potential of chronic intrathecal administration of clonidine has been studied by Gordh and colleagues.[63] They found that with doses of clonidine greater than those reported to produce clinical analgesia, there were no detectable neurotoxic changes noted with light electron microscopy.[63]

SYSTEMICALLY ADMINISTERED ANESTHETICS

Data on the effects of systemically administered anesthetics on spinal cord blood flow and metabolism are limited. It has been shown by Hickey and coworkers[28] that autoregulation of SCBF is intact under barbiturate anesthesia, with an autoregulatory range of approximately 60 to 120 mmHg demonstrated for both the brain and spinal cord. In the brain, barbiturates are known to decrease both CBF and cerebral metabolism. Using doses of barbiturates sufficient to produce EEG burst suppression, Hitchon and colleagues have noted a significant decrease in cervical and thoracic SCBF of 47 and 39 percent, respectively, from control values.[64]

Barbiturates also produce a decrease in local rates of spinal cord glucose utilization. This has been noted by Crosby and coworkers[65] to occur with the intravenous anesthetic pentobarbital. Interestingly, however, these investigators noted that the 10 to 20 percent reduction in spinal cord gray matter metabolism seen with pentobarbital was considerably less than the 20 to 50 percent depression in most brain structures. This study confirms the need to examine effects of anesthetic agents on both the brain and spinal cord, because even if the qualitative responses are similar, significant quantitative differences may exist. The intravenous anesthetic propofol also has been shown to decrease local glucose utilization in both the gray and white matter of the spinal cord.[66]

The inhalational agents halothane, enflurane, and isoflurane increase CBF. Halothane with nitrous oxide (1.5 MAC) produces large increases in CBF (166 percent of control values) while enflurane and isoflurane have a lesser effect.[67] Although less well documented, inhalational agents also appear to produce an increase in SCBF. Hoffman and coworkers evaluated regional CBF and SCBF in rats during isoflurane anesthesia.[68] They noted that 1.0 MAC isoflurane did not significantly change autoregulation or CBF in cortex or subcortex compared with awake values.[68] The midbrain and spinal cord, however, did show increases in blood flow and attenuation of autoregulation during 1.0 MAC isoflurane.[68] During 2.0 MAC isoflurane, CBF and SCBF were increased and autoregulation was attenuated in all regions, with the midbrain and the spinal cord showing the greatest changes.[68] Thus it appears that isoflurane produces dose-dependent cerebral vasodilation and loss of autoregulation that may be regionally specific. In terms of metabolism, the inhalational agents isoflurane, halothane, and enflurane reduce cerebral metabolic rate, the greatest reduction being associated with isoflurane. In the spinal cord, halothane reduces local glucose utilization, although the magnitude of the effect is less than that in the brain.[69] The effects of nitrous oxide on cerebral metabolism are more controversial, but it appears that there can be a substantial increase in cerebral metabolic rate if nitrous oxide is administered alone.[70] Nitrous oxide also increases spinal cord glucose utilization, with an effect quantitatively similar to that produced in brain (15 to 25 percent increases occur in most spinal cord laminae and cerebral structures).[65]

Another approach to the problem of evaluating anesthetic effects was carried out by Grissom and colleagues, who used a hydrophilic expansible mass implanted extradurally in a model of chronic spinal cord injury.[71] They investigated the responses to a 4-h exposure of either isoflurane, fentanyl-nitrous oxide, or ketamine hydrochloride 7 or 8 days postimplantation. Neurologic testing was conducted on an inclined plane, making the maximum angle at which an animal was able to maintain orientation perpendicular to the longitudinal midline. Scores were statistically modeled for each group to develop profiles of neurologic deficits, and neurologic outcomes were compared to a spinal cord injury reference group which received no postimplant anesthesia. The fentanyl group attained maximal recovery first ($p > .05$) but did not recover to a level different on the average from the reference group. The ketamine group demonstrated a poorer ($p > .05$) recovery level relative to the other anesthetics. Perhaps this may be due, in part, to the finding by Hickey and coworkers that ketamine abolishes CNS autoregulation.[72] Paradoxically, ketamine is also an N-methyl-D-aspartate (NMDA) receptor antagonist and as such has been shown to reduce neural tissue injury after hypoxic and ischemic injury.[73,74] Koike and colleagues[75] reported that neurologic deficit developed more rapidly in ketamine- and halothane-anesthetized rabbits than in control animals using an experimental spinal cord injury model. Perhaps a key physiologic factor with ketamine lies in its ability to increase CSF outflow resistance, and Mann and coworkers demonstrated that ketamine caused a 100 percent increase in the rats using an anesthetic dose.[76]

References

1. Brodal A: *Neurological Anatomy in Relation to Clinical Medicine,* 3d ed. New York, Oxford, Oxford University Press, 1981.
2. Brown AG: *Organization in the Spinal Cord. The Anatomy and Physiology of Identified Neurons.* Berlin, Springer-Verlag, 1981.
3. Adams RD, Victor M: *Principles of Neurology,* 2d ed. New York, McGraw-Hill, 1979.
4. Henneman E: Organization of the spinal cord and its reflexes. In Mountcastle VB (ed): *Medical Physiology,* vol 1, 14th ed. St Louis, Mosby, 1980.
5. Kobrine AI, et al: Spinal cord blood flow in the rhesus monkey in the hydrogen clearance method. *Surg Neurol* 1976; 2:197.
6. Hayashi N, et al: Local spinal cord blood flow and oxygen metabolism. In Davidoff RA (ed): *Handbook of the Spinal Cord,* Vols 2 and 3. New York, Marcel Dekker, 1984:817–830.
7. Rivlin AS, Tator CH: Regional spinal cord blood flow in rats after severe cord trauma. *J Neurosurg* 1978; 49:844.
8. Senter HJ, et al: An improved technique for measurement of spinal cord blood flow. *Brain Res* 1978; 149:197.
9. Bingham WG, et al: Blood flow in normal and injured monkey spinal cord. *J Neurosurg* 1975; 43:162.
10. Sandler AN, Tator CH: The effect of spinal cord trauma on spinal cord blood flow in primates. In Harper AM, et al (eds): *Blood Flow and Metabolism in the Brain: Proceedings of the 7th International Symposium on Cerebral Blood Flow and Metabolism.* Edinburgh, Churchill Livingstone, 1975:4.22–4.26.
11. Hayashi N, et al: Regional spinal cord blood flow and tissue oxygen content after spinal cord trauma. *Surg Forum* 1980; 31:461.
12. Kessler M: Oxygen supply to tissue in normoxia and in oxygen deficiency. *Microvasc Res* 1974; 8:283.
13. Leninger-Follert E, Hossman KA: Microflow and cortical oxygen pressure during and after prolonged cerebral flow. *Stroke* 1977; 8:351.
14. Lubbers DW: Regional cerebral blood flow and microcirculation. In Bain WH, Harper AM (eds): *Blood Flow through Organs and Tissues: Proceedings of an International Conference.* Baltimore, Williams & Wilkins, 1967:162–168.
15. Jellinger K: Comparative studies on spinal cord vasculature. In Cervos-Narvarro J (ed): *Pathology of Cerebral Microcirculation.* Berlin, Walter de Gruyter, 1974:45–58.
16. Hayashi N, et al: Local blood flow, oxygen tension and oxygen consumption in the rat spinal cord. I: Oxygen metabolism and neuronal function. *J Neurosurg* 1983; 58:516.
17. Gillilan LA: Veins of the spinal cord. *Neurology* 1970; 20:860.
18. Kindt GW: Autoregulation of spinal cord blood flow. *Eur Neurol* 1971–1972; 6:19.
19. Kindt GW, et al: Regulation of spinal cord blood flow. In Russell RWR (ed): *Brain and Blood Flow. Proceedings of the 4th International Symposium on the Regulation of Cerebral Blood Flow.* London, Pitman, 1971:401–409.
20. Griffiths IR, et al: Spinal cord blood flow measured by a hydrogen clearance technique. *J Neurol Sci* 1975; 26:529.
21. Flohr H, et al: Regulation of spinal cord blood flow. In Russell RWR (ed): *Brain and Blood Flow.* London, Pitman, 1971:406–409.
22. Marcus ML, et al: Regulation of total and regional spinal cord blood flow. *Circ Res* 1977; 41:128.
23. Kobrine AI, et al: Preserved autoregulation in the rhesus spinal cord after high cervical cord section. *J Neurosurg* 1976; 44:425.
24. Kobrine AI, et al: Spinal cord blood flow as affected by changes in systemic arterial blood pressure. *J Neurosurg* 1976; 44:12.
25. Griffiths IR: Spinal cord blood flow in dogs: The effect of blood pressure. *J Neurol Neurosurg Psychiatry* 1973; 36:914.
26. Kobrine AI, Doyle TF: Physiology of spinal cord blood flow. In Harper M, et al (eds): *Blood Flow and Metabolism in the Brain.* Edinburgh, London, New York, Churchill Livingstone, 1975:4.16–4.19.
27. Wullenweber R: First results of measurements of local spinal blood flow in man by means of heat clearance. In Bain WH, Harper AM (eds): *Blood Flow through Organs and Tissues.* Baltimore, Williams & Wilkins, 1967:176–183.
28. Hickey R, et al: Autoregulation of spinal cord blood flow: Is the cord a microcosm of the brain? *Stroke* 1986; 17:1183.
29. Kozniewska E, et al: Effects of endothelium-derived nitric oxide on cerebral circulation during normoxia and hypoxia in the rat. *J Cereb Blood Flow Metab* 1992; 12:311.
30. Kobrine AI, et al: Local spinal cord blood flow in experimental traumatic myelopathy. *J Neurosurg* 1975; 42:144.
31. Shalit MN: Carbon dioxide and cerebral circulatory control. III. The effects of brain stem lesions. *Arch Neurol* 1967; 17:342.
32. Haggendal E, Johansson B: Effects of arterial carbon dioxide

tension and oxygen saturation on cerebral blood flow autoregulation in dogs. *Acta Physiol Scand* 1966; 66:27.

33. Griffiths IR: Spinal cord blood flow after acute impact injury. In Harper M, et al (eds): *Blood Flow and Metabolism in the Brain.* Edinburgh, London, New York, Churchill Livingstone, 1975:4.27–4.29.

34. Griffiths IR: Spinal cord blood flow after acute experimental cord injury in dogs. *J Neurol Sci* 1976; 27:247.

35. Heistad DD, Marcus ML: Total and regional cerebral blood flow during stimulation of carotid baroreceptors. *Stroke* 1976; 7:239.

36. Bates D, Sundt TM Jr: The relevance of peripheral baroreceptors and chemoreceptors to regulation of cerebral blood flow in the cat. *Circ Res* 1976; 38:488.

37. Kennedy C, et al: Mapping of functional neural pathways by autoradiographic survey of local metabolic rate with [^{14}C]deoxyglucose. *Science* 1975; 187:850.

38. Olesen J: Contralateral focal increase of cerebral blood flow in man during arm work. *Brain* 1971; 94:635.

39. Risberg J, Ingvar DH: Patterns of activation in the grey and white matter of the dominant hemisphere during memorization and reasoning. *Brain* 1973; 96:737.

40. Sandler AN, Tator CH: Effect of acute spinal cord compression injury on regional spinal cord blood flow in primates. *J Neurosurg* 1976; 45:660.

41. Rivlin A, Tator CH: Regional spinal cord blood flow in rats after severe cord trauma. *J Neurosurg* 1978; 49:844.

42. Kobrine AI, Doyle TF: Histamine in spinal cord injury. In Harper M, et al (eds): *Blood Flow and Metabolism in the Brain.* Edinburgh, London, New York, Churchill Livingstone, 1975:4.30–4.31.

43. Porter SS, et al: Spinal cord and cerebral blood flow response to subarachnoid injection of local anesthetics with and without epinephrine. *Acta Anaesthesiol Scand* 1985; 29:330.

44. Dohi S, et al: The effect of subarachnoid lidocaine and phenylephrine on spinal cord and cerebral blood flow in dogs. *Anesthesiology* 1984; 61:238.

45. Dohi S, et al: Spinal cord blood flow during spinal anesthesia in dogs: The effects of tetracaine, epinephrine, acute blood loss and hyperemia. *Anesth Analg* 1987; 66:599.

46. Crosby G: Local spinal cord blood flow and glucose utilization during spinal anesthesia with bupivacaine in conscious rats. *Anesthesiology* 1985; 63:55.

47. Kozody R, et al: Subarachnoid bupivacaine decreases spinal cord blood flow in dogs. *Can J Anaesth* 1985; 32:216.

48. Kozody R, et al: Spinal cord blood flow following subarachnoid tetracaine. *Can J Anaesth* 1985; 32:23.

49. Kozody R, et al: Spinal cord blood flow following subarachnoid lidocaine. *Can J Anaesth* 1985; 32:472.

50. Cole DJ, et al: Spinal tetracaine decreases central nervous system metabolism during somatosensory stimulation in the rat. *Can J Anaesth* 1990; 37:231.

51. Kozody R, et al: The effect of subarachnoid epinephrine and phenylephrine on spinal cord blood flow. *Can J Anaesth* 1984; 31:503.

52. Cousins MJ, Mather LE: Intrathecal and epidural administration of opioids. *Anesthesiology* 1984; 61:276.

53. Hughes SC: Subarachnoid and epidural analgesics in obstetrics. In Barash PG (ed): *American Society of Anesthesiologists Refresher Courses,* vol 15. Philadelphia, Lippincott, 1987:65–78.

54. Chang HM, et al: Sufentanil, morphine, met-enkephalin, and κ-agonist (U-50, 488 H) inhibit substance P release from primary sensory neurons: A model for presynaptic spinal opioid actions. *Anesthesiology* 1989; 70:672.

55. Matsumiya N, Dohi S: Effects of intravenous or subarachnoid morphine on cerebral and spinal cord hemodynamics and antagonism with naloxone in dogs. *Anesthesiology* 1983; 59:175.

56. Kuroda Y, et al: Analgesic doses of epidural morphine do not affect local glucose utilization in the spinal cord in rats. *Anesth Analg* 1987; 66:1175.

57. Ossipov MH, et al: Antinociceptive interactions between alpha$_2$-adrenergic and opiate agonists at the spinal level in rodents. *Anesth Analg* 1989; 68:194.

58. Gordh T, et al: Effect of epidural clonidine on spinal cord blood flow and regional and central hemodynamics in pigs. *Anesth Analg* 1986; 65:1312.

59. Motsch J, et al: Addition of clonidine enhances postoperative analgesia from epidural morphine: A double-blind study. *Anesthesiology* 1990; 73:1067.

60. Huntoon M, et al: Epidural clonidine after cesarean section. Appropriate dose and effect of prior local anesthetic. *Anesthesiology* 1992; 76:187.

61. Eisenach JC, Grice SC: Epidural clonidine does not decrease blood pressure or spinal cord blood flow in awake sheep. *Anesthesiology* 1988; 68:335.

62. Crosby G, et al: Subarachnoid clonidine reduces spinal cord blood flow and glucose utilization in conscious rats. *Anesthesiology* 1990; 73:1179.

63. Gordh T, et al: Evaluation of the toxicity of subarachnoid clonidine, guanfacine, and a substrate p-antagonist on rat spinal cord and nerve roots: Light and electron microscopic observations after chronic intrathecal administration. *Anesth Analg* 1986; 65:1303.

64. Hitchon PW, et al: The response of spinal cord blood flow to high-dose barbiturates. *Spine* 1982; 7:41.

65. Crosby G, et al: A comparison of local rates of glucose utilization in spinal cord and brain in conscious and nitrous oxide- or pentobarbital-treated rats. *Anesthesiology* 1984; 61:434.

66. Cavazzuti M, et al: Brain and spinal cord metabolic activity during propofol anaesthesia. *Br J Anaesth* 1991; 66:490.

67. Eintrei C, et al: Local application of ^{133}xenon for measurement of regional cerebral blood flow (rCBF) during halothane, enflurane and isoflurane anesthesia in humans. *Anesthesiology* 1985; 63:391.

68. Hoffman WE, et al: Cerebral autoregulation in awake versus isoflurane-anesthetized rats. *Anesth Analg* 1991; 73:753.

69. Crosby G, Altlas S: Local spinal cord glucose utilization in conscious and halothane-anesthetized rats. *Can J Anaesth* 1988; 35:359.

70. Pellegrino DA, et al: Nitrous oxide markedly increases cerebral cortical metabolic rate and blood flow in the goat. *Anesthesiology* 1984; 60:405.

71. Grissom TE, et al: The effect of anesthetics on neurologic outcome during the recovery period of spinal cord injury in rats. *Anesth Analg* 1994; 79:66.

72. Hickey R, et al: Ketamine abolishes central nervous system autoregulation. *Anesth Rev* 1988; 15:77.

73. Marcoux FW, et al: Ketamine prevents ischemic neuronal injury. *Brain Res* 1988; 452:324.

74. Rigamonti DD, et al: Neuroprotective effects of ketamine in a model of peptide induced spinal cord injury: Anatomical and physiological correlates. In Domino E (ed): *Status of Ketamine in Anesthesiology.* Ann Arbor, NPP Books, 1990:563–577.

75. Koike M, et al: Adverse effects of some anesthetics on spinal-cord ischemic injury. *Anesthesiology* 1982; 57:A312.

76. Mann ES, et al: Differential effects of pentobarbital, ketamine hydrochlorformation rate and outflow resistance. In Shulamn K, et al (eds): *Intracranial Pressure,* 4th ed. Berlin, Springer-Verlag, 1980:466–471.

Chapter 32

ANESTHESIA AND SURGERY FOR SPINE AND SPINAL CORD PROCEDURES

CARIN HAGBERG

WILLIAM C. WELCH

MICHELLE BOWMAN-HOWARD

This chapter will cover all aspects of spine and spinal cord surgery excluding acute spinal cord injury (see chap. *33*). It will review the anatomy of the spine and spinal cord, its blood supply, and autoregulatory considerations. Neurosurgical aspects of the chapter include a classification of spine and spinal cord pathology ranging from congenital to acquired conditions, criteria for surgery, diagnostic methods, and surgical site/approach for these procedures. Finally, all aspects of the anesthetic management will be included, as well as possible perioperative complications and postoperative care of patients undergoing these procedures.

Anatomy

Spinal anatomy may be divided into three categories: the vertebral column, along with its attached muscles and ligaments; the spinal cord, along with its associated nerve roots and membranes; and the spinal cord vasculature.[1] Although all tissues that make up the spinal system are related, these categories are clinically useful.

VERTEBRAL COLUMN

The vertebral column is composed of 33 bones (vertebrae), which include 7 cervical, 12 thoracic, 5 lumbar, 5 sacral, and 4 coccygeal bones.[2] In adults, there are actually only 24 discrete vertebrae, since the 9 sacral and coccygeal vertebrae fuse early in development (Fig. 32-1).

The individual vertebrae are related by a fundamental plan, even though their shape varies considerably in different regions of the spine. The basic vertebral pattern is that of a ventral body and a dorsal neural arch surrounding the vertebral canal (Fig. 32-2). The neural arch is made up of a pedicle on either side, each supporting a lamina that passes posteromedially and joins to form a spinous process. The vertebral foramen is formed by the posterior body, pedicles, and laminae. The arch bears a posterior spine, lateral transverse processes, and superior and inferior articular facets.

There are 23 to 24 intervertebral disks which form

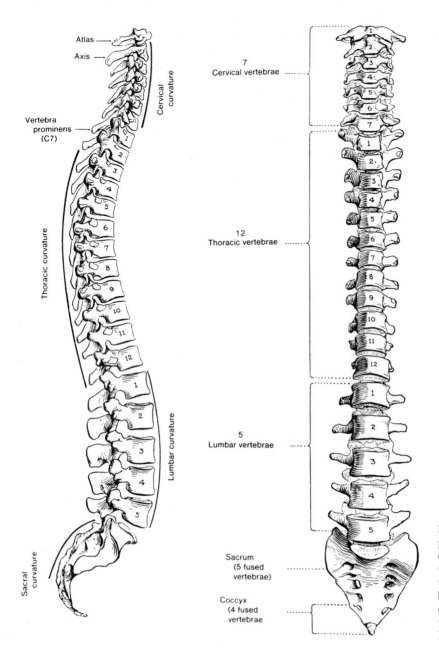

Atlas

Axis

Vertebra
prominens
(C7)

Cervical
curvature

Thoracic curvature

Lumbar curvature

Sacral
curvature

7
Cervical vertebrae

12
Thoracic vertebrae

5
Lumbar vertebrae

Sacrum
(5 fused
vertebrae)

Coccyx
(4 fused
vertebrae

Figure 32-1 The vertebral column showing 24 presacral vertebrae, sacrum, coccyx, and curvatures of the adult vertebral column. Note that the first coccygeal vertebra has fused with the sacrum. Most vertebral columns range between 72 and 75 cm in length. The vertebral column supports the skull and transmits the weight of the body through the pelvis to the lower limbs.

symphyses between the vertebral bodies. There are no disks between the occiput and the atlas, nor between the atlas and axis in the cervical region. Only remnants of disks occur within the sacrum and coccyx. The disks vary in shape, closely corresponding to the associated vertebral bodies, and permit a limited amount of movement between adjacent vertebrae. They are composed of an annulus fibrosus (outer portion) and the gelatinous nucleus pulposus (central portion) (Fig. 32-3). Clinical considerations include disk degeneration and disk herniation.

The vertebral column is stabilized by ligaments that run between the vertebral bodies, vertebral arches, transverse processes, and spinous processes (Fig.

32-4). The supraspinal ligament is the most superficial ligament. It joins adjacent spinous processes dorsally at their tips from C7 to the sacrum. In the cervical region, it forms the ligamentum nuchae. The interspinal ligaments run between spinous processes on their horizontal surfaces, and actually limit the range of motion of the vertebrae. The ligamentum flavum (yellow ligament) is composed of elastic tissue, unlike other ligaments, and stretches between adjacent laminae. Running the entire length of the vertebral bodies along their anterior and posterior aspects, respectively, are the tough anterior and posterior longitudinal ligaments. They extend from the occiput to the sacrum and provide stability to the vertebral column.

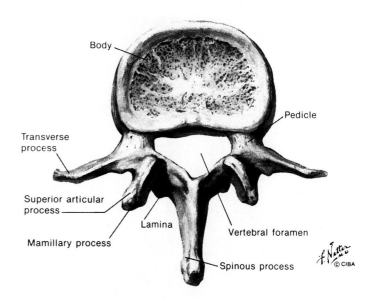

Figure 32-2   Superior view of 2d lumbar vertebra.

There are four normal curvatures of the vertebral column; these are due almost entirely to the shape of the intervertebral disks rather than the vertebral bodies. The cervical and lumbar curves are convex in a ventral direction (lordosis), whereas the thoracic and sacral curves are convex dorsally (kyphosis). When the vertebral column is reviewed laterally, the combination of these curves forms a characteristic sinusoidal shape (Fig. 32-1).

SPINAL CORD

The spinal cord is located in the upper two-thirds of the vertebral canal of the bony vertebral column.[2] It is an extension of the brain and a component of the central nervous system. It is continuous above with the medulla oblongata at the level of the foramen magnum and terminates as the conus medullaris at the level of the interspace between L1–2 in the adult and L3 in the infant (Fig. 32-5). The filum terminale is a prolongation of the pia mater and descends beyond the tip of the spinal cord to be attached to the back of the coccyx.

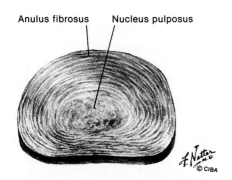

Figure 32-3   Intervertebral disk.

The spinal cord has two gross enlargements, the cervical and the lumbosacral, to accommodate the extra neurons that innervate the upper and lower limbs, respectively.

Any transverse section of the spinal cord reveals a central canal as well as a central core of gray matter surrounded by white matter (Fig. 32-6). The gray matter consists of nerve cell bodies, dendrites with their synapses, glial supporting cells, and blood vessels. The gray matter is butterfly-shaped and projects dorsal horns, ventral horns, and lateral horns. It is organized into nuclei, laminae, and a central gray area. The lateral horns contain the preganglionic neurons for the sympathetic division of the autonomic nervous system. The ventral horns contain the lower motor neurons for voluntary activity (alpha motor neurons) and smaller neurons that regulate muscle tone (gamma motor neurons). The central gray area contains a multitude of small motor neurons, many of which are associated with reflexes and some part of the spinoreticular tract. The surrounding white matter contains bundles of nerve axons organized into long ascending and descending tracts. The motor (descending) tracts are composed of upper motor neurons, which include the corticobulbar tract, the corticospinal tract, and the extrapyramidal pathways. These pathways mediate voluntary movement and control visceral sympathetic function. The sensory (ascending) tracts include the dorsal columns which convey touch and proprioception, the lateral spinothalamic tract which conveys sharp pain and temperature, the spinoreticulothalamic tract which conveys dull and diffuse pain, and finally, the spinocerebellar pathways which are responsible for proprioception and coordination.

The cord bears a deep longitudinal ventral median fissure, a narrower dorsal median sulcus and, on either

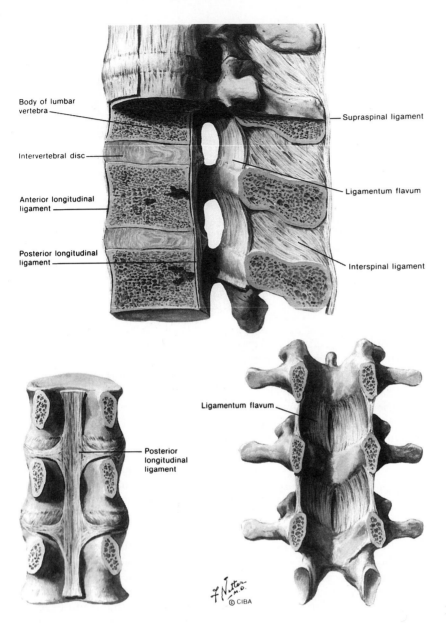

Figure 32-4 Ligaments of the spinal column.

side, a dorsolateral sulcus, along which the dorsal (sensory) nerve roots emerge (Fig. 32-6). These dorsal roots bear a ganglion which constitutes the first cell of the sensory nerves. The ventral (motor) nerve roots emerge serially along the ventrolateral aspect of the cord on either side (Fig. 32-7). At each intervertebral foramen, the ventral (anterior) and dorsal (posterior) nerve roots unite to form a spinal nerve, which subsequently splits into its ventral and dorsal primary rami, each transmitting both motor and sensory fibers.

There are 31 pairs of spinal nerves including eight cervical, twelve thoracic, five lumbar, five sacral and one coccygeal (Fig. 32-8). Only in the cervical region do the segments of the spinal cord correspond in position to the level of the corresponding vertebrae. C1 through C7 spinal nerves exit the canal superior to the corresponding vertebrae, whereas C8 exists inferior to it. Below the cervical region, each spinal nerve from a given cord segment travels inferiorly before exiting at the appropriate intervertebral foramen. Because the spinal cord is shorter than the spinal column, as the spinal segments progress caudally, there is an increasing distance that each nerve must travel to its intervertebral foramen. Below the termination of the cord, the lumbar and sacral nerve roots form the cauda equina (Fig. 32-5).

The spinal meninges are three individual membranes that surround the spinal cord; these are fundamentally similar to those of the brain (Fig. 32-9). The dura mater is a dense fibrous membrane that is the outermost meningeal layer and forms a sheath about the central nervous system. This layer begins at the

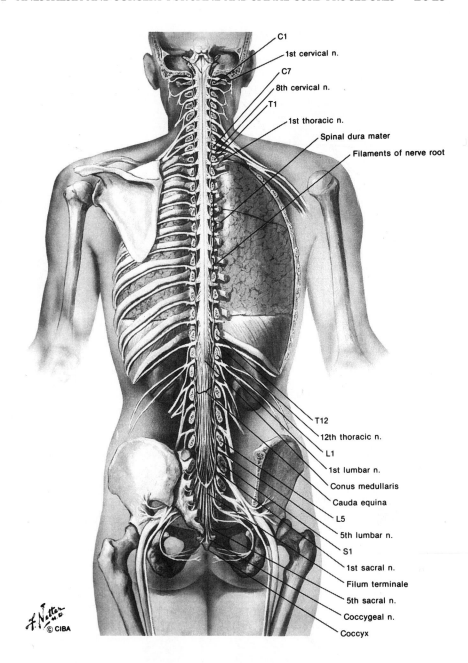

C1
1st cervical n.
C7
8th cervical n.
T1
1st thoracic n.
Spinal dura mater
Filaments of nerve root

T12
12th thoracic n.
L1
1st lumbar n.
Conus medullaris
Cauda equina
L5
5th lumbar n.
S1
1st sacral n.
Filum terminale
5th sacral n.
Coccygeal n.
Coccyx

Figure 32-5 Spinal cord in situ.

foramen magnum and extends to the level of the second sacral vertebrae, where it forms the coccygeal ligament. The dura defines the epidural space and subdural space. The arachnoid is a thin avascular membrane that forms the intermediate meningeal layer. Because the arachnoid is loosely adherent to the dura, there is a potential space (subdural space) between the two layers. Blood or pus may extravasate within this space. The arachnoid is attached to the underlying pia by numerous arachnoid trabeculae. The space between the arachnoid and pial layers defines the subarachnoid space. This space contains the cerebrospinal fluid (CSF), which suspends the central nervous system and nerve roots. Large blood vessels pass within this space.

The pia mater is a highly vascular membrane that forms the innermost meningeal layer and closely approximates both the brain and spinal cord. It contains the plexus of small blood vessels that supply the neural tissue.

SPINAL VASCULATURE

The spinal cord receives its blood supply from two distinct systems,[3] the anterior spinal artery and the paired posterior spinal arteries (Fig. 32-10). These small arteries usually arise as branches of the two vertebral arteries at the base of the brain stem and extend the full length of the spinal cord and form the posterior

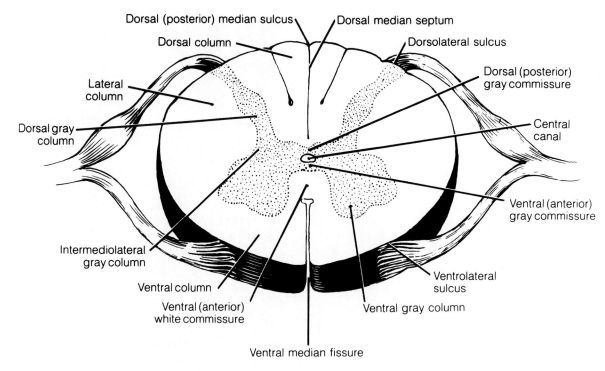

Dorsal (posterior) median sulcus
Dorsal median septum
Dorsal column
Dorsolateral sulcus
Lateral column
Dorsal (posterior) gray commissure
Dorsal gray column
Central canal
Ventral (anterior) gray commissure
Intermediolateral gray column
Ventrolateral sulcus
Ventral column
Ventral gray column
Ventral (anterior) white commissure
Ventral median fissure

Figure 32-6 Anatomy of the spinal cord.

spinal arteries. The anterior spinal artery lies in the anterior median sulcus and supplies the anterior two-thirds of the spinal cord. It usually originates in the upper cervical region and is fed by the two vertebral arteries as well as six to 10 anterior radicular arteries, the most important of which is the artery of Adamkie-wicz. As much as 50 percent of the entire spinal cord may depend on flow from this vessel.[4] It arises from a left-sided intercostal artery in 80 percent of individuals and usually enters the spinal cord between the eighth thoracic and third lumbar nerve roots.[3] There is often anatomic variation in the vascular anatomy of the spi-

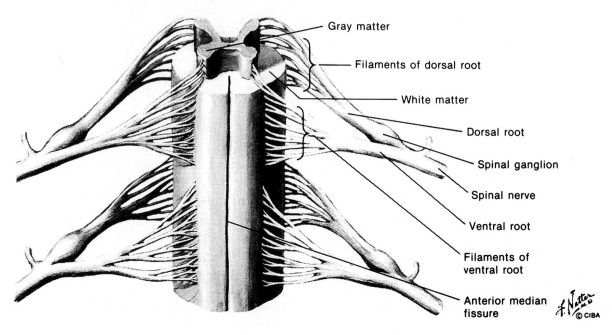

Gray matter
Filaments of dorsal root
White matter
Dorsal root
Spinal ganglion
Spinal nerve
Ventral root
Filaments of ventral root
Anterior median fissure

Figure 32-7 Anterior view of the spinal cord.

rior spinal artery, thus forming a plexus-like arrangement surrounding the cord.

Some areas of the spinal cord are more susceptible to ischemia than others if arterial blood supply is diminished. Particularly at risk are the "watershed" areas at the periphery of the territory supplied by the main contributory vessel.[7] For the anterior spinal artery segments, C3 to 5 and T12 to L2 are most vulnerable; for the posterior spinal arteries, segments C8 to T4 are most vulnerable. These zones are at risk if damage occurs to the vessels, perfusion pressure decreases, or general severe hypoxia occurs. The vascular anatomy of the spinal cord appears to be an important factor in the development of paraplegia as a complication of surgery. Because of its segmental blood supply, the anterior spinal artery territory is at risk if one of the main contributory vessels is damaged. Anterior spinal artery syndrome may result when injury to this artery occurs, rendering anterior-central cord ischemia.[8] Clinical manifestations of this syndrome include paraparesis or paraplegia along with dissociated sensory loss (i.e., loss of pain and temperature sensations, with preservation of position and vibration sense).[9] It may occur not only as a result of sustained hypoperfusion[10] (e.g., prolonged anesthesia-related hypotension), but also as a result of obstruction of the feeder vessels to the anterior spinal artery[11] (e.g., aortic cross-clamping), scoliosis correction,[12] disk herniation,[13,14] cervical spondylosis,[15,16] or vertebral trauma.[17-20] A myelogram is usually performed in order to exclude other lesions. Treatment varies according to the underlying mechanism involved, although general support should always be provided. Prognosis is often poor.[9]

The spinal veins resemble the related arteries in their distribution[21,22] (Fig. 32-11). There are two plexuses of veins, external and internal, which run the entire length of the vertebral column and anastomose freely with each other. Venous drainage occurs through radial veins of the spinal cord parenchyma. These radial veins drain into the coronal venus plexus or longitudinal veins on the spinal cord surface which drain into the external vertebral venous plexus. This external plexus, which lies in the fatty connective tissue of the epidural space, communicates with the smaller internal vertebral venous plexus that lies in the subarachnoid space by way of pedicular veins and drain into intervertebral veins. The vertebral venous plexus also communicates superiorly with the venous sinuses of the cranium and inferiorly with the venous sinuses of the deep pelvis. All venous drainage ultimately reaches the vena cava. Since this venous system is relatively devoid of valves, it can become engorged in certain physiologic or disease states. This is especially pronounced in obesity or pregnancy, where the increase in intra-abdominal

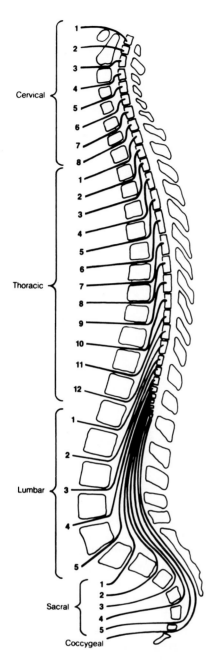

Figure 32-8 Schematic illustration of the relationship between the vertebral column, the spinal cord, and spinal nerves.

nal cord in individuals. Turnbull and coworkers[5] as well as Manners[6] noted postmortem findings of spinal cords having only one anterior radicular artery. Since variability is the rule, injuries or operations on the aorta or intercostal vessels may have widely different effects on different patients. The paired posterior arteries supply the posterior one-third of the spinal cord. They are fed from many radicular branches which anastomose freely with each other and with the ante-

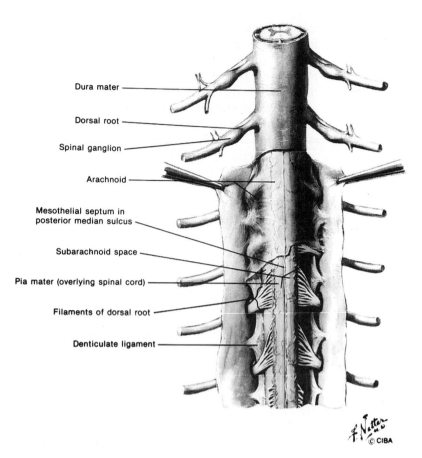

Dura mater

Dorsal root

Spinal ganglion

Arachnoid

Mesothelial septum in
posterior median sulcus

Subarachnoid space

Pia mater (overlying spinal cord)

Filaments of dorsal root

Denticulate ligament

Figure 32-9   Posterior view of the spinal cord.

pressure may obstruct venous flow through the inferior vena cava.

Physiology

BLOOD FLOW AND METABOLISM

Since noninvasive methods of measuring aspects of spinal cord physiology in humans are not available, concepts of spinal cord physiology are almost exclusively derived from animal research. Various techniques have been used including autoradiography,[23-26] radioactive microspheres[27-29] and clearance of heat,[30] [133]Xe,[31] or hydrogen.[31-36] Most studies suggest that the spinal cord blood flow (SCBF) is approximately 60 ml/100 g per min on average, which is similar to cerebral blood flow (CBF). Hayashi and coworkers[32] determined regional blood flow by placing microelectrodes in the spinal cord and using the hydrogen clearance method. This method measures the concentration of hydrogen by the oxidation of molecular hydrogen at the surface of a positively referenced platinum electrode. They found that the mean gray and white matter blood flow is 64.5 and 20.4 ml/100 g/min, respectively. Also, since the relative percentage of either gray matter

or white matter varies within various regions of the spinal cord (Fig. 32-12), the average blood flow for the cord as a whole will vary among cervical, thoracic, and lumbar regions (i.e., mean blood flow in the cervical and lumbar segments is approximately 40 percent higher than in the thoracic segments).[28]

Local metabolism of the spinal cord can be extrapolated from the measurement of local oxygen tension within the cord. Oxygen tensions and consumption are relatively independent of spinal level, despite the fact that gray matter has a higher metabolic demand than white matter.[33] As with the brain, spinal cord oxygen is based upon the balance of supply and demand. The relationship of oxygen consumption to blood flow is usually maintained at a consistent ratio. Coupling exists between regional SCBF and metabolism, which is demonstrated by the relatively higher SCBF in gray matter to meet its higher metabolic demand.[38] Marcus and coworkers[28] nicely illustrated a 50 percent increase in lumbosacral gray matter blood flow by electrically stimulating the sciatic and femoral nerves in lambs. The same concept applies to the overall metabolic rate of the spinal cord,[39] which is lower compared with that of the brain, and SCBF is proportionally lower than CBF.[40]

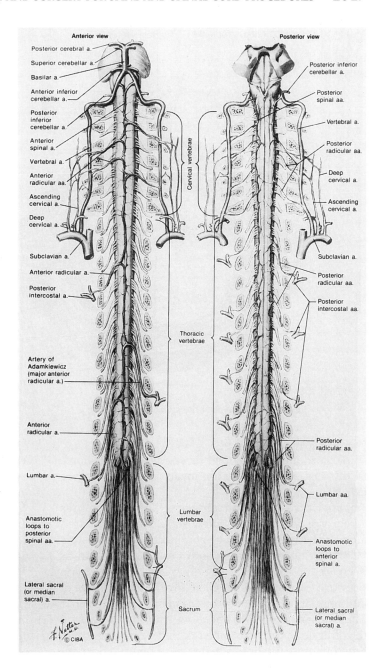

Figure 32-10   Arteries of the spinal cord.

REGULATION OF SPINAL CORD BLOOD FLOW

RESPONSE TO BLOOD PRESSURE

By using various techniques, animal studies have demonstrated that there is autoregulation of SCBF.[28–30,34–36,39,41–43] Both Kobrine and coworkers,[36] using hydrogen clearance in the monkey, and Hickey and associates,[29] while studying the rat spinal cord have shown that autoregulation in the cord mimics that in the brain. SCBF is well maintained between a mean arterial pressure of 60 to 120 mmHg. The limits of autoregulation are not as well defined in children. Below the lower limit and above the upper limit, autoreg-

ulation fails and blood flow becomes pressure-dependent. Despite this finding, some data[44] suggest that the spinal cord is less susceptible to ischemic damage as a result of reductions in regional blood flow than is the brain.

Studies have shown that autoregulation is a local phenomenon and not dependent on brain stem regulation.[35,37,41] The ability of the spinal circulation to autoregulate may be altered or eliminated by conditions that cause maximal vasodilation of the spinal vasculature, such as hypoxia[31] or severe hypercarbia,[31,43] as well as conditions that abolish vessel reactivity, such as

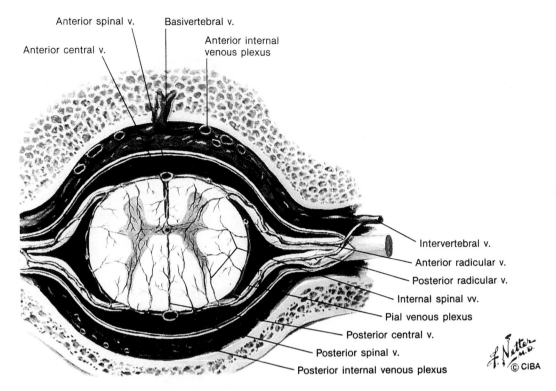

Figure 32-11   Veins of the spinal cord.

spinal cord injury.[26,45] Under these adverse conditions, SCBF varies linearly with mean arterial pressure (MAP).

Spinal cord perfusion pressure (i.e., MAP minus cerebrospinal fluid pressure), should be considered along the same lines as cerebral perfusion pressure. SCBF will not be affected until perfusion pressure is decreased to 40 to 50 mmHg.[4] If spinal cord perfusion pressure (SCPP) is sustained below the lower limits of autoregulation, spinal cord ischemia may occur.[46] Thus, it is imperative to not allow arterial hypotension to continue for any sustained period below the lower limit of autoregulation. The degree of neurologic damage is more dependent on the persistence than on the depth of the resulting ischemia. Factors other than

MAP, such as high CSF pressure or cord compression, can critically decrease local tissue perfusion. When CSF pressure rises to within 40 to 50 mmHg of MAP, SCBF will decrease.[47] This may occur during epidural anesthesia and thoracic aneurysm surgery. McCullough and coworkers[48] advocate monitoring CSF pressure with a lumbar subarachnoid catheter and draining CSF when pressures are excessive in order to maintain an adequate SCPP.

CSF pressure may also increase when sodium nitroprusside (SNP) is used to control blood pressure. Several authors[48] have shown that SNP, when used to control proximal hypertension during thoracic aortic cross clamping, increases the incidence of spinal cord ischemia. SNP increases CSF pressure and decreases

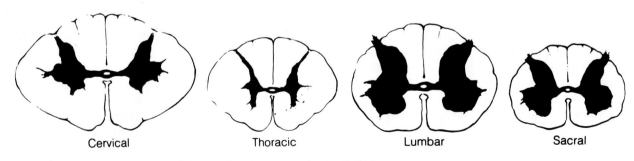

Figure 32-12   Transverse sections of the spinal cord at various levels. Black represents gray matter.

distal aortic pressure, thus decreasing SCPP. Recently, Simpson and associates[54] demonstrated that nitroglycerin has the same effects on the spinal cord as SNP.

RESPONSE TO ARTERIAL BLOOD GAS TENSIONS

SCBF, like CBF, is responsive to arterial blood gas tensions.[29,30,33,36,39,44,45] SCBF increases with hypercarbia and hypoxemia and decreases with hypocarbia.[30] When the two regions are compared, the absolute change in SCBF per unit change in carbon dioxide tension (between 20 to 80 mmHg) is less than the corresponding change in CBF, 0.5 ml/100 g per min per mmHg versus 1.0 to 1.5 ml/100 g per min.[40] Because baseline blood flow is lower in the spinal cord than in the brain, blood flow changes are similar for the two regions when expressed as percentage change. The ability of the spinal cord to respond to changes in Pa_{CO_2} may be reduced or even eliminated by various conditions such as spinal cord injury, low perfusion pressure and hypoxia. If SCBF is preserved, the CO_2 responsiveness of SCBF will be preseved with cord transection, indicating that brain stem centers are not responsible for mediating changes in SCBF with alterations in Pa_{CO_2}.[41,42]

RESPONSE TO TEMPERATURE

SCBF, like CBF, decreases with hypothermia.[52] It has been well documented that hypothermia protects against damage from cerebral ischemia, whereas hyperthermia worsens damage.[53] There are several proposed mechanisms for this protection, including decreased reperfusion hyperemia, improved glucose utilization, decreased blood-brain barrier permeability, and stabilization of lipid membranes.[54] Cooling has also been shown to be effective in the treatment of spinal cord injury when applied within 4 h of injury.[55] Indeed, Holier found that the "safe" ischemic time may be increased 51.5 min/°C reduction.[56]

EFFECTS OF ANESTHETIC AGENTS

Although few studies have addressed the effects of anesthetic agents on spinal cord physiology, it is assumed that these are similar to their effects in the brain. Thus, with the exception of ketamine, intravenous drugs most likely decrease SCBF and metabolism, while volatile anesthetics decrease metabolism but increase SCBF.

The metabolic effect of high-dose barbiturates on spinal metabolism was demonstrated by Hitchon and coworkers[57] by showing a significant reduction in cervical and thoracic SCBF as compared to controls. Thus, they suggest that barbiturate coma may even provide cord protection. Crosby and associates[58] also noted a decrease in spinal cord metabolism with the use of barbiturates, although to a lesser extent than cerebral metabolism. This may be explained by the fact that the

spinal cord has a much lower rate of blood flow and metabolism than the brain.

In general, the inhalational anesthetics produce dose-dependent increases in CBF, thus increasing cerebral blood volume and ICP. Hoffman and coworkers[59] recently noted similar findings in comparing regional CBF and SCBF in rats during various levels of isoflurane anesthesia. Other dose-related effects of inhalational anesthetics include a decrease in cerebral metabolic rate and loss of autoregulation, which they also verified in this study model. Although conflicting results of nitrous oxide (N_2O) on cerebral metabolism have been reported in the literature, the majority support the theory that N_2O is a cerebral vasodilator. Thus, administration of N_2O may increase SCBF. Also, Crosby and associates[58] demonstrated a similar effect of N_2O on glucose metabolism between the brain and the spinal cord.

Locally administered anesthetic agents, including local anesthetics, vasoconstrictors and narcotics have variable effects on SCBF. Studies have shown that subarachnoid local anesthetics do not have a uniform effects on SCBF[60-66] although it is evident that these studies differ in many aspects. Results of studies concerning the effects of local anesthetics on spinal metabolic activity, on the other hand, have consistently found a reduction in metabolic rate.[63,67]

Vasoconstrictive agents, including epinephrine and phenylephrine, affect SCBF differently. Contrary to popular belief, several studies[60,62,68] have found that various doses of subarachnoid epinephrine did not significantly change SCBF. However, epinephrine does prevent local anesthetic-induced vasodilatation when combined with a local anesthetic agent. Data concerning phenylephrine's effect on SCBF are conflicting.[61,68]

Although intrathecal and epidural narcotics have been used extensively in the clinical setting, little research has been performed concerning the use of these agents on SCBF and metabolism. Matsumiya and Dohi[69] found that systemically administered morphine significantly reduced both CBF and SCBF (approximately 73 percent), whereas intrathecally administered morphine had no effect on either. Thus, morphine requires involvement of supraspinal opiate receptors to alter SCBF. Fentanyl, on the other hand, affects both spinal metabolism and blood flow when administered intrathecally, epidurally, or intravenously.

The epidural administration of clonidine, an alpha-2 adrenoceptor agonist, has become very popular as an adjunct to epidural narcotics for postoperative pain relief, as it enhances analgesia. Gordh and coworkers[70] found a dose-dependent reduction in SCBF with epidural clonidine, whereas CBF was unaffected. Other studies have both negated and supported those findings.[71,72] The antinociceptive effect of clonidine has also been demonstrated when the drug is administeed intrathecally. Crosby and associates[72] demonstrated in rats that subarachnoid clonidine decreases both SCBF and glucose utilization, although the significance of this effect is unclear.

OPERATIVE PROCEDURE

SCBF may also be affected by the nature of the operative procedure, including type, duration, site, and surgical approach. In a review of the complications arising from use of the prone position, Anderson[73] reported damage to underlying major blood vessels causing extensive hemorrhage and spinal cord ischemia as a serious hazard during surgery on the spinal axis, although such injury may occur in any position. As mentioned previously, any reduction in MAP may cause diminished spinal cord blood flow. Anderson and coworkers[74] demonstrated in cats that the laminectomy procedure itself can cause a significant decrease in SCBF with exposure of the dura. They suspect that the mechanism for this effect was a temperature-induced vasoconstriction. Retraction necessary for surgical exposure may decrease SCBF by direct cord compression. Therefore, in the face of hypotension, whether unintentional or deliberate, excessive traction should be avoided.[75]

Classification of Spine and Spinal Cord Pathology

CONGENITAL

Congenital spinal cord and spinal column anomalies are seen in all patient populations. Physicians practicing in children's hospitals will encounter the greatest number of patients with congenital anomalies requiring neurosurgical or orthopaedic intervention. Further understanding of the natural history and pathophysiology of these lesions has encouraged physicians to intervene earlier rather than later in the hopes of preventing or limiting permanent disabilities. For these reasons, anesthesiologists must be knowledgeable about the relevant anatomy, associated congenital abnormalities, operative positions, surgical risks, and expected outcomes.

The most common congenital anomalies are the spinal dysrhaphic abnormalities. These include open and closed conditions, such as spina bifida occulta, meningocele, myelomeningocele, lipomyelomeningocele, diastematomyelia, and tethered cord. Dysrhaphic lesions are frequently found in conjunction with abnormalities of skeleton, renal defects, and abnormalities of the gastrointestinal system and other organ systems.[76] The most common and benign spinal dysrhaphic condition is spina bifida occulta. This lesion represents a failure of closure of the spinal canal. It occurs in approximately

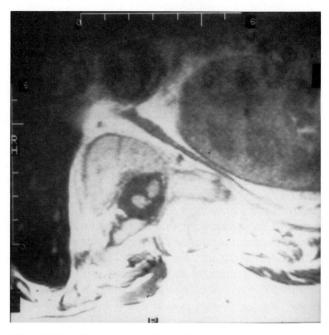

Figure 32-13 Diastematomyelia. Axial MR image through thoracic spinal cord demonstrating a split spinal cord consistent with diastematomyelia.

20 percent of the normal population and is frequently unrecognized. The diagnosis is often made incidentally when plain spine films are obtained for other reasons, such as lower back pain, and the lower lumbar lamina are noted to be incompletely fused. Although back pain and dysuria have been attributed to this lesion, there is little clinical support for the argument that milder forms of spina bifida occulta cause these symptoms.

Diastematomyelia is a rare condition. The term implies a splitting of the spinal cord with a bony spur or cleft occurring between the two hemicords (Fig. 32-13). The hemicords may share a dural covering or may have separate coverings. Diplomyelia implies the actual duplication of the spinal cord, and this may be associated with spinal column duplication as well. Both diastematomyelia and diplomyelia are associated with tethered spinal cord and bony and other abnormalities. Surgery is usually recommended because of its potential to correct or improve neurologic symptoms and possibly to prevent the development of late neurologic compromise.[77]

The tethered spinal cord syndrome is a clinical entity seen in both children and adults. The central etiology is a lesion that prevents normal upward mobility of the spinal cord. Tethering lesions incude scar tissue, a thickened filum terminale, tumors, bony clefts with diastematomyelia, and sinus tracts. The end result is fixed or progressive spinal cord dysfunction that probably occurs as a result of vascular, mechanical and metabolic factors.[78] Surgical correction of the underlying abnormality or release of the thickened filum is performed in most cases.

Meningocele is the failure of laminar fusion combined with the dura being exposed at the skin edge.[79] This lesion is recognized at birth and usually is associated with less severe neurologic deficits than those found in patients with meningomyelocele. The patient requires closure of the lesion to prevent fluid leakage and meningitis. The surgery is performed on a prone patient as described below.

Myelomeningocele and lipomyelomeningocele are more extreme examples of incomplete closure of the posterior elements. This lesion is thought to result from failure of neuropore closure at 26 days post-fertilization. The spinal cord fails to close at its terminus, and the conus medullaris is poorly formed. The terminal structure is called a neural placode and is visible through the skin of a newborn. Fatty elements may be contiguous with the neuroplacode, and this results in a lipomeningocele. The dura does not close over the placode, and cerebrospinal fluid usually leaks from the infant's back. This creates an immediate risk of meningitis and requires prompt surgical repair.

Myelomeningocele usually results in significant and permanent lumbosacral neurologic deficts, depending on the level of the lesion. For example, a high lumbar lesion might result in weakness of the iliopsoas musculature and paralysis of the remaining musculature. Sphincteric dysfunction is extremely common. The immediate goal of surgery is to obtain water-tight closure of the meninges without worsening of the neurologic deficits. Long-term goals are to prevent late neurologic complications due to neuro-placode adhesions with resultant tethered cord syndrome. The presence of a myelomeningocele should alert the physician to other systemic abnormalities. These include skeletal, gastrointestinal, pulmonary, cardiac, and other organ system anomalies.

Chiari malformations are a group of hindbrain abnormalities often associated with myelomeningocele. Specifically, over 90 percent of infants with myelomeningoceles will have Chiari malformations and associated hydrocephalus. Chiari malformations may be congenital or acquired. The pathologic substrate of the Chiari malformations is hindbrain abnormalities resulting in posterior fossa and other lesions. Four subtypes are generally recognized.

The severity of the Chiari malformations is variable. Low-lying cerebellar tonsils may be incidentally noted in adults (type I) receiving MRI scans for cervical or intracranial evaluation. In these cases, no active intervention may be required. More severe Chiari lesions are frequently identified with myelomeningocele (type II). These lesions are highly associated with hydrocephalus and will usually require ventriculoperitoneal shunting. Treatment of encephalocele may also be required with the type III lesions.

Syringomyelia is an abnormal cystic condition of the spinal cord. The cyst may be congenital and found in association with Chiari malformations and altered cerebrospinal fluid flow. Other etiologies include post-traumatic, vascular or post-hemorrhagic, tumor associated, disk-rupture associated,[80] inflammatory, or idiopathic (Fig. 32-14). The lesions are often separated and can be pathologically differentiated from dilatation of the central canal (hydromyelia) by the presence of non-ciliated, squamous epithelium lining the cavity.[81] The symptoms caused by the syrinx have a well-defined neuroanatomic basis. Specifically, white matter fibers of the spinal cord are compressed and dissected by the syrinx cavity as it expands anterior to the central canal.[81] This results in a "dissociated" or "cape-like" sensory loss of pain and temperature fibers over the shoulders and upper arms. Position and vibratory sense is preserved because of sparing of the dorsal columns. Eventually, the expanding lesions will cause upper and lower motor-type weakness. Syrinx cavities can extend into the brain stem (syringobulbia), with resultant lower cranial nerve palsies. The lesions also can involve the entire spinal cord (holocord syrinx) and cause neurologic deficits at each level.

Syringomyelic cavities can be asymptomatic or cause progressive neurologic deficits. Syringomyelic cavities will often contract following correction of spinal pathology (i.e., diskectomy, correction of kyphotic deformity). Direct or indirect drainage techniques include myelotomy with cyst-subarachnoid or cyst-peritoneal shunting, terminal cystostomy in cases of holocord syrinx, or ventriculo-peritoneal shunting.

Arteriovenous malformations (AVMs) are usually congenital abnormal communications between arteries or arterioles and veins. These lesions can be suspected or identified on myelography or MRI, but require spinal angiography for definitive diagnosis. Recently, attempts have been made to classify these rare lesions.[82] A basic distinction is made between intradural and extradural lesions. Intradural lesions can be subclassified as direct AV fistula, glomus, or juvenile lesions, depending on the type of blood flow pattern, structures involved, and location of the AVM nidus.

Dural AVMs are more common in older individuals. These lesions are supplied by dural branches of the intercostal and lumbar arteries. The lesions are located within the dural covering of the dorsal intercostal nerve root and spinal dura. Intradural AVMs are usually identified in younger patients. The lesions are fed by spinal cord medullary arteries, and the nidus is within the spinal cord or pia mater. The glomus sub-

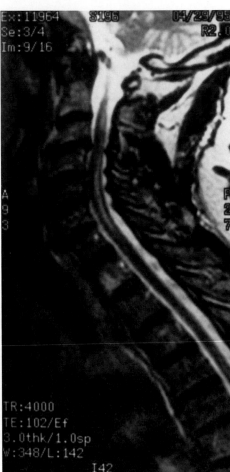

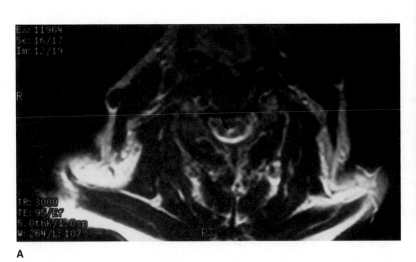

Figure 32-14 Syrinx. Axial (*A*) and sagittal (*B*) MR images through mid-cervical cord region identifying a small spinal cord syrinx (*arrow*).

type exhibits a consolidated mass of abnormal blood vessels located within the spinal cord itself. The juvenile AVM occupies the entire spinal cord level and is fed by large feeding vessels, which involve paraspinous structures including muscle and bone. These lesions are suspected when hemangiomatous-type skin changes are present in the cervical, thoracic, or lumbar regions.

Spinal AVMs can be found incidentally. More commonly, they present with such intermittent neurologic deficits as myelopathy, muscular weakness, sensory loss, or sphincteric disturbances, occasionally leading to the misdiagnosis of multiple sclerosis.[83] Rarely, they can cause radiculopathy.[84] These neurologic signs and symptoms are thought to be caused by progressive venous hypertension with associated spinal cord ischemia. Severe neurologic compromise can occur when vessels thrombose or bleed into the subarachnoid space causing spinal cord compression.

Scoliosis is the term used to describe complex spinal column rotatory and lateral curvatures with associated chest wall deformities.[85] The abnormal curvature is most common in the thoracolumbar region, and may be associated with sagittal vertebral deformities such as kyphosis and lordosis. The net effect of these deformities can be progressive cosmetic, respiratory, cardiac, and neurologic compromise.

Scoliosis is generally divided into three broad categories. Nonstructural scoliosis identifies abnormal curvatures that correct with side-bending, as confirmed on plain radiographs. These curves are usually postural or compensatory (leg-length discrepancy) in nature. Transient structural scoliotic curves are caused by underlying conditions, such as sciatica, intraabdominal and paraspinous infections, inflammatory processes, or hysteria. These nonphysiologic curves can be expected to resolve when the underlying condition is treated.

Structural scoliotic curves do not correct with side-bending. The most common etiology of these curves is idiopathic, possibly due to genetic influences. Idiopathic scoliosis is further subclassified as to age of onset. Infantile forms are identified before age three and frequently resolve spontaneously. Juvenile forms occur between age 3 and the onset of puberty. Adolescent forms are noted between age 10 and skeletal maturity. Generally, the younger the age of onset (excluding the infantile form), the more likely that the disease will progress and require treatment.

Congenital causes of structural scoliosis include the open and closed vertebral dysraphic conditions described above. There may be an associated neurologic deficit, such as that associated with myelomeningocele, and kyphotic deformities are also frequent. Vertebral anomalies such as hemivertebra may also contribute to the scoliotic curve. Extravertebral processes, such as congenital rib fusion, are also associated with this type of scoliosis.

Intramedullary tumors such as ependymoma and astrocytoma have been associated with structural scoliosis, as has neurofibromatosis. Other neurologic and muscular causes of structural scoliosis include cerebral palsy, poliomyelitis, muscular dystrophy, and Friedreich's ataxia.

Finally, mesenchymal conditions such as Marfan's syndrome, collagen vascular disorders, degenerative disease, trauma, and surgery have been associated with the development of structural scoliosis.

A direct complication of progressive scoliosis is respiratory compromise. This is associated with larger bony deformity (65 degree or greater primary curve as measured by the Cobb method). This compromise may result from restriction of normal ventilation by the abnormal rotation of the spine and rib cage. This may lead to impaired efficiency of the muscles of ventilation, with total lung capacity affected by a curvature greater than 60 degrees. Vital capacity may become impaired at curvatures of 90 degrees, with the development of secondary pulmonary hypertension and right ventricular hypertrophy.

The anesthetic team must also be aware of factors associated with the underlying cause of the scoliosis and the potential complications following treatment. For example, a patient with neurofibromatosis may have congenital defects involving the cardiac and genitourinary systems that can complicate the anesthetic technique. This same patient may undergo resection of multiple nerve root tumors and require surgical stabilization. Respiratory function might be compromised in the early postoperative period if multiple thoracic nerve roots were sacrificed, if pneumothorax or a CSF-pleural fistula developed, or if the patient experienced significant thoracic pain associated with the surgery. The associated disorders may have important anesthetic implications necessitating careful

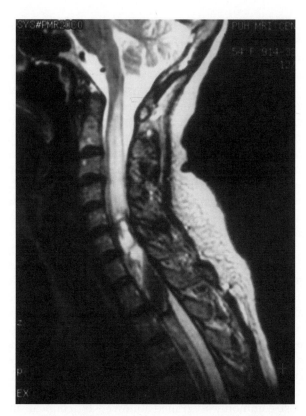

Figure 32-15 Intramedullary tumor. Mid-sagittal MR scan demonstrating an intramedullary, mixed-intensity lesion. A hemorrhagic ependymoma was completely resected through a cervical laminectomy.

preoperative assessment of the airway, pulmonary, and cardiac systems, and will require adequate cardiac, pulmonary, and neurologic monitoring throughout the perioperative period.

ACQUIRED

Acquired lesions of the spinal cord and column include tumors, infection, herniated nucleus pulposus, spinal stenosis, degenerative diseases, and trauma. Spinal cord tumors are classified by their etiology (e.g., primary or intrinsic lesions and secondary or metastatic lesions), anatomic location, and pathology. Symptoms usually develop slowly and progressively, and are manifested by proximal weakness, pain, sensory loss, radicular symptoms, and sphincteric dysfunction. Primary (intrinsic) spinal cord tumors arise from the substance of the spinal cord itself. They are termed intramedullary lesions and, by definition, are intradural (Fig. 32-15). These tumors are rare, accounting for approximately 15 percent of spinal neoplasms, often malignant, and include astrocytoma, ependymoma, ganglioglioma, oligodendroglioma, and hemangioblastoma.[86,87] These lesions are found most commonly in children and younger adults. Many of these tumors are associated with syrinx formation, which may also contribute to the patient's symptoms. Other types of intramedullary tumors include dermoids, epidermoids, teratomas, and, rarely, metastases.

The intradural, extramedullary tumors are relatively common, usually benign lesions. These include schwannoma, neurofibroma, and meningioma. They are most commonly identified in adults and in patients with neurofibromatosis, and occur with a higher frequency in the thoracic region. Malignant lesions in this location include metastases, filum terminale ependymoma, drop metastases from medulloblastoma, ependymoma or other tumors, and malignant degeneration of nerve sheath tumors.

Epidural tumors are most commonly metasatic.[88] The tumor cells travel into the epidural space surrounding the spinal cord or cauda equina either through direct spread or in the valveless venous channels (Batson's plexus). The tumors will often parasitize local vasculature or develop new collaterals, making resection difficult. Lung, breast, prostate, lymphoma, melanoma, renal, and gastrointestinal sources are most common. The lesion location is proportional to the number of vertebra, with thoracic region compression most commonly identified followed by cervical and lumbar region compression. Epidural tumors cause neurologic symptoms through compression of the dura and underlying neural tissue. Dural invasion is rare. Systemic malignancies can cause neurologic symptoms such as pain, weakness, and myelopathy through development of the paraneoplastic syndrome.

Vertebral hemangiomas are benign, extremely vascular bony lesions that may cause compression fractures, pain, or spinal cord compromise through epidural compression.[90] Other rare tumors such as chordoma can also cause epidural spinal cord compression.

Infections can occur in the same location and distribution as tumors. The symptoms will depend on the type of infection, virulence, immunologic status of the host, and treatment effectiveness. Bacterial infections are common, but viral, mycobacterial, and parasitic infections also occur, especially in compromised hosts.[91] Intramedullary infections are rare and are associated with transverse myelitis-type syndromes. These syndromes results in weakness, sensory loss, and sphincteric dysfunction, which may be permanent. Surgical biopsy may be required to establish an accurate diagnosis.

CSF infections or meningitis are usually bacterial, although fungal, viral, and postsurgical etiologies are frequently identified. By definition, these infections are subarachnoid and can be accessed via lumbar, cervical, or transventricular puncture. Neurosurgical patients undergoing posterior fossa surgery or resection of

dermoid, epidermoid, or craniopharyngioma tumors may experience a chemical meningitis with symptoms similar to bacterial infection.

Epidural infections are similar to metastatic tumors in that they both cause neurologic symptoms through spinal cord or cauda equina compression, and access the spinal canal through direct spread of Batson's plexus. Bacterial etiologies are most common, but mycobacterial infections must always be considered, especially in immunocompromised hosts. Surgical debridement and spinal stabilization may be required for adequate treatment.

Herniated nucleus pulposus is perhaps the most common diagnosis in a general neurosurgical practice. As discussed earlier, the intervertebral disk has a soft inner component (the nucleus pulposus, a notochord remnant) and a tough, fibrous outer layer (the annulus fibrosis). No fully accepted nomenclature for disk disorders exists. This has led to confusion when MRI and intraoperative pathology findings are described. The descriptive terms herniated nucleus pulposus, disk rupture, and disk herniation are probably synonymous to most clinicians. Each implies a tear in the annulus fibrosis with protrusion, extrusion, or free disk fragments present. Disk ruptures can occur superiorly and are called Schmorl's nodes. These may be an indication of degenerative disk changes and have been associated with painful conditions. Pure anterior or lateral disk ruptures are usually of little clinical significance but may cause swallowing difficulty in the cervical region. Posterior, posteriolateral, lateral, and far lateral disk ruptures may compress neural elements and cause radiculopathy, spinal cord compression, or cauda equina syndrome with loss of bowel and bladder control.

Patients with pain in a radicular distribution are initially treated with analgesics, rest, and anti-inflammatory agents. Persistence of symptoms, progression of neurologic deficits, or the presence of a significant neurologic deficit such as foot drop, cauda equina syndrome, on spinal cord compression with myelopathy dictates prompt surgical intervention.

Spinal stenosis is an anatomic condition such that inadequate canal volume exists to maintain normal neurologic function under physiologic conditions. The stenosis can be present throughout the spinal canal. It is frequently degenerative in nature, and is associated with facet hypertrophy and buckling of the ligamentum flavum. Congenital causes, such as short pedicular length or achondroplasia may also contribute to canal narrowing.

Cervical spinal stenosis is associated with myelopathy, which is frequently progressive and is described below. An important finding in these patients is that of Lhermitte sign. This electrical-like sensation occurs with neck extension or flexion and is indicative of posterior column lesions.[92] It is seen in patients with multiple sclerosis and severe cervical spinal cord compression.

Lumbar spinal stenosis, when clinically significant, most often causes neurogenic claudication. These patients have difficulty walking long distances. They describe proximal leg weakness, which is improved with lumbar flexion or rest. It is important and frequently difficult to distinguish neurogenic claudication from vascular claudication, and these lesions may both be present in the same patient.

The surgical treatment for either cervical or lumbar stenosis, when symptomatic, is decompression. This can be accomplished either anteriorly or posteriorly in the cerival region, and is performed posteriorly in the lumbar region. It is important to keep in mind that patients with cervical stenosis will often have lumbar stenosis, and vice versa.[93] The anesthetic team must prevent excessive cervical hyperflexion or hyperextension during intubation or surgery in this group of patients. We customarily limit cervical flexion such that the chin is no more than two fingerbreaths from the sternum during cervical decompression.

Degenerative conditions of spine include loss of disk height, vacuum disk changes, facet hypertrophy, reduced elasticity of intervertebral ligaments, degenerative spondylolisthesis (fracture of the pars interarticularis with intervertebral slippage), uncovertebral joint enlargement in the cervical region, osteophyte formation, and others. Many of these degenerative changes are common in asymptomatic adults. Pain syndromes may arise in association with these degenerative changes. Generally, nonsurgical treatments such as localized pain injections, facet blocks, epidural steroid injections, bracing, transcutaneous electrical nerve stimulation, ultrasound, and physical therapy are exhausted prior to surgical intervention.[94] Surgery can be used to correct certain specific conditions (e.g., fusion for spondylolisthesis) or it can be directed at neuropathic pain (e.g., insertion of spinal cord stimulator).

Trauma to the spinal cord and vertebral canal is a major cause of disability in the United States. Vertebral fractures are considered to be the result of forces acting individually or in combination with one another. These forces result in flexion, lateral flexion, extension, rotation, compression (axial loading), translation, or distraction.[95]

Traumatic injuries can occur anywhere in the spinal column from to the skull base to the coccyx. The cervical region is most commonly injured, followed by thoracolumbar coccyx. The cervical region is most commonly injured, followed by thoracolumbar fractures, especially the T12–L1 regions. The thoracic vertebral column proper is afforded increased protection from the rib cage and is least commonly injured. Approximately 15 percent of patients will have more than one vertebral column injury, and clinicans should assume that other fractures exist until adequate radiographs are available and an appropriate clinical examination can be performed. Children can experience spinal cord injuries without radiographic abnormalities (SCIWORA) due to physiologic ligamentous laxity.[96]

SPINAL CORD SYNDROMES: NEUROANATOMY AND CLINICAL PRESENTATION

The spinal cord is a delicate neuronal structure that begins at the skull base and extends to the L1-2 interspace in normal adults. The spinal cord itself is anatomically divided into gray and white matter. The gray matter is composed of neuronal cell bodies, dendrites, and glial cells. The central canal is located in the center of the gray matter and is lined with cuboidal or columnar cells. Axons and their oligodendroglial coverings comprise the white matter tracts. The cord is suspended within its arachnoid and dural coverings by the dentate ligaments which are composed of pia mater.

The lowest aspect of the spinal cord is termed the conus medullaris. Nerve roots exiting from this region of the spinal cord form the cauda equina and have a Schwann cell covering similar to peripheral nerves.[97]

Injury can occur at any level of the spinal cord, conus medullaris, and cauda equina. Mechanisms of injury include trauma, tumor, radiation, nutritional, degenerative changes, vascular, infection, iatrogenic, idiopathic, inflammatory, and others. A carefully obtained history, detailed neurologic examination, and appropriate radiographic studies allow the clinician to establish an accurate neurologic diagnosis and prognosis.

The involved location is identified as to spinal level and anatomic type. Radicular signs, specifically pain in a particular nerve root distribution, can provide excellent anatomic lesion localization. The clinician needs to remain cognizant, however, that nerve injury or irritation can result from intraspinal, foraminal, or extraforaminal lesions.

Myelopathic lesions indicate spinal cord dysfunction with neuropathologic changes from any of the causes noted above. The term is best defined clinically and is most common in the cervical region. Patients will frequently develop long tract (corticospinal and associated tract) signs such as spasticity, hyperreflexia, and Babinski responses.[98,99] Wasting of the intrinsic hand musculature, sensory loss from injury to the spinothalamic tracts and dorsal columns, and development of Lhermitte sign may also occur. The time course of the development of these signs is variable and depends on the etiology of the myelopathy and other factors.

Myelopathic findings do not localize lesion levels as specifically as radiculopathic changes, but the two are often found together in patients with spondylosis.

Complete spinal cord injuries result in total functional transection of the spinal cord, with loss of all sensory and motor modalities.[100] These lesions are usually traumatic, but can be the result of infection, vascular injury, malignancy, and other causes. A number of excellent articles have described the histologic, electrical, and clinical changes that occur with spinal cord injury.[101–104] These studies have shown that traumatic injuries cause tissue disruption and necrosis, cellular ischemia, gray and white matter hemorrhage, vascular edema, occlusion and reduced blood flow, and metabolic and electrical derangements. These events may contribute to secondary injury of the cord.

Spinal cord shock is a clinical condition commonly seen following significant spinal cord injury. The syndrome is manifested by flaccid, areflexic extremities, sensory loss, and loss of volitional rectal contraction. Autonomic dysfunction may be manifested by systemic hypotension with an inappropriately normal or low heart rate. Male patients may experience penile erection during the acute phase. Patients often require intravenous fluid resuscitation, central venous pressure monitoring, and urinary catheterization. Systemic vasopressor administration may be required to maintain adequate organ perfusion.

All efforts should be made to maintain adequate spinal cord perfusion, prevent further spinal cord compression, and reduce secondary spinal cord insults. High-dose methylprednisolone has become an accepted treatment for patients with spinal cord injury if they come to medical attention within eight hours of injury. The rationale behind its use is to stabilize membranes, reduce spinal cord edema, and maintain capillary blood flow.[105] The standard regimen includes a 30 mg/kg body weight intravenous bolus given over 15 minutes. This is followed with a continuous infusion of 5.4 mg/kg body weight each hour for 23 h.[106] Clinicians may continue steroids, such as dexamethasone, for some time afterwards. The risks of steroid use, including the development of gastric ulcers, wound infection, and others, should be weighed against the possible benefits in each individual case.[107]

Patient prognosis cannot be accurately determined until spinal shock is resolved. Return of spinal reflexes, such as the bulbocavernosus or clitoral reflexes, is an indication that spinal shock is resolving. Return of these reflexes can take hours to days.

Specific spinal cord syndromes can often be clinically recognized in patients who have suffered incomplete spinal cord injury. These syndromes have neuroanatomic correlations and will be reviewed below.[108,109]

A commonly recognized clinical spinal cord disorder

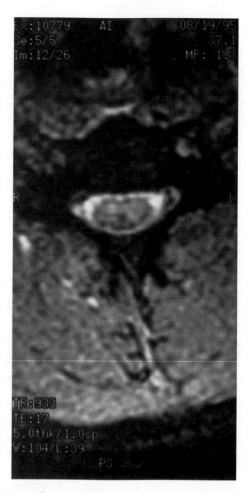

Figure 32-16 Central cord injury with spinal cord edema. T2-weighted mid-sagittal MR scan demonstrating edema in the cervical cord of a patient who experienced a hyperflexion-type injury.

is central cord syndrome. Elderly patients with narrow cervical spinal canals who suffer hyperextension of hyperflexion-type injuries are prone to this type of injury.[110] The clinical hallmark of this syndrome is weakness of the extremities, upper more so than lower extremities. Alterations in pain and temperature sensation, due to injury to the fibers as they cross the midline, also may be present. Centripetal injury to the central gray matter is the pathophysiologic event that explains the clinical, radiographic, and histopathologic findings (Fig. 32-16).

Acute and chronic central cord injuries can result in significant permanent neurologic disability. Difficulties with ambulation due to spasticity of the lower extremities, with permanent loss of the fine motor movements in the hands and normal bladder and bowel function, are common sequelae.[111] Both forms can also result in the development of syringomyelia, as discussed above.

The anterior cord syndrome is a neuropathologic and clinical entity that results from injury to all components of the spinal cord except the dorsal columns. This lesion results in loss of motor function and pain and temperature sensation, with preservation of vibratory and position sense. The injury may be the result of vascular (i.e., anterior spinal artery occlusion), traumatic, or other causes.

Posterior cord syndrome is an uncommon surgical entity. The neuropathologic correlate is loss of the dorsal spinal columns with preservation of the remainder of the cord. This results in the loss of both fine sensation and vibratory and position sense, with preservation of pain and temperature sensation. Although occlusion of the posterior spinal arteries might result in this syndrome, other causes, such as tabes dorsalis, B^{12} deficiency, multiple sclerosis, and paraneoplastic syndrome are more common.[112]

The Brown-Séquard or hemicord syndrome is a well described type of spinal cord injury with a good prognosis. The lesion represents functional hemisection of the spinal cord. This causes loss of ipsilateral motor function and position/vibratory sense from injury to the corticospinal tract and dorsal columns, respectively. Pain and temperature sensation is lost a few segments contralateral to and below the lesion due to the ipsilateral ascension of the fibers prior to their crossing over in the cord. A zone of ipsilateral anesthesia may also be present.[113] Brown-Sequard lesions may occur as a result of trauma, tumor, infection, syringomyelia, inflammation, and other conditions.

Conus medullaris syndromes occur as a result of injuries to the lowest aspect of the spinal cord. These lesions may also involve the lumbar nerve roots and usually cause areflexic bladder, bowel, and lower extremities.[114] Sacral reflexes may be preserved, depending on the level of injury within the conus. Rectal tone and perirectal sensation may also be reduced. This type of lesion is most commonly a result of traumatic or neoplastic etiologies in the authors' experience.

The cauda equina syndrome is peripheral nerve-type injury that occurs below the level of the conus medullaris. This lesion results in sensory, motor, bladder, and bowel dysfunction of a lower motor type. The lesion can be partial or complete. The prognosis for recovery is good if the underlying cause is rapidly corrected.

Criteria for Surgery

The criteria for recommended surgical intervention depend on the underlying disease process, rate of development of pain or neurologic deficits, expected longevity of the patient, surgical and anesthetic expertise, availability of effective nonsurgical alternative treatments, patient life-style considerations, and others. Neurosurgical intervention is undertaken for a number of reasons. The most common is to treat a condition that is causing progressive neurologic deficits, pain, or disability. Decompressive cervical surgery for progressive myelopathy would be an example of this. Conditions that have not responded well to nonsurgical alternatives may be considered for surgical intervention. Lumbar disk surgery for sciatic pain with minimal neurologic deficits is commonly performed for this reason.

Occasionally, surgery is performed to prevent the development of neurologic deficits. An example of this might be the untethering of a spinal cord in a child prior to a growth spurt. Rarely, neurosurgical intervention may be required to establish the diagnosis of a lesion. An example of this would be a transpedicular vertebral body biopsy to make a definitive histologic tumor diagnosis.

The following section is an outline of neurosurgical intervention for the more common disorders. Neither the categories nor the criteria for intervention are meant to be exhaustive. Rather, this is simply a guide to the common surgical indications for patients seen in a general neurosurgical practice.

CONGENITAL

Many congenital malformations, if noted at birth or in early childhood, require surgery to reverse or prevent the development of neurologic deficits and infectious complications or to improve rehabilitation potential.

The Chiari II malformation is usually found in combination with hydrocephalus and meningomyelocele at birth as described above. The initial procedures are closure of the meningomyelocele, if present, to avoid persistent CSF leakage and subsequent meningitis. Ventriculoperitoneal shunting is usually required to control hydrocephalus. These procedures may obviate the need for direct operative intervention on the hindbrain abnormalities. Evidence of continued brain stem compression (e.g., persistent spasticity or apneic spells) or alterations in CSF flow (e.g., progressive hydromyelia) are indications for posterior fossa decompression.[79] Chiari I malformations may require decompression for headache, progressive CSF flow abnormalities, spinal cord compression, or cranial nerve palsies.

The more severe spinal dysraphisms, such as meningocele and myelomeningocele, require surgery in the early perinatal period to stop CSF leakage. Hydromyelia and syringohydromyelia associated with the Chiari malformations usually respond to CSF-diverting procedures such as ventriculoperitoneal shunting. The development of progressive neurologic deficits such as weakness, spasticity, dissociated sensory loss, and bladder and bowel dysfunction in patients with adequately treated hydrocephalus is an indication for surgical treatment of the intramedullary fluid collection.

Other congenital spinal lesions, including dermal sinus tracts, diastematomyelia, lipomyelomeningocele, and thickened and tight filum terminale can cause tethered spinal cord. This condition results in back pain, progressive lower extremity weakness, spasticity, and bladder and bowel dysfunction. These lesions can be found in any age group, including the adult. Tethered spinal cord may be discovered incidentally as part of an evaluation for back pain, or it may be found following evaluation for progressive neurologic deficits. When discovered in childhood, surgery is usually recommended for the prevention of neurologic deficits that could reasonably be expected to occur if surgery were not performed. Surgery may be recommended if an adult is experiencing bladder or bowel dysfunction, difficulty with ambulation, worsening lower back pain, or progressive spasticity or spinal deformity.

The clinical presentation of patients with arteriovenous malformation is described above. These lesions often go undetected and frequently require thorough evaluation to establish the diagnosis. Occasionally, AVM lesions will be detected in patients who are evaluated for vascular skin changes of their lower back or poorly described neurologic symptoms. Intraspinal subarachnoid hemorrhages would be indications for urgent surgery. The development of progressive neurologic dysfunction, such as claudication, numbness, or weakness, or structural bone changes that may raise concerns of spinal instability would also be considered acceptable criteria for surgical intervention.

Transient structural scoliosis, such as that due to infection or disk rupture, will require intervention directed toward the underlying problem, although nonsurgical therapies may be adequate in selected cases. Surgical indications in idiopathic structural scoliosis are based on the known natural history of the disease.[115,116] Surgical indications include progressive curvature in a skeletally immature child or adolescent who does not respond to exercises and bracing. Curves greater than 50° generally require surgical correction. Patients may also require surgery to prevent pulmonary complications.

Degenerative scoliosis in the adult is associated with back pain and spinal stenosis. Progressive pain, nerve root compromise or neurogenic claudication are indications for surgery in healthy adults who do not respond to bracing, physical therapy, and other nonsurgical interventions.

ACQUIRED

Primary intramedullary spinal cord tumors, such as ependymoma, astrocytoma, and hemangioblastoma present with signs and symptoms of spinal cord dysfunction, pain, or radiculopathy. These lesions require surgical excision or biopsy for histopathologic identification, relief of symptoms, improvement of survival, and adjuvant treatment planning.[117] Extramedullary tumors, which are usually benign, require surgery if they are causing spinal cord dysfunction, progressive radiculopathy, or pain.

Secondary or metastatic spinal lesions may cause symptoms similar to the primary lesions. The secondary lesions also involve the spinal column and can cause bony or ligamentous instability. The generally recognized surgical criteria include pain not responsive to standard treatments, establishment of histopathologic diagnosis in cases where the primary is unknown, progressive kyphotic deformity, known tumor radioresistance, tumor recurrence following radiotherapy, bony compression of the cord, and rapid neurologic decline despite radiotherapy and steroid treatment.[88,118]

Infection can occur within the bone substance or disk space, in paraspinous structures, or in the intradural, intramedullary, or epidural spaces. Surgery may be required to obtain organisms for culture and antibiotic sensitivity testing. Open debridement and drainage of closed space infections is required to aid healing. This is applicable to patients with epidural infections, osteomyelitis, paraspinous infection, and disk space infection.[119,120] Other surgical indications for infectious processes include spinal cord decompression, removal of foreign bodies, correction of spinal deformity, and pain relief.[121]

Surgery for herniated nucleus pulposus is one of the most common procedures performed by neurologic surgeons. Immediate surgery is recommended in patients with known cervical disk rupture with myelopathy, cord syndrome, or progressive acute radicular symptoms. Patients with lumbar disk rupture and progressive, acute neurologic deterioration, such as foot drop or sensory loss, and patients with bladder or bowel dysfunction suggesting a cauda equina syndrome, also require emergent surgical diskectomy. Large thoracic disk ruptures with cord findings would prompt urgent surgical intervention as well.

Surgical indications for patients with cervical, thoracic, and lumbar disk ruptures and non-emergent conditions are less well defined. Most surgeons would recommend operative intervention for patients with persistent radicular pain and associated neurologic findings who have not responded favorably to nonsurgical measures such as bed rest, physical therapy, and possibly epidural or oral steroids. Patients whose pain impairs their ability to work or enjoy life and who have well-defined pathology with appropriate signs and symptoms may also be suitable surgical candidates.

Cervical spinal stenosis may cause spinal cord compression with associated ischemic cord changes.[122] The rationale behind surgery for cervical spondylotic (spondylitic) myelopathy is to reverse deficits such as myelopathy, and to prevent neurologic worsening in patients with progressive disease.[123] Patients who have progressive myelopathy and whose overall medical condition would allow them to undergo surgery are usually advised to undergo the decompressive procedures. Patients may also have associated radicular symptoms due to uncovertebral overgrowth. These patients are considered good surgical candidates as well.

Neurogenic claudication due to lumbar spinal stenosis may respond favorably to decompression with or without fusion. Lumbar spondylotic changes may reduce the space available for exiting nerve roots, causing nerve root entrapment symptoms similar to those seen with disk rupture. This radicular symptoms caused by this lateral recess syndrome often respond well to nerve root decompression.

Spinal cord and spinal column trauma frequently require surgical intervention for correction and stabilization. The major determinant as to whether a patient requires surgical intervention is the degree of instability caused by the traumatic event and underlying conditions. Surgeons attempt to determine the degree of spinal stability through the estimation of the mechanism of injury, forces involved, careful patient evaluation, and an accurate interpretation of radiographic studies.[124]

Anatomic and biomechanical theories have been developed to help assess spinal column stability.[125] A commonly applied theory divides the spinal support structures into two or three columns.[126,127] Injury to one (or two) columns may result in instability. Plain films are also used to determine stability. An atlanto-dens interval greater than 3.0 mm or extension of the C1 lateral masses 7.0 mm or more past the superior facet of the axis in the adult implies that the strong transverse ligament has been torn and that the C1–2 articulation is no longer stable.[128,129] Sagittal translation greater than 3.5 mm or angulation between adjoining vertebral bodies greater than 11 degrees also implies instability.[130,131]

The thoracic spine is reinforced by the rib cage and sternum. This area of the spinal column is relatively immobile. Instability is suggested when sagittal translation is noted to exceed 2.5 mm, angulation is greater than 5 degrees, many contiguous segments are involved, or neurologic dysfunction is present.[132]

The thoracolumbar region is a frequent site of spinal column injury, with flexion injuries being most common. Bony injuries in this area will frequently respond to external bracing, but may result in significant patient morbidity due to prolonged bed rest and limitation of activities. Ligamentous injuries usually require surgical intervention with fusion of the spinal unit to obtain adequate stability. Surgical intervention is often necessary in patients who have greater than 35 percent loss of vertebral body height, significant ligamentous or disk injuries, progressive kyphotic deformities, or neurologic deficits.

The lumbar spine is relatively flexible when compared to the thoracic spine. Flexion and axial compression-type injuries are commonly noted in this area. Surgery is usually warranted for patients with multicolumn injuries, significant burst-fractures, 3.0 mm or greater sagittal translation, or progressive deficits. Sacral fractures occasionally require surgical correction for nerve root entrapment or progressive neurologic deterioration, open injuries, and pelvic stability.

Surgical Site and Approach

Many surgical techniques have been developed during the 20th century. Greater understanding of spine biomechanics, anatomy, physiology, and anesthetic management have permitted surgeons to perform more advanced procedures. Many neurosurgical spine procedures are combined with fusion, often with surgical implants. The term fusion implies a union of bony elements or, in the case of the spine, vertebral segments or functional spinal units. Fusion is a healing process where the body uses osteogenic, osteoinductive, and matrix factors to create a bony bridge. This can be stimulated with the surgical introduction of bone decortication, bone support, and perhaps the addition of bone morphogenic proteins. This healing process is further augmented with immobilization. Immobilization can be obtained with external or internal orthoses, but these orthoses are no substitute for adequate surgical technique and the host factors that promote bone healing. Orthoses do provide immediate support and will frequently allow the patient to have early mobilization, which may reduce morbidity related to thromboembolism, skin breakdown and other problems.

CERVICAL

The cervical spine extends from the cranial base to the first thoracic vertebra. The first and second cervical vertebra have a unique anatomy that permits articulation with the skull base and subaxial cervical spine while allowing a great deal of movement. Their uniqueness requires separate surgical consideration. The traditional surgical approach to C1 and C2 has been posterior, through laminectomy. This approach is often combined with suboccipital surgery such as craniectomy or fusion for Chiari decompression or rheumatoid disease. The posterior approach is also commonly used for fusion purposes. The suboccipital bone can be exposed and used for fixation of surgical rectangles and other devices. The lamina of the vertebral bodies, when present, can also be used to anchor internal fixation devices such as Luque rectangles, Halifax clamps, Dewar tension bands, lateral mass plates, transarticular C1–2 screws, and others.[133–137]

While this approach provides excellent access to the posterior elements of the spinal column, it provides limited access to the lateral and anterior aspects of the spinal canal.[138] Surgical access to the odontoid for resection of bone or pannus formation is obtained through an anterior, transoral, transpharyngeal approach.[139] This surgery is usually performed by combined surgical teams with otolaryngologists providing the initial access. Intraoperative adjuncts including fluoroscopy and frameless stereotactic guidance may be utilized as well.[140]

Surgical access to the odontoid for screw fixation of odontoid fractures is provided by a retropharyngeal approach to avoid bacterial contamination of the instrumentation.[141] The foramen magnum, clivus, and ventral upper cervical spine for infection and tumor resection can be approached using lateral transcondylar and anterior retropharyngeal approaches.[142–144] Tracheostomy for airway management is often performed prior to these procedures.

The subaxial cervical spine is generally approached from either an anterior or posterior direction. The choice of surgical approach will depend on the vector of pathology, curvature of the spine, biomechanical considerations for postoperative stability, and the surgeon's experience and preference. Either approach may be acceptable for a particular type of pathology. For example, the goal of surgery for cervical stenosis is to relieve the spinal cord and nerve root compression. Most patients with this disease have anterior vectors of compression from uncovertebral joint overgrowth and disk/osteophyte complex formation. Posterior compression due to facet hypertrophy and buckling of the ligamentum flavum is frequently present. Anterior decompression at one or more levels, potentially performed with fusion, would be the choice of many surgeons in patients with primarily anterior vectors of cord compression or cervical kyphosis.

The technique of anterior cervical approaches in the subaxial spine begins with an anterior skin incision made in a vertical or transverse direction. Platysma is dissected and an interfascial muscular dissection is performed. The esophagus is retracted medially and the carotid artery is retracted laterally. Care is taken to protect these structures throughout the surgical procedure. The longus coli musculature is identified and pre-vertebral fascia is dissected, exposing the underlying vertebral bodies and disks. Disk is removed with pituitary forceps and spondylotic ridges are excised using curettes. Corpectomy, the partial removal of a vertebral body, can be performed to provide decompression of the anterior spinal canal. A fusion is performed as required. Platysma and skin are closed.

Posterior decompression is considered in patients with multilevel disease and normal cervical lordosis. The posterior approach is straightforward. A vertical skin incision is made and the cervical fascia is incised in the midline. The posterior spinous processes are identified and a subperiosteal dissection is performed. Lamina and ligamentum flavum is removed as necessary. The spinal cord and nerve roots are exposed. The foramina can be widened if necessary for the relief of radiculopathy. Lamina can be reattached for laminoplasty in younger patients.

Fusion of the cervical spine can be performed with or without the use of instrumentation from either an anterior or posterior approach. Anterior methods of fusion include diskectomy followed by the placement of autologous or bone bank bone into the interspace. Fusion after a corpectomy can be obtained with the placement of bone strut grafts, cylindrical titanium cages, or methylmethacrylate at the bone resection site. Anterior cervical plates can be placed over the grafts to provide increased biomechanical stability. Posterior fusion can be performed with posterior spinous process wiring, lateral mass plates, Halifax clamps, Luque rectangles, or other internal constructs (Fig. 32-17).

CERVICOTHORACIC

The cervicothoracic region is a transition between highly mobile cervical vertebra and relatively immobile thoracic vertebra. This region is easily approached posteriorly for the correction of dorsal pathology through a laminectomy. Anteriorly placed lesions are more difficult. The T1 vertebral body can often be accessed through an anterior cervical approach. This is less technically challenging in slender patients. Exposure of the T2–4 vertebral bodies may require removal of the upper sternum, disarticulation of the clavicle, splitting of the sternum, or other approaches.[145–147]

THORACIC

Posterior approaches to dorsal pathology are straightforward in the thoracic region and commonly used for tumor decompression, syringo-subarachnoid shunt insertion, sympathectomy, and other procedures. The posterior technique usually includes laminectomy, which provides excellent exposure of the dorsal and lateral spinal cord with little risk of instability. A number of lateral approaches to the spinal cord which are extrapleural and frequently transpedicular, have also been described.[148,149] These approaches usually begin with a paramedian incision and muscle dissection. The

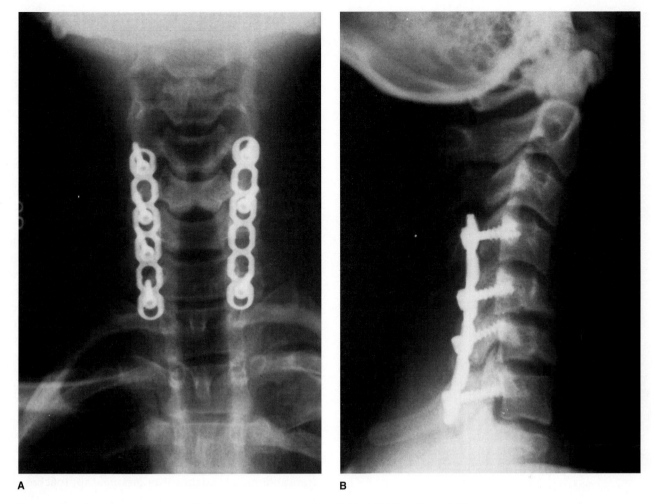

Figure 32-17   Lateral mass screws and plates. Same patient as Fig. 32-16. A-P (*A*) and lateral (*B*) views of an instrumented posterior cervical fusion construct using lateral mass plates and screws.

lateral spinal column is identified and the medical rib is removed. The pedicles can be entered, and anteriorly located pathology can be resected. Indications for this surgical approach includes ventral tumor resection, diskectomy, and vertebral body biopsy. Endoscopic devices can be used with most thoracic approaches to provide further spinal visualization.

Anterior thoracic spinal cord and spinal column structures can also be accessed via thoracotomy. Most spine surgeons work in conjunction with thoracic surgeons for these cases. With the patient in a lateral position, the surgery is performed in through a flank incision with one or two ribs removed and retracted. The lungs can be deflated with selected intubation, or they can be retracted. The pleura is identified and segmental vessels are ligated. Many surgeons temporarily clip the segmental vessels and observe the somatosensory evoked responses prior to ligating the vessels so as to avoid potential injury to the spinal artery of Adamkiewicz. The spinal pathology is located

and resected. This approach is used for central disk ruptures, tumors of the vertebral bodies, scoliosis, and kyphosis correction. Thoracoscopic procedures are also being developed as a minimally invasive means to perform diskectomy, sympathectomy, and corpectomy in select patients.

Thoracic fusion can be performed from an anterior or posterior approach or a combination of the two approaches. Posterior thoracic fusion is usually accomplished with rodding systems, rectangular constructs, or pedicle screws (Fig. 32-18). Lateral and anterior fusion constructs are performed with screw/rod instrumentation, plating systems, titanium cages, or bone strut grafts.

LUMBOSACRAL

Lumbosacral operations are the most commonly performed neurosurgical procedures. Lumbar diskectomy is effected with the patient in a lateral or prone position.

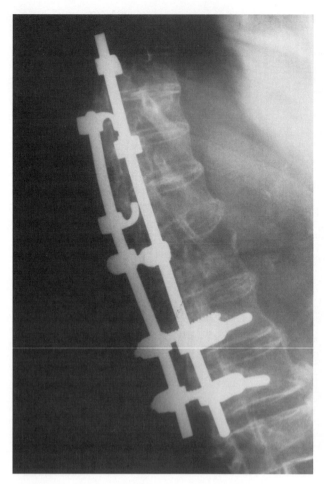

Figure 32-18 Thoracolumbar instrumentation. Oblique radiograph demonstrating a thoracic hook-claw rod construct utilizing upper lumbar pedicle screws.

A midline or paramedian incision is created and the lumbodorsal fascia is incised. Periosteal dissection exposes the laminae, which are removed as necessary to provide access to the thecal sac and nerve roots. The nerve roots are retracted medially to expose the posterior longitudinal ligament that covers the intervertebral disks. Diskectomy is performed by incising the ligament and removing disk material with forceps. The laminar resection can be extended to provide canal decompression in cases of spinal stenosis or posterior and lateral tumor resection. Tumor resection can be performed through canal decompression-type operations. The neural elements can be retracted more easily and safely during these procedures as the spinal cord has ended at L1–2. Tumor can be safely removed from lateral recesses using standard instruments, and transpedicular approaches can be considered in instances where the tumor is within the vertebral body. These operations can be combined with endoscopy for further anterior visualization.

The anterior spinal canal, vertebral bodies, and paraspinous structures can be accessed through transpedicular approaches. This procedure requires exposure of the facet and proximal transverse process, which are used for anatomic localization of the pedicle. The pedicle is entered and cancellous bone is removed. The medial pedicle wall is carefully removed and the nerve root and lateral and anterior thecal sac are observed. Preoperative angiography and embolization may be employed to help identify major arterial feeding vessels to tumors or arteriovenous malformations in this region. Embolization may enhance the safety of the operation by reducing intraoperative blood loss and operative time.[150,151]

The vertebral bodies can be exposed anteriorly through retroperitoneal or transabdominal approaches. The patient is placed in a supine or lateral position for these operations. A flank or midline incision allows dissection to the vertebral column. Retroperitoneal approaches reduce the risk of bowel injury but do carry a risk of ureteral injury. The retroperitoneal approach provides limited access to the lowest lumbar vertebral bodies. This approach can be used for sympathectomy procedures involving the lower extremities.[152]

Transabdominal operations offer excellent visualization of the vertebral bodies limited only by the major vessels. The abdominal contents are exposed and dissected, which places them at risk for injury. Both the transabdominal and the retroperitoneal approaches are used to resect anteriorly located pathology such as tumors or kyphotic deformities due to vertebral fractures. Complete intervertebral diskectomy can also be effected through these techniques.

Lumbar or lumbosacral fusions are performed following posterior or anterior exposure of the spine.[153,154] Posterior lumbar fusion requires exposure of the facet processes, laminae, and proximal transverse processes.[155] The fusion is performed after other procedures, such as canal decompression or tumor resection, are performed.[156] The articulating surfaces of the facet joints are decorticated to expose the underlying cancellous bone. Most surgeons also decorticate the transverse processes to obtain bilateral lateral fusion.[157] Cancellous bone, which is preferably obtained from the patient's iliac crest, is placed over the decorticated processes. Allograft and bone from posterior spinous processes or laminae can also be used for fusion.[158] The patients may be externally braced alone or an internal fusion construct may be placed. The fusion constructs employ metal rods or plates capable of withstanding multiple stress cycles without breakage. The vertebral bodies are connected with screws inserted into the bony pedicles, sub- or supralaminar hooks, sublaminar wires, pedicle hooks, or other devices.[159–161] These de-

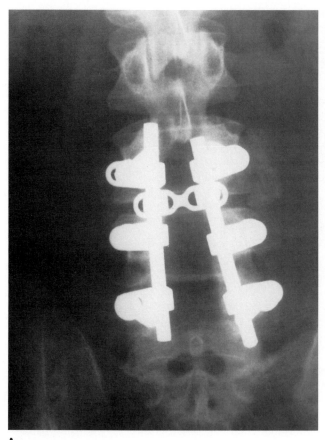
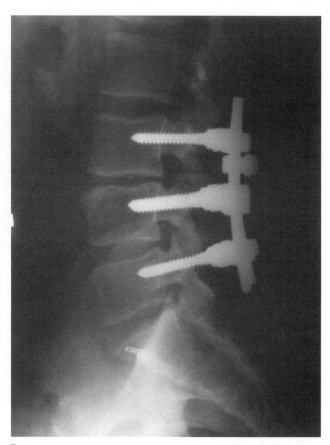

A   **B**

Figure 32-19   Lumbar pedicle screws. A-P (*A*) and lateral (*B*) radiographs of a segmental L3-L5 posterior lumbar fusion construct utilizing pedicle screw and rod instrumentation.

vices are connected to the rods, plates, rectangles, or other supports to reduce intervertebral movement and increase fusion rates.[162] Cores or strips of bone can be placed between intervertebral bodies from a posterior approach.[163] This posterior lumbar interbody fusion requires extensive diskectomy and nerve root retraction, but offers the potential advantage of anterior column support.[164,165]

Lumbar fusion can also be performed through the anterior approach as described above. Vertebral body (corpectomy) is performed and the disk is removed. A strut graft of bone is placed across the resection site and anchored into the vertebral bodies above and below. Bone screw and rod or bone plate instrumentation can be inserted into the anchoring vertebral bodies to obtain immediate stability (Fig. 32-19). Alternatively, the patient can be maintained in an external orthosis until the fusion is mature.

Diagnostic Methodology

Diagnostic radiology has become an extremely advanced science that allows precise localization and

characterization of spinal lesions prior to surgery. The basic radiographic study remains the plain radiograph, performed in anteroposterior and lateral views. These studies are the framework for future studies. They are necessary to define the number of lumbar vertebra and provide the required support of diagnoses such as spondylosis, infection, tumor erosion, Pott's disease, fracture, hemangioma, scoliosis, and others.[166] Oblique studies provide detailed views of the facet joints and pars interarticularis. Stress views, when necessary, provide confirmatory evidence of segmental spinal instability and transverse ligamentous laxity. Preoperative films are used for intraoperative comparison to confirm spinal level, identify fracture site, and to define pedicle bone anatomy.

CT scanning provides excellent bone imaging and helps to define bone and soft tissue abnormalities in the axial plane. Sagittal reformatting can be performed to enhance lesion interpretation. CT scanning is useful for measuring spinal canal and neuroforaminal diameter, it provides detailed anatomy of the facet joints, and can visualize acute hematoma formation with fair accuracy. A larger field of view during filming provides excellent definition of structures adjacent to the

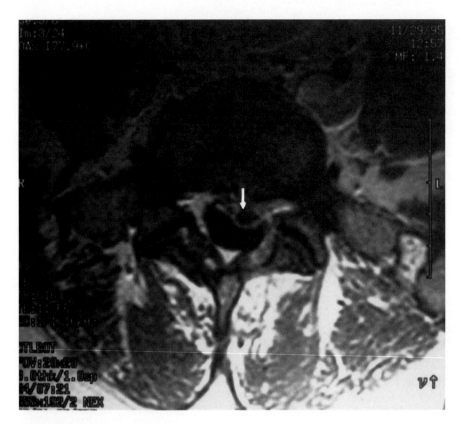

Figure 32-20 Recurrent lumbar disc herniation. Gd-enhanced axial lumbar MR scan with circumferential enhancement of recurrent disc herniation (*arrow*).

canal such as the muscles, kidneys, lymph nodes, and aorta. CT is particularly useful for surgical planning in patients with tumors causing direct metastatic compression of neural elements. A preoperative CT scan is required for fiducial registration with intraoperative guidance.[140]

Myelography, especially when combined with CT, can define pertinent spinal anatomy with precision. Myelography provides preliminary or confirmatory evidence of disk rupture, canal stenosis, traumatic or neoplastic subarachnoid block, root impingement, arachnoiditis, and other conditions. Tumor anatomy can be determined based on the vector of subarachnoid space compression. Myelography permits evaluation of the whole spinal column in a short time, usually with minimal patient discomfort. Intraoperative myelography can be used to confirm adequate canal decompression. Since myelography accesses the subarachnoid space, cerebrospinal fluid can be collected for culture and sensitivity, cell count glucose and protein determination, and cytologic evaluation for malignancy. Myelography also carries a small risk of neurologic deterioration.[167,168] We perform the spinal tap at the C1–2 interspace if complete block is suspected, and the patients are prepared for surgery prior to the puncture in case significant deterioration occurs.

MR scanning has become the standard of care in most institutions for preliminary and often definitive evaluation of the spine. MR scanners have become readily available and provide most of the advantages of myelography without the risk. The entire neuraxis can be scanned if necessary, with detailed views obtained for select regions. MRI has the advantage of imaging bone marrow well, which provides sensitive evidence of metastatic disease, osteomyelitis, and hemorrhage from compression fracture. This imaging modality is superior for imaging diskitis, syrinx formation, demyelinating disease, and cord edema. The addition of contrast agents such as gadolinium-DTPA provides increased sensitivity to intramedullary and other tumors, arachnoiditis, carcinomatous spread of tumor cells, recurrent disk herniation, and other conditions[169] (Fig. 32-20).

The disadvantages of MRI include lengthy data acquisition times, image degradation with patient movement, artifacts related to metallic implants, difficulty monitoring patients while they are in the scanner, and difficulty scanning patients on ventilators. Many patients are claustrophobic and cannot tolerate the enclosed MRI environment.

Special studies are obtained as needed. These studies include linear tomography, which is excellent at visualizing the dens and cervicomedullary junction (Fig. 32-21). 99m-Technetium bone scintigraphy and other nuclear medicine studies are employed for the evaluation of infection, blastic metastases, or inflammation.

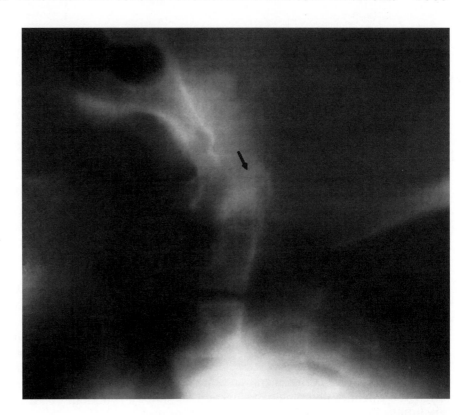

Figure 32-21   Linear tomography C1-2. Sagittal linear tomographs at the foramen magnum demonstrating basilar invagination and dens impaction (*arrow*).

Preoperative Assessment

ANESTHETIC CONSIDERATIONS

Preoperative evaluation and anesthetic management of the patient for spinal surgery must take into account the medical condition of the patient as well as the surgical procedure, including duration and surgical approach.[170] Most spinal surgical procedures will require general anesthesia because of the constraints of airway management, positioning, and duration of surgery. Factors to consider in preparing for spinal surgery include the patient's medical history and physical assessment, premedication, airway management, intraoperative monitoring and positioning, fluid requirements, special intraoperative requirements (i.e., the "wake-up" test), extubation, and postoperative pain control. The patient should be involved in the preoperative preparation, which includes patient education regarding monitoring, airway management, special intraoperative testing, and postoperative concerns including pain control and pulmonary toilet.

AIRWAY EVALUATION

Preoperative evaluation of the airway should include examination of the oropharynx with Mallampati classification, and range of motion of the neck with attention given to the elicitation of pain or other neurologic symptoms during manipulation.[171-173] Patients presenting for cervical spinal surgery should be discussed with the surgeon, and specific questions about instability, symptomatology, and the need for awake intubation as well as preoperative external stabilization should be reviewed.[174] Airway problems are most often encountered in patients with atlantoaxial subluxation, traumatic spinal cord injury combined with facial trauma, severe kyphoscoliosis or spinal deformity (i.e., rheumatoid arthritis, spastic contractures), and spine stabilization devices (i.e., cervical collar, "halo" traction).[175]

PULMONARY EVALUATION

A thorough history and physical examination should elicit the cardiopulmonary status of the patient. Patients most at risk for pulmonary dysfunction during spinal surgery include those with severe kyphoscoliosis (angle greater than 65 degrees),[174,176,177] arthritis, spinal deformities, cervical spinal cord injury, and neuromuscular disorders. Symptomatic patients with a history of noncardiogenic dyspnea, chronic cough, frequent pneumonias, or difficulty coughing should have pulmonary function tests and chest radiographs. Pulmonary function testing often reveals a restrictive pattern in patients with spinal deformities, (e.g., decreased FEV_1 and FVC). Vital capacity, expiratory reserve volume, and functional residual capacity are also often diminished in these patients. The patient with a cervical spinal cord injury may exhibit these abnormalities, with an even greater decrease in residual volume.[178,179]

CARDIAC EVALUATION

Cardiac function may be compromised by the underlying medical condition. Dysfunction is more likely to occur in patients with neuromuscular disorders (e.g., Duchenne's muscular dystrophy, myopathic disorders, and severe rheumatoid arthritis) and high cervical spinal cord injury. Patients with myopathies are more susceptible to cardiac dysrhythmias, decreased myocardial contractility, and malignant hyperthermia. Patients with rheumatoid arthritis may have cardiac abnormalities including rheumatoid nodules located within the cardiac conduction system, valvular lesions, or pericardial effusion.[179] Patients with high cervical or thoracic spinal cord injury are initially at risk for spinal shock and autonomic dysfunction with loss of sympathetic tone, impaired left ventricular function, and, later, autonomic hyperreflexia.[180,181]

NEUROLOGIC EVALUATION

Preoperatively, a thorough neurologic evaluation should be performed. Preexisting neurologic deficits should be carefully documented, especially if considering regional anesthesia. If general anesthesia is preferred, the extent of neurologic dysfunction may dictate intubation technique, monitoring, and choice of anesthetic agents.[182,183]

PHARMACOLOGY

Patients with spinal cord injuries and neurologic deficits may have altered pharmacokinetics due to muscle wasting, increased volume of distribution, and decreased serum albumin.[183] Patients with neuromuscular disease may have proliferation of extrajunctional acetylcholine receptors, with an exaggerated response to succinylcholine. The administration of succinylcholine to these patients may cause a massive release of potassium, which could lead to dysrhythmias, cardiac arrest, and death.[182] Patients who are paralyzed may also have delayed absorption from intramuscular injections due to decreased blood flow to these tissues.[170]

PATIENT PREPARATION

PATIENT EDUCATION

Both the patient and family should be included in the preoperative proceedings to help ensure cooperation and compliance during the perioperative period. This is especially important if an awake intubation or intraoperative "wake-up" test is required. It is also important to discuss placement of monitoring catheters and, when indicated, possible postoperative intubation and ventilatory support.

LABORATORY STUDIES

The preoperative work-up should be tailored to the patient and their general medical condition. Specific lab tests have been suggested for all patients undergoing spinal surgery, such as hemoglobin and hematocrit, white blood cell count, and urinalysis. Other tests might be indicated by history, including serum electrolytes, blood urea nitrogen, creatinine, prothrombin and partial thromboplastin times, platelet count, electrocardiogram, chest radiograph, arterial blood gases, and pulmonary function tests.[170] Patients receiving chronic diuretic therapy or those with possible renal dysfunction should have preoperative serum electrolytes and assessment of renal function. Any patient at risk for bleeding or extensive bone surgery should have clotting function evaluated. Those patients with pulmonary disease or dysfunction should have a baseline assessment of pulmonary function.

PREMEDICATION

The objectives for premedication include relief of anxiety, production of amnesia and/or sedation, control of pain, reduction of secretions, and aspiration prophylaxis. Medication may be administered by a variety of routes; however, most patients prefer either oral or intravenous, rather than intramuscular administration.[184]

Positioning

GOALS

A variety of positions are used for spinal surgery. The goals of positioning include not only providing adequate surgical exposure, but also maintaining normal anatomic positioning of the extremities (protects peripheral nerves) and head, avoiding abominal compression which may increase both venous return (increases surgical bleeding) and airway pressures (impairs ventilation), and finally, provides adequate padding (prevents ischemia and necrosis).[185] In patients with unstable cervical spine lesions or who are very obese, it may be safest to undergo an awake intubation followed immediately by positioning before general anesthesia is induced. The patient can verify that the position is comfortable and that the neurologic exam has not changed.[186]

COMMON POSITIONS

The most frequently used position is *prone* because it provides access to the posterior bony spinal elements and spinal cord. The head may be placed in a horseshoe headrest or upon padding. Care must be taken to maintain the neck in a neutral position if possible; however, the surgeon may require slight flexion or extension to achieve adequate surgical exposure. There should be no direct pressure on the eyes or periorbital area in order to prevent retinal ischemia and possible blindness. Also, the chin and nose should be well padded to prevent ischemia and ulceration.[185] Ischemia to the forehead and chin may be alleviated by periodically readjusting the head during the case. If the arms are flexed laterally during lumbar procedures, the brachial plexus is protected by maintaining an angle less than 90 degrees. Care should also be taken if the shoulders are displaced caudally during cervical procedures.[185] The breasts and male genitalia should be assessed for compression. The breasts should be displaced medially to the chest supports. The abdomen should move freely with each breath in order to avoid inadequate ventilation and high peak inspiratory pressures. The knees and feet should be adequately padded to prevent ischemic injury and pressure necrosis. It may be prudent to check peripheral pulses in the feet before finally draping the patient, and the use of an external compressive device to the legs may help prevent venous stasis. Patients who have undergone coronary revascularization procedures are particularly at risk for compression of the grafts against the chest wall in the prone position. They must be closely monitored for myocardial ischemia on the ECG, as myocardial damage may occur if corrective action is not taken.[187]

The *supine* position is used for anterior cervical procedures and occasionally as part of a 360-degree fusion of the lumbar spine. Care must be taken with neck extension, particularly in patients with neurologic symptoms and cervical spine lesions. The brachial plexus is also at risk in this position, especially when the shoulders are displaced caudally or if the arms lie posterior to the level of the trunk.[185]

The *lateral* position is useful for either a thoracotomy or flank dissection in order to obtain access to the anterior thoracolumbar spine. An axillary roll should be used to protect the dependent brachial neurovascular bundle, and the dependent arm should be continuously evaluated for adequate capillary refill and radial pulse. Often, the pulse oximeter is placed on this arm for this purpose. The other arm is usually placed on a well-padded tray or stand. The knees and ankles should be well padded in order to prevent ischemia since compression of the common peroneal nerve of the dependent knee may occur in this position. The dependent ear and eye should be free from folding and pressure, respectively. Restraining tapes and straps must also be assessed for possible pressure application leading to ischemia.[185]

The *sitting* position was used more commonly in the past for access to the posterior cervical spine, although it appears to be becoming popular again. The advantages of this position include better surgical access, decreased bleeding, and ease of hemostasis.[184,188] The major complications associated with this position include the possibility of venous air embolism, potential for greater hemodynamic instability (decreased venous return), quadriplegia and tongue swelling due to excessive neck flexion, sciatic nerve injury from inadequate sacral padding, and brachial plexus injury secondary to inadequate support for the arms.[185] It is important to remember that while monitoring blood pressure in this position, to subtract the gravitational gradient (approximately 12 to 20 torr) from the MAP at the heart level in order to accurately monitor SCPP.[188] In the standard sitting position, the cervical level of the spinal cord is approximately 15 to 25 cm above the heart.[189] If an arterial line is placed, the pressure transducer should be zero-referenced and positioned at this level. Also, neck flexion in this position should be cautioned since it may produce sufficient stretch of the spinal cord to alter autoregulation by mechanically affecting the spinal cord vasculature.[189]

HEAD POSITION

Head position is usually dictated by the surgical pathology and procedure; however, care must be taken to avoid hyperextension, hyperflexion and severe lateral rotation. Any restrictions of movement can best be judged during the preoperative assessment of the range of neck mobility. The patient's head and neck should not be maneuvered outside these limits once the general anesthesia is induced. If possible, the patient should be intubated in the neutral position. Hyperextension is most common in the prone position, and it may cause stretching and ischemia of the spinal cord. Hyperflexion is most common in the sitting position. It may cause decreased venous return from the head with resultant tongue swelling and intracranial hypertension and compression of the airway. After positioning, there should be two fingerbreaths of space between the chin and chest at maximal inspiration.[170]

Monitoring

PHYSIOLOGIC

Monitoring includes the routine monitors as specified by the American Society of Anesthesiologists.[190-195] More invasive monitoring may be required for lengthy procedures or those that have the potential for large blood loss, fluid shifts, or venous air embolism. It may also be indicated in those patients who have a complicated medical history, are hemodynamically unstable (i.e., spinal shock) or in procedures where special anesthetic techniques are used, including deliberate hypotension.[170] The placement of a Swan-Ganz catheter may

TABLE 32-1
Basic Monitoring Modalities for Spinal Surgery

Routine
  Precordial/Esophageal Stethoscope
  Noninvasive Blood Pressure
  Electrocardiogram
  Pulse Oximetry
  Oxygen Analyzer
  Exhaled Gas Analysis and Continuous End-Tidal CO_2 Analysis
  Temperature Probe
  Peripheral Nerve Stimulator
Invasive
  Urinary Catheter
  Arterial Pressure
  Central Venous Pressure
Neurophysiologic
  Wake-up Test
  Somatosensory Evoked Potentials
    Cortical
    Subcortical
  Motor Evoked Potentials
    Cortical Stimulation
    Spinal Cord Stimulation
  Awake Patient

---

be necessary for patients with severe cardiac or respiratory disease.

NEUROPHYSIOLOGIC

Monitoring of neurologic function is necessary during operations that may compromise the integrity of the spinal cord. Certain procedures place the spinal cord more at risk than others, including surgery for scoliosis correction, spinal cord tumor removal, or spinal fusion.[196–199] Four basic methods are used to assess spinal cord function: the wake-up test; somatosensory evoked potentials (SEP); motor evoked potentials (MEP); and the awake patient managed with local anesthesia and sedation (Table 32-1).

INTRAOPERATIVE WAKE-UP TEST

The intraoperative wake-up test is often used to assess spinal cord function during spinal instrumentation.[184,198,200–203] It is generally performed by decreasing anesthetic administration and requesting the patient to perform simple maneuvers (i.e., move the hands and feet), before completely emerging from the anesthetic. If necessary, the surgeon can reverse detrimental surgical interventions, possibly before permanent neurologic damage has occurred. If the motor demands are satisfactorily performed by the patient, the anesthetic is resumed and the operation is completed.[170,204] Some feel that this is the most obvious and best test of spinal cord function. One distinct advantage is the fact that no special equipment is required when used as the sole neurophysiologic monitor. The main disadvantage is

that it is only an intermittent monitor, as it can only evaluate motor and sensory function at the time it is applied. Therefore, the test should be applied in conjunction with more continuous forms of neurologic function monitoring. It is often used in conjunction with SEP monitoring and performed if and when abnormal SEP readings are obtained. Other disadvantages include increased blood loss, dislodgement of the endotracheal tube and intravenous lines, as well as patient discomfort and awareness. This technique is unsuitable in young children or the mentally incompetent.[205,206] Additionally, there is a remote possibility of venous air embolism in a patient who takes a sudden, deep inspiratory breath during awakening which may cause aspiration of air into the open vessels in the wound.[184]

SOMATOSENSORY EVOKED POTENTIALS (SEPs)

SEPs are elicited by typically electrically stimulating the median nerve (wrist) or posterior tibial nerve (ankle) and are detected by surface electrodes as transient potential differences.[207–209] Thus, the ascending dorsal columns,[210] which carry sensory input fibers, including proprioception and vibration from the periphery to the brain, can be monitored. Waveform peaks are described by polarity (positive/negative), amplitude (μV or nV), latency (msec) and distance separating the neural generators and recording electrodes (near-field/far-field). Injury or compromise of the neurologic pathway may be seen as an increase in latency or a decrease in amplitude of the waveforms. These potentials can also be affected by inhalation agents, bolus intravenous agents, ischemia, temperature, hypoxia, hypotension, anemia (hematocrit < 15 percent g/dl), hypercapnia, or other neurochemical depressants.[211–218] Disadvantages include the requirement for expensive equipment and specially trained personnel. Also, SEP monitoring reflects the electrophysiologic status of the posterior columns, not the anterior cord where the motor pathways course. Several recent case reports have also documented findings of postoperative neurologic impairment (i.e., paraplegia) while maintaining normal SEPs intraoperatively. Therefore, SEPs may not be predictive of postoperative motor dysfunction.[199,219–223]

Peripheral SEPs may also be measured by recording potentials from the epidural or intrathecal space, spinous processes, or even interspinous ligaments.[224–232] In comparison, spinal SEPs appear to be more stable and allow faster stimulation rates for cortical responses. On the other hand, epidural SEPs appear to be superior because of their safety, ease of performance, reliability, and higher amplitude recordings.[210] The wires are placed at the edge of the surgical site and project into the epidural space both rostrally and caudally.[225] This location avoids the surgical field and artifactual movements, which improves the quality of the recordings. Thirty to 50 percent attenuation of the evoked potentials when measured extradurally appears to be normal. However, a greater than 50 percent loss in amplitude or complete loss of one of the three negative peaks in the recording indicates probable postoperative neurologic sequelae. Each extremity should be stimulated separately, rather than simultaneously, to obtain a reading that best corresponds to outcome.[170,223]

Spinous process recordings can be significantly disrupted by surgical manipulation and blood or instrument electrode contact. The subdural recordings have only been used when the dura is opened by the surgeon.[208] Direct spinal cord stimulation and recording have been reserved for patients who show minimal response to peripheral nerve stimulation (e.g., Duchenne's muscular dystrophy and spinal muscular atrophy).[208] These potentials are not affected by anesthetic agents, but are sensitive to accidental cord compression or excessive traction during surgery. Cortical SEPs fluctuate in response to blood pressure changes, hypothermia, and general anesthesia, especially when drugs are administered in bolus fashion. Subcortical SEPs, on the other hand, are resistant to these nonsurgical factors.[208,209]

MOTOR EVOKED POTENTIALS (MEPs)

Motor evoked potentials are similar to SEP monitoring, but the functional integrity of the motor tracts is evaluated.[233] The motor cortex can be stimulated via bilateral scalp electrodes, or, alternatively, the spinal cord can be directly stimulated. Direct spinal cord electrical stimulation above the area at risk is the most common and only FDA-approved method of producing MEPs. The electrical potentials can then be measured at either the spinal cord, peripheral nerve, or muscle (electromyography).[234-238] Although virtually all anesthetic agents affect evoked potentials, transcranial stimulated MEPs are more sensitive than SEPs to nearly all types of anesthetics.[239-242] MEPs produced by spinal cord stimulation appear to be less sensitive to the effects of volatile anesthetics than are SEPs, but are just as sensitive to bolus infusions of intravenous drugs, hypothermia, hypoxia, and hypotension.[239-242] In the past, total intravenous anesthesia with ketamine or a combination of etomidate and narcotics has been advocated. Improved methods of stimulus application may allow for more variation in anesthetic technique. If the electrical potential is measured in the muscle, the use of neuromuscular blocking agents must be closely monitored. Although the effects of partial neuromuscular blockage on the sensitivity and specifically of MEP monitoring are unknown, neuromuscular blockade

must not be complete in order for muscle potentials to be recorded.[243-247] The impact of using MEPs on the effects of the cortex is unknown. There is theoretical concern that repetitive electrical or magnetic stimulation of the cortex could induce epileptic activity, neural damage, cognitive dysfunction, or memory impairment. Also, problems could potentially arise in patients with cardiac pacemakers or central venous catheters.

AWAKE PATIENT

Continuous assessment of the awake patient is extremely useful in any clinical setting in which CNS dysfunction may occur. Zigler and coworkers[248] described successful use of intravenous sedation combined with local anesthesia infiltration by the surgeon for posterior cervical stabilization procedures with fusion and iliac crest bone graft. They found that the patients not only tolerated the procedure well, but could communicate with the surgeon during crucial moments of spinal manipulation. Most of these procedures were performed on patients with traumatic posterior cervical instability resulting from flexion-compression-type injuries. Almost half of their patients had incomplete spinal cord injuries preoperatively, including Brown-Séquard, anterior and central cord syndromes. In this era of cost containment, such monitoring may become more popular. Although it does not require special equipment or technologists, it does require a skilled anesthesiologist who may select the appropriate patient and procedure. Awake neurologic monitoring may be difficult in uncooperative patients or lengthy procedures (e.g., longer than 3 h), since medications given to tolerate the procedure may decrease the sensitivity and specificity of the neurologic examination to detect injury.[249]

Anesthetic Management

REGIONAL ANESTHESIA

Although rarely chosen, local and regional techniques have been successfully used for spinal surgery.[170,250,251] From a medicolegal standpoint, it is generally agreed that regional techniques should be avoided in patients with preoperative neurologic deficits.

GENERAL ANESTHESIA

General anesthesia is most commonly used for spinal surgery for several reasons, including patient preference and the requirement for prolonged prone or uncomfortable positioning. Among other methods, a nitrous-narcotic based technique with low-dose inhalation agent supplementation can provide adequate amnesia and analgesia and not interfere with intraoperative neurologic monitoring, including a "wake-up" test. The combination of an inhalation agent in combination with an opioid technique may also provide a component of deliberate hypotension, which reduces intraoperative blood loss.

INDUCTION

Depending upon the stability of the cervical spine, an awake intubation may be indicated. If an awake intubation is necessary, the patient should be adequately prepared both mentally and physically. Once the patient has been informed of what to expect, an antisialagogue should be administered to enhance the mechanics of the procedure and to allow adequate topicalization of the airway. The patient should be carefully sedated in order to alleviate anxiety and permit cooperation. The patient undergoing an awake intubation should be able to answer questions and follow commands. They may also be able to help position themselves comfortably on the operating room table, even in the prone position, which may help minimize neurologic damage. Once the patient has been positioned and a brief neurologic evaluation has been performed, anesthetic induction may proceed.[186]

MAINTENANCE

As discussed earlier, a balanced anesthetic technique is most often used for patients undergoing spinal surgery, especially those having neurophysiologic monitoring or a "wake-up" test.[198,204] Muscle relaxants are used at the discretion of the anesthesiologist in collaboration with the surgeon and the neurologist monitoring neurophysiologic function. Some prefer not to use muscle relaxants so that nerve stimulation will indicate proximity to a nerve.[170] Blood pressure should be maintained close to or above the patient's lowest recorded awake MAP, in order to minimize the chance of spinal cord damage (i.e., maintain SCPP).

Intraoperative fluid administration regarding crystalloids and colloids remains an area of controversy. However, all agree that dextrose-containing fluids should be avoided because of the risk of a worse neurologic outcome in the presence of hyperglycemia during spinal cord ischemia.[252-254] Drummond and Moore[255] demonstrated in rabbits that plasma glucose concentrations as little as 40 mg/dl above normal profoundly worsen the injury. However, it remains controversial whether aggressive efforts to maintain a normal glucose are warranted. The type, duration, and extent of surgery may guide the approach to fluid administration and replacement.

METHODS TO MINIMIZE BLOOD LOSS

Methods for minimizing intraoperative blood loss include hemodilution, autologous blood donation, intra-operative blood salvage, and deliberate hypotension.[256-263] Hemodilution is performed by collecting blood from the patient and storing it during the operative procedure. The blood is replaced with crystalloid and or colloid, with a goal of achieving a hematocrit of 20 to 30 percent g/dl (varies with underlying medical condition). The stored blood is then reinfused intraoperatively or postoperatively.[264-266] Autologous blood donation allows healthy patients to predonate their own blood for future reinfusion. Intraoperative blood salvage uses a machine to collect blood from the surgical field. The blood is then processed and separated so that the red blood cells can be returned to the patient. Deliberate hypotension (DH) involves lowering arterial blood pressure to reduce blood loss, in addition to providing a better surgical field.[267-270] Any technique for DH should be easy to manage, devoid of toxicity, and quickly reversible. The desired drop in blood pressure is dependent on the patient's underlying medical condition and normal blood pressure, but generally the mean arterial pressure should be 50 to 65 mmHg.[266,271] A variety of medications have been used for this process including nitroglycerin, nitroprusside, inhalation anesthetics, beta-blockers, and calcium-channel blockers.[271] The mechanism of action of these drugs varies and results in a complex alteration in reflexes with subsequent changes in blood flow to various organs. During the use of DH, it is important to maintain organ perfusion and cardiac output, which is best accomplished by keeping venous filling pressures adequate during vasodilation.[266] Careful hemodynamic and spinal cord monitoring should be employed when using DH to assess organ function since the possibility of organ ischemia is a major concern. Sperry and co-workers[272] demonstrated that the choice of hypotensive technique may influence the extent of organ ischemia. Factors that contribute to venous bleeding should also be optimized, such as positioning, avoidance of PEEP, and avoidance of overhydration.

EXTUBATION

Extubation is usually performed in the operating room immediately following the surgical procedure. Since spinal surgery is performed with the patient in various positions, extubation techniques may vary. In addition to causing a smaller decrease in lung volumes, the prone position affords the advantage of allowing secretions to drain from the oral and nasal cavities. In order for extubation to be considered in this position, the patient should have normal airway anatomy that caused no problems with either ventilation or intubation. Although it is possible to reintubate a patient in the prone position, it may be difficult.

Postoperative ventilation may be indicated for patients with preoperative pulmonary dysfunction, high cervical spinal cord injury, hemodynamic instability, or in prolonged procedures with massive fluid shifts or persistent neuromuscular weakness. In any case where difficulty may be anticipated in reintubation (particularly a newly stabilized cervical spine), a conservative approach to extubation should be employed, with the patient fully awake. The use of a jet stylet during extubation of these patients may be considered. The jet stylet is a small, hollow, semirigid catheter that can be used as a means of ventilation (jet function) and/or as an intratracheal guide for reintubation (stylet function).[273] If endobronchial placement is avoided, this catheter is usually well tolerated by the patient until its use is no longer justified.

Postoperative Care

Postoperative care is administered along clinical pathways and individualized for each patient. The patient's preoperative status, surgical procedure, intraoperative complications, and pain tolerance are all considered in postoperative management.[274] In general, patients who undergo uncomplicated disk surgery, whether cervical or lumbar, can be expected to be discharged within one day. These patients are examined in the recovery room for resolution of preoperative pain and neurologic deficits. Patients who are relatively pain-free and who have stabilization or resolution of preoperative deficits are mobilized in the immediate postoperative period. Pain control is effected with intramuscular or oral agents. Cervical patients are braced for comfort. Discharge criteria include satisfactory ambulation, adequate oral tolerance, and normal urinary function. The most common complication in our experience, intraoperative cerebrospinal fluid leak, usually requires bed rest for 1 to 5 days.

Patients who have undergone more extensive posterior procedures, such as decompression, require longer hospitalization stays. These patients are generally older and may be at increased risk of postoperative complications. The more extensive procedures require longer incisions, greater muscle retraction, longer operative times, more bone removal, and greater blood loss. Early mobilization remains a priority to prevent the development of deep venous thrombosis (DVT), ileus, and pulmonary complications. Pain control is important so that patients can fully participate in physical therapy regimens. The patients are monitored closely for neurologic complications, and DVT prophylaxis is employed. Difficulty urinating in the early postoperative period is common, especially in men. This must be differentiated from early cauda equina syndrome. Straight catheterization is utilized when necessary, but

urinary function frequently returns to normal within a few days.

Anterior cervical procedures, which require neck dissection and retraction of the trachea, esophagus, and carotid arteries, are usually uncomplicated and create minimal pain for patients. These patients can have non-neurologic complications, such as esophageal injury, which may not be recognized immediately. They are observed for fever, difficulty swallowing, and expanding neck mass. Patients who have undergone multilevel cervical corpectomy with fusion require extremely careful observation within the hospital for at least three days. The surgery often requires extensive retraction and bone work, and the operation may not be completed until late in the day. When extubation is considered appropriate, the endotracheal tube is removed over a tube changer, and the patients are observed for respiratory compromise for a few more hours. Reintubation is extremely difficult or impossible should respiratory compromise occur. A tracheostomy kit is maintained at the bedside in case emergency airway control is required.

Lumbar fusion patients usually experience significant postoperative pain because of larger skin incision, muscular retraction, extensive bone dissection, and iliac crest autograft harvest. Patient-controlled analgesia pumps are routinely used for the first one to three days, after which patients are switched to intramuscular and oral agents. Incisions are carefully watched for the 5- to 7-day hospitalization, and drains are removed within 36 h.

Patients are fitted with external orthoses and are mobilized on the first postoperative day. The urinary catheter is removed when the patient is ambulating well, and physical and occupational therapy is begun. DVT prophylaxis, consisting of subcutaneous heparin, is administered after drains are removed.

Patients who have undergone thoracotomy for anterior disk resection or corpectomy, posterior extrapleural approaches to thoracic disk, transabdominal or retroperitoneal surgery for corpectomy, and other less common operations are monitored and treated on a highly individualized basis. The patients are observed for the complications unique to each procedure, especially pulmonary and gastrointestinal. Usually, two or three teams are following the patient, and care must be coordinated.

Complications

Complications are untoward events that prolong hospitalization. These events are becoming well defined as large series of patients are reported. Although every complication cannot be predicted or expected, certain events do occur with frequency and may be preventable. General perioperative complications include DVT, postoperative anemia, ileus, nausea and vomiting, dysuria, urinary tract infection, atelectasis, pneumonia, cardiac dysfunction, pancreatitis, major vessel injury, ureteral laceration, intraperitoneal injury, and wound infection. Although these complications can occur in any patient undergoing surgery, some of the complications are relatively common in spinal surgery patients and deserve further review.

DEEP VENOUS THROMBOSIS

Deep venous thrombosis is a well recognized clinical event that occurs in over 30 percent of neurosurgical and orthopaedic patients.[275] Risk factors for the development of DVT include advanced patient age, immobilization, prior DVT, hypercoagulability due to malignancy, oral contraceptives, hematologic disorders, and prolonged surgery with venous stasis.[276] DVT may occur in the deep veins of the leg or pelvis, causing leg edema and pain. Pulmonary embolism (PE) may occur as a result of DVT. PE may range in clinical severity from asymptomatic lesions to fatal events. Pneumatic stockings are widely employed to reduce the risk of DVT formation, as is subcutaneous heparin. Treatment of thrombotic events can include anticoagulation if the patient is felt to be a safe candidate. Alternatively, an inferior vena cava filter may be used in patients at high risk of recurrent PE or who are poor candidates for anticoagulation.

PULMONARY

Pulmonary complications, especially pneumonia, are common in spinal cord-injured patients.[277] Careful respiratory toilet, suctioning, intermittent positive pressure treatments, or ventilatory sighs may help reduce the incidence of pneumonia.[278]

WOUND INFECTION

Wound infections can occur in any patient who undergoes surgery. Fortunately, deep space infections, such as diskitis, occur in fewer than 1 percent of patients undergoing elective lumbar laminectomy and diskectomy.[279] Cervical disk operations have similar infection rates in our experience. More involved operations, such as fusions, have higher rates of infectious complications.[280,281] This is related to the implantation of spinal constructs, insertion of allograft or autograft bone, prolonged surgeries, and other factors.[282] Host factors such as poor nutrition, malignancy, steroid treatment, obesity, diabetes mellitus, concurrent infection, and local host factors all influence infection rates.[279] Most surgeons use prophylactic antibiotics for spinal surgery

in an effort to reduce perioperative infections, and this does seem to be beneficial.[283]

VESSEL INJURY

Injury to a major vessel, such as to the aorta, iliac arteries or veins, vertebral or carotid arteries occur with a very low frequency during spinal procedures.[284] Major vascular events occur most commonly during lumbar disk surgery. The event may be unrecognized by the surgeon and is considered only when the patient becomes hypotensive and tachycardiac. This represents a life-threatening condition that demands immediate attention. A vascular surgeon is called immediately, and the wound is packed. The patient is rotated to a supine position and the abdomen is prepared for laparotomy. The injured vessel is repaired and the lumbar incision is closed.

Injury to the carotid artery during lateral transcondylar approaches to the upper cervical region, anterior cervical diskectomy, or decompression can be repaired directly after the injury is visualized. Vertebral artery injury during these procedures requires further exposure, depending on the surgical approach. Dissection of the longus coli musculature and sacrifice of the artery[285] is generally required for vertebral artery injury during anterior cervical procedures. In summary, major vascular injuries need not be fatal if they are treated expediently and the patient remains in a stable physiologic condition.

The artery of Adamkiewicz is a segmental artery that usually arises from the left side of the aorta in the T7–L1 region. This artery is felt to be a dominant vessel which provides arterial supply to the thoracic spinal cord. Sacrifice of the artery without the development of cord ischemia is certainly possible, especially if segmental aortic arteries are disrupted unilaterally.[286] We routinely place temporary aneurysm clips on segmental vessels and monitor SSEP activity prior to permanent ligation of the vessels.

CEREBROSPINAL FLUID LEAKS

Cerebrospinal fluid leaks occur due to tears of both the dural and arachnoid membranes. These occur as a result of trauma, intraoperative tear, and other causes. Iatrogenic injury, in our experience, occurs in approximately 3 percent of patients undergoing lumbar laminectomy and diskectomy. This usually occurs during ligamentum flavum removal with the Kerrison punch. Iatrogenic injury during anterior or posterior cervical diskectomy occurs less frequently. More extensive procedures, including decompressive lumbar laminectomy, lumbar fusion, and reoperation for recurrent lumbar disk herniation carry higher rates of dural laceration. Patients with severe spinal trauma have very high rates of dural laceration and may have nerve roots extruded through the dural tears.[287,288]

Dural tears are usually found in association with laceration of the arachnoid membrane with resultant CSF leak. This is a potentially very serious complication that can result in meningitis, pseudomeningocele formation, or persistent CSF fistula. Intraoperatively, dural and arachnoid rents are identified if CSF fills the operative site and the dura wall becomes slack. Occasionally, the lumbar puncture site from a recent myelogram can be identified as a source of leakage. Infrequently, a small rent occurs and it goes unrecognized until the postoperative period, when clear, β_2-transferrin positive wound drainage is noted.

All attempts are made to completely repair the dural rent at the time of surgery. Surgeons usually can perform a primary closure with fine silk suture and reapproximation of the dura. Care is taken to prevent entrapment of the underlying nerve rootlets during this procedure, and multiple Valsalva maneuvers are performed to insure watertight closure. Repair of ventral and lateral tears, or tears that occur with extremely limited exposure such as in the cervicomedullary junction, are technically more difficult to close. In these circumstances, fascia lata or muscle may be used over the rent to obtain a seal. Occasionally, fibrin glue is used to seal the dura. The more superficial layers of the wound, including the fascia, subcutaneous layer and skin are closed meticulously to provide further protection against CSF fistula. The patients are routinely placed at bed rest for a period of 1 to 5 days following the surgery. Should CSF wound drainage continue, a subarachnoid drain may be placed to provide a low pressure conduit while the rent heals. Alternatively, the incision is re-explored in an attempt to locate and repair the leakage site.

NEUROLOGIC

Neurologic complications associated with spinal surgery include injuries to the nerve roots, spinal cord, sympathetic nervous system, lower cranial nerves, and cauda equina. Injuries to the peripheral nerves, especially the ulnar and lateral femoral cutaneous nerves, can occur as a result of body habitus, positioning, and surgical laceration during harvest of fascia lata or iliac crest bone graft. Neurologic complications can occur at any time during a patient's evaluation, transfer, surgery and postoperative course. An especially critical time is during patient positioning, as patients with pre-existing neurologic compromise or highly unstable injuries can experience worsening of their deficits during this time.[289,290] We routinely use SEP monitoring during positioning of patients with spinal cord find-

ings to prevent worsening of their preoperative deficits. Alternatively, some authors recommend the use of a "wake-up" test to determine neurologic function prior to proceeding with surgery.[291]

Spinal cord injury can occur during cervical, thoracic, or upper lumbar surgery. This may be the result of laminectomy, removal of soft tissue or ligamentum flavum, diskectomy, foraminotomy, corpectomy, correction of spinal cord deformity, insertion of pedicle bone screws, placement of sublaminar hooks, insertion of sublaminar wires, removal of tumor, insertion of spinal cord stimulators, development of intramedullary, subdural or epidural hematoma, and other causes.[292,293] The injury may occur as the result of direct injury, mechanical compression or vascular compromise. Any spinal cord injury pattern can result, but Brown-Séquard and central cord patterns are most common.

SEP monitoring is frequently employed to alert the surgical team of neurologic compromise, but false-positive and false-negative results are possible owing to the nature of the monitoring technique.[294,295] Combinations of motor and sensory modalities can be monitored in certain instances, but motor monitoring of the spinal cord has not become standard technique in most centers.[296] Significant changes in the evoked responses requires immediate attention of the surgical team. We reevaluate our last surgical maneuver, reduce the degree of spinal correction, and remove instrumentation if necessary. Steroids are immediately administered in an effort to reduce secondary neurologic injury.[106]

The cauda equina syndrome is described above. This lesion can be the result of surgical manipulation or trauma, bone compression, instrumentation, hematoma, and infection. The signs and symptoms must be recognized quickly and treated expeditiously, as resolution of neurologic deficits is possible.

Nerve root injury can occur as a result of direct surgical trauma, manipulation, entrapment in a dural rent, missed or recurrent disk herniation, hematoma, vascular compromise, bony compromise, or impingement from fusion instrumentation.[297-301] The injury can occur immediately or be delayed in onset. Fortunately, the nerve root is quite resilient to trauma, and oftentimes an injury is reversible if the compressive lesion is removed expeditiously. The development of a new root deficit in the immediate postoperative period is a cause for concern and further investigation. Plain radiographs are taken to evaluate bony lesions and instrumentation placement, but these studies can yield false-negative results.[302] CT scanning and possibly myelography may be required for further evaluation of the nerve root. Ultimately, the patient may require direct re-exploration of the surgical site for adequate root assessment.

The sympathetic nervous system can be injured during extensive dissections around the lumbosacral plexus. This complication is more frequent with bilateral dissections for sympathectomy or anterior lumbosacral dissection/fusion procedures.[303] Although impotence or sterility can occur in a male, the more common complication is retrograde ejaculation.[304,305]

Cranial nerves VII, IX, X, and XII may be exposed or injured during cervical surgery. They are at significant risk during anterior retropharyngeal or transcondylar approaches to the upper spinal canal.[143,144] The hypoglossal nerve may be repaired directly if the injury is identified.

The recurrent laryngeal nerve, which travels in the tracheoesophageal groove, and the vagus nerve, which travels in the carotid sheath, can be injured by laceration or trauma. This may not be recognized intraoperatively and can be a cause of hoarseness and dysphagia in the postoperative period. We have our ENT colleagues evaluate patients whose symptoms do not resolve in a month for vocal cord paralysis and esophageal dysmotility. Interestingly, hoarseness can improve, despite recurrent laryngeal nerve injury. All patients undergoing a procedure opposite a prior anterior cervical dissection should have preoperative vocal cord evaluations performed to prevent possible bilateral vocal cord paralysis.

AIR EMBOLISM

Air embolism occurs when air is entrained into either the venous or arterial systems. It usually occurs when there is a gradient greater than 5 cm between an open venous structure and the right atrium (reduced venous pressures), but it also can occur by infusion of air from an intravenous line. Venous pressures are reduced not only when the right atrium is positioned below the level of the wound, but also during spontaneous inspiration or intravascular depletion. Air embolism also may occur during the placement of a noncollapsible catheter with direct access to the right atrium.[170,306] A paradoxical air embolus occurs when air crosses from the venous to the arterial side. Clinical situations in which this may occur include intracardiac defects such as a patent foramen ovale, arteriovenous shunts in the pulmonary system, and increased pulmonary arterial pressure.

The clinical signs and symptoms depend on the volume and rate of air entrainment. A slow infusion of air will cause a gradual obstruction of the pulmonary outflow tract with bubbles, whereas a rapid injection of air causes accumulation of air in the right ventricle and formation of an "air lock." Therefore, clinical symptoms may include dysrhythmias, cardiovascular collapse, ventilation-perfusion abnormalities, pulmonary edema and/or increased pulmonary vascular re-

sistance.[178,187] A paradoxical air embolus may lead to ischemia or infarction of the heart, brain, and spinal cord.

The primary goal of monitoring for venous air embolism is its early identification. Other important considerations include prevention of further air entrainment, removal of air, preservation of normal hemodynamics and treatment of dysrhythmias, cardiovascular instability, ventilation-perfusion inequality, and pulmonary edema. Classically, a "mill-wheel" murmur has been described with venous air embolism, although this is a late sign. The most sensitive device for identifying air embolism is echocardiography; however, there are several disadvanages with this device. It is very expensive, often not readily available in the operating room, and requires extensive training and expertise to operate. The precordial Doppler is an inexpensive device that was first used to detect venous air embolism in 1968.[187,210] It is fairly reliable, although rare false-positive readings may occur. It is placed where cardiac sounds are heard best, usually at the right sternal border between the third to sixth intercostal spaces. Petts and Presson showed that positioning can be confirmed by injecting carbon dioxide or saline and that the use of air for this purpose should be contraindicated.[187] The precordial Doppler is limited in its use because of its sensitivity to interference and inability to reliably assess emboli size.[188]

Monitoring of exhaled gases includes measurement of end-tidal carbon dioxide and exhaled nitrogen. This method of air embolism detection is both specific and relatively fast. End-tidal carbon dioxide monitoring can be used to quantitate the size of an air embolism.[187] Emboli increase dead space by causing a drop in pulmonary blood flow and obstruction of pulmonary capillaries. Thus, carbon dioxide absorption into the alveoli is diminished until the air embolus is absorbed. End-tidal carbon dioxide monitoring will reveal a characteristic "wash-out" pattern on the capnograph.[307] The degree and duration of the diminished end-tidal carbon dioxide represents the size of the air embolus.[187,306] However, this type of monitoring is nonspecific, since decreased end-tidal carbon dioxide can also be seen in any situations causing sudden decreases in cardiac output.[190] If available, mass spectrometry may be utilized for detection of venous air embolism since nitrogen will appear in the expired gases, yet the disappearance of nitrogen is not always indicative of recovery.[187] If nitrogen is detected in this fashion, other possible causes of air entry such as system leaks or disconnections should be ruled out.

A late development of venous air embolism may be an increase in central venous pressure (CVP) and pulmonary artery pressure (PAP), which may occur after infusion of large air emboli. Changes in these variables mirror changes detected by end-tidal carbon dioxide monitoring. Central venous access may allow monitoring of the left-to-right gradient and permit the aspiration of air.

The best treatment of venous air embolism is prevention. The circumstances that commonly produce venous air embolism should be avoided if possible, such as when a vein is open at less than atmospheric pressure. If venous air embolism does occur, the surgeon should immediately be informed. The surgeon should flood the operative site with saline and pack the wound with saline-soaked sponges to prevent further air entrainment. The level of the wound should be lowered below the level of the heart; this will increase CVP and prevent further air entrainment. The CVP may also be increased by administering fluids or positive end-expiratory pressure (PEEP), although its use is controversial. Some argue that PEEP theoretically increases the incidence of paradoxical air embolism, yet studies have not confirmed this concern.[308] PEEP has been shown to increase paradoxical air embolism only if it is initiated during the procedure.[308] If air entrainment continues from the head, unilateral or bilateral jugular venous compression should be applied, thus increasing venous pressure at the site of air entrainment.[178]

If the patient is being maintained with a nitrous-oxygen mixture, many will advocate discontinuing nitrous oxide and administering 100 percent oxygen to prevent air bubble enlargement.[187] Some argue that enlargement occurs more quickly than can be prevented by discontinuing nitrous oxide, and this will help treat the hypoxia that may be associated with venous air embolism.[187] If possible, hemodynamic stability should be maintained. This may include cardiopulmonary resuscitation and administering drugs to support the circulation.[187]

Aspiration of air from the superior vena cava and right atrium should be included in the treatment, which is best accomplished by the use of a multiorificed right atrial catheter.[309] It can be correctly positioned by a variety of methods including ECG monitoring ("biphasic" p-wave on lead II), chest radiograph (catheter in midatrial position), and pressure wave measurements (right atrial pressure). Patients who have sustained a paradoxical air embolism and are symptomatic for cerebral, cardiac, or spinal cord ischemia may benefit from hyperbaric oxygen therapy. Administration or hyperbaric oxygen probably facilitates the reduction in size of air bubbles in order to enhance absorption into the circulation. If administered early enough, further ischemic damage may be prevented.

CARDIOVASCULAR COMPLICATIONS

Cardiovascular problems are most often seen with either venous air embolism (as described above) or in patients with chronic spinal cord injury. Patients with chronic spinal cord injury most often develop such cardiovascular complications as hypertension, dysrhythmias, or hypotension.[308] Hypertension is often associated with autonomic hyperreflexia, which can be prevented by maintaining deep general anesthesia or administering regional anesthesia. It can be treated with peripheral vasodilators such as alpha-adrenergic blockers, ganglionic blockers, or direct vasodilators. Dysrhythmias are also seen with autonomic hyperreflexia, such as sinus bradycardia, ectopic beats, and ST segment elevation.[308] Hypotension is often associated with induction in these patients, most likely due to intravascular volume depletion.

References

1. Albin M, et al: Anesthesia for spinal cord injury. *Probl Anesth* 1990; 4(1):138.
2. DeGroot J, Chusid J: *Correlative Neuroanatomy*, 20th ed 20. East Norwolk, CT, Appleton & Lange, 1988:32–52; 53–79.
3. Dommisse GF: The arteries, arterioles, and capillaries of the spinal cord. *Ann R Coll Surg Engl* 1980; 62:369.
4. Crosby G: *Practical aspects of spinal cord physiology.* In: Sperry R, et al (eds): *Anesthesia and the Central Nervous System.* Proc 38th Annual Postgraduate Course in Anesthesiology, Dordrecht. Kluwer Academic, London, 1993:17–25.
5. Turnbull IM, et al: Blood supply of the cervical cord in man. A microangiographic study. *J Neurosurg* 1966; 24:951.
6. Manners T: Vascular lesions in the spinal cord in the aged. *Geriatrics* 1966; 21:151.
7. Silver JR, Buxton PH: Spinal stroke. *Brain* 1974; 97:539.
8. Lazorthes G: Pathology, classification and clinical aspects of vascular disease of the spinal cord. In: Vinken PJ, Bruyn GW (eds): *Handbook of Clinical Neurology.* Amsterdam, North Holland 1972:492–506.
9. Netter F: The CIBA collection of Medical Illustrations Vol 1 Nervous System, Part II Neurologic and neuromuscular disorders. 1986:107.
10. Silver JR, Buxton PH: Spinal stroke. *Brain* 1974; 97:539.
11. Sandson TA, Friedman JH: Spinal cord infarction: Report of 8 cases and review of the literature. *Medicine* 1989; 68:282.
12. MacEwan GD, et al: Acute neurological complications in the treatment of scoliosis. A report of the Scoliosis Research Society. *J Bone Joint Surg* 1975; 57A:404.
13. Blackwood W: Discussion of vascular disease of the spinal cord. *Proc R Soc Med* 1958; 51:543.
14. Henson RA, Parsons M: Ischaemic lesions of the spinal cord: an illustrated view. *Am J Med* 1967; 36:205.
15. Hughes JT, Brownell B: Cervical spondylosis complicated by anterior spinal artery thrombosis. *Neurology* 1964; 14:1073.
16. Taylor AR, Aberd MB: Vascular factors in the myelopathy associated with cervical spondylosis. *Neurology* 1964; 14:62.
17. Ghaly R, et al: Effect of neuroleptanalgesia on motor potentials evoked by transcranial magnetic stimulation in primates. *Anesthesiology* 1991; 75:A595.
18. Grinker RR, Guy CC: Sprain of cervical spine causing thrombosis of anterior spinal artery. *JAMA* 1927; 88:1140.
19. Hughes JT: The pathology of vascular disorders of the spinal cord. *Paraplegia* 1965; 2:207.
20. Hughes JT: Vascular disorders. In: *Pathology of the Spinal Cord*, 2d ed. WB Saunders, Philadelphia, 1978:61–90.
21. Moore KL: *Clinically Oriented Anatomy*, 2d ed. Williams & Wilkins, Baltimore, 1985:565.

22. Netter F: *The CIBA collection of Medical Illustrations*, vol 1; *Nervous System, Part Anatomy and Physiology.* 1985:66.

23. Rivlin AS, Tator CH: Regional spinal cord blood flow in rats after severe cord trauma. *J Neurosurg* 1978; 49:844.

24. Senter HJ, et al: An improved technique for measurement of spinal cord blood flow. *Brain Res* 1978; 149:197.

25. Bingham WG, et al: Blood flow in normal and injured monkey spinal cord. *J Neurosurg* 1975; 43:162.

26. Sandler AN, Tator CH: The effect of spinal cord trauma on spinal cord blood flow in primates. In: Harper AM, et al (eds): *Blood Flow and Metabolism in the Brain: Proceedings of the 7th International Symposium on Cerebral Blood Flow and Metabolism.* Edinburgh, Churchill-Livingstone, 1975:4.22.

27. Smith DR, et al: Measurement of spinal cord blood flow by the microsphere technique. *Neurosurgery* 1978; 2:27.

28. Marcus ML, et al: Regulation of total and regional spinal cord blood flow. *Circ Res* 1977; 41:128.

29. Hickey R, et al: Autoregulation of spinal cord blood flow: Is the cord a microcosm of the brain? *Stroke* 1986; 17:1183.

30. Wullenweber R: First results of measurements of local spinal blood flow in man by means of heat clearance. In: Bain WH, Harper AM (eds): *Blood Flow through Organs and Tissues.* Baltimore, Williams & Wilkins, 1967:176.

31. Griffiths IR: Spinal cord blood flow in dogs: The effect of blood pressure. *J Neurol Neurosurg Psychiatry* 1973; 36:914.

32. Kobrine Al, et al: Spinal cord blood flow in the rhesus monkey by the hydrogen clearance method. *Surg Neurol* 1976; 2:197.

33. Hayashi N, et al: Local spinal cord blood flow and oxygen metabolism. In Austin GM (ed): *The Spinal Cord.* Charles C Thomas, Springfield, 1984:817–830.

34. Griffiths IR, et al: Spinal cord blood flow measured by a hydrogen clearance technique. *J Neurol Sci* 1979; 26:529.

35. Kobrine Al, et al: Preserved autoregulation in the rhesus spinal cord after high cervical cord section. *J Neurosurg* 1976; 44:425.

36. Kobrine Al, et al: Spinal cord blood flow as affected by changes in systemic arterial blood pressure. *J Neurosurg* 1976; 44:12.

37. Kobrine Al, Doyle TF: Physiology of spinal cord blood flow. In: Harper M, et al (eds): *Blood Flow and Metabolism in the Brain.* Churchill-Livingstone, London, 1975: 4.16–4.19.

38. Kennedy C, et al: Mapping of functional neural pathways by autoradiographic survey of local metabolic rate with [⁴C]deoxyglucose. *Science* 1975; 187:850.

39. Hayashi N, et al: Local blood flow, oxygen tension, and oxygen consumption in the rat spinal cord. *J Neurosurg* 1983; 58:516.

40. Sandler AN, Tator CH: Review of the measurement of normal spinal cord blood flow. *Brain Res* 1976; 118:181.

41. Kindt GW: Autoregulation of spinal cord blood flow. *Eur Neurol* 1971; 6:19.

42. Kindt GW, et al: Regulation of spinal cord blood flow. In: Russell RWR (ed): *Brain and Blood Flow.* Proceedings of the 4th International Symposium on the Regulation of Cerebral Blood Flow. Pitman, London, 1971:401–409.

43. Flohr H, Poll W, Brock M: Regulation of spinal cord blood flow. In Russell RWR (ed): *Brain and Blood Flow.* London, Pitman, 1971:406–409.

44. Sato M, Pawlik G, Heiss W-D: Comparative studies of regional CNS blood flow utoregulation and responses to CO₂ in the cat: effects of altering arterial blood pressure and Pa$_{CO_2}$ on rCBF of cerebrum, cerebellum, and spinal cord. *Stroke* 1984; 15:91.

45. Kobrine Al, et al: Local spinal cord blood flow in experimental traumatic myelopathy. *J Neurosurg* 1975; 42:144.

46. Griffiths IR: Spinal cord blood flow after acute experimental cord injury in dogs. *J Neurol Sci* 1976; 27:247.

47. Griffiths IR, et al: Spinal cord compression and blood flow: I. The effect of raised cerebrospinal fluid pressure on spinal cord blood flow. *Neurology* 1978; 28:1145.

48. McCullough JL: Paraplegia after thoracic aortic occlusion: Influence of cerebrospinal fluid drainage: experimental and early clinical results. *J Vasc Surg* 1988; 7:153.

49. Marini C, et al: Effect of sodium nitroprusside on spinal cord perfusion and paraplegia during aortic cross-clamping. *Ann Thorac. Surg* 1989; 47:379.

50. Cernaiann AC, et al: Effect of sodium nitroprusside on paraplegia during cross-clamping of the thoracic aorta. *Ann Thorac Surg* 1993; 56:1035.

51. Simpson JL, et al: Effect of nitroglycerine on spinal cord ischemia, during thoracic aortic cross clamping. *Anesthesiology,* 1994; 81(3A): A685.

52. Sakamoto T, Monafo WW: Regional blood flow in the brain and spinal cord of hypothermic rats. *Am J Physiol* 1989; 257:H785.

53. Minanisawg H, et al: The effect of mild hyperthermia and hypothermia on brain damage following 5, 10, and 15 minutes of forebrain ischemia. *Ann Neurol* 1990; 28:26.

54. Xue D, et al: Immediate or delayed mild hypothermia prevents focal cerebral infarction. *Brain Res* 1992; 587:66.

55. Albin MS: Resuscitation of the spinal cord. *Crit Care Med* 1978; 62:70.

56. Hollier LH: Protecting the brain and spinal cord. *J Vasc Surg* 1987; 5:524.

57. Hitchon PW, et al: The response of spinal cord blood flow to high-dose barbiturates. *Spine* 1982; 7:41.

58. Crosby G, et al: A comparison of local rates of glucose utilization in spinal cord and brain in conscious and nitrous oxide- or pentobarbital-treated rats. *Anesthesiology* 1984; 61:434.

59. Hoffman WE, et al: Cerebral autoregulation in awake versus isoflurane-anesthetized rats. *Anesth Analg* 1991; 73:753.

60. Porter SS, et al: Spinal cord and cerebral blood flow response to subarachnoid injection of local anesthetics with and without epinephrine. *Acta Anaesth Scand* 1985; 29:330.

61. Dohi S, et al: The effects of subarachnoid lidocaine and phenylephrine on spinal cord and cerebral blood glow in dogs. *Anesthesiology* 1984; 61:238.

62. Dohi S, et al: Spinal cord blood flow during spinal anesthesia in dogs: The effects of tetracaine, epinephrine, acute blood loss and hyperemia. *Anesth Analg* 1987; 66:599.

63. Crosby G: Local spinal cord blood flow and glucose utilization during spinal anesthesia with bupivacaine in conscious rats. *Anesthesiology* 1985; 63:55.

64. Kozody R, et al: Subarachnoid bupivacaine decreases spinal cord blood flow in dogs. *Can J Anaesth* 1985; 32:216.

65. Kozody R, et al: Spinal cord blood flow following subarachnoid tetracaine. *Can J Anaesth* 1985; 32:23.

66. Kozody R, et al: Spinal cord blood flow following subarachnoid lidocaine. *Can J Anaesth* 1985; 32:472.

67. Cole DJ, et al: Spinal tetracaine decreases central nervous system metabolism during somatosensory stimulation in the rat. *Can J Anaesth* 1990; 37:231.

68. Kozody R, et al: The effect of subarachnoid epinephrine and phenylephrine on spinal cord blood flow. *Can J Anaesth* 1984; 31:503.

69. Matsumiya N, Dohi S: Effects of intravenous or subarachnoid morphine on cerebral and spinal cord hemodynamics and antagonism with naloxone in dogs. *Anesthesiology* 1983; 59:175.

70. Gordh T, Feuk U, Norlen K: Effect of epidural clonidine on spinal cord blood flow and regional and central hemodynamics in pigs. *Anesth Analg* 1986; 65:1312.

71. Eisenach JC, Grice SC: Epidural clonidine does not decrease blood pressure or spinal cord blood flow in awake sheep. *Anesthesiology* 1988; 68:335.

72. Crosby G, et al: Subarachnoid clonidine reduces spinal cord blood flow and glucose utilization in conscious rats. *Anesthesiology* 1990; 73:1179.

73. Anderton JM: The prone position for the surgical patient: A historical review of the principles and hazards. *Br J Anaesth* 1991; 67:452.

74. Anderson DK, et al: Effects of laminectomy on spinal cord blood flow. *J Neurosurg* 1978; 48:232.

75. Albin M, et al: Clinical and experimental brain retraction pressure monitoring *Acta Neurol Scand* 1977; 56(suppl 64):522.

76. McLone DG, Dias MS: Normal and abnormal early development of the nervous system. In Cheek W (ed): *Pediatric Neurosurgery*, 3d ed. Philadelphia, WB Saunders, 1994:3–39.

77. Reigel DH, McLone DG: Tethered spinal cord. In Cheek WR (ed): *Pediatric Neurosurgery*, 3d ed. Philadelphia, WB Saunders, 1994:77–95.

78. Yamada S, et al: Pathophysiology of "tethered cord syndrome." *J Neurosurg* 1981; 54:494.

79. Reigel DH, Rothenstein D: Spina bifida. In Cheek WR (ed): *Pediatric Neurosurgery*, 3d ed. Philadelphia, WB Saunders, 1994:51–76.

80. Milhorat TH, et al: Surgical treatment of syringomyelia based on magnetic resonance imaging criteria. *Neurosurgery* 1992; 31:231.

81. Oakes WJ: Chiari malformations, hydromyelia, syringomyelia. In Wilkins RH, Rengachary SS, (eds): *Neurosurgery*. New York, McGraw-Hill, 1985; 406–415.

82. Rosenblum B, et al: Spinal arteriovenous malformations: A comparison of dural arteriovenous fistulas and intradural AVMs in 81 patients. *J Neurosurg* 1987; 67:795.

83. Symon L, et al: Dural arteriovenous malformations of the spine. Clinical features and surgical results in 55 cases. *J Neurosurg* 1984; 60:238.

84. Kohno M, et al: A cervical dural arteriovenous fistula in a patient presenting with radiculopathy. *J Neurosurg* 1996; 84:119.

85. Keim HA: Scoliosis. *Clin Symp* 1978; 30:1.

86. Russell DS, Rubinstein LJ: *Pathology of Tumors of the Nervous System*, 5th ed. Baltimore, Williams & Wilkins, 1989:95.

87. Connolly ES: Spinal cord tumors in adults. In Youmans JR (ed): *Neurological Surgery*, 2d ed. Philadelphia, W. B. Saunders, 1982:3196–3214.

88. Welch WC, Jacobs GB: Surgery for metastatic spinal disease. *J Neurooncol* 1995; 23:163.

89. Mancall EL: Paraneoplastic syndromes. In Rowland LP (ed): *Merritt's Textbook of Neurology*, 7th ed. Philadelphia, Lea & Febiger, 1984:708–709.

90. Fox MW, Onofrio BM: The natural history and management of symptomatic and asymptomatic vertebral hemangiomas. *J Neurosurg* 1993; 78:36.

91. Resnick DK, et al: Isolated toxoplasmosis of the thoracic spinal cord in a patient with acquired immunodeficiency syndrome. *J Neurosurg* 1995; 82:493.

92. Poser CM, et al: Demyelinating diseases. In Rowland LP (ed): *Merritt's Textbook of Neurology*, 7th ed. Philadelphia, Lea & Febiger, 1984:593.

93. Epstein NE, et al: Coexisting cervical and lumbar spinal stenosis: Diagnosis and management. *Neurosurgery* 1984; 15:489.

94. Carey TS, et al. The outcomes and costs of care for acute low back pain among patients seen by primary care practitioners, chiropractors, and orthopedic surgeons. *N Engl J Med* 1995; 333:913.

95. Bohlman HH, Ducker TB: Spine and spinal cord injuries. In Rothman RH, Simeone FA (eds): *The Spine*, 3d ed. Philadelphia, WB Saunders, 1992:973–1095.

96. Pang D, Wilberger JE: Spinal cord injury without radiographic abnormalities in children. *J Neurosurg* 1982; 57:114.

97. Cohen MS, et al: Anatomy of the spinal nerve roots in the lumbar and lower thoracic spine. In Rothman RH, Simeone FA (eds): *The Spine*, 3d ed. Philadelphia, WB Saunders, 1992:100–106.

98. Epstein JA, Epstein NE: The surgical management of cervical spinal stenosis, spondylosis, and myeloradiculopathy by means of the posterior approach. In The Cervical Spine Research Society (eds): *The Cervical Spine*, 2d ed. Philadelphia, JB Lippincott, 1989:625–644.

99. Montgomery DM, Brower RS: Cervical spondylotic myelopathy. Clinical syndrome and natural history. *Orthop Clin North Am* 1992; 23:487.

100. Waters RL, et al: Definition of complete spinal cord injury. *Paraplegia* 1991; 9:573.

101. Bohlman HH: Acute fractures and dislocations of the cervical spine: An analysis of 300 hospitalized patients and review of the literature. *J Bone Joint Surg* 1979; 61A:1119.

102. Ducker TB, et al: Experimental spinal cord trauma. I: Correlations of blood flow, tissue oxygen and neurologic status in the dog. *Surg Neurol* 1978; 10:60.

103. Ducker TB, et al: Experimental spinal cord trauma. II: Blood flow, tissue oxygen, evoked potentials in both paretic and plegic monkeys. *Surg Neurol* 1978; 10:64.

104. Panjabi MM, Wrathal JR: Biochemical analysis of spinal cord injury and functional loss. *Spine* 1988; 13:1365.

105. Meyer PR: Cervical Spine: Overview and conservative management. In Meyer PR (ed): *Surgery of Spine Trauma*. New York, Churchill-Livingstone, 1989; 341–395.

106. Bracken MD, et al: A randomized, controlled trial of methylprednisolone or naloxone in the treatment of acute spinal cord injury: Results of the Second National Acute Spinal Cord Injury Study. *N Engl J Med* 1990; 322:1405.

107. Demaria EJ, et al: Septic complications of corticosteroid administration after severe nervous system trauma. *Ann Surg* 1985; 202:248.

108. Crandall PH, Batsdorf U: Cervical spondylotic myelopathy. *J Neurosurg* 1966; 25:57.

109. Ferguson RJL, Kaplan LR: Cervical spondylitic myelopathy. *Neurol Clin* 1985; 3:373.

110. Marar BC: Hyperextension injuries of the cervical spine: The pathogenesis of damage to the spinal cord. *J Bone Joint Surg* 1974; 56A: 1655.

111. Stauffer ES: Rehabilitation of posttraumatic cervical spinal cord quadriplegia and pentaplegia. In The Cervical Spine Research Society (eds): *The Cervical Spine*, 2d ed. Philadelphia, JB Lippincott, 1989:521–525.

112. Miller JI, Parsa AT: Neurosurgical diseases of the spine and spinal cord: Surgical considerations. In Cottrell JE, Smith SD (eds): *Anesthesia and Neurosurgery*, 3d ed. St. Louis, CV Mosby, 1994:543–567.

113. Chusid JG: *Correlative Neuroanatomy and Functional Neurology*, 19th ed. Los Altos, Lange, 1985:229.

114. International Standards for Neurological and Functional Classification of Spinal Cord Injury, Revised 1992. Chicago, American Spinal Injury Association.

115. Weinstein S: Idiopathic scoliosis: Natural history. *Spine* 1986; 11:780.

116. Weinstein S, Ponsetti I: Curve progression in idiopathic scoliosis. *J Bone Joint Surg* 1993; 65:447.

117. Minehan KJ, et al: Spinal cord astrocytoma: Pathological and treatment considerations. *J Neurosurg* 1995; 83:590.

118. Grant R, et al: Metastatic epidural spinal cord compression: Current concepts and treatment. *J Neurooncol* 1994; 19:79.

119. Baker AS, et al: Spinal epidural abscess. *N Engl J Med* 1975; 293:463.

120. Kaufman DM, et al: Infectious agents in spinal epidural abscesses. *Neurology* 1980; 30:844.

121. Heller JG: Postoperative infections of the spine. In Rothman RH, Simeone FA (eds): *The Spine*, 3d ed. Philadelphia, WB Saunders, 1992:1817–1837.

122. Harkey HL, et al: Experimental chronic compressive cervical myelopathy: Effects of decompression. *J Neurosurg* 1995; 83:336.

123. Ebersold MJ, et al: Surgical treatment for cervical spondylitic myelopathy. *J Neurosurg* 1995; 82:745.

124. Pope MH, et al: Diagnosing instability. *Clin Orthop Rel Res* 1992; 279:60.

125. Kirkaldy-Willis WH: Presidential symposium on instability of the lumbar spine. Introduction. *Spine* 1985; 10:254.

126. Denis F: The three column spine and its significance in the classification of acute thoracolumbar spine injuries. *Spine* 1983; 8:817.

127. Rogers LF: Radiologic assessment of acute neurologic and vertebral injuries. In Meyer PR (ed): *Surgery of Spine Trauma*. New York, Churchill-Livingstone, 1989:185–277.

128. Fielding JW, et al: Tears of the transverse ligament of the atlas. *J Bone Joint Surg* 1976; 56:1683.

129. Spence KF, et al: Bursting atlanto-axial fracture associated with rupture of the transverse ligament. *J Bone Joint Surg Am* 1970; 52:543.

130. White AA, et al: Biomechanical analysis of clinical stability in the cervical spine. *Clin Orthop Rel Res* 1975; 109:85.

131. White AA, Panjabi MM: *Clinical Biomechanics of the Spine*, 2d ed. Philadelphia, JB Lippincott, 1990:277–378.

132. Hausfield JN: A biomechanical analysis of clinical stability in the thoracic and thoracolumbar spine (thesis). New Haven, Yale University School of Medicine, 1977.

133. Aldrich EF, et al: Halifax interlaminar clamp for posterior cervical fusion: A long-term follow-up review. *J Neurosurg* 1993; 78:702.

134. Lovely TJ, Carl A: Posterior cervical spine fusion with tension band wiring. *J Neurosurg* 1995; 83:631.

135. Marcotte P, et al: Posterior atlantoaxial facet screw fixation. *J Neurosurg* 1993; 79:234.

136. Jain VK, et al: Occipital-axis posterior wiring and fusion for atlantoaxial dislocation associated with occipitalization of the atlas. *J Neurosurg* 1993; 79:142.

137. Fehlings MG, et al: Posterior plates in the management of cervical instability: Long term results in 44 patients. *J Neurosurg* 1994; 81:341.

138. Fox MW, Onofrio BM: Transdural approach to the anterior soinal canal in patients with cervical spondylotic myelopathy and superimposed central soft disc herniation. *Neurosurgery* 1994; 34:634.

139. Menezes AH, VanGilder JC: Transoral-transpharyngeal approach to the anterior craniocervical junction. *J Neurosurg* 1988; 69:895.

140. Pollack IF, et al: Frameless stereotactic guidance-an intraoperative adjunct in the transoral approach for ventral cervicomedullary junction decompression. *Spine* 1995; 20:216.

141. Dickman CA, et al: Cannulated screws for odontoid screw fixation and atlantoaxial transarticular screw fixation. *J Neurosurg* 1995; 83:1095.

142. Sen CH, Sekhar LN: An extreme lateral approach to intradural lesions of the cervical spine and foramen magnum. *Neurosurgery* 1990; 27:197.

143. Babu RP, et al: Extreme lateral transcondylar approach: Technical improvements and lessons learned. *J Neurosurg* 1994; 81:49.

144. McAfee PC, et al. The anterior retropharyngeal approach to the upper part of the cervical spine. *J Bone Joint Surg* 1987; 69-A:1371.

145. An HS. Surgical exposure and fusion techniques of the spine. In: An HS, Cotler JM (eds): *Spinal Instrumentation*. Baltimore, Williams & Wilkins, 1992:11–18.

146. Nazzaro JM, et al: "Trap door" exposure of the cervicothoracic junction. *J Neurosurg* 1994; 80:338.

147. Sundaresan N, et al: An anterior surgical approach to the upper thoracic vertebra. *J Neurosurg* 1984; 61:686.

148. Larson SJ, et al: Lateral extracavitary approach to traumatic lesions of the thoracic and lumbar spine. *J Neurosurg* 1976; 45:628.

149. Lesoin F, et al: Posterolateral approach to tumors of the dorsolumbar spine. *Acta Neurochir* (*Wien*) 1986; 81:40.

150. Broaddus WC, et al: Preoperative superselective arteriolar embolization: A new approach to enhance resectability of spinal tumors. *Neurosurgery* 1990; 27:755.

151. Sundaresan N, et al: Treatment of spinal metastases from kidney cancer by presurgical embolization and resection. *J Neurosurg* 1990; 73:548.

152. Hardy RW, Bay JW: Surgery of the sympathetic nervous system. In Schmidek HH, Sweet WH (eds): *Operative Neurosurgical Techniques*, 2d ed. Orlando, Grune & Stratton, 1988:1271–1280.

153. Hutter, CG: Posterior intervertebral body fusion: A 25 year study. *Clin Orthop* 1983; 179:86.

154. Cotler JM, et al: Principles, indications, and complications of spinal instrumentation: A summary chapter. In: An HS, Cotler JM (eds): *Spinal Instrumentation*. Baltimore, Williams & Wilkins, 1992:435–456.

155. Wiltse LL: Surgery for intervertebral disc disease of the lumbar spine. *Clin Orthop* 1977; 129:22.

156. Steffee AD: The variable screw placement system with posterior lumbar interbody fusion. In: Lin PM, Gill K (eds): *Lumbar Interbody Fusion: Principles and Techniques in Spine Surgery*. Rockville, Aspen Publishers, 1989:81–93.

157. Steffee AD, Brantigan JW: The variable screw placement spinal fixation. Report of a prospective study of 250 patients enrolled in Food and Drug Administration clinical trials. *Spine* 1993; 18:1160.

158. Rish BL: A comparative evaluation of posterior lumbar interbody fusion for disc disease. *Spine* 1985; 10:855.

159. Esses SI, et al: Surgical anatomy of the sacrum: A guide for rational screw fixation. *Spine* 1991; 16:S283.

160. Mirkovic S, et al: Anatomic consideration for sacral screw placement. *Spine* 1991; 16:S289.

161. Louis R: Fusion of the lumbar and sacral spine by internal fixation with screw plates. *Clin Orthop* 1986; 203:18.

162. Zdeblick TA: A prospective, randomized study of lumbar fusion. *Spine* 1993; 18:983.

163. Wiltberger BR: The prefit dowel intervertebral body fusion as used in lumbar disc therapy: Preliminary report. *Am J Surg* 1953; 86:723.

164. Lin, PM: Posterior lumbar interbody fusion. In Schmidek HH, Sweet WH (eds): *Operative Neurosurgical Techniques*. Orlando, Grune & Stratton, 1988:1401–1420.

165. Christoferson LA, Selland B: Intervertebral bone implants following excision of protruded lumbar discs. *J Neurosurg* 1975; 42:401.

166. Henson RA, Urich H: Involvement of the vertebral column and spinal cord. In: Henson RA, Urich H (eds): *Cancer and the Nervous System: The Neurological Manifestations of Systemic Malignant Disease*. Blackwell Scientific, St. Louis, 1982:120–154.

167. Ruff RL, Lanska DJ: Epidural metastases in prospectively evaluated veterans with cancer and back pain. *Cancer* 1989; 63:2234.

168. Hollis PH, et al: Neurological deterioration after lumbar punc-

ture below complete spinal subarachnoid block. *J Neurosurg* 1986; 64:253.

169. Pomeranz SJ: Neoplasms of the spine: In Pomeranz SJ (ed.): *Craniospinal Magnetic Resonance Imaging.* Philadelphia, WB Saunders, 1989:513–540.

170. Marshall WK, Mostrom JL: Neurosurgical Diseases of the Spine and Spine Cord In: Cottrell JE, Smith DS (eds): *Anesthesia and Neurosurgery.* St. Louis, CV Mosby, 1993:569–603.

171. White AA, et al: Clinical instability in the lower cervical spine. *Spine* 1976; 1:15.

172. Johnson RM, Wolf JW: Stability in cervical spine. Research Society (eds): *The Cervical Spine.* Philadelphia, JB Lippincott, 1983:35–53.

173. White A, et al: Biomechanical analysis of clinical stability in the cervical spine. *Clin Orthop* 1975; 109:85.

174. Sinclair JR, Mason RA: Ankylosing spondylitis. The case for awake intubation. *Anaesthesia* 1984; 39:3.

175. Crosby ET: The adult cervical spine: Implications for airway management. *Can J Anaesth* 1990; 37:77.

176. Rodman GR, Schumacher R (eds): *Primer on Rheumatic Diseases,* 8th ed. Atlanta, Arthritis Foundation, 1983.

177. Fisher LR, et al: Relation between chest expansion, pulmonary function, and exercise tolerance in patients with ankylosing spondylitis. *Ann Rheum Dis* 1990; 49:921.

178. Porter S. *Anesthesia for Surgery of the Spine.* New York, McGraw-Hill, 1995.

179. Eisele JH: Connective tissue diseases. In Katz J, et al (eds): *Anesthesia and Uncommon Diseases.* Philadelphia, WB Saunders, 1990.

180. Bradford DS, et al: Scoliosis and kyphosis. In: Rothman RH, Simeone FA (eds): *The Spine.* Philadelphia, WB Saunders, 1980:316–439.

181. Andrews IC. Special considerations in the management of scoliosis. In Weekly Anesthesiology Update 1978:2:2.

182. Gronert GA, Theye RA: Pathophysiology of hyperkalemia induced by succinylcholine. *Anesthesiology* 1975; 43:4389.

183. Segal JL, Brunnemann SR: Clinical pharmacokinetics in patients with spinal cord injuries. *Clin Pharmacokinet* 1989; 17:109.

184. Loughnan BA, Hall GM: Spinal cord monitoring. *Br J Anaesth* 1989; 63:587.

185. Martin JT: Patient positioning. In Barash PG, et al (eds): *Clinical Anesthesia,* 2d ed. Philadelphia, JB Lippincott, 1992:709–736.

186. Lee C, et al: Neuroleptanalgesia for awake pronation of surgical patients. *Anesth Analg* 1977; 56:276.

187. Petts JS, Presson RG: A review of the detection and treatment of venous air embolism. *Anesthesiology Rev.* 1992; 19(4):13.

188. Michenfelder JD, et al: Neuroanesthesia. *Anesthesiology* 1969; 30:65.

189. Wilder, GL: Hypothesis: The etiology of midcervical quadriplegia after operation with the patient in the sitting position. *Neurosurgery* 1982; 11(4):530.

190. Barash P, et al: *Clinical Anesthesia,* 2d ed. New York, McGraw-Hill, 1992.

191. Calverley RK, et al: (eds): Introduction to anesthesia practice. *Clinical Anesthesia,* 2d ed. Philadelphia, JB Lippincott, 1992: 48–49.

192. American Society of Anesthesiologists: *Peer Review in Anesthesiology.* Park Ridge IL, 1989:14–16.

193. Eichhorn JH, et al: Standards for patient monitoring during anesthesia at Harvard Medical School. *JAMA* 1986; 256:1017.

194. American Society of Anesthesiologists: Directory 1994: 735–736.

195. ASA Standards for Basic Intraoperative Monitoring. American Society of Anesthesiologists. Approved October 21, 1986, last amended October 23, 1990; effective January 1, 1991.

196. MacKenzie CF, et al: Assessment of cardiac and respiratory function during surgery on patients with acute quadriplegia, *J Neurosurg* 1985; 62:843.

197. Machida M, et al: Spinal cord monitoring: electrophysiological measures of sensory and motor function during spinal surgery. *Spine* 1985; 10:407.

198. Vauzelle C, Stagnara P, Jouvinroux P: Functional monitoring of spinal cord activity during spinal surgery. *Clin Orthop* 1973; 93:173.

199. Ginsburg HH, et al: Postoperative paraplegia with preserved intraoperative somatosensory evoked potentials. *J Neurosurg* 1985; 63:296.

200. Marshall WK, Mostrom JL: Neurosurgical diseases of the spine and spinal cord: Anesthetic considerations. In Cottrell JE, Smith DS (eds): *Anesthesia and Neurosurgery,* 3d ed. St. Louis, Mosby-Year Book, 1994:568–603.

201. Vauzelle C, et al: Functional monitoring of spinal cord activity during spinal surgery. *Clin Orthop* 1973; 93:173.

202. Abbott TR, Bentley G: Intraoperative awakening during scoliosis surgery. *Anaesthesia* 1980; 35:298.

203. Eldar I, et al: Use of flumazenil for intraoperative arousal during spine fusion. *Anesth Analg* 1992; 75:580.

204. Abbott TR, Bentley G: Intraoperative awakening during scoliosis surgery. *Anaesthesia* 1980; 35:298.

205. Vauzelle C, et al: Functional monitoring of spinal cord activity during spinal surgery. *Clin Orthop* 1973; 93:173.

206. Sudhir KG, et al: Intraoperative awakening for early recognition of possible neurologic sequelae during Harrington-rod spinal fusion. *Anesth Analg* 1976; 55:526.

207. Friedman WA, et al: Electrophysiologic monitoring of the nervous system. In Stoelting RK, et al (eds): *Advances in Anesthesia.* Year Book, Chicago, 1988:231.

208. Morioka T, et al: Direct spinal versus peripheral nerve stimulation as monitoring techniques in epidurally recorded spinal cord potentials. *Acta Neurochir* 1991; 108:122.

209. Tamaki T, et al: The prevention of iatrogenic spinal cord injury utilizing the evoked spinal cord potential. *Int Orthop* 1981; 4:313.

210. Maroon JC, et al: Detection of minute venous air embolism with ultrasound. *Surg Gynecol Obstet* 1968; 127:1236.

211. Kobrine AL, et al: Correlation of spinal cord blood flow, sensory evoked response, and spinal cord function in subacute experimental spinal cord compression. *Adv Neurol* 1978; 20:389.

212. Albanese SA, et al: Somatosensory cortical evoked potential changes after deformity correction. *Spine* 1991; 15(8 suppl): S371.

213. Bennett MH: Effects of compression and ischemia on spinal cord evoked potentials. *Exp Neurol* 1983; 80:508.

214. Dasmahapatra HK, et al: Identification of risk factors for spinal cord ischemia by the use of monitoring of somatosensory evoked potentials during coarctation repair. *Circulation* 1987; 76(suppl III):III-14–III-18.

215. Hardy RW, et al: Effect of systemic hypertension on compression block of spinal cord. *Surg Forum* 1972; 23:434.

216. Shukla R, et al: Loss of evoked potentials during spinal surgery due to spinal cord hemorrhage. *Ann Neurol* 1988; 24:272.

217. Uematsu S, Uldarico R: Effect of acute compression, hypoxia, hypothermia and hypovolemia on the evoked potentials of the spinal cord. *Electromyogr Clin Neurophysiol* 1981; 21:229.

218. Lake CL: Evoked potentials. In: Lake CL (ed): *Clinical Monitoring.* Philadelphia, WB Saunders, 1990:757–800.

219. Molale M: False negative intraoperative somatosensory evoked potentials with simultaneous bilateral stimulation. *Clin Electroencephalogr* 1986; 17:6.

220. Friedman WA, Richards R: Somatosensory evoked potential

monitoring accurately predicts hemi-spinal cord damage: A case report. *Neurosurgery* 1988; 22:140.

221. Mostegl A, Bauer R: The application of somatosensory-evoked potentials in orthopedic spine surgery. *Arch Orthop Trauma Surg* 1984; 103:179.

222. Ginsburg HH, et al: Postoperative paraplegia with preserved intraoperative somatosensory evoked potentials: Case report. *J Neurosurg* 1985; 63:296.

223. Friedman WA, Grundy BL: Monitoring of sensory evoked potentials is highly reliable and helpful in the operating room. *J Clin Monit* 1987; 3:38.

224. Tamaki T, et al: The prevention of iatrogenic spinal cord injury utilizing the evoked spinal cord potential. *Int Orthop* 1981; 4:313.

225. Koyanagi I, et al: Spinal cord evoked potential monitoring after spinal cord stimulation during surgery of spinal cord tumors. *Neurosurgery* 1993; 33:451.

226. Abel MF, et al: Brainstem evoked potentials for scoliosis surgery: A reliable method allowing use of halogenated anesthetic agents. *J Pediatr Orthop* 1990; 10:208.

227. Britt RH, Ryan TP: Use of a flexible epidural stimulating electrode for intraoperative monitoring of spinal somatosensory evoked potentials. *Spine* 1986; 11:348.

228. Cohen BA, et al: Pudendal nerve evoked potential monitoring in procedures involving low sacral fixation. *Spine* 1991; 16(suppl):S375.

229. Fromme K, et al: Spinal cord monitoring during intraspinal extramedullary tumor operations (peroneal nerve evoked responses). *Neurosurg Rev* 1990; 13:195.

230. Jones SJ, et al: Sensory nerve conduction in the human spinal cord: Epidural recordings made during scoliosis surgery. *J Neurol Neurosurg Psychiatry* 1982; 45:446.

231. Nuwer MR: *Evoked Potential Monitoring in the Operating Room.* New York, Raven Press, 1986; 49–101.

232. Pelosi L, et al: Intraoperative recordings of spinal somatosensory evoked potentials to tibial nerve and sural nerve stimulation. *Muscle Nerve* 1991; 14:253.

233. Owen JH: Motor evoked potentials. In Salzman SK, (ed): *Neural Monitoring: The Prevention of Intraoperative Injury,* Humana Press, New Jersey, 1990:210–241.

234. Barker AT, et al: Noninvasive magnetic stimulation of human motor cortex (letter), *Lancet* 1985; I:1106

235. Levy WJ, et al: Motor evoked potentials from transcranial stimulation of the motor cortex in humans. *Neurosurgery* 1984; 15:287.

236. Levy WJ, York DH: Evoked potentials from the motor tracts in humans. *Neurosurgery* 1983; 12:422.

237. Levy WJ: Clinical experience with motor and cerebellar evoked potential monitoring. *Neurosurgery* 1987; 20:169.

238. Merton PA, et al: Scope of a technique for electrical stimulation of human brain, spinal cord, and muscle. *Lancet* 1982; II:597.

239. Ghaly R, et al: Effect of neuroleptanalgesia on motor potentials evoked by transcranial magnetic stimulation in primates. *Anesthesiology* 1991; 75:A595.

240. Kalkman CJ, et al: Effects of propofol, etomidate, midazolam and fentanyl on motor evoked responses to transcranial electrical or magnetic stimulation in humans. *Anesthesiology* 1992; 76:502.

241. Losasso TJ, et al: The effect of anesthetic agents on transcranial magnetic motor evoked potentials (TMEP) in neurosurgical patients. *Anesthesiology* 1991; 75:A1032.

242. Peterson R, Mongan P: Effect of intravenous anesthetics on neurogenic motor evoked potentials recorded at the spinal and sciatic level. *Anesthesiology* 1991; 75:A179.

243. Haghighi SS, et al: Depressive effect of isoflurane anesthesia on motor evoked potentials. *Neurosurgery* 1990; 26:993.

244. Taniguchi M, et al: Effects of four intravenous anesthetic agents on motor evoked potentials elicited by magnetic transcranial stimulation. *Neurosurgery* 1993; 33:407.

245. Jellinek D, et al: Effects of nitrous oxide on motor evoked potentials recorded from skeletal muscle in patients under total anesthesia with intravenously administered propofol. *Neurosurgery* 1991; 29:558.

246. Kalkman CJ, et al: Low concentrations of isoflurane abolish motor evoked responses to transcranial electrical stimulation during nitrous oxide/opioid anesthesia in humans. *Anesth Analg* 1991; 73:410.

247. Glassman SD, et al: Anesthetic effects on motor evoked potentials in dogs. *Spine* 1993; 18:1083.

248. Zigler J, et al: Posterior cervical fusion with local anesthesia: The awake patient as the ultimate spinal cord monitor. *Spine* 1987; 12:206.

249. Mahla ME: *Principles and Practice of Monitoring the Brain and Spinal Cord.* American Society of Anesthesiologists Refresher Course, 1995.

250. Ditzler JW, et al: Should spinal anesthesia be used in surgery for herniated intervertebral disk? *Anesth Analg* 1959; 38:118.

251. Rosenburg MK, Berner G: Spinal anesthesia in lumbar disc surgery: Review of 200 cases . . . with a case history. *Anesth Analg* 1965; 44:419.

252. Lanier WL, et al: The effects of dextrose infusion and head position on neurologic outcome after complete cerebral ischemia in primates: Examination of a model. *Anesthesiology* 1987; 66:39.

253. Pulsinelli WA, et al: Moderate hyperglycemia augments ischemic brain damage: a neuropathologic study in the rat. *Neurology* 1982; 32:1239.

254. Siemkowicz E, Hansen AJ: Clinical restitution following cerebral ischemia in hypo-, normo- and hyperglycemic rats. *Acta Neurol Scand* 1978; 58:1.

255. Drummond JC, Moore SS: The influence of dextrose administration on neurologic outcome after temporary spinal cord ischemia in the rabbit. *Anesthesiology* 1989; 70:64.

256. Bedford RF: Sodium nitroprusside hemodynamic dose-response during enflurane and morphine anesthesia. *Anesth Analg* 1979; 58:174.

257. Eckenhoff JE, Rich JC: Clinical experiences with deliberate hypotension. *Anesth Analg* 1966; 45:21.

258. Barbier-Böhm G, et al: Comparative effects of induced hypotension and normovolaemic haemodilution on blood loss in total hip arthroplasty. *Br J Anaesth* 1980; 52:1039.

259. Khambatta HJ, et al: Hypotensive anesthesia for spinal fusion with sodium nitroprusside. *Spine* 1978; 3:171.

260. Bailey TE Jr, Mahoney OM: The use of banked autologous blood in patients undergoing surgery for spinal deformity. *J Bone Joint Surg* 1987; 69-AL329.

261. Silvergleid AJ: Safety and effectiveness of predeposit autologous transfusion in preteen and adolescent children. *JAMA* 1987; 257:3403.

262. Nicholls MD, et al: Autologous blood transfusion for elective surgery. *Med J Aust* 1986; 144:396.

263. Stehling L: Autotransfusion and hemodilution. In: Miller RD (ed): *Anesthesia.* 3d ed. New York, Churchill-Livingstone, 1990:1501–1513.

264. Miller JI, Parsa AT: Neurosurgical diseases of the spine and spinal cord: Surgical considerations. In: Cottrell JE, Smith DS (eds): *Anesthesia and Neurosurgery.* St. Louis, Mosby, 1993: 543–567.

265. Martin E, et al: Acute limited normovolemic hemodilution: A method for avoiding homologous transfusion. *World J Surg* 1987; 11:53.

266. Kafer ER, et al: Automated acute normovolemic hemodilution

reduces blood transfusion requirements for spinal fusion. *Anesth Analg* 1986; 65:S76.

267. Thompson GE, et al: Hypotensive anesthesia for total hip arthroplasty: A study of blood loss and organ function (brain, heart, liver, kidney). *Anesthesiology* 1978; 48:91.

268. Ward CF, et al: Deliberate hypotension in head and neck surgery. *Head Neck Surg* 1980; 2:185.

269. Ahlerling TE, et al: Controlled hypotensive anesthesia reduces blood loss in radical cystectomy for bladder cancer. *J Urol* 1983; 129:953.

270. Sivarajan M, et al: Blood pressure, not cardiac output, determines blood loss during induced hypotension. *Anesth Analg* 1980; 59:203.

271. Miller ED Jr: Deliberate hypotension. In: Miller RD (ed) *Anesthesia*, 3d ed. Churchill-Livingstone, New York, 1990:1347–1367.

272. Sperry R, et al: The incidence of hemorrhage on organ perfusion during deliberate hypotension in rats. *Anesthesiology* 1992; 77:1171.

273. Benumof JL: Management of the difficult Adult Airway. *Anesthesiology* 1991; 75:1087.

274. Clinical pathway committee, University of Pittsburgh Medical Center, Lyda Dye, Case manager, 1995.

275. Powers SK, Edwards MSB: Prevention and treatment of thromboembolic complications in a neurosurgical patient. In Wilkins RH, Rengachary SS, (eds): *Neurosurgery* New York, McGraw-Hill, 1985:406.

276. Weinmann EE, Salzman EW: Medical Progress: Deep-vein thrombosis. *N Engl J Med* 1994; 331:1630.

277. McMichan JC, et al: Pulmonary dysfunction following traumatic quadriplegia. *JAMA* 1980; 243:528.

278. Cane RD, Shapiro BA: Pulmonary effects of acute spinal cord injury: Assessment and management. In Meyer PR (ed): *Surgery of Spine Trauma*. New York, Churchill-Livingstone, 1989:173.

279. Keller RB, Pappas AM: Infections after spinal fusion using internal fixation instruments. *Orthop Clin North Am* 1972; 3:99.

280. Horwitz NH, Curtin JA: Prophylactic antibiotics and wound infections following laminectomy for lumbar disc herniation: A prospective study. *J Neurosurg* 1975; 43:727.

281. Whitecloud TS, et al: Complications with the variable spinal plating system. *Spine* 1989; 14:472.

282. Sasso RC, Cotler JM, Thalgott JS: Transpedicular fixation with AE dynamic compression plates. In: An HS, Cotler JM, (eds): *Spinal Instrumentation*. Baltimore, Williams & Wilkins, 1992:257–280.

283. Meyer PR: Cervical Spine: Overview and conservative management. In Meyer PR (Ed): *Surgery of Spine Trauma*. New York, Churchill-Livingstone, 1989:625–715.

284. DeSaussure RL: Vascular injury coincidence to disc surgery. *J Neurosurg* 1959; 16:222.

285. Smith MD, et al: Vertebral artery injury during anterior decompression of the cervical: A retrospective review of 10 patients. *J Bone Joint Surg (Br)* 1993; 75B:410.

286. Stambough JL, Simeone FA: Vascular complications in spine surgery. In Rothman RH, Simeone FA (eds): *The Spine*, 3d ed. Philadelphia, WB Saunders, 1992:1877–1885.

287. Marshall LF: Cerebrospinal fluid leaks: Etiology and repair. In Rothman RH, Simeone FA (eds): *The Spine*, 3d ed. Philadelphia, WB Saunders, 1992:1892–1898.

288. Hadani FG, et al: Entrapped lumbar nerve root in pseudomeningocele after laminectomy: Report of three cases. *Neurosurgery* 1986; 19:405.

289. Przybylski GJ, Welch WC: Longitudinal atlanto-axial dislocation with type III odontoid fracture: A case report with review of the literature. *J Neurosurg* 1996; 84:666.

290. Rhee KJ, et al: Oral intubation in the multiply injured patient: The risk of exacerbation spinal cord damage. *Ann Emerg Med* 1990; 19:511.

291. Vauzelle P, et al: Functional monitoring of spinal cord activity during spinal surgery. *CORR* 1973; 93:173.

292. Abitol JJ, Garfin SR: Complications associated with posterior instrumentation of the spine. In: Rothman RH, Simeone FA (eds): *The Spine*, 3d ed, Philadelphia, WB Saunders, 1992:1846–1871.

293. Wilber RG, et al: Postoperative neurological deficits in segmental spinal instrumentation. *J Bone Joint Surg* 1984; 66:1178.

294. Ashkenaze D, et al: Efficacy of spinal cord monitoring in neuromuscular scoliosis. *Spine* 1993; 18:1627.

295. Fisher RS, et al: Efficacy of intraoperative neurophysiological monitoring. *J Clin Neurophysiol* 1995; 12:97.

296. Kothbauer K, et al: Intraoperative motor and sensory monitoring of the cauda equina. *Neurosurgery* 1994; 34:702.

297. West JL, et al: Results of spinal arthrodesis with pedicle screw-plate fixation. *J Bone Joint Surg* 1991; 73A:1179.

298. Pinto MR: Complications of pedicle screw fixation. *Spine* State of the art reviews. 1992; 6:45.

299. Rose RD, et al: Persistently electrified pedicle stimulation instruments (PEPSI) in spinal instrumentation: Technique and protocol development. *Spine*, in press.

300. Matsuzaki H, et al: Problems and solutions of pedicle screw plate fixation of lumbar spine. *Spine* 1990; 15:1159.

301. Vaccaro AR, et al: Transpedicular fixation of the spine using the variable screw placement system. In: An HS, Cotler JM (eds): *Spinal Instrumentation*. Baltimore, Williams & Wilkins, 1992:197–218.

302. Weinstein JN, et al: Spinal pedicle fixation: Reliability and validity of roentgenogram-based assessment and surgical factors on successful screw placement. *Spine* 1988; 13:1012.

303. Gybels JM, Sweet WH: Pain and headache. Sympathectomy for pain. In Gildenberg PL (ed): *Neurosurgical Treatment of Persistent Pain*, Vol 11. Basel, Karger, 1989:257–281.

304. Johnson RM, McGuire EJ: Urogenital complications of anterior approaches to the lumbar spine. *Clin Orthop* 1981; 154:114.

305. Johnson RM, et al: Surgical approaches to the spine. In Rothman RH, Simeone FA (eds): *The Spine* 3d ed. Philadelphia, WB Saunders, 1992:1607–1738.

306. English JB, et al: Comparison of VAE monitoring methods in supine dogs. *Anesthesiology* 1978; 48:425.

307. Kalenda Z: Capnography: A sensitive method of early detection of air embolism. *Acta Analg Bel* 1975; 23 Suppl:78.

308. Schonwald G, et al: Cardiovascular complications during anesthesia in chronic spinal cord injured patients. *Anesthesiology* 1981; 55:550.

309. Albin, MS: Air embolism. *Anesthesiol Clin North Am* 1993; 11:1.

Chapter 33

MANAGEMENT OF ACUTE CERVICAL SPINAL CORD INJURY

COLIN F. MACKENZIE

FRED H. GEISLER

Historical Background

The first record of spinal cord injury (SCI) appeared in the Edwin Smith Papyrus written 5000 years ago by an unknown Egyptian physician. In this document are descriptions of paralysis of all four extremities following trauma. The paralysis was associated with sensory loss, dribbling of urine, priapism, and involuntary semen emission.[1] Lord Nelson was the victim of a gunshot wound to the spine at the battle of Trafalgar; this caused paralysis at about T5. John Wilkes Booth, who assassinated President Abraham Lincoln, succumbed to a bullet wound of the cervical spinal cord, and President James Garfield died 79 days after a gunshot wound to the lower spine.[2] Until the 1940s, the medical profession did not progress beyond the ancient Egyptian verdict that SCI was "an ailment not to be treated." In World War I, mortality varied from 47 percent[3] to an overall mortality rate after 3 years of 80 percent.[2] Improvements occurred during World War II, but it was not until 1944 that specialized spinal cord treatment centers were instituted, initially in England. In 1945, an Army SCI center was established in Van Nuys, California; in 1950 it was transferred to the Veterans Administration (VA) Hospital at Long Beach, California.[4]

Epidemiology

Of 2011 patients with SCI treated at the VA Hospital at Long Beach between 1946 and 1965, 304 died (15 percent). The mortality rate among patients with cervical lesions was 12.4 percent. Age at injury was more important than the level or extent of other injuries. This unit, however, received relatively few patients within the first 2 months after injury.[5] In England, 608 patients with traumatic spine injury were admitted within 14 days to Stoke Mandeville Hospital, 62.5 percent of whom were transferred there within 48 h of injury. There were 229 cervical spine injuries; 27 of these patients died within 3 months, giving an early mortality rate of 11.8 percent.[6] Other SCI centers reported the beneficial effects of mechanical respirators in reducing mortality from respiratory failure among patients with acute quadriplegia.[7,8] Using standard life expectancy tables, the mortality rate of partial quadriplegia was reported to be twice the predicted rate; following complete quadriplegia it was almost 12 times the expected rate. Complete paraplegia was three times less likely to cause mortality than complete quadriplegia.[9]

It is only recently that reliable records were collected of the incidence of SCI and constructive efforts made in treatment and rehabilitation. Studies by Wilcox and coworkers[10] and a report to the National Paraplegic Foundation[11] identified an annual incidence of SCI between 25 and 12.4 per million population respectively. For 1971, US statistics estimate a 0.8/1000 incidence of complete or partial postinjury paralysis. These reports,

TABLE 33-1
Epidemiology of Acute Cervical Spine Injury

Cause	
Motor vehicle accidents (MVA)	40–50%
Falls (mostly older age group)	20%
Recreational activities	7–15%
Gunshot wounds	
Industrial and agricultural accidents	
Population and age	
Males, 15–34 years of age (4× more common than women)	
Site of injury	
C5–6 most frequent (see Fig. 33-1)	
Neurologic function after injury	
Quadriplegia	23.7%
Central cord	17.3%
Anterior cord syndrome	8.4%
Brown Séquard	4.9%
Other	3.7%
Intact	42.0%
Lifetime cost	
$750,000–$1 million	

however, excluded patients with transient paralysis or paresis and those who died before hospitalization.

An epidemiologic study of acute traumatic spinal SCI in 18 northern California counties during 1970 and 1971[12] found 619 persons with SCI among the 5.8 million residents, an annual incidence of 53.4 per million. The mortality rate was 25.8 per million, or 48.3 percent. Of the 299 persons who died, 235 were dead on arrival in the emergency room, and 64 died during hospitalization. Quadriparesis (incidence of 9.5 per million), the most frequent form of impairment, was more common in those injured in recreation-related activities, primarily diving accidents. Within the younger middle-aged population, acute SCI is more likely to occur from occupational injuries, whereas the older population are more likely to suffer SCI after falls at home. There appears to be a higher percentage of cervical SCI without bony injury in individuals over 50 years of age.[13] The incidence of quadriplegia was 3.2 per million. Men were 3.5 to 4.5 times more likely to have neurologic impairment and the 15 to 34 age group accounted for the single largest category with SCI. Over one-half (56 percent) of SCIs resulted from motor vehicle accidents (MVA). A summary of the epidemiology of acute SCI is shown in Table 33-1.

Meyer[14] estimated that about 4700 to 5500 new SCIs resulting in quadriplegia occur annually in the United States and that the majority occur as a result of MVAs; many are associated with drugs, particularly alcohol. The National Spinal Cord Registry[15,16] reports that 40 percent of spinal injuries are due to MVAs, 20 percent to falls, and the remaining 40 percent to gunshot wounds, recreational injuries, and industrial or agricultural accidents. The most frequent time of occurrence

of SCI is 12 midnight to 5 A.M. and 85 percent of the injured are men with a peak age range of 15 to 28 years. There is a rise in cervical spine injury in summer from diving accidents and in winter from skiing and snowmobile mishaps. The most frequent level of cervical spine injury is C5 to C6, corresponding to the area of greatest cervical spine mobility (Fig. 33-1).

In 1974, an estimated 5315 SCIs occurred as a result of MVAs in the United States; this corresponds to an average annual incidence of 25.1 per million population. Of the 3377 who survived to reach the hospital, 1091 were quadriplegics with either complete or incomplete lesions. The total direct and indirect cost of the 3377 motor vehicle-related spinal cord injured patients who survived was $828 million, giving an average cost per patient of $156,000 in 1974 dollars.[17] The annual cost in 1970 dollars for support and treatment of all SCIs was estimated by Young[18] at $2 billion.

It was estimated that in 1981 there were about 170,000 people suffering complete or partial paralysis as a result of traumatic SCI.[13] The 1982 National Head and SCI Survey indicated that roughly 10,000 new acute SCI patients with paraplegia and quadriplegia will be treated each year, of whom 4000 die before reaching a hospital and 1000 die during hospitalization.

Traumatic injuries consume a major amount of health care resources. Estimates place the total cost of traumatic injuries at 40 percent of all health care expenditures in the United States. Head and SCI have the highest morbidity, mortality, and cost to society of any disease among the youth of America. The death rate for these injuries is estimated at greater than 140,000 annually with over 60 million others seeking medical care.[19,20] An estimated $170 billion was spent in 1988 (the last year with published statistics). These figures include 10,000 to 12,000 SCIs each year with the majority of the victims being less than 30 years of age.[21–28] The 1991 lifetime cost of directly caring for a disabled SCI victim has been estimated to exceed $600,000.[29] Additional costs associated with SCI victims include lost wages and alterations necessary in their families for aiding in their care. The Oregon State Health Division has determined the following annual estimates for its population: 5 percent are involved in trauma; 0.825 percent have a major injury as defined by the Injury Severity Score (score >13); and 0.165 percent have a major injury to the head or spinal cord.[21]

The development of regional SCI centers as well as improved treatments have reduced the incidence of complete lesions from 65 to 45 percent. Survival for the paraplegic and quadriplegic patients has increased, putting a considerable financial burden on the community. First year hospital costs with acute SCI range from $35,000 to $100,000. The lifetime costs in the United

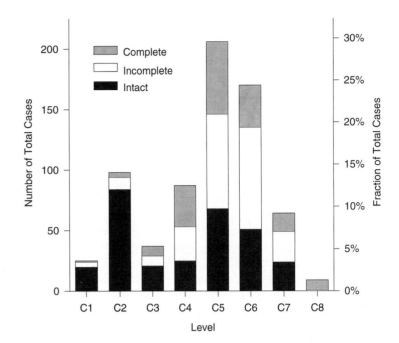

Figure 33-1   Distribution of neurologic status and frequency of cervical injury level among 696 cervical spine injury patients. [Data redrawn with permission from Meyer RP (ed): *Surgery of Spine Trauma*. New York, Churchill-Livingstone, 1989:23.]

States of acute SCI are estimated, most recently, at between $750,000 and $1 million. A summary of acute SCI statistics is shown in Table 33-2.

The mechanism of injury, mechanical damage, and clinical spectrum of SCI vary greatly. Some injuries involve massive transverse mechanical disruption of all neurologic tissue in the spinal cord. When this occurs, it is unlikely that any medical, surgical, or pharmacologic intervention can improve neurologic recovery and prevent lifelong disability. In most cases, the mechanical injury to the spinal cord is limited to contusion, and a portion of the nervous tissue damage results from secondary processes (i.e., the local biochemical derangement or the systemic hemodynamic consequences of injury). These secondary processes can be manipulated by medical or surgical therapy.

Treatment of cervical SCI is controversial in terms of the type and timing of medical and surgical therapy.

TABLE 33-2
Summary of Acute SCI Statistics 1914–1993 Showing Changes in Mortality, Incidence, Estimates, and Costs

1914–1918	World War I SCI acute mortality 47%, after 3 yrs, 80%
1946–1965	Of 2011 chronic SCI admitted to VA Hospital Long Beach over 20 yr (1946–1965): 15% (304) mortality. 229 acute cervical injuries at Stoke-Mandeville Hospital: 11.8% mortality within 3 months.
1965–1970	Incidence of SCI in Hawaii: 25 per million. Report to National Paraplegic Foundation: incidence 12.4 per million.
1970–1971	Acute SCI in 18 Northern California counties: incidence 53.4 per million, mortality rate was 48.3%, over 75% were dead on arrival to the emergency room. Incidence of quadriplegia 3.2 per million; of quadriparesis, 9.5 per million.
1974	Number of SCI occurring in MVAs: 5315 of which 3377 (63.5%) survived to reach hospital, one-third quadriplegic or quadriparetic.
1976	Estimate of 4700–5000 new SCI resulting in quadriplegia per year.
1981	Estimate of 170,000 people suffering complete or partial paralysis due to traumatic SCI.
1982	National Head and SCI Survey indicated roughly 10,000 acute SCI per year.
1988	Estimate of $170 billion spent in 1988 on traumatic SCI.
1991	Estimate of $600,000 lifetime cost of direct care for disabled SCI victim.
1993	Estimate of $35,000–$100,000 first year hospital costs with acute SI.
1993	Estimate of $750,000–$1 million lifetime cost of acute SCI.

Attention to initial resuscitation, the use of vasoactive agents within the first 72 h postinjury, and critical care management form the fundamental care plan for the victim of acute SCI.

Prevention of Acute SCI

The majority of the traumatic injuries are preventable; 70 percent of MVAs were a result of human error[30] and 91 percent of MVA-associated SCIs occurred in unrestrained passengers.[31] Because a cure for SCI neurologic deficits is unknown, elimination of these devastating injuries is the only current means to prevent the lifelong disability.[32] The medical treatments currently available are: (1) rehabilitation, which only enhances and adapts remaining neural function; (2) administration of high-dose methylprednisolone sodium succinate (MPSS) within 8 h of the acute SCI reported to have a relatively small increase in motor function[33–35]; (3) mechanical stabilization of fractures to prevent shifting of the vertebral fragments and resultant spinal cord reinjury[36,37]; and (4) intensive care management to optimize cardiopulmonary function in the acute postinjury period.[38–43] The programs for prevention of SCI are not only the first line for defense, but also the only true line of defense.

Motor vehicle accidents are the most common cause of SCI,[12,24–26] accounting for about 50 percent of all SCIs, with drugs or alcohol often a contributing factor.[44] Falls and diving injuries are the next most common causes.[45] Specifically, diving causes about 1000 SCIs per year, with 95 percent of these injuries resulting in quadriplegia.[46] Many SCIs result from violent assaults or gunshot wounds. Sports and recreational activity account for 7 to 15 percent of SCIs.[47,48] The exact frequency of each cause varies considerably in different geographic areas, seasons of the year, and socioeconomic groups.

Adolescents have a higher incidence of neurologic injury because of increased risks taken during that development stage.[12,24–26] Peer pressure, combined with poor judgment, are often the stimuli that result in an injury with potential lifelong disabilities. Children, aged 12 to 14 years, begin taking dares as a substitute for game playing.[49] During their high school years, adolescents undergo a period of self-centeredness with feelings of invulnerability.[50] Risky behavior is common in this age group because of their disregard for consequences and their limited experience.[51] When compared with adults, adolescents drive more at night, on weekends, drive faster, use shorter braking distances, and more frequently pass through an intersection on a yellow light.[52–54] Combined with risky behavior, adolescents wear safety belts less frequently, exposing them to greater potential injury.[55] This is also the period

in their life in which patterns are set for adult behavior and hence a prevention program can have potential long-term benefits.[56]

Three categories of techniques are used within the field of injury prevention: (1) automatic protection devices; (2) laws or rules that require a behavioral change; and (3) changing the risk-taking behavior.[32] Protection devices include side-impact protection panels, airbags, and automatic restraint systems in cars. The use of these devices does not require the cooperation of the individual for their function. Laws or rules require a behavioral change and include mandatory use of seat belts and motorcycle helmets, diving restrictions, and modifying the rules of sports games. Automobile seat belts reduce both injury and death by approximately 50 percent.[57] Persuading individuals to lessen the level of risk that they are willing to take is the most difficult, although the most effective, method of reducing SCI.

Prevention measures have been instituted in other areas when a contributing factor has been identified.[58] Athletic SCIs were studied with a registry system and high-risk activities identified. For football, this was found to be axial loading of the cervical spine.[59] Rule changes by the National Collegiate Athletic Association and the National Federation of State High School Associations were established to eliminate intentional use of the helmet to ram or strike the opponent.[60] Significant reductions in the SCI rate were noted after these rule changes were instituted.[59] Similarly, the Canadian Committee on Prevention of Spinal Injuries has adopted rule changes to decrease the incidence of injury in ice hockey.[61] SCIs resulting from use of the trampoline were analyzed and found to occur in skilled performers attempting a complex routine. Because adequate safeguards have not been developed for the trampoline, the Academy of Pediatrics has recommended that it be removed from school physical education classes and its use halted in competitive sports activity.[62] Other illustrations for prevention of SCI include advice on the management of breech presentation during childbirth[63] and the avoidance of SCI during occlusion of the descending thoracic aorta during surgery.[64,65]

The THINK FIRST® program was conceived in July 1990. The THINK FIRST Foundation was established and the National Head and SCI Prevention Program initiated. The foundation is composed of 21 members, 11 of whom are neurosurgeons nominated by the Executive Committee of the Congress of Neurological Surgeons and the Board of Directors of the American Association of Neurological Surgeons. The THINK FIRST program comprises four parts: (1) an educational program targeted at the teenager; (2) activities that reinforce the educational program; (3) raising public awareness of neurologic injury and its consequences;

and (4) working to establish registries and support public policies that enhance injury prevention measures and research. This program[32,66] reinforces prevention as a medical therapy and reminds us that it is an old concept rooted in the foundation of medicine with a quote from Louis Pasteur, "When meditating over a disease, I never think of finding a remedy for it, but instead, a means of preventing it."

The cornerstone of the THINK FIRST program[66] is the educational effort aimed at adolescents. The program discusses the devastating effects of risk taking and the vulnerability of the potential victim. The program deals directly with peer pressure, which is the major reason for risk taking. Adolescents are taught that they are in control of the consequences of their actions. The program is presented in school systems at large assemblies and in small classroom settings. An 18-minute film "Harm's Way" is first shown. This film presents interviews with youths after a neural injury has occurred and discusses the risk-taking behavior responsible for the accident and the subsequent consequences. A health care professional then reviews the definitions, types, and causes of neural injuries. The final third of the presentation is held with a youth following a posttraumatic injury in a discussion-and-answer session related to the personal account of the physical, emotional, and social consequences of the injury and subsequent disability. In some presentations of the program, a wheelchair obstacle course is set up in which students can experience wheelchair mobility or paramedics are present to discuss initial management and treatment of injury victims.

The reinforcement activities include posting of signs in high-risk areas where diving is potentially unsafe, school and community bulletin boards, school health fairs, and substance-free graduation events. These activities are an important adjunct to the primary education because it is not reasonable to assume that all adolescent behavior can be changed by a short assembly. Public awareness is important because most people are unaware of the vast magnitude of the current problem and the limited resources applied to combat it. Current estimates indicate the total federal research budget for all injuries was a relatively meager $160 million when compared to the $1400 million awarded by the National Cancer Institute and the $930 million by the National Heart, Lung, and Blood Institute. Local registries accumulate data relative to the target group of prevention programs and provide the basis for studies on the effectiveness of care and rehabilitation. Methods of prevention of acute SCI are summarized in Table 33-3.

The effects of the prevention programs can be measured in three ways: (1) assess the information retained after attending a program; (2) monitor changes in risk-

TABLE 33-3
Prevention of Cervical Spine Injury

1. Automatic protection devices, e.g., side-impact protection panels, airbags in motor vehicles
2. Laws, e.g., seat belt, helmet, random alcohol and drug testing
3. Identification of high-risk recreational activities, e.g., football, ice hockey, trampoline
4. Avoidance of medical causes, e.g., cross-clamp aorta and breech presentations
5. Education of teenagers and others about risk taking

taking behavior; and (3) determine whether the injury rate has decreased in populations exposed to the program.[32] Several studies regarding the efficacy of these programs have been published. In 1984, a Florida group noted that the SCI incidence had decreased in the counties using the THINK FIRST program relative to the nonparticipating counties.[46] A group from Oregon investigated changes in students' knowledge, attitude, and behavior following an educational assembly program.[67] They found that significant knowledge was retained by the students. However, this additional knowledge did not result in changes in attitude or observed behavior. They felt that a reinforcement program was necessary for an optimum prevention program.[67] A group from Missouri demonstrated an increase in both the awareness and the behavior of the participants. Furthermore, they found that several years after attending the program, the risk-taking attitudes were favorably modified, indicating that the information delivered at the program was retained.[68]

A Detroit group identified an increase in the number of gunshot SCI victims in their local community.[69] They questioned these patients for perceived causes. All the activities involved taking risks that placed them at the wrong place at the wrong time. This information led to a program to inform youths of the consequences of their potential risk-taking activities. A group from Australia also embarked on an SCI prevention program and concluded that the youths retained the information delivered at the program.[70,71] A global spine and head injury prevention project has been initiated to determine the causes of SCI in the third world countries.[72]

Current knowledge suggests that a substantial number of SCIs can be eliminated by prevention measures. No cure for devastating SCI exists either now or in the foreseeable future. It is commonly accepted that prevention is the best cure and should be vigorously pursued by all. Prevention programs are noted to have a beneficial effect on adolescents, the age group at greatest risk of SCI. Despite preventive measures that are available and effective in changing attitudes and lowering the injury rate, they do not enjoy widespread application.[73] Clearly these prevention programs deserve vigorous constant support to ensure their continued dissemination and use. It is hoped that the widespread use of prevention programs will reduce the number of patients who require therapy for SCI. SCI prevention will always be a better form of medical treatment than any intervention after an SCI has occurred.

Pathophysiology of Acute SCI

Although treatment of SCI varies between the North American preference (early stabilization) and the European preference (nonsurgical), neither approach has been proven scientifically better. A multicenter randomized study to examine the effect of timing of surgery has been proposed.[74] Despite differences in the specific medical and rehabilitative protocols, superior results occur at high-volume, specialized centers staffed with multidisciplinary teams consisting of experienced physicians, nurses, and paraprofessionals. The same multidisciplinary team manages the care phases including the initial diagnosis and acute treatment through rehabilitation and long-term follow-up of complications secondary to the injury.

Pathophysiologically, when the spinal cord is injured by either mechanical or ischemic insult, the damaged area begins centrally in the gray matter and spreads centrifugally outward as the force of the impact increases. Within the first 15 to 30 min, the central gray matter is disrupted and small hemorrhages appear. The damage appears to be primary and thus irreversible. However, the peripheral white matter tracts are a low metabolic demand region and their ultimate demise may take several hours to a few days. Animal experiments involving SCI indicate that spinal cord blood flow is a predictor of viability; the subjects with increased blood flow in the white matter tend to recover, whereas those with decreased blood flow in the white matter go on to physiologic transection of the spinal cord.[75] The pathophysiologic spinal cord changes located centrally have been verified by the imaging techniques of computed tomography (CT) scan, magnetic resonance imaging (MRI), and intraoperative ultrasound.[39,76]

The initial damaging blow creates a rapid complex series of anatomic and biochemical events. Subsequent scarring isolates the caudal spinal cord. SCI, like head injury, can be divided into primary and secondary damage. The primary neurologic damage results in the destruction of tissue from mechanical or ischemic insult between the time of injury and initial medical care. Although there is currently no way to alter this damage, nerve grafting may be considered to bridge

the damaged spinal cord segment. Secondary damage to the spinal cord occurs after the insult and is caused by a combination of delayed swelling, continuous mechanical reinjury to the injured spinal cord segment, anoxia, low perfusion to the injured spinal cord segment, and release of the endogenous factors. The chronic effects on total body physiologic homeostasis are more complex.[77] The cord pathology itself may be static after 2 or 3 months, but other organ systems undergo progressive changes. This discussion, however, will focus on the early bioelectrical, biochemical, hemodynamic, and cellular alterations that occur at the site of injury.

The majority of pathologic events begin and are most pronounced in the central gray matter of the spinal cord (Fig. 33-2).[78–80] The interconnecting fine mesh of gray substance is disrupted with the impact. Small vessels are torn, leading to disruption of vessel integrity and alterations in the local blood-brain barrier. Red and white blood cells appear in the capillary and venular perivascular spaces within 15 to 30 min after the blow. Small hemorrhages may occur with the initial damage and progress in size over the next 1 to 2 h. The endothelium of the vessels undergoes swelling and vacuolation, and ischemia and hemorrhage are clearly present in the central gray matter in routine histologic sections taken within 3 to 4 h after trauma.[81] Within a day of the initial injury and progressively over the next week there is an increase in gray matter necrosis. Changes in the white matter are not as great and occur after the changes in the central gray matter. In minor injuries, only the gray matter may reflect the pathology. The degree of damage is directly related to the severity of the initial impact and progresses from central to peripheral until it can involve the entire cord. Ample evidence supports the hypothesis that the total amount of destruction of the cord is related to the trauma inflicted with the initial blow.[78,81–83] The peripheral white matter carrying fiber tracts to and from the caudal spinal cord may show only edema and some distortion of perfusion. In severe injuries, the white matter will undergo demyelination. Damage within the gray matter causes reversible myotonal and dermatomal deficits at the level of the lesion, whereas the more caudal functions may be spared. In the case of cervical SCI, the patient presents with weak hands and strong legs—the "central cord syndrome."

These observations have prompted therapeutic efforts designed to minimize evolution of the pathologic changes. The initial segmental loss can be withstood because only a small portion of the total gray matter neuronal pool is involved. Segmental white matter loss causes flaccidity below the level of the lesion. Later, spastic quadriplegia or paraplegia ensues. If effective treatment could be initiated early, adjacent

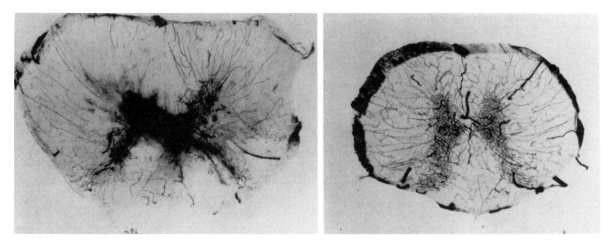

Figure 33-2 *Left.* Colloidal carbon angiogram of a cross section of a normal rat cord at the T1 level. Note the extensive microcirculation, especially in the gray matter. *Right.* Colloidal carbon angiogram 2 h after a moderately severe clip compression injury at T1 in the rat. There is extensive hemorrhage in the gray matter. Large areas of white and gray matter show loss of the microcirculation. (Reproduced with permission from Tator and Fehlings.[122])

white matter might be spared and irreversible paralysis avoided.

Electrical events measured after cord injuries support the progressive pathophysiologic hypothesis. Somatosensory evoked potentials (SSEPs)[83–89] can be used to assess the effects of graded cord trauma on function. Immediately after impact the animal (or human) is rendered paraplegic. There is complete loss of conduction (Fig. 33-3). Even after minor injuries, marked attenuation of SSEPs occurs; however, the wave form may recover rapidly in a few hours and can look normal within 1 week after injury. In animals damaged by an impact just sufficient to cause paralysis for 6 to 8 weeks, conduction loss occurs initially. More than one-half of the animals have return of conduction but not function at 3 h, then cord conduction again fails. The initial concussion impedes electrical impulse transmission. Electrical recovery may occur but fails in the long run due to progressive pathophysiologic involvement of the peripheral white matter.[86] Local segmental reflex activity may return transiently within 20 to 30 min after injury but disappears as gray matter disruption progresses.

Spinal cord metabolism is markedly depressed im-

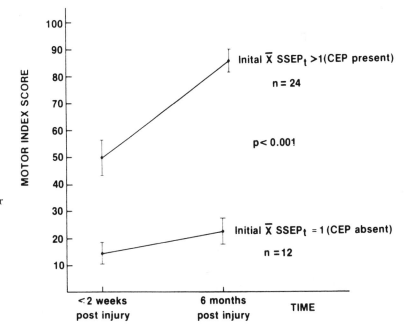

Figure 33-3 The relationship between the presence or absence of the initial mean posterior tibial somatosensory evoked potential (SSEP$_t$) obtained less than 2 weeks after injury and Motor Index score obtained at less than 2 weeks after injury and 6 months after injury. CEP, cortical evoked potential. (Reproduced with permission from Houldan DA, Rowed DW: Somatosensory evoked potentials and neurological grade as predictors of outcome in spinal cord injury. *J Neurosurg* 1990; 72:600.)

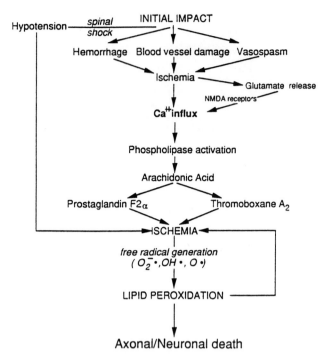

Figure 33-4 Biochemical cascade initiated by the primary event with acute spinal injury leading to neuronal/neuronal death. NMDA, *N*-methyl-D-aspartate. (Reproduced with permission from Lam AM: Acute spinal cord ischemia: Implications for anesthetic management. *Advances in Anesthesia*, vol 10. Chicago, Mosby-Year Book, 1993:247.)

mediately after initial blow.[90] Lactic acid buildup follows, consistent with local ischemia.[91,92] The ischemia triggers a biochemical cascade that itself may cause further spinal cord ischemia, which signals the onset of secondary injury leading to eventual infarctions of the spinal cord with permanent loss of function. The initial injury causes hemorrhage, ischemia, release of excitotoxic amino acids (glutamates) and an intracellular influx of calcium ions. The binding of glutamate to *N*-methyl-D-aspartate (NMDA) opens the receptor-gated channel and leads to a further increase in calcium flux. The intracellular accumulation of calcium then leads to activation of phospholipase and release of arachidonic acid and its metabolites of prostanoids and thromboxanes. These potent vasoconstrictors result in further ischemia and genesis of free radicals, causing lipid peroxidation and eventual destruction of neurones and axons (Fig. 33-4).

Local alterations in blood flow at the site of injury are important.[91,93–96] Histologic and microscopic flow studies demonstrate capillary and venular sludging and stasis. Circulation time is prolonged. Flame-shaped hemorrhages develop at capillary-venular junctions. Progressive traumatic dilatation of surface veins can be observed and may persist for 2 or 3 weeks.

Sludging and stasis in these vessels indicate the widespread circulatory effects of the trauma.[97]

The anterior 75 percent of the spinal cord is supplied by a single anterior spinal artery that arises from the vertebral artery and runs longitudinally for the length of the spinal cord. There are important contributions from the radicular vessels from the aorta via the intercostal arteries. The spinal cord segments between the radicular arteries receives its blood supply from above as well as below (Fig. 33-5). The two posterior spinal arteries that arise from the posterior branch of the vertebral arteries and also receive contributions from radicular vessels supply the posterior 25 percent of the spinal cord. In a postmortem review of 215 spinal

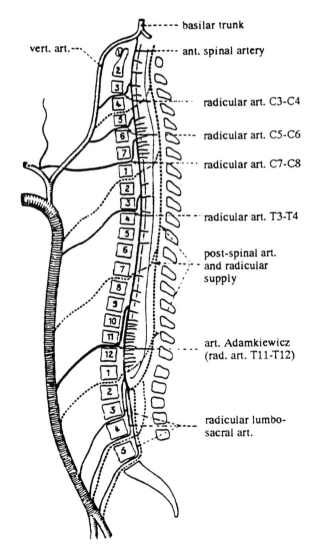

Figure 33-5 Vascular supply of the spinal cord circulation, illustrating the contributions from radicular arteries. (Reproduced with permission from Lam AM: Acute spinal cord ischemia: Implications for anesthetic management. *Advances in Anesthesia* vol. 10. Chicago, Mosby-Year Book, 1993:247.)

cords, Manners noted that this blood supply was variable. Forty-five (20.9 percent) of these had only one anterior radicular artery in the cervical cord.

Studies investigating the effects of varying perfusion pressure on spinal cord blood flow demonstrate that autoregulation is maintained between spinal cord perfusion pressure of 60 and 120 mmHg.[13] Below and above these pressures, spinal cord blood flow depends on perfusion pressure. Following acute SCI, autoregulation is changed or lost. Severe SCI results in marked decrease in spinal cord blood flow and loss of autoregulation. These autoregulatory responses may be particularly important in view of the tenuous blood supply of certain areas of the cord[98] (see Fig. 33-5). Jellinger noted that the "watershed" in blood supply to the cervical cord makes C6 most vulnerable to ischemia, because at this level blood flow splits in compartments flowing up and down the anterior spinal artery.[99] Hypotension below the lower limits of autoregulation should be prevented to protect the spinal cord from ischemic injury.

Vasomotor reactivity of the arterioles is altered with the impact.[36,100,101] Both distal and proximal segments of the spinal cord have transiently impaired responses to changes in arterial carbon dioxide tension; the caudal segment abnormality may persist for some time. The overall perfusion pattern of the injured cord may predict viability. For example, hyperemic spinal cord segments tend to recover, whereas segments with progressive ischemia do not.[91] Microangiographic studies of the injured spinal cord using barium microparticles confirm this pathologic process.[93,102] There is an initial ischemic phase lasting 5 to 15 min primarily involving the gray matter. Soon, ischemic and hemorrhagic lesions appear; the white matter vasculature dilates. The combination of central ischemia and peripheral hyperemia explains the measured increase in total spinal cord blood. Animals that have recovered after "injury" demonstrate hyperemia and increased vascularity. Presumably, the increased flow supports the reparative process.[86,103]

When tissue perfusion is reduced to ischemic levels, progressive necrosis occurs in the central gray matter[102] where the metabolic demands are five times that of white matter. The white matter pathology may reflect edema from the adjacent central gray matter damage. In the acute phase the cord appears normal on the outside when indeed there is ischemic, hemorrhagic, and necrotic central damage that is irreversible. Central cavitation and a traumatic syrinx may become evident at a later date in a small number of cases. Internal decompression to remove the damaged center in an attempt to preserve peripheral white matter function is a subject that has been previously reviewed.[104] Such operations were probably performed as early as 1905

by Cushing. Our limited clinical experience in removing the central hemorrhagic and necrotic center of the cord has not led to improved function sufficient enough to warrant such operative manipulations and indeed such procedures now have negative medicolegal implications.

Models and Biomechanics of Acute SCI

A variety of SCI models have been proposed and used in the laboratory.[105–125] The injury is produced with a weight drop, clip pressure, ischemia, and piston, and the assessment of the injury is made by histologic examination, ionic shifts, or behavioral ability weeks after the injury. However, no model has universal acceptance and it is doubtful that any animal model can fully simulate what happens in the clinical situation of a human SCI. Thus, the response to any drug therapy in animal models of SCI and the interpretation of the results may not be reproduced exactly in the human scenario. The forces of the trauma are unknown and totally uncontrolled; they vary from mild cord contusion with minimal neurologic deficit to severe cord contusion with complete transverse myelitis, and in rare cases, anatomic cord transection. Although the SCI can be the patient's only injury, typically in blunt trauma, as in an MVA, multiple body systems are often injured including the chest, brain, long bones, and abdomen.[126] These additional injuries can contribute to systemic hypoxia or hypotension, both of which aggravate the initial injury in the spinal cord.[38] Furthermore, the loss of sympathetic outflow in cervical SCI causes systemic hypotension from neurogenic shock.[39–43] In animal models, the thoracic cord is usually studied specifically to avoid the major cardiovascular problems related to neurogenic shock and their complicated medical treatments.

Alcohol and drugs are also present in a large percentage of human SCIs and may be an important modulator of the pathophysiologic response.[127–129] Clinically, patients with unstable spinal fractures have the potential for repeated mechanical trauma to the spinal cord during transport from the injury site to the hospital and in the hospital before stabilization. This repeated mechanical trauma is not accounted for in most animal models but was shown to be an important effect in one study.[39] The response to drug therapy after SCI can be measured in a variety of ways including histologic, chemical, and clinical recovery. Different methods of animal tissue analysis are sensitive to the gray or white matter protection after SCI. Sacrificing the animal at 24 h allows a large number of animals to be studied but obviously cannot directly measure the clinical recovery over the coming weeks to months. SCI models that sacrifice the animal shortly after the injury use an index of damage and measure the drug response to this early assessment of the total injury and then infer an ultimate recovery.

Survival of the spinal cord blood vessels and proper function of the microvascular perfusion to the spinal tissue minimizes the secondary damage to the spinal cord.[36,86,,91,97,130,131] Other factors that can affect the secondary injury in the spinal cord include the general physiology of the animal and cardiovascular parameters, blood pressure, cardiac output, nutritional status, oxygenation, and temperature. Ideally, all these factors would be controlled in an experimental animal model researching SCI.[132,133]

NEUROPROTECTION AND REGENERATION OF THE SPINAL CORD

Over the past decade, the study of central nervous system (CNS) tissue undergoing injury has disclosed a complex pathophysiologic response that is amenable to physiologic and drug manipulation. These studies have included the analysis of brain, spinal cord, and peripheral nerve tissues. This section provides a brief review of the CNS tissue responses to injury, with emphasis on SCI studies. Neuroprotection is a recent development in neuroscience and refers to the prevention or minimization of the secondary damage or self-destruction of a neuron following an injury. The basic conceptualization of neuroprotection occurred with the realization that a significant portion of the total injury is secondary, occurring after the primary insult and is, thus, potentially augmented by pharmacologic interventions.[122,134–139] Neuroprotection is often described in terms of manipulation of the excitotoxic process. Many insults may also have a penumbra of partial injury, which is potentially salvageable with therapy.

Neural regeneration refers to the actual growth of damaged neural elements with the reestablishment of functional synaptic connections and is currently not possible in the CNS tissue. Current research in the field of neural regeneration involves techniques of viable embryonic cell factors.[140,141] The field and techniques of neural regeneration will certainly expand over the coming years and will, one hopes, some day fulfill their potential of replacing nervous tissue lost in an injury with functional replacement tissue.

Much of the general knowledge of neuronal and nervous tissue physiology and pathophysiology has been derived from research of brain tissue in cell cultures and animal models. Many of these models study the specific concerns related to the unique cell types, neural function, local anatomy, and biomechanics of the spinal cord tissue. Recent advances in the pathophysiologic processes of nervous tissue and initiation

of clinical studies have led to a dramatic rise in the interest in neuroprotection and the potential of neuroregeneration as shown by multiple recent publications and conferences.

Both the brain and spinal cord can be damaged and result in cellular death from a variety of insults, which include trauma, stroke, hypoxia, surgical insults or manipulation, hypoglycemia, and neurotoxins. Despite the wide range of insults, many commonalities in the resultant delayed cellular death mechanism have been noted. Several agents elicit neuroprotective response in animals or cell culture models. These promising agents include steroids, gangliosides, endogenous opioid peptide antagonists, NMDA, glutamate antagonists, antioxidants, and calcium channel blockers (discussed later in this chapter). Combination therapy with these drugs is now in the early stages of investigation.[108] The first clinical studies investigating neuroprotective agents in acute SCI have recently been completed and suggest clinical applicability. Drugs that augment the depletion of neurotransmitters can also be used to manipulate the CNS pharmacologically as in L-dopa in Parkinson's disease and tacrine[142,143] in Alzheimer's disease. Human clinical studies are currently (February 1996) being conducted in head injuries and SCI, as well as stroke, to study the neuroprotective effects of several compounds.

A variety of strategies are available in the development of neuroprotective drug designs, affecting different points in the pathophysiologic processes of excitotoxicity.[140,144–147] It is not clear which interventions or what timing of multiple interventions will be most clinically useful in the treatment of SCI.

PRIMARY NEURONAL CELL CULTURES

Neuronal cell cultures have become a widely used model in the development of neuroprotective drugs and studying the pathophysiology underlying cell death.[148–153] These cultures are particularly well suited for studying cerebral ischemia. The primary neuronal cultures are usually derived from rats or mice with a variety of the CNS cell lines being used. The neurons adhere to the bottom of the culture dish after being applied in a dispersed cell culture. Processes start to form within a few hours and can develop cell bodies that assume the distinctive shape of their cell line.[154,155] Cell cultures with low densities allow morphologic investigation, whereas higher density cultures, which often form cell aggregates in a network of neurites with axons and dendrites, are used in pharmacologic studies. Typically, the cultured neurons undergo experimental damage and then the effect of a potentially neuroprotective drug is assessed.[156–160] The assessment of neural damage can be performed by simple microscopic examination to determine neural swelling, cell disintegration, or changes in the axon or dendrites. Additionally, several staining procedures and biochemical markers are used to quantify the extent of neuronal damage.[158,161–164] Most of the current neuroprotective drugs, with the exception of calcium antagonists, have an in vivo effect corresponding to that predicted with models in vitro. The primary neuronal cell cultures are useful for both basic research and screening of potential neuroprotective drugs.

Clinical Classification of Acute SCI

A detailed history is obtained as an indication of mechanism of injury and for medicolegal implications. Knowledge of the type of traumatic incident (i.e., MVA, diving, gunshot wound, or fall) identifies the mechanism of injury and often assists in determining the type of injury. The most common mechanisms of injury resulting in SCI include forced flexion (MVA or posterior blow), flexion with rotation (MVA), hyperextension (falls), and vertical compression (axial loading, diving accident). These mechanisms can occur singly or in combination. Penetrating wounds from gunshots or stabbings can pierce the spinal cord, causing mechanical disruption of the spinal cord tracts; a bullet passing near the spinal cord can cause cord concussion, producing a transient or permanent neurologic deficit.

Motor and sensory functions in all four extremities need to be clearly documented at the time of injury and on admission to the medical facility to provide a baseline for determining subsequent neurologic deterioration or improvement. Any complaint of neck or back pain or muscle spasm may indicate a spinal column injury without neurologic deficit. Patients with these conditions require serial radiologic and neurologic evaluations. If the cervical muscle spasm is severe and the neutral position radiologic studies demonstrate anatomic alignment, the flexion-extension lateral cervical radiographs are required several days postinjury to uncover any potential posterior ligamentous injury, because it may result in an unstable cervical spine once the muscle spasm subsides. Algorithms for evaluation of spine instability in the patient with multiple trauma and specific management for the patient with cervical spine injury without neurologic injury are outlined in Figs. 33-6 and 33-7.

The neurologic assessment is derived from a detailed motor and sensory examination. Of particular note are the pin sensations in the sacral dermatomes around the rectum and voluntary rectal tone. Their presence is synonymous with the presence of sacral sparing, which may be the only remaining neurologic function in an incomplete cervical spinal cord lesion. Its pres-

ence changes the patient category from complete to incomplete neurologic injury, an essential diagnostic distinction. Many patients with incomplete lesions tend to have partial recovery of neurologic function, whereas patients with complete spinal cord lesions do not have significant neurologic recovery.

Consistency of spinal cord assessment is important, particularly in noting subtle changes in sensation and motor function. The American Spinal Injury Association (ASIA) has developed a motor assessment system that provides a numerical grading system to document improvement or deterioration in function (Table 33-4).[165] Motor function is assessed by testing five key muscles on each side of the body on 0 to 5 scale (0 representing total paralysis and 5 representing normal function). The motor score is the sum of the strengths of all muscles (0 representing complete quadriplegia and 100 representing normal muscle function). Using this type of indexing, patient care providers can accurately and consistently document the patient's status.

The classification of cord injury can be anatomic or functional.[166] Anatomic classifications involve a description of the site of most severe damage to the cord. The most widely appreciated entity is the "central cord syndrome."[167] Central cord injury causes marked weakness and numbness of the hands and preservation of leg function. This clinical entity fits the experimental and clinical pathologic data that demonstrate marked damage within the central part of the cord after concussive cord injury.

Other anatomic injuries include the anterior and posterior cord syndromes (see Table 33-1). In the anterior cord syndrome, the anterior two-thirds of the spinal cord is damaged as a result of anterior spinal artery disruption.[168] With preservation of the posterior columns, position and vibration sense (proprioception) may be intact. In the posterior cord syndrome, all posterior and central aspects of the cord are damaged, only a few anterior white matter fiber tracts remain that carry pain and temperature past the damaged area. Bony cervical spine injury can produce all three lesions. A more uncommon anatomic injury is the Brown-Séquard syndrome due to hemisection of the spinal cord. This occurs rarely after trauma but was initially described in relation to a knife injury to the spinal cord. It results in loss of ipsilateral motor and proprioception and contralateral disruption of pain and temperature two or three dermatomes caudal to the lesion.

Although anatomic classifications are important in understanding pathophysiology, functional classifications as described by Guttman[169] and Frankel[23] are more useful when defining therapy for cord injured patients. Patients are graded as: (1) complete loss of all motor

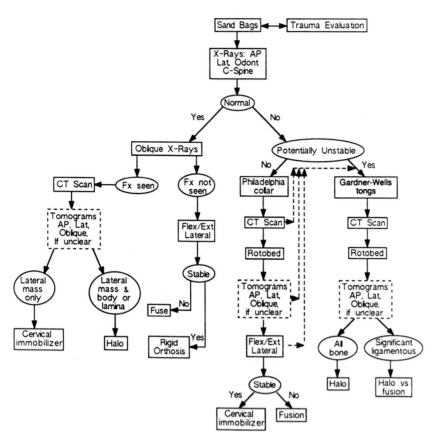

Figure 33-6 Algorithm for evaluating cervical spine instability in the patient with multiple trauma:

1. The portable lateral cervical radiograph must visualize the entire cervical spine and include all of C7. A bilateral facet dislocation of C7 on T1 may be missed unless the top of T1 is also seen. Visualizing down to T1 may require a "swimmer's view," pulling the shoulders down, or tomography.
2. To be considered normal the lateral radiograph must be 100 percent normal. Any degree of translational or angulation effect is considered abnormal under these circumstances.
3. Flexion-extension radiographs are performed when there is concern about possible ligamentous instability. They should be performed cautiously with only the patient moving the neck. These studies may be falsely normal shortly after injury due to cervical paraspinal muscle spasm.
4. Abnormal radiographic findings evaluated with additional diagnostic techniques including computed tomography, conventional tomography, and magnetic resonance imaging. (Reproduced by permission from Chestnut RM, Marshall LF: *Early Assessment, Transport and Management of Patients with Posttraumatic Spinal Instability*. Neurological Topic AANS, 1994:1.)

and sensory function, (2) loss of all motor function but preservation of some sensory function, (3) preservation of some motor function that is useless for ambulation and preservation of some sensory function, (4) preservation of motor function that is useful for functional purposes and possible ambulation, and (5) recovery to normal motor and sensory function. These functional descriptions allow for recovery comparisons related to various treatment modalities. Recently, more defined indices have been developed to grade motor function at many levels, which can be used to calculate recovery rates.[170] Using standard indices for motor function (0 equals none, 1 equals trace, 2 equals poor, 3 equals fair, 4 equals good, and 5 equals normal function), cord segments can be assigned an initial motor function and motor index from which recovery rates can be calculated. Sequential bilateral motor indices can be used to assess the effectiveness of therapy or the negative effects of systemic events (e.g., hypotension or hypoxia on spinal cord function). Classification can, however, be simple—a loss of motor or sensory function below the level of injury. Motor function may be assessed by muscle testing, usually on a 0 to 5 point scale. Sensory function (light touch and pin) C2 to S5 is tested as normal, decreased, or absent. Other, more standardized classifications include the ASIA motor score (Fig. 33-8) and the Frankel classification (see Table 33-4).

Experimental Therapeutics of Acute SCI

STEROIDS

For 18 years, several steroids or steroid-derived compounds have been studied for the treatment of CNS injury.[171–175] These steroids were investigated as potential agents to lessen the secondary injury after CNS insult. Several studies have indicated that glucocorticoids are ineffective in the treatment of secondary injury, whereas others reported improvement of neurologic recovery in experimental models with a high dose of MPSS in the range of 30 mg/kg.[144,176–182] Because this dose of steroid is far in excess of the physiologic dose, it has been hypothesized that the steroids work through other mechanisms, by inhibition of the posttraumatic lipid peroxidation (most cited)[130,176,182–188] or increased blood flow.[189–191] The efficacy of MPSS varies based on severity of the injury. Several clinical studies involving steroids have been concluded and reported a negative result in traumatic brain and SCI. One study by Gianotta and colleagues suggested reduced mortality in traumatic brain injury.[192]

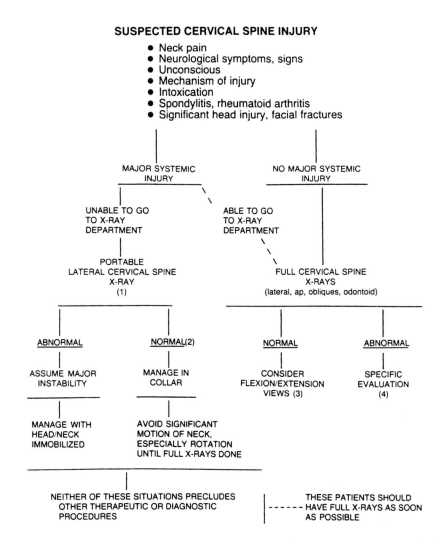

Figure 33-7 Algorithm for management of the patient with suspected cervical spine injury without neurologic deficit. (Reproduced by permission from Chestnut RM, Marshall LF: *Early Assessment, Transport and Management of Patients with Posttraumatic Spinal Instability.* Neurological Topic AANS, 1994:1.)

New compounds were developed to optimize the inhibitor activity of in vitro nervous tissue lipid peroxidation and to minimize the glucocorticoid activity.[184,193] These are nonglucocorticoid 21-aminosteroid compounds that have been generically termed *lazeroids.* These compounds build stabilized membranes and have activity as potent scavengers of lipid peroxy radicals.[194,195] Tirilazad mesylate, the 21-aminosteroid U74006F, has been demonstrated to be effective in a variety of CNS injury models,[195–210] which include cerebral ischemia, hypovolemic shock, cerebral vasospasm, subarachnoid hemorrhage, and traumatic SCI. Tirilazad significantly enhanced recovery of local motor function in a feline SCI model when administered 4 h after the injury. However, when the compound was not administered until 8 h after the injury, most of the protection effect preventing secondary injury was lost.[197] Tirilazad has also been investigated as a possible agent in the treatment of traumatic brain injury. Both the survival enhancement and early neurologic recovery in mice in a concussive head injury model were

reported.[210] Tirilazad altered both cerebral edema and local cation distribution in animal models with a traumatic brain injury and demonstrated significant postinjury reduction in mortality.[211,212] Currently, multicentered clinical trials that include tirilazad in one of the treatment arms are being conducted in the United States for both head injury and SCI.

ENDOGENOUS OPIOID PEPTIDE ANTAGONISTS

Endogenous opioid peptide receptors have been separated into mu, delta, kappa, and sigma subtypes.[213] Dynorphine is thought to be active at the kappa-receptor and β-endorphin is active at the mu receptors while leu- and met-enkephalin have greatest activity at the delta receptor.[214–216] Several experimental models have shown that endogenous opioid peptides augment the pathophysiology following SCI with a reported mechanism of action being alteration in microcirculatory blood flow at the injury site.[217–221] It is believed that

TABLE 33-4
Rating Scales for Neurologic Injury Assessment

Assessment of Neurologic Injury Using the ASIA Motor Score[165] and
Frankel Classification Grading System[23]

A. **Complete Neurologic Injury**—No motor function clinically detected below the level of injury.

B. **Preserved Sensation Only**—No motor function clinically detected below the level of injury; sensory function remains below the level of injury but may include only partial function (sacral sparing qualifies as preserved sensation).

C. **Preserved Motor Nonfunctional**—Some motor function is preserved below the level of injury, but is of no practical use to the patient.

D. **Preserved Motor Function**—Useful motor function below the level of the injury; patient can move lower limbs and walk with or without aid, but does not have a normal gait or strength in all motor groups.

E. **Normal**—No clinically detected abnormality in motor or sensory function with normal sphincter function; abnormal reflexes and subjective sensory abnormalities may be present.

For neurologic evaluations the ASIA Impairment Scale may be used:

Based on the International Standards for Neurologic and Functional
Classification by ASIA and the International Medical Society of Paraplegia (IMSOP)[165]

A. **Complete**—No motor or sensory function is preserved in sacral segments S4–5.

B. **Incomplete**—Sensory but no motor function is preserved below the neurologic level and extends through sacral segments S4–5.

C. **Incomplete**—Motor function is preserved below the neurologic level and the majority of key muscles below the neurologic level have a muscle grade < 3.

D. **Incomplete**—Motor function is preserved below the neurologic level and the majority of key muscles below the neurologic level have muscle grade ≥ 3.

E. **Normal**—Motor and sensory function are normal.

In addition to the ASIA motor and sensory scale a modified Benzel classification[499] can be used on follow-up to determine neurologic function:

Assessment of Neurologic Function at Follow-Up Examination
Using the Benzel Classification Scale[499]

I   No motor or sensory function is preserved in the sacral segments S4–5.

II   Sensory but no motor function is preserved in the sacral segments S4–5.

III   Motor function preserved below neurologic level and the majority of key muscles below neurologic level have grade <3/5. Patient is unable to walk.

IV   Some functional motor control below the level of injury that is significantly useful (i.e., assist in transfers). Patient is unable to walk.

V   Motor function allows walking with or without assistance, but significant problems secondary to lack of endurance or fear of falling limit patient mobility. Patient has limited walking ability.

VI   Ambulatory without assistance and without significant limitations other than one or both of the following: difficulty with micturition and dyscoordination. Patient has unlimited walking ability.

VII   Neurologically intact with the exception of minimal deficits that cause no functional difficulties.

dynorphine is the opioid peptide that is active in the modulation of secondary injury in traumatic SCI.[216,222,223] Dynorphine is elevated at the site of injury and can induce transient hind limb paralysis after intrathecal injection in a rat model and increase the kappa-receptor binding, which occurs following traumatic SCI. The opiate antagonists of the kappa-receptor lessen the neurologic and histologic deficits following experimental SCI, and pretreatment with dynorphine antisera lessens the neurologic damage. In animal models, the activation of dynorphine and the kappa-receptor system is active in secondary injury following traumatic brain injury.[224–226] Naloxone, a narcotic antagonist, was investigated in human SCI in the National

Acute Spinal Cord Injury Study 2 (NASCI 2) and reported as providing no clinical benefit.[33–35,227]

GANGLIOSIDES

Although no direct animal study has demonstrated the efficacy of the effects of gangliosides relative to SCI, many reports in the literature discuss enhancement of neurologic function after ganglioside administration.[228] Gangliosides are sialic acid-containing glycosphingolipids found in high concentrations in the membranes of nervous tissue, specifically at the synaptic areas.[229–231] GM-1, a monosialoganglioside, is active in the modulation of neuronal sprouting and growth as well as syn-

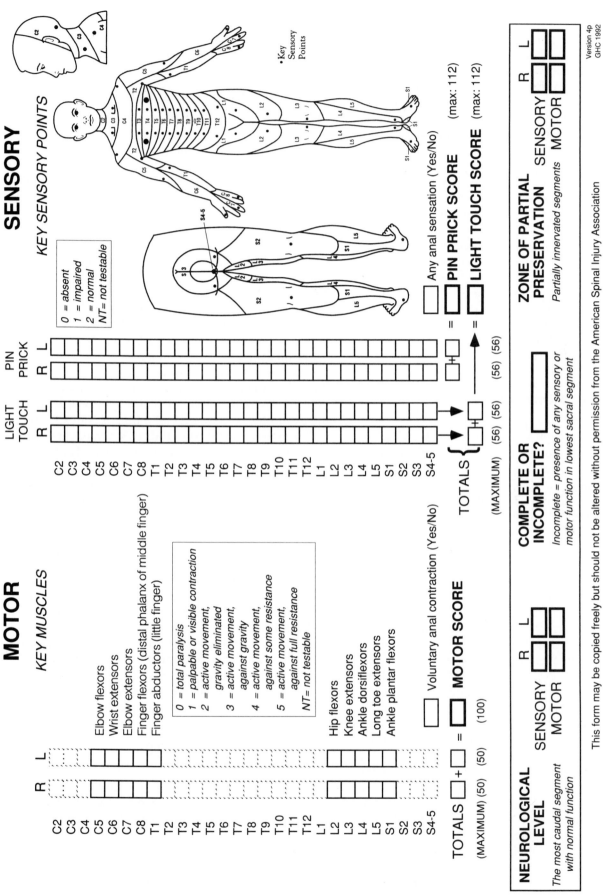

Figure 33-8 ASIA standard neurologic classification of spinal cord injuries. American Spinal Injury Association IM.[165]

aptic transmission, neuronal development, and plasticity.[230,232-254] Systemic administration of gangliosides improves the functional outcome of animals following a lesion in the brain tissue.[236,249,250,252,255-257] Furthermore, gangliosides are modulators of neurotransmitters because they alter the catecholamine neurotransmitter levels in cortical areas proximal to the transected pathway.[258] It is hypothesized that gangliosides augment the clinical effects of brain lesions by lessening the secondary injury of neuronal degeneration or increase the ability of the uninjured nervous tissue to reorganize itself into a functional state to replace the lost function of the injured tissue. It is postulated that GM-1 reduces the secondary damage after brain ischemia through a variety of mechanisms: it decreases the initial edema following the injury, restores the sodium-potassium pump adenosine triphosphatase (ATPase) activity, reduces NMDA-induced neurotoxicity, reduces the release of excitatory amino acid (EAA)-induced neurotoxicity, and enhances neural recovery and reorganization on a delayed basis.[258-263]

EXCITATORY AMINO ACID (EEA) ANTAGONISTS

Excitatory amino acids, glutamate and aspartate, are natural neurotransmitters in the CNS.[264] High concentration of EAA can result in increased neuronal firing, cell swelling, and eventual cell death.[265-268] Cell death in this manner has been termed *excitotoxin*.[269-271] The steps of neuronal cell death and excitotoxicity are described in Fig. 33-4. The release of large amounts of EAA neurotransmitters causes both an influx of sodium and chloride into the neuron, which produces acute cellular swelling and an influx of calcium leading to ultimate cell death.[148,272,273] It has also been reported that EAA cause increased hypoxia, cerebral ischemia, and hypoglycemia.[272,274-285] Four types of EAA receptors have been characterized based on responses to antagonists in ion channel measurements.[286-291] NMDA has been reported to correlate with the CNS region damaged by hypoxia, ischemia, or trauma.[292,293] Several pharmacologic antagonists to the NMDA receptor site are available. A positive drug effect has been reported both in vitro and in vivo with EAA receptor antagonists against hypoxia, ischemia, traumatic brain injury, and SCI.[110] The increase in the extracellular glutamate concentration appears to resolve in 1 to 2 h.[294-296] Thus, if the initiation of therapy is delayed for several hours, its clinical usefulness may be marginal or absent, even if the effect on immediate delivery of the NMDA antagonists would have been relatively large. Currently, no SCI clinical studies use these agents; however, ongoing clinical trials in Great Britain and the United States use the competitive NMDA antagonist CGS-19755 in traumatic brain injury. These compounds are potentially useful in the pharmacologic treatment of SCI.

CALCIUM CHANNEL BLOCKERS

The obstruction of blood flow causes ischemia and eventual stroke in neural tissue. A major obstruction of a cerebral vessel results in a cerebral stroke and microvascular dysfunction, which can cause local infarction. Without resumption of blood flow within minutes, the severely ischemic nervous tissue will be irreversibly damaged. There is a penumbra of low-flow tissue that has sufficient blood flow to maintain the viability but not the function of the nervous tissue.[297] If the blood flow in this area decreases below a critical value, 20 percent of normal, then irreversible damage will occur. However, if blood flow in this region is restored to normal, then this tissue can return to normal function. The decreased blood flow in the penumbra region causes a reduction in the adenosine triphosphate (ATP); when prolonged, it leads to dysfunction of the ATP-dependent processes, including the sodium-potassium pump that maintains cellular homeostasis. With failure there is an efflux of K^+ into the extracellular space and an influx of Na^+, Cl^- and Ca^{2+} into the cells.[298,299] The efflux of K^+ occurs first and can cause the release of neurotransmitters (EAA) that stimulate the NMDA receptors, causing additional influx of Na^+, Cl^-, and Ca^{2+}.[299,300] The intracellular free Ca^{2+} directly parallels the excitotoxic process of ischemic neuronal damage and ultimate cellular death. In the core of the ischemia zone, little protection is expected for calcium channel blockers, whereas, in the penumbral zone, the same blockers could attenuate the influx of Ca^{2+} and halt the destructive process. Nimodipine has been investigated in various animal models with mixed results.[301] However, strong evidence indicates that when nimodipine is given prophylactically or immediately after the insult, an effacious drug effect improves posttraumatic spinal cord blood flow.[302-306] The exact manner in which the calcium channel blockers will fit into the total treatment of injured nervous tissue remains to be defined.

FREE RADICAL SCAVENGERS AND ANTIOXIDANTS

An increase in free radicals occurs after CNS trauma and is believed to aggravate cerebral edema,[307] traumatic brain injury,[308] cerebral ischemia,[309-311] and spinal cord trauma.[127,196,312-316] An increase in the generation of free radicals has been studied with regard to intracellular calcium[223,300,317,318] and traumatic activation of the arachidonic acid cascade metabolites.[308,312] Free radicals are highly reactive and result in peroxidation of membrane phospholipids, which damage the neural membranes.[211] The free radicals can also directly damage the nervous tissue's vascular integrity and cause oxidation of cellular proteins and nucleic acids. Naturally occurring free radical scavengers are beneficial in controlling the secondary damage following CNS injury. For example, α-tocopherol (vitamin E) demonstrates a beneficial effect for neuroprotection in cerebral edema,[319,320] traumatic brain injury,[321,322] cerebral ischemia,[323–325] and spinal cord trauma.[105,176,326] The clinical usefulness of this treatment appears limited by the necessity to administer the α-tocopherol before the insult to the CNS tissue.

Other free radical scavengers including superoxide dismutase, polyethylene glycol, and dimethyl sulfoxide have been studied for potential beneficial effects following insult to the brain[319,327–330] and spinal cord.[331,332] Although it has been demonstrated that free radicals are involved in the pathologic process following CNS injury, it is not clear if pharmacologic manipulation of this process will be a part of the overall management of secondary injury. It is possible that the free radicals are end-stage markers of the damaged cascade process and manipulation will not greatly affect the underlying pathologic processes or ultimate recovery. However, a recent study with allopurinol, an inhibitor of xanthine oxidase, demonstrated in a rat SCI model that this treatment was not only efficacious but also showed a protective effect greater than observed with MPSS.[333]

Clinical Trials of Therapies for Acute SCI

There are three completed and two ongoing clinical drug trials for SCI. Results of the first National Acute SCI Study (NASCIS 1),[334,335] the second NASCIS (NASCIS 2),[33–35,171,227] and the Maryland GM-1 Ganglioside Study[336–340] have been completed and published. The NASCIS 3 and the Sygen® (GM-1) Acute SCI Study represent ongoing randomized, prospective studies that remain blinded.

NASCIS 1

The NASCIS 1 began entering patients in 1979 with the results published in 1984 and 1985.[334,335] This study compared the administration of two dosage regimens of intravenous (IV) MPSS for 10 days: 100 mg and 1000 mg. During the planning stage it was decided not to include a placebo group because many investigators believed that in some cases patients would be denied a potentially beneficial therapy. By design, the study was randomized, prospective, double-blinded, and multicentered. It required that the cord-injured patient be admitted to a participating center within 48 h of injury. In this study, an SCI was defined as any loss of motor or sensory function below the level of injury. Motor function was assessed by testing 14 muscles on each side of the body on a 0 to 5 point scale. Sensory function (light touch and pin) from C2 to S5 was assessed as normal, decreased, or absent. Neurologic examinations were performed on admission and then at 6 weeks, 6 months, and 1 year after injury. No difference in neurologic recovery of motor function or sensation was noted between the two treatment groups at 6 weeks and 6 months after injury. Wound infections of both trauma and operative sites were more prevalent in the high-dose regimen. With no placebo group, the results are consistent with either both treatment protocols being good or bad because the study demonstrated no difference between them. In a retrospective scrutiny of the study, it was noted that most patients were admitted late in the 48-h entry window, there was no uniform medical or surgical protocol used by all centers, and a detailed description of the medical care was not identified. The distribution of the initial severity of SCI between groups was not specified. Radiologic description and anatomic location of injury were not noted.

NASCIS 2

After completion of NASCIS 1, new animal SCI investigations involving MPSS revealed that very high doses were required for improvement after an SCI.[341–343] Treatment also needed to begin promptly, within minutes or a few hours, for the greatest effect. A mechanism of action for the neuroprotective effects of MPSS was thought to be a reduction in lipid peroxidation[176,186–188] and increased blood flow.[189–191] High doses of naloxone improved blood flow and motor ability up to 12 h after injury.[111,217]

The NASCIS 2 entered patients from May 1985 to December 1988 and the results were published in 1990.[33,35,227] This study compared placebo and MPSS (a 30 mg/kg bolus followed by 5.4 mg/kg per hour for 23 h) and naloxone (a 5.4 mg/kg bolus followed by 4.0 mg/kg per hour for 23 h). By design, this was a randomized, prospective, double-blinded, multicentered study. Randomization was performed within 12 h of injury and patients separated into two groups based on their entry time: less than 8 h or more than 8 h from injury. An SCI diagnosed by a physician was necessary for entry into this study; no initial degree of injury severity was required. Motor function was assessed by testing 14 muscles on each side of the body on a 0 to 5 point scale, and sensory function (light touch and pin) from C2 to S5 was assessed as normal, decreased, or absent. Neurologic examinations were obtained on admission and then at 6 weeks, 6 months, and 1 year after injury. Patients treated with MPSS within 8 h of injury had a significant increased recovery of neurologic function observed at 6 weeks, 6 months, and 1 year after the SCI injury. Patients treated after 8 h recovered less motor function in both the MPSS and naloxone groups compared with placebo. The medical complications were the same for all three groups. The total number of patients entered into the study was 487. However, the number of patients in the two groups used to determine the positive drug effect of MPSS was much less. There were 127 patients treated less than 8 h after injury—62 in the MPSS group and 65 in the placebo group. There were even fewer in the partial neurologic deficits subgroup—17 in the MPSS group and 22 in the placebo group, which contributed heavily to the changes in their group as a whole.

The results of NASCIS 2 have been criticized.[344-350] The dosage of MPSS used in NASCIS 2 was reported to be more effective than placebo. However, this may not be the optimum dose because only one dose was tested. As in NASCIS 1, no uniform medical or surgical protocol was used by all centers and a detailed description of the medical care was not collected. The distribution of the initial severity of SCI between groups was not specified in detail or within the subgroups in which improvement was reported. Radiologic description and types of bony injuries that produced the deficits were not specified. No functional scale of improvement was used in this study so the improvement in motor scores has an uncertain clinical usefulness. Additionally, the partial injury patients treated more than 8 h after injury had the same degree of neurologic recovery as patients treated less than 8 h after injury in the MPSS treatment group.[227] This raised the question as to whether the reported positive drug effect (i.e., the difference in recovery between the MPSS treatment group and the placebo group) was due mostly to a poor performance in the placebo group.[351] Others have questioned whether the true infection rate following this large dose of MPSS is increased in multitrauma patients.[352] NASCIS 2 reported no significant difference between the placebo and the MPSS groups for infection; however, it is believed that few multitrauma patients were admitted because the initial examination could not have been performed on these patients and hence the safety of MPSS in these high-risk patients remains unknown. Steroid psychosis has been reported from the NASCIS 2 dose and may place the patient at risk for a secondary injury.[353]

NASCIS 3

The NASCIS 3 has three parallel groups: (1) NASCIS 2 MPSS bolus and infusion for 23 h; (2) NASCIS 2 MPSS bolus and infusion for 48 h; and (3) NASCIS 2 MPSS bolus and infusion of tirilazad.[171]

MARYLAND GM-1 GANGLIOSIDE STUDY

The Maryland GM-1 Ganglioside Study was a prospective, randomized, placebo-controlled, double-blinded trial of GM-1 ganglioside involving major SCI. The patients were entered between January 1986 and May 1987, and the results published in 1991.[336,338-340,354] Of the 37 patients entered, 34 (23 cervical and 11 thoracic) completed the test drug protocol and the 1-year follow-up. The test drug protocol consisted of 100 mg monosialotetrahexosylganglioside (GM-1) sodium salt or placebo administered IV once a day for a total of 18 to 32 doses, with the first dose administered within 72 h of injury. All patients admitted to The Maryland Institute for Emergency Medical Services System in Baltimore with a spinal cord or column injury during the 16-month entrance period were considered for the study. The criteria for inclusion included: (1) patient consent obtained; (2) no contraindication to GM-1; (3) female patients surgically sterile or postmenopausal; (4) patient 18 years old; and (5) SCI with a major motor deficit of 3/5 in hands or legs.

The criteria for exclusion were: (1) patient had a premorbid major medical illness (i.e., end-stage diabetes, heart disease); (2) likelihood of patient being lost to follow-up; (3) patient involved in other experimental drug protocols; and (4) patient had significant damage to the cauda equina.

A standard medical protocol was used and included: (1) initial assessment and spinal immobilization; (2) medical management to correct neurogenic shock to optimize tissue perfusion and oxygenation; (3) 250 mg MPSS IV on admission and 125 mg every 6 h for 72 h; (4) continuous IV dopamine hydrochloride for most patients to reverse the neurogenic shock and maintain a normal to high-normal blood pressure; (5) prompt anatomic alignment of the spinal bony elements; (6) radiologic diagnostics (radiograph, myelogram, CT scan); (7) prompt surgical decompression of neural elements if closed spinal alignment failed to relieve the bony compression; and (8) stabilization of bony instability.[39] The ASIA motor score[355] and the Frankel classification grade[23] were used to assess the initial neurologic injury.

Comparison of the GM-1-treated patients and the placebo-treated patients revealed a significant drug effect with respect to change of two Frankel grades from entrance into the study to 1-year follow-up. The Cochran-Mantel-Haenszel chi squared analysis (34 patients) yielded a p value of .034, and the Fisher's exact test (two-tailed) (34 patients; 6 with one Frankel grade improvement counted as failures of treatment) had a p value of .014. The GM-1-treated patients also had a significant drug effect when compared to placebo-treated patients with respect to change in lower extremity ASIA motor score from entrance to 1-year follow-up and analysis of covariance with baseline ASIA

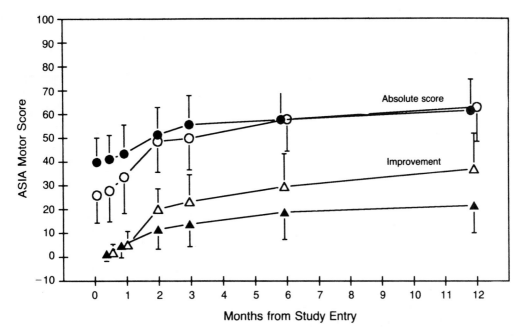

Figure 33-9   Improvement in mean ASIA motor score from entry to follow-up for all 34 patients completing the study, according to treatment group. The two lower curves show the improvement in the two groups after the ASIA motor scores were adjusted for the imbalance in scores at entry to allow direct comparison of the neurologic motor improvement. The error bars represent 95 percent confidence intervals. (Reproduced by permission from Geisler and coworkers.[340])

motor score (used to correct for baseline imbalance) had a *p* value of .047 (Figs. 33-9 and 33-10).

The proposed mechanism of recovery was hypothesized to be that GM-1 enhances function or potency of the damaged white matter passing through the level of the injury, thus allowing increased function at lower

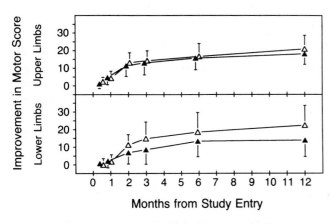

Figure 33-10   Improvement in ASIA motor scores for the upper and lower extremities over the 1-year study period in the 23 patients with cervical injuries who completed the study, according to treatment group. There was a trend toward a drug effect in the score for the upper extremities. Open triangles denote the 12 patients assigned to receive GM-1, and solid triangles the 11 patients assigned to placebo. The error bars represent 95 percent confidence intervals. (Reproduced by permission from Geisler and coworkers.[340])

levels.[230,233,235,237–239,243,246–250,252,254,356]   Animal experiments indicate that motor recovery occurs with only 5 percent of axons surviving through the injury site.[357] The enhanced motor function recovery of GM-1-treated patients may be related to increased survival of axons at the injury site, or possibly the GM-1 augmentation of the response of the neurons in the conus to the decreased input from the damaged white matter tracts passing through the injury site. This study formed the basis of the larger multicentered study using Sygen (GM-1) in the treatment of patients with acute SCI.

The Sygen (GM-1) Acute SCI Study sponsored by FIDIA Pharmaceutical Corporation (Washington, DC) is a prospective, double-blind, multicentered study stratified by injury level and severity, with three parallel groups: (placebo, low-dose GM-1, and high-dose GM-1) block-randomized by group 1 : 1 : 1 at each center. The low-dose GM-1 group had a loading dose of 300 mg followed by 100 mg/day for 56 days, and the high dose GM-1 group had a loading dose of 600 mg/day followed by 200 mg/day for 56 days.

The objectives of this study are to determine the efficacy and safety of two dose levels of GM-1 in the treatment of patients with acute SCI. The main statistical test planned is to determine whether the proportion of large improvers (defined later) is different between placebo and the two treatment groups.

Several planned secondary objectives of the Sygen (GM-1) SCI study include: (1) the effect on ultimate outcome based on radiologic injury analysis; (2) emergency medical technicians' arrival time at the injury scene; (3) emergency room arrival time; (4) hemodynamic resuscitation timing and parameters; (5) timing and type of surgery; (6) length of inpatient rehabilitation; (7) amount of continuous physical therapy in the follow-up period; (8) analysis of neurologic recovery in different anatomic regions; and (9) initial severities for different patterns of recovery.

The study is being conducted in 23 neurotrauma centers in North America with a total of 720 patients over a 3- to 4-year data collection period. Interim analyses are planned with the results reported to an extramural monitoring committee. This allows for early stopping of the study or an arm of the study for either a large drug effect or an increased complication rate of GM-1.

The inclusion criteria for this study are: (1) patient age 12 to 70 years; (2) restoration of blood pressure less than 8 h from injury; (3) major motor deficit from acute SCI score (sum of motor strength in the five ASIA motor groups of one leg ($\leq$ 15); (4) patient informed consent obtained; (5) MPSS therapy initiated within 8 h of injury (30 mg/kg bolus followed by 5.4 mg/kg per hour for 23 h); and (6) Sygen (GM-1) medication therapy initiated within 72 h of injury and after completion of the MPSS therapy.

The exclusion criteria were designed to ensure a group of SCI patients with a major injury were not contaminated with other confounding problems including: (1) SCI by direct penetration; (2) traumatic spinal cord anatomic transection; (3) major cauda equina or brachial or lumbar plexus injury; (4) significant head trauma or multitrauma; (5) significant systemic disease; (6) preexisting polyneuropathy or myelopathy; (7) inability to assess spinal cord function; (8) history of Guillain-Barré syndrome; (9) psychoactive substance use disorder in the 6 months before injury; (10) history of major depression, schizophrenia, paranoia, or other psychotic disorder; (11) pregnant or nursing women; (12) history of life-threatening allergic reaction; (13) inability to communicate effectively with the neurologic examiner; and (14) poor likelihood of patient being available for follow-up evaluation.

This study uses an initial or baseline neurologic evaluation as well as a detailed motor and sensory examination using the ASIA Impairment Scale (see Table 33-4). In addition to the ASIA motor and sensory scale, a modified Benzel classification scale is used at follow-up examination to determine neurologic function (see Table 33-4). A different scale is used in follow-up than in baseline evaluation because initially it is not possible to examine walking patients; often SCI victims have unstable spines and cannot be safely positioned verti-

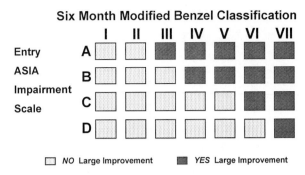

Test of Large Neurologic Improvement

Figure 33-11 The main statistical test used in the outcome evaluation is graphically presented. The patients are divided into *No* large improvement or *Yes* large improvement as determined by the difference between the entry ASIA impairment scale and the six-month modified Benzel classification.

cally. However, walking ability is important to include as a functional measure.

The main statistical test planned is to determine whether the proportion of patients with an increase of two grades between the initial Frankel grades A and B, Benzel follow-up grades, and patients with an increase of three grades between initial Frankel grades C and D and Benzel follow-up grades is different between placebo and the two drug treatment groups. This test is shown graphically in Fig. 33-11. A large improvement in the neurologic function between patients in the the two groups is clinically relevant because a large proportion of patients have an unexpected recovery. This test, if significant for drug effect, would demonstrate that the effect is not only statistically significant but also useful clinically.

A separate recovery pattern for the gray and white matter at the site of injury was first shown in the Maryland GM-1 SCI Study.[336–340] It was verified in an analysis of NASCIS 2.[358] These analyses demonstrated that white matter has more recovery potential than gray matter. It is hoped that the two ongoing drug trials will provide useful therapy to improve the ultimate neurologic function of the SCI victims and provide additional information on the nature and recovery patterns in SCI.

Respiratory Function after SCI

The degree of cardiac and respiratory function impairment that occurs following a SCI depends on the completeness and level of neurologic deficit and how recently the injury occurred. Preexisting cardiac and respiratory disease and other trauma sustained at the time of injury are also important factors.[359] In one center that admitted 2710 cord-injured patients (including cervical, thoracic, lumbar, and sacral SCIs), 26.2 percent had associated head and face injury, 16 percent had chest injury, 10 percent had injury of abdominal contents, and 8.5 percent had long bone or pelvic fractures. In diving accidents, SCI may be associated with near drowning. Appropriate resuscitation at the scene may then include external cardiac massage and mouth-to-mouth respiration. Blunt thoracic injury, sustained simultaneously with SCI in an MVA, may result in acute cardiorespiratory failure due to lung[359,360] and myocardial contusions.[361] Visceral hemorrhage may cause adbominal swelling, compromising diaphragmatic function, reducing circulating blood volume, and decreasing cardiac output.

If the patient is unconscious due to head injury, the airway should be maintained as the priority at the scene and during transportation. An esophagotracheal Combi-Tube can be passed once the neck is immobilized. This serves the dual purpose of protecting the airway when the cuff is inflated and allowing the lungs to be ventilated with a conventional resuscitator bag connection. This Combi-Tube is superior to the esophageal obturator. With the esophageal obturator, leakage of ventilation is not prevented by the face mask, which is difficult to seal. Rather, with the Combi-Tube a cuff is inflated in the oropharynx. The Combi-Tube does not require the skills necessary for tracheal intubation and in the unconscious patient can be inserted with limited movement of the neck. It is, therefore, ideally suited for airway management of the patient with suspected cervical spine injury. Use of the esophageal obturator has been abandoned because it has resulted in fatal complications including esophageal rupture and accidental tracheal intubation.[362] In the unconscious patient, a cricothyroidotomy provides emergency access to the airway, but it has the disadvantage of requiring surgical skill and results in no protection against regurgitation and aspiration of stomach contents. The conscious patient does not tolerate esophageal, nasopharyngeal, or oral airways; attempts to pass them result in resistance and neck movement. This should be avoided because the level of the lesion may ascend or an incomplete lesion may become complete.

Conscious patients may be helped by instruction in the use of diaphragmatic breathing because this is advocated as a means of achieving relaxation and coordinated breathing patterns.[363] Patients who cannot move their hands, arms, or legs (indicating no innervation below C4 level) require assisted ventilation at the scene and during transport. Mouth-to-mouth ventilation or, where available, use of a manual resuscitator, prevents CO_2 retention and alveolar collapse due to inadequate lung expansion. Adequate CO_2 removal is important to reduce further engorgement of the damaged cord. Where associated chest or abdominal injury

is present, additional O_2 should be delivered. Maintenance of the airway may be assisted by use of a nasopharyngeal catheter, which is usually adequately tolerated by conscious patients. The airway may be maintained in the dentulous patient by anterior displacement of the mandible and holding the jaw closed.

Patients who can shrug their shoulders and can outwardly rotate their arms (indicating an intact C5 innervation) and have no other associated cranial, thoracic, abdominal, or skeletal injury can breathe adequately provided they are not overly anxious. Anxiety results in inefficient usage of the innervated accessory muscles of respiration and the resulting tachypnea increases respiratory dead space. Neurologic deficit at C6 and below does not usually result in respiratory impairment during the acute phase unless there are associated injuries. The airway should then be managed as outlined above at the scene and during transportation.

The effects of spinal cord transection on respiratory function can be predicted from Fig. 33-12 that displays the spinal segmental innervation of the inspiratory and expiratory muscles of respiration.[364] The important muscles of expiration have thoracic segmental innervation; therefore, in cervical spinal cord transection, loss of expiratory function is to be expected and can be measured. The diaphragm is the principal muscle of inspiration and its movement accounts for more than two-thirds of the air that enters the lungs during quiet breathing.[365] The diaphragm is partially denervated with a C5 cord transection and there is gross impairment of respiratory function with a C4 level lesion. For acute SCI above C4, mechanical ventilatory support is usually mandatory in the acute phase. With a complete neurologic deficit in the cervical cord there is paralysis of the intercostal muscles, levatores costarum and serratus posterior superior, which elevate and abduct the ribs, enlarge the thorax, and facilitate the action of the other inspiratory muscles.[366]

Vital capacity may be as low as 100 ml following cervical SCI, but usual ranges are between 350 and 1000 ml. The average vital capacity of 30 motor complete quadriplegic patients (levels C3 to C7) reported in the literature is 1300 ml. Cervical spinal cord transection may reduce expiratory flow and expiratory reserve volume to 40 percent of predicted normals. Expiratory flow rates of 10 liters/s or 600 liters/min are required to produce an effective cough. Following cervical SCI at C5, expiratory flow may be as little as 2 liters/s (Fig. 33-13). This loss of expiratory power results in an increase in residual volume of 140 to 200 percent of predicted normal. The ineffective cough, inadequate expansion, and incomplete emptying of the lungs result in secretion retention and inadequate gas exchange. Respiratory function tests may be used as pre-

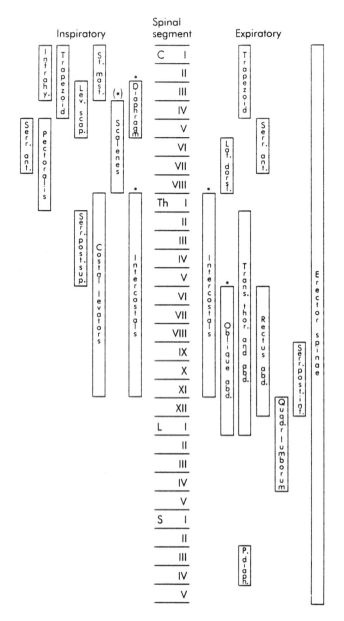

Figure 33-12 Spinal segmental innervation of the inspiratory muscles (*left*) and expiratory muscles (*right*). Muscles marked with asterisks are primary respiratory muscles, and those marked with asterisks in parentheses *may* be primary muscles. Other muscles are auxiliary. (Reproduced by permission from Fugl-Meyer.[364])

dictors of the need for mechanical ventilation and as an indicator of improvement following therapy. For example, a simple test such as vital capacity is useful to assess the patient's learning progress during the teaching of glossopharyngeal breathing. More sophisticated tests of pulmonary function such as specific airway conductance and lung compliance may be indicated to assess chest physiotherapy effectiveness in removal of retained lung secretions in quadriplegic patients. Serial measurements of respiratory function may be useful to determine the efficacy of a breathing exercise and retraining program (Table 33-5). Ledsome and Sharp[367] found that patients with C5 to C6 lesions had vital capacities of 30 percent of predicted and those with C4 level lesions had 21 percent of predicted vital capacities. A gradual improvement in vital capacity occurred 5 weeks and 3 months after injury. The almost doubling of vital capacity after 3 months was thought to be the result of spasticity and reflex contraction of the intercostal muscles resulting in improved expiratory flow.

Cardiovascular Function after SCI

CARDIAC MANAGEMENT AT THE SCENE AND DURING INITIAL HOSPITAL MANAGEMENT

In animals, the production of acute quadriplegia causes a brief mild rise in cardiac contractility, mean arterial pressure, and systemic vascular resistance, followed 6 to 8 min later by bradycardia, diminished cardiac contractility, and hypotension.[368] Albin and colleagues[369] found transient increases of intracranial pressure, arterial blood pressure, extravascular lung water, brain water, and a decrease in cerebral blood flow on production of acute quadriplegia in animals. Management of cardiac dysfunction immediately after SCI should include recording pulse rate, blood pressure, and the electrocardiogram (ECG). Patients with pulse rates below 50 beats per minute may benefit from IV atropine because this is reported to acutely elevate cardiac output and tissue O_2 delivery and reverse hypotension in the bradycardic quadriplegic patient who is in spinal shock (Fig. 33-14).[370] In addition, ephedrine 5 to 10 mg IV is a useful agent because it increases heart rate and cardiac contractility and acts as a temporizing measure having a longer duration of action than atropine. If bradycardia causing significant impairment of tissue O_2 delivery persists, a temporary pacemaker may be inserted to restore cardiac output or in preparation for upcoming surgery (Fig. 33-15).

Quadriplegic patients with associated injuries and hemorrhage should have an IV infusion started to restore circulating volume and maintain cardiac output. Use of a fluid challenge technique in association with close cardiorespiratory monitoring will avoid the hazards of overtransfusion and the resulting pulmonary edema while at the same time maintain optimum cardiac function and tissue oxygen delivery.[371] If IV infusion is not available, the quadriplegic patient with hemorrhagic and spinal shock may be managed once the neck is immobilized by tilting the whole patient

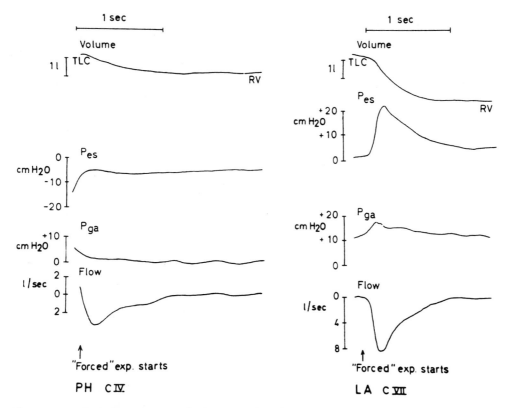

Figure 33-13   Typical registrations of volume, esophageal (P_{es}) and gastric (P_{ga}) pressures at a forced rate expiratory vital capacity maneuver from the total lung capacity (TLC) in a patient with high cervical and a patient with low cervical spinal cord transections. Expiratory flow are down. (Reproduced by permission from Fugl-Meyer.[364])

TABLE 33-5
Vital Capacity and Expiratory Volume of Quadriplegic Subjects before and after a Program of Pulmonary Therapy and Resistance Exercise[a]

Level	Sex	Age	VC 1 (ML)	VC 1 (%)	VC 2 (ML)	VC 2 (%)	Max VE 1 (Liters/Min)	Breaths/ Min	ML/ Breath	Max VE 2	Breaths/ Min	ML/ Breath
C5–6	F	26	2500	70	3400	96	18.3	35	523	25.6	32	800
C5–6	M	18	4000	84	4800	101	28.9	44	657	44.4	57	779
C4–5	F	17	1400	42	1600	49	10.8	38	284	22.3	58	384
C6–7	M	32	2700	59	3000	66	23.0	44	523	43.3	62	698
C5–6	M	24	2550	59	2700	63	20.4	45	453	35.7	39	915
C5–6	F	29	2100	62	2900	85	16.9	37	457	22.6	35	646
C5–6	M	19	2700	59	3500	77	19.4	38	511	48.9	39	1254
C6–7	M	25	3750	78	3900	82	27.0	28	964	48.3	33	1464
C4–5	M	17	1400	31	2000	44	13.0	30	433	20.4	35	583
C6–7	M	27	2100	51	3000	71	12.6	28	450	22.6	36	628
C5–6	M	20	3400	71	3900	82	22.4	28	800	35.9	35	1026
C7–8	M	32	2900	63	4200	92	40.4	50	808	62.6	62	1009
C4–5	M	26	2350	53	3000	70	21.0	29	724	32.3	30	1077
C5–6	F	33	2000	59	2800	82	11.6	20	580	16.4	25	656
C6–7	M	19	3200	74	4200	97	23.4	32	731	42.8	51	839

[a] VC1 and 2 denote vital capacity before and after the program, and Max VE 1 and 2 the volume of expired air before and after the program.

SOURCE: Walker J, Croney M: Improved respiratory function in quadriplegics after pulmonary therapy and arm ergometry. *N Engl J Med* 1987; 316:486; (letter), with permission.

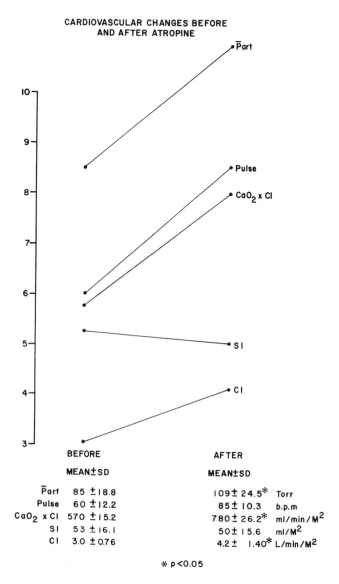

CARDIOVASCULAR CHANGES BEFORE
AND AFTER ATROPINE

	BEFORE MEAN±SD	AFTER MEAN±SD	
$\bar{P}$art	85 ±18.8	109± 24.5*	Torr
Pulse	60 ±12.2	85± 10.3	b.p.m
CaO_2 x CI	570 ±15.2	780± 26.2*	ml/min/M^2
SI	53 ±16.1	50± 15.6	ml/M^2
CI	3.0 ±0.76	4.2± 1.40*	L/min/M^2

* $p < 0.05$

Figure 33-14 Pulse, mean blood pressure (Part), cardiac (CI) and stroke (SI) indices and oxygen delivery (CaO_2 × CI) before and after atropine IV. (Reproduced by permission from Mackenzie and Ducker.[37])

head down on a stretcher or a flat wide surface. The use of Trendelenburg or head-down tilt is controversial[372] because it may have adverse effects on ventilation/perfusion relationships in the lung[373] and is reported to have no significant beneficial hemodynamic effects in the normal[374] or shocked patient.[375] Respiratory and cardiac function in spontaneously breathing quadriplegic patients differs from that in normal subjects. Ventilation/perfusion relationships and arterial oxygenation are more favorable in the supine than upright position.[376] In addition, quadriplegic patients are reported to have maximum vital capacity in the 20° head-down position.[377] Detrimental respiratory and cardiac effects have not been demonstrated in tilting hypovo-

lemic quadriplegic patients head down, but favorable respiratory effects are documented. The legs should not be elevated independently for fear of displacing lower spinal column fractures.

Military antishock trousers (MAST) are an alternative to fluid infusion at the scene or during transportation, because they have the advantage, as does placing the patient in the head-down position, of easy reversibility (deflating the trousers or placing the patient flat) should pulmonary edema occur. MAST may be used in conjunction with IV fluid administration for management of the quadriplegic patient with associated injuries and suspected hemorrhage.

CARDIAC MANAGEMENT DURING ANESTHESIA AND SURGERY

Cervical cord transection results in loss of the thoracolumbar outflow and sympathetic nervous system control over the heart and peripheral circulation; therefore, assessment of cardiac function is important in the acute phase of spinal shock. The hazards of surgery and anesthesia during spinal shock may be great unless the patient is adequately monitored to prevent decompensation. In the face of deficiencies in circulating volume, the quadriplegic patient is unable to maintain cardiac filling pressures by sympathetically induced constriction of the venous capacitance vessels, nor can blood pressure be maintained by arteriolar constriction. In the presence of overtransfusion, the normally innervated heart will respond with tachycardia and sympathetically induced increased contractility. The heart of the quadriplegic patient, however, is less able to deal with such an increase in venous return and acute pulmonary edema may develop. This is a well reported and common cause of death during the early course of acute quadriplegia. Wolman[378] performed autopsies on 44 patients with cervical spine injury. Thirty of the 44 died within 11 days of the onset of quadriplegia and 20 had severe pulmonary edema. Interruption of sympathetic innervation or respiratory failure was thought to be the possible mechanisms, although neurogenic and humoral influences on the pulmonary capillary were not excluded. Meyer and coworkers[379] reported that overreplacement of intravascular volume led to the sudden development of pulmonary edema in 4 of 9 quadriplegic patients.

The pulmonary artery catheter is important in monitoring the acutely quadriplegic patient. It may be used to assess reserve cardiac function and to optimize cardiac output and tissue perfusion, which may result in important long-term effects on recovery of neurologic function. Cardiac filling pressure trends and ventricular function curves are used as a guide to reserve cardiac function and the need for vasoactive drugs.[371] The

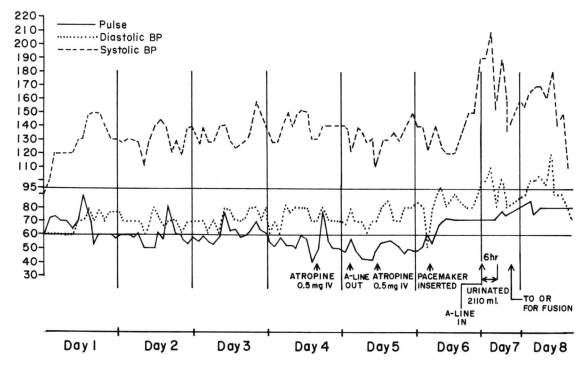

Figure 33-15 The pulse, systolic and diastolic blood pressure (BP) of a quadriplegic patient with a C5 to C6 spinal cord injury are shown from the time of admission (day 1) and including day 7 when spinal cord fusion occurred. Persistent bradycardia in the low 40 beats per minute responded to intravenous atropine on days 4 and 5. A transvenous pacemaker was inserted on day 6 before surgery. The increased heart rate to 70 beats per minute with pacing caused an increase in BP and resulted in marked increase in urinary flow (2110 ml in 6 h on day 7) suggesting improved perfusion of the kidneys. The pacing rate was changed and cardiac output measured intraoperatively, before establishing an optimal rate of 80 beats per minute on day 8.

change in cardiac contractility in response to a change in cardiac filling pressure enables the slope of an individual patient's ventricular function curve to be determined. Cardiac output and filling pressures are measured before and after central IV infusion of fluids at a rate of 50 ml/min in 250-ml increments until cardiac filling pressures rise and remain elevated at least 2 mmHg above baseline level before the fluid challenge. The Frank-Starling curve obtained may be used to objectively assess the need for fluid infusion, fluid restriction, or inotropic agents. The optimal value of filling pressure is the pulmonary capillary wedge pressure (PCWP) at the plateau value for left ventricular stroke work (Fig. 33-16). This method of fluid infusion is used to replace fluid loss during surgery or in the intensive care unit when a fluid deficit is known to exist.

There are four possible outcomes of the fluid challenge given at a rate of 50 ml/min (Fig. 33-17). The first is that cardiac filling pressure rises and continues to rise 5 min after infusion ceases. This indicates that the heart is unable to increase contractility in response to increased filling pressures and that it has limited

reserve function. In terms of the Starling function curve, this patient has been pushed onto the downward slope of the curve and cardiac failure has resulted. The treatment is to limit further fluid infusion, reduce myocardial depressants (such as the inhaled anesthetic agents), and, if this does not reverse the trend, consider giving continually acting inotropic agents such as isoproterenol or dopamine in low dosages.

The second possible outcome is that PCWP rises 3 to 4 mmHg above baseline but falls within 5 min to a level of 2 mmHg above the starting point. This response is interpreted as indicating that myocardial contractility is adequate for the prevailing vascular tone and increase in cardiac preload. The patient is, therefore, approaching the highest point on the Starling function curve, and any further increase in filling pressures will precipitate the situation found in the first outcome. The treatment is to increase fluids and maintain cardiac filling pressures within this range for optimum cardiac function and tissue oxygen supply.

The third possible outcome is that cardiac filling pressures do not change or rise immediately but then

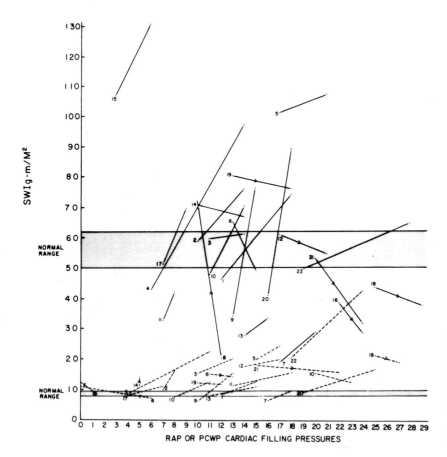

Figure 33-16 Left ventricular stroke work index (LVSWI) and right ventricular stroke work index (RVSWI) (g m/m²) before and after fluid challenge elevated pulmonary capillary wedge pressure (PCWP) by 2 mmHg. LVSWI is plotted against PCWP and RVSWI is plotted against right atrial pressure. Individual patient curves are represented by number. RVSWI is shown as a dashed line, LVSWI a continuous line. Arrows on the lines represent direction with fluid challenge. The dotted line represents RVSWI and solid lines values of LVSWI. Optimal left atrial filling pressure is defined as the PCWP at the plateau value for LVSWI; that is, patients #3, 5, and 13 are at optimal left atrial filling pressures, whereas patients #6, 12, 14, 16, 18, 19 and 21 show poor cardiac reserve (outcome #1 in Fig. 33-18) and impaired left ventricular function characteristic of acute quadriplegia. (Reproduced by permission from Mackenzie and coworkers.[371])

fall to the same baseline within 5 min of ceasing fluid infusion. This response indicates that the patient has considerable reserve cardiac function and that a greater circulating volume may be tolerated. Therefore, if this patient is hypotensive, oliguric, or has a low mixed venous oxygen partial pressure indicating inadequate tissue oxygen delivery, cardiac output should be increased by fluid infusion until the response seen in the second outcome is achieved. Inotropic agents, vasoconstrictors, and diuretics are not indicated and should be avoided. Rather, the inadequate tissue perfusion, hypotension, and oliguria should be reversed by increasing cardiac output with the infusion. The fourth outcome from fluid challenge is uncommonly seen and results in an initial lack of change in cardiac filling pressures but an increase in systemic arterial pressure and a fall in pulse rate. After infusion of 500 ml or more, cardiac filling pressures fall 2 to 3 mmHg below baseline and on measuring cardiac output this is found to be increased. The Starling function curve shifts to the left either as a result of systemic vasodilation due to rapid infusion of fluids or by slowing of heart rate with resulting improvement in myocardial perfusion and contractility. Further therapeutic intervention is usually not required because the increased cardiac output improves oxygen delivery and tissue perfusion.

The fluid challenge is diagnostic and therapeutic. By challenging the patient until cardiac filling pressures remain elevated, optimum circulating volume is achieved for the prevailing level of cardiac function and peripheral vascular tone. The PCWP should be elevated up to 18 mmHg in attempts to reverse hypo-

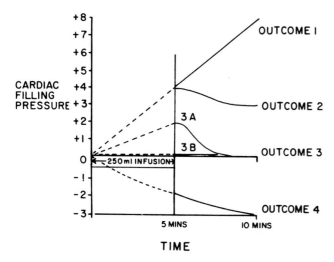

Figure 33-17 Outcome possibilities in response to fluid challenge. (Reproduced by permission from Mackenzie and coworkers.[371])

tension, oliguria, or low mixed venous oxygen tension before the addition of centrally acting inotropic agents.

Using the fluid challenge technique, cardiac function was assessed in 22 consecutively admitted quadriplegics[371] during operations for spine stabilization. All were monitored with indwelling arterial and pulmonary artery catheters and mechanically ventilated with the Engstrom 300 ventilator. The patients were quadriplegic as a result of trauma sustained an average of 4.8 days earlier. Sixteen patients had neurologically complete lesions, 4 had central cord injuries, and 2 had incomplete cervical lesions. Halothane was used as the anesthetic for 15 patients, droperidol/fentanyl for the others. Fluid challenge was given, using the technique described above, until PCWP was raised at least 2 mmHg above the baseline reading. The results demonstrated no difference between cardiopulmonary response to fluid challenge in those patients receiving halothane compared to droperidol/fentanyl and there were no differences between patients with complete or incomplete neurologic lesions. An average volume infusion of 520 ml (range 250 to 1500 ml) of plasma protein solution given in 12 min elevated PCWP from 13 to 17 mmHg. The Starling function curves for right and left heart function are shown in Fig. 33-16.

Following fluid challenge in the 22 patients studied, heart rate was unchanged. This suggests that the increased cardiac output obtained by fluid infusion was produced by a direct Starling response to increased myocardial fiber length. Right ventricular stroke work index (RVSWI) rose significantly ($p < .005$) from (mean $\pm$ standard deviation) 12 ± 4.9 before fluid challenge to 16 ± 7.0 g-m/m^2 after challenge and in all patients RVSWI was higher than or within the normal range ($8.8 \pm .5$ g-m/m^2) after fluid infusion. Left ventricular stroke work index (LVSWI), which rose from 52 ± 22.7 before to 65 ± 26.4 g-m/m^2 ($p < .03$) after fluid challenge, was still lower than normal (56 ± 6 g-m/m^2) in 6 of 22 patients (27 percent) despite fluid challenge. Cardiac index (normal = 3.2 ± 0.2 liter/min per meter squared) increased from 3.5 ± 1.16 to 4.2 ± 1.68 liter/min per meter squared ($p < .005$). The increased cardiac index was accompanied by a significant decrease in pulmonary vascular resistance.

There is a lower than normal systemic vascular resistance as a result of the loss of peripheral vascular tone found in acute quadriplegia. This is important because the low afterload reduces left ventricular work and may account for the normal cardiac index despite loss of sympathetic drive. Reversal of this favorable afterload reduction will decrease the already impaired function of the left heart. The use of peripheral vasoconstrictors is still advocated by some clinicians to "compensate" for the low systemic vascular resistance.[380] Vasoconstrictors that act peripherally with α-agonist activity, however, should not be used to "normalize" a low blood pressure for the patient in spinal shock because they increase afterload and cardiac work and reverse the favorable cardiac effects of low systemic vascular resistance. Respiratory function was unchanged despite average volume infusion of 520 ml, suggesting that rapid fluid infusion is well tolerated in spinal shock provided cardiac function is closely monitored. Fluid restriction and vasopressors should be avoided and emphasis placed on fluid replacement to maintain blood pressure, circulatory volume, renal function, and tissue oxygenation.

INOTROPIC AGENTS

Because of sympathetic denervation, myocardial contractility is reduced following SCI.[381] This limits the heart's ability to increase stroke volume and cardiac output. The impairment of cardiac function in quadriplegics can be compensated for by use of positive inotropic agents, which increase cardiac output in two ways. Centrally acting agents directly increase cardiac output, and peripherally acting drugs increase blood pressure and venous vascular tone. Increased venous vascular tone elevates cardiac filling pressures and arterial constriction increases left ventricular afterload. This combination of events may precipitate acute pulmonary edema. Isoproterenol, dobutamine, and dopamine in low dosages are examples of centrally acting inotropic agents; phenylephrine, methoxamine, and mephentermine act peripherally.

Isoproterenol, a β agonist, has positive inotropic and chronotropic actions that may make it the agent of choice in the bradycardic quadriplegic patient. Atropine 0.02 mg/kg had a rapid onset and short duration of action, lasting 10 to 15 min, making its use appropriate when acute changes in cardiac function occur. Ephedrine has positive inotropic and chronotropic actions as well as some peripheral effects. It has a longer duration of action than atropine. Dopamine has less chronotropic effect than isoproterenol and this may be advantageous because, in certain groups of patients such as those with myocardial ischemia or mitral stenosis, tachycardia may severely reduce myocardial perfusion or result in cardiac failure. Dopamine reportedly has advantages over other inotropic agents at low doses (5 μg/kg per min) because it is thought to improve renal perfusion selectively.[382]

Hypotension severe enough to cause reduced tissue perfusion (poor urinary output, reduction in mixed venous oxygen saturation, and lactic acidosis) is caused by decreased cardiac output, not decreases in systemic vascular resistance. The use of α-adrenergic agonists such as phenylephrine and methoxamine should be avoided because they further aggravate the lack of oxygen delivery to the tissues by causing vasoconstriction. Increased systemic vascular resistance results in elevation of left ventricular work and cardiac output may fall because myocardial oxygen supply is compromised. In patients undergoing spinal anesthesia, phenylephrine and methoxamine decrease cardiac output by increasing left ventricular afterload.[383,384] In the quadriplegic patient, left ventricular function is impaired (see Fig. 33-16).[371]

The favorable effects of reduction in ventricular afterload as a result of systemic vasodilatation following sympathectomy are reversed by the use of peripheral vasoconstrictors. In our opinion, α-adrenergic agents should be avoided completely and, in hypotensive quadriplegic patients, circulating volume should first be optimized by fluid challenge. If the patient remains hypotensive and oliguric and has a low mixed venous oxygen saturation following fluid administration and elevation of cardiac filling pressures to 18 mmHg, inotropic agents, not vasoconstrictors, are indicated. The object of fluid administration and inotropic support is to obtain mean arterial blood pressures of 80 to 90 mmHg in the recently admitted, previously normal adult SCI patient. Hypotension may have direct adverse effects on spinal cord perfusion.[95,101,381] Therefore, treatment of low blood pressure and inadequate spinal cord perfusion on admission is of extreme importance and may determine neurologic recovery.

The quadriplegic patient shows considerable fluctuation in blood pressure following SCI (see Fig. 33-15). Intervention with inotropic agents should occur only after fluid challenge and then should be related to specific guidelines. If reduced creatinine clearance (< 50 ml/min), decreased mixed venous oxygen saturation ($< 70\%$), lactic acidosis, or deterioration in the level of consciousness are resistant to fluid administration, there is inadequate tissue perfusion and a low cardiac output; inotropic support may be beneficial.

ATROPINE

The effect of atropine was studied in 10 acutely quadriplegic patients in spinal shock.[370] All had complete neurologic deficits at levels C4 to C8 and were mechanically ventilated. Sufficient IV atropine was given to raise pulse rate at least 5 beats per minute (0.5 to 1.5 mg). After arterial and pulmonary artery catheter insertion, cardiac index, intravascular pressures, and intrapulmonary shunt were measured before and within 5 min of the rise in pulse rate (see Fig. 33-14). Cardiac index rose significantly ($p < .05$) from 3.0 to 4.2 liters/min per meter squared. Pulmonary artery pressure and PCWP were unchanged after atropine, as were stroke index and systemic vascular resis-

tance. Pulmonary vascular resistance fell from 95 to 71 dynes/sec per cm[5], although this was not significant. Mean arterial pressure, however, rose significantly from 85 to 109 mmHg following atropine. Oxygen delivery (the product of arterial oxygen content and cardiac index) increased significantly from 570 to 780 ml/min per squared meter. The simplest explanation for these changes in the face of unchanged cardiac filling pressures, systemic vascular resistance and stroke volume is that this was a pure chronotropic effect—the increased heart rate causing increased cardiac output. These results in acutely quadriplegic patients are supported by the finding that atropine has no effect on peripheral vascular resistance or myocardial contractility when given to patients during high spinal anesthesia.[385] A large dose of IV atropine (0.04 mg/kg) was found to be an effective means of elevating blood pressure by investigators of the effects of spinal anesthesia[386,387] although there are reports that atropine is ineffective if physiologic doses (0.4 to 0.6 mg) are given.[79,388]

Intravenous atropine is indicated in quadriplegic patients who are bradycardic, acutely hypotensive, and in cardiac failure with pulmonary edema because atropine reverses hypotension and elevates cardiac output and tissue oxygen delivery. In the bradycardic quadriplegic patient atropine may be effective in reversing cardiac failure and may allow time for more definitive treatment by infusions of centrally acting inotropic agents[370] or insertion of a pacemaker. Atropine should be used with caution in patients with myocardial ischemia or valvular lesions where tachycardia may precipitate cardiac failure or severely compromise myocardial perfusion.

Current State of the Art Management

The diagnosis and acute management of SCI can be divided into six separate phases: (1) initial assessment and immobilization, (2) resuscitation and medical management, (3) radiologic diagnostics, (4) anesthesia management, (5) surgical therapy, and (6) postoperative critical care management.

INITIAL ASSESSMENT AND IMMOBILIZATION

The first care phase begins in the field. A patient with a possible SCI is identified using a high index of suspicion, an initial field screening, and a neurologic examination for motor and sensory deficits in all extremities. A protocol for splinting and immobilizing the spine is followed; the patient is placed on a backboard with the head and neck immobilized in a neutral position with a cervical collar and tape. A spine board can be slipped behind the victim in a car seat prior to extraction. The major goal is to reduce the risk of neurologic deterioration from repeated mechanical insults to the spinal cord; flexion of the neck offers the greatest potential for additional damage. A cervical collar is routinely used on patients with serious head injuries because as many as 4 percent of these victims will have an unsuspected cervical spine fracture. Failure to recognize this may have devastating consequences for the patient.

Maintenance of an airway and adequate ventilation during assessment and transport must supersede total neck immobilization. Jaw thrust and slight head extension can improve oxygenation while occipital-C1 movement should not provoke damage to lower cervical areas (C3 through C7).[389] Reluctance to move the neck of a potential SCI patient with respiratory embarrassment may result in inadequate ventilation and eventual respiratory arrest. In response to this apparent dilemma, many emergency medical service protocols include field or immediate emergency room tracheal intubation of a patient with identified airway compromise. When the patient requires intubation, in-line manual stabilization facilitates placement of the endotracheal tube without compromising the spinal cord.

Bony alignment of the spinal column is reestablished by alleviating direct mechanical compressive forces on the spinal cord or roots. This goal is accomplished with Gardner-Wells cervical traction or Halo vest immobilization. By relieving the pathologically increased tissue pressure within hours of injury, along with the treatment of neurogenic shock, tissue perfusion is enhanced at the site of spinal cord damage and may improve neurologic outcome.

Patients with acute SCIs should proceed directly to an SCI center, not just the nearest hospital. Regional SCI centers are described later in this chapter. The receiving center should be equipped for SCI patients and include skull tongs (e.g., Gardner-Wells) and Halo rings that can be attached to a vest and cast (skeletal fixation permits immediate reduction). A frame to hold the patient (e.g., Stryker Manufacturing Co., Kalamazoo, Michigan) must also be available. A circle electric bed in the acute setting is contraindicated because of the cardiovascular instability. After skeletal traction, serial radiographs or image intensification radiologic equipment are essential to ensure appropriate realignment of the damaged spine.

RESUSCITATION AND MEDICAL MANAGEMENT

The second care phase involves the medical support necessary to reverse the physiologic changes that occur

as a consequence of a cervical SCI. A severe cervical SCI physiologically interrupts the outflow of the entire sympathetic nervous system as it passes through the cervical spinal cord before it exits in the thoracic region. This interruption causes loss of vascular tone and of the body's inability to maintain normal blood pressure. Patients in neurogenic shock typically present with hypotension and bradycardia, a state differing from that of hypovolemic hypotension associated with blood loss from other injuries because of the absence of tachycardia. The hypotension associated with the neurogenic shock of SCI usually can be reversed with fluids (see below) and small doses of dopamine (3 to 5 g/kg per min), which can be adjusted to maintain a mean blood pressure of 80 to 90 mmHg in a previously normal, young healthy individual. Cardiopulmonary-vascular management details have been covered in a previous section.

INITIAL MEDICAL MANAGEMENT

Although treatment priorities for the multitrauma patient mandate management of life-threatening injuries as the first priority, the displaced spinal column can often be reduced rapidly with cervical traction and stabilized while any required multisystem diagnostic studies take place. The initial management goals are to preserve the neurologic function present on arrival and to reverse the presenting neurologic deficits. All patients, despite the severity of the initial injuries, are presumed to have incomplete SCIs with a potential for recovery until serial neurologic examinations conducted after 72 h document irrecoverable motor or sensory loss.

These goals also include maintaining arterial blood gases and vital signs in the normal range. A patient presenting clinically with a C5 quadriplegia requires close respiratory status monitoring (tidal volume, vital capacity, and negative inspiratory force). Such a patient often has adequate spontaneous breathing immediately after the injury but will then tire or may undergo a change in neurologic level within 4 to 12 h, requiring intubation and mechanical ventilatory assistance. Serial monitoring of respiratory parameters provides early identification of these impending problems for appropriate intervention before a major respiratory crisis occurs (Table 33-6).

Patients with cervical SCI are managed initially by a traumatology/anesthesiology team, which performs the initial resuscitation, immediate interventions, and multitrauma evaluation. Medical management includes a lateral cervical spine radiograph with at least one view showing inferior to C7.[390] After the diagnosis of a cervical fracture or SCI, the patient is maintained in cervical traction during the entire admission phase,

TABLE 33-6
Indication for Intubation and Mechanical Ventilation in Acute Quadriplegia

Intubation Criteria	Value Indicating Need for Intubation
Maximum expiratory force	$< +20$ cmH$_2$O
Maximum inspiratory force	< -20 cmH$_2$O
Vital capacity	< 15 ml/fkg or < 1000 ml
Pa$_{O_2}$/Fi$_{O_2}$	< 250
Chest x-ray	Atelectasis or infiltrate

SOURCE: Mackenzie and Ducker,[37] with permission.

including all radiologic studies. Concurrently, consultations from the neurosurgery, orthopedic, and critical care teams are obtained. If a cervical fracture/dislocation or SCI is identified, a complete radiologic investigation of the entire spinal column is performed in addition to the lateral cervical spinal x-ray.

Two large-bore IV catheters, a Foley catheter, and a nasal gastric tube are inserted in each SCI patient. A pulmonary artery catheter is also inserted in an SCI patient with neurologic deficit who requires surgery and anesthesia. A baseline laboratory work-up is conducted including a complete blood count, electrolytes, amylase, coagulation profile, blood type and cross match, urinalysis, arterial blood gas, and electrocardiogram.

In addition to diagnosing the SCI, an initial diagnostic work-up of a patient with multitrauma will aid in identifying other life-threatening injuries. Such injuries involve the brain, chest, and abdomen and are often occult.[391] In addition to a physical examination, a lateral C-spine, chest, and pelvis roentgenograms are obtained. A head CT scan and a diagnostic peritoneal lavage or CT scan of the abdomen complete the initial diagnostic assessment.[390,392] Typically, patients with cervical SCI resulting from industrial accidents or MVAs incur multisystem injuries, whereas victims of diving injuries do not.[390] If a cervical fracture/dislocation is identified and is potentially reducible with traction, Gardner-Wells or Halo traction is applied and rapid bony reduction or realignment with progressively increasing weights under radiographic control is performed. After obtaining optimal closed reduction of the cervical fracture/dislocation, as determined by x-ray film, a C1 to C2 iohexol myelogram is performed (Fig. 33-18), followed by a CT myelogram. MRI or cervical tomograms can image the injury and may be used instead of the CT myelogram. The initial reduction is performed on a Stryker frame. The patient undergoes CT scanning on a board (OSI Transport Board, Orthopedic Systems, Inc. [OSI], Union City, CA) capable of maintaining cervical alignment and traction during transport and the scan, thus minimizing the likeli-

hood of additional mechanical damage to the spinal cord. Bone and soft tissue compressing the spinal cord or roots, as determined by the CT myelogram, are surgically removed on an emergent basis, at which time internal stabilization and fusion are also performed.

SECONDARY INTERVENTIONS

Patients without mechanical compression of nervous tissue on the CT myelogram are maintained with external stabilization until internal stabilization (Fig. 33-19) is performed or definitive external stabilization (Halo vest or Yale brace) is applied; these secondary interventions typically occur 1 to 2 days after injury unless other injuries preclude cervical surgery. Rapid stabilization allows safe, early mobilization and decreases medical complications secondary to immobilization.

During the first 72 h following an SCI, the patient's mean arterial blood pressure is maintained between 80 and 90 mmHg with optimization of circulating volume and the cardiac output maintained in a normal to high-normal (1.5 times the normal output) range.[40] Inotropic support with dopamine or dobutamine may be necessary after fluid infusion to attain these physiologic

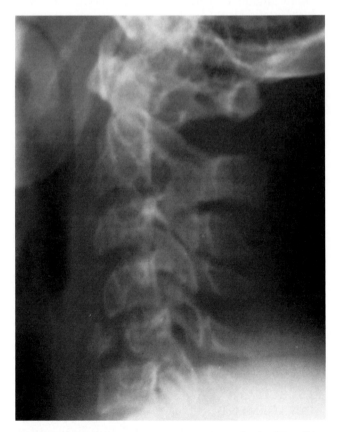

Figure 33-18 Initial emergency room radiograph of a C5 to C6 fracture/dislocation with the post inferior C5 body fragment in the spinal canal causing continued spinal canal compression.

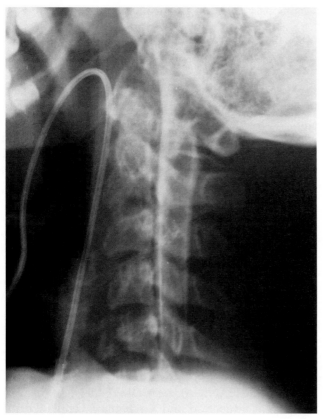 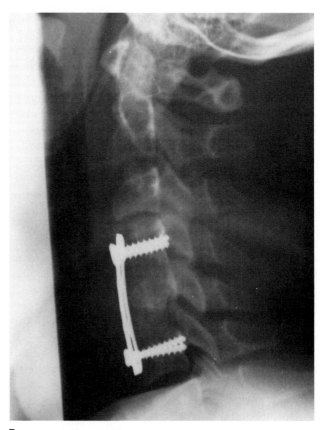

A   B

Figure 33-19 *A*. A mini myelogram in the prone position after tong traction reduction of the C5 body fragments. Note relatively good alignment of the C5 body compared to the prereduction radiograph in Fig. 33-18A. *B*. CT myelogram of C4 to C6 internal stabilization with anterior plate screw construct and autograft in C5 region anteriorly. Note anatomic alignment of C4 to C6 area.

goals. The hyperdynamic cardiac output enhances spinal cord perfusion during the neurogenic shock state, which begins at the time of injury. The augmented cardiovascular parameters are carefully monitored and maintained throughout induction of anesthesia or during surgery in patients requiring early spinal decompression or emergency surgery. The patient receives MPSS in a 30 mg/kg bolus followed by 5.4 mg/kg per h for 23 h.[33,35,227]

RADIOLOGIC DIAGNOSTICS

The third care phase involves detailed, diagnostic radiologic procedures to define the bony damage and to verify decompression of the spinal cord and nerve roots. Patients undergo an MRI or a cervical myelogram via a C1 to C2 puncture with a water-soluble contrast agent, followed by a high-resolution CT scan including sagittal reconstruction. The initial radiologic evaluation is occasionally supplemented with MRI. The CT myelogram provides superb bony detail of the fracture site and the anatomic relation of fractured or dislocated fragments to the spinal cord, whereas the

MRI provides better images of anterior disks, posterior ligamentum flava, or spinal cord contusion.[45]

The bony injuries may be classified into flexion, flexion compression, compression, extension, and the rare distraction injury. All require different positioning and weight traction. The neurologic deficit may be less if reduction is achieved rapidly. Few patients will not realign and in these operative reduction is required to achieve canal restoration.

ANESTHESIA MANAGEMENT

PREOPERATIVE CONSIDERATIONS

During spinal shock, which lasts from 3 days to 6 weeks following the onset of quadriplegia,[393] anesthesia may be especially hazardous because of impaired cardiac and respiratory function. The adequacy of ventilation should be assessed preoperatively by arterial blood gas measurement and pulmonary function testing. If the patient has evidence of hypoxemia (on mask oxygen) or hypercarbia, tracheal intubation may be indicated preoperatively. Many quadriplegic patients, when seen preoperatively, will already be in a critical care unit because of respiratory difficulties and may be mechanically ventilated and have a tracheostomy. All quadriplegic patients, whether they are in respiratory failure or not, should have respiratory function assessed preoperatively (see below). These simple measurements act as a baseline and can easily be monitored postoperatively and used as an indicator of progress toward weaning from mechanical ventilation.

An ECG should be taken because myocardial ischemia may be present in the elderly quadriplegic or even in the younger population who may have suffered hypoxemia from, for example, near drowning following a diving accident. In quadriplegic patients who have shown cardiovascular instability, evidenced by hypotension, hypertension, bradycardia, or arrhythmias, it is advisable to make an assessment of reserve cardiac function preoperatively and to optimize circulating volume. In persistently bradycardic patients, a pacemaker may be useful in increasing cardiac output and improving cardiac reserve without use of infused inotropic agents (see Fig. 33-15).

Pulmonary artery and radial artery catheterization is advisable for monitoring of all quadriplegic patients undergoing general anesthesia during the spinal shock period. Circulating volume can be optimized for each patient, the volume given depending on cardiac function and peripheral vascular tone. During elevation of cardiac filling pressures by infusion through the right atrial line in these mechanically ventilated patients, pulmonary artery pressure and ventilator end-inspiratory pressure (lung/thorax compliance) should be continuously monitored. Acute elevation of either parameter is considered to be indicative of development of cardiac failure and pulmonary edema, and fluid infusion is terminated. Fluids can be administered appropriately when cardiac function is monitored with a pulmonary artery or central venous catheter. The central venous pressure that provides optimum cardiac function can be determined when the patient has a pulmonary artery catheter in position and this can be used as a baseline for volume loading should oliguria or other evidence of impaired tissue perfusion occur postoperatively, after removal of the pulmonary artery catheter. Unless sepsis or hypoxemia occurs, it is unusual to require pulmonary artery catheterization outside the perioperative period.

The patient should be informed preoperatively of the procedure to be undertaken and should have a chance to ask questions. This is difficult in an intubated and mechanically ventilated patient. Sign language and phrasing of standard questions asked by other patients preoperatively may help. If the patient has a tracheostomy, a speaking attachment allows phonation. If the patient is very apprehensive, premedications such as midazolam may be indicated. In the spon-

taneously breathing quadriplegic patient it is advisable to give premedicant drugs only when their effects can be closely monitored. Respiratory and cardiac depression resulting from opiates and sedatives prescribed as premedicants may prove fatal unless the impairment is recognized by someone able to take appropriate supportive action. This usually means that premedicant drugs are avoided in spontaneously breathing quadriplegics until the patient reaches the operating room, where IV midazolam may be given and its effects observed by the anesthesiologist. Atropine should be given as a premedicant especially if the patient has a pulse rate less than 70 beats per minute because the myocardial depressant effects of anesthetic agents may be reversed by atropine. Doses reportedly as high as 0.04 mg/kg IV may be required to elevate the pulse rate,[386,387] although we have found 0.02 mg/kg to be satisfactory.[370] The operative procedure and patient positioning should be discussed and planned with the surgeon preoperatively and baseline values of pulse, intravascular pressures, and ECG obtained before induction of anesthesia.

INDICATIONS FOR TRACHEAL INTUBATION AND MECHANICAL VENTILATION

Tracheal intubation and mechanical ventilation may be necessary because cervical spine neurologic deficits result in inadequate alveolar ventilation causing carbon dioxide retention. In addition, because respiratory function is subnormal and there is loss of the ability to cough effectively, there is incomplete clearance of secretions from the lungs and the potential for respiratory complications is greatly increased. Oxygenation may, therefore, be compromised. To assess the need for tracheal intubation and mechanical ventilation, simple respiratory function tests may be measured and values established to determine when intubation is required. Guidelines that may be used as indications for intubation in the acutely quadriplegic patient are given in Table 33-6.

Arterial oxygen should be greater than 60 mmHg on room air, and oxygen should be given to maintain Pa_{O_2} around 100 mmHg. A chest x-ray should show no signs of atelectasis or infiltrate. Intrapulmonary shunt may be assessed by determining the PaO_2/ fraction inspired oxygen (FiO_2) ratio. If this value is less than 250 (equivalent to about 15 percent shunt) and Pa_{CO_2} rises above 45 mmHg, tracheal intubation should be performed and mechanical ventilation instituted. Atelectasis appearing on chest x-ray within 12 h of cord transection usually means the patient will require mechanical ventilation. Poor respiratory function as outlined in Table 33-6 usually means that within 12 to 24 h the patient will require mechanical ventilation. These criteria may be used as predictors of this trend rather than waiting for respiratory distress to occur.

TECHNIQUES FOR TRACHEAL INTUBATION

Controversy exists concerning the techniques that should be used to intubate the trachea in a patient with cervical spine injury. The cervical spine will usually be stabilized with sandbags or a soft or hard collar or the patient may be in neck traction with tongs or a Halo ring. The techniques used to intubate the trachea in patients with cervical spine injury depend on the general condition of the patient, the neurologic deficit, and on how recently the spine injury occurred. There is no single acceptable technique of tracheal intubation for all patients with cervical spine injuries.

Weiss[80] advocates nasotracheal intubation for cervical cord-injured patients. Rocco and Vandam[394] maintained the head in the neutral position and intubated the trachea under topical anesthesia with a Thomas collar still in place. Sokoll[395] differentiates beween those patients having complete spinal cord transection with fractures of the vertebral body or lamina in whom modest extension is permissible to facilitate tracheal intubation, and patients with fractures of the odontoid process in whom extension of the neck may be fatal. For odontoid fractures, Sokoll suggests nasotracheal intubation with sedation and topical anesthesia. In patients with a cervical fracture but intact or only partially compromised neurologic function, Sokoll advocates topical anesthesia of the nose, pharynx, larynx, and upper trachea and sedation before blind nasal or fiberoptic laryngoscope-assisted intubation of the trachea. Pitts[380] generally concurs with the assessment of intubation techniques advocated by Sokoll, stressing the important fact that most unstable cervical spine injuries become worse with neck flexion and are generally improved with gentle axial traction or neck extension. In the nonemergency "elective intubation," it appears that nasal intubation under topical anesthesia performed with the patient awake is the technique of choice. Neurologic function may then be assessed before and after the tracheal tube is secured in place and the patient appropriately positioned for induction of general anesthesia or other elective intervention.

The spinal cord-injured patient who is in acute respiratory distress or shock, or who has suffered other injuries, should not undergo heavy sedation and prolonged efforts to provide adequate topical anesthesia for awake intubation. In our experience, when attempts are made to perform awake intubation in the shocked, recently admitted, cervical spine-injured patient who may also be under the influence of alcohol and have a full stomach, neck movement is increased and incomplete anesthesia results in a high frequency of vomiting and aspiration. Topical anesthesia has been abandoned

TABLE 33-7
Bullard Laryngoscopy: Neck Extension Compared to Conventional Blades and Time for Intubation Compared to Flexible Fiberoptic Bronchoscopy

Laryngoscope Blade	Head Extension
Bullard	2°
Macintosh	10°
Miller	11°
Time for Intubation (s)	
Bullard	46.1 ± 10.98 (SD) sec ($p < .01$)
Fiberoptic	99.3 ± 48.32 sec

SOURCE: From Hastings et al. *Anesthesiology* 1995; 82:859–869, with permission, and from Cohn A, Zornow MH: *Anesth Analg* 1995; 81:1283–6, with permission.

for the initial intubation in such patients. Rather, following preoxygenation and application of cricoid pressure,[396] intubation is performed using succinylcholine after administration of a sleep dose of barbiturate. If difficulty is encountered in intubation because of weighted traction, a second person, preferably a neurosurgeon, assists by reducing the traction weight until the trachea can be intubated. In our hands, this technique has been used successfully for many years without producing any alterations in neurologic function. In the patient without traction, the front half of the collar is removed to allow application of cricoid pressure and a second person holds the head in the neutral position and applies in-line neck stabilization. These techniques are not recommended for novice laryngoscopists. Someone experienced in tracheal intubation should perform the laryngoscopy. Similarly, operators of fiberoptic laryngoscopes are advised not to use the apparatus on cervical spine-injured patients for the first time. Once mastered, fiberoptic laryngoscopy is now a useful technique that may be used with topical anesthesia for emergency intubation of the trachea in an otherwise stable patient. The Bullard laryngoscope in expert hands can achieve tracheal intubation more rapidly than fiberoptic bronchoscopy with only 2° head extension (Table 33-7). The Bullard laryngoscope or the Upsher modification may be an alternative in some of the above scenarios to avoid removal of cervical traction if the patient can be satisfactorily mask ventilated.

Induction of anesthesia may be unnecessary or contraindicated for the unconscious recently injured patient with spinal cord trauma or those in severe shock with an unrecordable blood pressure. In these circumstances, after preoxygenation and application of cricoid pressure, succinylcholine alone is used to facilitate rapid tracheal intubation with a cuffed tube by the oral route. Nasal intubation is not used in emergencies because, unless there is extensive preintubation use of effective mucosal vasoconstrictors such as cocaine, bleeding is precipitated by passage of a nasal tube. This further complicates visualization of the larynx. An orotracheal tube can be changed to a nasal tube under controlled, ideal circumstances of optimum oxygenation at some future time after the patient is stabilized. Prolonged nasal intubation for the spinal cord-injured patient is not often used in our institution because of the relatively high incidence of purulent sinusitis associated with nasotracheal and nasogastric tubes.[397] Rather, tracheostomy is used as the means of access and protection of the airway once the need for anterior spinal surgery is excluded. If the spine is approached anteriorly in the presence of a tracheostomy there is likely to be contamination of the surgical wound from the colonized airway because the surgical incision is in such close proximity to the tracheostomy stoma.

INDUCTION AND MAINTENANCE OF ANESTHESIA: TECHNIQUES AND PRECAUTIONS

Several reports in the literature have addressed cardiovascular collapse following IV succinylcholine in patients and animals with spinal cord and neural injury.[398–403] Stone and coworkers[400] reported that a C6 spine-injured quadriplegic developed cardiac arrest when succinylcholine was injected IV 46 days after SCI. The patient's serum potassium level was increased from 4.6 to 11.6 mEq/liter within 2 min of succinylcholine administration. The same authors found that, in laboratory animals with transected spinal cords, hyperkalemia after succinylcholine infusion was significant after 14 days and highly significant 28 days following spinal cord transection.[401]

Tobey[403] reported on the effects of continuous infusion of succinylcholine in four paraplegic patients, 44 to 85 days after injury. Serum potassium increased from 7.3 to 13.6 mEq/liter within 2 min of infusion of as little as 20 mg succinylcholine. One patient had a cardiac arrest and was successfully resuscitated. Tobey[403] concluded that succinylcholine should not be used in paraplegics within 24 to 48 h of injury. Tobey and colleagues[402] found that, in 23 patients with peripheral nerve injuries, potassium increased following succinylcholine, but not following gallamine or *d*-tubocurarine. Curare prior to succinylcholine reduced the potassium rise, but did not suppress it.

The mechanism for the sensitivity to acetylcholine or drugs having a cholinergic agonist activity, such as succinylcholine, is probably related to the changes in muscle membrane following denervation. The pharmacologic receptor area of the end plate at the neuromuscular junction is hypertrophied and spreads into the muscle as extra junctional receptors. Sensitivity to depolarizing muscle relaxants such as succinylcholine is developed over a period of several weeks[404] and may be increased 10^4 to 10^5 times normal. In addition to hypertrophy and increased sensitivity of the end plate, there is a decreased reentry permeability to potassium in denervated muscle.[405] These factors appear to account for the dramatic hyperkalemia found clinically. The spread and hypertrophy of cholinergic receptor is first detectable at about 3 to 4 days after injury and reaches its peak 7 to 14 days later.[395,398] The duration of the hypersensitivity to succinylcholine is not well documented. Smith[406] reported cardiac arrest following *d*-tubocurarine pretreatment and succinylcholine given to a quadriplegic patient 6 months after injury. It is generally recommended that succinylcholine be avoided and not be given until at least 8 months after injury. Nowadays, alternatives such as rocuronium give rapid-onset muscular relaxation and may be used to replace succinylcholine in all SCI patients requiring rapid sequence induction of anesthesia with tracheal intubation.

Most anesthesiologists would avoid succinylcholine up to at least 8 months after SCI and then it would only be used with nondepolarizing relaxant pretreatment and when no alternative techniques were available. Besides the uncertainty of duration of this sensitivity, there is also a confusion about the onset. From the literature, it appears clear that the chance of succinylcholine causing hyperkalemia increases from the third postinjury day.[395,398,405,407] It seems appropriate, therefore, to avoid the use of succinylcholine in quadriplegic patients between 3 days and at least 8 months following paralysis.

Induction agents commonly used include thiopental (2.5 to 4.0 mg/kg), propofol (2.0 to 2.5 mg/kg), etomidate (0.3 mg/kg), or ketamine (1 to 2 mg/kg). Maintenance agents such as nitrous oxide, halothane, enflurane, isoflurane, or desflurane all appear to be satisfactory and have the advantage over IV agents in that, should hypotension occur, they are rapidly excreted through the lungs after reduction of the inspired concentration. Rapid excretion is proportional to blood/gas solubility (desflurane > isoflurane > enflurane > halothane).

Halothane is reported to be a good agent for controlling the hypertension associated with autonomic hyperreflexia in quadriplegic and paraplegic patients.[408,409] Enflurane and isoflurane may prove to be as effective as halothane for anesthetic management. Circulating volume status and cardiac function should be assessed intraoperatively as described earlier in the chapter. Some individuals may be unduly sensitive to inhalational agents. Reduction of inspired concentration, however, produces a rapid improvement in left

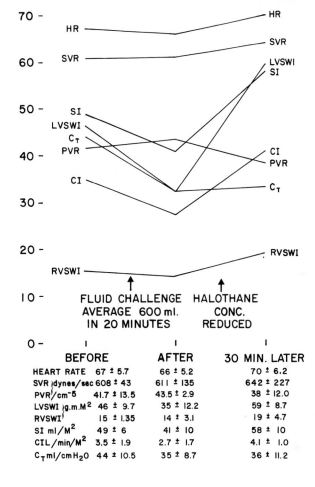

MEAN CHANGE IN CARDIORESPIRATORY PARAMETERS OF 3 QUADRIPLEGIC PATIENTS FOLLOWING FLUID CHALLENGE AND SUBSEQUENT REDUCTION IN HALOTHANE CONCENTRATION

	BEFORE	AFTER	30 MIN. LATER
HEART RATE	67 ± 5.7	66 ± 5.2	70 ± 6.2
SVR (dynes/sec)	608 ± 43	611 ± 135	642 ± 227
PVR/cm^{-5}	41.7 ± 13.5	43.5 ± 2.9	38 ± 12.0
LVSWI g.m.M^2	46 ± 9.7	35 ± 12.2	59 ± 8.7
RVSWI	15 ± 1.35	14 ± 3.1	19 ± 4.7
SI ml/M^2	49 ± 6	41 ± 10	58 ± 10
CIL/min/M^2	3.5 ± 1.9	2.7 ± 1.7	4.1 ± 1.0
C$_T$ml/cmH$_2$O	44 ± 10.5	35 ± 8.7	36 ± 11.2

Figure 33-20   Change in heart rate, systemic vascular resistance (SVR) and pulmonary vascular resistance (PVR), left (LVSWI) and right (RVSWI) ventricular stroke work indices, cardiac (CI) and stroke (SI) indices, and lung/ thorax compliance (C$_T$) before and after fluid challenge during 0.5% halothane anesthesia and 30 min after reduction of halothane from 0.5 to 25%. (Reproduced by permission from Mackenzie and Ducker.[37])

and right heart function as shown in three patients in Fig. 33-20.

INTRAOPERATIVE MONITORING

Cervical spinal cord-injured patients in the spinal shock phase require specialized monitoring for anesthesia (Table 33-8); an arterial line and pulmonary ar-

TABLE 33-8
Intraoperative Monitoring and Equipment for Management of Acute SCI Patient in Spinal Shock

Electrocardiograph	Urinary catheter
Invasive arterial blood pressure	Airway pressure
Pulmonary artery catheterization	Blood warmer/external warmer
Cardiac output computer	Humidifier
Temperature	Arterial and venous blood gases
End-tidal CO$_2$	Somatosensory evoked potentials
Pulse oximeter	

tery catheter are inserted preoperatively. These enable beat-to-beat determination of intravascular pressures, frequent arterial and mixed venous blood gas analysis, and cardiac output determination. In stable, chronically injured patients, arterial and pulmonary artery catheterization is not normally necessary for elective surgery. ECG, end-tidal carbon dioxide and pulse oximeter monitors, urine output by indwelling catheter, and temperature are monitored during anesthesia.

Somatosensory and cortical evoked potentials provide a noninvasive, objective, sensitive, and reproducible method to assess conduction through a spinal cord injury. Alteration in wave pattern, amplitude, and latency can be used to assess neurologic function. Evoked potentials (EPs) are generated by the nervous system in response to brief stimuli. Somatosensory evoked potentials (SSEPs) are produced by electrical stimulation of a peripheral nerve (i.e., posterior tibial or median nerve) with recording of the electrical potential along the signal pathway. The pathway includes the nerve, posterior columns of the spinal cord, medial lemniscus, thalamus, and somatosensory cortex in the brain. Cortical or motor evoked potentials (CEPs) stimulate the motor cortex either by an electrical or magnetic stimulus and produce potentials through the anterior spinal cord, nerves, and muscles excited by the stimulus.

Evoked potentials are used for diagnosis, monitoring, and prognosis in SCI. Information not obtainable from a clinical neurologic examination can be accumulated using EPs. Patients unable to cooperate with a physical examination due to associated injuries can be evaluated with EPs; the severity and anatomic level of an SCI can be assessed using SSEP. SSEP absence after trauma has a high correlation with complete spinal cord transection. Acquisition of the SSEP below the level of the SCI confirms adequate stimulation and the presence of an interruption of the pathway. Anatomic level localization can be obtained through segmental sensory stimulation. For example, patients with a low cervical SCI with an intact median and absent posterior tibial nerve SSEP will have a lesion level below C6 to C7. Segmental stimulation may indicate sacral sparing in a "complete" SCI despite being unable to elicit posterior tibial nerve SSEP. Incomplete spinal cord lesions may show SSEP fluctuations. Sequential SSEP monitoring detects acute changes in an incomplete lesion that allows for prompt therapeutic intervention to preserve neuronal function. Interventions that may be attempted include increasing blood pressure, ensuring adequate oxygenation, and reevaluating spinal cord integrity. Perot has documented SSEP changes 3 to 6 days after SCI related to spinal cord edema not associated with a change in the patient's clinical status.

General anesthesia prohibits examination of the functional integrity of the spinal cord. The SSEP decreases the necessity for frequent wake-up tests during surgery. Intact posterior column function does not guarantee intact anterior motor spinal cord function. However, the incidence of false-negative SSEP (SSEP remains stable despite immediate postoperative neurologic deficit) is extremely rare. SSEPs do not predict future neurologic outcome but are a monitor of the current status of posterior spinal cord function. SSEP evidence of postoperative improvment may not occur immediately and can be quite delayed; therefore, SSEP should not be a criterion for judging operative success.[410]

In the operating room, if significant SSEP changes occur (i.e., 50 percent decrease of amplitude), the surgeons should be notified and a cause for the changes elicited. At our institution, to differentiate surgical, anesthetic, and technical etiology for EP changes, cortical and subcortical potentials are monitored above and below the lesion. If a technical event occurs, such as a stimulating electrode becoming loosened, all potentials

are affected. Anesthetic events are typically seen in the cortical measurements. An attempt should be made to maintain a constant anesthetic milieu by avoiding bolus drug administration in favor of infusion techniques. A surgical event, such as overdistraction of the spinal cord by instrumentation, affects all potentials above the lesion. Response to therapeutic measures may be documented using SSEP. For example, if the surgeon was manipulating instrumentation, then the distraction should be relaxed, and the EPs reevaluated. If identification and correction of the problem do not correct the SSEP changes, then a wake-up test may be performed (see below).

The use of SSEPs for prognosis in SCI has been inconsistent. Patients with improved SSEPs within 1 week of trauma, associated with a decreasing latency and increasing amplitude, showed a high probability of future clinical improvement. Patients without an elicited SSEP (complete spinal cord transection) obviously have an unfavorable prognosis. The major limitation to the use of SSEP in SCI is due to the anatomic and vascular dissociation between the posterior ascending sensory and anterior descending motor tracts. CEPs are postulated as reliable indicators of neurologic motor function. Stimulation of the anterior spinal cord or motor cortex produces a large initial positive component from direct activation of pyramidal cells followed by three to four waves caused by interneuron activity in the ventral gray matter. Direct stimulation used experimentally has been supplanted by a transcranial technique of electrical or magnetic stimulation. CEP correlates well with histologic damage to the spinal cord and is an accurate measurement of the degree of motor recovery. In clinical practice, where SSEP and CEP have differed, CEP has proven more accurate in predicting motor function. Transection of the spinal cord obviously abolishes CEP.[410]

At present, the clinical use of CEP is limited by the unproven safety of repeated transcortical stimuli. Direct cortical stimulation causes gliosis and neuronal loss adjacent to the stimulation electrode but no major neuronal damage has been ascribed due to the transcranial technique. Investigators have noted hypertension, tachycardia, and visual changes during transcranial stimulation. Clearly, CEP is a better monitor for motor function after an SCI but, at present, monitoring of the anterior spinal cord is not an innocuous reality.

The possibility of motor injury without sensory evoked response alteration means that in some centers wake-up tests are used to evaluate motor neurologic function. However, in cervical spine surgery the head is pinned or immobilized on a head rest so that any movement of the patient during such a test could cause cervical vertebral movement and cord injury. In addition, if the patient is prone there is a potentially disastrous risk of extubation. Apart from those risks, including that of emotional distress for the patient (although they may be amnesic of such tests), the only benefit is a single confirmation that motor function is intact. The wake-up test does not exclude the possibility that subsequent damage from surgical or anesthetic maneuvers occurs after anesthesia is reinduced. As an alternative to the wake-up test, the patient may be intubated awake and positioned for surgery before repeat evaluation to confirm lack of change in neurologic function. Anesthesia is then induced. Again this only provides a single viewpoint to confirm that tracheal intubation and patient positioning did not alter motor function.

The prone position or placing the patient head up or down on a Stryker frame may produce significant changes in cardiorespiratory function, which should be monitored. Because the quadriplegic patient has lost the normal compensatory vasoconstrictor mechanisms to maintain cardiac filling, rapid head elevation greater than 20° during the spinal shock period, especially in an anesthetized patient, may cause a sudden decrease in cardiac filling pressures, a resulting fall in cardiac output, and even cardiac arrest. Because of loss of sympathetic cardiac innervation associated with lesions above the level of T1, the steep head-down position may precipitate acute myocardial failure with pulmonary edema. These movements should be monitored carefully, for example, when a myelogram requires marked changes in posture to determine whether there is spinal cord compression.

SURGICAL THERAPY OF CERVICAL FRACTURES

The fifth phase includes a potential urgent surgical decompression of mechanically compressed neurologic elements. Radiologic studies will identify elements that were not decompressed by the anatomic bony alignment procedure of phase three. The majority of the cases are bilateral locked facets that cannot be reduced with traction. Additional cases of anterior disk dislocation in the spinal canal or bone fragments will be noted. Although most surgeons agree that the deteriorating neurologic status with a mass lesion causing compression requires urgent removal if possible, not all surgeons agree with the timing of surgery in a patient with a stable neurologic deficit.

TIMING OF SURGICAL INTERVENTION

Both the use and timing of surgical intervention in cervical SCI remains controversial because no conclusive scientific evidence has been presented for either aspect. Surgical decompression or internal stabilization occurs in one-half to three-quarters of all patients in

acute hospitalization in North America.[411,412] These incidence studies were both prospective[412] and retrospective.[412] In the United Kingdom and Australia, the nonsurgical treatment of acute SCI using postural reduction and prolonged bed rest are the standard, with surgery reserved only for the most extreme cases.[413–417]

A series of nonrandomized studies have reported that urgent fracture reduction did not improve outcome.[418,419] However, no randomized, prospective study relative to surgical timing has been conducted. NASCIS 2 was a randomized, prospective study that compared two drugs with placebo.[33,35,227] When the investigators post hoc analyzed their data for effects of the timing of surgery, they recommended a trial specifically designed to answer this question because their data could not. Currently, a multicenter randomized prospective study relative to the timing of surgery is being proposed by the neurosurgery community with Dr. Charles Tator as the principal investigator. After receiving funding, results are not expected before 1999.

Persistent compression on the spinal cord after an acute SCI is a potential contributor to the secondary injury mechanism described earlier. The outcome following SCI is determined by many factors including impact force, duration of compression, and physical displacement.[420–425] Laboratory experiments have also demonstrated that the outcome is inversely related to both the force of impact and the time period of compression.[420,421] Multiple clinical accounts of unexpected recoveries following urgent surgical or closed reduction decompression of the spinal cord also exist.[426–429] Although these accounts provide a basis to hypothesize that urgent surgical decompression will aid some individuals, the fraction who will benefit and the extent of the favorable outcome remain unknown.

Some physicians believe deferred surgical treatment is most advantageous for the patient because no benefit from urgent surgery has been demonstrated and because increased complication rates, especially respiratory, have been reported with urgent surgery.[23,417,430–432] The advocates of urgent surgery have not produced data indicating improved outcome, but have reported faster mobilization and transfer to a rehabilitation center.[429,433,434] In the past 10 years, the diagnostic and surgical options have significantly improved with the advent of rapid CT, MRI, intraoperative ultrasound,[39] and internal stabilization, which allow complete decompression of the spinal canal. There is also better understanding and control of systemic blood pressure and cardiac output during neurogenic shock in the acute phase of the injury, allowing the safe use of anesthesia during this period. Hypotension during the induction of anesthesia or during the surgery is deleterious to the injured spinal cord and can even damage a normal spinal cord.[40] Furthermore, the most recent analysis of complications following early surgical intervention actually reported lower rates of complications. This suggests that improvements in clinical management have decreased the complication rate, making urgent surgery a safe clinical choice with the potential to improve outcome.[434]

MECHANICAL STABILIZATION OF THE UNSTABLE CERVICAL FRACTURE

Mechanical stabilization of the spinal column is necessary to obtain vertical stability and prevent reinjury of the spinal cord from repeated movement. The stabilization technique is individualized for each fracture and its expected instability. The techniques include internal stabilization (see Fig. 33-19), external splinting, and prolonged cervical traction.

A patient may deteriorate postoperatively due to direct operative trauma to the spinal cord. Poor technique or poor judgment in choice of instruments may lead to direct injury. Fortunately these occurrences are rare. On the other hand, rarely will these patients show immediate improvement. Consequently, preoperative and postoperative examinations must be performed. If the patient is worse postoperatively or if the patient deteriorates after operation, diagnostic studies must be done to pinpoint the etiology.

Recurrent compression may occur due to bony malalignment, hematoma, swelling, or delayed abscess formation. Ischemia can occur with compression or edema or from reduced circulating blood volume and poor perfusion pressure. Breakdown of the wound can lead to leakage of cerebrospinal fluid and, in turn, contribute to wound infection and even meningitis. Certain wounds will require revision. Recurrent compression is the greatest fear. Postoperative hematomas, although rare, may cause deterioration over a few hours. Rapid identification of the hematoma and operative removal are necessary.

POSTOPERATIVE CRITICAL CARE MANAGEMENT

LONG-TERM VENTILATORY MANAGEMENT

In quadriplegic or paretic states, interval measurements of the simple pulmonary function tests outlined in Fig. 33-13 and Table 33-9 are an appropriate monitor of progression for the patient who requires mechanical ventilation. In our experience, controlled mechanical ventilation with a time-cycled, volume-preset ventilator was used, initially, for all high cervical spine injuries because this mode of ventilation provides optimum inflation of the lung at all times. Intermittent mandatory ventilation or assisted ventilation has the

TABLE 33-9
Weaning Criteria for Removal from Mechanical Ventilation

Weaning Criteria	Acceptable Value
Maximum inspiratory force	>-20 cmH$_2$O
Maximum expiratory force	$>+20$ cmH$_2$O
Vital capacity	>1000 ml
Expiratory flow	>10 liters/s (level dependent)
Pa$_{O_2}$/Fi$_{O_2}$	>250
Vd/Vt	>0.55
Lung thorax compliance	>30 ml/cmH$_2$O

SOURCE: Mackenzie and Ducker,[37] with permission

disadvantage that lung expansion is inadequate because of the spontaneous breaths between the mandatory or assisted cycles. Inadequate lung expansion, in the early stages of quadriplegia, may give rise to undesirable respiratory complications such as atelectasis, pneumonitis, and pneumonia. The role of high-frequency jet ventilation or oscillation remains unresolved. Advocates of these forms of mechanical ventilation claim good patient tolerance and lack of secretion retention and aspiration as important benefits.[435,436]

Serial pulmonary function testing determines when weaning from mechanical ventilation may be indicated. Vital capacity and maximum inspiratory and expiratory pressures are indicators of the ability to maintain spontaneous ventilation. With more sophisticated equipment for measurement of flow, the efficacy of the patient's cough can be determined by measuring expiratory flow. Expiratory flow rates of 10 liters/s or 600 liters/min are required to produce an effective cough (see Fig. 33-13). Intrapulmonary shunt can be approximated by Pa$_{O_2}$/FiO$_2$ or the alveolar-arterial oxygen difference and, together with measurement of dead space (Vd/Vt), may be used to assess the adequacy of gas exchange. Lung/thorax compliance can be easily calculated at the bedside[437] and indicates the pressure changes that the patient has to generate for each breath. Some values used in weaning adult quadriplegic patients are shown in Table 33-9.

It must be stressed that it is essential that the quadriplegic patient is adequately prepared for removal from mechanical ventilation both physically and mentally. The physical requirements include adequate nutrition and metabolic status. Supplementary hyperalimentation may be necessary and the patient should be in electrolyte balance.[7] Infection may be masked because of the lack of temperature control in quadriplegic patients and should be treated. Fluid management must be optimized so that the patient is neither volume underloaded or overloaded in relation to cardiac and renal function. Lastly, mechanical impairments to breathing such as gastric distension, too tight a Halo vest, or inappropriate positioning should be avoided during spontaneous breathing. Psychologically, the patient should be prepared by reassurance that help is at hand should breathing difficulty occur and by an explanation of what to expect during the weaning process.

Progressive reduction in rates of intermittent mandatory ventilation may be beneficial for C3 to C4 level quadriplegics as a means of gradually reducing chronic ventilator dependence. Some chronic cervical cord-injured patients find that cuirass ventilators, negative pressure jackets, or rocking beds enable them to remain out of hospital by providing support when respiration is impaired during sleep. There is an increasing number of ventilator-dependent quadriplegic patients who, with family support, are able to be discharged from hospital.

LONG-TERM VENTILATOR SUPPORT BY DIAPHRAGM PACING IN QUADRIPLEGIA

The phrenic nerves originate from the C4 roots, and the spinal cord centers for motor neurons are located opposite the C1 to C3 bony levels. A complete SCI at these levels can destroy the diaphragm function, requiring the patient to be on permanent ventilator support. In recent years it has been possible to use electrical stimulation of the phrenic nerves to pace the diaphragm in many quadriplegic patients with respiratory paralysis. The successful use of this pacer requires that sufficient cell bodies and functional axons of the phrenic nerve have survived. The cerebral drive signal can be totally disrupted as it is replaced by the pacing signal. Nonventilator breathing provides a tremendous increase in independence and psychological advantage for the patient. Ventilator-dependent patients typically are unable to go outside or even leave their rooms. A review of the history of phrenic pacing is presented by Tibballs.[438]

Full-time ventilator support was reported[439] in 13 of 37 patients and at least half-time support in 10 others. There were only 2 deaths among these 23 patients. In 14 patients pacing was not possible and 8 of these died. Average follow-up was 26 months and the longest paced patient was at 60 months. These authors felt that damage to the phrenic nerves by either the initial trauma or the surgical intervention of electrode placement was the major reason for failure. Damage to the phrenic nerve from the electrical stimulation was not noted to be a problem.

Another study[440] consisting of 23 patients, whose ages ranged from 17 to 63, reported 14 patients with unilateral phrenic nerve implantation and 9 with bilateral implants. The surgery was performed between 12 and 16 weeks from injury. The exciting electrode was placed on the cervical phrenic nerve in 13 patients and on the thoracic phrenic nerve in 10 patients. The indication for the procedure was inability to wean the patient from ventilator support. Inability to stimulate the phrenic nerve implantation occurred in 3 patients even though they had preoperative testing indicating a good response. In this group, 8 patients were ventilator independent, 9 patients required the ventilator at night only, 3 patients had part-time ventilator independence, and 3 patients received no benefit from the procedure. Three patients in this study required additional surgery to repair implant components.

CHEST PHYSIOTHERAPY

Both spontaneously breathing and mechanically ventilated patients need prophylactic chest physiotherapy to prevent atelectasis and the development of pneumonia.[441,442] Because the quadriplegic patient has decreased vital capacity, total lung capacity, expiratory reserve volume, and forced expiratory volume at 1 s, pulmonary complications are common.[364,442–447] In addition, paralysis of the trunk and extremity muscles makes patients unable to turn themselves and cough, and diaphragm function is limited by abdominal muscle and intercostal muscle paralysis. During the first 3 months following acute traumatic quadriplegia, death is most frequently due to pulmonary complications[448,449]; chest physiotherapy is reported to be highly successful in reducing pulmonary complications in these patients.[442,450] Chest physiotherapy includes postural drainage, chest wall percussion and vibration, tracheal suctioning, and breathing exercises. Specific active and passive range of motion exercises are also performed.[451]

The quadriplegic patient may be mechanically ventilated or breathing spontaneously in traction, a Halo vest, or a body cast. Chest physiotherapy varies in each of these situations. Pulmonary function is influenced by body position in the spontaneously breathing quadriplegic patient and is different from that in normal subjects. Spontaneously breathing quadriplegic patients have increased inspiratory capacity and tidal volume in the supine position and maximum vital capacity in the 20° head-down position.[364,376,377] Optimum lung function for quadriplegic patients is, therefore, not in the sitting position as it is for normal subjects. In the acute phase following injury, chest physiotherapy management is facilitated by use of a bed that allows a patient to be turned and positioned for postural drainage, chest percussion, and vibration. The Stryker frame is best for mechanically ventilated or spontaneously breathing patients with cervical cord transection or spine injury because it can be positioned head up, head down, prone, or supine and percussion and vibration can be performed over most lung segments. Cervical traction is maintained throughout positioning. Loss of traction in the head-down position is prevented by securing the patient's ankles to the frame by padded straps[450] or the feet may be placed in padded boots.[377] The Rotorest bed electronically rotates from side to side and is advocated by some for use in the spine-injured patient. This may be of benefit for quadriplegic patients at home or in a chronic facility where there is insufficient help for adequate turning of patients. The Rotorest bed only allows access to 4 of the 11 postural drainage positions; it complicates many nursing procedures and may cause decubitus ulcers and tissue breakdown from the shoulder straps due to movements with continuous rotation.[451] In comparison, 7 of the 11 postural drainage positions can be obtained with a Stryker frame, skin integrity can be assessed easily over the whole body, and bony prominences may be protected. The hydraulic Stryker frame enables positioning for chest physiotherapy to be carried out by one person.

Medical and paramedical personnel working with the quadriplegic patient must be aware that rapid changes in body position may have cardiac as well as respiratory effects. During spinal shock, head elevation causes a sudden decrease in cardiac filling pressures and this results in a fall in cardiac output and may cause cardiac arrest. Equally, acute change into the head-down position, because of loss of sympathetic cardiovascular innervation, may precipitate acute myocardial failure with pulmonary edema. In spinal shock and until vasomotor tone returns, these movements must be performed gradually and with careful monitoring of arterial and venous pressures. Ace wraps around the lower extremities, abdominal binders, G-suits, or MAST may be used to minimize orthostatic hypotension.

If the quadriplegic patient has copious secretions, long periods of head-down positioning may be necessary. Copious secretions may occur if tracheitis develops following prolonged tracheal intubation and the use of corticosteroids, or if the patient has preexisting sputum-producing lung disease. In spontaneously breathing patients who have a poor cough in whom there is no access to the trachea through a tube to allow secretions to be adequately suctioned, drainage of secretions into the oropharynx is assisted by up to 120 min of head-down postural drainage.[450] In the prone position, movement of the abdomen should not be restricted. Adequate diaphragm excursion should occur and may be helped by placing a roll under the iliac crest or cutting a larger hole in the Stryker frame canvas.

Once pulmonary status is stabilized and the patient is weaned from a mechanical ventilator, a Halo vest enables cervical spine stabilization to be maintained.

When the Halo vest is worn, chest physiotherapy may be given in all postural drainage positions. By releasing one side of the vest with the patient in the lateral position, percussion and vibration can be carried out over the anterior, lateral, and posterior chest wall. In the prone position, the jacket is unfastened on both sides to allow percussion over the posterior basal and superior segments of the lower lobes. All personnel should be aware that the Halo vest must be closed before a position change, and must not be released while the patient is being positioned. The Halo vest allows for optimal management for patients with minimal neurologic deficit and respiratory impairment, because the patient can be mobilized early for gait training and generalized muscle strengthening exercises.

Body casts, which are an alternative to the Halo vest, usually compromise respiratory function because of their rigidity and restriction of access for chest physiotherapy maneuvers. However, if they are adapted by cutting large windows, chest therapy may be given to specific lung segments, chest movement is not compromised, and pressure sores from the cast can be easily evaluated and treated.

COUGH

Cough can be improved in quadriplegic patients by glossopharyngeal breathing. Teaching the patient to inspire to total lung capacity, forcefully exhale, with the abdominal muscles supported to prevent relaxation and distension during expiration, improves cough. In C5 lesions and below, the patient can be taught to carry out this maneuver independently. Huffing may also be used to increase cough effectiveness in the nonintubated spontaneously breathing quadriplegic patient. Huffing is a series of short expiratory blasts, interrupted by pauses, produced after a single maximal inspiration. If secretions were mobilized into the larger airways by other techniques, such as postural drainage and chest wall percussion and vibration, huffing, which results in rapid changes in airflow, oscillates the secretions and so may mechanically simulate a normal cough.[452,453] Huffing does not cause glottic closure and generates a lower intrathoracic pressure than coughing.[453,454] This may help decrease small airway closure associated with forced expiration.[455]

BREATHING EXERCISES

Guttman[456] advocates breathing exercises to improve function in the remaining innervated respiratory muscles, such as the sternocleidomastoid, trapezius, levator scapula, and platysma. These muscles may be exercised and used to increase the anteroposterior diameter of the chest and, hence, tidal volume. Diaphragmatic breathing exercises may be helpful. Although, in normal subjects, the effects of breathing exercises could not be correlated with altered diaphragmatic function,[457] it appears that quadriplegic patients are capable of taking deeper breaths and coughing more effectively after instruction in breathing exercises.[445] While teaching diaphragmatic breathing exercises, expiration is controlled to avoid increased airway resistance resulting from a forceful expiration.[453,454] Diaphragmatic breathing exercises are well described elsewhere, and the techniques for teaching are enumerated by Ciesla.[451]

Chest physiotherapy is instituted prophylactically with emphasis on areas of the lungs showing involvement clinically and on chest x-ray. No benefit was found in the use of bronchodilators for the quadriplegic patient.[458] Intermittent positive-pressure breathing and mucolytic agents by aerosol do not appear to be any more effective than adequate humidification in liquefying lung secretions.[459] Mucolytic agents may cause bronchoconstriction.[460–462] Mechanical aids to lung expansion have recently been critically evaluated,[463] and, although incentive inspiratory spirometry was generally favored over expiratory spirometry, which was condemned,[464] this technique still needs to be compared in terms of cost and effectiveness to deep breathing alone and deep breathing in conjunction with the chest physiotherapy techniques outlined above. Incentive spirometry, blow bottles, and intermittent positive-pressure breathing have limited use in mechanically ventilated patients.

GLOSSOPHARYNGEAL BREATHING

Dail[465] published the first report of the beneficial effect of glossopharyngeal breathing in a paralyzed polio patient. The technique was termed glossopharyngeal breathing or frog breathing by Dail and colleagues[466] because it uses the muscles of the mouth, pharynx, and larynx as a respiratory pump to inflate the lungs in a similar manner to the respiratory movements of the frog and other amphibia. The use of glossopharyngeal breathing is reported in many patients with paralysis following poliomyelitis and in acute quadriplegia.[467–471] The benefits include an increase in vital capacity from 11 to 50 percent of predicted normal by use of an average of 20 glossopharyngeal strokes of 80 ml each[472] and an increase in duration of breathing without mechanical assistance from 1 min to over 3 h, on the average. Maximal glossopharyngeal breathing resulted in increased lung volume and better cough and mucous clearance than unaided breathing.[466] Lung/thorax compliance and peak expiratory flow were increased by glossopharyngeal breathing.[468] Glossopharyngeal breathing also helps speech by allowing longer phrases to be formed in one large breath.

Dail and coworkers,[466] who reported the largest series (100 patients), found that glossopharyngeal breathing was used by 69 patients to assist breathing, to stretch their chest, improve cough, and as an aid in talking. Forty-two of these patients depended on glossopharyngeal breathing to be free of mechanical ventilatory support. Murphy and associates[473] measured lung/thorax compliance and found that this was increased by glossopharyngeal breathing in all the patients studied, whether they could generate glossopharyngeal breaths more than 40 percent or less than 20 percent of predicted total lung capacity. They found that the patients used glossopharyngeal breathing to speak loudly, cough effectively, and increase the scope or intensity of their physical or social activities. Even though the patient is a good glossopharyngeal breather, however, the cough effort is still diminished because of impaired function of the abdominal muscles and diaphragm.[468] Glossopharyngeal breathing cannot be performed during sleep[469,472]; therefore, the quadriplegic patient will require mechanical ventilatory support for sleeping. It is difficult for eating and glossopharyngeal breathing to be carried out simultaneously, but use of the accessory muscles of respiration while masticating and glossopharyngeal breathing after swallowing is reported.[469] Patients may take from one day to several months to master the technique of glossopharyngeal breathing.[473] Once mastered, the technique takes several weeks before strength and endurance are increased sufficiently to cough effectively.

In 23 traumatic quadriplegics injured at levels C4 to C7, vital capacity averaged 60 percent of predicted normal and was increased to 81 percent of normal by use of glossopharyngeal breathing. The ability to improve respiratory function was thought to allow a greater range of rehabilitation because it produced sufficient respiratory function for increased metabolic demands.[470] In 14 patients with C5 to C7 cord transections, breath-holding time, maximum breathing capacity, maximum expiratory flow, and vital capacity were all increased by use of glossopharyngeal breathing. It took 1 to 6 weeks for these quadriplegic patients to learn the technique, to cough productively, and to shout loudly enough to gain the attention of a nurse at the far end of a hospital corridor.[471]

In summary, glossopharyngeal breathing is a breathing substitute that may be used by quadriplegic patients. It requires none of the ordinary muscles of respiration and no mechanical equipment. It increases vital capacity, lung/thorax compliance, and expiratory flow and improves cough.

HYPERREFLEXIC SYNDROMES

Following spinal shock, which is an areflexic state, recovery begins with return of the bulbocavernosus, cremasteric, and Babinski reflexes. As spasticity develops, uncontrolled *hyperreflexic spasms of muscles* occur.

TABLE 33-10
Signs and Symptoms of Autonomic Hyperreflexia

Hypertension	Nausea
Bradycardia	Blurred vision
Dysrhythmia—heart block, ex-trasystoles	Muscle fasiculation
	Convulsion
Sweating (below lesion)	Loss of consciousness
Piloerection (below lesion)	
Headache	*In General*
Shortness of breath	Vasoconstriction (below lesion)
Flushed face and neck	Vasodilation (above lesion)

SOURCE: Schreibman and Mackenzie,[410] with permission.

This mass reflex is probably caused by the hyperactive spinal reflexes controlling muscle tone. In the quadriplegic patient it is thought these mass reflexes cause muscle contraction by multiple level spinal reflex arcs in response to stimuli below the level of SCI. Cervical cord transection functionally separates the nuclei in the brainstem and hypothalamus from the thoracolumbar spinal sympathetic outflow. This causes spinal reflex activity from several segments below the level of the lesion with no inhibition by the higher centers.[474]

Autonomic hyperreflexia is characterized by acute generalized sympathetic acivity in response to an endogenous or exogenous stimulus below the level of spinal cord transection. Head and Riddoch[475] noted reflex responses in traumatic paraplegics during World War I and found that cutaneous, proprioceptive, and visceral stimuli triggered this reflex response. Many stimuli are incriminated as precipitants of autonomic hyperreflexia including cold[476] and hot cutaneous stimuli,[477] urinary catheterization, bladder irrigation, urinary retention, enemas,[475] gastric distension,[478] and acute pyelitis.[477] In addition, rectal examination or manual disimpaction together with muscle stretching, positioning, or any surgical procedures performed without adequate anesthesia on the bowel or bladder or below the level of SCI, may precipitate autonomic hyperreflexia.[479]

Symptoms of autonomic hyperreflexia include severe headache, sweating, nasal obstruction, desire to vomit, blurring of vision; the person may complain of feeling flushed (Table 33-10). The signs of autonomic hyperreflexia are hypertension, bradycardia, arrhythmias, sweating, and gooseflesh. Sweating rarely extends below T10 and is most marked at the level of the lesion.[479] Below the level of transection, sweating is more likely to be part of the general sympathetic response.[480] There is cutaneous vasodilatation above and vasoconstriction below the SCI.[394] Additional signs that may occur include changes in skin and rectal temperature, convulsions or loss of consciousness, cessa-

tion of respiration, visual field defects, and signs of cerebrovascular accident.[475,478,479,481] In the SCI patient with a lesion above T7, hypertension, resulting from autonomic hyperreflexia during surgery performed below the level of the spinal cord lesion without anesthesia, occurs in 65 to 85 percent of patients.[482] Hypertension is seen in 65 to 85 percent despite compensation upper extremity vasodilation and is accompanied by baroreceptor-medicated bradycardia. In high levels of SCI if sympathetic innervation of the heart is included in the autonomic efferent activity, tachycardia can result.

The original explanation of autonomic hyperreflexia was proposed by Kurnick[481] in which he described the neural pathways in relation to stimulation of the bladder. The afferent limb of the reflex is the pelvic nerves, posterior columns, and spinothalamic tract. The efferents are the autonomic fibers to blood vessels and viscera. From Guttman and Whitteridge's[478] observations, the splanchnic outflow T5 to T11 is probably the most important. Somatic efferent nerves may also be involved. Vasoconstriction and visceral contraction apear below the level of SCI and muscle spasms may occur.[394] The massive vasoconstriction below the level of the lesion is associated with a rise in plasma norepinephrine and dopamine hydroxylase.[481] Normally, hypertension that follows peripheral vasoconstriction results in stimulation of the carotid and aortic arch baroreceptors, resulting in vasodilation, bradycardia, and a fall in blood pressure. In the quadriplegic patient, because there is loss of inhibition of the spinal reflex by the higher centers, vasodilation does not occur and the hypertension is not relieved. The rise in blood pressure then results in stimulation of the afferents that pass in the ninth and tenth cranial nerves from the aortic and carotid baroreceptors to the vasomotor center. Efferents from the vasomotor center pass in the tenth cranial nerve, causing bradycardia. Cardiac arrhythmias may result from this vagal hyperactivity.[474] There is a rise in plasma norepinephrine but not epinephrine.[483] Dopamine hydroxylase is also elevated, suggesting that sympathetic overactivity is the cause of the cardiovascular changes.[484] Plasma renin does not rise and there appears to be no change in secretion from the adrenal medulla.

Garnier and coworkers[485] showed a 47 to 68 percent increase in blood pressure in four quadriplegics when 2 to 5 μg/min norepinephrine was infused, whereas this same dose produced insignificant changes in normal controls. This suggests that denervation hypersensitivity in adrenergic structures distal to the site of transection causes the autonomic hyperreflexia; or that vascular supersensitivity may exacerbate the problem of autonomic hyperreflexia.[486]

Autonomic hyperreflexia should be anticipated before it occurs and preparations should be made to treat hypertension. If autonomic hyperreflexia occurs during surgery, the precipitating cause should be stopped immediately while therapy is initiated. Autonomic hyperreflexia occurs during surgery performed below the level of the spinal cord lesion without anesthesia in 65 to 85 percent of patients.[474,481] Patients at risk for developing autonomic hyperreflexia are protected from intraoperative hypertension by either general or spinal anesthesia. Topical anesthesia, sedation, or no anesthesia did not prevent hypertension.[482] Local anesthesia is reported to be effective if used in adequate dosages long enough before the procedure. Comarr[487] suggests that 60 to 99 ml 0.25% pontocaine instilled into the bladder 20 min before the cystoscopy is an effective means of preventing autonomic hyperreflexia. Spinal[487–489] and epidural anesthesia[490,491] prevent autonomic hyperreflexia, but there are difficulties associated with determining sensory levels in quadriplegic patients. Spinal or epidural anesthesia may cause severe hypotension when given to patients with chronic cord injury,[474] but this may be prevented by adequate prior volume replacement.[491]

In the intensive care unit or chronic facility, autonomic hyperreflexia may occur in association with a nonsurgical stimulus and use of anesthesia then is inappropriate. Pharmacologic means of prevention and control include the use of ganglionic blockers, α-adrenergic anatagonists, and nitric oxide donor drugs acting directly on the vessel wall such as sodium nitroprusside.[394,481,489,491] Arrhythmias resulting from autonomic hyperreflexia may be controlled with β-blocking agents.[408] Stimuli known to provoke the response should be avoided and sedation may be helpful to control the patient's anxiety.

REGIONAL SCI CENTERS

Patients with acute SCIs should not be taken to the nearest hospital. Within any state, there should be a designated hospital or hospitals where neurosurgeons and critical care physicians are immediately available to treat these injured persons. Although it is rare, immediate realignment of fracture dislocations has led to functional recovery. A designated center is essential for these few patients.

There are 35 patients per million per year who will suffer these injuries; any area that has a population near a million should, therefore, designate a center where expertise in the resuscitation and treatment of these victims is immediately available. The medical and economic consequences of permanent quadriplegia or paraplegia are so devastating that anything less than an all-out medical effort for these victims can no longer be justified.

Obviously, it is most important that such a center be staffed by dedicated personnel and physicians to manage the acute circumstance. Rehabilitation specialists are essential for long-term management.[492] Urologists, orthopedic surgeons, critical care physicians, physical and occupational therapists, and specialized social workers are all important in coordinating the total rearrangement of life-style necessary after cord damage. The concept of specialized care for patients with SCI was instituted in the 1940s.[478] These early SCI centers emphasized that rehabilitation services should not be separated from the initial treatment of SCI. Evidence confirms the benefits of early admission to an SCI center including reduced hospital length of stay, decreased patient care costs, reductions in associated complications, and less mortality.[493–496] As a result of changes in therapy and admission to regional SCI centers, there has been a significant decrease in the proportion of patients with complete neurologic injuries.[493,497,498] This decrease has been attributed to improved first aid, evacuation, and transportation to the specialized care of regional SCI units,[497,498] although other factors are likely to have played a part. Meyers and Greesan[498] state that the amount of time between onset of a SCI and receipt of acute spine injury care is possibly the most important measurable influence on eventual neurologic outcome.

Earlier in this chapter we detailed the therapies that are under investigation for pharmacologic management. Maintenance or restoration of spinal cord perfusion is critical. Early administration or pharmacologic agents that reduce cord edema, antagonize or block mediators that result in reperfusion injury is mandatory for these agents to have beneficial effects. Rapid institution of optimum cardiac and respiratory management is essential to minimize multiorgan dysfunction and reduce morbidity. Early reduction and stabilization of bony injury is the cornerstone of preventing further neurologic deficit during the first few hours after injury. All these initial management issues are expedited by delivery of the SCI patient to a regional SCI center where the staff are experienced in managing such patients. The equipment necessary for critical resuscitation and stabilization is at hand and the SCI center is staffed 365 days a year with experts in SCI management.

In addition to management benefits occurring within 12 h of SCI, there are other advantages of admission to a regional SCI center. Physical therapy and rehabilitation treatment can begin within 24 h of SCI. Based on a review of patients admitted early or late to a regional SCI center, Oakes and coworkers support the practice of initiating rehabilitation soon after injury.[495] Quadriplegics who were admitted to regional SCI centers early and began rehabilitation on average 3 days after cervical trauma had a significantly shorter hospital stay (by 66 days) compared to those admitted late. They had similar findings for paraplegics who had their hospital stay decreased by an average 38.5 days. For both the quadriplegic and paraplegic patients it was time spent in the acute care facility that differed, while total time in rehabilitation was similar for both groups regardless of early or late admission to the regional SCI center.

The advantages of implementing physical therapy early are that it allows conscious patients to assist in their own care very early, which appears to help both patients and family adjust to SCI. The physical contact that occurs during therapy may diminish some of the sensory deprivation that occurs in intensive care units and is compounded by the sensory loss occurring with SCI. Involvement of physical therapists in the care team during the acute phase ensures that realistic goals are established within a few days of injury. The objects of such physical therapy involvement early in SCI management are to prevent secondary respiratory complications (with chest physiotherapy), avoid contractures (with range of motion and mobilization techniques), and maintain conditioning of function muscle groups (with exercise programs). These factors are all essential to decrease hospitalization time and costs.

Conclusion

The treatment of cervical SCI remains controversial in terms of the type and timing of medical and surgical therapy. Basic physiologic support combines mechanical reduction and stabilization, thereby allowing maximum recovery of neurologic function. Attention to initial resuscitation and the use of fluid challenge and inotropic agents to maintain cardiac output and mean blood pressure within the first 72 h following injury are fundamental. Pharmacologic agents such as steroids and GM-1 gangliosides are undergoing controlled, prospective clinical trials to determine their efficacy. It is probable that in the future other pharmacologic agents will be tested to block mediators of the secondary injury occurring after spinal cord trauma.

Acknowledgments

The authors wish to acknowledge the contributions of the many people who helped make this work a reality. They include Alice Eissele, Paul Delaney, Renée Kahn, and Sue Tavitas for their extensive typing, editing, and management of references.

References

1. Breasted JH: *The Edwin Smith Surgical Papyrus.* Chicago: University of Chicago Press, 1930.

2. Guttman L: Historical background. In Guttman L (ed): *Spinal Cord Injuries: Comprehensive Management and Research,* 2nd ed. London: Blackwell, 1976.

3. Vellacott PN, Webb-Johnson AE: Spinal injury with retention of urine. The avoidance of catheterization. *Lancet* 1919; 1:733.

4. Bors E: The spinal cord injury center of the Veterans Administration Hospital. *Paraplegia* 1967; 5:126.

5. Nyquist RH, Bors E: Mortality and survival in traumatic myelopathy during nineteen years from 1946–1966. *Paraplegia* 1967; 5:22.

6. Guttman L, Frankel H: The value of intermittent catheterization in the early management of traumatic paraplegia and tetraplegia. *Paraplegia* 1966; 4:63.

7. Cheshire DJE, Coats DA: Respiratory and metabolic management in acute tetraplegia. *Paraplegia* 1966; 4:1.

8. Silver JR, Gibbon NOK: Prognosis in tetraplegia. *BMJ* 1968; 4:79.

9. Jousse AT, et al: Follow up study of life expectancy and mortality in traumatic transverse myopathy. *Can Med Assoc J* 1968; 98:770.

10. Wilcox NF, et al: A statistical analysis of 423 consecutive patients admitted to the Spinal Cord Injury Center, Rancho Los Amigos Hospital, January 1, 1964–December 31, 1967. *Paraplegia* 1970; 8:27.

11. Sharman GJ, Owen KA: Spinal cord injury—A report to the National Paraplegia Foundation, 1970.

12. Kraus JF, et al: Incidence of traumatic spinal cord lesions. *J Chron Dis* 1975; 28:471.

13. Sloan TB, et al: Anesthetic management of the patient with acute spinal cord injury. In Stoelting RK (ed): *Advances in Anesthesia.* St. Louis: CV Mosby, 1991:55.

14. Meyer PR: Illinois EMS and spinal cord injury: The midwest regional spinal cord injury care system. In Cowley RA (ed): *Collected Papers in EMS and Traumatology* 1976:306.

15. Ducker TB, Perot PL: Newsletter III: National Spinal Cord Registry. *Medical University Press,* Charleston, 1973:1.

16. Lewis ED, et al: Regulation of plasma potassium in hyperkalemic periodic paralysis. *Neurology* 1979; 29:1131.

17. Smart CN, Sanders CR: Motor vehicle related spinal cord injuries. *Insurance Institute for Highway Safety.* Washington, D.C. 1975.

18. Young J: Development of system of spinal cord injury management with correlation to the development of other esoteric health care systems. *Ariz Med* 1979; 27:1.

19. National Center for Health Statistics. *Advance Report of Final Mortality Statistics, 1985.* 1987.

20. National Center for Health Statistics. *Current Estimates from the National Health Interview Survey, United States, 1985.* 1986.

21. Baker SP, et al: *The Injury Fact Book.* New York: Oxford University Press, 1992.

22. Bracken MB, et al: Incidence of acute traumatic hospitalized spinal cord injury in the United States, 1970–1977. *Am J Epidemiol* 1981; 113:615.

23. Frankel HL, et al: The value of postural reduction in the initial management of closed injuries of the spine with paraplegia and tetraplegia, Part I. *Paraplegia* 1969; 7:179.

24. Griffin MR, et al: Traumatic spinal cord injury in Olmsted County, Minnesota, 1935–1981. *Am J Epidemiol* 1985; 121:884.

25. Kalsbeek WD, et al: The National Head and Spinal Cord Injury Survey: Major findings. *J Neurosurg* 1989; 53:S19.

26. Kraus JF: Epidemiology of head injury. In Cooper PR (ed): *Head Injury.* Baltimore, MD: Williams & Wilkins, 1987:1.

27. Le CT, Price M: Survival from spinal cord injury. *J Chronic Dis* 1982; 35:487.

28. Thomas JP: Introduction. In Young JS, et al. (eds): *Spinal Cord Injury Statistics: Experience of the Regional Spinal Cord Injury*

Systems. Phoenix, AZ: Good Samaritan Medical Center, 1982:1–10.

29. Public Health Service. *Healthy People 2000.* National health promotion and disease prevention objectives—full report with commentary. Public Health Service, No. PHS 91-50212. Washington, DC: U.S. Department of Health and Human Services, 1991.

30. Council on Scientific Affairs. Automobile-related injuries, components, trends, prevention. *JAMA* 1983; 249:3216.

31. Schmidt G, et al: *Fact Pack, Prevention of Head and Spinal Cord Injury Facts.* Tallahassee, FL, Florida Interagency Office of Disability Prevention, 1989.

32. Eyster EF, Watts C: An update of the National Head and Spinal Cord Injury Prevention Program of the American Association of Neurological Surgeons and the Congress of Neurological Surgeons. THINK FIRST. *Clin Neurosurg* 1992; 38:252.

33. Bracken MB, et al: Methylprednisolone or naloxone treatment after acute spinal cord injury: 1-year follow-up data. Results of the second National Acute Spinal Cord Injury Study. *J Neurosurg* 1992; 76:23.

34. Bracken MB: Treatment of acute spinal cord injury with methylprednisolone: Results of a multicenter, randomized clinical trial. *J Neurotrauma* 1991; 8:S47.

35. Bracken MB, et al: A randomized, controlled trial of methylprednisolone or naloxone in the treatment of acute spinal cord injury. Results of the second National Acute Spinal Cord Injury Study. *N Engl J Med* 1990; 322:1405.

36. Ducker TB, Kindt GW: The effect of trauma on the vasomotor control of spinal cord blood flow. *Curr Topics Surg Res* 1971; 163.

37. Mackenzie CF, Ducker TB: Cervical spinal cord injury. In Matjasko J, Katz J (eds): *Clinical Controversies in Neuroanesthesia and Neurosurgery.* Orlando, FL, Grune & Stratton, 1986:77.

38. Dolan EJ, Tator CH: The effect of blood transfusion, dopamine, and gamma hydroxybutyrate on post-traumatic ischemia of the spinal cord. *J Neurosurg* 1982; 56:350.

39. Geisler FH: Acute management of cervical spinal cord injury. *Md Med J* 1988; 37:525.

40. Guha A, et al: Spinal cord blood flow and systemic blood pressure after experimental spinal cord injury in rats. *Stroke* 1989; 20:372.

41. Piepmeier JM, et al: Cardiovascular instability following acute cervical spinal cord trauma. *Cent Nerv Syst Trauma* 1985; 2:153.

42. Tator CH: Hemodynamic issues and vascular factors in acute experimental spinal cord injury. *J Neurotrauma* 1992; 9:139.

43. Tator CH: Review of experimental spinal cord injury with emphasis on the local and systemic circulatory effects. *Neurochirurgie* 1991; 37:291.

44. Carter RE Jr.: Traumatic spinal cord injuries due to automobile accidents. *South Med J* 1977; 70:709.

45. Stover SL, Fine PR: *Spinal Cord Injury: The Facts and Figures* National Spinal Cord Injury Statistical Center, The University of Alabama at Birmingham, 1986.

46. Shaw LR, et al: The Florida approach to spinal cord injury prevention. *Rehabil Lit* 1984; 45:85.

47. Kraus JF, Conroy C: Mortality and morbidity from injuries in sports and recreation. *Annu Rev Public Health* 1984; 5:163.

48. Maiman D, et al: Diving associated spinal cord injuries during drought conditions: Wisconsin, 1988. *MMWR* 1988; 37:453.

49. Jessor R, Cited by Lewis CE: Peer pressure and risk-taking behaviors in children. *Am J Public Health* 1984; 74:580.

50. Lewis CE, Lewis MA: Peer pressure and risk-taking behaviors in children. *Am J Public Health* 1984; 74:580.

51. Irvin C, Millstein S: Biopsychosocial correlates of risk-taking behavior during adolescence. *J Adolesc Health Care* 1986; 7:S82.

52. Baker SP, et al: *The Injury Fact Book.* Lexington, MA: DC Heath & Company, 1984:219.

53. Finn P, Bragg BWE: Perception of the risk of accident by young and older drivers. *Accid Anal Prev* 1986; 18:289.

54. Matthews ML, Moran AR: Age differences in male drivers' perception of accident risk in the role of perceived driving ability. *Accid Anal Prev* 1986; 18:299.

55. Committee on Trauma Research Commission on Life Sciences NR, Institute of Medicine. Injury in America: A Continuing Public Health Problem. 1985.

56. Jessor R: Adolescent development and behavioral health. In Matarazzo J et al. (eds): *Behavioral Health: A Handbook of Health Enhancement and Disease Prevention.* New York: John W. Wiley, 1984:69.

57. National Highway Traffic Safety Administration. Fatal Accident Reporting Systems, 1987. 1988.

58. Torg JS: Epidemiology, pathomechanics, and prevention of athletic injuries to the cervical spine. *Med Sci Sports Exerc* 1985; 17:295.

59. Torg JS, et al: Cervical quadriplegia resulting from axial loading injuries: Cinematographic, radiographic, kinematic, and pathologic analysis. Proc Amer Orthopaedic Soc for Sports Med, Interim Meeting, Atlanta, GA, Feb 8–9, 1984.

60. National Collegiate Athletic Association: National Collegiate Athletic Association Football Rules, Changes and/or Modifications. January 23, 1976. Rule 2, Section 24; Rule 9, Section 1, Article 2-L; Rule 9, Section 1, Article 2-N. 1976.

61. Tator CH, Edmonds VE: National survey of spinal injuries in hockey players. *Can Med Assoc J* 1984; 130:875.

62. American Academy of Pediatrics. Committee on Accident and Poison Prevention and Committee on Pediatric Aspects of Physical Fitness, Recreation, and Sports. Policy Statement. Trampolines. *Pediatrics* 1981; 67:438.

63. Bhagwanani SG, et al: Risks and prevention of cervical cord injury in the management of breech presentation with hyperextension of the fetal head. *Am J Obstet Gynecol* 1973; 115:1159.

64. Laschinger JC, et al: Evolving concepts in prevention of spinal cord injury during operations on the descending thoracic and thoracoabdominal aorta. *Ann Thorac Surg* 1987; 44:667.

65. Molina JE, et al: Adequacy of ascending aorta-descending aorta shunt during cross claiming of the thoracic aorta for prevention of spinal cord injury. *J Thorac Cardiovasc Surg* 1985; 90:126.

66. Eyster EF, Watts C: The National Head and Spinal Cord Injury Prevention Program. *J Med Assoc Ga* 1989; 78:333.

67. Neuwelt EA, et al: Oregon Head and Spinal Cord Injury Prevention Program and Evaluation. *Neurosurgery* 1989; 24:453.

68. Frank R, et al: A preliminary study of a traumatic injury prevention program. *Psych Health* 1992; 6:129.

69. Weingarden SI, Graham PM: Targeting teenagers in a spinal cord injury prevention program. *Paraplegia* 1991; 29:65.

70. Wigglesworth EC: Towards prevention of spinal cord injury: The role of a national register. *Paraplegia* 1988; 26:389.

71. Yeo JD, Walsh J: Prevention of spinal injuries in Australia. *Paraplegia* 1987; 25:221.

72. Alexander E Jr: Global spine and head injury prevention program (SHIP). *Surg Neurol* 1992; 38:478 (editorial).

73. Rice DR, et al: Potential savings from injury prevention. In: *Cost of Injury in the United States: A Report to Congress.* San Francisco, CA: Institute for Health and Aging, University of California and Injury Prevention Center, The Johns Hopkins University 1985; 5:111.

74. Tator CH. Personal communication. 1994.

75. Carol MP, Ducker TB: Spinal cord injury and spinal shock syndrome. In Siegel JH (ed): *Trauma: Emergency Surgery and Critical Care.* New York, Churchill Livingstone, 1987:947.

76. Mirvis SE, Geisler FH: Intraoperative sonography of cervical spinal cord injury: Results in 30 patients. *Am J Roentgenol* 1990; 155:603.

77. Scarff JE: Injuries of the vertebral column and spinal cord. In Brock S (ed): *Injuries of the Brain and Spinal Cord and Their Coverings.* New York: Springer-Verlag, 1960:530.

78. Ducker TB, Lucas JT: Recovery from spinal cord injury. In Seeman P, Brown GM (eds): *Frontiers in Neurology & Neuroscience Research.* Toronto: University of Toronto Press, 1974:142.

79. Ward RJ, et al: Experimental evaluation of atropine and vasopressors for treatment of hypotension of high subarachnoid anesthesia. *Anesth Analg* 1966; 45:621.

80. Weiss MH: Critical care of the neurosurgical patient. In Berk JL, Sampliner JE (eds): *Handbook of Critical Care,* 2nd ed. Boston, Little, Brown, 1982:490.

81. Ducker TB, et al: Pathological findings in acute experimental spinal cord trauma. *J Neurosurg* 1971; 35:700.

82. Ducker TB: Experimental injury of the spinal cord. In Braakman R (ed): *Handbook of Clinical Neurology.* New York, Elsevier, 1976:9.

83. Rawe SE, et al: The histopathology of experimental spinal cord trauma. *J Neurosurg* 1978; 48:1002.

84. D'Angelo CM, et al: Evoked cortical potentials in experimental spinal cord trauma. *J Neurosurg* 1973; 38:332.

85. Dorfman LJ, et al: Use of cerebral evoked potentials to evaluate spinal somatosensory function in patients with traumatic and surgical myelopathies. *J Neurosurg* 1980; 52:654.

86. Ducker TB, et al: Experimental spinal cord trauma II. Blood flow, tissue oxygen, evoked potentials in both paretic and plegic monkeys. *Surg Neurol* 1978; 10:71.

87. Greenberg RP, Ducker TB: Evoked potentials in the clinical neurosciences. *J Neurosurg* 1982; 56:1.

88. Perot PL: The clinical use of somatosensory evoked potentials in spinal cord injury. *Clin Neurosurg* 1972; 20:367.

89. Singer JM, et al: Changes in evoked potentials after experimental cervical spinal cord injury in the monkey. *Exp Neurol* 1970; 29:449.

90. Tator CH: Spinal cord cooling and irrigation for treatment of acute cord injury. In Popp AJ (ed): *Neural Trauma,* New York, Raven Press, 1979:363.

91. Ducker TB, et al: Experimental spinal cord trauma I. Correlation of blood flow, tissue oxygen and neurologic status in the dog. *Surg Neurol* 1978; 10:60.

92. Locke GE, et al: Ischemia in primate spinal cord injury. *J Neurosurg* 1971; 34:614.

93. Dohrman GJ, et al: Spinal cord blood flow patterns in experimental traumatic paraplegia. *J Neurosurg* 1973; 38:52.

94. Dohrman GJ, et al: The microvasculature in transitory traumatic paraplegia. An electron microscopic study in the monkey. *J Neurosurg* 1971; 35:263.

95. Kobrine AL, et al: Spinal cord blood flow as affected by changes in systemic arterial blood pressure. *J Neurosurg* 1976; 44:12.

96. Sandler AN, Tator CH: Effect of acute spinal cord compression injury on regional spinal cord blood flow in primates. *J Neurosurg* 1976; 45:660.

97. Assenmacher DR, Ducker TB: Experimental traumatic paraplegia. The vascular and pathological changes seen in reversible and irreversible spinal-cord lesions. *J Bone Joint Surg* 1971; 53:671.

98. Hickey R, et al: Autoregulation of spinal cord blood flow: Is the cord a microcosm of the brain? *Stroke* 1986; 17:1183.

99. Jellinger K: Spinal cord arteriosclerosis and progressive vascular myelopathy. *J Neurol Neurosurg Psychiatry* 1967; 30:195.

100. Hukuda S, et al: Effects of hypertension and hypercarbia on spinal cord tissue oxygen in acute experimental spinal cord injury. *Neurosurgery* 1980; 6:639.

101. Senter HJ, Venes JL: Loss of autoregulation and post-traumatic ischemia following experimental spinal cord trauma. *J Neurosurg* 1979; 50:198.

102. Fairholm DJ, Turnbull IM: Microangiographic study of experimental spinal cord injuries. *J Neurosurg* 1971; 35:277.

103. Kobrine AL, et al: Local spinal cord blood flow in experimental traumatic myelopathy. *J Neurosurg* 1975; 42:144.

104. Benes V: *Spinal Cord Injury.* Baltimore, Williams & Wilkins, 1968.

105. Anderson DK, et al: Pretreatment with alpha tocopherol enhances neurologic recovery after experimental spinal cord compression injury. *J Neurotrauma* 1988; 5:61.

106. Behrmann DL, et al: Spinal cord injury produced by consistent mechanical displacement of the cord in rats: Behavioral and histologic analysis. *J Neurotrauma* 1992; 9:197.

107. Choi DW: Comment: Modeling for drug development in spinal cord injury. *J Neurotrauma* 1992; 9:135.

108. Constantini S, Young W: The effects of methylprednisolone and the ganglioside GM1 on acute spinal cord injury in rats. *J Neurosurg* 1994; 80:97.

109. Dolan EJ, et al: The effect of spinal distraction on regional spinal cord blood flow in cats. *J Neurosurg* 1980; 53:756.

110. Faden AI, et al: N-methyl-D-aspartate antagonist MK801 improves outcome following traumatic spinal cord injury in rats: Behavioral, anatomic, and neurochemical studies. *J Neurotrauma* 1988; 5:33.

111. Faden AI, et al: Endorphins in experimental spinal injury: Therapeutic effect of naloxone. *Ann Neurol* 1981; 10:326.

112. Finkelstein SD, et al: Experimental spinal cord injury: Qualitative and quantitative histopathologic evaluation. *J Neurotrauma* 1990; 7:29.

113. Goldberger ME, et al: Criteria for assessing recovery of function after spinal cord injury: Behavioral methods. *Exp Neurol* 1990; 107:113.

114. Holtz A, et al: Neuropathological changes and neurological function after spinal cord compression in the rat. *J Neurotrauma* 1990; 7:155.

115. Kakulas BA: Pathology of spinal injuries. *Cent Nerv Syst Trauma* 1984; 1:117.

116. Kwo S, et al: Spinal cord sodium, potassium, calcium, and water concentration changes in rats after graded contusion injury. *J Neurotrauma* 1989; 6:13.

117. Lemke M, Faden AI: Edema development and ion changes in rat spinal cord after impact trauma: Injury dose-response studies. *J Neurotrauma* 1990; 7:41.

118. Lucas JH: In vitro models of mechanical injury. *J Neurotrauma* 1992; 9:117.

119. Midha R, et al: Assessment of spinal cord injury by counting corticospinal and rubrospinal neurons. *Brain Res* 1987; 410:299.

120. Stokes BT, Reier PJ: Fetal grafts alter chronic behavioral outcome after contusion damage to the adult rat spinal cord. *Exp Neurol* 1992; 116:1.

121. Stokes BT: Experimental spinal cord injury: A dynamic and verifiable injury device. *J Neurotrauma* 1992; 9:129.

122. Tator CH, Fehlings MG: Review of the secondary injury theory of acute spinal cord trauma with emphasis on vascular mechanisms. *J Neurosurg* 1991; 75:15.

123. Tator CH, et al: Effect of acute spinal cord injury on axonal counts in the pyramidal tract of rats. *J Neurosurg* 1984; 61:118.

124. Tator CH: Acute spinal cord injury: A review of recent studies of treatment and pathophysiology. *Can Med Assoc J* 1972; 107:143.

125. Young W: Rapid quantification of tissue damage for assessing acute spinal cord injury therapy. *J Neurotrauma* 1992; 9:151.

126. Meguro K, Tator CH: Effect of multiple trauma on mortality and neurological recovery after spinal cord or cauda equina injury. *Neurol Med Chir (Tokyo)* 1988; 28:34.

127. Anderson TE: Effects of acute alcohol intoxication on spinal cord vascular injury. *Cent Nerv Syst Trauma* 1986; 3:183.

128. Ridella SA, Anderson TE: Compression of rat spinal cord in vitro: Effects of ethanol on recovery of axonal conduction. *Cent Nerv Syst Trauma* 1986; 3:195.

129. Zink BJ, et al: Effects of ethanol in traumatic brain injury. *J Neurotrauma* 1993; 10:275.

130. Hall ED, Wolf DL: Post-traumatic spinal cord ischemia: Relationship to injury severity and physiological parameters. *Cent Nerv Syst Trauma* 1987; 4:15.

131. Nelson E, et al: Spinal cord injury. The role of vascular damage in the pathogenesis of central hemorrhagic necrosis. *Arch Neurol* 1977; 34:332.

132. Faden AI: Comment: Need for standardization of animal models of spinal cord injury. *J Neurotrauma* 1992; 9:169.

133. Guha A, Tator CH: Acute cardiovascular effects of experimental spinal cord injury. *J Trauma* 1988; 28:481.

134. Cotman CW, et al: Enhancing the self-repairing potential of the CNS after injury. *Cent Nerv Syst Trauma* 1984; 1:3.

135. Gorio A, et al: Neuronal decay of function and degeneration are prevented by processes secondary to membrane preservation. *Cent Nerv Syst Trauma* 1987; 4:135.

136. Hogan EL, et al: Calcium-activated mediators of secondary injury in the spinal cord. *Cent Nerv Syst Trauma* 1986; 3:175.

137. Trump BF, et al: Mechanisms of cellular injury and death. *J Neurotrauma* 1988; 5:215.

138. Young W: Secondary injury mechanisms in acute spinal cord injury. *J Emerg Med* 1993; 11:S13.

139. Young W: Secondary CNS injury. *J Neurotrauma* 1988; 5:219.

140. Bernstein JJ: Regeneration and grafting. *J Neurotrauma* 1988; 5:229.

141. Yant RWJ: Update on the American Paralysis Association's research program for CNS regeneration. *Cent Nerv Syst Trauma* 1987; 4:63.

142. Knapp MJ, et al: A 30-week randomized controlled trial of high-dose tacrine in patients with Alzheimer's disease. *JAMA* 1994; 271:985.

143. Winker MA: Tacrine for Alzheimer's disease. Which patient, what dose? *JAMA* 1994; 271:1023 (editorial).

144. Braughler JM, et al: Interactions of lipid peroxidation and calcium in the pathogenesis of neuronal injury. *Cent Nerv Syst Trauma* 1985; 2:269.

145. Faden AI, Salzman S: Pharmacological strategies in CNS trauma. *Trends Pharmacol Sci* 1992; 13:29.

146. Nockels R, Young W: Pharmacologic strategies in the treatment of experimental spinal cord injury. *J Neurotrauma* 1992; 1:S211.

147. Steward O: Reorganization of neuronal connections following CNS trauma: Principles and experimental paradigms. *J Neurotrauma* 1989; 6:99.

148. Choi D, et al: Glutamate neurotoxicity in cortical cell culture. *J Neurosci* 1987; 7:357.

149. Dichter MA: Rat cortical neurons in cell culture: Culture methods, cell morphology, electrophysiology, and synapse formation. *Brain Res* 1978; 149:279.

150. Heuttner JE, Baughman RW: Primary culture of identified neurons from the visual cortex of postnatal rats. *J Neurosci* 1986; 6:3044.

151. Messer A: The maintenance and identification of mouse cerebellar granule cells in monolayer culture. *Brain Res* 1977; 130:1.

152. Rothman S: Synaptic release of excitatory amino acid neurotransmitter mediates anoxic neuronal death. *J Neurosci* 1984; 4:1884.

153. Scott BS: Adult neurons in cell culture: Electrophysiological characterization and use in neurobiological research. *Progr Neurobiol* 1982; 19:187.

154. Banker GA, Cowan WM: Further observations on hippocampal neurons in dispersed cell culture. *J Comp Neurol* 1979; 187:469.

155. Mattson MP, Kater SB: Development and selective neurodegeneration in cell cultures from different hippocampal regions. *Brain Res* 1989; 490:110.

156. Choi DW, et al: Pharmacology of glutamate neurotoxicity in cortical cell culture: Attenuation by NMDA antagonists. *J Neurosci* 1988; 8:185.

157. Krieglstein J, et al: Cultured neurons for testing cerebroprotective drug effects in vitro. *J Pharmacol Meth* 1988; 20:39.

158. Novelli A, et al: Glutamate becomes neurotoxic via the N-methyl-D-asparate receptor when intracellular energy levels are reduced. *Brain Res* 1988; 451:205.

159. Peruche B, et al: Cultured neurons for testing antihypoxic drug effects. *J Pharmacol Meth* 1990; 23:63.

160. Seif el Nasr M, et al: Neuroprotective effect of memantine demonstrated in vivo and in vitro. *Eur Pharmacol* 1990; 185:19.

161. Atkinson DE: The energy charge of the adenylate pool as a regulatory parameter. Interaction with feed-back modifiers. *Biochemistry* 1968; 7:4030.

162. Goldberg MP, et al: N-methyl-D-asparate receptors mediate hypoxic neuronal injury in cortical culture. *J Pharmacol Exp Ther* 1987; 243:784.

163. Lysko PG, et al: Excitatory amino acid neurotoxicity at the N-methyl-D-asparate receptor in cultured neurons. *Brain Res* 1989; 499:258.

164. Pauwels PJ, et al: Effects of antimycin, glucose deprivation, and serum on cultures of neurons, astrocytes, and neuroblastoma cells. *J Neurochem* 1985; 44:143.

165. American Spinal Injury Association IM: International Standards for Neurologic and Functional Classification of Spinal Cord Injury. Chicago, 1992.

166. Michaelis LS, Braakman R: Current terminology and classification of injuries of spine and spinal cord. In Vinken PJ, Bruyn GW (eds): *Handbook of Clinical Neurology*. Amsterdam, North Holland, 1976:145.

167. Schneider RC, et al: The syndrome of acute central cervical cord injury with special reference to mechanisms involved in hyperextension injuries of cervical spine. *J Neurosurg* 1954; 11:546.

168. Schneider RC: The syndrome of anterior spinal cord injury. *J Neurosurg* 1955; 12:95.

169. Guttman L: Classification of spinal fractures. In Guttman L (ed): *Spinal Cord Injuries: Comprehensive Management and Research*. London, Blackwell, 1976:107.

170. Ducker TB, et al: Recovery from spinal cord injury. *Clin Neurosurg* 1983; 30:495.

171. Bracken MB: Pharmacological treatment of acute spinal cord injury: Current status and future projects. *J Emerg Med* 1993; 11:S43.

172. Cooper PR, et al: Dexamethasone and severe head injury. *J Neurosurg* 1979; 51:307.

173. Gudeman SK, et al: Failure of high-dose steroid therapy to influence intracranial pressure in patients with severe head injury. *J Neurosurg* 1979; 51:301.

174. Shapira Y, et al: Dexamethasone and indomethacin do not affect brain edema following head injury in rats. *J Cereb Blood Flow Metab* 1988; 8:395.

175. Tornheim PA, McLaurin RL: Effect of dexamethasone on cerebral edema from cranial impact in the cat. *J Neurosurg* 1978; 48:220.

176. Anderson DK, et al: Lipid hydrolysis and peroxidation in

injured spinal cord: Partial protection with methylprednisolone or vitamin E and selenium. *Cent Nerv Syst Trauma* 1985; 2:257.

177. Braughler J, Hall E: Correlation of methylprednisolone pharmacokinetics in cat spinal cord with its effect on (Na+-K+)ATPase, lipid peroxidation and motor neuron function. *J Neurosurg* 1981; 56:838.

178. Braughler JM, Lainer MJ: The effects of large doses of methylprednisolone on neurologic recovery and survival in the Mongolian gerbil following three hours of unilateral carotid occlusion. *Cent Nerv Syst Trauma* 1986; 3:153.

179. Hall ED, Yonkers PA: Comparison on two ester pro-drugs of methylprednisolone on early neurologic recovery in a murine closed head injury model. *J Neurotrauma* 1989; 6:163.

180. Hall ED: High-dose glucocorticoid treatment improves neurological recovery in head-injured mice. *J Neurosurg* 1985; 62:882.

181. Hall ED, et al: Effects of a single large dose of methylprednisolone sodium succinate on experimental posttraumatic spinal cord ischemia. Dose-response and time-action analysis. *J Neurosurg* 1984; 61:124.

182. Hall ED, Braughler JM: Glucocorticoid mechanisms in acute spinal cord injury: A review and therapeutic rationale. *J Neurosurg* 1982; 18:320.

183. Braughler JM, Hall ED: High dose methylprednisolone and a CNS injury. *J Neurosurg* 1988; 64:985.

184. Braughler JM, et al: Novel 21-aminosteroids as potent inhibitors of iron-dependent lipid peroxidation. *J Biol Chem* 1987; 262:10434.

185. Hall E, Braughler J: Role of lipid peroxidation in post-traumatic spinal cord degeneration—A review. *J Neurotrauma* 1986; 3:281.

186. Hall ED: The neuroprotective pharmacology of methylprednisolone. *J Neurosurg* 1992; 76:13.

187. Hall ED: Inhibition of lipid peroxidation in CNS trauma. *J Neurotrauma* 1991; 8:S31.

188. Hall ED, Braughler JM: Effects of intravenous methylprednisolone on spinal cord lipid peroxidation and (Na$^+$ + K$^+$)ATPase activity. Dose response analysis during 1st hour after contusion injury in the cat. *J Neurosurg* 1982; 57:247.

189. Anderson D, et al: Microvascular perfusion and metabolism in injured spinal cord after methylprednisolone treatment. *J Neurosurg* 1983; 56:106.

190. Means ED, et al: Effect of methylprednisolone in compression trauma to the feline spinal cord. *J Neurosurg* 1981; 55:200.

191. Young W: Blood flow, metabolic and neurophysiological mechanisms in spinal cord injury. In Becker D, Povlishock J (eds): *Central Nervous System Trauma Status Report*. Rockville, MD, National Institutes of Health, 1985:463.

192. Gianotta SL, et al: High dose glucocorticoids in the management of severe head injury. *Neurosurgery* 1984; 15:497.

193. Braughler JM, et al: A new 21-aminosteroid antioxidant lacking glucocorticoid activity stimulates adrenocorticotropin secretion and blocks arachidonic acid release from mouse pituitary tumor (AtT-20) cells. *J Pharmacol Exp Ther* 1988; 244:423.

194. Braughler JM, Pregenzer JF: The 21-aminosteroid inhibitors of lipid peroxidation: Reactions with lipid peroxy and phenoxy radicals. *Free Rad. Biol Med* 1989; 7:125.

195. Hall ED: Effects of the 21-aminosteroid U74006F on post-traumatic spinal cord ischemia in cats. *J Neurosurg* 1988; 68:462.

196. Anderson D, et al: Effects of treatment with U74006F on neurological outcome following experimental spinal cord injury. *J Neurosurg* 1988; 69:562.

197. Anderson DK, et al: Effect of delayed administration of U74006F (tirilazad mesylate) on recovery of locomotor function after experimental spinal cord injury. *J Neurotrauma* 1991; 8:187.

198. Hall E, et al: 21-aminosteroid lipid peroxidation inhibitor U74006F protects against cerebral ischemia in gerbils. *Stroke* 1988; 19:997.

199. Hall E: Beneficial effects of the 21-aminosteroid U74006F in acute central nervous system trauma in hypovolemic shock. *Acta Anaesthesiol Belg* 1987; 38:421.

200. Hall ED, et al: New pharmacological treatment of acute spinal cord trauma. *J Neurotrauma* 1988; 5:81.

201. Hall ED, Travis MA: The effects of the nonglucocorticoid 21-aminosteroid U74006F on acute cerebral hypoperfusion following experimental subarachnoid hemorrhage. *Exp Neurol* 1988; 102:244.

202. Hall ED, Braughler JM: Role of lipid peroxidation in post-traumatic spinal cord degeneration: A review. *Cent Nerv Syst Trauma* 1986; 3:281.

203. Natak JE, et al: Effect of the aminosteroid U74006F after cardiopulmonary arrest in dogs. *Stroke* 1988; 19:1371.

204. Perkins WJ, et al: Effect of a 21-aminosteroid oxygen radical scavenger on neurological outcome following complete cerebral ischemia in dogs. *J Neurosurg Anesth* 1989; 1:118.

205. Steinke DE, et al: A trial of the 21-aminosteroid U74006F in a primate model of chronic cerebral vasospasm. *Neurosurgery* 1989; 24:179.

206. Travis MA, et al: Attenuation of post-hemorrhagic and post-ischemic cerebral hypoperfusion by the 21-aminosteroid U74006F. *Soc Neurosci Abstr* 1987; 13:114.

207. Vollmer DG, et al: Effect of the nonglucocorticoid 21-aminosteroid U74006F. *Surg Neurol* 1989; 31:190.

208. Young W, et al: Pharmacological therapy of acute spinal cord injury: Studies of high dose methylprednisolone and naloxone. *Clin Neurosurg* 1988; 34:675.

209. Zuccarello M, et al: Effect of the 21-aminosteroid U-74006F on cerebral vasospasm following subarachnoid hemorrhage. *J Neurosurg* 1980; 71:98.

210. Hall ED, et al: Effects of the 21-aminosteroid U74006F on experimental head injury in mice. *J Neurosurg* 1988; 68:456.

211. Hall ED, et al: Biochemistry and pharmacology of lipid antioxidants in acute brain and spinal cord injury. *J Neurotrauma* 1992; 9(suppl 2):S425.

212. McIntosh TK, et al: The novel 21-aminosteroid U74006F attenuates cerebral edema and improves survival after brain injury in the rat. *J Neurotrauma* 1992; 9:33.

213. Zukin RS, Zukin SR: Multiple opiate receptors: Emerging concepts. *Life Sci* 1981; 29:2681.

214. Cox B: Endogenous opioid peptides: A guide to structures and terminology. *Life Sci* 1982; 31:1655.

215. Faden AI: Role of thyrotropin-releasing hormone and opiate receptor antagonists in limiting central nervous system injury. *Adv Neurol* 1988; 47:531.

216. Faden AI: Neuropeptides and central nervous system injury. *Arch Neurol* 1986; 43:501.

217. Faden AI, et al: Opiate antagonist improves neurologic recovery after spinal injury. *Science* 1981; 211:493.

218. Faden AI, et al: Thyrotropin-releasing hormone improves neurologic recovery after spinal trauma in cats. *J Engl J Med* 1981; 305:1063.

219. Flamm ES, et al: Experimental spinal cord injury: Treatment with naloxone. *Neurosurgery* 1982; 10:227.

220. Holaday JW, Faden AI: Naloxone acts as central opiate receptors to reverse hypotension, hypothermia and hypoventilation in spinal shock. *Brain Res* 1980; 189:295.

221. Young W, et al: Effect of naloxone on post-traumatic ischemia in experimental spinal contusion. *J Neurosurg* 1981; 55:209.

222. Faden AI, et al: Opiate-receptor antagonist nalmefene improves neurological recovery after traumatic spinal cord injury

in rats through a central mechanism. *J Pharmacol Exp Ther* 1988; 245:742.

223. Panter SS, et al: Alteration in extracellular amino acids after traumatic spinal cord injury (see comments). *Ann Neurol* 1990; 27:96.

224. Hayes RL, et al: Effects of naloxone on systemic and cerebral responses to experimental concussive brain injury in cats. *J Neurosurg* 1983; 58:720.

225. McIntosh TK, et al: The effects of naloxone hydrochloride treatment after experimental traumatic brain injury in the rat. *J Cereb Blood Flow Metab* 1991; 11(suppl 2):S734.

226. Robinson SE, et al: The effect of naloxone pretreatment on behavioral responses to concussive brain injury in the rat. *Neurosci Abstr* 1988; 2:1254.

227. Bracken MB, Holford TR: Effects of timing of methylprednisolone or naloxone administration on recovery of segmental and long-tract neurological function in NASCIS 2. *J Neurosurg* 1993; 79:500.

228. Bose B, et al: Ganglioside-induced regeneration and reestablishment of axonal continuity in spinal cord-transected rats. *Neurosci Lett* 1986; 63:165.

229. Fishman PH, Brady RO: Biosynthesis and function of gangliosides. *Science* 1976; 164:906.

230. Ledeen RW: Ganglioside structures and distribution: Are they localized at the nerve ending? *J Supramol Struct* 1978; 8:1.

231. Weigandt H: Glycosphingolipids. *Adv Lipid Res* 1971; 9:249.

232. Agnati LF, et al: Gangliosides increase the survival of lesioned nigral dopamine neurons and favor the recovery of dopaminergic synaptic function in striatum of rats. *Acta Physiol Scand* 1983; 119:347.

233. Ceccareli B, et al: Effects of brain gangliosides in functional recovery in experimental regeneration and reinnervation. In Porcellati G, et al. (eds): *Advances in Experimental Medicine and Biology*. New York, Plenum Press, 1976; 71:275.

234. Di Gregorio F, et al: The influence of gangliosides on neurite growth and regeneration. *Neuropediatrics* 1984; 15:93.

235. Epstein N, et al: Gastrointestinal bleeding in patients with spinal cord trauma. Effects of steroids, cimetidine, and minidose heparin. *J Neurosurg* 1981; 54:16.

236. Fass B, Ramirez J: Effects of ganglioside treatments on lesion induced behavioral impairments and sprouting in the CNS. *J Neurosci Res* 1984; 14:445.

237. Gorio A: Gangliosides as a possible treatment affecting neuronal repair process. *Adv Neurol* 1988; 47:523.

238. Gorio A: Ganglioside enhancement of neuronal differentiation, plasticity, and repair. *CRC Crit Rev Clin Neurobiol* 1986; 2:241.

239. Gorio A, et al: Gangliosides and their effects on rearranging peripheral and central neural pathways. *Cent Nerv Syst Trauma* 1984; 1:29.

240. Gorio A, et al: Motor nerve sprouting induced by ganglioside treatment. *Brain Res* 1980; 197:236.

241. Karpiak SE, et al: Ganglioside treatment: Reduction of CNS injury and facilitation of functional recovery. *Brain Inj* 1982; 1:161.

242. Kojima H, et al: GM1 ganglioside enhances regrowth of noradrenaline nerve terminals in rat cerebral cortex lesioned by neurotoxin 6-hydroxydopamine. *Neuroscience* 1984; 13:1011.

243. Ledeen RW: Biology of gangliosides: Neuritogenic and neuronotrophic properties. *J Neurosci Res* 1984; 12:147.

244. Roison FJ, et al: Ganglioside stimulation of axonal sprouting in vitro. *Science* 1981; 214:577.

245. Rybak S, et al: Gangliosides stimulate neurite outgrowth and induce tubuline mRNA accumulation in neural cells. *Biochem Biophys Res Commun* 1983; 116:974.

246. Sabel BA: Anatomic mechanisms whereby gangliosides induce brain repair: What do we really know. In Stein D, Sabel B (eds): *Pharmacological Approaches to the Treatment of Brain and Spinal Cord Injury*. New York, Plenum Press, 1988:67.

247. Sabel BA, et al: Reduction of anterograde degeneration in brain damaged rats by GM1-gangliosides. *Neurosci Lett* 1987; 77:360.

248. Sabel BA, Stein DG: Pharmacological treatment of central nervous system injury. *Nature* 1986; 323:493.

249. Sabel BA, et al: Gangliosides minimize behavioral deficits and enhance structural repair after brain injury. *J Neurosci Res* 1984; 12:429.

250. Sabel BA, et al: GM1 ganglioside treatment facilitates behavioral recovery from bilateral brain damage. *Science* 1984; 225:340.

251. Skaper SD, Leon A: Monosialogangliosides, neuroprotection and neuronal repair processes. *J Neurotrauma* 1992; 9:S507.

252. Toffano G, et al: Effects of gangliosides on the functional recovery of damaged brain. *Adv Exp Med Biol* 1984; 174:475.

253. Toffano G, et al: GM1-ganglioside stimulates the regeneration of dopaminergic neurons in the central nervous system. *Brain Res* 1983; 261:163.

254. Walker MD: Acute spinal cord injury. *N Engl J Med* 1991; 324:1885 (editorial).

255. Karpiak S: Ganglioside treatment improved recovery of alternation behavior after unilateral entorhinal lesion. *Exp Neurol* 1983; 81:330.

256. Ramirez JJ, et al: Ganglioside treatments reduce locomotor hyperactivity after bilateral lesions of the entorhinal cortex. *Neurosci Lett* 1987; 75:283.

257. Ramirez JJ, et al: Gangliosides induce enhancement of behavioral recovery after bilateral lesions of the entorhinal cortex. *Brain Res* 1987; 414:85.

258. Shigemori M, et al: Effect of monosialoganglioside (GM1) on transected monoaminergic pathways. *J Neurotrauma* 1990; 7:89.

259. Carolei A, et al: Monosialoganglioside GM1 in cerebral ischemia. *Cerebrovasc Brain Metab* 1991; 3:134.

260. Karpiak S, Mahadik S: Reduction of cerebral edema with GM1-ganglioside. *J Neurosci Res* 1984; 12:485.

261. Karpiak SE, Li YS, Mahadik SP: Acute ganglioside effects limit CNS injury. In Stein DG, Sabel BA (eds): *Pharmacological Approaches to the Treatment of Brain and Spinal Cord Injury*. New York, Plenum Press, 1988:219.

262. Nicoletti F: Gangliosides attenuate NMDA receptor-mediated excitatory amino acid release in cultured cerebellar neurons. *Neuropharmacology* 1989; 28:1283.

263. Ramirez JJ, et al: Enhanced recovery of learned alternation in ganglioside-treated rats after unilateral entorhinal lesions. *Behav Brain Res.* 1991; 43:99.

264. McLennan H: Receptors for the excitatory amino acid in the mammalian CNS. *Prog Neurobiol* 1983; 20:251.

265. Coyle J: Neurotoxic action of kainic acid. *J Neurochem* 1983; 41:1.

266. Lucas DR, Newhouse JP: The toxic effect of sodium glutamate on the inner layers of the retina. *Arch Ophthalmol* 1957; 158:193.

267. Olney JW: Neurotoxicity of excitatory amino acids. In McGeer EG (ed): *Kainic Acid as a Tool in Neurobiology*. New York, Raven Press, 1978:95.

268. Olney JW: Glutamate-induced retinal degeneration in neonatal mice: Electron microscopy of the actively evolving lesion. *Science* 1969; 164:719.

269. Olney JW, et al: Cytotoxic effects of acidic and sulphur-containing amino acid on the infant mouse central nervous system. *Exp Brain Res* 1971; 14:61.

270. Rothman SM, Olney JW: Excitotoxicity and the NMDA receptor. *Trends Neurosci* 1987; 10:299.

271. Rothman SM, Olney JW: Glutamate and the pathophysiology of hypoxic-ischemic brain damage. *Ann Neurol* 1986; 19:105.

272. Choi D: Calcium-mediated neurotoxicity: Relationship to specific channel types and its role in ischemic damage. *Trends Neurosci* 1989; 11:21.

273. Choi D: Ionic dependence of glutamate neurotoxicity. *J Neurosci* 1987; 7:369.

274. Benveniste H: The excitotoxic hypothesis in relation to cerebral ischemia. *Cerebrovasc Brain Metab Rev* 1991; 3:213.

275. Benveniste H, et al: Ischemic damage in hippocampal CA1 is dependent on glutamate release and intact innervation from CA_3. *J Cereb Blood Flow Metab* 1990; 59:1.

276. Buchan AM: Do NMDA antagonists protect against cerebral ischemia: Are clinical trials warranted? *Brain Metab Rev* 1990; 2:1.

277. Ferriero DM, et al: Selective sparing of NADPH-diaphorase neurons in neonatal hypoxia-ischemia. *Ann Neurol* 1988; 24:670.

278. Ikonomidou C, et al: Hypobaric-ischemic conditions produce glutamate-like cytopathology in infant rat brain. *J Neurosci* 1989; 9:1693.

279. Kochhar A, et al: Glutamate antagonist therapy reduces neurologic deficits produced by focal central nervous system ischemia. *Arch Neurol* 1988; 45:148.

280. Kohmura E, et al: Hippocampal neurons become more vulnerable to glutamate after subcritical hypoxia: An in vitro study. *Blood Flow Metab* 1990; 10:877.

281. Meldrum B: Possible therapeutic applications of antagonists of excitatory amino acid transmitters. *Clin Sci* 1985; 68:113.

282. Onodera H, et al: Excitatory amino acid binding sites in the rat hippocampus after transient forebrain ischemia. *J Cereb Blood Flow Metab* 1989; 9:623.

283. Tombaugh GC, Sapolsky RM: Mechanistic distinctions between excitotoxic and acidotic hippocampal damage in an *in vitro* model of ischemia. *J Cereb Blood Flow Metab* 1990; 10:527.

284. Westerberg E, et al: Dynamic changes of excitatory amino acid receptors in the rat hippocampus following transient cerebral ischemia. *J Neurosci* 1989; 9:798.

285. Wieloch T: Hypoglycemia-induced neuronal damage prevented by an *N*-methyl-*D*-asparate antagonist. *Science* 1985; 230:681.

286. Ault B, et al: Selective depression of excitatory amino acid induced depolarizations by magnesium ions in isolated spinal cord preparations. *J Physiol* 1980; 307:413.

287. Cox JA, et al: Excitatory amino acid neurotoxicity at the *N*-methyl-*D*-asparate receptor in cultured neurons: Role of the voltage-dependent magnesium block. *Brain Res* 1989; 499:267.

288. Fagg G: *L*-glutamate, excitatory amino acid receptors and brain function. *Trends Neurosci* 1985; 2:207.

289. Mayer ML, et al: Voltage-dependent block by Mg^{++} of NMDA receptors in spinal cord neurons. *Nature* 1984; 261:263.

290. Nowak L, et al: Magnesium gates glutamate-activated channels in mouse central neurons. *Nature* 1984; 307:462.

291. Stanfield PR: Intracellular Mg^{2+} may act as a cofactor in ion channel function. *Trends Neurosci* 1988; 11:475.

292. Choi D: Methods for antagonizing glutamate neurotoxicity. *Cerebrovasc Brain Metab Rev* 1990; 2:105.

293. Choi D: The role of glutamate neurotoxicity in hypoxic-ischemic neuronal death. *Annu Rev Neurosci* 1990; 13:171.

294. Faden AI, et al: The role of excitatory amino acids and NMDA receptors in traumatic brain injury. *Science* 1989; 244:798.

295. Katayama Y, et al: Preoperative determination of the level of spinal cord lesions from the killed end potential. *Surg Neurol* 1988; 29:91.

296. Nilsson P, et al: Changes in cortical extracellular levels of energy-related metabolites and amino acids following concussive brain injury in rats. *J Cereb Blood Flow Metab* 1990; 10:631.

297. Seisjo BK: Mechanisms of ischemic brain damage. *Crit Care Med* 1988; 16:954.

298. Miller AJ: Multiple calcium channels and neuronal function. *Science* 1987; 235:46.

299. Seisjo BK: Historical overview: Calcium, ischemia and death of brain cells. *Ann N Y Acad Sci* 1988; 522:638.

300. Young W: The post-injury response in trauma and ischemia. Secondary injury or protective mechanisms? *J Neurotrauma* 1987; 4:27.

301. Feuerstein G, et al: Calcium channel blockers and neuroprotection. In Marangos PJ, Lal H (eds): *Emerging Strategies in Neuroprotection*. Birkhauser, 1994:129.

302. Fehlings MG, et al: The effect of nimodipine and dextran on axonal function and blood flow following experimental spinal cord injury. *J Neurosurg* 1989; 71:403.

303. Guha A, et al: Improvement in post-traumatic spinal cord blood flow with a combination of a calcium channel blocker and a vasopressor. *J Trauma* 1989; 29:1440.

304. Guha A, et al: Effect of a calcium channel blocker on posttraumatic spinal cord blood flow. *J Neurosurg* 1987; 66:423.

305. Ross IB, et al: Effect of nimodipine or methylprednisolone on recovery from acute experimental spinal cord injury in rats. *Surg Neurol* 1993; 40:461.

306. Ross IB, Tator CH: Further studies of nimodipine in experimental spinal cord injury in the rat. *J Neurotrauma* 1991; 8:229.

307. Chan P, Fishman R: Transient formation of superoxide radicals in polyunsaturated fatty acid induced brain swelling. *J Neurochem* 1980; 35:1004.

308. Kontos H, Povlishock J: Oxygen radicals in brain injury. *J Neurotrauma* 1986; 3:257.

309. Demopoulos HB, et al: Oxygen free radicals in central nervous system ischemia and trauma. In Autor AP (ed): *Pathology of Oxygen*. London, Academic Press, 1982:127.

310. Kontos HA: Oxygen radicals in cerebral vascular injury. *Circ Res* 1985; 57:508.

311. Lundgren J, et al: Acidosis-induced ischemic brain damage: Are free radicals involved? *J Cereb Blood Flow Metab* 1991; 11:587.

312. Hall ED, Wolf DL: A pharmacological analysis of the pathophysiological mechanisms of post-traumatic spinal cord ischemia. *J Neurosurg* 1986; 64:951.

313. Hsu C, et al: Increased thromboxane level in experimental spinal cord injury. *J Neurol Sci* 1986; 74:289.

314. Hsu C, et al: Alterations of thromboxane and protacyclin levels in experimental spinal cord injury. *Neurology* 1985; 35:1003.

315. Pielronigra DD, et al: Loss of ascorbic acid from injured feline spinal cord. *J Neurochem* 1983; 41:1072.

316. Xu J, et al: Xanthine oxidase in experimental spinal cord injury. *J Neurotrauma* 1991; 8:11.

317. Kontos HA: Oxygen radicals in central nervous system damage. *Chem Biol Interact* 1989; 72:229.

318. Seisjo B, Wieloch T: Brain injury: Neurochemical aspects. In Becker DP, Povlishock J (eds): *Central Nervous System Trauma Status Report*. Bethesda, MD, National Institute of Neurological and Communicative Disorders and Stroke, National Institutes of Health, 1985:513.

319. Chan P, et al: Protective effects of liposome-entrapped superoxide dismutase on post-traumatic brain edema. *Ann Neurol* 1987; 21:540.

320. Yoshida S, et al: Compression-induced brain edema: Modification by prior depletion and supplementation of vitamin E. *Neurology* 1983; 33:166.

321. Clifton GL, et al: Effect of D_1a-tocopheryl succinate and polyethylene glycol on performance tests after fluid percussion brain injury. *J Neurotrauma* 1989; 6:71.

322. Hall ED, Yonkers PA: Mechanisms of neuronal degeneration

secondary to central nervous system trauma or ischemia. *J Neurotrauma* 1989; 6:227 (letter).

323. Abe K, et al: Strong attenuation of ischemic and postischemic brain edema in rats by a novel free radical scavenger. *Stroke* 1988; 19:480.

324. Yamamoto M, et al: A possible role of lipid peroxidation in cellular damage caused by cerebral ischemia and the protective effect of a-tocopherol administration. *Stroke* 1983; 14:977.

325. Yoshida S, et al: Postischemic cerebral lipid peroxidation in vitro: Modification by dietary vitamin E. *J Neurochem* 1985; 44:1593.

326. Saunders RD, et al: Effects of methylprednisolone and the combination of a-tocopherol and selenium on arachidonic acid metabolism and lipid peroxidation in traumatized spinal cord tissue. *J Neurochem* 1987; 49:24.

327. Forsman M, et al: Superoxide dismutase and catalase failed to improve neurologic outcome after complete cerebral ischemia in the dog. *Acta Anaesthesiol Scand* 1988; 32:152.

328. Liu TH, et al: Polyethylene-glycol-conjugated superoxide dismutase and catalase reduce ischemic brain injury. *Am J Physiol* 1989; 256:H589.

329. Martz D, et al: Dimethyl thiourea reduces ischemic brain edema without affecting cerebral blood flow. *J Cereb Blood Flow Metab* 1990; 10:352.

330. Matsumiya N, et al: Conjugated superoxide dismutase reduces extent of caudate injury after transient focal ischemia in cats. *Stroke* 1991; 22:1193.

331. Coles JC, et al: Role of radical scavenger in protection of spinal cord during ischemia. *Ann Thorac Surg* 1986; 41:555.

332. Lim KH, et al: Prevention of reperfusion injury of the ischemic spinal cord: Use of recombinant superoxide dismutase. *Ann Thorac Surg* 1986; 42:282.

333. Roy R, et al: Allopurinol minimizes histological changes in spinal cord injury. *Scientific Program of the 62nd Annual Meeting of the American Association of Neurological Surgeons.* 1994:124.

334. Bracken MB, et al: Methylprednisolone and neurological function 1 year after spinal cord injury. Results of the National Acute Spinal Cord Injury Study. *J Neurosurg* 1985; 63:704.

335. Bracken MB, et al: Efficacy of methylprednisolone in acute spinal cord injury. *JAMA* 1984; 251:45.

336. Geisler FH: GM-1 ganglioside and motor recovery following human spinal cord injury. *J Emerg Med* 1993; 11:S49.

337. Geisler FH, et al: Past and current clinical studies with GM-1 ganglioside in acute spinal cord injury. *Ann Emerg Med* 1993; 22:1041.

338. Geisler FH, et al: GM-1 ganglioside in human spinal cord injury. *J Neurotrauma* 1992; 9:S407.

339. Geisler FH, et al: Correction: Recovery of motor function after spinal-cord injury—A randomized, placebo-controlled trial with GM-1 ganglioside. *N Engl J Med* 1991; 325:1659 (letter).

340. Geisler FH, et al: Recovery of motor function after spinal-cord injury—A randomized, placebo-controlled trial with GM-1 ganglioside. *N Engl J Med* 1991; 324:1829.

341. Braughler JM, Hall ED: Lactate and pyruvate metabolism in injured cat spinal cord before and after a single large intravenous dose of methylprednisolone. *J Neurosurg* 1983; 59:256.

342. Hall E, et al: Effects of a single large dose of methylprednisolone sodium succinate on posttraumatic spinal cord ischemia: Dose-response and time-action analysis. *J Neurosurg* 1984; 61:124.

343. Hall E, Braughler J: Glucocorticoid mechanisms in acute spinal cord injury: A review and therapeutic rational. *Surg Neurol* 1988; 18:320.

344. Bracken MB: Methylprednisolone in the management of acute spinal cord injuries. *Med J Aust* 1990; 153:368 (letter).

345. Bracken MB: Steroids after spinal cord injury. Methylpredniso-

lone in the management of acute spinal cord injuries. *Lancet* 1990; 336:279 (letter).

346. Ducker TB, et al: Spinal cord injury and glucocortical steroid therapy: Good news and bad. *J Spinal Disord* 1990; 3:433.

347. Hanigan WC, Anderson RJ: Commentary on NASCIS-2. *J Spinal Disord* 1992; 5:125.

348. Rosner MJ: Methylprednisolone for spinal cord injury. *J Neurosurg* 1992; 77:324 (letter/comment).

349. Rosner MJ: National acute spinal cord injury study of methylprednisolone or naloxone. *Neurosurgery* 1991; 28:628 (letter).

350. Taylor TK, Ryan MD: Methylprednisolone in the management of acute spinal cord injuries. *Med J Aust* 1990; 153:307.

351. Rosner MJ: Treatment of spinal cord injury. *J Neurosurg* 1994; 80:954 (letter).

352. Galandiuk S, et al: The two-edged sword of large-dose steroids for spinal cord trauma. *Ann Surg* 1993; 218:419.

353. Travlos A, Hirsch G: Steroid psychosis: A cause of confusion on the acute spinal cord injury unit. *Arch Phys Med Rehabil* 1993; 74:312.

354. Geisler FH, et al: GM-1 ganglioside in human spinal cord injury. *J Neurotrauma* 1992; 9:S517.

355. Anonymous: Standards for neurological and functional classification of spinal cord injury. Proceedings endorsed by the International Medical Society of Paraplegia Annual Meeting, Barcelona, Spain, September 7, 1992. American Spinal Injury Association, International Medical Society of Paraplegia. 1994.

356. DiGregorio F, et al: The influence of gangliosides on neurite growth and regeneration. *Neuropediatrics* 1994; 15:93.

357. Young W: Recovery mechanisms in spinal cord injury: Implications for regenerative therapy. In Seil FJ (ed): *Neural Regeneration and Transplantation.* New York, Alan R. Liss, 1989:157.

358. Boyeson MG, Harmon RL: Effects of trazodone and desipramine on motor recovery in brain-injured rats. *Am J Phys Med Rehabil* 1993; 72:286.

359. Meinecke FW: Frequency and distribution of associated injuries in traumatic paraplegia and tetraplegia. *Paraplegia* 1968; 5:196.

360. Roscher R, et al: Pulmonary contusion. *Arch Surg* 1974; 109:508.

361. Sutherland GR, et al: Anatomic and cardiopulmonary responses to trauma with associated blunt chest injury. *J Trauma* 1981; 21:1.

362. Smith JP, et al: The esophageal obturator airway. *JAMA* 1983; 250:1081.

363. Brach BB, et al: 33-Xenon washout patterns during diaphragmatic breathing. Studies in normal subjects and patients with chronic obstructive pulmonary disease. *Chest* 1977; 71:735.

364. Fugl-Meyer AR: Effects of respiratory muscle paralysis in tetraplegic and paraplegic patients. *Scand J Rehabil Med* 1971; 3:141.

365. Altose MD: Pulmonary mechanics. In Fishman AP (ed): *Pulmonary Diseases and Disorders.* New York, McGraw-Hill, 1980:359.

366. Agostoni E: Action of respiratory muscles. In Fenn WO, Rhan H (eds): *Handbook of Physiology.* American Physiology Society, Washington, DC, 1964:377.

367. Ledsome JR, Sharp JM: Pulmonary function in acute cervical cord injury. *Am Rev Respir Dis* 1981; 124:41.

368. Tibbs PA, et al: Studies of experimental cervical spinal cord transection. Part I. Hemodynamic changes after acute cervical spinal cord transection. *J Neurosurg* 1978; 49:558.

369. Albin MS, et al: Brain and lungs at risk after cervical spinal cord transection: Intracranial pressure, brain water, blood-brain barrier permeability, cerebral blood flow, and extravascular lung water changes. *Surg Neurol* 1985; 24:191.

370. Mackenzie CF, Shin B: Cardiac effects of atropine in bradycardic quadriplegics during spinal shock. *Crit Care Med* 1981; 9:150.

371. Mackenzie CF, et al: Assessment of cardiac and respiratory function during surgery on patients with acute quadriplegia. *J Neurosurg* 1985; 62:843.

372. Sibbald WJ, et al: The Trendelenberg position: Hemodynamic effects in hypotensive and normotensive patients. *Crit Care Med* 1979; 7:218.

373. Reed JH, Wood EH: Effect of body position on vertical distribution of pulmonary blood flow. *J Appl Physiol* 1970; 218:303.

374. Wilkins RW, et al: The acute circulatory effects of the head-down position (negative G) in normal man with a note on some measures designed to relieve cranial congestion in this position. *J Clin Invest* 1950; 29:940.

375. Taylor J, Weil H: Failure of the Trendelenberg position to improve circulation during clinical shock. *JAMA* 1967; 124:1005.

376. Haas F, et al: Time related posturally induced changes in pulmonary function in spinal cord injured man. *Am Rev Respir Dis* 1978; 117:344.

377. Cameron GS, et al: Diaphragmatic respiration in the quadriplegic patient and the effect of position on his vital capacity. *Ann Surg* 1955; 141:451.

378. Wolman L: The disturbance of circulation in traumatic paraplegia in acute and late stages: A pathological study. *Paraplegia* 1965; 2:213.

379. Meyer GA, et al: Hemodynamic responses to acute quadriplegia with or without chest trauma. *J Neurosurg* 1971; 34:168.

380. Pitts LH: The management of cervical and spinal cord trauma. *American Society of Anesthesiology Annual Refresher Course Lecture* 1981; 121:4.

381. Dolan EJ, Tator CH: The treatment of hypotension due to acute experimental spinal cord compression injury. *Surg Neurol* 1980; 13:380.

382. Horowitz D, et al: Increased blood pressure responses to dopamine and norepinephrine produced by monoamine oxidase inhibitors in man. *J Lab Clin Med* 1960; 56:747.

383. Li TH, et al: Methoxamine and cardiac output in nonanesthetized man and during spinal anesthesia. *Anesthesiology* 1965; 26:21.

384. Smith NT, Corbascio AN: The use and misuse of pressor agents. *Anesthesiology* 1970; 33:58.

385. Greene NM: *Physiology of Spinal Anesthesia*. Baltimore, Williams & Wilkins, 1981.

386. Greene NM, Bachaud RG: Vagal components of the chronotropic response to baroreceptor stimulation in man. *Am Heart J* 1971; 82:22.

387. O'Rourke GW, Greene NM: Autonomic blockade and the resting heart rate in man. *Am Heart J* 1970; 80:469.

388. Graves CL, et al: Intravenous fluid administration as therapy for hypotension secondary to spinal anesthesia. *Anesth Analg* 1968; 47:548.

389. Cowley RA, et al: An economical and proven helicopter program for transporting the emergency critically ill and injured patient in Maryland. *J Trauma* 1973; 13:1029.

390. Anonymous: *Shock Trauma/Critical Care Handbook*. Rockville, MD, Aspen, 1986.

391. Soderstrom CA, et al: The diagnosis of intraabdominal injury in patients with cervical cord trauma. *J Trauma* 1983; 23:1061.

392. Soderstrom CA, Brumback RJ: Early care of the patient with cervical spine injury. *Orthop Clin North Am* 1986; 17:3.

393. Guttman L: Patterns of reflex disturbances. In Guttman L (ed): *Spinal Cord Injuries: Comprehensive Management and Research*, 2d ed. London, Blackwell, 1976:243.

394. Rocco AG, Vandam LD: Problems in anesthesia for paraplegics. *Anesthesiology* 1959; 20:348.

395. Sokoll MD: Anesthetic management of patients with spinal cord injuries. Lecture. *American Society of Anesthesiology Annual Refresher Course, St Louis,* 1980; 131:1.

396. Sellick BA: Cricoid pressure to control regurgitation of stomach contents during induction of anaesthesia. *Lancet* 1961; 2:404.

397. Caplan ES, Hoyt NJ: Nosocomial sinusitis. *JAMA* 1982; 247:639.

398. John DA, et al: Onset of succinylcholine induced hyperkalemia following denervation. *Anesthesiology* 1976; 45:294.

399. Snow JC, et al: Cardiovascular collapse following succinylcholine in a paraplegic patient. *Paraplegia* 1973; 11:109.

400. Stone WA, et al: Succinylcholine—Danger in the spinal cord injured patient. *Anesthesiology* 1970; 32:168.

401. Stone WA, et al: Succinylcholine-induced hyperkalemia in dogs with transected sciatic nerves or spinal cords. *Anesthesiology* 1970; 32:515.

402. Tobey RE, et al: The serum potassium response to muscle relaxants in neural injury. *Anesthesiology* 1972; 37:332.

403. Tobey RE: Paraplegia, succinylcholine and cardiac arrest. *Anesthesiology* 1970; 32:359.

404. Axelsson J, Thesleff S: A study of supersensitivity in denervated mammalian skeletal muscle. *J Physiol* 1957; 149:178.

405. Harris EJ, Nicholls JG: The effect of denervation on the rate of entry of potassium into the frog muscle. *J Physiol* 1956; 131:473.

406. Smith RB: Hyperkalemia following succinylcholine administration in neurological disorders: A review. *Can Anaesth Soc J* 1971; 18:199.

407. Quimby CW, et al: Anesthetic problems of the acute quadriplegic patient. *Anesth Analg* 1973; 52:333.

408. Alderson JD, Thomas DG: The use of halothane anesthesia to control autonomic hyperreflexia during trans-urethral surgery in spinal cord injury patients. *Paraplegia* 1975; 13:183.

409. Drinker AS, Helrich M: Halothane anesthesia in the paraplegic patient. *Anesthesiology* 1963; 24:399.

410. Schreibman DL, Mackenzie CF: The trauma victim with acute spinal cord injury. In Matjasko MJ, Shin B (eds): *Problems in Anesthesia*, 3rd ed. Philadelphia, JB Lippincott, 1994:459.

411. Ahn JH, et al: Current trends in stabilizing high thoracic and thoracolumbar spinal fractures. *Arch Phys Med Rehab* 1984; 65:366.

412. Tator CH, et al: Comparison of surgical and conservative management in 208 patients with acute spinal cord injury. *Can J Neurol Sci* 1987; 14:60.

413. Bedbrook G: Recovery of spinal cord function. *Paraplegia* 1980; 18:315.

414. Ducker TB, Saul TS: The poly-trauma and spinal cord injury. In Tator CH (ed): *Early Management of Acute Spinal Cord Injury*. New York, Raven Press, 1982:53.

415. Duh M, et al: The effectiveness of surgery on the treatment of acute spinal cord injury and its relation to pharmacological treatment. *Neurosurgery* 1935; 35:240.

416. Guttman L: *Spinal Cord Injuries: Comprehensive Management and Research*. London, Blackwell, 1976.

417. Guttman L: Initial treatment of traumatic paraplegia and tetraplegia. In Anonymous (ed): *Spinal Injuries Symposium*. Edinburgh, Morrison & Gibb, Ltd., Royal College of Surgeons, 1963:80.

418. Dall DM: Injuries of the cervical spine. II. Does anatomical reduction of the bony injuries improve the prognosis for spinal cord recovery? *S Afr Med J* 1972; 46:1083.

419. Harris P, et al: The prognosis of patients sustaining severe cervical spine injury (C2–C7 inclusive). *Paraplegia* 1980; 18:324.

420. Dolan EJ, et al: The value of decompression for acute experimental spinal cord compression injury. *J Neurosurg* 1980; 53:749.

421. Guha A, et al: Decompression of the spinal cord improves

recovery after acute experimental spinal cord compression injury. *Paraplegia* 1987; 25:324.

422. Hung TK, et al: Stress strain relationship and neurological sequelae of uniaxial elongation of the spinal cord of cats. *Surg Neurol* 1975; 15:471.

423. Noyes DH, Bresnahan JC: Correlation between spinal cord lesion volume and impact parameters. *Proc Biophys Soc* 1981; 33:H12.

424. Panjabi MM: Experimental spinal cord trauma. A biomechanical viewpoint. *Paraplegia* 1987; 25:217.

425. Rivlin AS, Tator CH: Effect of duration of acute spinal cord compression in a new acute cord injury model in the rat. *Surg Neurol* 1978; 10:38.

426. Gillingham J: Early management of spinal cord trauma. *J Neurosurg* 1976; 44:766 (letter).

427. Hall ED, et al: Correlation between attenuation of posttraumatic spinal cord ischemia and preservation of tissue vitamin E by the 21-aminosteroid U74006F: Evidence for an in vivo antioxidant mechanism. *J Neurotrama* 1989; 6:169.

428. Sussman BJ: Early management of spinal cord trauma. *J Neurosurg* 1976; 44:766 (letter).

429. Wolf A, et al: Operative management of bilateral facet dislocation. *J Neurosurg* 1991; 75:883.

430. Braakman R: Some neurological and neurosurgical aspects of injuries of the lower cervical spine. *Acta Neurochir (Wien)* 1970; 22:245.

431. Heiden JS, et al: Management of cervical spine cord trauma in Southern California. *J Neurosurg* 1975; 43:732.

432. Marshall LF, et al: Deterioration following spinal cord injury. A multicenter study. *J Neurosurg* 1987; 66:400.

433. Horsey WJ, et al: Experience with early anterior operation in acute injuries of the cervical spine. *Paraplegia* 1977; 15:110.

434. Wilberger JE: Diagnosis and management of spinal cord trauma. *J Neurotrauma* 1991; 8:S21.

435. Klain M, et al: Is jet ventilation without a cuffed tube safe? *Anesth Analg* 1982; 61:195.

436. Sjostrand UH, Erikkson A: High rates and low volumes in mechanical ventilation—Not just a matter of ventilatory frequency. *Anesth Analg* 1980; 59:567.

437. Mackenzie CF, et al: Changes in total lung/thorax compliance following chest physiotherapy. *Anesth Analg* 1980; 59:207.

438. Tibballs J: Diaphragmatic pacing: An alternative to long-term mechanical ventilation. *Anaesth Intensive Care* 1991; 19:597.

439. Glenn WW, et al: Long-term ventilatory support by diaphragm pacing in quadriplegia. *Ann Surg* 1976; 183:566.

440. Miller JI, et al: Phrenic nerve pacing of the quadriplegic patient. *J Thorac Cardiovasc Surg* 1990; 99:35.

441. Mackenzie CF: Clinical usage and chest physiotherapy indications for acute lung pathology. In Mackenzie CF (ed): *Chest Physiotherapy in the Intensive Care Unit,* 2nd ed. Baltimore, Williams & Wilkins, 1989:53.

442. McMichan JC, et al: Pulmonary dysfunction following traumatic quadriplegia. *JAMA* 1980; 243:528.

443. Bake B, et al: Breathing patterns and regional ventilation distribution in tetraplegic patients and in normal subjects. *Clin Sci* 1972; 42:117.

444. Bergofsky EH: Mechanisms for respiratory insufficiency after cervical cord injury. *Ann Intern Med* 1964; 61:435.

445. Haas A, et al: Impairment of respiration after spinal cord injury. *Arch Phys Med Rehabil* 1965; 46:399.

446. Odry A, et al: Alterations in pulmonary function in spinal cord injured patients. *Paraplegia* 1975; 13:101.

447. Stone DJ, Keltz H: The effect of respiratory muscle dysfunction on pulmonary function. *Am Rev Respir Dis* 1963; 88:621.

448. Bellamy R, et al: Respiratory complications in traumatic quadriplegia. *J Neurosurg* 1973; 39:596.

449. Cheshire DJE: Respiratory management in acute traumatic tetraplegia. *Paraplegia* 1964; 1:252.

450. Ciesla N: Chest physiotherapy for special patients. In Mackenzie CF (ed): *Chest Physiotherapy in the Intensive Care Unit,* 2nd ed. Baltimore: Williams & Wilkins, 1989:251.

451. Ciesla N: Postural drainage, positioning and breathing exercises. In Mackenzie CF (ed): *Chest Physiotherapy in the Intensive Care Unit,* 2nd ed. Baltimore: Williams & Wilkins, 1989:93.

452. Frownfelter DL: *Chest Physical Therapy and Pulmonary Rehabilitation.* Chicago: Year Book Medical Publishers, 1978.

453. Hietpas BG, et al: Huff coughing and airway patency. *Respir Care* 1979; 24:710.

454. Gaskell DV, Webber BA: *The Brompton Hospital Guide to Chest Physiotherapy.* London, Blackwell, 1973.

455. Marshall R, Holden WS: Changes in calibre of the smaller airways in man. *Thorax* 1963; 18:54.

456. Guttman L: Respiratory disturbances. In Guttman L (ed): *Spinal Cord Injuries: Comprehensive Management and Research,* 2nd ed. London, Blackwell, 1976:209.

457. Wade L: Movements of the thoracic cage and diaphragm in respiration. *J Physiol* 1954; 124:193.

458. Fugl-Meyer AR: Injuries to the spine and spinal cord. In Braakman R (ed): *Handbook of Clinical Neurology.* New York, Elsevier, 1976:335.

459. Imle PC: Adjuncts to chest physiotherapy. In Mackenzie CF (ed): *Chest Physiotherapy in the Intensive Care Unit,* 2nd ed. Baltimore, Williams & Wilkins, 1989:281.

460. Bernstein IL, Ausdenmoore RW: Iatrogenic bronchospasm occurring during clinical trials of a new mucolytic agent, acetylcysteine. *Dis Chest* 1964; 46:469.

461. Rao S, et al: Acute effects of nebulization of N-acetylcysteine on pulmonary mechanics and gas exchange. *Am Rev Repir Dis* 1970; 102:17.

462. Waltemath CL, Bergman NA: Increased respiratory resistance provoked by endotracheal administration of aerosols. *Am Rev Respir Dis* 1973; 108:520.

463. National Heart Lung and Blood Institute (NHLBI). Proceedings of the 1979 Conference on the Scientific Basis of In-hospital Respiratory Therapy. *Am Rev Respir Dis* 1980; 122:161.

464. Pontoppidan H: Mechanical aids to lung expansion in nonintubated surgical patients. *Am Rev Respir Dis* 1980; 122:109.

465. Dail CW: Glossopharyngeal breathing by paralyzed patients: Preliminary report. *Calif Med* 1951:75.

466. Dail CW, et al: Clinical aspects of glossopharyngeal breathing. *JAMA* 1955; 158:445.

467. Aidran GM, et al: Cineradiographic studies of glossopharyngeal breathing. *J Radiol* 1959; 32:322.

468. Feigelson CI, et al: Glossopharyngeal breathing as an aid to the coughing mechanism in the patient with chronic poliomyelitis in a respirator. *N Engl J Med* 1956; 254:611.

469. Kelleher WH, Parida RK: Glossopharyngeal breathing, its value in respiratory muscle paralysis of poliomyelitis. *BMJ* 1957; 2:740.

470. Metcalf VA: Vital capacity and glossopharyngeal breathing in traumatic quadriplegia. *Phys Ther* 1966; 46:835.

471. Montero JC, et al: Effects of glossopharyngeal breathing on respiratory function after cervical cord transection. *Arch Phys Med Rehab* 1967; 48:650.

472. Affeldt JE, et al: Glossopharyngeal breathing: Ventilation studies. *J Appl Physiol* 1955; 18:111.

473. Murphy AJ: Glossopharyngeal breathing in the management of the chronic poliomyelitic respirator patient. *Arch Phys Med Rehab* 1956; 37:631.

474. Desmond J: Paraplegia: Problems confronting the anesthesiologist. *Can Anaesth Soc J* 1970; 17:435.

475. Head M, Riddoch G: The autonomic bladder, excessive sweat-

ing and some other reflex conditions in gross injuries of the spinal cord. *Brain* 1917; 40:188.

476. Johnson B, et al: Autonomic hyperreflexia: A review. *Mil Med* 1975; 140:345.

477. Bors E: The challenge of quadriplegia. *Bull L A Neurol Soc* 1956; 21:105.

478. Guttman L, Whitteridge D: Effects of bladder distension on autonomic mechanisms after spinal cord injuries. *Brain* 1947; 70:361.

479. Guttman L: Disturbances of the bladder and urinary tract. In Guttman L (ed): *Spinal Cord Injuries: Comprehensive Management and Research,* 2nd ed. London, Blackwell, 1976; 352:67.

480. List CF, Pimenta AD: Sweat secretion in man: Spinal reflex sweating. *Arch Neurol Psych* 1944; 51:501.

481. Kurnick NB: Autonomic hyperreflexia and its control in patients with spinal cord lesions. *Ann Intern Med* 1956; 44:678.

482. Lambert DH, et al: Anesthesia and the control of blood pressure in patients with spinal cord injury. *Anesth Analg* 1982; 61:344.

483. Mathias CJ, et al: Plasma catecholamines during paroxysmal neurogenic hypertension in quadriplegic man. *Circ Res* 1976; 39:304.

484. Mathias CJ, et al: Dopamine beta-hydroxylase during hypertension from sympathetic nervous overactivity in man. *Cardiovasc Res* 1976; 10:176.

485. Garnier B, et al: Vergleichende Untersuchungen uber die Wirkungen einer endogenen vegetativen Erregung und intravenos verabreichten Noradrenalins beim Paraplegiker. *Cardiologia (Basel)* 1964; 44:167.

486. Debarge O, et al: Plasma catecholamines in tetraplegics. *Paraplegia* 1974; 12:44.

487. Comarr AE: The practical urological management of the patient with spinal cord injury. *Br J Urol* 1959; 31:1.

488. Broecker BH, et al: Low spinal anesthesia for the prevention of autonomic dysreflexia in the spinal cord injury patients. *J Urol* 1979; 122:366.

489. Ciliberti BJ, et al: Hypertension during anesthesia in patients with spinal cord injuries. *Anesthesiology* 1954; 15:275.

490. Eggers GWN, Baker JJ: Ventricular tachycardia due to distension of the urinary bladder. *Anesth Analg* 1969; 6:963.

491. Ravindran RS, et al: Experience with the use of nitroprusside and subsequent epidural anesthesia in a pregnant quadriplegic patient. *Anesth Analg* 1981; 60:61.

492. Imle PC: Physical therapy for acute spinal cord injury. *Phys Ther Pract* 1994; 3:1.

493. Buchanan LE, et al: Spinal cord injury: A ten-year report. *Pa Med* 1990; 93:36.

494. Donovan WH, Carter RE: Incidence of medical complications in spinal cord injury: Patients in specialized compared with non specialized centers. *Paraplegia* 1984; 22:282.

495. Oakes DD, et al: Benefits of early admission to a comprehensive trauma center for patients with spinal cord injury. *Arch Phys Med Rehabil* 1990; 71:637.

496. Tator CH: Acute management of spinal cord injury. *Br J Surg* 1990; 77:485.

497. Duncan EG, et al: Treatment in a specialized unit improves three measures of outcome after acute spinal cord injury: Statistical analysis of 552 cases. *Surg Forum* 1987; 38:501.

498. Meyers PR, Greesan GT: Management of acute spinal cord injured patients by the midwest regional spinal cord injury system. *Top Acute Care Trauma Rehabil* 1987; 1:1.

499. Benzel EC, Larson SJ: Functional recovery after decompressive spine operation for cervical spine fractures. *Neurosurgery* 1987; 20:742.

Chapter 34

MANAGEMENT OF ACUTE HEAD INJURY

ANTHONY M. AVELLINO

ARTHUR M. LAM

H. RICHARD WINN

Closed head injury is a term used to define all nonmissile blunt head injuries excluding open compound skull fractures. There are a number of classification schemes that have been designed, for the purpose of triage and management, to grade patients according to their initial neurologic status and history. In common with many institutions, we use the initial post-resuscitation Glasgow Coma Scale (GCS) to grade the severity of closed head injury into three groups (GCS range: 3 to 15): mild (GCS 13 to 15), moderate (GCS 9 to 12), and severe (GCS <8).[1] The GCS is known to have low interobserver variability and high reliability when used by health care personnel whether medical, nursing, or paramedical.[2] The GCS provides a quantitative measure of level of consciousness based on best eye opening, best motor response, and best verbal response (Table 34-1). In this chapter we will discuss the initial evaluation and resuscitation, operative and anesthetic management, aggressive intensive care monitoring, and management of post-injury systemic and concomitant problems of acute head injury. These measures are aimed at preventing secondary injury and optimizing conditions for brain recovery and improved outcome.

Epidemiology

Trauma is the leading cause of death for persons under 45 years of age in the United States.[3] It is estimated that about half of the 148,480 injury-related deaths in the United States in 1990 involved damage to the brain.[4] The overall mortality was found to be three-fold higher in patients with head injury compared to those without head injury.[5]

The overall annual head injury-associated death rate in the United States has been estimated to range between 16.9 to 30 per 100,000 U.S. residents.[6,7] It is estimated that head injury accounts for one-third of all injury deaths in the United States. The overall annual incidence of head injury is estimated to be in the range of 200 per 100,000 U.S. residents. The peak incidence of brain injury in the United States is in young people aged 15 to 24 with males three times more often affected than females, regardless of ethnicity.[7] Infants and elderly (>70 years old) patients also have a higher incidence compared to other age groups. In the United States, the largest proportion of *closed head injuries* is generally caused by transport-related accidents (e.g., motor vehicle accidents including pedestrians, motor-

TABLE 34-1
Glasgow Coma Scale

	Score
Eye opening	
Spontaneous	4
To speech	3
To pain	2
None	1
Best verbal response	
Oriented	5
Confused	4
Inappropriate	3
Incomprehensible	2
None	1
Best motor response	
Obeys commands	6
Localizes pain	5
Withdraws from pain	4
Flexes to pain	3
Extends to pain	2
None	1

cyclists, occupants, and bicyclists), followed by falls, sports/recreation-related injuries, and assaults and firearms.[8] In 1992, however, firearm-related causes (*open head injury*) were the largest single cause of death associated with head injury in the United States.[7] Of all head injury hospitalizations, it appears that mild head injury accounts for 60 to 80 percent of cases, moderate for 10 to 20 percent, and severe for 10 percent.[4,9–13]

Pathophysiology of Head Injury

CONCEPT OF PRIMARY AND SECONDARY INJURY

Major advances have been made in the clinical neuropathologic and experimental studies of brain damage in human head injury. The pathology of brain damage from head injury can be divided into two main stages: primary and secondary damage. The first stage involves the primary damage that occurs at the moment of impact or injury. The second stage involves the production of vascular and hematologic events that cause reduction and alteration in cerebral blood flow leading to hypoxia and ischemia. These hypoxia- and ischemia-induced abnormalities of cellular chemistry lead to cell death, and ultimately, necrosis of neurons, glia, and endothelial cells.

PRIMARY INJURY

MECHANISM OF INJURY
Gennarelli and colleagues characterized the primary stage of human brain injury into contact and acceleration/deceleration mechanisms.[14] Contact in-

juries are described as injuries resulting from an object striking the head with resultant effects of scalp laceration, skull fractures, extradural hematoma, surface contusions, and/or cortical lacerations. In contrast, acceleration/deceleration injuries result from angular inertial momentum that produces shear, tensile, and compressive strains as seen with motor vehicle accidents, falls from considerable heights, and assaults with resultant effects of acute subdural hematoma, diffuse axonal injury, multiple petechial hemorrhages, and/or primary rupture of extra- and intracranial vessels.

Scalp lacerations are important to recognize acutely as they can be sources of considerable blood loss, especially in infants. Skull fractures can be divided into three categories: simple linear fracture, compound depressed fracture without dural laceration, and penetrating depressed skull fracture with associated dural tear. Skull fractures can serve as potential routes for intracranial infections from rhinorrhea or otorrhea, and are often associated with an increased incidence of post-traumatic epilepsy. Contusions and lacerations of the brain surface occur predominantly in the frontal and temporal poles where the brain rests on bony protuberances. Histologically, they are most severe at the crests of gyri in adults, and in the subcortical white matter and outer cortical layers in young infants.[15] Diffuse axonal injury,[16] also known as "shear injury,"[17] which is the most severe degree of primary damage, refers to the "shearing" of nerve fiber axons. Macroscopically, there are focal structural lesions located in the corpus callosum and one or both dorsolateral quadrants of the rostral brainstem which are typically hemorrhagic at early stages, and cystic gliotic scars at later stages. Microscopically, there are initially axonal bulbs or retraction balls throughout the subcortical white matter and basal ganglia (Fig. 34-1). Clusters of microglia in the white matter and long-tract Wallerian degeneration occur later. Multiple petechial hemorrhages in the brain are lesions predominately seen in the rostral brainstem, and occur in patients dying within minutes or hours after injury.

SECONDARY INJURY

CHANGES IN CEREBRAL BLOOD FLOW
Neuropathologic examinations in fatal human head injury victims have repeatedly documented the high incidence of ischemic changes.[18,19] Recent studies have confirmed that alterations in cerebral blood flow (CBF) occur acutely soon after impact. It has been observed that an ischemic state (CBF less than 18 ml/100 g brain per min) occurs 0.7–4 h after injury in 30 percent of severe head-injured patients using stable xenon enhanced computed tomography. The presence of early

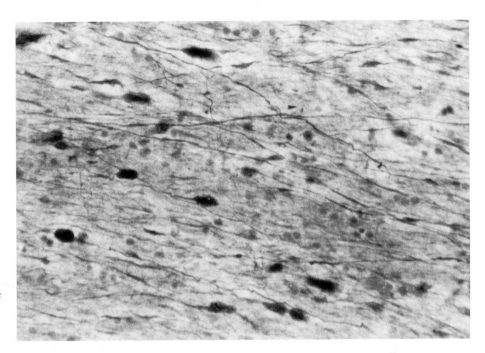

Figure 34-1 Photomicrograph of section taken from corpus callosum of a severely head-injured patient which demonstrates axon retraction balls. Palmgren, ×69.

ischemia was correlated with a poor clinical outcome. In contrast, after 18 h, there was a significantly lower incidence of patients (less than 5 percent) with evidence of ischemia.[20-23] Consequently, earlier studies performed more than 24 h after initial injury failed to document significant cerebral ischemia.[24] This acute reduction appears to be a direct response to the impact and not related to, although it can be aggravated by, systemic hypotension.

SYSTEMIC FACTORS CONTRIBUTING TO SECONDARY INJURY

The injured brain is vulnerable to the occurrence of other insults such as hypoxemia and hypotension, and both clinical and experimental studies have documented the deleterious effects of these added insults on outcome.[25-28] Results from the Traumatic Coma Data Bank have emphasized the importance of systemic hypotension as a major factor contributing to secondary injury.[29,30]

Hypertension and Hypotension

The complex interaction between systemic and cerebral hemodynamics determines the net cerebral perfusion. Under normal circumstances, the cerebral perfusion pressure (CPP) is the difference between mean arterial pressure (MAP) and intracranial pressure (ICP), and, within the physiologic limits of 50 to 150 mmHg, the homeostatic mechanism of autoregulation maintains CBF at a relatively constant level. (*See also* Physiologic Considerations, *below.*) However, after brain injury, with decrease in intracranial compliance (increase in elastance) and increase in ICP, the homeostatic defen-

sive mechanism fails. Thus, systemic hypotension and hypertension can aggravate brain injury in two ways: (1) With defective autoregulation, hypotension decreases CPP and may lead to cerebral ischemia.[31] Conversely hypertension may result in the development of vasogenic edema and further increase ICP. (2) With intact or preserved autoregulation, systemic hypotension causes compensatory vasodilation with secondary increase in cerebral blood volume (CBV), which leads to an increase in ICP. This results in a further reduction in CPP, providing a feedback for further vasodilation and continuation of the vicious cycle. This has been referred to as the vasodilatory cascade[32] (Fig. 34-2). Conversely an elevated or normal blood pressure will have a salutory effect on CBV and ICP, initiating the vasoconstriction cascade. Management based on these principles has resulted in favorable outcome in patients with severe head injury with CGS ≤ 7.[32]

Hyperglycemia

The association of hyperglycemia with poor neurologic outcome has been documented both in adult and pediatric head injuries.[33,34] Although no prospective clinical studies have been performed, there is abundant experimental evidence to support the concept of hyperglycemia aggravating ischemic insults to the central nervous system.[35,36] This is based on the premise that the availability of abundant glucose during ischemia leads to the development of lactic acidosis which is injurious to neurons.[37,38]

Hypoxemia and Hypercapnia

In addition to the obvious deleterious effects of hypoxemia leading to tissue hypoxia, and the occurrence

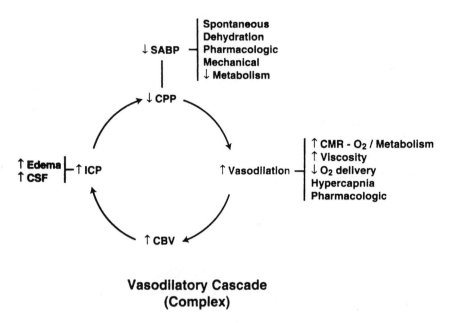

Vasodilatory Cascade (Complex)

Figure 34-2 The complex vasodilatory cascade model illustrating how reducing cerebral perfusion pressure (CPP) [systemic arterial blood pressure (SABP) − intracranial pressure (ICP)] may stimulate cerebral autoregulatory vasodilation, with an increase in cerebral blood volume (CBV) and ICP. If the SABP component remains unchanged, CPP will further decrease and the cycle will continue until the vasodilation is maximum or an SABP response occurs. The cascade may also be initiated at any point; for example, hypoxemia may stimulate cerebral vasodilation and initiate the cascade. Drugs, dehydration, or ventilator settings affecting the systemic blood pressure may stimulate the cascade from the systemic side. CSF, cerebrospinal fluid; CMR-O_2, cerebral metabolic rate for oxygen. (From Rosner et al.,[32] with permission.)

of respiratory acidosis from hypercapnia, both disturbances cause cerebral vasodilation with increases in CBV and ICP. Both conditions are frequently present in patients with severe head injury.[39]

Coagulopathy

The brain is rich in tissue thromboplastin, which, when released as a result of the injury, may lead to disseminated intravascular coagulation and intracerebral hemorrhage. The presence of clotting abnormalities in traumatic brain injury (TBI) severely worsens the prognosis.[40]

THE BIOCHEMICAL CASCADE

Secondary damage occurs following the direct trauma or events initiated by the initial trauma leading to ischemia and hypoxia. This ischemic and hypoxic insult results in secondary biochemical events that involve the pathologic activation of neurotoxic processes. These include release of excitotoxic amino acids, generation of highly reactive superoxide and free radicals, lipid peroxidation, and influx of calcium, which result in a cellular damage cascade (Figs. 34-3 and 34-12). The end result of this cellular damage cascade is edema and neuronal death, which may lead to increased intracranial pressure and further ischemic and hypoxic cell damage. In addition, the primary injury, such as intracranial hemorrhage, may act as a "space-occupying" lesion that increases ICP and decreases CPP, thus potentiating secondary damage if left untreated. For example, neuropathologic studies have demonstrated that infarction was more common in the cerebral hemisphere underlying an acute intracranial extracerebral hematoma or the hemisphere ipsilateral to an intracere-

bral hematoma than in the contralateral hemisphere.[41] These findings were corroborated in an animal model of acute subdural hematoma where it was observed that there is a marked reduction in cerebral blood flow and metabolism in the brain underlying the hematoma.[42] Moreover, in this model there was a profound increase in glucose utilization in the hippocampus bilaterally which may activate excitatory neuronal projections. This agrees with the more than 80 percent ischemic hippocampal damage found after fatal human head injury.[18,19]

CEREBRAL AUTOREGULATION AND CO_2 REACTIVITY

The cerebral circulation is a dynamic one and influenced by multiple control mechanisms. (See also "Physiologic Considerations," below). Two major homeostatic mechanisms, namely, autoregulation and CO_2 reactivity, may be impaired by head injury. Cerebral autoregulation, the ability of the cerebral vascular resistance to change in response to changes in mean systemic blood pressure within the range of 50 to 150 mmHg, is often impaired by brain injury. Although significant impairment is more likely to occur with severe injury, there are no clinical predictors of this impairment. Moreover, patients with mild to moderate head injury may also suffer from loss of autoregulation, as demonstrated in a recent investigation in which 8 out of 31 such patients had impaired autoregulation.[43] The interaction between systemic blood pressure and ICP has already been mentioned above, and its significance was recently documented by Bouma and coworkers.[44]

On the other hand, CO_2 reactivity is more robust, and is almost always preserved, although the response

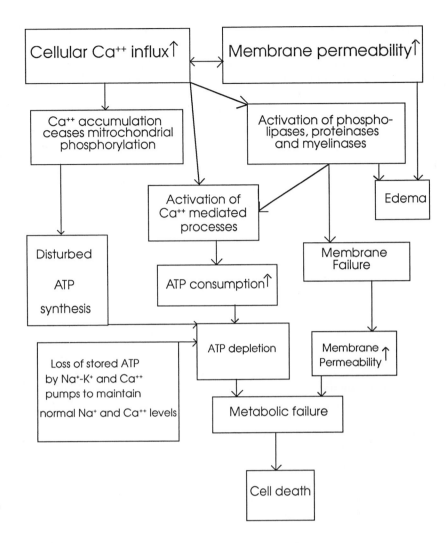

Figure 34-3 The effects of membrane permeability changes and increased intracellular calcium.

may be reduced in severe head injury.[45,46] The absence of CO_2 reactivity is a poor prognostic sign and is indicative of complete vasomotor paralysis. For this reason, these patients generally do not respond to barbiturate therapy.[47]

CEREBRAL EDEMA

Traumatic brain swelling and edema, with the resultant increase in brain volume, may lead to increased ICP and secondary damage, and ultimately herniation and death. In general, a swollen brain may be caused by either an increase in CBV as seen in early stages following head injury, or increase in brain tissue water content as seen in later stages. An increase in CBV may occur from arterial dilatation due to simultaneous impaired autoregulation and increase in arterial pressure, intact autoregulation and systemic hypotension, brainstem influences, or venous obstruction. An increase in brain tissue water content as seen with cerebral edema can be classified into five theoretical types: vasogenic, cytotoxic, hydrostatic, hypoosmotic, and interstitial.

Vasogenic Edema

Vasogenic edema results from physical disruption of brain tissue with impairment of the blood-brain barrier. It is formed largely in the gray matter, but does spread into the white matter.[48] The pathophysiology of clinically significant vasogenic edema involves: (1) increase in capillary permeability, (2) increase in transmural capillary pressure, and (3) retention of the extravasated fluid in the interstitial space.

First, an increase in capillary permeability may result from damage to endothelial membranes, activation of transendothelial pinocytosis, and disruption of tight endothelial junctions. Damage to the endothelial membranes by direct injury or secondary edemagenic substances is probably the most likely mechanism. In an experimental head injury model, increased pinocytosis was shown in cerebral vessels located in the midline of the brainstem, but it was not associated with significant brain edema.[49] Numerous edemagenic substances that can cause cerebral edema have been characterized. Bradykinin,[50] histamine,[51] arachidonic acid,[52] superoxide and hydroxyl radicals,[53] and oxygen free radicals[54] have been shown to increase cerebral edema formation experimentally.

Second, an increase in the capillary transmural pressure by elevation of body temperature and hypercapnia has been shown experimentally to increase the rate and extent of brain edema formation by relaxing precapillary resistance vessels.[55]

Third, retention of extravasated fluid appears to be mediated by the electrical charge of the protein molecule.[56] For example, albumin, an anionic protein that readily passes through the damaged blood-brain barrier, is subsequently cleared just as readily by pericytes and other cells. In contrast, IgG fraction, a cationic protein, remains within the interstitial space by adherence to anionic binding sites.[51] The complexity of the pathogenesis of vasogenic edema is highlighted by the fact that administration of steroids improves the process in chronic subdural hematomas as well as brain neoplasms. Edema adjacent to focal contusions, intracerebral hemorrhages, chronic subdural hematomas, and brain neoplasms are all representative examples of vasogenic edema.

Cytotoxic Edema

Cytotoxic edema is primarily caused by failure of cell membrane pump mechanisms due to the lack of energy secondary to a reduction of CBF to critical threshold levels which impairs the sodium potassium-ATPase pump. It is an intracellular process affecting astrocytes and neurons.[48,57] The resultant ischemic process produces a cascade of biochemical reactions consisting of an increase in potassium in the extracellular space and accumulation of calcium intracellularly, which lead to irreversible cell damage from membrane dysfunction. In the baboon, it has been shown that the amount of flow reduction and its duration correlated with the rate and extent of cytotoxic brain edema formation.[58] Mechanisms that produce focal or global ischemia / hypoxia, such as infarctions, may lead to the formation of cytotoxic edema.

Hydrostatic Edema

Hydrostatic edema is caused by an increase in the transmural vascular pressure (i.e., the hydrostatic pressure gradient between the intravascular and extravascular space), which leads to an accumulation of extracellular fluid.[59] Loss of cerebral autoregulation may also lead to an abruptly increased transmural pressure at the capillary bed.[60] An example would be the formation of diffuse edema of the ipsilateral cerebral hemisphere after acute subdural hematoma evacuation; the sudden reduction in ICP results in an abrupt increase in the cerebral vascular transmural pressure.

Hypoosmotic Edema

Osmotic brain edema is a complex process, and results from a critical fall in serum osmolality and hypona-

tremia.[61-63] Hyponatremia at serum sodium levels less than 125 mmol / liter may tip the osmotic balance causing cerebral edema. At a given sodium level, it has been shown that females are more likely to suffer brain swelling compared to men, presumably due to the differential effects of sex hormones.[64]

Interstitial Edema

Interstitial brain edema is caused by high-pressure obstructive hydrocephalus whereby CSF infiltrates the periventricular tissues by high hydrostatic pressure within the ventricular system.[65] In acutely head-injured patients, this type of edema rarely occurs, but may occur as a complication of head injury. When it does occur, this perifocal edema, secondary to mass effect, posthemorrhage, or arterial dilatation, may produce brain ischemia and neuronal dysfunction. It has been proposed that either substances in the edema fluid or products of the ischemic cellular cascade may be responsible for the vascular and neuronal dysfunction that occur.[51]

After head injury, the brain is frequently swollen in the early stages. This initial cerebral swelling is due to an increase in cerebral blood volume, largely in the high capacitance venous compartments[66] and not brain tissue water content. Neurogenic factors by brainstem stimulation or release of vasoactive substances in the cerebral circulation may account for this initiation.[51] Therefore, impaired cerebral autoregulation, brainstem influences on arterial dilatation, or venous obstruction may increase vascular or congestive brain swelling. In later stages, however, if cerebral edema becomes critical, ICP increases and cerebral perfusion pressure decreases, leading to further ischemic as well as vasogenic and cytotoxic brain edema.

Initial Evaluation and Resuscitation

The management of the acute head-injured patient is a comprehensive process that begins at the scene and continues through transport to the emergency room where definitive neurosurgical care occurs. The main goals are to prevent ischemic and hypoxic brain injury thereby optimizing outcome.

PREHOSPITAL CLINICAL EVALUATION

The initial evaluation and prehospital management of a patient with an acute head injury involves an aggressive multisystem and multidisciplinary team approach. It is estimated that up to 20 percent of trauma victims die secondary to inadequate treatment at the scene or en route to a medical facility. Therefore, it is important to begin aggressive assessment and treatment at the scene.[67] Ideally, the initial stabilization begins at the scene by emergency medical technicians or during transit to the hospital by paramedics. The initial evaluation at the accident scene should include a brief, but directed: (1) adequate history of the accident from the patient or an observer at the scene to assess the mechanism of injury; (2) assessment of vital signs; (3) mini-neurologic exam of level of consciousness using the GCS and identification of focal neurologic deficits; (4) recognition and stabilization of associated injuries; (5) documentation of past medical history; and (6) consideration of the presence of substance abuse. The primary goal of prehospital management is to begin proper aggressive management and treatment in the field to prevent secondary insults from hypoxia and ischemia.

Advanced trauma and basic life support using the "ABC" system should be followed in rapidly assessing and initiating life-support measures to assure the airway (A), breathing (B), and circulation (C) to provide adequate ventilation and maintenance of blood pressure. An open functional airway is necessary for adequate oxygenation to prevent hypoxia; placement of large-bore intravenous lines allows for adequate fluid resuscitation to prevent hypotension (to keep systolic blood pressure greater than 100 mmHg) and for the administration of pharmacologic agents such as vasopressors, steroids, mannitol, and others. Stabilization of the cervical spine is important as all patients with head injuries should be assumed to have a cervical spine injury until proved otherwise. Other associated injuries also need to be assessed and treated. If there is evidence of elevated ICP as indicated by clinical pupillary asymmetry or lateralizing neurologic signs, then emergent ICP treatment should be initiated by hyperventilation and/or administration of osmotic diuretic agents such as mannitol (rapid infusion bolus infusion of 1 g/kg) with or without furosemide (10-mg boluses intravenously) if there is no evidence of hemodynamic instability.

EMERGENCY ROOM CLINICAL EVALUATION

GENERAL MEASURES

Once in the emergency room, the trauma team should proceed in a rapid and thorough manner with the diagnostic and therapeutic maneuvers begun in the prehospital management. In the emergency room the primary goals are: (1) stabilization of the airway, ventilation, oxygenation, and blood pressure; (2) establishment of an anatomic diagnosis; (3) further assessment of other systemic injuries, as many severe head-injured patients have multiple injuries; and (4) the prioritization of investigative procedures and management of injuries. Initial x-rays of the lateral cervical spine, chest, and pelvis are obtained to rule out spinal column injury, pulmonary abnormalities, and pelvic fractures. A nasogastric tube and Foley catheter are placed for decompression of the stomach and evaluation of urine output, respectively. Routine blood chemistries are obtained and should include complete blood count, electrolyte levels (including BUN, creatinine, and glucose), arterial blood gas, full coagulation profile, serum ethanol level, and urine toxicology screen.

TOXIC DRUG EFFECTS

The two most common recreational drugs associated with trauma are ethanol and cocaine. They are present in over 50 percent of patients who are admitted as a result of trauma[68] or who have died from trauma.[69] The effects of these toxins often confound the effects of head injury.

Individuals impaired by ethanol may have (1) depressed respiratory rate, (2) thrombocytopenia, and/or (3) induced hypoglycemia. In experimental head injury, alcohol causes systemic hypotension and reduction in CBF and exacerbates neuronal injury.[70,71] Clinical studies appear to support these findings.[72] In contrast, cocaine-intoxicated patients may have (1) tachycardia, hypertension, diaphoresis, agitation, or euphoria[73]; (2) induced cerebral vasospasm[74]; (3) hypertensive hemorrhage, often from aneurysms[75]; (4) severe hyperthermia; and/or (5) prolonged seizures.[76] Pharmacologic treatment of cocaine-induced effects may be needed, for example, naloxone (0.4 mg intravenous), benzodiazepines for agitation, and sodium nitroprusside for hypertension.[76]

Intoxication by drugs can affect the adequate evaluation of the acute head-injured patient. For example, intoxication from drugs may skew the evaluation of pupillary reactions, and lead to inadequate and prolonged treatment. Some examples include abnormally small pupils from opiate use; abnormally large pupils from cocaine, amphetamine, atropine, and glutethimide use; and equal midposition and nonreactive pupils from ethanol and barbiturate use.

NEUROLOGIC EVALUATION

Documentation of the neurologic exam is of utmost importance and should be repeated frequently to detect signs of deterioration. The neurologic assessment should include: (1) level of consciousness as determined by the GCS, (2) pupillary assessment, (3) brain stem reflexes, (4) identification of focal or lateralizing neurologic signs, and (5) external evaluation of the head for signs of a scalp laceration, open depressed skull fracture, penetrating wound, hemotympanum, otorrhea, rhinorrhea, mastoid ecchymosis (Battle's sign, signifying a middle cranial fossa fracture), and periorbital ecchymosis (raccoon eyes, signifying an anterior cranial fossa fracture). Pupillary assessment should include size and reactivity to light; and a greater than 1-mm difference between the two sides is abnormal. In the face of severe hypotension, drug or alcohol intoxication, or facial trauma, however, the pupillary exam is unreliable as an index of a focal lesion as bilaterally dilated and fixed pupils may result from inadequate cerebral vascular perfusion. In patients who are pharmacologically paralyzed, pupillary light responses are not affected. The rapid assessment of neurologic function is used to classify patients into categories of mild, moderate, and severe head injury.

Meticulous attention to the fundamental principles of advanced life support and resuscitation is needed to avoid secondary cardiopulmonary abnormalities that can further potentiate traumatic injuries leading to cell death and poor outcome.

RADIOLOGIC EVALUATION

After medical and hemodynamic stabilization of the acute head-injured patient, diagnostic studies are performed and may include a computed tomography (CT) scan of the head without contrast, skull and spine radiographs, carotid angiography, and brain magnetic resonance imaging. At our institution, a head CT scan is obtained acutely in all patients with any history of loss of consciousness to assess for surgically treatable mass lesions. According to the American College of Surgeons Advanced Trauma Life Support guidelines, "all patients with head injury except 'trivial' need a head CT scan at some time." Initial CT scanning has been shown to be highly predictive of the risk of subsequent deterioration, development of elevated ICP, as well as death in the recent report from the findings of the National Traumatic Coma Data Bank Cohort (TCDB).[77] This report showed that the overall risk of dying after severe head injury with any CT abnormality was 40 percent; the risk increases to 50 percent with bilateral diffuse swelling, and 60 percent with a mass lesion.[77]

Until the late 1980s, controversy existed over the most appropriate radiologic evaluation in minor head-injured patients, primarily the relative merits of skull x-rays versus head CT scanning. In 1987, skull x-rays were obtained in 53 percent of low-risk patients (defined as asymptomatic, mild headache, dizziness, and/or scalp injury) in a prospective study of 7035 head-injured patients. Skull fractures were identified in 0.4 percent of cases and were not associated with any evidence of intracranial injury. Therefore, this multidisciplinary panel concluded that skull x-rays are rarely helpful after minor head injury.[78]

The usefulness of magnetic resonance imaging (MRI) in the acute setting remains to be proved. However, it is most useful in identifying nonhemorrhagic diffuse axonal injuries, brainstem hemorrhage, small or chronic subdural hematomas, and when the neurologic exam does not explain the injury based on head CT scan.[79,80]

HYPOXEMIA AND AIRWAY MANAGEMENT

In the recent TCDB cohort, hypoxemia ($Pa_{O_2} \le$ 60 mmHg during resuscitation) was documented in 22.4 percent of patients and was associated with a 28 percent mortality rate and a 21.7 percent poor outcome rate (i.e., severe or vegetative state).[81] In addition, over 50 percent of patients not intubated and who arrived in the ER breathing spontaneously have been shown to have hypoxemia.[82] In acute head-injured patients, the threshold for the clinical decision to intubate should be low as both hypoxemia and hypercapnia cause cerebral vasodilation and increased ICP which may lead to decreased CPP and further ischemic damage. All patients with diminished protective airway reflexes require tracheal intubation for adequate ventilation and oxygenation to prevent cerebral hypoxia. This also applies to patients with a depressed level of consciousness or intoxicated with alcohol or other CNS depressants, or in patients at risk of airway compromise secondary to an expanding hematoma in the neck or pharynx.

A functional airway can be accomplished by clearing the mouth and oropharynx of foreign bodies such as vomitus, secretions, blood, dentures, and loose teeth, accompanied by chin lift, jaw thrust, and suctioning maneuvers. Orotracheal intubation is frequently indicated and, in difficult patients, transtracheal jet ventilation or cricothyroidotomy may be necessary. Factors that must be considered when contemplating tracheal intubation include the risk of an associated cervical spine injury (10 percent in high speed trauma victims[83]), laryngeal fractures, midface injury or CSF rhinorrhea, and/or oropharyngeal and tracheal reflex sympathetic stimulation that may increase blood pressure and ICP. The preferred method is orotracheal intubation with in-line stabilization of the cervical spine since it has been shown to have a good safety record without adverse neurologic events.[84-86] In the head-injured patient, orotracheal intubation is best accomplished with rapid sequence induction using 3 to 5 mg/kg thiopental and 1 to 2 mg/kg of succinylcholine.[76,86,87,88] In addition, the intravenous administration of lidocaine (1.5 mg/kg) prior to intubation, diminishes reflex cardiovascular effects and attenuates the increased ICP effects,[88,89] probably as a result of its cerebrovasoconstrictive effect.[89] Thiopental, a short-acting barbiturate, may cause significant hypotension following intravenous administration, especially in the volume depleted trauma patient, thus it must be used with caution.[90] Propofol has similar cerebral and systemic effects as thiopental.[91] Etomidate, 1 to 2 mg/kg, causes less cardiovascular depression and may be a better alternative.[92] Although succinylcholine and the mechanical stimulation associated with laryngoscopy and orotracheal tube placement may increase ICP, heart rate, and mean blood pressure, this response is transient and the risk is balanced by the benefit of being able to establish the airway quickly and efficaciously.[76,93,94] Moreover, Kovarik and coworkers recently reported that neurologically injured patients do not respond to the administration of succinylcholine with increase in ICP and cerebral blood flow.[95] Succinylcholine, however, may cause life-threatening hyperkalemia in patients with head injury or neurologic deficits, although not within 24 h of the acute injury.[96] Cricothyroidotomy may be needed in patients where major facial or upper airway trauma has occurred. However, complications from cricothyroidotomy have been reported to be as high as 32 percent in the emergency setting compared with 6 to 8 percent in the elective setting, especially in children, where a high incidence of postsurgical stenosis has been reported.[97-99] Therefore, this technique should only be used as a last resort.

Other related injuries that cause hypoxemia and hypercapnia should also be ruled out. These include acute cardiac failure, airway obstruction, chest wall injuries, tension pneumo- or hemothorax, cardiac tamponade, diaphragmatic paralysis from a high cervical cord injury, aspiration, pulmonary contusion, and drug overdose. Oxygenation may also be compromised by aspiration, neurogenic pulmonary edema, or the development of adult respiratory distress syndrome (ARDS). Frequent arterial blood gases are essential to assess adequacy of oxygenation, ventilation, and acid-base status. Airway control has multiple purposes in the acute head-injured patients including avoidance of hypoxemia and hypercapnia, as well as lowering ICP. In patients with moderate or severe head injury, elevated ICP may lead to cerebral ischemia as well as posttraumatic vasogenic edema. As carbon dioxide is one of the most potent cerebral vasodilators, judicious hyperventilation leading to hypocapnia will result in cerebral vasoconstriction and decreased ICP.

HYPOTENSION AND FLUID RESUSCITATION

In an earlier study, hypotension (systolic blood pressure less than 85 mmHg) was associated with a 35.3 percent mortality rate.[100] More recently, in the TCDB cohort, hypotension (systolic blood pressure less than 90 mmHg during resuscitation) occurred in 11.4 percent of patients and was associated with a 50 percent mortality rate and a 17.1 percent poor outcome rate (i.e., severe or vegetative state).[81] In the absence of brainstem injury, the cause of hypotension in an adult trauma patient is seldom due to a head injury, and is

most likely due to extracranial bleeding or a cervical or high thoracic spinal cord injury. A patient with a spinal cord injury is usually bradycardic compared to patients in hypovolemic shock who are tachycardic. It is of utmost importance to avoid hypotension and to maintain an arterial systolic blood pressure greater than 100 mmHg to provide the optimal level of cerebral perfusion. The assumption that "excessive" amounts of fluid during resuscitation in a multitraumatized patient with head injury is detrimental has not been well documented clinically. This assumption had primarily been based on laboratory studies investigating the effects in the initial 6-h period following experimental head injury. In contrast, clinically, maximal brain swelling and increasing ICP usually occur after 24 h.[101] In fact, aggressive fluid resuscitation in multitraumatized patients with head injury has not led to increased ICP or clinical neurologic deterioration.[102] The fluids of choice during resuscitation are crystalloid solutions such as 0.9% normal saline or other isotonic fluids. Hypotonic fluids are avoided as they may precipitate brain edema secondary to decreased serum osmolality and sodium levels. These patients should be maintained in a euvolemic state with a normal cardiac output. It may prove necessary to supplement fluid resuscitation with vasopressors as well as inotropic and chronotropic agents. Glucose-containing solutions should generally be avoided. In severe head-injured patients, recent studies suggest that hyperglycemia is associated with a poor prognosis.[33,34] The excessive glucose load during ischemia promotes anaerobic metabolism and leads to acidosis, vasoparalysis, and cell damage. Hypertonic solutions such as 3% saline have been shown to be efficacious in resuscitation without causing an increase in ICP,[103] although at present there is insufficient data to justify its routine use. The use of colloid or crystalloid solutions are further discussed below under *Management Considerations.*

It is most important, irrespective of fluid used, to adequately fluid-resuscitate a hypotensive multitraumatized patient to increase the chance of survival. If stabilization of vital signs does not occur after administration of 1 to 2 liters of fluid, then blood should be given. However, if more than 10 units of blood must be given, then clotting factors such as platelets should also be given to reduce the risk of coagulopathy. The development of rapid infusion devices has also been shown to facilitate fluid management in the severely hypotensive head-injured patient.[104]

Operative Management

SURGICAL APPROACH

The decision to operate on a head-injured patient is based on both the neurologic condition and radiologic investigations. At our institution, changes on the CT scan provide guidance for surgical intervention. Surgery is indicated in the presence of intracranial mass lesions such as epidural hematoma and acute subdural hematoma, midline shift of greater than 5 mm, significant mass effect, compressed basilar cisterns, and/or compressed or increased ventricular size. Although these are specific head CT findings, the decision for operative intervention must also be individualized and the risks and benefits of surgery must be carefully weighed for each patient. The decision for operative intervention should be made as quickly as possible, as some studies suggest that the sooner the intracranial mass lesion is evacuated the better the chances of a good outcome.[105] The primary goal of surgical intervention is to remove mass lesions that may increase ICP and decrease CPP, and therefore lead to further ischemic and hypoxic secondary damage.

SUBDURAL HEMATOMA

Generally, an acute subdural hematoma (ASDH) is defined as a hematoma in the subdural space (i.e., between the inner layer of the dura and the arachnoid layer) that occurs up to 72 h after injury.[106–109] The incidence of ASDH is difficult to determine as there has been disagreement in the definition of ASDH. However, in the TCDB cohort, a 24 percent incidence of ASDH was reported, which is consistent with a 1981 series of 366 patients that showed a 22 percent rate.[105] In most series, males outnumber females 2 to 4 times,[110–113] and ASDH most commonly occurs during the fifth and sixth decades.[105] Falls and assaults are more likely to cause ASDH than motor vehicle accidents and occupational injuries.[105,113,114]

ASDH results from the tearing of surface or bridging vessels from acceleration-deceleration injuries or by accumulation around a parenchymal laceration. However, the majority of ASDHs are caused by tearing of the parasagittal bridging veins located over a convexity which drain the surface of the hemisphere into the dural venous sinuses.[114,115] The magnitude of impact damage and the degree of injury are highest with ASDH compared to other traumatic mass lesions, thus making this type of lesion more lethal. Frequently, the magnitude of injury secondary to the mechanism of ASDH leads to coexisting parenchymal damage and more than half are associated with intracranial lesions such as parenchymal contusions.[105,116] In the TCDB cohort, there was a 50 percent mortality rate in patients with an ASDH that required evacuation.[117]

The clinical presentation of patients with ASDH depends on the severity of brain injury sustained at the time of impact and the rate of growth of the ASDH. The signs and symptoms of presentation may range from minimal neurologic deficits to a comatose state.

The most common clinical signs are motor deficits and anisocoria.[115] On CT scan, the classic appearance is a high-density crescentic-shaped lesion deforming the surface of the brain (Fig. 34-4).

In symptomatic patients, the treatment should be rapid surgical evacuation. The goals of surgical evacuation are clot removal, hemostasis of the hemorrhagic source, and, in a minority of cases, the resection of nonviable and necrotic brain tissue. The operation is performed through a large craniotomy flap situated over the hematoma and contused brain.

EPIDURAL HEMATOMA

The incidence of traumatic epidural hematomas (EDHs) has been reported to range from 0.2 to 6 percent of all patients with head injury.[118–125] In most series, males outnumber females by between 3 and 5 to 1.[123–128] These hematomas usually occur in young adults during the second and third decades of life,[126,127] and are rare before age 2 and after age 60, because the dura is more adherent to the inner table of the skull in these age groups.[118,123,126] Traffic accidents and falls are the most frequent cause of trauma in patients with EDH.[124–126]

EDH is a collection of blood that lies between the inner table of the skull and the periosteal outer layer of the dura. It is usually caused by a skull fracture and the resultant underlying tear in a meningeal vessel. However, EDH can occur without a fracture. EDH is not caused by an acceleration-deceleration mechanism, which is often the precipitating event with ASDH. The underlying meningeal vessel tear may be from the middle meningeal artery (half of cases), the middle meningeal vein (one-third of cases), the dural sinuses (less than 10 percent of cases), or diploic veins (in patients with a chronic EDH where the diploic veins cause diffuse dural bleeding).[122,128,129]

The clinical signs and symptoms are wide and varied depending on time from injury, hematoma size and growth, and presence of other associated intra- and/or extracranial injuries. The clinical presentation may range from only nausea and vomiting to pupillary dilatation, hemiparesis, and decerebration.[115] On CT scan, the classic appearance is a high-density biconvex- or lenticular-shaped lesion adjacent to the skull (Fig. 34-5). The operative mortality for patients with acute EDH is directly related to the level of consciousness at the time of surgery. For example, in patients who are awake and neurologically intact, the mortality is close to zero regardless of the size or location of the hematoma. In contrast, in patients who had deteriorated to coma, the mortality increases to about 40 percent.[130] In the TCDB cohort, there was a 17.8 percent mortality rate in patients with an acute EDH that required evacuation.[117]

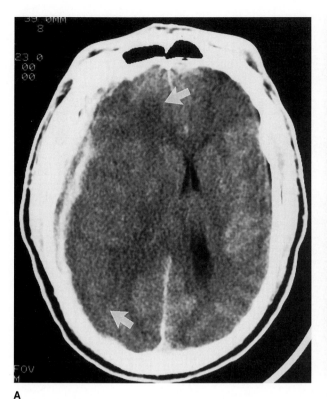

A

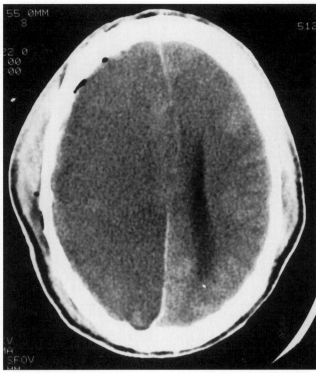

B

Figure 34-4   Herniation and infarction. If the shift is great enough or if there is direct injury to vessels at the base of the skull or in the neck, there can be secondary infarction within the brain following head trauma. *A.* This axial CT section shows the linear collections of hyperdense and isodense blood-layering within the right subdural space, consistent with a hyperacute SDH. There is subfalcine herniation with flattening of the right lateral ventricle, effacement of the third ventricle, and effacement of sulci in the right hemisphere. On this initial image, there is only a faint suggestion of a loss of differential density between gray and white matter in the inferior frontal and superior temporal lobes (*arrows*). This subtle loss of gray-white differentiation is a sign of early infarction. *B.* Axial CT scan obtained 24 h later, following evacuation of the subdural hematoma. There is generalized loss of gray-white differentiation throughout the right hemisphere, most notably when right and left hemispheres are compared. The right-sided ventricular structures and the right-sided sulci are totally compressed. The entire right hemisphere has infarcted with compression of the right internal carotid artery secondary to herniation.

The treatment ranges from operative evacuation for symptomatic patients to conservative management for asymptomatic patients. In the majority of patients, operative intervention is the most appropriate approach based on the relative risks and benefits of nonoperative treatment, costs of prolonged hospitalization, and the need for repetitive head CT scans. Evacuation of the EDH is performed through a craniotomy, preferably a large flap, over the hematoma, to provide complete exposure of the EDH. The goals of surgical evacuation are clot removal, meticulous hemostasis of the lacerated meningeal vessel, and prevention of reaccumulation using numerous dural tack-up sutures.

ACUTE INTRACEREBRAL HEMATOMAS AND CONTUSIONS

It is often difficult to differentiate between a space-occupying intracerebral hematoma and a hemorrhagic cerebral contusion. In the TCDB cohort, the incidence of a combined intracerebral lesion and a hemorrhagic contusion was 13 percent. They most commonly occur in patients between 21 to 40 years of age, and are more frequent in men than in women.[111,131] Motor vehicle accidents, followed by falls and assaults, were the most common causes. Intracerebral hematomas are frequently located in the frontal and temporal lobes.[115,132,133] The majority occur when the moving head strikes a fixed object (e.g., when the frontal and temporal poles are traumatized by the irregular bony floor of the frontal and middle cranial fossas).[134] They can also occur from blows to the head where the depressed fracture causes an underlying hematoma or contusion, and from penetrating wounds such as missiles and knives.[134]

Since these lesions often coexist with extracerebral hematomas, the clinical signs and symptoms can be

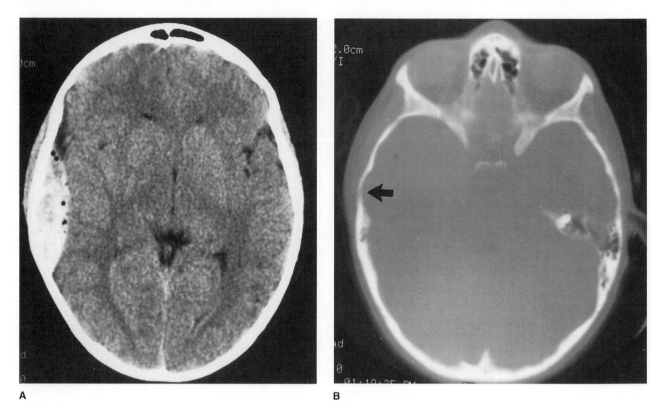

A   **B**

Figure 34-5   Epidural hematoma. Epidural hematomas are commonly associated with skull fracture and are seen as biconvex or lenticular collections of blood lying superficial to the brain. The presence of intracranial air in a patient with a closed head injury leads to a presumptive diagnosis of a fracture into an air-containing space, such as the mastoid air cells or the sinuses. *A*. Axial CT scan showing mixed iso- to hyperdense collection in the epidural space of the right middle cranial fossa. Several small low-attenuation foci caused by intracranial air are seen at the margin of the collection. The medial surface of the collection is bowed away from the skull. The mixture of iso- to hyperdensity within the EDH suggests that the injury is active and that clot formation is incomplete. *B*. Axial CT section obtained more inferiorly in the same patient. The section, displayed using bone windows, shows a linear fracture in the right temporal bone (*arrow*). The EDH was immediately adjacent to the fracture.

quite variable, and the patient presentation may range from lucid to comatose states. The diagnosis is best established by head CT scan. These CT-detected findings may vary from homogeneous well-delineated areas of high density (e.g., hematoma) to heterogeneous, poorly defined, mixed-density lesions surrounded by a low-density zone signifying edema (e.g., contusion) that can reach considerable size. The treatment is based on the neurologic status of the patient, location of the lesion, and evidence of uncontrollable ICP. In a symptomatic patient where the lesion causes elevated ICP, mass effect, and midline shift of the brain, a large craniotomy flap is performed over the lesion to evacuate the hematoma and to resect the surrounding traumatized nonviable brain. However, in patients with deep white matter or basal ganglia lesions which frequently represent diffuse axonal injuries, nonoperative management of increased ICP is the preferred treatment, although stereotactic evacuation of the clot

may be useful. In the TCDB cohort, there was a 26.8 percent mortality rate in patients with an intracerebral hematoma that required evacuation.[117]

PENETRATING INJURIES

Missile injuries are caused by a variety of objects such as knives, bullets, and pointed instruments that produce local damage, but little rotational or angular injury as there is little movement of the head. Upon arrival to the emergency room, the rapid assessment of the following should occur: (1) overall medical condition, (2) neurologic status, (3) evaluation of the entrance and exit wounds of the penetrating injury, and (4) lateral skull x-ray to evaluate the presence and location of the penetrating object. CT scan is critical to determine the missile tract and to rule out coexistent hematomas (subdural/epidural or intracranial hematoma). The operative goals for treatment of cerebral penetrating injuries are generally: (1) debridement of penetrating tract for evacuation of nonviable and ne-crotic brain, (2) hemostasis, (3) removal of retained fragments of bone and/or metal fragments where fea-sible and without causing further brain damage, (4) wound culture and sensitivity, and (5) primary watertight dural and scalp closure.[115] Prophylactic anti-biotics against gram-positive organisms, as well as pro-phylactic anticonvulsants should be administered to minimize the incidence of brain abscess[135] and sei-zures,[136,137] respectively.

Anesthetic Management

IMMEDIATE PREPARATION

Upon arrival in the operating room, a preoperative evaluation must be obtained (if not already completed) and should include a brief and rapid assessment of the patient's airway; cervical spine clearance; breathing; circulating status; associated injuries; GCS; preexisting illnesses; allergies; medications; past medical, surgical, and anesthesia history; circumstances of the injury; and associated toxic drug use. Appropriate laboratory data should be available and must include hematocrit, coagulation profile, electrolytes, glucose, BUN, and creatinine. Adequate intravenous access must be estab-lished. The primary anesthetic objectives are: (1) to con-tinue the initial resuscitation and maintenance of ex-isting vital organ function; (2) to avoid hypotension (arterial systolic blood pressure less than 100 mmHg), hypoxemia (PaO_2 less than 60 mmHg), and elevated ICP; (3) to prevent failure of other organ systems; (4) to correct coagulation abnormalities and/or fluid and electrolyte imbalances; and (5) to prevent the occur-rence of seizures (see Fig. 34-7). The main goal of anes-thetic management is directed at the avoidance of sec-ondary brain injury which may be caused by inadequate cerebral blood flow secondary to arterial hypotension, elevated ICP, excessive hyperventilation, and/or hypoxemia. Basic brain physiology, anesthetic principles, and management considerations of patients with acute head injury will be discussed.

PHYSIOLOGIC CONSIDERATIONS

INTRACRANIAL CONTENTS

The skull is a rigid container of fixed volume, and the brain bulk (80 percent), blood volume (5 percent), and cerebrospinal fluid (CSF) (15 percent) make up the intracranial contents. According to the Monroe-Kellie doctrine, the intracranial volume is equal to the volume of the brain bulk, blood, CSF, and other mass lesions. Therefore, an increase in the volume of one of these compartments can increase ICP and result in a reduc-tion in CPP and possibly a reduction in CBF if autoreg-ulation is not intact or if the CPP is below the limit of autoregulation.

INTRACRANIAL COMPLIANCE/ELASTANCE

The magnitude of increase in ICP with expansion of any of the intracranial compartments is dependent on the compliance (or, more accurately, the elastance) of the system. There is only a small buffering capacity; CSF can be displaced caudally to the lumbar space and venous vessels may be compressed. Once this capacity is exhausted, ICP will rise, and transtentorial or brain stem herniation may occur. As it is difficult to measure brain volume and CBV, the elastance has been esti-mated experimentally or clinically by measuring the volume-pressure response (change in ICP in response to the addition of 1 to 2 ml of saline into the CSF space via a ventriculostomy catheter) or derivation of the pressure volume index (PVI). The PVI is the volume of saline injected or withdrawn that would result in a 10-fold change in ICP,[138] and is calculated as:

$$PVI = \frac{\Delta V}{\log \frac{p_f}{p_i}}$$

where ΔV = volume of saline injected or withdrawn, p_f = final ICP, p_i = initial ICP. The normal PVI is 25 ml, and is frequently found to be decreased in patients with traumatic brain injury.[139] A decrease to 18 ml is indicative of significant decrease in compliance, and a value of 13 ml is considered to be a critical threshold, which carries a bad prognosis.[139] CSF is normally se-creted from the choroid plexus by active transport and its rate is not influenced by ICP. Its absorption via the subarachnoid granules into the venous circulation occurs passively and the rate is linearly related to the ICP. Either increase in CSF formation or resistance to absorption will lead to an elevation of ICP.

CBV AND CBF

Although the compliance of the system can be esti-mated from the CSF compartment, it is frequently the increase in CBV compartment that results in elevation of ICP in patients with head injury.[66] This leads to various therapeutic maneuvers to decrease CBF. It should be emphasized that although there is a general correlation between CBF and CBV, as decrease in vas-cular resistance will lead to increase in both, this is not always true. For instance, venous obstruction will lead to an increase in CBV, but a decrease in CBF. In con-trast, autoregulatory response to increase in MAP will result in vasoconstriction with a decreased CBV, but an unchanged CBF. This concept is particularly im-portant in view of the elucidation of ischemia as a cause of secondary injury in head trauma.

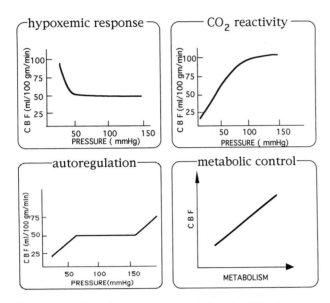

Figure 34-6 Normal regulatory control of cerebral blood flow (CBF). Pa_{CO_2} is by far the most influential determinant of CBF under physiologic conditions.

As mentioned elsewhere in this textbook, CBF averages 50 ml/100 g brain per min in an unanesthetized, normothermic human. Although the brain accounts for only 2 percent of total body weight, it receives about 15 percent of the cardiac output and consumes 20 percent of the oxygen supply. In an anesthetized patient, cessation of EEG activity occurs with a CBF less than 15 to 18 ml/100 g per min. The normal brain can usually tolerate a 50 percent reduction in CBF before significant irreversible damage occurs. However, an injured brain may require better perfusion. Major factors that influence CBF are shown in Fig. 34-6. Of these factors, autoregulation and CO_2 reactivity deserve special attention. As mentioned above, autoregulation may be impaired in patients with head injury while CO_2 reactivity is usually preserved. Hyperventilation is thus one of the most effective mechanisms in controlling CBV and ICP. It is estimated that CBF changes by 3 to 4 percent, and CBV by 1 percent per mmHg change in Pa_{CO_2}.[140]

CPP is the driving force in maintaining adequate CBF. In a patient with intact autoregulation, the CBF is maintained constant over a CPP range of 50 to 150 mmHg. In head-injured patients, anesthetic agents and therapeutic measures should ideally maintain a CPP greater than 70 mmHg for maintenance of adequate CBF to avoid the potential occurrence of ischemia.

FLOW-METABOLISM COUPLING

The cerebral metabolic rate of oxygen (CMR_{O_2}) is determined by the product of CBF and arteriovenous oxygen difference (AVD_{O_2} = 6 to 7 vol% at a Pa_{CO_2} of 40 mmHg). The use of jugular venous catheters to measure the AVD_{O_2} provides an estimate of CBF. Thus a high AVD_{O_2} implies a low CBF, and vice versa. CMR_{O_2} averages about 3.2 ml/100 g brain per min. When CBF decreases below critical values, cerebral oxygen extraction increases, but CMR_{O_2} only changes when oxygen delivery is severely compromised. Because flow is normally coupled to metabolism, inadequate analgesia/anesthesia in a head-injured patient may lead to cerebral stimulation, with resultant increase in flow/metabolism, vasodilation, and subsequent increase in ICP. Although it has been suggested that brain injury may reduce anesthetic requirement,[141] most studies have not substantiated this.[142,143]

CBF, CPP, CMR_{O_2}, and ICP are important parameters to optimize in order to achieve effective anesthetic goals.

EFFECTS OF ANESTHETIC AGENTS ON CEREBRAL PHYSIOLOGY

The choice of anesthetic agents and other adjunctive drugs is based on consideration of their effects on CBF, CMR_{O_2}, autoregulation, and CO_2 reactivity (Table 34-2). Their use should be tailored to each patient to optimize cerebral physiologic dynamics, with the ultimate goal of maintaining CPP and avoiding ischemia and hypoxemia. However, caution should be exercised in the selection and administration of drugs to avoid oversedation so that a complete neurologic exam may be obtained in the immediate postoperative period.

INTRAVENOUS AGENTS

Intravenous agents such as barbiturates, propofol, and etomidate produce cerebral vasoconstriction and reduction in CBF, secondary to a decrease in CMR_{O_2}. Thus, their effectiveness in reducing CBF, and hence CBV and ICP, is dependent on the preexisting cerebral metabolic activity. With onset of electrical silence in EEG, additional doses of barbiturates produce no further reduction in flow or change in ICP. All three agents, when given in adequate dosages, can result in electrically silent EEG. Barbiturates and propofol are cardiovascular depressants, and therefore may reduce MAP. Thus, it is important to monitor CPP when using these agents, and support with vasopressors may be necessary. Etomidate causes less cardiovascular depression and is the drug of choice when hypovolemia and/or cardiovascular disease is suspected. However, its use has not been popular because of the concern that it suppresses the adrenocortical hormonal response to stress.[144] Nevertheless, it has been used to cause maximal cerebral metabolic suppression during aneurysm surgery.[145] Benzodiazepines have only minor effects on the cerebrovascular system, causing only a slight

TABLE 34-2
Summary of the Cerebral Actions of Commonly Used Anesthetic Agents

Agents	CBF	CMR_{O_2}	Autoregulation	CO_2 Reactivity
Thiopental	↓↓	↓↓	↔	↔
Propofol	↓↓	↓↓	↔	↔
Etomidate	↓↓	↓↓	↔	↔
Halothane	↑↑ [a]	↔	↓ [a]	↔/↑
Isoflurane	↔/↑ [a]	↓	↓ [a]	↔/↑
Desflurane	↔/↑ [a]	↓	↓ [a]	↔/↑
Sevoflurane	↔/↑ [a]	↓	↓ [a]	↔/↑
Nitrous oxide	↑	↔/↑	↔	↔

[a] Dose-related changes.

reduction in metabolism and flow. Thiopental, propofol, and etomidate can all be used as induction agents, as well as for maintenance of anesthesia. If immediate evaluation of neurologic function is an important concern, then propofol is the preferred drug because of the short recovery time from redistribution.

All intravenous agents preserve autoregulation in normal individuals and have negligible influence on the cerebrovascular response to CO_2.[146-149] The influence of these agents on these homeostatic mechanisms in patients with brain injury and/or impaired autoregulation is unknown. Because of the reduction in CBF with these agents, when measured in absolute terms, CO_2 reactivity is reduced.

VOLATILE AGENTS
Volatile anesthetics include halothane, enflurane, isoflurane, and the two new agents, desflurane and sevoflurane. Although similar in action, differences among them exist to influence the choice of anesthetic for the patient with substantial brain injury. Volatile agents are generally considered to be cerebral vasodilators and cause increase in CBF in a dose-related manner. Although these agents are also said to uncouple flow and metabolism since they may increase flow while reducing metabolism, recent evidence suggests that flow-metabolism coupling persists during volatile anesthesia, but the balance may be shifted with a higher flow at a given metabolic rate.[150,151] All volatile anesthetic agents have intrinsic cerebrovasodilatory action, and potentially can increase CBF. However, any simultaneous reduction in CMR_{O_2} may lead to a coupled reduction in flow. Thus, the overall effect reflects a balance between the direct vasodilatory and the indirect flow-metabolism coupling-mediated vasoconstriction.[151] At low doses, halothane has negligible effect on CMR_{O_2} and therefore no indirect influence on flow; hence it is the most potent cerebral vasodilator.

Isoflurane is a potent cerebral metabolic depressant and therefore the least cerebral vasodilating. The effect of enflurane is intermediate between isoflurane and halothane. With the exception of a lower blood-gas solubility, and therefore a quicker onset and offset, the cerebrovascular and metabolic profile of the two recently introduced agents, desflurane and sevoflurane, are indistinguishable from isoflurane. Halothane and enflurane are seldom used in the management of patients with brain injury. Although their administration may facilitate control of systemic blood pressure, it is done at the expense of undesirable effects on the brain. Because of the uncertainty regarding their cerebrovascular action (partly dependent on the background cerebral metabolic activity) and thus the potential for increasing CBF and CBV, volatile agents should always be used with caution, if at all, and only in low doses in patients with brain injury. If brain swelling is noted intraoperatively, it is prudent either to discontinue the volatile agents or to reduce the dose to 0.5 minimum alveolar concentration (MAC) or less and only when mild to moderate hyperventilation can be accomplished.

All volatile anesthetics impair autoregulation in a dose-related manner; autoregulation is preserved at 0.5 MAC but abolished at 1.5 MAC and above.[146] This is another reason for limiting use of volatile anesthetics to low doses. Cerebrovascular response to CO_2 is not altered significantly by volatile anesthetic agents. In absolute terms, it is actually enhanced since CBF tends to be unchanged or higher during volatile anesthesia.

NITROUS OXIDE
Nitrous oxide is a potent cerebrovasodilator, whether used alone or in combination with volatile agents.[152] The resultant increase in ICP has been well documented.[153,154] It has negligible effects on autoregulation and CO_2 reactivity. Its cerebral vasodilatory effects are

minimal when used in combination with intravenous anesthetic agents such as thiopental, propofol, or benzodiazepines.[149,153,155] However, when administered to patients whose EEG has been rendered silent with propofol, nitrous oxide will cause cerebral vasodilation as evidenced by an immediate increase in blood flow velocity.[156] With the introduction of desflurane and sevoflurane, both with blood-gas solubility similar to nitrous oxide, it no longer stands as the sole inhaled agent with the apparent advantage of quick onset and rapid elimination. Although there are no outcome studies to demonstrate its deleterious effect, considering the availability of the more potent agents with a better cerebral vascular profile, nitrous oxide should probably not be used in patients with brain injury and/or elevated ICP.

NARCOTICS

Narcotics such as morphine have negligible direct effects on the cerebral circulation and metabolism. However, they may cause cerebral vasodilation from histamine release and systemic hypotension. The cerebrovascular and metabolic actions of the synthetic narcotics, including fentanyl, sufentanil, and alfentanil, are more complex. Various reports have documented increases in ICP when some or any of these agents are administered to patients with increased ICP.[157,158] This has been variously attributed to increases in CBF,[159,160] although such actions have never been clearly documented in humans. In volunteers, sufentanil does not cause an increase in CBF.[161] Similarly, when administered to patients maintained on low-dose isoflurane anesthesia and systemic blood pressure is supported, alfentanil does not increase CBF velocity or jugular bulb oxygen saturation.[162] Reviewing the literature, it is clear that there is no conclusive evidence demonstrating direct cerebral vasodilatory action of any of the synthetic narcotics. However, all three agents can and do cause systemic hypotension. As demonstrated elegantly by Rosner and coworkers[32] and Bouma and colleagues,[44] in patients with preserved cerebral autoregulation, such systemic hypotension would lead to compensatory cerebral vasodilation with resultant increase in CBV and ICP. It is conceivable that the systemic effects of the synthetic narcotics explain the conflicting reports on ICP. Recent work done by Werner and coworkers have corroborated this explanation. When systemic blood pressure is maintained, ICP does not increase when sufentanil is administered to patients with head injury.[163] Irrespective of the mechanism, these observations underscore the importance of administering these agents cautiously, in small increments, and, when necessary, with support of the systemic blood pressure with vasopressors. Fentanyl has the least propensity to result in systemic hypotension,

and is therefore generally the preferred narcotic. The new ultra-short acting narcotic, remifentanil, when approved for use in neurosurgical patients, may be particularly suitable for use in the neurosurgical patient because of its short half-life.[164,165] Narcotics have no clinically significant effects on autoregulation or CO_2 reactivity.

KETAMINE

Ketamine can increase CBF and CMR_{O_2}. It is therefore traditionally avoided in patients with neurologic disease, and specifically in patients with head injury. However, as a noncompetitive *N*-methyl-D-aspartate antagonist, it has been shown to ameliorate neuronal injury both in vivo[166] and in vitro.[167] There is a resurgence of interest in its use in neurosurgical patients.[168] A number of studies suggest that the increase in CBF and ICP observed with ketamine is secondary to either an increase in Pa_{CO_2} or systemic blood pressure or both.[169] Albanese and coworkers have recently reported that ketamine given in doses of 1 mg/kg and 5 mg/kg to ventilated head-injured patients did not cause increases in cerebral blood flow velocity or ICP.[170] As an induction agent, it maintains cardiovascular stability, particularly in a hypovolemic patient. Thus, theoretically it may be beneficial in a patient with concomitant head injury and systemic injury complicated with significant blood loss. Its actual use in this setting, however, must await further investigation of its physiologic effects, as well as accumulation of data from clinical trials.

MUSCLE RELAXANTS

Nondepolarizing muscle relaxants such as vecuronium, rocuronium, and pancuronium have no effect on CBF, CMR_{O_2}, or ICP. In contrast, succinylcholine may increase ICP, CBF, and CMR_{O_2} under some circumstances.[171,172] The mechanism of succinylcholine-induced increase in ICP has been extensively studied by Lanier and coworkers. They concluded that the stimulation of the gamma motor neurons during depolarization causes antidromic conduction resulting in cerebral stimulation and a coupled increase in CBF.[173] Accordingly, this action is blocked by the administration of an appropriate dose of a nondepolarizing muscle relaxant. However, the same authors reported that this cerebral stimulation is also absent in dogs made globally ischemic prior to the administration of succinylcholine. Kovarik and coworkers have since made similar observations in patients with neurologic disease and report that succinylcholine causes neither increase in CBF velocity nor increase in ICP in patients maintained mildly hypocapnic in the intensive care unit.[95] Thus, in the acute setting where rapid sequence intubation and prompt institution of controlled ventilation are indicated, succinylcholine remains the drug of choice. Rocuronium, in high doses (1.0 to 1.2 mg/kg), has an onset time comparable to succinylcholine, and is a suitable alternative.

VASOACTIVE AGENTS

Agents used to control blood pressure may alter ICP. Generally, adrenergic agonists such as dopamine, phenylephrine, and ephedrine, adrenergic antagonists such as labetolol, esmolol, and propranolol, and ganglionic blocking drugs such as trimetaphan have little effect on CBF, and therefore do not affect CBV and ICP. However, direct-acting vasodilators including nitroglycerin, sodium nitroprusside, and hydralazine decrease cerebrovascular resistance, and thus increase CBV and possibly ICP.[174,175] Thus, beta-adrenergic antagonists should be the agents of choice when it is necessary to reduce the systemic blood pressure pharmacologically. The potent vasodilating agents should only be used when ICP monitoring is in place.[176]

CSF FORMATION AND ABSORPTION

Anesthetic agents may influence CSF formation and absorption. Although this is not a major consideration in the acute treatment of patients with traumatic brain injury undergoing craniotomy, this may become important in patients with increased ICP undergoing extracranial procedures. Intravenous agents have negligible effects on the CSF compartment. However, halothane and enflurane increase CSF by increasing formation or decreasing absorption, whereas isoflurane has no significant effect.[177]

MONITORING

Intraoperatively, the cardiovascular, respiratory, and central nervous systems require continuous anesthetic monitoring. In addition to routine pulse oximetry, capnography, and electrocardiography, monitoring should include an arterial catheter for direct blood pressure monitoring as well as intermittent blood gases and electrolyte analysis. A urinary catheter is mandatory. In addition to two large-bore intravenous catheters, central venous pressure or pulmonary artery pressure monitoring may be desirable. The benefits of extensive monitoring, however, must be balanced against the risks of causing delay to the surgical procedure, which could be life-threatening. Thus, it is prudent to allow emergency evacuation of intracranial hematomas to proceed as quickly as possible while monitoring is being established.

Time permitting, the insertion of a jugular bulb catheter may provide important information, allowing measurement of jugular venous oxygen saturation, calculation of arteriovenous oxygen content difference,

and estimation of the balance between CBF and CMR_{O_2}. In addition, it allows optimization of the degree of hyperventilation.[178] Since hyperthermia increases the rate of brain metabolism and the levels of carbon dioxide, temperature should be monitored closely and, if elevated, normalized with surface cooling blankets and antipyretics as needed. In experimental studies, hyperthermia has been shown to increase cerebral edema by up to 40 percent,[55] and CMR_{O_2} increases about 4 to 5 percent per each degree Celsius. The head should be in the neutral position and elevated 15 to 30 degrees above the heart to avoid cerebral venous outflow obstruction which will provide a reduction in ICP without any concomitant compromise of cardiac function.[179,180]

MANAGEMENT CONSIDERATIONS

FLUID MANAGEMENT

In patients with head injury, fluid management can be complicated. Many head-injured patients have concurrent multisystem injury and evidence of hypovolemia. It is important to maintain an adequate circulating intravascular volume at all times to prevent hypotension (systolic arterial blood pressure less than 100 mmHg) and to maintain CPP. In a recent study of 17 patients who experienced intraoperative hypotension, an 82 percent mortality rate was reported.[181] Intravascular volume should be maintained and replaced using glucose-free isotonic crystalloid solutions (0.9% normal saline), albumin (5%), and/or blood products, guided by blood pressure, heart rate, urine output, central venous pressure, and/or pulmonary artery occlusion pressure. In an adult, hemoglobin concentrations greater than 10 g/dl and a hematocrit concentration around 30% should also be maintained to optimize oxygen transport. Traditionally, fluid restriction has been advocated to reduce brain water content and prevent the development of cerebral edema.[182] This, however, may not be possible because of other associated injuries. Moreover, in experimental studies vigorous fluid resuscitation did not have major adverse effects on either the injured or uninjured brain in the posttrauma period.[183,184] Furthermore, inotropes and vasopressors may be needed to increase systolic arterial pressure as the clinical situation dictates.

Colloid versus Crystalloid

The movement of water and solutes from the intravascular space to interstitial and intracellular space is governed by the hydrostatic, osmotic, and oncotic pressures. Because of the tight junctions present in the cerebral capillary endothelium, except when the blood-brain barrier is disrupted, electrolytes cannot enter the brain's extracellular space. Although colloids (albumin or hetastarch) have higher oncotic pressure and theoretically could reduce cerebral edema, the oncotic pressure is a small driving force compared to the osmotic pressure. Hence, in experimental studies a decrease in osmolality without change in oncotic pressure always results in cerebral edema, whereas a decrease in oncotic pressure without change in osmotic pressure has no effect on ICP and brain water content.[184-187] It would appear that maintaining osmotic pressure is more important than maintaining oncotic pressure, at least in the normal brain. In head-injured patients with an impaired blood-brain barrier the movement of water across the blood-brain barrier becomes less predictable and may become a function of hydrostatic pressure rather than osmotic gradients. Colloid fluids, such as albumin, hetastarch, and plasmanate (5% plasma protein fraction), can expand the intravascular volume more efficiently, but, should the blood-brain barrier become disrupted, more cerebral edema may develop as high-molecular-weight particles can accumulate intracerebrally. However, colloids have been shown to be beneficial in some experimental studies and are favored by some clinicians.[188] Tomita and coworkers reported that continuous oncotic therapy for two weeks with 25% albumin in patients with closed-brain injury with cerebral contusions safely reduced contusional brain edema.[189] Thus, the use of crystalloid versus colloid solutions remains controversial in head injury.

If colloid is to be used, albumin is probably preferred although it is expensive. The use of hetastarch in head-injured patients demands a word of caution since it can cause or aggravate coagulopathy. Although this may be prevented in previously normal patients by limiting the dose to 1000 ml or less in one setting or 20 ml/kg per day,[190] its use in neurosurgical patients remains risky as subclinical or evolving coagulopathy may not be recognized.[191] A recent study on the use of hetastarch for hypervolemic therapy after subarachnoid hemorrhage could not establish a safe dose for its usage.[192] Pentastarch, with a lower molecular weight than hetastarch (264,000 versus 450,000) may have less effect on coagulation.[193]

Hypertonic Solutions

Hypertonic crystalloid solutions, such as 0.9%, 3%, or 7.5% normal saline, increase the plasma osmotic pressure and thus remove water from the brain interstitial space. Vassar and coworkers reported that the infusion of a small volume of 7.5% normal saline solution early in resuscitation of hypotensive multitrauma patients improved survival rates in a human prospective, double-blind, randomized clinical trial.[194] Hypertonic solutions have also been shown to improve ICP, cerebral edema, and cerebral blood flow in a variety of experimental models. For example, hypertonic saline (3% or 7% normal saline) has been found to be useful in maintaining systemic perfusion without raising ICP during resuscitation of hemorrhagic or endotoxic shock associated with experimental head injury.[195-199] Hypertonic saline (7.5%) appears to be as effective as 20% mannitol in reducing ICP in experimental head injury with the added advantage of rapid cardiovascular resuscitation.[200] In addition, the use of small-volume resuscitation with hypertonic, hyperoncotic solutions has been shown to expand extracellular fluid volume, increase CVP, improve cardiac output without significantly raising mean arterial blood pressure, and transiently increase CBF in an experimental hemorrhagic shock model in dogs.[201] However, clinical studies assessing the use of hypertonic saline in humans remain limited.[103] Thus, isotonic solutions without dextrose are those most frequently in use for fluid replacement in head-injured patients. In the setting of combined head injury and hemorrhagic shock, or in the presence of hyponatremia, hypertonic saline (3% or 7.5%) may be indicated. In contrast, hypotonic solutions, such as 0.45% normal saline, lactated Ringer's, or D_5W, should be avoided as they decrease plasma osmotic pressure and increase cerebral edema even in normal brain.

The composition and osmotic/oncotic pressure of various intravenous fluids are listed in Tables 34-3 and 34-4.

CARDIORESPIRATORY MANAGEMENT

In patients with isolated head trauma, especially young adults, life-threatening arrhythmias, other EKG abnormalities, hypertension, tachycardia, and increased cardiac output have been reported to develop, presumably due to sympathetic system catecholamine discharge.[202,203] Cerebral edema may worsen and cause further ischemic and hemorrhagic complications. In the setting of extreme hypertension (e.g., MAP > 130 to 140 mmHg), esmolol (500 μg/kg in divided doses intravenously) and propranolol (0.5- to 1.0-mg boluses intravenously) (beta-adrenergic blocker), phentolamine (alpha-adrenergic blocker), and labetolol (5- to 10-mg boluses intravenously) (alpha- and beta-adrenergic blocker) are effective in decreasing systemic blood pressure in patients with elevated ICP with no effect on CBF. Vasodilators such as nitroglycerin and sodium nitroprusside should probably not be used unless ICP is being monitored as they may increase ICP.[174,175] The classic Cushing reflex of systemic hypertension, bradycardia, and respiratory irregularities secondary to an elevated ICP may also occur, and its treatment is controversial as the elevated blood pressure helps to maintain cerebral perfusion.

Ventilation should be adjusted to maintain adequate oxygenation and provide mild to moderate hypo-

TABLE 34-3
Electrolyte Compositions of Crystalloid and Colloid Fluids

Fluids	Osmolarity (mosm/liter)	Na (mEq/liter)	Cl (mEq/liter)	K (mEq/liter)	Ca/Mg (mEq/liter)	HCO_3^- (mEq/liter)	Glucose (g/liter)	pH	Kcal	Oncotic pressure (mmHg)
PLASMA	289	141	103	4–5	5/2	26		7.4		21
CRYSTALLOID										
Plasma-Lyte®	294	140	98	5	0/3			7.4		0
0.9% NS	308	154	154					5.0		0
0.45% NS	154	77	77							0
3% NS	1027	513	513							0
7.5% NS	2567	1283	1283							0
LR	273	130	109	4	2.7/0	28		6.5	<10	0
D5LR	525	130	109	4	2.7/0	28	50	5.0	180	0
D5W	252						50	4.0	170	0
D5NS	560	154	154				50	4.0	170	0
D5 0.45% NS	406	77	77				50	4.0	170	0
Mannitol (20%)	1098							5.0		0
COLLOID										
6% Hetastarch	310	154	154					5.5		30
5% Albumin	290	145 ± 15								20
Plasmanate®	270–300	145	100	0.25				6–7		21

NOTE: NS = normal saline; LR = Lactated Ringer's; plasmanate = 5% plasma protein fraction.

capnia (Pa_{CO_2} = 30 to 35 mmHg). In patients with hypoxemia (Pa_{O_2} < 60 mmHg), PEEP may be used, and in general PEEP less than 10 cmH$_2$O does not increase ICP appreciably, particularly in patients with poor pulmonary compliance.[204,205] However, institution of ICP monitoring would further increase the safety of the use of PEEP.

ICP MANAGEMENT

The treatment for management of intraoperative elevated ICP (ICP > 20 mmHg) or brain swelling are (1) hyperventilation, (2) diuretics, (3) discontinuing inhalational anesthetics, (4) barbiturate administration, (5) sedation and paralytic agents administration, (6) head elevation and repositioning, (7) control of temperature in normothermic range, (8) external ventricu-

TABLE 34-4
Characteristics of Colloid Fluids

Colloid Fluid	COP (mmHg)	Potency[a]
5% Albumin	20	1.3:1
25% Albumin	70	4:1
6% Hetastarch	30	1.3:1

[a] Relative increase in vascular volume (ml) per ml infused colloid.

NOTE: COP, colloid osmotic pressure.

lostomy CSF drainage, and (8) surgical decompression by hemicraniectomy and/or temporal or frontal lobectomy.

Cerebral Blood Volume

In most instances, the CBV is the compartment that can be most easily and rapidly altered. Hyperventilation to a Pa_{CO_2} of 25 to 30 mmHg reduces brain volume by decreasing cerebral blood volume through cerebral arteriolar vasoconstriction. Because of the generally preserved CO_2 reactivity in head-injured patients, hyperventilation can lead to an acute reduction in CBF, CBV, and ICP. This is potentially life-saving as it may alert impending herniation and improve CPP. On the other hand, it is now recognized that hyperventilation by itself can produce cerebral ischemia. In 27 severely head-injured patients, Cold documented that the number of brain regions with flow <20 ml/100 g per min was increased when normocapnia was replaced with hypocapnia.[206] Therefore, acute hyperventilation is indicated to effect immediate reduction in ICP, but chronic hyperventilation should be avoided. Moreover, Muizelaar and colleagues have demonstrated in a small clinical series of patients with severe head injury that chronic hyperventilation was associated with an adverse outcome.[207] Jugular venous oxygen saturation (Sjv_{O_2}) monitoring, if available, may help to detect global ischemia (but not regional ischemia) and allows optimal adjustment of Pa_{CO_2}. In the absence of Sjv_{O_2} monitoring, Pa_{CO_2} should not be maintained below 25 mmHg. If aggressive hyperventilation is necessary to control ICP, it is prudent to transfuse if the hematocrit is low, and to increase the inspired oxygen concentration to maximize oxygen delivery to the brain.[208] Administration of vasoconstricting anesthetic agents such as thiopental or propofol will also increase cerebral vascular resistance and reduce CBV. Thiopental is a potent cardiovascular depressant and may cause significant hypotension. It is usually given as a 5 mg/kg intravenous loading dose over 1 to 2 min followed by a continuous infusion of 5 to 10 mg/kg per h and titrated to control ICP in the absence of cardiovascular complications. Pentobarbital may also be used at a 10 mg/kg loading dose over 30 min and 5 mg/kg every 1 h for 3 h, followed by maintenance doses of 1 mg/kg per h adjusted to achieve serum levels of 3 to 5 mg/dl and to control ICP. In patients with poor cardiovascular function, it may be necessary to administer vasopressor therapy with a phenylephrine or dopamine infusion. Although the use of barbiturate coma for head injury remains controversial, a recent prospective randomized multicenter trial showed a clear benefit in reducing ICP in a subset of patients after all other conventional means of ICP control had failed.[209] Although most efforts are directed towards reducing CBV by arterial vasoconstriction, it should be recognized that good cerebral venous drainage is of equal importance to minimize any increase in the cerebral venous blood volume. Mannitol may also reduce CBV by reflex compensatory vasoconstriction as a result of the transient increase in CBF.[210]

Adequate anesthetic/analgesic and paralytic agents should be used to decrease ICP by decreasing agitation and somatic stimulation.

Brain Bulk and CSF

Mannitol (osmotic diuretic) and/or furosemide (loop diuretic) are used frequently for the rapid reduction of ICP. Twenty percent mannitol (osmolality 1098) at a dose of 0.25 to 1.0 g/kg is given as a rapid intravenous infusion. Effective action occurs within 10 to 15 min and lasts for up to 4 h.[211] Complicating effects of mannitol include (1) hemodynamic instability (hypotension followed by hypertension), (2) fluid overload and congestive heart failure in patients with poor myocardial function, (3) dehydration, (4) electrolyte disturbances, (5) hyperosmolality, and (6) acute renal failure over a 2- to 5-day period if it occurs. When using mannitol, serum osmolality and electrolyte levels should be measured frequently. When serum osmolality equals or exceeds 320 mosm, mannitol should be discontinued to avoid the potential complications of acute renal tubular

injury, hyponatremia, hyperkalemia, metabolic acidosis, and mental status deterioration.[212,213]

The rapid action of mannitol (as with hypertonic saline), may also be due to a decrease in CSF formation.[214–216] Furosemide, a loop diuretic, is also used to reduce ICP by inducing a systemic diuresis and decreasing CSF production.[217–219] It is initially given at a large dose of 0.5 to 1.0 mg/kg alone, or at a lower dose of 0.15 to 0.30 mg/kg in combination with mannitol. It has been demonstrated that combined treatment of furosemide and mannitol has a synergistic action, and prolongs the effect of lower doses of mannitol, but may lead to more electrolyte abnormalities and severe dehydration.[220,221] In patients with impaired cardiac function, furosemide may be preferable to mannitol.

Steroids have been administered to patients with severe head injury, but numerous studies have failed to support the hypothesis that steroids improve ICP and promote a favorable outcome.[222,223]

ANESTHETIC REGIMEN FOR THE BRAIN-INJURED PATIENT

Although there are no outcome data available to define the ideal anesthetic for the brain-injured patient, appropriate choices can be made based on sound physiologic and pharmacologic principles. The regimen must also take into consideration the overall plan and postoperative management of the patient. For the severely brain-injured patient who would require postoperative intensive care, continuous thiopental (3 to 6 mg/kg per h) or propofol (200 to 250 μg/kg per min) infusion supplemented with narcotics provides an excellent anesthetic. Nitrous oxide should be avoided. Isoflurane, or sevoflurane, if desired to allow better control of systemic blood pressure, should only be used in low doses ($\leq$0.5 MAC), and only when mild to moderate hyperventilation has been implemented. If unexpected brain swelling occurs, it is always prudent to discontinue nitrous oxide and/or volatile agents if any is in use at the time. For the less severely injured patient, such as a conscious or slightly drowsy patient with an epidural hematoma, the anesthetic regimen must balance the benefits of a completely intravenous-based anesthetic with optimal brain conditions versus the risk of a potential delay in emergence. Many anesthesiologists would favor the use of a propofol-based anesthetic, as it results in cerebral vasoconstriction and is compatible with an early recovery. (A simple algorithm is shown in Fig. 34-7.)

Intraoperative Complications

The main intraoperative complications that may occur include difficulties in hemostasis, control of severe

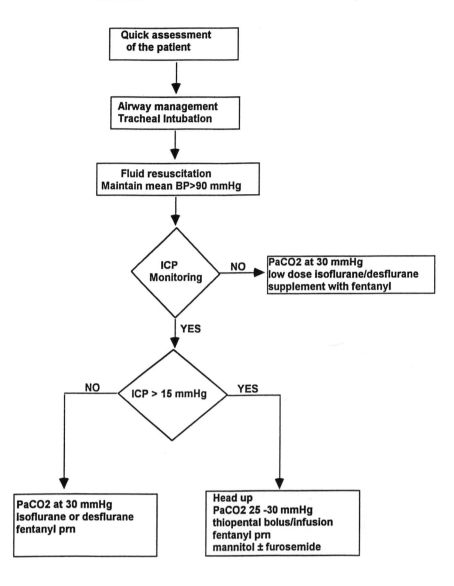

Figure 34-7   Simple algorithm for the anesthetic management of an acutely head-injured patient.

BLEEDING

Even though arterial bleeding may occur secondary to bone fragments, venous bleeding is the most common source of hemorrhage during trauma craniotomies. This venous bleeding may be abundant and difficult to control as intracranial venous pressure increases in association with increasing ICP. The best treatment for controlling venous hemorrhage in this situation is to reduce the ICP. The venous bleeding may also occur secondary to venous obstruction, therefore it is important to ascertain that the internal jugular veins are not compromised from neck compression by a tight collar or excessive turning. A systemic contributing factor to the hemostasis problem is the occurrence of hypothermia.[224] Not only does hypothermia occur fre-

quently in a patient suffering from trauma, intentional hypothermia is also advocated by some to decrease brain injury. Recent studies using thromboelastography have demonstrated that even mild hypothermia interferes with normal coagulation.[225,226] The benefits of hypothermia therefore must be balanced against the associated risks. In a hypothermic patient with uncontrolled bleeding, it is prudent to restore normothermia in addition to correcting any existing coagulation deficits as determined with conventional laboratory measurements. Platelets and fresh frozen plasma should be transfused as needed.

SEVERE BRAIN SWELLING

A close cooperation between the anesthesiologist and the surgeon is of utmost importance to achieve optimal results. In this setting, the surgeon can pack the area to reduce bleeding, while the anesthetist can reduce brain volume by hyperventilation, intravenous mannitol, and administration of barbiturates. Body, head, and neck position should again be checked to ensure good venous drainage. The head should be elevated and not rotated to avoid jugular vein compromise, recognizing that this may increase the risk of venous air embolism. Barbiturate therapy with thiopental or pentobarbital may also be pursued in extremely severe cases, provided the patient is hemodynamically stable. In selected patients with uncontrollable ICP, a decompressive hemicraniectomy may be an option. If these complications do occur intraoperatively, it is important to obtain a head CT directly from the operating room.

SUDDEN HYPOTENSION

Many patients harboring intracranial hematoma have increased intracranial pressure which may invoke the Cushing's response, resulting in increased sympathetic tone and vascular resistance. The patient may exhibit the classic response with systemic hypertension and bradycardia. These signs, however, are often modified by the general sympathetic response to trauma and the blood volume status. More often than not, however, the patient may exhibit tachycardia/hypertension when normovolemic, and tachycardia/normotension when hypovolemic. To prevent the development of catastrophic hypotension upon decompression, appropriate steps must be taken. A high index of suspicion about the presence of this reflex must be maintained in any patient suspected to have elevated ICP, either based on CT or history. Adequate venous access and fluid resuscitation must be accomplished before decompression occurs. Finally, good communication between the surgeon and the anesthesiologist is essential, as acute resuscitation may be required upon decompression of the cranium.

Nonoperative and Postoperative Intensive Care Unit Management

The major goals of intensive care management of a head-injured patient are aimed at maintaining an adequate CPP and normalizing ICP to prevent secondary injury. The prompt recognition and treatment of systemic complications such as hypotension, hypoxemia, electrolyte disturbances, coagulation abnormalities, seizures, hyperthermia, and infection must be achieved. Routine management should include (1) pulmonary toilet, (2) deep vein thrombosis prophylaxis with elastic compression stockings and intermittent pneumatic compression devices, and (3) nutritional assessment. Physiologic monitoring should

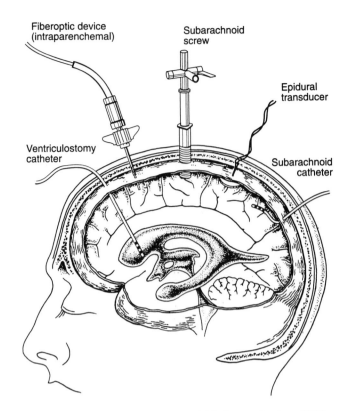

Figure 34-8 Different modalities available for monitoring of ICP.

include an ICP monitor, arterial and central venous catheter, pulse oximetry, foley catheter for urine output, and nasogastric tube. Close communication and a team approach must be maintained between all consulting services and the nursing staff to clearly define each patient's needs and goals.

In addition to standard ICP monitoring, the introduction of other adjuncts, including continuous jugular venous oximetry and CBF velocity monitoring by transcranial Doppler ultrasonography (TCD), provides more physiologic information and may prove useful in optimizing therapy to improve outcome.

ICP MONITORING

The value of ICP monitoring in the care of the head-injured patient is well established in North America. Devices used to measure ICP include: intraventricular catheter, subarachnoid bolt, epidural transducers, subdural catheter, and a fiberoptic intraparenchymal monitor (Camino Fiberoptic Intracranial Pressure Monitoring Systems, Camino Laboratories, San Diego, CA) (Fig. 34-8). All clinically available ICP monitor systems have their recognized advantages and disadvantages. The intraventricular catheter and the fiberoptic intraparenchymal device are the most commonly used. We routinely place the monitor on the

TABLE 34-5
Summary of Formulas and Values

1. $CE_{O_2} = Sa_{O_2} - SjV_{O_2}$
   Normal = 24–40%
   Hyperemia = <24%
   Low flow (ischemia) = >40%
2. $AVD_{O_2} = CBF_{O_2}/CBF$
   Normal = 5–7.5 vol%
   Hyperemia = <5 vol% (narrow AVD_{O_2})
   Low flow = >7.5 vol% (wide AVD_{O_2})
3. SjV_{O_2}
   Normal = 60–80%
   Hyperemia = >90%
   Low flow = <50–54%

same side of the intracranial pathology as a pressure differential may exist between the ipsilateral and contralateral side as has been reported with subarachnoid bolts.[227] ICP monitoring is essential in patients with elevated ICP to tailor appropriate treatment. Treatment should be initiated when ICP is greater than 20 mmHg for more than 5 min. The various treatment modalities are aimed at preventing secondary brain ischemia and brain herniation. They have been outlined above in the "ICP Management" section.

JUGULAR VENOUS OXIMETRY

Ischemic brain damage is common in patients dying from closed head injury. Venous blood sampling from the jugular bulb using a retrograde jugular catheter can be used to determine the jugular venous oxygenation saturation (SjV_{O_2}). Thus, jugular bulb catheterization allows detection of cerebral venous desaturation resulting from a decrease in CBF/CMR_{O_2}, by measuring arterial blood gases and hematocrit ($AVD_{O_2} = CMR_{O_2}/CBF$). Cerebral venous desaturation reflects either increased extraction or inadequate blood flow for the metabolic need. It is a reflection of global CBF and desaturation may be defined as (1) none when SjV_{O_2} > 50%; (2) mild when 45% < SjV_{O_2} < 50%; and (3) severe when SjV_{O_2} < 45%.[178,228,229] AVD_{O_2} is the actual ratio of cerebral metabolism to CBF, and can be calculated from the difference between the arterial oxygen content (Hb × 1.39 × hemoglobin O_2 saturation) + (Pa_{O_2} × 0.0031) and SjV_{O_2} content. Cerebral extraction of oxygen (CE_{O_2}) is another parameter that has been used to quantify the demand/supply ratio to the brain. With a stable hemoglobin, and neglecting the contribution of dissolved oxygen, $CE_{O_2} = Sa_{O_2} - SjV_{O_2}$. In the absence of hypoxemia, Sa_{O_2} is generally equal to unity, therefore $CE_{O_2} = 1 - SjV_{O_2}$ (Table 34-5).

In a patient with a stable hemoglobin content, the measurement of SjV_{O_2} is indicative of changes in the oxygen delivery-to-requirement ratio, and allows quantification of cerebral hemodynamic reserve. For example, a low SjV_{O_2} simply indicates that there is an increase in oxygen extraction which may be an early warning sign of possible ischemia. In a recent study on acute brain-injured patients, continuous monitoring of cerebral oxygenation was clinically useful in identifying impaired cerebral oxygenation even when CPP was normal.[230] The measurement of SjV_{O_2} and AVD_{O_2} allows the optimization of the global cerebral hemometabolic requirements by altering ICP treatment protocols. Various treatments and physiologic situations have different effects on CE_{O_2}, AVD_{O_2}, and SjV_{O_2} (Table 34-6). In adults, monitoring AVD_{O_2} will help detect episodes of cerebral ischemia (>7.5 vol%) and hyperemia (<5 vol%). For example, when ICP therapy such as excessive hyperventilation (Pa_{CO_2} = 20 to 25 mmHg) is employed, a SjV_{O_2} below 50% indicates cerebral ischemia occurring as a complication of therapy. In this setting, decreasing the hyperventilation has in some cases improved cerebral perfusion and decreased ICP. Gopinath and coworkers have reported that desaturation below 50% in severely head-injured patients was associated with a poor neurologic outcome.[231]

However, there are limitations to SjV_{O_2} monitoring. It is invasive and it is a global estimate of adequacy of flow; and as focal ischemia is compatible with a normal SjV_{O_2}, it might lead to a false sense of security. It is also influenced by the hemoglobin concentration, and anemia may cause desaturation because of the limitation on oxygen-carrying capacity. Jugular bulb venous oxygen saturation can be determined either with intermittent sampling or with continuous fiberoptic oximetry. The latter is clearly preferred in the intensive care unit setting as it provides continuous monitoring in a potentially unstable patient with changing cerebral hemodynamics. However, the current generation of fiberoptic oximeters has a high incidence of malfunction rate, and frequent recalibration and confirmation are often required. An algorithm for fiberoptic oximetry used by Sheinberg and coworkers is shown in Fig. 34-9.

TABLE 34-6
ICP and Treatment Effects on CE_{O_2}, AVD_{O_2}, and SjV_{O_2}

	CE_{O_2}	AVD_{O_2}	SjV_{O_2}
↑ ICP (low flow)	↑	↑	↓
Hyperemia	↓	↓	↑
Mannitol	↓	↓	↑
Barbiturates	↔ or ↑	↔ or ↑	↔ or ↓
Hyperventilation	↑	↑	↓

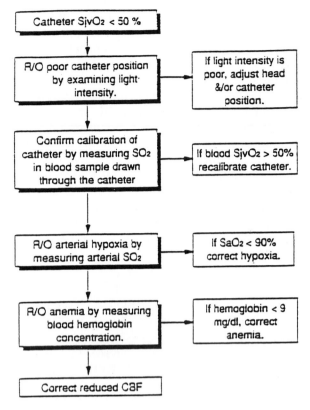

Figure 34-9 Algorithm for diagnosing the cause of jugular venous desaturations. Sjv_{O_2} = jugular venous oxygen saturation; R/O = rule out; SO2 = venous, arterial oxygen saturation; CBF = cerebral blood flow. (From Sheinberg et al,[228] with permission.)

TRANSCRANIAL DOPPLER MONITORING

Transcranial Doppler (TCD) monitoring is a noninvasive way to measure systolic, diastolic, and mean velocity of flow in the major intracranial arteries. Using a 2 mHz pulsed Doppler, the ultrasound can penetrate the temporal bone to allow insonation of the anterior, middle, and posterior cerebral arteries. The most commonly insonated artery is the middle cerebral artery (MCA). Not only is it the easiest artery to insonate, but it also carries 75 to 80 percent of the ipsilateral carotid artery blood flow. The TCD can be used for a variety of diagnostic purposes in the management of the head-injured patient. These include (1) as a noninvasive monitor of cerebral blood flow, (2) diagnosis of posttraumatic vasospasm, and (3) an indirect estimate of ICP or CPP. The current equipment available is easy to use, but skill and training are still required. In addition, a limiting factor to its use is the absence of a transtemporal ultrasonic window in some segment of the population, particularly elderly females.

1. *Indirect measurement of flow.* Provided that the vessel diameter stays constant, change in flow velocity is directly proportional to change in flow. Although the flow velocity cannot be converted into an absolute CBF value, relative and directional changes are considered to be valid indices of corresponding CBF changes. In addition, the pulsatility index (PI), a dimensionless variable and an estimate of the cerebral vascular resistance, can be derived from differences in systolic-diastolic flow velocity divided by mean flow.[232] A similar estimate, the resistance index, is derived from difference in systolic-diastolic flow velocity divided by systolic flow velocity. With the use of an anchoring device, either a headband or face frame,[233] continuous monitoring of MCA flow velocity is possible and provides a practical and noninvasive alternative to conventional CBF methods such as xenon-133 inhalation techniques for the assessment of therapeutic responses to various modalities.

2. *Diagnosis of vasospasm.* The recording of variables such as velocity and PI can be invaluable in patients with changing CPP and ICP. For example, a decreased MCA mean velocity may be due either to elevated ICP

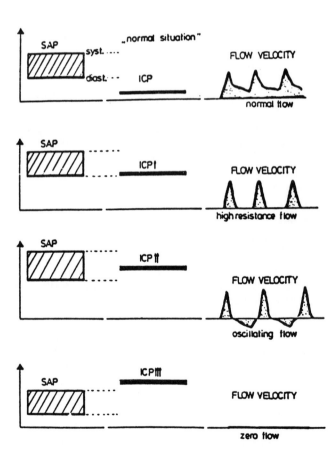

Figure 34-10 Relationships between systemic arterial blood pressure (SAP), intracranial pressure (ICP), and flow velocity as measured in the middle cerebral artery by transcranial Doppler ultrasonography (TCD). In all displayed TCD spectra, upward deflections indicate blood flow toward the Doppler probe, whereas downward deflections appear with flow directions away from the probe. (From Hassler et al,[236] with permission.)

or low arterial pressure. In contrast, an increase in MCA mean velocity (>100 cm/s) may indicate either cerebral hyperemia or posttraumatic vasospasm. The latter is now recognized to be an important factor in the development of secondary injury. Considered a rare complication before the advent of TCD, vasospasm is now known to occur in 20 to 40 percent of patients with traumatic brain injury.[234,235] The time course is similar to what occurs in subarachnoid hemorrhage from a ruptured cerebral aneurysm. The onset is between 48 and 72 h, peaks in 4 to 5 days, and usually subsides by 7 to 10 days.[234] To distinguish vasospasm from hyperemia, the ipsilateral extracranial carotid artery is insonated and the ratio of Vmca/Veica is calculated. A ratio exceeding 3 is considered to be consistent with vasospasm. Sjv_{O_2} monitoring, if available, would also aid in the diagnosis as a decreased AVD_{O_2} or high Sjv_{O_2} would be consistent with hyperemia and not vasospasm.

3. *Indirect estimate of ICP and CPP.* The change in TCD waveform with increase in ICP and decrease in CPP has been characterized and documented (Fig. 34-10).[236] An initial decrease in diastolic velocity, leading to an increased PI, is followed by disappearance of diastolic flow. The onset of retrograde diastolic flow or oscillating flow signifies the presence of intracranial circulatory arrest (see Chap. 38). Quantifying this change in waveform with PI, most studies have demonstrated a good direct correlation between ICP and PI, and an inverse relationship between CPP and PI.[237] The predictive value, however, is relatively low. Hence, it is a qualitative estimate rather than a quantitative measurement of ICP and CPP.

CLINICAL EXPERIENCE IN THE USE OF TCD

In a recent study, TCD monitoring was used to monitor the hyperemic state by an increased mean velocity and a decrease in PI prior to the development of acute cerebral edema which led to an adjustment in therapy to minimize the secondary insult related to elevated ICP.[238]

Simultaneous measurements of flow velocity, CPP, and jugular venous oxygen saturation obtained from a retrograde jugular catheter may be valuable in evaluating various modalities of treatment. In a recent study of 22 patients, the simultaneous recording of PI and Sjv_{O_2} was studied under changing CPP conditions. It was demonstrated that a sharp decrease in Sjv_{O_2} occurred when the CPP fell below the critical threshold of 68 mmHg. Similarly, an increasing PI occurred when the CPP fell below 71 mmHg.[31,239]

Knowledge regarding the integrity of the autoregulatory mechanism and CO_2 reactivity can be valuable in identifying patients at risk of developing secondary ischemia from reduced cerebral perfusion caused by a decrease in blood pressure or increased ICP, and conversely, patients at risk of developing secondary hemorrhages and vasogenic edema from a sudden increase in blood pressure. TCD can be used to assess dynamic cerebral autoregulation by observing the temporal response in cerebral blood flow velocity to a transient decrease in blood pressure.[240-242] Knowledge of these responses may play important roles in determining the optimal management therapy in a head-injured patient.

Organ Systemic Effects and Complications in Neurointensive Care Unit

The management of head-injured, multiple-traumatized patients is challenging as they are often the most ill, with many systemic complications in addition to head injury. The delayed systemic sequelae of head injury are diverse and may complicate management. The systemic effects include cardiovascular problems (shock, arrhythmias, and ECG changes), pulmonary problems (airway obstruction, hypoxemia, pneumonia, neurogenic pulmonary edema, and adult respiratory distress syndrome), fluid and electrolyte abnormalities (syndrome of inappropriate ADH secretion and diabetes insipidus), hematologic abnormalities (disseminated intravascular coagulopathy), gastrointestinal problems (gastric ulcers), and complications from infection, seizures, and toxic drugs. The systemic sequelae are both a direct result of the initial injury and indirect complications from the head injury.

CARDIOVASCULAR SYSTEM

The stimulation of the sympathetic nervous system plays an important role in the autonomic dysregulation underlying cardiac abnormalities. Life-threatening alterations in cardiac rate, rhythm, and conduction can occur after head trauma.[203] In addition, a variety of ECG changes have occurred such as high-amplitude P waves, increased QRS voltage, Q waves, prolonged QT interval, shortened QT interval, depressed ST segments, elevated ST segments, T wave flattening, T wave inversion, tall and peaked T waves, notched T waves, U waves, pulsus alternans, and U wave alternans.[30] The most common cardiac arrhythmia following head trauma is supraventricular tachycardia which has been associated with elevated sympathetic activity and correlated with elevated CK-MB fractions.[244] The most common cardiovascular effects of head trauma are listed in Table 34-7.

Treatment of hemodynamically unstable cardiac arrhythmias is imperative; it may require fluid resuscita-

TABLE 34-7
Cardiovascular Effects of Head Trauma

Hyperdynamic cardiovascular state
  Hypertension
    Increased cardiac output
    Increased intracranial pressure (Cushing response)

  Cardiac arrhythmias
    Bradycardia
    Nodal rhythms
    Sinus tachycardia
    Sinus arrhythmia
    Atrial fibrillation
    Premature ventricular contraction
    Heart block
    Ventricular tachycardia (*torsade de pointes* arrhythmia)

  Electrocardiogram changes of myocardial ischemia
    Peaked P waves
    Prolonged QT intervals, corrected for heart rate
    Depressed ST segments
    Inverted / flattened T waves
    Prominent U waves

  Focal areas of myocardial necrosis

Hypotension
  Uncommon, must rule out other causes
  May occur with brain decompression

tion as well as administration of vaspressors and inotropic and / or chronotropic agents. In contrast, hemodynamically stable cardiac abnormalities can be followed with a rule-out myocardial infarction protocol.

The importance of hypertension and hypotension have already been discussed above, and the treatment principles are no different than in the intraoperative period.

PULMONARY SYSTEM

Hypoxemia has particularly detrimental effects in head-injured patients as the injured brain is vulnerable to secondary injury. Therefore, it is important to prevent hypoxemia and to treat promptly should it occur. In patients with head injuries, the cause of hypoxemia is multifactorial and may result from either direct lung injury and / or neurogenic effects secondary to head injury (Table 34-8). Important factors that affect the pulmonary system include (1) a depressed level of consciousness leading to abnormal respiratory patterns, (2) infection including pneumonia, and (3) impaired pulmonary function with alteration of ventilation-perfusion (V/Q) relationship.

ABNORMAL RESPIRATORY PATTERNS

The respiratory rate (RR) and depth are altered in about 60 percent of head-injured patients.[30] Tachypnea (RR > 25/min), dyspnea, irregular breathing, and Cheyne-Stokes respiration pattern may change over time and occur with nearly equal frequency.[245] Usually, hypoventilation and hypercapnia occur only as a terminal event.

PNEUMONIA

Pneumonia is the most frequent pulmonary complication in head-injured patients, because airway protective reflexes are compromised, resulting in aspiration of oral pharyngeal secretions.[246] In the TCDB cohort, pneumonia was an independent predictor of poor outcome.[30] Loss of consciousness, distended stomach, sedation, and paralytics all contribute to loss of airway protective reflexes. In head-injured patients with increased ICP, routine chest physiotherapy and postural drainage are often not possible, and therefore the chances of nosocomial infection, atelectasis, pulmonary embolus, and acute respiratory distress syndrome are increased. An increase in the incidence of pneumonia has been correlated with use of an ICP monitor,[247] the use of barbiturates for elevated ICP, corticosteroid use,[248,249] and histamine type 2 blockers.[250]

Nosocomial pneumonia in ICU patients may be separated into an early and a late phase. Half of the ICU pneumonias occur during the early phase of up to 5 days after admission, and relate to oropharyngeal aspiration. In a recent study, 41 percent of patients following closed head injury developed pneumonia with the majority occurring during the first 3 days.[251] The predominant organisms are gram-positive organisms such as *Staphylococcus aureus, Streptococcus pneumonia,* and *Haemophilus influenzae.*[252] In contrast, late-onset pneumonia occurs after 5 days and correlates with the overall health status of the patient, atelectasis, gastric pH neutralization, and duration of mechanical ventilation. Gram-negative organisms such as enteric bacteria and *Pseudomonas* are the most predominant.[253]

TABLE 34-8
Pulmonary Effects of Head Trauma

Pulmonary etiologies
  Flail chest
  Pneumothorax
  Hemothorax
  Pulmonary contusion
  Aspiration
  Atelectasis
  Cardiogenic pulmonary edema
  Fat embolism syndrome
  Adult respiratory distress syndrome (ARDS)
  Pneumonia

Neurogenic etiologies
  Abnormal respiratory patterns
  Reduced functional residual capacity
  Neurogenic alterations in ventilation/perfusion matching
  Neurogenic pulmonary edema

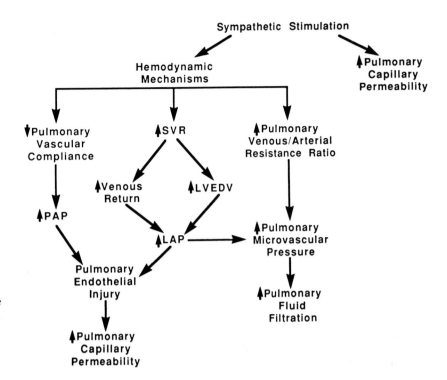

Figure 34-11 Hypothesized mechanism in the pathogenesis of neurogenic pulmonary edema. SVR, systemic vascular resistance; PAP, pulmonary artery pressure; LVEDV, left ventricular end-diastolic volume; LAP, left atrial pressure.

Prophylactic antibiotics alone have not been shown to be effective in lowering the morbidity or mortality during the early or late phases of pneumonia.[252,254] The diagnosis of pneumonia is difficult, but any patient with fever, leukocytosis, and a new or progressive infiltrate on chest x-ray should be suspected of having pneumonia and treated. Antibiotics should be selected on the basis of sputum culture and sensitivities, and chest physiotherapy, postural drainage, and nasotracheal suctioning should be performed as vigorously as the patient's condition allows.

IMPAIRED PULMONARY FUNCTION
There is a spectrum of impaired pulmonary functions associated with acute brain injury, including neurogenic pulmonary edema (NPE). NPE often, but not always, occurs after an acute elevation in ICP. The pathophysiology remains unclear, but is characterized by marked pulmonary vascular congestion, intraalveolar hemorrhage, and a protein-rich edema fluid (Fig. 34-11). During the Vietnam war, it was reported that 85 percent of combat casualties who died from a severe isolated head injury demonstrated pulmonary pathology that was not due to direct lung injury, aspiration, or cardiogenic-related causes.[255]

Neurogenic pulmonary edema can be classified into an early and a late form. The early form occurs within minutes to several hours, frequently after a convulsion, but also occurs with head trauma and subarachnoid hemorrhage.[30] It is characterized by dyspnea, tachypnea, hypoxemia, tachycardia, rales, fever, hypoxia, and mild leukocytosis. On chest x-rays, there are bilateral and central fluffy infiltrates without cardiomegaly, pleural effusion, or dense consolidations. The clinical and radiologic findings usually disappear within 24 to 48 h. Severe systemic and pulmonary hypertension may occur transiently.[256] In contrast, the delayed form presents 12 h to several days after injury, and is most commonly caused by head injury.[257] The delayed form has not been associated with episodes of increased systemic or pulmonary hypertension.[258]

The mechanism of NPE is related to a massive sympathetic adrenergic discharge which results in increased pulmonary microvascular hydrostatic pressure and pulmonary capillary permeability (Fig. 34-11).[259] Pathologic factors responsible for the development of NPE include (1) left arterial hypertension, (2) systemic hypertension, (3) pulmonary venoconstriction, (4) reduction in pulmonary vascular compliance, and (5) physical opening of capillary tight junctions by sympathetic innervation to endothelial cells and their contractile elements.[259–261]

The treatment of NPE is directed at reducing ICP, along with supportive measures of ventilatory assistance including PEEP, head elevation, use of diuretics, sedation, and blockade of sympathetic hyperactivity.[262]

FLUID AND ELECTROLYTES

In the TCDB cohort, electrolyte disturbances were the most common extracranial complication.[263] The usual maintenance fluid volume should be about 2500 to

3000 ml/day, and/or to maintain a central venous pressure of 6 to 8 mmHg, and/or urine output between 0.5 to 1.0 ml/kg per h. The most important electrolyte abnormality in head-injured patients is sodium imbalance leading to hyponatremia or hypernatremia as well as hyperglycemia.

HYPONATREMIA

Hyponatremia is defined as a serum sodium less than 135 meq/liter. Hyponatremia has been associated with further deterioration of brain injury[264]; therefore, early recognition and treatment are important. Unfortunately, in the patient with a severe head injury, hyponatremia may occur quickly and be exacerbated by mannitol treatment for elevated ICP. When evaluating a patient with hyponatremia, the volume status should be carefully assessed as serum sodium is a marker for disturbances in free-water balance. Volume status is evaluated by measuring serum and urine electrolytes and osmolarity, renal function, urine output, nasogastric output, and other fluid intake and output. Hyponatremia may be divided into three types based on volume status: isovolemic, hypovolemic, and hypervolemic.

Isovolemic hyponatremia involves the syndrome of inappropriate secretion of antidiuretic hormone (SIADH). The syndrome may be caused by drugs, hypoaldosteronism, hypothyroidism, polydipsia, iatrogenic water intoxication, and hyperosmolar states as seen with hyperglycemia (glucose > 180 mg/dl) and mannitol treatment. It usually begins 3 to 15 days after injury, and may last up to 10 to 15 days with appropriate therapy. Enhanced secretion of ADH can also be caused by intracranial hypertension after head trauma, hypoxia, stress, and hypercapnia, as well as by pharmacologic agents such as barbiturates, halothane, morphine, and nicotine.[265] In contrast, pharmacologic agents such as ethanol, naloxone, and phenytoin can inhibit ADH secretion. The hallmark of SIADH is inappropriately concentrated urine (urine osmolality greater than 100 mosm/liter) in the face of hypotonic plasma (plasma osmolality below 290 mosm/liter). In patients not taking diuretics, the following criteria must be met: (1) serum sodium less than 135 mmol/liter, (2) serum osmolarity less than 280 mosm/liter, (3) urine osmolarity greater than serum osmolarity, and (4) inappropriately high urine sodium of greater than 40 meq/liter.[30] Fluid restriction of 800 to 1000 ml of free water intake per 24 h is the treatment for mildly to moderately symptomatic patients and the abnormalities can be safely corrected over a 48-h period. However, in severe hyponatremia (serum sodium less than 120 meq/liter), rapid correction of serum sodium can lead to central pontine myelinolysis.[266,267] In this setting, an increase in the serum sodium at a rate of 1 to 2 meq/liter per h until a level of 130 meq/liter is reached is the recommended treatment protocol. In the head-injured patient requiring fluid resuscitation, SIADH may be treated with demeclocycline (300 mg p.o. every 6 h) which inhibits ADH action,[268] or fluorocortisone (0.1 to 0.2 mg p.o. per day).[30] An alternative for the correction of mild to moderate hyponatremia is the administration of intravenous urea and normal saline, which allows adequate hydration with a concomitant hyponatremic diuresis.[269]

Hypovolemic hyponatremia occurs secondary to cerebral salt wasting or from iatrogenic replacement of salt and water losses with hyponatremic solutions. Cerebral salt wasting is characterized by inappropriate natriuresis or renal sodium wasting. Treatment of cerebral salt wasting involves volume and sodium replacement with 0.9% normal saline as well as the judicious use of 3% saline.

Hypervolemic hyponatremia may be caused by cirrhosis, congestive heart failure, and renal failure. Hyponatremia in this setting is caused by a dilutional effect of excess extracellular volume leading to a fictitiously low serum sodium. Treatment is directed at the underlying pathologic process.

HYPERNATREMIA

Hypernatremia is defined as a serum sodium over 145 meq/liter. It may be iatrogenic or secondary to diabetes insipidus. The most common cause of hypernatremia in the intensive care unit is the loss of hypotonic fluids. However, diabetes insipidus may occur in a small percentage of head-injured patients from inadequate ADH secretion.

Diabetes insipidus (DI) can be divided into two categories, central and nephrogenic. Central DI can occur with either minor or severe closed head injury.[270] Clinically, DI presents with polyuria, polydipsia, hypernatremia, high serum osmolality, and dilute urine. The onset is usually evident within 24 h of the inciting event. Central DI secondary to trauma is usually self-limiting and transient. Its development following severe head injury is associated with a poor prognosis as it reflects severe disruption of the brainstem.[30] Treatment of central DI generally involves replacement of free water, or in severe cases the administration of aqueous desmopressin acetate (DDAVP, 2 to 4 μg I.V. every 8 to 12 h or 5 to 10 units s.c. every 4 to 6 h). In alert patients, the thirst mechanism can compensate for the volume loss without treatment.

HYPERGLYCEMIA

Hyperglycemia is frequently present in patients with severe head injury, and is correlated with a poor outcome.[33,271] Experimental studies consistently demonstrate that moderately elevated blood glucose levels in the presence of cerebral ischemia have a deleterious effect on neurologic recovery.[35,272,273] These deleterious effects correlate with increased levels of tissue lactate and decreased levels of phosphorylated high-energy compounds.[274,275] This may be related to the decreased production of adenosine after cerebral ischemia and reperfusion during hyperglycemia,[276] as adenosine appears to have several cerebroprotective functions including cerebral vasodilation,[277] depression of neuronal activity and glutamate release,[278,279] and inhibition of neutrophil activation.[280]

COAGULATION

Coagulopathy frequently develops in patients with severe head injury,[281,282] and may lead to further extra- or intracranial hemorrhagic complications. In a recent study of 253 patients with closed head injury, it was shown that the risk of developing a delayed brain injury including diffuse brain swelling, intracranial hematoma, contusion/infarction, or subarachnoid hemorrhage/intraventricular hemorrhage on head CT, was 85 percent in those with at least one abnormal coagulation study, compared to 31 percent for those without a coagulation abnormality.[282] Following head injury, disseminated intravascular coagulopathy (DIC) may occur as a consequence of the intravascular activation of the intrinsic and/or extrinsic pathways of the coagulation system. Presumably brain tissue thromboplastin, when released into the systemic circulation, activates the extrinsic clotting cascade, whereas endothelial injury activates the intrinsic clotting cascade.[283] It has been suggested that the magnitude of brain parenchymal damage correlates with plasma fibrinogen degradation product levels.[40,284] Evidence of DIC is characterized by elevated prothrombin time, partial thromboplastin time, and fibrin degradation product levels, as well as decreased plasma fibrinogen levels and platelet counts.

The treatment of DIC is early detection and correction of the underlying pathologic process. Supportive treatment and replacement of clotting factors with fresh-frozen plasma, cryoprecipitate, platelet concentrates, and blood may be required.

According to the 1994 task force of the College of American Pathologists,[285] the following are practice parameters for the use of fresh-frozen plasma (FFP), cryoprecipitate, and platelets. The clinical indications for FFP are: (1) history of coagulopathy with increased prothrombin time and activated partial thromboplastin time, (2) massive blood transfusions, (3) reversal of warfarin effect, (4) deficiency of antithrombin III, and (5) hypoglobulinemic states. The starting dose is 2 packs except when 5 to 6 units of platelets are being infused which are equivalent to 1 pack of FFP. The

clinical indications for platelets are: (1) decreased platelet production with or without increased platelet destruction (especially with counts below 50,000/mm^3), (2) enhanced platelet destruction such as DIC, and (3) platelet dysfunction. The starting dose should be given to increase the platelet count to above 50,000/mm^3, and one unit increases the count by about 5000 to 10,000/mm^3. The clinical indications for cryoprecipitate are: (1) hypofibrinogenemia, (2) von Willebrand's disease, (3) hemophilia A, and (4) fibrin surgical adhesive. Fibrinogen levels higher than 100 mg/dl are desirable, and an empirical rule is to give 1 unit of cryoprecipitate for every 5 to 10 kg of body weight.

GASTROINTESTINAL SYSTEM

Gastric ulcerations, gastroparesis, and swallowing disorders are common gastrointestinal complications in head-injured patients.

Gastric ulcerations can occur within 24 h and are evident by endoscopic exam in over 75 percent of head-injured patients.[286-289] The mechanism of gastric ulcerations includes mucosal barrier disruption, increased mucosal permeability, excessive gastric acid secretion, and defects in mucosal microcirculation. Although sucralfate and antacids sucralfate and antacids are both comparable in reducing the incidence of stress ulcer bleeding,[290] sucralfate (1 g p.o. every 6 h), a cytoprotective agent which maintains the mucosal barrier integrity without altering gastric pH, is the treatment of choice for prophylaxis. If significant hemorrhage occurs, then endoscopy and surgical intervention are warranted.

Gastroparesis is common following severe head injury, and these patients often have difficulty in tolerating enteral feedings during the first 14 days after injury.[291] The mean duration from injury to successful initiation of full-strength enteral feeding has been reported to be 11.5 days.[292] It is important early on to initiate a bowel program to avoid excessive straining. In addition, the administration of metoclopramide has been shown to improve gastric emptying.[293]

The most common swallowing disorder following traumatic head injury is the delayed triggering of the swallowing reflex. Other swallowing disorders such as dysfunction of oromotor control, pharyngeal peristalsis, and airway reflex protection mechanisms may also occur.[294] Adequate evaluation by a speech pathologist is warranted if these disorders occur.

INFECTION

Predisposing factors that increase the incidence of infection in acute head-injured patients include wound contamination, mechanical ventilation, steroid therapy, and catheter contamination. In posttrauma patients, numerous impairments of immune mechanisms have been reported. These include alterations in immunoglobulin and complement concentrations, decreased functional activity of granulocytes, and phagocyte inhibition.[295–297]

SEIZURES

Posttraumatic seizures may occur early or late; early posttraumatic seizures occur during the first week and late posttraumatic seizures occur after the first week. The incidence of early posttraumatic seizures following head injury is estimated at between 1.9 to 4.6 percent.[298,299] In contrast, late posttraumatic seizures occur in 1.6 to 5 percent of all head-injured patients and up to 15 percent of severely head-injured patients.[298–300] The main risk factor for early seizures appears to be an anatomic lesion such as an intracranial hematoma. Thus, the incidence of early and late posttraumatic seizures for patients with an intracranial hematoma are 25 and 35 percent, respectively.[298] Control of seizures may be accomplished by both short-acting agents in the acute setting (e.g., Lorazepam 0.2 mg/kg) and/or long-acting anticonvulsants (e.g., phenytoin 20 mg/kg). Unfortunately phenytoin prophylaxis for posttraumatic seizures in patients with severe head injury is only effective for one week, and does not prevent delayed seizure.[300] The policy at our institution is to treat all head-injured patients for 7 days after a head injury with intravenous or p.o. phenytoin (adults: loading bolus of 1 g or 20 mg/kg followed by 300 mg per day; children: loading bolus of 10 mg/kg followed by 5 mg/kg per day).

Promising New Therapies

Improved understanding of the pathophysiology and biochemistry of head injury and neuronal death has made it possible to develop a rational and targeted approach based on blockade of specific pathways or combination thereof. Although a dramatic breakthrough has not occurred, these potentially promising therapies have given a glimpse into the future. Some of the physiologic and pharmacologic therapies currently being investigated are summarized in Fig. 34-12.

GLUCOCORTICOID AND NONGLUCOCORTICOID THERAPY

The role of glucocorticoid and nonglucocorticoid lipid antioxidant therapy has been extensively studied with controversial results. Despite early enthusiasm,[301–303] subsequent clinical trials failed to demonstrate any beneficial effect of steroids in central nervous system

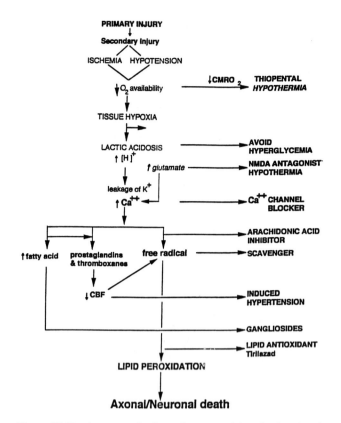

Figure 34-12 A proposed schematic summarizing the functional abnormalities of traumatic brain injury and illustrating the potential therapeutic approaches using pharmacologic means.

trauma.[222,223,249,304] With the recent demonstration that high-dose methylprednisolone improves outcome after acute human spinal cord injury,[305] there has been renewed interest in the use of steroids in head injury. More potent lipid antioxidants devoid of glucocorticoid action (21-aminosteroids) appear to be promising.[306,307] Tirilazad mesylate, which has no direct effect on cerebral blood flow and metabolism in healthy humans,[308] is currently undergoing clinical trials in head injury and subarachnoid hemorrhage.

EXCITATORY AMINO ACID ANTAGONISTS

Excitatory amino acids play an important role in the development of delayed neuronal necrosis after hypoxic or ischemic insults.[309,310] Energy depletion after brain ischemia results in synaptic accumulation of glutamate release as well as the failure of cellular reuptake of glutamate.[310,311] This high concentration of extracellular glutamate stimulates glutamate receptors of the *N*-methyl-D-aspartate (NMDA) subtype which, via receptor-gated channels, allows intracellular calcium influx.[309,310] Intracellular accumulation of calcium activates phospholipase with generation of free radicals and destruction of membrane proteins and lipids, with eventual neuronal death.[312] Elevated levels of gluta-mates have been recovered from CSF of patients with severe head injury.[313] Thus, blockade of NMDA recep-tors with specific antagonists or noncompetitive ion channel blockers may provide cerebral protection.[314] The opportunities for using this therapy in head trauma have been reviewed by Zauner and Bullock.[315] Experimentally, NMDA receptor antagonists that can penetrate the blood-brain barrier have the most thera-peutic potential in the treatment of brain injury. One of the most investigated drugs is dizocilpine maleate (MK-801) which is a noncompetitive NMDA receptor antagonist. In experimental head injury, Shapira and coworkers and McIntosh and coworkers observed im-provement in both neurologic status and brain edema in MK-801 treatment groups.[316,317] Although Buchen and Pulsinelli attributed the beneficial effects of MK-801 to the concurrent development of hypothermia,[318] numerous studies on other noncompetitive and com-petitive glutamate antagonists have repeatedly demon-strated the cerebroprotective potential.[311] Ketamine, an-other noncompetitive NMDA-antagonist, given to rats 1 h after experimental head injury, also decreased hem-orrhagic necrosis of the brain, and improved neuro-logic score.[166]

Clinically, using the technique of microdialysis, Zauner and Bullock reported that in patients with un-controllable ICP, prolonged secondary insults, or cere-bral blood flow below the ischemic threshold, there was a massive release of excitatory amino acids. In contrast, in stabilized patients with severe head injury in the ICU, the excitatory amino acid level was not increased.[315] Clinical trials of NMDA antagonists for head injury and stroke are currently underway.[319]

FREE RADICAL SCAVENGERS

Free radicals are produced during ischemia and reper-fusion from dissociation of the mitochondrial electron transport chain because of the lack of oxygen as a terminal electron acceptor. The most important free radical produced is the superoxide radical which at-tacks proteins and polyunsaturated phospholipids in membranes, and disrupts cellular functioning and leads to neuronal death.[320,321] Under normal circum-stances, free radicals generated are scavenged by su-peroxide dismutase (SOD) to form hydrogen peroxide and oxygen, the capacity of which is overwhelmed during ischemia. In a phase II clinical trial Muizelaar and coworkers reported that polyethylene glycol con-jugated-SOD given to severe head-injured patients (GCS < 8) is safe, and there was a trend toward im-proved neurologic outcome. Further evaluations are clearly indicated.[321]

SYSTEMIC HYPOTHERMIA

This is perhaps the most promising of all the therapies currently undergoing clinical trials. The clinical appli-cation of hypothermic therapy began in 1944 when Field and coworkers showed that hypothermia sig-nificantly decreased cerebral oxygen consumption.[322] Michenfelder further clarified the mechanism of hypothermia and the relationship to the cerebral meta-bolic rate, explaining its protective effect in brain in-jury. Maximal cerebral protection, however, is only achieved during profound hypothermia to a tempera-ture of 15 to 18°C, when isoelectric EEG occurs.[323] Thus the benefits of profound hypothermia are balanced by impracticality, as well as by the risks of the inherent associated systemic complications. Recent studies have focused on the use of mild to moderate hypothermia for cerebral protection. In rodent models of global ischemia, moderate hypothermia (30 to 33°C) during and after ischemia significantly diminished neuronal loss.[324,325] In related studies, mild to moderate hypother-mia suppressed the release of toxic neurotransmitter glutamate and glycine.[326,327] Thus, it appears the cere-broprotective effect of mild to moderate hypothermia is based more on suppression of release of toxic neuro-transmitters than on a direct effect on cerebral metab-olism.

A phase II clinical trial of moderate hypothermia (32 to 33°C) within 6 h of injury for 48 h in 46 patients with severe head injury suggested that this degree of hypothermia is safe and is associated with a trend toward improved neurologic outcome.[328] Two other small clinical trials have demonstrated the potential therapeutic effects of moderate hypothermia.[329,330] Mar-ion and coworkers randomized 40 consecutive patients with severe head injury to either normothermia or hy-pothermia (32 to 33°C) for 24 h. Although the trend toward better outcome in the hypothermia group was not statistically significant, ICP, CBF, and CMR_{O_2} were all lower in the hypothermia group. No difference in the incidence of complications was observed between the two groups.[329] Shiozake and coworkers randomized 33 severely head-injured patients whose ICP was greater than 20 mmHg and resistant to conventional therapy of hyperventilation and barbiturates to either normothermia or mild hypothermia (34°C). Not only did ICP decrease, in concert with the reduction in CBF and CMR_{O_2}, survival was improved (50 percent versus 18 percent).[330] A randomized, multicenter trial de-signed to enroll 500 patients is now underway, but the results will not be available until 1997 or later.

INDOMETHACIN

Although the use of indomethacin is limited by the potential complication of hemorrhage, this nonsteroid anti-inflammatory agent is the only one of its class that has a profound effect on cerebral hemodynamics. In a small series of five severely head-injured patients with elevated ICP refractory to therapy, Jensen and coworkers administered an intravenous bolus of indomethacin 30 mg/kg followed by a continuous infusion of 30 mg/h for 7 h and were able to reduce the ICP to below 20 mmHg in all.[331] The mechanism appears to be based on cerebral vasoconstriction as indomethacin causes a profound reduction in CBF. Unfortunately this is not accompanied by a change in cerebral metabolic rate; thus, indomethacin uncouples the normal flow-metabolism coupling favoring the development of ischemia.[332] In patients with refractory ICP secondary to hyperemia, however, it may represent a potentially useful therapy.

LUND THERAPY

Recently, the "Lund concept" of posttraumatic brain edema therapy has been introduced into clinical practice in Sweden.[333] In severely head-injured patients, there is presently no pharmacologic treatment to repair the disrupted blood-brain barrier or the impaired cerebral autoregulation. This therapy is based on the assumption that extracellular brain edema, caused by an impaired blood-brain barrier and cerebral autoregulation, is an important component of posttraumatic cerebral swelling and is easier to approach therapeutically than intracellular edema. The aim of this therapy is to keep ICP at a safe level until repair of the blood-brain barrier and cerebral autoregulation is restored to prevent brain herniation and to minimize ischemic secondary brain injury. Although the essential components of the "Lund Therapy" can be considered standard (decrease in cerebral metabolism; thermal and glucose regulation; reduction of cerebral blood volume by hyperventilation or barbiturate coma; maintenance of colloid osmotic pressure), the use of induced hypotension to reduce capillary hydrostatic pressure to decrease cerebral edema stands in stark contrast to the conventional emphasis on maintenance of cerebral perfusion pressure.[333,334] The use of a cerebral venous vasoconstrictor, dihydroergotamine, to reduce cerebral blood volume also represents a novel therapy.[335] Their early clinical experience with this therapy in 52 patients appears to be promising, but clearly more studies are needed to confirm its efficacy.

Conclusion

The injury mechanisms of head injury are complex with multiple pathologic pathways and biochemical cascades. Identification of these pathophysiologic and biochemical mechanisms allows development of effective interventions to prevent or minimize secondary injury and development of pharmacologic therapy targeted to specific gateways to interrupt the injury process. Many of the current concepts based on these considerations are reviewed in this chapter. It is recognized that as our knowledge base increases, therapies will change accordingly. Although the mortality of head injury remains unacceptably high, it is hoped that better characterization of the injury mechanisms and future advances in pharmacotherapy may lead to improved neurologic outcome and the overall management results.

Acknowledgment

The authors would like to thank Jennifer Avellino for help in preparing the manuscript.

References

1. Jennett B, Teasdale G: Aspects of coma after severe head injury. *Lancet* 1977; 1:878.
2. Jennett B, Bond M: Assessment of outcome after severe brain damage. *Lancet* 1975; 1:480.
3. U.S. Department of Health, Education, and Welfare: Facts of life and death. Publication # (HRS) 74-1222. Rockville, MD, National Center for Health Statistics, 1974.
4. National Center for Health Statistics: Births, marriages, divorces, and deaths for 1990. Monthly Vital Statistics Report, vol. 39, No. 12, Public Health Services, 1991, Hyattsville, MD.
5. Gennarelli TA, et al: Mortality of patients with head injury and extracranial injury treated in trauma centers. *J Trauma* 1989; 29:1193.
6. Sosin DM, et al: Head injury-associated deaths in the U.S. from 1979–1986. *JAMA* 1989; 262:2251.
7. Sosin DM, et al: Trends in death associated with traumatic brain injury, 1979 through 1992. *JAMA* 1995; 273:1778.
8. Kraus JF: Epidemiology of head injury. In Cooper PR (ed): *Head Injury*, 3d ed. Baltimore, Williams & Wilkins, 1993:1.
9. Jennett B, MacMillan R: Epidemiology of head injury. *Br Med J* 1981; 282:101.
10. Rimel RW, et al: Moderate head injury: Completing the clinical spectrum of brain trauma. *Neurosurgery* 1982; 11:344.
11. Whitman S, et al: Comparative head trauma experience in two socioeconomically different Chicago-area communities: A population study. *Am J Epidemiol* 1984; 119:570.
12. Kraus JF, Nourjah P: The epidemiology of mild, uncomplicated brain injury. *J Trauma* 1988; 29(12):1637.
13. Leroux PD, Grady MS: Epidemiology of head injury. In Lam AM (ed): *Anesthetic Management of Acute Head Injury*. New York, McGraw-Hill, 1995:1.
14. Gennarelli TA, et al: Influence of the type of intracranial lesion on outcome from severe head injury. *J Neurosurg* 1982; 56:26.
15. Lindenberg R, Freytag E: Morphology of brain lesions from blunt trauma in infancy. *Arch Pathol* 1969; 87:298.
16. Adams JH, et al: Diffuse axonal injury in head injury: Definition, diagnosis, and grading. *Histopathology* 1989; 15:49.
17. Strich SJ: Shearing of nerve fibers as a cause of brain damage due to head injury. *Lancet* 1961; 2:443.

18. Graham DI, et al: Ischemic brain damage in fatal non-missile head injuries. *J Neurol Sci* 1978; 39:213.

19. Graham DI, et al: Ischaemic brain damage is still common in fatal non-missile head injury. *J Neurol Neurosurg Psychiatry* 1989; 52:346.

20. Bouma GJ, et al: Cerebral circulation and metabolism after severe traumatic brain injury: The elusive role of ischemia. *J Neurosurg* 1991; 75:685.

21. Bouma GJ, et al: Ultra-early evaluation of regional cerebral blood flow in severely head-injured patients using xenon-inhanced computerized tomography. *J Neurosurg* 1992; 77:360.

22. Muizelaar JP, Schroder ML: Overview of monitoring of cerebral blood flow and metabolism after severe head injury. *Can J Neurol Sci* 1994; 21:S6.

23. Marion DW, et al: Acute regional cerebral blood flow changes caused by severe head injuries. *J Neurosurg* 1991; 74:407.

24. Obrist WD, et al: Cerebral blood flow and metabolism in comatose patients with acute head injury. *J Neurosurg* 1984; 61:241.

25. Miller JD, Becker DP: Secondary insults to the injured brain. *J Royal Coll Surg (Edinburgh)* 1982; 27:292.

26. Gentleman D: Causes and effects of systemic complications among severely head injured patients transferred to a neurosurgical unit. *Int Surg* 1992; 77:297.

27. Fearnside MR, et al: The Westmead Head Injury Project outcome in severe head injury. A comparative analysis of prehospital, clinical and CT variables. *Br J Neurosurg* 1993; 7:262.

28. Jenkins LW, et al: Increased vulnerability of the mildly traumatized rat brain to cerebral ischemia: The use of controlled secondary ischemia as a research tool to identify common or different mechanisms contributing to mechanical and ischemic brain injury. *Brain Res* 1989; 477:211.

29. Marmarou A, et al: Impact of ICP instability and hypotension on outcome in patients with severe head trauma. *J Neurosurg* 1991; 75:S59.

30. Chesnut RM: Medical complications of the head-injured patient. In Cooper PR (ed): *Head Injury,* 3d ed. Baltimore, Williams & Wilkins, 1993:459.

31. Chan K-H, et al: The effect of changes in cerebral perfusion pressure upon middle cerebral artery blood flow velocity and jugular bulb venous oxygen saturation after severe brain injury. *J Neurosurg* 1992; 77:55.

32. Rosner MJ, et al: Cerebral perfusion pressure: Management protocol and clinical results. *J Neurosurg* 1995; 83:949.

33. Lam AM, et al: Hyperglycemia and neurological outcome in patients with head injury. *J Neurosurg* 1991; 75:545.

34. Michaud LJ, et al: Elevated initial blood glucose levels and poor outcome following severe brain injuries in children. *J Trauma* 1991; 31:1356.

35. Pulsinelli WA, et al: Moderate hyperglycemia augments ischemic brain damage: A neuropathologic study in the rat. *Neurology* 1982; 32:1239.

36. Lanier WL, et al: The effects of dextrose infusion and head position on neurologic outcome after complete cerebral ischemia in primates: Examination of a model. *Anesthesiology* 1987; 66:39.

37. Gardiner M, et al: Influence of blood glucose concentration on brain lactate accumulation during severe hypoxia and subsequent recovery of brain energy metabolism. *J Cereb Blood Flow Metab* 1982; 2:429.

38. Nedergaard M: Transient focal ischemia in hyperglycemic rats is associated with increased cerebral infarction. *Brain Res* 1987; 408:79.

39. Pfenninger EG, Lindner KH: Arterial blood gases in patients with acute head injury at the accident site and upon hospital admission. *Acta Anaesthesiol Scand* 1991; 35:1378.

40. Olson JD, et al: The incidence and significance of hemostatic abnormalities in patients with head injuries. *Neurosurgery* 1989; 24:825.

41. MacPherson P, Graham DI: Correlation between angiographic findings and the ischemia of head injury. *J Neurol Neurosurg Psychiatry* 1978; 41:122.

42. Inglis FM, et al: Ischaemic brain damage associated with tissue hypermetabolism in acute haematoma: Reduction by a glutamate antagonist. *Acta Neurochirurgica* 1990; 5(Suppl):277.

43. Jeunger E, et al: Cerebral autoregulation in patients with mild and moderate head injury. *Stroke* 1996; 27:796 (abstr).

44. Bouma GJ, et al: Blood pressure and intracranial pressure-volume dynamics in severe head injury: Relationship with cerebral blood flow. *J Neurosurg* 1992; 77:15.

45. Cold GE: Cerebral blood flow in acute head injury. The regulation of cerebral blood flow and metabolism during the acute phase of head injury, and in significance for therapy. *Acta Neurochir Suppl(Wien)* 1990; 49:1.

46. Marion DW, Bouma GJ: The use of stable xenon-enhanced computed tomographic studies of cerebral blood flow to define changes in cerebral carbon dioxide vasoresponsivity caused by a severe head injury. *Neurosurgery* 1991; 29:869.

47. Schalen W, et al: Cerebral vasoreactivity and the prediction of outcome in severe traumatic brain lesions. *Acta Anaesthesiol Scand* 1991; 35:113.

48. Klatzo I: Presidential address: Neuropathological aspects of brain edema. *J Neuropath Exp Neurol* 1967; 26:1.

49. Povlishock JT, et al: Vascular permeability alterations to horseradish peroxidase in experimental brain injury. *Brain Res* 1978; 153:223.

50. Wahl M, et al: Mediators of blood-brain barrier dysfunction and formation of vasogenic brain edema. *J Cereb Blood Flow Metabl* 8:621, 1988

51. Miller JD: Traumatic brain swelling and edema. In Cooper PR (ed): *Head Injury,* 3d ed. Baltimore, Williams & Wilkins, 1993:331.

52. Chan PH, et al: Induction of brain edema following intracerebral injection of arachidonic acid. *Ann Neurol* 1983; 63:235.

53. Kontos HA, Wei EP: Superoxide production in experimental brain injury. *J Neurosurg* 1986; 64:803.

54. Ikeda Y, Long DM: The molecular basis of brain injury and brain edema: The role of oxygen free radicals. *Neurosurgery* 1990; 27:1.

55. Clasen RA, et al: Experimental study of relation of fever to cerebral edema. *J Neurosurg* 1974; 41:576.

56. Houthoff HJ: Pathobiology of the blood brain barrier and brain edema. In Cohadon F, et al (eds): *Traumatic Brain Edemas.* Padova, Fidia Research Series No. 8, Liviana Press, 1987:1.

57. Astrup J: Energy requiring cell functions in the ischemic brain. *J Neurosurg* 1982; 56:482.

58. Bell BA, et al: CBF and time thresholds for the formation of ischemic cerebral edema and effect of reperfusion in baboons. *J Neurosurg* 1985; 62:31.

59. Schutta HS, et al: Brain swelling produced by injury and aggravated by arterial hypertension. *Brain* 1968; 91:281.

60. Langfitt TW, et al: Cerebral vasomotor paralysis produced by intracranial hypertension. *Neurology* 1965; 15:622.

61. Stern WE, Coxon RV: Osmolality of brain tissue and its relation to brain bulk. *Am J Physiol* 1964; 206:1.

62. Arieff AI: Hyponatremia, convulsions, respiratory arrest and permanent brain damage after elective surgery in healthy women. *N Engl J Med* 1986; 314:1529.

63. Arieff AI: Hyponatremia associated with permanent brain damage. *Adv Intern Med* 1987; 32:325.

64. Fraser CL, et al: Sex differences result in increased morbidity from hyponatremia in female rats. *Am J Physiol* 1989; 256:R880.

65. Fishman RA: Brain edema. *N Engl J Med* 1975; 293:706.

66. Marmarou A, et al: Contribution of CSF and vascular factors to elevation of ICP in severely head-injured patients. *J Neurosurg* 1987; 66:883.

67. Miller JD, et al: Further experience in the management of severe head injury. *J Neurosurg* 1981; 54:289.

68. Rivara FP, et al: Drug use in trauma victims. *J Trauma* 1989; 29:462.

69. Tardiff K, et al: An analysis of cocaine positive fatalities. *J Forensic Sci* 1989; 34:53.

70. Albin MS, Bunegin L: An experimental study of craniocerebral trauma during ethanol intoxication. *Crit Care Med* 1986; 14:841.

71. Zink BJ, et al: Effects of ethanol in traumatic brain injury. *J Neurotrauma* 1993; 10:275.

72. Ronty H, et al: Cerebral trauma and alcohol abuse. *Eur J Clin Invest* 1993; 23:182.

73. Goldfrank LR, Hoffman RS: The cardiovascular effects of cocaine. *Ann Emerg Med* 1991; 20:165.

74. Levine SR, et al: Cerebrovascular complications of the use of the "crack" form of alkaloidal cocaine. *N Engl J Med* 1990; 323:699.

75. Wojak JC, Flamm ES: Intracranial hemorrhage and cocaine use. *Stroke* 1987; 18:712.

76. Delaney KA, Goldfrank LR: Initial management of the multiply injured or intoxicated patient. In Cooper PR (ed): *Head Injury*, 3d ed. Baltimore, Williams & Wilkins, 1993:43.

77. Eisenberg HM, et al: Initial CT findings in 753 patients with severe head injury. A report from the NIH traumatic coma data bank. *J Neurosurg* 1990; 73:688.

78. Masters ST, et al: Skull x-ray examinations after head trauma. Recommendations by a multidisciplinary panel and validation study. *N Engl J Med* 1987; 316:84.

79. Gentry LR, et al: Prospective comparative study of intermediate-field MR and CT in the evaluation of closed head trauma. *AJNR* 1988; 9:91.

80. Gentry LR, et al: MR imaging of head trauma: Review of the distribution and radiopathologic features of traumatic lesions. *AJNR* 1988; 9:101.

81. Chestnut RM, et al: The role of secondary brain injury in determining outcome from severe head injury. *J Trauma* 1993; 34:216.

82. Frost EA, et al: Pulmonary shunt as a prognostic indicator in head injury. *J Neurosurg* 1979; 50:768.

83. Mahoney BD, Ruiz E: Acute resuscitation of the patient with head and spinal cord injuries. *Emerg Med Clin North Am* 1983; 1:583.

84. Majernick TG, et al: Cervical spine movement during orotracheal intubation. *Ann Emerg Med* 1986; 15:417.

85. Rhee KJ, et al: Oral intubation in the multiply injured patient: The risk of exacerbating spinal cord damage. *Ann Emerg Med* 1990; 19:511.

86. Talucci RC, et al: Rapid sequence induction with oral endotracheal intubation in the multiply injured patient. *Am Surg* 1988; 54:185.

87. Grande CM, et al: Appropriate techniques for airway management of emergency patients with suspected spinal cord injury. *Anesth Analg* 1988; 67:714.

89. Roberts DJ, et al: Neuromuscular blockade for critical patients in the emergency department. *Ann Emerg Med* 1986; 15:152.

89. Donegan JF, Bedford RF: Intravenously administered lidocaine prevents intracranial hypertension during endotracheal suctioning. *Anesthesiology* 1980; 52:516.

90. Kastrup J, et al: Intravenous lidocaine and cerebral blood flow: Impaired microvascular reactivity in diabetic patients. *J Clin Pharmacol* 1990; 30:318.

91. Pinaud M, et al: Effects of propofol on cerebral hemodynamics and metabolism in patients with brain trauma. *Anesthesiology* 1990; 73:404.

92. Moss E, et al: Effect of etomidate on intracranial pressure and cerebral perfusion pressure. *B J Anaesth* 1979; 51:347.

93. Marsh ML, et al: Succinylcholine-intracranial pressure effects in neurosurgical patients. *Anesth Analg* 1980; 59:550.

94. Forbes AM, Dally FG: Acute hypertension during induction of anesthesia and endotracheal intubation in normotensive man. *Br J Anaesth* 1970; 42:618.

95. Kovarik DW, et al: Succinylcholine does not change intracranial pressure, cerebral blood flow velocity, or the electroencephalogram in patients with neurologic injury. *Anesth Analg* 1994; 78:469.

96. Frankville DD, Drummond JC: Hyperkalemia after succinylcholine administration in a patient with closed head injury without paresis. *Anesthesiology* 1987; 67:264.

97. Brantigan CO, Grow JB: Cricothyroidotomy: Elective use in respiratory problems requiring tracheotomy. *J Thorac Cardiovasc Surg* 1976; 71:72.

98. Esses BA, Jafek BW: Cricothyroidotomy: A decade of experience in Denver. *Ann Otol Rhinol Laryngol* 1987; 96:519.

99. McGill J, et al: Cricothyroidotomy in the emergency department. *Ann Emerg Med* 1982; 11:361.

100. Klauber MR, et al: Determinants of head injury mortality: Importance of the low risk patient. *Neurosurgery* 1989; 24:31.

101. Wilberger JE: Emergency care and initial evaluation. In Cooper PR (ed): *Head Injury*, 3d ed. Baltimore, Williams & Wilkins, 1993:27.

102. Scalea T, et al: Fluid resuscitation in head injury. In *American Association for the Surgery of Trauma Abstract Book*. New York, American Association for the Surgery of Trauma, 1989.

103. Fisher B, et al: Hypertonic saline lowers raised intracranial pressure in children after head trauma. *J Neurosurg Anesthesiol* 1992; 4:4.

104. Haglund MM, et al: Rapid infusion system for neurosurgical treatment of massive intraoperative hemorrhage. *J Neurotrauma* 1994; 11:623.

105. Seelig JM, et al: Traumatic acute subdural hematoma. Major mortality reduction in comatose patients treated within four hours. *N Engl J Med* 1981; 304:1511.

106. McKissock W, et al: Subdural hematoma. A review of 389 cases. *Lancet* 1960; 1:1365.

107. McLaurin RL, Tutor FT: Acute subdural hematoma. Review of ninety cases. *J Neurosurg* 1961; 18:61.

108. Talalla A, Morin MA: Acute traumatic subdural hematoma: A review of one hundred consecutive cases. *J Trauma* 1971; 11:771.

109. Stone JL, et al: Traumatic subdural hygroma. *Neurosurgery* 1981; 8:542.

110. Cooper PR, et al: Hemicraniectomy in the treatment of acute subdural hematoma: A re-appraisal. *Surg Neurol* 1976; 5:25.

111. Jamieson K, Yelland J: Traumatic intracerebral hematoma. Report of 63 surgically treated cases. *J Neurosurg* 1972; 37:528.

112. Rosenorn J, Gjerris F: Long-term follow-up review of patients with acute and subacute subdural hematomas. *J Neurosurg* 1978; 48:345.

113. Stone JL, et al: Acute subdural hematoma: Progress in definition, clinical pathology, and therapy. *Surg Neurol* 1983; 19:216.

114. Gennarelli TA, Thibault LE: Biomechanics of acute subdural hematoma. *J Trauma* 1982; 22:680.

115. Cooper PR: Post-traumatic intracranial mass lesions. In Cooper PR (ed): *Head Injury*, 3d ed. Baltimore, Williams & Wilkins, 1993:275.

116. Fell DA, et al: Acute subdural hematomas. Review of 144 cases. *J Neurosurg* 1975; 42:37.

117. Marshall LF, et al: The outcome of severe closed head injury. *J Neurosurg* 1991; 75:S28.

118. Jamieson KG, Yelland JDN: Extradural hematoma. Report of 167 cases. *J Neurosurg* 1968; 29:13.

119. Galbraith SL: Age-distribution of extradural hemorrhage without skull fracture. *Lancet* 1973; 1:1217.

120. Foulkes MA, et al: The traumatic coma data bank: Design, methods, and baseline characteristics. *J Neurosurg* 1991; 75:S8.

121. Kvarnes TL, Trumpy JH: Extradural hematoma. Report of 132 cases. *Acta Neurochir* 1978; 41:223.

122. Cordobes F, et al: Observations on 82 patients with extradural hematoma. Comparison of results before and after the advent of computerized tomography. *J Neurosurg* 1981; 54:179.

123. Phonprasert C, et al: Extradural hematoma: Analysis of 138 cases. *J Trauma* 1980; 20:679.

124. Heiskanen O: Epidural hematoma. *Surg Neurol* 1975; 4:23.

125. Rivas JJ, et al: Extradural hematoma, analysis of factors influencing the courses of 161 patients. *Neurosurgery* 1988; 23:44.

126. Baykaner K, et al: Observation of 95 patients with extradural hematoma and review of the literature. *Surg Neurol* 1988; 30:339.

127. Bricolo AP, Pasut LM: Extradural hematoma: Toward zero mortality. A prospective study. *Neurosurgery* 1984; 14:8.

128. Weinman D, Muttucumaru B: Extradural hematoma. *Ceylon Med J* 1969; 14:60.

129. Pozzati E, et al: Subacute and chronic extradural hematomas: A study of 30 cases. *J Trauma* 1980; 20:795.

130. Seelig JM, et al: Traumatic acute epidural hematoma: Unrecognized high lethality in comatose patients. *Neurosurgery* 1984; 15:617.

131. Papo I, et al: Traumatic cerebral mass lesions: Correlations between clinical, intracranial pressure, and computed tomographic data. *Neurosurgery* 1980; 7:337.

132. Gurdjian ES, Gurdjian ES: Cerebral contusions: Re-evaluation of the mechanism of their development. *J Trauma* 1976; 16:35.

133. Schonauer M, et al: Space occupying contusions of cerebral lobes after closed brain injury. Considerations about 51 cases. *J Neurosurg Sci* 1979; 23:279.

134. Courville CB: Traumatic intracerebral hemorrhages. With special reference to the mechanisms of their production. *Bull Los Angeles Neurol Soc* 1962; 27:22.

135. Nagib MG, et al: Civilian gunshot wounds to the brain: Prognosis and management. *Neurosurgery* 1986; 18:533.

136. Crockard HA: Bullet injuries of the brain. *Ann Roy Coll Surg Engl* 1974; 55:111.

137. Gordon DS: Missile wounds of the head and spine. *Br Med J* 1975; 1:614.

138. Marmarou A, et al: Compartmental analysis of compliance and outflow resistance of the cerebrospinal fluid system. *J Neurosurg* 1975; 43:523.

139. Maset AL, et al: Pressure-volume index in head injury. *J Neurosurg* 1987; 67:832.

140. Grubb RL, et al: The effects of changes in Pa_{CO_2} on cerebral blood volume, blood flow, and vascular mean transit time. *Stroke* 1974; 5:630.

141. Archer DP, et al: The influence of cryogenic brain injury on the pharmacodynamics of pentobarbital: Evidence for a serotonergic mechanism. *Anesthesiology* 1991; 75:634.

142. Todd MM, et al: A focal cryogenic brain lesion does not reduce the minimum alveolar concentration for halothane in rats. *Anesthesiology* 1993; 79:139.

143. Shapira Y, et al: Influence of traumatic head injury on halothane MAC in rats. *Anesth Analg* 1992; 74:S282.

144. Fragen KJ, et al: Effects of etomidate on hormonal responses to surgical stress. *Anesthesiology* 1984; 61:652.

145. Batjer HH: Cerebral protective effects of etomidate: Experimental and clinical aspects. *Cerebrovas Brain Metab Rev* 1993; 5:17.

146. Strebel S, et al: Dynamic and static cerebral autoregulation during isoflurane, desflurane, and propofol anesthesia. *Anesthesiology* 1995; 83:66.

147. Stephan H, et al: The effect of sufentanil on cerebral blood flow, cerebral metabolism and the CO_2 reactivity of the cerebral vessels in man. *Anaesthesist* 1991; 40:153.

148. Strebel S, et al: Cerebral vasomotor responsiveness to carbon dioxide is preserved during propofol and midazolam anesthesia in humans. *Anesth Analg* 1994; 78:884.

149. Eng C, et al: The influence of propofol with and without nitrous oxide on cerebral blood flow velocity and CO_2 reactivity in humans. *Anesthesiology* 1992; 77:872.

150. Lam AM, et al: Change in cerebral blood flow velocity with onset of EEG silence during inhalation anesthesia in humans: Evidence of flow-metabolism coupling? *J Cereb Blood Flow Metab* 1995; 15:714.

151. Hanson TD, et al: The role of cerebral metabolism in determining the local cerebral blood flow effects of volatile anesthetics: Evidence of persistent flow-metabolism coupling. *J Cereb Blood Flow Metab* 1989; 9:323.

152. Lam AM, et al: Nitrous oxide-isoflurane anesthesia causes more cerebral vasodilation than an equipotent dose of isoflurane in humans. *Anesth Analg* 1994; 78:462.

153. Phirman JR, Shapiro HM: Modification of nitrous oxide induced intracranial hypertension by prior induction of anesthesia. *Anesthesiology* 1977; 46:150.

154. Lam AM, Mayberg TS: Use of nitrous oxide in neuroanesthesia, why bother! *J Neurosurg Anesthesiol* 1992; 4:285.

155. Hoffman WE, et al: The effects of midazolam on cerebral blood flow and oxygen consumption and its interaction with nitrous oxide. *Anesth Analg* 1986; 65:729.

156. Matta BF, Lam AM: Nitrous oxide increases cerebral blood flow velocity during pharmacologically induced EEG silence in humans. *J Neurosurg Anesthesiol* 1995; 7:89.

157. Marx W, et al: Sufentanil, alfentanil and fentanyl: Impact on cerebrospinal fluid pressure in patients with brain tumors. *J Neurosurg Anesthesiol* 1989; 1:3.

158. Sperry RJ, et al: Fentanyl and sufentanil increase intracranial pressure in head trauma patients. *Anesthesiology* 1992; 77:416.

159. Milde LN, et al: Effects of sufentanil on cerebral circulation and metabolism in dogs. *Anesth Analg* 1990; 70:138.

160. Trindle MR, et al: Effects of fentanyl versus sufentanil in equianesthetic doses on middle cerebral artery blood flow velocity. *Anesthesiology* 1993; 78:454.

161. Mayer N, et al: Sufentanil does not increase cerebral blood flow in healthy human volunteers. *Anesthesiology* 1990; 73:493.

162. Mayberg TS, et al: The effect of alfentanil on cerebral blood flow velocity and intracranial pressure during isoflurane-nitrous oxide anesthesia in humans. *Anesthesiology* 1993; 78:288.

163. Werner C, et al: Effects of sufentanil on cerebral hemodynamics and intracranial pressure in patients with brain injury. *Anesthesiology* 1995; 83:721.

164. Glass P, et al: Preliminary pharmacokinetics and pharmacodynamics of an ultra-short-acting opioid: Remifentanil (GI87084B). *Anesth Analg* 1993; 77:1031.

165. Kapila A, et al: Measured context-sensitive half-times of remifentanil and alfentanil. *Anesthesiology* 1995; 83:968.

166. Shapira Y, et al: Therapeutic time window and dose response of the beneficial effects of ketamine in experimental head injury. *Stroke* 1994; 25:1637.

167. Rothman SM, et al: Ketamine protects hippocampal neurons from anoxia in vitro. *Neuroscience* 1987; 21:673.

168. Mayberg TS, et al: Ketamine does not increase cerebral blood

flow velocity or intracranial pressure during isoflurane/nitrous oxide anesthesia in patients undergoing craniotomy. *Anesh Analg* 1995; 81:84.

169. Schwedler M, et al: Cerebral blood flow and metabolism following ketamine administration. *Can Anaesth Soc J* 1982; 29:222.

170. Albanese J, et al: Effects of intravenous ketamine on cerebral hemodynamics in head trauma patients. *Anesthesiology* 1994; 81:A201.

171. Minton MD, et al: Increases in intracranial pressure from succinylcholine: Prevention by prior nondepolarizing blockade. *Anesthesiology* 1986; 65:165.

172. Stirt JA, et al: "Defasciculation" with metocurine prevents succinylcholine-induced increases in intracranial pressure. *Anesthesiology* 1987; 67:50.

173. Lanier WL, et al: Cerebral stimulation following succinylcholine in dogs. *Anesthesiology* 1986; 64:551.

174. Ghani GA, et al: Effects of intravenous nitroglycerin on the intracranial pressure and volume response. *J Neurosurg* 1983; 58:562.

175. Griswold WR, et al: Nitroprusside-induced intracranial hypertension. *JAMA* 1981; 246:2679.

176. Olsen KS, et al: Effect of labetalol on cerebral blood flow, oxygen metabolism and autoregulation in healthy humans. *Br J Anaesth* 1995; 75:51.

177. Artru AA: New concepts concerning anesthetic effects on intracranial dynamics: Cerebral spinal fluid and cerebral blood volume. *ASA Annual Refresher Course Lecture* 1987; 133.

178. Matta BF, et al: A critique of the intraoperative use of jugular venous bulb catheters during neurosurgical procedures. *Anesth Analg* 1994; 79:745.

179. Durward QJ, et al: Cerebral and cardiovascular responses to changes in head elevation in patients with intracranial hypertension. *J Neurosurg* 1983; 59:938.

180. Feldman Z, et al: Effect of head elevation on intracranial pressure, cerebral perfusion pressure, and cerebral blood flow in head injured patients. *J Neurosurg* 1992; 76:207.

181. Pietropaoli JA, et al: The deleterious effects of intraoperative hypotension on outcome in patients with severe head injuries. *J Trauma* 1992; 33:403.

182. Shenkin HA, et al: Restricted fluids intake: Rational management of the neurosurgical patient. *J Neurosurg* 1976; 45:432.

183. Tommasino C, et al: The effects of fluid resuscitation on brain water content. *Anesthesiology* 1982; 57:A109.

184. Warner DS, Boehland LA: Effects of iso-osmolal intravenous fluid therapy on post-ischemic brain water content in the rat. *Anesthesiology* 1988; 68:86.

185. Kaieda R, et al: Acute effects of changing plasma osmolality and colloid oncotic pressure on the formation of brain edema after cryogenic injury in the rabbit. *Neurosurgery* 1989; 24:671.

186. Zornow MH, et al: The acute cerebral effects of changes in plasma osmolality and oncotic pressure. *Anesthesiology* 1987; 67:936.

187. Poole GV, et al: Cerebral hemodynamics after hemorrhagic shock: Effects of the type of resuscitation fluid. *Crit Care Med* 1986; 14:629.

188. Tranmer BI, et al: Effects of crystalloid and colloid infusions of intracranial pressure and computerized electroencephalographic data in dogs with vasogenic brain edema. *Neurosurgery* 1989; 25:173.

189. Tomita H, et al: High colloid oncotic therapy for contusional brain edema. *Acta Neurochir* 1994; 60(Suppl):547.

190. Claes Y, et al: Influence of hydroxyethyl starch on coagulation in patients during the perioperative period. *Anesth Analg* 1992; 75:24.

191. Cully MD, et al: Hetastarch coagulopathy in a neurosurgical patient. *Anesthesiology* 1987; 66:706.

192. Trumble ER, et al: Coagulopathy with the use of hetastarch in the treatment of vasospasm. *J Neurosurg* 1995; 82:44.

193. Strauss RG, et al: Pentastarch may cause fewer effects on coagulation than hetastarch. *Transfusion* 1988; 28:257.

194. Vassar MJ, et al: Prehospital resuscitation of hypotensive trauma patients with 7.5% NaCl versus 7.5% NaCl with added dextran. A controlled trial. *J Trauma* 1993; 34:622.

195. Battistella FD, Wisner DH: Combined hemorrhagic shock and head injury: Effects of hypertonic saline [7.5%] resuscitation. *J Trauma* 1991; 31:182.

196. Gunnar W, et al: Cerebral blood flow following hypertonic saline resuscitation in an experimental model of hemorrhagic shock and head injury. *Braz J Med Biol Res* 1989; 22:287.

197. Prough DS, et al: Effects on intracranial pressure of resuscitation from hemorrhagic shock with hypertonic saline versus lactated Ringer's solution. *Crit Care Med* 1985; 13:407.

198. Prough DS, et al: Effects on cerebral hemodynamics of resuscitation from endotoxic shock with hypertonic saline versus lactated Ringer's solution. *Crit Care Med* 1995; 13:1040.

199. Prough DS, et al: Regional cerebral blood flow following resuscitation from hemorrhagic shock with hypertonic saline. Influence of a subdural mass. *Anesthesiology* 1991; 75:319.

200. Freshman SP, et al: Hypertonic saline (7.5%) versus mannitol: A comparison for treatment of acute head injuries. *J Trauma* 1993; 35:344.

201. Prough DS, et al: Hypertonic/hyperoncotic fluid resuscitation after hemorrhagic shock in dogs. *Anesth Analg* 1991; 73:738.

202. Clifton GL, et al: Circulatory catecholamines and sympathetic activity after head injury. *Neurosurgery* 1981; 8:10.

203. McLeod AA, et al: Cardiac sequelae of acute head injury. *Br Heart J* 1982; 47:221.

204. Burchiel KJ, et al: Intracranial pressure changes in brain-injured patients requiring positive end-expiratory pressure ventilation. *Neurosurgery* 1981; 8:443.

205. Cooper KR, et al: Safe use of PEEP in patients with severe head injury. *J Neurosurg* 1985; 63:552.

206. Cold GE: Does acute hyperventilation provoke cerebral oligaemia in comatose patients after acute head injury? *Acta Neurochir (Wien)* 1989; 96:100.

207. Muizelaar JP, et al: Adverse effects of prolonged hyperventilation in patients with severe head injury: A randomized clinical trial. *J Neurosurg* 1991; 75:731.

208. Matta BF, et al: The influence of arterial oxygenation on cerebral venous oxygen saturation during hyperventilation. *Can J Anaesth* 1994; 41:1041.

209. Eisenberg HM, et al: High dosage barbiturate control of elevated intracranial pressure in patients with severe head injury. *J Neurosurg* 1988; 69:15.

210. Muizelaar JP, et al: Mannitol causes compensatory cerebral vasoconstriction and vasodilatation in response to blood viscosity changes. *J Neurosurg* 1983; 59:822.

211. Wise BL, Chater N: The value of hypertonic mannitol solution in decreasing brain mass and lowering cerebrospinal-fluid pressure. *J Neurosurg* 1962; 19:1038.

212. Feig PN, McCurdy DK: The hypertonic state. *N Engl J Med* 1977; 297:1449.

213. Dorman HR, et al: Mannitol-induced acute renal failure. *Medicine* 1990; 69:153.

214. Donato T, et al: Effect of mannitol on cerebrospinal fluid dynamics and brain tissue edema. *Anesth Analg* 1994; 78:58.

215. Foxworthy JC, Artru AA: Cerebrospinal fluid dynamics and brain tissue composition following intravenous infusions of hypertonic saline in anesthetized rabbits. *J Neurosurg Anesthesiol* 1990; 2:256.

216. Sahar A, Tsipstein E: Effects of mannitol and furosemide on the rate of formation of cerebrospinal fluid. *Exp Neurol* 1978; 60:584.

217. Domer FR: Effects of diuretics on cerebrospinal fluid formation and potassium movement. *Exp Neurol* 1969; 24:54.

218. Cottrell JE, et al: Furosemide- and mannitol-induced changes in intracranial pressure and serum osmolality and electrolytes. *Anesthesiology* 1977; 47:28.

219. Clasen RA, et al: Furosemide and pentobarbital in cryogenic cerebral injury and edema. *Neurology* 1974; 24:642.

220. Schettini A, et al: Osmotic and osmotic loop diuresis in brain surgery: Effects on plasma and CSF electrolytes and ion excretion. *J Neurosurg* 1982; 56:679.

221. Wilkinson HA, Rosenfeld S: Furosemide and mannitol in the treatment of acute experimental intracranial hypertension. *Neurosurgery* 1983; 12:405.

222. Gudeman S, et al: Failure of high-dose steroid therapy to influence intracranial pressure in patients with severe head injury. *J Neurosurg* 1979; 51:301.

223. Dearden NM, et al: Effect of high-dose dexamethasone on outcome from severe head injury. *J Neurosurg* 1986; 64:81.

224. Ferrara A, et al: Hypothermia and acidosis worsen coagulopathy in the patient requiring massive transfusion. *Am J Surg* 1990; 160:515.

225. Stapelfeldt WH, et al: Effect of temperature on the thromboelastogram: Role of preexisting patient hypothermia. *Anesthesiology* 1995; 83:A283.

226. Felfernig M, et al: Influence of hypothermic therapy on whole blood coagulation in patients with severe head injury. *Anesthesiology* 1995; 83:A284.

227. Weaver DD, et al: Differential intracranial pressure in patients with unilateral mass lesions. *J Neurosurg* 1982; 56:660.

228. Sheinberg M, et al: Continuous monitoring of jugular venous oxygen saturation in head-injured patients. *J Neurosurg* 1992; 76:212.

229. Cruz J, et al: Cerebral oxygenation monitoring. *Crit Care Med* 1993; 21:1242.

230. Cruz J, et al: Continuous monitoring of cerebral oxygenation in acute brain injury: Injection of mannitol during hyperventilation. *J Neurosurg* 1990; 73:725.

231. Gopinath SP, et al: Jugular venous desaturation and outcome after head injury. *J Neurol Neurosurg Psychiatry* 1994; 57:717.

232. Aaslid R, et al: Non-invasive transcranial Doppler ultrasound recording of flow velocity in basal cerebral arteries. *J Neurosurg* 1982; 58:769.

233. Lam AM: Intraoperative transcranial Doppler monitoring. *Anesthesiology* 1995; 82:1536.

234. Weber M, et al: Evaluation of post-traumatic cerebral blood flow velocities by transcranial Doppler ultrasonography. *Neurosurgery* 1990; 27:106.

235. Martin NA, et al: Posttraumatic cerebral arterial spasm: Transcranial Doppler ultrasound, cerebral blood flow, and angiographic findings. *J Neurosurg* 1992; 77:575.

236. Hassler W, et al: Transcranial Doppler ultrasonography in raised intracranial pressure and in intracranial circulatory arrest. *Neurosurgery* 1988; 68:745.

237. Homburg AM, et al: Transcranial Doppler recordings in raised intracranial pressure. *Acta Neurol Scand* 1993; 87:488.

238. Muttaqin Z, et al: Hyperaemia prior to acute cerebral swelling in severe head injuries: The role of transcranial Doppler monitoring. *Acta Neurochir* (Wien) 1993; 123:76.

239. Chan KH, et al: Multimodality monitoring as a guide to treatment of intracranial hypertension after severe brain injury. *Neurosurgery* 1993; 32:547.

240. Aaslid R, et al: Cerebral autoregulation dynamics in humans. *Stroke* 1989; 20:45.

241. Aaslid R, et al: Assessment of cerebral autoregulation dynamics from simultaneous arterial and venous transcranial Doppler recordings in humans. *Stroke* 1991; 22:1148.

242. Newell DW, et al: Comparison of flow and velocity during dynamic autoregulation testing in humans. *Stroke* 1994; 25:793.

243. President's Commission on the Study of Ethical Problems in Medicine and Biomedical and Behavioral Research: Guidelines for the determination of death. Report of the medical consultants on the diagnosis of death to the President's Commission for the Study of Ethical Problems in Medicine and Biomedical and Behavioral Research. *JAMA* 1981; 246:2184.

244. Cruickshank JM, et al: Stress/catecholamine-induced cardiac necrosis. Reduction by beta 1-selective blockade. *Postgrad Med* 1988; 83 (Spec. Report):140.

245. North JB, Jennett S: Abnormal breathing patterns associated with acute brain damage. *Arch Neurol* 1974; 31:338.

246. Demling R, Riessen R: Pulmonary dysfunction after cerebral injury. *Crit Care Med* 1990; 18:768.

247. Craven DE, et al: Risk factors for pneumonia and fatality in patients receiving continuous mechanical ventilation. *Am Rev Respir Dis* 1986; 133:792.

248. Braun SR, et al: Role of corticosteroids in the development of pneumonia in mechanically ventilated head-trauma victims. *Crit Care Med* 1986; 14:198.

249. Braakman R, et al: Megadose steroids in severe head injury. Results of a prospective double-blind clinical trial. *J Neurosurg* 1983; 58:326.

250. Driks MR, et al: Nosocomial pneumonia in intubated patients given sucralfate as compared with antacids or histamine type-2 blockers. *N Engl J Med* 1987; 317:1376.

251. Hsieh AH-H, et al: Pneumonia following closed head injury. *Am Rev Respir Dis* 1992; 146:290.

252. Stoutenbeek CP, et al: The effect of oropharyngeal decontamination using topical nonabsorbable antibiotics on the incidence of nosocomial respiratory tract infections in multiple trauma patients. *J Trauma* 1987; 27:357.

253. Salata RA, et al: Diagnosis of nosocomial pneumonia in intubated, intensive care unit patients. *Am Rev Respir* 1987; 135:426.

254. Mandelli M, et al: Prevention of pneumonia in an intensive care unit: A randomized multicenter clinical trial. Intensive Care Unit Group in Infection Control. *Crit Care Med* 1989; 17:501.

255. Simmons R, et al: Respiratory insufficiency in combat casualties (pulmonary edema following head injury). *Ann Surgery* 1969; 170:39.

256. Colice G: Neurogenic pulmonary edema. *Clin Chest Med* 1985; 6:473.

257. Katsurada K, et al: Respiratory insufficiency in patients with severe head injury. *Surgery* 1973; 73:191.

258. Fein IA, Rackow EC: Neurogenic pulmonary edema. *Chest* 1982; 81:318.

259. Malik AB: Mechanisms of neurogenic pulmonary edema. *Circ Res* 1985; 57:1.

260. Stein PM, et al: Total body vascular capacitance changes during high intracranial pressure. *Am J Physiol* 1983; 245:947.

261. Rosell S: Neuronal control of microvessels. *Annu Rev Physiol* 1980; 42:359.

262. Colgan FS, et al: Protective effects of beta blockade on pulmonary function when intracranial pressure is elevated. *Crit Care Med* 1983; 11:368.

263. Piek J, et al: Extracranial complications of severe head injury. *J Neurosurg* 1992; 77:901.

264. Sterns RH, et al: Osmotic demyelination syndrome following correction of hyponatremia. *N Engl J Med* 1986; 314:1535.

265. Gaufin L, et al: Release of antidiuretic hormone during mass-

induced elevation of intracranial pressure. *J Neurosurg* 1977; 46:627.

266. Messert B, et al: Central pontine myelinolysis. Considerations on etiology, diagnosis, and treatment. *Neurology* 1979; 29:147.

267. Norenberg MD, et al: Association between rise in serum sodium and central pontine myelinolysis. *Ann Neurol* 1982; 11:128.

268. Maxon HR, Rutsky EA: Vasopressin-resistant diabetes insipidus associated with short-term demethylchlortetracycline (Declomycin) therapy. *Milit Med* 1973; 138:500.

269. Reeder RF, Harbaugh RE: Administration of intravenous urea and normal saline for the treatment of hyponatremia in neurosurgical patients. *J Neurosurg* 1989; 70:201.

270. Leramo OB, Rao AB: Diplopia and diabetes insipidus secondary to type II fracture of the sella turcica: Case report. *Can J Surg* 1987; 30:53.

271. Young B, et al: Relationship between admission hyperglycemia and neurologic outcome of severely brain-injured patients. *Ann Surg* 1989; 210:466.

272. Ginsberg MD, et al: Deleterious effect of glucose pretreatment on recovery from diffuse cerebral ischemia in the cat. 1. Local cerebral blood flow and glucose utilization. *Stroke* 1980; 11:347.

273. Hoffman WE, et al: Brain lactate and neurologic outcome following incomplete ischemia in fasted, nonfasted, and glucose-loaded rats. *Anesthesiology* 1990; 72:1045.

274. Ibayashi S, et al: Cerebral blood flow and tissue metabolism in experimental cerebral ischemia of spontaneously hypertensive rats with hyper, normo and hypoglycemia. *Stroke* 1986; 17:261.

275. Welsh FA, et al: Deleterious effect of glucose pretreatment on recovery from diffuse cerebral ischemia in the cat. *Stroke* 1980; 11:355.

276. Hsu SSF, et al: Influence of hyperglycemia on cerebral adenosine production during ischemia and reperfusion. *Am J Physiol* 1991; 261 (Heart Circ Physiol 30):H398.

277. Winn HR, et al: The role of adenosine in the regulation of cerebral blood flow. *J Cereb Blood Flow Metab* 1981; 1:239.

278. Coradetti R, et al: Adenosine decreases aspartate and glutamate release from rat hippocampal slices. *Eur J Pharmacol* 1984; 104:19.

279. Phillis JW, et al: A potent depressant action of adenine derivatives on cerebral cortical neurones. *Eur J Pharmacol* 1975; 30:125.

280. Cronstein BN, et al: Adenosine: A physiologic modulator of superoxide anion generation by human neutrophils. Adenosine acts via an A2 receptor on human neutrophils. *J Immunol* 1985; 135:1366.

281. Clark JA, et al: Disseminated intravascular coagulation following cranial trauma. Case Report. *J Neurosurg* 1980; 52:266.

282. Stein SC, et al: Delayed brain injury after head trauma: Significance of coagulopathy. *Neurosurgery* 1992; 30:160.

283. Astrup T: Assay and content of tissue thromboplastin in different organs. *Thromb Diath Haemorrh* 1965; 14:401.

284. Ueda S, et al: Correlation between plasma fibrin-fibrinogen degradation product values and CT findings in head injury. *J Neurol Neurosurg Psychiatry* 1985; 48:58.

285. Fresh-Frozen Plasma, Cryoprecipitate, and Platelets Administration Practice Guidelines Development Task Force of the College of American Pathologists: Practice parameter for the use of fresh-frozen plasma, cryoprecipitate, and platelets. *JAMA* 1994; 271:777.

286. Kamada T, et al: Gastrointestinal bleeding following head injury: A clinical study of 433 cases. *J Trauma* 1977; 17:44.

287. Kamada T, et al: Acute gastroduodenal lesions in head injury: An endoscopic study. *Am J Gastroenterol* 1977; 68:249.

288. Kamada T, et al: Gastric mucosal hemodynamics after thermal or head injury: A clinical application of reflectance spectraphotometry. *Gastroenterology* 1982; 83:535.

289. Brown TH, et al: Acute gastritis occurring within 24 hours of severe head injury. *Gastrointest Endosc* 1989; 35:37.

290. Borrero C, et al: Comparison of antacid and sucralfate in the prevention of gastrointestinal bleeding in patients who are critically ill. *Am J Med* 1985; 79(Suppl 2C):62.

291. Young B, et al: The effect of nutritional support on outcome from severe head injury. *J Neurosurg* 1987; 67:668.

292. Norton JA, et al: Intolerance to enteral feeding in the brain-injured patient. *J Neurosurg* 1988; 68:62.

293. Jackson MD, Davidoff G: Gastroparesis following traumatic brain injury and response to metoclopramide therapy. *Arch Phys Med Rehabil* 1989; 70:553.

294. Weaver JP, Ward JD: Closed head injury. In Apuzzo ML (ed): *Brain Surgery: Complication Avoidance and Management*. New York, Churchill Livingstone, 1993:1351.

295. Passwell JH, et al: The effects of protein malnutrition on macrophage function and the amount of affinity and antibody response. *Clin Exp Immunol* 1974; 17:491.

296. Van Woerkom TCAM, et al: Biochemical and ultrastructural aspects of the inhibited phagocytosis by neutrophil granulocytes in acute brain-damaged patients. *J Neurol Sci* 1977; 31:223.

297. Renk CM, et al: Comparison between in-vitro lymphocyte activity and metabolic changes in trauma patients. *J Trauma* 1982; 22:134.

298. Jennett B: *Epilepsy after Nonmissile Injuries,* 2d ed. Chicago, Year Book Medical Publishers, 1975.

299. Annegers JF, et al: Seizures after head trauma: A population study. *Neurology* 1980; 30:683.

300. Temkin NR, et al: A randomized, double-blind study of phenytoin for the prevention of post-traumatic seizures. *N Engl J Med* 1990; 323:497.

301. Korbine AI, Kempe LG: Studies in head injury. II. Effect of dexamethasone on traumatic brain swelling. *Surg Neurol* 1973; 1:38.

302. Yamaguchi M, et al: Steroid treatment of brain edema. *Surg Neurol* 1975; 4:5.

303. Giannotta SL, et al: High-dose glucocorticoids in the management of severe head injury. *Neurosurgery* 1984; 15:497.

304. Cooper PR, et al: Dexamethasone and severe head injury. A prospective double blind study. *J Neurosurg* 1979; 51:307.

305. Bracken MB, et al: A randomized, controlled trial of methylprednisolone or naloxone in the treatment of acute spinal cord injury. *N Engl J Med* 1990; 322:1405.

306. Hall ED, et al: Biochemistry and pharmacology of lipid antioxidants in acute brain and spinal cord injury. *J Neurotrauma* 1992; 9:S425.

307. Thomas PD, et al: Inhibition of superoxide generating NADPH oxidase of human neutrophils by lazaroids [21-aminosteroids and 2-methylaminochromans]. *Biochem Pharmacol* 1993; 45:241.

308. Olsen KS, et al: The effect of Tirilazad mesylate (U74006F) on cerebral oxygen consumption, and reactivity of cerebral blood flow to carbon dioxide in healthy volunteers. *Anesthesiology* 1993; 79:666.

309. Choi DW: Calcium-mediated neurotoxicity: Relationship to specific channel types and role in ischemic damage. *Trends Neurosci* 1988; 11:465.

310. Rothman SM, Olney JW: Glutamate and the pathophysiology of hypoxic-ischemic brain damage. *Ann Neurol* 1986; 19:105.

311. Faden AI, et al: The role of excitatory amino acids and NMDA receptors in traumatic head injury. *Science* 1989; 244:798.

312. Siesjo BK, Bengtsson F: Calcium fluxes, calcium antagonists, and calcium-related pathology in brain ischemia, hypoglycemia, and spreading depression: A unifying hypothesis. *J Cereb Blood Flow Metab* 1989; 9:127.

313. Baker AJ, et al: Excitatory amino acids in cerebrospinal fluid

following traumatic brain injury in humans. *J Neurosurg* 1993; 79:369.

314. Cotman CW, Iverson LL: Excitatory amino acids in the brain-focus on NMDA receptors. *TINS* 1987; 10:263.

315. Zauner A, Bullock R: The role of excitatory amino acids in severe brain trauma: Opportunities for therapy: A review. *J Neurotrauma* 1995; 12:547.

316. Shapira Y, et al: Protective effect of MK-801 in experimental brain injury. *J Neurotrauma* 1990; 3:131.

317. McIntosh TK, et al: The *N*-methyl-D-aspartate receptor antagonist MK-801 prevents edema and improves outcome after experimental brain injury in rats (abstract). In Hoff, Betz (eds): Seventh International Symposium on ICP and Brain Injury. Ann Arbor, MI, University of Michigan Press, 1988:199.

318. Buchan A, Pulsinelli WA: Hypothermia but not the *N*-methyl-D-aspartate antagonist, MK-801, attenuates neuronal damage in gerbils subjected to transient global ischemia. *J Neurosci* 1990; 10:311.

319. Bullock R: Strategies for neuroprotection with glutamate antagonists. *Ann NY Acad Sci* 1995; 765:272.

320. Freeman BA, Crapo JD: Biology of disease. Free radicals and tissue injury. *Lab Invest* 1982; 47:412.

321. Muizelaar JP: Cerebral ischemia-reperfusion injury after severe head injury and its possible treatment with polyethyleneglycol-superoxide dismutase. *Ann Emerg Med* 1993; 22:1014.

322. Field J, et al: Effect of temperature on the oxygen consumption of brain tissue. *J Neurophysiol* 1944; 7:117.

323. Michenfelder JD: *Anesthesia and the Brain.* New York, Churchill Livingstone, 1988:23.

324. Busto R, et al: Small differences in intraischemic brain temperature critically determine the extent of ischemic neuronal injury. *J Cereb Blood Flow Metab* 1987; 7:729.

325. Clifton GL, et al: Marked protection by moderate hypothermia after experimental traumatic brain injury. *J Cereb Blood Flow Metab* 1991; 11:114.

326. Busto R, et al: Effect of mild hypothermia on ischemia-induced release of neurotransmitters and free fatty acids in rat brain. *Stroke* 1989; 20:904.

327. Baker AJ, et al: Hypothermia prevents ischemia-induced increase in hippocampal glycine concentration in rabbits. *Stroke* 1991; 22:666.

328. Clifton GL, et al: A phase II study of moderate hypothermia in severe brain injury. *J Neurotrauma* 1993; 10:263.

329. Marion DW, et al: The use of moderate therapeutic hypothermia for patients with severe head injuries: A preliminary report. *J Neurosurg* 1993; 79:354.

330. Shiozake T, et al: Effect of mild hypothermia on uncontrollable intracranial hypertension after severe head injury. *J Neurosurg* 1993; 79:363.

331. Jensen K, et al: The effects of indomethacin on intracranial pressure, cerebral blood flow and cerebral metabolism in patients with severe head injury and intracranial hypertension. *Acta Neurochir (Wien)* 1991; 108:116.

332. Jensen K, et al: The effect of indomethacin upon cerebral blood flow in healthy volunteers. The influence of moderate hypoxia and hypercapnia. *Acta Neurochir (Wein)* 1993; 124:114.

333. Asgeirsson B, et al: The Lund concept of post-traumatic brain oedema therapy. *Acta Anaesthesiol Scand* 1995; 39:103.

334. Asgeirsson B, et al: Effects of hypotensive treatment with alpha 2-agonist and beta 1-antagonist on cerebral haemodynamics in severely head injured patients. *Acta Anaesthesiol Scand* 1995; 39:347.

335. Grande PO: The effects of dihydroergotamine in patients with head injury and raised intracranial pressure. *Intensive Care Med* 1989; 15:523.

Chapter 35

PEDIATRIC NEUROANESTHESIA

BRUNO BISSONNETTE

DEREK C. ARMSTRONG

JAMES T. RUTKA

The child is not simply a small adult. At birth the central nervous system (CNS) development is incomplete and will not be mature until the end of the first year of life. Because of this delay in CNS maturation, several specific pathophysiologic and psychological differences ensue.

Anesthesia for pediatric neurosurgical procedures presents an interesting challenge to the anesthesiologist.[1] Although one has little control over the patient's primary lesion, the selection of an anesthetic technique designed to protect the perilesional area and the recognition of perioperative events and changes may well have a profound effect in the reduction or prevention of significant morbidity. Current neuroanesthetic practice is based on the understanding of cerebral physiology and how it can be manipulated for patient benefit in the face of intracranial pathology. The anesthesiologist in the field of pediatric neuroanesthesia must face the added challenge of the physiologic differences between developing children and their adult counterparts. In addition to the common problems of administering anesthesia to the general pediatric population, special considerations must be given to the effects of anesthesia on the CNS of children with neurologic disease.

The practice of anesthesia for pediatric neurosurgery requires some knowledge of neuroembryology and development, neuroanatomy, and neurophysiology. This chapter reviews the basic concepts necessary for a better clinical management and understanding of the anesthetic problems related to children with neurologic disease. It is also accompanied, for the benefit of the neuroanesthesiologist, by information on neuroradiologic procedures. A section on general anesthetic management of specific neurosurgical conditions is presented to facilitate the management of the particular problems encountered by the specialist pediatric neuroanesthesiologist.

Neuroembryology and Development

The CNS is the first to begin and probably the last to complete its development in human maturation. To understand the various disorders encountered in pediatric neurologic practice, the time sequences for the major events in CNS development are important. The nature of several neurologic disorders will be related to a specific developmental stage of the CNS.

The CNS development begins from a relatively simple single layer of cells into a very complex multilayered central structure that eventually connects it with every part of the body. The processes by which the CNS will eventually develop follow three steps: (1)

TABLE 35-1
Phases and Stages of Neural Development During Gestation

Phases	Stages	Age (days)	Outcome
1 Neurulation	7	16–18	Brain, spinal cord through L2–4
2 Canalization	13–20	30–52	Sacral, coccygeal segments
3 Retrogressive differentiation	18–birth	46–birth	Filum terminale

SOURCE: Modified from Lemire and coworkers, with permission.[8]

neurulation, (2) canalization, and (3) retrogressive differentiation.

NEURULATION

EARLY STAGE

The process by which the neural tube initially folds is called *neurulation*. This occurs very early in the development of the embryo and it is vitally important. Although this process has been well studied, many of its mechanisms remain unclear. Several factors have been identified as possible determinants involved in the process of neurulation.[2]

Neural tube differentiation is part of a long process of neurologic development that occurs in the first 56 to 60 days following fertilization of the ovum.[3–6] Table 35-1 indicates the stages of development. The nervous system does not appear until stage 6 or the second week of gestation. Primary orientation of the embryo arises when the primitive streak and Hensen's node are present. Shortly thereafter (stage 7), a cellular process (the notochord) is found extending rostrally from Hensen's node. Over the next 2 days, when there are six to seven somites, fusion of the neural folds occurs (stage 10). The initial site of fusion is at the level of the third or fourth somite, which correlates with the future rhombencephalon (hindbrain) region.[7] By early stage 11 the young embryo possesses fused neural folds to the level of the colliculi rostrally. The primordia of the thalamus and corpus striatum distort the terminal hole and may be involved in its closure. At this time the only contact between the neuroectoderm and the amniotic cavity is through the posterior neuropore.

LATER DEVELOPMENT OF THE NEURAL TUBE

Cerebral cortex and cerebullum development is correlated with developmental stage in Fig. 35-1. Following closure of the anterior neuropore in stage 11, there is an interval before the first indication of differentiation of the telencephalon (forebrain). In stage 15, bilateral cerebral vesicles appear and their connections with the existing neural tube later become the foramina of Monro. The midline lamina terminalis forms a keel to these enlarging structures and by stage 17, areas that will become frontal and parietal lobes are identifiable. Primordia of the occipital lobe become present at stage 19 and the temporal pole appears at stage 23.

At this early stage, however, these poles bear no resemblance to their final form. The main differentiation of the cerebral cortex occurs throughout the gestational period but mainly during the third trimester.[8] The external surfaces of the developing brain can provide some information in regard to gestational age. Fissures and sulci develop. A majority of the cortical surface becomes buried as the gyri are formed. The primordium of cortical gray matter is formed when a layer of neuroblasts derived mainly from pyramidal cells migrates into the marginal zone during stage 22. The progressive formation of upper and lower fibers divides the caudate nucleus from the putamen and the globus pallidus at stage 23.

The deep cerebral nuclei, which are derived from the diencephalon (midbrain), appear at different stages. The thalamic structure begins to appear at stage 15 with a separate lateral part becoming identifiable later. The anlage of the cerebellum may be found when the pontine and cervical flexures begin to form during stage 13. Interestingly, most of the early development of the cerebellum occurs about 1 month after the embryonic period begins even though at that time, the paired cerebellar primordia have not acquired a recognizable pattern. The development of the cerebral cortex and the white matter is relatively primitive by the time of transition from embryo to fetus. This supports the concept that the brain grows mainly during the later phases of gestation and will be continued postnatally.

CANALIZATION AND RETROGRESSIVE DIFFERENTIATION

The process of formation of the neural tube caudal to that formed by neurulation is called *canalization* and consists of the development of the lower lumbar, sacral, and coccygeal segments. A proliferation of cells occurs in neural tube wall in this region. This "secondary" phase of caudal neural tube development with the associated vertebrae is in excess of segments that are needed. The processes involved in the formation of the filum terminale and the cauda equina is the

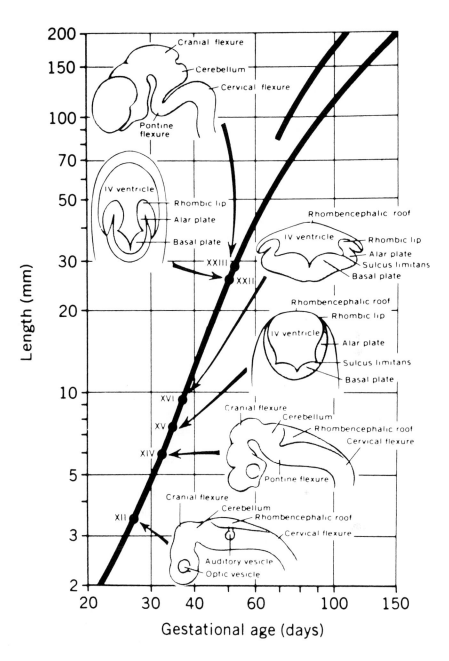

Figure 35-1 Early development of human cerebellum as correlated with developmental stage (Roman numerals), gestational age, and crown-rump length. (Reproduced by permission from Lemire and coworkers.[8])

result of the *retrogressive differentiation*.[9] It consists of a degenerative process that remodels the excess segments formed by canalization. It eventually brings the conus medullaris to its adult level, which is opposite to L1 to L2.

Any developmental defect of the CNS can be referred to as a *neural tube defect*. The classification of neurulation defects fall into these general categories: (1) those involving the brain and spinal cord, (2) those involving the brain alone, and (3) those involving the spinal cord alone. For example, in the early developmental stages, when both the brain and the spinal column fail to undergo proper neurulation, a condition

of total dysrhaphism (or craniorachischis) results. If the brain alone fails to close then anencephaly develops.

In the later stage of development many malformations of the brain can occur and have clinical relevance for the pediatric anesthesiologist. Microencephaly is a small brain enclosed in a small skull. In itself, it is seldom a neurosurgical problem, but forms of craniosysnostosis or encephalocele have to be considered in the differential diagnosis. Congenital hydrocephaly, an increase in the amount of cerebrospinal fluid (CSF) in the cranial cavity, is a common complication. A variety of cortical malformations are the result of neuronal migration and some may be visible on the surface.[10]

Schizencephaly (clefts in the cerebral wall), *pachygyri* (sparse, broad gyri), and *polymicrogyria* are all anomalies strongly associated with migrational abnormalities. *Lissencephaly*, or smooth brain, is a severe anomaly that may be produced by either migrational anomalies or earlier disruptions in neurogenesis. *Agenesis of the corpus callosum*, which is not believed to be a migrational anomaly is, however, often associated with such anomalies and it may be complete or partial. Caudally defective neurulation results in myelocele if the lesion is flat or meningomyelocele if an enlarged subarachnoid space dorsal to the dysplastic cord is present. In summary, the correlation of these anatomic locations with the probable stages in which they arise is shown in Table 35-1.

VENTRICULAR SYSTEM AND CEREBROSPINAL FLUID PATHWAY

At the time of closure of the posterior neuropore in stage 12, the ventricular system is closed and consists of that within the prosencephalon, diencephalon, mesencephalon, rhombencephalon (metencephalon, nyelencephalon), and central canal of the spinal cord. During stage 14 the rhombencephalic roof becomes thinner and in stage 15 the evaginations of the cerebral hemispheres develop. This demarcates the anlage of the lateral ventricles, the third ventricle, and the foramen of Monro. By stage 20, the cerebral hemispheres have overlapped the diencephalon and at this stage the lateral ventricles are the largest of the ventricular system. At about this stage a perforation of the roof of the fourth ventricle occurs thereby creating the foramen of Magendie.[11] The foramina of Luschka do not form until some $2\frac{1}{2}$ months later. Within the cranium, the aqueduct of Sylvius narrows as the tectum and tegmentum enlarge. The actual volume within the lateral, third, and fourth ventricles becomes somewhat reduced as the choroid plexuses differentiate and the brain substance increases. The central canal of the spinal cord is normally obliterated after birth by the cellular proliferation with the spinal cord. Thus, the ventricular system terminates at the obex in the caudal floor of the fourth ventricle. The disturbed embryology of the caudal cerebellum in the spina bifida–Arnold Chiari malformation complex frequently alters this normal course of events. It causes the central canal to remain enlarged and patent to the point of causing symptomatic hydrosyringomyelia.

CEREBROVASCULAR DEVELOPMENT

There are five periods in the development of the cerebral vasculature.[12] The first period corresponds to stage 8 or 9 where there are neither arteries nor veins. The primordial endothelium-lined channels then form a plexiform network that eventually, during the second period (stages 10 to 13), differentiates into arteries and veins. This provides the initial circulation to the head. Direct connections with the primitive aortic system supply on the arterial side and the venous drainage join the jugular system. At stage 19, corresponding to the fourth period and leading into fetal life, there is separation of the arterial and venous systems. The final period extends beyond birth and consists of late histologic changes in vascular walls transforming them into the adult form. It is believed that most of vascular malformations occur before the embryo attains a length of 40 mm and that is before the arterial walls thicken. This is a structural defect in the formation of the primitive arteriolar-capillary network.[13]

Neuroanatomy

The CNS is unique in its vulnerability to trauma, hypoxia, ischemia, and other pathophysiologic phenomena. The management of these events by up-to-date techniques in cerebral protection, resuscitation, and monitoring is as important as the provision of excellent anesthesia in the operating room. For this reason a knowledge of normal CNS anatomy and physiology is essential for the neuroanesthesiologist.

CRANIOSPINAL COMPARTMENT

The craniospinal compartment is limited by the calvarium and the vertebral column. It is a single continuous space well developed to protect the vulnerable neural tissue of the brain and the spinal cord. However, the compliance of the system is low due to a lack of distensibility within the subdural space. The contents of this space include the brain parenchyma (neurons, glial tissue and the interstitial fluid), CSF (10 percent) and the cerebral blood volume (10 percent). The consequences of an increase in volume of any of these compartments by, for example, a tumor growth, hydrocephalus, or hemorrhage, will result in compression of vital tissue and displacement of adjacent structures. The change in volume will produce a rapid rise in intracranial pressure (ICP).

The brain at birth weighs about 335 g and provides about 10 to 15 percent of total body weight. It grows rapidly in the first year of life. It doubles in weight within 6 months and finally reaches 900 g by 1 year. At the end of the second year it weighs 1000 g and will reach adult weight (1200 to 1400 g) by about 12 years of age. The weight ratio of CNS to the total body in adulthood is about 2 percent.[14] The calvarium at birth consists of ossified plates covering the dura mater, which are separated by fibrous sutures and the

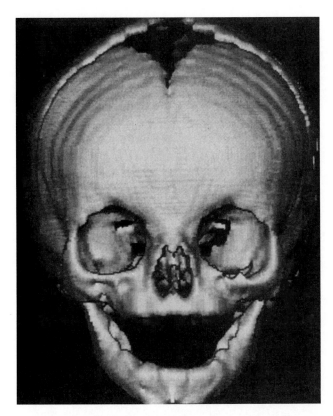

Figure 35-2   Three-dimensional image constructed from a computed tomography-scan of a 9-month-old infant showing craniofacial contours. The small size of the face relative to the cranium is evident. The open anterior fontanelle is easily seen. The coronal and the metopic sutures are also visualized.

fontanelles (Fig. 35-2). Two fontanelles are identifiable at birth. The posterior fontanelle closes during the second or third month and the anterior fontanelle closes usually at the age of 10 to 16 months.[14] The fontanelle does not totally ossify until the teenage years.[14]

However, it should be noted that even before closure of the fibrous fontanelle, the ability to accommodate to an acute increase in ICP is limited if not nonexistent. The distensibility of the dura mater and the osteofibrous cranium resembles that of a leather bag and offers a high resistance to an acute rise in pressure.[15] Slow pressure rises can to a certain point be accommodated by expansion of the fontanelle and separation of the suture lines.[16] Palpation or application of skin transducer on the fontanelles may be used clinically to assess ICP.[17,18] The intracranial space is separated into two major compartments by a layer of dura called the tentorium cerebelli.

SUPRATENTORIAL COMPARTMENT

The supratentorial compartment is the largest compartment of the craniospinal space and its size is determined by the calvaria and the tentorium cerebelli (Fig.

35-3). The two hemispheres are separated by the falx cerebri. Each hemisphere consists of three lobes (frontal, temporal, and parieto-occipital) each of which has several complex and specialized functions. Lesions of the temporal and parieto-occipital lobes have more serious clinical consequences than lesions in the frontal lobe.

The diencephalon forms the central part of the supratentorial compartment and is the rostral end of the brain stem. It consists of the thalamus, hypothalamus, epithalamus, and subthalamus and it surrounds the third ventricle. It is vulnerable to involvement from neoplasms or ischemia. The impairment of blood supply is often due to compression by the hemispheric masses.

In neuroanesthesia, intracranial procedures are described as supratentorial or infratentorial according to their location. It is important to note that the supratentorial compartment includes both the anterior and the middle cranial fossa. The anterior cranial fossa is occupied by the inferior part and anterior extremities of the frontal lobe. The tentorium is a tent-shaped dural septum that forms a roof over the posterior cranial fossa intervening between the supratentorial compartment and the cerebellum. Between the anteriomedial parts of the right and left leafs of the tentorium is an oval opening called the tentorial incisura (notch). It allows the brain stem to pass from the middle cranial fossa to the posterior cranial fossa (see Fig. 35-3).

Clinically, if a severe primary injury to the brain results in gross hemorrhage or edema both the inferior edge of the falx cerebri (a large sickle-shaped vertical formation of dura in the longitudinal fissure between the two cerebral hemispheres) and the tentoria incisura become important sites of secondary injury. These clinical consequences are caused by a differential pressure being created across the tentoria incisura, which may lead to herniation of the brain stem and other vital structures. This could lead to cerebral ischemia by impingement of the anterior cerebral artery. If the pressure increases even more, this structure will finally herniate through the tentoria incisura such as the diencephalic brain stem, cerebral peduncles, oculomotor nerve, and the posterior communicating artery. Because the medial aspect of the temporal lobe sits in the medial cranial fossa on either side of the tentoria incisura, the uncus will herniate with the following clinical consequences: contralateral hemiplegia, ipsilateral large irregular poorly reactive pupil, and posturing problem.

INFRATENTORIAL COMPARTMENT

The posterior cranial fossa is the largest and the deepest of all three cranial fossae. It contains the cerebellum, the pons, and the medulla oblongata. The skull cov-

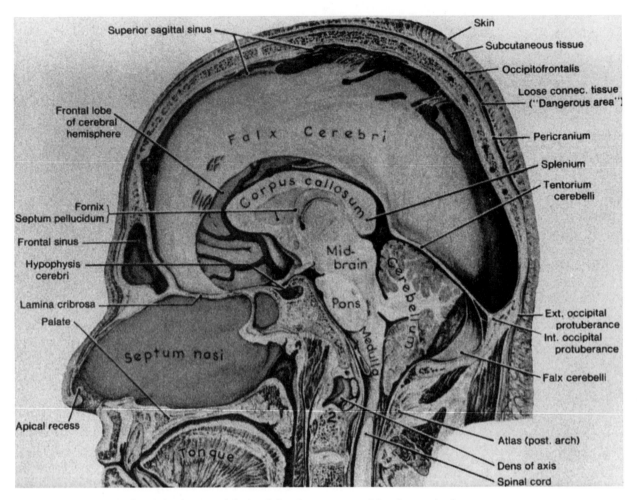

Figure 35-3 Drawings of a median section of the head showing supratentorial and posterior fossa structures. (Modified with permission from Moore KL: *Clinically Oriented Anatomy.* Baltimore, Williams & Wilkins, 1985.)

ering the posterior fossa is formed largely by the inferior and anterior parts of the occipital bone.

The clinical consequences of injury or disease in the posterior cranial fossa may be devastating due to its physical compression of many vital structures such as the reticular system, cardiac and respiratory centers, and cranial nerves. The cerebellum occupies most of the posterior cranial fossa. It is mainly concerned with motor functions that regulate posture, muscle tone, and coordination. Midline or bilateral lesions on the cerebellum may cause permanent injury such as unsteady gait, hypotonia, and tremor.

From a clinical standpoint, the cerebellar tonsils, which are posteroinferior prolongations of cerebellar tissues, are of considerable importance. Pressure differentials produced by posterior cranial fossa pathology cause herniation of the cerebellar tonsils through the foramen magnum. It results in a syndrome called the "pressure cone" phenomenon, which is commonly fatal. The neuroanesthesiologist should keep in mind

that the identification of increasing posterior cranial fossa pressure leading eventually to herniation may be relatively subtle and often requires a high index of suspicion for diagnosis.

SPINAL CANAL COMPARTMENT

The spinal cord, which represents a significant proportion of CNS volume, lies in the vertebral canal. It is a cylindrical structure that is slightly flattened anteriorly and posteriorly where the vascularization predominates. The spinal cord is a continuation of the medulla, which is the inferior part of the brainstem. The spinal cord in adults is usually 42 to 45 cm in length and ends opposite to the intervertebral disk between L1 and L2, but may terminate anywhere between T12 and L3. At birth, after retrogressive differentiation is accomplished, the spinal cord ends at the intervertebral space of L3 (Fig. 354A–C). As the body grows, the end of the spinal cord will reach the adult level at 8 years of age (Fig. 35-4*D*). However, the intradural space is

Pediatric Anesthesia

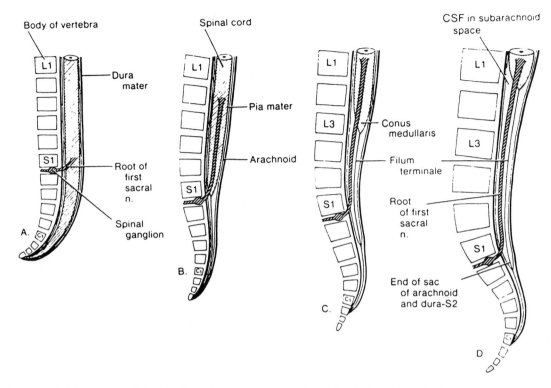

Figure 35-4 The position of the inferior end of the spinal cord in relation to the vertebral column and meninges at various stages of development. *A,* 8 weeks; *B,* 24 weeks; *C,* newborn; *D,* 8-year-old-child and adult. (Reproduced by permission from Moore KL: *Clinically Oriented Anatomy.* Baltimore, Williams & Wilkins, 1985.)

much longer than the spinal cord and it ends at S2 (Fig. 35-4*D*). The spinal cord occupies approximately the two-thirds of the entire vertebral space. The total space is occupied by the CSF. The L2 to S2 segments, therefore, consist of a reservoir of CSF. This may provide a relief mechanism during an increase in ICP such as tumor growth. However, it must be remembered that the spinal compartment is larger than the posterior cranial fossa and its greater compliance associated with the slight distensibility of the spinal dura mater and the compressibility of the venous plexuses set the stage for transforaminal tonsil herniation. Therefore, it must be remembered that an acute decompression of the spinal compartment by lumbar puncture may readily precipitate such herniation.

VASCULAR ANATOMY

The brain is supplied by an extensive system of branches from two pairs of vessels, the internal carotid and the vertebral arteries. Each contributes to the circulus arteriosus cerebri (circle of Willis). It is formed by the posterior cerebral artery, the posterior communicating artery, the internal carotid siphon, the anterior cerebral artery, and the anterior communicating artery. Although this structure seems to be designed to prevent cerebral infarction in the event of occlusion of one of these vessels, it is unfortunate that in most cases insufficient blood is supplied by these collateral routes. In the typical cerebral arterial circle there is usually an exchange of blood between the cerebral arteries via the anterior and posterior communicating arteries. Twenty-eight percent of individuals lack at least one anastomotic component of the circle of Willis with the anterior communicating artery being most frequently absent.

The venous drainage of the brain is achieved mainly by the venous sinuses of the dura mater. These sinuses and lacunae are venous channels located between the dura mater and the periosteum lining the cranium. The venous sinuses are lined with endothelium that is continuous with that of the cerebral veins that enter them. These sinuses have no values and no muscle in their walls. The brain is insensitive to pain but the cerebral dura mater shows nociceptive responses, especially around the venous sinuses of the dura. Several sinuses form the venous drainage system and some more important than others for the anesthesiologist.

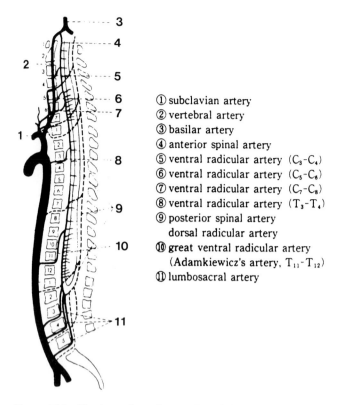

① subclavian artery
② vertebral artery
③ basilar artery
④ anterior spinal artery
⑤ ventral radicular artery (C_3-C_4)
⑥ ventral radicular artery (C_5-C_6)
⑦ ventral radicular artery (C_7-C_8)
⑧ ventral radicular artery (T_3-T_4)
⑨ posterior spinal artery
  dorsal radicular artery
⑩ great ventral radicular artery
  (Adamkiewicz's artery, T_{11}-T_{12})
⑪ lumbosacral artery

Figure 35-5 Blood supply to the spinal cord. (Reproduced by permission from Goto and Crosby.[64])

The *superior sagittal sinus*, which travels in the midline, is a particularly important anesthetic consideration during the surgical correction of a craniosynostosis or during a morcellation craniectomy. In about 60 percent of cases, the superior sagittal sinus ends by becoming the *right transverse sinus*. The transverse sinus runs above the tentorium cerebelli laterally to the *sigmoid sinus*. The sigmoid sinus is so named because of its S-shaped course in the posterior cranial fossa. It eventually enters venous enlargements called the superior bulbs of the internal jugular veins. All the venous sinuses of the dura mater deliver most of their blood to the sigmoid sinuses and then to the internal jugular vein with the exception of the inferior petrosal sinuses, which enter these veins directly. Finally, the *occipital sinus*, which is the smallest, lies along the foramen magnum to communicate with the internal vertebral plexus. The *cavernous sinuses*, large and short, surround the sella turcica. They join the inferior petrosal sinuses, which drains into the transverse sinus.

SPINAL CORD VASCULAR ANATOMY

The spinal cord vascular anatomy is comprised of essentially separate anterior and posterior circulations with both arising from the vertebral arteries and supplemented by intercostal and lumbar vessels from the descending aorta (Fig. 35-5). The ventral two-thirds of

the spinal cord, which includes the corticospinal tracts and motor neurons, is supplied by a single anterior spinal artery. The dorsal one-third of spinal cord parenchyma, which transmits sensations of proprioception and light touch, is supplied by paired posterior spinal arteries that actually form a plexus-like arrangement on the surface of the cord.[19] However, there is essentially no collateral flow between the anterior and the posterior circulations.

The anterior spinal artery is of great clinical importance because it supplies motor neurons and tracts. Some of its branches run circumferentially on the ventrolateral surface of the cord to supply white matter tracts, whereas sulcal branches penetrate the cord parenchyma and divide in ventral gray matter. The anterior spinal artery is of uneven caliber and not functionally continuous throughout its length. The blood flow to the ventral spinal cord in some patients may be heavily dependent on collateral flow through radicular arteries arising from the aorta. These radicular vessels are unpaired and typically arise from intercostal or lumbar arteries on the left side of the aorta. Only six to eight of the 62 radicular vessels present during development will persist into adult life and 45 percent of the population have fewer than five (generally one to two cervical, two or three thoracic, and one or two lumbar). The large distance between these radicular vessels leaves watershed areas at the upper thoracic and lumbar levels where the spinal cord is particularly vulnerable to ischemia. For this reason, the great radicular artery of Adamkiewicz, which arises from the aorta between the eighth thoracic and third lumbar nerve roots and supplements flow to the ventral portion of the distal thoracic spinal cord and lumbar enlargement, is a particularly important collateral vessel. It provides up to 50 percent of the entire spinal cord blood flow and thus is of critical importance during aortic or spinal surgery or following spinal trauma.

The venous outflow of the spinal cord is divided into two systems called the vertebral venous plexuses.[20] An internal and an external plexus communicate with each other and with both segmental systemic veins and the portal system.

The *internal plexus* consists of thin-walled, valveless veins in basketwork pattern, which surround the dura mater of the spinal cord and the posterior longitudinal ligament. This plexus communicates through the foramen magnum with the occipital and basilar sinuses. At each spinal segment, the plexus receives veins from the spinal cord and a basilar-vertebral vein from the body of a vertebra. The plexus in turn is drained by intervertebral veins, which pass through the intervertebral and sacral foramina to the vertebral, intercostal, lumbar, and lateral sacra veins.

The *external plexus* is formed by the veins coming

out of each vertebral body, which join to develop the anterior vertebral plexus. The veins passing through the ligamenta flava form the posterior vertebral plexus.

Neurophysiology

To understand the effects of anesthetic agents on the CNS, this section reviews the physiology of the energetics of cerebral metabolism, cerebral blood flow (CBF), CSF dynamics, and spinal cord blood flow.

ENERGETICS OF CEREBRAL METABOLISM

An analysis of the structure, physiology, and function of the human brain represents one of the most complex of all biologic problems. A major aspect of this complexity is the myriad synaptic connections, voltage- and ligand-gated into channels, and intracellular second messenger systems that mediate interneuronal communications.[21] The energy required to maintain and regulate these systems is considerable. At the age of 8 years and for the rest of one's life the brain weighs a mere 2 percent of the total body weight but consumes more than 20 percent of the entire adenosine triphosphate (ATP) produced in the body. Under normal conditions, the main substance used for energy production in the brain is glucose.[22] In the presence of oxygen, D-glucose is the sole or major source of metabolic fuel that is necessary to generate high-energy intermediates from the Krebs cycle. This biochemical process generates ATP from adenosine diphosphate (ADP) and inorganic phosphate and produces NADH from nicotinamide-adenine dinucleotide (NAD^+).

Glucose depletion rapidly leads to coma and eventually to brain death. It is surprising that the brain stores minuscule amounts of glucose and glycogen while muscle tissue stores 10 times and the liver tissue 100 times as much glycogen per unit of mass. The glycogen storage capacity of the brain is sufficient to provide less than 3 minutes of normal rates of ATP consumption. Therefore, the brain is entirely dependent on blood circulation for the 120 g of glucose it requires each day. Neonatal mammals have much greater glycogen stores and this may explain why they seem more resistant to longer periods of oxygen deprivation. The overall metabolic rate for the brain tissue of children (mean age, 6 years) is markedly higher for oxygen than the adult rate (5.8 versus 3.5 ml O_2 min per 100 g of brain tissue) and for glucose (6.8 versus 5.5 mg glucose min per 100 g).[22]

In the absence of oxygen the glycogen will proceed through the anaerobic glycolysis pathway, which will transform the pyruvate to lactate-regenerating NAD^+.

This energy production is accompanied, unfortunately, by the generation of hydrogen ions, which decrease the intracellular pH, eventually altering conductivity and viability. When the oxygen supply to a neuron is reduced to a minimum, the decrease will trigger survival mechanisms that will reduce or slow the fall in ATP levels until reestablishment of cerebral perfusion and substrates intake is improved. These include: (1) the utilization of phosphate phosphocreatinine stores (a high-energy phosphate that can donate its energy passively to maintain ATP), (2) the production of ATP at low levels by anaerobic glycolysis, and (3) a rapid cessation of spontaneous electrophysiologic activity reducing the energy demand by 50 percent.[23]

CEREBRAL BLOOD FLOW AND CEREBRAL BLOOD VOLUME

Cerebral blood flow is a variable readily altered by the anesthetist and, to the extent that CBF is related to cerebral blood volume, allows for reduction in ICP with modification in CBF. Although intracranial pathology may alter or even paradoxically reverse this relationship, it is, for the most part, the clinician's most useful tool in attempting to control ICP. Global CBF in children between the ages of 3 and 12 years is higher than adults and is maintained around 100 ml/100 g per min.[24,25] Infants and small children between the age of 6 to 40 months have demonstrated a CBF of about 90 ml/100 g per min.[26] However, reported values for CBF in premature infants and newborns appear to be about 40 to 42 ml/100 g per min.[27,28] The CBF in gray matter is higher than that in white matter and areas of predominant brain activity in children shift as they develop.[29] Regional areas in the brain that exhibit high levels of metabolic activity will have higher levels of blood flow. In this supply and demand relationship, as the cerebral metabolic rate of oxygen consumption (CMR_{O_2}) increases or decreases cerebral vasoconstriction or vasodilatation will occur, altering CBF in an attempt to fulfill the current demand for oxygen utilization. This phenomenon is known as *autoregulation* and experimental evidence suggests that changes in local adenosine concentration in response to changes in lactate levels are responsible for this vasoactivity. As CMR_{O_2} rises, as in fever or during seizure activity, CBF will increase with a concomitant increase in cerebral blood volume, and ICP will potentially increase. Conversely, hypothermia and certain anesthetic agents, which decrease CMR_{O_2}, will cause a reduction in CBF. During hypothermia, CMR_{O_2} and CBF decrease on the order of 7 percent per degree centigrade.[30]

Global CMR_{O_2} measured in children aged 3 to 12 years is 5.2 ml O_2/100 g brain mass per min, substantially greater than that measured in adults.[24,25] The

CMR_{O_2} in anesthetized newborns and infants is 2.3 ml $O_2/100$ g brain mass per min.[25] The above discussion has looked at changes in CBF from the demand side, yet important relationships exist on the supply side as well. Cerebral blood flow will autoregulate to maintain a constant O_2 delivery over a wide range of perfusion pressures. Adults maintain a constant CBF over a range of mean arterial pressures (MAPs) between 60 and 150 mmHg.[31] Autoregulatory thresholds for infants and children are not well known and neonatal animal models suggest that the lower limit for autoregulation may be around 40 mmHg with a suggested limit at 90 mmHg.[32,33] Although it is not possible to calculate the effect of hypotension or hypertension on CBF, it seems reasonable to assume that neonates with MAPs below 60 mmHg also autoregulate but at lower blood pressures. Induced hypotension in infants seems to be well tolerated.[34]

Above and below the limits for autoregulation CBF changes passively with blood pressure. Blood pressure alone is an insufficient measure of cerebral perfusion. Cerebral perfusion pressure (CPP) is described as the MAP minus the central venous pressure (CVP) or in the case of the intact cranium is MAP minus ICP when ICP exceeds CVP. Again, on the supply side, anemia, hemodilution, or drugs that alter the rheologic properties of blood can increase O_2 delivery by decreasing viscosity. Adenosine levels will fall, venoconstriction will occur, and cerebral blood volume will decrease in the face of an overall constant CBF; this concept is known as *blood viscosity autoregulation.* Autoregulation is impaired or abolished by hypoxia,[35,36] vasodilators[37,38] and high concentrations of volatile anesthetics.[39] However, as in adults, hyperventilation has been reported to restore autoregulation in the neonate.[40] Intracranial pathology as the result of trauma, areas of inflammation surrounding tumor, abscess, or sites of focal ischemia exhibit altered autoregulation.[41] As demonstrated, autoregulation is easily impaired or lost in the newborn and it may lead to the development of intraventricular hemorrhage, CNS damage, or death.[42]

The cerebrovascular reactivity to hypocarbia is the anesthetist's most useful tool in reducing CBF. In adults, CBF varies linearly with Pa_{CO_2} between 20 and 80 mmHg. A 1 mmHg fall in Pa_{CO_2} results in a 4 percent decrease in CBF. As Pa_{CO_2} falls, CSF pH rises and periarteriolar changes in pH are reflected in vasoconstriction. Chronic hyperventilation will result in slow movement of bicarbonate ions out of the CSF with normalization of CSF pH and CBF within 24 h.[30] Sudden increases in Pa_{CO_2} after chronic hyperventilation of more than 24 h can result in cerebral vasodilatation and increases in ICP.[43]

Previous studies have suggested that the immature brain is relatively unresponsive to small changes in Pa_{CO_2},[44] and a recent publication on fetal rabbit brain demonstrated that CBF responded to changes in Pa_{CO_2}.[45] A study in anesthetized infants and children using transcranial Doppler sonography has demonstrated that CBF velocity changes logarithmically and directly with end-tidal Pet_{CO_2}.[46] It suggests that the vasodilatory effect of CO_2 on the cerebral vasculature may be reached at a much lower Pa_{CO_2} than in adults. The cerebral vascular response to hypoxia is not well studied in children. Adults show no change in CBF until Pa_{O_2} falls below 50 mmHg, at which time CBF begins to increase exponentially.

CEREBROSPINAL FLUID

Most of the CSF (50 to 80 percent) is produced by the choroid plexuses lining the ventricular system. Extrachoroidal sites of production are not well identified, but studies suggest the brain's ependymal surface as well as the brain parenchyma itself are possible sites of production.[47–49] Under normal circumstances CSF production and absorption exist in equilibrium, with a mean production rate in children of 0.35 ml/min.[50] The composition of CSF differs from that of plasma, which suggests that it is the product of active secretion via a Na^+/K^+-dependent ATPase pump. Cerebrospinal fluid from the ventricular system exits from the fourth ventricle through the foramina of Magendie and Luschka into the subarachnoid space surrounding the brain and spinal cord. The main absorption of CSF is thought to occur in the arachnoid villi that project into the veins and sinuses of the brain. The exact mechanism of resorption is unknown and both passive and active transport mechanisms have been proposed. Even the choroid plexus itself has been suggested as a possible site of absorption.[51] Under normal conditions the ICP is much more dependent on CBF and cerebral blood volume than CSF production. Reduction of CSF production by one-third has been shown to reduce ICP by only 1.1 mmHg.[52] It is therefore not surprising that drugs, such as acetazolamide, that reduce CSF production have a minimal effect on ICP and become significant only in the patients whose intracranial compliance curve lies to the right. In this group of patients anesthetic agents that increase CSF production or decrease CSF absorption should be avoided.

INTRACRANIAL PRESSURE

Uncontrolled increases in ICP constitute one of the most deleterious pathophysiologic derangements facing the anesthetist and efforts to control ICP are fundamental. In general the cranium can be viewed as a closed space, occupied by brain mass (70 percent), extracellular fluid (10 percent), blood volume (10 percent), and CSF (10 percent). Increases in the volume of any one of these must be offset by a reduction in the others to maintain an overall constant volume. The brain mass itself is relatively incompressible and changes in CSF volume serve as the primary buffer to increases in the other volumes. The point at which increases in intracranial volume can no longer be offset results in an increase in ICP. An idealized pressure/volume relationship can be described and represents the intracranial compliance curve. Intracranial pressure has been measured in neonates and infants.[53,54] Normal ICP in adults lies between 8 and 18 mmHg and ICP in children usually lies in the range of 2 to 4 mmHg. Newborns normally have a positive ICP on the day of birth but subsequently may actually exhibit subatmospheric ICP in early life.[53] Because newborn babies usually lose weight in association with salt and water loss during the first few days after birth, the brain contributes to this loss by reducing the intracerebral volume, which is reflected by a smaller head growth during this period of time.[53] It is postulated that negative ICP may promote intraventricular hemorrhage, especially in premature infants weighing less than 2500 g.

Although the cranium is most easily viewed as a rigid space, the pediatric patient with open fontanelles or suture lines may be able to compensate for a *slow* increase in intracranial volume by expansion of the skull. Suture lines, bridged by fibrous connective tissue, are relatively difficult to separate and cannot compensate for acute increases in intracranial volume. In the older child, as in the adult, the skull is considered a rigid nonexpandable container in which the pressure depends on the total volume of brain substance, interstitial fluid, CSF, and blood. A patient may have a normal ICP yet be at a noncompliant point on the curve and a small change in volume will result in a large and potentially dangerous increase in ICP. This is of course an idealized relationship and evidence suggests that the intracranial compliance curve is a smooth logarithmic curve accounted for by the buffering of intracranial mass by the compliance of cerebral blood vessels and a pressure-driven increase in CSF absorption.[55-57] A review of the pressure/volume intracranial compliance curve demonstrates that with initial volume changes in one compartment, compensation is possible allowing only a small change in pressure.[58] The pressure/volume index (PVI) is an assessment of this compliance such that

$$PVI = \Delta V / \log_{10}(P_p / P_o)$$

where ΔV is the volume of the fluid bolus, P_p is the peak ICP after bolus injection and P_o is the baseline ICP. In normal adults about 25 ml is required to raise baseline ICP by a factor of 10, whereas in infants, the normal PVI is 10 ml because PVI is proportional to the neural axis volume.[59] Therefore, the ICP in infants and children rises much faster than it does in adults, which explains why a child can progress from neurologically well to moribund in 30 min.

Intervention on the part of the anesthetist lies in the ability to shift the patient's intracranial compliance curve to the right, change the slope of the patient's curve, or move the patient to a position on the left along his own curve.

SPINAL CORD BLOOD FLOW

The use of Doppler flowmetry in medecine has simplified certain methodological problems that researchers and clinicians have encountered with the measure of spinal cord blood flow. Until recently, nearly all data available concerning spinal cord circulation physiology were obtained from the body of literature on animal studies. Within the limits of the Doppler technology and the determination of flow velocities, it is interesting to see that the rate of flow inferred with these measurements correlates well with those determined in cats.[60] Animal data suggest, nevertheless, that the spinal cord blood flow is controlled by the same factors and operates according to the same general physiologic principles as the brain.[61,62] It is known, however, that the spinal cord blood flow is lower because the absolute spinal metabolism is lower than the brain. The blood flow to spinal gray matter is about 50 percent that of cerebral cortex and the flow to the white matter is lower still, which is approximately one-third of the rate of the spinal gray matter.[63] Metabolic rate in the spinal cord is proportionally lower so the ratio of supply to demand is probably similar to that of brain.

REGULATION

The concept of spinal cord perfusion pressure (SCPP) (SCPP = MAP − extrinsic pressure on the cord) is clinically useful because it describes factors that affect the adequacy of spinal perfusion.[64] Pressure exerted by local extrinsic mechanical compression[65] such as tumor, hematoma, spinal venous congestion, and increased intraspinal fluid pressure can be important determinants of the SCPP. Because spinal blood flow is maintained constant by vasodilating or vasoconstricting its vasculature to accommodate changes in MAP,[61,62] it suggests that blood pressure is not a determining factor in spinal cord perfusion. The limits of spinal cord blood flow autoregulation are inconsistent in the literature and a range of 60 to 150 mmHg is often quoted. However, a lower limit of 45 mmHg[66] and an upper limit of 180 mmHg[67] have been suggested. Several conditions will affect this autoregulatory mechanisms and include: (1) blood pressure exceeding these limits,[68] (2) severe hypoxia,[69] (3) hypercapnia,[69] and (4) trauma that abolishes vascular reactivity.[67]

Epidural anesthesia may affect the spinal fluid pressure. The administration of 10 ml of solution into the epidural space increases CSF pressure,[70] but this effect is transient and probably has little significance on the SCPP. Much like the cerebral circulation, the spinal cord vasculature is very reactive to changes in oxygenation and carbon dioxide levels. Like the cerebral vasculature, the spinal cord does not respond to change in Pa_{O_2} until it decreases below about 60 mmHg when the spinal cord blood flow increases sharply.[69] Many investigators have suggested that the spinal cord blood flow is linear between 20 and 80 mmHg with an absolute change in spinal cord blood flow of about 0.5 to 1.0 ml/100 g per minute per mmHg change in Pa_{CO_2},[63] whereas the cerebral circulation changes approximately 1 to 2 ml/100 g per min per mmHg change in Pa_{CO_2}.[71] This difference probably reflects baseline differences in the absolute rate of spinal blood flow and CBF rather than differences in the sensitivities of the two vascular systems to carbon dioxide.

Neuropharmacology

GENERAL PRINCIPLES

Evidence from animal data has suggested that the lethal dose for many medications in 50 percent of the animals (LD_{50}) is significantly lower in the neonatal and infancy period compared to the adult.[72] It is essential for the pediatric anesthesiologist to know that the sensitivity of the human newborn to most of the sedatives, hypnotics, and narcotics is increased and that it is probably related to an increased brain immaturity (incomplete myelination and blood-brain barrier) as well as increased permeability for some medications, namely the lipid-soluble drugs, which are largely used in anesthesia.[73] In addition, the use of volatile anesthesic agents is influenced by the age of the patient. The minimum alveolar concentration (MAC) in the neonate (0 to 31 days) is much lower than infants aged 30 to 180 days.[74] Although there is an increase in anesthetic requirement in infancy, it must be emphasized that there is a smaller margin of safety between adequate anesthesia and severe cardiopulmonary depression in the infant and child compared to the adult.[75] Therefore, dosages must be appropriately calculated and therapeutic effects must be monitored to avoid inadvertent adverse clinical consequences and prolonged effects.

In addition to this basic knowledge of the effect of anesthetic drugs on the CBF, CMR_{O_2}, and the CSF dynamics are essential to the neuroanesthetist. The lim-

ited amount of data in infants and children relating to the effects of drugs on neurophysiology may persuade the pediatric neuroanesthetist to assume that the effects are the same as those observed in adults. This section discusses the general principles.

INHALATIONAL ANESTHETIC AGENTS

All currently used inhalational anesthetic agents have a variable degree of cerebrovascular effects.

NITROUS OXIDE

Despite substantial investigations, the effect of nitrous oxide on cerebral circulation remains controversial.[76] The variability of the effects of nitrous oxide on CBF and ICP in different reports is probably due to differences in experimental species and background anesthesia. It is suggested that in subanesthetic doses such as 60% to 70%, it causes excitement and cerebral metabolic stimulation, which is accompanied by increase in CBF.[77-80] Because nitrous oxide is not an adequate anesthetic in the absence of other inhalational agents such as halothane and isoflurane or intravenous anesthetics, all studies reporting an increase in CBF with nitrous oxide were accomplished with concurrent uses of such medications. A recent study in infants and children showed that 70% nitrous oxide in oxygen with fentanyl/diazepam/caudal epidural anesthesia increased CBF significantly when compared with an air/O_2 mixture.[81] This increase in CBF was not associated with significant changes in MAP, heart rate, or cerebrovascular resistance and it was suggested that nitrous oxide may have a direct effect on mitochondrial cerebral metabolic activity. In an animal study, it was shown that CMR_{O_2} increased without any alterations in arterial blood pressure and heart rate.[78] It was hypothesized that these results may be attributed to direct effects of nitrous oxide on cerebral metabolism.[78] Clinically, nitrous oxide can increase CBF and ICP in adults and children.[78,81,82] Barbiturates and hypocapnia in combination may prevent these increases. There are indications that, even given individually, barbiturates, benzodiazepines, and morphine are effective in reducing the effect of nitrous oxide on CBF.[83,84]

In contrast, the use of a volatile agent may add to the increase in CBF obtained from nitrous oxide.[85] Although nitrous oxide is commonly used in neuroanesthesia, it would seem prudent in event of encountering a "tight" brain intraoperatively to discontinue its administration. Furthermore, because of its ability to increase CMR_{O_2}, it would be unwise to continue its administration in face of a jeopardized cerebral perfusion.

HALOTHANE

Halothane is a cerebral vasodilator that decreases cerebrovascular resistance and increases CBF in a dose-dependent fashion.[86-88] In pediatric neuroanesthesia, halothane remains an excellent anesthetic agent and is thus widely used. It is commonly used in combination with hyperventilation. Halothane is a potent vasodilator and its effect seems to be maximal even at 1.0 MAC. It has been shown, using an animal model, that between normocapnia and hypercapnia either at 0.5 MAC or 1.0 MAC halothane concentrations, no additional vasodilatation was caused by increasing the level of carbon dioxide.[89] In children, using a transcranial Doppler and with a similar anesthetic technique, it was reported that at normocapnia CBF velocity changed between 0.5 MAC and 1.0 MAC, but failed to show any further increases at 1.5 MAC.[90] It was also observed that despite decreasing the halothane concentration from 1.5 MAC and 0.2 MAC, an increased CBF velocity was maintained for approximately 30 to 45 min.[91] This halothane response was called a hysteresis phenomenon on the cerebral vasculature. This finding could be important in patients with raised ICP. In animal studies halothane decreased cerebrovascular resistance, increased CBF, and increased ICP.[92] Many human studies have reported these findings.[86,93,94] Finally, a recent study in children showed that the cerebrovascular reactivity to carbon dioxide during halothane anesthesia (0.5 or 1.0 MAC) was preserved, but the vasoconstrictive effect of 20 mmHg of carbon dioxide at 1.0 MAC halothane was not as strong as observed at 0.5 MAC halothane.[95] Therefore, if ICP is not being monitored, halothane should be avoided in patients known to have reduced intracerebral compliance until the dura is open and halothane effects on the brain can be observed.

ISOFLURANE

Isoflurane is the most popular of the volatile anesthetics for neuroanesthesia. Its popularity is based on the fact that it affects CBF less than halothane does at equivalent MAC doses[87,96] and on the belief that it may provide cerebral protection.[97] Cerebral autoregulation is less affected by isoflurane than halothane.[87] Also, isoflurane does not change CSF production as does enflurane[98] and it reduces the resistance to reabsorption of CSF.[98] Studies in children suggest that isoflurane has minimal effects on the cerebrovascular reactivity to carbon dioxide.[95] They showed that during normocapnia, varying the concentration of isoflurane between 0.5 MAC and 1.5 MAC in a loop fashion did not change CBF velocity.[99] Furthermore, they were unable to show any time-response effect of 1.0 MAC of isoflurane CBF velocity in anesthetized children over 90 min.[100] These results are similar to those of previous investigators using isoflurane in comparable concentrations.[101,102] However, despite their dissimilar effects on CBF, isoflurane and halothane increase ICP equally in an animal model of brain injury.[103,104] This is probably because isoflurane and halothane increase cerebral blood volume to a similar degree.[105]

ENFLURANE

Enflurane increases CBF to a maximum of 8 to 37 percent depending on the concentration used, which is less than the effect of halothane.[106-108] Enflurane reduces CMR_{O_2} to a degree similar to that of halothane.[106] Enflurane in high concentration disrupts autoregulation but does not affect cerebrovascular reactivity to carbon dioxide. No available data describe the effects of enflurane in pediatric anesthesia. Two undesirable effects of enflurane in neuroanesthesia render it unsuitable. First, it increases the rate of secretion of CSF production[109] and it increases the resistance to reabsorption of CSF, the latter effect to a greater extent than that observed with halothane.[110] Second, and by far the most important disadvantage of enflurane, is its ability to induce seizure-like electroencephalographic (EEG) activity demonstrated by high-voltage spike waves with burst suppression (2.0 MAC).[111]

SEVOFLURANE

Sevoflurane is similar to isoflurane with respect to its effects on CBV, CMR_{O_2}, and ICP in adults.[112] As yet, no data are available in children. In rats, sevoflurane induces substantially smaller increases in ICP than isoflurane.[113] Furthermore, it is suggested that sevoflurane has a protective effect during incomplete ischemia compared to fentanyl with nitrous oxide.[114]

DESFLURANE

In an animal study desflurane increased CBF and decreased CMR_{O_2}.[115] One MAC desflurane increased ICP significantly in neurosurgical patients with supratentorial mass lesions despite the institution of hypocapnia.[116] There are no available data for desflurane in children.

INTRAVENOUS ANESTHETICS

BARBITURATES

Barbiturates decrease CBF and CMR_{O_2} in a dose-dependent manner[117,118] and are efficient in reducing ICP. A major problem with barbiturates is that they can significantly reduce myocardial contractility, systemic blood pressure, and therefore, CPP. In nonclinical doses (10 to 55 mg/kg), thiopental can produce an isoelectric EEG and decrease the CMR_{O_2} by 50 percent.[118] Barbiturates may be useful in preventing an increase in ICP[119] during laryngoscopy and tracheal intubation due to their vasoconstricting effect on the cerebral vasculature and reduction in CBF. Cerebral autoregulation and cerebrovascular reactivity to carbon dioxide is preserved with barbiturates. The production and reabsorption of CSF is not altered by administration of such drugs.[120] Barbiturates are also effective in controlling epileptiform activity with the exception of methohexital, which may activate seizure foci in patients with temporal lobe epilepsy.[121]

ETOMIDATE
Etomidate reduces CBF (34 percent) and CMR_{O_2} (45 percent).[122] Etomidate has a direct vasoconstrictive effect on cerebral vasculature even before the metabolism is suppressed.[123] Cerebrovascular reactivity to carbon dioxide is maintained.[122] Its advantage over barbiturates is that it does not produce cardiovascular depression. However, two disadvantages to its use are its suppression of the adrenocortical response to stress[124] and the fact that it may trigger myoclonic activities especially after prolonged infusion.[125]

DROPERIDOL
Droperidol is a cerebral vasoconstrictor leading to a reduction in CBF (40 percent in dogs) without changing the CMR_{O_2}.[126] Failure to lower CMR_{O_2} despite reduction in CBF could be undesirable in patients with cerebral vascular disease or increased ICP. The combination of fentanyl and droperidol has little effect on CBF.[127]

PROPOFOL
Propofol is a rapidly acting agent that reduces CBF and CMR_{O_2}.[128] It can reduce ICP but its ability to reduce MAP may jeopardize CPP.[129] There are no data available for children.

BENZODIAZEPINES
Benzodiazepines have been reported to decrease CBF and CMR_{O_2} by approximately 25 percent.[130-132] The reduction of CBF is though to be related to the decrease in CMR_{O_2}. Benzodizepines can reduce ICP. Flumazenil is a benzodiazepine antagonist that has been reported to reverse the beneficial effects of the benzodiazepines on CBF, CMR_{O_2}, and ICP.[130] It thus may cause detrimental effects to patients with high ICP or abnormal intracranial elastance.

OPIOIDS
Opioid anesthetics cause a minor reduction or have no effect on CBF, CMR_{O_2}, and ICP when compared with conditions of a nonstimulated brain.[132] However, if the patient is experiencing pain, opioids can cause a modest reduction in these variables by an indirect effect on the sympathetic system.[133] The use of fentanyl with nitrous oxide in neuroanesthesia is associated with decreases in CBF and CMR_{O_2} of 47 percent and 18 percent, respectively.[106] The cerebrovascular reactivity to carbon dioxide as well as the cerebral autoregulation is

preserved with narcotics. Finally, fentanyl does not have any effects on CSF production but data suggest that it reduces CSF reabsorption by at least 50 percent.[110,134] It has been shown in an animal model that fentanyl does not affect neonatal cerebral circulation.[135] Controversies exist with narcotics such as alfentanil and sufentanil. In patients with brain tumors, alfentanil increases CSF pressure.[136] This effect was less than that observed with sufentanil but greater than that observed with fentanyl. Alfentanil has the greatest effect on MAP and CPP.[137] Controversy surrounds the use of sufentanil in neuroanesthesia because some studies reported a decrease in CBF and CMR_{O_2},[138] whereas other authors suggest an increase in CBF and ICP.[137-139]

KETAMINE
Ketamine is a potent cerebral vasodilator capable of increasing CBF by 60 percent in the presence of normocapnia.[140] It effects on the CMR_{O_2} are negligible. Patients with increased ICP due to hydrocephalus or other pathology have been reported to have suffered clinical deterioration after administration of ketamine.[141] Although it is suggested that ketamine may have some cerebral protective effects, it remains contraindicated in neuroanesthesia.

MUSCLE RELAXANTS
Muscle relaxants have little effect on cerebral circulation.

Succinylcholine produces an initial fall in ICP followed by a rise above baseline levels, especially in patients with a decrease in intracranial compliance. This is caused by a subsequent increase in CBF.[142-144] Mechanisms suggested to explain this increase in ICP probably relate to cerebral stimulation from increases in afferent muscle spindle activity.[144] This increase in ICP and CBF associated with succinylcholine is reduced by prior administration of deep general anesthetics or by pretreatment with nondepolarizing muscle relaxants.[145] However, pediatric patients with increased ICP will benefit more from rapid control of the airway with hyperventilation following successful tracheal intubation than the slight increase in ICP caused by succinylcholine. It is important to remember that life-threatening hyperkalemia can ensue after administration of succinylcholine in patients with closed head injury without motor deficits,[146] severe cerebral hypoxia,[147] subarachnoid hemorrhage,[148] cerebrovascular accident with loss of brain substance,[149] and paraplegia.[150]

Pancuronium and *atracurium* in the presence of halothane have been shown to have no effect on cerebral blood volume, ICP, or CMR_{O_2}.[151] Large doses of *d*-tubocurarine, atracurium, or metocurine may cause transient cerebrovascular dilatation due to the histamine release and therefore could be responsible for a slight increase in ICP. However, this association with a decrease in MAP may compensate for this change in intracerebral blood volume.[152] *Vecuronium* is an agent known for its cardiovascular stability and its relatively short duration of action. In a study of patients with reduction in intracranial compliance, vecuronium caused a slight decrease in ICP, which was probably associated with a concomitant decrease in CVP.[153]

Pathophysiology of Intracranial Pressure

When the blood supply to the brain is compromised, the consequences are usually related to ischemia and damage to the neurons. The brain is the organ most sensitive to ischemic damage.[23] To understand the rationale of the therapy used to protect the brain against hypoxic-ischemic damage, it is essential for the anesthesiologist to appreciate the pathophysiologic mechanisms that are associated with such an insult.

The central event precipitating cellular damage is a reduced production of energy (ATP) due to the blockade of the oxidative phosphorylation at the respiratory chain of the mitochondrion. The production of ATP depends entirely on the supply of glucose. The activity of the ATP-dependent ion pumps is reduced and the intracellular levels of electrolytes such as sodium and calcium increase, whereas potassium levels decrease. These ion changes cause the neurons to depolarize and release excitatory amino acids such as glutamate and aspartate, which are responsible for the increase in local acidosis. The increase in glutamate favors further neuronal depolarization and calcium entry through the *N*-methyl-D-aspartate (NMDA) receptor channel. The high intracellular calcium level leads to an increase in the activity of the proteases and phospholipases as well as activating the Haber-Weiss reaction through the iron anions pathways.[154] This increased phospholipase activity results in the production of free radical and lipid peroxidation, which leads to the release of free fatty acid and membrane destruction. Ischemia can either be global or focal in nature. Although the mechanisms of neuronal damage are similar in both cases, there are important distinctions between the two. In focal ischemia three anatomohistologic factors are identifiable. First, the region affected does not receive blood flow and responds the same as globally ischemic tissue. Second, a transitional zone called the penumbra receives collateral blood flow but though salvageable, remains vulnerable to ischemia. It is dependent on the reestablishment of this vulnerable perfusion. Third, the surrounding region is well perfused and normal.

Brain trauma may cause permanent physical neuronal damage. The mechanism can be either brain herniation or the severing of blood vessels in brain tissue, both of which will lead to ischemia. In these circumstances it is important to prevent the ischemia that will be related to the release of vasoconstrictive substances during reperfusion.[155,156] Again, calcium influx resulting from the trauma has been implicated as a trigger for the damage.[157]

The hemorrhage often associated with trauma may increase ICP by changing the intracranial blood volume leading to a decrease in CPP. Furthermore, the extravasated blood can cause additional damage by increasing the release of free radicals due to the release of iron from the hemoglobin.

These pathophysiologic events associated with brain damage may be ameliorated by vigorous treatment. Procedures that may help protect against ischemic brain damage include maintaining ATP levels (either by increasing substrate uses or reducing the metabolic rate), blocking the ionic flux across the cell membrane, limiting free radical production or increasing the efficiency of scavenging mechanisms, and avoiding the production of acidic metabolites such as glutamate and aspartate that favor neuron depolarization and destruction. Most importantly, CBF and the delivery of oxygen to the tissues must be maintained.

Hydrocephalus is characterized by an increased volume of CSF within the ventricular system and is, with few exceptions, caused by obstruction of CSF circulation or reduced reabsorption. The obstruction may lie within the ventricles themselves, within the subarachnoid space, or at sites of CSF egress or absorption. Patients with obstructive hydrocephalus and blocked access to the arachnoid villi appear to have alternative sites of CSF absorption. There is evidence of some lymphatic-type drainage, as well as transependymal absorption.[158] Many classifications of hydrocephalus have been proposed. Inherent in all is the recognition of the degree to which ICP is increased and an understanding of the pathophysiology responsible. Increased ICP may occur without hydrocephalus and conversely, hydrocephalus may exist without increased ICP.

In the newborn period and especially in premature infants, hydrocephalus is usually secondary to intraventricular hemorrhage. Other causes are aqueductal stenosis or an Arnold-Chiari malformation, the two often coexisting. Bleeding into the subependymal germinal matrix may extend into the ventricle causing a primary blockage to CSF flow. Secondarily, an obliterative arachnoiditis may form that will obstruct CSF flow even after resorption of the primary bleed.[159,160] In the neonate, hydrocephalus may exist despite a normal ICP. The increase in CSF volume is compensated for by a decrease in brain mass up to the compliance limit of immature brain tissue. An Arnold-Chiari malformation is common and it consists of an array of abnormalities mainly in the posterior fossa and cervical region. The brain stem is displaced downward and, together with an abnormal vermis, extends below the foramen magnum and into the cervical canal. The fourth ventricle becomes compressed and its foramina may become obstructed. The cranial nerves may be stretched or entrapped secondary to this downward displacement, causing a variety of bulbar symptoms. Hydrocephalus is present in some 90 percent of cases. Other diseases of childhood may predispose to hydrocephalus through several mechanisms. The mucopolysaccharidoses are often characterized by an obliteration of the subarachnoid space and achondroplastic children can present with hydrocephalus caused presumably by occipital bone growth and impediment to venous outflow.[161,162] In a similar manner, any condition that causes significant cranial deformity can lead to hydrocephalus. In childhood, the most common cause of hydrocephalus is a brain tumor.

BRAIN TUMORS

Malignant disease is second only to trauma as a cause of death in children less than 15 years of age.[163] After leukemia, the second most common neoplasms of childhood, primary brain tumors, are responsible for 20 percent of all cancers in children and for 20 percent of childhood cancer deaths.[164] Tumor incidence is slightly higher for males than females (1.2 : 1), but this sexual predominance merely reflects the normal population sex ratio.[165,166] For the year 1991, in the United States, the annual projected incidence is approximately 3.1 / 100,000 among children under 15 years of age.[167] In comparison, the rate of head injuries requiring surgery ranges from 150 to 400 / 100,000 depending on age and sex.[168]

Two-thirds of all childhood brain tumors arise in the posterior fossa with an unfortunate predisposition for midline structures. Thus, they are frequently associated with obstructive hydrocephalus. The usual history includes headache and vomiting over days or weeks. Medulloblastomas (comprising 15 to 20 percent of CNS tumors in children) are usually found growing adjacent to or within the fourth ventricle. Ependymomas, more common in the pediatric age group, are also most frequently found in the fourth ventricle. Posterior fossa tumors should be suspected in all children who present with increased ICP or cranial nerve symptomatology. Choroid plexus papillomas appear to be the only pathologic cause of CSF overproduction causing hydrocephalus.

Brain tumors are expanding space-occupying lesions that lead eventually to a significant increase in ICP and to a reduction in CPP; the cascade of events associated with brain ischemia has been discussed above. Vessels associated with these tumors that do not autoregulate, contribute to peritumoral vasogenic edema, which further elevates ICP. Ultimately, untreated brain masses will lead to brain stem herniation and death.

The anesthesiologist has an important role in the management of children with brain tumors. Before surgical excision, the vasogenic edema surrounding the tumor can be reduced significantly by the administration of dexamethasone. Brain bulk may be reduced by dehydration using mannitol, hypertonic saline, and furosemide. In addition to its effect of promoting diuresis, furosemide may secondarily decrease ICP by reducing CSF production and reducing CVP through peripheral venodilatation. The administration of osmotically active agents is discussed in the section on fluid management.

COMPLICATIONS OF ELEVATED INTRACRANIAL PRESSURE

It is usual to consider the cranial space as a closed box. However, it is divided into distinct spaces with the cerebral hemispheres divided by the falx cerebri and the posterior fossa elements separated from the hemispheres by the tentorium cerebelli. Shifts of intracranial contents occur when asymmetrical increases in pressure create gradients across the falx, the tentorium, and the foramen magnum. Tentorial herniation (the uncal syndrome) results in typical eye and motor signs as the diencephalon moves backward through the tentorial notch. Compression of the superior colliculus results in the vertical gaze palsy (sunset sign). When a mass effect occurs within one compartment, extrusion of brain from one compartment to another begins when the limits of compensation or buffering have been exceeded. As a mass expands in one hemisphere, one anterior cerebral artery may be compressed as brain tissue gains access into the opposite hemisphere under the falx cerebri. Resulting ischemia produces further edema and swelling. Herniation at this level often disrupts cortical pathways to the contralateral limbs and bladder sphincter. Compression of the posterior cerebral artery against the tentorium results in hemianopsia. Calcarine infarction may arise from bilateral compression of these basal arteries and may lead to irreversible blindness.[169] Protrusion of the parahippocampal gyrus (uncus) of the temporal lobe beneath the tentorium cerebelli and through the tentorial hiatus presents with signs of brain stem compression, progressive obtunding of reflexes, ipsilateral pupillary dilatation, and contralateral hemiparesis, and if uncontrolled will lead to cardiorespiratory arrest. Midbrain compression in children is associated with hypertonic extension of the upper arms and legs (doggy paddling arms and cycling legs), opisthotonus, decerebrate rigidity, decorticate posturing, and hypotonia. Further compression of the midbrain results in coma, hypertension, bradycardia, tachypnea, and periodic respirations. As the ICP increases on the medullary respiratory center, bradypnea will be replaced by apnea.[169]

Distortion within the posterior fossa due to a mass effect may obstruct the flow of CSF and result in obstructive hydrocephalus. Even without herniation, increases in ICP may result in global or regional cerebral ischemia. As ICP increases and approaches MAP, the CPP falls below critical levels. This will result in tissue hypoxia, cellular injury, or death; swelling from increased brain edema as fluid shifts to compensate for disturbed electrolyte balance; and a vicious cycle of increasing brain volume and ICP. Herniation from the posterior fossa usually involves the cerebellar tonsils that protrude through the foramen magnum. This causes compression of the medullary cardiorespiratory centers. Loss of upward gaze (sunset sign), projectile vomiting, miotic fixed pupils, and central hyperventilation are suggestive of posterior fossa hypertension. Failure of vocal cord abduction may result in inspiratory stridor. Gross displacement of the brain (and the final manifestation of severe posterior fossa hypertension) compresses the vascular supply to the medulla as it protrudes through the foramen magnum. The result is Cushing's triad of tachypnea, hypertension, and bradycardia, eventually leading to apnea and death.[170]

General Anesthetic Considerations

In the following sections, the anesthetic management of most frequent pediatric neurosurgical procedures will be discussed. The concepts common to most of these surgical procedures are reviewed in this section; the discussion of specific surgical and anesthetic considerations follows.

PREOPERATIVE ASSESSMENT OF THE NEUROSURGICAL PATIENT

In recent years exciting advances have occurred in the preoperative assessment of the neurosurgical patient because of both an increased understanding of cerebral pathophysiology and improved diagnostic imaging techniques.

The cornerstone of the assessment of cerebral function rests on the history and physical examination. The preoperative anesthetic workup of the neurosurgical patient includes assessments of ICP, the function of vital respiratory and cardiovascular centers that can

be affected in the neuropathologic process either in the brain stem or the spinal cord, and the specific disturbance in neurologic function.[171]

Central to the neuroanesthetic management is the preoperative recognition of intracranial hypertension and major neurologic deficits. History and physical findings of intracranial hypertension differ somewhat according to age group.

In general, the clinical presentation of the patient with intracranial hypertension varies with its time course from the initial increase in ICP. Sudden massive increases in ICP may cause coma. In a subacute case, however, a history of headache on awakening is suggestive of vasodilatation caused by hypercapnia during sleep due to reduced intracranial compliance. Vomiting is a common clinical sign. Neonates and infants often present with a history of increased irritability, poor feeding, or lethargy. A bulging anterior fontanelle, dilated scalp veins, cranial enlargement or deformity, or lower extremity motor deficits are common signs of increased ICP in this age group.[172] Increased ICP presenting in childhood is frequently caused by tumor. As ICP reaches critical levels, vomiting, decreased level of consciousness, and evidence of herniation may develop. Other symptoms include double vision due to oculomotor or gaze palsies (sunset sign), dysphonia, dysphagia, or gait disturbance. Injury to the third cranial nerve may result in ptosis. Injury to the sixth cranial nerve produces a strabismus from a loss of abduction. Nausea and vomiting usually occur and older children will complain of morning headache. Papilledema and absent venous pulsation of the retinal vessels may be present on fundoscopy.[59,169-173]

Neurogenic pulmonary edema is a clinical syndrome presenting with acute hypoxia, pulmonary congestion, pink frothy protein-rich pulmonary edema, and radiologic evidence of pulmonary infiltrates.[174,175] It is associated with a variety of intracranial pathologies including hemorrhage,[176,177] head trauma,[178] and seizure disorders.[179] The mechanism responsible for the activation of the sympathetic system and the vagal centers that lead to pulmonary edema seems to be related to ischemia of the medulla and distortion of the brainstem.[180,181] Auscultation of the patient's lungs may determine whether aspiration has occurred. Assessment of cranial nerve function and the patient's ability to protect the airway must be evaluated. During the preoperative assessment of a neurologic patient, one cannot exclude the possibility of spinal cord dysfunction. Disturbances of neurologic function arising from injury of the cervical spinal cord may affect the respiratory and cardiovascular centers. This is discussed further in the section on spinal cord injury.

Laboratory tests may yield evidence of syndrome of inappropriate antidiuretic hormone (SIADH) as well as

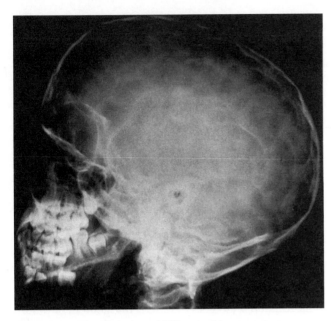

Figure 35-6 Chronic increased ICP caused by premature universal suture stenosis shows extensive "beaten copper" or "thumb printing" signs on a lateral projection.

electrolyte abnormalities or volume contraction from protracted vomiting. Diabetes insipidus may result in hypernatremia.[182] Disturbances in metabolism such as hypo- and hyperglycemia may occur. The preoperative history and chart review may reveal the need for steroid supplementation in patients with a suppressed adrenal axis from prior steroid therapy aimed at reducing tumor edema. Neurosurgical patients may also be receiving anticonvulsant medication. Recognition of their seizure history as well as any potential drug interaction is important. Patients with a suprasellar tumor such as craniopharyngioma frequently have pituitary dysfunction and should have a complete endocrine evaluation that includes thyroid and adrenal function studies.

Four imaging modalities that aid in the assessment of intracranial hypertension are skull x-rays, ultrasonography, computed tomography (CT) scan and magnetic resonance imaging (MRI). Skull x-rays may show the "beaten copper sign" (Fig. 35-6) and splitting of the sagittal sutures caused by chronic increased ICP and universal suture stenosis. In infants and young children, the cranial sutures should not exceed 2 mm and should not have bridges or closures.[183] Ultrasonography of the brain is useful in premature infants and neonates because it is relatively inexpensive, does not require sedation, and can be performed at the bedside through the fontanelle. The real-time sector scanner can visualize virtually all parts of the brain.[184]

In the past two decades, the development of CT scanning and MRI has revolutionized the investigation of brain disease. It is essential for anesthesiologists to become familiar with these modalities of preoperative assessment and insist on reviewing them before proceeding with the anesthetic management. The preoperative evaluation of these laboratory reports will facilitate the identification of the neuroanesthetic considerations and will help in the design of the anesthetic technique most appropriate to use in these surgical procedures.

PREMEDICATION

The routine use of sedation in pediatric neurosurgical patients is best avoided. Sedatives and narcotics should not be given to nonmonitored children because the drugs may precipitate respiratory depression with consequent hypercarbia or loss of airway integrity.

Exceptions to this rule include patients with intracranial vascular lesions (with no increase in ICP) who may benefit from some degree of sedation to avoid precipitating a preoperative hemorrhage. For small children, we suggest the use of pentobarbital 4 mg/kg or chloral hydrate in a dose of 50 mg/kg administered orally or rectally 1 hour before surgery. Emotional preparation is essential and this can be accomplished by both the anesthesiologist and the parents working together. In older children, a simple explanation of what may be expected before induction of anesthesia will reduce the element of surprise and the incidence of hemodynamic responses in a threatening environment.

PATIENT POSITIONING

The planning of a successful anesthetic includes the preparation of the operating table with proper equipment to protect the patient after positioning. The anesthesiologist's preoperative visit should contribute helpful information regarding management and positioning.

Although patient positioning in neurosurgery depends on the procedure, the general principles remain the same. The eyes must be securely taped closed and if the patient is prone, the face and other vulnerable areas should be padded with foam sheeting to prevent the adverse effects of localized pressure. Ventilation may be compromised by incorrect positioning and it is mandatory to ensure that chest excursions remain adequate, especially if the patient is prone. This may be achieved by using suitable bolsters or a frame, which, when place under the chest and pelvic girdle, allows the abdomen to hang free facilitating respiratory movements during intermittent positive-pressure ventilation (IPPV). The endotracheal tube should be taped securely, realizing that in the prone position secretions may loosen the tape. Usually a 10° head-up tilt is advisable to improve cerebral venous return and reduce venous congestion. Rotation of the head to one side may kink the jugular vein system and reduce venous return. This may be avoided by rotating the trunk to maintain the axial position. During any surgical procedure, the anesthesiologist must be able to inspect the endotracheal tube and anesthetic circuit connection and have access for possible endotracheal suctioning. In addition, it is desirable to observe a body part such as a hand or foot during the surgery to assess peripheral perfusion and adequacy of gas exchange.

MONITORING

Over the past decade, neuromonitoring has increased in importance and is now contributing to improve the neurosurgical outcome.[185] Recent technological progress now allows noninvasive monitoring of bioelectric signals, cerebral perfusion, and flow velocity, brain tissue oximetry, and ICP.

Basic monitoring for pediatric anesthesia consists of a precordial/esophageal stethoscope, electrocardiography (ECG), noninvasive blood pressure, temperature, pulse oximetry, and capnometry. A radial pulse Doppler allows for continuous monitoring of peripheral perfusion on a beat-to-beat basis and provides a noninvasive measurement of blood pressure. It is especially useful in neontal anesthesia. Neuromuscular blockade monitoring by a peripheral nerve stimulator is desirable. A urinary catheter is usually in place for long surgical procedures and mandatory if osmotic diuretics are administered. (Monitoring for specific operations is discussed in the section "Specific Anesthetic Considerations.")

GENERAL PRINCIPLES OF INDUCTION OF ANESTHESIA

The selection of the anesthetic technique and recognition of perioperative events may have a profound effect on the reduction or prevention of significant morbidity. The age of the pediatric population ranges from the premature neonate at one extreme to the 16-year-old young adult. Knowledge of normal physiology in these differing age groups is essential. Neonatal anesthesia differs significantly from that in the older child and adult, particularly regarding the respiratory system, the cardiovascular system, and thermoregulation.[186] An understanding of these differences may directly influence the neurosurgical outcome.

Anesthesia in a patient with elevated ICP is fraught with danger. Following induction of anesthesia, rapid control of the airway by tracheal intubation and hyperventilation will help to lower the ICP. The systemic hypertension usually associated with laryngoscopy may be discouraged by the use of intravenous lidocaine at induction of anesthesia. However, it is important to note that the possibility of cardiac arrhythmias and arrest associated with the administration of lidocaine 2 mg/kg has been reported in the small infant.[187] Intravenous lidocaine may be followed by major disturbances in cardiac rhythm and rate. Caution must be used and small doses should decrease the potential for adverse effects.

A rapid sequence technique involving the administration of thiopental, atropine, and succinylcholine followed by carefully applied cricoid pressure and manual hyperventilation is recommended. In October 1994, a controversy erupted on the routine use of succinylcholine in children and adolescents. This controversy was based on a few cases reported with cardiac arrest and hyperkalemia.[188] It has been shown that the use of this muscle relaxant has passed the test of time in hundreds of thousands of infants and children without a single death attributable to it.[189] The benefit of this fast-acting relaxant in pediatric anesthesia and the availability of intravenous calcium to treat hyperkalemic responses provides succinylcholine with an essential role in the airway management of these small patients.[189] Furthermore, it has also been shown that the association of thiopental and succinylcholine reduces the incidence of complications described with this muscle relaxant.[190]

A recent study has shown that cricoid pressure and manual ventilation can be performed without insufflation of the stomach.[191,192] This provides protection of the airway in cases of recent feeding or delayed gastric emptying often associated with increased ICP. For tracheal intubation, muscular relaxation can be achieved using succinylcholine or vecuronium. The rapidity with which succinylcholine produces satisfactory intubing conditions outweighs its small incremental effect on ICP, and it is used routinely in pediatric neuroanesthesia. However, vecuronium 0.4 mg/kg has produced excellent intubing conditions which are comparable to succinylcholine.[193]

Patients without ready intravenous access may be induced by means of a small butterfly needle that can be inserted with minimal patient stress or hemodynamic fluctuation. Failing this, it is probably less injurious in children with raised ICP to perform a skillful inhalation induction than it is to subject them to a difficult intravenous placement or an awake intubation, especially in the small infant. A recent study has reported an increase in ICP in infants subjected to an awake tracheal intubation.[194] It was suggested that the rise in anterior fontanelle pressure seen in the awake group may be attributed to a reduction of the venous outflow from the cranium, thereby increasing cerebral blood volume and subsequently the ICP.

Anesthesia is best maintained with nitrous oxide in oxygen, isoflurane, and a suitable muscle relaxant. Intermittent positive pressure ventilation is provided by a mechanical ventilator. Hypoventilation and hypercarbia are best avoided. An intravenous narcotic may be used in children, with special attention to the small children. Deep levels of anesthesia are not needed and are contraindicated in children.

FLUID MANAGEMENT AND INTRACRANIAL PRESSURE CONTROL

FLUID MANAGEMENT

It is essential for the neuroanesthesiologist to understand the basic physiologic principles of fluid movement and electrolyte balance in neonates, infants, and children to administer the proper fluid regimen during a neurosurgical procedure.[195] Management of fluid administration in the neurosurgical patient will depend on the type of pathology or brain insult being treated. A frequent manifestation of these insults is brain edema with a resultant increase ICP.

Edema formation results from an inequality of the net movement of fluid between the intra- and extracellular compartments. It is the result of the influences of the pressure gradients between the hydrostatic, osmotic, and colloid oncotic pressures and the properties of the barrier that separate them.[196] The blood-brain barrier is composed of capillary endothelial cells that are connected in continuous fashion by tight junctions. This system forms a barrier that excludes polar hydrophilic molecules. The property of this endothelium differs in the brain in comparison with the rest of the body. In most non-CNS tissue the tight junction between the endothelial cells is 65 Å, whereas in the CNS there is a 7 Å gap. In the brain, the size of these junctions is sufficiently small in preventing protein and sodium to traverse freely. Essential molecules such as glucose and amino acids cross the blood-brain barrier by means of carrier energy-mediated transport systems. Only water can freely communicate on both side of the membrane. This passive movement of water is regulated by the oncotic, osmotic, and hydrostatic pressure changes across the barrier. The colloid oncotic pressure is a relatively weak driving force. A reduction of 50 percent of the colloid oncotic pressure (normal 20 mmHg) will result in a pressure gradient across the membrane that is less than that caused by a transcapillary osmolarity difference of 1 mosm/liter. The effect of a reduction in the colloid oncotic pressure in the brain will not have the same impact as that observed in the bowel. This is because the brain's extracellular space is poorly compliant due to its network of glial cells and discourages edema formation even in presence of a severe colloid oncotic pressure gradients. The administration of Ringer's lactate alone will lead eventually to hemodilution with reduction of plasma osmolarity (osmolarity: 273 mosm/liter), which would encourage cerebral edema.[97]

The safe approach in the choice of fluid to be administered must be dictated by the neuropathologic process involved. Ultimately, it should be oriented toward the logical principle of maintaining an isovolemic, iso-osmolar, and relatively iso-oncotic intravascular volume. For example, a patient with increased ICP or brain mass requires a fluid administration regimen that must balance adequate intravascular volume against any effort to dehydrate the brain mass, yet in a patient undergoing a ventricular shunt or repair of myelomeningocele, fluid management is directed mainly at replacement of third-space losses.

The ability to maintain an osmolar gradient is possible only in areas where the blood-brain barrier is intact. Under normal circumstances, osmotic diuretics and plasma expanders such as albumin are excluded. Unfortunately, areas that might benefit the most from dehydration therapy, such as tumor edema, exhibit blood-brain barrier incompetence. Agents of high osmolality accompanied by water may move into these tissues and increase the edema.[198]

Any efforts to dehydrate the brain are complicated by the requirement of maintaining adequate circulating blood volume. In many neurosurgical procedures, a substantial portion of the blood loss is onto the drapes and thus difficult to measure. Furthermore, the addition of large amounts of irrigation solution renders it very difficult to assess blood loss accurately. The initial phase of any neurosurgical procedure produces blood loss, especially during the scalp incision. Infiltration of the scalp with bupivacaine 0.125% with 1:200,000 epinephrine has been reported to reduce blood loss and contribute to reduce hemodynamic responses (increase heart rate and blood pressure) during incision.[199] In all cases, bupivacaine blood level remained within therapeutic range.[200] Procedures, such as resection of a vascular malformation may require massive volume replacement. The ultilization of large-bore intravenous access and the availability of blood products will be part of any appropriate initial planning. It must be noted that urine output in the face of aggressive diuresis is a misleading indicator of adequate volume replacement and that CVP monitoring may be more useful.

There is no single perfect protocol for fluid replacement in neurosurgical patients with increased ICP. Most anesthetists begin osmotic diuretic therapy at the beginning of anesthesia and measure the resulting diuresis. As surgery and blood loss progress, volume replacement usually consists of a mixture of crystalloid associated with colloid solutions to maintain the isovolemic, iso-osmolar, and iso-oncotic intravascular volume. After an initial 20 ml/kg of crystalloid solution, the authors recommend the use of a mixture of normal saline with albumin 5% in a ratio of 3:1. Maintenance of cerebral perfusion should represent the optimal goal of fluid therapy. The brain that has sustained a recent insult (primary lesion) is vulnerable to so-called secondary insult (penumbra area) by a minor episode of hypotension, hypoxia, or ischemia.

These conditions may be related to mechanical insults[201] such as excessive retraction pressures[202] or simply ischemia (hemodynamic instability).[203] Rapid administration of normal saline (10 ml/kg) has little effect on cerebral blood volume and ICP but may be enough to reinstitute hemodynamic stability.[204] The administration of blood products should be indicated only on the basis of hemodynamic instability associated with diminution of oxygen-carrying capacity.

Finally, pediatric patients (particularly neonates and infants) present the additional problem of glucose homeostasis. Dextrose-containing solutions are associated with a poorer neurologic outcome and are, where possible, best avoided unless the presence of hypoglycemia has been confirmed.[205,206] Stressed neonates have reduced glycogen stores and patients from the intensive care unit may have high glucose loads in their parenteral nutrition. Abrupt cessation of high dextrose solutions can precipitate an insulin-induced hypoglycemia. In these patients, blood glucose levels should be determined frequently and normoglycemia maintained.[195]

DIURETICS TO REDUCE INTRACRANIAL PRESSURE
Hypertonic Saline
Some investigators have suggested that successful extracellular volume dehydration can be accomplished by raising serum osmolality using hypertonic saline (3%).[207] In the literature of resuscitative fluid therapy, hypertonic saline has received considerable interest and has been shown to be effective for volume resuscitation, resulting in less cerebral edema or ICP elevation.[208] In the infancy period, the relationship between cerebrovascular fragility and hypernatremia limits the use of this solution. Furthermore, until more studies are available to prove the benefit of a solution with such an elevated osmolality with its consequences on renal function, myocardial contractility, and neuronal integrity, it would be wise to avoid hypertonic saline.

Mannitol
Mannitol (20% solution) remains the most popular diuretic used to reduce ICP and provide brain relaxation. Small doses, such as 0.25 to 0.5 g/kg are adequate to raise osmolality by 10 mosm, which has been shown to be capable of reducing cerebral edema and ICP.[209,210]

Its action begins within 10 to 15 min and will remain effective for at least 2 h. Mannitol-induced vasodilatation affects intracranial and extracranial vessels and can transiently increase cerebral blood volume and ICP while simultaneously reducing systemic blood pressure.[211] In particular, children may show transient hemodynamic instability (first 1 to 2 min) caused by the rapid administration of mannitol[212] so it is preferred that it be given at a rate no greater than 0.5 g/kg over 20 to 30 min. Subsequently, this period of hypotension will be followed by an increase in cardiac index, blood volume, and pulmonary capillary wedge pressure, which all reach peak values 15 min after infusion.[213] Thus, mannitol should be administered with caution to children with congestive heart failure (CHF). This change in intravascular volume lasts for about 30 min after which the central hemodyamic changes return to normal levels. The administration of furosemide immediately before mannitol would seem to be an appropriate choice to increase venous capacitance and reduce the transient increase in intravascular volume, at the same time providing more effective dehydration. There is, however, a danger in producing too profound dehydration with severe electrolyte imbalance.[214] Larger doses produce a longer duration of action but there is no evidence that it is capable of further reducing the ICP.[209] In the presence of cerebral ischemia, larger doses of mannitol up to 2.0 g/kg may be used.[215] Mannitol increases CBF[216,217] and cardiac output[218] probably through its reduction in blood viscosity (rheology)[219] or because of its increase in intravascular volume. It has also been suggested that mannitol may cause autoregulatory vasoconstriction.

Loop Diuretics
Loop diuretics such as furosemide and ethacrynic acid may be useful in reducing brain edema by inducing a systemic diuresis, decreasing CSF production,[220] and resolving cerebral edema by improving cellular water transport.[221,222] Furosemide can reduce ICP without a transient increase in cerebral blood volume or blood osmolality. It is, however, not as effective as mannitol.[221] The initial pediatric dose of furosemide should be 0.6 to 1.0 mg/kg if administered alone[221] or 0.3 to 0.4 mg/kg if administered with mannitol.[220] It has been suggested that secondary brain injury may be reduced by the administration of ethacrynic acid through a decrease in glial swelling.[223] Raising serum osmolality above 320 mosm may precipitate acute renal failure and a falling serum osmolality. Rebound intracranial hypertension may result after a period of aggressive dehydration.

Corticosteroids
Corticosteroids are an important part of the therapeutic regimen in neurosurgical patients with raised ICP.

They reduce edema around brain tumors but may require hours or days to produce an effect.[224] However, the administration of dexamethasone preoperatively or even at induction of anesthesia frequently causes neurologic improvement that can precede the ICP reduction. It has been suggested that this is in response to a partial restoration of normal blood-brain barrier.[225]

TEMPERATURE HOMEOSTASIS

Although hypothermia reduces the $CMRO_2$, it frequently contributes to further complications. Delayed drug clearance, slow reversal of muscle relaxants, decreased cardiac output, conduction abnormalities, attenuated hypoxic pulmonary vasoconstriction, altered platelet function, electrolyte abnormalities, and postoperative shivering may occur.[186] Intraoperative vasoconstriction produced by hypothermia reverts to vasodilatation and redistribution of body heat on rewarming with a subsequent fall in core temperature.[226]

Neonates and infants are at greatest risk of hypothermia due to their large surface area relative to body mass. Despite a warm operating room environment, body temperature falls immediately after induction of anesthesia due to internal redistribution of body heat from the central compartment to the periphery.[186] As body heat loss continues, pediatric patients trigger a series of thermoregulatory responses in an attempt to limit further the cooling.[226] These responses include vasoconstriction and nonshivering thermogenesis in an attempt to rewarm. In the paralyzed and ventilated patient, an increase in body temperature and a rise in end-tidal carbon dioxide concentration at constant minute ventilation may occur.[227,228] This phenomenon may not be readily apparent because it is usually overwhelmed by the effect of cold fluid administration. Temperature monitoring is essential but the actual site for the probe is less important than its reliability.[229] For this reason, we usually select esophageal or rectal placement. During induction of anesthesia and placement of intravenous lines and monitors, a large body surface area is exposed. Although the heat gain to the patients is minimal, premature infants and small infants should be placed under radiant heat lamp and extremities may be covered in plastic wrap. Dry inspired gases should be warmed and humidified with a heat exchanger.[230,231] However, one must remember that the use of warmed fresh gases will falsely increase the esophageal temperature by 0.35°C.[232] Although the usefulness of warming blankets has been questioned, they cover a substantial body surface area and appear to work well as long as they are positioned both above and below the patient. Blood warmers should always be used if substantial fluid replacement is required.

Rewarming measures such as a convective-force warmed air system can be used in the postoperative period if severe hypothermia has occurred.

VENOUS AIR EMBOLISM

Venous air embolism is one of the most serious complications of anesthesia and surgery. It may occur whenever the operative site is elevated above the heart and the risk increases as the height difference increases. Classically, it is associated with posterior fossa surgery in the sitting position but it is not confined to this procedure. It has been reported in infants and children during several procedures involving the skull such as morcellation of the cranial vault or craniectomy for craniosysnostosis and during spinal cord procedure.[233,234] It is reported to have occurred with the patient in the lateral position.[235] The incidence of venous air embolism has been reduced considerably by the use of the prone position for posterior fossa surgery[236] and the abandonment of spontaneous ventilation in major neuroanesthesia.

Air entrainment occurs when a number of conditions are met, including: (1) venous pressure at the operative site that is below atmospheric pressure, (2) a vein that is open to the atmosphere, and (3) a vein that is prevented from collapsing. It most commonly occurs during the first hour of surgery. The most frequent sites of air entrainment are the cranial diploic veins, emissary veins, and intracranial venous sinuses, which are kept open by their dural attachment. It is important to note that venous air embolism can also occur from veins in muscles as well as from the puncture site of the multipoint head holder often used in children over 3 years of age.[237,238] Detection of venous air embolism depends entirely on the sensitivity of the monitors used. Reports suggest a widely variable incidence.[239,240] The introduction of the highly sensitive precordial Doppler has increased the reported incidence, which may be as high as 58 percent in adult patients undergoing posterior fossa surgery in a sitting position.[241] Less than half the cases of detected emboli produce systemic hypotension.[242] In pediatric neurosurgery the incidence of detectable air emboli is about 33 percent,[243] but systemic complications occur in more than half the cases. Although children are not more prone to air emboli than adults, they are more susceptible to it. For example, the incidence of air embolism during craniosysnostoisis repair in supine infants may be as high as 67 percent.[233] It may explain why, without any obvious reason, a patient's blood pressure remains low for a period of time. In addition, the increase in right-sided pressure[244] may cause air to pass from the right side of the heart into the left via a septal defect[245] causing paradoxical air embolus. Anatomically, some 27 percent of patients have a patent foramen ovale and are therefore potentially at risk. It is reported that air may reach the systemic circulation without the presence of an intracardiac septal defect.[246] The consequences of which are cerebral or myocardial infarction.

It is essential to take all measures to avoid this potentially disastrous complication. Meticulous avoidance of a gradient and the routine use of positive-pressure ventilation are mandatory. On detection of air entrainment, the anesthesiologist must: (1) advise the neurosurgeon to stop surgery, flood the surgical field, and compress the jugular veins to prevent further ingree of air; (2) ventilate with 100% oxygen; (3) attempt to withdraw air through the central venous catheter; (4) treat any hemodynamic consequences; and (5) if hemodynamic instability persists, turn the patient to a left-side down position. When venous air is detected during craniotomy in children, the success related to aspiration of this air is between 38 and 60 percent.[243] Intravenous fluids,[247] appropriate antiarrhythmic agents, and inotropic agents or vasopressors may be necessary and should be administered as needed. Nitrous oxide must be discontinued because its diffusional properties increase size of the embolus several fold causing further physiologic compromise.[248] Some authors have proposed that a positive end-expiratory pressure (PEEP) of 10 cmH$_2$O might decrease the rate of entry by increasing venous pressure, but other investigators have demonstrated that 10 cmH$_2$O is not enough to elevate the venous pressure such that it would prevent air entry.[249] The use of PEEP may cause paradoxical air embolism. However, in an animal model it has been demonstrated that the use of 8 cmH$_2$O did not increase the right atrial pressure to a level greater than the left atrial pressure.[250]

Special Considerations

NEURORADIOLOGY

Children and infants, unlike their adult counterparts, frequently require general anesthesia or constant sedation with appropriate monitoring for neuroradiologic diagnostic or interventional therapeutic procedures. Anesthetic management has become *sine qua non* in complex diagnostic procedures in infants and children. In the present and in the future, the diagnosis of disease involving the CNS in the pediatric age group will depend almost entirely on the radiologic evaluation. These procedures have become longer and more complex and would not be possible without adequate anesthetic management and patient control.

Imaging diagnostic techniques involving the CNS include MRI, myelography, CT scanning, and cerebral angiography. Historically, cerebral angiography and air encephalography were the only neuroradiological procedures available. In air encephalography, air or carbon dioxide was injected into the subarachnoid space and the brain and spinal cord thereby defined, the gas acting as a contrast agent to delineate the adjacent soft tissues. Because of the many side effects, this test fortunately belongs to memory. Contrast agents for intrathecal or intravenous injection have improved significantly the neuroimaging quality and are far more physiologically compatible than their former predecessors. Diagnostic tests, however, frequently require injection of contrast agent by the intravenous, intraarterial, or intrathecal route and remain at least to some degree "invasive." This is particularly true of cerebral angiography and its recent development, interventional neuroangiography. The neuroanesthetist must therefore be aware of, and familiar with, the purpose of the procedure and the means by which it will be performed, including injection of contrast and other pharmacologic agents, postural change requirements, and any functional testing the procedure may involve.

All children undergoing the neurodiagnostic procedures mentioned do not necessarily have to be anesthetized. The length of the procedure and the degree of pain and anxiety provoked by it in part give rise to the need for neuroanesthetic support and control.

Although cerebral angiography requires general anesthetic management, many CT scans, myelographic and MRI investigations may not require anesthesia. A typical patient requiring an anesthetic is the infant or young child who cannot cooperate or with whom other methods of management, including sedation, have failed.

In addition to the complete discussion of risks and benefits of the procedure with the parent or guardian, the need to establish a friendly rapport with the child cannot be overstated. This is the first line of management and control for any diagnostic procedure and is an essential skill for the health care worker dealing with children. With supportive reassurance most children will be cooperative even through long and painful procedures. When support and encouragement fail to overcome anxiety or inability to cooperate, sedation by the radiologist may be necessary and, in fact, deemed elective with infants and younger children. Diagnostic tests and interventional procedures in recent years have become more complicated and longer lasting, and may involve pain and discomfort. With MRI, the patient must remain absolutely motionless for periods of up to an hour. Patient management during such procedures has become correspondingly challenging and increasingly the anesthetist plays a role. Patient management for diagnostic tests has been guided by the American Academy of Pediatrics[251] and the American Society of Anesthesiologists. With patient safety the leading issue, routines and protocols have been established regarding sedation decisions, drug usage, and patient monitoring during and after the procedure. Drug choice for patient management in the radiology department depends on whether the sedation is required for a diagnostic, painless procedure or an interventional procedure likely to be associated with nociceptive stimulation.

DIAGNOSTIC PROCEDURES

For painless procedures, chloral hydrate or pentobarbital have become the most commonly used, depending on the age of the child. With infants under 1 to 2 months of age, particularly the newborn, it is preferred not to give a sedative agent at all, but instead to feed the child, thereby inducing postprandial slumber.

Chloral hydrate is the drug of choice for infant to age 6 months. A dose of 50 to 80 mg/kg orally is used, to a maximum of 2 g for older children. If sedation has not occurred at 45 min to 1 h after the initial dose, a further dose of 20 to 40 mg/kg may be given.

For children between 5 and 25 kg pentobarbital is the drug of choice. Although the usual route for pentobarbital administration had been intramuscular, the intravenous route is currently preferred. The onset of sedation with intravenous pentobarbital is normally immediate, making this route the preferred one, especially in a busy pediatric department. The intramuscular dose is 6 mg/kg for a child under 15 kg and 5 mg/kg for a child over 15 kg. The maximum intramuscular dose is 200 mg. If sedation has not occurred in 1 h after the initial intramuscular dose, for the child under 15 kg, 2 mg/kg is given, and for the child over 15 kg, 2.5 mg/kg is repeated to complete the sedation. If this fails, no further medication is given, and the sedation is considered a failure. When pentobarbital is used intravenously, an initial dose of 5 mg/kg is drawn up to a maximum dose of 150 mg, and diluted in 10 ml saline. The first half of the 10 ml is given over 30 s, with a 1-min wait to see the sedative effect of this initial dose. A further 2.5 ml may then be given over 30 s followed after a 1-min interval with the remaining 2.5 ml administered over 30 s. This is a dependable technique. One or 2 mg/kg may be given in addition if the initial 5 mg/kg does not provide sedation. Sedation is most likely to be successful if the child is relatively sleep deprived. Occasionally, this dose may fail to sedate the patient and in rare instances, the child may become paradoxically excited from which state sedation may then occur rapidly, or the state of excitement may remain until recovery from the sedation occurs. The excitement is likely due to a sensation of agitated depression, the child resisting the overwhelming and probably disorienting feeling of rapidly falling into sleep. The sedation may then be completed with midazolam, but most radiologists are unhappy about going beyond recommended doses and mixing sedative drugs. The advice and help of the anesthetist is invaluable in such a situation where drug doses and combinations are managed with greater confidence.

The anesthetist is also essential in the management of difficult children weighing over 25 kg. Most children in this age group are cooperative and not fearful, but it is likely to be impossible to manage fear and motion in the mentally challenged older child whose intellectual age may be significantly below the chronological age. Sedation failure is more likely to occur with the intramuscular route because the onset of sedation may require up to 45 min. If there is agitation, the period of agitation will last longer. If intravenous contrast material is to be given during the examination, then an intravenous route should be established at the beginning rather than after a child is sedated via the intramuscular route because the child may be disturbed by the contrast injection, causing the sedation to fail. The sedation in these older children is managed by an anesthetist with the current drug of choice being propofol. It is administered by infusion following an induction dose and it is titrated according to the level of sedation required to allow the procedure. A dose as low as 50 μg/kg per min can be used for the CT scan or MRI examination, whereas up to 200 μg/kg per min might be needed for interventional neuroradiology requiring endotracheal intubation. Sedation with propofol reverses almost immediately after the infusion is ended.

INTERVENTIONAL PROCEDURES

Interventional procedures require some medication for pain in addition to that needed for sedation. Further, local anesthesia is likely to be required for skin entry for biopsy, tube placement, and so on. For infants under 6 months, oral chloral hydrate is the routine. For patients 5 to 25 kg intravenous pentobarbital at 3 mg/kg followed 5 min later by intravenous meperidine, 1 mg/kg provides sedation and pain management. A supplemental dose of pentobarbital, 3 mg/kg, and meperidine, 1 mg/kg, may later be needed. For children over 25 kg, intravenous diazepam at a dose of 0.1 mg/kg may be used, followed 5 min later by intravenous meperidine, 1 mg/kg. Midazolam may be used alone at a dose of 0.05 mg/kg intravenously, which may be repeated once. Midazolam may be used orally instead at a dose of 0.3 to 0.5 mg/kg in the child over 20 kg and a dose of 0.5 to 0.75 mg/kg in the child under 20 kg. A pentobarbital and midazolam combination may also be used intravenously for interventional procedures. Flumazenil should be available for reversal of excessive sedation caused by a benzodiazapine. At our institution, these drugs are ordered by the radiologist for diagnostic or interventional procedures and given by a trained and experienced nurse at the beginning of the procedure. The radiologist should be in the adjacent area when chloral hydrate and intramuscular or intravenous pentobarbital is given by the nurse, but should be in the room if there are any concerns, if the dose needed for sedation reaches a high level, or for drug combinations, and should be ready to begin the procedure immediately after sedation occurs.

Parents and older children should be fully informed of the nature of the test or procedure and informed consent given. For outpatients, information sheets are mailed to parents, and when they confirm their appointment, the test is further described. Feeding instructions are essential. NPO guidelines are included in the preoperative preparations. Solid food or milk are not allowed within 6 h of the procedures, whereas clear fluid can be given up to 2 h preceding the procedure. If the NPO guidelines are not adhered to, an elective procedure is deferred until later in the day if possible, or rescheduled. CT scanning of the abdomen and gastrointestinal tract, however, require oral contrast to demonstrate the bowel. This contravenes the NPO guideline but is taken as an accepted risk for the procedure.

PATIENT MANAGEMENT

The need for sedation is assessed for each child. Diagnostic imaging studies, in particular CT, MRI, nuclear medicine studies, and interventional procedures, require significantly longer periods of sedation than before. Children under age 6 years, unable to hold still for the time required, will almost certainly require sedation. Those 6 years or older would likely be able to hold still and not require sedation. Older children who are developmentally impaired will likely need sedation. Any movement during the acquisition of the image data would be unacceptable because it would destroy the image being obtained and require repeating the process with the consequence of further prolonging the scan and exposure to unnecessary stress. The use of oral and rectal preparations including chloral hydrate in older children is not appropriate because the onset of action is unpredictable and the sedation is not deep enough to prevent motion. This sedative agent should be replaced by intramuscular or preferably intravenous agents for adequate complex imaging studies to be performed.

As the nurse assesses the child for the appropriateness of sedation, the physical status classification of the American Society of Anesthesiologists provides a fundamental guide:

Class I—Normal healthy patient

Class II—Patient with mild systemic disease

Class III—Patient with severe systemic disease that limits activity but is not incapacitating

Class IV—Patient with incapacitating disease that is a constant threat to life

Class V—Moribund patient not expected to survive 24 h with or without surgery

Patients in classes I and II would electively undergo radiologically managed sedation as well as most patients in class III. In this class, the decision between radiologic and anesthetic management should be tailored for each individual patient. Patients in classes IV and V are managed by the anesthesia or intensive care staff.

The assessment should include the fasting status of the child, current medications being used, allergies, and past and present medical diagnoses. Certain contraindications may have to be considered. Relative contraindications include the neonatal period, children with small mouths or restricted mouth opening, porphyria, severe asthma, raised ICP, brainstem lesions including tumors and Leigh's disease, airway limitation by musculoskeletal abnormalities restricting or compromising chest movement, neck extension restriction such as Klippel-Feil syndrome, CNS depression, upper respiratory tract infection, a history of apnea, impaired liver and renal function, and drug sensitivity. Absolute contraindications include severe respiratory depression, laryngotracheomalacia, and airway lesions such as obstructing masses in the upper or lower airway.

Consent should cover a description or "disclosure" of the procedure, including "tangible" or reasonable risks, the benefits, and the alternatives. Legally the general consent signed on admission to hospital is not sufficient. The American Academy of Pediatrics[251] indicates that a "documented informed consent" is needed. Consent for sedation may be obtained either as part of the consent for the study or as a separate consent. Written documentation of the verbal discussion with the parents must be part of the progress note or in the sedation record. Anesthetist input into the sedation discussion and consent has been proposed[252] as he or she will in the future play an expanding role in patient management for procedures in the department of radiology.

A comprehensive sedation record should be made to be entered into the patient's chart along with the written consent. The sedation record should include:

1. Preprocedural assessment including chart review, physical systems review, and assessment of the need for sedation

2. Consent(s) for sedation and procedure

3. The drug or drugs used, route, dose, effect, and adverse effect if any
4. Vital signs during and after the procedure
5. Assessment and record of the discharge criteria

Patient monitoring for the procedure is performed by the nurse. During the procedure, vital signs are monitored every 5 min and every 15 min following the procedure. The monitoring includes ongoing oxygen saturation, which should remain above 95% on room air. Heart rate, respiratory rate, and blood pressure are monitored. However, it is important to limit disturbances to the sedated child. The vital signs are recorded on the sedation record. The pulse oximeter is set to alarm at 90% oxygen saturation. Saturation may fall below this level, usually during induction, which will be monitored until spontaneous resolution or by the administration of oxygen by face mask. The cause is most likely due to tongue relaxation and obstruction of the airway at this level, relieved by neck extension and jaw thrust. If the oxygen saturation does not maintain above 95%, oxygen may be given by mask during the study. The adverse effects of pentobarbital should always be kept in mind. These include cardiorespiratory depression, circulatory collapse, bronchospasm in asthmatics, allergic reaction, severe CNS depression, nausea, vomiting, coughing, and laryngospasm. Because of its low pH, intravenous pentobarbital is painful unless diluted in 5 to 10 ml saline. Occasionally, paradoxical excitement may occur, which appears to respond better to the addition of a benzodiazepine such as midazolam for successful sedation.

There should be an adequately staffed and equipped recovery area for the continued monitoring of patients recovering from sedation. The decision for discharge is made approximately 2 h after the beginning of sedation. The child should be awake or rousable, should be able to sit unaided, and should be able to drink, indicating return of protective reflexes. Vital signs must have returned to their presedation baseline. To prevent further or ongoing sedation and possible respiratory arrest after discharge, the child is allowed to leave only after these criteria are met.

Sedation is a major consideration in every busy pediatric radiology unit for efficient and safe patient management. Radiologists and radiology department nurses should be familiar with the particular needs for sedation in the pediatric group. Their sedation familiarity and training should include intravenous access, patient need and assessment for sedation, procedure explanation and consent discussion, narcotic and other sedative drug administration, and sedation and monitoring recording. They should be trained in cardiopulmonary life support techniques for children and should be thoroughly familiar with the sedative agents in routine use in their department. They should also be prepared to manage allergic response to medication or contrast agents and should be familiar with the use of airway and life support equipment, which should be maintained in the induction and imaging room. Oxygen delivery systems should include cannuli and clear masks. Ambu bags of various sizes for positive-pressure ventilation, suction apparatus with rigid Yankauer suction tips, and oral airways of different sizes should be immediately available, as well as intubation equipment. This includes endotracheal tubes, 3 to 6 mm uncuffed and 5.5 to 9 mm cuffed, laryngoscope and blades, number 1, 2, and 3 straight and number 3 curved. Emergency drugs include naloxone for narcotic reversal, diphenhydramine for minor allergic response, and epinephrine and hydrocortisone for moderate and severe allergic response. For cardiorespiratory arrest, atropine, succinylcholine, calcium chloride, sodium bicarbonate, and lidocane must be kept on the emergency resuscitation tray. Intravenous solutions including 0.9% sodium chloride, lactated Ringer's, 5% dextrose, and 18- to 24-gauge intravenous catheters are part of the basic equipment.

The radiologist and nurse should be familiar with the techniques and problems of airway management and able to identify signs of early and late airway complications. They should be familiar with the use of an Ambu bag for IPPV and in an emergency should be able to formally secure the airway by means of intubation. In such an emergency, anesthesia should immediately take over management of the airway and at all times an anesthetist should be available for routine consultation, urgent help, or for management if such an emergency occurs. An active pediatric radiology department therefore requires the essential interaction with the anesthesia department and should not carry out these procedures without such help. The anesthetist is essential in the decision making for assessment and planning for sedation; management of sedation, particularly with drug combinations for prolonged painful interventional procedures; and for any patient management-related emergency in the radiology department.

MAGNETIC RESONANCE IMAGING

In recent years MRI has acquired widespread use and has become the dominant imaging modality in diagnostic investigation. It is used in parallel with or frequently instead of CT scanning, with universal application both in children as well as adults in the investigation of the brain and spinal cord, surrounding CSF spaces, and adjacent musculoskeletal structures.

Magnetic resonance imaging uses radiofrequencies in the non-ionizing lower end of the electromagnetic spectrum. Hydrogen ions or protons, abundant in the body, act as micromagnets aligned within a static magnetic field which are anatomically localized by a gradient coil while they coherently interact with a radiofrequency coil. The slice and matrix technology of MRI displays two-dimensional images of a three-dimensional object on the display screen. The static magnet is largely responsible for the immense weight of an MRI unit and many units are for this reason separated from the remainder of the radiology department. There are no known injurious aspects of the intense magnetic field, but because of the strength of the magnetic field, no ferromagnetic objects or equipment can be stored or used within the same room as the magnet. Just as for CT scanning, younger patients and many older patients will require sedation for the MR scan. The scan time for MRI is routinely 30 to 45 min, during which time the child must lie still. Added to this challenge is the length of the MRI tunnel or gantry where the patient must lie, physically isolated from parent or guardian. In addition to these practical difficulties, no ferromagnetic monitoring equipment may be kept in the room with the magnet. Sedations are managed by the radiologist and nurse with the same indications and protocols as for CT scanning. For the many patients who require anesthetic management for their MR scan, intravenous propofol is used routinely. It is infused slowly using an injection pump. The anesthetist remains with the injection pump in the control room, with propofol being injected through a volumetric pump system attached to the patient with four lengths of 60-inch extension tubing joined end to end (Fig. 35-7). Propofol doses of 50 to 100 μg/kg per min will provide light anesthesia without the need for tracheal intubation, ensuring also a rapid awakening allowing postanesthetic recovery to be undertaken in the radiology recovery room. The patient can then be transferred back to the ward or simply return home as an outpatient admission.

Metallic objects implanted within or attached to patients should be nonferromagnetic because they cause two types of problems. The first is the production of artifact and image distortion caused by prostheses such as braces, metallic clips, or spinal rods or screws. The second is caused when such objects are ferromagnetic; they will tend to induce motion or torque in the magnetic field. This involves in particular aneurysm clips.[253] Most implants are held with sufficient force, however, to prevent movement or dislodgment.[254] Some cochlear implants are ferromagnetic and the type should be determined before the patient undergoes MR scanning. If there is concern about an embedded metallic foreign body, plain film x-rays should be obtained before the MRI procedure.[255] With halo vests induced current may occur in the ring portion made from electrically conductive material according to Faraday's law.[256] The pa-

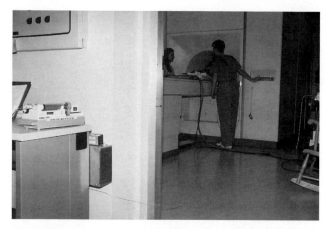

Figure 35-7   MRI with anesthetic management. The injection pump containing propofol is located in the control room on the left, its extension tubing running along the floor to the intravenous line in the patient's left arm. The patient is in position on the MR table with usual monitor applied. The anesthesiologist and the technologist complete positioning for the scan. Oxygen is administered by face mask, laryngeal mask airway, or nasal prongs according to individual need. The patient's vital signs including heart rate, respiratory rate, blood pressure, and oxygen saturation are displayed on a monitor that is viewed by the attending anesthesiologist through the window of the control room.

tient's tissue may be involved in forming such a current loop, with possible burn or electrical injury. Any implanted devices that are electrically, magnetically, or mechanically activated should be fully assessed before the patient undergoes MR scanning.

The images are unsurpasssed in their soft-tissue definition and MRI has acquired universal use in the imaging of the CNS and the craniospinal axis. Particularly in children, MRI has become an indispensible diagnostic tool for congenital and traumatic lesions, lesions associated with infection, neoplasm, and other diseases. In addition, MRI may demonstrate CSF pulse motion and MR spectroscopy may be used to determine substrate concentrations within lesions such as infarcts and tumors.

MYELOGRAPHY

As a diagnostic tool, the myelogram provides information about the vertebral column and the associated structures of the nervous system. The function of the vertebral column is to provide for locomotion and to protect the spinal cord. Anatomic causes of these functional disturbances may be amply demonstrated with myelography. The vertebrae of the spine may be examined and in particular the contents of the spinal canal. These include the spinal cord, the surrounding subarachnoid space, the meninges, and the epidural fat within the spinal canal. The spinal canal is therefore conveniently divided into three compartments—the

TABLE 35-2
Iodine Concentration and Osmolality

Name	Iohexol Conc. mg/ml	Iodine Conc. mg/ml	Osmolality mOsm/kg H_2O
Omnipaque 140	302	140	322
Omnipaque 180	388.3	180	408
Omnipaque 240	517.7	240	520
Omnipaque 300	647.1	300	672
Omnipaque 350	755.0	350	844

epidural, the intradural extramedullary space, and the intramedullary space within the cord itself. Both congenital anomalies or acquired diseases in the structures in or around the spinal canal may give rise to a compression syndrome, and although most myelograms are done electively, acute spinal cord compression needs to be investigated on an urgent basis. Myelography has been largely replaced by MR scanning of the spine, but it remains the examination of choice in some instances, particularly in the demonstration of injuries to the brachial plexus nerve roots. It is considered an invasive test because a contrast agent is introduced into the subarachnoid space to render it radiographically opaque for imaging. Contrast media for myelography have evolved from the earliest oil-soluble (CSF-insoluble lipiodol), through water-soluble ionic contrast agents to the water-soluble non-ionic contrast omnipaque. This latter group is the most physiologically compatible and the pharmacologic molecule does not disassociate into free ions as the ionic contrasts do. It is available in various iodine concentrations from 140 to 350 mg I/ml (Table 35-2). The higher concentrations are hyperosmolar, which will cause an osmotic gradient. Although it may be a concern in certain situations such as cerebral angiography, the concentration used for myelography remains low at 180 mg I/ml. The volume of dye injected is determined by the age of the patient (Table 35-3).

Anesthesia is required for myelography in infants

TABLE 35-3
Volume of Dye Determined by Patient's Age

COMPLETE MYELOGRAPHY DOSAGE TABLE		
	Iohexol	
Age	Conc. mg/ml	ml
<2 mo	180	1–3
2 mo–2 y	180	2–4
3–7 y	180	4–8
8–12 y	180	7–12
13–17 y	180	8–14

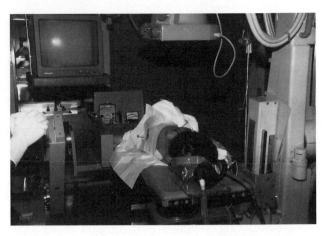

Figure 35-8 Myelography with anesthesia. The anesthetized child lies in a decubitus position facing the anesthesiologist, allowing the neuroradiologist access to perform the myelographic puncture. After the intrathecal contrast is injected, a single film is taken to document the needle position, then the needle is removed, and the child is turned into a supine position for further filming. Verbal communication between the anesthesiologist and the neuroradiologist is essential at all times to manage properly the movement of the head and neck.

and younger children up to the age of 6 years and occasionally in older children. With children above this age, myelography is routinely done without anesthesia and rapport and cooperation are required to reassure the child throughout the procedure. Sedation is not routinely used. Occasionally the older child who is uncooperative because of pervading anxiety or developmental delay will need anesthesia assistance for myelography.

The myelogram routinely consists of two parts, the introduction of contrast and initial plain film imaging, followed by cross-sectional CT scanning with the contrast spread through the subarachnoid space. The first part is done under fluoroscopic control and the second in the CT scan room. This sequence necessitates movement of the patient from one table to another under anesthesia. It requires close attention to management and control of the patient. Because the patient is intubated, myelography is routinely begun in a decubitus instead of prone position as is the routine for adult conscious myelography (Fig. 35-8). The decubitus position with the patient facing the anesthetist provides easy access to the airway tube, which is normally orotracheal. This position allows the radiologist on the other side of the myelographic table access to the patient's back. The spine should be flexed as much as possible so that the spinous processes may be easily palpated and the intraspinous space is opened maximally. The position should be as close as possible to a true decubitus because rotation of the pelvis forward or backward will alter the required trajectory of the needle entry. The patient's head should be supported on a ring or sponges to exclude downward lateral flexion. This prevents the myelographic contrast from running freely into the intracranial space if the myelographic table is angled head down. Instead, supporting the head so that there is slight upward lateral flexion allows the collection of the contrast easily in the cervical spine without loss into the intracranial space. Intracranial spillage reduces the spinal concentration of contrast. With iohexol, adverse systemic reactions have been extremely rare, but are more likely with careless intracranial spillage. Headache, nausea, and vomiting may occur, but these may be due to CSF pressure change instead, and usually occur 1 to 10 h after the procedure, subsiding within 24 h. Convulsions have been reported in less than 0.1 percent, caused by careless spillage and diffusion into the intracranial subarachnoid fluid. Finally, evidence of rare complications such as transient cranial palsies and behavior changes have been reported.

The procedure should be performed with the myelographic table in a slightly head-up position. In addition to the prevention of intracranial flow of the contrast agent, the slight head-up position facilitates confirmation of needle introduction into the subarachnoid space. In this position the hydrostatic pressure at the caudal end of the arachnoid space is increased, and CSF return is more brisk and more determinate of subarachnoid space entry. The slight head-up table position is also justified by the need to control contrast diffusion through the subarachnoid space. The ability to collect and hold the subarachnoid contrast in the region of entry is a skill that may require table angle and patient position change and is essential for diagnostic quality imaging.

In preparation for the procedure, the skin of the back is scrubbed and draped. Local anesthetic is not normally used with anesthetized patients, but the anesthetist may often request it according to the level of anesthesia and for postoperative purposes. Notably, pain sensory endings are concentrated in the dermis of the skin and the periosteum of the vertebral arches. The dura contains a lesser concentration of sensory endings. If the needle comes against a nerve root after subarachnoid entry a sensory pain stimulus is referred down the leg in that distribution. With this sensory map, only the immediate subcutaneous tissue and secondarily the periosteum need be anesthetized, but this latter should normally be avoided with careful myelography. It is debatable whether the needle for local anesthetic is less painful than the needle for myelography for which anesthesia is being acquired. Depending on the child's age the needle length may be $1\frac{1}{2}$, $2\frac{1}{2}$, or $3\frac{1}{2}$ in., and though previously 20-gauge needles were used, currently 22- or 25-gauge needles are preferred. Both needles have an angled bevel and therefore can be

maneuvered easily. Their introduction from the skin to the subarachnoid space is performed under fluoroscopic guidance. When the latter indicates correct positioning, the needle stylet is removed and clear CSF return indicates entry into the subarachnoid space. The puncture will be nontraumatic if done slowly and a bloody return that clears indicates passage through an epidural vein, either dorsal or ventral to the dural sac. If the CSF return becomes completely clear, then the contrast may be introduced, but the needle may need to be repositioned if this does not occur. Myelography should be deferred in patients with hemophilia or other bleeding diathesis. Sterile technique as a precaution against spinal meningitis cannot be overstated. The contrast solution is administered under fluoroscopic guidance. Occasionally improper or incomplete entry into the subarachnoid space may occur, indicated by a slower than expected CSF return. The bevel of the needle is then located half in the subarachnoid space and half in the subdural space. CSF will return, but the contrast when injected may preferentially flow into the subdural space, ruining the myelogram as a diagnostic test. The myelogram may also be spoiled if the needle is withdrawn from the subarachnoid space and reintroduced. The meningeal puncture will allow contrast leak, either into the subdural space or into the epidural space, with decompression of the subarachnoid space. A film is normally taken in lateral projection with the needle in position to document the level of entry and the free flow of contrast from the needle.

The contrast may be held for filming in the lumbar curve or introduced into the thoracic or cervical curves of the spine to suit the region of interest for filming. The patient may therefore have to be moved from the decubitus position into a supine or even prone position and the table angle may need to be changed to manage the contrast movement. The anesthetist must be aware of the any intended patient position changes in which case, he or she will assume the leadership of this period of manipulation. For cervical spine myelography the table may need to be tipped head down, but the problem of intracranial spillage may be prevented by head flexion and support to collect the omnipaque in the cervical subarachnoid space. Such maneuvering of the head and neck is also the domain of the anesthetist. Although the craniocaudal position of the orotracheal tube tip may not change significantly even with strong head flexion, the elasticity of the tube may cause it to press against the posterior tracheal wall, disturbing the patient, depending on the depth of anesthesia. With head-down positioning, another concern in anesthetic management may arise. The diaphragm may be displaced upward by the heavy abdominal viscera, lung aeration sometimes causing gas exchange disturbances. Venous return from the legs and trunk will

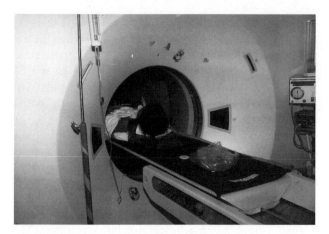

Figure 35-9 Myelography with anesthesia. After contrast introduction into the spinal canal and initial filming the child is transferred to the CT table. CT imaging completes the myelogram. The child is positioned in the CT gantry for imaging and vital signs are displayed from monitors easily seen by the anesthesiologist.

initially increase, with positive ionotropic and chronotropic effects. The trachea may move upward leading to a rise of the carnia with the consequence that the orotracheal tube may become occluded against it, or enter one of the main bronchi, preferentially the right lower bronchus. The anesthetist must be informed of the maneuver intended and be responsible for the movement of the head and neck as the body is moved.

Imaging with CT is the routine for myelography and initial plain films may therefore be kept at a minimum. The child must be transferred from the fluoroscopic room to the CT scan room. This requires a maneuver from the fluoroscopic table to the transporting stretcher and to the CT scan table. A portable oxygen supply and pulse oximeter are needed for transfer; while in the CT room the anesthetic cart these is used.

The time needed in the fluoroscopy room is approximately 30 min in addition to anesthetic induction period and in the CT scan room another 30 min is routinely needed for imaging. The anesthetic recovery is achieved in the postanesthetic recovery room.

For CT imaging, the child is placed supine, body toward the gantry because it is the spinal region that is to be imaged. The anesthetist has free access to the child's head and face (Fig. 35-9). The anesthetic gas delivery system and connections to the orotracheal tube are supported with towels or sponges and fixed in position. The child and the anesthetic equipment are displaced as a single unit into or out of the gantry. The whole spine may be the region of interest or the latter may consist of a small part of the spine only. The arms lying on the side of the body may decrease the image quality. When the thoracic or lumbar spine is imaged, the child's arms are fixed in position beside

the head, whereas for imaging the cervical spine, the arms and shoulders are pulled gently downward. The thickness of the CT scan slice may vary from 1.5 to 10 mm, and the slices may be done contiguously or with space in between each slice.

Currently, myelography is used predominantly in the investigation of birth, motor vehicle accident brachial plexus injuries, and in patients in whom metal spinal devices and implants render MRI useless (Fig. 35-10). The radiologist monitors the scans as they are done so that the anesthetist may know how soon the procedure will be ended. The child then recovers and is taken to the postanesthesia room where he or she remains for 2 h in a 30° or greater head-up position as a continued precaution against intracranial diffusion of contrast.

COMPUTED TOMOGRAPHY SCANNING

Performing CT scans in infants and children does not usually require anesthesia assistance. After explanation of the procedure by the nurse or technologist, most children will allow the scan to be performed without difficulty. Most older children do not need to be sedated or anesthetized for their CT scan. Their cooperation, however, must include the ability to lie absolutely still while the scanning is being done. The time needed for scanning currently is 1 s for every scan slice although with older machines it has been significantly longer.

Younger children and infants are unable to cooperate

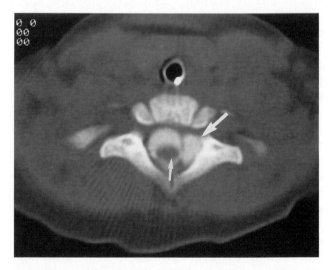

Figure 35-10 The CT myelogram. The cross-sectional image through the cervical spine demonstrates myelographic contrast surrounding the spinal cord (*small arrow*) in a patient with a traumatic brachial plexus palsy that occurred at birth. The brachial plexus nerve root avulsion has torn the dural sac or nerve root sheath, allowing CSF to leak into the epidural space creating a pseudomeningocele. This has been filled and demonstrated by the myelographic contrast (*large arrow*).

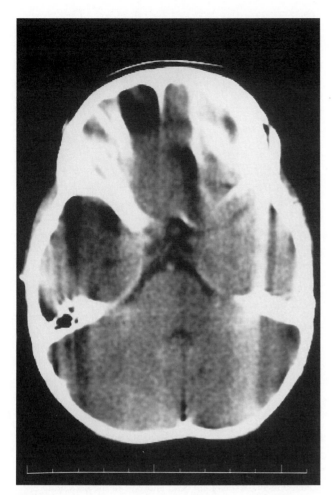

Figure 35-11   Image degredation during CT scanning. The patient moved while the scan was being acquired causing the extensive bright and dark straight line artifacts and the inability to resolve gray and white matter within the brain.

and remain absolutely still during scanning. Movement during scanning causes degradation of the image with loss of sharpness and "ghost" images scattered over the main image (Fig. 35-11). When this occurs and the artifact produced by body movement cannot be compensated for by an image clean-up algorithm called *segmentation*, then the slice must be repeated. There is no guarantee that the child will not move again on the second attempt.

Despite faster scan times, CT scanning may require a longer overall procedure time because of greater complexity of the nature of the scan. Sedation or anesthetic management, therefore, becomes a central issue for the child to be motionless throughout the period of scanning (Fig. 35-12). Neonates may be scanned without sedation, after feeding; infants up to 10 kg or 12 months of age routinely are sedated with chloral hydrate. Children up to the age of 6 years are routinely sedated with intravenous pentobarbital. Above this age, sedation is not normally necessary except in the

older patients who are developmentally delayed. The sedation of children for CT scans is routinely managed by the radiology staff and nurses in the department. Anesthetic consultation to assist or take over management is sometimes necessary. In the nonurgent situation, the anesthetist may be asked electively to manage an older developmentally delayed child or to take over the sedation of a child in whom a full dose of pentobarbital has failed to achieve sedation either with the current sedation or at a previous attempt.

Scan techniques are addressed or tailored to the clinical problem for which the child is referred. The scan may be done at several angles, including axial and coronal scanning for different projections of the organ or tissue being studied. The slice may be varied in thickness from 1 to 10 mm depending on the size of the object of interest and the resolution of the image desired. With patient positioning and angulation of the CT gantry, many parts of the body can be scanned at any angle from the axial to the coronal plane. Intra-

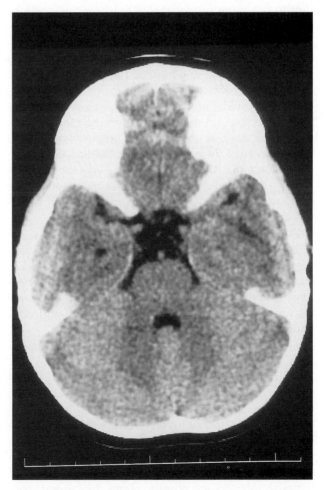

Figure 35-12   The scan repeated while the patient was motionless is free of artifacts with better demonstration of cerebellar gray matter and white matter. Cessation of motion is vitally important for the timely acquisition of diagnostic quality images.

venous contrast may be injected to enhance tissue contrast and highlight the difference between normal and abnormal tissues. Contrast injection is an essential component in enhancing the demonstration of any abnormality and may be used, depending on the clinical history, during the first CT scan and for all follow-up scans on some patients. The contrast agent used routinely is iohexol. This contrast agent is a non-ionic water-soluble contrast medium excreted unchanged by the kidneys.[257,258] Eighty to 90 percent of the injected dose is excreted in the first 24 h, with peak urine concentrations occurring the first hour.[259,260] The different concentrations are reported in Table 35-2. With impaired renal function, excretion by the kidneys is delayed but can be compensated by intrahepatic elimination through bile excretion. As a non-ionic contrast medium, remaining unionized after injection, iohexol is undoubtedly the safest of the contrast media. It is less likely to cause patient discomfort, changes in physiologic parameters, and less histamine release and complement activation than ionic contrast agents. In addition to CT scanning, iohexol is used for angiography and for myelography. Because it does not ionize, it is less likely than ionic contrast media to cause osmolality-related disturbances. Its use is contraindicated in patients with renal and hepatic function impairment. As with other foreign substances, in particular iodinated compounds, allergic and anaphylactic reactions may rarely occur.[261] In this situation the radiologist is dependent on the anesthetist or intensivist for best management of the acute situation. Water-soluble contrast agents may cause hypertensive crisis with pheochromocytoma, red cell sickling in homozygous sickle cell anemia, and renal failure in patients with multiple myeloma.

Computed tomography scanning is routinely applied to the entire spectrum of abnormalities involving the CNS such as congenital malformations (Fig. 35-13), trauma, infections, degenerative diseases, and neoplasms of the brain and the spinal cord. It is also used for musculoskeletal investigation and head and neck anomalies (Fig. 35-14).

CEREBRAL ANGIOGRAPHY

The radiologic investigation of the arterial and venous systems of the head and neck and particularly of the intracranial space has evolved and refined from previous techniques. It now involves direct needle puncture of the carotid and vertebral arteries to the transfemoral puncture technique. From conventional filming techniques to digital subtraction angiography, from old hyperosmolar ionic contrast agents to current nonionic contrast agents of much lower osmolarity, the role of cerebral angiography in the diagnostic armamentarium has changed. Previously it was the primary

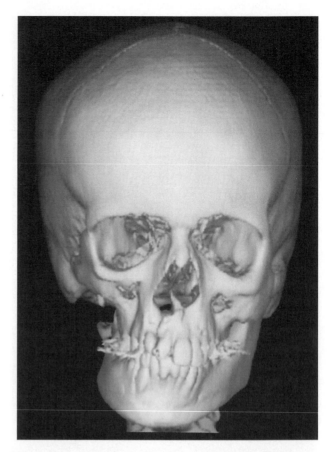

Figure 35-13 Three-dimensional imaging of the craniofacial skeleton in a patient with right lateral facial dysplasia. The area scanned includes the entire head and part of the neck and requires that the patient be completely motionless during the scanning to prevent image artefacts from occurring. The regular lines extending from the teeth are artefacts due to metallic teeth fillings.

means of investigation of the intracranial anatomy and pathology, but current cross-sectional imaging including CT, MRI, and MR angiography can demonstrate intracranial vascular anatomy quite clearly, and the role of cerebral angiography has consequently changed. The arteries and veins demonstrated by CT scanning and MRI are the large proximal branches (Fig. 35-15). However, cerebral angiography retains its role in the demonstration of the smaller, more distal branches and when precise anatomic information such as arterial and venous wall disease is suspected, as in arteritis or vasculitis. It is also needed for precise demonstration of abnormal vasculature associated with a tumor, arteriovenous malformation (AVM), or dural fistula involving the intracranial space. Transcatheter techniques remain and will become more important in the future for therapeutic intervention in interventional neuroradiology. There are several concerns for the neuroradiologist, the first being that the risks of the procedure be justified by the benefit of

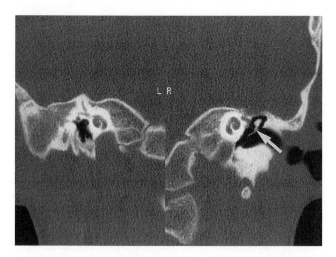

Figure 35-14   Imaging of the petrous bones. Most patients with craniofacial deformities have a narrow slice high-resolution petrous bone study at the time of initial imaging. This patient with lateral facial dysplasia has a small right middle ear cavity and no bones of the ossicular chain are recognized, as they are on the left side (*arrow*).

obtaining precise anatomic information for planning of treatment, surgery, or endovascular interventional management.

Needle and catheter passage through an arterial wall may cause damage; this, however, has become more unlikely with currently available materials and with skilled puncture technique. A sheath system is introduced through which the catheter is passed. The sheath remains motionless while the catheter is advanced, moved back, or rotated within the protection of the sheath. If the sheaths were not used, the catheter movement could induce severe arterial spasm at the point of entry, combined with vascular intimal separation, which could cause local thrombosis as well as vasospasm. During the course of the angiogram if the catheter system is large enough to occlude the artery, the thrombus may extend antegrade and retrograde so that after the angiogram, a large thrombus is left in situ. Associated with persistent vasospasm, both complications may together cause significant limb ischemia. The catheter system should not occlude the arterial lumen and a sheath over the catheter should always be used. Multiple attempts at arterial entry with accidental femoral vein puncture at the same time may cause arteriovenous fistula formation. Movement of the catheter tip through the arterial system is very unlikely to cause vascular intimal epithelial damage, but advancement of the catheter should always be with a soft guidewire protruding beyond the catheter tip to guard against this possibility. Catheter tip injury is unlikely in children with smooth intimal endothelium, but in adults with arthrosclerotic plaques, the

tip may lodge under a plaque, elevate it, eventually setting it free or creating local thrombosis by obstruction.

Throughout the angiogram, meticulous care must be taken to prevent the introduction of air bubbles into the catheter system or allow thrombus to form within the catheter system. Either of these ejected into the internal carotid or vertebrobasilar systems will cause immediate stroke by small or large vessel occlusion (Fig. 35-16 and 35-17). Prevention of the introduction of air requires the diligence and skill of the neuroradiologist, while thrombus formation is prevented by frequently flushing the catheter system with heparinated saline. Systemic heparinization is the routine in some angiographic centers.

Contraindications include recent surgery or spontaneous intracranial hemorrhage within the previous 7 days. In a patient with a bleeding diathesis, heparin is not given. Hypertension is a relative contraindication. If the transfemoral catheter is large and occludes the femoral artery or renders blood flow through it static, the patient should be heparinized to prevent extensive femoral artery thrombosis. In their workup for anesthesia, patients in addition to routine hematocrit, have

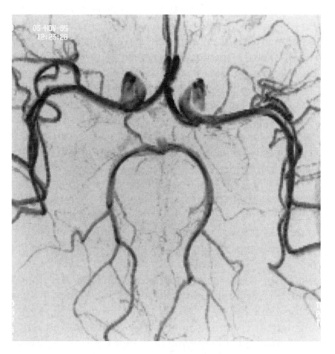

Figure 35-15   MRI angiography. Anatomic and functional information concerning the intracranial blood vessels can be acquired by MRI angiography, without the injection of a contrast medium. The arterial system or the venous system may be selectively imaged. The images provide good demonstration of the large and intermediate size vessels, but the small distal branches are not demonstrated by this technique.

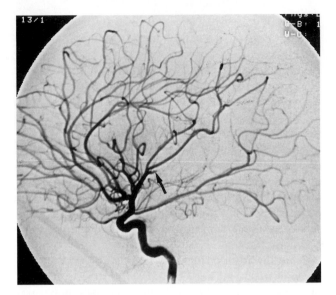

Figure 35-16 Complications of neuroangiography. An abrupt termination of a middle cerebral branch is seen (*arrow*) due to embolization of thrombus or air from the catheter during angiography. Careless catheter system maintenance and failure to exclude air from the system will cause clot or bubbles to be ejected from the catheter tip.

their prothrombin time, protracted thromboplastin time, and platelet count routinely performed to unmask a bleeding tendency. Various protocols for heparin anticoagulation are used. A dose of 100 units/kg is given intravenously after the femoral artery has been catheterized, with no further dose being given unless the angiogram lasts longer than 4 h. Heparin activity is not normally tested during the angiogram and if a repeat dose is to be given, it is 50 percent of the initial dose. If the cerebral angiogram ends sooner than expected and especially if the patient is hypertensive or has had a large catheter system placed in the femoral artery, there will likely be difficulty with femoral artery compression; at this point heparin may be reversed with protamine at a dose of 1 mg/100 units active heparin left. Following the procedure, the patient should lie flat and not flex the hip for 6 h, during which time the femoral, popliteal, and pedal pulses should be palpated at hourly intervals. Sepsis because of breach of sterile technique should not be discounted as an impossibility, either locally at the skin entry site or systemically.

Contrast volume is not normally an issue and while 2 to 3 ml/kg is the normal range for CT scan, a patient with adequate renal function may receive up to 6 ml/kg total contrast dose during the course of the angiogram. It is normally spread over 1 to 3 h. The non-ionic water-soluble contrast agents currently used have a much lower osmolarity than others used previously. Total volume of contrast and heparinized saline for

flushing may become a problem and require meticulous conservation in neonates and infants with poor cardiovascular reserve. This situation is typically seen in a child with a cerebrovascular malformation causing cardiac decompensation.

Diagnostic cerebral angiography and interventional neuroangiography are the most invasive and potentially dangerous procedures in which the Neuroradiologist and neuroanesthetist will be involved together. Neuroanesthesia is considered essential for neuroangiography in children. It is very unlikely that their anxiety will be allayed and they will not be able to lie still for the period of time required. Complete cessation of movement during angiographic exposures is necessary during digital subtraction angiography or the contrast injection and image acquisition will be degraded and made useless. Even motion due to respiration may affect the quality of the images. General anesthesia with tracheal intubation, neuromuscular relaxation, and IPPV allowing control period of apnea on the neuroradiologist's request are used during angiographic filming.

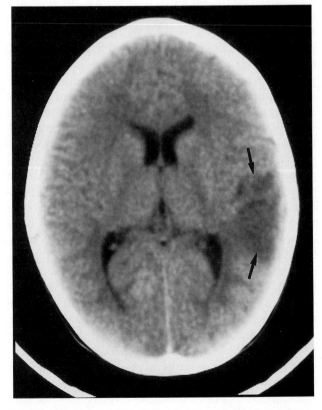

Figure 35-17 Complications of neuroangiography. Image shows the consequence of the branch occlusion illustrated in Fig. 35-16. A defined area of low attenuation in the left parietal region (*arrow*) shows local cerebral edema caused by ischemia due to the occlusion of the feeding arterial branch. The patient suffered a persistent right hemiparesis. Every precaution must be taken to prevent such a complication during neuroangiography.

Ventilatory control of carbon dioxide concentration is also essential for high-quality imaging. Patients are subjected to moderate hyperventilation before filming to induce a degree of hypocapnia, which causes intracranial vasoconstriction. The advantage of a constricted artery bed during cerebral angiography is to allow the maintenance of the contrast bolus at a much greater or stronger concentration than if the vasculature were dilated. In addition, intracranial vasoconstriction in response to hypocapnia only occurs with normal unaffected vascular territories. It will contribute to accentuate the difference between these and damaged or otherwise abnormal vessels such as those forming the circulation within a tumor.[262–264] Hypocapnia and vasoconstriction induced in the presence of an anesthetic will affect directly the quality of the investigation. However, though hypocapnia is normally desirable during cerebral angiography, it may be dangerous in patients with occlusive intracranial vascular disease, such as those with the Moyamoya disease, whose cerebral perfusion may be marginally adequate prior to vasoconstriction and cerebral ischemia may occur during induced hypocapnia. Despite general anesthesia, infiltration of local anesthetic around the femoral artery puncture site may be advisable to allay pain in the area and discomfort and distress during recovery.

The neuroanesthetist is essential for the performance of high-quality cerebral angiography in children and should be fully informed by the neuroradiologist as to the reason and nature of the investigation, the disease process to be investigated, and any change in patient status that may occur during the angiogram. The neuroanesthetist should be entirely familiar with the equipment in the angiographic suite and the space availability. The radiology theater should be equipped for anesthetic support and management with the same requirement as the operating room, including complete monitoring capability and equipment for emergency situations. Patient monitoring should include blood pressure, ECG, temperature probe, and oxygen saturation monitoring devices on the limbs, not on the leg in which the femoral artery is being catheterized or on the patient's arm near the radiologist, because these may become compressed or dislodged or be read erroneously. Access by the neuroanesthetist becomes difficult after the patient is draped and under the fluoroscopic equipment (Fig. 35-18). For extended diagnostic and for all interventional neuroangiographic procedures, the patient's bladder should be catheterized. Adequate body support including arms and legs and protection for the eyes should be achieved immediately after anesthetic induction, to protect against pressure or other injury.

Cerebral angiography is most frequently performed

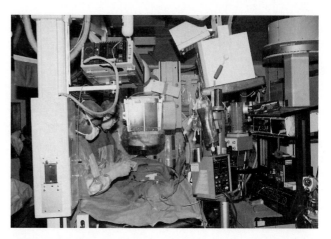

Figure 35-18   The busy angiography room. In the foreground are the anesthetic table, the blood pressure monitor and the table support, while in the background are the ceiling mounted fluoroscopic television monitors and in the center over the patient's head, the image intensifier tube. Access to the patient by the anesthesiologist would require the neuroangiographer to slide the table to the left of the picture. Patient monitoring equipment should not be placed on the arm or leg adjacent to the neuroangiographers to prevent compression or dislodgment.

in patients with vascular diseases such as AVMs, arteriovenous fistula, varix of the vein of Galen, vascular aneurysms and for studies of hemorrhage and stroke. It is also performed to diagnose and assess the state of cerebral vasculitis and vasculopathy such as Moyamoya and in the blood supply to neoplastic diseases involving the brain, the meninges, and skull.

In the investigation of patients with seizures to determine their candidacy for neurosurgical resection, a Wada test is part of the workup in view of seizure surgery. The Wada test is performed in the angiography suite. The transfemoral catheter is placed into each internal carotid artery and amobarbital injected into each internal carotid artery in turn to determine hemisphere dominance and speech center location. This may be difficult because the child must be awake and cooperative to undergo a battery of memory and object recognition tests. With the amobarbital injection the transient hemiplegia is monitored, EEG leads monitor brain electrical activity, and the ability to respond verbally to questions and commands is examined. In addition to the neuroradiologist, neuroanesthetist, radiology nurses, and technologists, the neurologist, psychologist, and EEG technologist are in the room as well.[265]

Patients may also undergo angiography as part of investigation for radiosurgery. Radiosurgery has been used for inoperable AVMs. Their size should be under 3 cm and they may need to be reduced in size by embolization before being accepted for radiosurgery.[266] Transfemoral cerebral angiography is performed with

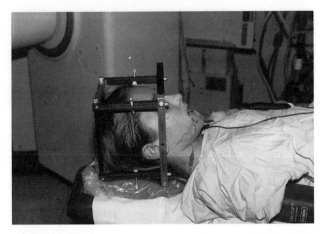

Figure 35-19 Stereotactic radiosurgery. For radiosurgical treatment of brain arteriovenous malformations and small solid lesions, the patient undergoes cerebral angiography and CT scanning for localization of the lesion. The stereotactic localization frame has been attached to the patient's skull in preparation for the cerebral angiogram. The frame is rigidly attached by four pins to the outer table of the skull.

the head of the patient in a stereotactic localizor frame rigidly attached to the skull by four fixing pins screwed into the outer table of the skull (Fig. 35-19). The AVM is thereby stereotactically localized. The patient is transferred from the angiography suite with the stereotactic frame in position to the radiosurgery suite, where the location of the AVM has been computed for targeting by radiosurgery (Fig. 35-20).

INTERVENTIONAL NEUROANGIOGRAPHY

Interventional neuroangiography has become a rapidly expanding field in which the neuroangiographic modality extends to therapeutic procedures. Also known as therapeutic neuroangiography, surgical neu-

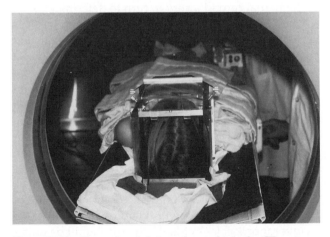

Figure 35-20 The patient is being advanced into the CT gantry with the stereotactic frame in position. The X and Y coordinates of localizers in the Plexiglas plates as well as those of the target lesion are computed for localization for radiosurgical ablation.

roangiography, or endovascular neurosurgery, its basic principles as a treatment modality are based on an approach to the lesion from within the vascular bed.[267–269] The goal of interventional neuroradiology in performing a procedure may be definitive, adjunctive (i.e., presurgery or preradiotherapy), or palliative (as intraarterial chemotherapy for an intraoperable brain tumor).[270] In addition to the essential interaction between the neuroanesthetist and the neuroradiologist, there are frequently particular considerations and precise ways in which the neuroanesthetist may contribute both to the safety and outcome of the patient care and the procedure. Intentional hypercapnia may be required in the endovascular therapy of dural and extradural AVMs and in venous malformations of the head and neck. Hypercapnia increases intracranial circulation, cerebral blood volume, and the rate of venous return from the intracranial space, protecting the intracranial and adjacent veins from any embolic agent that may drain toward these veins. Intentional hypertension will assist in cerebral perfusion in the presence of occlusive cerebrovascular disease such as vasospasm or other cause for arterial constriction. This technique will also facilitate cerebral perfusion when balloon occlusion of a carotid artery for intracranial aneurysm is performed, increasing blood flow across the circle of Willis. Deliberate hypotension is helpful when AVMs are being treated to decrease the flow velocity across the AVM, so that tissue adhesive N-butyl cyano-acrylate (NBCA) glue for embolization will polymerize within the lesion rather than beyond on the venous side. The same technique is of benefit during the management of ruptured cerebral aneurysms or those that rupture during an interventional attempt to occlude them. It is also useful for the intracranial hemorrhage that may follow dissolution of clot by locally infused thrombolytic agents.

Airway swelling may follow interventional management of tumors or mass lesions in the head and neck after both endovascular and percutaneous therapy. Hemorrhage into the airway from epistaxis may also present difficulty during endovascular treatment for this problem.

As an alternative to anesthesia, intravenous sedation with limited monitoring or having an anesthetist on call is almost always inadequate. General anesthesia is the only appropriate management, particularly in children. The anesthetic technique may be modified to neuroleptanalgesia when consciousness is required for response and neurologic testing. The risks associated with interventional neuroangiography include those discussed in diagnostic neuroangiography and the particular danger of the lesion for which the interventional procedure is being undertaken.[271]

Interventional neuroradiology has established a

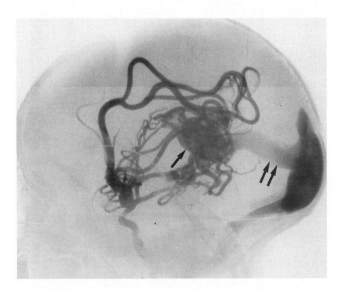

Figure 35-21 Vein of Galen varix. A lateral view of an internal carotid artery injection demonstrates emptying of anterior cerebral branches (*upper*), the middle cerebral (*middle*), and posterior cerebral (*lower*) arteries into the vein of Galen that is abnormally expanded to become a varix (*arrow*), which drains into the straight sinus (*double arrow*) and the confluence of sinuses. The effect of this complex congenital arteriovenous connection is the premature dumping of arterial blood into the venous compartment, there being no capillary resistance bed. Blood flow is preferential through the malformation because of the pressure sump or dump effect, and arterial supply to the surrounding brain, as can be seen from the angiogram, is severely compromised. The hyperdynamic outflow state frequently causes cardiac failure and death in the first days of life. Treatment is by endovascular occlusion of the feeding branches using glue or coils. This undertaking is extremely difficult because of the patient's size and frequently a decompensating cardiovascular status. These patients should be treated urgently, before hyperdynamic output failure begins.

unique niche in the treatment of AVMs and fistulae, both congenital and posttraumatic, vein of Galen varices, and aneurysms (Fig. 35-21). AVMs of the brain may be treated exclusively by endovascular therapy or may be reduced by this technique before surgery or radiotherapy. Arteriovenous fistulae are typically found in the dural coverings of the brain. Posttraumatic fistulae commonly involve the internal carotid artery within the cavernous sinus.[272-275]

Current technology has allowed extensive development of sophisticated intravascular devices. Coaxial catheter systems allow microcatheters to be advanced into the distal branches of the intracranial and extracranial circulation and through these microcatheters various embolizing agents may be deployed. Platinum coils of various sizes may be deposited into arterial branches to cause occlusion or into the lumen of an aneurysm.

Previously, occlusive coils were electrolytically detached from the microcatheter. Currently, they are re-

leased from the catheter simply by rotating their locking device after ejection from the catheter. Tissue adhesive NBCA glue has become largely the occlusive agent of choice for occlusion of the feeding branches of AVM and arteriovenous fistulae. NBCA is a monomer that polymerizes on exposure to charged particles in ionic solution—blood and saline. It is prevented from polymerizing within the introducing catheter by prior flushing with 5% glucose. The NBCA is mixed with tantalum powder and ethiodol (lipiodol), a non-ionizing oil-based contrast agent. These opacify the NBCA so that it may be observed during its deposition. The ratio of ethiodol to NBCA in the mixture controls the polymerization time from a fraction of a second to greater than a second. Microparticles may be injected instead through the catheter. The intention with this technique is to lodge them in the microvaculature of the lesion leading to an occlusion within the small vessel diameter. Such particles of polyvinyl alcohol (PVA) are 50 to 1000 μm in diameter and once deposited, render the lesion avascular, and are suitable for embolizing tumors or AVMs. Their effect, unlike NBCA however, is not permanent and revascularization may occur in days to weeks. The PVA technique is useful for presurgical obliteration of a tumor or AVM. Detachable balloons may also be introduced through catheter systems and are used in the treatment of aneurysms. They are deposited either within the aneurysm lumen or in the parent vessel proximal to the aneurysm or within the arteriovenous fistulae.[276-279] The sequence of the intravascular obliteration of an AVM is demonstrated in Fig. 35-22.

Interventional techniques have also been used extensively in the endovascular obliteration of neoplasms and other lesions involving the extracranial head an neck. AVMs frequently involve the face, and arteriovenous fistulae may involve the vertebral arteries. Neoplasms may be benign or malignant, the nasopharyngeal angiofibroma being an important example in the adolescent age group. Transcatheter PVA particle embolization is used in AVMs and neoplasms and in the treatment of epistaxis whether anterior from the nostril, Little's area, the nasal turbinate or posterior from the nasopharynx and oropharynx. Epistaxis may also be associated with hypertension, coagulopathy, trauma, vascular dysgenesis, or in the adult, atherosclerosis. PVA particle embolization of AVMs and neoplasms is usually preoperative, whereas the occlusion of arteriovenous fistula balloon placement technique represents the definitive technique. When preoperative endovascular obliteration of vascular or mass lesions is undertaken, intraoperative blood loss and operating time are significantly decreased. Other vascular lesions found in children include the hemangioma, which is initially proliferative, then involutive after approxi-

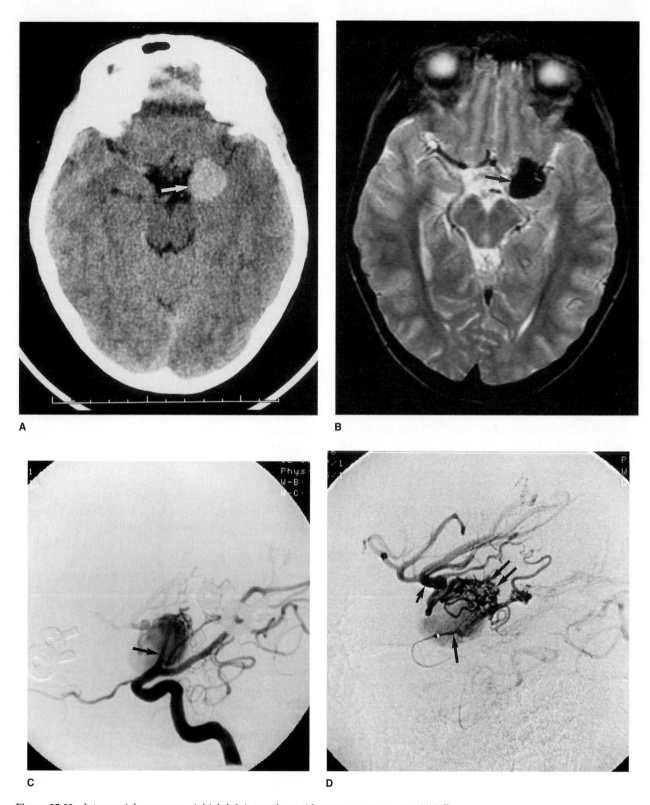

A

B

C

D

Figure 35-22 Intracranial aneurysm. A high left internal carotid artery aneurysm was initially demonstrated on a contrast-enhanced CT scan in the lateral recess of the suprasellar cistern. *A.* The lumen of the aneurysm filled with contrast, giving it its high CT attenuation. Cross-sectional MRI demonstrated a large signal void within the aneurysm, (*B*) indicating that the aneurysm contained flowing blood (*arrow*). *C.* Neuroangiography with contrast injection into the left internal carotid artery demonstrated the lumen of the aneurysm, with the jet of contrast through the neck of the aneurysm (*arrow*). *D.* Superselective internal carotid angiography with the catheter tip at the anterior choroidal artery (*single arrow*) demonstrates the collateral flow through the basal ganglia perforators (*double arrows*) to the middle cerebral artery (*short arrow*) beyond. The development of collaterals was due to the compression and occlusion of the terminal internal carotid artery and proximal middle cerebral artery by the mass effect of the aneurysm.

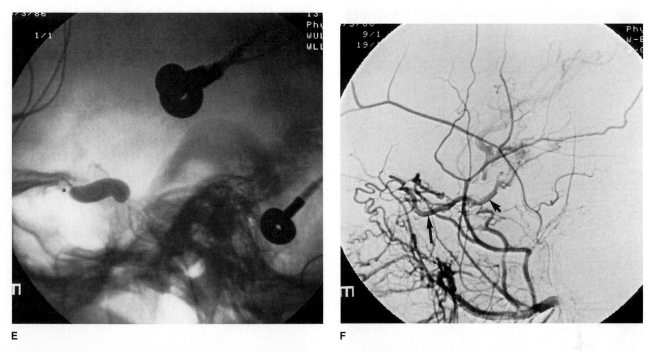

Figure 35-22 (*Continued*) *E.* A balloon placed in the cavernous portion of the internal carotid artery after test occlusion reduced the blood flow velocity, causing the aneurysm to thrombose. *F.* The middle cerebral artery continues to be fed via the basal ganglia perforators from the internal carotid artery (*short arrow*). This in turn is fed via the ophthalmic (*long arrow*), which itself is fed by middle meningeal and internal maxillary branches of the external carotid system.

mately 2 years of age. No vascular treatment is required, although it may become a dangerous lesion if eyelid closure or airway compromise occurs. In contrast to the AVMs and arteriovenous fistulas, venous and lymphatic malformations are low-flow or slow-flow vascular lesions. Treatment is by means of percutaneous sclerosis of their endovascular space, by the injection of USP grade 95% ethanol. This destroys the endothelium, obliterating the endovascular space. The amount of alcohol injected is limited to less than 1 ml/kg. It is opacified by mixing with metrizamide powder. The mixture is injected percutaneously through an 18- or 20-gauge angiocath needle after venous or lymphatic fluid return has proven successful entry into the venous or lymphatic space. Alcohol injection may cause hypoglycemia and symptoms of intoxication including agitation after the procedure. Percutaneous alcohol injection requires anesthesia or deep sedation with analgesia for pain management. To control and reduce swelling, intravenous dexamethasone is given after the beginning of the anesthetic technique for the following 3 days at a dose of 4 mg three times a day intravenously or orally. Swelling after the alcohol injection can be intense and concern regarding the airway patency should be discussed before the procedure.

The discipline of interventional neuroradiology in the pediatric population can only have developed with the help of the neuroanesthetist. His or her active coop-

eration in preemptive patient management is essential, particularly with respect to brain protective measures, as well as in the anesthetic management of patients with poor cardiovascular reserve or other reasons for instability. Professional and mutual interaction between the neuroradiologist and neuroanesthetist will continue to benefit the children and advance the discipline of interventional neuroradiology. To increase patient safety, neuroanesthetic support and patient management are essential to successful neurodiagnostic and neurointerventional procedures.

SKULL ABNORMALITIES

The most frequent skull anomalies encountered in pediatric anesthesia are the craniosynostosis (Fig. 35-23) and the craniofacial dysmorphism (Fig. 35-24).

CRANIOSYNOSTOSIS
Sagittal Synostosis

Sagittal synostosis accounts for approximately half of all craniosynostoses. Occasional cases are familial suggesting a genetic predisposition, and males predominate in most reported series. With fusion of the sagittal suture, the skull becomes scaphocephalic in appearance resulting in an elongated anteroposterior dimension. The frontal and occipital bones frequently demonstrate marked degrees of bossing. The biparietal

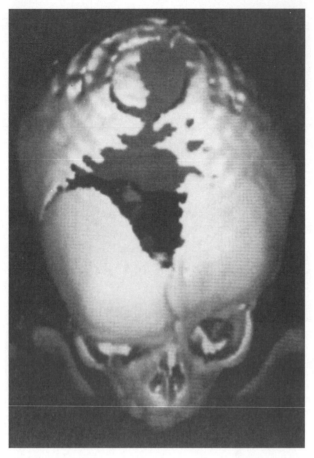

Figure 35-23 Three-dimensional CT scan of a 6-month-old infant shows the cranial vault contours. The asymmetrical deformity of the skull is due to premature synostosis of the coronal and metopic sutures.

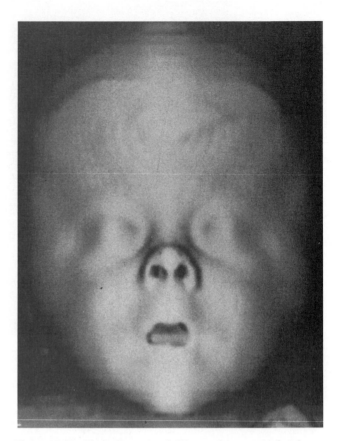

Figure 35-24 Three-dimensional CT scan shows craniofacial contours of an infant with Crouzon's syndrome.

dimension is characteristically reduced. Clinically, a palpable midline sagittal bony ridge is found extending from the anterior to the posterior fontanelle. The anterior fontanelle may be small or absent. In most instances, underlying brain development and neurologic examinations are normal. Operative intervention is directed toward releasing the affected suture at an early age (< 6 months).

A multitude of neurosurgical procedures have been proposed for sagittal synostosis ranging from the relatively straightforward "strip craniectomy" with or without interposed Silastic sheeting wrapped around the cut bone edges, to multiple suture craniectomies performed in conjunction with generous cranial vault osteotomies (Fig. 35-25). Each procedure has its relative merits.

Coronal Synostosis

Coronal synostosis is the second most common single suture synostosis accounting for approximately 20 percent of all craniosynostoses. When unilateral, patients have a characteristic flattening of the forehead on the

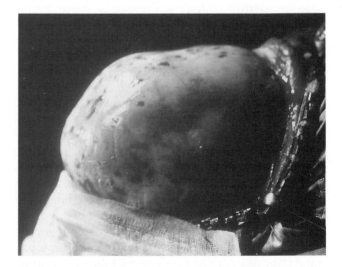

Figure 35-25 Intraoperative photograph of patient with sagittal synostosis undergoing total cranial vault reconstruction. The entire cranial vault has been exposed. Such wide exposures frequently lead to blood loss, which must be matched with adequate intravenous fluid replacement throughout the case.

side of the involved suture, ipsilateral elevation of the supraorbital bar, and contralateral bulging of the forehead. Typically, the nose deviates away from the stenotic suture (see Fig. 35-23). Bilateral coronal synostosis is a frequent finding in patients with inherited craniofacial dysmorphic syndromes such as Apert, Crouzon (see Fig. 35-24), and Saethre-Chotzen syndrome. Concomitant fusion of the frontoethmoidal sutures may lead to narrowing of the nasal airway in some of these patients and pose special airway risks of which the neuroanesthesiologist should be aware.

When unilateral, coronal synostosis may be treated early in infancy (< 6 months of age) by a lateral canthal advancement procedure. Patients with bilateral coronal synostosis and older infants with unilateral coronal synostosis (> 6 months) will require anterior cranial vault reshaping and bilateral canthal advancements. This latter procedure requires more neurosurgical time and leads to more blood loss in all infants than does a simple unilateral canthal advancement. As with sagittal synostosis procedures, anterior cranial vault reshaping mandates removal of the anterior cranial vault over the anterior sagittal sinus in the midline.

Multiple Suture Synostosis
Multiple suture synostosis unassociated with craniofacial dysmorphism accounts for approximately 7 percent of all cases of craniosynostoses. The head shape varies with respect to the sutures involved (see Fig. 35-23). Total cranial vault reshaping may be required for the best cosmetic result. To perform this procedure during one anesthetic, the entire cranial vault must be exposed, frequently with the patient prone and the neck greatly extended, and the head supported in a head rest or a specially designed bean-bag head holder. Such extension of the neck mandates close observation of the endotracheal tube throughout the surgical procedure. Blood loss from multiple suture craniectomies and craniotomies may be extensive.

Special anesthetic considerations for infants with craniosynostosis include:

1. Increased ICP
2. Massive blood loss
3. Venous air embolism

Children and infants undergoing craniectomy should be examined for evidence of increased ICP and induction of anesthesia should proceed as discussed previously in this chapter. The degree of blood loss is increased in patients with multiple strip craniectomies which are usually reserved for older infants (> 6 months) who have thicker bone tables. Blood loss either during or after surgery may become clinically significant. As a safe anesthetic conduct, cross-matched

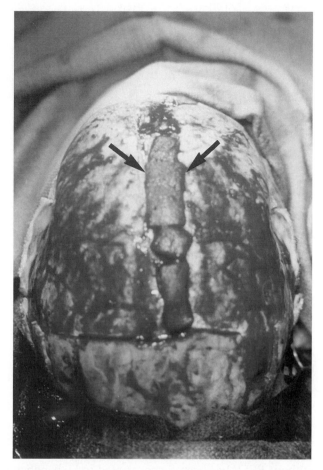

Figure 35-26 Intraoperative photograph shows exposed cranial dura after the entire sagittal suture has been removed. Gelfoam strips are placed over the sagittal sinus to control blood loss (*arrows*). Blood loss can continue from the exposed dura and from the bone edges once cut.

blood should always be available in the operating theater because blood replacement therapy is most often used. Communication with the surgical team is essential at all times. Neuroanesthesiologists caring for such infants must pay special attention to the time when the neurosurgeon is removing the midline fused sagittal suture from the sagittal sinus (Fig. 35-26) because it is during this maneuver that brisk venous bleeding[280] and air embolism can occur.[235] Most craniosynostosis surgery is performed in children between 2 and 6 months of age, a period that coincides with physiologic anemia. Transfusion may therefore be required to maintain an acceptable hemoglobin level. Simple suture craniectomy in the young child with normal ICP does not require arterial line placement. However, during surgical procedure for children with elevated ICP and those undergoing extensive multiple suture procedures, the use of an indwelling arterial catheter is highly recommended. It is our usual practice to use induced hypotension during these procedures. Deliberate hypoten-

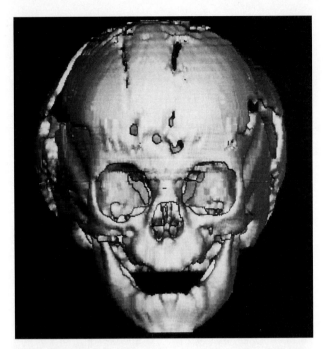

Figure 35-27 Postoperative three-dimensional CT scan of same patient as Fig. 35-24 following total cranial vault reconstruction. The biparietal diameter is now widened. The osteotomies are well appreciated in the frontal and temporal regions. The overall cosmetic appearance is highly satisfactory.

sion using halothane and controlled ventilation without PEEP has been demonstrated to be beneficial for children undergoing craniectomy for unilateral or bilateral craniosynostosis. In one study, estimated blood loss was decreased from 111 to 89 ml (mean) for all ages and from 133 to 72 ml (mean) for infants between 8 and 32 weeks of age compared with the normotensive control group.[281] Because bleeding can be early and brisk, it is mandatory that neuroanesthesiologists do not begin the surgical procedure until adequate intravenous access for fluid and blood replacement has been obtained. The problem of air embolism has been dealt with earlier in this chapter.

CRANIOFACIAL PROCEDURES

Special considerations for craniofacial procedures include:

1. Difficult intubation
2. Blood loss
3. Extubation and airway edema

Many craniofacial procedures require frontal bone advancement or reshaping (Fig. 35-27) and as such constitute intracranial surgery. Efforts to reduce brain bulk are often helpful to the surgeon. Occasionally a lumbar subarachnoid drain is placed for continuous CSF drainage.

Intubation

Patients undergoing craniofacial procedures present a multiplicity of intubation problems that can include mandibular hypoplasia, immobile neck or trachea, macroglossia, and poor mouth opening. Few children will tolerate awake laryngoscopy or awake fiberoptic intubation. The mainstay of induction in the difficult pediatric airway is an inhalational technique even in the presence of raised ICP. As previously described in this chapter, the utilization of an inhalational agent combined with manual assisted-ventilation will maintain or even reduce carbon dioxide, which will contribute to limited changes in ICP. After successful induction, direct laryngoscopy or fiberoptic intubation (in endotracheal tubes > 4.0 mm) can usually be accomplished. In the older child or teenager, local anesthesia combined with neuroleptanesthetic technique may be used. Help should always be available for difficult intubations as well as equipment for surgically securing the airway. After the endotracheal tube is placed, it should be wired to the mandible by the surgeon and the patient's eyes lubricated and sewn closed with a tarsorrhaphy stitch. Mono-bloc procedures require intraoperative replacement of the tube nasally.

Blood Loss

Craniofacial surgery often includes multiple suture craniectomies, dissection of large skin flaps as well as facial bone repositioning, resulting in copious blood loss in the order of a half to several blood volumes.[282] Rapid blood transfusion may lead to a rapid increase in potassium, which in very small children is recognized as a serious potential complication.[283,284] A hypotensive anesthetic technique is frequently used to reduce blood loss. These patients should receive placement of at least two large-bone intravenous lines along with an arterial line and urinary catheter placement. Central line placement is often helpful for managing fluid replacement and aspiration of intracardiac air should air embolism occur. Patients in whom air embolism is likely require precordial Doppler monitoring. Mangement of air embolism has been discussed.

Extubation and Airway Edema

Patients undergoing facial procedures below the orbits frequently have significant edema of their upper airway structures. In our institution, patients having extensive frontal craniotomies remain intubated, sedated, and ventilated with subarachnoid drains in place for 24 to 48 h postoperatively in an effort to reduce CSF leakage through the dura prior to extubation. The patient should be fully awake and carefully suctioned to remove any clots and residual blood in the oropharynx before the tracheal tube is removed.

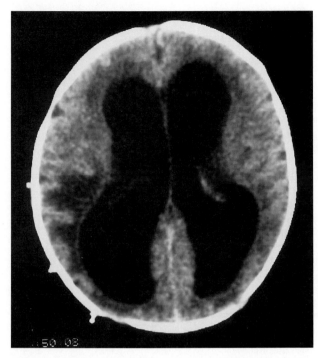

Figure 35-28 Axial CT scan of newborn baby with gross ventriculomegaly and hydrocephalus. The ICP is high and periventricular edema is evident.

HYDROCEPHALUS

Hydrocephalus is a congenital or acquired pathologic condition with many variations, but it is always characterized by an increase in the amount of CSF that is or has been under increased pressure (Fig. 35-28) It may be found at any period of life.[285] It is classified according to its three basic physiologic processes as outlined in Table 35-4.

NEUROSURGICAL TREATMENT

The most common neurosurgical operation for hydrocephalus today is the ventriculoperitoneal shunt (Fig. 35-31). For this procedure, the neurosurgeon makes an incision over the posterior parietal region for occipital horn entry (or straddling the coronal suture for frontal horn placed catheters) and an incision in the abdominal wall. The two incisions are joined with a device known as a *shunt passer,* which is tunneled subcutaneously so that the shunt itself can be laid to rest in a subcutaneous trough traveling from one incision to the other. The shunt passer may compromise the ventilation of small infants with hydrocephalus, and so the time that it remains in situ by the neurosurgeon should be minimized. Cannulation of the ventricle with a ventricular catheter is straightforward. CSF frequently comes through a well-placed catheter under high pressure. Compromised vital signs of children with intracranial hypertension frequently return to normal rapidly once

decompression of the ventricle is accomplished. The ventricular catheter is connected to the peritoneal catheter (which usually contains a pressure-regulating valve) and the peritoneal catheter is then placed in the abdomen.

Ventriculoperitoneal shunts are prone to malfunction and a shunt revision is a common operation in pediatric neurosurgery. In 80 percent of instances, a proximal or ventricular catheter obstruction is found at the time of revision. It is usually a simpler matter to replace the obstructed ventricular catheter with a new catheter. Occasionally, the peritoneal catheter is obstructed and must be replaced (10 percent of cases). Rarely, both ventricular and peritoneal catheters will need to be replaced.

Three types of ventricular shunts are in current use, the ventriculoperitoneal, ventriculoatrial, and ventriculopleural shunts. Each has its indications and anesthetic implications. Often, as the pediatric patient grows, the shunt must be revised and replaced secondary to malfunction or removed due to infection. Shunt procedures are common in both severely neurologically impaired children as well as otherwise healthy patients. These children may present to the operating room several times and may request a specific induction technique. It must be stated that the patient presenting for CSF shunting procedures may exhibit a broad spectrum of symptoms and clinical signs varying from an apparently healthy child with minimal disability to a seriously ill comatose patient for whom surgery is urgent.

Preanesthetic assessment must include:

1. **Level of consciousness:** Patients presenting for primary shunting, shunt revision, or malfunction may exhibit severe elevations in ICP, which require aggressive treatment.
2. **Full stomach:** Evidence of vomiting or delayed gastric emptying are indications to induce anesthesia by a rapid sequence technique.
3. **Coexisting pathology:** Does the child have evidence of other significant organ system compromise, such as the child with cerebral palsy who frequently aspirates?
4. **Age-related pathophysiology:** Is the patient likely to present problems with apnea, poor pulmonary compliance, or immature renal function?

MONITORING

Routine monitoring has been discussed. Arterial line placement is usually reserved for the patient with uncontrolled ICP and hemodynamic instability.

PREINDUCTION

A shunt scan is useful in determining the site of malfunction. In patients with increased ICP secondary to

TABLE 35-4
Classification of Hydrocephalus

I. Excessive production of CSF
   A. Choroid plexus papilloma

II. Obstruction of CSF pathways[a]
   A. Obstruction within the ventricular system
      i. Lateral ventricular (atrium, body, foramen of Monro)
      ii. Third ventricular
      iii. Aqueductal (congenital stenosis, mass lesions) (Fig. 35-29)
      iv. Fourth ventricular (Dandy-Walker) (Fig. 35-30)
   B. Obstruction within the subarachnoid space
      i. Basal cisterns (Chiari I malformation, postinfectious)
      ii. Convexity

III. Decreased absorption of CSF
   A. Obstruction at the arachnoid villus (plugging by tumor cells, protein, blood, bacteria, etc.)
   B. Obstruction at the major dural venous sinuses (thrombus, hematologic malignancies, infection)
   C. Obstruction at extracranial venous sinuses (achondroplasia)

[a] Common causes of CSF block:
1. Infectious—abscess, meningitis, encephalitis
2. Neoplastic—astrocytoma, ependymoma, choroid plexus papilloma, oligodendroglioma, medulloblastoma, meningioma
3. Vascular—AVM, aneurysm
4. Congenital—arachnoid cysts, colloid cysts, Chiari malformation, encephalocele

shunt malfunction, the ICP may be lowered acutely by tapping the proximal reservoir. Infiltration of the skin with local anesthetic allows the tap to proceed with minimal trauma to the patient. The needle may then be left in place to monitor ICP during induction. In the patient at risk for emesis at induction, placement of gastric suctioning may precipitate coughing and bucking with an undesirable elevation in ICP. Severely neurologically compromised children often have gastrostomy tubes and opening these before induction is a recommended precaution.

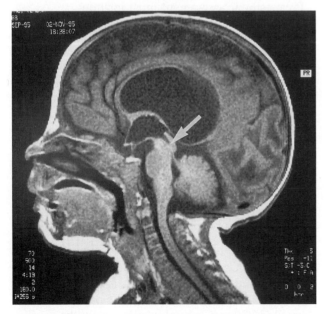

Figure 35-29 Hydrocephalus is the result of congenital aqueductal obstruction. The proximal aqueduct and third ventricle are dilated, the distal aqueduct being closed, due to congenital failure of cannulation (*arrow*), and the fourth ventricle distally is not dilated.

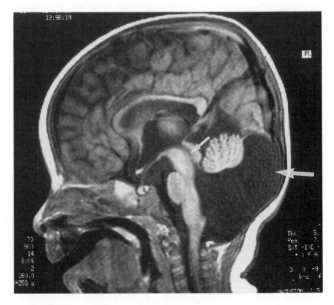

Figure 35-30 Hydrocephalus is due to Dandy-Walker malformation. The aqueduct connecting the third to fourth ventricle (*small arrow*) is visible and patent, while the fourth ventricle where the foramina of Magendie and Luschka have failed to fenestrate, has expanded significantly to become a large posterior fossa cystic mass (*large arrow*) beginning in intrauterine life.

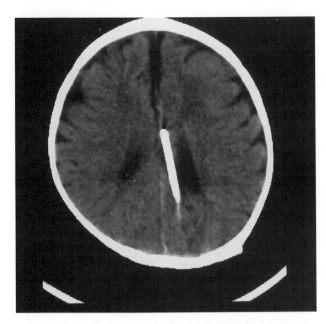

Figure 35-31   Same patient as in Fig. 35-28 with ventriculoperitoneal shunt in place 4 months postoperatively. The shunt catheter is seen coursing into the right lateral ventricle. The ventricles are now normal in size. The brain appears normal by comparison.

INDUCTION AND INTUBATION

Many patients with hydrocephalus have undergone multiple surgical procedures and this should be recognized at induction of anesthesia. In the child without clinical evidence of elevated ICP, induction may proceed by mask or intravenously and we usually allow children their preference. On the other hand, children with increased ICP and delayed gastric emptying are usually induced intravenously following preoxygenation, with thiopentone, atropine, lidocaine, narcotic, and a nondepolarizing muscle relaxant. Cricoid pressure is applied and the patient hyperventilated at low peak inspiratory pressures. Laryngoscopy is a potent stimulus in increasing ICP and the trachea is orally intubated as smoothly as possible.

MAINTENANCE

The anesthetic considerations of maintenance of anesthesia are:

1. Positioning
2. Ventilation
3. Anesthetic agents
4. Muscle relaxants
5. Fluid management
6. Maintenance of body temperature

Patients are placed in a supine position with the head turned, or in a slightly lateral position. Compromised patients should be placed in a 30 degree head-up position with minimal neck rotation or flexion to improve venous drainage. Patients often have their shunt tubing placed posteriorly before coursing to the abdomen, and those patients placed in a lateral position should have an axillary roll in place and all extremities padded.

After securing the airway, patients with increased ICP are hyperventilated to a Pa_{CO_2} between 25 and 30 mmHg. Patients with normal ICP are maintained at normocapnia. Spontaneous ventilation should be avoided in patients with ventriculopleural shunts to reduce the risk of pneumothorax and in those with ventriculoatrial shunts to avoid air embolism during placement or whenever the cranium is opened. Neonates and infants with poor pulmonary compliance or at risk for apnea under anesthesia are mechanically ventilated.

Anesthesia is usually maintained with a combination of nitrous oxide in oxygen together with low concentrations of isoflurane and minimal narcotic supplementation. Although nitrous oxide increases CBF in anesthetized pediatric patients,[81] it has been suggested that this increase in CBF and CMR_{O_2} caused by nitrous oxide is effectively blunted by hyperventilation and pretreatment with thiopentone. Halogenated anesthetics increase CBF, cerebral blood volume, and ICP in a dose-dependent manner with isoflurane having less adverse effect than halothane.[90,95,101,102,285] They are therefore used in low concentrations in patients with elevated ICP. Muscle relaxation is usually maintained with vecuronium or atracurium if the procedure is to be of short duration.

Ventricular shunt procedures usually do not result in significant blood or third-space losses and fluid management centers around replacement of intravascular volume lost from emesis, dehydration, or diuresis induced by drugs to manage a patient presenting with high ICP.

Maintenance of body temperature is important during shunt procedures despite their relatively short duration. A large body surface area is exposed and prepared, particularly for ventriculoperitoneal shunting, and infants may cool rapidly.[229] Techniques to maintain temperature homeostasis were described previously.

EMERGENCE

Anesthetic considerations for emergence are:

1. Elimination of anesthetics
2. Reversal of neuromuscular blockade
3. Delayed gastric emptying

Prior to extubation of the trachea, adequate time for elimination of the anesthetic agents should be allowed and adequate reversal of neuromuscular blockade ensured. Although not providing absolute insurance against regurgitation, gastric suctioning before extubation should be performed in patients who may have gastric contents. The patient should be fully awake with an appropriate gag reflex to protect the airway against emesis on emergence. Unfortunately, some patients coming for shunt procedures are severely neurologically impaired and have poor airway control under the best of circumstances.

POSTOPERATIVE MANAGEMENT

The anesthetic considerations for postoperative care are similar to those required for any general anesthetic. They include:

1. Oxygen and respiration
2. Maintenane of body temperature
3. Analgesia

Supplemental oxygen should be given and respiratory pattern and adequacy assessed. Neurosurgical patients in general and preterm infants less than 50 weeks postgestational age in particular are liable to have abnormal respiratory patterns or apnea. Hypothermic patients should be rewarmed before extubation.

Analgesics should be used judiciously and under close supervision in neurologically impaired patients. Generous use of local anesthetic skin infiltration at the time of surgery can substantially reduce the requirement for postoperative analgesia. Patients without neurologic impairment before surgery can be given a routine postoperative pain regimen.

INTRACRANIAL TUMORS

Neoplasms of the CNS account for a major proportion of all solid tumors in children younger than 15 years of age[286] and, in fact, constitute the second most common cancer in childhood after leukemia.[164] Table 35-5 presents the classification of pediatric brain tumors. Treatment of childhood primary malignant brain tumors has not resulted in a comparable dramatic increases in survival seen for example with the recent advances in the treatment of childhood leukemia.[164] The survival of children with tumors of the CNS has improved significantly over the last several decades, but much remains to be accomplished especially in those less than 2 to 3 years of age at the time of diagnosis. From the viewpoint of the anesthesiologist, intracranial brain tumors are divided according to the localization of the tumor. The following section describes an anesthetic approach for supratentorial and posterior fossa craniotomies. Special aspects of anesthesia will be discussed for the surgical excision of craniopharyngioma.

TABLE 35-5
Classification of Pediatric Brain Tumors

I. Central Neuroepithelial Tumors
   Astrocytoma—low and high grade
   Astroblastoma
   Oligodendroglioma
   Ependymoma
   Subependymoma
   Ependymoblastoma
   Medulloblastoma (primitive neuroectodermal tumor—PNET)
   Neuroblastoma
   Ganglioglioma
   Choroid plexus papilloma and carcinoma

II. Meningeal Tumors
   Meningiomas
   Primary meningeal sarcoma
   Primary leptomeningeal melanoma

III. Developmental Tumors
   Dermoid tumor
   Epidermoid tumor
   Craniopharyngioma
   Rathke's cleft cyst
   Intracranial lipoma
   Hamartoma

IV. Germ Cell Tumors
   Germinoma
   Embryonal carcinoma
   Endodermal sinus tumor
   Choriocarcinoma
   Teratoma

V. Vascular Tumors
   Capillary telangiectasia
   Arteriovenous malformation
   Cavernous malformation
   Venous angioma

SUPRATENTORIAL CRANIOTOMY

Supratentorial lesions account for about half of all pediatric brain neoplasms. For reasons that presumably relate to embryogenesis, pediatric brain tumors often arise from midline structures including the hypothalamus, epithalamus and thalamus, and basal ganglia (Fig. 35-32). They tend to impinge on the ventricular system, resulting in obstructive hydrocephalus. Other supratentorial lesions are the hemispheric masses that are more common during the first year of life.[165] In infants, their frequency among all intracranial neoplasms is approximately twice as high compared to the overall incidence in children, that is 37 percent compared to 16 to 24 percent.[166] The relative incidence of hemispheric tumors is also higher after the age of 8 to 10 years.[287]

Anesthetic Considerations

1. Increased ICP: Estimate the degree of rise in ICP; review the CT scan and MRI film.

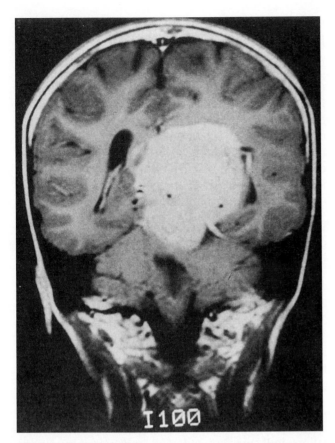

Figure 35-32 Midsagittal nuclear MRI demonstrates a midline glioma in a child. The black rounded spots within the tumor represent the basal cerebral arteries.

2. Full stomach: Delayed gastric emptying occurs in the patient with raised ICP.
3. Electrolyte and fluid: Hydration state and electrolyte balance may be altered in the child with intracranial pathology and SIADH.
4. Age-related pathophysiology: Anesthetic considerations are identical to those discussed in earlier sections.
5. Positioning: The head should be elevated not more than 10° from horizontal; ensure that venous return is not obstructed.

Monitoring

To the routine monitoring previously described the use of invasive monitoring should be considered. All patients in our institution receive arterial line placement for hemodynamic monitoring and blood chemistry sampling. Patients in whom blood loss will be significant, those with expected hemodynamic instability, or those at increased risk for air embolism receive central venous catheters. The use of a urinary catheter is mandatory because of the duration of the surgical procedure and the use of diuretic drugs.

Preinduction

Determination of the degree to which ICP is elevated in patients undergoing craniotomy is essential. Patients with large mass lesions, significant tumor edema, or obstruction to CSF outflow will require an anesthetic approach aimed at reducing ICP. Some children may undergo ventriculostomy placement prior to their definitive surgical procedure and can be managed in the manner discussed in the earlier sections. Preoperative neurologic deficits should be evaluated and documented. Intracranial pathology of many kinds, such as tumor or inflammation, can present with SIADH. The child may show evidence of hyponatremia, low serum osmolality, high urine osmolality, and oliguria. Edema is rarely present. Preoperative treatment usually includes fluid restriction.

Induction and Intubation

Unlike children with normal ICP, induction followed by a minimally stimulated rapidly secured airway and hyperventilation is of paramount importance in the patient with significantly elevated ICP. Induction generally proceeds as discussed in the section on hydrocephalus, with intravenous thiopental, lidocaine, narcotic, and a nondepolarizing muscle relaxant. Cricoid pressure is applied and the patient hyperventilated with low peak inspiratory pressures to avoid inflation of the stomach. Laryngoscopy should proceed as smoothly as possible. Some anesthetists prefer nasotracheal intubation for patients in whom postoperative ventilation is expected or in small infants in whom the tube may be better stabilized.

Maintenance

The considerations for maintenance of anesthesia include:

1. Ventilation
2. Positioning
3. Anesthetic agents and muscle relaxants
4. Fluid management
5. Maintenance of body temperature

Patients with increased ICP are generally ventilated to a Pa_{CO_2} between 25 and 30 mmHg. Occasionally a very "tight brain" with uncontrollable hypertension can require lower levels of Pa_{CO_2}. Caution must be exercised, because vasoconstriction induced by extreme hyperventilation may decrease CPP leading to ischemia or alternatively shifting blood flow to hyperemic brain with impaired autoregulation. PEEP is generally avoided to facilitate cerebral venous drainage. The use of PEEP may also decrease MAP and this should be considered in patients with decreased CPP. In patients with impaired oxygenation, small amounts of PEEP may be gradually increased to the minimum necessary to correct hypoxia so that there will be the least possible obstruction to venous return.

Pediatric patients are usually placed supine for supratentorial procedures, with the head elevated slightly to facilitate venous drainage. Extremities should be well padded and the eyes protected from injury. Care must be taken to avoid undue flexion, extension, or rotation of the neck. Prone positioning is discussed in Chap. 29.

Discussion of the specific pharmacology of each anesthetic agent is beyond the scope of this text. Agent selection should be based on the wide compilations of clinical and laboratory data. We select one of two techniques; neuroleptanalgesia or a balanced inhalational approach. The neurolept technique combines nitrous oxide, a synthetic short-acting narcotic (usually fentanyl citrate) and a nondepolarizing muscle relaxant with either a benzodiazepine or droperidol. With a balanced approach, sub-MAC concentrations of isoflurane are used with nitrous oxide, fentanyl, and a nondepolarizing muscle relaxant. While any nondepolarizing muscle relaxant is likely to be acceptable for the neurosurgical patient, in the small infant it may be preferable to use pancuronium for its vagolytic properties and lack of histamine release, which could potentially increase ICP.

Fluid management for the patient undergoing craniotomy can be problematic. Patients with increased ICP usually receive dehydration therapy using mannitol. This increases the possibility of intravascular volume collapse especially in light of the substantial blood loss that often accompanies the skin incision and excision of the bone flap. CVP monitoring can be a valuable aid and volume expansion is usually effected by colloid solutions such as 5% albumin. Simple craniotomy in patients without significantly increased ICP and in procedures with manageable blood loss frequently receive crystalloid replacement only.

Body temperature should be maintained as described previously.

Emergence

Anesthetic considerations for emergence include:

1. Elimination of anesthetic agents
2. Reversal of neuromuscular blockade
3. Delayed gastric emptying
4. Increased ICP

The decision to extubate the trachea at the end of the procedure is made on the basis of the success of the surgical intervention, smoothness of the intraoperative course, normalization of ICP, age of the patient, the degree of residual neurologic deficit, and how these

factors will affect respiration and airway protection. Patients without adequate respiratory effort will retain carbon dioxide with the potential for increased ICP. A gag reflex should be present for airway protection. Children who remain sedated and who hyperventilate in the postoperative period should be suspected of having increased ICP. Neonates with poor pulmonary compliance or an immature respiratory drive may remain intubated postoperatively. Barring any adverse complications such as these, the child can be extubated awake after reversal of the neuromuscular blockade and elimination of the anesthetic agents.

Postoperative Management

Considerations for postoperative management after supratentorial craniotomy include:

1. Oxygen and respiration
2. Temperature homeostasis
3. Analgesia
4. Neurologic assessment
5. Hypertension
6. Seizures

As with any postsurgical patient, supplemental oxygen should be administered and the adequacy of respiration assessed. Patients requiring postoperative ventilation will require sedation and possibly muscle relaxation to avoid agitation and increased ICP. Body temperature should be maintained at a normal level. The use of local anesthetic skin infiltration intraoperatively or a cervical superficial plexus blockade at the end of the procedure can reduce the requirement for postoperative analgesics. A balance between patient comfort and the ability to follow the patient's neurologic status must be sought. An obtunded patient must be investigated for increased ICP or other surgically correctable pathology such as intracranial bleeding.

The most common contributor to postoperative increased ICP is uncontrolled hypertension. When postoperative pain control has been achieved, blood pressure may be controlled with the use of vasodilators. β-Blocking drugs have been used successfully, particularly labetolol with its combined β- and α-blocking properties and because it does not normally cross the blood-brain barrier.[288]

Seizures frequently occur in the immediate postoperative period. Many surgeons place their patients on preoperative anticonvulsants and continue these postoperatively. Phenobarbital appears to be the most frequently used drug and phenytoin or other medications are added for refractory patients.

CRANIOPHARYNGIOMA

Craniopharyngiomas are the most common intracranial tumors of nonglial origin in the pediatric population.[289,290] Despite their benign histologic appearance, craniopharyngiomas commonly cause progressive neurologic deterioration and death because of their propensity to involve critical structures in the suprasellar regions such as the hypothalamus, optic nerves, and pituitary stalk. The optimum method of management of patients with craniopharyngiomas remains controversial, with proponents for radical removal, radiation therapy, or a combination of these modalities.

Craniopharyngiomas may be subdivided on the basis of their location into three main types: sellar, prechiasmatic, and retrochiasmatic. Patients with sellar craniopharyngiomas usually present with headaches and endocrine dysfunction. Patients with prechiasmatic tumors have reduced visual acuity, field cuts, and optic atrophy. Those with retrochiasmatic tumors frequently develop obstructive hydrocephalus and demonstrate signs and symptoms of raised ICP with papilledema.

Patients with craniopharyngiomas are imaged preoperatively with MR and CT scans. CT scans are superior to MRI in demonstrating intratumoral calcification. Prior to surgery, all patients undergo formal neuro-ophthalmologic, neuroendocrinologic, and if possible, neuropsychological assessments. These assessments are then repeated in the early and late postoperative period.

The first approach to all craniopharyngiomas should be attempted total removal. Total removal can be achieved in over 65 percent of patients. For sellar and prechiasmatic craniopharyngiomas, a unilateral, right subfrontal approach is used. Retrochiasmatic tumors are removed in the same manner, except that we fashion the bone flap so as to permit a combined subfrontal-pterional approach by removing the lateral sphenoid wing.

Seizures are frequently seen in the immediate postoperative period, so all patients receive prophylactic anticonvulsants for 5 to 10 days. Steroids are given perioperatively in high doses until a complete endocrine reassessment can be completed. Diabetes insipidus becomes apparent on the second or third postoperative day in 90 percent of patients and is successfully managed with desmopressin acetate (DDAVP).

Special anesthetic considerations for craniopharyngioma surgery include:

1. Positioning
2. Hypopituitarism
3. Diabetes insipidus
4. Altered insulin requirement
5. Hyperthermia
6. Seizures

A craniopharyngioma is a benign encapsulated tumor of the hypophysis cerebri (Fig. 35-33). Children

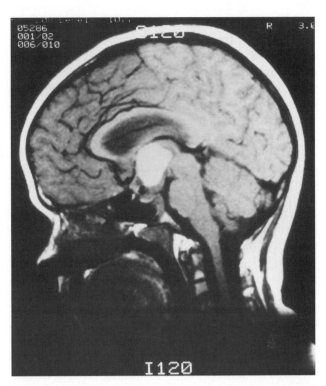

Figure 35-33 Mid-sagittal nuclear MRI showing a high signal mass lesion filling the suprasellar cistern (craniopharyngioma). The mass is extending from the pituitary fossa and it herniates into the third ventricle.

frequently present with symptoms of endocrine failure, visual disturbances, or hydrocephalus as the tumor grows beyond the sella turcica and compresses the optic chiasm or other midline structures. The transphenoidal approach to this tumor is rarely used in pediatric patients and a majority of resections are performed by way of a frontal craniotomy. Anesthesia for craniopharyngioma and hypothalamic tumor surgery is similar to that for supratentorial craniotomy.

Preoperative evaluation of the child with craniopharyngioma is focused on the recognition of the presence of hydrocephalus and the types of endocrine dysfunction that could affect anesthetic management. Children may present with symptoms of hypothyroidism, growth hormone deficiency, corticotropin deficiency or diabetes insipidus.[291] Hormone replacement may be necessary both preoperatively and postoperatively with thyroid hormone and corticosteroids.

Diabetes insipidus is a complication of pituitary surgery. It may also be associated with other cerebral pathology such as head injury and is secondary to the disruption of antidiuretic hormone (ADH)-secreting cells. Rarely present preoperatively, it frequently presents in the immediate postoperative period beginning 4 to 6 h after completion of surgery. It may occasionally become evident intraoperatively. Characteristically, patients produce a large quantity of dilute urine in association with a rising serum osmolality and low urine osmolality (usually < 200 mosm/liter). The easiest and most appropriate test at the bedside is to determine the urine specific gravity, which will, in the presence of diabetes insipidus, be lower than 1.002 with the patient becoming hypernatremic and hypovolemic. When the diagnosis of diabetes insipidus is established, fluid therapy should begin. The appropriate regimen is determined by the patient's hourly urine output. Maintenance fluids should be administered together with three-quarters of the previous hour's urine output. The choice of fluid to be administered is determined by the patient's electrolyte levels. The fluid loss consists of urine that is low in sodium content. Therapy consists therefore, of fluid replacement with hypotonic solutions such as half-normal saline with D_5W and replacement of lost electrolytes. Hyperglycemia and superimposed osmotic diuresis may occur if a large volume of D_5W is used. It is now routine to administer vasopressin or one of its analogues such as DDAVP in an early stage. If administered intraoperatively, the aqueous solution of DDAVP, although free of cardiovascular side effects, may occasionally produce hypertension. Postoperatively the intranasal route is often used, and the dose of DDAVP is 0.05 to 0.3 ml/day divided into two doses (5 to 30 μg/day). If the intravenous route is chosen the dose should be one-tenth of the intranasal dose also divided into two doses daily. Vasopression can also be administered through an infusion and the rate is 0.5 mU/kg per h. The rate must be adjusted until the desired antidiuresis is achieved.

Additionally, the postoperative management should include the administration of steroid, thyroid, mineralocorticoid, and sex hormone supplements. Insulin-dependent diabetic patients may have reduced insulin requirements after surgery. Their blood glucose levels must be closely monitored and their insulin regimens altered.[292]

Other problems arising in the postoperative period include seizures and hyperthermia. Adequate surgical exposure requires significant retraction of the frontal lobes and anticonvulsant prophylaxis may begin intraoperatively and be continued into the postsurgical period. Injury to the hypothalamic thermoregulatory mechanisms may result in hyperthermia. Efforts should be made to maintain normothermia and reduce the risk of hypermetabolic cell injury.

POSTERIOR FOSSA SURGERY

Posterior fossa tumors (Fig. 35-34) occur more frequently in children than in adults and 50 to 55 percent of all pediatric brain tumors are infratentorial.[293] The four common types include medulloblastoma (30 percent), cerebellar astrocytoma (30 percent), brainstem

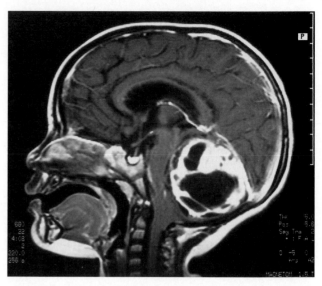

Figure 35-34 Sagittal MRI scan with gadolinium of 3-year-old girl with a large posterior fossa tumor. The tumor fills the posterior fossa and is causing some brainstem compression. At surgery, the tumor was removed through a posterior fossa craniotomy and proved to be a low-grade cerebellar astrocytoma.

glioma (30 percent), and ependymoma (7 percent). The remaining 3 percent include acoustic neuroma (Fig. 35-35), meningioma, ganglioglioma, and so forth. Cerebellar astrocytomas have no sex predilection but medulloblastoma occurs more frequently in males.[294] The common symptoms of a posterior fossa tumor in children are due to hydrocephalus, which is present in 90 percent of children with medulloblastoma and in virtually all children with cerebellar astrocytoma (see Fig. 35-12).[295]

The most frequent nontumoral posterior fossa procedure is decompression for Arnold-Chiari malformation with obex occlusion (Fig. 35-36). The Arnold-Chiari malformation is a comlex developmental anomaly characteristically presenting with downward displacement of the inferior cerebellar vermis into the upper cervical spinal canal with elogation of the medulla oblongata and the fourth ventricle. Preoperatively, the anesthesiologist should pay particular attention to the neurologic symptoms such as cerebellar dysfunction, evidence of upper airway obstruction (inspiratory stidor), cardiovascular instability, and increased ICP.

Anesthetic Considerations

1. Age-related pathophysiology
2. ICP: Associated symptomatic hydrocephalus external ventricular drain after induction of anesthesia. The maintenance of cerebral perfusion is essential. In addition, mannitol, furosemide, and corticosteroids may be given.
3. Full stomach: Posterior fossa pathology increases the

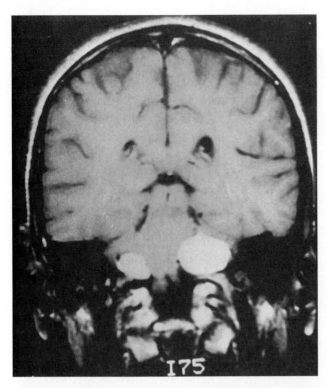

Figure 35-35 Coronal nuclear MRI through the brainstem and cerebellar pontine shows large round bilateral tumors indicating the presence of acoustic neuromas in a patient with neurofibromatosis.

gastric emptying in children and makes the patient prone to regurgitation at induction.

4. Associated preexisting problems: *Cardiovascular system*: some patients may be hypertensive as a response to brainstem compression. *Pulmonary system*: recurrent aspiration pneumonia is a common occurrence. *Nervous system*: central sleep apnea occurs and may persist postoperatively.
5. Air embolism
6. Airway management: Arnold-Chiari malformation or brainstem compression may cause upper airway dysfunction with inspiratory stridor.
7. Fluid and electrolytes: Preoperative attempt to reduce ICP may generate electrolyte imbalance and intravascular volume contraction.
8. Premedication: Discussed previously.

Preoperative Evaluation and Induction of Anesthesia

The preinduction assessment is similar to that described previously. It is important to reinforce that every neuroanesthesiologist should always be familiar with the radiologic findings before proceeding with the anesthetic induction.

The induction of anesthesia must be aimed at preserving CPP, avoiding an increase in ICP, and providing an appropriate depth of anesthesia. The choice of anesthetic is not as crucial as the manner in which the medications are administered. A combination of thiopental, atropine, and a nondepolarizing muscle relaxant, associated with a narcotic such as fentanyl, constitute the authors' anesthetic preferences. Succinylcholine can be used safely[296] unless the patient shows signs of severe ICP with hemodynamic instability. To minimize the possibility of kinking and obstruction, a reinforced armored orotracheal tube may be used. Although many neuroanesthesiologists prefer a nasotracheal tube for better stability and fixation, we prefer an oral tracheal tube with soft bite block to eliminate epistaxis and possible infection.

Maintenance

As with induction of anesthesia, no single anesthetic technique has been shown to be superior[297] and the maintenance regimen must be tailored to the need of the patient and the requirement of the surgical procedure. After skin preparation, local anesthetic (bupivacaine 0.125% with epinephrine 1:200,000) should be infiltrated along the incision line[199] and anesthesia depth should be increased with fentanyl or isoflurane. The aim is to provide a "slack brain," which will reduce the amount of retractor pressure and allow adequate cerebral perfusion. A nondepolarizing muscle relaxant is given and the ICP is reduced by mannitol preceded by furosemide. During the initial surgical approach, the IPPV is adjusted to maintain the Pa_{CO_2} in the range of 25 to 28 mmHg.

Patient Positioning

Three common patient positions are used for posterior fossa tumor operations. The prone position is used in 55 percent of all procedures, the sitting position in 30 percent, and the lateral position in 15 percent.[295] At our institution, all surgical procedures in the posterior cranial fossa or the upper cervical spine are performed in the prone position (Fig. 35-37)[298] with the patient lying on U bolsters or a Relton frame.[299] It is the anesthesiologist's responsibility to apply special care during positioning with regard to ventilation, pressure points, and ensuring that flexion of the head does not occlude jugular venous drainage nor displace the endotracheal tube to an endobronchial position. The method of head fixation depends on the age of the patient (thickness of the skull) and also to the preference of the surgeon. Horse-shoe head rests are appropriate but the face of the patient must be padded carefully with special attention to the eyes. In children greater than 3 years of age, the multipin head holder using 30 to 40 lb of tension per pin is preferable. Infiltration of the pin sites with local anesthetic will reduce nociceptive responses.

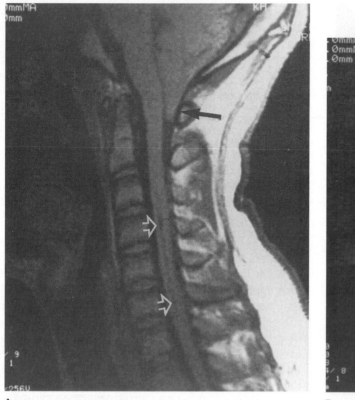

A

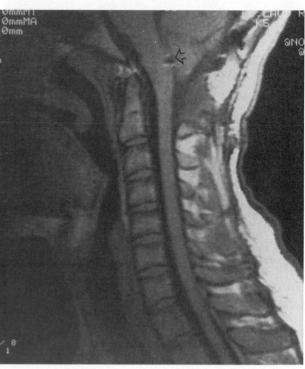

B

Figure 35-36 *A.* Mid-sagittal nuclear MRI of an Arnold-Chiari I malformation showing the cerebellar tonsil engaged through the foramen Magnum (*black arrow*) and the association of a cervicospinal syringomyelia (*open white arrows*). *B.* Posterior fossa decompression with occlusion of the obex using fat (*open black arrow*). The cervicospinal syrinx has disappeared.

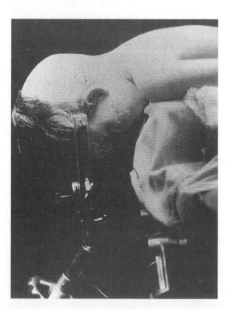

Figure 35-37 Posterior fossa surgery in the prone position. The patient is positioned on U bolsters or frame to facilitate pulmonary ventilation; pressure points must be carefully padded and the anesthesiologist must pay special attention to the flexion of the head to avoid occlusion of jugular venous drainage. Particular care must also be given to the endotracheal tube.

Monitoring

Monitoring for posterior fossa surgery is basically the same as in supratentorial craniotomy with the important exception of the precordial Doppler for detection of air embolism and the occasional use of sensory-evoked potentials for intramedullary or brainstem tumor.

Emergence and Recovery

The need for prompt awakening is mandatory but must be combined with the need for a hemodynamically stable and unstimulated patient during extubation. An understanding of the pathologic process will indicate the correct airway management postoperatively (e.g., tracheal intubation is essential postoperatively following resection of intramedullary tumor). In cases where extubation is appropriate, the preoperative administration of narcotics associated with lidocaine 0.5 to 1.0 mg/kg in infants and children will facilitate the emergence by reducing coughing and straining, which could otherwise lead to a hypertensive episode and intracerebral bleeding. Postoperative pain management can usually be achieved with codeine with or without acetaminophen. The necessity to avoid medication that affects the sensorium or the pupils is important.

CEREBROVASCULAR ANOMALIES

Arteriovenous malformations are uncommon congenital or acquired lesions that provide an important anesthetic challenge mainly in infants and children.[300] Congenital AVMs and arterial aneurysms arise from an abnormal development of the arteriocapillary network connecting the arterial and venous systems. These vascular malformations consist of large arterial feeding vessels that lead to dilated communicating vessels and finally to veins, which are easily identifiable because they carry arterialized blood. Flow of blood through the low resistance arteriocapillary circuitry results in progressive distension and dilatation of the entire venous system of the brain and cranium.[34] Several specific vascular anomalies are known in the pediatric population such as those involving the posterior cerebral artery and the great vein of Galen (see Fig. 35-21). They usually present clinically in the newborn period with CHF.[300] The saccular dilatation of the vein of Galen may be associated with hydrocephalus due to the obstruction of the aqueduct of Sylvius.[301] Although moyamoya disease in not neurologically classified as an AVM, similar anesthetic considerations apply.[34,302] Moyamoya disease is a chronic occlusive cerebrovascular disease of the basal cerebral arteries, which leads to severe dilatation of perforating arteries at the base of the brain to form the so-called moyamoya vessel.[303,304] It is important to note that moyamoya has been reported to be associated with progressive myopathy.[305] Most AVMS go undetected until the fourth or fifth decade of life and only 18 percent present below the age of 15 years. Cerebral injury may ensure due to one or more causes:

1. Hemorrhage with thrombosis and infarction
2. Compression of adjacent neural structures
3. Parenchymal ischemia caused by "steal" of blood flow to the low-resistance network
4. CHF and hypoperfusion
5. Surgical disruption or diversion of the blood flow.

Patients with AVMs may undergo radiologically controlled embolization of the arterial blood supply or stereotactic radiosurgery as definitive or adjunctive therapy. Surgical clipping of feeding vessels may be performed as a single or staged procedure.

ANESTHETIC CONSIDERATIONS

Considerations for patients undergoing AVM resection are:

1. Preexisting pathophysiology: Does the patient present with increased ICP or CHF? Does the patient have associated congenital defects?
2. Age-related pathophysiology: Will organ system immaturity have an impact on the anesthetic technique?
3. Blood loss: The possibility of massive blood loss is real. Appropriate precautions must be taken.
4. Ventilation pattern: The indication for hyperventilation in the patient with vascular anomalies becomes a contraindication with moyamoya disease.

MONITORING

Routine monitoring has been described previously. Patients undergoing AVM resection should have at least two large-bore intravenous catheters with blood pumps in place before surgery. Intravenous solutions should be warmed from the beginning of the procedure. Arterial line placement is essential. CVP monitoring is always used on all but the smallest AVMs. Urinary catheter placement is mandatory following induction of anesthesia.

PREINDUCTION

Symptomatology varies with the age at which the disease presents.[300] Older children most commonly present with evidence of subarachnoid hemorrhage or intraventricular hemorrhage. Over 70 percent of pediatric patients presenting with spontaneous subarachnoid hemorrhage have AVMs as the causative etiology. Seizure is the presenting symptom in approximately 25 percent of patients. The neonatal presentation of cerebral AVM is the most challenging because it is often associated with CHF.

The low-resistance pathway of the AVM results in volume overload and signs of right heart failure. The CHF rarely presents in utero and patency of the ductus arteriosis may supply a pressure release for the right ventricle by pumping into the low-resistance placental circulation. The demand for increased cardiac output as well as increased pulmonary blood flow as pulmonary vascular resistance decreases may precipitate left ventricular failure. The low resistance of the cerebral AVM results in a low systemic diastolic pressure combined with an increased left ventricular end-diastolic pressure from overload. Coronary perfusion pressure is thus reduced and myocardial ischemia ensues.[160] Right-to-left ductal shunting may occur and can divert a majority of descending aortic blood flow to the cerebral circulation. Thus, cardiac failure in these infants is secondary to both pressure and volume overload and present with a picture similar to persistent fetal circulation.[306,307] Physical examination will show signs of left or right heart failure such as tachypnea, tachycardia, cyanosis, pulmonary edema, hepatomegaly, and

ECG changes. Laboratory studies will provide evidence of severe electrolyte imbalances that are the inevitable result of aggressive diuretic therapy. Neonates in severe CHF receive digoxin therapy and may well require tracheal intubation with mechanical ventilation and continuous intravenous inotropic support. Patients without evidence of CHF can be premedicated to reduce agitation and hypertension prior to induction.

INDUCTION AND INTUBATION

Central to induction of anesthesia in children with AVM without CHF is prevention of hypertension during laryngoscopy. Inhalation or intravenous induction may be performed in the child without evidence of increased ICP. Incremental doses of intravenous induction agent and narcotic are given along with lidocaine prior to laryngoscopy. A nondepolarizing muscle relaxant is recommended. Neonates in CHF will have intravenous access in place before induction. Extreme caution must be observed because many anesthetic agents used during induction (including lidocaine) are myocardial depressants and may precipitate cardiovascular collapse.[187] Oral or nasal intubation may proceed as the anesthetist prefers.

MAINTENANCE

Considerations for maintenance of anesthesia include:

1. Positioning
2. Ventilation
3. Anesthetic agents
4. Blood loss and fluid management
5. Temperature maintenance

Positioning for surgery depends on the site of the malformation. The AVMs most commonly receive their blood supply from the middle meningeal artery distribution and are approached by supratentorial craniotomy.

All patients are mechanically ventilated for control of Pa_{CO_2}. Patients with hydrocephalus may require some degree of hyperventilation until the pressure is relieved. It is our practice to maintain normocarbia in children undergoing AVM resection based on the assumption that hypocarbia will decrease CBF in normal vessels and shunt additional blood flow to the low-resistance malformed vessels. This could result in ischemia of brain parenchyma and increase bleeding from the AVM.

Anesthetic agents selected for maintenance are similar to those used for any intracranial procedure. In the absence of CHF, a hypotensive technique may be used at time of ligation of the AVM using drugs such as trimethaphan, nitroprusside, nitroglycerin, or high concentrations of isoflurane. We have found a phentol-

amine infusion to be particularly useful, easily titrateable, and predictable. Neonates in CHF are usually on inotropic support and cannot tolerate hypotensive anesthesia. Vasoactive drugs should be infused via central lines if possible.

Fluid management in these patients is difficult. Neonates may not tolerate fluid loads at all and children with contracted intravascular compartments resulting from attempts at brain dehydration may experience rapid circulatory collapse following brisk intraoperative bleeding.

Maintaining body temperature can be difficult in children especially during massive transfusion.[308] It may be beneficial to allow the patient's core temperature to decrease to 34°C to provide the beneficial cerebral protective effect of mild hypothermia.[309–311] A recent study using canine model of transient, complete cerebral ischemia demonstrated that even small, clinically relevant changes in temperature (1° or 2°C) resulted in significant alterations in both postischemic neurologic function and cerebral histopathology.[312] Assuming that these results are transferable to humans, it suggests that, in patients at imminent risk for ischemic neurologic injury, body temperature should be closely monitored. Further, the clinician should aggressively treat all episodes of hyperthermia until the patient is not longer at risk for ischemic neurologic injury.

EMERGENCE

Considerations for emergence from anesthesia include:

1. Elimination of anesthetic agents
2. Reversal of neuromuscular blockade
3. Assessment of airway patency and respiration

Patients without a history of CHF may be extubated following the elimination of anesthetic agents and reversal of neuromuscular blockade. Patients with a likelihood of significant neurologic deficit, extensive resection, brain retraction, or cerebral edema remain sedated and intubated into the postoperative period.

POSTOPERATIVE MANAGEMENT

The basic anesthetic considerations for postoperative care have been discussed. More specific to the postoperative management of these patients are:

1. Cerebral edema
2. CHF
3. Hypertension
4. Vasospasm

Cerebral edema resulting from the lesion or secondary to the surgical procedure may require further therapeutic intervention such as continuous mechanical ventilatory support and pharmaceutical adjuncts. As such, the transfer to the intensive care unit is indicated. It is not unusual for the patient with severe AVM to return to full consciousness following surgical removal after several days only. During this period of time, close neurologic observation is required to detect possible clinical deterioration.

Although the AVM obliteration reduces the right-to-left shunt, the patient with preoperative CHF usually remains in a precarious medical state in the postoperative period and requires transfer to an intensive care unit for observation and continuous therapy. The necessity to not only maintain adequate CPP, but to reduce the cardiac overload as well, makes the management rather difficult.

In conjunction with analgesics, antihypertensive therapy may be required to avoid sudden increases in blood pressure, which could precipitate rebleeding.

Vasospasm is not a common postoperative complication of cerebrovascular surgery but must be considered with neurologic deterioration. The pathogenesis of vasospasm is poorly understood but its early diagnosis is crucial for the future outcome of the patient. The detection and prevention of vasospasm are essential during postoperative care. The use of transcranial Doppler sonography is helpful in the diagnosis of this complication. The treatment of vasospasm is limited but the use of calcium blocker agents has received interesting attention.

SURGERY FOR EPILEPSY

Specific anesthetic considerations for surgical procedure for the relief of epilepsy include:

1. The awake patient
2. Analgesia
3. Airway maintenance

The conduct of an anesthetic for excision of a seizure focus is most challenging. It requires a sedated patient who is cooperative to identify the precise surgical site using preoperative cortical EEG (Fig. 35-38). Neuroleptanalgesia remains the technique of choice, although propofol total intravenous anesthesia has gained popularity recently. Anesthesia is induced with a neuroleptic agent such as droperidol together with fentanyl. The analgesic state is maintained by serial doses of fentanyl citrate. No additional droperidol should be given following the induction dose because it will impair the patient's ability to cooperate in the identification of the speech and motor area. The administration of N_2O in O_2 by loosely fit mask or soft nasopharyngeal cannulae can be used as adjunct to the intravenous analgesia until cortical mapping is performed. The use of nasopharyngeal cannulae makes

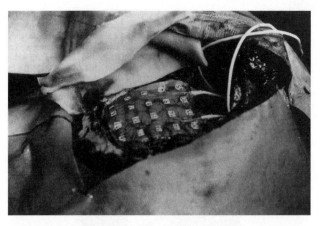

Figure 35-38   Electrocortography. The use of neuroleptanesthesia is essential for cortical EEG mapping during surgery for epilepsy. Cortical mapping is an integral part of this surgical procedure to detect the epileptic focus.

the measurement of end-tidal carbon dioxide possible and the administration of fresh gases to the patient more efficient. Arterial and central line placement is accomplished with local anesthetic infiltration. Generous local anesthetic infiltration is performed during placement of the multipin head holder and prior to skin incision.[199] Analgesia is supplemented throughout the procedure with additional doses of fentanyl in a dose sufficient to keep the respiratory rate between 8 and 16 breaths per minute. Verbal encouragement may be necessary to achieve this.

We have found this technique acceptable in children above 4 years of age. Younger patients are usually unable to cooperate and require tracheal intubation and general anesthesia. Limitations of the neuroleptanalgesia technique include: (1) restlessness in children who must remain motionless for a long period in an uncomfortable position; (2) breakthrough pain during dural manipulation and electrocautery; and (3) poor cooperation in the psychologically disturbed child with seizure disorder.

MYELODYSPLASIA

Hydrocephalus is accompanied by abnormalities in the spinal column and spinal cord in some 70 percent of hydrocephalic infants.[313] Myelodysplasia refers to an abnormality in the fusion of the embryologic neural groove that normally closes in the first month of gestation. Failure of neural tube closure results in the saclike herniation of meninges (meningocele) or a herniation containing neural elements (myelomeningocele). The spinal cord is often tethered caudally by the sacral roots resulting in orthopedic or urologic symptoms in later childhood if it is not surgically corrected (Fig. 35-39). Myelomeningoceles most commonly occur in the

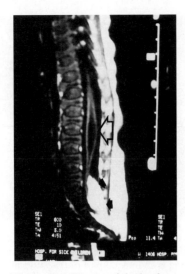

Figure 35-39 Mid-sagittal CT scan of the lumbosacral spine demonstrated a lipomyelomeningocele. The spinal cord lies abnormal and low due to its tethering at the site of the lipomeningocele (*white arrow*). A large syrinx is seen throughout the length of the cord (*open black arrow*).

lumbosacral region but failure of rostral fusion of the neural groove can result in their formation at any level in the neuraxis. Most children with meningomyelocele with also have an associated Arnold-Chiari type II acquired malformation (Fig. 35-40); therefore, hydrocephaly will develop and become part of the anesthetic considerations. An encephalocele is most frequently found in the occipital/suboccipital or nasal area (Fig. 35-41). Anencephaly represents a defect in anterior closure of the neural groove.

Exposed CNS tissue places the patient at extreme risk of infection, which is the single most common cause of death.[314] Patients younger than 1 year old have a greater risk of infection than older children. Myelomeningocele and meningitis have the higher infection rate among other etiologies.[314,315] Studies have demonstrated the incidence of infection is related to the length of time the lesion remains unrepaired. The incidence of ventriculitis is directly proportional to the speed with which the myelomeningocele is surgically repaired. It is less than 7 percent if the surgical repair is performed within 48 h of birth and 37 percent in those taken care after that time.[315,316] A further reason to avoid delay in closure is the likelihood of progressive neural damage with eventual decrease in the motor function.[317] For these reasons, myelodysplasia is regarded as a surgical emergency and most neonates will present for closure in the first 24 h of life.

NEUROSURGICAL CONSIDERATIONS
Early neurosurgical repair of a myelomeningocele will lead to the restoration of a more normal configuration of the spine, which will facilitate the care and future handling of the back of the child. Although techniques of closure vary somewhat, a standard five-layer closure is usually performed first with the reconvolution of the spinal cord by closing the pia-arachnoid with a running suture. This is followed by closure of the dura, iliocostal fascia, subcutaneous tissue, and finally skin. Occasionally, for widely splayed and deformed laminae, a kyphectomy may be performed to help restore the bony contour of the spine. With open neural tube defects, the skin is always deficient and significant undermining of subcutaneous skin flaps is required. This may lead to the creation of large potential spaces into which occult bleeding may occur about which the neuroanesthesiologist must be aware during the dissection. In addition, for very large skin defects, myocutaneous flaps may need to be raised and swung over the repaired neural tube. The elevation of such flaps will add considerable anesthetic time to a typically short procedure, and in such instances, the anesthesiologist will need to gauge the anesthetic procedure accordingly.

ANESTHETIC CONSIDERATIONS

1. Coexisting disease: Additional pathology may accompany myelodysplasia (Arnold-Chiari, hydrocephalus).

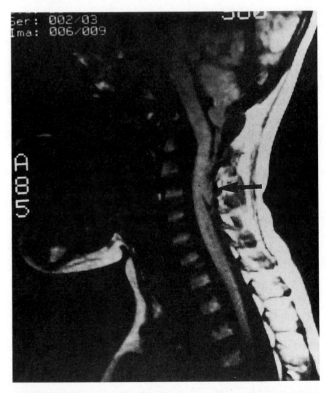

Figure 35-40 Mid-sagittal nuclear MRI demonstrates an Arnold-Chiari malformation type II. The cerebellar tonsils can be seen as low as the fifth cervical vertebral body within the cervical spinal canal (*black arrow*).

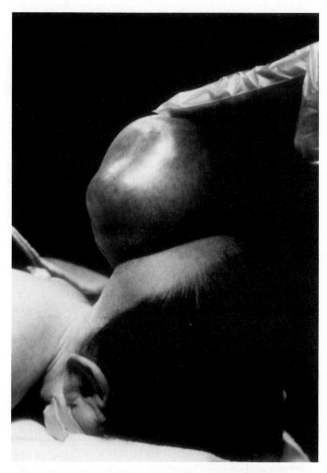

Figure 35-41   Preoperative demonstration of large occipital encephalocele. The patient is prone. The encephalocele is covered with atrophic skin and contains both CSF and dysgenetic brain tissue. Large encephaloceles such as this one will frequently require that the infant is intubated in the lateral position to prevent direct pressure on the sac and its contents.

2. Age-related pathophysiology: Discussed previously.
3. Airway management: Encephaloceles may present particular difficulty in control of the airway.
4. Positioning: Protection of the neuroplaque
5. Volume status: High third-space losses from the skin defect
6. Potential for hypothermia: Exposure of large body surface area and loss of third-space fluid

MONITORING

Routine monitoring is included. Blood loss can be insidious especially if the sac is large and significant undermining of skin, relaxing incisions, or grafting is required for closure. Blood transfusion may become necessary. Patients with encephaloceles who must undergo craniotomy for repair should have an arterial line placed for blood pressure and hemoglobin measurement. A central venous line may become indicated

for a nasal encephalocele that is commonly repaired with the patient in a semi-sitting position.

PREINDUCTION

Infants presenting for repair of meningomyeloceles rarely exhibit increased ICP. The majority of myelodysplatic patients have an associated Arnold-Chiari malformation and may have an associated hydrocephalus, which will not always require ventricular shunt placement. Preoperatively, these children show varied neurologic deficits depending on the level of the lesion. Seventy-five percent of all lesions occur in the lumbosacral region, with lesions above T4 usually resulting in total paraplegia and lesions below S1 allowing ambulation. The legs are severely affected by lesions between L4 and S3.[316,318] Prior to induction of anesthesia, volume status of the patient should be assessed in light of the large potential third-space losses from the exposed myelomeningocele.

INDUCTION AND INTUBATION

Patients with lumbosacral or thoracic myelomeningoceles may be induced either in the left lateral position or alternatively supine with the sac protected with a cushioned ring. A majority of patients can be induced intravenously with thiopental, atropine, and a muscle relaxant before tracheal intubation. Awake laryngoscopy and tracheal intubation after giving atropine intravenously is an alternative technique. Either a nondepolarizing muscle relaxant or succinylcholine may be used safely.[319] Caution should be observed when inducing patients with nasal encephalocele because airway obstruction is common and poor mask fit may be encountered.

MAINTENANCE

The anesthetic considerations for maintenance of anesthesia are:

1. Positioning
2. Ventilation
3. Anesthetic agents
4. Muscle relaxants
5. Fluid management
6. Maintenance of body temperature

After intubation, the patient should be turned to the prone position avoiding injury to the exposed neural tissue (Fig. 35-42). Chest and hip rolls are then placed to ensure that the abdomen hangs free to facilitate ventilation and reduce intra-abdominal pressure, which may potentially increase bleeding from the epidural plexus. Because most of these children have an Arnold-Chiari malformation with cervical neurologic considerations, care should be taken to avoid excessive

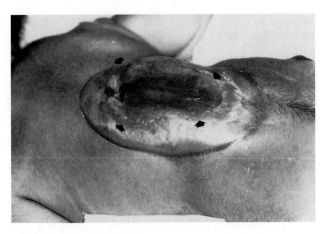

Figure 35-42   Myelomeningocele. The central darker nonepithelial region represents the neuroplaque (unprotected neural tissue) (*black arrows*).

rotation of the neck. Extremities should lie in a relaxed position and be well padded.

Mechanical ventilation is used in these patients and attention must be paid to the risk of barotrauma in the immature lung. Premature infants (especially those < 32 weeks and < 1500 g) are at increased risk of retinopathy of prematurity[320] and lung injury from prolonged exposure to high oxygen concentrations[321] and if possible, the forced inspired oxygen is adjusted in these patients to maintain a Pa_{O_2} of 60 to 70 mmHg and a saturation of 90% to 95%.

Anesthesia can be maintained with a variety of agents. Narcotics and ketamine should be avoided because they have been associated with a high incidence of postoperative apnea in neonates. Neurosurgeons may require selective nerve stimulation to identify neural structures. In this circumstance, muscle relaxants are contraindicated.

Blood loss is usually not excessive and fluid management is directed toward replacement of third-space losses. Should closure of the wound be extensive and blood loss greater than 10 percent of circulating blood volume adequate intravenous access for transfusion must be in place.

The large area of exposed tissue and the liberal use of surgical preparation solutions increase the risk of hypothermia in these patients. Active measures to prevent this have been described. Care must be taken to prevent drying or thermal injury to the exposed neural tissue by the use of radiant heat lamps.

EMERGENCE
Anesthetic considerations for emergence include:

1. Elimination of anesthetic agents
2. Reversal of neuromuscular blockade
3. Assessment of airway patency

Neonates at risk for apnea after anesthesia, patients with severe central neurologic deficits, or those undergoing craniotomy for encephalocele repair should have their tracheas extubated fully awake after elimination of the anesthetic agents and adequate reversal of muscle relaxants. Patients with repair of nasal encephaloceles may have residual obstruction or blood in the oropharynx. It may be necessary to delay extubation in these cases.

POSTOPERATIVE MANAGEMENT
Basic anesthetic considerations for the postoperative period have been discussed.

SPINAL CORD SURGERY

The most common diseases that require surgery on the spinal cord are herniated disks, spondylosis, syringomyelia, primary or metastatic tumors, hematomas or abscesses, and trauma. In all cases, compression of the spinal cord may produce ischemia,[322] interstitial edema, and venous congestion[323] and interfere with nerve transmission.[65,324] Maintaining SCPP and reducing cord compression are the crucial considerations in our clinical management.

Despite apparently optimal surgical and anesthetic management, devastating neurologic complications still occur during spinal surgery. Intraoperative monitoring of spinal cord function is an essential part of a safe anesthetic. Methods for monitoring the integrity of spinal cord function intraoperatively include: (1) the wake-up test, (2) somatosensory evoked potentials (SSEP), and (3) motor evoked potentials (MEP). The wake-up test remains the traditional method for assessing spinal cord function during corrective procedures on the spinal column. Its main advantage is that it assesses anterior spinal cord (i.e., motor) function, but its limitations are that it does so only at one point in time. The use of evoked potential monitors, though still not routine, is gaining popularity. SSEP monitoring involves the generation of electrical potentials within the neuraxis by stimulation of peripheral nerves such as the median nerve at the wrist or the posterior tibial nerve at the ankle. If transmission is intact, a signal is recorded from the scalp or at various sites along the neural pathway. The electrical signals are thought to arise from axonal action potentials and graded postsynaptic potentials during propagation of the impulse from the periphery to the brain.[325] The technique has limitations in that it applies only to the sensory nervous system. The appeal of MEP in which the motor cortex is stimulated by a transcranial electric current or a pulsed magnetic field generated by a coil placed over the scalp has generated increased interest.[326–328]

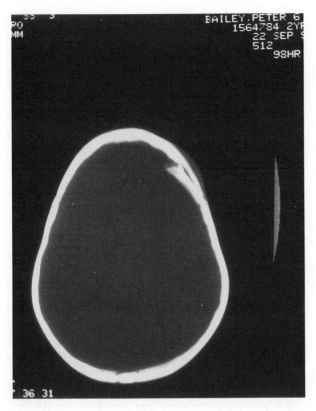

Figure 35-43 Depressed skull fracture in the left frontal region.

HEAD INJURY

Head trauma is a major cause of morbidity and mortality in the pediatric population.[329] Skull fractures (Fig. 35-43 and Table 35-6) are found in over one-fourth of all children who present at hospitals with head injuries[330] and in more than half the fatal cases of head trauma in childhood.[331] The incidence of posttraumatic intracranial hematomas varies considerably in children because only a minority of children with head injuries will become candidates for surgical decompression and treatment.[332] Despite this low incidence, failure to recognize the presence of a hematoma may transform an otherwise mild injury into a fatal or permanently disabling one. This medical complication must be recognized early and treated aggressively.

TABLE 35-6
Classification of Skull Fractures in Children

I. Linear

II. Depressed

III. Open (linear or depressed)[a]

III. Basal Skull Fracture[b]

[a] Open skull fractures generally mandate an anesthetic and neurosurgery for irrigation and debridement of involved tissues.

[b] One should not intubate with a nasal tube a patient suspected of having a basal skull fracture involving the anterior cranial fossa floor.

TABLE 35-7
Traumatic Pediatric Intracranial Hemorrhages

Epidural hematoma

Subdural hematoma

Subarachnoid hemorrhage

Intracerebral hematoma

Intraventricular hemorrhage

Head injury encompasses many different forms of trauma to the skull and brain, and the pathophysiologic events following head injury are subdivided into intracranial hematomas (epidural, subdural, intracerebral) (Table 35-7) brain contusion, brain edema, and systemic effects of head injury. There is a significant difference between adult and children with respect to the pattern of injury sustained. Adults suffer more hematomas than children, but diffuse cerebral edema occurs more often in the pediatric population.[333]

Epidural hematoma is most frequently caused by arterial bleeding from a middle meningeal artery torn in the course of a deceleration injury, but these children do not necessarily show an overlying skull fracture. Epidural hematomas comprise 25 percent of all intracranial hematomas in the pediatric population and are one of the true neurosurgical emergencies (Fig. 35-44). The clinical presentation in the adult population is described as a period of lucidity between an initial loss of consciousness and later neurologic deterioration. In children, the initial alteration in the state of consciousness reported in adults is often not seen. When a child is

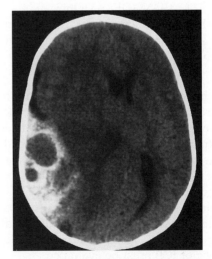

Figure 35-44 Axial CT scan of an acute epidural hematoma in 2-year-old boy causing mass effect and shift of brain from right to left. The ventricles are pushed across the midline. Acute epidural hematomas such as this are life-threatening emergencies that demand the swift activation of a skilled team of neuroanesthesiologists and neurosurgeons.

lucid and old enough to complain verbally, increasing headache will continue until the patient becomes confused or lethargic. However, the rapid development of hemiparesis, posturing, and pupillary dilatation is also typical and may confuse the diagnosis. The pathologic process is explained by a rapid expansion of the hematoma leading to a herniation of the temporal lobe downward through the tentoria incisura. One of the earliest signs is anisocoria resulting from loss of the pupilloconstrictor innervation of the oculomotor nerve. This herniation will eventually lead to a syndrome of rostrocaudal deterioration that is classically associated with Cushing's triad of bradycardia, slowed and irregular breathing, and widened pulse pressure.[170] Although the relationship between the degree of brain shift and the level of consciousness has been confirmed, the role of uncal herniation in the syndrome has been questioned.[334]

Subdural hematoma is associated with cortical damage due to parenchymal contusion and blood vessel laceration. The mass effect of the contused and edematous brain may prompt surgical removal of the hematoma if the brain region involved is not functionally important. Recent studies using positron emission tomography have demonstrated that in patients with brain contusion the cerebral metabolism and blood flow were reduced by 50 percent.[335] Severe edema and ICP will often lead to persistent neurologic deficits in the postoperative period (Fig. 35-45).

Intracerebral hematoma is rare but carries a poor prognosis. Intraparenchymal hematoma does not require surgery for fear of damaging viable brain tissue.

ANESTHETIC CONSIDERATIONS

The anesthesiologist usually sees these children during the early stages of trauma care. There are several considerations:

1. Resuscitation and stabilization: Airway, breathing, and circulation are the essential component of the initial clinical assessment. The traumatized patient may often have a variety of physiologic disturbances such as acid-base and electrolytes imbalance. Glucose homeostasis and body temperature control may be disturbed.
2. Neurologic status: The use of the Glasgow coma scale provides a baseline from which subsequent changes can be evaluated. Symptomatology leading to the presence of ICP must be evaluated.
3. Associated injuries: Pediatric trauma is often associated with high-velocity energy transfer that leads to associated injuries to the neck, chest, and abdominal organs.
4. Full stomach: Evidence of vomiting may suggests

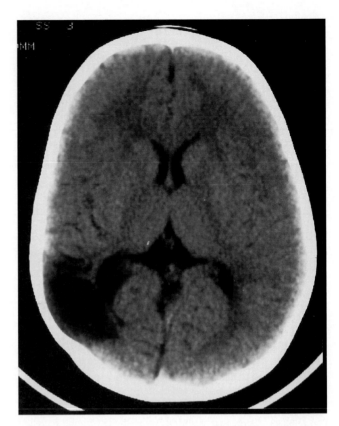

Figure 35-45 Axial CT scan several months after the evacuation of the epidural hematoma showing successful resolution of the midline shift. A small area of occipital brain infarction in the territory of the posterior cerebral artery is seen. This child had a complete recovery without neurologic deficit.

pulmonary aspiration and respiratory complications.
5. Age-related pathophysiology

MONITORING

Routine monitoring has been discussed earlier. Arterial catheter and central venous line placement are indicated. A urinary bladder catheter should be inserted unless contraindicated by an associated bladder neck injury. Central body temperature should be monitored at all times.

PREINDUCTION

Computed tomography scan remains the procedure of choice during the first 72 h for the evaluation of the patient with head injury. The management of an elevated ICP is paramount to a safe anesthetic. However, adequate hemodynamic resuscitation and stabilization must be achieved to maintain adequate CPP and brain tissue oxygenation.

INDUCTION AND INTUBATION

Providing a patent airway is an essential part of the management of the patient with head injury. Although the airway may not be compromised by the injury in a patient with a changing level of consciousness, it is appropriate to proceed with tracheal intubation to protect the lungs against aspiration of stomach contents or secretions and to provide ventilatory support as part of the management of increased ICP. Because the association of head injury and neck injury in infants and children is important, it is mandatory that ventilatory assistance be accomplished with minimal manipulation. Stabilization of the head by an assistant with axial traction is indicated. Until proven otherwise, a cervical spine fracture is always to be considered in the management of a patient with head injury and should be treated accordingly. Therefore, the use of the Sellick maneuver is contraindicated. Patients not already on ventilatory support but undergoing evacuation of intracranial hematoma should be hemodynamically stable before induction of anesthesia. After a difficult airway has been ruled out, induction of anesthesia should proceed in a rapid sequence fashion with atropine, thiopentone, lidocaine, and either succinylcholine or a nondepolarizing muscle relaxant such as vecuronium. Ketamine remains contraindicated. Induction of anesthesia for patients with a suspected difficult airway may require a two-person technique. Depending on the age of the patient, the use of volatile anesthetic with assisted ventilation or the use of neuroleptanesthesia with topical anesthesia to the larynx is recommended.

MAINTENANCE

The anesthetic considerations for maintenance of anesthesia are similar to those previously described in the supratentorial section above. Evacuation of intracranial hematomas usually involves a craniotomy for exploration without opening of the dura mater. However, it must be noted that large hematomas may, on evacuation, cause a sudden release of ICP with consequent upward movement of the brainstem through the tentoria incisura. The consequences may be transient hemodyamic instability associated with cardiac arrhythmias.

EMERGENCE
AND POSTOPERATIVE MANAGEMENT

Patients with severe head injury will remain intubated for ventilatory support and control of the elevated ICP due to cerebral edema. The transfer to an intensive care unit is indicated for continued care.

CERVICAL SPINAL CORD INJURY

Because isolated cervical spine injury is rare in the pediatric population compared to adults, all children with a severe head injury should be treated as candi-

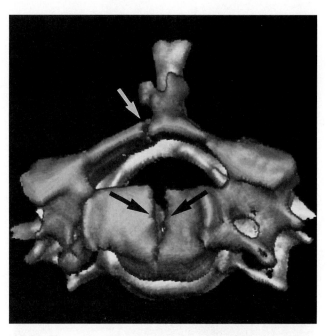

Figure 35-46 Three-dimensional CT scan demonstrates the effect of high-velocity cervical spine fracture in a teenage boy. The C5 vertebral body has been compressed and demonstrates a sagittal split (*black arrows*). There is also a fracture of the right posterior lamina of C5 (*white arrow*). Such a cervical spine injury must be construed as highly unstable until proven otherwise. All cervical spine precautions must be undertaken before, during, and after intubating patients with these injuries.

dates for cervical spine injury until proven otherwise. Their management requires similar strategies as those provided for the adults. The mechanism of injury of high cervical cord is associated with high-velocity injuries to the cranium in children (Fig. 35-46). The classical representation of cord injury or disruption may be the patient discovered without respiratory efforts and usually in cardiac arrest or profound hypotension leading subsequently to death from hypoxic/ischemic encephalopathy with or without a serious traumatic brain injury.[336] In this study, all patients with absence of vital signs had confirmation on a lateral view x-ray of the neck of the presence of high cervical cord luxation. The physician not aware of this clinical scenario might think that this situation is related only to blood loss due to intraabdominal, pelvic, or thoracic injury or even devastating cerebral injury with loss of brain stem function but not the cervical spine!

The state-of-the-art management of pediatric patients with unstable spinal cord fractures in the operating room now mandates the use of a tracheal intubation performed during constant sedation or neuroleptic anesthesia ensuring the patient's cooperation during positioning while under continuous evoked potential monitoring. The continuous recording of the evoked potentials is essential immedi-

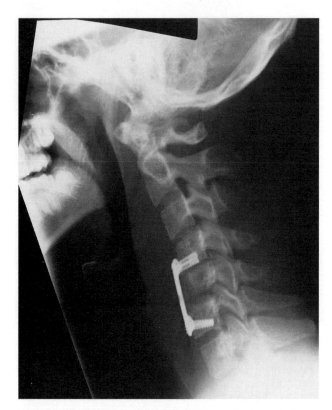

Figure 35-47 Lateral cervical spine x-ray postinstrumentation of the cervical spine with an anterior vertebral body plate and screws. The titanium plate is applied through an anterior cervical exposure. In many instances, the application of such plates obviates the need for a halo crown and vest.

ately before positioning to obtain a baseline recording. After the patient is positioned prone and demonstrates ability to move the extremeties to command and after the evoked potentials are constant with the prepositioning recording, the patient can be safely anesthetized.

Stabilization of the cervical spine can now be safely performed in the pediatric age group at surgery using bone graft, wires, or titanium plating systems (Figs. 35-47 and 35-48). Intraoperative evoked potentials should be used throughout the procedure until the patient is turned supine and extubated and can follow commands.

ANESTHETIC CONSIDERATIONS AND MANAGEMENT

Some cervical spine injury victims may have signs of brain shift and elevated ICP. The anesthetic considerations for these patients include:

1. Resuscitation and stabilization of cardiopulmonary function
2. ICP reduction and improvement of cerebral perfusion

3. Cervical spine injury: stabilization and management
4. Cardiovascular and metabolic disturbances
5. Acute respiratory distress syndrome
6. Associated injuries and identification of the central rostrocaudal deterioration and uncal herniation
7. Age-related problems
8. Fluid therapy guided by the usual requirements for trauma victims avoiding lactated Ringer's solution in favor of iso-osmolar solutions such as normal saline
9. Monitoring, including arterial line, central venous line, urinary catheter
10. Coagulopathy activated by brain tissue thromboplastin release must be often corrected
11. Treatment of diabetes insipidus is mandatory (see craniopharyngioma).
12. SIADH based on the finding of hyponatremia in the absence of hypovolemia or sodium retention, urine sodium above 40 meq/liter[337]

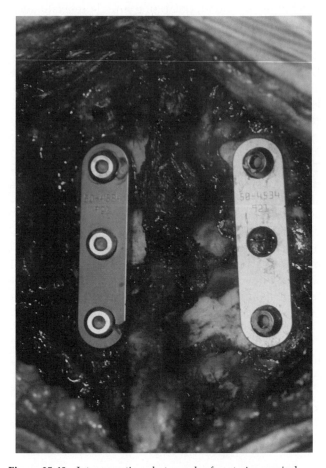

Figure 35-48 Intraoperative photograph of posterior cervical spine and lateral mass plates. These titanium plates are applied from a posterior cervical exposure with the patient placed prone on the table. The plates are placed over the lateral masses of the cervical vertebrae, and the screws are placed so as to hold the plates firmly attached to the lateral masses.

13. Hyperglycemia occurs frequently in head-injured patients and is thought to be a good indicator of the severity of the injury and a predictor of outcome.[338] It is advisable to prevent the increase in glucose and avoid the neurologic deficit associated with this problem.[339]

References

1. Kleinman S, Bissonnette B: Management of successful pediatric neuroanesthesia. In Bissonnette B (ed): *Cerebral protection, Resuscitation and Monitoring: A Look into the Future of Neuroanesthesia. Anesthesiology Clinics of North America.* Philadelphia, WB Saunders, 1992:537–563.

2. Karfunkel P: The mechanisms of neural tube formation. *Int Rev Cytol* 1974; 38:245.

3. Streeter G: Developmental horizons in humans embryos. Description of age group XIII, embryos about 4 or 5 millimeters long and age group XIV, period of indentation of the lens vesicle. *Contrib Embryol* 1942; 31:211.

4. Streeter G: Developmental horizons in human embryos. Description of age group XV, XVI, XVII and XVIII, being the third issue of a survey on the Carnegie collection. *Contrib Embryol* 1948; 32:133.

5. Streeter G: Developmental horizons in human embryos (fourth issue). A review of the histogenesis of bone and cartilage. *Contrib Embryol* 1949; 33:149.

6. Streeter G: Developmental horizons in human embryos. Description of age groups XIX, XX, XXI, XXII, XXIII, being the fifth issue of a survey of the Carnegie collection. *Contrib Embryol* 1951; 34:165.

7. Heuser C, Corner G: Development horizons in human embryos. Description of age group X, 4 to 12 somites. *Contrib Embryol* 1975; 36:29.

8. Lemire R, Loeser J, Leedh R, Alvord E: *Normal and Abnormal Development of the Normal Nervous System.* New York, Harper & Row, 1975.

9. Streeter G: Factors involved in the formation of the filum terminale. *Am J Anat* 1919; 25:1.

10. Kandt R, et al: The central nervous system: Basic concepts. In Gregory G (ed): *Pediatric Anesthesia.* New York, Churchill-Livingstone, 1986;164–181.

11. Brocklehurst G: The development of the human cerebrospinal fluid pathway with particular reference to the roof of the fourth ventricle. *J Anat* 1969; 105:467.

12. Streeter GL: The development alterations in the vascular system of the brain of the human embryo. *Contrib Embryol* 1918; 8:5.

13. Padget D: The cranial venous system in man in reference to development, adult configuration and relation to the arteries. *Am J Anat* 1956; 98:307.

14. Milhorat T: Circulation of the cerebrospinal fluid. In McLaurin R, et al (eds): *Pediatric Neurosurgery. Survey of the Developing Nervous System. Section of Pediatric Neurosurgery of the American Society of Neurological Surgeons.* Philadelphia, WB Saunders, 1989;170–180.

15. Harris M, Stone D: Anesthesia for increased intracranial pressure in pediatrics. *Problems in Anesthesia* 1980; 4:67.

16. Lofgren J, Zwetnow NN: Cranial and spinal components of the cerebrospinal fluid pressure-volume curve. *Acta Neurol Scand* 1973; 49:575.

17. Hill A, Volpe J: Measurement of intracranial pressure using the Ladd intracranial pressure monitor. *J Paediatr* 1984; 98:974.

18. Hill A: Intracranial pressure measurements in the newborn. *Clin Perinatol* 1985; 12:161.

19. Ross RT: Spinal cord infarction in disease and surgery of the aorta. *Can J Neurol Sci* 1985; 12:289.

20. Batson O: The vertebral vein system. *Am J Roentgenol* 1957; 78:195.

21. Bickler P: Energetics of cerebral metabolism and ion transport. In Bissonnette B (ed): *Cerebral Protection, Resuscitation and Monitoring: A Look into the Future of Neuroanesthesia. Anesthesiology Clinics of North America.* Philadelphia, WB Saunders, 1992:563–575.

22. Sokoloff L: Circulation and energy metabolism of the brain. In Siegel G, et al (eds): *Basic Neurochemistry: Molecular, Cellular and Medical Aspects.* New York, Raven Press, 1989:565–591.

23. Siesjo BK: Cell damage in the brain: A speculative synthesis. *J Cereb Blood Flow Metab* 1981; 1:155.

24. Kennedy C, Sokoloff L: An adaptation of nitrous oxide method to the study of the circulation in children: Normal values for cerebral blood flow and cerebral metabolic rate in childhood. *J Clin Invest* 1957; 36:1130.

25. Settergren G, et al: Cerebral blood flow and exchange of oxygen, glucose ketone bodies, lactate, pyruvate and amino acids in anaesthetized children. *Acta Paediatr Scand* 1980; 69:457.

26. Mehta S, et al: Energy metabolism of brain in human protein-calorie malnutrition. *Pediatr Res* 1977; 11:290.

27. Younkin DP, et al: Noninvasive method of estimating human newborn regional cerebral blood flow. *J Cereb Blood Flow Metab* 1982; 2:415.

28. Cross KW, et al: An estimation of intracranial blood flow in the new-born infant. *J Physiol (Lond)* 1979; 289:329.

29. Ogawa A, et al: Regional cerebral blood flow with age: Changes in rCBF in childhood. *Neurol Res* 1989; 11:173.

30. Rosomoff H, Holaday D: Cerebral blood flow and cerebral oxygen consumption during hypothermia. *Am J Physiol* 1954; 179:85.

31. Lassen NA, Christensen MS: Physiology of cerebral blood flow. *Br J Anaesth* 1976; 48:719.

32. Hernandez MJ, et al: Autoregulation of cerebral blood flow in the newborn dog. *Brain Res* 1980; 184:199.

33. Purves MJ, James IM: Observations on the control of cerebral blood flow in the sheep fetus and newborn lamb. *Circ Res* 1969; 25:651.

34. McLeod ME, et al: Anaesthesia for cerebral arteriovenous malformations in children. *Can Anaesth Soc J* 1982; 29:299.

35. Tweed A, et al: Impairment of cerebral blood flow autoregulation in the newborn lamb by hypoxia. *Pediatr Res* 1986; 20:516.

36. Ong BY, et al: Acidemia impairs autoregulation of cerebral blood flow in newborn lambs. *Can Anaesth Soc J* 1986; 33:5.

37. Hennes HJ, Jantzen JP: Effects of fenoldopam on intracranial pressure and hemodynamic variables at normal and elevated intracranial pressure in anesthetized pigs. *J Neurosurg Anesthesiol* 1994; 6:175.

38. Barry D, Strandgaard S: Acute effects of antihypertensive drugs on autoregulation of cerebral blood flow in spontaneously hypertensive rats. *Prog Appl Microcirc* 1985; 8:206.

39. Van Aken H, Van Heimelrijck J: Influence of anesthesia on cerebral blood flow and cerebral metabolism: An overview. *Agressologie* 1991; 32:303.

40. Gregory G, et al: Hyperventilation restores autoregulation in the cerebral circulation in the neonate. *Anesthesiology* 1983; 59:427.

41. Lassen NA: Control of cerebral circulation in health and disease. *Circ Res* 1974; 34:749.

42. Lou HC, et al: Impaired autoregulation of cerebral blood flow in the distressed newborn infant. *J Pediatr* 1979; 94:118.

43. Muizelaar JP, et al: Pial arteriolar vessel diameter and CO_2

reactivity during prolonged hyperventilation in the rabbit. *J Neurosurg* 1988; 69:923.

44. Hidaka A, et al: Influence of maternal hyperoxia or hypercarbia on the hemodynamics of the placenta and fetal brain. *Nippon Sanka Fujinka Gakkai Zasshi* 1986; 38:1754.

45. Yamashita N, et al: CO_2 reactivity and autoregulation in fetal brain. *Childs Nerv Syst* 1991; 7:327.

46. Pilato MA, et al: Transcranial Doppler: Response of cerebral bloodflow velocity to carbon dioxide in anaesthetized children. *Can J Anaesth* 1991; 38:37.

47. Milhorat TH: Failure of choroid plexectomy as treatment for hydrocephalus. *Surg Gynecol Obstet* 1974; 139:505.

48. Pollay M: Formation of cerebrospinal fluid. Relation of studies of isolated choroid plexus to the standing gradient hypothesis. *J Neurosurg* 1975; 42:665.

49. Hammock MK, Milhorat TH: Recent studies on the formation of cerebrospinal fluid. *Dev Med Child Neurol* 1973; (suppl):27–34.

50. Rubin RC, et al: The production of cerebrospinal fluid in man and its modification by acetazolamide. *J Neurosurg* 1966; 25:430.

51. Milhorat TH, et al: Cerebrospinal fluid production by the choroid plexus and brain. *Science* 1971; 173:330.

52. Cutler RW, et al: Formation and absorption of cerebrospinal fluid in man. *Brain* 1968; 91:707.

53. Welch K: The intracranial pressure in infants. *J Neurosurg* 1980; 52:693.

54. Raju TN, et al: Intracranial pressure monitoring in the neonatal ICU. *Crit Care Med* 1980; 8:575.

55. Kosteljanetz M: Pressure-volume conditions in patients with subarachnoid and/or intraventricular hemorrhage. *J Neurosurg* 1985; 63:398.

56. Chopp M, et al: Hydraulic model of the cerebrovascular bed: An aid to understanding the volume-pressure test. *Neurosurgery* 1983; 13:5.

57. Marmarou A, et al: Contribution of CSF and vascular factors to elevation of ICP in severely head-injured patients. *J Neurosurg* 1987; 66:883.

58. Shapiro HM: Intracranial hypertension: Therapeutic and anesthetic considerations. *Anesthesiology* 1975; 43:445.

59. Shapiro K, Marmarou A: Mechanism of intracranial hypertension in children. In McLaurin R, et al (eds): *Pediatric Neurosurgery.* Philadelphia, WB Saunders, 1989:338–352.

60. Lindsberg PJ, et al: Validation of laser-Doppler flowmetry in measurement of spinal cord blood flow. *Am J Physiol* 1989; 257:H674–80.

61. Hickey R, et al: Autoregulation of spinal cord blood flow: Is the cord a microcosm of the brain? *Stroke* 1986; 17:1183.

62. Marcus ML, et al: Regulation of total and regional spinal cord blood flow. *Circ Res* 1977; 41:128.

63. Sandler AN, Tator CH: Review of the effect of spinal cord trauma on the vessels and blood flow in the spinal cord. *J Neurosurg* 1976; 45:638.

64. Goto T, Crosby G: Anesthesia and the spinal cord. In Bissonnette B (ed): *Cerebral Protection, Resuscitation and Monitoring: A Look into the Future of Neuroanesthesia. Anesthesiology Clinics of North America.* Philadelphia, WB Saunders, 1992:493–521.

65. Griffiths IR, et al: Spinal cord blood flow and conduction during experimental cord compression in normotensive and hypotensive dogs. *J Neurosurg* 1979; 50:353.

66. Rubinstein A, Arbit E: Spinal cord blood flow in the rat under normal physiological conditions. *Neurosurgery* 1990; 27:882.

67. Guha A, et al: Spinal cord blood flow and systemic blood pressure after experimental spinal cord injury in rats. *Stroke* 1989; 20:372.

68. Griffiths IR: Spinal cord blood flow in dogs: 1. The effect of blood pressure. *J Neurol Neurosurg Psychiatry* 1973; 36:914.

69. Griffiths IR: Spinal cord blood flow in dogs. 2. The effect of the blood gases. *J Neurol Neurosurg Psychiatry* 1973; 36:42.

70. Usubiaga JE, et al: Effect of saline injections on epidural and subarachnoid space pressures and relation to postspinal anesthesia headache. *Anesth Analg* 1967; 46:293.

71. Lassen N: Cerebral and spinal cord blood flow. In Cottrell J (ed): *Anesthesia and Neurosurgery.* St. Louis, CV Mosby, 1986:1–22.

72. Goldenthal EI: A compilation of LD_{50} values in newborn and adult animals. *Toxicol Appl Pharmacol* 1971; 18:185.

73. Kupferberg H, Way E: Pharmacologic basis for the increased sensitivity of the newborn rat to morphine. *J Pharmacol Exp Ther* 1963; 141:105.

74. Lerman J, et al: Anesthetic requirements for halothane in young children 0–1 month and 1–6 months of age. *Anesthesiology* 1983; 59:421.

75. Cook DR, et al: The inspired median effective dose, brain concentration at anesthesia and cardiovascular index for halothane in young rats. *Anesth Analg* 1981; 60:182.

76. Shapiro H: Anesthesia effects upon cerebral blood flow, cerebral metabolism and the electroencephalogram. In Miller R (ed): *Anesthesia.* New York, Churchill Livingstone, 1986:1264.

77. Sakabe T, et al: Cerebral effects of nitrous oxide in the dog. *Anesthesiology* 1978; 48:195.

78. Pelligrino DA, et al: Nitrous oxide markedly increases cerebral cortical metabolic rate and blood flow in the goat. *Anesthesiology* 1984; 60:405.

79. Theye RA, Michenfelder JD: The effect of nitrous oxide on canine cerebral metabolism. *Anesthesiology* 1968; 29:1119.

80. Todd MM: The effects of Pa_{CO_2} on the cerebrovascular response to nitrous oxide in the halothane-anesthetized rabbit. *Anesth Analg* 1987; 66:1090.

81. Leon JE, Bissonnette B: Transcranial Doppler sonography: Nitrous oxide and cerebral blood flow velocity in children [published erratum appears in *Can J Anaesth* 1992; 39:409]. *Can J Anaesth* 1991; 38:974.

82. Moss E, McDowall DG: ICP increases with 50% nitrous oxide in oxygen in severe head injuries during controlled ventilation. *Br J Anaesth* 1979; 51:757.

83. Hoffman WE, et al: The effects of midazolam on cerebral blood flow and oxygen consumption and its interaction with nitrous oxide. *Anesth Analg* 1986; 65:729.

84. Phirman JR, Shapiro HM: Modification of nitrous oxide-induced intracranial hypertension by prior induction of anesthesia. *Anesthesiology* 1977; 46:150.

85. Sakabe T, et al: Cerebral responses to the addition of nitrous oxide to halothane in man. *Br J Anaesth* 1976; 48:957.

86. Wollman H, et al: Cerebral circulation of man during halothane anesthesia: Effects of hypocarbia and of *d*-tubocurarine. *Anesthesiology* 1964; 25:180.

87. Todd MM, Drummond JC: A comparison of the cerebrovascular and metabolic effects of halothane and isoflurane in the cat. *Anesthesiology* 1984; 60:276.

88. Albrecht RF, et al: Cerebral blood flow and metabolic changes from induction to onset of anesthesia with halothane or pentobarbital. *Anesthesiology* 1977; 47:252.

89. Manohar M, Goetz TE: Cerebral, renal, adrenal, intestinal, and pancreatic circulation in conscious ponies and during 1.0, 1.5, and 2.0 minimal alveolar concentrations of halothane-O_2 anesthesia. *Am J Vet Res* 1985; 46:2492.

90. Lazzell V, et al: Effect of halothane on the cerebral blood flow in infants and children. A hysteresis phenomenon. *Anesthesiology* 1989; 71:A327.

91. Lazzell V, Bissonnette B: Transcranial Doppler: Effect of halo-

thane on cerebral hemodynamics in children. *Anesthesiology* 1989; 71:A332.

92. Madsen JB, et al: Cerebral blood flow, cerebral metabolic rate of oxygen and relative CO_2-reactivity during craniotomy for supratentorial cerebral tumours in halothane anaesthesia. A dose-response study. *Acta Anaesthesiol Scand* 1987; 31:454.

93. Christensen MS, et al: Cerebral vasodilatation by halothane anaesthesia in man and its potentiation by hypotension and hypercapnia. *Br J Anaesth* 1967; 39:927.

94. Adams RW, et al: Halothane, hypocapnia, and cerebrospinal fluid pressure in neurosurgery. *Anesthesiology* 1972; 37:510.

95. Leon JE, Bissonnette B: Cerebrovascular responses to carbon dioxide in children anesthetized with halothane and isoflurane. *Can J Anaesth* 1991; 38:817.

96. Drummond JC, Todd MM: The response of the feline cerebral circulation to Pa_{CO_2} during anesthesia with isoflurane and halothane and during sedation with nitrous oxide. *Anesthesiology* 1985; 62:268.

97. Newberg LA, Michenfelder JD: Cerebral protection by isoflurane during hypoxemia or ischemia. *Anesthesiology* 1983; 59:29.

98. Artru AA: Effects of enflurane and isoflurane on resistance to reabsorption of cerebrospinal fluid in dogs. *Anesthesiology* 1984; 61:529.

99. Leon J, Bissonnette B: Does cerebrovascular hysteresis exist under isoflurane anaesthesia. *Can J Anaesth* 1991; 72:S160.

100. Bisonnette B, Leon JE: Cerebrovascular stability during isoflurane anaesthesia in children. *Can J Anaesth* 1992; 39:128.

101. Algotsson L, et al: Cerebral blood flow and oxygen consumption during isoflurane and halothane anesthesia in man. *Acta Anaesthesiol Scand* 1988; 32:15.

102. Eintrie C, et al: Local application of 133 Xenon for measurement of regional cerebral blood flow (rCBF) during halothane, enflurane, and isoflurane anesthesia in humans. *Anesthesiology* 1985; 63:391.

103. Archer DP, et al: Cerebral blood volume is increased in dogs during administration of nitrous oxide or isoflurane. *Anesthesiology* 1987; 67:642.

104. Scheller MS, et al: The intracranial pressure effects of isoflurane and halothane administered following cryogenic brain injury in rabbits. *Anesthesiology* 1987; 67:507.

105. Artru AA: Relationship between cerebral blood volume and CSF pressure during anesthesia with isoflurane or fentanyl in dogs. *Anesthesiology* 1984; 60:575.

106. Michenfelder JD, Cucchiara RF: Canine cerebral oxygen consumption during enflurane anesthesia and its modification during induced seizures. *Anesthesiology* 1974; 40:575.

107. Sakabe T, et al: Cerebral circulation and metabolism during enflurane anesthesia in humans. *Anesthesiology* 1983; 59:532.

108. Artru AA: Relationship between cerebral blood volume and CSF pressure during anesthesia with halothane or enflurane in dogs. *Anesthesiology* 1983; 58:533.

109. Artru AA, et al: Enflurane causes a prolonged and reversible increase in the rate of CSF production in the dog. *Anesthesiology* 1982; 57:255.

110. Artru AA: Effects of halothane and fentanyl anesthesia on resistance to reabsorption of CSF. *J Neurosurg* 1984; 60:252.

111. Lebowitz MH, et al: Enflurane-induced central nervous system excitation and its relation to carbon dioxide tension. *Anesth Analg* 1972; 51:355.

112. Scheller MS, et al: The effects of sevoflurane on cerebral blood flow, cerebral metabolic rate for oxygen, intracranial pressure, and the electroencephalogram are similar to those of isoflurane in the rabbit. *Anesthesiology* 1988; 68:548.

113. Lu G, et al: Cerebral vasodilating effect of sevoflurane vs. isoflurane. *Anesthesiology* 1990; 73:A625.

114. Werner C, et al: The effects of sevoflurane on neurological outcome from incomplete ischemia in rats. *J Neurosurg Anesthesiol* 1991; 3:237.

115. Lutz LJ, et al: The cerebral functional, metabolic, and hemodynamic effects of desflurane in dogs. *Anesthesiology* 1990; 73:125.

116. Muzzi DA, et al: The effect of desflurane and isoflurane on cerebrospinal fluid pressure in humans with supratentorial mass lesions. *Anesthesiology* 1992; 76:720.

117. Pierce E, et al: Cerebral circulation and metabolism during thiopental anesthesia and hyperventilation in man. *J Clin Invest* 1962; 41:1664.

118. Michenfelder JD: The interdependency of cerebral functional and metabolic effects following massive doses of thiopental in the dog. *Anesthesiology* 1974; 41:231.

119. Shapiro HM, et al: Rapid intraoperative reduction of intracranial pressure with thiopentane. *Br J Anaesth* 1973; 45:1057.

120. Mann J, et al: Differential effects of pentobarbital, ketamine hydrochloride and enflurane anesthesia on cerebrospinal fluid formation rate and outflow resistance in the rat. *Neurosurgery* 1979; 2:482.

121. Rockoff MA, Goudsouzian NG: Seizures induced by methohexital. *Anesthesiology* 1981; 54:333.

122. Renou AM, et al: Cerebral blood flow and metabolism during etomidate anaesthesia in man. *Br J Anaesth* 1978; 50:1047.

123. Milde LN, et al: Cerebral functional, metabolic, and hemodynamic effects of etomidate in dogs. *Anesthesiology* 1985; 63:371.

124. Fragen RJ, et al: Effects of etomidate on hormonal responses to surgical stress. *Anesthesiology* 1984; 61:652.

125. Laughlin TP, Newberg LA: Prolonged myoclonus after etomidate anesthesia. *Anesth Analg* 1985; 64:80.

126. Michenfelder JD, Theye RA: Effects of fentanyl, droperidol, and innovar on canine cerebral metabolism and blood flow. *Br J Anaesth* 1971; 43:630.

127. Sari A, et al: The effects of thalamonal on cerebral circulation and oxygen consumption in man. *Br J Anaesth* 1972; 44:330.

128. Van Hemelrijck J, et al: Effect of propofol on cerebral circulation and autoregulation in the baboon. *Anesth Analg* 1990; 71:49.

129. Pinaud M, et al: Effects of propofol on cerebral hemodynamics and metabolism in patients with brain trauma. *Anesthesiology* 1990; 73:404.

130. Fleischer JE, et al: Cerebral effects of high-dose midazolam and subsequent reversal with Ro 15-1788 in dogs. *Anesthesiology* 1988; 68:234.

131. Nugent M, et al: Cerebral metabolic, vascular and protective effects of midazolam maleate: comparison of diazepam. *Anesthesiology* 1982; 56:172.

132. Jobes DR, et al: Cerebral blood flow and metabolism during morphine-nitrous oxide anesthesia in man. *Anesthesiology* 1977; 47:16.

133. Drummond J, Shapiro H: Cerebral physiology. In Miller R (ed): *Anesthesia.* New York, Churchill Livingstone, 1990:621.

134. Artru AA: Effects of halothane and fentanyl on the rate of CSF production in dogs. *Anesth Analg* 1983; 62:581.

135. Yaster M, et al: Effects of fentanyl on peripheral and cerebral hemodynamics in neonatal lambs. *Anesthesiology* 1987; 66:524.

136. Jung R, et al: Cerebrospinal fluid pressure in anesthesized patients with brain tumors: Impact of fentanyl vs. alfentanil. *J Neurosurg Anesthesiol* 1989; 1:136.

137. Marx W, et al: Sufentanil, alfentanil and fentanyl: Impact on cerebrospinal fluid pressure in patients with brain tumors. *J Neurosurg Anesthesiol* 1989; 1:3.

138. Young WL, et al: A comparison of the cerebral hemodynamic effects of sufentanil and isoflurane in humans undergoing carotid endarterectomy. *Anesthesiology* 1989; 71:863.

139. Milde LN, et al: Effects of sufentanil on cerebral circulation and metabolism in dogs. *Anesth Analg* 1990; 70:138.

140. Takeshita H, et al: The effects of ketamine on cerebral circulation and metabolism in man. *Anesthesiology* 1972; 36:69.

141. Shapiro H, et al: Ketamine anesthesia in patients with intracranial pathology. *Br J Anaesth* 1972; 44:1200.

142. Ducey JP, et al: A comparison of the effects of suxamethonium, atracurium and vecuronium on intracranial haemodynamics in swine. *Anaesth Intensive Care* 1989; 17:448.

143. Cottrell JE, et al: Intracranial and hemodynamic changes after succinylcholine administration in cats. *Anesth Analg* 1983; 62:1006.

144. Lanier WL, et al: Cerebral stimulation following succinylcholine in dogs. *Anesthesiology* 1986; 64:551.

145. Minton MD, et al: Increases in intracranial pressure from succinylcholine: Prevention by prior nondepolarizing blockade. *Anesthesiology* 1986; 65:165.

146. Frankville DD, Drummond JC: Hyperkalemia after succinylcholine administration in a patient with closed head injury without paresis. *Anesthesiology* 1987; 67:264.

147. Tong TK: Succinylcholine-induced hyperkalemia in near-drowning. *Anesthesiology* 1987; 66:720.

148. Iwatsuki N, et al: Succinylcholine-induced hyperkalemia in patients with ruptured cerebral aneurysms. *Anesthesiology* 1980; 53:64.

149. Cooperman LH: Succinylcholine-induced hyperkalemia in neuromuscular disease. *JAMA* 1970; 213:1867.

150. John DA, et al: Onset of succinylcholine-induced hyperkalemia following denervation. *Anesthesiology* 1976; 45:294.

151. Lanier WL, et al: The cerebral effects of pancuronium and atracurium in halothane-anesthetized dogs. *Anesthesiology* 1985; 63:589.

152. Vesely R, et al: The cerebrovascular effects of curare and histamine in the rat. *Anesthesiology* 1987; 66:519.

153. Rosa G, et al: Effects of vecuronium bromide on intracranial pressure and cerebral perfusion pressure. A preliminary report. *Br J Anaesth* 1986; 58:437.

154. Siesjo BK: Cerebral circulation and metabolism. *J Neurosurg* 1984; 60:883.

155. Bruce D: Management of severe head injury. In Cottrell J, Turndorf H (ed): *Anesthesia and Neurosurgery*. St. Louis, CV Mosby, 1986:150–160.

156. Archer D, Priddy R: Anesthetic management of patients with head injury. In Bissonnette B (ed): *Cerebral Protection, Resuscitation and Monitoring: A Look into the Future of Neuroanesthesia, Anesthesiology Clinics of North America*. Philadelphia, WB Saunders, 1992:603–619.

157. Young W, Koreh I: Potassium and calcium changes injured spinal cords. *Brain Res* 1986; 365:42.

158. Casley-Smith J, et al: The prelymphatic pathways of the brain as revealed by cervical lymphatic obstruction and the passage of particles. *Br J Exp Pathol* 1976; 57:179.

159. Chaplin ER, et al: Posthemorrhagic hydrocephalus in the preterm infant. *Pediatrics* 1980; 65:901.

160. Jedeikin R, et al: Cerebral arteriovenous malformation in neonates. The role of myocardial ischemia. *Pediatr Cardiol* 1983; 4:29.

161. Pierre-Kahn A, et al: Hydrocephalus and achondroplasia. A study of 25 observations. *Childs Brain* 1980; 7:205.

162. Friedman WA, Mickle JP: Hydrocephalus in achondroplasia: A possible mechanism. *Neurosurgery* 1980; 7:150.

163. Li F: Cancers in children. in Schottenfeld D, Fraumeni J (eds): *Epidemiology and Prevention*. Philadelphia, WB Saunders, 1982:1012.

164. Gold E: Epidemiology of brain tumors. *Rev Cancer Epidemiol* 1982; 1:245.

165. Farwell JR, et al: Central nervous system tumors in children. *Cancer* 1977; 40:3123.

166. Farwell JR, et al: Intracranial neoplasms in infant. *Arch Neurol* 1978; 35:533.

167. Crist WM, Kun LE: Common solid tumors of childhood. *N Engl J Med* 1991; 324:461.

168. Rivara F, Mueller B: The epidemiology and prevention of pediatric head injury. *J Head Trauma Rehabil* 1986; 1:7.

169. Brown J: The pathological effects of raised intracranial pressure. *Clin Dev Med* 1991; 38:113.

170. Cushing H: Some experimental and clinical observations concerning the states of increased intracranial pressure. *Am J Med Sci* 1902; 124:375.

171. Brown K: Preoperative assessment of neurologic function in the neurosurgical patient. In Bissonnette B (ed): *Cerebral Protection, Resuscitation and Monitoring: A Look into the Future of Neuroanesthesia. Anesthesiology Clinics of North America*. Philadelphia, WB Saunders, 1992:645–657.

172. Gascon G, Leech R: Medical evaluation. In Leech R, Brunback R (eds): *Hydrocephalus: Current Clinical Concepts*. St. Louis, CV Mosby, 1991:105.

173. Jennett WB: Raised intracranial pressure. In Jennett WB (ed): *Introduction to Neurosurgery*, 3d ed. London, W Heineman Medical Books, 1977:3.

174. Bekemeyer WB, Pinstein ML: Neurogenic pulmonary edema: new concepts of an old disorder. *South Med J* 1989; 82:380.

175. Milley JR, et al: Neurogenic pulmonary edema in childhood. *J Pediatr* 1979; 94:706.

176. Carlson RW, et al: Pulmonary edema following intracranial hemorrhage. *Chest* 1979; 75:731.

177. Ciongoli AK, Poser CM: Pulmonary edema secondary to subarachnoid hemorrhage. *Neurology* 1972; 22:867.

178. Baigelman W, O'Brien JC: Pulmonary effects of head trauma. *Neurosurgery* 1981; 9:729.

179. Terrence CF, et al: Neurogenic pulmonary edema in unexpected, unexplained death of epileptic patients. *Ann Neurol* 1981; 9:458.

180. Colice G: Neurogenic pulmonary edema. *Clin Chest Med* 1985; 6:473.

181. Malik AB: Mechanisms of neurogenic pulmonary edema. *Circ Res* 1985; 57:1.

182. Shucart WA, Jackson I: Management of diabetes insipidus in neurosurgical patients. *J Neurosurg* 1976; 44:64.

183. Hodges FI: Pathology of the skull. In Tavaras J (ed): *Radiology Diagnosis—Imaging—Intervention: Neuroradiology and Radiology of the Head and Neck*. Philadelphia, JB Lippincott, 1989:123.

184. Grant E, Richardson J: Infant and neonatal neurosonography technique and normal anatomy. In Tavaras J (ed): *Radiology Diagnosis—Imaging—Intervention: Neuroradiology and Radiology of the Head and Neck*. Philadelphia, JB Lippincott, 1989:453.

185. Wilder-Smith O, et al: Neuromonitoring in anesthesia. [French]. *Ann Fr Anesth Reanim* 1995; 14:95.

186. Bissonnette B, Davis P: Thermal regulation—Physiology and perioperative management in infants and children. In Motoyama E, Davis P (eds): *Smith's Anesthesia for Infants and Children*, 6th ed. St. Louis, Mosby-Year Book, 1996:5.1–5.20.

187. Garner L, et al: Heart block after intravenous lidocaine in an infant. *Can Anaesth Soc J* 1985; 32:425.

188. Rosenberg H, Gronert GA: Intractable cardiac arrest in children given succinylcholine. *Anesthesiology* 1992; 77:1054.

189. Lerman J, et al: Succinylcholine warning. *Can J Anaesth* 1994; 41:165.

190. Lazzell VA, et al: The incidence of masseter muscle rigidity after succinylcholine in infants and children. *Can J Anaesth* 1994; 41:475.

191. Moynihan RJ, et al: The effect of cricoid pressure on preventing

gastric insufflation in infants and children. *Anesthesiology* 1993; 78:652.

192. Salem MR: Cricoid pressure for preventing gastric insufflation in infants and children. *Anesthesiology* 1994; 80:1182.

193. Sloan MH, et al: Pharmacodynamics of high-dose vecuronium in children during balanced anesthesia. *Anesthesiology* 1991; 74:656.

194. Millar C, Bissonnette B: Awake intubation increases intracranial pressure without affecting cerebral blood flow velocity in infants. *Can J Anaesth* 1994; 41:281.

195. Bissonnette B: Fluid therapy. In Wolf A (ed): *Handbook of Neonatal Anaesthesia*. London, WB Saunders, 1995:110–132.

196. Drummond J: *Fluid Management for Neurosurgical Patients*. Philadelphia, JB Lippincott, 1992.

197. Korosue K, et al: Comparison of crystalloids and colloids for hemodilution in a model of focal cerebral ischemia. *J Neurosurg* 1990; 73:576.

198. Kaieda R, et al: Acute effects of changing plasma osmolality and colloid oncotic pressure on the formation of brain edema after cryogenic injury. *Neurosurgery* 1989; 24:671.

199. Hartley E, et al: Scalp infiltration with bupivacaine in pediatric brain surgery. *Anesth Analg* 1991; 73:29.

200. St. Louis P, et al: Determination of bupivacaine in plasma by high-performance liquid chromatography. Levels after scalp infiltration in children. *Clin Biochem* 1991; 24:463.

201. Ishige N, et al: The effect of hypoxia on traumatic head injury in rats: Alterations in neurologic function, brain edema, and cerebral blood flow. *J Cereb Blood Flow Metab* 1987; 7:759.

202. Albin MS, et al: Brain retraction pressure during intracranial procedures. *Surg Forum* 1975; 26:499.

203. Araki T, et al: Neuronal damage and calcium accumulation following repeated brief cerebral ischemia in the gerbil. *Brain Res* 1990; 528:114.

204. Ravussin P, et al: The effects of rapid infusions of saline and mannitol on cerebral blood volume and intracranial pressure in dogs. *Can Anaesth Soc J* 1985; 32:506.

205. Lanier WL, et al: The effects of dextrose infusion and head position on neurologic outcome after complete cerebral ischemia in primates: Examination of a model. *Anesthesiology* 1987; 66:39.

206. Pulsinelli WA, et al: Increased damage after ischemic stroke in patients with hyperglycemia with or without established diabetes mellitus. *Am J Med* 1983; 74:540.

207. Smerling A: Hypertonic saline in head trauma: A new recipe for drying and salting. *J Neurosurg Anesthesiol* 1992; 4:1.

208. Gunnar W, et al: Head injury and hemorrhagic shock: Studies of the blood brain barrier and intracranial pressure after resuscitation with normal saline solution, 3% saline solution, and dextran-40. *Surgery* 1988; 103:398.

209. Marshall LF, et al: Mannitol dose requirements in brain-injured patients. *J Neurosurg* 1978; 48:169.

210. Nath F, Galbraith S: The effect of mannitol on cerebral white matter water content. *J Neurosurg* 1986; 65:41.

211. Ravussin P, et al: Changes in CSF pressure after mannitol in patients with and without elevated CSF pressure [published erratum appears in *J Neurosurg* 1989; 70:662]. *J Neurosurg* 1988; 69:869.

212. Cote CJ, et al: The hypotensive response to rapid intravenous administration of hypertonic solutions in man and in the rabbit. *Anesthesiology* 1979; 50:30.

213. Rudehill A, et al: Effects of mannitol on blood volume and central hemodynamics in patients undergoing cerebral aneurysm surgery. *Anesth Analg* 1983; 62:875.

214. Schettini A, et al: Osmotic and osmotic-loop diuresis in brain surgery. Effects on plasma and CSF electrolytes and ion excretion. *J Neurosurg* 1982; 56:679.

215. Suzuki J, et al: Use of balloon occlusion and substances to protect ischemic brain during resection of posterior fossa AVM. Case report. *J Neurosurg* 1985; 63:626.

216. Jafar JJ, et al: The effect of mannitol on cerebral blood flow. *J Neurosurg* 1986; 64:754.

217. Meyer FB, et al: Treatment of experimental focal cerebral ischemia with mannitol. Assessment by intracellular brain pH, cortical blood flow, and electroencephalography. *J Neurosurg* 1987; 66:109.

218. Warren SE, Blantz RC: Mannitol. *Arch Intern Med* 1981; 141:493.

219. Muizelaar JP, et al: Mannitol causes compensatory cerebral vasoconstriction and vasodilation in response to blood viscosity changes. *J Neurosurg* 1983; 59:822.

220. Pollay M, et al: Effect of mannitol and furosemide on blood-brain osmotic gradient and intracranial pressure. *J Neurosurg* 1983; 59:945.

221. Cottrell JE, et al: Furosemide- and mannitol-induced changes in intracranial pressure and serum osmolality and electrolytes. *Anesthesiology* 1977; 47:28.

222. Clasen RA, et al: Furosemide and pentobarbital in cryogenic cerebral injury and edema. *Neurology* 1974; 24:642.

223. Bourke R, et al: Studies on the formation of astroglial swelling and its inhibition by clinically useful agents. In Popp A, et al (eds): *Neural Trauma*. New York, Raven Press, 1979:95.

224. Galicich J, French L: Use of dexamethasone in the treatment of brain tumors and brain surgery. *American Practitioner* 1961; 12:169.

225. Bouzarth WF, Shenkin HA: Possible mechanisms of action of dexamethasone in brain injury. *J Trauma* 1974; 14:134.

226. Bissonnette B: Temperature and anesthesia. In Lerman J (ed): *New Developments in Pediatric Anesthesia. Anesthesiology Clinics of North America*. Philadelphia, WB Saunders, 1991:849–872.

227. Bissonnette B, Sessler DI: The thermoregulatory threshold in infants and children anesthetized with isoflurane and caudal bupivacaine. *Anesthesiology* 1990; 73:1114.

228. Bissonnette B, Sessler DI: Thermoregulatory thresholds for vasoconstriction in pediatric patients anesthetized with halothane or halothane and caudal bupivacaine. *Anesthesiology* 1992; 76:387.

229. Bissonnette B: Temperature monitoring in pediatric anesthesia. *Int Anesthesiol Clin* 1992; 30:63.

230. Bissonnette B, Sessler DI: Passive or active inspired gas humidification increases thermal steady-state temperatures in anesthetized infants. *Anesth Analg* 1989; 69:783.

231. Bissonnette B, et al: Passive and active inspired gas humidification in infants and children. *Anesthesiology* 1989; 71:350.

232. Bissonnette B, et al: Intraoperative temperature monitoring sites in infants and children and the effect of inspired gas warming on esophageal temperature. *Anesth Analg* 1989; 69:192.

233. Harris MM, et al: Venous air embolism and cardiac arrest during craniectomy in a supine infant. *Anesthesiology* 1986; 65:547.

234. Harris MM, et al: Venous embolism during craniectomy in supine infants. *Anesthesiology* 1987; 67:816.

235. Joseph M, et al: Venous air embolism during repair of craniosynostosis in the lateral position. *Anesth Rev* 1985; 12:46.

236. Meridy HW, et al: Complications during neurosurgery in the prone position in children. *Can Anaesth Soc J* 1974; 21:445.

237. Wilkins RH, Albin MS: An unusual entrance site of venous air embolism during operations in the sitting position. *Surg Neurol* 1977; 7:71.

238. Cabezudo JM, et al: Air embolism from wounds from a pin-type head-holder as a complication of posterior fossa surgery in the sitting position. Case report. *J Neurosurg* 1981; 55:147.

239. Michenfelder JD, et al: Air embolism during neurosurgery. An

evaluation of right-atrial catheters for diagnosis and treatment. *JAMA* 1969; 208:1353.

240. Marshall WK, Bedford RF: Use of a pulmonary-artery catheter for detection and treatment of venous air embolism: a prospective study in man. *Anesthesiology* 1980; 52:131.

241. Black S, et al: Outcome following posterior fossa craniectomy in patients in the sitting or horizontal positions. *Anesthesiology* 1988; 69:49.

242. Michenfelder JD, et al: Evaluation of an ultrasonic device (Doppler) for the diagnosis of venous air embolism. *Anesthesiology* 1972; 36:164.

243. Cucchiara RF, Bowers B: Air embolism in children undergoing suboccipital craniotomy. *Anesthesiology* 1982; 57:338.

244. Deal CW, et al: Hemodynamic effects of pulmonary air embolism. *J Surg Res* 1971; 11:533.

245. Gronert GA, et al: Paradoxical air embolism from a parent foramen ovale. *Anesthesiology* 1979; 50:548.

246. Marquez J, et al: Paradoxical cerebral air embolism without an intracardiac septal defect. Case report. *J Neurosurg* 1981; 55:997.

247. Colohan AR, et al: Intravenous fluid loading as prophylaxis for paradoxical air embolism. *J Neurosurg* 1985; 62:839.

248. Munson ES: Effect of nitrous oxide on the pulmonary circulation during venous air embolism. *Anesth Analg* 1971; 50:785.

249. Bedford R: Perioperative venous air embolism. *Seminars in Anesthesia,* 1987; 6:163.

250. Pearl RG, Larson CJ: Hemodynamic effects of positive end-expiratory pressure during continuous venous air embolism in the dog. *Anesthesiology* 1986; 64:724.

251. American Academy of Pediatrics Committee on Drugs: Guidelines for monitoring and management of pediatric patients during and after sedation for diagnostic and therapeutic procedures. *Pediatrics* 1992; 89:1110.

252. Nelson MJ: Guidelines for the monitoring and care of children during and after sedation for imaging studies. *Am J Roentgenol* 1993; 160:581.

253. Kanal E, Shellock FG: MR imaging of patients with intracranial aneurysm clips. *Radiology* 1993; 187:612.

254. Shellock FG, et al: MR imaging and metallic implants for anterior cruciate ligament reconstruction: Assessment of ferromagnetism and artifact. *J Magn Reson Imaging* 1992; 2:225.

255. Shellock FG, Kanal E: Policies, guidelines, and recommendations for MR imaging safety and patient management. SMRI Safety Committee. *J Magn Reson Imaging* 1991; 1:97.

256. Shellock FG, Slimp G: Halo vest for cervical spine fixation during MR imaging. *Am J Roentgenol* 1990; 154:631.

257. Mutzel W, et al: Biochemical-pharmacologic properties of iohexol. *Acta Radiol Suppl* 1980; 362:111.

258. Aakhus T, et al: Tolerance and excretion of iohexol after intravenous injection in healthy volunteers. Preliminary report. *Acta Radiol Suppl* 1980; 362:131.

259. Edelson J, et al: Pharmacokinetics of iohexol, a new nonionic radiocontrast agent, in humans. *J Pharm Sci* 1984; 73:993.

260. Higgins CB, et al: Evaluation of the hemodynamic effects of intravenous administration of ionic and nonionic contrast materials. Implications for deriving physiologic measurements from computed tomography and digital cardiovascular imaging. *Radiology* 1982; 142:681.

261. Shehadi WH, Toniolo G: Adverse reactions to contrast media: A report from the Committee on Safety of Contrast Media of the International Society of Radiology. *Radiology* 1980; 137:299.

262. Ferrer-Brechner T, Winter J: Anesthetic considerations for cerebral computer tomography. *Anesth Analg* 1977; 56:344.

263. Glauber DT, Audenaert SM: Anesthesia for children undergoing craniospinal radiotherapy. *Anesthesiology* 1987; 67:801.

264. Brann C, Janik D: Anesthesia in the radiology suite. *Problems in Anesthesia* 1992; 6:413.

265. Wada J, Rassmussen T: Intracarotid injection of sodium amytal for the lateralization of cerebral speech dominance: Experimental and clinical observations. *J Neurosurg* 1960; 17:266.

266. Dawson RC 3d: Treatment of arteriovenous malformations of the brain with combined embolization and stereotactic radiosurgery: results after 1 and 2 years. *Am J Neuroradiol* 1990; 11:857.

267. Barnwell SL: Interventional neuroradiology. *West J Med* 1993; 158:162.

268. Bryan RN: Remarks on interventional neuroradiology. *Am J Neuroradiol* 1990; 11:630.

269. Martin N: Neurosurgery and interventional neuroradiology. In Vinuela F, et al (eds): *Interventional Neuroradiology: Endovascular Therapy of the Nervous System.* New York, Raven Press, 1992:193–201.

270. Young WL, Pile SJ: Anesthetic considerations for interventional neuroradiology. *Anesthesiology* 1994; 80:427.

271. O'Mahony BJ, Bolsin SN: Anaesthesia for closed embolisation of cerebral arteriovenous malformations. *Anaesth Intensive Care* 1988; 16:318.

272. Picard L, et al: Spontaneous dural arteriovenous fistulas. *Siemen Intervent Radiol* 1987; 4:219.

273. Debrun GM, et al: Indications for treatment and classification of 132 carotid-cavernous fistulas. *Neurosurgery* 1988; 22:285.

274. Halbach VV, et al: Treatment of vertebral arteriovenous fistulas. *Am J Roentgenol* 1988; 150:405.

275. Halbach VV, et al: Transvenous embolization of direct carotid cavernous fistulas. *Am J Neuroradiol* 1988; 9:741.

276. Fox AJ, et al: Use of detachable balloons for proximal artery occlusion in the treatment of unclippable cerebral aneurysms. *J Neurosurg* 1987; 66:40.

277. Linskey ME, et al: Aneurysms of the intracavernous carotid artery: A multidisciplinary approach to treatment. *J Neurosurg* 1991; 75:525.

278. Higashida RT, et al: Treatment of intracranial aneurysms with preservation of the parent vessel: Results of percutaneous balloon embolization in 84 patients. *Am J Neuroradiol* 1990; 11:633.

279. Strother CM, et al: Thrombus formation and structure and the evolution of mass effect in intracranial aneurysms treated by balloon embolization: Emphasis on MR findings. *Am J Neuroradiol* 1989; 10:787.

280. Meyer P, et al: Blood loss during repair of craniosynostosis. *Br J Anaesth* 1993; 71:854.

281. Diaz JH, Lockhart CH: Hypotensive anaesthesia for craniectomy in infancy. *Br J Anaesth* 1979; 51:233.

282. Davies D, Munro I: The anesthetic management and intraoperative care of patient undergoing major facial osteotomies. *Plast Reconstr Surg* 1975; 55:50.

283. Brown KA, et al: Hyperkalaemia during massive blood transfusion in paediatric craniofacial surgery. *Can Anaesth Soc* 1990; 37:401.

284. Brown KA, et al: Hyperkalaemia during rapid blood transfusion and hypovolaemic cardiac arrest in children. *Can J Anaesth* 1990; 37:401.

285. Matson D: *Neurosurgery of Infancy and Childhood.* Springfield, IL, Charles C. Thomas, 1969.

286. Duffner PK, et al: Pediatric brain tumors: An overview. *CA Cancer J Clin* 1985; 35:287.

287. Childhood Brain Tumor Consortium. A study of childhood brain tumors based on surgical biopsies from ten North American institutions: Sample description. *J Neurooncol* 1988; 6:9.

288. Sperry RJ, et al: The influence of hemorrhage on organ perfusion during deliberate hypotension in rats. *Anesthesiology* 1992; 77:1171.

289. Gilles FH, et al: Epidemiology of seizures in children with

brain tumors. The Childhood Brain Tumor Consortium. *J Neurooncol* 1992; 12:53.

290. Childhood Brain Tumor Consortium. The epidemiology of headache among children with brain tumor. Headache in children with brain tumors. *J Neurooncol* 1991; 10:31.

291. Keon T, Templeton J: Diseases of the endocrine system. In Katz J, Steward D (eds): *Anesthesia and Uncommon Pediatric Diseases*. Philadelphia, WB Saunders, 1987:311.

292. Ravin MB, Feinberg G: Anesthetic management of hypophysectomy. *NY State J Med* 1968; 68:776.

293. Rorke L, Schut L: Introductory survey of pediatric brain tumors. In McLaurin R, et al (eds): *Pediatric Neurosurgery. Survey of the Developing Nervous System. Section of Pediatric Neurosurgery of the American Society of Neurological Surgeons*. Philadelphia, WB Saunders, 1989:335–337.

294. Chatty EM, Earle KM: Medulloblastoma. A report of 201 cases with emphasis on the relationship of histologic variants to survival. *Cancer* 1971; 28:977.

295. Albright AL, et al: Current neurosurgical treatment of medulloblastomas in children. A report from the Children's Cancer Study Group. *Pediatr Neurosci* 1989; 15:276.

296. Stirt JA, et al: "Defasciculation" with metocurine prevents succinylcholine-induced increases in intracranial pressure. *Anesthesiology* 1987; 67:50.

297. Todd MM, et al: A prospective, comparative trial of three anesthetics for elective supratentorial craniotomy. Propofol/fentanyl, isoflurane/nitrous oxide, and fentanyl/nitrous oxide. *Anesthesiology* 1993; 78:1005.

298. Humphreys RP, et al: Advantages of the prone position for neurosurgical procedures on the upper cervical spine and posterior cranial fossa in children. *Childs Brain* 1975; 1:325.

299. Relton JE, Hall JE: An operation frame for spinal fusion. A new apparatus designed to reduce hemorrhage during operation. *J Bone Joint Surg Br* 1967; 49:327.

300. Millar C, et al: Cerebral arteriovenous malformations in children. *Can J Anaesth* 1994; 41:321.

301. McLeod ME, et al: Anaesthetic management of arteriovenous malformations of the vein of Galen. *Can Anaesth Soc J* 1982; 29:307.

302. Bingham RM, Wilkinson DJ: Anaesthetic management in Moyamoya disease. *Anaesthesia* 1985; 40:1198.

303. Ausman JI, et al: Cerebrovascular occlusive disease in children: A survey. *Acta Neurochir (Wien)* 1988; 94:117.

304. Rovira M, et al: Etiology of moya moya disease acquired or congenital. *Acta Radiol Suppl* 1976; 347:229.

305. Coakham HM, et al: Moya-moya disease: Clinical and pathological report of a case with associated myopathy. *J Neurol Neurosurg Psychiatry* 1979; 42:289.

306. Cumming GR: Circulation in neonates with intracranial arteriovenous fistula and cardiac failure. *Am J Cardiol* 1980; 45:1019.

307. Levy AM, et al: Congestive heart failure in the newborn infant in the absence of primary cardiac disease. *Am J Cardiol* 1970; 26:409.

308. Bissonnette B: Temperature monitoring in pediatric anesthesia. In Pullerits J, Holtzman R (eds): *Anesthesia Equipment for Infants and Children. International Anesthesiology Clinics*. Boston, Little, Brown, 1992:63–81.

309. Dietrich WD, et al: The importance of brain temperature in alterations of the blood-brain barrier following cerebral ischemia. *J Neuropathol Exp Neurol* 1990; 49:486.

310. Busto R, et al: Effect of mild hypothermia on ischemia-induced release of neurotransmitters and free fatty acids in rat brain. *Stroke* 1989; 20:904.

311. Busto R, et al: The importance of brain temperature in cerebral ischemic injury. *Stroke* 1989; 20:1113.

312. Wass CT, et al: Temperature changes of ≥ 1 degree C alter functional neurologic outcome and histopathology in a canine model of complete cerebral ischemia. *Anesthesiology* 1995; 83:325.

313. Leech R, Myelodysplasia, Arnold-Chiari malformation and hydrocephalus. In Leech R, Brumbaric R (eds): *Hydrocephalus: Current Clinical Concepts*. St. Louis, Mosby-Year Book, 1991:129.

314. Ersahin Y, et al: Cerebrospinal fluid shunt infections. *J Neurosurg Sci* 1994; 38:161.

315. Laurence K: The natural history of spina bifida cystica: Detailed analysis of 407 cases. *Arch Dis Child* 1964; 39:41.

316. Lorber J: Results of treatment of myelomeningocele. An analysis of 524 unselected cases, with special reference to possible selection for treatment. *Dev Med Child Neurol* 1971; 13:279.

317. Charney EB, et al: Management of the newborn with myelomeningocele: Time for a decision-making process. *Pediatrics* 1985; 75:58.

318. Lorber J: Some paediatric aspects of myelomeningocele. *Acta Orthop Scand* 1975; 46:350.

319. Dierdorf SF, et al: Failure of succinylcholine to alter plasma potassium in children with myelomeningocoele. *Anesthesiology* 1986; 64:272.

320. Flynn J: Retinopathy of prematurity. In Martyn L (ed): *Pediatric Ophthalmology. Pediatric Clinics of North America*. Philadelphia, WB Saunders, 1987:1487–1516.

321. Bryan MH, et al: Pulmonary function studies during the first year of life in infants recovering from the respiratory distress syndrome. *Pediatrics* 1973; 52:169.

322. Sandler AN, Tator CH: Effect of acute spinal cord compression injury on regional spinal cord blood flow in primates. *J Neurosurg* 1976; 45:660.

323. Kato A, et al: Circulatory disturbance of the spinal cord with epidural neoplasm in rats. *J Neurosurg* 1985; 63:260.

324. Kobrine AI, et al: Correlation of spinal cord blood flow, sensory evoked response, and spinal cord function in subacute experimental spinal cord compression. *Adv Neurol* 1978; 20:389.

325. Grundy B: Evoked potential monitoring. In Britt C (ed): *Monitoring in Anesthesia and Critical Care Medicine*. New York, Churchill Livingstone, 1990:461.

326. Maertens de Noordhout A, et al: Magnetic stimulation of the motor cortex in cervical spondylosis. *Neurology* 1991; 41:75.

327. Lam A: Do evoked potentials have any value in anesthesia? In Bissonnette B (ed): *Cerebral Protection, Resuscitation and Monitoring: A Look into the Future of Neuroanesthesia. Anesthesiology Clinics of North America*. Philadelphia, WB Saunders, 1992:657–683.

328. Grundy BL: Intraoperative monitoring of sensory-evoked potentials. *Anesthesiology* 1983; 58:72.

329. Bruce DA, et al: Outcome following severe head injuries in children. *J Neurosurg* 1978; 48:679.

330. Hardwood-Nash D: Fractures of the petrous and tympanic parts of the temporal bone in children: A tomographic study of 35 cases. *Am J Roentgenol Radium Ther Nucl Med* 1970; 110:598.

331. Freytag E: Autopsy findings in head injuries from blunt forces. Statistical evaluation of 1,367 cases. *Arch Pathol* 1963; 75:402.

332. Hendrick BE, et al: Head injuries in children: A survey of 4465 consecutive cases at the Hospital for Sick Children, Toronto, Ontario, Canada. *Clin Neurosurg* 1964; 11:46.

333. Bruce DA, et al: Diffuse cerebral swelling following head injuries in children: The syndrome of "malignant brain edema." *J Neurosurg* 1981; 54:170.

334. Ross DA, et al: Brain shift, level of consciousness, and restoration of consciousness in patients with acute intracranial hematoma. *J Neurosurg* 1989; 71:498.

335. Langfitt TW, et al: Computerized tomography, magnetic resonance imaging, and positron emission tomography in the

study of brain trauma. Preliminary observations. *J Neurosurg* 1986; 64:760.

336. Bohn D, et al: Cervical spine injuries in children. *J Trauma* 1990; 30:463..

337. Narins RG: Therapy of hyponatremia: Does haste make waste? *N Engl J Med* 1986; 314:1573.

338. Young B, et al: Relationship between admission hyperglycemia and neurologic outcome of severely brain-injured patients. *Ann Surg* 1989; 210:466.

339. Pulsinelli WA, et al: Moderate hyperglycemia augments ischemic brain damage: A neuropathologic study in the rat. *Neurology* 1982; 32:1239.

Neurologic Assessment and Monitoring

Integral to appropriate therapy of neurosurgical-neurologic intensive care unit (neuroICU) patients is diagnosis and ongoing assessment to determine the onset of treatable neurologic deterioration. The mainstay of neurologic assessment is history and examination. In addition, a variety of techniques are available for serial or continuous assessment of cerebral perfusion and metabolism. All such techniques aim to detect the onset of cerebral ischemia, which is to say the occurrence of insufficient supply of metabolic substrates to meet metabolic demands. Such techniques necessarily entail assessment of cerebral perfusion, cerebral electrical activity, and, finally, cerebral oxygenation. In addition, another extremely important tool in neurologic assessment of the neuroICU patient is imaging technology, which can provide information about both physiology and structure.

NEUROLOGIC EXAMINATION

A detailed description of neurologic examination techniques are beyond the scope of this chapter. However, for most purposes in the neuroICU, a rapid neurologic assessment is sufficient to establish baseline conditions and detect changes in neurologic status.[1-3] Figure 36-1 is a schematic outline of the major motor and sensory pathways.[1] The major sensory pathways ascend as they cross the midline, synapse in the thalmus and in the contralateral sensory area of the cerebral cortex. The corticospinal tract and other motor pathways synapse in the spinal cord. Lesions above the synapse produce upper motor neuron deficits and lesions below it produce lower motor neuron deficits, which produce different clinical signs[1] (Table 36-1).

A brief neurologic examination can be performed as described by Goldberg.[1] Mental status is assessed by orientation to person, place, and time. General mental status is determined by assessing general information, such as, who is the president, obtaining a description of some current events, assessing spelling ability for simple words, and asking the patient to add or subtract serial 3s or 7s. In addition, the patient can be asked to recall three objects several minutes after the examiner mentions them. Attention is tested by asking the patient to recall a series of numbers or to spell "world" backward.

Cranial nerves can be assessed as follows:

I (Olfactory)—test each side with a mild agent such as soap or tobacco.

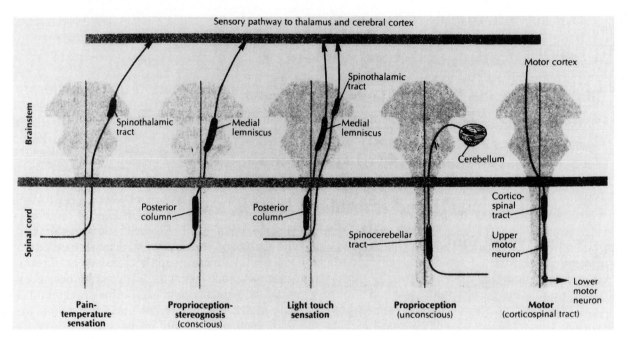

Figure 36-1 Schematic outline of the major motor and sensory pathways. (Reproduced by permission from Goldberg S. The Four Minute Neurologic Exam, MedMaster, 1992[1])

II (Optic)—Near and far visual acuity and gross visual fields are assessed. Ophthalmoscopic examination is performed.

III, IV, VI (Oculomotor, trochlear, abducens)—Pupillary light response. Lateral and vertical gaze are assessed.

V (Trigeminal)—Assessment of touch sensation in both sides of the face is performed in all three trigeminal divisions. In addition, corneal blink reflex can also be assessed.

VII (Facial)—Symmetrical smile assessment is performed. In addition, brow wrinkling can be assessed to determine central versus peripheral seventh nerve function.

VIII (Auditory)—Ability to hear fingertips moving is assessed. Lateralizing the sound of a tuning fork placed over the mid-forehead can localize a hearing deficit.

IX, X (Glossopharyngeal, Vagus)—Gag reflex is assessed with a tongue blade or tonsil tip suction device.

XI (Accessory)—Bilateral shoulder elevation (trapexius) and head-turning (sternocleidomastoid) strength is assessed.

XII (Hypoglossal)—The patient is asked to extrude the tongue. If there is weakness on one side of the tongue, the tongue will deviate to that side.

Motor examination is performed by assessing pronator drift of the upper extremity. Hand grasps and toe and foot dorsiflexion as well as the major flexors and extensors of the upper and lower extremities are assessed. In addition, assessment of individual muscles can also be assessed and graded (Table 36-2).

Sensation is assessed by stimulation with a pin on the hand and feet with determination of the patient's ability to distinguish between sharp or dull sensation.

TABLE 36-1
Clinical Findings With Upper And Lower Motor Neuron Deficits

Upper Motor Neuron Deficit	Lower Motor Neuron Deficit
Spastic weakness	Flaccid weakness
No significant muscle atrophy	Significant atrophy
No fasciculations/fibrillations	Fasciculations/fibrillations
Hyperreflexia	Hyporeflexia
Babinski reflex may be present	No babinski reflex

SOURCE: Reproduced by permission from Goldberg S. The Four Minute Neurologic Exam, MedMaster, 1992.[1]

TABLE 36-2
Grading of Muscle Strength

Grade	Examination
0	No evidence of muscle contraction
1	Slight contraction but no joint motion
2	Complete horizontal motion (i.e., without gravity)
3	Barely complete motion against gravity
4	Complete motion against gravity and some resistance
5	Complete motion against gravity and full resistance

The examination should be done in a repetitive manner because patients can report both stimuli as sharp bilaterally and then some 10 s later report to only one side as sharp indicating a subtle deficit on the dull side. A similar maneuver is performed on the cheeks for cranial nerve V and the dorsum of the feet. It is important to note that this examination technique has been associated with the spread of infectious diseases[4] and thus, a new pin or other sharp device should be used for each assessment with every effort made to not elicit bleeding. Light touch sensation is tested in a similar manner using the touch of a finger in the place of a pin.

Coordination is assessed by finger-to-nose and heel-to-shin testing and assessment of rapid alternating movements of the hand and or foot. This aspect of the examination tests cerebellar and basal ganglia function because these structures play an important role in coordination. Deep tendon reflexes are assessed in the biceps, triceps, patella, and Achilles. The Babinski reflexes are assessed by stroking the lateral foot. In addition to test for meningeal irritation, the Kernig (elevation of straightened lower extremity) and Brudzinski (head flexion by examiner) tests are performed.

Procedures performed in evaluation of the comatose patient include determination of viable vital signs and assessment of hand drop over the head when nonphysiologic coma is suspected. Pupil size and response to light are assessed. Pinpoint pupils imply a pontine lesion or drug effect, whereas large pupils can suggest a structural lesion, hypoxia, or a drug effects. Uncal herniation will produce a unilateral pupillary enlargement with ptosis and inferior-lateral position due to third cranial nerve lesion. Eye movements are assessed by first evaluating eye position. In destructive cerebral lesions, the eyes deviate toward the side of the lesion. Assessment of the oculocephalic (doll's eye) reflex is performed by turning the head suddenly to one side. The eyes tend to lag behind when the patient has lethargy or is semicomatose, but they move with the head in the awake state and when brainstem centers are impaired. Further indication of brainstem impairment is present when the corneal and gag responses are absent and when there is extensor or flexor posturing. Response to noxious stimulus is assessed peripherally by stimulating the sternum or nail beds or centrally by supraorbital pressure. The Babinski reflex is assessed.

The neurologic examination, by its nature, is a nonparametric subjective assessment tool. Interobserver reliability has been assessed and been found to be variable.[5-7] However, it has been determined that the availability of a clinical history significantly enhances the consistency of the neurologic examination.[7] Accordingly, some clinicians and investigators use quantitative or semiquantitative methods to document neurologic status and reliably follow trends. Quantitative

TABLE 36-3
Glasgow Coma Scale

Item	Factor	Score
Best motor response	Obeys	6
	Localizes	5
	Withdraws (flexion)	4
	Abnormal flexion	3
	Extensor response	2
	Nil	1
Verbal response	Oriented	5
	Confused conversation	4
	Inappropriate words	3
	Incomprehensible sounds	2
	Nil	1
Eye opening	Spontaneous	4
	To speech	3
	To pain	2
	Nil	1

methods have been used for general neurologic sensory assessment,[8-10] pupillary assessment,[11] and overall clinical neurologic examination.[10,12] Others have devised techniques to quantitatively document and trend neurologic function after spinal cord injury.[13,14] In addition, a variety of scales have been published to similarly quantitate neurologic function for clinical and research purposes. Such scales have been oriented to head trauma,[15,16] stroke,[17-21] sedation assessment,[21a] and general assessment.[21b] The best known of these scales is the Glasgow coma scale (GCS) (Table 36-3),[15,16,21] which has achieved widespread use in semiquantitation of the neurologic status in patients after head trauma. The GCS may also be used in nontrauma settings. The primary advantage is simplicity. However, there is no sensory component to the examination and verbal assessment is lost with substantial decrement in the score if a patient is intubated. If the patient is intubated and awake this may produce an artifactual decrease.

CEREBRAL BLOOD FLOW

PHYSIOLOGY

The flow of blood to the brain is finely regulated to provide substrates according to the needs of neural tissue. This coupling occurs via several mechanisms. The cerebral vasculature is extensively innervated with a wide variety of neurotransmitter-containing nerves that appear to work in close concert with the endothelium and neural metabolism. In addition, viscosity, blood pressure, and humorally released substances also play an important role in maintenance of appropriate cerebral blood flow (CBF).[22-24]

Based on CBF observations with mannitol it has been suggested that there is viscosity autoregulation present in the brain.[25,26] Mannitol-induced decreased viscosity results in a decrease in cerebral blood volume (CBV) as cerebral vessels constrict to maintain CBF constant. However, the observation that pentoxifylline *increases* CBF presumably due to a decrease in viscosity suggests that the concept of viscosity autoregulation may not be well understood.[27] It is of interest that Cavestri and coworkers[26] reported that rheologic changes had no effect on CBF in subjects less than 45 years old, whereas those older did show changes in flow with variations in viscosity. Their conclusion was that rheologic autoregulation occurs in youth and that it may diminish with age.

A wide variety of nerve types innervate the cerebral vasculature. These include nerves containing amines, peptides, neuropeptide Y, norepinephrine, acetylcholine, epinephrine, vasoactive intestinal peptide, peptide histidine, isoleucine, substance P, neurokinin A, calcitonin, gene-related peptide, cholecystokinin, dynorphin B, galanin, gastrin-related peptide, antidiuretic hormone (ADH), neurotensin, somatostatin, glutamate, serotonin, enkephalin, dopamine, and prostanoids.[28-40] These neurotransmitters confer vasoconstriction or vasodilation on the cerebral vasculature. The neurons innervating the cerebral vessels arise from numerous areas. These anatomic loci include intracranial ganglia,[34,40] the spinal cord,[41] other extracranial nerves,[39] or intracerebral nuclei.[36] Neural metabolic factors also clearly have an important role in fine tuning of local CBF. Such products of metabolism as lactate and P_{CO_2} to decrease pH, nitric oxide, and other factors contribute to this aspect of autoregulation.[23,38,42-44] Such a notion is reinforced by observations of coupled variations in CBF with extremity movements or thought processes.[23,42] It is thought that nitric oxide is an important component of this neural metabolic fine tuning of local CBF.[38,43,44] Indeed, it has been suggested that hypercapnia-mediated increased CBF occurs by way of nitric oxide.[38]

The endothelium of cerebral blood vessels appears to be a central component of blood flow regulation by way of innervation or neural metabolism.[35,40,43,45,46-50] There are several examples of the dependence of neural and metabolic factors on endothelium to exert effects on CBF. Tachykinin effects on CBF are removed with removal of the endothelium.[33] Endothelium has been suggested as one of the areas where hypertension may have CBF effects.[46,47] Angiotensin-converting enzyme (ACE) has been observed immunohistochemically in brain endothelium.[35,51] In addition, endothelin, a potent vasoconstrictor, and prostanoids reportedly arise from human brain endothelial cells in response to exogenous stimuli.[49,50]

The vasodilator acetylcholine requires an intact endothelium to function.[40] Nitric oxide is an example of a metabolic mediator depending on endothelium with a rather complex interaction. It is thought that activation of receptors by the excitatory amino acid glutamate is a major stimulus for NO release, resulting in vasodilatation to produce local flow-metabolism coupling. It is of interest that NO synthase-containing nerves innervate large cerebral blood vessels and arterioles, further supporting this notion.[38] However, Kontos[48] suggests that the actual mediator, formerly known as endothelium-derived relaxation factor, in cerebral arterioles is not NO but is an NO-containing compound, nitrosothiol, which activates guanylate cyclase. Overall, it is clear that the endothelium exerts an important influence on cerebral vascular tone via synthesis and release of vasoactive factors. Relaxing factors include nitric oxide and prostacyclin. Endothelial-derived contracting factors include cyclo-oxygenase products of arachidonic acid and endothelins.[50]

In addition to innervation and neural metabolic control of cerebral circulation, remote influences are exerted by way of blood pressure and humorally mediated influences. Blood pressure has long been known to have an impact on the cerebral circulation. Alterations in blood pressure result in changes in cerebral vascular resistance (CVR) to maintain CBF constant within the range of physiologic blood pressures. At the extremes, however, blood pressure changes result in a linear pressure-dependent change in flow. This relationship is altered by chronic hypertension shifting the relationship to higher pressures. This has been observed in a dynamic manner in correlation with transcranial Doppler blood flow velocity (BFV) measurements.[52] Humoral mechanisms also have important effects on the regulation of CBF and the effect of chronic hypertension.[46,47]

Overall it appears that metabolism and CBF are tightly coupled although CBF is heterogeneous. Short-term dynamic coupling is thought to be mediated by local vasoactive factors. Conversely, long-term homeostatic coupling is thought to be mediated by capillary density changes developed in response to local metabolic activity.[45]

Chronic propranolol at low doses has no effect on CBF although at high doses it does increase CBF.[53] Similarly, intravenous labetalol has no effect on CBF.[54] In general, data indicate no significant effect of β-adrenergic agonist or antagonist administration on CBF.[53-56] Information suggests that endogenous local catecholamine release may have more pronounced influence on CBF[57] and that an intact blood-brain barrier (BBB) is required for there to be minimal CBF effects of catecholamines.[58]

Cerebral blood flow is exquisitely sensitive to changes of P_{CO_2} with a linear fluctuation in CBF reported with changes in P_{CO_2}.[59-63] This sensitivity of CBF to P_{CO_2} is the underlying physiology supporting the use of CO_2 changes to provocatively change CBF through inhibition of carbonic anhydrase with acetazolamide[64-67] or through induced alterations in minute ventilation or inspired CO_2 to changed P_{CO_2}.[68]

Oxygen level is an essential aspect of maintenance of CBF. Ordinarily, the CBF remains relatively constant with variations in P_{O_2} as long as arterial oxygen saturation is greater than 95%. However, with decrements in P_{O_2} the CBF increases substantially in a compensatory manner to maintain oxygen supply.[69]

Sleep is a normal physiologic function that has significant influences on CBF in the progression through the various stages of sleep. It has been observed that slow wave sleep is associated with lower CBF, whereas rapid eye movement (REM) sleep is associated with high CBF.[70] Although not exactly the same, Madsen and Vorstrup's data[71] indicated that REM CBF is similar to that awake, whereas light sleep and deep sleep (non-REM) is associated with only a 10 percent decrease in CBF.

Aging is another important factor in evaluating CBF. In general it has been observed that the highest CBF occurs in childhood (5 to 10 years old) with lower CBF at younger ages and a progressive decline in CBF as the individual ages.[72-75] This is thought to be associated with decreases in brain tissue.[74] Moreover, the decrease of CBF is reportedly associated with a decrease of CO_2 reactivity.[72]

PATHOPHYSIOLOGY

The aforementioned considerations in normal cerebrovascular physiology are altered in a variety of pathologic conditions. Most importantly, normal physiology will be disrupted with chronic hypertension and ischemic cerebrovascular disease.

Numerous reports document the shift of the lower limit of pressure autoregulation with chronic hypertension.[76] The anatomic basis for this is thought to be vascular hypertrophy and remodeling of the microcirculation.[76] CO_2 reactivity is reportedly maintained with chronic hypertension.[62] However, responses to humoral effectors are altered in chronic hypertension due to decreased endothelial responses.[46,47] Because of the shift of the autoregulation curve to higher pressures, there is always concern that decreasing blood pressure will result in ischemia.[77] A variety of studies have examined the effects of blood pressure reduction on CBF.[78-82] Generally, ACE inhibitors and calcium antagonists seem to be able to bring blood pressure down in this condition without producing dramatic decreases in CBF.[78,82]

Occlusive cerebral vascular disease produces decrements in CBF such that aerobic metabolism may not be supported, with a consequent decrement in neuronal function and risk of neuronal injury or death. However, a more subtle manifestation of occlusive cerebral vascular disease is a decrease in cerebrovascular reserve. That is, a compromise in vascular inflow results in compensatory vasodilatation such that, at the microcirculatory level and at a given systemic blood pressure, there will be a greater degree of vasodilatation than there would be otherwise resulting in normal blood flow. When this occurs, the lower limit of the pressure autoregulation curve is increased such that flow varies linearly with pressure at a higher blood pressure than normal. The functional consequence of this is that ordinary perturbations that are well tolerated through physiologic vasodilation will not be tolerated if further vasodilation cannot be achieved. Thus, decreases in blood pressure or oxygen supply may not be tolerated such that a stroke may arise. The abnormality of CO_2 reactivity in occlusive cerebral vascular disease has been documented in a number of reports.[68,83-86] In addition, to avoid the awkwardness of CO_2 administration systems and the discomfort that it may cause, acetazolamide has been used as an alternate means to increase cerebrospinal fluid (CSF) CO_2 to assess changes in CBF.[87,88] Moreover, this technique has occasionally been used in an effort to define prognosis of ICU patients.[89]

A variety of collateral routes are available for maintaining CBF in focal ischemic situations. Leptomeningeal anastomoses are an example of one means of maintaining flow when larger primary and secondary flow becomes compromised.[90] In addition, anastomoses of the cerebral venous system play a role in the collateral circulation.[91] The circle of Willis clearly provides the major collateral route with carotid occlusion.[92] In addition to these routes, brain capillary density also develops in accordance with demands[44] as may occur in Moyamoya disease.[93]

MEASUREMENT

A number of measurement technologies have evolved over the years to evaluate CBF. Generally, the methods entail assessment of washin or washout of a tracer substance or bulk flow measurement. Methods described include stable xenon computed tomography (CT) CBF,[94-96] technecium-labeled red blood cell techniques,[97] thermodilution techniques,[98] xenon 133 methods,[99,100] ultrasonic volume flow,[101] positron emission tomography (PET),[102,103] single photon emission computed tomography (SPECT),[60,104-107] AV_{O_2} difference assessment,[108,109] radioisotope measurement of brain-blood turnover,[110] forehead thermography,[111] thermal diffusion flowmetry,[112] planar gamma camera images CBF/cerebral blood volume determination,[113] laser Doppler flowmetry,[114] and ultrafast CT with iodinated contrast.[115]

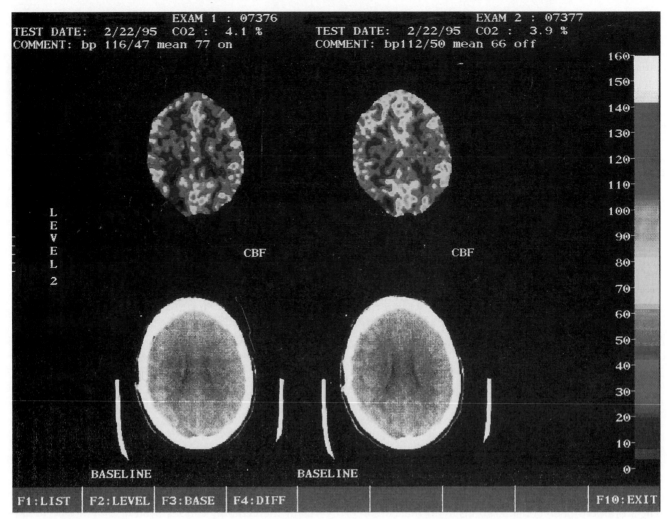

A

Figure 36-2 Stable xenon-CT cerebral blood flow (CBF). Stable xenon is inhaled by the subject over a circumscribed period of time with concurrent monitoring of end-tidal CO_2 and end-tidal xenon during which serial CT scans are acquired. Xenon is radiopaque and taken up into the brain in proportion to blood flow. Thus, changes in CT density reflect uptake of xenon and permit calculation of blood flow in each pixel of the two-dimensional image across the brain. CBF scale is on the right in ml/100g/min. CT images are indicated in the lower figures and CBF maps in the upper figures. This technique can be used to assess effects of therapy. Two examples of this are shown. *A.* The patient, who had sustained a subarachnoid hemorrhage, had CBFs determined with (on) and without (off) phenylephrine infusions. CBF decreased with phenylephrine infusion.

The methods most commonly used in neuroICU patients are as follows.

Stable Xenon CTCBF (XeCTCBF)

With this technique, the subject may inhale from 26% to 33% stable xenon. The xenon is rapidly taken up into the blood, transported to the brain, and taken up into the brain. End-tidal xenon is recorded continuously and assumed to be arterial. Xenon is radiopaque; thus, changes in radiodensity with serial CT scanning can be used to calculate CBF throughout the brain (Fig. 36-2). The method computes solubility (λ) throughout the brain and then uses the adjusted λ for all CBF

calculations. This results in more valuable data in patients with disease states where λ may not be uniform throughout the brain. The technique has been criticized because of pharmacologic effects of xenon. Xenon inhalation effects reportedly include decreasing CO_2 and augmenting CBF.[116] However, using multiple early images and weighting calculations to the early portion of the washin curve has eliminated the effect of flow activation on CBF calculation.[94–96,117] In addition, in evaluation of CBF in normals, the flow values obtained with XeCTCBF are clearly consistent with those obtained with other methods suggesting that potential bias induced by xenon inhalation is not a significant

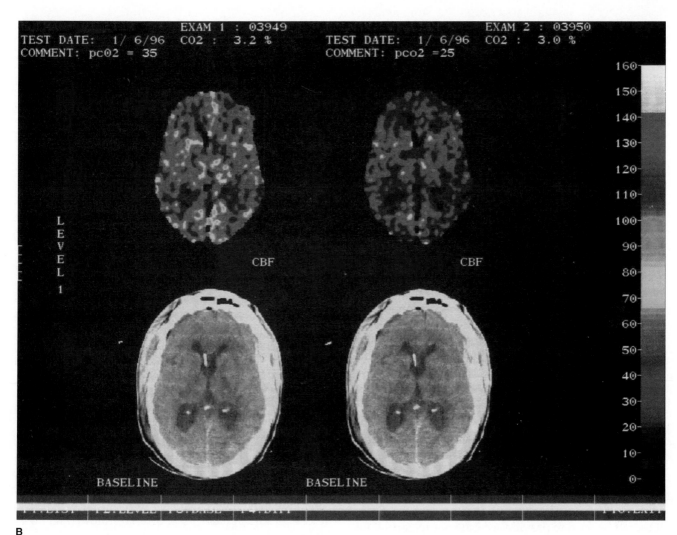

B

Figure 36-2 (*Continued*) *B.* P_{CO_2} was altered in a patient with head trauma. Decreasing P_{CO_2} from 35 to 25 mmHg was associated with a significant decrease in CBF, particularly in white matter areas and some cortical areas.

factor. Many of the patients who are undergoing CBF assessment are having it done to assess areas of low blood flow. Thus, regardless of concerns about potential CBF increasing effects, XeCTCBF has been shown to be a versatile and useful tool especially in the evaluation of low blood flow conditions. Moreover, because studies can be repeated at 20-min intervals reactivity challenge testing of therapies can be performed. The fact that it can be readily given while a patient is in the CT scan is a major advantage because it can be obtained in the course of obtaining structural information during CT scanning.

Radioactive Xenon

These methods have been widely used by either inhalation, intravenous injection, or intraarterial injection.[99,100,118,119] All such methods eliminate considerations about xenon effects on CBF because only trace amounts of xenon are administered. However, the CBF values are obtained from gamma counters located at specific loci on the scalp, recording CBF in only one dimension. In conditions of low flow this technology can be problematic, missing low flow deep in the brain or conversely missing low flow on the cortex because of persistent flow in deeper structures (look-through phenomenon).[120]

Positron Emission Tomography

The use of positron emission tomography (PET) can provide rapid CBFs with only small amounts of tracer providing information in three dimensions, although without the regional resolution or quantitation provided by XeCTCBF. It is performed using $H_2^{15}O$, which is rapidly distributed throughout the brain in proportion to CBF and is then rapidly washed out permitting serial flows to be obtained. Radiation limits the number of repetitive studies that can be done. In addition, it is a technology available in only a few major medical centers, predominately for research purposes. In addition, PET entails transporting the patient, who generally requires CT for structural information, to another imaging suite, in addition to CT.[102,103]

Single Photon Emission Computed Tomography

This methodology has achieved relatively widespread use. It entails administration of a tracer (HMPAO), which is radioactive and is distributed through the brain in proportion to flow. Once in the brain it remains for several hours. Accordingly, the tracer can be injected in the ICU during an event and at relative leisure. The CBF signal can then be acquired shortly thereafter, after transporting the patient to the nuclear scanner to acquire the signal. SPECT suffers generally from a lack of quantitation without the resolution available with XeCTCBF. There is, however, no concern about the possibility of tracer effects on CBF. It does require transport to an imaging suite distinct from CT and it cannot be easily repeated to assess the effects of therapeutic interventions. Recently, reports have described methods that provide better quantitation of SPECT.[68,106,107] This may represent an advance that will make this technology much more useful in the neuroICU.

AV$_{O_2}$ Difference

This measurement is based on the Fick equation. Given a stable cerebral metabolic rate, changes in AV$_{O_2}$ difference of oxygen will represent changes in CBF. Thus, it cannot be used to provide accurate nor regional CBF and it does depend on accurate insertion of a catheter into the jugular bulb. However, it can be used at the bedside in a serial manner to provide information regarding adequacy of CBF relative to cerebral metabolic rate (CMR).[108,109] The primary problem with data acquired with AV$_{O_2}$ difference techniques arises in situations of heterogeneous CBF. It is a global measure and its information can be misleading when hyperemic areas overshadow ischemic areas of the brain.

Laser Doppler Flowmetry

This technique uses the Doppler principle with laser light. However, it is invasive, requiring placement of a probe directly on the cortex or dura, and is very positional. However, when it works well, it provides continuous second-to-second information regarding CBF in the area insonated. By its nature, it provides only regional information.[114]

In the evaluation of CBF it is important to consider the effects of concomitant drug use. A large number of reports have detailed the effects on CBF of many of the drugs used in the neuroICU. This knowledge is too large for this chapter to provide a comprehensive overview.

TRANSCRANIAL DOPPLER

Transcranial Doppler ultrasonography (TCD) uses reflected ultrasound from basal cerebral arteries and the Doppler principle to determine the velocity of blood (cm/s) in a given insonated artery. It provides real-time dynamic information regarding BFV, providing a continuous waveform, similar to that obtained with intraarterial blood pressure monitoring. An example is shown in Fig. 36-3 of TCD recordings during a difficult anesthetic induction sequence. Insonated arteries include the proximal arteries of the circle of Willis. The reproducibility of TCD recordings depends on a constant angle of the transducer insonating a given vessel. This is an important operator-dependent factor. This factor is minimized as the insonation angle becomes more parallel to the vessel being examined. Another important factor in interpreting BFV measurements is the vessel diameter. Decreases in vessel caliber can increase BFV in the face of decreasing CBF. In addition, hematocrit, P$_{CO_2}$, and blood pressure can also influence BFV, although this may actually be a reflection of changes in CBF.[121,122]

It is important to note that TCD is not a quantitative flow monitor in ml/100 g per minute. Rather it provides information, which can be useful, regarding the presence and character of flow. In some situations TCD changes may reflect changes in CBF, particularly in those of abrupt changes in arterial inflow (Fig. 36-4). It has several uses in the neuroICU. These uses include assessment of vasospasm, vascular reactivity, increased intracranial pressure (ICP), brain death, arterial patency, flow direction, emboli, and hyperemia.

Transcranial Doppler ultrasonography is an excellent early indicator of the presence of vasospasm before the onset of a clinically evident ischemic deficit. These observations are based on the physical principle that, with narrowing of a basal cerebral artery, BFV would increase, even as flow decreased. Thus, TCD has found a routine place in many neuroICUs as a screening tool for the occurrence of vasospasm.[123-126] However, subsequent studies, perhaps related to increased use of nimodipine, have shown that increased velocity in patients with subarachnoid hemorrhage (SAH) is associated with hyperemia more often than it is associated with vasospasm.[127] In addition, TCD can miss distal spasm, thus giving a false sense of safety. Thus, TCD, although still possibly of value as a rough screening tool, has insufficient sensitivity and specificity to be the sole criterion to make important therapeutic decisions in SAH. It still may be used as a trend once it is established that a patient clearly is in vasospasm or is

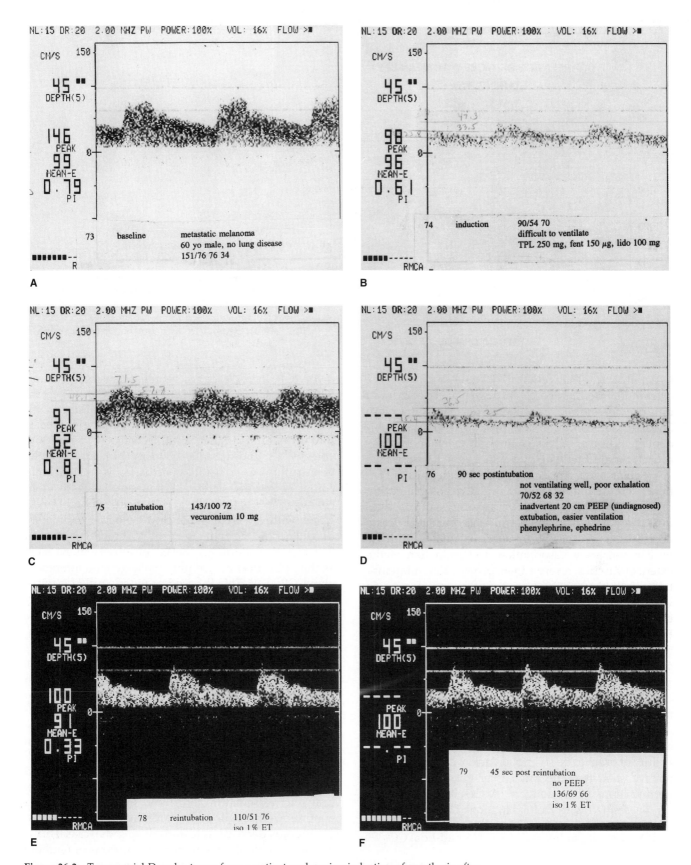

Figure 36-3 Transcranial Doppler traces from a patient undergoing induction of anesthesia after which difficult ventilation was encountered. *A.* Baseline, awake tracing. Mean blood flow velocity is 99 cm/s. *B.* Thiopental induction with some ventilation difficulty. *C.* Intubation. *D.* Postintubation with discovery of inadvertent 20 cmH₂O positive end-expiratory pressure (PEEP). Patient was extubated subsequently. *E.* Reintubation with no PEEP. *F.* 45 s after intubation.

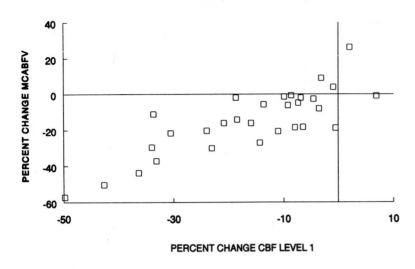

CORRELATION OF XeCBF WITH MEAN BFV DURING BTO

Figure 36-4 Scatter plot showing change in middle cerebral artery (MCA) blood flow velocity (MCA BFV) as a function of change in MCA distribution of CBF during balloon test occlusion. $r^2 = 0.733$ ($p < .0001$). (Reproduced by permission from Kofke and coworkers.[143a])

hyperemic. Alternatively it may be used to assess the extent of vasodilatory cerebrovascular reserve, and thus provide indirect information regarding how close a vasospastic condition is to producing clinically evident symptoms.[128-130] It is unclear whether this approach can differentiate hyperemia versus vasospasm.

Vascular reactivity is an important measure in patients with a brain insult. Normally, autoregulating cerebral vasculature implies the existence of vasodilatory reserve, which can permit the brain to tolerate decreases in perfusion pressure, oxygen, or glucose by compensatory vasodilation. Determination of the extent of vascular reserve, then, provides a semiquantitative indicator of the severity of injury to a given vascular bed. Reactivity assessment is done by manipulation of either perfusion pressure or carbon dioxide. For a given change in mean arterial pressure, within the normal autoregulatory range, there should be no change in BFV. A change in flow velocity indicates abnormal autoregulation.

Carbon dioxide reactivity can be assessed by increasing inspired CO_2 or by increasing tissue CO_2 via administration of acetazolamide. BFV normally should increase 3 to 4 percent per mmHg increase in Pa_{CO_2}. Failure of brain to do so implies lack of cerebrovascular reserve such that the brain may not tolerate minor perturbations in O_2 delivery. A CO_2 reactivity index can be defined with CO_2 inhalation[131]:

$$CO_2 \text{ reactivity index} = (V2-V1)/(\Delta \text{ end-tidal } CO_2)$$

Normal CO_2 reactivity index is 1.78 ± 0.48 (SD). In patients with cerebrovascular disease this index was found to vary from 0.15 to 2.6.[494] Failure of brain to demonstrate a normal increase in BFV with CO_2 increase implies the presence of maximal vasodilation.

As ICP increases or cerebral perfusion pressure (CPP) decreases, the character of the TCD waveform changes, becoming more "spiky" in appearance with increased pulsatility[132,133] (Fig. 36-5). This is the basis for the definition of the pulsatility index [(systolic flow velocity − end-diastolic velocity)/(mean diastolic velocity)].[134] As diastolic perfusion is increasingly compromised, the cerebral circulation takes on more characteristics of the higher resistance peripheral circulation with lower diastolic flow velocity. Ultimately diastolic flow velocity is zero as cerebral perfusion becomes discontinuous. Based on observations such as this, TCD may be useful to make general inferences about CPP.[135,136] This is based predominantly on retrospective reports, having not yet been assessed prospectively in a large number of patients to determine whether TCD could be used to reliably and noninvasively determine the CPP in a given patient.

Increases in ICP into the 20 to 30 mmHg range, although of epidemiologic significance, have not been shown to have substantial physiologic significance in terms of a dangerous decrement in CBF. As ICP increases, cerebral vasodilation occurs in a compensatory fashion and the actual CBF tends to be not in the ischemic range at lower ICPs.[132] However with further ICP increases approaching diastolic arterial pressure[133] and infringing on the critical closing pressure of the cerebral microvasculature,[137,138] flow, which ordinarily is continuous throughout the cardiac cycle, becomes discontinuous decreasing to zero during diastole. This is consistent with the theoretical conclusions of Giulioni and colleagues[132] wherein they suggest, based on considerations of intracranial elastance and vasomotor tone, that systolic increase and diastolic decrease in BFV should occur when ICP reaches the "breakpoint" value. They suggest that the Gosling pulsatility index

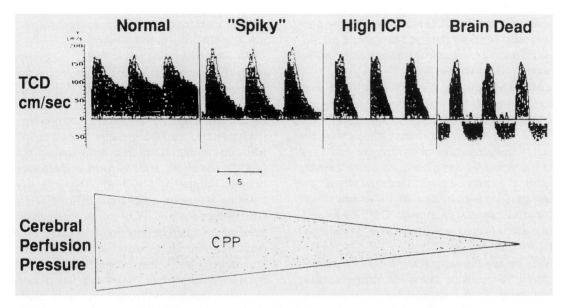

Figure 36-5 Progression of TCD waveforms with after head injury from intact CBF and normal-appearing TCD waveform to intracranial hypertension sufficient to induce intracerebral circulatory arrest. Schematic of decreasing cerebral perfusion pressure (CPP) indicated in the lower panel. (Reproduced by permission from Hassler and coworkers.[133])

should be a useful indicator of high ICP. ICP in such situations of zero diastolic flow theoretically should be in the 40 to 60 mmHg range.[137,138] Indeed, an ICP of 48 mmHg is the average level at which patients progressing to brain death have been observed initially to sustain a high ICP, systolic spike pattern with the oscillating pattern developing at 62.5 mmHg.[139] Hassler and coworkers[133] clearly showed the relationship between ICP and phasic blood pressure and how TCD waveform can reflect ICP encroachment on diastolic flow when ICP exceeds diastolic pressure. Their hypothesis, moreover, fits in quite well with observations of similar high ICP waveforms with aortic insufficiency[140] (Fig. 36-6) and hypotension[141,141a] (Fig. 36-7).

It is of theoretical interest that TCD waveforms might contain information suggesting high ICP that is not high enough to produce zero diastolic velocity. This concept is supported by recent reports of an exponential correlation between ICP and pulsatility index.[135] An ICP of 40 mmHg produced, on average, a pulsatility index of about 1.5 with the lowest pulsatility index at that ICP approximately 1.3. In a rabbit cisternal infusion high ICP model mean BFV and CBF remained relatively unchanged (and correlated, $r = 0.86$) with increasing ICP until perfusion pressure decreased to about 40 mmHg. Below this level, at which calculated vascular resistance increased due to high ICP, BFV decreased with continued decrease in perfusion pressure.[142] Such data suggest, in the absence of vasospasm, that the onset of decreasing mean BFV with increasing ICP implies that perfusion pressure has decreased to below the lower limit of autoregulation.

As cerebral perfusion pressure progressively decreases to sustained levels associated with no CBF, brain death ensues. With TCD this manifests as diastolic reversal of flow presumably due to blood "bouncing" backward off an edematous brain[133] (see Fig. 36-5). Thus, TCD may be useful as a screening tool for brain death. However, it is important to consider the diastolic blood pressure when making such assess-

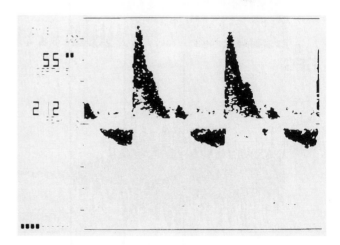

Figure 36-6 TCD findings in a 25-year-old man without cerebrovascular disease but with severe aortic insufficiency. The waveform was obtained before induction of anesthesia for replacement of an infected aortic valve. The patient also had a double outlet single ventricle and pulmonary atresia, and previously had undergone a Blalock-Taussig shunt procedure. Blood pressure was 196/34, heart rate 104, hematocrit 44%, Sa_{O_2} 85%. Figure provided courtesy ML Dong, McKeesport Hospital, McKeesport, PA and reproduced by permission from Kofke.[140])

ments. A strikingly similar TCD waveform can be generated in a totally sentient patient with aortic insufficiency and diastolic pressure low enough to be in the range of normal ICP (see Fig. 36-6).[140]

Occasionally a patient may be admitted to the neuroICU after having had a procedure to the middle cerebral or internal carotid arteries. In such cases TCD has been used to confirm continued patency of the blood vessel.[143] Because clinical symptoms may not occur until the vessel is completely occluded or may not occur at all, TCD may be used to indicate when flow in the monitored vessel is changed in an unwanted manner. Data indicate that changes in CBF due to arterial occlusion are reflected in changes in TCD-detected flow velocity[143a] (see Fig. 36-4).

Emboli can be readily detected with TCD. This is most commonly a relevant question during cardiac or carotid surgery. In the neuroICU, TCD can help determine the adequacy of anticoagulation in patients with artificial cardiac valves or patients with tenuous proximal vascular patency. However, it has been observed that emboli are very common in some situations, without obvious neurologic sequelae. Thus, determination that a given frequency of emboli in a given patient warrants major changes in therapy is presently a matter of clinical judgement.

As a bedside diagnostic test TCD can provide important information regarding the direction of blood flow in the vessels of the circle of Willis. Such information can be helpful in making inferences regarding the extent and source of collateral circulation.

Hyperemia can be a major problem in some clinical conditions, as after arteriovenous malformation (AVM) resection, after carotid endarterectomy, with hepatic failure, and systemic hypertension. Given a baseline value or calibration of a TCD value with a CBF determination, TCD can be used to ascertain the presence of a cerebral hyperfusion syndrome. This has been reported after carotid endarterectomy by Stieger and colleagues[144] and Lindegaard and coworkers.[145] Such syndromes risk the occurrence of normal perfusion pressure breakthrough, wherein cerebral edema or hemorrhage can occur, despite the presence of normal blood pressure. After carotid endarterectomy, cerebral hyperemia is thought to predispose to postoperative cerebral hemorrhage, presumably as a consequence of impaired cerebral autoregulation.[146] Thus, TCD might be useful to judge the cerebral risk and titrate the need for aggressive prevention or treatment of systemic hypertension.

In the neuroICU, TCD can be used as a tool for making intermittent, serial diagnostic assessments or it can be used as a continuous monitor. As a diagnostic tool it is used to assess the cerebral vasculature intermittently. TCD data are highly operator dependent. Thus, problems can arise due to different people obtaining the signals. Insofar as possible TCD data should be acquired by the same person daily with the person acquiring the information recorded in the record.

Training is required to acquire and identify a signal from a cerebral artery. Once acquired, however, maintaining acquisition of a good signal for monitoring purposes can be challenging. Minor changes in the angle of insonation can result in loss or degradation of the signal. Thus, well trained and motivated nurses are needed to use TCD successfully as a monitor in the neuroICU. It is most optimally used for monitoring purposes when data are acquired hourly, or with each neuro check, thus providing a useful trend indicator over hours.

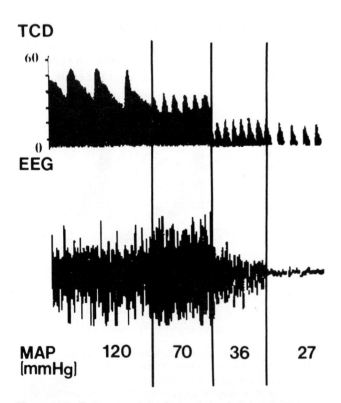

Figure 36-7 Patient sustaining hemorrhage during surgery. *Top,* compressed TCD observations; *middle,* compressed raw electroencephalographic (EEG) findings; *bottom,* mean arterial pressure. (Figure provided and modified with permission from C. Werner, Munich, Germany.)

ELECTROENCEPHALOGRAPHY AND EVOKED POTENTIALS IN THE NEUROICU

ELECTROENCEPHALOGRAPHY

Electroencephalography (EEG) provides a means to assess the electrical potential between two sites in the brain as reflected by recording electrodes, typically applied to the scalp. Electrodes can also be placed intra-

EEG

↓

Sort
and
Measure

↓

Smooth

↓

Compress
and
Suppress

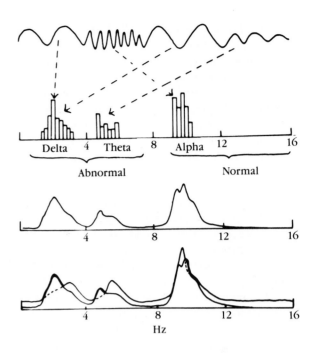

Figure 36-8 Computerized processing of a raw EEG signal to produce a Fourier-transformed series of wave forms.

cranially but for most neuroICU purposes it is used with scalp electrodes, which reflect cortical activity. The electrical activity recorded is a summation of highly complex functional activity in the underlying brain. The EEG waves represent a summation of the extracellular current fluctuations from the underlying superficial cortical layers. Surface negative waves represent a summation of excitatory postsynaptic potentials, whereas surface positive waves indicate the summation of inhibitory postsynaptic potentials in underlying cortex.[147] It can be recorded as a raw unprocessed continuous recording or the signals can undergo computerized processing to allow data to be presented in a more compact fashion. One commonly used method of more efficiently presenting the EEG data is Fourier analysis also known as power spectrum analysis.[148] This analytic procedure analyzes the sinusoidal wave content in the EEG signal, determining the summed amplitudes at each frequency of sinusoidal waves contained in the EEG signal (Fig. 36-8). This results in compact presentation of the EEG data, enhancing the ability of the human observer to detect subtle changes in amplitude or frequency content of an EEG signal, thus facilitating detection of important physiologic events (see Chap. 6). Uses of EEG as a monitor in the neuroICU include detection of cerebral hypoxic/ischemic conditions similar to that in the operating room[149,150] (Chap. 27). In addition, it can be used to detect seizure activity and titrate sedative drugs or anticonvulsant therapy. The primary limitation of EEG is that it does not reliably reflect events in tissue below the cortex, as the EEG signal reflects predominantly cortical activity.

EVOKED POTENTIALS

Evoked potentials (EPs) have been used for many years in the outpatient and operating room setting. They can be helpful diagnostically to localize the site of a functional disturbance in patients with neurologic disorders. In addition, EPs can be used to continuously confirm functional integrity of neurologic structures when surgery places a specific neurologic tract at risk. EPs have found use in ICUs, primarily for one-time diagnostic testing. However, there is interest in the use of EPs as brain monitors in the critically ill. Although intuitively apparent, no reports conclusively demonstrate the clinical usefulness of EPs when they are used as a neuroICU monitor.

The primary effect of diseases on EPs is either to increase the latency or decrease the amplitude of the evoked waveforms. The disease states commonly seen in the neuroICU that produce these effects are ischemia and anatomic mechanical disruption of a neural pathway. To use EPs as a monitoring tool, one presupposes that a given EP signal or signal change will prompt an alarm and attending diagnostic/therapeutic interventions. However, lacking extensive experience with EPs used in this fashion, it is sometimes difficult for one to declare with certainty when an alarm condition exists. Moreover, in the neuroICU there may be considerable variability in the signal obtained, rendering alarm conditions from EPs even more enigmatic. It has been suggested that changes in EPs should be regarded as indicative of a pathologic continuum with abrupt changes more significant than gradual changes.[151,152] For brain stem EPs, the following have been suggested as graded alarm criteria[516]:

1. A trend of sequentially and additive small changes
2. Excessive variablity
3. Increased latency > 0.5 ms or amplitude decrements > 30 percent—mild concern
4. Increased latency > 1.0 ms or amplitude decrements > 50 percent—heightened concern
5. Increased latency > 1.5 ms or amplitude decrements > 80 percent—great concern
6. Complete loss—great concern; abrupt is worse than gradual.

For somatosensory EPs, data from carotid endarterectomy reports suggesting a 50 percent decrement in amplitude warrant great concern. Patients with such changes intraoperatively were found postoperatively to have sustained neuropsychologic deficits[154,155] (see Chap. 7).

In the neuroICU, EPs have been used for a variety of indications. These include monitoring for global or focal ischemia, intracranial hypertension, and vasospasm, postoperative monitoring of the still-anesthetized patient, screening for brain death, and obtaining prognostic information.[156]

IMAGING IN THE NEUROICU

In addition to the numerous indicators of cerebral function, anatomy is an essential element of the data base in characterizing many neurologic disorders. Such information is provided with respect to bone, brain tissue, CSF, and vascular anatomy. The modalities used to acquire such information include skull radiograph, CT, magnetic resonance imaging (MRI), and angiography.

Skull radiography is used to assess extent of bony injury to the skull and cervical spine with trauma, assess the sella turcica, and ascertain location of jugular bulb catheters.

Computed tomography uses x-rays circumferentially applied to the skull with computerized analysis of absorption to derive tomographic information about bony structures as well as the brain. It provides excellent information about ventricular size, edema, qualitative BBB dysfunction, and hemorrhage. Occasionally it can be used to detect intraarterial thrombosis although the sensitivity is not very reliable used for this purpose. Recent advances in CT technology have resulted in the newest generation of CT scanners, so called helical CT. This provides images that can be rotated in three dimensions on the CT screen as desired by the viewer. Combined with intravascular contrast agents, this method can be used to provide detailed three-dimensional images of the vascular anatomy, so-called CT angiography (CTA). In addition, three-dimensional images can be provided of the CSF anatomy also.

Magnetic resonance imaging uses pulses of radiowaves to orient nuclei in a given configuration. Subsequent relaxation of these nuclei results in pulses of radio energy the orientation of which allows highly detailed images of the structures containing the precessing nuclei. MRI can be used to make detailed assessment of gray matter, white matter, CSF, edema, and BBB function (with gadolinium contrast infusion). In addition, magnetic pulsing of blood entering the brain can result in images of the intracranial vasculature, so called MR angiography (MRA).

Angiography is used as the optimal method for assessing intracranial vascular anatomy. It is the gold standard for assessing aneurysms, AVMs, and other abnormalities in arterial and venous anatomy.

Imaging technology is increasingly being used to provide information about physiology. Both MRI and CT technology are being developed to provide dynamic CBF information. MRI can provide important biochemical information and PET can be used for definition of receptor distribution and glucose and oxygen utilization. All of these techniques are at varying levels of development relevant to neuroICU applications (see Chap. 24).

General Care of the NeuroICU Patient

NUTRITION

Although the brain does not participate in mechanical work, osmotic work, or extensive biosynthesis, processes that use large amounts of energy, it undergoes almost as high a rate of oxidative metabolism as some of these high energy-using tissues do. The CMR_{O_2} of rat brain is about 4.4 μmol/min per gram. This is comparable to the oxygen used by the heart (8.7 μmol/min per gram), kidney (7 to 13 μmol/min per gram), or liver (5.5 μmol/min per gram). In primates, the larger brain/body weight ratio results in an even larger percentage of total oxygen consumption by the central nervous system (CNS).

Neural tissue has little stored endogenous fuel, relying almost solely on continuous blood-borne supply of nutrients. The brain normally is dependent primarily on glucose for its energy source with a steep blood-brain gradient for glucose. There may be a very small contribution of amino acids and short-chain amino acids. Ketone bodies are important fuels in situations of starvation stress. Glucose uptake is regulated by both carrier-mediated and diffusional mechanisms. Amino acid uptake is regulated by carrier-mediated transport. Both types of transport result in a dependence of brain concentrations on blood concentrations. Thus, major alterations in blood glucose or amino acids result in corresponding alterations in brain concentrations of these substances. In addition, the usual effects of insulin in controlling uptake of glucose and amino acids are less pronounced for the brain. The carrier-mediated functions generally require an intact BBB to function properly. Thus, areas of the brain without a BBB such as the pituitary gland or areas of injury are more likely to have more reliance on diffusional influx of nutrients.[157]

Nutritional management in some patients can be an essential factor necessary for survival. After the initial neurologic insult the incidence of death from extracranial causes such as sepsis increases dramatically.[158] Bodily defense mechanisms against such secondary insults as septicemia, pneumonia, and meningitis rely heavily on adequate nutritional support.[159]

Assessment of nutritional needs in the neuroICU patient is similar to methods used for other types of critically ill patients. The Harris-Benedict equation provides a satisfactory method to develop an initial estimate of basal energy expenditure (BEE) based on weight and gender.

$$BEE \text{ (men)} = 66.47 + 13.75W + 5.00H - 6.76A$$
$$BEE \text{ (women)} = 655.10 + 9.56W + 1.85H - 4.68A$$

where W = weight (kg), H = height (cm), and A = age (years).

This initial caloric estimate is then adjusted with a multiplier based on a qualitative assessment of factors that may be altering the baseline caloric needs. Head trauma patients can have a 1.5 to twofold increase in metabolic needs associated with massive nitrogen loss. Similar hypermetabolism can also occur in patients with seizures. In addition, hypermetabolic conditions associated with many neurologic conditions can also result in increased caloric needs. In contrast, some neuroICU patients may be receiving high doses of CNS depressant drugs, have high spinal cord lesions, or be comatose, with a significant decrease in metabolic needs. All of these factors should be considered in deciding what a given patient's initial nutrition needs are.

Continued assessment of nutritional status as an indication of trends in a patient's nutritional status can be obtained from serial assessment of visceral protein levels, physical examination, and weight. Other more sophisticated measures of nutrition such as calorimetry or nitrogen balance can also be obtained for problematic cases. A discussion of such techniques is beyond the scope of this chapter.

On admission to the neuroICU, virtually all patients receive nothing by mouth until they have undergone neurologic evaluation or have recovered from the initial event to adequately self-feed. If after about 3 days, self-nutrition is not likely, enteral nutrition is started, usually via gastric or duodenal tube. Even in patients receiving high doses of CNS depressants or neuromuscular blockade, the enteral approach should be attempted, provided bowel sounds are present. If enteral nutrition is not successful, as judged by high residual volume (> 50 ml/2 h) with repeated attempts and with metoclopramide, then parenteral nutrition is implemented via a centrally placed venous catheter.

Patients receiving nutritional therapy require increased monitoring for metabolic complications, which can be particularly deleterious in the neuroICU patient. Such complications include abnormalities in glucose, sodium, magnesium, and phosphate. Hyperglycemia is thought to exacerbate some forms of ischemic brain damage, whereas hypoglycemia may not be tolerated if cerebrovascular reserve is compromised. In addition, hypoglycemia, hyponatremia, and hypophosphatemia can cause seizures, a potentially devastating complication in some neuroICU patients. Hyponatremia will exacerbate edema as can overaggressive treatment of hypernatremia. Magnesium is thought to have a role in blocking the N-methyl-D-aspartate (NMDA)-gated sodium channel and may have anticonvulsant properties; thus low magnesium should also be avoided. Finally, catheter-related sepsis can also be devastating because it is known to decrease CBF while increasing CMR and disrupting the BBB.[160] In addition, it can decrease blood pressure in a manner that may not be well tolerated by the brain with abnormal cerebrovascular reserve.

DEEP-VEIN THROMBOSIS PROPHYLAXIS

Deep-vein thrombosis (DVT) formation is encouraged by a number of clinical situations, many of which predispose to the widely accepted pathogenetic factors: stasis, vessel wall injury, and hypercoagulability. Numerous clinical factors have been identified that predispose to DVT. Such factors include recent surgery; malignancy; immobilization; trauma; acute stroke; acute myocardial infarction; previous DVT; pregnancy; estrogen use; deficiencies of antithrombin III, protein C, or protein S; nephrotic syndrome; congestive heart failure; obesity; age above 40 years; disseminated intravascular coagulation; anticardiolipin antibody; lupus anticoagulant; dysfibrinogenemia; and vasculitis. Many of these factors occur commonly in neuroICU patients, placing them into a high-risk category for the development of DVT.[161] The primary concern with respect to DVT is the potential for pulmonary embolism.

Methods to prevent DVT include the use of intermittent pneumatic compression devices, elastic compression stockings, early ambulation, physical therapy, and anticoagulation therapy. Several of these methods have been proven to effectively prevent the formation of

TABLE 36-4
Recommendations For Deep-Vein Thrombosis Prophylaxis in High-Risk Situations

Type of Patient	Therapy
Elective gynecologic or general surgery and immobilized > 48 h	Low-dose heparin (5000 U SQ q12h) or intermittent pneumatic compression
Elective urologic or major knee surgery	Intermittent pneumatic compression
Elective hip surgery	Titrated heparin to keep aPTT high-normal Coumadin to prolong PT to INR 2–3
Hip fracture	Coumadin to prolong PT to INR 2–3

NOTE: aPTT, activated partial thromboplastin time; INR, International Normalized Ratio; PT, prothrombin time.
SOURCE: Adapted with permission from DeGeroria and coworkers.[161]

DVT in nonneurologic conditions, such as postoperative gynecologic, urologic, or orthopedic procedures (Table 36-4). In neurologic or neurosurgical patients there is the concern that anticoagulation will predispose to intracranial hemorrhage, although published reports do not support this[162–164] with reports of anticoagulation in stroke patients indicating an efficacious effect in preventing DVT.[165,166] In neurosurgical patients, intermittent pneumatic compression appears to effectively decrease the incidence of DVT.[167] Ambulation is to be encouraged as soon as possible in neuroICU patients but this is often not possible. Thus, DVT prophylaxis in the neuroICU generally comprises passive motion physical therapy, elastic compression stockings, intermittent pneumatic compression, and low-dose anticoagulation (if CT scanning shows no intracranial hemorrhage).

GASTRIC ULCER PROPHYLAXIS

NeuroICU patients, like other critically ill patients, are at risk of gastric ulceration. The genesis of such ulcers is thought to be related to increased gastroduodenal acidity in a stressed patient in whom gastric mucosal defense mechanisms are suboptimal. Preventive treatment is used on all neuroICU patients and consists of therapy with either H_2 antagonists, antacids, sucralfate, or enteral feeding.

EXTERNAL VENTRICULAR DRAIN MANAGEMENT

An external ventricular drain (EVD; ventriculostomy) may be placed to provide drainage for hydrocephalus or provide a means to measure ICP. Such drains require meticulous attention to their position relative to the patient and sterility. A typical drainage setup is shown in Fig. 36-9. A drainage level relative to the midbrain is ordered if drainage is desired when ICP reaches a certain level. Alternatively the EVD can be maintained clamped, with pressure monitored. In such cases the EVD will be drained if ICP reaches a sustained level beyond a prescribed threshold.

When the drain is open there are several important considerations. If the drain is kept too high and the patient cannot drain CSF sufficiently, hydrocephalus or elevated ICP will result. If the drain is too low, excessive drainage can occur. If this allows gradients to arise, a herniation syndrome, usually across the midline (if the drain is contralateral from a mass lesion), can result. In addition, if there is an unruptured cerebral aneurysm, too low placement can produce an increase in transmural gradients across the aneurysm and encourage rupture. Too low a placement can encourage formation of a subdural hematoma as the brain retracts from the skull and tension is placed on bridging veins.

It remains an unresolved problem what to do about abrupt brief and normal increases in ICP as may occur with coughing or other causes of a Valsalva maneuver. Such events result in a brief overflow of CSF, followed then by a period of low ICP, which might encourage aneurysmal bleeding or subdural hematoma.

When the EVD is clamped, constant monitoring must be used to detect when the ICP is above the predetermined threshold, which indicates the need for drainage. When it is clamped and in the monitoring mode, the usual arterial line flush system used for most pressure-monitoring purposes must never be attached.

Infection is a major concern with an EVD. Published data indicate that the risk of EVD infection rises dramatically after 5 days of placement.[168,169] Antibiotic infusions intrathecally have been used but have not been documented to decrease the infection rate, and possibly actually encourage growth of resistant organisms. Subcutaneous tunneling of the EVD catheter is one method that may be effective to decrease the incidence of infection. Because of these concerns most neurosurgeons change EVDs weekly or more often. Alternatively, some monitor white blood cell counts in the CSF to assess for occurrence of infection, although the necessary violation of the system to obtain such information may actually increase the infection rate.

SEDATION

Sedation is particularly problematic in the neuroICU patient. The act of sedating a patient with a brain insult results in obfuscation of the ability to assess the very problem for which the neuroICU admission is required. Inability to adequately assess progress of the

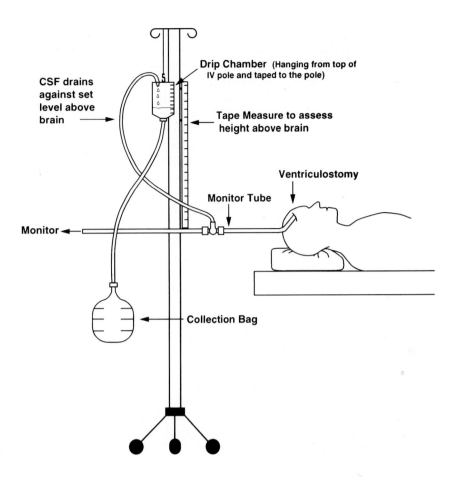

CSF drains against set level above brain →

Drip Chamber (Hanging from top of IV pole and taped to the pole)

Tape Measure to assess height above brain

Ventriculostomy

Monitor Tube

Monitor ←

Collection Bag

Figure 36-9   External ventricular drainage system (EVD).

illness can result in a prolonged neuroICU stay and morbidity related to undiagnosed, treatable neurologic deterioration. Thus, sedation in the neuroICU has traditionally been withheld except in situations where the patient's agitation results in a danger to himself or herself or inability to undergo diagnostic or nursing procedures.

When sedation is used, preference should be given to the use of drugs that can be reversed or drugs with a short duration of action. Thus, drugs such as fentanyl (or congeners), midazolam, thiopental, or propofol are reasonable drugs to use. The precise means of administering these drugs is a subject of controversy. They can be given as bolus or infusion, and given as needed or on a schedule. In addition, the choice of drug can also be subject to clinical judgment.

Giving a drug as a bolus when needed has the advantage of ensuring that a patient has a return to baseline level of consciousness before further administration of drug, ensuring that prolonged excessive use does not occur. However, such a paradigm makes it more likely that the patient will have bouts of hypertension and other agitation-related problems, which can be deleterious.

Giving a drug as a titrated infusion risks the patient slowly creeping into an overdose if scrupulous assessment is not frequently performed. In addition, the drug can accumulate in body tissues, such that a longer period of time is needed to allow the drug to be eliminated from the body. Conversely, such a scheme will ensure that the adverse events for which the drug is prescribed are less likely to occur.

Opioid drugs are readily reversed and have little hemodynamic side effects. In addition, their antitussive side effects can be put to good use in intubated patients. In these patients, opioids can also blunt any dyspnea related to being on a ventilator. Opioids thus have a number of characteristics making them ideal for neuroICU patients. However, in both animal and human studies, opioids have been reported in high doses (> 20 μg/kg fentanyl in humans or equivalent in animals) to cause epileptiform activity on EEG[170–172] and there are numerous studies suggesting that opioids may be deleterious in cerebral ischemia.[173,174] The relevance of these observations to the typical neuroICU patient is unclear.

Benzodiazepines can be reversed although reversal risks the production of seizures.[175] As with most γ-aminobutyric acid (GABA)ergic drugs, there may be brain-protective side effects. However, they seem to have a more pronounced effect to decrease blood pressure and can produce disorientation. In some patients benzodiazepines can exacerbate agitation. Benzodiazepines can accumulate in tissues making arousal time quite prolonged if given for prolonged periods.

Propofol is an excellent new addition to the list of drugs that can be satisfactorily used for neuroICU sedation but there is no way to reverse its action. However, it is generally so short-lived, that even with high doses given over long periods, rather quick arousal times occur with its use. It does have a tendency to decrease blood pressure. There have been concerns about proconvulsant properties of propofol,[176] although their relevance to neuroICU use is not clear. Recent very carefully controlled studies indicate that the proconvulsant properties of propofol are no worse than those of thiopental.[177] It probably has brain-protective properties[178] because it is a potent GABAergic drug[179] and many drugs with such properties are protective in some situations. It cannot be given in patients with triglyceride intolerance because it is in a triglyceride emulsion vehicle.

Thiopental is occasionally used for neuroICU sedation. There is no reversal agent for it. Given over a short period (i.e., hours) this is generally not problematic due to its short duration because of redistribution. However, with prolonged use, it accumulates in tissues making arousal time quite prolonged. It may have brain protective properties and can be used to keep ICP down.[180,181]

New technology is becoming available by which precise titration of sedative drugs may be practical using processed EEG. This is presently experimental but holds promise as a practical and feasible manner to titrate sedative drugs in the neuroICU.

AIRWAY MANAGEMENT

In situations where ICP is increased, concerns in airway management include full stomach, concurrent medical/surgical problems, an awareness that hypercapnea and hypoxemia may be poorly tolerated, and the potential to increase ICP or worsen cerebral edema. Thus, a reasonable approach is to use heavy sedation or intravenous anesthetics often combined with neuromuscular blockade with rapid intubation. The specific drugs chosen depend on the patient's baseline condition and hemodynamic stability. If blood pressure increases to too high a level, ICP may increase due to distention of vasoparalyzed vasculature and brain edema may be exacerbated. If blood pressure decreases to too low a level then cerebral ischemia may occur. In situations where cerebrovascular reserve may be compromised, hypoxemia will be more likely to cause neuronal injury. Hypercapnea and hypoxemia will also exacerbate intracranial hypertension.

Syndromes with decreased level of consciousness or physiologic or anatomic disruption of gas exchange generally indicate the need for airway protection. In such situations, the need to use ICP-reducing but CNS-depressing drugs such as fentanyl or thiopental require consideration of the consequences as to the ability to follow neurologic examination versus desirable hemodynamic or ICP effects. Although it is widespread practice to use such intravenous anesthetics to secure the airway in unconscious patients with high ICP, no scientific studies have been published that show that outcome is altered based on their use or the selection of any specific intubation protocol. Clinicians generally use information regarding occurrence of unacceptable or desirable side effects to guide decision making.

Syndromes with depressed neuromuscular function require careful consideration in the selection of neuromuscular-blocking agents. There are many syndromes wherein succinylcholine use can produce life-threatening hyperkalemia.

GAS EXCHANGE

Cerebrovascular reserve is compromised in many intracranial pathologic processes. Normally the brain compensates for decrements in supply of oxygen and substrates by vasodilating to maintain or increase flow. Animal experiments indicate that it is possible to produce a condition in which cerebrovascular reserve is compromised with increased tendency to cerebral infarction. For example, occlusion of one carotid artery or moderate hypoxemia individually does not produce symptoms because cerebral vasodilatation occurs as a compensation mechanism. Indeed, some contend that arterial hypoxemia, occurring with normal cerebral vascular compensatory mechanisms, does not cause brain damage. One contributing factor to this notion is that hypoxic myocardial dysfunction produces organismic death such that isolated neuronal injury cannot occur. However, add hypoxemia to carotid occlusion, or vice versa, and a stroke occurs because compensatory mechanisms, already fully utilized, cannot accommodate the further decrease in O_2 supply.[182] Examples of variants of this situation abound clinically.[87,88] Such examples of attenuated cerebrovascular reserve include cerebral edema, hypoxemia, carotid stenosis, and peri-infarct penumbra. In each of these situations, although not easy to quantitate, it is clear that added compromise of O_2 supply to the brain will risk neuronal injury.

Pa_{CO_2} has a profound impact on CBF. Normally CBF varies linearly with Pa_{CO_2} between 20 and 60 mmHg.[59–63,89] Pa_{CO_2}-mediated changes in CBF occur with corresponding changes in cerebral blood volume. Thus, in situations of abnormal intracranial compliance where small changes in intracranial volume have large

ICP effects, decreased Pa_{CO_2} decreases ICP and increased Pa_{CO_2} increases ICP.

The primary concern with elevated ICP is that it may be associated with cerebral oligemia. These effects of Pa_{CO_2} on ICP are paradoxical. That is, decreased Pa_{CO_2} decreases ICP, but at the expense of decreasing CBF[183] (Fig. 36-10), the very entity that is desired to be maintained. Conversely, allowing hypercapnea to occur, although associated with increased ICP, is associated with increased CBF. These observations pertain to normally autoregulating tissue. Thus, the CBF effects in injured brain tissue may be as desired, although this can be unpredictable. For example, allowing Pa_{CO_2} to increase CBF in autoregulating brain areas by increasing ICP, may compromise flow in injured, already fully dilated areas. Conversely, decreasing ICP in normally autoregulating areas, may produce an inverse steal effect in injured regions of the brain. The concern is that this increased blood flow in injured areas may constitute a hyperperfusion syndrome and exacerbate edema. In addition, data from head trauma studies indicate that routine use of hyperventilation can worsen outcome.[184]

Finally, despite observations that hyperglycemia worsens ischemic brain damage, recent evidence indicates that mild acidosis can be protective in the brain.[185,186] This is thought to be due to antagonism of the NMDA glutamate receptor. If these initial in vitro studies are relevant to clinical care then hyperventilation, in addition to decreasing CBF, may have adverse biochemical effects.

TEMPERATURE

Temperature management can be critical in the neuroICU. In animal models hyperthemia has been shown to have deleterious effects on outcome after cerebral ischemia,[187] head trauma,[187] and seizure.[188] Conversely, mild hypothermia has been shown to be protective.[189,190] It is of interest that the extent of hypothermia required to produce protection is modest, in the 32° to 36°C range or possibly even less. The extent of protection is not adequately explained by reduction in CMR,[191] suggesting that hypothermia has additional beneficial effects such as decreased free radical production or reduction in neurotransmitter neurotoxicity.[192] In a multicenter trial with head trauma, moderate hypothermia in preliminary reports confers cerebral protection when applied within 6 h of insult and maintained for 24 to 48 h.[189] No clinical trials have assessed hypothermia in humans with cerebral ischemia or seizure, although a recent survey of neuroanesthesiologists in North America indicated that it is now routinely used during neurosurgery.[193]

Such observations indicate that in the absence of conclusive trials for nontraumatic neurologic conditions, a minimal approach would be to aggressively treat and prevent the occurrence of fever. Such an approach requires a therapeutic paradigm almost as aggressive as that used to institute hypothermia. For induced hypothermia, an order is written to maintain temperature at a given level. Similarly, an order can be written to maintain temperature at 37.5°C using cooling blankets and antipyretic drugs.

BLOOD PRESSURE MANAGEMENT

Blood pressure management is an important issue in most neuroICU patients. Concern exists that systemic hypertension may exacerbate cerebral edema or intracranial hemorrhage or have deleterious cardiopulmonary effects such as pulmonary edema or myocardial ischemia. Conversely, blood pressure decreases can lead to insufficient perfusion even at a pressure in the normal range of autoregulation. Moreover, mild blood pressure decreases have been implicated in the genesis of plateau waves. Several important principles apply to management of blood pressure in neuroICU patients and follow.

HYPERTENSION

When blood pressure is elevated a central question that must be addressed initially is whether the pressure is elevated due to normal homeostatic mechanisms to maintain adequate perfusion. For example, with conditions of inadequate brainstem perfusion, a compensatory hyperadrenergic state may occur resulting in increased blood pressure, thus maintaining sufficient perfusion to maintain aerobic metabolism in the brainstem. If a decision is made to decrease blood pressure, then brainstem failure and death may ensue.

Animal data with cerebral ischemia models provide strong support for the notion that sympatholytic drugs should be used to decrease blood pressure if cerebral ischemia is a possibility. Compared to hemorrhagic-induced hypotension, ischemic damage was decreased with the use of ganglionic blockade with hexamethonium,[194] central adrenergic blockade with α-2 agonists,[195] and ACE inhibition.[196] Hemorrhaged controls sustained an increase in exogenous catecholamine concentrations. To test the hypothesis that these catecholamines contributed to brain damage, some of the animals treated with hexamethonium also received intravenous catecholamine infusions. Reversal of the hexamethonium brain protective effect was observed in these animals (Fig. 36-11).[194] Similarly, brain protection has been observed in laboratory studies with preischemic[197] and preseizure[198] treatment with reserpine, a drug that depletes presynaptic catecholamine stores. Finally, there is a report by Neil-Dwyer and coworkers[199] wherein subarachnoid hemorrhage patients received therapy with phentolamine/propranolol com-

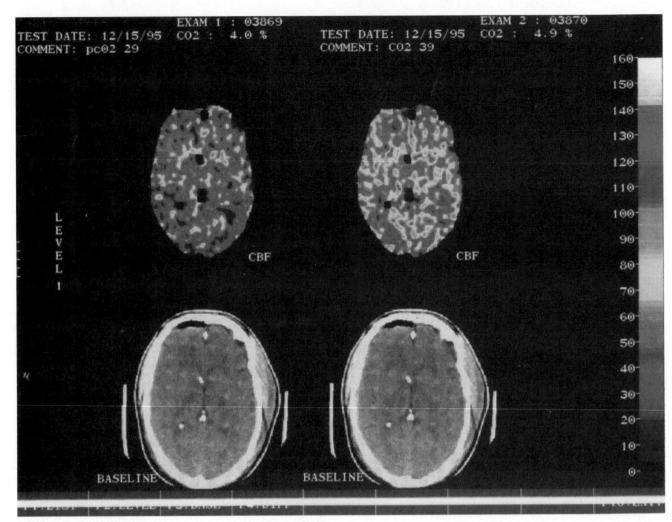

A

Figure 36-10 Effects of hyperventilation on cerebral blood flow (CBF). Two examples of disparate effects of hyperventilation on CBF. Both figures are stable xenon CBFs in head trauma patients, with and without hyperventilation. CBF scale is indicated on the right in ml/100 g per minute and P_{CO_2} is indicated above each study. CT images are indicated in the lower figures and CBF maps in the upper figures. A. P_{CO_2} was decreased from 39 to 29 mmHg. The baseline scan (*right*) shows hyperemia and the hyperventilated scan (*left*) shows CBFs of approximately 30 ml/100 g per minute, probably acceptable flows.

pared to no sympatholytic therapy (see Fig. 36-27). Subjects who received sympatholytic therapy had significantly better neurologic outcome than controls. In addition, β-adrenergic blocking drugs have not been reported to produce cerebral vasodilatation or increase ICP.[200–202]

Calcium channel antagonist drugs, which also may have brain-protective effects, are also available for antihypertensive therapy. Drugs available include verapamil, diltiazem, nifedipine, nimodipine, and nicardipine. Nimodipine and nicardipine, developed specifically for brain protection purposes, have been assessed in numerous studies with several reports of

their conferring protection versus ischemic brain damage.[203–209] They become reasonable choices for antihypertensive drugs based solely on these observations. They are vasodilators and can increase ICP.[210,211] As vasodilators, they may be expected to produce compensatory catecholamine release,[212] and, based on the previous discussion, this may obviate some of their protective qualities.

Peripheral vasodilators such as nitroprusside, nitroglycerin, and hydralazine all have the potential to induce cerebral vasodilatation and thus cause hyperemic intracranial hypertension.[213–216] Moreover, they are associated with compensatory increase in peripheral cat-

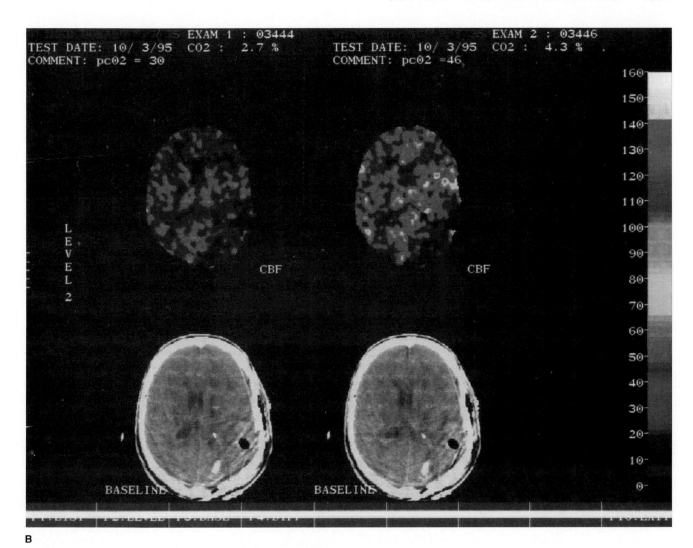

B

Figure 36-10 (*Continued*) *B.* P_{CO_2} was decreased from 46 to 30 mmHg. The baseline CBF (*right*) had only marginally acceptable CBF. The effect of hyperventilation (*left*) was to produce widespread areas of CBF less than 20 ml/100 g per minute, probably unacceptable flows.

echolamines and renin,[212] factors that may make is-chemic brain damage worse.[194,197] However, the lack of bradycardia and bronchoconstriction associated with their use may make them the optimal choice in some patients with these conditions. If such a drug is chosen and the patient is at risk of neurologic deterioration from ischemia or high ICP, close clinical observation is indicated. Any deterioration would mandate discontinuation of the drug. Such concerns are important for deciding amongst these three drugs. Although hydralazine is convenient to use, it cannot be reversed at the receptor and its effects can last hours. Thus, it may be preferable to use nitroprusside in such situations because adverse effects can be treated quickly simply by discontinuing the infusion.

The choice of antihypertensive agent in a patient at risk of cerebral ischemia is not straightforward. Thera-peutic urgency, sympatholytic and brain protective side effects, and potential to increase ICP are all important considerations in the choice of antihypertensive drug (Table 36-5).

If it is deemed that blood pressure has to be lowered quickly (within minutes), trimethophan in boluses is very effective and can be titrated safely. Trimethaphan, 1 mg/ml, can be given intravenously with the dosage doubled every few minutes until the desired effect is achieved. Once the blood pressure is reduced a maintenance regimen of trimethaphan or another drug can then be started. Alternatively, if it is already mixed, an infusion of sodium nitroprusside can be started. Nitroprusside has a variety of deleterious side effects elaborated on previously. However, it is perhaps the most potent and reliable antihypertensive drug available. Nicardipine can also be mixed, 0.1 mg/ml, and

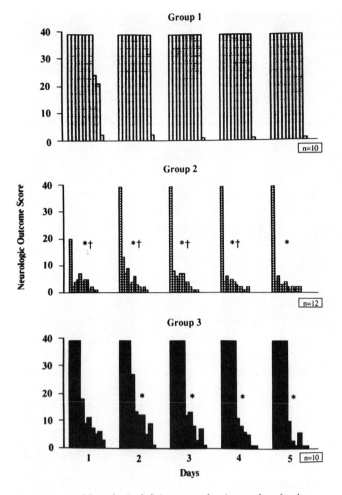

Figure 36-11 Neurologic deficit scores after incomplete focal cerebral ischemia in rats over a 5-day examination period. Each bar represents the neurologic score for each rate (* $p < .05$ versus group 1; † $p < .05$ versus group 3). The rats are ranked according to total outcome score in descending order (0 = normal). Cerebral ischemia was induced with occlusion of one carotid artery with hemorrhagic hypotension. Group 1 rats received no vasoactive drugs; group 2 rats received preischemic hexamethonium, and group 3 rats received hexamethonium plus intravenous epinephrine and norepinephrine. Protection was conferred by hexamethonium in a catecholamine-reversible manner. (Reproduced by permission from Werner et al.[194])

given in a fashion similar to trimethaphan, starting at 0.1 mg intravenously to effect a fast, temporary blood pressure reduction.

Plateau waves, first reported by Lundberg[217] and associated with neurologic deterioration, were demonstrated by Risberg to be associated with cerebral vasodilation.[218] Rosener and colleagues reported that mild decreases in blood pressure to the 60 to 80 mmHg range can be associated with plateau waves.[219] Presumably, the decrease in blood pressure prompts vasodilatation in normally autoregulating tissue. The increase in cerebral blood volume, which is an exponential function versus cerebral perfusion pressure,[219] superimposed on the exponential ICP versus intracranial vol-

ume relationship, is then associated with an explosive hyperemic increase in ICP producing a plateau wave (see Figs. 36-14, 36-15, and 36-16). This introduces the concern with use of any antihypertensive agent, aside from specific, direct cerebrovascular effect, that normal autoregulation may also increase ICP as cerebral perfusion pressure decreases to about 80 mmHg or below.

Clearly, any time hypotensive therapy is used in a patient with altered intracranial compliance, edema, or ischemia, close and recurrent observation is mandatory. Deterioration should prompt consideration of one of the above processes occurring with corrective therapy then introduced with reconsideration of the need to decrease blood pressure.

HYPOTENSION AND INDUCED HYPERTENSION

When any patient is hypotensive, efforts should also be ongoing to ascertain its cause. In head trauma patients, consideration needs to be given to other injuries with hemorrhage or spinal shock. Loss of blood flow to the brainstem can similarly be associated with hypotension, which can be difficult to treat. In addition, usual nonneurologic causes of hypotension in an ICU (e.g., pneumothorax, sepsis, and cardiogenic causes) should also be considered.

When therapy to increase blood pressure is contemplated, as may be done with vasospasm, the need for it must be seriously considered because excessive increases in blood pressure can exacerbate cerebral edema.[220–224] This presumably occurs in brain areas with dysautoregulation and BBB disruption, such that increasing blood pressure, rather than producing vasoconstriction and no change in regional CBF (rCBF), causes vascular distension, increased rCBF, and transudation of fluid across the damaged BBB. In addition, increases in blood pressure risk producing or exacerbating intracranial hemorrhage.

TABLE 36-5
Antihypertensive Drugs

Drug	Potential to Increase ICP	Brain Protective Side Effects	Sympatholytic
Nitroprusside	+++	0	0
Nitroglycerin	++	0	0
Hydralazine	+++	0	0
Enalopril	+	++	+
Trimethophan	0	+++	+++
Labetalol	0	+	+++
Propranolol	0	+	+++
Esmolol	0	+	+++
Nifedipine	++	+	0
Nicardipine	++	+++	0
Clonidine		+++	+++

Catecholamines used to increase blood pressure are neurotransmitters or are chemically similar to neurotransmitters. It is thus to be expected that if they cross the BBB that neural effects will occur secondary to their use. Normally, exogenously administered catecholamines do not cross the BBB and have no effect on CBF or metabolism.[58] However, catecholamine infusion in the presence of BBB disruption leads to increased blood flow and metabolism.[225] In patients with SAH, catecholamine infusions produce a variety of disparate and unpredictable effects on CBF[226] and adrenergic blockade confers neurologic protection.[199] Finally, catecholamines have direct neurotoxic potential as indicated by data showing neurotoxicity with application directly to the cortex in vivo.[227] Unfortunately, catecholamines are the only clinically accepted routine means to increase blood pressure pharmacologically in neuro-ICU patients.

Increased preload to the heart is one nonpharmacologic method to increase blood pressure. With crystalloid or colloid infusion this is generally associated with hemodilution. The effects of this on a given patient's status should be considered when this is contemplated. The hemodilution may improve flow to areas where microcirculation is compromised. However, it may be associated with increased CBV and hyperemic intracranial hypertension if hematocrit decreases excessively with compensatory vasodilatation.

Whether to use crystalloid or colloid for this purpose remains controversial. The BBB is functionally an osmometer.[228–233] Thus, the added trivial increase in osmolarity with colloid is not a sufficient reason to use it. Thus, it makes sense and is supported by animal studies that isoosmolar or slightly hyperosmolar fluids should be used to decrease the possibility of increasing brain edema secondary to fluid administration.

GLUCOSE

Hyperglycemia has been associated with exacerbation of brain damage with both head trauma and cerebral ischemia.[234–237] It is, however, not a straightforward issue. Clearly, neuronal damage after global cerebral ischemia is exacerbated with hyperglycemia.[235,238–241] Some studies have suggested that a blood glucose over 120 mg/dl is deleterious in stroke patients.[234] However, subsequent studies have suggested a threshold of around 180 mg/dl with subhuman primates subjected to global ischemia.[241] Clearly, blood glucose greater than 400 mg/dl causes striking worsening of neurologic outcome with global ischemia.[235,240]

With focal cerebral ischemia, it is a good deal less clear. Animal and human studies have shown the brain damage is worsened, not affected, or lessened with hyperglycemia.[234,242–259] One report by Prado and co-

workers,[256] using rats, suggested that the discriminating factor whether brain damage is worsened with hyperglycemia concerns itself with collateral flow. Areas of the brain with minimal collaterals were not affected or were improved with hyperglycemia. Brain areas with a continued trickle of flow sustained worsened brain damage. Presumably, the continued substrate supply in oligemic (not ischemic) areas allowed greater accumulation of organic acids in the cells leading to worsening of brain damage.[236,247] Unfortunately, these observations are difficult to apply clinically to patients with focal ischemia.

Even if low levels of hyperglycemia were deleterious, it would not be straightforward to treat. A too aggressive therapy of hyperglycemia would impose a risk of hypoglycemia, with deleterious effects imposed by that. Thus, it seems that a reasonable approach is to aim for a blood glucose level of approximately 200 mg/dl in all hyperglycemic patients at risk of cerebral ischemia. Blood glucose should not be allowed to undergo wide variations in its concentration to avoid having it swing to under 100 mg/dl or above 400 mg/dl. Thus, an insulin infusion with frequent glucose assessment should be used in patients at risk of cerebral anaerobic metabolism who develop hyperglycemia greater than 225 mg/dl. An infusion titrated to keep blood glucose about 200 mg/dl should be instituted.

Hyperglycemia has not been shown to have deleterious or protective effects in two animal models of status epilepticus.[260,261] The model used by Swan and colleagues[261] produced limbic system damage, whereas Kofke and coworkers[260] used a model producing substantia nigra damage. Nigral damage in this model is associated with hypermetabolic lactic acidosis,[262] which should have been exacerbated with hyperglycemia. The fact that nigral damage was not exacerbated with hyperglycemia suggests that metabolic acidosis may not be an important factor in the development of brain damage after seizure.

SODIUM

HYPERNATREMIA

Hypernatremia can occur in neuroICU patients from nonketotic diabetic coma, dehydration from lack of fluid intake or diuretic use, inappropriate hypertonic fluid administration, diabetes insipidus, or panhypopituitarism.[263,264] It can be associated with thirst, irritability, seizures, intracranial hemorrhage, or coma, although the rate of increase in the sodium is thought to be an important factor in the clinical presentation. For example, a sodium of 170 meq/liter can be associated with little neurologic symptomatology if the rise occurs over a prolonged period.

When diuretics are given, especially when they are

aggressively given for intracranial hypertension, it is essential that electrolytes be followed frequently so corrective measures can be taken early. Once hypernatremia occurs its treatment is compounded by effects of decreasing osmolarity on brain water and ICP; thus early treatment and detection are important.

Diabetes insipidus can occur when disease processes affect the pituitary or its vascular supply. It should be expected when urine output is inappropriately increased in the appropriate clinical situation. Commonly the urine output can increase abruptly to greater than a liter an hour and be associated with severe hypernatremia with hypovolemic hypotension. Diagnosis of diabetes insipidus is based on continued output of dilute urine in the context of hypotonic serum. Specific gravity of urine will be close to 1.001 with osmolarity less than 200 despite serum osmolarity that may be greater than 320 mosm.

In the hypovolemic patient, which is the usual scenario, therapy is directed as replacement of the total body water (TBW) deficit:

$$\text{TBW deficit} = 0.6 \times \text{Weight (kg)} - (140/[\text{Na}^+]_p) \times 0.6 \times \text{Weight (kg)}$$

The water deficit is replaced over 24 to 48 h at a rate no faster than 1 to 2 mEq/liter per h. Hypernatremia should be treated slowly to avoid complications from overzealous treatment such as seizures and cerebral edema.[265–267] If the patient is both hypervolemic and hypernatremic, furosemide combined with dilute crystalloid solution can be administered to decrease plasma volume and sodium.

HYPONATREMIA

Hyponatremia can occur due to the syndrome of inappropriate secretion of antidiuretic hormone (SIADH), the so-called syndrome of cerebral salt wasting, or inappropriate free water administration. SIADH is generally associated with hypervolemia and cerebral salt wasting with hypovolemia. Both syndromes may be associated with elevated urinary sodium concentrations making differentiation beween the two syndromes difficult in routine clinical practice.[268,269]

Severe symptoms require an urgent approach to treatment. In such cases 3% saline with furosemide can increase the sodium concentration rapidly. However, rapidly increasing sodium concentration can produce permanent neurologic damage due to central pontine myelinolysis.[270–272] Thus, such emergent therapy should be reserved for only the most critical type of situation. If the hyponatremia is not associated with such serious neurologic deterioration, and if the patient is judged to be hypervolemic or an element of induced hypovolemia is thought to be safe, then fluid restriction is an initial reasonable approach. If however, hypovolemia is thought to be already present or hypovolemia is not thought to be optimal (as with vasospasm after a subarachnoid hemorrhage), then sodium can be added in a titrated manner to the patient's diet or fluids. One to 4 g of sodium can be added to the enteral diet. Alternatively, or in addition, the patient can have all intravenous fluids consist of 0.9% saline. Finally, 3% saline can be infused, starting at about 10 ml/h and titrated upward as indicated by serial plasma sodium assessments. Generally, the rate of correction of plasma sodium should not exceed 2.5 meq/liter per h and the total daily increment should not exceed 20 meq/liter.[273]

The more urgent the situation, the more frequently plasma sodium should be evaluated. It should be assessed hourly for urgent situations, every 4 to 8 h for moderate situations, and daily for routine observation or nonthreatening abnormalities in sodium concentration.

HYPERPERFUSION SYNDROMES

In a variety of clinical situations CBF may be inappropriately increased for a given blood pressure. In the extreme case of such situations, vasoparalysis is present and CBF is thought to become more or less a linear function of blood pressure. Such hyperperfusion syndromes may occur early in severe hepatic encephalopathy,[274] 2 to 3 days after severe head injury,[275–278] after resection of large AVMs,[279,280] after carotid endarterectomy of severely stenotic lesions with poor collaterals,[281,282] probably after arterial thrombolysis, and during administration of cerebral vasodilators.

Aggarwal and coworkers[274] have systematically examined cerebral hemodynamics and metabolism in severe hepatic encephalopathy and during recovery after hepatic transplantation. They have identified phases that are traversed in the course of going from normal cerebral physiology to brain death. Patients initially demonstrate extremely elevated CBF at normotension. This is usually followed by hyperemic intracranial hypertension, edema with oligemic intracranial hypertension, and then intracranial circulatory arrest and brain death. The data clearly suggest that the hyperemia is deleterious and may be contributing to the development of subsequent cerebral edema. This is supported by observations that the cerebral edema can be prevented through the use of barbiturates and hyperventilation during the hyperemic phase.

Several workers, in the course of examining cerebrovascular physiology after head trauma, have observed that patients with severe head injury initially have normal or low blood flow. This is followed a few days later by hyperemia, which is associated with intracranial hypertension.[278]

The concept of normal perfusion pressure breakthrough has been suggested for the hyperperfusion syndrome that occurs after resection of large AVMs. The pathogenesis of this is thought to be related to the chronic arterial hypotension proximal to the AVM. The larger the AVM, the lower the intracranial blood pressure the patient has lived with, with the cerebral vasculature essentially downregulating the CBF-mean arterial pressure (MAP) autoregulatory relation. Removing the AVM abruptly exposes the cerebral arterial vessels and arterioles to pressure never before experienced. Thus, despite the blood pressure being within normal limits, the pressure-naive vasculature is unable to autoregulate and the physiology of malignant hypertension may arise with cerebral edema or hemorrhage. This is an attractive hypothesis that seems to make physiologic sense. However, observations of Young and coworkers[280,283–286] indicate that autoregulation of the vascular bed after AVM resection is generally intact, indicating that vasoparalysis due to chronic hypotension is not the most important contributor to normal perfusion pressure breakthrough.

One cause of neurologic deterioration after carotid endarterectomy is distal cerebral edema or hemorrhage. This is rare but the presence of a throbbing headache suggests that it may be present in a given patient. Blood flow studies reveal such patients to have hyperemia associated with removal of a large proximal obstruction. Although normotension is usually well-tolerated, hypertension probably increases the risk of hemorrhage, especially if there was a preoperative infarction. Similar to the AVM situation, vasculature that had acclimated to low proximal pressure now is presented with pressure that is much higher, although within the normal range.[281,282]

After thrombolysis of a cerebral artery one important source of morbidity is edema or hemorrhage of the reperfused territory. With the reperfusion of the ischemic tissue, hyperemia occurs for a period of time. If sustained, this suggests that irreversible endothelial damage has occurred and that the patient is at risk for secondary edema or hemorrhage.

Vasodilators such as nitroprusside are frequently used in patients with severe hypertension. When CBF is measured it is noted that such vasodilators increase CBF substantially. In addition, they are known to cause a pronounced increase in ICP. The extent of this ICP elevation and hyperemia decreases as blood pressure is lowered. This notion is supported by observations during neurosurgery wherein cerebral swelling is noted when nitroprusside is started but with its use for induced hypotension during neurosurgery, the brain is flaccid. Thus, cerebral vasodilators can produce a

cerebral hyperperfusion syndrome. However, their use has not yet been reported to be associated with exacerbation of cerebral edema or hemorrhage.

All of the above syndromes describe a clinical course in humans consisting of inappropriate hyperemia for a given blood pressure followed by cerebral edema or hemorrhage. This suggests that the failure to autoregulate to pressure results in exposure of arterioles and capillaries to unacceptably high pressure. This then results in disruption of the BBB with consequent transudation of fluid and blood.

NEUROGENIC PULMONARY EDEMA AND MYOCARDIAL ISCHEMIA

Many neurologic processes are associated with a hyperdynamic state characterized by elevated plasma catecholamine concentrations. Examples include intracranial hypertension, ischemic syndromes, transtentorial herniation, SAH, status epilepticus, and midbrain ischemic or excitatory syndromes. In many of these situations pulmonary edema, myocardial ischemia, and myocardial infarction reportedly are frequent concomitants of the primary neurologic process.[287–315] Indeed, the cardiopulmonary dysfunction can exacerbate brain damage in many of these situations.

Neurogenic pulmonary edema can occur with a fulminant onset in association with neurologic syndromes associated with a hyperdynamic hyperadrenergic state.[301,302,306] This association leads to the notion that high afterload and increased myocardial oxygen consumption produce myocardial dysfunction, which is probably ischemic in origin. This is supported by reports that hearts obtained from brain dead donors can have areas of subendocardial necrosis,[312] despite there being no coronary artery disease. Moreover, abnormal electrocardiograms (ECG), increased creatine phosphokinase (CPK), and myocardial wall motion abnormalities are reported after SAH and increased ICP.[300,303–305,309] Animal models have duplicated the clinical observations.[316–318] Thus, the overall picture that emerges from the numerous reports examining neurogenic pulmonary edema and myocardial ischemia is one wherein the neurologic process compromises blood flow to cause excitation in catecholaminergic centers in the brain responsible for cardiovascular regulation. This results in a massive release of catecholamines into the circulation, causing profound increases in pulmonary and systemic afterload, myocardial ventricular distension, and increased resistance to ejection of blood. These processes associated with increased myocardial oxygen consumption, are combined with coronary vasoconstriction (similar to Prinzmetal's angina). The combination of increased oxygen consumption with decreased supply leads to diastolic dysfunction. This, in turn, promotes rapid accumulation of fluid in the lungs and the clinical appearance of "flash" pulmonary edema. The entire process can be short lived as the neurologic process settles down.

However, there can be residual effects on myocardial function, manifest as either a myocardial stun or infarction. In addition, fluid accumulated in the lung can take some time to resorb. By the time invasive monitoring is established, pulmonary capillary wedge pressure (PCWP) may be normal, leading the clinician to conclude that the pulmonary edema is noncardiogenic. All of the evidence discussed so far is concordant with the notion that the pulmonary edema has a high pressure hydrostatic basis. The only data suggesting otherwise are the common clinical observation of low PCWP and suggestions that pulmonary permeability may be affected by catecholamines or neural factors related to pulmonary innervation. It has been suggested that the reflection coefficient, possibly due to the mechanical effects of very high hydrostatic pressure, can be altered by neural influences in the lung.[299,308,319,320] If such is the case then hyperadrenergic conditions may, in addition to the aforementioned effects on the heart, also exacerbate the pulmonary edema by making it easier for water to filter into the pulmonary parenchyma. Such a notion is supported by reports of high protein in pulmonary edema fluid and low PCWP in patients with neurogenic pulmonary edema.[308,313]

Intracranial Hypertension

PHYSIOLOGY

The brain, spinal cord, CSF, and blood are encased in the skull and vertebral canal, thus constituting a nearly incompressible system (Fig. 36-12). In a totally incompressible system pressure would vary linearly with increased volume. However, there is capacitance in the system, thought to be provided by the intervertebral spaces. Once this capacitance is exhausted the ICP increases dramatically with increased intracranial volume.

Based on the relationship:

$$CBF = (MAP - ICP)/CVR$$

the concern is raised that increasing ICP is associated with decrements in CBF. However, the effect of increasing ICP on CBF is not straightforward as MAP may increase with ICP elevations,[321] and cerebral vascular resistance (CVR) adjusts with decreasing cerebral perfusion pressure (increasing cerebral blood volume) to maintain CBF until maximal vasodilatation occurs.[218,219,322,323] This is thought to occur at cerebral per-

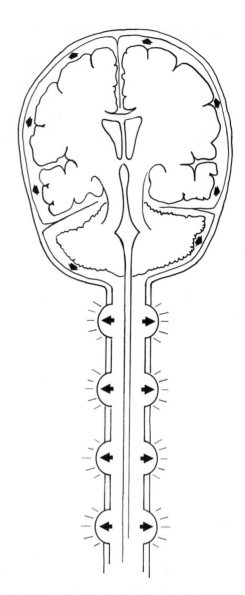

Figure 36-12 The brain, spinal cord, and blood are encased in the skull and vertebral canal, thus constituting a nearly incompressible system. System capacitance is thought to be provided via intervertebral spaces.

fusion pressure less than 50 mmHg although considerable interindividual heterogeneity in this value exists.[324] Thus, increasing ICP is often associated with vasodilatation or increasing MAP to maintain CBF.

Normal ICP is less than 10 mmHg.[2] ICP greater than 20 mmHg is generally associated with escalation of ICP-reducing therapy.[325,326] However, this is an epidemiologically derived number. Head trauma studies have indicated that patients with an ICP greater than 20 mmHg generally do not do well.[325] However, physiologically, simply elevating ICP to far greater than 20 mmHg is not necessarily associated with decrements in CBF, provided the above-noted compensatory mechanisms occur.[327]

Nonetheless, increasing ICP due to mass lesions or obstruction of CSF outflow can exhaust compensatory mechanisms. When this occurs, compromise of CBF does eventually occur. Initially, abnormality arises in distal runoff of the cerebral circulation. As the process continues, compromise of diastolic perfusion arises. With this the normally continuous (through systole and diastole) cerebral perfusion becomes discontinuous (Fig. 36-5).[133] Further compromise of cerebral perfusion pressure results in anaerobic metabolism, exacerbation of edema, and ultimately intracranial circulatory arrest.[133,328] Thus, when ICP increases it is important to detect it and ascertain whether this lethal sequence of events may be beginning to occur.

FACTORS THAT EXACERBATE INTRACRANIAL HYPERTENSION

The skull and vertebral canal contain the brain and spinal cord, CSF, and blood. With an abnormal condition, masses due to blood (hematoma) or neoplasia may also occupy space. When the volume of one or more of these compartments enlarges sufficiently to exhaust normal capacitive compensatory mechanisms, ICP begins to rise. Further increases in volume of one or more of these compartments then leads to the sequence of events associated with increasing ICP described above.[329,330]

BRAIN
The brain normally occupies about 80 percent of the contents of the skull. Brain volume can be increased by edema. The two types of edema are cytotoxic or vasogenic, referring to edema produced by cellular processes or vascular processes, respectively.[331] The edema can then act to increase ICP. Edema can be heterogeneously distributed such that pressure gradients can occur leading to a variety of herniation syndromes.[332]

CEREBROSPINAL FLUID
About 800 ml CSF is produced daily.[333] CSF is produced in the choroid plexus and absorbed in the arachnoid villi. As such an equilibrium exists between production and absorption. Disruption of this equilibrium can lead to increased ICP with hydrocephalus, the condition wherein there is an excess of fluid in all or part of the CSF system in the brain. Hydrocephalus is generally categorized as communicating or noncommunicating. In communicating hydrocephalus, the CSF circulation between the site of CSF production and absorption is intact. However, abnormally decreased absorption or increased production results in increased CSF accumulation. In noncommunicating hydrocephalus, the pathways are blocked such that CSF cannot circulate to the convexity of the brain to be absorbed. This results in accumulation of CSF in the ventricles, producing distension.[334]

BLOOD
Blood volume (CBV) is an important contributor to variations in ICP, in part due to the wide variations in CBV which can occur with normal physiologic homeostasis and with the effects of drugs and disordered physiology. When CBV increases due to increased CBF, this can produce a dramatic increase in ICP if intracranial compliance is abnormal. However, unlike ICP increases due to CSF, edema, or tumor in which decreased CBF is an expected adverse result, this variety of ICP increase is produced by increased CBF, with unclear significance.

Another mechanism of increased CBV occurs with obstruction of venous outflow. This results in CBV-mediated increased ICP, but without increased CBF.[335]

MASSES
The fourth cause of increased ICP is pathologic masses. These can be in the form of hematoma or neoplastic tumors. In both cases the faster the onset of the mass effect, the more acute the rise in ICP. Evidently there are compensatory mechanisms in intracranial compliance, which can allow quite large slow-growing masses to arise in the brain without elevated ICP. Similar size masses, arising acutely, are associated with quite large, symptomatic increases in ICP.

TWO TYPES OF INTRACRANIAL HYPERTENSION

There are two types of intracranial hypertension, categorized according to CBF as hyperemic or oligemic (Fig. 36-13). In the normal state, increases in CBF are not associated with increased ICP, as the normal capacitive mechanisms absorb the increased intracranial volume. However, in the situation of disordered intracranial compliance, small increases in intracranial volume produce increases in ICP. When CBV increases then intracranial contents increase to thereby increase ICP in a noncompliant system.[219]

This, however, suggests an important issue, that elevated ICP has traditionally been considered to be a concern because it indicates that cerebral perfusion might be jeopardized. It is unclear whether it is appropriate to be concerned about high ICP inducing intracranial oligemia when the cause of the high ICP is intracranial hyperemia. There have been no detailed examinations of this question although there have been some studies that allow reasonable inferences about the significance of hyperemic intracranial hypertension.

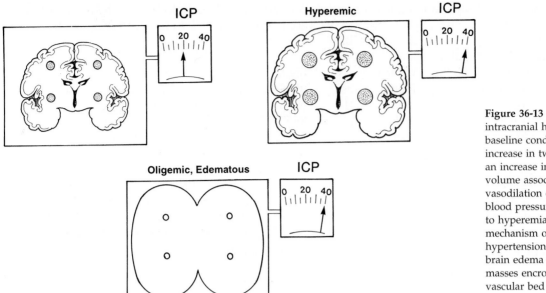

Figure 36-13 Two types of intracranial hypertension. From a baseline condition ICP can increase in two ways. One is via an increase in cerebral blood volume associated with reflex vasodilation due to moderate blood pressure decreases or due to hyperemia. The second mechanism of intracranial hypertension is via malignant brain edema or other expanding masses encroaching on the vascular bed to produce intracranial ischemia.

For many years it has been known that brief noxious stimuli briefly increase ICP in the setting of decreased intracranial compliance. Recent studies have reported that such situations are associated with hyperemia, strongly suggesting that hyperemic intracranial hypertension is not a dangerous situation.[336] However, it is reasonable to be concerned about such hyperemia for three reasons. First, elevated ICP due to hyperemia in one portion of the brain may increase ICP to compromise CBF in other areas of the brain in which rCBF is marginal. Secondly, increased pressure in one area of the brain may produce gradients that might lead to a herniation syndrome. Thirdly, there is theoretical concern that inappropriate hyperemia may predispose the brain to worsened edema or hemorrhage as occurs with other hyperperfusion syndromes. Thus, hyperemic intracranial hypertension has a theoretical potential to be deleterious but this has yet to be conclusively demonstrated. For brief periods, as may occur during intubation or other limited noxious stimuli, it is suggested that it may not be problematic.[337]

In contrast, oligemic intracranial hypertension is associated with compromised cerebral perfusion.[496] This is supported by the high mortality observed in head trauma patients in whom ICP rises due to brain edema after head injury with decrements in CBF.[276,325] TCD and CBF studies on these patients have demonstrated that CBF is low and perfusion is discontinuous during the cardiac cycle.[133,276] Moreover, jugular venous bulb data indicate that O_2 extraction is markedly increased, suggesting anaerobic metabolism.[276] In this setting noxious stimuli can further increase the ICP, thus producing the situation of hyperemic on oligemic intracranial hypertension. Presumably in this setting the hyperemic rise in ICP acts to further compromise rCBF in areas of brain edema.

BLOOD PRESSURE EFFECTS ON INTRACRANIAL PRESSURE— PLATEAU WAVES

In 1960, Lundberg[217] monitored ICP in hundreds of patients, identifying characteristic pressure waves. One of these waves has been identified as plateau waves and are known to be associated with increased cerebral blood volume[218] (Fig. 36-14). Such waves occur when the ICP abruptly increases to nearly systemic levels for about 15 to 30 min, occasionally accompanied by neurologic deterioration. Rosner and Becker[219] synthesized data, which convincingly suggest that intracranial blood volume dysautoregulation is responsible for plateau waves. They induced mild head trauma in cats and subsequently intensively monitored the animals after the insult. With normal fluctuations in blood pressure, while in the normal range, they observed that mild blood pressure decrements to approximately 70 to 80 mmHg preceded the development of plateau waves (Fig. 36-15). Cerebral blood volume in normally autoregulating brain tissue dilates with decreasing blood pressure and, moreover, the increase in CBV is nonlinear. There is an exponential increase in CBV as blood pressure decreases to below 80 mmHg (Fig. 36-16).[219a] A small decrease in blood pressure, although in the normotensive range, produces exponential increases in CBV in a setting of abnormal intracranial compliance with the ICP at the elbow of the ICP/intracranial volume relation. Thus, a small decrease in blood pressure introduces an exponential CBV change

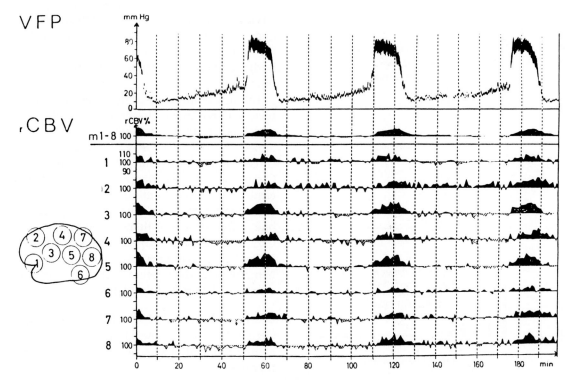

VFP

rCBV

Figure 36-14   Simultaneous recordings of regional cerebral blood volume (rCBV) and ventricular fluid pressure (VFP) during three consecutive plateau waves. The rCBF was measured in eight regions over the left hemisphere. The mean changes in the eight regions are shown in the uppermost curve of the rCBF diagram. Note that the rCBV and VFP curves show a very similar course during the three waves.[210] (Reproduced by permission from Risberg and coworkers.[218])

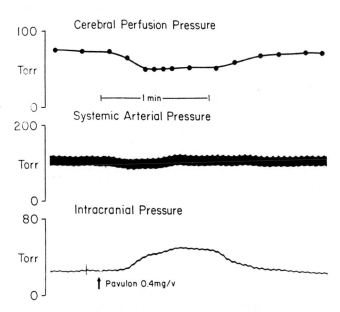

Figure 36-15   In an animal head trauma model a trivial-appearing and transient decrease in systemic arterial blood pressure in the setting of borderline cerebral perfusion pressure (CPP) precipitates sufficient cerebral vasodilatation to markedly increase the ICP. Restoration of CPP is associated with abolition of the plateau wave. (Reproduced by permission from Rosner and Becker.[219])

on an exponential ICP relation such that ICP will increase abruptly and to a significant extent. Plateau waves spontaneously resolve with a hypertensive response or with hyperventilation which will act to oppose the increase in CBV. Clearly, to develop a plateau wave there must be a portion of the brain with normally reactive vasculature in the setting of other brain areas with a mass effect and elevated ICP, which is a situation of heterogeneous autoregulation. In addition to preventing and treating plateau waves, such data indicate that it is probably important to maintain MAP in patients with high ICP in the 80 to 100 mmHg range.

Conversely, hypertension can also increase ICP. Within the normal autoregulatory range and normal ICP, changes in blood pressure have no effect on ICP. However, with brain injury and associated vasoparalysis, blood pressure increases mechanically produce cerebral vasodilation to increase ICP[219b] (Fig. 36-17).

It thus appears that both increasing and decreasing blood pressure can increase ICP, suggesting the presence of a CPP optimum for ICP. This is probably about 80 to 100 mmHg, although this has not been definitively determined experimentally (Figs. 36-18 and 36-19).

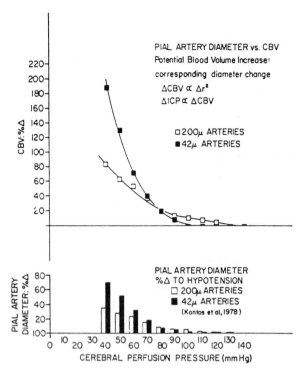

Figure 36-16 Vasodilatation occurs at a logarithmic rate as CPP is reduced. ICP will increase at a proportional rate within each pressure range with the most rapid increase occurring below a CPP of 80 mmHg. (Reproduced by permission from Rosner and Becker.[219a])

TREATMENT OF INTRACRANIAL HYPERTENSION

The general goals in treating intracranial hypertension are to promote adequate oxygen and nutrient supply by maintaining adequate CPP, oxygenation, and glucose supply (without hyperglycemia). The clinical strategy is to diagnose and treat the underlying cause, avoid exacerbating factors, and reduce ICP. Underlying causes include masses (tumors and hematomas), hydrocephalus, cerebral edema, and cerebrovascular dilatation.

Therapy of intracranial hypertension is primarily directed at removing the etiology insofar as possible, which is not always feasible. In such cases therapy is aimed at controlling ICP, hoping that the primary cause of the intracranial hypertension will resolve. Controlling ICP is thus a supportive maneuver, intended to preserve viable neuronal tissue until the high ICP situation resolves. Therapeutic maneuvers involve one of five classes of therapy including: a decrease of CBV, a decrease of CSF volume, resection of dead or injured brain tissue, resection of nonneural masses of hematomas and the removal of the calvarium to permit unopposed outward brain swelling.

CEREBRAL BLOOD VOLUME REDUCTION
Cerebral blood volume can be decreased with hyperventilation, CBF-decreasing drugs, mannitol, or hypothermia.

Hyperventilation
Hyperventilation can acutely reduce CBF and CBV to reduce ICP.[59,338–341] However, CBF returns to its original state within hours in a normal situation.[59,341] It is thus unclear why sustained decreases in ICP can be achieved with hyperventilation. Hyperventilation is performed in the intubated patient by increasing tidal volume or rate.

Hyperventilation has several adverse effects. Hyperventilation introduces a risk of decreasing CBF to a dangerous level[183] (see Fig. 36-10). In a recent study in trauma patients, routine hyperventilation was associ-

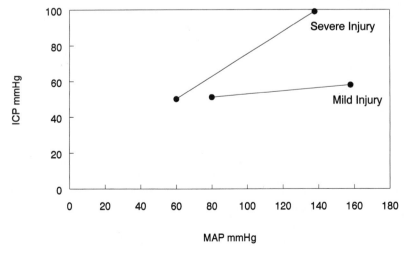

ICP response to hypertension with head injury

Figure 36-17 Blood pressure changes within the normal autoregulatory range normally have no effect on ICP. However, with brain injury, increases in MAP produce increases in ICP with this effect more pronounced with more severe injury. Presumably, this effect is due to distension of vasoparalyzed blood vessels with a consequent increase in cerebral blood volume. (Graph produced from data of Matakas and coworkers.[219b])

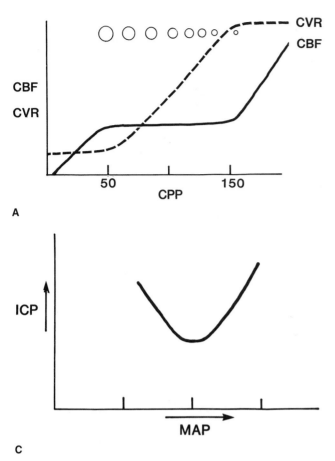

A

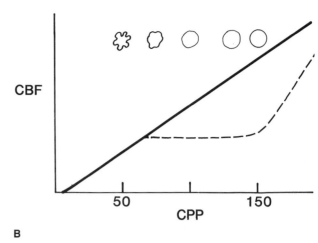

B

Figure 36-18   Cerebral perfusion pressure (CPP) versus CBF and cerebrovascular resistance (CVR). *A.* Blood flow is normally maintained constant through changes in CVR, depicted as changes in vascular diameter (and therefore cerebral blood volume [CBV]) in the figure. CBV varies inversely with CPP. *B.* With vasoparalysis due to injury CVR does not change with CPP variations such that CBF and CBV vary directly with CPP. *C.* In the situation of decreased intracranial compliance both of these factors in *A* and *B* may interact to increase ICP. Normally autoregulating tissue as in *A* will predispose to CBV-mediated ICP elevation with decreasing blood pressure, whereas vasoparalyzed tissue (*B*) will predispose to CBV-mediated ICP elevations with increasing blood pressure, leading to the notion of an ICP optimum (probably about 80 to 100 mmHg) with varying CPP.

C

ated with worse neurologic outcome at 3 and 6 months after the injury (Fig. 36-26).[184] The reason for this is uncertain and presently no one has demonstrated that anaerobic metabolism occurs with hyperventilation in this setting. It will produce alkalemia and increased affinity of oxygen for hemoglobin. In addition it will decrease seizure threshold.[342] Another important con-

cern is the potential for hyperventilation to produce only a transient effect (Fig. 36-20), or produce a para-doxical increase in ICP (Fig. 36-21). The causes of these effects are likely multifactorial but may include normal CSF pH regulation processes[341] or normal effects of CBF autoregulation similar to plateau waves.[219] Finally, on discontinuation of hyperventilation, a paradoxical

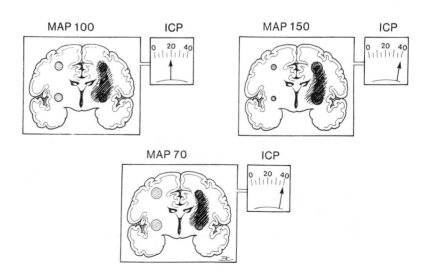

Figure 36-19   In the setting of heterogeneous autoregulation in the brain, conditions may predispose to CBV-mediated increases in ICP with both increases or decreases in blood pressure.

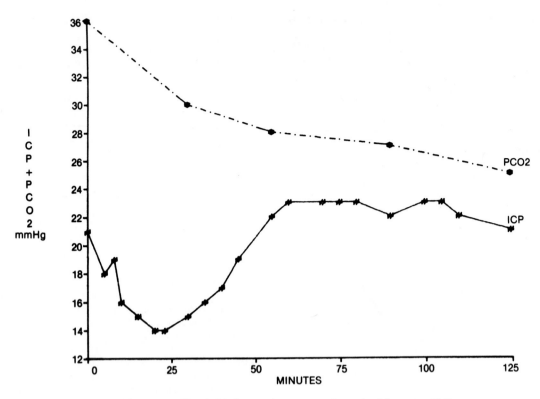

Figure 36-20 Typical temporal profile of ICP change after acute and sustained hyperventilation. Despite slight further lowering of P_{CO_2}, ICP has returned to its original level by 1 h. (Reproduced by permission from Ropper.[342a])

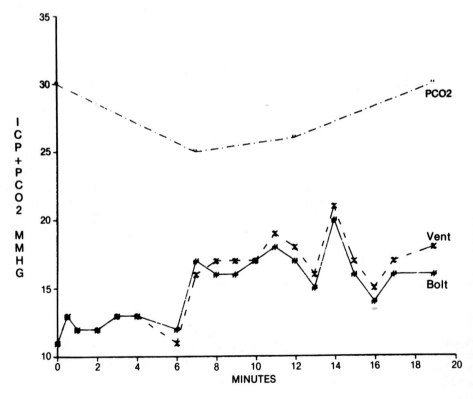

Figure 36-21 Paradoxical rise in ICP induced by mechanical hyperventilation, presumably due to mechanical pressure effects predominating over hypocarbic cerebral vasoconstriction. It is likely that hyperventilation induced a decrease in blood pressure, which resulted in an opposing reflex increase in cerebral blood volume. "Bolt" refers to subarachnoid screw, "vent" to ventricular catheter. (Reproduced by permission from Ropper.[342a])

CSF acidosis can occur.[59,341] These adverse effects indicate that hyperventilation should not be used routinely prophylactically. Nonetheless, it can be an effective means to decrease ICP if the patient has hyperemic intracranial hypertension which can be determined by use of jugular bulb oximetry.[343] High ICP associated with a low AVD_{O_2} across the brain (3 to 4 vol%) is thought to indicate that hyperventilation can be safely used. In an emergent situation, even if the nature of the high ICP (oligemic versus hyperemic) is not known hyperventilation should be used to keep ICP down or reverse a herniation syndrome or plateau wave until more definitive diagnosis or therapy can be performed.

Cerebral Blood Volume-Decreasing Drugs

Cerebral blood flow-decreasing (and therefore CBV-decreasing) drugs that can decrease ICP include barbiturates,[344-346] benzodiazepines,[347] etomidate,[348,349] and propofol.[346,350] Notably, all are CNS depressants. Thus, their use indicates acceptance on the part of the clinician to lose a reliable neurologic examination. Unlike hyperventilation, these agents decrease CBF coupled to CMR. Thus, the CBF decreases should not provide a milieu for anaerobic metabolism. Lidocaine also decreases CBF and CMR to decrease ICP although with a less pronounced decrement in neurologic function.[351,352] Mannitol's immediate effects are also thought to be mediated by reduction in CBV.[25]

BARBITURATES Barbiturates decrease ICP by decreasing CBF, CBV, CMR, and seizure activity.[344-346] Barbiturate therapy will usually decrease ICP. Failure for barbiturates to lower ICP is a bad prognostic sign. Ultrashort barbiturates, such as thiopental or methohexital, can be helpful in the intubated patient for acute increases in ICP. In addition barbiturates can be used when intracranial hypertension is refractory to other treatments. Moreover, barbiturates have the advantage of decreasing the amount of mannitol needed, thus decreasing mannitol-related side effects. In addition, by blunting shivering they can facilitate use of hypothermia therapy and they can be helpful to blunt the rise in ICP secondary to suctioning and other nursing procedures.

There are several adverse effects of prolonged barbiturate therapy for high ICP. Barbiturates blunt the neurologic examination. Thus, a growing intracranial mass lesion or other neurologic exacerbation may not be obvious until it causes an increase in ICP or increasing barbiturate requirement to maintain normal ICP. Hypotension and respiratory depression may occur. Blood pressure may need to be pharmacologically supported and intubation and mechanical ventilation are mandatory. Dysfunction of the alimentary tract may occur making it difficult to use enteral nutrition. Ther-

moregulation is disturbed. Hypothermia may occur inadvertently and infection may be masked due to lack of fever. Finally, physical addiction and tolerance may occur making it difficult to discontinue barbiturate treatment without seizure.

Thiopental can be given 1 to 4 mg/kg in boluses and repeated as needed to control ICP and is subsequently infused as needed. Pentobarbital is given in a loading dose of 3 to 5 mg/kg over 30 to 60 min, followed by 1 mg/kg per h, with the infusion adjusted as needed to control ICP. EEG can be used concurrently to assist in titration. Infusion can be increased until a burst-suppression pattern arises on EEG. Increasing the barbiturate dose beyond that needed to produce burst suppression is unlikely to provide further decreases in ICP as further decrements in CMR are not thought to occur at a dose beyond that needed for burst suppression.[353] Alternatively, serum pentobarbital levels can be monitored, aiming for a 30 to 50 μg/ml blood level. Discontinuation of barbiturate therapy can be considered when: there is no decrease in ICP with barbiturate loading; despite an initial favorable response, intracranial hypertension recurs despite maximal barbiturate therapy; or ICP has remained less than 15 mmHg for more than 24 to 48 h. In the latter case barbiturates should be weaned with continued ICP monitoring.

ETOMIDATE Etomidate decreases ICP by decreasing CBF and CMR.[348,349] It does not have as potent hemodynamic effects as the barbiturates such that it can decrease ICP without decreasing CPP as much as occurs with thiopental. It is not suitable for prolonged infusion to control ICP due to inhibition of adrenal corticosteroid synthesis[354] unless steroids are concomitantly administered. Nonetheless it can be used for brief periods as an adjunct in ICP control, especially if there is hemodynamic concern. The dose is 0.1 to 0.3 mg/kg intravenously.

PROPOFOL Although propofol has some ICP-reducing properties,[346,350] it also decreases blood pressure significantly.[355] Thus, its use for elevated ICP is generally limited to taking advantage of it as a side effect in selecting propofol as a sedative in the neuroICU.

LIDOCAINE Lidocaine decreases ICP by decreasing CBF and CMR but without as much CNS depression as barbiturates.[351,352] It is not as potent or reliable as barbiturates in decreasing ICP but it can be useful to decrease ICP when there is hemodynamic instability or when barbiturates are thought to be not tolerated hemodynamically. It can be useful before airway manipulations.[352] It is not typically used in prolonged therapy of intracranial hypertension. Rather, it is most useful given 0.5 to 1.5 mg/kg for acute treatment of high

ICP, particularly if associated with airway manipulation.

MANNITOL Mannitol, long a mainstay of the therapy of elevated ICP, probably works via a dual mechanism. Initially, accounting for its prompt action, it decreases blood viscosity.[25,352a] The effect of this is to prompt vasoconstriction in normally autoregulating brain areas to decrease CBV and secondarily, ICP. Subsequently, it may induce a further decrease in ICP through fluid shifts from brain to blood in areas with intact BBB,[356-358] although this may be limited through generation of intracellular iodogenic osmoles[359,360] equalizing transmembrane osmolar gradients.

Unfortunately, mannitol can have delayed effects to increase ICP. This can occur by four mechanisms. First, as a potent diuretic, mannitol can have a secondary effect to decrease blood volume, thus decreasing cardiac output and blood pressure. This can result in reflex increases in CBV, which can increase ICP.[219] Second, the increased urine output can elevate the hematocrit, thus opposing the initial mannitol-induced decrease in viscosity.[361] Third, mannitol can cross the BBB in an unpredictable manner, with the possibility introduced of rebound increase in ICP, similar to that observed with urea.[361,362] Fourth, there is a theoretical possibility of generation of increased intracellular osmolarity, via so-called idiogenic osmoles, which may predispose to rebound increase in brain volume with discontinuation of mannitol.[359,360] These complications of mannitol are probably lessened if urine output is replaced with balanced crystalloid infusion and if, once blood osmolarity is increased, it is not allowed to decrease to the prior level unless clinical improvement indicates that weaning of ICP-reducing therapy is appropriate.

CEREBROSPINAL FLUID DRAINAGE

Volume of CSF can be reduced by removal through ventricular drain. This can be effected by setting the drainage at a prescribed level above the midbrain or prescribing that the drain be opened anytime ICP exceeds 20 to 25 mmHg. Leaving a drain open risks excessive CSF drainage when the patient coughs or with drain manipulation in the course of routine nursing procedures. Excessive and abrupt decrease in local pressure around the drain can produce intracranial gradients, leading to a herniation syndrome. Leaving the drain clamped and monitored, however, risks the development of untreated intracranial hypertension.

RESECTION OF BRAIN TISSUE

Resection of brain tissue is occasionally used for malignant intracranial hypertension. Due to its proximity to the brainstem one approch is to resect part of the temporal lobe in an effort to avert a herniation syn-

$$\text{Low PEEP} \rightarrow \downarrow\text{CO} \rightarrow \downarrow\text{BP} \rightarrow \uparrow\text{CBV} \rightarrow \uparrow\text{ICP}$$

$$\text{High PEEP} \rightarrow \uparrow\text{CVP} \rightarrow \uparrow P_{SS} > \text{ICP} \rightarrow \uparrow\text{ICP}$$

Figure 36-22 Two mechanisms of PEEP-mediated increases in ICP. Addition of PEEP decreases cardiac output (CO) and blood pressure (BP) leading to a reflex increase in CBV. If cerebral perfusion pressure is marginal with heterogeneous autoregulation this can lead to further increases in ICP. Conversely, to increase sagittal sinus pressure (P_{SS}) to an extent sufficient to further increase ICP, which is already elevated, PEEP levels at or greater than the ICP must be applied.

drome.[363] An alternative approach suggested specifically for malignant intracranial hypertension due to stroke is to resect dead and swelling infarcted tissue, leaving noninfarcted tissue intact.[364]

RESECTION OF NONNEURAL MASSES OR HEMATOMAS

When clinical examination indicates a global decrement in level of consciousness, indicating elevated ICP, and imaging studies indicate the presence of a mass lesion, then urgent surgical removal of the mass is thought to be indicated.[363]

SURGICAL REMOVAL OF SKULL AND DURA

Decompressive craniectomy is somewhat controversial when used to allow brain swelling without intracranial hypertension after a large stroke. However, there is laboratory support for it and encouraging anecdotal evidence in patients describing its use.[365-368]

POSITIVE END-EXPIRATORY PRESSURE AND INTRACRANIAL HYPERTENSION

Positive end-expiratory pressure (PEEP) can increase ICP in two ways. The first is through impedance of cerebral venous return to increase cerebral venous pressure and ICP. The second is through decreased blood pressure and reflex increase in CBV to increase ICP (Fig. 36-22). Data from Huseby and colleagues[372] suggest that cerebral venous effects occur only with very high PEEP.

Shapiro and Marshall[369] demonstrated increases in ICP in head-injured humans with intracranial hypertension with application of PEEP (Fig. 36-23). Examination of their data indicates that the most profound decreases in CPP occurred in patients with PEEP-induced decrements in MAP consistent with the notion put forth by Rosner and Becker[219] that decreases in blood pressure increase CBV to increase ICP. Aidinis and coworkers[370] in studies in cats confirmed these observations in a more controlled setting. In addition, they assessed the role of pulmonary compliance, finding that decreased pulmonary compliance with oleic acid injections results in less of an effect of PEEP to increase ICP. Such observations indicate in situations where PEEP is likely to be needed, often accompanied by decrements in pulmonary compliance, that any adverse effects on ICP are less likely to be manifest. This may be related to observations that hemodynamic effects of PEEP are less apparent with noncompliant lungs[371] such that hypotensive-mediated increases in CBV do not occur.

The intuitive notion that PEEP increases cerebral venous pressure to increase ICP is not as straightforward as some may indicate. For PEEP to increase cerebral venous pressure to levels that will increase ICP, the cerebral venous pressure must equal, at least, the

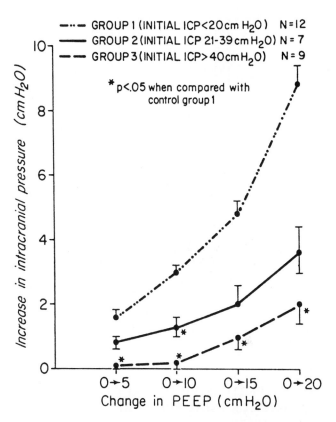

Figure 36-24 Increases in intracranial pressure (ICP) with positive end-expiratory pressure (PEEP) in dogs. Values are mean ± standard error of the mean. Group 1 included 12 animals with initial ICP less than 20 cm H_2O; group 2 included 7 animals with initial ICP of 21 to 39 cm H_2O; group 3 included 9 animals with initial ICP greater than 40 cm H_2O. Blood pressure was maintained constant in all animals. Note that with blood pressure maintained constant that the most significant increases in PEEP occur in the animals with the lowest starting PEEP level. (Reproduced by permission from Huseby and coworkers.[372])

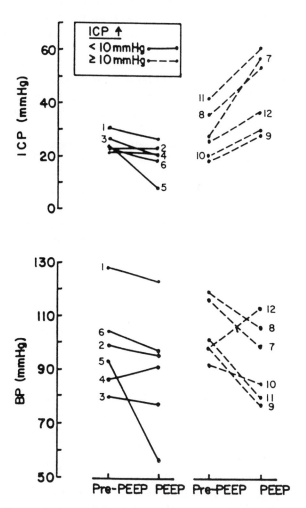

Figure 36-23 Intracranial pressure (ICP) and arterial blood pressure (BP) before and with the application of PEEP (4 to 8 cmH_2O) in severely head-injured patients. The patients are arbitrarily divided into two groups: those with an ICP increase equal to or above 10 mmHg, and those with ICP gains below 10 mmHg. Note that PEEP-induced blood pressure decreases appear to be more marked in patients sustaining larger ICP increases. (Reproduced by permission from Shapiro and Marshall.[369])

ICP. Thus, the higher the ICP, the higher PEEP must be to have such a direct hydraulic effect on ICP. This concept was shown by Huseby and associates[372] in dog studies, in which PEEP was increased progressively with different starting levels of ICP (Fig. 36-24). It is important to note that they prevented PEEP-induced decrements in blood pressure, thus avoiding any reflex increases in CBV. They suggested an hydraulic model to better conceptualize this (Fig. 36-25). Thus, for example, if all of a 10 cmH_2O PEEP application were transmitted to the cerebral vasculature, which is unlikely given the decreased pulmonary compliance associated with the need for such PEEP, then ICP will only be affected if it is 10 cmH_2O or less (7.7 mmHg) with it increasing to a level no higher than the applied PEEP. Such observations are consistent with the notion that there is a Starling resistor regulating cerebral venous outflow.[373]

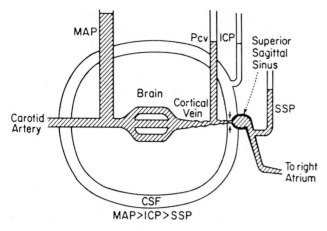

Figure 36-25 Schematic illustration of the intracranial space during raised intracranial pressure (ICP). The arrows indicate the position of the hypothesized Starling resistor. Here, the mean arterial pressure (MAP) is greater than ICP, which is greater than sagittal sinus pressure (SSP). Cortical vein pressure (Pcv) cannot fall below ICP, and thus flow is dependent on MAP-ICP, and independent of small changes in SSP. (Reproduced by permission from Huseby and coworkers.[372])

ANTIHYPERTENSIVE THERAPY EFFECTS ON INTRACRANIAL PRESSURE

Intracranial pressure can also be influenced by nonanesthetic drug administration, particularly antihypertensive drugs. In general, vasodilator drugs such as nitroprusside,[214,215,374a] nitroglycerin,[216] and nifedipine[211] can be expected to increase ICP. Conversely nonvasodilator antihypertensive drugs, generally sympatholytic drugs such as trimethophan,[374a] or β-adrenergic blocking drugs such as esmolol or labetalol,[201,202] can be expected to have little or no effect on ICP. The rise in ICP due to vasodilators is caused by increased CBF with attendant increase in CBV. The increase in ICP thus does not threaten ischemia. There is the possibility that herniation and hyperperfusion syndromes can occur and may be problematic. There has been a report of neurologic deterioration with nitroprusside use despite no change in blood pressure.[215] Another consideration in the use of vasodilators is the propensity to reflexly increase plasma catecholamines.[212] Such increases in plasma catecholamines may be deleterious to the marginally perfused brain.[194,195,199]

Postoperative Neurosurgical Care

After an uncomplicated neurosurgical procedure a patient is generally admitted to an ICU or intermediate care unit for observation, primarily to evaluate any neurological changes that may occur. However, some complications relevant to the specific procedure or the patient's medical history may also warrant close observation and intervention if needed. Ropper and Kennedy[374] nicely summarized the concerns after specific common neurosurgical procedures (Table 36-6).

During this observation period neurologic deterioration mandates immediate evaluation of the etiology and complicating this assessment can be residual anesthetic effects. In patients without underlying neurologic problems, emergence from anesthesia can be associated with a myriad of abnormal neurologic signs.[374,375] Moreover, in patients who had a previous neurologic deficit, even if not apparent on induction of anesthesia, it can reappear during the emergence period after anesthesia.[376] It is thus important, in the first few hours after a neurosurgical procedure to make decisions based on intraoperative events and the overall picture of the patients condition. For example, a patient with a newly appearing Babinski reflex who is otherwise awake and well appearing in the first hour after anesthesia probably does not have a structural lesion. Conversely, the same patient with a globally depressed sensorium that cannot be accounted for by amount of anesthetics administered should be cause of some concern.

A primary concern after any neurosurgical procedure is intracranial hematoma formation.[377,377a] This has been reported to occur in 2.2 percent of patients of whom 88 percent develop their hematomas within 6 h of surgery.[377] It is thus thought to be important to prevent abrupt or severe increases in venous or arterial pressure during this postoperative period. In addition to decreasing the likelihood of hematoma formation, such therapy should also attenuate predisposition to edema formation in the operative site.

Neurologic and Neurosurgical Disorders

HEAD TRAUMA

PATHOPHYSIOLOGY

Head trauma results in widespread abnormalities in brain anatomy, perfusion, metabolism, and function. With closed head trauma, to which this discussion will be limited, the initial impact results in mechanical disruption of the integrity of cellular and supporting tissue membranes.[378-380] Subsequently, numerous secondary phenomena result, which can worsen the patient's condition.[381-385] As a consequence of the trauma, blood and edema fluid accumulate as normal compartmentation is disrupted. Consequent to vascular disruption and the accumulating edema, secondary ischemia then assumes primary pathophysiologic importance. As ischemia develops, a variety of adverse biochemical processes occur. Many of these processes occur due to

TABLE 36-6
Neurosurgical Procedures and Main Associated Complications

Operation	Complication Immediate	Complication 24–48 h	Management
Craniotomy/tumor	Cerebral edema Cerebral hemorrhage Subdural hemorrhage	Subgaleal CSF leak Vasospasm	Avoid hypertension Slow steroid taper Fluid restriction CT and clinical follow-up ICP monitoring when indicated

Aneurysmectomy	Stroke from vascular
	  manipulation or clip
		Vasospasm
		Cerebral edema
			Blood pressure and aggressive
			  fluid management
			Clinical monitoring

AVM resection	Hemorrhage	Cerebral edema	Avoid excessive hypertension Fluid restriction if no vasospasm
Transsphenoidal hypophysectomy	Diabetes insipidus	Diabetes insipidus Nasal CSF leak Visual loss	Monitoring visual acuity Preoperative endocrine evaluation and postoperative replacement
Carotid endarterectomy	Hypotension	Hypotension Myocardial infarction Neck hematoma	Avoid blood pressure extremes ECG Watch for neck swelling
Tracheotomy	Hypocarbia Bleeding Airway occlusion Cuff leak		Adjust ventilator
Cerebellopontine angle tumor	Epidural hematoma	Hydrocephalus Apnea Aspiration	Follow-up CT Clinical monitoring

SOURCE: Adapted with permission from Ropper and Kennedy.[374]

the mechanical disruption and secondarily are exacerbated by ischemia and (indicating a positive feedback cycle) worsen the sequelae of ischemia. These biochemical events include release of free radicals[386] with lipid peroxidation, excitatory amino acid release,[387–389] inflammatory mediators,[390] metabolic acidosis,[391,392] and others that worsen the neurologic outcome. As time progresses, microcirculatory disturbances occur related to edema and BBB disruption and abnormalities in substances that regulate blood flow. In addition, it is thought that areas of vasospasm may occur, perhaps related to the presence of free blood in the CSF or locally around parenchymal blood vessels.[393]

From an overview perspective, CBF goes through phases with time after a head injury.[276–278,381,394,395] Initially it is depressed, subsequently becoming hyperemic. After that it returns to normal with resolution of membrane abnormalities or it progresses to zero with infarction as hyperemia probably exacerbates the edema.

With edema and hemorrhage, the intracranial volume of blood and brain tissue can increase. This results in increasing ICP.[325,385,394] Regional or global ICP will increase progressively with worsening edema re-

sulting in lower CBF and an oligemic form of intracranial hypertension that clearly can lead to permanent brain damage. Also, in patients with head injury, cerebral dysautoregulation with altered intracranial compliance will result in hyperemia manifesting as high ICP, causing in this case hyperemic intracranial hypertension. Hyperemic intracranial hypertension is exacerbated by increased blood pressure (producing distension of injured vasculature), fever, cerebral stimulants, cerebral vasodilators, and noxious/painful stimuli. Hyperemic intracranial hypertension probably does not have the same dire significance as the oligemic type with respect to whole brain function as it indicates globally elevated CBF. However, the intracranial hypertension, if elevated enough, may produce regional exacerbation of the brain damage ultimately sustained in edematous brains areas with tenuous perfusion. Moreover, the pathophysiology of hyperperfusion may exacerbate the damage.

Mechanical effects of the injury on brain structure have a major impact on the ultimate outcome. The categories of structural abnormalities include penetrating injury, hematoma effects, contusion, and white matter shear. The specific effects of such anatomic disruption depend to a great extent on the anatomic location. Isolated cortical or white matter lesions tend to produce focal deficits. Injuries to the midbrain and hindbrain, or diffusely and bilaterally to the cerebral hemispheres, tend to have global effects on level of consciousness. Penetrating injury produces irreversible structural abnormalities. The effects of contusion and hematoma produce abnormalities that may resolve to an extent with resolution of the lesion. White matter shear occurs as a result of inertia between brain tissue, thereby disrupting neural circuitry.[396,397] Such lesions may be suggested by the presence of petechial lesions on CT scan. They may not be evident and the diagnosis may then depend on the extent of clinical improvement being less than expected based on initial imaging studies.

PRESENTATION

The history generally indicates that the patient is a trauma victim. Details may indicate the level of consciousness at the scene of the injury, which compared to the level of consciousness in the hospital, can be diagnostically helpful.

Patients are usually scored according to the GCS (see Table 36-3). A score less than 8 indicates a severe head injury. A score above 12 indicates a mild head injury. The lowest GCS of 3 indicates a moribund patient.

On admission important issues to consider, because they indicate immediately treatable problems, include:

- Adequacy of gas exchange
- Other injuries
- Presence of intracranial problems that require immediate treatment
  - Increased ICP
  - Hematoma
  - Massive edema
  - Hydrocephalus
- Metabolic abnormalities
- Concurrent chronic medical problems

Initial diagnostic procedures are directed to determination of the presence of such problems. The admission data base should include[398]:

- Examination of airway and chest, arterial blood gases, chest radiograph. Respiratory failure significantly worsens the outcome after head injury.[399]
- Studies as indicated by the history and examination to diagnose concurrent injuries. In particular, concern regarding stability of the cervical spine is generally warranted. In addition, conditions that may produce abnormal gas exchange or perfuson pressure should be considered because these problems can lead to secondary exacerbation of head injury.

- Neurologic evaluation includes neurologic examination, optimally in the absence of sedation or neuromuscular blockade, CT scan, and cervical spine radiographs.
- Blood should be drawn to determine electrolytes, hematocrit, hemoglobin, PT, PTT, and platelets.
- History should indicate concurrent medical problems and chronic medications being taken. An ECG should be obtained if cardiac contusion or coronary artery disease are suspected.

THERAPY

Primary Disease

Neurosurgical therapy is generally indicated for several consequences of head trauma. An EVD is placed if hydrocephalus is present or there is need to monitor ICP/drain CSF. If a hematoma is present it may need to be drained if it is epidural or of a size large enough to produce high ICP or a herniation syndrome. Brain edema that is regional and producing intractable oligemic intracranial hypertension may require resection for the patient to survive.[363]

CCM Considerations

Primary considerations in critical care medicine (CCM) management of the head-injured patient are to control gas exchange, temperature, blood pressure, ICP, glucose, and electrolytes. Aspects in the management of these problems specifically relevant to head injury follow.

AIRWAY MANAGEMENT   Important concerns in airway management of the head trauma patient include: concurrent airway/cervical spine injury, hemodynamic status, level of consciousness (and presumed presence of high ICP), a presumed full stomach, and adequacy of gas exchange. In general, endotracheal intubation is required according to routine indications for respiratory failure. In addition, if GCS is 8 or less, neurologic considerations will indicate the need for endotracheal intubation because of inability to protect the airway or respiratory dysrhythmias.

Once the decision is made to perform endotracheal intubation the decisions that need to be made are:

- Nasotracheal versus orotracheal intubation versus tracheostomy
- Whether and which CNS depressant drugs are needed
- Whether neuromuscular blockade is required

Usually these decisions in a given patient require the use of considerable clinical judgment. Often, reasonable arguments can be made in favor of quite different choices and the clinician is often best off using the "do what is least bad" philosophy in determining the optimal decisions.

Nasotracheal intubation has been recommended if spinal cord injury is a possibility.[400] The rationale is that avoidance of laryngoscopy decreases the likelihood of exacerbation of spinal cord injury and decreases the likelihood of laryngoscopy-induced intracranial hypertension. However, to perform nasotracheal intubation without laryngoscopy neuromuscular blockade cannot be used and only minimal sedation can be used lest apnea or gastric aspiration occur. Unfortunately, this results in a patient likely to be uncooperative, turning his or her head from side to side, thus eliminating any advantage in terms of cervical spine stability. In addition, some head trauma patients have basilar skull fractures that may not be readily apparent on presentation. Insertion of tubes into the nasopharynx risks the devastating complication of an intracranial placement of the tube. Finally, a smaller endotracheal tube is likely to be used and sinusitis becomes a part of the differential in considering fever when the patient is admitted to the ICU, such that many practitioners routinely change a nasotracheal tube to an oral tube when such patients are admitted to the ICU, thus subjecting the patient to another airway manipulation. In general, orotracheal intubation is preferred. Tracheostomy is usually reserved for patients in whom nasal or oral intubation cannot be performed.

To facilitate the intubation generally some sort of anesthetic drug is used. In the patient who is responsive, this is done for comfort purposes and to ensure optimal conditions for laryngoscopy and intubation. For these patients and those with severe depression of consciousness many of the CNS depressants, such as thiopental and etomidate, have primary effects to reduce ICP, which increases (due to hyperemia) with laryngoscopy and intubation.[336] To prevent extreme increases in blood pressure, which also may be deleterious, fentanyl or a congener are also commonly administered.

Because a full stomach is also usually a consideration, either succinylcholine or rocuronium is used to facilitate a rapid sequence induction. The problem of hyperkalemia following the use of succinylcholine in the head-injured patient should always be considered. When a rapid sequence induction approach is used, the precise drug dose is a judgment. If there are certain to be no other injuries, one can err on the high dose side and then treat any postintubation decrease in blood pressure with pressors or fluid until the anesthetic drug effects subside. If there is any doubt about the presence of other injuries, lower doses should be used. As hypertension occurs with laryngoscopy and intubation, it can then be treated with increased doses of anesthetic drug as needed.

GAS EXCHANGE   As in any situation in which there is a decrease in cerebrovascular reserve, decreases in Pa_{O_2}, which otherwise can be well tolerated through vasodilatation, risk exacerbation of brain damage presumably due in large part to the lack of normal compensatory mechanisms. This is undoubtedly an important contributing reason that head-injured victims who are found unconscious and hypoxic at the scene very seldom do well. Thus, every effort to avoid hypoxemia is indicated, including continuous pulse oximetry, supplemental oxygen to increase fraction of inspired oxygen (FiO_2), and PEEP.

Hyperventilation has for years been a routine aspect of the care of patients with head trauma, but a quite low CBF can be produced with this technique (see Fig. 36-10).[183] Although biochemical evidence of hyperventilation-mediated anaerobiasis is lacking, there has been one important report that neurologic outcome is altered in patients who undergo routine hyperventilation after head injury[184] (Fig. 36-26). If an acute increase in ICP occurs and a herniation syndrome is occurring or is likely, temporary hyperventilation should be used. In addition, some authors advocate the use of hyperventilation with severe head injury, but with guidance from jugular bulb oximetry or direct measures of CBF.[67,95,401–403] Such an approach is suggested to ensure that hyperventilation is not used for oligemic intracranial hypertension but that it may be entirely appropriate when titrated to O_2 extraction for hyperemic intracranial hypertension.

TEMPERATURE   Temperature has recently been demonstrated to be an extremely important factor in outcome after head injury. Every effort should be made to avoid fever. In addition, early observations indicate a reasonable likelihood that hypothermia induced to 32 to 34°C improves outcome after head injury. A multi-institutional randomized study is presently ongoing and indicates a protective effect of moderate hypothermia.[189]

Hypothermia is induced in the intubated patient through application of external cooling, such as hypothermia blankets and application of ice packs. Centrally measured temperature must be used to guide temperature management. Because there is usually continued decrease in temperature, the active cooling measures should be less aggressively applied as the temperature goal is neared with no cooling applied once 33 to 34°C is achieved. The reason for this caution is that overshoot in cooling tends to result in metabolic acidosis and arrhythmias.

Just as hypothermia can be protective, multiple animal studies have clearly demonstrated the adverse effects of hyperthermia with brain injury.[187] Every effort must be used to prevent and treat fever with a liberal

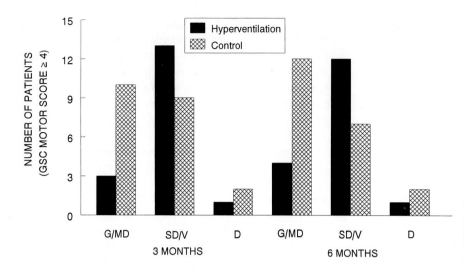

Figure 36-26 Head trauma patients were randomized to receive hyperventilation or normoventilation. Outcome was worse in hyperventilated patients. (Graph made from data of Muizelaar and coworkers.[184])

threshold for antipyretic therapy, about 38.2°C. When this threshold is reached, acetaminophen and external cooling are used to get central temperature into a normal range.

In addition to controlling temperature, the cause of the fever should be sought and treated. Cultures should be obtained and vascular catheters changed as indicated. If the fever is due to sepsis, this may further compromise neural function through an inappropriate decrease in CBF and BBB disruption.[404]

BLOOD PRESSURE   Blood pressure issues are similar to those discussed earlier in the context of high ICP. To avoid plateau waves, it is reasonable to maintain MAP about 80 to 100 mmHg.

GLUCOSE   Hyperglycemia in humans is reportedly associated with worse outcome after head injury.[237] There have been no controlled studies in animals in support of this. As head injury worsens, it is associated with an increase in stress and glucose levels rise. It is therefore difficult to ascertain whether the hyperglycemia contributed to the poorer outcome, or whether it was simply an epiphenomenon. Focal ischemia is thought to be an important aspect of the pathogenesis of head trauma. As severe hyperglycemia may be deleterious with focal cerebral ischemia, it seems reasonable to aim for a blood glucose of around 200 mg/dl in hyperglycemic head-injured patients.

ELECTROLYTES   Electrolytes can become abnormal with head injury. The stress response including elevated catecholamines, corticotropin, and ADH can result in fluid retention with an excessive retention of water over sodium, making hyponatremia a common occurence. In addition, cerebral salt wasting may also occur in head trauma.[405] With this, there is release of a natriuretic factor that produces loss of sodium in the urine.[268,406] In addition, SIADH can also occur with head trauma in association with fluid retention.[407] The occurrence of hyponatremia will decrease osmolarity to thus predispose the brain to increased edema. Every effort should be made to monitor and prevent hyponatremia. The only way to differentiate SIADH from salt wasting is by blood volume determination.[268,406] This can be estimated with invasive hemodynamic monitoring, although this has not been shown to be an effective way to differentiate these two hyponatremic syndromes. One effective clinical approach is to treat hyponatremia empirically with diuretics and sodium therapy as needed, addressing intravascular fluid volume and sodium concentration independently.

If injuries affect the pituitary gland or hypothalamus, diabetes insipidus can occur with head trauma. It should be suspected when urine output increases inappropriately to greater than 500 ml/h. A dilute urine is elaborated in the context of plasma hyperosmolarity with hypernatremia, which can be quite profound and seemingly abrupt. In this situation, prompt recognition can be life-saving. Diabetes insipidus can be treated with DDAVP or vasopressin.

Osmolarity is an important consideration in head trauma. Hypo-osmolar conditions should be avoided because they may predispose to cerebral edema.[230,231,233] In addition, a hyperosmolar state is often iatrogenically induced if ICP is high. Most clinicians decrease or discontinue mannitol therapy when serum osmolarity increases to 320 to 330 mosm.

Fluid management in head trauma is not straightforward. Some literature suggests that fluid restriction is helpful in decreasing the severity of cerebral edema. However, such an approach can modestly decrease blood pressure and may predispose a patient with heterogenously distributed CBF autoregulation to plateau waves.[219] In addition, fluid restriction may produce hemoconcentration, thereby compromising microcirculatory flow in at-risk areas of the brain. We generally aim for a normovolemic condition.

SPINAL CORD INJURY (also see Chap. 33)
PATHOPHYSIOLOGY
Automobile accidents, diving injuries, and gunshot wounds account for most spinal cord injuries. Injuries generally occur due to the mobility of the vertebrae relative to one another. About half of such injuries occur in the C4 to C7 region.[408] The clinical situations generally are associated with a predisposition to other injuries.[409] With spinal cord injury, manifestations of such injuries may be masked by effects of spinal cord disruption.

Injuries to the spinal cord produce approximately 12,000 new paraplegic or quadriplegic patients per year.[410] Loss of neural input from above the cervical cord results in respiratory muscle weakness or paralysis, loss of voluntary muscle control and tone, and cardiovascular dysautoregulation. Thus, cervical spinal cord trauma produces significant physiologic alterations in many organ systems. Life-threatening problems can arise that include respiratory failure, shock, and hypothermia.[410,411]

PRESENTATION
Patients with high cervical injury develop many serious manifestations of spinal interruption. These include respiratory insufficiency, hemodynamic instability, and poikilothermia.

Respiratory insufficiency occurs secondary to interruption of innervation of the intercostal muscles and the diaphraghm. Intercostal muscle denervation occurs in relation to the dermatomal level of the cord interruption. Complete loss of intercostal function occurs with lesions above C5. The phrenic nerve arises from cervical levels C3 to C5. Thus, partial interruption occurs C3 to C5 and complete interruption of diaphragmatic innervation occurs above C3.

Cervical cord lesions produce compromise of sympathetic outflow from the T1 to L2 spinal segments, leading to a state of spinal shock. This typically manifests with hypotension, bradycardia and decreased systemic vascular resistance. Bradycardia may be present. The patient will not be able to develop a tachycardic response to hypovolemia. Moreover, the unopposed vagal tone can result in severe bradycardia with maneuvers that produce vagal stimulation, such as oropharyngeal stimulation, ocular pressure, or a deep breath.

The loss of motor neural control results in loss of shivering as an important component of thermoregulation. Consequently poikilothermia can be problematic.[412]

Occasionally, cord edema progresses cephalad. This results in worsening of presenting deficits and can result in life-threatening respiratory compromise if the ascension of the deficit is not detected.

THERAPY[409-411]
Primary Disease
Further injury to the traumatized spinal cord is avoided by maintaining normal body anatomy as closely as possible. The neck-cervical spine must be stabilized using a halo thoracic vest, Gardner-Wells tongs, or Crutchfield tongs. Surgery with anterior or posterior fusion of the spine with an external fixation device may be required.

In the neuroICU, problems concerning spine stabilization are continually observed by the nursing staff. Alignment is assessed with radiologic studies. It is important that movement of the patient be performed with the patient as a single unit. This log-rolling technique requires two to three people to perform appropriately.

Serial assessment of neurologic status with accurate charting of the motor and sensory levels is mandatory the first 48 h after the injury to manage any worsening of the patient's status due to lesional ascension.[413] Neurologic checks should be performed hourly for the first 24 h. If the level is stable, the frequency can be decreased to every 2 h for the next 2 to 3 days. Any change in level at any time manadates an increase in frequency of the checks and evaluation by a neurosurgeon for the need for surgical intervention. If the deficit below a cord lesion remains complete for 24 h then irreparable cord damage may be present and recovery will usually not occur.

By comparing the level of vertebral injury with the level of paraplegia or quadriplegia, the component of the deficit due to nerve root damage can be separated from deficit due to the cord. Importantly, deficits due to nerve root injury can persist for weeks and still recover. Return of reflex activity below the level of the lesion, but without return of motor power, is not considered a good prognostic sign. If there is some return of sensation or some return of motor function in areas innervated by segments below the lesion within 24 h of the injury then some cord function has been spared in the area of the injury and recovery may occur.

Evidence in animals and humans indicates that administration of glucocorticoids early after spinal cord injury can confer an element of protection.[414,415] Thus, within 8 h after injury methylprednisolone should be given as a bolus of 30 mg/kg body weight, followed by infusion at 5.4 mg/kg per h for 23 h after the injury.[415] This may encourage a modest improvement in neurologic scoring, with minimal functional improvement.

CCM Considerations

AIRWAY MANAGEMENT   Endotracheal intubation is emergently indicated to maintain gas exchange if no diaphragmatic or intercostal function is present. Intubation may be only urgently indicated if there is incomplete diaphragmatic function. Intubation may also be indicated due to other injuries or the need for surgery.

Options to consider in airway management with cervical cord injury due to a cervical spinal vertebral injury are oral versus nasal intubation, direct laryngoscopy versus bronchoscopy or other indirect method, and what local anesthetics or CNS depressant drugs to use.

Oral intubation is generally preferred for several reasons. A larger tube is generally used for oral intubation than nasal intubation. This decreases the likelihood of inspissation of secretions in the tube, which can be life threatening, and makes it easier to perform therapeutic fiberoptic bronchoscopy, which is often required in these patients for atelectasis. If a head injury accompanies the cervical-spine injury, nasal intubation risks an intracranial intubation if a basilar skull fracture is present. Finally, an intubated quadriplegic is destined to have serial and potentially major problems with infection. The presence of an indwelling nasotracheal tube will make sinusitis a serious consideration in the differential diagnosis of sepsis. In such a situation the tube will need to be changed to an oral tube anyway. If the patient by that time has undergone surgical fixation of the cervical spine or has a halo thoracic vest in place, changing the tube to an oral one can be extremely difficult and dangerous. One primary advantage of nasal intubation is that it can usually be performed without the need for laryngoscopy and its attendant possibility of misalignment of the unstable cervical spine.

Fiberoptic intubation has been reported to be effective and safe with cervical-spine injury[416] and if time permits, it is the preferred method to secure the endotracheal tube. Its use decreases the risk of cervical spine displacement if the patient is cooperative. However, if the patient is not cooperative and is not yet in a halo vest, and cannot be made cooperative by sedation, then the movement of the patient can result in spinal displacement. If the intubation is emergent or the patient cannot remain immobile, then oral intubation with direct laryngoscopy and in-line immobilization is the method of choice.

Direct largyngoscopy should be done by the most experienced person available. This method has been assessed in large numbers of patients with cervical-spine injuries with no new neurologic deficits occurring secondary to endotracheal intubation.[417,418] Nonetheless others' observations indicate that a small amount of vertebral movement occurs with this procedure.[419–421] In-line immobilization should be done to minimize this.[422] Notably, this procedure should not be done with the assistant providing traction, rather he or she should simply be immobilizing the head and neck as a unit as much as possible. These patients should be considered to have full stomachs. Thus, cricoid pressure is generally used. However, the cricoid ring abuts the cervical-spine (C4 to C5) and may cause displacement of an injured vertebra.[419] Thus, the amount of pressure should be modulated somewhat if the injury is or may be near the cricoid ring.

Options in use of anesthetic drugs include topical agents, sedation, general anesthesia, and neuromuscular blockade. Observations of Suderman and colleagues indicate that the choice of anesthesia versus awake or oral versus nasal intubation had no discernible effect on incidence of neurologic deficits, which were quite low.[423] It thus appears that the primary goal is to proceed in a deliberate and careful manner. If the patient is to be intubated without substantial CNS depression, a topical agent is mandatory and can be accomplished safely.[423,424] This should include anesthesia of the oropharynx, larynx, and trachea. This is often not sufficient to have the patient remain cooperative with neck immobility. However, with the halo-immobilized patient this can be reasonable to try and followed by an awake laryngoscopy to see if the larynx can be visualized, which is rather unusual, but occasionally can be done, in which case the endotracheal tube can then be inserted.

The first principle in use of anesthetic drugs to facilitate intubation is that one always maintains ability to ventilate the patient and this cannot be guaranteed with the patient in a halo traction device. Thus, heavy sedation should not be used and during the intubation process the patient in a halo device must always be spontaneously breathing. If a halo is not in place, manual mask ventilation is easier to perform and laryngoscopy can be done in a more or less routine manner, such that the great majority of patients can be successfully intubated, given good intubating conditions. In such cases rapid sequence induction can be performed. One can induce hypnosis with thiopental or etomidate and analgesia with fentanyl or a congener.[423] Neuromuscular blockade is controversial because of situations where the need for rapid intubation signified the use of succinycholine, a depolarizing muscle relaxant known to cause life-threatening hyperkalemia because of changes in the muscle membrane following denervation.[425] Fortunately, the recent appearance of the rapid-acting nondepolarizing agent, rocuronium, has allowed one to replace succinylcholine in the acute spinal cord injury case requiring a rapid sequence induction with tracheal intubation.[426] Because of the predisposition to bradycardia with endotracheal intubation, pretreatment with atropine may be helpful.

GAS EXCHANGE   A cervical cord lesion produces paralysis of the intercostal muscles with decrements in vital capacity and other measures of pulmonary function.[427] Thus the patient must rely entirely on diaphragmatic function for spontaneous ventilation. If the lesion is above C6, diaphragmatic weakness will arise, with it progressively worse as the lesion ascends until it is above C3 at which point there is no diaphragmatic function. With cervical cord lesions compromised or inadequate ventilation can occur with decreased vital capacity, retention of secretions, poor cough, and decreased pulmonary compliance. Moreover, the efficiency of breathing may be further compromised by paralytic ileus. All of these problems partially or wholly may result in the need for the patient to undergo endotracheal intubation and mechanical ventilation.

Chest physical therapy should be instituted early to lessen the likelihood of respiratory complications. Some clinicians use automatic beds to produce sequential patient turning. If chest physical therapy is not effective in clearing secretions, fiberoptic bronchoscopy may be required to prevent atelectasis and pneumonia.

Because the lesion can ascend, the caretaker must be vigilant to serially and accurately monitor respiratory function. A quadriplegic with compromised but compensated ventilatory function, with ascension of the lesion can develop severe ventilatory dysfunction requiring mechanical ventilatory assistance. In this respect it becomes essential that hypoxemia or hypercapnea be avoided due to concerns that cord edema may be exacerbated, initiating a positive feedback cycle such that hypoxemia begets worsened edema, which then exacerbates respiratory function. Ventilatory rate, vital capacity (normal 65 to 75 ml/kg), maximum negative inspiratory force (normal 75 to 100 cmH$_2$O), chest auscultation, Sa$_{O_2}$ by oximetry, and arterial blood gases should be followed serially to assess trends. Vital capacity should initially be checked hourly. If vital capacity is less than 15 ml/kg, negative inspiratory force is less than 25 cmH$_2$O, or there is difficulty clearing secretions, especially if trends suggest gradual deterioration, intubation should be carefully performed before the onset of frank pulmonary insufficiency. With the onset of mechanical ventilation, with the lack of sympathetic autoregulatory mechanisms, the decreased venous return produced by positive-pressure ventilation may result in hypotension.

Pulmonary embolism is a significant risk. In the study of Wilson and colleagues,[428] although comprising only 4 percent of all trauma admissions, spinal cord injury accounted for 31 percent of all pulmomary emboli in the total trauma population (2525 patients). A sequential compression device should be used. Subcutaneous heparin is controversial and is thought to be suboptimal.[428] Some clinicians prophylactically perform an insertion of a vena cava filter in all patients with an acute complete spinal cord injury.[428]

Pulmonary infection is a major concern in quadriplegic patients.[427,429] Surveillance for pulmonary dysfunction must be ongoing. Unfortunately, the signs can be rather subtle because fever may not be apparent in this poikilothermic physiologic situation and the white blood cell count may be artifactually elevated due to concurrent steroid therapy. Tracheal aspirates using Gram's stain and cultures obtained two to three times per week and serial chest radiographs may provide the only clues of early infection. Trends in leukocyte counts can also be followed to monitor an infection process.

TEMPERATURE   Disordered temperature regulation results from lesions above T8.[412] Hypothermia to less than 35°C can occur initially after cervical cord injury due to vasodilatation and dissipation of heat. However, hyperthermia can occur with high ambient temperature or humidity, or it may indicate presence of infection. Hyperthermia occurs due to inability to dissipate heat through normal mechanisms of sweating, vasodilatation, and behaviors to dissipate heat (e.g., removing a blanket).

Passive warming measures are usually sufficient for mild hypothermia. When hypothermia is more severe (e.g., < 35°C) more active measures such as a heating blanket, warming the room, humidified inspired gases, or gastric lavage with warm fluid may be required. Similarly, hyperthermia is managed by keeping the patient uncovered and using a cooling blanket, sponge baths, and fan. When severe (> 40°C), ice water lavage or packing the patient in ice may be needed.

BLOOD PRESSURE MANAGEMENT   Compromise of sympathetic outflow from T1 to L2 spinal segments results in cardiovascular dysautoregulation. Hypotension is a major concern as low perfusion pressure for the cord may exacerbate edema and lead to ascension of the lesion.[413] Monitoring is needed to assess the patient and guide therapy. A bladder catheter, arterial cannula, ECG, and central venous catheter are usually used. If pulmonary edema is present, the patient is oliguric or hypotensive despite high central venous pressure (CVP) or high fluid infusion, or there is concern for other reasons about pulmonary edema (e.g., chest radiograph indications, rales, mycoardial/pulmonary contusion), then a pulmonary artery catheter is indicated. Fluids should be infused and titrated to produce a MAP usually greater than 60 mmHg with urine output greater than 0.5 ml/kg/per h. CVP or PCWP can be used to decide on an upper safe end point for fluid infusion. If the patient is hypotensive despite the presence of adequate preload, then vasopressor infusion may be needed to ensure adequate perfusion pressure. Centrally acting inotropes such as isoproterenol, doputamine, and dopamine in low doses can be reasonably used and adjusted to maintain adequate perfusion pressure with adequate urine output. If bradycardia is problematic,[430] atropine may be the only vasoactive drug needed to maintain adequate perfusion pressure and can also be used to prevent bradycardia due to suctioning or other vagotonic maneuvers.

In the acute phase ECG changes consistent with subendocardial ischemia have been reported in both clinical and laboratory reports with transections at or above C5 to C6. Other ECG changes also can occur, including sinus pause, shifting sinus pacemaker, atrial fibrillation, ventricular extrasystoles, ventricular tachycardia, and ST-T segment changes.[431,432]

As the patient survives the acute phase, spinal shock ultimately subsides and such intensive support of the circulation becomes unnecessary. However, about a month after the injury, the patient becomes susceptible to autonomic dysreflexia.[433] This syndrome manifests with paroxysmal hypertension, sweating, facial flushing, headache, and nasal congestion. When severe, retinal or cerebral hemorrhage can occur. It is precipitated by autonomic sensory input from stimuli such as defecation, bladder distension, or muscle spasms. The precipitating causes must be prevented. Thus the bladder must be maintained empty with regular intermittent catheterization or continuous catheterization, fecal impaction must be prevented with regular bowel care (including laxatives, suppositories, and stool softeners as needed), and muscle relaxants such as benzodiazepines, dantrolene, or spinal baclofen should be used.

GLUCOSE   Drumond and Moore[434] reported exacerbation of spinal cord lesions with moderate hyperglycemia in a rabbit laboratory model. It thus seems prudent to maintain blood glucose at about 200 mg/dl in hyperglycemic patients.

ELECTROLYTES AND FLUIDS   In the acute phase, gastrointestinal ileus will result in the need for a nasogastric tube to empty the stomach, reducing the risk of aspiration, decreasing mechanical interference with breathing by distended bowel, and preventing gastric distension from aerophagia, a common problem with spinal cord injury. Ileus contraindicates the use of enteral nutrition. This can be tolerated for a few days. If the ileus resolves during this period enteral nutrition,

with elemental formulations if necessary, should be started. If enteral nutrition is not tolerated than parenteral nutrition may be needed until the ileus resolves.

BRAIN TUMORS
PATHOPHYSIOLOGY
The incidence of primary brain tumors has been estimated to be 15/100,000 and of secondary brain tumors 46/100,000. The symptoms that will lead a patient to seek medical help or result in the need for intensive observation or care are related to straightforward principles of physics and physiology. Such factors result in high ICP or local effects causing a neurologic deficit. When consciousness is decreased so that neuroICU admission is needed, a tumor may contribute to this by uncal transtentorial herniation, direct infiltration of the reticular activating system, hydrocephalus, seizures with a postictal condition, and intratumor bleeding.[435] Further exacerbating the effects of tumor mass is the common occurrence with brain tumors of peritumor vasogenic edema.[436]

PRESENTATION
Patients present to the neuroICU preoperatively when a tumor produces a decrement in consciousness or seizures, or is in a location that jeopardizes critical structures. However, the more common presenting scenario is usually after intracranial surgery.

As ICP increases patients will be noted to sustain personality or behavioral changes, headaches, papilledema, and vomiting. Twenty to 50 percent of patients with brain tumors will develop seizures.[436]

THERAPY
Primary Disease
Intracranial tumors generally require resection when they become symptomatic or if a malignancy is suspected. Preoperative therapy to reduce ICP or other mass effects may be used. These include steroids for vasogenic edema and mannitol or furosemide to reduce ICP.

Postoperatively, the major neurologic concerns are hematomas, brain edema, hydrocephalus, and retractor-mediated deficits. Postoperative neurologic deterioration can be caused by any of these and mandates urgent CT scan to elucidate the cause and need for neurosurgical intervention. If a hematoma occurs, it is most likely to occur in the first 6 h after surgery and to be in the operative site.[377,377a] Notably, posterior fossa procedures, if followed by hematoma, can lead to abrupt and severe neurologic deterioration. In such cases, the most urgent approach to therapy possible is required because such patients may recover if decompression occurs quickly but will die if brainstem ischemia occurs for too long a period.[437] Such considerations justify the occasional practice of performing a decompressive opening of the surgical wound in the neuroICU.

CCM Considerations

AIRWAY MANAGEMENT   In the patient with increasing ICP due to tumor, considerations for airway management are similar to those previously discussed for airway management with high ICP.

After supratentorial tumor surgery patients usually arrive extubated. If reintubation is required, consideration should be given to the possibility that ICP is elevated due to one of the above-noted causes and that systemic hypertension from laryngoscopy may worsen the problem if the patient is suffering from a hypertension-induced hematoma. After posterior fossa surgery, there may be problems with respiratory dysrhythmias or cranial nerve dysfunction such that the patient may not be able to protect the airway. If this is a concern, such patients may remain intubated electively to determine whether routine postoperative brain edema will produce or worsen such problems. If by postoperative day 1 or 2 such problems have not occurred, extubation can usually be safely performed.

GAS EXCHANGE   Areas of the brain with postoperative edema can be expected to have decreased cerebrovascular reserve. In such situations the normal vasodilatory response to anemia or hypoxia may be compromised such that neuronal injury could occur. It thus is essential that hypoxemia be avoided in these patients and that pulse oximetry be used to ensure Sa_{O_2} greater than 94%. Similarly, anemia to a hematocrit below 30% should be avoided.

Causes of hypoxemia in this setting include fluid overload, pulmonary embolism, and atelectasis. Fluid overload is uncommon because many of these patients receive intraoperative diuretics to improve surgical exposure. Pulmonary embolism occurs with high frequency in brain tumor patients.[438,439] If pulmonary embolism or DVT occurs there is some disagreement whether anticoagulation or vena caval interruption (with filter) is more appropriate,[439,440] although oral anticoagulation appears to be safe.[439] Brain tumor patients should receive treatment with a sequential compression device and subcutaneous heparin. Atelectasis can occur consequent to surgical position or intraoperative misplacement of the endotracheal tube. If this occurs, chest physical therapy may be required. This is usually sufficient to treat the problem. Fiberoptic bronchoscopy is seldom required.

BLOOD PRESSURE MANAGEMENT   Postoperative hypertension commonly occurs in these patients. Such hypertension may predispose to the development of postoperative hematoma. Thus, control of blood pressure is very important after tumor resection. After evaluating and treating or ruling out other causes of postoperative hypertension such as hypercarbia, bladder distension, shivering, or pain, therapy directed to treat high blood pressure is indicated. If there was significant decompression of tumor such that ICP is thought to be low, vasodilator drugs such as nitroprusside or hydralazine can be used. If there is concern that the ICP may still be high or is at risk of being high, then such drugs should be avoided if possible. Generally adequate treatment of hypertension is achieved with labetalol, nifedipine, or nicardipine.

GLUCOSE   Because of concerns about ischemic pathophysiology, hyperglycemic patients should have blood sugar maintained at about 200 mg/dl.

ELECTROLYTES AND FLUIDS   During surgery for intracranial tumor diuretics may have been given. Such therapy often produces abnormalities in sodium, potassium, and osmolarity. Thus, on arrival in the neuroICU these electrolytes should be evaluated and treated as needed.

PITUITARY TUMORS

PATHOPHYSIOLOGY
Pituitary tumors usually arise as discrete nodules in the anterior part of the gland. Tumors less than 1 cm in diameter are known as microadenomas and those larger as adenomas. Medical problems arise when the tumor enlarges enough to produce a significant effect, or more commonly, when the neoplastic tissue secretes pituitary hormones free of normal homeostatic autofeedback control.

PRESENTATION
Pituitary adenomas come to medical attention because of headache, visual abnormalities, or endocrine disturbances. Fifty percent of patients with pituitary adenomas complain of headache. Endocrine symptoms are attributable to oversecretion of anterior pituitary hormones—prolactin, somatotropin, adrenocorticotropin, gonadotropin, growth hormone, or thyrotropin or to hormonal hyposecretion. Oversecretion of the posterior hormone vasopressin can also occur. Growth of the tumor can result in visual abnormalities due to compression of the optic chiasm. This typically produces a bitemporal hemianopsia. Finally, on rare occasion an adenoma can produce pituitary apoplexy, hemorrhage into the pituitary tumor, which can be lead to a life-threatening loss of pituitary hormones.[441]

Patients with pituitary tumors typically are admitted

to the neuroICU because of mass effect of a very large tumor causing intracranial hypertension or pituitary apoplexy, or postoperatively after resection. Pituitary apoplexy presents with the acute onset of headache, opthalmoplegia, bilateral amaurosis, and decreased level of consciousness with possible subarachnoid hemorrhage, pleocytosis, and elevated protein in the CSF.

THERAPY

Primary Disease

Many smaller pituitary tumors can be treated pharmacologically or with radiation. If such therapy is not effective or there are immediate concerns regarding mass effects surgery becomes the principal therapy. A transsphenoidal approach is used if the tumor is small enough and positioned appropriately to safely permit it. If the tumor has significant suprasellar extension then a frontal craniotomy is usually performed.

CCM Considerations

Postoperatively, the usual postcraniotomy concerns are present. In addition, careful observation for the development of diabetes insipidus is indicated. If undetected, this can lead to life-threatening hypernatremia and when detected prompt therapy is required.

The awake patient will generally complain of severe thirst.[442] In the noncommunicative patient, the first sign may be profound diuresis, often in excess of 1 liter/h. In association with this the patient will develop progressive hypernatremia, which can exceed 170 meq/liter, with hypovolemia. Other signs of hyponatremia include restlessness, irritability, ataxia, increased muscle tone, hyperreflexia, seizures, and intracranial hemorrhage.[443]

In general, diabetes insipidus can be diagnosed when, in the face of hyperosmolar serum (mOsm > 285) the urine specific gravity is close to 1.000 and urine osmolarity is less than 200 mOsm with little or variable sodium in the urine.[444] Incomplete diabetes insipidus can also occur, a situation wherein intermediate urine and serum electrolytes will be found.[444,445]

In the appropriate setting where diabetes insipidus is a possibility, serial plasma sodium concentrations should be determined every 6 h. If the sodium is elevated or is rising, the frequency should be increased. If the patient is diuresing in the 1 liter/h range, then hourly sodium levels are required until an elevated serum sodium develops, whereupon urine osmolality and specific gravity should be obtained with simultaneous serum sodium and osmolality to establish the diagnosis safely and unequivocally.

After pituitary surgery, patients are at high risk to develop temporary or permanent diabetes insipidus.[265,446,447] Half of patients develop transient diabetes lasting 3 to 5 days, 33 percent develop permanent diabetes insipidus and 33 percent develop a triphasic course. Initially a substantial diuresis occurs, which lasts 12 to 24 h. Subsequently, as ADH previously synthesized is released, the diabetes will appear to resolve with a risk of iatrogenic hyponatremia secondary to treatment of the initial diabetes insipidus. Subsequently this phase may recede as fully established diabetes insipidus appears, which may or may not be permanent.[448]

Other causes of postoperative polyuria should also be considered, notably diuresis induced by mannitol, excessive fluids, or hyperglycemia. However in these conditions, the urine specific gravity and osmolarity will be higher than is observed with diabetes insipidus.

Once the diagnosis of diabetes insipidus has been made, therapy is indicated with either DDAVP or vasopressin. DDAVP is given 1 to 4 μg every 12 to 24 h intravenously, subcutaneously, or intramuscularly. The specific dosage interval can be determined by the resumption of polyuria. Vasopressin, 5 to 10 units intramuscularly is given every 4 to 6 h or as dictated by the occurrence of polyuria. To avoid overtreatment some authors have suggested a continuous infusion of low-dose vasopressin, a regimen thought to be more titratable. Therapeutic effects last only 3 h after cessation of infusion.[449,450]

Other concerns after pituitary surgery are related to loss of adrenocortical function. Prophylactic use of stress steroid coverage is indicated using hydrocortisone 100 mg every 8 h.

If pituitary surgery was for acromegaly, the sequelae of prolonged growth hormone secretion should be considered. These include airway abnormalities, hypertension, cardiomegaly, glucose intolerance, and fluid balance abnormalities. If not fully awake at the end of surgery, such patients should be allowed to fully awaken from anesthesia in the neuroICU. Only when fully awake should extubation be performed. If intubation attempts were traumatic such that airway edema is a concern, extubation should be performed over a bronchoscope or endotracheal tube changer. Hypertension may predispose such patients to blood pressure lability, although a recent retrospective review at our institution suggested this is not a major intraoperative problem. Careful consideration of a given patient's preoperative cardiovascular function is nonetheless indicated to assess for evidence of ventricular dysfunction, which may make fluid management more difficult.

STROKE

Stroke is the third leading cause of death in the United States. For every patient who dies of a stroke there are about 13 survivors who carry on with the effects of their loss of neural tissue.[451] The 2-year incidence of stroke is 10/1000 and the incidence due to atherothrombotic brain infarction is 4.4/1000.[451] Some of the risk factors for atherothrombotic stroke are hypertension, left ventricular hypertrophy, cigarette use, elevated lipids, obesity, and polycythemia.[451]

SUBARACHNOID HEMORRHAGE
Pathophysiology

INCIDENCE Autopsy studies indicate that as many as 5 percent of people may harbor aneurysms.[452] Data from the cooperative aneurysm study suggest that about 80 percent of SAHs arise from aneurysmal rupture.[453] Estimates of the incidence of SAH vary from 3.9 to 19.4/100,000 per year,[454–457] accounting for 6 percent of all strokes.[458] Mortality from SAH differs considerably among reports, varying from 3 to 5 percent in patients in good clinical condition to as high as 68 percent, with the overall mortality probably in the range of 23 percent.[452,455–460] Of the survivors over half sustain major disability, with 64 percent of those returning home never again attaining their premorbid quality of life.[461]

Several types of aneurysms can rupture. The types of aneurysms are classified as saccular, atherosclerotic, mycotic, traumatic, and dissecting.[452] The risk of rupture for an unruptured incidental aneurysm seems to increase as the diameter of the aneurysm exceeds 10 mm angiographically. Giant aneurysms are greater than 25 mm and comprise 5 percent of all aneurysms.[462] Finally, multiple aneurysms occur in 13 percent of the cases.[463,464]

ICTUS The initial bleed is associated with a transient increase in ICP to systemic levels. This has two predominant effects. The first is to produce a decrement in level of conscious with unconsciousness occurring in 45 percent. Usually the loss of consciousness is brief but in 10 percent of cases it can last for days.[465] The second effect of the elevated ICP may be to stop the egress of blood from the arterial rupture to promote clot formation.

Subsequent to the bleed a complex series of events can occur. These include rebleeding, hydrocephalus, and vasospasm, which can lead to a delayed neurologic deficit. In addition extracranial complications can also contribute to postbleed morbidity and contribute to neurologic problems.

REBLEED The probability of rebleeding is about 4 percent the first day after the bleed and about 1.5 percent per day thereafter. Overall the incidence of rebleeding is reportedly 19 percent the first 2 weeks, 64 percent by the end of the first month, and 78 percent by the end of 8 weeks postbleed.[466–470] Several predisposing

TABLE 36-7
Predisposing Factors for Rebleeding From a Ruptured Aneurysm During the First 14 Days After Subarachnoid Hemorrhage

Female gender

Advanced age (> 70 years)

Short interval after SAH (days 0–1)

Poor neurologic grade

Poor medical condition

Moderate to severe systolic hypertension (170–240 mmHg)

Lumbar puncture in the presence of intracranial hypertension

Ventriculostomy to relieve intracranial hypertension associated with systemic hypertension

Infusion of mannitol to relieve ICP associated with intracranial hypertension

Abrupt interruption of antifibrinolytic therapy inducing a rebound in plasma fibrinolytic activity

Intubation without adequate anesthesia or sedation

SOURCE: Reproduced by permission from Espinosa and coworkers.[466]

factors for rebleeding have been identified.[470] These include female gender, admission within the first day after SAH (implying that survival outside the hospital for longer periods selects more stable patients), poor neurologic grade, poor general medical condition, and systolic blood pressure greater than 170 mmHg. Other factors have also been identified based on theoretical considerations or observations and are listed in Table 36-7.

The occurrence of a rebleed is associated with a mortality rate varying in reports from 48 to 78 percent.[466,471]

HYDROCEPHALUS Based on temporal considerations, hydrocephalus can be divided into three categories: acute, subacute, and delayed[472,475,475a] (Table 36-8). The ventricular dilation arises secondary to the effects of fresh blood in the CSF, which can fill the ventricles, blocks the aqueduct of Sylvius, fills and obstructs the fourth ventricle, fills the subarachnoid cisterns, or blocks the arachnoid villi. This results in obstruction of CSF circulation or reabsorption leading to hydrocephalus, increased ICP, and a depressed level of consciousness.

Intraventricular hemorrhage in association with

TABLE 36-8
Acute Hydrocephalus After Subarachnoid Hemorrhage

Category	Time of Onset After SAH	Presentation
Acute	Hours	Abrupt coma
Subacute	Few days	Gradual decline in mental status
Delayed	Weeks to years	Dementia, gait apraxia, bladder incontinence

SAH is associated with substantially worse outcome when hydrocephalus occurs.[473,474] The etiology of this is obstruction of egress of CSF from the ventricles and obstruction of absorption in the choroid plexus. The likelihood of hydrocephalus correlates with the amount of blood evident on CT scan.[475a] The overall mortality when hydrocephalus occurs is reportedly 64 percent.[474] Even with ventricular drainage mortality can remain quite high.[474] Most such patients are admitted with a poorer neurologic grade. The morbidity is related to herniation and to decrements in CBF, which may already be compromised. Hydrocephalus can occur at any time after SAH. Acutely, it occurs in 20 percent,[475a] and subacutely or chronically, it occurs in 15 to 20 percent of patients.[466] Permanent CSF diversion is required in 5 to 10 percent of patients after SAH.[466]

VASOSPASM   Three to 21 days after SAH, post-SAH vasospasm may occur. The peak incidence is between days 6 and 8 after SAH with duration of up to 2 weeks.[476,477] The actual incidence of post-SAH vasospasm varies in the literature with reports between 15 and 76 percent. The true incidence is probably somewhere in between, in the 30 to 40 percent range.[466,478-488] Delayed cerebral ischemia due to delayed vascular narrowing remains one of the most frightening and devastating causes of stroke in a patient otherwise doing well recovering from SAH and surgery. Of the patients developing vasospasm, about 30 percent will sustain an ischemic deficit due to the vasospasm[489] with about 7 to 17 percent going on to develop permanent neurologic deficit or dying.[476,478,490]

The pathogenesis of vasospasm has been correlated clinically with the amount of blood in the basal cisterns adhering to basal cerebral arteries.[475a,475-477,491-495] In further support of this are observations that in vivo and in vitro application of blood to cerebral arteries produces contraction of the vessels.[496-498] Many studies have been reported examining the many components of blood for their potential to produce vasospasm.[496] Many of these components do cause spasm although no single spasmogen has been identified as the sole culpable substance. Similarly, numerous studies have examined many of the chemicals in the blood, determining that many can cause spasm of cerebral arteries in the experimental situation.[496] Other potential contributors to vasospasm include mechanical wall disruption, inflammation, and free radicals.[496]

The cerebral vasculature maintains the appropriate vascular tone through the interplay of numerous factors. Important in this homeostasis is the balance between endothelin and nitric oxide. Endothelin is a potent vasoconstrictor and nitric oxide is a short-lived potent vasodilator. Oxyhemoglobin binds nitric oxide. Thus, with degradation of the erythrocytes in the CSF,

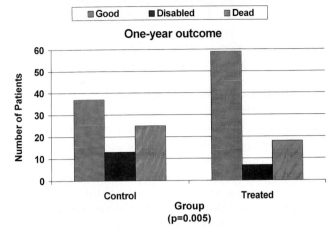

Figure 36-27   Subarachnoid hemorrhage patients were randomly treated with propranolol or placebo. Neurologic outcome was better in patients undergoing β blockade. (Graph made from data of Neil-Dwyer and coworkers.[199])

the basal cerebral arteries are exposed to oxyhemoglobin, which may bind nitric oxide, resulting in spasm.[496,499] Further support for this is in studies wherein intracarotid nitric oxide infused into the vasospastic artery of a monkey relieves the spasm.[500]

Serum catecholamine levels increase dramatically after SAH, notably peaking at the same time as the peak incidence of vasospasm after SAH.[302,306,311,315,501-505] This leads to the notion that hypothalamic injury with excess catechlamine release may be an important factor in the genesis of post-SAH spasm.[311,501,506] Several lines of evidence further support this hypothesis:

The cerebral vasculature is invested somewhat with adrenergic nerves. With SAH, the adrenergic receptors in the cerebral vessels decrease in quantity.[507,508] This suggests that denervation hypersensitivity may be occurring such that the increase in humoral catecholamines with SAH produces spasm in hyperreacting vessels.

Treatment of humans with SAH with β- and α-adrenergic antagonists is associated with an improvement in neurologic outcome (Fig. 36-27)[199] and ECG abnormalities.[307]

Catecholamine release after SAH is sufficient to produce ECG abnormalities[287,289-292,306,307,309,501,509,510] with ventricular wall motion abnormalities[304,305,511] and myocardial injury.[293,294,312,314]

In animal models, selective destruction of hindbrain adrenergic nuclei with cephalad projections prevents the development of vasospasm.[316-318] Moreover, laboratory studies indicate an important role for vasopressin in vasospasm because vasospasm cannot be produced in vasopressin-deficient rats.[512]

Subarachnoid hemorrhage is associated with a decrease in rCBF and $CMRO_2$ even with a good clinical grade and without angiographic vasospasm.[496,513–515] Nonetheless, many studies have shown a relationship between decreased rCBF and the presence of vasospasm, particularly when vasospasm is severe or there are focal deficits.[514–519] The decrease in rCBF is accompanied by an increase in CBV,[514] suggesting that the large vessel constriction is accompanied by small vessel dilatation. The lack of normal chemoregulation to a CO_2 challenge supports this notion.[516]

Data indicate that the vasospasm-mediated decreased rCBF and accompanying decrease in CMR are uncoupled.[517] The extent of the uncoupling of vascular control from metabolic needs is so severe that decrements in rCBF sufficient to cause ischemic stroke can occur.[466,520,521] In SAH nonsurvivors, as many as 45 percent of such patients developed a stroke after the SAH.[521–524] Thus, vasospasm represents an extreme form of cerebral dysautoregulation—one severe enough to persist despite persistent and severe anaerobic metabolism. It is thus clear that the genesis of vasospasm is extremely complex and appears to be multifactorial.

SEIZURES During the acute phase after SAH about 3 to 5 percent of patients develop seizures.[525] Moreover, 13 to 15 percent go on to develop epilepsy as a chronic complication of their SAH with the incidence increasing to 30 percent when the SAH arises from a middle cerebral artery aneurysm, presumably because of proximity to the temporal lobe. In addition, the incidence increases from 5 percent in those without neurologic deficit to 41 percent in those with neurologic deficits.[526]

EXTRACRANIAL COMPLICATIONS A variety of extracranial complications arise as direct consequences of the SAH. These include abnormalities in cardiovascular, pulmonary, endocrine, and electrolyte homeostasis. Many of these abnormalities can be traced to the post-SAH hyperadrenergic state or disordered functioning of the hypothalamus.

Systemic hypertension is common after SAH[527] and is most likely related to elevated catecholamines and renin secondary to hypothalamic disturbance.[287,288] Other causes include intracranial hypertension, preexisting essential hypertension, seizures, vomiting, pain, bladder distension, agitation, or vasospasm. Hypertension, in addition to predisposing to rebleeding, is associated with a higher incidence of vasospasm and death.[528]

Cardiac arrhythmias are observed in almost all patients after SAH[289,290] and ECG changes suggestive of myocardial ischemia occurs in 50 to 80 percent of patients after SAH.[287,289,290–292,306,307,309] The arrhythmias can

TABLE 36-9
Electrocardiographic Abnormalities After Subarachnoid Hemorrhage

Prominent P waves	ST segment elevation or depression
Prolonged or shortened PR interval	Prominent or inverted U waves
Broad, inverted or flattened T waves	Pathologic Q waves
QT prolongation or shortening	S in V_1 and R in V_5 combined > 35 mm
	Rhythm disturbances

SOURCE: Adapted by permission from Adams and Love.[527]

be severe or life threatening in 20 percent.[289,290] A rather diverse array of ECG changes can occur (Table 36-9) with many of them indicative of myocardial ischemia. It is likely that these changes represent more than simple artifact. Ventricular wall motion abnormalities consistent with myocardial ischemia have been observed after SAH, particularly with worsened neurologic grade.[304,305,511] In addition, CPK isoenzyme elevations indicative of myocardial infarction have been reported[293,294] and at postmortem examination myocardial necrosis has been documented in association with SAH.[529]

Neurogenic pulmonary edema is a rare complication of SAH, having been ascribed to the brief period of severe intracranial hypertension associated with the initial bleed or the postbleed surge in catecholamines.[295–299,308,313,320] It has also been suggested that post-SAH increases in blood-borne vasogenic substances occur. These substances lead to increased permeability of the pulmonary vasculature such that pulmonary edema occurs at lower hydrostatic pressures than normal.[295]

After SAH, abnormalities in fluid and sodium homeostasis occur in about 33 percent of patients.[530] Both hypovolemia and hyponatremia are commonly observed. The clinical presentation may appear consistent with SIADH. In the past, such patients typically were treated with fluid restriction,[531,532] which in retrospect would be expected to aggravate the more recently discovered hypovolemia and increase blood viscosity, both undesirable after SAH. More recent studies indicate that both fluid and sodium are lost after SAH,[268,269,406,530,533] indicating that the hyponatremia is not a straightforward issue of dilution of sodium due to excessive water retention. Declines in blood volume have been observed using tracer techniques.[264,530,533] In addition, the kidney is unable to retain sodium,[264,534] consistent with observed increases in atrial natriuretic factor,[534,535] constituting the so-called cerebral salt-wasting syndrome.[268,406,527,534] Atrial natriuretic factor levels in plasma peak 3 days after SAH and then fall by 7 days after the SAH.

Hypokalemia occurs frequently after SAH and is most likely due to vomiting, elevated circulating catecholamines, corticosteroids, renin, or diuretic use.[510]

Fever is a common concomitant condition with SAH.[536-538] The etiology of it is unclear. Nonetheless, fever can be one indicator of developing vasospasm.[538] Unfortunately, SAH patients commonly have undergone instrumentation of the vasculature, bladder, brain, or trachea, all of which may independently cause an infection with accompanying fever. In addition, these patients may have other potential causes of fever including DVT, biliary stasis, and multiple drug administrations. The presence of fever in this patient group is made more serious by the fact that fever seriously exacerbates the consequences of cerebral ischema,[187] as may occur with vasospasm.

Presentation

RISK FACTORS   Predisposing factors to SAH from aneurysmal or nonaneurysmal causes include systemic hypertension, athersclerosis, pregnancy, endocarditis with cerebral emboli, blood dyscrasias or bleeding diathesis, brain tumors, cigarette smoking, coarctation of the aorta, polycystic kidney disease, fibromuscular dysplasia, and intracranial infections.[452,466,539-544]

ICTUS   The most characteristic symptom of an SAH is a sudden, severe, unremitting headache unlike any other in the prior experience of the patient. Consciousness is lost transiently in 45 percent of cases and the patient may remain unconscious for days in 10 percent.[465] In addition the patient may report nausea, vomiting, neck or back pain, dizziness/vertigo, fatigue, diplopia, and photophobia. In about a third of the cases a sentinel hemorrhage will have occurred previously, an event associated with an increase in mortality by 14 percent (29 to 43 percent).[545,546]

CLASSIFICATION   There are two primary methods of grading SAH: clinical appearance and CT scan. The first clinical grading system was introduced by Botterell and colleagues in 1956.[547] This was subsequently modified by Hunt and Hess, meeting with widespread clinical application[548] (Table 36-10). The CT classification by Fisher,[549] based on amount and location of blood on CT scan, has become useful in prediction of likelihood of vasospasm after SAH (Table 36-11).

DELAYED NEUROLOGIC DETERIORATION   After admission with SAH, a patient is subject to sustain a secondary neurologic deterioration due primarily to one of three causes: rebleed, hydrocephalus, and vasospasm. It is important to consider other causes also. These include seizures, hyponatremia, hypocalcemia, hypotension, hypoxemia, sepsis, and drug-induced CNS depression.[527,550]

Recurrent hemorrhage is a leading cause of death and moribidity after SAH, effectively doubling the mortality rate.[551,552] Of unclipped aneurysms 4 percent rebleed in the first 24 h.[553] Twenty to 33 percent rebleed in the first 2 weeks after SAH,[554,555] and 50 percent rebleed in the first 6 months after SAH.[556] Rebleeding typically presents with an abrupt worsening of neurologic condition with a new headache. The neurologic change, unfortunately, usually consists of a decline in level of consciousness. Extensor posturing may arise if not already present.[557] If the patient already has a depressed sensorium, signs may include hemodynamic changes, respiratory dysrhythmias, increased ICP, or an abrupt increase in CSF drainage from the EVD with an increase in blood in CSF.

Acute hydrocephalus presents in the first hours after the initial SAH. It often presents with an abrupt increase in ICP associated with the abrupt onset of coma. With increased time after SAH, the signs of hydrocephalus are less abrupt and pronounced. Thus, hydrocephalus occurring days after the SAH may present with only a subtle decline in mental status or with only a minor focal neurologic deficit.

Among patients with SAH, a group of patients at risk for subsequent development of *vasospasm* can be identified.[527] This group includes women and patients with worse neurologic grade, ECG changes, hydrocephalus, Fisher grade 3 CT scan, and systemic hypertension.[549,558-567] Moreover, ischemic complications of vasospasm are more likely if the patient is hyponatremic, dehydrated, or hypotensive.

The peak times for occurrence of vasospasm are between days 4 and 10 after SAH. The vasospasm can occur and be totally asymptomatic using ordinary clinical examination techniques. However, serial assessment of rCBF may indicate a regional oligemic condition not yet severe enough to produce a neurologic deficit detectable by routine bedside methods.[568] In addition, BFV assessed by TCD may also indicate an increase in velocity, indicating that the proximal basal cerebral artery is narrowing.[569] Several studies have indicated that TCD used in this manner can predict the development of occult vasospasm and thus predict whether clinically evident vasospasm is likely to occur.[175-178,180] However, a recent study by Clyde[127] at our institution, after the routine use of nimodipine, indicates that measurement is most correlated with blood flow, such that high BFV, rather than indicating spasm with low flow, often indicates the presence of hyperemia.

The clinical manifestation of this gradual process can, however, be rather abrupt or it can be insidious with minor transient changes waxing and waning over hours. Patients may complain of increased headache, or develop fever, meningismus, seizures, decreased

TABLE 36-10
Classification of Patients With Intracranial Aneurysms According to Surgical Risk

Grade[a]	Criteria	Perioperative Mortality (%)[b]
0	Unruptured aneurysm	
1	Asymptomatic, or minimal headache and slight nuchal rigidity	0–5
2	Moderate to severe headache, nuchal rigidity, no neurologic deficit other than cranial nerve palsy	2–10
3	Drowsiness, confusion, or mild focal deficit	10–15
4	Stupor, moderate to severe hemiparesis, possibly early decerebrate rigidity, and vegetative disturbances	60–70
5	Deep coma, decerebrate rigidity, moribund appearance	70–100

[a] The original classification has been revised to include grade 0 for patients who have unruptured aneurysms and grade 1a for patients who have a stable residual neurologic deficit who are past the period of acute cerebral reaction.

[b] Surgical mortality rates vary among institutions

Serious systemic disease such as hypertension, diabetes, severe atherosclerosis, chronic pulmonary disease, and severe vasospasm seen on arteriography result in placement of the patient in the next less favorable category.

SOURCE: Reproduced by permission from Hunt and Hess.[548]

mentation, or focal neurologic deficits. A new deficit may be nothing more than a minor pronator drift or it may present with hemiplegia, aphasia, behavioral change, or loss of consciousness, depending on the neurologic functions performed by brain territory subserved by vasospastic vessels.[558,559,563] This ischemic process can lead to infarction and permanent neurologic deficit.

Therapy

PRIMARY DISEASE   A number of diagnostic studies are required to confirm the occurrence of an aneurysmal SAH. First consideration in the diagnosis of SAH is a consistent history and physical examination. CT scan will usually show SAH. However, in a small number of cases (1 to 12 percent), the CT scan will be negative.[570] If the history suggests SAH with a negative CT scan then a lumbar puncture must be done to positively rule out the possibility of a small SAH. It is essential that a small SAH not be missed because such a bleed could be a sentinal hemorrhage such that a

TABLE 36-11
Computed Tomography Scan Grading
of Subarachnoid Hemorrhage

Grade	Criteria
1	No blood detected
2	Diffuse deposition or thin layer with all vertical layers of blood; interhemispheric, insular cistern, ambient cistern, < 1 mm thick
3	Localized clots or vertical layers of blood > 1 mm thick
4	Diffuse or no subarachnoid blood but with intracerebral or intraventricular blood

SOURCE: Reproduced by permission from Fisher and coworkers.[549]

rebleed could seriously exacerbate the patient's outcome. After SAH is established, then cerebral angiography is required to establish whether the source of the SAH is a ruptured aneurysm. About 5 to 10 percent of SAH patients have a negative angiogram.

With a diagnosis of SAH, intracranial surgery and clipping of the aneurysms is generally the most appropriate therapy. Left unclipped the incidence of rebleeding is quite high.[553–556] Thus, the only reasons for an aneurysm to not be clipped are medical instability, technical difficulty, or patient/family refusal. In situations where definitive surgery is not feasible other techniques may be used such as proximal arterial ligation or endovascular occlusion using interventional neuroradiologic techniques. The timing of surgery has been the source of some controversy. For a period of time the consensus was that surgery should be delayed until after the risk of vasospasm had subsided and acute edema had subsided to improve operating conditions. In support of this were studies indicating that operative morbidity and mortality when surgery was delayed, was generally quite good.[556a] However, delaying surgery leaves the patient at risk of rebleed during a phase of the disease wherein hypertension will be induced or occur spontaneously and other medical complications of the SAH may increase the likelihood of rebleed. Although the operative statistics may be quite good when surgery is delayed, the overall outcome of delaying surgery appears to be better if surgery is performed in the first few days after SAH and before the onset of vasospasm.[571–582] A large epidemiologic study on the timing of aneurysm surgery, involving 3521 patients, supports the notion that early surgery can improve outcomes, especially in patients from grades I to IV.[583,584]

A major consideration in the care of a patient after

SAH is prediction and prompt detection and accurate diagnosis of neurologic deterioration. The overriding rationale for this is that neurologic deterioration can herald an individual's subsequent permanent disability and there are good therapeutic options for the usual causes of post-SAH neurologic deterioration.

The mainstay of detection is serial neurologic examinations by nursing and medical staff. Physicians generally perform such examinations once to twice a day or when notified by nursing staff. NeuroICU nurses then provide the monitoring function by performing detailed neurologic assessment serially every 1 to 2 h with documentation of a standardized examination protocol.

Serial daily TCD examinations have been reported to be helpful in detecting the onset of vasospasm prior to symptomatic ischemia.[569,585,586] However, recent evaluation of TCD compared to rCBF[127,587,588] indicates that the sensitivity and specificity of the measure may be inadequate to make major medical decisions, although it may still be useful as a noninvasive screening tool. In particularly unstable cases, TCD can be used continuously or hourly, although this is expensive and has not been validated.

The EEG and EPs have been used to provide minute-to-minute monitoring of neurologic function in patients at particular risk of vasospasm.[156] Occasionally such monitoring can be used to detect changes[589–593] (see Fig. 36-29). Because a short period of severe focal cerebral ischemia can lead to stroke,[594] it is conceivable that cerebral ischemia, sufficient to produce brain damage, could occur between serial examinations. Thus, it seems, intuitively obvious that continuous electrophysiologic monitoring should be able to provide early warning if cerebral ischemia as it does in the operating room. However, such an approach is expensive and has not undergone scrutiny in a randomized controlled trial.

Near infrared spectroscopy ("brain oximetry") will hopefully be useful to detect vasospasm-induced decrements in brain blood oxygen saturation and thus provide an early warning of decreased cerebrovascular reserve or the onset of anaerobic metabolism. However, this is a new monitor that requires further study to validate its use in this setting.

Computed tomography scans are obtained on admission and generally periodically after surgery to evaluate for ventricular size and edema. In addition, in some institutions, serial CBF studies are done to evaluate for early vasospasm. Such studies are done using stable XeCTCBF, xenon 133, or SPECT methodology. XeCTCBF and Xenon-133 CBF provide quantitative information and the ability to observe the response to therapies.

Neurologic deterioration mandates an urgent evaluation for the cause (Table 36-12). Hypoxemia, and sodium abnormalities should be evaluated. Concurrently, a CT scan is obtained to evaluate for hydrocephalus or rebleeding. If these are not present, an urgent CBF is obtained to confirm the presence of ischemia. One approach is to initiate vasopressor support to increase blood pressure immediately after the onset of the neurologic deficit. The patient then undergoes XeCTCBF to validate the diagnosis of ischemia (versus hydrocephalus or bleeding) and to assess the need for the vasopressors to increase CBF. If CBF assessment indicates that ischemia is likely, an arteriogram can be obtained to confirm the presence of vasospasm and plan interventional angiography.

REBLEED The diagnosis of rebleeding should not be made solely on clinical grounds because this has been found to result in the wrong diagnosis in about one-third of patients.[550] CT scan is the best diagnostic study. Rebleeding often heralds a catastrophe. Thus, major efforts are warranted to prevent rebleeding. The most effective measure is early clipping of the aneurysm.

TABLE 36-12

Diagnostic Studies That May Be Useful in the Evaluation of Patients With Neurologic Deterioration After Aneurysmal Subarachnoid Hemorrhage

Procedure	Evaluating For
Computed tomography	Rebleeding, infarction edema, hydrocephalus
EEG	Seizures
Transcranial Doppler	Vasospasm, elevated ICP
CBF	Ischemia, response to therapy
Arteriography	Vasospasm, therapeutic options
CSF examination	Rebleeding, infection
Arterial blood gases	Hypoxemia, acidosis
Chest x-ray	Pneumonia, pulmonary embolus, pulmonary edema
ECG	Arrhythmia, myocardial ischemia
Blood glucose	Hyper- or hypoglycemia
Serum sodium	Hyper- or hyponatremia
Serum calcium	Hyper- or hypocalcemia
Serum magnesium	Hyper- or hypomagnesemia
Serum phosphate	Hypophosphatemia
Cultures urine, blood, sputum, CSF	Infection
White blood cell count and differential	Infection
Drug levels	Excessive doses of sedatives, anticonvulsants
Toxin screen	Unknown CNS depressant ingestion

SOURCE: Adapted with permission from Adams and Love.[527]

Prior to clipping (and prior to vasospasm) every effort should be made to keep blood pressure below hypertensive levels and the patient calm. This is generally done with bed rest, titrated administration of β-adrenergic blocking drugs, or phenobarbital. Other measures occasionally used include antifibrinolytic therapy and proximal vessel ligation.[527] Carotid ligation is rarely done because of concerns regarding risk of secondary ischemic stroke. Its use is limited generally to giant aneurysms or aneurysms in or near the cavernous sinus. If it is required, preocclusion balloon test occlusion of the carotid artery with examination and CBF assessment is a suitable means to assess the safety of carotid occlusion.[595] Enforced bed rest has been studied.[596] The results suggested a benefit of this approach, but they were not conclusive. Antifibrinolytic therapy in the past was used to prevent lysis of the aneurysmal clot to decrease rebleeding.[527] Both ε-aminocaproic acid and tranexamic acid were used. A randomized placebo-controlled trial, a nonrandomized trial, and other reports assessing the efficacy of antifibrinolytic therapy showed a significantly decreased incidence of rebleeding. However, mortality was not altered because such therapy was associated with a higher incidence of ischemic stroke.[597–599] Thus, antifibrinolytic therapy is seldom used presently. However, the possibility remains that a role may be found for it given during the few-hour interval between angiography and operation, when early surgery is performed. Antifibrinolytic agents should not be used in patients who are pregnant or who have DVT, coagulation disorders, or renal insufficiency.[446] Important side effects include increased bleeding tendency after discontinuation, diuresis, diarrhea, abdominal discomfort, nausea, rash, and dizziness.[600,601]

HYDROCEPHALUS A depression in level of consciousness indicates the need for CT scan. If hydrocephalus is present ventriculomegaly will be evident. This is best discerned by comparing the scan with earlier scans. In this situation an external ventricular drain is indicated.[527,602–604] Once inserted the shunt is subject to several problems. The pressure at which drainage is allowed must be carefully assessed and controlled. If there is a large amount of ventricular blood the shunt can become occluded. Such occlusion can present with recurrent depression and acute hydrocephalus. Some clinicians are using intraventricular thrombolytic therapy to maintain shunt patency as a lifesaving maneuver. Finally, infections are a serious concern after a shunt has been in place for 5 days or more.[168,169] Most neurosurgeons try to remove or replace an EVD by 7 days after insertion.

Once an EVD is in place it is monitored daily for amount of fluid drained and white cell count. After initial insertion, the EVD is set to drain at a prescribed fluid pressure based on the hydraulic arrangement of the drainage tubing (Fig. 36-9). Initially, to treat ventriculomegaly the drainage is set at 0 to 10 cmH$_2$O. Too low a pressure will risk rebleeding if there is an unclipped aneurysm. Too high a level will interfere with resolution of ventriculomegaly and drainage of blood out of the CSF. Over the next several days the level of drainage is gradually increased as permitted by maintenance of a stable neurologic examination, low CSF drainage amount, and constant normal ventricular size on serial CT scans. Drainage approaching 300 ml of fluid indicates that substantial obstruction to circulation is persisting and the patient is unlikely to tolerate having the drainage level elevated. During this period the slightest change in mental status warrants a repeat CT scan to assess for ventricular size. With successfully achieving a drainage level of 30 cmH$_2$O above the midbrain with a small amount of daily drainage and no change in neurologic status, the drain is clamped. If neurologic status and ventricular size remain stable then the EVD can be removed. If this does not occur then the drain will need to be changed between 5 and 10 days after insertion or when there is evidence of increased leukocytes in the CSF. The CSF, which already has peripheral blood in it, can be expected to have a ratio of red/white cells of about 500:700. If this ratio decreases substantially then there is evidence of inflammation or infection further indicating the need to change the EVD system.

SYMPTOMATIC VASOSPASM The classical diagnostic signs of symptomatic vasospasm are focal neurologic deficit with elevated BFV on TCD in the appropriate vessels and decreased rCBF in the appropriate vascular distribution. However, all of these signs need not be present. If spasm is predominantly in distal vessels then both TCD and angiography may miss it with the only evidence of spasm being focal neurologic deficit, decreased rCBF, or both.

A wide variety of approaches to the management of vasospasm have been examined. Wilkins has divided this rather active area into reports in both animals and humans based on eight categories (Table 36-13).

Surgical procedures may have a role in the prevention of vasospasm. Taneda[579] reported a reduction in incidence of vasospasm from 25 to 11 percent with early surgery compared to a 10-day delay in surgery. In addition, others have advocated extensive irrigation of cisterns and removal of as much clot as possible as another means to reduce the indigence of vasospasm.[605–607] However, this can be technically difficult or impossible and efforts to remove subarachnoid clot can lead to ischemic injuries also.[606]

TABLE 36-13
Partial Listing of Agents and Procedures of Potential Value in the Prevention and Treatment of Cerebral Vasospasm

Category	Drug Class or Procedure
1. Dilate cerebral arteries or antagonize constriction	A. Sympathomimetics B. α-adrenergic Blockers C. β-adrenergic Blockers D. Acute adrenergic denervation E. Parasympathomimetics F. Postganglionic cholinergic blockers G. Serotonin antagonists H. Nitrites I. Phosphodiesterase inhibitors J. Nonsteroidal antiinflammatory agents K. Prostaglandin agents L. Antiplatelet agents M. Adenosine compounds N. Free Radical Scavengers O. Local anesthetics P. Calcium Antagonists Q. Papaverin and analogs R. Miscellaneous drugs
2. Improvement of rheology and oxygen delivery and anti-ischemia and anti-edema drugs	A. Hemodilution B. Perfluorochemicals C. Opiate antagonists D. Barbiturates E. Steroids F. Miscellaneous drugs
3. Antifibrinolysis	A. ε-aminocaproic Acid B. Tranexamic acid C. Gabexate mesylate
4. Neutralize vasospastic effects of subarachnoid blood	A. Haptoglobin intracisternal B. Antithrombin III topical C. Sodium nitrite subarachnoid D. Plasmin intracisternal E. Early operation with mechanical removal of blood F. Drainage of subarachnoid spaces G. Ventriculosternal irrigation H. Tissue plasminogen activator intracisternal
5. Treat intracranial acidosis	A. Bicarbonate
6. Increase blood pressure and cardiac output	A. Intravascular volume expansion with blood or blood products B. Induced arterial hypertension C. Increased cardiac output
7. Interrupt sympathetic innervation	A. Cervical sympathectomy B. Stereotactic lesions of monaminergic pathways C. Adrenalectomy
8. Other Procedures	A. Postponement of procedure until spasm resolved B. External decompression to decrease ICP C. Dilation of spastic arteries with intravascular balloon catheter D. EC-IC bypass

SOURCE: Adapted by permission from Wilkins.[496] Procedures described performed in animal models and humans. Not all are suitable for clinical application.

Nimodipine, an enterally administered calcium channel blocker, is the only drug thus far found to be clinically efficacious in prospective randomized trials in the treatment of vasospasm. It has been found to prevent or reduce ischemic deficits by 40 to 70 percent.[608–614] Based on these data it is generally recommended that all SAH patients receive nimodipine 30 to 60 mg enterally every 4 to 6 h for 2 to 3 weeks after SAH. Its use is associated with hypotension, which can oppose any helpful therapeutic effects. If this occurs fluid administration may be increased, especially if hypovolemia is suspected, or the same daily dose can be given over smaller intervals or the overall dose can be reduced.

Nicardipine is a calcium channel blocker that can be given intravenously. It has been studied for vasospasm with preliminary studies indicating a lower than expected incidence of angiographic narrowing associated with its use.[615] In one controlled study,[616] it was associated with a lower incidence of vasospasm and lower incidence for a requirement for hypertensive hypervolemic therapy drugs, although both treated and control groups had similar final neurologic outcomes.

Tirilazad is a potent in vitro inhibitor of free radical-mediated lipid peroxidation.[617–619] This is thought to be the primary action of the drug in animal models of cerebral ischemia.[617–619] In animal SAH models tirilazad has decreased the severity and incidence of post-SAH vasospasm.[620,621] The drug is presently undergoing clinical trials with encouraging results.[622] These studies suggest that adverse effects which may be a concern include venous irritation, rhabdomyopathy, cardiomyopathy, and hepatic toxicity.

Hypervolemic, hypertensive, hemodilution (HHH) therapy has also been used. Hypovolemia with contraction of circulating blood volume has been reported after SAH.[264,268] Moreover, several investigators have suggested that this decrease in circulating blood volume is an important factor (or perhaps an epiphenomenon) in the development of delayed ischemic deficits after SAH.[264,406,530] In addition, the onset of vasospasm sufficient to attenuate cerebrovascular reserve creates a situation where CBF becomes a function of CPP.[268,623–625] Moreover, as luminal size decreases the viscosity becomes an important factor in determination of CBF. From such observations has arisen the use of HHH therapy to prevent and actively treat delayed cerebral ischemia due to vasospasm. It is now consistently applied to patients after SAH. HHH therapy has been reported to increase rCBF and ameliorate ischemic deficits due to post-SAH vasospasm.[626–631]

Hypervolemia is generally induced with infusion of 5% albumin 75 to 125 ml/h plus 250 to 500-ml infusions to maintain CVP or pulmonary artery wedge pressure (PAWP) about 10 to 14 mmHg. Notably, the PAWP often does not correlate with CVP,[211,212] such that titrating fluid infusions to CVP may result in unacceptable left ventricular pressures and risk pulmonary edema or pleural effusion. This may be related to observed ventricular wall motion abnormalities or ECG changes suggestive of ischemia, both of which may predispose to myocardial diastolic dysfunction.[287,291–294,529] Thus, pulmonary artery catheterization should be performed in any SAH patient undergoing HHH therapy.

The physiologic basis for why an increase in blood volume would increase rCBF is obscure. However, the infusion of erythrocyte-free solutions may cause a decrease in hematocrit, which decreases viscosity of blood.[632] Such hemodilution is known to increase rCBF due to decreased viscosity. Animal studies indicate that the optimal hematocrit is 33 percent, that is, O_2-carrying capacity is not compromised until hematocrit decreases to below this level.[632] This concept has been applied to clinical care in determining the end point for hemodilution therapy.[633] Venesection is performed only after hypervolemia has been achieved and the hematocrit is still too high.

Increasing preload will tend to increase blood pressure. In addition, as vasospasm worsens patients tend to spontaneously increase blood pressure. If despite these two factors tending to increase blood pressure, delayed cerebral ischemia arises, then hypertensive therapy is indicated. Such therapy has been reported to increase rCBF[629] and ameliorate ischemic deficits.[634] Hypertensive therapy is instituted with titrated infusion of a vasopressor intravenously. The end point is reversal of neurologic deficits. This may require a blood pressure as high as 240 mmHg systolic. The blood pressure end point may be attenuated somewhat if there is evidence of inability of the heart to tolerate the hypertension. It is to be expected that afterload increase will decrease cardiac output. If cardiac output decreases sufficiently to compromise splanchnic flow (as indicated by decreasing urinary output or increasing lactate), PCWP increases to threaten pulmonary edema, or ischemic changes arise on ECG, then the therapy should be altered to include an inotrope or it should be abandoned in favor of another approach (e.g., angioplasty). The specific drug chosen varies among investigators and physicians but includes phenylephrine, dopamine, dobutamine, and norepinephrine.[265] Although catecholamine-based pressor therapy is reported to occasionally reverse neurologic deficits, their cerebrovascular and metabolic effects in this situation are unclear. Darby and coworkers[226] measured rCBF throughout the brain using stable XeCTCBF, reporting that rather heterogeneous effects occurred with dopamine infusion intravenously. Many areas of the brain sustained significant decreases in rCBF. However, areas of the brain with baseline low flow, presum-

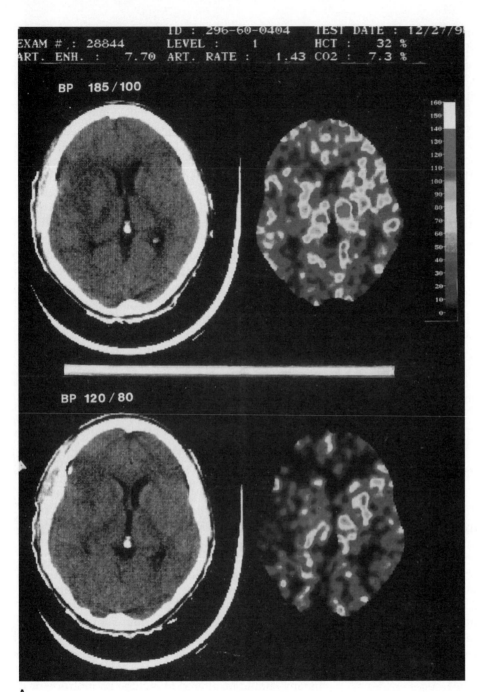

Figure 36-28 Effects of dopamine infusion on cerebral blood flow (CBF). Two examples of disparate effects of dopamine infusion on CBF in subarachnoid hemorrhage patients with vasospasm. CBF scale is indicated on the right in ml/100 g per min. CT images are indicated in the left figures and CBF maps in the right figures. Blood pressures before and after dopamine infusion are indicated. *A.* Dopamine infusion is associated with a general increase in CBF, whereas in (*B*) it is associated with a decrease in CBF.

ably vasospastic areas, tended to increase rCBF with dopamine infusion. When catecholamines cross the BBB, which is disrupted with vasospasm,[635–638] they have been reported in animals to produce hypermetabolism and hyperemia.[639] Conversely, catecholamines given with an intact BBB have no significant effect on CBF[640] (Fig. 36-28). Therefore, although there are numerous anecdotes of symptomatic improvement with vasopressor therapy, there is a theoretical basis for concern regarding effects of catecholamine therapy on overall outcome.

An important consideration in implementation of hypertensive therapy is appropriate treatment of ICP. Elevated ICP will reduce CPP. Thus, if there is any evidence of brain edema or hydrocephalus placement of an EVD can be an important component of HHH therapy.

Institution of HHH therapy often results in brady-

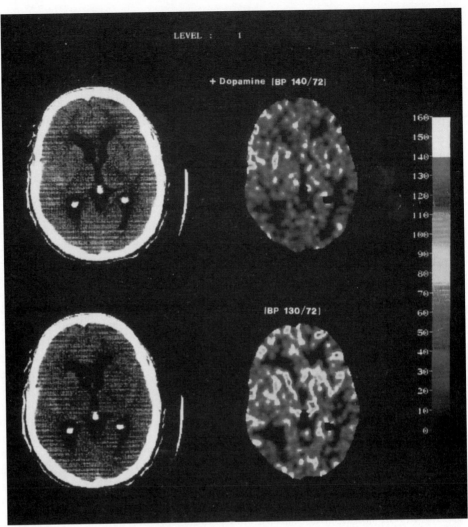

LEVEL : 1

+ Dopamine [BP 140/72]

[BP 130/72]

Figure 36-28 (*Continued*)

B

cardia or urine output increases sufficiently to prevent the desired increase in preload. Atropine (1 mg intramuscularly every 3 to 4 h) or vasopressin (5 units intramuscularly to keep urine outless less than 200 ml/h) may be required.[634]

The basis for the use of HHH therapy is the many anecdotes and case series reporting improvement in rCBF or neurologic deficits in patients acting as their own controls. It is important to note, however, that this therapy remains without prospective randomized trials documenting its effect on overall outcome after SAH. There are neurologic and systemic complications associated with the use of HHH therapy, which may undo therapeutic effects.

This therapy should be used either prophylactically[641] or in the setting of active ischemia without infarction. If infarction is present some evidence suggests that HHH therapy may cause deterioration.[634] Hemorrhagic infarction has been reported with HHH

therapy.[643] In addition, there may be an increased risk of rebleeding if therapy is implemented prior to clipping the aneurysm.[644] This risk is removed if early surgery is performed.[645–647]

These patients require intensive care with invasive hemodyamic monitoring including central venous or pulmonary artery monitoring and intraarterial catheter placement for arterial blood gas and blood pressure monitoring. Such monitors are associated with a risk of septicemia, which itself may predispose to decreased blood pressure and decreased rCBF.[404] Moreover, the heavy-handed administration of fluids in a setting wherein pulmonary vascular permeability may be decreased and myocardial diastolic function may be abnormal will predispose a patient to pulmonary edema and pleural effusion. If such complications result in a need for prolonged endotracheal intubation and mechanical ventilation that might otherwise have not occurred, then the patient will be at increased risk for pneumonia. All of these pulmonary complications will risk the occurrence of hypoxemia, which, in the setting of decreased cerebrovascular reserve, may be expected to predispose a patient to stroke. Overall, the incidence of systemic complications associated with HHH therapy are 7 to 17 percent pulmonary edema, 2 percent myocardial infarction, 3 to 35 percent dilutional hyponatremia, and 3 percent coagulopathy.[633,641,647,648] A host of other iatrogenic complications secondary to the intensive care required for HHH may also negatively influence outcome. These include urinary tract infection, pneumothorax, carotid artery puncture, agitation-induced rebleed, and barotrauma to name but a few.

In patients refractory to conventional treatment with HHH therapy, transluminal angioplasty has been shown to effectively reverse angiographic evidence of vasospasm of proximal accessible vessels in 75 percent of patients.[649] If vasospasm is present in distal vessels then intra-arterial papaverine has been infused and associated with a favorable reversal of vasospasm.[649,650] However, papaverine can transiently produce neurologic deterioration during infusion and manifest, depending on the vascular territory infused as seizure (personal observation), hemiparesis, pupillary changes, unconsciousness, increased ICP, or cardiovascular collapse.[650–654] Because of the morbidity associated with HHH therapy and increasing experience with these procedures, there appears to be a trend to earlier use of angioplasty or papaverine infusion.

In patients too unstable or with too severe of a grade to safely undergo intracranial surgery, occlusion of the aneurysm with coils to induce an intraaneurysmal clot can be used. This is particularly helpful if the patient develops vasospasm and the need for HHH therapy. The coils can then act to protect the aneurysm lumen from the high pressures associated with HHH therapy and thus reduce the risk of rebleeding.[655,656]

SEIZURE   A patient reported to have had a "seizure" should be given consideration for having had this symptom. However, the decerebrate posturing that can occur with a rebleed episode should also be thought of. True seizures occur in only 3 to 5 percent of patients.[525] If a seizure occurs, this is most likely deleterious to a patient with SAH in terms of cerebral hypermetabolism and extracranial effects such as hypertension and hypoxemia. Thus, it is common practice to give all SAH patients an anticonvulsant, either phenytoin 300 to 400 mg/day or phenobarbital, 120 to 240 mg/day (with adjustments based on blood levels). Prior to clipping, phenobarbital has the added advantage of providing an element of sedation at a time that agitation and hypertension are to be avoided. Thereafter phenytoin, because it is less sedating, tends to be used.

CCM Considerations

AIRWAY MANAGEMENT   With worsening grade of SAH, patients tend to have difficulty with airway protection from secretions or vomitus and may develop respiratory dysrhythmias. Thus, endotracheal intubation may be required as such signs arise. These changes may occur secondary to brain edema, hydrocephalus, vasospasm, rebleeding, or seizure. Often, the decision to intubate is a judgment in a patient who is lethargic but arousable. In such patients the trachea may be intubated simply to ensure that angiography can be performed safely. In such situations where there is time, it is optimal to have an intra-arterial cannula placed before intubation. In cases where hypoxemia or aspiration are immediate concerns, or the patient is not ventilating properly, the priority is given to securing the airway over all other issues.

The goals in endotracheal intubation of an SAH patient with an unclipped aneurysm (presumed or known) are maintenance of normal blood pressure, prevention of aspiration from a presumed full stomach, and avoidance of hypoxemia, hypercapnea, and hypocapnea. Both phenylephrine infusion and trimethaphan for bolus injection should be prepared prior to intubation. Topical anesthesia and sedation can be used if the patient is cooperative. The advantage of this is that the airway remains reasonably well protected. However, the expected disadvantage is hypertension with a risk of rebleeding.[657] Fast-acting or short-acting antihypertensive drugs may be needed. Intravenous boluses of trimethaphan can be used effectively for this purpose, 1 mg initially, and increased as indicated and tolerated. The alternate approach is to use a rapid sequence induction with fentanyl 1 to 5 μ/kg followed by thiopental, 3 to 5 mg/kg, and succinylcholine 1 to 1.5 mg/kg. This can be a heavy-handed pharmacologic approach, usually producing a decrease in blood pressure. However, hypertension is seldom a problem, thereby minimizing the major concern of intubation-induced rebleeding. A phenylephrine infusion can be used if blood pressure decreases unacceptably. Another disadvantage of this approach is that the airway is unprotected if intubation cannot be quickly achieved.

If the aneurysm has been clipped already then the concerns about hypertension are not so severe. If vasospasm is present, perhaps contributing to the need for intubation, hypertension should not be so aggressively treated or prevented. Lower doses of induction drugs can be used if a general anesthetic approach is chosen or topical anesthesia with sedation may be chosen. Nonetheless, phenylephrine or trimethaphan should still be readily available.

GAS EXCHANGE   Gas exchange due to pulmonary edema can occur due to neurogenic causes or secon-

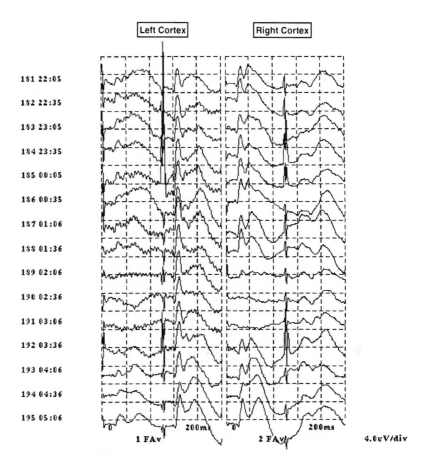

Figure 36-29 Effects of fever on evoked potentials in a patient with vasospasm. A 55-year-old white woman day 8 after subarachnoid hemorrhage underwent somatosensory evoked potential monitoring because she was thought to be at high risk for vasospasm. Stimulation was done sequentially to the left arm and then the right arm. Left cortex recordings show the potentials from the right hand stimulation as the second, more pronounced waveform, whereas right cortex recordings show the potentials from the left hand stimulations as the first, more pronounced, waveform. Concomitant nursing records indicate rectal temperature 37.5°C at midnight, 38.5°C at 2 A.M. and 37.7°C at 4 A.M. indicating fever as a factor contributing to the loss of evoked potentials from 1:30 to 3:30 A.M. No concomitant neurologic deficit was noted.

dary to HHH therapy. In addition, difficulties can arise secondary to inability to protect the airway or respiratory dysrhythmias. Neurogenic pulmonary edema will occur rarely.

TEMPERATURE   Fever occurs very commonly with SAH, particularly at about the time of worsening vasospasm.[536–538] A significant proportion of fevers are thus central in origin. However, these patients typically are heavily instrumented via Foley catheter, EVD, vascular catheters, or endotracheal intubation and thus are at risk of a variety of infections. Each fever requires evaluation for infection from each of these instrumented sources. In addition, fever itself is a major concern for any patient at risk of cerebral ischemia (Fig. 36-29). Thus fever above 38.2°C should be aggressively treated with acetaminophen, aspirin, and cooling blankets. In addition, if vasospasm with ischemic deficit is thought to be a significant risk, efforts can be made to continuously treat any temperature above 37° to 37.5°C using the same approach used to induce hypothermia but aiming for a higher temperature.

In cases where vasospasm is refractory to all therapy, hypothermia may occasionally be induced to about 34°C as a protective measure. This has not under-

gone experimental evaluation in this specific clinical setting.

BLOOD PRESSURE MANAGEMENT   SAH is known to be accompanied by a hyperadrenergic state.[287,289–292,307–309,501–506] This is undoubtedly one contributing factor to hypertension associated with SAH. Early after SAH, with an unclipped aneurysm, there is concern that this will predispose to rebleed. In addition ample data in animal studies indicate that catecholamines can cause neurologic sequelae.[194–197] Thus, if there are no medical contraindications, sympatholytic drugs should be used to treat hypertension. Such drugs include β-adrenergic blocking drugs, trimethaphan, clonidine, and ACE inhibitors. In addition, because of limited data suggesting brain protective effects, nicardipine or nimodipine may be advantageously used in this setting.

If surgery occurs early (before vasospasm is present), systolic blood pressure can be treated immediately postoperatively when it exceeds about 160 mmHg. However, as the likelihood of vasospasm increases, blood pressure should not be treated unless there is concern about it being tolerated by the heart, lungs, or kidneys, perhaps about 240 mmHg systolic pressure or 150 mmHg MAP. Many patients develop blood pressure in this range spontaneously. If hypertensive therapy is to be used there is not a consensus regarding the most appropriate pressor to use. There is a theory that increasing cardiac output will increase CBF, supporting the use of dobutamine and dopamine. However, the physiologic basis for this is not clear. An alternative approach is to use primarily vasoconstrictor drugs such as phenylephrine or norepinephrine, based on the notion that rCBF in vasospastic areas will vary primarily as a function of perfusion pressure. However, it is possible that each drug, which is a neurotransmitter or neurotransmitter analogue, may have unique effects on the cerebral vasculature independent of blood pressure or cardiac output effects, which also vary according to permeability of the BBB. This notion is supported by observations by Darby and colleagues[226] of highly disparate rCBF effects within the brain of individual subjects with SAH and between subjects with SAH. Further work is needed to properly decide the most appropriate drug to use and to ascertain whether outcome is actually improved with catecholamine infusion with SAH.

GLUCOSE   As with other ischemic states, hyperglycemia should be avoided. If blood glucose is greater than 200 mg/dl, an insulin infusion is justified to maintain blood glucose at a steady level around 200 mg/dl.

ELECTROLYTES AND FLUIDS   Hyponatremia is a common problem with SAH.[264,268,406,530,533] This hyponatremia is not a simple dilutional problem amenable to therapy by fluid restriction. Even if it were, one would not prescribe fluid restriction in a condition where hemodilution is desired and hypovolemia is a common concomitant condition. Thus, patients tend to receive generous infusions of fluids and if sodium is low their intake is supplemented with sodium intravenously or enterally. Generally, intravenous supplementation can be accomplished simply by changing all parenteral solutions to 0.9% sodium chloride. If the enteral route is chosen, 1 to 4 g sodium can be added to tube feeding daily. Finally, 3% saline can be infused, starting at about 10 ml/h and titrated upward as indicated by serial plasma sodium assessments. Generally the rate of correction of plasma sodium should not exceed 2.5 meq/liter per h and the total daily increment should not exceed 20 meq/liter.[273]

Hypernatremia also occurs, usually as an iatrogenic problem, best treated by decreasing sodium intake. However, with anterior communicating aneurysms particularly, one must be observant for diabetes insipidus, which would also include the presence of polyuria or dilute urine.

INTRACEREBRAL HEMATOMA
Pathophysiology
Multiple epidemiologic studies performed after the advent of CT scanning indicate that the incidence of intracerebral hematoma (ICH) is about 12 to 15/100,000 and constitutes about 8 to 13 percent of all strokes.[658-660] Below the age of 45 the incidence is less than 2/100,000. With each 10 years above that the incidence progressively increases to 350/100,000 for those 80 years old or greater.[660] In the Rochester 32-year study ICH increased with age, male gender, and hypertension. With time and better control of hypertension the incidence of ICH decreased, indicating that hypertension is a controllable risk factor for ICH.[658,659] The use of anticoagulants increases the risk of ICH sixfold.[611]

With the onset of blood leaking from an intracranial vessel, blood accumulates locally under arteriolar pressure, injuring adjacent vessels, which then leak, destroying parenchyma locally, displacing intact neural structures, and dissecting away from the initial bleeding site. High arterial pressure and atrophied brain will promote enlargement of the hematoma and local tissue pressure combined with elevating ICP will tend to limit the size of the enlarging hematoma.[662] This bleeding focus has been described pathologically as fibrin globes or bleeding globes.[663,664] The bleeding is thought to generally be an abrupt monophasic event usually occurring and ending within minutes.[664-666] Symptoms and signs are then due to increased ICP, disruption of local neural function, and brain edema.[662] However, recent anecdotes and reports of series indicate that secondary enlargement of the hemorrhage can occur.[664,667,668]

Specific vascular abnormalities that may contribute to or cause ICHs have been identified although the presence of other factors is still a possibility. Fibrinoid necrosis, lipohyalinosis, and microaneurysms of brain blood vessels have been implicated. Fibrinoid necrosis refers to observations of fibrin-platelet masses seen primarily at the interface between hematoma and surrounding brain tissue. Such fibrin globes seem to cover areas of disruptions in small arteries.[669,670] Lipohyalinization is a degenerative process in which there is subintimal accumulation of lipid and proteinaceous material in the walls of small arteries associated with focal necrosis and inflammation.[671,672] Charcot-Bouchard miliary microaneurysms are also seen in patients with ICH and also are associated with lacunar infarcts.[663,673]

Intracerebral hematomas have been categorized pathologically based on size as petechial, small, large, and massive. An ICH is considered massive when it is greater than 3 cm in the cerebrum, 2 cm in the cerebellum, and 1 cm in the brainstem.

TABLE 36-14
Anatomic Site, Frequency, and Etiologies
of Intracerebral Hematomas

Location	Frequency	Usual Etiologies
Caudate/Putamen	35–50%	Hypertension
Subcortical white matter	30%	AVM, saccular aneurysm, neoplasm, blood dyscrasia, drug abuse, amyloid angiopathy, hypertension
Cerebellum	16%	Hypertension, AVM, blood dyscrasia
Thalamus	10–15%	Hypertension
Pons	5–12%	Hypertension, AVM

AVM, arteriovenous malformation

The primary risk factor for developing an ICH is hypertension.[664,669] Its frequency as a preexisting condition has been reported in 72 to 81 percent of ICH.[674,675] This is further supported by observations of left ventricular hypertrophy in ICH patients[676–678] and significantly higher admission blood pressures in ICH patients compared to other types of stroke.[665] However, other conditions may also predispose to ICH. These include blood dyscrasias, vascular malformations, and tumors, accounting for about 25 percent of ICH.[679] Others have suggested that hypertension accounts for only half of ICH[680,681] not three-quarters as earlier reported.[674,675] Amyloid angiopathy accounts for most lobar hemorrhages.[682]

The anatomic location of ICH has been described in a number of reports.[664,669] The approximate frequencies are as shown in Table 36-14. The anatomic location is thought to provide some etiologic information also (Table 36-15).

Presentation

The presenting neurologic symptoms and signs of ICH are related to location of the ICH, headache, vomiting, seizures, and altered sensorium.[662,664] The specific nature and severity of these symptoms and signs vary in proportion to the size of the bleed. Vomiting will occur in 50 to 75 percent of ICH.[662] Headache does not occur with small ICH, but with large ICH with intracranial hypertension or ICH sufficient to produce brain tissue shifts affecting the meninges, headaches will occur.[271] Depressed level of consciousness, related to intracranial hypertension, occurs in 60 percent of ICH and of these two-thirds of the patients are comatose.[683–685] Seizures are uncommon with the onset of ICH, occurring in 7 to 14 percent of patients with ICH.[661,664,684] Seizures are associated with lobar extension of the hematoma to involve cortical structures.[662,664]

In most cases symptoms occur during activity, with onset during sleep extremely rare.[686,687] Neurologic signs are in relation to ICH location (see Table 36-15). The abruptness of the deficits relate to the speed with which the hematoma grows. This will depend on the size and location of the arteries involved. Thus, in rapidly developing bleeds, deficits may arise over seconds to minutes. More commonly, the deficits may develop over 10 to 30 min as the hematoma enlarges. Thus, most patients on presentation will have the maximal size hematoma with any progression of signs due to edema.[662,684,688,689] However, there are occasions where the hematoma enlargement may continue for hours after the initial bleed.[664,667,668,688,689]

Therapy

PRIMARY DISEASE   In addition to history and physical examination, the primary diagnostic procedure is CT and MRI scanning. Lumbar puncture with examination of CSF can provide important contributory information but is dangerous and is seldom done anymore with the advent of imaging and the recognized risk of uncal or tonsillar herniation.[664] Angiography is also used as supplemental diagnostic procedure when the etiology of the ICH is in doubt, for example, nonhypertensive hemorrhage, multiple ICH, or atypical sites to look for AVM or tumor.[664]

The managment of ICH is controversial. Some authors recommend an aggressive operative approach, whereas others prefer a nonsurgical approach.[451] It is now generally recommended that patients with smaller hematomas who are alert with small ICH be treated medically, but those with larger or expanding ICH should undergo angiography (to rule out a vascular abnormality such as AVM or aneurysm) and imaging with surgical removal of the ICH.[451] There are a variety of pros and cons to the surgical approach. Large hematomas can be associated with local tissue damage. Conversely, small hematomas, which have only dissected through white matter planes locally, can resorb without injuring anything. Performing surgery could thus induce brain tissue injury that otherwise would not have occurred. However, if the ICH is large enough to produce high ICP then decompression, by decreasing ICP, can prevent secondary brain damage from compromised CPP and herniation. Thus, the judgment whether to operate revolves largely about the hematoma's mass effect in compromising blood flow to still-viable brain tissue.[451] This assessment is becoming even further complicated by the introduction of non-craniotomy methods of clot removal such as percutaneous aspiration with or without stereotactic guidance, local fibrinolysis, and endoscopic evacuation.[451]

TABLE 36-15
Classic Signs of Intracerebral Hematoma Based on Site of Bleeding

	Motor/Sensory Signs	Oculomotor Signs	Pupils	Alertness	Behavioural Signs
Basal Ganglia-Putamen	Contralat hemiparesis, hemisensory loss hemianopia	Conjugate deviation to same side; conjugate gaze palsy to other size	Normal	Normal if small lesion	Aphasia (L), left neglect (R)
Thalamus	Contralat sensory > motor loss; hemianopia sometimes	Conjugate dev to same or opp side; eyes down or down and in; ocular skew; vertical gaze palsy; hyperconvergence "pseudo VIth' palsy	Both small and poorly reactive; ipsilateral smaller	Reduced	Confusion; poor memory; aphasia (L), left neglect (R)
Cerebral lobes					
Frontal	Contralat weakness, abnormal reasoning, abulia				Aphasia, inertia
Paracentral	Contralat weakness, numbness, ataxia				Broca or global aphasia
Parietal	Contralat limb ataxia, visual neglect, visual deficits, paresthesia				Spatial disorientation (R), conduction aphasis (L)
Temporal	Early stupor/uncal herniation (IIIrd n palsy), contralat sup quadrantaniopia, auditory/visual neglect	IIIrd n palsy	Enlarged with IIIrd n palsy	Decreased with herniation	Wernicke-type aphasia
Occipital	Contralateral visual field deficit, contralat sensory loss if parietal spread				Spatial disorientation (R), alexia without agraphia (L)
Pons	Quadriparesis; decerebrate movements	Bilateral, horiz gaze paresis; preserved vertical reflex movements; ocular bobbing	Small, reactive pupils	Coma	
Cerebellum	Gait ataxia, leaning to side of lesion; ipsilateral limb incoordination sometimes	Ipsilateral VIth or conjugate gaze paresis; nystagmus sometimes	Small reactive pupils; at times, ipsilateral pupil smaller	Stupor with larger lesions	

SOURCE: Adapted with permission from Caplan.[662]

CCM Considerations

AIRWAY MANAGEMENT   Endotracheal intubation is required when the hematoma has resulted in sufficient decrement in consciousness that the patient cannot protect the airway or sustain adequate gas exchange. Concerns in airway management are similar to those with intracranial hypertension. In a situation where a hematoma has produced parenchymal compression locally, it is not obvious whether extra efforts are required to ensure that hypertension does not occur. In addition, the morbidity of a decrease in blood pressure

with anesthetics used to facilitate intubation is equally unclear. A reasonable approach is to use a general anesthetic with trimethaphan or phenylephrine available, proceeding as described for SAH but with lower doses of anesthetic drugs.

Once intubation is performed it seems appropriate to ensure that excessive coughing does not occur. If the ICH is due to an AVM there is a good likelihood that the bleeding arose from the venous side of the AVM[690] and coughing-induced increased venous pressure may predispose to enlargement of the ICH.

GAS EXCHANGE   Issues are similar to those described for intracranial hypertension. The role of hyperventilation is controversial for two reasons. First, there is concern that excessive hyperventilation will predispose CO_2-reactive brain to CBF decrements sufficient to induce anaerobic metabolism.[183,184] Second, there is concern that decreasing tissue pressure will predispose to extension of the ICH.

TEMPERATURE   Fever occurs commonly with ICH[691] as it does with intracranial processes. Considerations are similar to those for SAH and intracranial hypertension. Fever is to be avoided and normothermia aggressively maintained.

BLOOD PRESSURE MANAGEMENT   Blood pressure management in a patient with ICH, particularly if the ICH is due to hypertension, is controversial and enigmatic. If the ICH is due to hypertension then it seems logical to control blood pressure. However, if ICP is high, drugs used to control blood pressure may increase ICP while decreasing blood pressure, possibly compromising CPP dangerously.[211] In addition, if the hematoma has compressed the brain tissue from which the bleed arose and there is a fibrin clot on the bleeding source, it seems unlikely that the high blood pressure being recorded peripherally is actually relevant to the cerebral microcirculation from which the bleed arose. In support of this notion are the observations that ICH seldom enlarges. It thus seems that the most appropriate course of treatment is to treat blood pressure when it is very high, that is, greater than about 180 to 200 mmHg systolic or 130 to 140 mmHg mean. Any blood pressure reduction should be accompanied by careful neurologic assessment and discontinuation of antihypertensive therapy if deterioration occurs in temporal association with blood pressure reduction.

GLUCOSE   Concerns in glucose management are similar to those with high ICP and focal cerebral ischemia previously discussed.

ELECTROLYTES AND FLUIDS   Issues are similar to those with high ICP.

ISCHEMIC STROKE
Pathophysiology
Data from animal models of ischemia have provided some insight into the pathogenesis of neuronal death with cerebral ischemia. The primary event is energy failure. With cessation of total brain flow in normal subjects, consciousness is lost within 7 s, with cessation of EEG activity occurring by 10 s.[629] In canine models, brain adenosine triphosphate (ATP) is depleted to less than 20 percent of baseline by 5 min of no blood flow.[693]

Recirculation after ischemic periods as long as 60 min in animal models is associated with return of brain high-energy phosphates to greater than 90 percent of baseline.[694–697] However, this restoration of energy metabolism does not correlate with functional recovery.[697,698] Such observations led to a search for other causes of neurologic deficit after cerebral ischemia. Pathologic studies have indicated that there is a heterogeneous susceptibility among neurons to ischemia-mediated death. Specifically, selectively vulnerable neurons have been identified and in rodents a hierarchy of vulnerability has been identified (CA1 = inferior colliculus > 3d and 5th layers of neocortex = striatum = CA3 = medial geniculate = substantia nigra). Furthermore, these neurons have been observed to die hours to days after the ischemic insult, leading to the concept of delayed maturation of a lesion with postischemic continuation of potentially reversible pathophysiologic processes a possibility.[699–703] Subsequent reports indicated that most of the ischemia-susceptible neurons are innervated by glutamatergic fibers. Such observation clearly suggested a relationship between glutamate-mediated synaptic transmission and postischemic neuronal death.

Ischemia is associated with a massive increase in excitatory neurotransmitters.[704] The most injurious is thought to be dicarboxylic amino acids such as glutamate. Other neurotransmitters, however, may also play a role. Neurotransmitter release stimulates metabotropic G-coupled receptors and agonist-gated iontropic receptors. Metabotropic receptors activate α phospholipase C, which results in production of phospholipid-derived second messengers, inositol 1,4,5-triphosphate (IP3) and diacylglycerol (DAG). DAG stimulates protein kinase C (PKC) and IP3 leads to a further increase in intracellular calcium from intracellular stores. Ionotropic receptors permit sodium, which can promote cellular swelling, and calcium to enter. Thus, massive increases in intracellular calcium occur due to both exogenous and endogenous entry. The calcium allows activation of calcium-dependent protein kinase. This overall process leads rapidly to activation of a variety of enzyme systems, which cause a cellular response, including alterations in gene expression. This gene expression can take hours to arise and likely accounts for the delay in observable injury in selectively vulnerable neurons.[699–709] However, if the severity of the ischemia is substantial enough in terms of duration or decrement in flow, then the cells will simply die acutely with maturation obviously becoming a not very important issue.[699] A host of intranuclear events occur consequent to cerebral ischemia. They include elaboration of immediate early genes, heat shock proteins, and amyloid precursor protein.[699] There are undoubtedly a host of other genetic responses yet to be determined.

With focal ischemia, increased intracellular osmolarity arises. In addition, vascular and cell membranes may become disrupted,[710,711] or even disintegrate.[699] The combination of these factors sets the stage for brain edema. With perfusion of the border zones around the ischemic zone, peri-infarct edema arises.[712,713] This can further compromise perfusion of this already marginally perfused zone. Indeed, in this low flow area perfusion may be insufficient to prevent anaerobic metabolism, yet be sufficient to supply substrates for edema such as sodium and glucose.[714,715] There may also be a contribution of neutrophils and an inflammatory response to this edema.[715]

A variety of other factors also contribute to the neurochemical pathogenesis of cerebral infarction. They include factors that increase vascular permeability such as interleukin-1, bradykinin, serotonin, histamine, arachidonic acid, and free radicals. Many of these mediators may be released locally by neutrophils.[699]

Ischemic infarcts in the brain are due to one of three mechanisms of vascular insufficiency: cerebral arterial hypotension (hemodynamic infarct), embolism, and thrombosis. Cerebral arterial hypotension occurs with systemic hypotension with CPP less than 60 mmHg. However, it can also occur with focal intracranial stenosis(es) such that a patient who is normotensive may sustain intracranial hypotension. One notable situation where this occurs is in the hypertensive patient undergoing antihypertensive therapy who develops ischemic signs as blood pressure is normalized. Cerebral embolism arises from clots originating in the left chamber of the heart, aorta, carotid artery, or from venous thromboembolism with right-to-left passage through the heart. Thrombotic stroke arises when a thrombosis arises in an otherwise patent artery. Typically, the vessel is previously stenotic from athersclerosis and the low flow state, with perhaps nonlaminar flow predisposing to coagulation, results in thrombotic occlusion of the artery with ischemia to distal tissues.[716]

Presentation

Patients with ischemic stroke, particularly those with thrombotic stroke, often present with a prior history that includes risk factors for stroke, including hypertension, smoking, heart disease, and diabetes. In addition, a history of transient ischemic attacks commonly can be obtained, particularly with thrombotic stroke. Patients will present with focal signs that usually come on abruptly and may have progressed from the time of onset.

The clinical categories of ischemic stroke are atherothrombotic, cardioembolic, or lacunar. However, 30 to 40 percent of patients cannot be readily categorized and are considered to have infarction of unknown origin. Atherothrombotic strokes occur secondary to arteriosclerotic narrowing of a cerebral vessel with superimposed development of a thrombus, which can then propagate distally. Less commonly symptoms arise from the narrowing of the lumen without thrombus formation. Another way that atherothrombotic mechanisms produce stroke is via proximal thrombosis throwing emboli distally. Atherothrombotic strokes are thought to account for two-thirds of ischemic strokes.[717] Cardioembolic strokes are associated with cardiac conditions that predispose to intracardiac thrombosis and embolization. Such conditions include atrial fibrillation, recent myocardial infarction, ventricular aneurysms, dilated cardiomyopathy, mitral or aortic valve disease, or septal defect that can allow a right-to-left shunt.

Embolism is suggested when there are multiple brain infarcts in different arterial territories. Most of these infarcts involve cortical structures with a predilection for involvement of the middle cerebral artery vascular territory. Cardioembolic strokes are thought to account for about one-third of ischemic strokes.[717] Lacunar strokes, a subcategory of atherothrombotic stroke, are small infarcts caused by occlusion of small penetrating arteries of the brain that tend to branch at 90° from the parent artery and supply the deep white and gray matter of the cerebral hemispheres.

Ischemic stroke has a variety of presentations that vary according to the vascular territory being disrupted[724] (Table 36-16). The brain's vascular supply can be divided into the anterior circulation arising from the carotid artery, and the posterior circulation arising from the vertebrobasilar arteries. Strokes due to internal carotid artery occlusion can be due to low flow or distal embolus and can present with a spectrum of symptoms varying from infarction of the entire anterior cerebral artery (ACA) and middle cerebral artery (MCA) territories to silent occlusion. MCA symptoms vary according to which MCA division(s) have been occluded. *Superior division MCA* stroke usually presents with hemiparesis (face and arm more than leg), hemisensory loss, mutism or motor aphasia, and dysarthria. *Inferior division MCA* stroke may present with Wernicke's aphasia (left hemisphere) without hemiparesis, homonymous hemianopia, neglect, dressing apraxia, and constructional apraxia (right hemisphere). *MCA stem* occlusion produces contralateral hemiplegia, hemisensory loss, global aphasia, homonymous hemianopia, and gaze preference. ACA occlusion is produced by embolus or thrombus, producing contralateral weakness and sensory loss in the foot and leg more than arm, grasp reflex, incontinence, and transcortical motor aphasia. *Posterior cerebral artery* (PCA) occlusion causes contralateral homonymous hemianopia, sensory loss, hemiparesis (usually transient), and memory loss. In dominant hemisphere PCA in-

TABLE 36-16
Ischemic Stroke Signs and Symptoms by Site

Site	Signs and Symptoms
Internal carotid artery	No signs/sxs with adequate collaterals Wide range of contralateral deficits depending on collaterals and mechanism: monoparesis, hemiparesis, sensory deficit, language difficulty. Ipsilateral transient monocular blindness
Middle cerebral artery	M1 occlusion: Contralateral hemiplegia, hemisensory deficit, homonymous hemianopsia; gaze preference, and aphasia (dominant stroke) and nondominant parietal syndrome (nondominant stroke). If surface collaterals intact may see only motor or no deficit. Distal occlusions produce partial syndromes
Anterior cerebral artery	Contralateral leg weakness and sensory deficit. May see some involvement of proximal muscles of contralateral arm. Cognitive impairment. Grasp responses
Vertebral artery	Lateral medullary infarct (also from occlusion of PICA): vertigo, nausea, vomiting, dysphagia, ipsilateral cerebellar ataxia, ipsilateral Horner's syndrome, decreased pain/temperature sensation ipsilateral face and contralateral legs/arms and trunk.
Basilar artery	Variable severity of deficits; none, TIAs, brainstem infarction. Dizziness, vertigo, nystagmus, locked in, coma, cranial nerve palsies
Posterior cerebral artery	Contralateral homonymous visual field deficit. Alexia without agraphia (dominant hemisphere). Thalamic sensory loss with proximal lesion. Sometimes transient hemiplegia.

Onset of signs and symptoms is usually abrupt but not always. The deficits can either progress or remit in the first 24 h.

farcts, a syndrome of alexia (inability to read) without agraphia (inability to write) may occur. *Basilar artery* occlusion produces brainstem signs such as cranial nerve palsies, gaze palsies, internuclear opthalmoplegia (paresis for eye adduction), bilateral long tract signs (motor or sensory), and cerebellar ataxia. Lower and midbasilar arterial occlusions are usually due to thrombosis and in the upper basilar embolus is more common.

Coma in association with stroke is an important stroke subset in the neuroICU. Coma tends to occur when there is loss of function of both cerebral hemispheres or the reticular activating system in the midbrain and upper pons. Thus, strokes producing decrements in flow to these areas depress consciousness. Bilateral cerebral ischemia is uncommon on presentation with focal ischemia of only one hemisphere unless there is hypotension, previous infarction of the other hemisphere, or emboli to both hemispheres. Such patients tend to appear responsive in their sensorium. However, if the stroke is large enough and significant poststroke swelling occurs, then elevations in ICP can compromise perfusion to the brainstem or other hemisphere leading to a comatose state. Conversely, patients with significant basilar ischemia involving the reticular activating system may present initially comatose and remain so unless there is early recanalization of the obstructed artery. Patients presenting with cerebellar hemorrhage or infarction, however, may present in a responsive condition. However, the cerebellum can swell. There is little space for edema formation in the posterior fossa and obstructive hydrocephalus can arise secondary to occlusion of the fourth ventricle. Thus, a limited amount of swelling can precipitiously lead to a comatose state after cerebellar infarction or hemorrhage.

Coma can also be produced by nonischemic events with stroke. One of the most significant of these is seizures. Such an occurrence can appear to be quite occult if the patient is having nonconvulsive seizure activity or the seizure was not witnessed and the patient is exhibiting a postictal depression of consciousness. Other causes of coma that may be seen with stroke include sepsis, electrolyte disturbances, hyperosmolar states, hypoglycemia, Wernicke's encephalopathy, hepatic encephalopathy, and toxic ingestion.[718]

Therapy

PRIMARY DISEASE   Stroke is recently identified as a medical emergency. Thus, efforts are underway to increase public awareness of signs and symptoms of stroke to expedite entry of stroke patients into the emergency medical system with urgent institution of diagnostic and therapeutic procedures. Immediate management includes initially evaluation of the airway, gas exchange, and circulation with resuscitative treatment instituted as needed. Immediate diagnostic procedures include ECG, chest radiograph, complete blood count, platelet count, PT, PTT, electrolytes, blood glucose, arterial blood gas, and if needed, alcohol and toxicology screen. Intravenous access is obtained and oxygen is administered. A soon as possible thereafter, a noncontrast CT scan is performed. Additional diagnostic studies that may be performed include MRI, arteriography, and ultrasonography, CT angiography, conventional angiography, MRI angiography, echocardiography, Holter monitoring, cholesterol, triglycerides, fasting blood sugar, VDRL, erythrocyte sedimentation rate, blood culture, antinuclear antibodies, anticardiolipin antibody, lupus anticoagulant, antithrombin III, protein S, protein C, and activated protein C resistance (factor V Leiden mutation).

About 17 percent of stroke patients require intensive care.[719] Reasons for neuroICU admission include unstable neurologic status, embolic middle cerebral or carotid occlusion, basilar system stroke, septic/multiple emboli, elevated ICP, and proposed interventional therapy such as thrombolysis or hypervolemic hemodilution. Nonneurologic problems may also be present. Such problems that may result in need for neuroICU admission include arrhythmias, myocardial infarction, hemodynamic instability, aspiration pneumonia, inability to protect the airway, or severe underlying medical problems. The *primary concern* in stroke therapy is maintenance of normal physiologic homeostasis. This is discussed in more detail under CCM considerations. Notable in this regard is blood pressure management. In general, hypertension associated with stroke should not be treated aggressively unless there is clinical concern that other morbidity will be produced by the elevated blood pressure.

Therapeutic maneuvers directed primarily to the neurologic problems include recurrent assessment of neurologic function and physiologic parameters that are important to normal neurologic functioning. Other primary neurologic therapies that may be used include anticoagulation, ICP management, seizure prophylaxis and control, reperfusion therapy, and a variety of other investigational techniques. In addition, there are situations where a neurosurgical approach is warranted. Therapies found so far not to be helpful in clinical studies, despite theoretical advantages or efficacy in animal studies, include steroids, opiate antagonists, vasopressors, vasodilators, hemodilution, brain oxygenating drugs, and therapies aimed at reducing cerebral metabolism.[720] Nonetheless, continued investigation of some of these modalities may find subsets of patients in whom efficacy may be demonstrated.

About 20 percent of ischemic stroke patients sustain worsening of the initial deficit within 4 days of the onset of symptoms.[721] It is likely that such progression of a stroke is secondary to enlargement of the clot causing the stroke, thus providing a logical rationale for the use of heparin. However, other factors such as increasing peri-infarct edema or metabolic disturbances may also contribute to secondary worsening as may hemorrhagic conversion of the infarct. Thus use of anticoagulation is not entirely straightforward. Anticoagulation with heparin has not yet been demonstrated in controlled scientific clinical trials to improve outcome.[720–724] This is particularly true if an infarction has become established and there is no ongoing or threatened worsening of stroke signs and symptoms. In a small prospective randomized trial of heparin for ischemic stroke (125 patients) no efficacy was observed with heparin use, nor were there any complications from it.[725] Nonetheless, heparin continues to be recommended for smaller strokes, vertebrobasilar circulation strokes, cardioembolic strokes with known atrial fibrillation, mural thrombus, MCA stenosis or tight carotid stenosis, or strokes that appear to be in evolution.[721,723,724,726] The rationale for this continued use is that these are subgroups of patients in whom heparin use may be helpful, such as those with recent carotid occlusion, or risk for early, recurrent embolus, acknowledging that administering heparin to all stroke patients probably will not be proven efficacious.

The primary morbidity contraindicating the routine use of anticoagulation is the possibility of hemorrhagic conversion of an ischemic stroke. In the setting of an anticoagulated patient this can result in a precipitous life-threatening deterioration of the patient. Hemorrhagic conversion occurs reportedly in 5 to 30 percent of strokes with a mortality of 1 percent.[720–722,727] This appears to be related to the size of the stroke and the timing of heparin use. Large hemispheric strokes, particularly when the entire MCA distribution including the lenticulostriates are involved, carry the greatest risk of parenchymal hemorrhage with anticoagulation. Heparin appears to be quite safe with small strokes. Conversely anticoagulation in large cardioembolic strokes is associated with a higher (18 percent) incidence of hemorrhage but may reduce the incidence of recurrent embolism.[723,728] This risk of repeated cardioembolic ischemia, if the source of the embolism is left untreated, makes the decision to anticoagulate in such a situation controversial and subject to judgment.[721] If anticoagulation is contemplated there must be certainty (based on CT scan) that there is no intracranial hemorrhage.[721] Anticoagulation with heparin does reduce significantly the incidence of DVT in stroke patients.[722]

Another complication of heparin use is thrombocytopenia, which occurs in 5 percent of patients receiving heparin.[721] In addition, there is a risk in about 0.5 percent of patients receiving heparin of heparin-induced thrombosis associated with severe thrombocytopenia.[721] Such a complication should be expected to exacerbate the stroke.

Elevated intracranial pressure can be a cause of delayed deterioration after stroke. Indeed, a patient may be admitted fully conscious with a large deficit related to hemispheric ischemia and be dead within days due to swelling of the infarcted brain and surrounding tissue. In general, the larger the stroke the greater the chance of intracranial hypertension. Thus, patients with strokes involving the entire vascular supply of one carotid artery or MCA should be admitted to an area where recurrent neurologic assessment can be performed. In addition, malignant brain edema may occur more readily in younger patients in whom there is less intracranial room for swelling. Swelling sufficient to produce a decrement in consciousness warrants use of ICP-reducing therapy. Consideration should be given to surgical approaches to relief of elevated ICP as discussed below.

It is estimated that 4 to 10 percent of stroke patients will develop seizures secondary to the stroke.[729–731] These seizures occur without effects noted of age, sex, or side of the stroke. Fifty-sixty percent of seizures occur in the first 24 h after the onset of the stroke, 7 to 8 percent by the end of the first month and the remainder occur later. About 50 percent of the seizures are grand mal, that is, tonic-clonic, convulsions. Simple partial seizures occur in 37 to 47 percent and status epilepticus in 6 to 8 percent.[729] The occurrence of a hemorrhage tends to increase the incidence of seizure. Infarct-associated seizure occurs when the infarct involves the cortex in the parietal lobe or motor cortex. When a seizure occurs after a stroke it is associated with an increase in mortality from 21 to 31 percent.[729] Presently, data from head trauma studies do not support the routine use of prophylactic anticonvulsant therapy. However, if a seizure should occur, then aggressive management of the seizure and continued anticonvulsant therapy as with any patient with epilepsy is appropriate.[366,729]

Reperfusion therapy is being used in an uncontrolled and controlled fashion in many medical centers. There have been numerous anecdotes and clinical trials of this approach to the management of acute stroke in both the anterior and posterior intracranial circulations.[727,732–735] Outcome measures have been inconstant, including clinical outcome and recanalization. In addition, there has been wide variation in the timing of therapy. When treatment is started earlier, a better outcome occurs. A recent meta-analysis of thrombolysis therapy for stroke indicated that the procedure

should be an effective technique.[727] Six randomized trials were examined. After removing studies without CT scan availability to remove hemorrhagic strokes, they found that thrombolytic therapy was associated with a 37 percent reduction of the probability of death and a 56 percent reduction of the probability of death or deterioration. A recent multi-institutional study of tissue plasminogen activator (tPA) for acute ischemic stroke indicated a protective effect in terms of neurologic disability but not mortality with an increased incidence of hemorrhage (6.4 versus 0.6 percent).[736] A major concern with thrombolytic therapy is that it may produce hemorrhagic transformation of a bland ischemic stroke, leading to ICH and worse disability or death. Wardlaw and Warlow[727] analyzed this comparing it with the best estimate of the natural rate of hemorrhagic conversion, reportedly about 5 percent.[737] Their analysis of 55 reports of 1781 patients undergoing thrombolysis therapy for stroke indicated an overall incidence of hematoma of 5 percent. They noted a 5 percent incidence of hematoma with use of streptokinase, 3 percent with urokinase, and 8 percent for tPA. This incidence of postthrombolysis hematoma appears to be related to the depth of ischemia prior to reperfusion.[738] Moreover, recent studies indicate that there may be a false-positive rate of apparent CT-confirmed hemorrhage, as dye extravasation is common after intraarterial infusion, thus mimicking a hematoma on CT scan.[739] These promising data indicate that thrombolysis therapy is safe and efficacious. A therapeutic window is suggested from these studies and earlier investigations indicating the time-dependent nature of the outcome after focal temporary ischemia. Thus, stroke patients in whom such therapy is being contemplated must undergo transportation and evaluation in the most urgent manner. The data suggest that treatment must be instituted within 3 h of the onset of symptoms and much more preferably, within 2 h of symptom onset. Anecdotes suggest that complete recovery is possible when recanalization occurs promptly, as may occur with in-hospital strokes.[740]

Urokinase is the most commonly used thrombolytic agent because of its low cost and lack of allergic reactions. Urokinase is administered intra-arterially in the angiography suite, whereas streptokinase and tPA are administered intravenously. Intravenous tPA can be given sooner and is expected to act in a highly clot-specific manner. However, the dose of tPA that produces clot lysis is not yet well defined, whereas many studies show efficacy with urokinase and streptokinase.

Neurosurgery is indicated on an urgent basis in a few subsets of stroke patients. Procedures that may be used include urgent revascularization, strokectomy, decompressive craniectomy, cerebellar resection, and external ventricular drain placement. Revascularization (i.e., carotid endarterectomy or extracranial-intracranial bypass) is occasionally performed when the onset time has been brief, usually indicating an in-hospital stroke and endovascular reperfusion techniques are not feasible.[741] It may also be indicated when the patient has progressive stroke in the presence of known ulcerating intraarterial plaque or when there are fluctuating symptoms of hemodynamic origin and systemic perfusion-augmenting therapy is not thought to be appropriate. Decompressive craniectomy is somewhat controversial. It is used for malignant intracranial hypertension and involves resection of the skull and dura to allow unopposed outward brain swelling without intracranial hypertension after a large stroke. However, there is laboratory support for it and encouraging anecdotal evidence in humans describing its use.[365-368] Strokectomy has recently been described for malignant brain dema after ischemic stroke as a lifesaving alternative to temporal lobe resection.[364] Cerebellar decompression can be dramatically lifesaving when the deterioration is detected and decompression occurs in a timely manner.[366,742] *Ventriculostomy placement* can be performed if ICP is thought to be increasing and ICP-reducing therapy is to be used titrated versus ICP measurements. In addition, it can be used to remove CSF in an elevated ICP state or if hydrocephalus arises, as can occur after cerebellar infarction.

A variety of promising therapies are presently being evaluated for stroke. Such therapies are based on the rather extensive literature reporting a variety of important pathogenetic processes thought to be susceptible to treatment to prevent or reverse the effects of blood flow cessation or interruption. Therapies being studied include thrombolysis, anticoagulation, calcium channel antagonists, free radical scavengers, excitatory amino acid antagonists, and others. A detailed review of this is beyond the scope of this chapter.

CCM Considerations

AIRWAY MANAGEMENT AND GAS EXCHANGE   Data in laboratory studies clearly indicate that hypoxemia in the presence of cerebrovascular occlusion, which otherwise is asymptomatic, leads to cerebral infarction. Thus, borderline degrees of hypoxemia, which otherwise may be tolerated via compensatory mechanisms, in the setting of compromised cerebrovascular reserve as occurs with stroke syndromes, may produce or exacerbate the stroke. It follows, therefore, that every effort should be made to avoid hypoxemia in stroke patients. Continuous pulse oximetry should be used and if there is any doubt about oxygenation, supplementary oxygen should be administered.[366] If there are any reservations about the ability of the patient to protect the airway, particularly if due to decreased level of consciousness, endotracheal intubation should be considered.

Endotracheal intubation should be effected using a technique that preserves the CPP even if elevated. This can be achieved with sedation and topical anesthesia of the airway. Use of thiopental and neuromuscular blockade can also be done safely but lower doses of thiopental than usual should be used with additional doses given if an unacceptable rise in blood pressure occurs. The physician should be prepared to administer phenylephrine or other pressor agent after intubation until the CNS-depressant drug effects subside. This may mean infusing a pressor to maintain a hypertensive pressure if the patient's preintubation blood pressure was elevated. Because the patient may require that blood pressure to maintain blood flow to other areas of the brain or in the ischemic penumbra, it is essential that intubation not be associated with a decrease in blood pressure, which may compromise blood flow in such at-risk brain areas.

Hyperventilation should not be routinely used in stroke patients due to concerns that this may decrease blood flow in regions with marginal perfusion. Such concerns are based on observations of low rCBF in head trauma patients with hyperventilation[743] and data indicating exacerbation of neurologic insult in hyperventilated head trauma patients.[184] Hyperventilation as an ineffective treatment for stroke was reported in 1973.[744-746] Conversely, hypoventilation has also been reported to be deleterious to recovery of ischemic tissue.[747]

TEMPERATURE   Hypothermia has been shown to be protective in numerous animal models of stroke[748-752] although its use for 48 h after stroke in a primate stroke model was associated with exacerbation of brain damage.[753] Although it has achieved widespread use in the controlled setting of the operating room,[193] hypothermia is not yet proven appropriate for stroke patients. However, these data clearly underscore the importance of preventing and aggressively treating fever in stroke patients.[366]

BLOOD PRESSURE MANAGEMENT   Laboratory studies have provided evidence that an ischemic stroke produces a central ischemic core around which there is an ischemic penumbra, where flow is perfusion pressure dependent via collateral vessels. This dependence of flow on blood pressure is supported by clinical observations in stroke patients.[753a] Such data suggest that it may not be safe to decrease blood pressure in a stroke patient without strong indications to do so. There are a variety of theoretical and demonstrated pros and cons to antihypertensive therapy with stroke. These are rather complex considerations that have been recently reviewed in detail by Powers.[754] The overall conclusion of his review is that data are presently indefinite regarding antihypertensive therapy in stroke. He suggests that present data indicate that blood pressure reduction is accompanied by a real risk of producing further ischemic damage. Thus, blood pressure should only be reduced when there is thought to be a risk of hypertensive encephalopathy or cardiovascular compromise due to hypertension (e.g., myocardial ischemia or low output state with preexisting ventricular dysfunction).[366,754] If blood pressure reduction is contemplated agents used should be short lived, readily reversible, and not prone to increase ICP.[366] Sympatholytic drugs are preferred because they may confer some neuronal preservation.[194-196] If a vasodilator is used, nicardipine should be a primary consideration due to potential for brain protective side effects.[204,207-209]

Similar to intracranial hemorrhage, ischemic stroke has also been reported to be associated with ECG changes.[300,312,755,756] In addition, stroke is associated with a significantly increased incidence of cardiac arrhythmias, with ventricular ectopy being most common.[757,758] These ECG changes indicate a poorer prognosis.[759] In addition, 11 percent of patients with ECG changes develop elevations in cardiac isoenzymes,[760] an observation associated with a doubling of mortality.[366] These observations are probably related to stroke-induced elevations of blood catecholamines.[307,755,761] It is thus apparent that these ECG changes in stroke patients are not mere artifact. Any stroke patient who presents with ECG changes should have CPK isoenzymes determined and be monitored continuously for cardiac arrhythmias.

GLUCOSE   Hyperglycemia has been convincingly demonstrated to be deleterious with global complete and incomplete cerebral ischemia.[235,236,238-240,242,247,747,762] Data in animals suggest that hyperglycemic exacerbation of ischemic brain damage occurs as a stepwise function, that is, a continuum of increases in blood glucose are associated with discrete, incremental worsening of brain damage.[236,238] The exact mechanism is unclear. However, laboratory studies indicate an important role for brain tissue acidosis.[236,747]

However, data with focal cerebral ischemia are conflicting.[247] Laboratory and clinical studies show that hyperglycemia worsens,[234,244,248-250,253,258] has no effect,[245,763] and improves[251,252,257,259] brain damage after focal ischemia. In addition recent evidence suggests that hyperglycemia on presentation may predispose to hemorrhagic conversion of an ischemic stroke.[242,246] Unfortunately, patients with the highest blood glucose concentrations have been reported to have the highest cortisol levels, suggesting that the initial stroke severity is the primary factor and stroke-mediated stress is the cause of the hyperglycemia, thus producing a self-fulfilling correlation of hyperglycemia with worse stroke.[243-245]

Prado and colleagues[256] report a series of studies with both incomplete and complete focal ischemia in the same animals. They observed that areas of focal incomplete ischemia sustained worse injury with hyperglycemia, whereas no effect of hyperglycemia was apparent in brain areas without collateral low blood flow. As the numerous conflicting reports are from a variety of clinical scenarios and laboratory models and hyperglycemic exacerbation clearly is related to accumulation of lactate, it seems attractive to conclude that focal ischemia is subject to hyperglycemic exacerbation if there is residual low flow.

A synthesis of these conflicting data lead to the recommendation that severe hyperglycemia be avoided in patients with stroke. If blood sugar is above 200 mg/dl it seems warranted to administer insulin to keep the blood glucose concentration about 200 mg/dl.[366] Efforts to further decrease blood glucose may not be helpful, indeed may be harmful, and predispose to iatrogenic hypoglycemia, which clearly is not expected to improve outcome. If insulin is required, it should be given as an infusion with frequent assessment of blood glucose concentration during the acute phase of the stroke to avoid wide variations in blood glucose concentration, which typically occur when intermittant insulin coverage is provided to react to undesirably elevated blood glucose levels.

ELECTROLYTES AND FLUIDS   Hemodilution is commonly used in the operating room and for SAH. The physiologic basis for such practice is that a modest decrease in hematocrit will decrease viscosity and flow will increase to more than compensate for the decrease in oxygen-carrying capacity produced by the hemoglobin concentration decrease. Animal studies indicated that hemodilution should be an effective therapy for stroke.[764-766] Thus, clinical trials were performed in a large number of patients with stroke to assess the efficacy of hemodilution. Results have been conflicting, showing improvement,[767-771] no effect,[772-775] and deterioration as well as increased mortality,[776] leading to the general consensus that hemodilution is not an effective therapy for stroke. However, there have been concerns that hemodilution in these studies was not performed effectively,[777,778] early enough,[776,777] or in the appropriate subset of stroke patients.[778] Goslinga and coworkers[778] report a method of inducing hemodilution guided by PCWP measurements. Patients who were dehydrated on admission received only appropriate rehydration and patients who were not dehydrated received hemodilution. Both subgroups showed improvement. This report suggests that hemodilution titrated to an individual patient's hemodynamic condition may be a safe, efficacious manner to induce hemodilution.

Hyponatremia can exacerbate any cerebral edema and in so doing may extend the area of infarction. Thus, decreases in sodium should prompt more aggressive monitoring for hyponatremia and treatment titrated to the serum sodium level.

NEUROMUSCULAR DISORDERS

GUILLIAN-BARRÉ SYNDROME

Pathophysiology

The incidence of Guillain-Barré syndrome (GBS) is approximately 1 to 1.5 cases per 100,000 per year. It is an acute inflammatory polyneuropathy of unknown etiology. In about two-thirds of the patients an acute viral syndrome precedes the symptoms by 1 to 3 weeks. Weakness is thought to arise secondary to immune-mediated inflammation of the peripheral nerves. Immunologic mechanisms are thought to include both antibody- and cell-mediated immune mechanisms leading to damage to peripheral nerve myelin.[779-784]

Presentation

Most patients with GBS present with a several day to weeks' course of ascending weakness, hypotonia, and areflexia typically preceded by a viral syndrome. In 90 percent the peak of the illness occurs within 10 to 14 days. The generalized symmetrical weakness is often accompanied by mild sensory symptoms and pain. Pain occurs in more than half the patients and presents as a muscular pain with tenderness. Paresthesias are also common, occurring in about 80 percent of patients, but usually are transient. Left untreated the weakness can ascend to produce respiratory failure and death. The widespread demyelination can also affect cranial nerves, typically involving the facial nerve and to a lesser extent the third, fifth, and ninth nerves. In addition, autonomic nerves can be affected leading to dysfunction of important nerves such as vagal, glossopharyngeal, and preganglionic sympathetic nerves.

The speed of onset and severity of symptoms can be variable. Several variants of the typical presentation are recognized. Fisher's syndrome is a form of GBS presenting with opthalmoplegia, ataxia, and areflexia. In other variants, patients may present with pure sensory loss with areflexia, pure motor GBS, pure pandysautonomia, polyneuritis cranialis, pharyngeal-cervical-brachial dysfunction, and paraparesis.[785-787]

Diagnosis is based on the presence of a constellation of findings. Features thought to be required to make the diagnosis include relatively symmetric and progressive muscle weakness, areflexia, and absence of other causes of acute neuropathy. Presenting features thought to be strongly supportive of the diagnosis of GBS include progression over days to 4 weeks, only mild sensory symptoms, cranial nerve involvement, absence of fever with the onset of neuritic signs, autonomic dysfunction, increased CSF protein concentration in the presence of few or no cells, electrodiagnostic findings supportive of demyelination, and recovery beginning 2 to 4 weeks after cessation of progression.

Therapy

PRIMARY DISEASE   The two primary therapies used for GBS are plasmapheresis and immunoglobulin administration.[783,784]

Several randomized trials support the early use of plasmapheresis during the rapidly evolving phase of GBS. Patients treated within 2 weeks of onset show a decreased hospitalization time and decreased severity of the syndrome. Young patients tend to respond to plasmapheresis better than older patients. It is generally not warranted for mild forms of the syndrome. Thus, it tends to be used when difficulty arises with walking, maintaining a normal vital capacity, or bulbar dysfunction. The plasmapheresis regimen advocated removes 250 ml/kg in four to six treatments on alternate days with fluid removed replaced with saline and 5% albumin or fresh frozen plasma.[783,788,789]

Morbidity from plasmapheresis is related to vascular cannulation, bacteremia, citrate intoxication, hypotension, cardiac arrhythmias, and anticoagulation-related morbidity. It is estimated that lethal complications have occurred in 3/10,000 procedures.[783]

Recently, intravenous administration of immune globulin (0.4 g/kg/per day for 5 days) has been reported to be as effective as plasmapheresis for GBS.[790] Concern has been expressed that the plasmapheresis control gorup did more poorly than expected, thus possibly producing a false-positive result.[783] However, immunoglobulin therapy has fewer side effects than plasmapheresis and is thought to be indicated when plasmapheresis is contraindicated or does not appear to be effective.[783]

CCM Considerations

The primary reason for neuroICU admission in GBS is respiratory failure due to weakness of respiratory muscles or bulbar dysfunction leading to inability to protect the airway from oral or gastric secretions. The course of GBS is substantially lengthened if a patient is ill enough to require intensive care with hospital stays lasting months. However, given suitable intensive care about 80 to 90 percent of these patients recover with little or no disability.[791] Mortality is 1 to 5 percent.[786] Major neuroICU complications include tracheostomy (50 percent), pneumonia (25 percent), urinary tract infections (20 percent), phlebitis, pulmonary embolism (2 percent), and psychological depression.[791]

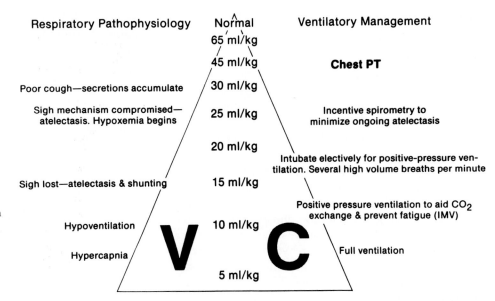

Respiratory Pathophysiology   Normal   Ventilatory Management
                                     65 ml/kg
                                     45 ml/kg   Chest PT
Poor cough—secretions accumulate   30 ml/kg

Sigh mechanism compromised—   25 ml/kg   Incentive spirometry to
  atelectasis. Hypoxemia begins   minimize ongoing atelectasis

                                     20 ml/kg
                                                     Intubate electively for positive-pressure ven-
                                                     tilation. Several high volume breaths per minute
Sigh lost—atelectasis & shunting   15 ml/kg

                                                     Positive pressure ventilation to aid CO₂
                                                     exchange & prevent fatigue (IMV)

Hypoventilation   10 ml/kg

Hypercapnia   **V   C**   Full ventilation

                                     5 ml/kg

Figure 36-30 The continuum of pathophysiologic abnormalities with progressively increasing muscle weakness and corresponding therapy. Note that hypoxemia generally precedes hypercapnea. (Reproduced by permission from Ropper.[791])

Turning is essential to prevent pulmonary complication, decubiti, and pressure nerve palsies.

AIRWAY MANAGEMENT   The primary concerns for endotracheal intuation are the patient's sensorium, presence of gag, extent of systemic weakness, presence of autonomic dysfunction, and presence of a full stomach. If autonomic dysfunction is present, it may be most prudent to assume that a full stomach is present. If endotracheal intubation is required, the need for neuromuscular blockade may be decreased by the patient's overall weakness and the presence of bulbar weakness, lessening the gag response. However, sensation and sensorium are usually sufficiently intact to indicate the need for an amnestic or hypnotic drug as indicated by the patient's baseline awareness and anxiety and hemodynamic stability (see below—this is not ensured). With such a demyelinating syndrome it is to be expected that there may be postsynaptic upregulation of nicotinic cholinergic receptor at the neuromuscular junction. Such physiology should predispose a subject to succinylcholine-induced hyperkalemia.[792] This is supported by case reports of succinylcholine-associated cardiac arrest in GBS patients.[792,793] Thus, if neuromuscular blockade is required to facilitate endotracheal intubation a rapid-onset nondepolarizing neuromuscular blocking drug such as vecuronium or rocuronium should be used. A reasonable alternative is to use topicalization, reassurance, and sedation. GBS patients typically are cooperative, having had time to be educated about their disease, resulting in a cooperative patient, despite the urgent circumstance.

GAS EXCHANGE   As muscle weakness progresses a continuum of abnormalities in gas exchange arise as depicted in Fig. 36-30. Initially, coughing is compro-

mised resulting in accumulation of secretions. Subsequently, as weakness progresses to a vital capacity of about 25 ml/kg, atelectasis arises and the alveolar-arterial gradient increases. Thus, the first important abnormality that may be observed is not hypercapnea, but rather, a decrement in pulse oximetry readings concurrent with decreases in vital capacity. As vital capacity further decreases tachypnea is no longer sufficient to compensate for the low vital capacity then resulting in hypoventilation and hypercapnea.

It thus becomes essential to detect and then treat these respiratory abnormalities. On hospital admission, the nonintubated GBS patient should undergo serial vital capacity determinations every 2 to 4 h during the day and 4 to 6 h at night until it stabilizes. This has been found to be an excellent modality for predicting the need for mechanical ventilatory support.[794] As vital capacity decreases to 15 ml/kg endotracheal intubation is indicated,[791,794] followed by mechanical ventilation to maintain normal gas exchange. If the syndrome has not resolved within 2 weeks and the patient continues to have a low vital capcity, then tracheostomy is generally performed for patient comfort and safety and to prevent laryngeal injury. Weaning efforts can be started once improvement begins and the vital capacity increases to 7 ml/kg with extubation considered when the patient is easily breathing without ventilatory assistance, typically when vital capacity is greater than 10 to 15 ml/kg.

An important component of respiratory care with GBS is aggressive and meticulous attention to details of respiratory management. This includes use of chest physical therapy, frequent turning, maintenance of thin secretions with aerosolized saline, and avoidance of systemic dehydration. In addition, some authors advocate the routine use of systemic anticoagulation with heparin infusion to increase the PTT 2 to 2.5 times normal.[783,791]

BLOOD PRESSURE MANAGEMENT   Autonomic dysautonomia can pose a significant challenge in the management of GBS. Manifestations of dysautonomia include sinus tachycardia (37 percent), urinary retention (27 percent), paroxysmal hypertension (24 percent), orthostatic hypotension (19 percent), constipation (14 percent), ileus (9 percent), and heart rate lability (8 percent).[795] Less common but significant cardiovascular abnormalities include life-threatening arrhythmias, ECG changes, creatinine phosphokinase elevations. Reduced RR interval with severe hypertension may predict life-threatening arrhythmias.[796] Hypotension can be clinically significant with blood pressure low enough to produce syncope.[797,798] Conversely, hypertension can be severe enough to produce or cause concern for sudden death, SAH, seizures, pulmonary edema, or hypertensive encephalopathy.[791]

Continuous monitoring for ECG and blood pressure abnormalities is mandatory. Each abnormality is treated as it occurs. Thus, sustained hypertension is treated with a parenteral antihypertensive agent such as nitroprusside or a β-adrenergic blocking drug. Persistent hypotension, after evaluating for other causes not due to dysautonomia (e.g., gastrointestinal bleed) can be managed with a titrated infusion of phenylephrine or dopamine, assisted by pulmonary artery pressure readings. Arrhythmias are treated with appropriate antiarrhythmic drugs. Symptomatic bradycardia may require use of a pacemaker.[791] Ischemic changes on ECG are treated as nonartifactual signs of ischemia. Anti-ischemic therapy such as nifedipine, β-adrenergic blockade, or nitrates should be considered. GBS patients can be sensitive to vasoactive drugs. Thus, treatment should be initiated cautiously in a titrated manner with attention to untoward effects.

ELECTROLYTES AND FLUIDS   Hyponatremia can occur with GBS. SIADH has been associated with GBS.[791,799] This usually responds to fluid restriction. Similarly, natriuresis has also been identified but apparently is less common than SIADH.

PAIN MANAGEMENT   Pain can be a significant problem in GBS. Comfort measures are important in management, including use of lambskins, frequent position changes, and close attention to avoidance of cold in the extremities. Nonsteroidal anti-inflammatory agents may be tried and if ineffective supplemented with opioid drugs. Epidural opiates have been used for pain in GBS.[783]

MYASTENIA GRAVIS (also see Chap. 13)
Pathophysiology
Myasthenia gravis (MG) is a syndrome characterized by reduction in nicotinic cholinergic receptors at the neuromuscular junction due to autoimmune mechanisms.[800–802] It is frequently associated with thymoma (10 percent). Indeed, one important reason for neuroICU admission is postoperatively after thymoma resection. Its incidence is 2 to 4/100,000 per year and prevalence is estimated to be 4 to 8/100,000.[803,804]

Presentation
Patients typically give a history of fluctuating weakness, more prominent in the evening or at night. Closer questioning may reveal that the patient has had difficulty with sustained muscular contraction. Sustained gaze away from the midline causes diplopia or there is inability to perform functions above the head, for example. Difficulty chewing or swallowing can also occur. Myasthenic crisis or cholinergic crisis results in the need for intensive care as does the need for surgery with readjustment of MG medications perioperatively. Myasthenic crisis is estimated to occur in 2 percent of patients.[803,804]

The signs and symptoms can be variable along a continuum of severity. This has resulted in development of a staging system to describe where on this continuum a given patient is[805]:

  I. Ocular myasthenia
 II. A. Mild generalized myasthenia with slow progression; no crises; drug responsive
     B. Moderate generalized myasthenia; severe skeletal and bulbar involvement but no crises; drug response less than satisfactory
III. Acute fulminating myasthenia; rapid progression of severe symptoms with respiratory crises and poor drug response; high incidence of thymoma; high mortality
IV. Late severe MG, same as III but progression over 2 years from class I to II.

Myasthenic crisis occurs when weakness is severe enough to produce symptomatic dyspnea or difficulty with swallowing and airway protection. The crisis may be precipitated by emotional distress, infection, or other stress. Conversely, patients being treated for myasthenia may develop cholinergic crisis due to decreasing needs for medication or inadvertent overdose. When this occurs, patients may have sialorrhea, bronchorrhea, diarrhea, colic, nausea, vomiting, bradycardia, miosis, diaphoresis, and muscle fasciculations and weakness, unresponsive to anticholinesterase treatment. Generally, symptoms are aggravated by a small test dose of edrophonium or neostigmine.

Diagnosis is made primarily by history supplemented by electromyogram, anti-AChR antibody assay, and edrophonium (Tensilon) test. The edrophonium test is performed by administration sequentially of 2 mg, then 3 mg, then 5 mg edrophonium separated by 45 s, followed by assessment of levator palpebrae or extraocular muscle. If the patient has MG, improvement in muscular function should be apparent within 5 min. If the patient has cholinergic crisis the weakness should worsen. Edrophonium may precipitate respiratory failure when weakness is due to over- rather than undertreatment. Precautions should be taken beforehand to deal with this possibility.

Therapy

PRIMARY DISEASE   Treatment options in MG include administration of anticholinesterases, immunosuppressants, and corticosteroids; thymectomy; and plasmapheresis. Pyridostigmine (Mestinon) is the most commonly used anticholinesterase, 15 to 90 mg orally every 6 h. Its use risks a cholinergic crisis. Thymectomy is suggested in most MG patients under 50 years old who are not responding well to conservative therapy. Prednisone is given 40 to 45 mg/day. It may be followed initially by worsening of symptoms, which improve after 7 to 10 days. If this is not effective, immunosuppression with azathioprine, 2.5 mg/kg per day, can be added to decrease the number of receptor antibodies. Plasmapheresis can be used to achieve temporary remission. This is particularly useful for myasthenic crisis.[804] Myasthenic crisis can also be treated initially with an intravenous infusion of neostigmine 0.5 to 1 mg/h or pyridostigmine 0.1 to 0.5 mg/h, with the infusion slowly increased and titrated to the patient's strength. Atropine should also be given 0.5 mg subcutaneously, three to five times daily.[803]

CCM Considerations

Patients with MG need critical care when they develop myasthenic crisis or require surgery. After surgery, anticholinesterase requirements may change and their use is complicated further by the use of neuromuscular blocking drugs during surgery or complicating effects of anesthetic and other drugs given perioperatively.

Patients presenting with myasthenic crisis may report a variety of warning signs preceding the crisis episode. These signs include rapid fluctuations in the severity of the weakness, continued reduction of daily activities, loss of body weight, steady increase in anticholinesterase dose, head dropping, progressive dysarthria and shortness of breath, febrile infections, especially involving the respiratory tract, and ingestion of medications that may impair neuromuscular transmission (Table 36-17).

AIRWAY MANAGEMENT   Insofar as possible, neuro-

TABLE 36-17
Therapeutic Agents That May Worsen Myasthenia Gravis

Class of Drug	Specific Agents
Antibiotics	Gentamicin, tobramycin, streptomycin, polymixin B, clindamycin, lincomycin, tetracycline, sufonamides
Antiepileptic drugs	Phenytoin, carbamazepine, trimethadione, quinine, others
Antiarrhythmics	Local anesthetics (lidocaine), procainamide, verapamil, propranolol, others
Antirheumatic drugs	Muscle relaxants, D-Penicillamine, chloroquine, resochine, quinine, others
Antipsychotic drugs	Lithium, chlorpromazine
Tranquilizers	Diazepam, opioids
Hormones	Corticosteroids, triiodthyronine, thyroxine
Laxatives	Magnesium salts
Hypnotics	Barbiturates, others

SOURCE: Reproduced by permission from Toyka and Mullges.[803]

muscular-blocking drugs should be avoided in patients with MG. Thus, the optimal means to achieve suitable intubation conditions is sedation and the use of topical anesthesia of the airway. Local anesthetic have been implicated in worsening of MG but not as dramatically as neuromuscular-blocking drugs.

GAS EXCHANGE   Patients presenting with a history suggestive of myasthenic crisis require close observation for imminent respiratory failure. Serial vital capacity measurements should be made every 2 to 4 h or more frequently if acute changes in status are occurring. Observation is also required for other signs of imminent respiratory failure, which include inability to swallow secretions, dyspnea, orthopnea, inability to hold the head up or off the bed, and increased alveolar-arterial gradient. In this setting if vital capacity has decreased to 10 to 15 ml/kg and the patient is not responding to anticholinesterase therapy then endotracheal intubation is indicated.

TEMPERATURE   Infection is a major exacerbating condition with MG. Thus, any infection should be treated aggressively, avoiding aminoglycosides if possible. Because infections are a major iatrogenic problem in the neuroICU, surveillance for infection is essential with every effort made to instrument the patient as little as possible.

ELECTROLYTES AND FLUIDS   Potassium and magnesium should be monitored and maintained in the normal range because abnormalities in their levels are associated with exacerbation of MG.

PERIOPERATIVE MANAGEMENT Differing approaches have been used in managing MG after surgery. Some advocate use of intravenous neostigmaine perioperatively, titrated to muscle strength because the severity of MG may vary after surgery. Others advocate discontinuing anticholinesterase therapy perioperatively, electively ventilating the patient for a few days after surgery, and then, after fluctuations in stress and perioperative medications have worn off, reinstitute the patient's anticholinesterase therapy.

STATUS EPILEPTICUS (see Chaps. 19, 20, 21)

PATHOPHYSIOLOGY

In over 50% of cases status epilepticus is the initial seizure event. It affects 50,000 to 60,000 people annually in the United States and carries a mortality rate of 3 to 10 percent.

Status epilepticus is defined as more than 30 min of continuous seizure activity, or two or more sequential seizures without full recovery of consciousness between seizures.[806,807] An urgent approach to seizure control is supported by observations of seizure-associated brain damage in humans[808] and by animal studies showing uncontrolled status epilepticus for 20 min or longer to be associated with neuronal damage.[809,810] Thus, generalized convulsive status epilepticus is considered to be a neurologic emergency.

Classification

The classification of seizures (both epileptic and nonepileptic) has changed during the last several decades. More precise delineations have been facilitated by the development of specialized epilepsy centers throughout the world. These centers use closed-circuit monitoring combined with scalp or intracranial EEG to record and review in detail the components of seizures. The most recent and widely accepted classification of epileptic seizures was published in 1981.[811] In addition to spontaneous epileptic seizures, alcohol withdrawal and exogenous toxins can also induce seizures. There are also "pseudoseizures," which have no EEG correlate and represent either conscious malingering or, more frequently, a psychiatric condition such as conversion disorder.[812] Differentiating between epileptic seizures, toxin-evoked seizures, and pseudoseizures may require expert skills and sophisticated resources.

Epilepsies are much more difficult to classify than seizures and will not be discussed. Interested readers are referred to a recent textbook by Engel.[813] A classification of seizures is presented in Table 36-18.

PARTIAL SEIZURES   A *partial seizure* is one that has a local or focal onset within the brain. The first type of clinically relevant partial seizure is the *simple partial*

TABLE 36-18
Classification of Seizures

I. Partial seizures
  A. Simple
  B. Complex
  C. Partial onset with generalization
II. Generalized seizures
  A. Inhibitory
    1. Absence
    2. Atomic
  B. Excitatory
    1. Myoclinic
    2. Clonic
    3. Tonic
III. Pseudoseizures
IV. Nonepileptic seizures

seizure. The term "simple" implies no detectable alteration in consciousness during the seizure. Electrographically, these seizures have a limited distribution in the brain, consistent with the notion that bilateral cerebral or reticular activating system involvement is required to alter consciousness. Simple partial seizures have frequently been termed "auras." When seizures spread into multiple areas of the brain and alter consciousness (no matter how slight) they are classified as *complex partial seizures.* Also termed "psychomotor" or "temporal lobe" seizures, complex partial seizures involve automatisms, different degrees of unresponsiveness, and are followed by amnesia. The final type of seizure in this category is *partial onset with generalization.* This seizure starts focally in one part of the brain and then spreads to involve much of the brain and brain stem, producing convulsive seizures. *Convulsive seizures* are usually either clonic or tonic, and once they occur, they are behaviorally indistinguishable from those with a primarily generalized onset. A simple partial seizure can progress to a complex partial seizure and then to a convulsion.

GENERALIZED SEIZURES   A generalized seizure occurs when the EEG shows simultaneous involvement of both cerebral hemispheres. The term "generalized seizures" implies that they have no focal onset; however, some types are multifocal or have a partial onset that cannot be resolved by present technology. Therefore, operationally, it is best to just categorize these seizures as generalized. This group can be divided into two major categories: *inhibitory* generalized seizures, which produce predominantly negative phenomenon and include absence seizures (petit mal seizures) and atonic seizures (during which the patient loses muscle tone and falls down), and (2) *excitatory* seizures, which produce positive phenomenon and include myoclonic, clonic, and tonic seizures.

PSEUDOSEIZURES   Pseudoseizures may mimic any of the previously mentioned partial or generalized seizures. If a patient's behaivor is clearly outside the range of that expected with a true seizure, this differentiation may be important. As many as 17 percent of patients admitted to an epilepsy unit turned out to have pseudoseizures.[812]

NONEPILEPTIC SEIZURES   Nonepileptic seizures caused by alcohol withdrawal or other exogenous toxins usually occur as generalized tonic or clonic seizures. However, some patients may have underlying brain damage that produces an area of decreased seizure threshold so that a partial onset may occur. Consequently, such patients may have multifocal seizures or focal motor seizures without having true epilepsy. Status epilepticus of these different types can occur in people who do not have epilepsy.

Pathogenesis of Seizure

Epilepsy is a rather heterogeneous disease with a diverse array of pathogenetic mechanisms. Seizures can arise as a result of abnormalities in (1) regulation of neural circuits, (2) the balance between excitation and inhibition, (3) extracellular potassium homeostasis, and (4) genes. This will be briefly overviewed. Several excellent recent reviews provide a more detailed summary.[814–817] Many of the mechanisms suggested for the genesis of seizures are hypotheses. However, they have been proposed in the context of ample experimental support to make them credible.

The CNS exists in a delicate equilibrium between depression and excitation. Pathologic processes that disrupt this can lead to seizure. This is the overriding concept that seems to be common to all of the theories of the pathogenesis of epilepsy.

ANATOMIC CIRCUIT MECHANISMS   Seizure activity is generated and propagated by specific neural circuits. These circuits often exist in a state of interactive modulation of their respective functions. That is, an excitatory pathway, in addition to sending afferents to a given structure, may also be modulated by another structure that will then modulate the originating excitatory source. One example of this in rat models is the substantia nigra. Available evidence indicates that the substantia nigra acts as a gating mechanism to modulate, via GABAergic efferents, excitation in other brain structures.[818,819]

Uncontrolled seizure produces selective neuronal loss that, one theory suggests, leads to disruption of the inhibitory-excitatory balance to favor subsequent recurrent seizures. Hippocampal sclerosis has long been associated with epilepsy. Resection of this injured area of the hippocampus substantially decreases sei-

zure tendency. This suggests that an initial seizure damages the hippocampus, which then leads to further seizures and worse hippocampal damage, further predisposing to seizure. Thus, a single inciting clinical event, such as a febrile seizure, could lead to this positive feedback cycle and epilepsy.[820]

Two theories have been suggested that could account for this phenomena of seizures begetting epilepsy. The first is the "dormant basket cell hypothesis."[821] Temporal lobe seizure leads to selective loss of excitatory cells in the hippocampus. These cells excite GABAergic interneurons to modulate the effects of the exciting afferent cell and other excitatory cells in the hippocampus. Thus, the paradoxical effect may arise wherein loss of excitatory cells results in more excitation due to synaptic dysinhibition. The second hypothesis, the "mossy fiber sprouting hypothesis," holds that increased dentate granule cell excitability is due to pathologic rearrangement of neuronal circuitry consequent to seizure-induced damage.[822,823] With the loss of the mossy cell, the granule cell, rather than synapsing with the mossy cell, synapses on itself in a positive manner such that the granule cell is more prone to have an increased response to an excitatory input[814] (Fig. 36-31). The anatomic basis for this observation has been reported in animal models[823–826] and in specimens from humans with epilepsy.[823,826,827]

LOCAL IMBALANCE BETWEEN EXCITATION AND INHIBITION   Excitation/inhibition imbalance is basically the mechanism of epileptogenesis with neuronal circuit abnormalities. Several mechanisms are important at the level of neurotransmitters and receptors, which can contribute to this imbalance. Enhanced function of the NMDA receptor has been identified in some animal models[828] and is thought to be related to a novel NMDA receptor type.[828] Consistent with these observations in animals are reports of enhanced excitatory amino acid receptor function in tissue from epileptic humans.[829] Conversely, experimental evidence indicates that the efficacy of GABA stimulation to increase chloride conductance decreases in kindled rats.[830] Similar observations, decreased GABA-A and benzodiazepine receptor binding and reduced benzodiazepine receptors, have also been made in humans with epilepsy.[831] Microdialysis studies indicate that there is increased release of excitatory amino acids in animal models[832] and in humans with epilepsy.[833] However, it is unclear if these observations are causative or are an effect of seizures.

EXTRACELLULAR POTASSIUM   The role of potassium in epilepsy has been very nicely reviewed and synthesized by McNamara.[814] Elevated extracellular potassium has been observed in in vivo seizure models in

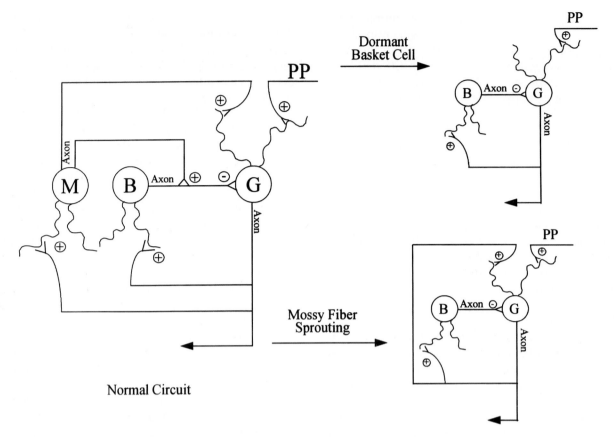

Figure 36-31 Simplified schematic of hypotheses suggested explaining increased dentate cell excitability in epilepsy and epilepsy models. Normal anatomic circuitry is depicted on the left showing mossy cells (M) providing excitatory input to the GABAergic inhibitory basket cells (B) and granule cells (G). In the dormant basket cell hypothesis, seizure-induced damage to mossy cells decreases activity of basket cells making granule cells more susceptible to excitation. In the mossy fiber sprouting hypothesis seizure-induced damage to mossy cells results in granule cells synapsing on themselves making granule cells more susceptible to excitation (Adapted by permission from McNamara[814] and reproduced by permission from Kofke and coworkers.[814a])

animals.[834,835] Whether such increases in extracellular potassium are causative of seizure or an epiphenomenon has been questioned.[836] In vitro studies have suggested that elevated extracellular potassium may be an important contributor to initiation and propagation of seizure.[837] The evidence is most supportive of the notion that high extracellular potassium is an important contributor to propagation of seizure, for example, after an interictal spike. The theory proposed suggests that a variety of epileptogenic events occur consequent to elevated extracellular potassium.[837] These consequences include: (1) partial depolarization, shifting the membrane potential closer to the spike threshold; (2) decreasing postburst after hypolarization, which normally limits repetitive firing; (3) reduction of the GABA-B component of the inhibitory postsynaptic potential (IPSP), which is mediated by potassium efflux,[838,839] while reducing the GABA-A component of the IPSP[840]; (4) swelling of cells via re-

duced potassium efflux,[841] further increasing extracellular potassium concentration through decreased size of the extracellular space[842] and further increasing neuronal synchronization[814]; and (5) depolarization induced by extracellular potassium promoting NMDA receptor activation.[843]

GENES   Inherited forms of epilepsy account for at least 20 percent of all patients with epilepsy.[844] Several animal models of genetic epilepsy identifying a variety of gene mutations that can cause epilepsy have been described. Indeed there are reports localizing some epilepsies in humans to a specific chromosome.[845] Studies of twins with epilepsy with a 65 percent concordance for penetrance of an epilepsy phenotype provide further support for the notion that there is a strong genetic influence on the development of epilepsy.[815] Several other studies of human and animal epilepsy have also been reported.[815] These studies clearly indicate that the genesis of epilepsy can be multifactorial and that several genetic abnormalities most certainly underlie the predisposition to develop epilepsy.

PRESENTATION

The term convulsion refers generally to generalized tonic-clonic motor seizures. A variety of presentations may be associated with this. The patient may notice feeling different or apathetic, depressed, or irritable. Other prodromes have also been associated with subsequent seizure, such as morning myoclonic jerks or headache. On over half the patients there is a remembered apparent precipitant such as jerking or palpitation, or an unusual feeling in the epigastic area. This aura is a simple complex seizure that is about to generalize. However, a seizure can also occur abruptly without prodromal warning. The initial motor signs of a generalized tonic-clonic seizure, as described by Adams,[846] are "a brief flexion of the trunk, an opening of the mouth and eyelids, and upward deviation of the eyes. The arms are elevated and abducted, the elbows semiflexed, and the hands pronated. These are followed by a more protracted extension phase, involving first the back and neck, then the arms and legs. There may be a piercing cry as the whole musculature is seized in a spasm and air is forcibly emitted through the closed vocal cords. Since the respiratory muscles are caught up in the tonic spasm, breathing is suspended, and after some seconds the skin and mucous membranes become cyanotic. The pupils are dilated and unreactive to light. The bladder may empty at this stage or later, during the postictal coma. This is the *tonic phase* of the seizure that lasts for 10 to 20 s."

"There then occurs a transition from the tonic to the *clonic phase* of the convulsion. At first there is a mild generalized tremor, which is in effect a repetitive relaxation of the tonic contraction. It begins at a rate of 8 per second and coarsens to 4 per second and then rapidly gives way to brief violent flexor spasms that come in rhythmic salvos and agitate the entire body. The face becomes violaceous and contorted by a series of grimaces and often the tongue is bitten. Autonomic signs are prominent: the pulse is rapid, blood pressure is elevated, pupils are dilated, and salivation and sweating are abundant; bladder pressure may increase sixfold during this phase. The clonic jerks decrease in amplitude and frequency over a period of about 30 s. The patient remains apneic until the end of the clonic phase, which is marked by a deep inspiration." If seizures stop the patient then enters the postictal phase characterized by varying degrees of altered consciousness. This may last minutes to hours. If another seizure recurs prior to return of consciousness and more than 30 min have passed the patient has technically begun to suffer not from an isolated seizure but rather from status epilepticus.

THERAPY

Primary Disease

To prevent brain damage,[808–810,847] seizures should be stopped as soon as possible, certainly within 60 min and, more optimally, within 30 min.[807–810,847] Treatment must be given within the first few minutes to prevent systemic, hypoxic, and cardiovascular complications. Subsequent antiseizure treatment should be effective within 20 to 30 min. Thus, attention should be given first to the basic life support ABCs (airway, breathing, circulation) and then to effective therapy to stop seizure activity.[806,807]

There are many different approaches to the management of convulsive status epilepticus. One of many methods of treatment is shown in Table 36-19. There has been controversy regarding which drug should be used initially for status epilepticus. Initial drug choices include phenobarbital,[807] phenytoin,[848] and a benzodiazepine.[849] Numerous studies have been published comparing different approaches to the initial management of status epilepticus. General principles have been outlined.[806,807] Seizures should be stopped as soon as possible, neuromuscular-blocking agents should not be used as primary anticonvulsant drugs, and therapy-induced hypoventilation, hypoxemia, and hypotension should be avoided. Benzodiazepines can be administered initially if convulsions are ongoing because of their reliability and prompt onset, followed by a longer-acting anticonvulsant such as phenobarbital or phenytoin.[806,807] Phenobarbital and phentoin can also reasonably be used as primary anticonvulsants, although they may require a somewhat longer time to be effective. Phenytoin, although generally effective, is sometimes awkward to administer and requires 15 to 20 min to effectivley control seizures in most patients.[848] Studies comparing phenobarbital or phenytoin with diazepam have shown diazepam to be effective but short lived,[850] and to be associated more often with endotracheal intubation.[851]

The primary advantage of benzodiazepines is that they are usually effective.[852–854] In addition, some evidence in animals suggests that postseizure maturation of damage in one area of the brain unrelated to the limbic system may be favorably altered with benzodiazepines,[855] although the clinical relevance of this is unclear. Many considerations influence the choice of benzodiazepine. Midazolam and diazepam have a shorter onset time than lorazepam, although lorazepam generally has a longer duration of action with a lower likelihood of severe respiratory depression, making it the preferred agent of some authors.[856] Diazepam has been reported to be effective rectally[857] and midazolam to be effective intramuscularly.[852] Both benzodiazepines have been used effectively as continuous infusions.[858,859] However, benzodiazepines should not be used alone for control of status epilepticus. A

TABLE 36-19
Timetable for the Treatment of Status Epilepticus

Time, min	Action
0–5	—Diagnose status epilepticus by observing continued seizure activity or one additional seizure. —Give oxygen by nasal cannula or mask; position patient's head for optimal airway patency; consider intubation if respiratory assistance is needed. —Obtain and record vital signs at onset and periodically thereafter; control any abnormalities as necessary; initiate ECG monitoring. —Establish an IV; draw venous blood samples for glucose level, serum chemistries, hematology studies, toxicology screens, and determinations of antiepileptic drug levels.
6–9	If hypoglycemia is established or a blood glucose determination is unavailable, administer glucose; in adults, give 100 mg of thiamine first, followed by 50 ml of 50% glucose by direct push into the IV; in children, the dose of glucose is 2 ml/kg of 25% glucose.
10–20	Administer either 0.1 mg/kg of lorazepam at 2 mg/min or 0.2 mg/kg of diazepam at 5 mg/min by IV; if diazepam is given, it can be repeated if seizures do not stop after 5 min; if diazepam is used to stop the status, phenytoin should be administered next to prevent recurrent status.
21–60	If status persists, administer 15–20 mg/kg of phenytoin no faster than 50 mg/min in adults and 1 mg/kg per min in children by IV; monitor ECG and blood pressure during the infusion; phenytoin is incompatible with glucose-containing solutions—the IV should be purged with normal saline before the phenytoin infusion.
>60	—If status does not stop after 20 mg/kg of phenytoin, give additional doses of 5 mg/kg to a maximal dose of 30 mg/kg. —If status persists, give 20 mg/kg of phenobarbital IV at 100 mg/min; when phenobarbital is given after a benzodiazepine, the risk of apnea or hypopnea is great and assisted ventilation is usually required. —If status persists, give anesthetic doses of drugs such as phenobarbital or pentobarbital or other anesthetic drugs; ventilatory assistance and vasopressors are virtually always necessary. —Appropriate anesthetic drugs include midazolam, thiopental, ketamine, etomidate, and isoflurane. Pros and cons of their use described in the text.

[a] Time starts at seizure onset. Note that a neurologic consultation is indicated if the patient does not wake up, convulsions continue after the administration of a benzodiazepine and phenytoin, or confusion exists at any time during evaluation and treatment.

NOTE: Anesthetic management guidelines are the opinion of the authors and are not based on randomized clinical trials.

SOURCE: Adapted by permission from The Epilepsy Foundation of America's Working Group on Status Epilepticus.[807]

longer-acting anticonvulsant such as phenytoin or phenobarbital should be given concomitantly to ensure long-term control of seizures once the effects of benzodiazepines wear off.

Concomitant with efforts to control seizures are efforts to diagnose and treat a reversible cause. Status epilepticus may be associated with preexisting epilepsy (often with reduction of antiepileptic drug intake), an acute progressive neurologic insult, or systemic metabolic disturbance, or no precipitating cause may be identified. Precipitants of status epilepticus may include meningitis, head trauma, postischemic-anoxic encephalopathy, hypoglycemia, electrolyte imbalances (hyponatremia, hypocalcemia), eclampsia, drug intoxication, fever, tumor, remote neurologic insults such as stroke, cerebral palsy, or trauma, or congenital abnormalities.[807] Idiopathic causes account for about one-third of cases.[807]

Anesthetic Considerations

After all standard therapy has failed or has been determined to have unacceptable side effects, or if frequent seizures result in acidosis despite anticonvulsant therapy, most neurology textbooks recommend consulting an anesthesiologist for administration of general anesthesia to manage status epilepticus. Under these circumstances, what anesthetic should the anesthesiologist administer? Unfortunately, no controlled clinical studies exist to answer this question adequately. Several clinical series have been published, however, reporting experience with different anesthetic approaches. Anesthetic agents and adjuvants that have been used successfully to stop seizures include pentobarbital,[860-862] thiopental,[863] benzodiazepines,[852,854,856-859] isoflurane,[864-866] etomidate,[867] propofol,[868] ketamine,[869] enflurane,[870] halothane,[866,870] and althesin.[871]

In a situation where general anesthesia is needed, patient outcome is thought to correlate more with the underlying disease than with success in stopping seizures,[865] as initiation of general anesthesia is usually significantly delayed once seizures have begun. Such a therapeutic approach generally involves significant respiratory and hemodynamic side effects that require intubation, mechanical ventilation, and some cardiovascular monitoring or therapy. Moreover, prolonged use of high doses of barbiturates has been associated with barbiturate tolerance,[864,872] which may exacerbate the underlying seizure problem. Administration of volatile anesthetics outside the operating room is fraught with logistic problems including staffing and gas scavenging issues.[864–866] In addition, the neurochemical effects of such prolonged anesthetic use have never been evaluated. One study using animals suggests that prolonged anesthetic use can result in substantial increases in brain glycogen after only a few hours.[873] Moreover, the potential for prolonged volatile anesthesia to be organotoxic or induce tolerance is unknown.

The foregoing information suggests that a specific approach may be appropriate when general anesthesia is being considered for status epilepticus. It is important to understand that this approach is a synthesis of data from animal studies and clinical reports and that there have been no randomized clinical trials. Once it is clear that routine anticonvulsant therapy is not maintaining the patient seizure free, benzodiazepine therapy should be escalated. Continuous EEG monitoring is helpful at this point to assist in titration of therapy and evaluate for the possibility of continued nonconvulsive status epielpticus. Midazolam can be administered as an infusion titrated versus motor seizure and EEG. If this is ineffective, thiopental or pentobarbital should be added. It is common that patients in this situation require pressors or fluids to maintain blood pressure. If this is a major consideration in a given patient, then intravenous etomidate[867] or ketamine,[869] which are better tolerated hemodynamically, can be used instead of high-dose barbiturate or benzodiazepine therapy. However, the experience with these drugs is not as extensive as with benzodiazepines and barbiturates and unknown problems may arise. If etomidate is used it is advisable to concomitantly administer glucocorticoids to avoid sequelae of etomidate-induced adrenal suppression.[874]

If such therapy with intravenous anesthetics is ineffective or there is concern about the risk of further cardiovascular depression, then isoflurane anesthesia should be administered to attain control of seizures. It is useful when there are cardiovascular concerns because the option is retained to treat adverse hemodynamic effects by rapidly decreasing the blood concentration. In addition, volatile anesthetics have advantages related to being able to continuously titrate them to maintain anticonvulsant levels specific to EEG activity. They are the only anticonvulsants with which this can be done. In one patient,[865] monitoring end-tidal volatile anesthetic concentration facilitated titration of the anticonvulsant anesthetic against EEG once the patient's seizure tendency appeared to subside after organophosphate ingestion. In another patient, isoflurane use facilitated withdrawal of a prolonged barbiturate infusion on which the patient was suspected to be dependent.[864] Thus, volatile anesthetics may have a role in closely titrating anticonvulsant therapy for

seizures in situations wherein the duration of use can reasonably be expected to be short lived.

One study described the neuropathologic effects of anesthetic choice on seizure-induced brain damage.[855] Isoflurane, thiopental, ketamine, and midazolam were assessed in rats undergoing mercaptopropionic acid or flurothyl-induced seizures. Midazolam use resulted in less damage in the substantia nigra after seizures. No protective effect was found with isoflurane or thiopental, and although a protective effect was suggested with ketamine, it was statistically insignificant. Unfortunately, this study revealed nothing about the anesthetic effects on seizure-induced damage in the limbic system. The ketamine data, however, are supported by other reports of the anticonvulsant or neuroprotective effects of ketamine in the limbic system during seizure in rodents.[875–878]

The standard approach to managing seizures with a general anesthetic is to use as little anesthetic as possible, while observing closely for cessation of seizure and hemodynamic compromise. Such patients must be tracheally intubated and mechanically ventilated. EEG should be monitored throughout anesthetic administration. If thiopental is used, 50 to 500 mg intravenously can be given as a loading dose (in an adult) followed by an intravenous infusion. After the loading dose, the infusion rate can be initially set at 500 to 1000 mg/h and decreased thereafter to the lowest rate feasible. Repeated boluses might be needed initially or throughout to maintain close titration. A similar algorithm can be used with equipotent doses of other intravenous drugs. If isoflurane is used, it should be started at 0.2% to 0.3% inspired concentration and increased over 10 to 20 min as indicated by EEG and as tolerated hemodynamically. The anesthesiologist should be prepared to educate neuroICU nurses and primary service physicians at the bedside about the effects of isoflurane. An anesthesia machine is usually used to administer isoflurane. A satisfactory scavenging system can usually be fashioned with the suction system in the neuroICU. As this is a rather unusual therapy to use in neuroICU, it is the authors' opinion that continuous bedside presence of an anesthesia caregiver be maintained.

Determining the endpoint to guide anesthetic drug titration can be enigmatic because bursts occurring in a burst-suppression pattern on EEG can resemble epileptiform discharges. The decision should be made jointly with the referring neurologist or epileptologist. Once seizures are controlled, and if the etiology is still unclear, reversible causes should be sought and corrected, after which anesthesia should be stopped. Otherwise, the anesthetic dose should be decreased periodically to permit assessment. If seizures continue to recur on anesthetic discontinuation, an ethical decision must be made. This decision must consider the many unknown effects and logistic and economic issues related to prolonged anesthetic administration, as opposed to the effects of allowing seizures to continue or withdrawing life support.

CCM Considerations

Status epilepticus can produce a variety of systemic abnormalities of concern.[807,879,880]

AIRWAY MANAGEMENT AND GAS EXCHANGE   Status epilepticus by definition includes unconsciousness. With this, airway and gas exchange can become compromised, particularly if vomiting has occurred. Consequently, hypoxemia and hypercarbia can arise. If the patient has a brief seizure followed by a postictal phase with easy breathing and normal pulse oximetry, simple administration of oxygen is generally sufficient unless there is vomiting, in which case endotracheal intubation should be performed. If status epilepticus has developed, particularly if CNS-depressant drugs are being given or there are copious secretions, endotracheal intubation should be performed. Generally, a potent hypnotic such as thiopental and neuromuscular-blocking drugs should be administered to provide suitable intubating conditions. This is made necessary by the involuntary movements associated with the seizure. If the seizures are nonmotor then other approaches can be considered. Patients chronically receiving anticonvulsant therapy will be somewhat tolerant to fentanyl and higher than normal fentanyl doses, although still titrated, may be needed. In addition, the effects of fentanyl[881] and nondepolarizing neuromuscular blockade[882–885] are shortened on patients previously being treated with anticonvulsants.

TEMPERATURE   Status epilepticus generally is associated with hyperthermia. This is thought to exacerbate the seizure-induced brain damage.[188] Every effort should be made to maintain normothermia.

BLOOD PRESSURE MANAGEMENT   Hypertension usually occurs early in status epilepticus. With time, however, blood pressure generally decreases and may fall to hypotensive levels. If seizures are continuing such a decrease in blood pressure, perhaps normally well tolerated, may be associated with exacerbation of the neurologic sequelae of prolonged seizure. There is theoretical concern that overzealous use of antihypertensive drugs, despite the presence of normotension, may provide insufficient substrate supply in a hypermetabolic brain.[886] Brady- and tachyarrhythmias can occur as can cardiac arrest.

GLUCOSE   Hypoglycemia can arise as either a cause or result of status epilepticus. As the duration of uncontrolled seizures increases, hyperglycemia will tend to occur as a secondary phenomenon. Insulin secretion induced by this, possibly combined with exhaustion of glycogen stores, can then result in secondary hypoglycemia. Assessment of glucose is indicated. Animal studies indicate that, unlike cerebral ischemia, hyperglycemia is not deleterious with status epilepticus.[887,888] Thus, aggressive maintenance of normoglycemia, particularly because hypoglycemia is a known risk, seems to be not warranted unless the blood glucose level is quite high.

ELECTROLYTES AND FLUIDS   Seizures can be associated with renal dysfunction.[879] An important contributing factor is rhabdomyolysis, which can occur with prolonged seizure. A variety of metabolic abnormalities can arise with status epilepticus. These abnormalities include acidosis, hyperkalemia, hypoglycemia, hyponatremia, and hyperkalemia. Appropriate laboratory studies are required with treatment of any abnormalities as they occur.

MENINGITIS/ENCEPHALITIS

PATHOPHYSIOLOGY

Bacterial meningitis occurs when pathogenic virulence factors overcome host defense mechanisms.[889] The barriers traversed by an invading bacterium include mucosa, intravascular space, BBB, and CSF. Clinical symptoms of meningitis arise predominantly from the inflammatory response of the host. Components of bacteria walls appear to be very important in provoking this response.[889,890] This inflammatory response includes the appearance of substantial polymorphonuclear leukocytes in the infected region. Inflammatory mediators such as interleukin-1, interleukin-6, and tumor necrosis factor are elaborated and the BBB permeability increases.[889–891] Brain edema develops with intracranial hypertension.[892,893] CBF initially increases and subsequently decreases with deterioration of cerebrovascular autoregulation.[894,895]

Virtually any bacterium can produce meningitis. However, the most common causative organisms are *Streptococcus pneumoniae, Haemophilus influenzae, Nisseria meningitidus, Escherichia coli,* and *Listeria monocytogenes.*[889] These and other less common organisms gain entry to the CNS predominantly via the bloodstream. However, infections can also arise from middle ear infections, sinusitis, congenital neuroectodermal defects, craniotomy sites, or skull fractures.[896]

PRESENTATION

The generally recognized clinical signs of early bacterial meningitis are fever, severe headache, generalized motor seizures, altered mental status, and neck stiff-

TABLE 36-20
Presenting Signs of Bacterial Meningitis in Adults[897]

Percentage	Sign
95	Fever (≥37.7°C or 100°F) at presentation
99	Fever within 24 h of admission
88	Nuchal rigidity
11	Rash (73% of whom had meningococcal meningitis)
79	Altered mental status
51	Confusion or lethargy
22	Responsive only to pain
6	Unresponsive to any stimuli
29	Focal seizure or focal deficits
23	Seizures
7	Focal seizures
13	Generalized seizures

ness. Brudzinski sign (flexion of the hip in response to flexion of the neck) and Kernig sign (inability to extend the legs) may also be present but not reliably, particularly if the patient is very young or stuporous.[896] A recent study summarized in 493 patients the presentation and course of adults with bacterial meningitis.[897] Only two-thirds of the patients showed the classic triad for meningitis of fever, nuchal rigidity, and altered mental status, although every patient had at least one of these signs. A summary of the findings are listed in Table 36-20.

Typical CSF findings include elevated opening pressure, pleocytosis, elevated protein, decreased glucose concentration, and positive culture. However, these findings are not a constant in all patients with bacterial meningitis. In community-acquired meningitis: opening pressure is 140 mmH$_2$O or greater in 91 percent, white cell count is above 100/mm^3 in 90 percent, percent neutrophils is over 20 in 98 percent, total protein is greater than 46 in 96 percent, glucose is less than 40 mg/dl in 50 percent, CSF is gram positive in 60 percent, and CSF is culture positive in 73 percent. In patients with nosocomial meningitis opening pressure is 140 mmH$_2$O or greater in 77 percent, white cell count is above 100/mm^3 in 83 percent, percent neutrophils is over 20 in 98 percent, total protein is greater than 46 in 94 percent, glucose is less than 40 mg/dl in 45 percent, CSF is gram positive in 46 percent, and CSF is culture positive in 83 percent.[897] Counterimmunoelectrophoresis can be additionally done on the CSF. This sensitive technique permits identification of bacterial antigens in the CSF in a very short period of time.[896]

During the course of meningitis a variety of neurologic complications can arise.[896a] CNS complications include arterial or venous ischemia/infarction, cerebral edema, hydrocephalus, abscess, subdural empyema or effusion, diabetes insipidus, and SIADH. Systemic complications include routine ICU complications but in addition include septic shock, disseminated intravascular coagulation, adult respiratory distress syndrome, septic arthritis, or rhabdomyolysis.

Initial therapeutic decisions may be based on the likelihood of a given bacterium producing the patient's infection. Clinical scenarios have been associated with different pathogens. *Meningococcus* meningitis typically occurs with a very fast onset accompanied by a purpuric, petechial, or ecchymotic rash and cardiovascular collapse. It may occur in the setting of a known epidemic. *Pneumococcus* meningitis is commonly preceded by infection of the sinuses, ears, lungs, or heart valves, or appears in patients who are alcoholic or have undergone prior splenectomy. In addition, it is associated with recurrent meningitis, dermal sinus tracts, sickle cell anemia, and basilar skull fracture. *H. influenzae* meningitis usually occurs in children after infections of the respiratory tract. *Staphylococcus* infection should be considered when meningitis occurs after a neurosurgical procedure.[896]

THERAPY
Primary Disease
Bacterial meningitis should be attended to diagnostically and therapeutically in an emergent manner. It is a potentially reversible disease process that is fatal in 20 percent of the cases.[897] The initial therapy should include immediate antibiotic administration in a dose sufficient to enter the CNS in bactericidal concentrations. The initial choice of antibiotic is typically based on the history and Gram stain. After definitive cultures are available, the antibiotic may be changed as appropriate. Which of the three most common types of bacteria may be involved are outlined above. *Pneumococcus* or *meningococcus* meningitis should be treated with penicillin; *H. influenzae* meningitis with chloramphenicol, ampicillin (if ampicillin resistance has been ruled out), or a third-generation cephalosporin (cefotaxime, cefoperazone, ceftizoxime); and *staphylococcus* meningitis with a penicillinase-resistant penicillin (oxacillin or nafcillin) or vancomycin. Therapy should be continued for 2 weeks or longer if the source infection is known and is persisting (e.g., sinus infection).

CCM Considerations
AIRWAY MANAGEMENT Concerns for airway management are related to the potential for elevated ICP and sinus infection. Thus, intubation should be performed using methods thought to not adversely affect ICP. In addition, transnasal intubation is relatively contraindicated due to possible development of sinusitis.

Such a development would obfuscate somewhat efforts to elucidate the cause of the meningitis.

GAS EXCHANGE   If the source of the meningitis is a pulmonary infection, then pneumonia may be an added concern with potential for inadequate gas exchange and exacerbation of the neurologic injury.

TEMPERATURE   Fever is a very common effect of meningitis. Because ischemic complications also occur with meningitis and fever can exacerbate the effects of ischemia, it becomes essential that fever be vigorously treated.

BLOOD PRESSURE MANAGEMENT   Blood pressure management should be similar to that with elevated ICP and stroke. However, there is the additional concern that sepsis-related abnormalities in cardiovascular homeostasis may occur. Sepsis-induced decreases in blood pressure can turn an area of cerebral ischemia into an area of cerebral infarction. Thus, careful attention to maintenance of suitable perfusion pressure is essential.

GLUCOSE   Due to problems with high ICP and cerebral ischemia, hyperglycemia should be avoided. However, no studies have specifically examined the role of glucose in the pathogenesis of brain damage after meningitis.

ELECTROLYTES AND FLUIDS   Serial assessment of sodium and fluid balance is essential to detect and treat diabetes insipidus or SIADH should either syndrome arise.

References

1. Goldberg S: *The Four-Minute Neurologic Exam.* Miami, Med-Master, 1992.
2. Rimel RW, Tyson GW; The neurologic examination in patients with central nervous system trauma. *J Neurosurg Nurs* 1979; 11:148.
3. Pitts LH: Neurological evaluation of the head injury patient. *Clin Neurosurg* 1982; 29:203.
4. Scott M: Infectious hazards of neurologic tests. *N Engl J Med* 1969; 280:904.
5. Tomasello F, et al: Assessment of inter-observer differences in the Italian multicenter study on reversible cerebral ischemia. *Stroke* 1982; 13:32.
6. Marr JA, Reid B: Spinal cord testing: Auditing for quality assurance. *J Neurosci Nurs* 1991; 23:101.
7. Vogel HP: Influence of additional information in interrater reliability in the neurologic examination. *Neurology* 1992; 42:2076.
8. Halar EM, et al: Sensory perception threshold measurement: An evaluation of semiobjective testing devices. *Arch Phys Med Rehabil.* 1987; 68:499.
9. Mills RJ, Renfrew S: Measurement of pain threshold by thermal contact. *Lancet* 1971; 1:738.
10. Ropper AH, et al: Computer-guided neurologic assessment in the neurologic intensive care unit. *Heart Lung* 1981; 10:54.
11. Lord-Feroli K, Maguire-McGinty M: Toward a more objective approach to pupil assessment. *J Neurosurg Nurs* 1985; 17:309.
12. Stern PH: Quantitative clinical neurological examination. *Neurology* 1970; 20:419.
13. Klose KJ, et al: University of Miami Neuro-Spinal Index (UMNI): A quantitative method for determining spinal cord function. *Paraplegia* 1980; 18:331.
14. Botsford DJ, Esses SI: A new scale for the clinical assessment of spinal cord function. *Orthopedics* 1992; 15:1309.
15. Teasdale G, Jennett B: Assessment and prognosis of coma after head injury. *Acta Neurochir (Wien)* 1976; 34:45.
16. Saloman M, et al: Calculated recovery rates in severe head trauma. *Neurosurgery* 1981; 8:301.
17. Cote R, et al: The Canadian Neurological Scale: A preliminary study in acute stroke. *Stroke* 1986; 17:731.
18. Adams RJ, et al: Graded neurologic scale for use in acute hemispheric stroke treatment protocols. *Stroke* 1987; 18:665.
19. Collin C, Wade D: Assessing motor impairment after stroke: A pilot reliability study. *J Neurol Neurosurg Psychiatry* 1990; 53:576.
20. Orgogozo JM, et al: A unified form for neurological scoring of hemispheric stroke with motor impairment. *Stroke* 1992; 23:1678.
21. Clifton GL, et al: Outcome measures for clinical trials involving traumatically brain-injured patients: Report of a conference. *Neurosurgery* 1992; 31:975.
21a. Hansen-Flaschen J, et al: Beyond the Ramsay scale: Need for a validated measure of sedating drug efficacy in the intensive care unit. *Crit Care Med* 1994; 22:732 (editorial).
21b. Crosby L, Parson LC: Clinical neurologic assessment tool: Development and testing of an instrument to index neurologic status. *Heart Lung* 1989; 18:121.
22. Ursino M: Mechanisms of CBF regulation. *Crit Rev Biomed Eng* 1991; 18:255.
23. Kuschinsky M: Coupling of blood flow and metabolism in the brain. *J Basic Clin Physiol Pharmacol* 1990; 1:1991.
24. Meyer JS, et al: Effects of alpha adrenergic blockade on autoregulation and chemical vasomotor control of CBF in stroke. *Stroke* 1973; 4:187.
25. Muizelaar JP, et al: Effect of mannitol on ICP and CBF and correlation with pressure autoregulation in severely head-injured patients. *J Neurosurg* 1984; 61:700.
26. Cavestri R, et al: Influence of erythrocyte aggregability and plasma fibrinogen concentration on CBF with aging. *Acta Neurol Scand* 1992; 85:292.
27. Bowton DK, et al: Pentoxifylline increases CBF in patients with cerebrovascular disease. *Stroke* 1989; 20:1662.
28. Hanko JH, et al: Neuropeptide Y induces and modulates vasoconstriction in intracranial and peripheral vessels of animals and man. *J Auton Pharmacol* 1986; 6:117.
29. Owman C, et al: Pharmacological in vitro analysis of amine-mediated vasomotor functions in the intracranial and extracranial vascular beds. *Blood Vessels* 1978; 15:128.
30. Uddman R, Edvinsson L: Neuropeptides in the cerebral circulation. *Cerebrovasc Brain Metab Rev* 1989; 1:230.
31. Hardebo JE, et al: Excitatory amino acids and cerebrovascular tone. *Acta Physiol Scand* 1989; 136:483.
32. Parsons AA: 5-HT receptors in human and animal cerebrovasculature. *Trends Pharmacol Sci* 1991; 12:310.
33. Jansen I, et al: Tachykinins (substance P, neurokinin A, neuropeptide K, and neurokinin B) in the cerebral circulation: Vaso-

motor responses in vitro and in situ. *J Cereb Blood Flow Metab* 1991; 11:567.

34. Owman C: Peptidergic vasodilator nerves in the peripheral circulation and in the vascular beds of the heart and brain. *Blood Vessels* 1990; 27:73.

35. Paulson OB, Waldemar G: Role of the local renin-angiotensin system in the autoregulation of the cerebral circulation. *Blood Vessels* 1991; 28:231.

36. Sato A, Sato Y: Regulation of regional CBF by cholinergic fibers originating in the basal forebrain. *Neurosci Res* 1992; 14:242.

37. Toda N, Okamura T: Cerebral vasoconstrictor mediators. *Pharmacol Ther* 1993; 57:359.

38. Faraci FM, Brian JE Jr: Nitric oxide and the cerebral circulation. *Stroke* 1994; 25:692.

39. Garnett ES, et al: Regional CBF in man manipulated by direct vagal stimulation. PACE Pacing Clin Electrophysiol 1992; 15:1579.

40. Suzuki N, Hardebo JE: The cerebrovascular parasympathetic innervation. *Cerebrovasc Brain Metab Rev* 1993; 5:33.

41. Meglio M, et al: Spinal cord stimulation and cerebral haemodynamics. *Acta Neurochir (Wien)* 1991; 111:43.

42. Decety J, et al: The cerebellum participates in mental activity: Tomographic measurements of regional CBF. *Brain Res* 1990; 535:313.

43. Iadecola C, et al: Nitric oxide synthase inhibition and cerebrovascular regulation. *J Cereb Blood Flow Metab* 1994; 14:175 (review).

44. Kuschinsky W, Paulson OB: Capillary circulation in the brain. *Cerebrovasc Brain Metab Rev* 1992; 4:261.

45. Kuschinsky W: Coupling of function, metabolism, and blood flow in the brain. *Neurosurg Rev* 1991; 14:163.

46. Faraci FM, et al: Cerebral circulation: Humoral regulation and effects of chronic hypertension. *J Am Soc Nephrol* 1990; 1:53.

47. Faraci FM, Heistad DD: Regulation of cerebral blood vessels by humoral and endothelium-dependent mechanisms. Update on humoral regulation of vascular tone. *Hypertension* 1991; 17:917.

48. Kontos HA: Nitric oxide and nitrosothiols in cerebrovascular and neuronal regulation. *Stroke* 1993; 24:I115.

49. Spatz M, et al: Vasoconstrictive peptides induce endothelin-1 and prostanoids in human cerebromicrovascular endothelium. *Am J Physiol* 1994; 266:C654.

50. Faraci FM: Regulation of the cerebral circulation by endothelium. *Pharmacol Ther* 1992; 56:1.

51. Waldemar G, Paulson OB: Angiotensin converting enzyme inhibition and cerebral circulation—a review. *Br J Clin Pharmacol* 1989; 28(suppl 2):177S.

52. Giller CA: The frequency-dependent behavior of cerebral autoregulation. *Neurosurgery* 1990; 27:362.

53. Globus M, et al: The effect of chronic propranolol therapy on regional CBF in hypertensive patients. *Stroke* 1983; 14:964.

54. Pearson RM, et al: Comparisons of effects on CBF of rapid reduction in systemic arterial pressure by diazoxide and labetalol in hypertensive patients: Preliminary findings. Br J Clin Pharmacol 1979; 8(suppl 2):195S.

55. Griffith DN, et al: The effect of beta-adrenergic receptor blocking drugs on CBF. *Br J Clin Pharmacol* 1979; 7:491.

56. Olesen J, et al: Isoproterenol and propranolol: Ability to cross the blood-brain barrier and effects on cerebral circulation in man. *Stroke* 1978; 9:344.

57. Guell A, et al: Effects of a dopaminergic agonist (pirlbedil) on CBF in man. *J Cereb Blood Flow Metab* 1982; 2:255.

58. Oleson J: The effect of intracarotid epinephrine, norepinephrine, and angiotensin on the regional CBF in man. *Neurology* 1972; 22:978.

59. Raichle ME, et al: CBF during and after hyperventilation. *Arch Neurol* 1970; 23:3.

60. Greenberg JH, et al: Local cerebral blood volume response to carbon dioxide in man. *Circ Res* 1987; 43:324.

61. Iliff LD, et al: Cerebrovascular carbon dioxide reactivity and conductance in patients awake and under general anesthesia. *Neurology* 1976; 26:835.

62. Tominaga S, et al: Cerebrovascular CO_2 reactivity in normotensive and hypertensive man. *Stroke* 1976; 7:507.

63. Skinhoj E: Regulation of CBF as a single function of the interstitial pH in the brain. A hypotheses. *Acta Neurol Scand* 1966; 42:604.

64. Lassen NA, et al. Effects of acetazolamide on CBF and brain tissue oxygenation. *Postgrad Med J* 1987; 63:185.

65. Sullivan HG, et al: The rCBF response to Diamox in normal subjects and cerebrovascular disease patients. *J Neurosurg* 1987; 67:525.

66. Vorstrup S, et al: Effect of acetazolamide on CBF and cerebral metabolic rate for oxygen. *J Clin Invest* 1984; 74:1674.

67. Yonas H, Pindzola RR: Physiological determination of cerebrovascular reserves and its use in clinical management. *Cerebrovasc Brain Metab Rev* 1994; 6:325 (review).

68. Bushnell DL, et al: Evaluation of cerebral perfusion reserve using 5% CO_2 and SPECT neuroperfusion imaging. *Clin Nucl Med* 1991; 16:263.

69. Shimojyo S, et al: The effects of graded hypoxia upon transient CBF and oxygen consumption. *Neurology* 1968; 18:127.

70. Sawaya R, Ingvar DH: CBF and metabolism in sleep. *Acta Neurol Scand* 1989; 80:481.

71. Madsen PL, Vorstrup S: CBF and metabolism during sleep. *Cerebrovasc Brain Metab Rev* 1991; 3:28.

72. Reich T, Rusinek H: Cerebral cortical and white matter reactivity to carbon dioxide. *Stroke* 1989; 20:453.

73. Chiron C, et al: Changes in regional CBF during brain maturation in children and adolescents. *J Nucl Med* 1992; 33:696.

74. Strandgarrd S: CBF in the elderly: Impact of hypertension and antihypertensive treatment. *Cardiovasc Drugs Ther* 1991; 6:1217.

75. Martin AJ, et al: Decreases in regional CBF with normal aging. *J Cereb Blood Flow Metab* 1991; 11:684.

76. Heistad DD, Baumbach GL: Cerebral vascular changes during chronic hypertension: Good guys and bad guys. *J Hypertens Suppl* 1992; 10:S71.

77. Graham DI: Ischemic brain following emergency blood pressure lowering in hypertensive patients. *Acta Med Scand Suppl* 1983; 678:61.

78. Bertel O, et al: Effects of antihypertensive treatment on cerebral perfusion. *Am J Med* 1987; 82:29.

79. Minematsu K, et al: Effects of angiotensin converting enzyme inhibitor (captopril) on CBF in hypertensive patients without a history of stroke. *Clin Exp Hypertens A* 1987; 9:551.

80. Goldberg HI, et al: Patterns of cerebral dysautoregulation in severe hypertension to blood pressure reduction with diazoxide. *Acta Neurol Scand* 1977; 64:64.

81. Kindt GW, et al: Factors influencing the autoregulation of the CBF during hypotension and hypertension. *J Neurosurg* 1967; 26:299.

82. Paulson OB, Waldemar G: ACE inhibitors and CBF. *J Hum Hypertens* 1990; 4:69072.

83. Thompson SW: Reactivity of CBF to CO_2 in patients with transient cerebral ischemic attacks. *Stroke* 1971; 2:273.

84. McHenry LC Jr, et al: Regional CBF. Response to carbon dioxide inhalation in cerebrovascular disease. *Arch Neurol* 1972; 27:403.

85. Clifton GL, et al: Cerebrovascular CO_2 reactivity after carotid artery occlusion. *J Neurosurg* 1988; 69:24.

86. Levine RK, et al: Blood flow asymmetry in carotid occlusive disease. *Angiology* 1992; 43:100.

87. Schroeder T: Cerebrovascular reactivity to acetazolamide in carotid artery disease. Enhancement of side-to-side CBF asymmetry indicates critically reduced perfusion pressure. *Neurol Res* 1986; 8:231.

88. Hojer-Pedersen E: Effect of acetazolamide on CBF in subacute and chronic cerebrovascular disease. *Stroke* 1987; 18:887.

89. Schalen W, et al: Cerebral vasoreactivity and the prediction of outcome in severe traumatic brain lesions. *Acta Anaesthesiol Scand* 1991; 35:113.

90. Widner W, et al: Collateral circulation in the posterior fosa via leptomeningeal anastomoses. *Am J Roentgenol Radium Ther Nucl Med* 1965; 95:831.

91. Mikhailov SS, Kagan II: The anastomoses of the venous system of the brain and their role in the collateral circulation. *Folia Morphol* 1968; 16:10.

92. Hegedus SA, Shackelford RT: Carbon dioxide and obstructed CBF. Correlation between CBF, crossfilling, and neurological findings. *JAMA* 1965; 191:279.

93. Haltia M, et al: Spontaneous occlusion of the circle of Willis (Moyamoya syndrome). *Clin Neuropathol* 1982; 1:11.

94. Good WF, Gur D: Xenon-enhanced CT to the brain: Effect of flow activation on derived CBF measurements. *AJNR Am J Neuroradiol* 1991; 12:83.

95. Yonas H: Use of xenon and ultrafast CT to measure CBF. *AJNR Am J Neuroradiol* 1994; 15:794.

96. Kashiwagi S, et al: The washin/washout protocol in stable xenon CT CBF studies. *AJNR Am J Neuroradiol* 1992; 13:49.

97. Britton KE, et al: CBF in hypertensive patients with cerebrovascular disease: technique for measurement and effect of captopril. *Nucl Med Commun* 1985; 6:251.

98. Dublin AB, et al: Carotid blood flow response to Conray-60: Diagnostic implications. *AJNR Am J Neuroradiol* 1983; 4:274.

99. Obrist WD, et al: Regional CBF estimated by 133-xenon inhalation. *Stroke* 1975; 6:245.

100. Obrist WD, et al: A subtraction method for determining CBF by xenon-133 inhalation. *Neurology* 1970; 20:411.

101. Miyamori I, et al: Effects of a calcium entry blocker on cerebral circulation in essential hypertension. *J Clin Hypertens* 1987; 3:528.

102. Kanno I, et al: Optimal scan time of oxygen-15-labeled water injection method for measurement of CBF. *J Nucl Med* 1991; 32:1931.

103. Iida H, et al: Rapid measurement of CBF with positron emission tomography. *Ciba Found Symp* 1991; 163:3.

104. Maier-Hauff K, et al: CBF measurements with HMPAO- and HiPOM-SPECT in brain tumors: Basic rCBF studies. *Psychiatry Res* 1989; 29:341.

105. Hayashida K, et al: Validation of eliminate vascular activity on 99Tcm-HMPAO brain SPECT for regional CBF (rCBF) determination. *Nucl Med Commun* 1991; 12:545.

106. Pupi A, et al: An analysis of the arterial input curve for technetium-99m-HMPAO: Quantification of rCBF using single-photon emission computed tomography. *J Nucl Med* 1991; 32:1501.

107. Murase K, et al: Kinetic behavior of technetium-99m-HMPAO in the human brain and quantification of CBF using dynamic SPECT. *J Nucl Med* 1992; 33:135.

108. Schmidt JF: Changes in human CBF estimated by the (A-V) O_2 difference method. *Dan Med Bull* 1992; 39:335.

109. Cruz J, et al: Continuous monitoring of cerebral hemodynamic reserve in acute brain injury: Relationship to changes in brain swelling. *J Trauma* 1992; 32:629.

110. Oldendorf WH, Kitano M: Radioisotope measurement of brain blood turnover time as a clinical index of brain circulation. *J Nucl Med* 1967; 8:570.

111. Karpman HL, Sheppard JJ: Effect of papaverine hydrochloride on CBF as measured by forehead thermograms. *Angiology* 1975; 26:592.

112. Dickman CA, et al: Continuous regional cerebral blood low monitoring in acute craniocerebral trauma. *Neurosurgery* 1991; 28:467.

113. Merrick MV, et al: Parametric imaging of cerebral vascular reserves. 1. Theory, validation and normal values. *Eur J Nucl Med* 1991; 18:171

114. Frerichs KU, Feurestein GZ: Laser-Doppler flowmetry. A review of its application for measuring cerebral and spinal cord blood flow. *Mol Chem Neuropathol* 1990; 12:55.

115. Gould RG: Perfusion quantitation by ultrafast coomputed tomography. *Invest Radiol* 1992; 27(suppl 2):S18.

116. Hartmann A, et al: Effect of stable xenon on region CBF and the electroencephalogram in normal volunteers. *Stroke* 1991; 22:182.

117. Yonas H, et al: Effects of xenon inhalation on CBF: Relevance to humans of reported effects in the rat. *J Cereb Blood Flow Metab* 1985; 5:613.

118. Obrist WD, et al: Determination of regional CBF by inhalation of 133-Xenon. *Circ Res* 1967; 20:124.

119. Obrist WD, Wilkinson WE: Regional CBF measurement in humans by xenon-133 clearance. *Cerebrovasc Brain Metab Rev* 1990; 2:283 (review).

120. Skyhoj Olsen T, et al: Focal cerebral ischemia measured by the intra-arterial 133-xenon method. Limitations of 2-dimensional blood flow measurements. *Stroke* 1981; 12:73.

121. Otis SM: Pitfalls in transcranial Doppler diagnosis. In Babikian VL, Wechsler LR (eds): *Transcranial Doppler Ultrasonography*, St. Louis, Mosby, 1993:39–50.

122. Tegeler CH, Eicke M: Physics and principles of transcranial Doppler ultrasonography. In Babikian VL, Wechsler LR (eds): *Transcranial Doppler Ultrasonography*, St. Louis, Mosby, 1993:3–10.

123. Sloan MA: Detection of vasospasm following subarachnoid hemorrhage. In Babikian VL, Wechsler LR (eds): *Transcranial Doppler Ultrasonography*, St. Louis, Mosby, 1993:105–127.

124. Harders AG, Gilsbach JM: Time course of blood velocity changes related to vasospasm in the circle of Willis measured by transcranial Doppler ultrasound. *J Neurosurg* 1987; 66:718.

125. Seiler RW, et al: Cerebral vasospasm evaluated by transcranial ultrasound correlated with clinical grade and CT-visualized subarachnoid hemorrhage. *J Neurosurg* 1986; 64:594.

126. Caplan LR: Transcranial Doppler ultrasound: Present status. *Neurology* 1990; 40:696.

127. Clyde BL, et al: The relationship of transcranial Doppler velocity to stable xenon/CT cerebral blood flow following aneurysmal subarachnoid hemorrhage. *Neurosurgery* 1996 (in press).

128. Hassler W, Chioff F: CO_2 reactivity of cerebral vasospasm after aneurysmal subarachnoid hemorrhage. *Acta Neurochir* 1989; 98:167.

129. Hiramatsu K, et al: The evaluation of cerebrovascular reactivity to acetazolamide by transcranial Doppler ultrasound after subarachnoid hemorrhage. *Stroke* 1990; 21(suppl 1):1.

130. Shinoda J, et al: Acetazolamide reactivity on CBF in patients with subarachnoid hemorrhage. *Acta Neurochir* 1991; 109:102.

131. Miller JD, et al: Carbon dioxide reactivity in the evaluation of cerebral ischemia. *Neurosurgery* 1992; 30:518.

132. Giulioni M, et al: Correlations among intracranial pulsatility, intracranial hemodynamics, and transcranial Doppler wave form: Literature review and hypothesis for future studies. *Neurosurgery* 1988; 22:807.

133. Hassler W, et al: Transcranial Doppler ultrasonography in raised intracranial pressure and in intracranial circulatory arrest. *J Neurosurg* 1988; 68:745.

134. DeWitt LD, et al: Transcranial Doppler ultrasonography: Normal values. In Babikian VL, Wechsler LR (eds): *Transcranial Doppler Ultrasonography*. St. Louis, Mosby, 1993:29–38.

135. Homburg AM, et al: Transcranial Doppler recordings in raised intracranial pressure. *Acta Neurol Scand* 1993; 87:488.

136. Goraj B, et al: Correlation of intracranial pressure and transcranial Doppler resistive index after head trauma. *AJNR Am J Neuroradiol* 1994; 15:1333.

137. Early CB, et al: Dynamic pressure-flow relationships in the monkey. *J Neurosurg* 1974; 41:590.

138. Dewey RC, et al: Experimental cerebral hemodynamics. Vasomotor tone, critical closing pressure, and vascular bed resistance. *J Neurosurg* 1974; 41:597.

139. Thomas K, et al: Physiological correlation of transcranial Doppler waveform patterns in brain dead patients. Proceedings of the 5th International Symposium and Tutorials on Intracranial Hemodynamics: Transcranial Doppler CBF and Other Modalities. The Institute of Applied Physiology and Medicine, Seattle, WA, 1991.

140. Kofke WA: Transcranial Doppler ultrasonography in anesthesia. In Babikian VL, Wechsler LR (eds): *Transcranial Doppler Ultrasonography*. St. Louis, Mosby, 1993:190–215.

141. Serra VS, et al: Abnormal transcranial Doppler pattern in a pregnant woman during orthostatic hypotension. *Lancet* 1991; 337:1296.

141a. Werner C, et al: Transcranial Doppler sonography indicates critical brain perfusion during hemorrhagic hypotension in dogs. *Anesth Analg* 1991; 74:S247.

142. Barzo P, et al: Measurements of regional CBF and blood flow velocity in experimental intracranial hypertension: Infusion via the cisterna magna in rabbits. *Neurosurgery* 1991; 28:821.

143. Giller CA, et al: The transcranial Doppler appearance of acute carotid artery occlusion. *Ann Neurol* 1992; 31:101.

143a. Kofke WA, et al: Middle cerebral artery blood flow velocity and stable xenon-enhanced computed tomographic blood flow during balloon test occlusion of the internal carotid artery. *Stroke* 1995; 26:1603.

144. Steiger JH, et al: Results of microsurgical carotid endarterectomy: A prospective study with transcranial doppler and EEG monitoring, and elective shunting. *Acta Neurochir* 1989; 100:31.

145. Lindegaard KF, et al: Variations in middle cerebral artery blood flow investigated with noninvasive transcranial blood velocity measurements. *Stroke* 1987; 18:1025.

146. Piepgras DG, et al: Intracerebral hemorrhage after carotid endarterectomy. *J Neurosurg* 1988; 68:532.

147. Rodichok LD: Basic scalp electroencephalography. In Russell GB, Rodichok LD (eds): *Primer of Intraoperative Neurophysiologic Monitoring*. Boston, Butterworth-Heinemann, 1995:65–80.

148. Rabiner LJ, Gold B: *Theory and Application of Digital Signal Processing*. Englewood, Cliffs, NJ, Prentice-Hall, 1975.

149. Michenfelder JD, et al: Isoflurane when compared to enflurane and halothane decreases the frequency of cerebral ischemia during carotid endarterectomy. *Anesthesiology* 1987; 67:336.

150. Messick JM Jr, et al: Correlation of regional CBF (rCBF) with EEG changes during isoflurane anesthesia for carotid endarterectomy: Critical rCBF. *Anesthesiology* 1987; 66:344.

151. Friedman WA, et al: Intraoperative brain-stem auditory evoked potentials during posterior fossa microvascular decompression. *J Neurosurg* 1985; 62:552.

152. Raudzens PA, Shetter AG: Intraoperative monitoring of brain-stem auditory evoked potentials. *J Neurosurg* 1982; 57:341.

153. Nuwer MR: *Evoked Potential Monitoring in the Operating Room*. New York, Raven Press, 1986.

154. Brinkman SD, et al: Neuropsychological performance one week after carotid endarterectomy reflects intraoperative ischemia. *Stroke* 1984; 15:497.

155. Cushman L, et al: Neuropsychological impairment after carotid endarterectomy correlates with intraoperative ishemia. *Cortex* 1984; 20:403.

156. Crippen DW: Noninvasive neurologic monitoring. In Levine RL, Fromm RE Jr (eds). *Critical Care Monitoring, From Pre-Hospital to the ICU*. St. Louis, Mosby, 1995:233–264.

157. Hawkins R: Cerebral energy metabolism. In McCandless DW (ed): *Cerebral Energy Metabolism and Metabolic Encephalopathy*. New York, Plenum Press, 1985:3–23.

158. Pazzaglia P, et al: Clinical course and prognosis of acute posttraumatic coma. *J Neurol Neurosurg Psychiatry* 1975; 38:149.

159. Gadisseux P, Ward JD: Nutritional support of head-injured patients. In Becker DP, Gudeman SK (eds): *Textbook of Head Injury*. Philadelphia, Saunders, 1989:241–254.

160. Ekstrom-Jodal B, et al: Cerebral blood flow and oxygen uptake in endotoxic shock. An experimental study in dogs. *Acta Anaesth Scand* 1982; 26:163.

161. DeGerogia MA, et al: Prophylaxis of deep venous thrombosis. In Hacke W, et al: (eds): *Neurocritical Care*. Berlin, Springer-Verlag, 1994:162–166.

162. Cerrato D, et al: Deep vein thrombosis and low-dose heparin prophylaxix in neurosurgical patients. *J Neurosurg* 1978; 49:378.

163. Powers SK, Edwards MSB: Prophylaxis of thromboembolism in the neurosurgical patient: A review. *Neurosurgery* 1982; 10:509.

164. Barnett HG, et al: Saety of mini-dose heparin administration for neurosurgical patients. *J Neurosurg* 1977; 47:27.

165. McCarthy ST, Turner J: Low-dose subcutaneous heparin in the prevention of deep-vein thrombosis and pulmonary emboli following acute stroke. *Age Ageing* 1986; 15:84.

166. McCarthy ST, et al: Low-dose heparin as a prophylaxis against deep-vein thrombosis after acute stroke. *Lancet* 1977; 2:800.

167. Black PM, et al: External pneumatic calf compression reduces deep venous thrombosis in patients with ruptured intracranial aneurysms. *Neurosurgery* 1986; 18:25.

168. Mayhall CG, et al: Ventriculastomy-related infections. *N Engl J Med* 1984; 310:553.

169. Paramore CG, Turner DA: Relative risks of ventriculostomy infection and morbidity. *Acta Neurochir* 1994; 127:79.

170. Tempelhoff R, et al: Fentanyl-induced electrocortographic seizures in patients with complex partial epilepsy. *J Neurosurg* 1992; 77:201.

171. Kearse LA Jr, et al: Epileptiform activity during opioid anesthesia. *Electroenceph Clin Neurophysiol* 1993; 87:374.

172. Kofke WA, et al: Alfentanil-induced hypermetabolism, seizure, and neuropathology in rats. *Anesth Analg* 1992; 75:953.

173. Kofke WA, et al: Opioid neurotoxicity: Fentanyl-induced exacerbation of forebrain ischemia in rats. *Anesthesiology* 1994; 81:A820.

174. Baskin DS, Hosobuchi Y: Naloxone reversal of ischaemic neurological deficits in man. *Lancet* 1981; 2:272.

175. Haverkos GP, et al: Fatal seizures after flumazenil administration in a patient with mixed overdose. *Ann Pharmacother* 1994; 28:1347.

176. Mäkelä JP, et al: Seizures associated with propofol anesthesia. *Epilepsia* 1993; 34:832.

177. Samra SK, et al: Effects of propofol sedation on seizures and intracranially recorded epileptiform activity in patients with partial epilepsy. *Anesthesiology* 1995; 82:843.

178. Kochs E, et al: The effects of propofol on brain electrical activity, neurologic outcome, and neuronal damage following incomplete ischemia in rats. *Anesthesiology* 1992; 76:245.

179. Jewett BA, et al: Propofol and barbiturate depression of spinal nociceptive neurotransmission. *Anesthesiology* 1992; 77:1148.

180. Selman WR, et al: Barbiturate-induced coma therapy for focal

cerebral ischemia. Effect after temporary and permanent MCA occlusion. *J Neurosurg* 1981; 55:220.

181. Eisenberg HM, et al: High-dose barbiturate control of elevated intracranial pressure in patients with severe head injury. *J Neurosurg* 1988; 69:15.

182. Levine S: Anoxic-ischemic encephalopathy in rats. *Am J Pathol* 1960; 36:1.

183. Stringer WA, et al: Hyperventilation-induced cerebral ischemia in patients with acute brain lesions: Demonstration by xenon-enhanced CT. *Am J Neuroradiol* 1993; 14:475.

184. Muizelaar JP, et al: Adverse effects of prolonged hyperventilation in patients with severe head injury: A randomized clinical trial. *J Neurosurg* 1991; 75:731.

185. Leahy JC, et al: Chronic mild acidosis specifically reduces functional expression of N-methyl-D-aspartate receptors and increases long-term survival in primary cultures of cerebellar granule cells. *Neuroscience* 1994; 63:457.

186. Ebine Y, et al: Mild acidosis inhibits the rise in intracellular Ca^{2+} concentration in response to oxygen-glucose deprivation in rat hippocampal slices. *Neurosci Lett* 1994; 168:155.

187. Dietrich WD: The importance of brain temperature in cerebral injury. *J Neurotrauma* 1992; 9(suppl)2:S475.

188. Blennow G, et al: Epileptic brain damage: The role of systemic factors that modify cerebral energy metabolism. *Brain* 1978; 101:687.

189. Marion DW, et al: The use of moderate therapeutic hypothermia for patients with severe head injuries: A preliminary report. *J Neurosurg* 1993; 79:354.

190. Ginsberg MD, et al: Therapeutic modulation of brain temperature: Relevance to ischemic brain injury. *Cerebrovasc Brain Metab Rev* 1992; 4:189.

191. Nemoto EM, et al: Effect of mild hypothermia on active and basal cerebral oxygen metabolism and blood flow. *Adv Exp Med Biol* 1994; 361:469.

192. Busto R, et al: Effect of mild hypothermia on ischemia-induced release of neurotransmitters and free fatty acids in rat brain. *Stroke* 1989; 20:904.

193. Craen RA, et al: Current anesthetic practices and use of brain protective therapies for cerebral aneurysm surgery at 41 North American centers. *J Neurosurg Anesthesiol* 1994; 6:303.

194. Werner C, et al: Ganglionic blockade improves neurologic outcome from incomplete ischemia in rats: Partial reversal by exogenous catecholamines. *Anesthesiology* 1990; 73:923.

195. Hoffman WE, et al: Dexmedetomidine improves neurologic outcome from incomplete ischemia in the rat. Reversal by the alpha 2-adrenergic antagonist atipamezole. *Anesthesiology* 1991; 75:328.

196. Werner C, et al: Captopril improves neurologic outcome from incomplete cerebral ischemia in rats. *Stroke* 1991; 22:910.

197. Busto R, et al: Cerebral norepinephrine depletion enhances recovery after brain ischemia. *Ann Neurol* 1985; 18:329.

198. Kofke WA, et al: Opioid neurotoxicity: Role of neurotransmitter systems. *J Neurosurg Anesthesiol* 1995; 7:321 (abstr).

199. Neil-Dwyer G, et al: Beta-blockade benefits patients following a subarachnoid hemorrhage. *Eur J Clin Pharmacol* 1985 28(suppl):25.

200. Schroeder T, et al: Effect of labetalol on CBF and middle cerebral arterial flow velocity in healthy volunteers. *Neurol Res* 1991; 13:10.

201. Orlowski JP, et al: Labetalol to control blood pressure after cerebrovascular surgery. *Crit Care Med* 1988; 16:765.

202. Van Aken H, et al: Effect of labetalol on intracranial pressure in dogs with and without intracranial hypertension. *Acta Anaesth Scand* 1982; 26:615.

203. Kakarieka A, et al: Clinical experiences with nimodipine in cerebral ischemia. *J Neural Trans Suppl* 1994; 43:13 (review).

204. Rosenbaum D, et al: Early treatment of ischemic stroke with a calcium antagonist. *Stroke* 1991; 22:437.

205. Anonymous: A multicenter trial of the efficacy of nimodipine on outcome after severe head injury. The European Study Group on Nimodipine in Severe Head Injury. *J Neurosurg* 1994; 80:797.

206. Pickard JD, et al: Effect of oral nimodipine on cerebral infarction and outcome after subarachnoid haemorrhage: British aneurysm nimodipine trial. *BMJ* 1989; 298:636.

207. Kucharczyk J, et al: Nicardipine reduces ischemic brain injury. Magnetic resonance imaging/spectroscopy study in cats. *Stroke* 1989; 20:268.

208. Alps BJ, et al: Comparative protective effects of nicardipine, flunarizine, lidoflazine and nimodipine against ischaemic injury in the hippocampus of the Mongolian gerbil. *Br J Pharmacol* 1988; 93:877.

209. Grotta J, et al: The effect of nicardipine on neuronal function following ischemia. *Stroke* 1986; 17:213.

210. Bedford RF, et al: Adverse impact of a calcium entry-blocker (verapamil) on intracranial pressure in patients with brain tumors. *J Neurosurg* 1983; 59:800.

211. Hayashi M, et al: Treatment of systemic hypertension and intracranial hypertension and intracranial hypertension in cases of brain hemorrhage. *Stroke* 1988; 19:314.

212. Stanek B, et al: Plasma catecholamines, plasma renin activity and haemodynamics during sodium nitroprusside-induced hypotension and additional beta-blockage with bunitrolol. *Eur J Clin Pharmacol* 1981; 19:317.

213. Overgaard J, Skinhoj E: A paradoxical cerebral hemodynamic effect of hydralazine. *Stroke* 1975; 6:402.

214. Griswold WR, et al: Nitroprusside induced intracranial hypertension. *JAMA* 1981; 246:2679.

215. Marsh ML, et al: Changes in neurologic status and intracranial pressure associated with sodium nitroprusside administration. *Anesthesiology* 1979; 51:336.

216. Dohi S, et al: The effects of nitroglycerin on cerebrospinal fluid pressure in awake and anesthetized humans. *Anesthesiology* 1981; 54:511.

217. Lundberg N: Continuous recording and control of ventricular fluid pressure in neurosurgical practice. *Acta Psychiatr Neurol Scand* 1960; 36(suppl 149):1.

218. Risberg J, et al: Regional cerebral blood volume during acute rises in the intracranial pressure (plateau waves). *J Neurosurg* 1969; 31:303.

219. Rosner MJ, Becker DP: Origin and evolution of plateau waves. Experimental observations and a theoretical model. *J Neurosurg* 1984; 50:312.

219a. Rosner MJ, Becker DP: The etiology of plateau waves: A theoretical model and experimental observations. In Ishii S, et al: *Intracranial Pressure V.* New York, Springer-Verlag, 1983:301.

219b. Matakas F, et al: Increase in cerebral perfusion pressure by arterial hypertension in brain swelling. A mathematical model of the volume-pressure relationship. *J Neurosurg* 1975; 42:282.

220. Meinig G, et al: Induction of filtration edema by extreme reduction of cerebrovascular resistance associated with hypertension. *Eur Neurol* 1972; 8:97.

221. Langfitt TW, et al: The pathophysiology of brain swelling produced by mechanical trauma and hypertension. *Scand J Clin Lab Invest Suppl* 1968; 102.

222. Marshall WJ, et al: Brain swelling caused by trauma and arterial hypertension. Hemodynamic aspects. *Arch Neurol* 1969; 21:545.

223. Schutta HS, et al: Brain swelling produced by injury and aggravated by arterial hypertension. A light and electron microscopic study. *Brain* 1968; 91:281.

224. Marshall WJ, et al: The pathophysiology of brain swelling produced by mechanical trauma and hypertension. *Surg Forum* 1968; 19:431.

225. MacKenzie ET, et al: Influence of endogenous norepinephrine on CBF and metabolism. *Am J Physiol* 1976; 231:489.

226. Darby JM, et al: Acute CBF response to dopamine-induced hypertension after subarachnoid hemorrhage. *J Neurosurg* 1994; 80:857.

227. Stein SC, Cracco RG: Cortical injury without ischemia produced by topical monoamines. *Stroke* 1982; 13:74.

228. Hindman BJ, et al: Differential effect of oncotic pressure on cerebral and extracerebral water content during cardiopulmonary bypass in rabbits. *Anesthesiology* 1990; 73:951.

229. Kaieda, R, et al: Prolonged reduction in colloid oncotic pressure does not increase brain edema following cryogenic injury in rabbits. *Anesthesiology* 1989; 71:554.

230. Kaieda R, et al: Acute effects of changing plasma osmolality and colloid oncotic pressure on the formation of brain edema after cryogenic injury. *Neurosurgery* 1989; 24:671.

231. Zornow MH, et al: Acute cerebral effects of isotonic crystalloid and colloid solutions following cryogenic brain injury in the rabbit. *Anesthesiology* 1988; 69:180.

232. Tommasino C, et al: Cerebral effects of isovolemic hemodilution with crystalloid or colloid solutions. *Crit Care Med* 1988; 16:862.

233. Zornow MH, et al: The acute cerebral effects of changes in plasma osmolality and oncotic pressure. *Anesthesiology* 1987; 67:936.

234. Pulsinelli WA, et al: Increased damage after ischemic stroke in patients with hyperglycemia with or without established diabetes mellitus. *Am J Med* 1983; 74:540.

235. Siemkowicz E: Hyperglycemia in the reperfusion period hampers recovery from cerebral ischemia. *Acta Neurol Scand* 1981; 64:207.

236. Rehncrona S, et al: Brain lactic acidosis and ischemic cell damage: 1. Biochemistry and neurophysiology. *J Cereb Blood Flow Metab* 1981; 1:297.

237. De Salles AA, et al: Hyperglycemia, cerebrospinal fluid lactic acidosis, and CBF in severely head-injured patients. *Neurosurgery* 1987; 21:45.

238. Li PA, et al: The influence of plasma glucose concentrations on ischemic brain damage is a threshold function. *Neurosci Lett* 1994; 177:63.

239. Warner DS, et al: Insulin-induced normoglycemia improves ischemic outcome in hyperglycemic rats. *Stroke* 1992; 23:1775.

240. Siemkowicz E, Gjedde A: Post-ischemic coma in rat: Effect of different pre-ischemic blood glucose levels on cerebral metabolic recovery after ischemia. *Acta Physiol Scand* 1980; 110:225.

241. Lanier WL, et al: The effect of dextrose infusion and head position on neurologic outcome after complete cerebral ischemia in primates: Examination of a model. *Anesthesiology* 1987; 66:39.

242. Broderick JP, et al: Hyperglycemia and hemorrhagic transformation of cerebral infarcts. *Stroke* 1995; 26:484.

243. Murros K, et al: Serum cortisol and outcome of ischemic brain infarction. *J Neurol Sci* 1993; 116:12.

244. Murros K, et al: Blood glucose, glycosylated haemoglobin, and outcome of ischemic brain infarction. *J Neurol Sci* 1992; 111:59.

245. Matchar DB, et al: The influence of hyperglycemia on outcome of cerebral infarction. *Ann Intern Med* 1992; 117:449.

246. de Courten-Myers GM, et al: Hemorrhagic infarct conversion in experimental stroke. *Ann Emerg Med* 1992; 21:120.

247. Sieber FE, Traystman RJ: Special issues: Glucose and the brain. *Crit Care Med* 1992; 20:104 (review).

248. Yip PK, et al: Effect of plasma glucose on infarct size in focal cerebral ischemia-reperfusion. *Neurology* 1991; 41:899.

249. Vazquez-Cruz J, et al: Progressing cerebral infarction in relation to plasma glucose in gerbils. *Stroke* 1990; 21:1621.

250. Kushner M, et al: Relation of hyperglycemia early in ischemic brain infarction to cerebral anatomy, metabolism, and clinical outcome. *Ann Neurol* 1990; 28:129.

251. Kraft SA, et al: Effect of hyperglycemia on neuronal changes in a rabbit model of focal cerebral ischemia. *Stroke* 1990; 21:447.

252. Zasslow MA, et al: Hyperglycemia decreases acute neuronal ischemic changes after middle cerebral artery occlusion in cats. *Stroke* 1989; 20:519.

253. de Courten-Myers G, et al: Hyperglycemia enlarges infarct size in cerebrovascular occlusion in cats. *Stroke* 1988; 19:623.

254. Duverger D, MacKenzie ET: The quantification of cerebral infarction following focal ischemia in the rat: Influence of strain, arterial pressure, blood glucose concentration, and age. *J Cereb Blood Flow Metab* 1988; 8:449 (review).

255. Nedergaard M: Mechanisms of brain damage in focal cerebral ischemia. *Acta Neurol Scand* 1988; 77:81 (review).

256. Prado R, et al: Hyperglycemia increases infarct size in collaterally perfused but not end-arterial vascular territories. *J Cereb Blood Flow Metab* 1988; 8:186.

257. Ginsberg MD, et al: Hyperglycemia reduces the extent of cerebral infarction in rats. *Stroke* 1987; 18:570.

258. Nedergaard M: Transient focal ischemia in hyperglycemic rats is associated with increased cerebral infarction. *Brain Res* 1987; 408:79.

259. Nedergaard M, Astrup J: Infarct rim: Effect of hyperglycemia on direct current potential and [14C]2-deoxyglucose phosphorylation. *J Cereb Blood Flow Metab* 1986; 6:607.

260. Kofke WA, et al: Substantia nigra damage after flurothyl-induced seizures in rats worsens after post seizure recovery: No exacerbation with hyperglycemia. *Neurol Res* 1993; 15:333.

261. Swan JH, et al: Hyperglycemia does not augment neuronal damage in experimental status epilepticus. *Neurology* 1986; 36:1351.

262. Ingvar M, et al: Metabolic alterations underlying the development of hypermetabolic necrosis in the substantia nigra in status epilepticus. *J Cereb Blood Flow Metab* 1987; 7:103.

263. Oh MS, Carroll HJ: Disorders of sodium metabolism: Hypernatremia and hyponatremia. *Crit Care Med* 1992; 20:94 (review).

264. Hund EF, et al: Disturbances of water and electrolyte balance. In Hacke W, et al: *Neurocritical Care*, Berlin, Springer-Verlag, 1994:917–927.

265. Petrozza PH, Prough DS: Postoperative and intensive care. In Cottrell JE, Smith DS (eds): *Anesthesia and Neurosurgery*, 3d ed. St. Louis, Mosby, 1994:625–660.

266. Black PL, et al: Incidence and management of complications of transphenoidal operation for pituitary adenomas. *Neurosurgery* 1987; 20:920.

267. Bland RD, Shoemaker WC: Probability of survival as a prognostic and severity of illness score in critically ill surgical patients. *Crit Care Med* 1985; 13:91.

268. Maroon JC, Nelson PB: Hypovolemia in patients with subarachnoid hemorrhage: Therapeutic implications. *Neurosurgery* 1979; 4:223.

269. Solomon RA, et al: Depression of circulating blood volume in patients after subarachnoid hemorrhage: Implications for the management of symptomatic vasospasm. *Neurosurgery* 1984; 15:354.

270. Adams RD, Victor M: The acquired metabolic disorders of the nervous system. In Adams RD, Victor M (eds): *Principles of Neurology*, 5th ed. New York, McGraw-Hill, 1993:877.

271. Burcar PJ, et al: Hyponatremia and central pontine myelinolysis. *Neurology* 1977; 27:223.

272. Laureno R, Kapp BI: Pontine and extrapontine myelinolysis

following rapid correction of hyponatremia. *Lancet* 1988; 1:1439.

273. Berl T: Treating hyponatremia: Damned if we do and damned if we don't [clinical conference]. *Kidney Int* 1990; 37:1006 (review).

274. Aggarwal S, et al: Cerebral hemodynamic and metabolic changes in fulminant hepatic failure: A retrospective study. *Hepatology* 1994; 19:80.

275. Cold GE: The relationship between cerebral metabolic rate of oxygen and CBF in the acute phase of head injury. *Acta Anaesthesiol Scand* 1986; 30:453.

276. Jaggi JL, et al: Relationship of early CBF and metabolism to outcome in acute head injury. *J Neurosurg* 1990; 72:176.

277. Bouma GJ, Muizelaar JP: CBF, cerebral blood volume, and cerebrovascular reactivity after severe head injury. *J Neurotrauma* 1992; 9(suppl 1):S333.

278. Sharples PM, et al: CBF and metabolism in children with severe head injury. Part 1: Relation to age, Glasgow coma score, outcome, intracranial pressure, and time after injury. *J Neurol Neurosurg Psychiatry* 1995; 58:145.

279. Batjer HH, et al: Cerebrovascular hemodynamics in arteriovenous malformation complicated by normal perfusion pressure breakthrough. *Neurosurgery* 1988; 22:503.

280. Young WL, et al: [133]Xe blood flow monitoring during arteriovenous malformation resection: A case of intraoperative hyperperfusion with subsequent brain swelling. *Neurosurgery* 1988; 22:765.

281. Reigel MM, et al: Cerebral hyperperfusion syndrome: A cause of neurologic dysfunction after carotid endarterectomy. *J Vasc Surg* 1987; 5:628.

282. Schroeder T, et al: Cerebral hyperperfusion following carotid endarterectomy. *J Neurosurg* 1987; 66:824.

283. Young WL, et al: The effect of arteriovenous malformation resection on cerebrovascular reactivity to carbon dioxide. *Neurosurgery* 1990; 27:257.

284. Young WL, et al, Columbia University AVM Project: Cerebral hyperemia after AVM resection is related to "break-through" complications but not to feeding artery pressure. *Anesth Analg* 1995; 80:S573 (abstr).

285. Young WL, et al, Columbia University AVM Study Project: Evidence for adaptive autoregulatory displacement in hypotensive cortical territories adjacent to arteriovenous malformations. *Neurosurgery* 1994; 34:601.

286. Young WL, et al: Pressure autoregulation is intact after arteriovenous malformation resection. *Neurosurgery* 1993; 32:491.

287. Marion DW, et al: Subarachnoid hemorrhage and the heart. *Neurosurgery* 1986; 18:101.

288. Neil-Dwyer G, et al: Plasma renin activity in patients after a subarachnoid hemorrhage: A possible predictor of outcome. *Neurosurgery* 1980; 7:578.

289. DiPasquale G, et al: Torsade de pointes and ventricular flutter-fibrillation following spontaneous cerebral subarachnoid hemorrhage. *Int J Cardiol* 1988; 18:163.

290. Estanol Vidal B, et al: Cardiac arrhythmias associated with subarachnoid hemorrhage: Prospective study. *Neurosurgery* 1979; 5:675.

291. Gascon P, et al: Spontaneous subarachnoid hemorrhage simulating acute transmural myocardial infarction. *Am Heart J* 1983; 105:511.

292. Stober T, Kunze K: Electrocardiographic alterations in subarachnoid hemorrhage: Correlation between spasm of the arteries of the left side of the brain and T inversion and QT prolongation. *J Neurol* 1982; 227:99.

293. Fabinyi G, et al: Myocardial creatin kinase isoenzyme in serum after subarachnoid hemorrhage. *J Neurol Neurosurg Psychiatry* 1977; 40:818.

294. Neil-Dwyer G, et al: β-blockers, plasma total creatinine kinase and creatine kinase myocardial enzymes, and the prognosis of subarachnoid hemorrhage. *Surg Neurol* 1986; 25:163.

295. Touho H, et al: Neurogenic pulmonary edema in the acute stage of hemorrhagic cerebrovascular disease. *Neurosurgery* 1989; 25:762.

296. Wauchob TD, et al: Neurogenic pulmonary edema. *Anaesthesia* 1984; 39:529.

297. Weisman SJ: Edema and congestion of the lungs resulting from intracranial hemorrhage. *Surgery* 1939; 6:722.

298. Simmons RL, et al: Respiratory insufficiency in combat casualties: II. Pulmonary edema following head injury. *Ann Surg* 1969; 170:39.

299. Schell AR, et al: Pulmonary edema associated with subarachnoid hemorrhage. *Arch Int Med* 1987; 147:591.

300. Myers MG, et al: Cardiac sequelae of acute stroke. *Stroke* 1982; 13:838.

301. Myers MG, et al: Plasma norepinephrine in stroke. *Stroke* 1981; 12:200.

302. Minegishi A, et al: Plasma monoaminergic metabolites and catecholamines in subarachnoid hemorrhage. Clinical implications. *Arch Neurol* 1987; 44:423.

303. Jachuck SJ, et al: Electrocardiographic abnormalities associated with raised intracranial pressure. *BMJ* 1975; 1:242.

304. Davies KR, et al: Cardiac function in aneurysmal subarachnoid hemorrhage: A study of electrocardiographic and echocardiographic abnormalities. *Br J Anaesth* 1991; 67:58.

305. Pollick C, et al: Left ventricular wall motion abnormalities in subarachnoid hemorrhage: An echocardiographic study. *J Am Coll Cardiol* 1988; 12:600.

306. Cruickshank JM, et al: Possible role of catecholamines, corticosteroids, and potassium in production of electrocardiographic abnormalities associated with subarachnoid hemorrhage. *Br Heart J* 1974; 36:697.

307. Cruickshank JM, et al: The effect of oral propranolol upon the ECG changes occurring in subarachnoid hemorrhage. *Cardiovasc Res* 1975; 9:236.

308. Theodore J, Robin ED: Pathogenesis of neurogenic pulmonary oedema. Lancet 1975; 2:749.

309. Brouwers PJAM, et al: Serial electrocardiographic recordings in aneurysmal subarachnoid hemorrhage. *Stroke* 1989; 20:1162.

310. Malik AB: Pulmonary vascular response to increase in intracranial pressure: Role of sympathetic mechanisms. *Am J Physiol* 1977; 42:335.

311. Loach AB, Benedict CR: Plasma catecholamine concentration associated with cerebral vasospasm. *J Neurol Sci* 1980; 45:261.

312. Kolin A, Norris JW: Myocardial damage from acute cerebral lesions. *Stroke* 1984; 15:990.

313. Colice GL: Neurogenic pulmonary edema. *Clin Chest Med* 1985; 6:473.

314. Feibel JH, et al: Myocardial damage and cardiac arrhythmias in cerebral infarction and subarachnoid hemorrhage: Correlation with increased systemic catecholamine output. *Trans Am Neurol Assoc* 1976; 101:242.

315. Dilraj A, et al: Levels of catecholamine in plasma and cerebrospinal fluid in aneurysmal subarachnoid hemorrhage. *Neurosurgery* 1992; 31:42.

316. Svengaard NA, et al: Subarachnoid hemorrhage in the rat: Effect on the development of cerebral vasospasm of lesions in the central serotonergic and dopaminergic systems. *Stroke* 1986; 17:86.

317. Svengaard NA, et al: Subarachnoid haemorrhage in the rat: Effect on the development of vasospasm of selective lesions of the catecholamine systems in the lower brain stem. *Stroke* 1985; 16:602.

318. Delgado TJ, et al: Subarachnoid hemorrhage in the rat: CBF

and glucose metabolism after selective lesions of the catecholamine systems in the brainstem. *J Cereb Blood Flow Metab* 1986; 6:600.

319. Hakim TS, et al: Effects of sympathetic nerve stimulation on lung fluid and protein exchange. *Am J Physiol* 1979; 47:1025.

320. Fein IA, Rachow EC: Neurogenic pulmonary edema. *Chest* 1982; 81:318.

321. Cushing H: Concerning a definite regulatory mechanism of the vaso-motor centre which controls blood pressure during cerebral compression. *Johns Hopkins Hosp Bull* 1901; 12:290.

322. Greenberg JH, et al: Local cerebral blood volume response to carbon dioxide in man. *Circ Res* 1978; 43:324.

323. Sakai F, et al: Regional cerebral blood volume and hematocrit measured in normal human volunteers by single photon emission computed tomography. *J Cereb Blood Flow Metab* 1985; 5:207.

324. Strandgaard S, et al: Autoregulation of brain circulation in severe arterial hypertension. *BMJ* 1973; 3:507.

325. Miller JD, et al: Significance of intracranial hypertension in severe head injury. *J Neurosurg* 1977; 47:503.

326. Lundberg N, et al: Continuous recording of ventricular fluid pressure in patients with severe acute traumatic brain injury. A preliminary report. *J Neurosurg* 1965; 22:581.

327. Giulioni M, et al: Correlations among intracranial pulsatility, intracranial hemodynamics, and transcranial Doppler wave form: Literature review and hypothesis for future studies. *Neurosurgery* 1988; 22:807.

328. Greitz T, et al: Aortocranial and carotid angiography in determination of brain death. *Neuroradiology* 1973; 5:13.

329. Langfitt TW, et al: Cerebral vasomotor paralysis produced by intracranial hypertension. *Neurology* 1965; 15:622.

330. Langfitt TW, et al: Transmission of increased intracranial pressure. I. Within the craniospinal axis. *J Neurosurg* 1964; 21:989.

331. Klatzo I: Neuropathological aspects of brain edema. *J Neuropathol Exp Neurol* 1967; 24:1.

332. Hartmann A, et al: General treatment strategies for elevated intracerebral pressure. In Hacke W, et al (eds): *Neurocritical Care.* Berlin, Springer-Verlag, 1994:101–115.

333. Guyton AC: Basic Neuroscience, Anatomy and Physiology. Philadelphia, Saunders, 1987.

334. von Haken MS, Aschoff AA: Acute obstructive hydrocephalus. In Hacke W, et al (eds): *Neurocritical Care.* New York, Springer-Verlag, 1994:869.

335. Bederson JB, et al: Intracranial venous hypertension and the effects of venous outflow obstruction in a rat model of arteriovenous fistula. *Neurosurgery* 1991; 29:341.

336. Kofke WA, et al: Transcranial Doppler ultrasonography with induction of anesthesia for neurosurgery. *J Neurosurg Anesthesiol* 1994; 6:89.

337. Michenfelder JD. The 27th Rovenstein Lecture: Neuroanesthesia and the achievement of professional respect. *Anesthesiology* 1989; 70:695.

338. Lassen NA: Control of cerebral circulation in health and disease. *Circ Res* 1974; 34:749.

339. Shapiro HM: Intracranial hypertension: Therapeutic and anesthetic considerations. *Anesthesiology* 1975; 43:445.

340. Shenkin HA, Bouzarth WF: Clinical methods of reducing intracranial pressure. *N Engl J Med* 1970; 282:1465.

341. Raichle ME, Plum F: Hyperventilation and CBF. *Stroke* 1972; 3:566 (review).

342. Chater SN, Simpson KH: Effect of passive hyperventilation on seizure threshold in patients undergoing electroconvulsive therapy. *Br J Anaesth* 1988; 60:70.

342a. Ropper AH: Treatment of intracranial hypertension. In Ropper AH, et al (eds): *Neurological and Neurosurgical Intensive Care,* 3d ed. New York, Raven Press, 1993:31.

343. Cruz J, et al: Continuous monitoring of cerebral oxygenation in acute brain injury: Injection of mannitol during hyperventilation. *J Neurosurg* 1990; 73:725.

344. Pierce EC, et al: Cerebral circulation and metabolism during thiopental anesthesia and hyperventilation in man. *J Clin Invest* 1962; 41:1664.

345. Marshall LF, et al: Pentobarbital therapy for intracranial hypertension in metabolic coma. Reye's syndrome. *Crit Care Med* 1978; 6:1.

346. Hartung HJ: Intracranial pressure after propofol and thiopental administration in patients with severe head trauma. *Anaesthetist* 1987; 36:285.

347. Larsen R, et al: The effects of midazolam on the general circulation, the CBF and cerebral oxygen consumption in man. *Anaesthetist* 1981; 30:18.

348. Renou AM, et al: CBF and metabolism during etomidate anaesthesia in man. *Br J Anaesth* 1978; 50:1047.

349. Prior JGL, et al: The use of etomidate in the management of severe head injury. *Intensive Care Med* 1983; 9:313.

350. Vandesteene A, et al: Effect of propofol on CBF and metabolism in man. *Anaesthesia* 1988; 43(suppl)42.

351. Sakabe T, et al: The effects of lidocaine on canine metabolism and circulation related to the electroencephalogram. *Anesthesiology* 1974; 40:433.

352. Yano M, et al: Effect of lidocaine on ICP response to endotracheal suctioning. *Anesthesiology* 1986; 64:651.

352a. Muizelaar JP, et al: CBF is regulated by changes in blood pressure and in blood viscosity alike. *Stroke* 1986; 17:44.

353. Michenfelder JD: The interdependency of cerebral functional and metabolic effects following massive doses of thiopental in the dog. *Anesthesiology* 1974; 41:231.

354. Preziosi P, Vacca M: Adrenocortical suppression and other endocrine effects of etomidate. *Life Sci* 1988; 42:477 (review).

355. Skues MA, Prys-Roberts C: The pharmacology of propofol. *J Clin Anesth* 1989; 1:387 (review).

356. Reichenthal E, et al: The ambivalent effect of early and late administration of mannitol in cold-induced brain oedema. *Acta Neurochir Suppl* 1990; 51:110.

357. Rosenberg GA, et al: Selective effect of mannitol-induced hyperosmolality on brain interstitial fluid and water content in white matter. *Metab Brain Dis* 1988; 3:217.

358. Bell, BA, et al: Brain water measured by magnetic resonance imaging. Correlation with direct estimation and changes after mannitol and dexamethasone. *Lancet* 1987; 1:66.

359. Chan PH, Fishman RA: Elevation of rat brain amino acids, ammonia and idiogenic osmoles induced by hyperosmolality. *Brain Res* 1979; 161:293.

360. Pollock AS, Arieff AI: Abnormalities of cell volume regulation and their functional consequences. *Am J Physiol* 1980; 239:F195.

361. Kofke WA: Mannitol: Potential for rebound intracranial hypertension? *J Neurosurg Anesth* 1993; 5:1 (editorial; comment).

362. Rudehill A, et al: Pharmacokinetics and effects of mannitol on hemodynamics, blood and cerebrospinal fluid electrolytes, and osmolality during intracranial surgery. *J Neurosurg Anesth* 1993; 5:4.

363. Gudeman SK, et al: Indications for operative treatment and operative technique in closed head injury. In Becker DP, Gudeman SK (eds): *Textbook of Head Injury.* Philadelphia, Saunders, 1989;138–181.

364. Kalia KK, Yonas H: An aggressive approach to massive middle cerebral artery infarction. *Arch Neurol* 1993; 50:1293.

365. Kondziolka D, Fazl M: Functional recovery after decompressive craniectomy for cerebral infarction. *Neurosurgery* 1988; 23:143.

366. Adams HP, et al: Guidelines for the management of patients with acute ischemic stroke. A statement for health care profes-

sionals form a special writing group of the stroke council, American Heart Association. *Stroke* 1994; 25:1901.

367. Fisher CM, Ojemann RG: Bilateral decompressive craniectomy for worsening coma in acute subarachnoid hemorrhage. Observations in support of the procedure. *Surg Neurol* 1994; 41:65.

368. Forsting M, et al: Decompressive craniectomy for cerebral infarction. An experimental study in rats. *Stroke* 1995; 26:259.

369. Shapiro HM, Marshall LF: Intracranial pressure responses to PEEP in head-injured patients. *J Trauma* 1978; 18:254.

370. Aidinis SJ, et al: Intracranial responses to PEEP. *Anesthesiology* 1976; 45:275.

371. Harken AH, et al: The hemodynamic response to positive end-expiratory ventilation in hypovolemic patients. *Surgery* 1974; 76:786.

372. Huseby JS, et al: Effects of positive end-expiratory pressure on intracranial pressure in dogs with intracranial hypertension. *J Neurosurg* 1981; 55:704.

373. Luce JM, et al: A Starling resistor regulates cerebral venous outflow in dogs. *J App Physiol* 1982; 53:1496.

374. Ropper AH, Kennedy SK: Postoperative neurosurgical care. In Ropper AH: *Neurological and Neurosurgical Intensive Care,* 3d ed. New York, Raven Press, 1993:185.

374a. Turner JM, et al: Intracranial pressure changes in neurosurgical patients during hypotension induced with sodium nitroprusside or trimetaphan. *Br J Anaesth* 1977; 49:419.

375. Rosenberg H, et al: Neurologic changes during awakening from anesthesia. *Anesthesiology* 1981; 45:125.

376. Thal G, et al: Exacerbation or unmasking of focal neurologic deficits by sedative medication. *J Neurosurg Anesthesiol* 1993; 5:291 (abstr).

377. Kalfas IH, Little JR: Postoperative hemorrhage: A survey of 4992 intracranial procedures. *Neurosurgery* 1988; 11:337.

377a. Taylor WA, et al: Timing of postoperative intracranial hematoma development and implications for the best use of neurosurgical intensive care. *J Neurosurg* 1995; 82:48.

378. Nevin C: Neuropathologic changes in the white matter following head injury. *J Neuropathol Exp Neurol* 1967; 26:77.

379. Nilsson B, et al: Experimental head injury in the rat. Part 1: Mechanics, pathophysiology, and morphology in an impact acceleration trauma model. *J Neurosurg* 1977; 47:241.

380. Povlishock JT: Experimental studies of head injury. In Becker DP, Gudeman SK (eds): *Textbook of Head Injury.* Philadelphia, Saunders, 1989: .

381. Muttaqin Z, et al: Hyperaemia prior to acute cerebral swelling in severe head injuries: The role of transcranial Doppler monitoring. *Acta Neurochir* 1993; 123:76.

382. Wald SL, et al: The effect of secondary insults on mortality and long-term disability after severe head injury in a rural region without a trauma system. *J Trauma* 1993; 34:377.

383. Wahl M, et al: Mediators of vascular and parenchymal mechanisms in secondary brain damage. *Acta Neurochir Suppl* 1993; 57:64 (review).

384. Graham DI, et al: Quantification of primary and secondary lesions in severe head injury. *Acta Neurochir Suppl* 1993; 57:41.

385. Unterberg A, et al: Long-term observations of intracranial pressure after severe head injury. The phenomenon of secondary rise of intracranial pressure. *Neurosurgery* 1993; 32:17.

386. Braughler JM, Hall ED: Involvement of lipid peroxidation in CNS injury. *J Neurotrauma* 1992; 9(suppl)1:S1 (review).

387. Kanthan R, Shuaib A: Clinical evaluation of extracellular amino acids in severe head trauma by intracerebral in vivo microdialysis. *J Neurol Neurosurg Psychiatry* 1995; 59:326.

388. Palmer AM, et al: Traumatic brain injury-induced excitotoxicity assessed in a controlled cortical impact model. *J Neurochem* 1993; 61:2015.

389. Hayes RL, et al: Neurotransmitter-mediated mechanisms of traumatic brain injury: Acetylcholine and excitatory amino acids. *J Neurotrauma* 1992; 9(suppl)1:S173 (review).

390. Kochanek PM: Ischemic and traumatic brain injury: Pathobiology and cellular mechanisms. *Crit Care Med* 1993; 21(9 suppl):S333.

391. Marmarou A: Intracellular acidosis in human and experimental brain injury. *J Neurotrauma* 1992; 9(suppl)2:S551 (review).

392. Hovda DA, et al: Secondary injury and acidosis. *J Neurotrauma* 1992; 9(suppl)1:S47 (review).

393. Martin NA, et al: Postraumatic cerebral arterial spasm: Transcranial Doppler ultrasound, CBF, and angiographic findings. *J Neurosurg* 1992; 77:575.

394. Obrist WD, et al: CBF and metabolism in comatose patients with acute head injury. Relationship to intracranial hypertension. *J Neurosurg* 1984; 61:241.

395. Muizelaar JP: Cerebral blood flow, cerebral blood volume, and cerebral metabolism after severe head injury. In Becker DP, Gudeman SK (eds): *Textbook of Head Injury.* Philadelphia, Saunders, 1989:221–240.

396. Maxwell WL, et al: Ultrastructural evidence of axonal shearing as a result of lateral acceleration of the head in non-human primates. *Acta Neuropathol* 1993; 86:136.

397. Povlishock JT: Traumatically induced axonal injury: Pathogenesis and pathobiological implications. *Brain Pathol* 1992; 2:1 (review).

398. Narayan RK: Emergency room management of the head-injured patient. In Becker DP, Gudeman SK (eds): *Textbook of Head Injury.* Philadelphia, Saunders, 1989:23–66.

399. Miller JD, et al: Further experience in the management of severe head injury. *J Neurosurg* 1981; 54:289.

400. Collicott PE, et al: Advanced trauma life support course for physicians. American College of Surgeons, 1984:155.

401. Cruz J: An additional therapeutic effect of adequate hyperventilation in severe acute brain trauma: Normalization of cerebral glucose uptake. *J Neurosurg* 1995; 82:379.

402. Cruz J, et al: Cerebral oxygenation monitoring. *Crit Care Med* 1993; 21:1242 (review).

403. Johnson DW, et al: Stable xenon CT CBF imaging: Rationale for and role in clinical decision making. *Am J Neuroradiol* 1991; 12:201 (review).

404. Ekstrom-Jodal B, et al: CBF and oxygen uptake in endotoxic shock. An experimental study in dogs. *Acta Anaesth Scand* 1982; 26:163.

405. Kawajiri K, et al: Cerebral salt wasting syndrome secondary to head injury: A case report. *No Shinkei Geka* 1992; 20:1003.

406. Nelson PB, et al: Hyponatremia in intracranial disease: Perhaps not the syndrome of inappropriate secretion of antidiuretic hormone (SIADH). *J Neurosurg* 1981; 55:938.

407. Gaufin L, et al: Release of ADH during mass-induced elevation of ICP. *J Neurosurg* 1977; 46:627.

408. Ransohoff J, et al: Mechanisms of injury and treatment of acute spinal cord trauma. In Cottrell JE, Turndorf H (eds): *Anesthesia and Neurosurgery,* St. Louis, Mosby-Yearbook, 1980:361–386.

409. Albin MS, et al: Spinal cord injury—epidemiology, emergency care, and acute care: Advances in pathophysiology and treatment. *Curr Probl Surg* 1980; 17:190.

410. Luce JM: Medical management of spinal cord injury. *Crit Care Med* 1985; 13:126 (review).

411. Anderson DK, et al: Spinal cord injury and protection. *Ann Emerg Med* 1985; 14:816 (review).

412. Schmidt KD, Chan CW: Thermoregulation and fever in normal persons and in those with spinal cord injuries. *Mayo Clin Proc* 1992; 67:469 (review).

413. Tator CH, Fehlings MG: Review of the secondary injury theory of acute spinal cord trauma with emphasis on vascular mechanisms. *J Neurosurg* 1991; 75:15 (review).

414. Ducker TB, Zeidman SM: Spinal cord injury. Role of steroid therapy. *Spine* 1994; 19:2281 (review).

415. Bracken MB, et al: A randomized, controlled trial of methylprednisolone or naloxone in the treatment of acute spinalcord injury. Results of the Second National Acute Spinal Cord Injury Study. *N Engl J Med* 1990; 322:1405.

416. Sidhu VS, et al: A technique of awake fibreoptic intubation. Experience in patients with cervical spine disease. *Anaesthesia* 1993; 48:910.

417. Scannell G, et al: Orotracheal intubation in trauma paients with cervical fractures. *Arch Surg* 1993; 128:903 (discussion 905).

418. Criswell JC, et al: Emergency airway management in patients with cervical spine injuries. *Anaesthesia* 1994; 49:900.

419. Donaldson WF 3d, et al: A methodology to evaluate motion of the unstable spine during intubation techniques. *Spine* 1993; 18:2020.

420. Gajraj NM, et al: Cervical spine movement during orotracheal intubation: Comparison of the Belscope and Macintosh blades. *Anaesthesia* 1994; 49:772.

421. Fitzgerald RD, et al: Excursions of the cervical spine during tracheal intubation: Blind oral intubation compared with direct laryngoscopy. *Anaesthesia* 1994; 49:111.

422. Heath KJ: The effect of laryngoscopy of different cervical spine immobilisation techniques. *Anaesthesia* 1994; 49:843.

423. Suderman VS, et al: Elective oral tracheal intubation in cervical spine-injured adults. *Can J Anaesth* 1991; 38:785.

424. Meschino A, et al: The safety of awake tracheal intubation in cervical spine injury. *Can J Anaesth* 1992; 39:114.

425. Smith RB: Hyperkalemia following succinylcholine administration in neurological disorders. A Review. *Can Anaesth Soc J* 1971; 18:199.

426. Wierda JM, et al: Pharmacokinetics and pharmacokinetic/dynamic relationship of rocuronium bromide in humans. *Eur J Anaesth Suppl* 1994; 9:66.

427. McKinley AC, et al: Pulmonary function, ventilatory control, and respiratory complications in quadriplegic subjects. *Am Rev Respir Dis* 1969; 100:526.

428. Wilson JT, et al: Prophylactic vena cava filter insertion in patients with traumatic spinal cord injury: Preliminary results. *Neurosurgery* 1994; 35:234.

429. Silver JR, Moulton A: The physiological and pathological sequelae of paralysis of the intercostal and abdominal muscles in tetraplegic patients. *Paraplegia* 1969; 7:131.

430. Dixit S: Bradycardia associated with high cervical spinal cord injury. *Surg Neurol* 1995; 43:514.

431. Greenhoot JH, et al: Experimental spinal cord injury: Electrocardiographic abnormalities in fuchsinophilic myocardial degeneration. *Arch Neurol* 1972; 26:524.

432. Kopaniky DR: Pathophysiology and management of spinal cord trauma. In Frost E (ed): *Clincal Anesthesia in Neurosurgery*, 2d ed. Boston, Butterworth-Heinemann, 1991.

433. Kewalramani LS: Autonomic dysreflexia in traumatic myelopathy. *Am J Phys Med* 1980; 59:1 (review).

434. Drummond JC, Moore SS: The influence of dextrose administration on neurologic outcome after temporary spinal cord ischemia in the rabbit. *Anesthesiology* 1989; 70:64.

435. Marshall SB, et al: *Neuroscience Critical Care*. Philadelphia, Saunders, 1990.

436. Adams RD, Victor M: *Principles of Neurology*, 5th ed. New York, McGraw-Hill, 1993.

437. Stone JL, et al: Epidural hematomas of the posterior fossa. *Surg Neurol* 1979; 11:419.

438. Muchmore JH, et al: Deep vein thrombophlebitis and pulmonary embolism in patients with malignant gliomas. *South Med J* 1989; 82:1352.

439. Altschuler E, et al: The risk and efficacy of anticoagulant therapy in the treatment of thromboembolic complications in patients with primary malignant brain tumors. *Neurosurgery* 1990; 27:74.

440. Olin JW, et al: Treatment of deep vein thrombosis and pulmonary emboli in patients with primary and metastatic brain tumors. Anticoagulant or inferior vena cava filter? *Arch Intern Med* 1987; 147:2177.

441. Adams RD, Victor M: Intracranial neoplasms. In Adams RD, Victor M (eds): *Principles of Neurology*, 5th ed. New York, McGraw-Hill, 1993:554–598.

442. Robertson GL: Thirst and vasopressin function in normal and disordered states of water balance. *J Lab Clin Med* 1983; 101:351.

443. Arieff AI: Central nervous system manifestations of disordered sodium metabolism. *Clin Endocrinol Metab* 1984; 13:269.

444. Miller M, et al: Recognition of partial defects in antidiuretic hormone secretion. *Ann Intern Med* 1970; 72:721.

445. Marshall SB, et al: *Neuroscience Critical Care*. Philadelphia, Saunders, 1990:296–298.

446. Seckl JR, et al: Neurohypophyseal peptide function during early postoperative diabetes insipidus. *Brain* 1987; 110:737.

447. Verbalis JG, et al: Postoperative and post-traumatic diabetes insipidus. In Czernichow P, Robinson AG (eds): *Diabetes Insipidus in Man: Frontiers of Hormone Research*, vol 13. Basel, Karger, 1984:247–265.

448. Robinson AG: DDAVP in the treatment of central diabetes insipidus. *N Engl J Med* 1976; 294:507.

449. Chauveau ME: Pathology of posterior pituitary. In Pinsky MR, Dhainaut JF A (eds): *Pathophysiologic Foundations of Critical Care*. Baltimore, Williams & Wilkins, 1993:910–916.

450. Chanson P, et al: Management of early postoperative diabetes insipidus with parenteral desmopressin. *Acta Endocrinol (Copenh)* 1988; 117:513.

451. Wolf, et al: Epidemiology of stroke. In Barnett HJM, et al (eds). *Stroke: Pathophysiology, Diagnosis, and Management*, 2d ed. New York, Churchill Livingstone, 1992:3–28.

452. Mohr JP, et al: Intracranial aneurysms. In Barnett HJM, et al (eds): *Stroke: Pathophysiology, Diagnosis, and Management*, 2d ed. New York, Churchill Livingstone, 1992:617–644.

453. Sahs AL: Preface. In Sahs AL, et al (eds): *Aneurysmal Subarachnoid Hemorrhage. Report of the Cooperative Study*. Baltimore, Urban and Schwarzenberg, 1981:xvii.

454. Peerless SJ, Yasargil MG: Adrenergic innervation of the cerebral blood vessels in the rabbit. *J Neurosurg* 1971; 35:148.

455. Pritz MB, et al: Treatment of patients with neurological deficits associated with cerebral vasospasm by intravascular volume expansion. *Neurosurgery* 1978; 3:364.

456. Ohno K, et al: A review of 102 consecutive patients with intracranial aneurysms in a community hospital in Japan. *Acta Neurochir (Wien)* 1988; 94:23.

457. Fodstad H, et al: Tranexamic acid in the preoperative management of ruptured intracranial aneurysms. *Surg Neurol* 1978; 10:9.

458. Mohr JP, Kase CS: Cerebral vasospasm. *Rev Neurol* 1983; 139:99.

459. Popovic EA, Siu K: Ruptured intracranial aneurysms: A 12-month prospective study. *Med J Aust* 1989; 150:492.

460. Martelli N, et al: Cerebromeningeal hemorrhage: Analysis of autopsies performed over a 10-year period. *Arq Neurospiquiatr* 1988; 46:166.

461. Ropper AH, Zervas NT: Outcome one year after subarachnoid hemorrhage from cerebral aneurysm. *J Neurosurg* 1984; 60:909.

462. Morley TP, Barr HWK: Giant intracranial aneurysms: Diagnosis, course, and management. *Clin Neurosurg* 1968; 16:73.

463. Fairbaum B: ''Twin'' intracranial aneurysms causing subarachnoid hemorrhage in identical twins. *BMJ* 1973; 1:210.

464. Sakoda K, et al: A study of the treatment of multiple aneurysms. *Hiroshima J Med Sci* 1989; 38:151.

465. Findlay JM, et al: Arterial wall changes in cerebral vasospasm. *Neurosurgery* 1989; 25:736.

466. Espinosa F, et al: Nonoperative treatment of subarachnoid hemorrhage. In Yeomans JR (ed): *Neurological Surgery*, 3d ed. Philadelphia, Saunders, 1990:1661–1688.

467. Fodstad H, et al: Antifibrinolysis with tranexamic acid in aneurysmal subarachnoid hemorrhage. A consecutive controlled clinical trial. *Neurosurgery* 1981; 8:158.

468. Kassell NF, Boarini DJ: Perioperative care of the aneurysm patient. *Contemp Neurosurg* 1984; 6:1.

469. Kassell NF, Torner JC: Epidemiology of intracranial aneurysms. *Int Anesthesiol Clin* 1982; 20:13.

470. Torner JC, et al: Preoperative prognostic factors for rebleeding and survival in aneurysm patients receiving antifibrinolytic therapy: Report of the cooperative aneurysm study. *Neurosurgery* 1981; 9:506.

471. Nishioka H, et al: Cooperative study of intracranial aneurysms and subarachnoid hemorrhage: A long-term prognostic study. II. Ruptured intracranial aneurysms managed conservatively. *Arch Neurol* 1984; 41:1142.

472. Heros RC: Acute hydrocephalus after subarachnoid hemorrhage. *Stroke* 1989; 20:715.

473. McNealy DE, Plum F: Brainstem dysfunction with supratentorial mass lesions. *Arch Neurol* 1962; 7:26.

474. Mohr G, et al: Intraventricular hemorrhage from ruptured aneurysm. Retrospective analysis of 91 cases. *J Neurosurg* 1983; 58:482.

475. vab Gijn J, et al: Acute hydrocephalus after aneurysmal subarachnoid hemorrhage. *J Neurosurg* 1985; 63:355.

475a. Black PMcL: Hydrocephalus and vasospasm after subarachnoid hemorrhage from ruptured intracranial aneurysms. *Neurosurgery* 1986; 18:12.

476. Kassell NF: The natural history and treatment outcome of SAH: Comments derived from the national cooperative aneurysm study. In Battye R (ed): *Calcium Antagonists: Possible Therapeutic Use in Neurosurgery*. New York, Raven Press, 1983:24.

477. Weir BK: Pathophysiology of vasospasm. *Int Anesthesiol Clin* 1982; 20:39.

478. Ropper AH, Zervas NT: Outcome one year after subarachnoid hemorrhage from cerebral aneurysm. Management, morbidity, and functional status in 112 consecutive good-risk patients. *J Neurosurg* 1984; 60:909.

479. Schucart WA, et al: Epsilon-aminocaproic acid and recurrent subarachnoid hemorrhage: A clinical trial. *J Neurosurg* 1980; 53:28.

480. Gurus IN, et al: The value of computerized tomography in aneurysmal subarachnoid hemorrhage. *J Neurosurg* 1984; 60:763.

481. Hayward RD: Subarachnoid hemorrhage of unknown aetiology: A clinical and radiological study of 51 cases. *J Neurol Neurosurg Psychiatry* 1977; 40:926.

482. Herdt D Jr, et al: Combined arterial and arterivenous aneurysms of the spinal cord. *Radiology* 1971; 99:589.

483. Pritz MB, et al: Treatment of patients with neurological deficits associated with cerebral vasospasm by intravascular volume expansion. *Neurosurgery* 1978; 3:364.

484. Senguptu RP, et al: Use of epsilon-aminocaproic acid (EACA) in the preoperative management of ruptured intracranial aneurysms. *J Neurosurg* 1976; 44:479.

485. Allcock JM, Drake CG: Ruptured intracranial aneurysms: The role of arterial spasm. *J Neurosurg* 1965; 22:21.

486. Suzuki J, et al: Early operation for ruptured intracranial aneurysms: Study of 31 cases operated on within the first four days of ruptured aneurysm. *Neurol Med Chir (Tokyo)* 1978; 18:82.

487. Mohr JP, Kase CS: Cerebral vasospasm. *Rev Neurol* 1983; 139:99.

488. Tannenbaum H, et al: Therapeutic considerations in the treatment of vasospasm in aneurysms. *Acta Neurochir* 1980; 52:158.

489. Sundt TM Jr: Management of ischemic complications after subarachnoid hemorrhage. *J Neurosurg* 1974; 43:418.

490. Winn HE, et al: The assessment of the natural history of single cerebral aneurysms that have ruptured. In Hopkins LN, Long DM (eds): *Clinical Management of Intracranial Aneurysms*. New York, Raven Press, 1982:1.

491. Espinosa F, et al: A randomized placebo-controlled double-blind trial of nimodipine after SAH in monkeys. Part 1. Clinical and radiological findings. *J Neurosurg* 1984; 60:1167.

492. Espinosa F, et al: A randomized placebo-controlled double-blind trial of nimodipine after SAH in monkeys. Part 2: Pathological findings. *J Neurosurg* 1984; 60:1176.

493. Kistler JP, et al: The relation of cerebral vasospasm to the extent and location of subarachnoid blood visualized by CT scan. A prospective study. *Neurology* 1983; 33:424.

494. Silver AJ, et al: CT of subarachnoid hemorrhage due to ruptured aneurysm. *AJNR Am J Neuroradiol* 1981; 2:13.

495. Pasqualin A, et al: Role of computed tomography in the management of vasospasm after subarachnoid hemorrhage. *Neurosurgery* 1984; 15:344.

496. Wilkins RH: Cerebral vasospasm. *Crit Rev Neurobiol* 1990; 6:51.

497. Wilkins RH: Intracranial vascular spasm in head injuries. In Vinken PJ, Bruyn GW (eds): *Handbook of Clinical Neurology*, vol 23. *Injuries of the Brain and Skull. Part I.* Amsterdam, North-Holland, 1975:163.

498. Echlin FA: Spasm of basilar and vertebral arteries caused by experimental subarachnoid hemorrhage. *J Neurosurg* 1965; 23:1.

499. Kanamaru K, et al: Inhibition of endothelium dependent relaxation by hemoglobin and cerebrospinal fluid from patients with aneurysm subarachnoid hemorrhage: A possible mechanism and relation to cerebral vasospasm. In Wilkins RH (ed): *Cerebral Vasospasm: Proceedings of the Charlottesville Conference Held April 29–May 1, 1987.* New York, Raven Press, 1988:163.

500. Afshar JK, et al: Effect of intracarotid nitric oxide on primate cerebral vasospasm after subarachnoid hemorrhage. *J Neurosurg* 1995; 83:118.

501. Wilkins RH: Hypothalamic dysfunction and intracranial arterial spasm. *Surg Neurol* 1975; 4:472.

502. Peerless SJ, Griffiths JC: Plasma catecholamines following subarachnoid hemorrhage. In Smith RR, Robertson JT (eds): *Subarachnoid Hemorrhage and Cerebrovascular Spasm*. Springfield, IL, Charles C. Thomas, 1975:148.

503. Cruickshank JM, et al: Electrocardiographic changes and their prognostic significance in subarachnoid hemorrhage. *J Neurol Neurosurg Psychiatry* 1974; 37:755.

504. Cruickshank JM, et al: Possible role of catecholamines, corticosteroids, and potassium in production of electro-cardiographic abnormalities associated with subarachnoid hemorrhage. *Br Heart J* 1974; 36:697.

505. Neil-Dwyer G, et al: Their urinary catecholamine and plasma cortisol levels in patients with subarachnoid haemorrhage. *J Neurol Sci* 1974; 22:375.

506. Crompton MR: Hypothalamic lesions following the rupture of cerebral berry aneurysms. *Brain* 1963; 86:301.

507. Fraser RAR, et al: Noradrenergic mediation of experimental cerebrovascular spasm. *Stroke* 1970; 1:356.

508. Peerless SJ, Kendall MJ: The innervation of the cerebral blood vessels. In Smith RR, Robertson JT (eds): *Subarachnoid Hemor-*

rhage and Cerebrovascular Spasm. Springfield, IL, Charles C. Thomas, 1975:38.

509. Wilkins RH, et al: Intracranial arterial spasm: A clinical analysis. *J Neurosurg* 1968; 29:121.

510. Cruickshank JM, et al: Possible role of catecholamines, corticosteroids, and potassium in production of electrocardiographic abnormalities associated with subarachnoid hemorrhage. *Br Heart J* 1974; 36:697.

511. Kono T, et al: Left ventricular wall motion abnormalities in patients with subarachnoid hemorrhage: neurogenic stunned myocardium. *J Am Coll Cardiol* 1994; 24:636.

512. Svendgaard NA, et al: Catecholaminergic and peptidergic systems underlying cerebral vasospasm: CBF and CMRgl changes following an experimental subarachnoid hemorrhage in the rat. In Wilkins RH (ed): *Cerebral Vasospasm: Proceedings of the Charlottesville Conference Held April 29–May 1, 1987.* New York, Raven Press, 1988:178.

513. Wilkins RH: The role of intracranial arterial spasm in the timing of operations for aneurysms. *Clin Neurosurg* 1977; 24:185.

514. Grubb RL Jr, et al: Effects of subarachnoid hemorrhage on cerebral blood volume, blood flow, and oxygen utilization in humans. *J Neurosurg* 1977; 46:446.

515. Powers WJ, Grubb RL Jr: Hemodynamic and metabolic relationships in cerebral ischemia and subarachnoid hemorrhage. In Wood JH (ed): *CBF: Physiologic and Clinical Aspects.* New York, McGraw-Hill, 1987:387.

516. Ishii R: Regional CBF in patients with ruptured intracranial aneurysms. *J Neurosurg* 1979; 50:587.

517. Powers WJ, et al: Regional CBF and metabolism in reversible ischemia due to vasospasm: Determination by positron emission tomography. *J Neurosurg* 1985; 62:539.

518. Weir B, et al: Regional CBF in patients with aneurysms: Estimation by xenon 133 inhalation. *Can J Neurol Sci* 1978; 5:301.

519. Weir B: *Aneurysms Affecting the Nervous System*, Baltimore, Williams & Wilkins, 1987.

520. Robertson EG: Cerebral lesions due to intracranial aneurysms. *Brain* 1949; 72:150.

521. Wilson G, et al: The pathologic anatomy of ruptured cerebral aneurysms. *J Neurosurg* 1954; 11:128.

522. Crompton MR: The pathogenesis of cerebral infarction following the rupture of cerebral berry aneurysms. *Brain* 1964; 87:491.

523. Tomlinsons BE: Brain changes in ruptured intracranial aneurysms. *J Clin Pathol* 1959; 12:391.

524. Birse SH, Tom ML: Incidence of cerebral infarction associated with ruptured intracranial aneurysms: A study of 8 unoperated cases of anterior cerebral aneurysms. *Neurology* 1960; 10:101.

525. Kassell NF, Boarini DJ: Perioperative care of the aneurysm patient. *Contemp Neurosurg* 1984; 6:1.

526. Keranen T, et al: Late epilepsy after aneurysm operations. *Neurosurgery* 1985; 17:897.

527. Adams HP, Love BB: Medical management of aneurysmal subarachnoid hemorrhage. In Barnett HJM, et al (eds): *Stroke: Pathophysiology, Diagnosis, and Management*, 2d ed. New York, Churchill Livingstone, 1992:1029–1054.

528. Disney L, et al: Trends in blood pressure, osmolality, and electrolytes after subarachnoid hemorrhage from aneurysms. *Can J Neurol Sci* 1989; 16:299.

529. Koskelo P, et al: Subendocardial hemorrhage and ECG changes in intracranial bleeding. *BMJ* 1964; 1:1479.

530. Wijdicks EFM, et al: Hyponatremia and cerebral infarction in patients with ruptured intracranial aneurysms: is fluid restriction harmful? *Ann Neurol* 1985; 17:137.

531. Crowell RM, Zervas NT: Management of intracranial aneurysms. *Med Clin North Am* 1979; 63:695.

532. Peerless SJ: Pre- and postoperative management of cerebral aneurysms. *Clin Neurosurg* 1979; 26:209.

533. Widjicks EFM, et al: Volume depletion and natriuresis in patients with a ruptured intracranial aneurysm. *Ann Neurol* 1985; 18:211.

534. Diringer M, et al: Plasma atrial netriuretic factor and subarachnoid hemorrhage. *Stroke* 1988; 19:1119.

535. Rosenfeld JV, et al: The effect of subarachnoid hemorrhage on blood and CSF atrial natriuretic factor. *J Neurosurg* 1989; 71:32.

536. Jourdan C, et al: [Hyperthermia in meningeal hemorrhage. Contribution of daily determination of inflammation proteins]. Hyperthermie au cours des hemorragies meningees. Apport du dosage quotidien des proteines de l'inflammation. *Agressologie* 1990; 31:380.

537. Simpson RK Jr, et al: Neurogenic hyperthermia in subarachnoid hemorrhage. *South Med J* 1989; 82:1577.

538. Rousseaux P, et al: Fever and cerebral vasospasm in ruptured intracranial aneurysms. *Surg Neurol* 1980; 14:459.

539. Chason JL, Hindman WM: Berry aneurysms of the circle of Willis: Results of a planned autopsy study. *Neurology* 1958; 8:41.

540. Stehbens WE: Etiology of intracranial berry aneurysms. *J Neurosurg* 1989; 70:823.

541. Fox JL: *Intracranial Aneurysms*, New York, Springer-Verlag, 1983.

542. Chester AC, et al: Polycystic kidney disease. *Am Fam Physician* 1977; 16:94.

543. Mettinger KL: Fibromuscular dysplasia and the brain: II. Current concept of the disease. *Stroke* 1982; 13:53.

544. Longstreth WT, et al: Cigarette smoking, alcohol use, and subarachnoid hemorrhage. *Stroke* 1992; 23:1242.

545. Leblanc R, Winfield JA: The warning leak in subarachnoid hemorrhage and the importance of its early diagnosis. *Can Med Assoc J* 1984; 131:1235.

546. Okawara S: Warning signs prior to rupture of an intracranial aneurysm. *J Neurosurg* 1973; 38:575.

547. Botterell EH, et al: Hypothermia, and interruption of carotid, or carotid and vertebral circulation in the surgical management of intracranial aneurysms. *J Neurosurg* 1956; 13:1.

548. Hunt WE, Hess RM: Surgical risk as related to time of intervention in the repair of intracranial aneurysms. *J Neurosurg* 1968; 28:14.

549. Fisher CM, et al: Relation of cerebral vasospasm to subarachnoid hemorrhage visualized by computed tomographic scanning. *J Neurosurg* 1980; 6:1.

550. Vermeulen M, et al: Causes of acute deterioration in patients with a ruptured intracranial aneurysm. *J Neurosurg* 1984; 60:935.

551. Adams HP Jr, et al: Early management of aneurysmal subarachnoid hemorrhage: A report of the Cooperative Aneurysm Study. *J Neurosurg* 1981; 54:141.

552. Ingall TJ, et al: Has there been a decline in subarachnoid hemorrhage mortality? *Stroke* 1989; 20:718.

553. Kassell NF, Torner JC: Aneurysmal rebleeding: A preliminary report from the Cooperative Aneurysm Study. *Neurosurgery* 1983; 13:479.

554. McKissock W, et al: Middle cerebral aneurysms: further results in the controlled trial of conservative and surgical treatment of ruptured intracranial aneurysms. *Lancet* 1962; 2:417.

555. Nibbelink DW, et al: Intracranial aneurysms and subarachnoid hemorrhage—report of a randomized treatment study: IV. A. Regulated bed rest. *Stroke* 1977; 8:202.

556. Jane JA, et al: The natural history of aneurysms and arteriovenous malformations. *J Neurosurg* 1985; 62:321.

556a. Drake CG: Management of cerebral aneurysm. *Stroke* 1981; 12:273.

557. van Crevel H: Pitfalls in the diagnosis of rebleeding from intracranial aneurysm. *Clin Neurol Neurosurg* 1980; 82:1.

558. Chyatte D, Sundt TM Jr: Cerebral vasospasm after subarachnoid hemorrhage. *Mayo Clin Proc* 1984; 59:498.

559. Heros RC, et al: Cerebral vasospasm after subarachnoid hemorrhage: An update. *Ann Neurol* 1983; 14:599.

560. Kassell NF, et al: Cerebral vasospasm following aneurysmal subarachnoid hemorrhage. *Stroke* 1985; 16:562.

561. Weir B, et al: Time course of vasospasm in man. *J Neurosurg* 1978; 48:173.

562. Black PMcL: Hydrocephalus and vasospasm after subarachnoid hemorrhage from ruptured intracranial aneurysms. *Neurosurgery* 1986; 18:12.

563. Hijdra A, et al: Delayed cerebral ischemia after aneurysmal subarachnoid hemorrhage: Clinicoanatomic observations. *Neurology* 1986; 36:329.

564. Fraser J, et al: Prediction of cerebral vasospasm with subarachnoid hemorrhage due to ruptured intracranial aneurysm by computed axial tomography. *Neurosurgery* 1980; 6:686.

565. Kistler JP, et al: The relation of cerebral vasospasm to the extent and location of subarachnoid blood visualized by CT scan: A prospective study. *Neurology* 1983; 33:424.

566. Pasqualin A, et al: Role of computed tomography in the management of vasospasm after subarachnoid hemorrhage. *Neurosurgery* 1984; 15:344.

567. Sano H, et al: Prospection of chronic vasospasm by CT findings. *Acta Neurochir* 1982; 63:23.

568. Yonas H: Cerebral blood measurements in vasospasm. *Neurosurg Clin North Am* 1990; 1:307 (review).

569. Sekhar LN, et al: Value of transcranial Doppler examination in the diagnosis of cerebral vasospasm after subarachnoid hemorrhage. *Neurosurgery* 1988; 22:813.

570. van der Wee N, et al: Detection of subarachnoid haemorrhage on early CT: Is lumbar puncture still needed after a negative scan? *J Neurol Neurosurg Psychiatry* 1995; 58:357.

571. Sundt TM Jr, et al: Results and complications of surgical management of 809 intracranial aneurysms in 722 cases. *J Neurosurg* 1982; 56:753.

572. Hunt WE, Miller CA: The results of early operation for aneurysm. *Clin Neurosurg* 1976; 24:208.

573. Kori S, Suzuki J: Early intracranial operation for ruptured aneurysms. *Acta Neurochir* 1979; 46:93.

574. Sano K, Saito I: Timing and indication of surgery for ruptured intracranial aneurysms with regard to cerebral vasospasm. *Acta Neurochir* 1978; 41:49.

575. Bolander HG, et al: Retrospective analysis of 162 consecutive cases of ruptured intracranial aneurysms: Total mortality and early surgery. *Acta Neurochir* 1984; 70:31.

576. Hugenholtz H, Elgie R: Considerations in early surgery on good-risk patients with ruptured intracranial aneurysms. *J Neurosurg* 1982; 56:180.

577. Kassell NF, et al: Overall management of ruptured aneurysm: Comparison of early and late operation. *Neurosurgery* 1981; 9:120.

578. Ljunggren B, et al: Early management of aneurysmal subarachnoid hemorrhage. *Neurosurgery* 1982; 11:412.

579. Taneda M: Effect of early operation for ruptured aneurysms on prevention of delayed ischemic symptoms. *J Neurosurg* 1982; 57:622.

580. Weir B, Aronyk K: Management mortality and the timing of surgery for supratentorial aneurysms. *J Neurosurg* 1981; 54:146.

581. Yamamoto I, et al: Early operation for ruptured intracranial aneurysms: Comparative study with computed tomography. *Neurosurgery* 1983; 12:169.

582. Ohman J, Heiskanen O: Timing of operation for ruptured supratentorial aneurysms: A prospective randomized study. *J Neurosurg* 1989; 70:55.

583. Kassell NF, et al: The International Cooperative Study on the timing of aneurysm surgery. I. Overall management results. *J Neurosurg* 1990; 73:18.

584. Kassell NF, et al: The International Cooperative Study on the timing of aneurysm surgery. II. Surgical results. *J Neurosurg* 1990; 73:34.

585. Harders AG, Gilsbach JM: Time course of blood velocity changes related to vasospasm in the circle of Willis measured by transcranial Doppler ultrasound. *J Neurosurg* 1987; 66:718.

586. Grossett DG, et al: Use of transcranial Doppler sonography to predict development of a delayed ischemic deficit after subarachnoid hemorrhage. *J Neurosurg* 1993; 78:183.

587. Laumer R, et al: Cerebral hemodynamics in subarachnoid hemorrhage evaluated by transcranial Doppler sonography. Part 1. Reliability of flow velocities in clinical management. *Neurosurgery* 1993; 33:1.

588. Steinmeier R, et al: Cerebral hemodynamics in subarachnoid hemorrhage evaluated by transcranial Doppler sonography. Part 2. Pulsatility indices: Normal reference values and characteristics in subarachnoid hemorrhage. *Neurosurgery* 1993; 33:10.

589. Jordan KG: Continuous EEG and evoked potential monitoring in the neuroscience intensive care unit. *J Clin Neurophysiol* 1993; 10:445 (review).

590. Dauch WA: Prediction of secondary deterioration in comatose neurosurgical patients by serial recording of multimodality evoked potentials. *Acta Neurochir* 1991; 111:84.

591. Nau HE, Rimpel J: Multimodality evoked potentials and electroencephalography in severe coma cases. Clinical experiences in a neurosurgical intensive care unit. *Intensive Care Med* 1987; 13:249.

592. Symon L, et al: Central conduction time as an index of ischaemia in subarachnoid haemorrhage. *J Neurol Sci* 1979; 44:95.

593. Labar DR, et al: Quantitative EEG monitoring for patients with subarachnoid hemorrhage. *Electroencephalogr Clin Neurophysiol* 1991; 78:325.

594. Yonas H, et al: Stable xenon-enhanced CT measurement of CBF in reversible focal ischemia in baboons. *J Neurosurg* 1990; 73:266.

595. Steed DL, et al: Clinical observations on the effect of carotid artery occlusion on CBF mapped by xenon computed tomography and its correlation with carotid artery back pressure. *J Vasc Surg* 1990; 11:38.

596. Nibbelink DW, et al: Randomized treatment study: Regulated bed rest. In Sahs AL, et al (eds): *Aneurysmal Subarachnoid Hemorrhage. Report of the Cooperative Study.* Baltimore, Urban and Schwarzenberg, 1981:27.

597. Vermeulen M, et al: Antifibrinolytic treatment. I Subarachnoid Hemorrhage. *N Engl J Med* 1984; 311:432.

598. Kassell NF, et al: Antifibrinolytic therapy in the acute period following aneurysmal subarachnoid hemorrhage: preliminary observations from the Cooperative Aneurysm Study. *J Neurosurg* 1984; 61:225.

599. Ramirez-Lassepas M: Antifibrinolytic therapy in subarachnoid hemorrhage caused by ruptured intracranial aneurysm. *Neurology* 1981; 31:316.

600. Glick R, et al: High dose ε-aminocaproic acid prolongs the bleeding time and increases rebleeding and intraoperative hemorrhage in patients with subarachnoid hemorrhage. *Neurosurgery* 1981; 9:398.

601. Green D, et al: Clinical and laboratory investigation of the effects of ε-aminocaproic acid on hemostasis. *J Lab Clin Med* 1985; 105:321.

602. Heros RC: Acute hydrocephalus after subarachnoid hemorrhage. *Stroke* 1989; 20:715.

603. Kusske JA, et al: Ventriculostomy for the treatment of acute hydrocephalus following subarachnoid hemorrhage. *J Neurosurg* 1973; 38:591.

604. Yasargil MG, et al: Hydrocephalus following spontaneous subarachnoid hemorrhage: Clinical features and treatment. *J Neurosurg* 1973; 39:474.

605. Ohta H, et al: Extensive evacuation of subarachnoid clot for prevention of vasospasm: Effective or not? *Acta Neurochir* 1982; 63:111.

605a. Young B, et al: Relationship between admission hyperglycemia and neurologic outcome of severely brain-injured patients. *Ann Surg* 1989; 210:466.

606. Wakabayashi T, Fujita S: Removal of subarachnoid blood clots after subarachnoid hemorrhage. *Surg Neurol* 1984; 21:533.

607. Mizukami M, et al: Prevention of vasospasm by early operation with removal of subarachnoid blood. *Neurosurgery* 1982; 10:301.

608. Allen GS, et al: Cerebral arterial spasm: A controlled trial of nimodipine in patients with subarachnoid hemorrhage. *N Engl J Med* 1983; 308:619.

609. Mee E, et al: Controlled study of nimodipine in aneurysm patients treated early after subarachnoid hemorrhage. *Neurosurgery* 1988; 22:484.

610. Neil-Dwyer G, et al: Early intervention with nimodipine in subarachnoid hemorrhage. *Eur Heart J* 1988; 8:41.

611. Petruk KC, et al: Nimodipine treatment in poor grade aneurysm patients: Results of a multicenter double-blind placebo-controlled trial. *J Neurosurg* 1988; 68:505.

612. Pickard JD, et al: Effect of oral nimodipine on cerebral infarction and outcome after subarachnoid hemorrhage. British Aneurysm Nimodipine Trial. *BMJ* 1989; 298:636.

613. Terttenborn D, Dycka J: Prevention and treatment of delayed ischemic dysfunction in patients with aneurysmal subarachnoid hemorrhage. *Stroke* 1990; 21(suppl):85.

614. Jan M, et al: Therapeutic trial of intravenous nimodipine in patients with established cerebral vasospasm after rupture of intracranial aneurysm. *Neurosurgery* 1988; 23:154.

615. Flamm ES, et al: Dose-escalation study of intravenous nicardipine in patients with aneurysmal subarachnoid hemorrhage. *J Neurosurg* 1988; 68:393.

616. Haley EC, Torner JC, Kassell NF, and participants. Cooperative randomized study of nicardipine in subarachnoid hemorrhage. Preliminary report. In Sano K, et al (eds): *Cerebral Vasospasm. Proceedings of the Fourth International Conference on Cerebral Vasospasm.* Tokyo, University of Tokyo Press, 1990:519.

617. Althaus JS, et al: The use of salicylate hydroxylation to detect hydroxyl radical generation in ischemic and traumatic brain injury. Reversal by tirilazad mesylate (U-74006F). *Molec Chem Neuropathol* 1993; 20:147.

618. Hall ED: Neuroprotective actions of glucocorticoid and nonglucocorticoid steroids in acute neuronal injury. *Cell Molec Neurobiol* 1993; 13:415 (review).

619. Hall ED, et al: Effects of tirilazad mesylate on postischemic brain lipid peroxidation and recovery of extracellular calcium in gerbils. *Stroke* 1991; 22:361.

620. Zuccarello M, et al: Effect of the 21-aminosteroid U-74006F on cerebral vasospasm following subarachnoid hemorrhage. *J Neurosurg* 1989; 71:98.

621. Steinke DE, et al: A trial of the 21-aminosteroid U74006F in a primate model of chronic cerebral vasospasm. *Neurosurgery* 1989; 24:179.

622. Haley EC Jr, et al: Phase II trial of tirilazad in aneurysmal subarachnoid hemorrhage. A report of the Cooperative Aneurysm Study. *J Neurosurg* 1995; 82:786.

623. Ishii R: Regional CBF in patients with ruptured intracranial aneurysms. *J Neurosurg* 1979; 50:587.

624. Levy ML, et al: Cardiac performance enhancement from dobutamine in patients refractory to hypervolemic therapy for cerebral vasospasm. *J Neurosurg* 1993; 19:494.

625. Levy ML, Giannotta SL: Cardiac performance indices during hypervolemic therapy for cerebral vasospasm. *J Neurosurg* 1991; 75:27.

626. Awad IA, et al: Clinical vasospasm after subarachnoid hemorrhage: Response to hypervolemic hemodilution and arterial hypertension. *Stroke* 1987; 18:365.

627. Brown FD, et al: Treatment of aneurysmal hemiplegia with dopamine and mannitol. *J Neurosurg* 1978; 49:525.

628. Kassell NF, et al: Treatment of ischemic deficits from vasospasm with intravascular volume expansion and induced arterial hypertension. *Neurosurgery* 1982; 11:337.

629. Muizelaar JP, Becker DP: Induced hypertension for the treatment of cerebral ischemia after subarachnoid hemorrhage. Direct effect on CBF. *Surg Neurol* 1986; 25:317.

630. Otsubo H, et al: Normovolaemic induced hypertension therapy for cerebral vasospasm after subarachnoid hemorrhage. *Acta Neurochir* 1990; 103:18.

631. Solomon RA, et al: Prophylactic volume expansion therapy for the prevention of delayed cerebral ischemia after early aneurysm surgery. Results of a preliminary trial. *Arch Neurol* 1988; 45:325.

632. Wood JM, Kee DB: Hemorrheology of the cerebral circulation in stroke. *Stroke* 1985; 16:765.

633. Awad IA, et al: Clinical vasospasm after subarachnoid hemorrhage: Response to hypervolemic hemodilution and arterial hypertension. *Stroke* 1987; 18:365.

634. Kassell NF, et al: Treatment of ischemic deficits from vasospasm with intravascular volume expansion and induced arterial hypertension. *Neurosurgery* 1982; 11:337.

635. Germano A, et al: Blood-brain barrier permeability changes after experimental subarachnoid hemorrhage. *Neurosurgery* 1992; 30:882.

636. Nakagomi T, et al: Blood-arterial wall barrier disruption to various sized tracers following subarachnoid haemorrhage. *Acta Neurochir (Wien)* 1989; 99:76.

637. Doczi T, et al: Blood-brain barrier damage during the acute stage of subarachnoid hemorrhage, as exemplified by a new animal model. *Neurosurgery* 1986; 18:733.

638. Doczi T: The pathogenetic and prognostic significance of blood-brain barrier damage at the acute stage of aneurysmal subarachnoid hemorrhage. Clinical and experimental studies. *Acta Neurochir (Wien)* 1985; 77:110.

639. MacKenzie ET, et al: Influence of endogenous norepinephrine on CBF and metabolism. *Am J Physiol* 1976; 231:489.

640. Olesen J: The effect of intracarotid epinephrine, norepinephrine, and angiotensin on the regional CBF in man. *Neurology* 1972; 22:978.

641. Swift DM, Solomon RA: Unruptured aneurysms and postoperative volume expansion. *J Neurosurg* 1992; 77:908.

642. Eng CC, Lam AM: Cerebral aneurysms: Anesthetic considerations. In Cottrell JE, Turndorf H (eds): *Anesthesia and Neurosurgery.* St. Louis, Mosby-Yearbook, 1980:376–406.

643. Terada T, et al: Hemorrhagic infarction after vasospasm due to ruptured cerebral aneurysm. *Neurosurgery* 1986; 18:415.

644. Kaku Y, et al: Superselective intra-arterial infusion of papaverine for the treatment of cerebral vasospasm after subarachnoid hemorrhage. *J Neurosurg* 1992; 77:842.

645. Solomon RA, et al: Prophylactic volume expansion therapy for the prevention of delayed cerebral ischemia after early

aneurysm surgery: Results of a preliminary trial. *Arch Neurol* 1988; 45:325.

646. Solomon RA, et al: Early aneurysm surgery and prophylactic hypervolemic hypertensive therapy for the treatment of aneurysmal subarachnoid hemorrhage. *Neurosurgery* 1988; 23:699.

647. Buckland MR, et al: Anesthesia for cerebral aneurysm surgery: Use of induced hypertension in patients with symptomatic vasospasm. *Anesthesiology* 1988; 69:116.

648. Hasan D, et al: Effect of fluid intake and antihypertensive treatment on cerebral ischemia after subarachnoid hemorrhage. *Stroke* 1989; 20:1511.

649. Newell DW, et al: Angioplasty for the treatment of symptomatic vasospasm following subarachnoid hemorrhage. *Neurosurgery* 1989; 71:654.

650. Clouston JE, et al: Intraarterial papaverine infusion for cerebral vasospasm after subarachnoid hemorrhage. *Am J Neuroradiol* 1995; 16:27.

651. Barr JD, et al: Transient severe brain stem depression during intraarterial papaverine infusion for cerebral vasospasm. *Am J Neuroradiol* 1994; 15:719.

652. McAuliffe W, et al: Intracranial pressure changes induced during papaverine infusion for treatment of vasospasm. *J Neurosurg* 1995; 83:430.

653. Mathis JM, et al: Transient neurologic events associated with intraarterial papaverine infusion for subarachnoid hemorrhage-induced vasospasm. *Am J Neuroradiol* 1994; 15:1671.

654. Hendrix LE, et al: Papaverine-induced mydriasis. *Am J Neuroradiol* 1994; 15:716.

655. Guglielmi G, et al: Endovascular treatment of posterior circulation aneurysms by electrothrombosis using electrically detachable coils. *J Neurosurg* 1992; 77:515.

656. Casasco A, et al: [Giant intracranial aneurysm. Elective endovascular treatment using metallic coils]. Aneurysms gigantes intracraniens. Traitement endovasculaire electif par des spires metalliques. *Neuro-Chirurgie* 1992; 38:18 (review).

657. Eng CC, et al: The diagnosis and management of a perianesthetic cerebral aneurysmal rupture aided with transcranial Doppler ultrasonography. *Anesthesiology* 1993; 78:191.

658. Frankowski RF: Epidemiology of stroke and intracerebral hemorrhage. In Kaufman HH (ed): *Intracerebral Hematomas*, New York, Raven Press, 1992:1.

659. Broderick JP, et al: Incidence rates of stroke in the eighties: The end of the decline in stroke? *Stroke* 1989; 20:577.

660. Brott T, et al: Hypertension as a risk factor for spontaneous intracerebral hemorrhage. *Stroke* 1986; 17:1078.

661. Furlan AJ, et al: The decreasing incidence of primary intracerebral hemorrhage: A population study. *Ann Neurol* 1979; 5:367.

662. Caplan LR: Clinical features of spontaneous intracerebral hemorrhage. In Kaufman HH (ed): *Intracerebral Hematomas*. New York, Raven Press, 1992:31.

663. Fisher CM: Pathological observations in hypertensive cerebral hemorrhage. *J Neuropathol Exp Neurol* 1971; 30:536.

664. Kase CS, et al: Intracerebral hemorrhage. In Barnett HJM, et al (eds): *Stroke: Pathophysiology, Diagnosis, and Management*, 2d ed. New York, Churchill Livingstone, 1992:561–616.

665. Ojemann RG, Mohr JP: Hypertensive brain hemorrhage. *Clin Neurosurg* 1976; 23:220.

666. Herbstein DJ, Schaumburg HH: Hypertensive intracerebral hematoma: An investigation of the initial hemorrhage and rebleeding using chromiun 51-labeled erythrocytes. *Arch Neurol* 1974; 30:412.

667. Broderick JP, et al: Ultraearly evaluation of intracerebral hemorrhage. *J Neurosurg* 1990; 72:195.

668. Fehr MA, Anderson DC: Incidence of progression or rebleeding in hypertensive intracerebral hemorrhage. *J Stroke Cerebrovasc Dis* 1991; 1:111.

669. Kaufman HH, Schochet SS: Pathology, physiology, and modeling. In Kaufman HH (ed): *Intracerebral Hematomas*. New York, Raven Press, 1992:13.

670. Fisher CM: Cerebral miliary aneurysms in hypertension. *Am J Pathol* 1971; 66:313.

671. Feigin I, Prose P: Hypertensive fibrinoid arteritis of the brain and gross cerebral hemorrhage. *Arch Neurol* 1959; 1:98.

672. Ooneda G, et al: Morphogenesis of plasmatic angionecrosis as the cause of hypoertensive intracerebral hemorrhage. *Virchows Arch Pathol Anat* 1973; 361:31.

673. Rosenblum WI: Miliary aneurysms and "fibrinoid" degeneration of cerebral blood vessels. *Hum Pathol* 1977; 8:133.

674. Mohr JP, et al: The Harvard Cooperative Stroke Registry: A prospective registry. *Neurology* 1978; 28:754.

675. Furlan AJ, et al: The decreasing incidence of primary intracerebral hemorrhage: A population study. *Ann Neurol* 1979; 5:367.

676. Brewer DB, et al: A necropsy series of non-traumatic cerebral hemorrhages and softenings, with particular reference to heart weight. *J Pathol Bacteriol* 1968; 96:311.

677. Mutlu N, et al: Massive cerebral hemorrhage: Clinical and pathological correlations. *Arch Neurol* 1963; 8:74.

678. Stehbens WE: *Pathology of the Cerebral Blood Vessels.* St. Louis, Mosby, 1972.

679. McCormick WF, Rosenfield DB: Massive brain hemorrhage: A review of 144 cases and an examination of their causes. *Stroke* 1973; 4:946.

680. Brott T, et al: Hypertension as a risk factor for spontaneous intracerebral hemorrhage. *Stroke* 1986; 17:1078.

681. Schutz H, et al: Age-related spontaneous intracerebral hematoma in a German community. *Stroke* 1990; 21:1412.

682. Gilles S, et al: Cerebral amyloid angiopathy as a cause of multiple intracerebral hemorrhages. *Neurology* 1984; 34:730.

683. Hier DB, et al: Hypertensive putaminal hemorrhage. *Ann Neurol* 1977; 1:152.

684. Mohr JP, et al: The Harvard Cooperative Stroke Registry: A prospective registry. *Neurology* 1978; 28:754.

685. Wiggins WS, et al: Clinical and computerized tomographic study of hypertensive intracerebral hemorrhage. *Arch Neurol* 1978; 35:832.

686. Fisher CM: Pathological observations in hypertensive cerebral hemorrhage. *J Neuropathol Exp Neurol* 1971; 30:536.

687. Fisher CM, et al: Acute hypertensive cerebellar hemorrhage: Diagnosis and surgical treatment. *J Nerv Ment Dis* 1965; 140:38.

688. Broderick J, et al: Ultra-early evaluation of intracerebral hemorrhage (ICH). *Stroke* 1989; 20:158.

689. Kelly R, et al: Active bleeding in hypertensive intracerebral hemorrhage: Computed tomography. *Neurology* 1982; 32:852.

690. Miyasaka Y, et al: An analysis of the venous drainage system as a factor in hemorrhage from arteriovenous malformations. *J Neurosurg* 1992; 76:239.

691. Rudy TA, et al: Hyperthermia produced by simulated intraventricular hemorrhage in the cat. *Exp Neurol* 1978; 58:296.

692. Rossen R, et al: Acute arrest of cerebral circulation in man. *Arch Neurol Psychiatry* 1943; 50:510.

693. Michenfelder JD, Theye RA: The effects of anesthesia and hypothermia on canine cerebral ATP and lactate during anoxia produced by decapitation. *Anesthesiology* 1970; 33:430.

694. Hossmann K-A, Sato K: The effect of ischemia on sensorimotor cortex of the cat. Electrophysiological, biochemical, and electronmicroscopical observations. *Z Neurol* 1970; 198:33.

695. Kleihues P, et al: Purine nucleotide metabolism in the cat brain after one hour of complete ischemia. *J Neurochem* 1974; 23:417.

696. Kleihues P, et al: Resuscitation of the monkey brain after 1 hour complete ischemia. III. Indications of metabolic recovery. *Brain Res* 1975; 95:61.

697. Ljunggren B, et al: Cerebral metabolic state following complete compression ischemia. *Brain Res* 1974; 73:291.

698. Hinzen DH, et al: Metabolism and function of dog's brain recovering from longtime ischemia. *Am J Physiol* 1972; 223:1158.

699. Kogure K, Kato H: Neurochemistry of stroke. In Barnett HJM, et al (eds): *Stroke: Pathophysiology, Diagnosis, and Management*, 2d ed. New York, Churchill Livingstone, 1992:69–102.

700. Araki T, et al: Selective neuronal vulnerability following transient cerebral ischemia in the gerbil: Distribution and time course. *Acta Neurol Scand* 1989; 80:548.

701. Kirino T: Delayed neuronal death in the gerbil hippocampus following ischemia. *Brain Res* 1982; 239:57.

702. Pulsinelli WA, et al: Temporal profile of neuronal damage in a model of transient forebrain ischemia. *Ann Neurol* 1982; 11:491.

703. Kofke WA, et al: Striatal extracellular dopamine levels are not increased by hyperglycemic exacerbation of ischemic brain damage in rats. *Brain Res* 1994; 633:171.

704. Benveniste H: The excitotoxin hypothesis in relation to cerebral ischemia. *Cerebrovasc Brain Metab Rev* 1991; 3:213.

705. Choi DW, et al: Glutamate neurotoxicity in cortical cell culture. *J Neurosci* 1987; 7:357.

706. Coyle JT, et al: Excitatory amino acid neurotoxins: Selectivity, specificity, and mechanisms of action. *Neurosci Res Prog Bull* 1981; 19:331.

707. Fisher SK, Agranoff BW: Receptor activation in inositol lipid hydrolysis in neural tissues. *J Neurochem* 1987; 48:999.

708. Siesjo BK, Bengtsson F: Calcium fluxes, calcium antagonists, and calcium-related pathology in brain ischemia, hypoglycemia, and spreading depression: A unifying hypothesis. *J Cereb Blood Flow Metab* 1989; 9:127.

709. Nishizuka Y: The role of protein kinase C in cell surface signal transduction and tumor promotion. *Nature* 1984; 308:693.

710. Furukawa K, et al: Post-ischemic alterations of spontaneous activities in rat hippocampal CA1 neurons. *Brain Res* 1990; 530:257.

711. Suzuki R, et al: The effects of 5-minutes ischemia in Mongolian gerbils. II. Changes of spontaneous neuronal activity in cerebral cortex and Ca1 sector of hippocampus. *Acta Neuropathol (Berl)* 1983; 60:217.

712. Gotoh O, et al: Ischemic brain edema following occlusion of the middle cerebral artery in the rat. I. The time course of the brain water, sodium, and potassium contents and blood-brain barrier permeability to 125 I-albumin. *Stroke* 1985; 16:101.

713. Kogure K, et al: The role of hydrostatic pressure in ischemic brain edema. *Ann Neurol* 1981; 9:273.

714. Kato H, et al: Greater disturbance of water and ion homeostasis in the periphery of experimental focal cerebral ischemia. *Exp Neurol* 1987; 96:118.

715. Shiga Y, et al: Neutrophil as a mediator of ischemic edema formation in the brain. *Neurosci Lett* 1991; 125:110.

716. Garcia JH, et al: Pathology of stroke. In Barnett HJM, et al (eds): *Stroke: Pathophysiology, Diagnosis, and Management*, 2d ed. New York, Churchill Livingstone, 1992:125–146.

717. Grotta JC: Acute stroke management: Diagnosis. (Part I). In Grotta JC, et al (eds): *Stroke: Clinical Updates* 1993; 3:17. National Stroke Association, Englewood, CO.

718. Frank JI, Biller J: Coma in focal cerebrovascular disease: An overview. In Grotta JC, et al (eds): *Stroke: Clinical Updates* 1992; 3:9. National Stroke Association, Englewood, CO.

719. Brott T, et al: General therapy of acute ischemic stroke. In Hacke W, et al (eds): *Neurocritical Care*, New York, Springer-Verlag, 1994:553–577.

720. WHO Task Force on Stroke and Other Cerebrovascular Disorders: Recommendations on stroke prevention, diagnosis, and therapy. *Stroke* 1989; 20:1407.

721. Rothrock JF, Hart RG: Antithrombotic therapy in cerebrovascular disease. *Ann Intern Med* 1991; 11:885.

722. Sandercock PAG, et al: Antithrombotic therapy in acute ischemic stroke: An overview of the completed randomized trials. *J Neurol Neurosurg Psychiatry* 1993; 56:17.

723. Marshall RS, Mohr JP: Current management of ischaemic stroke. *J Neurol Neurosurg Psychiatry* 1993; 56:6.

724. Adams RD, Victor M: Cerebrovascular diseases. In Adams RD, Victor M (eds): *Principles of Neurology*, 5th ed. New York, McGraw-Hill, 1993:669.

725. Duke RJ, et al: Intravenous heparin for the prevention of stroke progression in acute partial stable stroke. *Ann Intern Med* 1986; 105:825.

726. Fisher CM: The "herald hemiparesis" of basilar artery occlusion. *Arch Neurol* 1988; 45:1301.

727. Wardlaw JM, Warlow CP: Thrombolysis in acute ischemic stroke: Does it work? *Stroke* 1992; 23:1826.

728. The Cerebral Embolism Study Group: Immediate anticoagulation of embolic stroke: A randomized trial. *Stroke* 1983; 14:668.

729. Bladin CF, Willmore J: Seizures after stroke. In Grotta JC et al (eds): *Stroke: Clinical Updates* 1994; 5:5. National Stroke Association, Englewood, CO.

730. Gupta SR, et al: Postinfarction seizures. A clinical study. *Stroke* 1988; 19:1477.

731. Shinton RA, et al: The frequency, characteristics and prognosis of epileptic seizures at the onset of stroke. *J Neurol Neurosurg Psychiatry* 1988; 51:273.

732. Barr JD, et al: Acute stroke intervention with intraarterial urokinase infusion. *J Vasc Interv Radiol* 1994; 5:705.

733. Brott T, et al: Thrombolytic therapy for stroke. *Curr Opin Neurol* 1994; 7:25 (review).

734. Jungreis CA, et al: Intracranial thrombolysis via a catheter embedded in the clot. *Stroke* 1989; 20:1578.

735. Hacke W, et al: Intra-arterial thrombolytic therapy improves outcome in patients with acute vertebrobasilar occlusive disease. *Stroke* 1988; 19:1216.

736. The NINDS Stroke Study Group: Tissue plasminogen activator for acute ischemic stroke. *N Engl J Med* 1995; 333:1581.

737. Hornig CR, et al: Hemorrhagic cerebral infarction—A prospective study. *Stroke* 1986; 17:179.

738. Ueda T, et al: Evaluation of risk of hemorrhagic transformation in local intra-arterial thrombolysis in acute ischemic stroke by initial SPECT. *Stroke* 1994; 25:298.

739. Wildenhain SL, et al: CT after intracranial intraarterial thrombolysis for acute stroke. *Am J Neuroradiol* 1994; 15:487.

740. Barr JD, et al: Intraoperative urokinase infusion for embolic stroke during carotid endarterectomy. *Neurosurgery* 1995; 36:606.

741. Furlan AJ, et al: Special aspects in the treatment of severe hemispheric brain infarction. In Hacke W, et al (eds): *Neurocritical care*, New York, Springer-Verlag, 1994:578–595.

742. Chen H-J, et al: Treatment of cerebellar infarction by decompressive suboccipital craniectomy. *Stroke* 1992; 23:957.

743. Marion DW, et al: Hyperventilation therapy for severe traumatic brain injury. *New Horizons* 1995; 3:439.

744. Simard D, Paulson OB: Artificial hyperventilation in stroke. *Trans Am Neurol Assoc* 1973; 98:309.

745. Christensen MS, et al: Cerebral apoplexy (stroke) treated with or without prolonged artificial hyperventilation. 2. Cerebrospinal fluid acid-base balance and intracranial pressure. *Stroke* 1973; 4:620.

746. Christensen MS, et al: Cerebral apoplexy (stroke) treated with or without prolonged artificial hyperventilation. 1. Cerebral circulation, clinical course, and cause of death. *Stroke* 1973; 4:568.

747. Katsura K, et al: Acidosis induced by hypercapnia exaggerates ischemic brain damage. *J Cereb Blood Flow Metab* 1994; 14:243.

748. Meden P, et al: Effect of hypothermia and delayed thrombolysis in a rat embolic stroke model. *Acta Neuro Scand* 1994; 90:91.

749. Colbourne F, Corbett D: Delayed and prolonged post-ischemic hypothermia is neuroprotective in the gerbil. *Brain Res* 1994; 654:265.

750. Maher J, Hachinski V: Hypothermia as a potential treatment for cerebral ischemia. *Cerebrovasc Brain Metab Rev* 1993; 5:277 (review).

751. Dietrich WD, et al: Intraischemic but not postischemic brain hypothermia protects chronically following global forebrain ischemia in rats. *J Cereb Blood Flow Metab* 1993; 13:541.

752. Kader A, et al: The effect of mild hypothermia on permanent focal ischemia in the rat. *Neurosurgery* 1992; 31:1056.

753. Michenfelder JD, Milde JH: Failure of prolonged hypocapnia, hypothermia, or hypertension to favorably alter acute stroke in primates. *Stroke* 1977; 8:87.

753a. Meyer JS, et al: Impaired neurogenic cerebrovascular control and dysautoregulation after stroke. *Stroke* 1973; 4:169.

754. Powers WJ: Acute hypertension after stroke: The scientific basis for treatment decisions. *Neurology* 1993; 43:461.

755. Dimant J, Grob D: Electrocardiographic changes and myocardial damage in patients with acute cerebrovascular accidents. *Stroke* 1977; 8:448.

756. Goldstein D: The electrocardiogram in stroke with relationship to pathophysiological type and comparison with prior tracings. *Stroke* 1979; 10:253.

757. Myers MG, et al: Cardiac sequelae of acute stroke. *Stroke* 1982; 13:838.

758. Norris JW, et al: Cardiac arrhythmias in acute stroke. *Stroke* 1978; 9:394.

759. Lavy S, et al: The effect of acute stroke on cardiac functions as observed in an intensive care unit. *Stroke* 1974; 5:775.

760. Norris JW, et al: Serum cardiac enzymes in stroke. *Stroke* 1979; 10:548.

761. Myers MG, et al: Plasma norepinephrine in stroke. *Stroke* 1981; 12:200.

762. Warner DS, et al: Temporal thresholds for hyperglycemia-augmented ischemic brain damage in rats. *Stroke* 1995; 26:655.

763. Derouesne C, et al: Infarcts in the middle cerebral artery territory. Pathological study of the mechanisms of death. *Acta Neurol Scand* 1993; 87:361.

764. Hartmann A, et al: Hemodilution in cerebral infarcts. *Arzneimittelforschung* 1991; 41:348.

765. Lyden PD, et al: Hemodilution with low-molecular-weight hydroxyethyl starch after experimental focal cerebral ischemia in rabbits. *Stroke* 1988; 19:223.

766. Wood JH, et al: Hypervolemic hemodilution in experimental focal cerebral ischemia. Elevation of cardiac output, regional cortical blood flow, and ICP after intravascular volume expansion with low molecular weight dextran. *J Neurosurg* 1983; 59:500.

767. Staedt U, et al: Haemodilution in acute ischaemic stroke comparison of two haemodilution regimens. *Neurol Res* 1992; 14:152.

768. Strand T: Evaluation of long-term outcome and safety after hemodilution therapy in acute ischemic stroke. *Stroke* 1992; 23:657.

769. Koller M, et al: Adjusted hypervolemic hemodilution in acute ischemic stroke. *Stroke* 1990; 21:1429.

770. Anonymous: Hypervolemic hemodilution treatment of acute stroke. Results of a randomized multicenter trial using pentastarch. The Hemodilution in Stroke Study Group. *Stroke* 1989; 20:317.

771. Strand T, et al: A randomized controlled trial of hemodilution therapy in acute ischemic stroke. *Stroke* 1984; 15:980.

772. Asplund K: Randomized clinical trials of hemodilution in acute ischemic stroke. *Acta Neurol Scand Suppl* 1989; 127:22.

773. Anonymous: Multicenter trial of hemodilution in acute ischemic stroke. Results of subgroup analyses. Scandinavian Stroke Study Group. *Stroke* 1988; 19:464.

774. Anonymous: Haemodilution in acute stroke: Results of the Italian Haemodilution Trial. Italian Acute Stroke Study Group. *Lancet* 1988; 1:18.

775. Anonymous: Multicenter trial of hemodilution in acute ischemic stroke. I. Results in the total patient population. Scandinavian Stroke Study Group. *Stroke* 1987; 18:691.

776. Mast H, Marx P: Neurological deterioration under isovolemic hemodilution with hydroxyethyl starch in acute cerebral ischemia. *Stroke* 1991; 22:680.

777. Koltringer P, et al: Hypervolemic haemodilution and completed stroke: How important is the application time for its effect? *Neurol Res* 1992; 14(2 suppl):171.

778. Goslinga H, et al: Custom-tailored hemodilution with albumin and crystalloids in acute ischemic stroke. *Stroke* 1992; 23:181.

779. Waksman BH, Adams RD: Allergic neuritis: An experimental disease of rabbits induced by the injection of peripheral nervous tissue and adjuvants. *J Exp Med* 1955; 102:213.

780. Brostoff SW, et al: Induction of experimental allergic neuritis with a peptide from myelin P2 basic protein. *Nature* 1977; 268:752.

781. Hartung H-P, et al: Serum interleukin-2 concentrations in Guillain-Barré syndrome and chronic idiopathic demyelinating polyneuropathy: Comparison with other neurological diseases of presumed immunopathogenesis. *Ann Neurol* 1991; 30:48.

782. Koski CL, et al: Clinical correlation with anti-peripheral nerve myelin antibodies in Guillain-Barré syndrome. *Ann Neurol* 1986; 19:573.

783. Hund EF, et al: Acute inflammatory polyneuropathy (Guillain-Barré syndrome). In Hacke W, et al (eds): *Neurocritical Care.* New York, Springer-Verlag, 1994:773–787.

784. Adams RD, Victor M: Diseases of the peripheral nerves. In Adams RD, Victor M (eds): *Principles of Neurology*, 5th ed. New York, McGraw-Hill, 1993:1117.

785. Ropper AH: Current concepts: The Guillain-Barré syndrome. *N Engl J Med* 1992; 326:1130.

786. Ropper AH, et al: *Guillain-Barré Syndrome.* Philadelphia, Davis, 1991.

787. Hughes RAC. *Guillain-Barré Syndrome*, London, Springer, 1990.

788. McKhann GM, Griffin JW: Plasmapheresis and the Guillain-Barré syndrome. *Ann Neurol* 1987; 22:762.

789. McKhann GM, et al: Plasmapheresis and Guillain-Barré syndrome: Analysis of prognostic factors and the effect of plasmapheresis. *Ann Neurol* 1988; 23:347.

790. van der Meche FGA, Schmitz PIM and the Dutch Guillain-Barré Study Group: A randomized trial comparing intravenous immune globulin and plasma exchange in Guillain-Barré syndrome. *N Engl J Med* 1992; 326:1123.

791. Ropper AH: Critical care of Guillain-Barré syndrome. In Ropper AH (ed): *Neurological and Neurosurgical Intensive Care*, 3d ed. New York, Raven Press, 1993:363–382.

792. Fergusson RJ, et al: Suxmethonium is dangerous in polyneuropathy. *BMJ* 1981; 282:298.

793. Feldman JM: Cardiac arrest after succinylcholine administration in a pregnant patient recovered from Guillain-Barré syndrome. *Anesthesiology* 1990; 72:942.

794. Chevrolet JC, Deleamont P: Repeated vital capacity measurements as predictive parameters for mechanical ventilation

need and weaning success in the Guillain-Barré syndrome. *Am Rev Respir Dis* 1991; 144:814.

795. Traux BT: Autonomic disturbances in Guillain-Barré syndrome. *Semin Neurol* 1984; 4:462.

796. Winer JB, Hughes RAC: Identification of patients at risk of arrhythmias in the Guillain-Barré syndrome. *Q J Med* 1988; 68:735.

797. Dalos NP, et al: Cardiovascular autonomic dysfunction in Guillain-Barré syndrome. Therapeutic implications of Swan-Ganz monitoring. *Arch Neurol* 1988; 45:115.

798. Ropper AH, Wijdicks EFM: Blood pressure fluctuations in the dysautonomia of Guillain-Barré syndrome. *Arch Neurol* 1990; 27:337.

799. Posner JB, et al: Hyponatremia in acute polyneuropathy. *Arch Neurol* 1967; 17:530.

800. Drachman DB: Myasthenic antibodies cross-link acetylcholine receptors to accelerate degradation. *N Engl J Med* 1978; 298:136.

801. Fambrough DM, et al: Neuromuscular junction in myasthenia gravis: Decreased acetylcholine receptors. *Science* 1973; 182:293.

802. Patrick J, Lindstrom JP: Autoimmune response to acetylcholine receptor. *Science* 1973; 180:871.

803. Toyka KV, Mullges W: Myasthenia gravis and Lambert-Eaton myasthenic syndrome. In Hacke W, et al (eds): *Neurocritical Care,* New York, Springer-Verlag, 1994:807–815.

804. Adams RD, Victor M: Myasthenia gravis and episodic forms of muscular weakness. In Adams RD, Victor M (eds): *Principles of Neurology,* 5th ed. New York, McGraw-Hill, 1993:1252.

805. Osserman KE: *Myasthenia Gravis.* New York, Grune & Stratton, 1958.

806. Delgado-Escueta AV, et al: Current concepts in neurology: Management of status epilepticus. *N Engl J Med* 1982; 306:1337.

807. Treatment of convulsive status epilepticus. Recommendations of the Epilepsy Foundation of America's Working Group on Status Epilepticus. *JAMA* 1993; 270:854.

808. Corsellis JA, Bruton CJ: Neuropathology of status epilepticus in humans. *Adv Neurol* 983; 34:129.

809. O'Connell BK, et al: Neuronal lesions in mercaptopropionic acid-induced status epilepticus. *Acta Neuropathol* 1988; 77:47.

810. Towfighi J, et al: Substantia nigra lesions in mercaptopropionic acid induced status epilepticus: A light and electron microscopic study. *Acta Neuropathol* 1989; 77:612.

811. From the Commission on Classification and Terminology of the International League Against Epilepsy. Proposal for revised clinical and electroencephalographic classification of epileptic seizures. *Epilepsia* 1981; 22:489.

812. Lelliott PT, Fenwick P: Cerebral pathology in pseudoseizures. *Acta Neurol Scand* 1991; 83:129.

813. Engel J Jr: *Seizures and Epilepsy.* Philadelphia, Davis, 1989.

814. McNamara JO: Cellular and molecular basis of epilepsy. *J Neurosci* 1994; 14:3413.

814a. Kofke WA, et al: Anesthetic implications of epilepsy. I. Epilepsy, Status Epilepticus and Epilepsy Surgery. *J Neurosurg Anesth* (in press).

815. Loscher W: Basic aspects of epilepsy. *Curr Opin Neurol Neurosurg* 1993; 6:223.

816. Jeffreys JGR: Experimental neurobiology of epilepsies. *Curr Opin Neurol* 1994; 7:113.

817. Dichter MA: Emerging insights into mechanisms of epilepsy: Implications of new antiepileptic drug development. *Epilepsia* 1994; 35(suppl 4):S51.

818. Gale K: GABA and epilepsy: Basis concepts from preclinical research. *Epilepsia* 1992; 33(suppl 5):S3.

819. Garant DS, Gale K: Substantia nigra-mediated anticonvulsant actions: Role of nigral output pathways. *Exp Neurol* 1987; 97:143.

820. Sagar HJ, Oxbury JM: Hippocampal neuron loss in temporal lobe epilepsy: Correlation with early childhood convulsions. *Ann Neurol* 1987; 22:334.

821. Sloviter RS: Feedforward and feedback inhibition of hippocampal principal cell activity evoked by perforant path stimulation: GABA-mediated mechanisms that regulate excitability in vivo. *Hippocampus* 1991; 1:31.

822. Nadler JV, et al: Selective reinnervation of hippocampal area CA1 and the fascia dentata after destruction of CA3-CA4 afferents with kainic acid. *Brain Res* 1980; 182:1.

823. Tauck DL, Nadler JV: Evidence of functional mossy fiber sprouting in hippocampal formation of kainic acid-treated rats. *J Neurosci* 1985; 5:1016.

824. Sutula T, et al: Synaptic reorganization in the hippocampus induced by abnormal functional activity. *Science* 1988; 239:1147.

825. Cavazos JE, et al: Mossy fiber synaptic reorganization induced by kindling: Time course development, progression, and permanence. *J Neurosci* 1991; 11:2795.

826. Sutula TP: Reactive changes in epilepsy: Cell death and axon sprouting induced by kindling. *Epilepsy Res* 1991; 10:62.

827. Sutula T, et al: Mossy fiber synaptic reorganization in the epileptic human temporal lobe. *Ann Neurol* 1989; 26:321.

828. Martin D, et al: Kindling enhances sensitivity of CA3 hippocampal pyramidal cells to NMDA. *J Neurosci* 1992; 12:1928.

829. Avoli M: Excitatory amino acid receptors in the human epileptogenic neocortex. *Epilepsy Res* 1991; 10:33.

830. Tietz EI, Chiu TH: Regional GABA-stimulated chloride uptake in amygdala kindled rats. *Neurosci Lett* 1991; 123:269.

831. McDonald JW, et al: Altered excitatory and inhibitory amino acid receptor binding in hippocampus of patients with temporal lobe epilepsy. *Ann Neurol* 1991; 29:529.

832. Minamato Y, et al: In vivo microdialysis of amino acid neurotransmitters in the hippocampus in amygdaloid kindled rats. *Brain Res* 1992; 573:345.

833. Ronneengstrom E, et al: Intracerebral microdialysis of extracellular amino acids in the human epileptic focus. *J Cereb Blood Flow Metab* 1992; 12:873.

834. Moody WJ, et al: Extracellular potassium activity during epileptogenesis. *Exp Neurol* 1974; 42:248.

835. Fisher RS, et al: The role of extracellular potassium in hippocampal epilepsy. *Arch Neurol* 1976; 33:76.

836. Lux HD, et al: Ionic changes and alterations in the size of the extracellular space during epileptic activity. In Delgado-Escueta AV, et al (eds): *Advances in Neurology* 1986, vol 44, *Basic Mechanisms of the Epilepsies.* New York, Raven Press, 1986:619.

837. Traynelis SF, Dingledine R: Potassium-induced spontaneous electrographic seizures in the rat hippocampal slice. *J Neurophysiol* 1988; 59:259.

838. Dutar P, Nicoll RA: A physiological role for $GABA_B$ receptors in the central nervous system. *Nature* 1988; 332:156.

839. Solis JM, Nicoll RA: Pharmacological characterization of GABAB-mediated responses in the CA1 region of the rat hippocampal slice. *J Neurosci* 1992; 12:3466.

840. Chamberlin NL, Dingledine R: GABAergic inhibition and the induction of spontaneous epileptiform activity by low chloride and high potassium in the hippocampal slice. *Brain Res* 1988; 445:12.

841. Dietzel I, et al: Transient changes in the size of the extracellular space in the sensorimotor cortex of cats in relation to stimulus-induced changes in potassium concentrations. *Exp Brain Res* 1980; 40:432.

842. Hablitz JJ, Heinemann U: Alterations in the microenvironment during spreading depression associated with epileptiform activity in the immature cortex. *Dev Brain Res* 1989; 46:243.

843. Dingledine R, et al: Excitatory amino acids in epilepsy. *Trends Pharmacol Sci* 1990; 11:334.

844. McNamara JO: The neurobiological basis of epilepsy. *Trends Neurosci* 1992; 15:357.

845. Dumer M, et al: Localization of idiopathic generalized epilepsy on chromosome 6p in families of juvenile myoclonic epilepsy patients. *Neurology* 1991; 41:1651.

846. Adams RD, Victor M: Epilepsy and other seizure disorders. In Adams RD, Victor M (eds): *Principles of Neurology*, 5th ed. New York, McGraw-Hill, 1993:273.

847. Nevander G, et al: Status epilepticus in well-oxygenated rats causes neuronal necrosis. *Ann Neurol* 1985; 18:281.

848. Wilder BJ: Efficacy of phenytoin in treatment of status epilepticus. *Adv Neurol* 1983; 34:441.

849. Tassinari CA, et al: Benzodiazepines: Efficacy in status epilepticus. *Adv Neurol* 1983; 34:465.

850. Nicol CF, et al: Parenteral diazepam in status epilepticus. *Neurology* 1969; 19:332.

851. Orr RA, et al: Diazepam and intubation in emergency treatment of seizures in children. *Ann Emerg Med* 1991; 20:1009.

852. Mayhue FE: Im Midazolam for status epilepticus in the emergency department. *Ann Emerg Med* 1988; 17:643.

853. Treiman DM: Pharmacokinetics and clinical use of benzodiazepines in the management of status epilepticus. *Epilepsia* 1989; 30:S4.

854. Treiman DM: The role of benzodiazepines in the management of status epilepticus. *Neurology* 1990; 40:32.

855. Kofke WA, et al: Effects of anesthetics on neuropathologic sequelae of status epilepticus in rats. *Anesth Analg* 1993; 77: 330.

856. Chiulli DA, et al: The influence of diazepam or lorazepam on the frequency of endotracheal intubation in childhood status epilepticus. *J Emerg Med* 1991; 9:13.

857. Seigler RS: The administration of rectal diazepam for acute management of seizures. *J Emerg Med* 1990; 8:155.

858. Bell HE, Bertino JS Jr: Constant diazepam infusion in the treatment of continuous seizure activity. *Drug Intelligence and Clinical Pharmacology* 1984; 18:965.

859. Crisp CB, et al: Continuous infusion of midazolam hydrochloride to control status epilepticus. *Clin Pharmacol* 1988; 7:322.

860. Goldberg MA, McIntyre HB: Barbiturates in the treatment of status epilepticus. *Adv Neurol* 1983; 34:499.

861. Young RS, et al: Pentobarbital in refractory status epilepticus. *Pediatr Pharmacol* 1983; 3:63.

862. Lowenstein DH, et al: Barbiturate anesthesia in the treatment of status epilepticus: Clinical experience with 14 patients. *Neurology* 1988; 38:395.

863. Brown AS, Horton JM: Status epilepticus treated by intravenous infusion of thiopentone sodium. *BMJ* 1967; 1:27.

864. Kofke WA, et al: Prolonged low flow isoflurane anesthesia for status epilepticus. *Anesthesiology* 1985; 62:653.

865. Kofke WA, et al: Isoflurane for refractory status epilepticus: A clinical series. *Anesthesiology* 1989; 71:653.

866. Ropper AH, et al: Comparison of isoflurane, halothane, and nitrous oxide in status epilepticus. *Ann Neurol* 1986; 19:98 (letter).

867. Yeoman P, et al: Etomidate infusions for the control of refractory status epilepticus. *Intensive Care Med* 1989; 15:255.

868. MacKenzie SJ, et al: Propofol infusion for control of status epilepticus. *Anaesthesia* 1990; 45:1043.

869. Fisher MM: Use of ketamine hydrochloride in the treatment of convulsions. *Anaesth Intensive Care* 1974; 2:266.

870. Opitz A, et al: General anesthesia in patients with epilepsy and status epilepticus. *Adv Neurol* 1983; 34:531.

871. Tzeng JI, et al: Status epilepticus controlled by althesin infusion (a case report). *Ma Tsui Hsueh Tsa Chi* 1986; 4:229.

872. Osorio I, Reed RC: Treatment of refractory generalized tonic-clonic status epilepticus with pentobarbital anesthesia after high-dose phenytoin. *Epilepsia* 1989; 30:464.

873. Brunner EA, et al: The effect of volatile anesthetics on levels of metabolites and on metabolic rate in rat brain. *J Neurochem* 1971; 18:2301.

874. Wagner RL, et al: Inhibition of adrenal steroidogenesis by the anesthetic etomidate. *N Engl J Med* 1984; 310:1415.

875. Clifford DB, et al: Ketamine, phencyclidine, and MK-801 protect against kainic acid-induced seizure-related brain damage. *Epilepsia* 1990; 31:382.

876. Sagratella S, et al: An investigation on the mechanism of anticonvulsant action of ketamine and phencyclidine on convulsions due to cortical application of penicillin in rabbits. *Pharmacol Res* 1985; 17:773.

877. Velisek L, et al: Effects of ketamine on metrazol-induced seizures during ontogenesis in rats. *Pharmacol Biochem Behav* 1989; 32:405.

878. Veliskova J, et al: Ketamine suppresses both bicuculline- and picrotoxin-induced generalized tonic-clonic seizures during ontogenesis. *Pharmacol Biochem Behav* 1990; 37:667.

879. Glaser GH: Medical complications of status epilepticus. *Adv Neurol* 1983; 34:395.

880. Oxbury JM, Whitty CWM: Causes and consequences of status epilepticus in adults. *Brain* 1971; 94:733.

881. Tempelhoff R, et al: Anticonvulsant therapy increases fentanyl requirements during anaesthesia for craniotomy. *Can J Anaesth* 1990; 37:327.

882. Tempelhoff R, et al: Resistance to atracurium-induced neuromuscular blockade in patients with intractable seizure disorders treated with anticonvulsants. *Anesth Analg* 1990; 71:665.

883. Liberman BA, et al: Pancuronium-phenytoin interaction: A case of decreased duration of neuromuscular blockade. *Int J Clin Pharmacol Ther Toxicol* 1988; 26:371.

884. Szenohradszky J, et al: Interaction of rocuronium (ORG 9426) and phenytoin in a patient undergoing cadaver renal transplantation: a possible pharmacokinetic mechanism? *Anesthesiology* 1994; 80:1167.

885. Ornstein E, et al: Accelerated recovery from doxacurium-induced neuromuscular blockade in patients receiving chronic anticonvulsant therapy. *J Clin Anesth* 1991; 3:108.

886. Blennow G, et al: Influence of reduced oxygen availability on cerebral metabolic changes during bicuculline-induced seizures in rats. *J Cereb Blood Flow Metab* 1985; 5:439.

887. Swan JH, et al: Hyperglycemia does not augment neuronal damage in experimental status epilepticus. *Neurology* 1986; 36:1351.

888. Kofke WA, et al: Substantia nigra damage after flurothyl-induced seizures in rats worsens after post seizure recovery: No exacerbation with hyperglycemia. *Neurol Res* 1993; 15:333.

889. Quagliarello V, Scheld WM: Bacterial meningitis: Pathogenesis, pathophysiology, and progress. *N Engl J Med* 1992; 327:864.

890. Tuomanen E, et al: The relative role of bacterial cell wall and capsule in the induction of inflammation in pneumococcal meningitis. *J Infect Dis* 1985; 151:535.

890a. Waage A, et al: Local production of tumor necrosis factor α, interleukin 1, and interleukin 6 in meningococcal meningitis: Relation to the inflammatory response. *J Exp Med* 1989; 170:1859.

891. Quagliarello VJ, et al: Morphologic alterations of the blood-brain barrier with experimental meningitis in the rat: tempo-

ral sequence and role of encapsulation. *J Clin Invest* 1986; 77:1084.

892. Fishman RA: Brain edema. *N Engl J Med* 1975; 293:706.

893. Saukkinen K, et al: The role of cytokines in the generation of inflammation and tissue damage in experimental gram positive meningitis. *J Exp Med* 1990; 171:439.

894. Tureen JH, et al: Loss of cerebrovascular autoregulation in experimental meningitis in rabbits. *J Clin Invest* 1990; 85: 577.

895. Pfister HW, et al: Microvascular changes during the early

phase of experimental bacterial meningitis. *J Cereb Blood Flow Metab* 1990; 10:914.

896. Adams RD, Victor M: Nonviral infections of the nervous system. In Adams RD, Victor M (eds): *Principles of Neurology*, 5th ed. New York, McGraw-Hill, 1993:599.

896a. Pfister H-W, Roos KL: Bacterial meningitis. In Hacke W, et al (eds): *Neurocritical Care*, New York, Springer-Verlag, 1994.

897. Durand ML, et al: Acute bacterial meningitis in adults. A review of 493 episodes. *N Engl J Med* 1993; 328:21.

PHYSIOLOGIC CHANGES WITH AGING IN THE CENTRAL NERVOUS SYSTEM

ROSEMARY HICKEY

TOD B. SLOAN

The central and peripheral nervous systems deteriorate steadily after 50 years of age. Because of the intimate relation between the functioning of the nervous system and the functioning of other body systems, aging of the central nervous system (CNS) has been postulated to be a major contributor to aging of the body as a whole.[1]

Studies of aging have been confounded by two problems. First, there are marked interspecies variations, and contradictory findings are not uncommon. Second, within species there are marked differences between individuals. Despite these confounding factors, some generalizations can be made. First, there is a consistent deterioration of the central and peripheral nervous systems with age. In some individuals these changes appear to start early (age 50 to 60 years), while in others the processes are delayed until later (age 70 to 80 years). It is unclear what causes this variability with age: however, hereditary factors, the presence of medical diseases (such as cardiovascular disease and diabetes), and perhaps the individual's behavior (physical and mental activity) all appear to alter the rate of degeneration.

When degeneration begins, it primarily affects the frontal and temporal lobes. However, different individuals show changes in different regions of the nervous system with different time sequences, causing a wide spectrum of functional and neurologic changes. These changes create an imbalance in the functioning of the nervous system, with a net suppression of some responses and an exaggeration of others. Overall, function deteriorates.

This chapter reviews the changes associated with aging that occur in the neural structures at macroscopic and microscopic levels in the CNS and the peripheral nervous system (PNS), the neurochemical and biochemical changes of aging, the functional changes which occur, and the resulting alterations in the neurologic examination that distinguish older from younger individuals. Finally, an overview of alterations in response to inhalational, intravenous, and local anesthetics is given.

Changes in CNS Morphology with Age

GROSS ANATOMIC CHANGES

Vertebrate brains follow a consistent pattern of development from conception through maturation to senescence. Since neural cells do not appear to divide once they are formed, some researchers believe that neural cells are programmed to deteriorate with age.

According to the traditional view, several anatomic changes in the brain are characteristic of aging (Table 37-1). While this view has been questioned,[2] brain weight appears to decrease starting at age 40, reaching about 93 percent of the weight at age 20 by age 80. The decrease in brain volume results in widening and deepening of the sulci with a decrease in the width of the gyri and an increase in ventricular size. The former changes are most dramatic in the frontal lobes.[3] There is also neuronal loss in the cortex, with a reduction in lipids and water content. A concomitant increase in glial cells and glial cell processes occurs, and this may explain increases in protein, RNA, and DNA as a fraction of overall brain weight.[3,4] In addition, the meninges thicken and the choroid plexus deteriorates.[5]

TABLE 37-1
Gross Anatomic Changes

Decline in brain weight

Widening and deepening of sulci

Decrease in width of gyri

Increase in ventricular size

Thickening of meninges

Deterioration of choroid plexus

MACROSCOPIC CHANGES IN NEURONS

A variety of macroscopic changes occur in neural cells, particularly in the frontal and temporal lobes (Table 37-2). The neuronal cell populations that appear to decrease with age include granular cells, cerebellar Purkinje cells, ganglion cells, cells in layer VI of the cerebral cortex (notably in the temporal lobe), and the pyramidal cells in layer III of the frontal lobe. Studies have revealed a 20 percent loss of nerve cells in individuals who are mentally healthy over age 70 (compared with persons age 19 to 28).[5] There is increased loss in diseases of aging: senile dementia, 35 to 38 percent (at age 79); Alzheimer's disease, 50 percent (at age 67). Overall, the areas affected first appear to be regions of phylogenetically younger CNS formations. Neurons in subcortical regions and in the vital areas of the brainstem do not appear to decline in number, but a selective depopulation of melanin-containing neurons in the locus ceruleus and substantia nigra has been noted. This loss may be related to cell degeneration resulting from free radical formation, since melanin exists in a free radical form.[6]

Individual neurons become elongated, somewhat irregular, and occasionally lobulated with aging. A generalized degeneration of axons occurs, especially in myelinated axons, because of a diffuse degeneration of myelin sheaths.[5] Spinal roots, for example, show a decrease in the number of myelinated fibers. The remaining axons may have a smaller diameter of the axis cylinder and myelin sheath. Degeneration of myelin results in an alteration of its normal functions,

TABLE 37-2
Neuronal Changes

Macroscopic neuronal changes
  Decrease in cortical neurons
  Increase in glial cells
  Decrease in myelinated axons
Microscopic neuronal changes
  Loss of Nissl substance
  Increase in lipofuscin and intracellular deposits
  Nuclear atrophy with morphological changes
  Granulation or fragmentation of mitochondria

which include (1) promotion of the rate of impulse transmission, (2) enhancement of repetitive impulse transmission capacity over a given time period, and (3) conservation of nerve function energy. Thus, with aging, there is a loss of the coordination of function by myelinated axons.[7]

Within individual axons, neural dendrites appear to degenerate, with an overall loss of dendrite numbers. In some cases, arborization (branching) is more prevalent and neurofibrillary tangles occur.[5] The number of synapses per neuron decreases.[3] Extracellular heuristic plaques (sensile plaques) occur in the elderly and appear to consist of a central amyloid core surrounded by degenerating neuronal processes (mainly presynaptic terminals and degenerating cellular organelles and reactive astrocytes) and an outer layer of glial cells.[4] These normal cellular changes of aging are more extensive with dementia.[8]

CHANGES IN NEURON INTERACTIONS

Neurons do not appear to age without affecting adjacent neurons. When a neuron dies, the metabolism and activity of adjacent neurons increase sharply. This may be part of the neural adaptation to the process of aging. Neighboring cells increase their surface area, nuclear volume, number of nucleoli, and contact with blood vessels. These adaptive changes probably help maintain the functional capacity of the CNS in the face of declining neuron numbers.[1,9]

Regression of neuronal dendrites reduces cell-to-cell communication, since it leads to a decrease in the number of synapses (95 percent of the receptor surface of cortical neurons is in the dendrites).[4] Pre- and postsynaptic neurons are also altered with age; this may be related to changes in neurotransmitters (see below). Coincident with the dendrite decrease, an age-related increase in the number of terminal branches with endplates is seen (terminal sprouting). Therefore, despite the decrease in dendrite numbers, there is no net denervation.[10]

MICROSCOPIC CHANGES IN NEURONS

On microscopic examination of aging neurons, a general loss of Nissl substance (basophilic RNA-containing chromophil substance) and ribosomes is seen. A variety of organelle changes are also observed, as well as deposits of copper, iron, melanin, and pigments. Nuclear changes occur, including atrophy, changes in definition, and alterations in staining characteristics. Mitochondria and the Golgi apparatus become granulated or fragmented. There is an increase in lipofuscin ("wear and tear pigment," "senility pigment," "chromolipid"), a pigment that is thought to

TABLE 37-3
Changes in Cellular Biochemistry and Physiology

Decreased cerebral blood flow

Loss of vascular autoregulation and responsiveness to neuronal demand and hypercapnia

Decreased cellular oxygen and glucose metabolism

Altered sodium and potassium homeostasis

Alterations in calcium homeostasis

be associated with aging. Its accumulation is the only constant cytologic change that correlates with age, and different neuron pools accumulate the lipofuscin pigment at different rates. It has been postulated that accumulation correlates with the activity of oxidative enzymes in individual cells.[5] Lipofuscin is thought to result from the oxidation of lipids polymerized with protein and unsaturated peptides. It appears in granules that are believed to be end-stage liposomes with indigestible cellular debris.[4,6]

Biochemical, Neurochemical, and Physiologic Changes

CEREBRAL BLOOD FLOW AND METABOLISM

A variety of cellular biochemical and physiologic changes occur with aging (Table 37-3). Cerebral blood flow (CBF) with advancing age has been extensively studied.[11-13] There is disagreement about the meaning of the decline in CBF observed. Before 1960, it was commonly believed that senility is due to inadequacies of CBF. However, it is now appreciated that CBF is reduced in proportion to brain mass and metabolism.[14] A reduction in CBF is paralleled by a reduction in the cerebral metabolism of oxygen and glucose (CMR_{O_2} and CMR_{Glc}). In general, CBF is reduced by 28 percent at age 80, with more dramatic reductions in patients who exhibit intellectual deterioration. Greater changes in CBF are also seen in diseases such as dementia. In addition, individuals with diabetes, hypertension, and atherosclerotic disease clearly demonstrate CBF reductions with advancing age.[15] With advancing age, the normal rise in regional CBF associated with local neuronal activity is blunted.[15] A loss of autoregulation also may occur in these individuals,[3] and CBF may show a reduced responsiveness to hypercapnia.[16]

Age-related changes in metabolism appear to be heterogeneous. There are marked regional variations throughout the brain, although more impressive changes are consistently seen in the frontal and temporal lobes.[8] It has been postulated that these changes are due to atherosclerotic deterioration of blood vessel walls. As blood vessels become sclerotic and thickened,

the blood supply is impaired.[1,3] CBF and CMR_{O_2} are deeply intertwined, but it appears that cerebrovascular changes may be the causative agent in reductions of both, making cerebrovascular disease a primary force in the aging process. Indeed, elderly individuals without cerebrovascular disease appear to have normal CBF.[3]

With the decrease in metabolism associated with aging, there is a decreasing supply of energy for the maintenance of cell membrane function. This leads to a slowing of the outflow of sodium from cells and of the inflow of potassium. As a result, the electrochemical potential capability of the nerve cell and its capacity for prolonged activity are limited.[1] The loss of energy may also contribute to decreases in axoplasmic flow of RNA, protein, amino acids, and other substances in neurons, leading to decreases in peripheral nerve function and consequent alterations in the organs innervated by those nerves.[1]

CALCIUM METABOLISM

Disordered calcium ion homeostasis has been suggested to be a contributor to the aging process, with intracellular calcium levels reported to be increased in some studies and decreased in others. Studies in the hippocampus (notably CA1 cells) clearly document changes consistent with increased intracellular levels of calcium caused by reduced cellular clearance.[10] The brain may be vulnerable to injury from altered calcium homeostasis, since many neuronal processes are calcium-regulated or calcium-facilitated. In general, aging reduces calcium movement across membranes, impairing uptake and elimination; diminishes cytosolic free calcium; and alters the binding of calcium and calcium stores. Pharmacologic treatments that promote the entry of calcium into cells seem to reverse some of these effects.[17]

Uptake of calcium appears to occur through two types of cell membrane calcium channels. The fast calcium channels close quickly (1 s) after stimulation and probably play a role in neurotransmitter release. The slow channels remain open longer (15 to 30 s) and probably play a role in prolonged cell depolarization as in tetanic stimulation. The affinity of calcium-binding sites in some areas declines with aging, while an increase in binding sites may be seen in other areas. The net effect may be a decline in the rapid phase of synaptosomal calcium uptake.[17] Membrane depolarization stimulates calcium uptake, which normally facilitates neurotransmitter release. With the decline in calcium uptake associated with aging, neurotransmitter release is inhibited.

Nerve cell membranes have two calcium pumps to remove calcium and maintain the level of cytosolic

TABLE 37-4
Effects of Altered Neuronal Calcium

Altered cell membrane structure and function
Altered cellular protease activity
  Increased accumulation of intracellular deposits
  Decrease in oxidative metabolism
Reduced calcium-mediated neurotransmitter release
Reduced axoplasmic transport
Reduced synaptic neurotransmitter release

calcium. A sodium-calcium exchanger is driven by external sodium levels moving down their transmembrane electrochemical gradient. Calcium-magnesium ATPase is an adenosine triphosphate (ATP) energy-driven and magnesium-dependent pump. With age, the function of the sodium exchange channel declines about 15 percent as a result of decreased calcium affinity. A similar change in affinity is seen in the ATPase pump. As a consequence of these changes, aging impairs the ability of neurons to remove calcium and maintain intracellular calcium homeostasis.[17]

In general, calcium binding to the plasma membranes increases with age in neural as well as nonneural tissues.[17] Age-related changes in negatively charged binding sites, sialidase activity, membrane fluidity, or gangliosides (a major binding material) could increase the affinity of binding sites.[17] Calcium binding to the cell membrane may alter the cell's structure, fluidity, and ability to communicate with other cells. Aging also alters calcium-coupled receptors, and the cell membrane may be hampered in its ability to transduce the external signals which normally bind to these receptors.[17] Altered neuronal calcium levels may also mediate other effects (Table 37-4) through altered cellular protease activity.

NEUROTRANSMITTERS

A variety of changes occurs in neurotransmitter function with aging. Calcium-dependent neurotransmitter release declines with age, probably as a result of reduced calcium uptake. Calcium reduction may also reduce axoplasmic transport in cells by inhibiting microtubule movement of transport vesicles.[17] Aging decreases calmodulin activity, which in turn results in an alteration of the various enzymes and cellular processes that are activated by calcium-protein binding (e.g., calmodulin). This may cause a reduction in the usual enhancement of neurotransmitter release from synaptic vesicles.[17]

In addition, an age-related "leakage" of neurotransmitters appears to occur which may be due to altered calcium levels or to displacement of calcium from membrane gangliosides.[17] This leakage phenomenon

has been seen with acetylcholine, dopamine, and glutamate and could cause a minor depolarization of the postsynaptic membrane. Total brain quantities of these neurotransmitters and norepinephrine are also decreased with age.[4] Serotonin has been documented to be decreased in the caudate nucleus. These progressive but uneven declines are probably due to a general decrease in the enzymatic functions of oxidation and phosphorylation. The net effect appears to be a decrease in the amount of neurotransmitters released upon stimulation, resulting in effective synaptic depression.[10]

The progressive imbalance between various neurotransmitter systems in the brain with aging leads to altered neural system function (Table 37-5).[18] In addition to the decline in the release of various neurotransmitters, there are decreases in receptor binding of neurotransmitters. This decline is thought to result from a reduction in the number of receptors rather than from reduced receptor affinity. In addition, the CNS appears to be less able to increase the number of receptors (supersensitivity) when diminished stimulation occurs. Hence, the aged CNS has diminished neurotransmitter-mediated responsiveness. Specifically, this effect has been well described for both beta-adrenergic and acetylcholine receptors.[18] This altered activity of the brain's cholinergic system probably contributes to the declining cognitive and memory functions of older age.[9] The reduction in cholinergic function may be due to several causes, including a decrease in neuronal uptake of choline (the precursor), a drop in synthesis by choline acetyltransferase (CAT), a decline in acetyl-

TABLE 37-5
Proposed Functional Consequences of Altered Neurotransmitter Systems in Aging

Neurotransmitter	Functional change
Cholinergic system	
General decrease	Decline in cognition and memory
Reduced sympathetic and parasympathetic ganglia function	Blunted cardiovascular reflexes
Dopaminergic system	
Reduced anterior pituitary release of prolactin and luteinizing hormone	Senescence of estrous cycles
Reduced activity in basal ganglia	Senile gait, posture, and tremor
Norepinephrine system	
Reduced gonadotropin secretion	Endocrine senescence
Reduced sympathetic function	Blunted cardiovascular reflexes
General decrease	Depression
Serotonin system	
General decrease	Depression

cholinesterase, and diminution of receptor binding sites.[3,18,19] It is unclear if the altered acetylcholine system accounts for the increased susceptibility of older individuals to the effects of anticholinergics such as scopolamine.

Dopamine levels may decline with age because of a decrease in tyrosine hydroxylase (the enzyme responsible for the initial synthetic step for tyrosine), and increases in monoamine oxidase (responsible for dopamine metabolism) also contribute to this decline. In addition, the receptor population for dopamine declines. These changes in dopamine may be linked to several functional changes that occur with aging. For example, dopamine is believed to regulate the anterior pituitary release of prolactin and luteinizing hormone, and a reduction in this neurotransmitter or its receptors could cause senescence of estrous cycles. An age-related loss of dopaminergic function in the basal ganglia has been postulated to be the cause of abnormalities in gait and posture, which may accelerate degenerative changes in joints. Both factors may contribute to the senile gait and increased tendency toward falling seen in the elderly. Basal ganglia changes also may be responsible for a senile tremor that occurs in all limb positions. This sets the tremor apart from the tremor of Parkinson disease (maximal with limb in repose) or cerebellar damage (maximal with limb approaching a target). Senile tremor is rarely a functional problem; it is interesting that it can usually be treated with beta blockers.[6,9]

Norepinephrine and dopamine share some synthetic and catabolic enzymes; therefore, it is not surprising that norepinephrine levels also decrease with aging. Adrenergic receptors, as was discussed above are also reduced. Since norepinephrine is thought to play a role in gonadotropin secretion, reduced levels may be related to endocrine senescence.[19]

Although dopamine and norepinephrine levels fall with advancing age, serotonin levels appear to be rather constant.[5] The activities of gamma-aminobutyric acid (GABA) and its synthetic enzyme glutamic acid decarboxylase are reduced by age in a number of areas of the cortex. In contrast, GABA receptor-binding sites may be increased.[9] This may contribute to an alteration in the response to agents which act through GABA-mediated channels (e.g., benzodiazepines and barbiturates).

CELLULAR NEUROPHYSIOLOGY

In addition to neurotransmitter changes, cellular neuroelectrophysiology is altered with age (Table 37-6). Although membrane potentials are not altered, action potential duration increases as a result of the reduced membrane activity in ion transport noted above. In-

TABLE 37-6
Alterations in Cellular Electrophysiology

Cellular
  Increased action potential duration
  General decrease in excitability
  Decreased peripheral nerve conduction velocity
Imbalance of inhibitory and facilitory influences
  Altered reflex responses
Reduced peripheral nerve function
Electroencephalogram
  Slowing: generalized and focal
  Hypersynchronization and spindle activity
Evoked potentials
  Increased latency

terneuron thresholds for spinal reflexes also change. In general, electrical excitability is decreased. However, some areas become more excitable, and this may explain the lowered threshold for seizure activity seen with a number of convulsant drugs.[1] Changes in excitability also lead to altered reflex activity, resulting in modification of the functional state of other organs innervated by autonomic pathways. In general, the difference between the most and least excitable structures decreases with age, and CNS responses to widely different stimuli become more generalized and stereotypical.

A variety of changes occur in descending facilitory and inhibitory neural pathways. Some reflex responses are activated, while others are inhibited.[1] In general, the most important manifestation of change in the CNS is a weakening of inhibition at the various levels of its organization. Since inhibitory influences play an important role in coordinating and integrating CNS function, this leads to overall changes in reflex activity and a disorganization of highly coordinated activities.[1]

NEUROENDOCRINE FUNCTION

The homeostasis of the entire organism is altered by changes in the neurohumoral system that maintains the internal milieu (Table 37-7). Therefore, disturbances leading to altered blood pressure, blood sugar, and acid-base balance are tolerated less well than they are in young individuals. This can lead to pathologic processes that would not occur in younger individuals whose bodies are confronted with otherwise innocuous stimuli.[1]

The function of the hypothalamic-pituitary system is modified with age, altering peripheral organ function: Some organs increase their activity, while others decrease it. Many investigators believe that changes in hypothalamic function are a leading cause of aging

TABLE 37-7
Autonomic and Homeostatic Changes

Decreased anterior hypothalamic activity

Decreased sensitivity of hypothalamus to inhibitory hormones

Increased threshold of vagal and sympathetic nerves

Altered sympathetic and parasympathetic function

Reduced control and responsiveness of cardiovascular tone

Reduced temperature regulation

Orthostatic hypotension

Chronic constipation

Decreased sympathetic function (slowed heart rate and decreased blood pressure)

in the entire body. In general, anterior hypothalamic activity appears to decrease with age, but this is not uniform. In addition, the anterior hypothalamus becomes less responsive to hormonal control. This dysfunction of the anterior hypothalamus leads to changes in peripheral organ systems, tending to send the whole body out of homeostatic control.[1] In addition, a decrease in the sensitivity of the hypothalamic system to the inhibitory action of various hormones (particularly estrogen and corticosteroids) may lead to hypertension, atherosclerosis, obesity, and diabetes.[1]

One of the most typical characteristics of aging is a reduction in the power of the organism to adapt to environmental changes. The response to stress of various types is less effective. For example, age changes in the hypothalamic-pituitary-adrenal axis lead to reductions in the ability to respond to external stresses such as cold, pain, and immobilization. In addition, changes in the levels of catecholamines and stimulation of the limbic system are tolerated less well. This leads to an altered ability to regular body temperature during heating and cooling.[1]

The unequal aging process of brain structures which regulate the cardiovascular and respiratory systems leads to circulatory pathology and altered cardiovascular and ventilatory responses. Weakening of nervous control of the cardiovascular system is a general phenomenon. For example, the thresholds for stimulation of the vagus and sympathetic nerves are raised, causing hemodynamic changes. Aging results in a reduction in the excitability of the sympathetic and parasympathetic ganglia caused by reductions in the synthesis and hydrolysis of acetylcholine. As a consequence, significant CNS changes are not as vigorously translated into peripheral changes in cardiovascular tone.[1] As a result, responses to surgical pain may be blunted so that hypotension occurs with minimal anesthesia or in the face of hypovolemia. As neural control of the periphery by the CNS weakens, there are also changes

in sensitivity to humoral factors. Many reactions in old age become prolonged and protracted.[1] Therefore, mild cardiovascular disturbances such as blood loss may be poorly tolerated.

Behavioral and Functional Changes

Normal functional changes in the geriatric nervous system are a result of aging of the neural systems, as was described above (Table 37-8). Some functions decline, others appear to be unaffected, and still others improve with age. Several clearly definable functions decline with age and are responsible for dependency.[3] In individuals over 65 years of age, 93 percent of those dependent on others for care have problems identifiable as neurologic disease. Among those who are disabled, 48 percent have neurologic disease. Among individuals disabled by neurologic disease, the most common causes are movement disorders (20.5 percent), dementia (16.4 percent), and strokes or transient ischemic attacks (TIAs) (16 percent).[20]

BEHAVIOR AND MEMORY

Most types of behavior slow with age. There is a 15 to 20 percent increase in reaction time between 20 and 60 years of age.[3] This increase appears to be due primarily to a change in neural processing, with a general slowing of the speed of response. The increased reaction time appears to affect most activities, including task-oriented responses.[3]

Alterations in behavior may also be due in part to changes in memory and learning. Dysfunction in learning and memory is repeatedly shown in psychometric studies of older individuals and is a common complaint in the elderly.[3] The most strikiing change in memory is reduced information retrieval. Of interest,

TABLE 37-8
Behavioral and Functional Changes

Slowed reaction time

Dysfunction in learning

Reduced information retrieval (especially short-term memory)

Slower peripheral information acquisition time

Decrease in intelligence

Decline in language skills

Depression

Decreased sensory function

    Reduced visual sensitivity to short wavelengths

    High-frequency hearing loss

    Decreased proprioception and vibration

there is no decline in the ability to recognize items, even when recognition requires memorization.[3]

The speed and consistency of short-term memory appear to decline most with age.[3] Learning appears to change in the elderly; individuals learn better when learning patterns have some element of previously learned material (i.e., already in memory). As a consequence, the elderly may have trouble coping in new environments where they must adapt to situations that were not previously encountered.[21] The elderly require more trials to learn lists, and this may be related to difficulty in encoding items in memory. The elderly appear to be forgetful in everyday activities, probably as a consequence of difficulty with memory retrieval.[3] Above age 70, memory retrieval deficits (identified as errors in naming objects) become more noticeable. By age 75 years, 25 percent of the elderly show memory deficits (50 percent do so by age 80).[4] The acquisition speed for environmental information is slowed, and this also contributes to the decline in learning and memory.

INTELLIGENCE, COGNITION, AND EMOTION

A variety of changes in cognition, personality, and emotion occur normally with age.[21] Intelligence appears to decline linearly, beginning as early as adolescence.[3] Cognitive function declines with age.[3] Information processing is clearly affected, with changes in both peripheral and central information.[3] Language skills such as naming and defining begin to decline after age 70, but this appears to be related to forgetting rather than to lack of understanding.[21] Emotional problems of many varieties increase with age; the most common is depression. A variety of studies suggest that this may be related to altered levels of neurotransmitter substances (notably norepinephrine and serotonin), neuronal sodium accumulation, and possibly altered hormonal levels.[18] Studies are not clear, however, since reductions in motivation are commonly seen in the elderly, resulting from behavioral slowness. This leads to dependence on group opinion and may be interpreted as depression.[3]

SENSORY FUNCTION

Normal changes with aging generally result in the deterioration of sensory modalities (distal extremities), with muscle wasting, a decline in strength, and an absence of or decrease in tendon reflexes.[@2] Visual acuity appears to decline, with increases in light threshold, a decrease in visual task performance, and a reduction of the ability to appreciate shorter wavelengths. These changes are thought to be related primarily to processes in the eye.[3] A loss of auditory acuity also occurs

TABLE 37-9
Common Neurologic Changes in the Elderly

Cognition	
Memory	Modest decline in short-term memory
Verbal intelligence	Decline after seventh decade
Processing speech	Decline with age
Sensory, Motor	
Vision	Smaller pupils, slow reactivity, progressive limitation of upward gaze, presbyopia (loss of lens elasticity)
Hearing	Decreased acuity at high frequencies (presbycusis)
Vibratory sense	Decline in function of distal extremities
Spinal reflexes	Ankle jerks decreased or absent, increased primitive reflexes (glabella, palmomental, snout)
Gait/posture	Slowed, forward-flexed, and mildly unsteady
Motor	Decline in grip strength and mild state of extrapyramidal dysfunction

with age. This appears to be related to changes in the ear, although the decline in speech perception is probably due to central changes.[3] These changes are reflected in diagnostic electrophysiologic studies (see below).

PERIPHERAL NERVOUS SYSTEM FUNCTION

By age 50 years, 20 percent of individuals have abnormal neurologic findings on examination (Table 37-9). Common changes include reduced rate and amount of motor activity, impaired fine coordination and agility, slowed reaction time, slowed and narrowed perception, decreased vibratory sense in the feet and toes, and reduced Achilles tendon reflexes. Patients 55 to 75 years of age constitute the largest group of individuals with peripheral neuropathy. The most commonly cited causes are diabetes, malignancy, alcohol, drugs, demyelination, autoimmune diseases, and nutritional deficiencies. Aging itself is responsible for loss and damage of the component nerve fibers (motor, sensory, and autonomic).[22]

A variety of changes cause a decrease in the information transmitted along nerve pathways to peripheral locations. These changes include a decline of nerve endings and receptors, a decrease in the number of neurons in the brain, and a reduction in the number of fibers in nerve trunks. Changes in metabolism and transport mechanisms within nerve cells and slowing of the velocity of impulse conduction also contribute.[1] It has been estimated that about 25 percent of lumbosacral anterior horn cells and spinal sensory ganglia are lost with aging.[4] This appears to correlate with reductions in reaction time. It is of note that individuals who exercise regularly have faster reaction times. A variety of evidence suggests that the decline in physical activity parallels the decline in mental activity.[3]

Loss of motor and sensory axons is most prominent in the legs. This results in a reduction in conduction velocity in sensory nerves to the greatest extent and in motor neurons to a lesser extent. There is a progressive fall in the number of functional motor sites in the peripheral nervous system over age 60, and the majority of the remaining fibers innervate slow (type 1) muscles.[9] Motor and sensory nerve conduction velocity slows after age 60, particularly in the distal parts of axons.[9] The decline in physical fitness and athletic ability appears to be related to aging of the CNS,[3] with a decrease in conduction velocity contributing to a slowed response time.[4] Proprioceptive and vibratory senses are reduced, probably as a result of peripheral changes.[3]

AUTONOMIC FUNCTION

Age-related changes in the autonomic nervous system produce a functional neuropathy that may result in clinical disease by altering the maintenance and integration of visceral functions or by causing subclinical changes that diminish the safety margin for physiological insults (Table 37-7). Deterioration in the autonomic nervous system leads to difficulties with homeostasis as organ coordination is lost. Autonomic dysfunction is due to a variety of causes, including dysfunction in the dorsal nucleus of the vagus, hypothalamus, intermediolateral columns of the spinal cord, and sympathetic ganglia,[23] as well as altered sensivitity of the baroreceptors, decreases in compliance of the blood vessels, loss of fibers, and slowed nerve conduction velocity.[24]

These autonomic changes lead to several disturbances. Postural hypotension, which is uncommon in middle age (1 percent), is far more common in old age (18 percent of those over 65 years of age).[24] Diminished sympathetic function is thought to occur, and this may explain a decrease in heart rate and blood pressure in the absence of vascular disease. The reduced sympathetic function may be due to a decrease in norepinephrine in the neural system, decreased receptor responsiveness, axonal degeneration (thought to be due to loss of postganglionic sympathetic neurons), decreased vasoreceptor sensitivity, and decreased adrenergic responsiveness of the heart.

Blood pressure is normally regulated by the autonomic nervous system through alterations in vascular tone and myocardial function. This occurs via sensors in the vasoreceptors of the great vessels and the carotid sinus, with neural input to the brainstem through the glossopharyngeal nerve and carotid sinus nerves. Me-

diation occurs through the nuclei of the tractus solitarius and the paramedian nuclei, with efferents to higher centers and to preganglionic sympathetic cells of the spinal cord. Postganglionic fibers of sympathetic and parasympathetic nature then radiate to the vascular system.[24] Autonomic dysfunction leads to impaired activity of this complex system, impaired thermoregulation (caused by impairment of sweating and diminished vasoconstriction upon cooling), and chronic constipation (disordered bowel motility).

EEG/EVOKED POTENTIALS

A variety of electrophysiological changes occur in the brain, paralleling functional and neurophysiologic changes (Table 37-6). A general slowing in the electroencephalogram (EEG) has been observed.[3] This frequency change appears to be related to general activity and health: older individuals may have predominant frequencies in the theta range [4 to 7 hertz (Hz)], resembling the slow record of childhood, with more active individuals having frequencies in the alpha range (8 to 12 Hz), similar to younger adults. The generalized EEG slowing is also associated with the reduced CBF and CMR_{O_2} seen with aging.[3] More diffuse slowing, with ventral replacement of normal EEG activity, is most common in patients with dementia or psychiatric disease and has a strong relation with significant intellectual deterioration.[3]

In addition to the generalized EEG changes, focal slowing occurs, with localized sharp waves or spikes which are not normally associated with epileptiform discharges. These focal changes are seen most commonly in the temporal lobes.[3] EEG changes of hypersynchronization and spindle activity or disorganization probably can be explained by alterations in the number and properties of neurons, reduction of CBF, changes in cortical-subcortical relations, and a reduction in the flow of afferent impulses.[1]

Consistent with decreased proprioception, somatosensory evoked potentials are commonly increased in latency. Auditory evoked potentials usually are not altered unless there is high-frequency hearing loss. Visual evoked responses usually show a decline in amplitude of the cortical waves that may be related to a decrease in attention.[6]

Changes in Anesthetic and Analgesic Requirements

The decline in CNS function associated with aging is accompanied by a reduced anesthetic and analgesic requirement. Although the precise neuroanatomic basis for these changes is unknown, many of the anatomic and functional changes described above have been theorized to play a role. For example, the gradual decline in cortical neuron density and the decrease in synaptic transmission may play a role. The reduction in neuronal density is accompanied by a decline in hemispheric CBF and CMR_{O_2}. Also theorized to play a role is the age-related decrease in the rate of synthesis of, and the corresponding reduction in the brain levels of, neurotransmitters. A reduction in the number of receptor sites and a decrease in the sensitivity to biogenic amines (e.g., catecholamines) also have been proposed as an explanation for the greater sensitivity of elderly patients to the depressant effects of drugs that act on the CNS. In the peripheral nervous system, the reduction in the axonal population and the deterioration of the myelin sheath may contribute to the progressive slowing of peripheral motor and sensory nerve conduction velocities seen with advancing age.

The reduced anesthetic requirements for geriatric patients apply to inhalational, intravenous, and local anesthetics. Although alterations in many other systems may affect these requirements, this discussion will focus primarily on the CNS effects of these drugs.

INHALATIONAL DRUGS

The MAC (minimum alveolar concentration of a drug that prevents movement on skin incision in 50 percent of patients) decreases with advancing age. This has been shown repeatedly for different inhalational agents. Gregory and associates[25] noted that the MAC of halothane is highest in the newborn and lowest in the elderly. Studying halothane in different age groups, Nicodemus and coworkers[26] found that halothane is 1.28 and 1.12 times more potent in producing anesthesia in adults than it is in the 0- to 6-month and 6- to 24-month age groups, respectively. Stevens and associates[27] studied patients 19 years of age and older and noted a reduction in isoflurane MAC with increasing age. The MAC of the newer inhalational agents desflurane and sevoflurane has also been shown to be age-related. Rampil and colleagues[28] noted that for patients between the third and fifth decades, the desflurane anesthetic requirement declined to 83 percent of third-decade MAC. Smaller MAC values of sevoflurane have also been noted in elderly patients[29] compared with the values reported for children and adults.[30–32]

To test the thesis that aging has a general effect on the anesthetic requirement for all agents, Munson and associates[33] compared the age-related changes in halothane and isoflurane MAC to those found with cyclopropane, an anesthetic with solvent and pharmacologic properties significantly different from those of halothane and isoflurane. They noted that the slope of the relation between MAC and age for cyclopropane

paralleled those previously noted for halothane and isoflurane. These results were consistent with the thesis that aging has a general effect on the anesthetic requirement for all agents. To obtain a rough estimate of MAC in geriatric patients, the published MAC value of inhalational agents is decreased by 4 percent for every decade of age over 40 years.[34] For example, the MAC of halothane in an 80-yer-old is obtained by multiplying by 84 percent, which was derived from the formula [100% − (4% × 4 decades)] times the published halothane MAC value of 0.76, to equal 0.64.[34]

INTRAVENOUS DRUGS

The apparent sensitivity of the CNS to intravenous drugs is also increased in elderly patients. Both pharmacodynamic (plasma concentration–drug response relation) and pharmacokinetic (drug uptake, tissue distribution, hepatic metabolism, and renal elimination) factors may play a role, the balance of which depends on the particular drug involved.

For thiopental sodium and etomidate, the dose required to reach a uniform EEG endpoint decreases significantly with increasing age.[35,36] However, it has been suggested that the increased sensitivity to these drugs with aging relates more to differences in pharmacokinetic than to pharmacodynamics. For example, a reduction in the initial distribution volume for both thiopental and etomidate in an elderly patient results in higher serum concentrations after a given dose.[35,36] This contributes to the lower dose requirements in elderly patients. An increase in the volume of distribution at steady state has been shown for thiopental sodium, producing an increase in the terminal elimination half-life.[37] A decrease in the clearance of etomidate is consistent with the decline in hepatic blood flow in the elderly, since etomidate clearance depends on hepatic blood flow.[36]

The plasma concentration of diazepam required to achieve a desired pharmacologic effect is lower in elderly patients (pharmacodynamic response).[38] A prolonged terminal elimination half-life of diazepam reflects an increased volume of distribution (pharmacokinetic response). Sensitivity to midazolam is also increased in elderly patients. For example, a dose of 0.3 mg/kg was adequate for anesthetic induction in 100 percent of unpremedicated elderly patients (age 60 years or over), whereas 0.5 mg/kg did not adequately induce anesthesia in 40 percent of young unpremedicated patients.[39] Elimination half-life is longer and total clearance of midazolam is reduced in elderly versus young males.[40]

The dose requirement of narcotics decreases significantly in the elderly. The dose requirement of fentanyl or alfentanil decreases 50 percent from age 20 to age

89.[41] The alteration in dose requirement is primarily a function of altered brain sensitivity (pharmacodynamic response). Elderly patients have an increased brain sensitivity to fentanyl and alfentanil, as demonstrated by a study relating spectral edge frequency to narcotic serum concentrations.[41] Some changes in pharmacokinetic parameters have also been noted, including a decrease in plasma clearance and an increase in terminal elimination half-life.[42,43]

LOCAL ANESTHETICS

Reduced requirements for local anesthetics may be seen in elderly patients. For example, there is a greater segmental spread of local anesthetic in elderly patients undergoing epidural anesthesia.[44] Serum levels of local anesthetics are increased, and thus it is suggested that the dose of local anesthetic for epidural anesthesia should be reduced in an elderly patient. Similarly, for spinal anesthesia, it has been demonstrated that the time to maximum spread is shorter and the sensory spinal blockade is slightly higher in older patients.[45] A number of reasons have been postulated for reduced local anesthetic requirements, including (1) progressive occlusion of the intervertebral foramina with increasing age so that local anesthetic solutions injected epidurally have a greater longitudinal spread, (2) reduced vertebral column height lowering dose requirements for spinal anesthesia, (3) deterioration of myeline sheaths, (4) decreased CNS neuronal population, (5) decreased number of axons in peripheral nerves, and (6) alterations in the pharmacokinetics of local anesthetics in elderly patients.

Summary

The rate of normal aging differs among individuals, with variability among individuals in regard to the specific effects. A global decrease in neural function is a general process. However, the hallmark of aging neural function is the development of processes that lead to an imbalance in the various systems that control neural and visceral functioning. In general, older individuals share (1) reduced short-term memory, (2) a need for basing learning patterns on previously learned material, (3) a tendency to depression, (4) reduced visual, auditory, and peripheral nerve function, (5) altered gait and tremor with loss of fine motor coordination, and (6) reduced homeostatic control, making them more susceptible to physiologic disturbances that would be easily accommodated by a younger individual. The decline in CNS function in elderly patients is accompanied by a reduction in requirements for inhalational, intravenous, and local anesthetics. This may be due to alterations in pharmacodynamic and/or pharmacokinetic responses. The greater sensitivity to anesthetic agents may lead to decreased dose requirements, slowed onset, prolonged duration of action, and exaggerated side effects.

References

1. Frol'kis VV, Bezrukov VV: Aging of the central nervous system. *Hum Physiol* 1978; 78:478.
2. Duckett S: The normal aging human brain. In Duckett S (ed): *The Pathology of the Aging Human Nervous System.* Philadephia, Lea & Febiger, 1991:1–19.
3. Long DM: Aging in the nervous system. *Neurosurgery* 1985; 17:348.
4. Boss BJ: Normal aging in the nervous system: Implications for SCI nurses. *SCI Nurs* 1991; 8:42.
5. Berlin M, Wallace RB: Aging and the central nervous system. *Exp Aging Res* 1976; 2:125.
6. Morris JC, McManus DQ: The neurology of aging: Normal versus pathologic change. *Geriatrics* 1991; 46:47.
7. Knobler RL: Demyelinating disorders of the aged brain. In Duckett S (ed): *The Pathology of the Aging Human Nervous System.* Philadelphia, Lea & Febiger, 1991:317–335.
8. Duara R, et al: Changes in structure and energy metabolism. of the aging brain. In Finsh CE, Schneider EL (eds): *Handbook of the Biology of Aging,* 2d ed. New York: Van Nostrand Reinhold, 1985:595–616.
9. Hubbard BM, Squier M: The physical ageing of the neuromuscular system. In Tallis R (ed): *The Clinical Neurology of Old Age.* Chichester, J Wiley, 1989:3–26.
10. Smith DO: Cellular and molecular correlates of aging in the nervous system. *Exp Gerontol* 1988; 23:399.
11. Gustafson L, et al: Presenile dementia: Clinical symptoms, pathoanatomical findings and cerebral blood flow. In Meyer JS, Lechner H, Reivich M (eds): *Cerebral Vascular Disease.* Amsterdam, Excerpta Medica, 1976:5–9.
12. Gustafson L, et al: Speech disturbances in presenile dementia related to local cerebral blood flow abnormalities in the dominant hemisphere. *Brain Lang* 1978; 5:103.
13. Gustafson T, Risberg J: Regional cerebral blood flow measurements by the ^{133}Xe inhalation techniques in differential diagnosis of dementia. *Acta Neurol Scand* 1979; 72:546.
14. Strehler BL: Fundamental mechanisms of neuronal aging. In Cervos-Navarro J, Sarkander H-I (eds): *Brain Aging: Neuropathology and Neuropharmacology.* New York, Raven Press, 1983:75–95.
15. Arnold KG: Cerebral blood flow in geriatrics—a review. *Age Ageing* 1981; 10:5.
16. Deshmukh VD, Meyer JS: *Noninvasive Measurement of Regional Cerebral Blood Flow in Man.* New York, S P Medical Scientific Books, Spectrum, 1978.
17. Gibson GE, Peterson C: Calcium and the aging nervous system. *Neurobiol Aging* 1987; 8:329.
18. Samorajski T: Normal and pathologic aging of the brain. In Enna SJ, Samorajski T, Beer B (eds): *Brain Neurotransmitters and Receptors in Aging and Age-Related Disorders.* New York, Raven Press, 1981:1–12.
19. Rogers J, Bloom FE: Neurotransmitter metabolism and function in the aging central nervous system. In Finch CE, Schneider EL (eds): *Handbook of the Biology of Aging,* 2d ed. New York, Van Nostrand Reinhold, 1985:645–691.
20. Broe GA: The neuroepidemiology of old age. In Tallis R (ed): *The Clinical Neurology of Old Age.* Chichester, UK, Wiley, 1989:51–65.

21. Binks M: Changes in mental functioning associated with normal ageing. In Tallis R (ed): *The Clinical Neurology of Old Age*. Chichester, UK, Wiley, 1989:27–39.

22. Vital C, Vital A: Peripheral neuropathy. In Duckett S (ed): *The Pathology of the Aging Human Nervous System*. Philadelphia, Lea & Febiger, 1991:393–432.

23. Gray F, Poirier J, Scaravilli F: Parkinson's disease and Parkinsonian syndromes. In Duckett S (ed): *The Pathology of the Aging Human Nervous System*. Philadelphis, Lea & Febiger, 1991: 179–199.

24. Lye M: Autonomic dysfunction and abnormal vascular reflexes. In Tallis R (ed): *The Clinical Neurology of Old Age*. Chichester, UK, Wiley, 1989:191–211.

25. Gregory GA, et al: The relationship between age and halothane requirement in man. *Anesthesiology* 1969; 30:488.

26. Nicodemus HF, et al: Median effective doses (ED_{50}) of halothane in adults and children. *Anesthesiology* 1969; 31:344.

27. Stevens WC, et al: Minimum alveolar concentrations (MAC) of isoflurane with and without nitrous oxide in patients of various ages. *Anesthesiology* 1975; 42:197.

28. Rampil IJ, et al: Clinical characteristics of desflurane in surgical patients: Minimum alveolar concentration. *Anesthesiology* 1991; 74:429.

29. Nakajima R, et al: Minimum alveolar concentration of sevoflurane in elderly patients. *Br J Anaesth* 1993; 70:273.

30. Katoh T, Ikeda K: Minimum alveolar concentration of sevoflurane in children. *Br J Anaesth* 1992; 68:139.

31. Katoh T, Ikeda K: The minimum alveolar concentration (MAC) of sevoflurane in humans. *Anesthesiology* 1987; 66:301.

32. Scheller MS, et al: MAC of sevoflurane in humans and the New Zealand white rabbit. *Can J Anaesth* 1988; 35:153.

33. Munson ES, et al: Use of cyclopropane to test generality of anesthetic requirement in the elderly. *Anesth Analg* 1984; 63:998.

34. Hilgenberg JC: Inhalational and intravenous drugs in the elderly patient. *Semin Anesth* 1986; V:44.

35. Homer TD, Stanski DR: The effect of increasing age on thiopental distribution and anesthetic requirement. *Anesthesiology* 1985; 62:714.

36. Arden JR, et al: Increased sensitivity to etomidate in the elderly: Initial distribution versus altered brain response. *Anesthesiology* 1986; 65:19.

37. Jung D, et al: Thiopental disposition as a function of age in female patients undergoing surgery. *Anesthesiology* 1982; 56:263.

38. Reidenberg MM, et al: Relationship between diazepam dose, plasma level, age, and central nervous system depression. *Clin Pharmacol Ther* 1978; 23:371.

39. Gamble JAS, et al: Evaluation of midazolam as an intravenous induction agent. *Anaesthesia* 1981; 36:868.

40. Greenblatt DJ, et al: Effect of age, gender and obesity on midazolam kinetics. *Anesthesiology* 1984; 61:27.

41. Scott JC, Stanski DR: Decreased fentanyl and alfentanil dose requirements with age: A simultaneous pharmacokinetic and pharmacodynamic evaluation. *J Pharmacol Exp Ther* 1987; 240:159.

42. Helmers H, et al: Alfentanil kinetics in the elderly. *Clin Pharmacol Ther* 1984; 36:239.

43. Bentley JB, et al: Influence of age on the pharmacokinetics of fentanyl. *Anesth Analg* 1982; 61:171.

44. Finucane BT, et al: Influence of age on vascular absorption of lidocaine from the epidural space. *Anesth Analg* 1987; 66:843.

45. Racle JP, et al: Spinal analgesia with hyperbaric bupivacaine: Influence of age. *Br J Anaesth* 1988; 60:508.

BRAIN DEATH, VEGETATIVE STATE, DONOR MANAGEMENT, AND CESSATION OF THERAPY

THOMAS W. K. LEW

AKE GRENVIK

Coma and Its Sequelae

Consciousness may be defined as a "state of awareness of the self and the environment" and requires two intact physiologic components: wakefulness or arousability, and cognition or content of consciousness.[1] Obtundation and stupor represent increasing grades of altered responsiveness, culminating in coma, which is a state of unarousable unresponsiveness with absence of purposeful response to external stimuli and inner need.[1] To distinguish from states of transient unconsciousness (e.g., syncope, concussion), coma must persist for at least 1 h.[2] Most acute states of altered consciousness are associated with impairment of arousal mechanisms, making assessment of cognitive function difficult. In contrast, some chronic states of altered consciousness have no impairment of wakefulness but are associated with selective or complete absence of cognition (e.g., dementia and vegetative state). The cerebrum provides for cognition and self-excitation, while the brain stem and thalamus provide the activating mechanism.[3] Corticothalamocortical loop impulses also contribute to arousal mechanisms. Therefore, injury to the cerebral hemispheres or the diencephalon, or both, contribute to a depressed level of consciousness. Coma may be secondary to structural or nonstructural causes. Structural lesions, which may be traumatic or nontraumatic in nature, lead to progressive compression or shift of contents in the supra- or infratentorial compartments, resulting in disruption to the brain stem hypothalamic activating mechanisms. Classical supratentorial herniation syndromes have been described by Plum and Posner, outlining successive pathologic and clinical stages.[1] Nonstructural metabolic or toxic encephalopathies diffusely depress brain stem and cerebral arousal mechanisms. The onset of coma may be abrupt, such as after a severe anoxic insult, or insidious, following a period of confusion and inattention (e.g., Wernicke's encephalopathy).

The sequelae to coma may be (1) recovery, with absence or varying degrees of disability, (2) vegetative state, with total loss of cognition but preserved hypothalamic and brain stem function, or (3) brain death, with total loss of cerebral and brain stem function. Death may also occur from acute nonneurologic complications. Two other distinct clinical entities are described. In the locked-in syndrome, severe paralysis of the voluntary motor system leads to an inability to communicate.[1,2,4] This condition usually follows injury to the descending corticospinal and corticobulbar pathways at or below the level of the pons but may also be associated with diseases of the peripheral motor nerves or neuromuscular junction. Akinetic mutism is characterized by pathologically slowed or nearly absent bodily movement and loss of speech following subacute bilateral damage to the paramedian mesencephalon, basal diencephalon, or inferior portions of the frontal lobes[1,2] (see Table 38-1).

This chapter reviews the diagnosis and management of brain death and the persistent vegetative state, and outlines the perioperative management of the brain-dead cadaveric organ donor. Because it is also in the realm of the neurointensive care and neuroanesthetic practice to frequently manage patients presenting with devastating and often unsalvageable injuries, the ethical and medical issues relating to cessation of therapy are also discussed.

TABLE 38-1
Characteristics of the Persistent Vegetative State and Related Conditions

Condition	Self Awareness	Sleep-Wake Cycles	Motor Function	Experience of Suffering	Respiratory Function	EEG Activity	Cerebral* Metabolism	Prognosis for Neurologic Recovery
Persistent vegetative state	Absent	Intact	No purposeful movement	No	Normal	Polymorphic delta or theta, sometimes slow alpha	Reduced by 50% or more	Depends on cause (acute traumatic or nontraumatic injury, degenerative or metabolic condition, or developmental malformation)
Coma	Absent	Absent	No purposeful movement	No	Depressed variable	Polymorphic delta or theta	Reduced by 50% or more (depends on cause)	Usually recovery, persistent vegetative state, or death in 2 to 4 weeks
Brain death	Absent	Absent	None or only reflex spinal movements	No	Absent	Electrocerebral silence	Absent	No recovery
Locked-in syndrome	Present	Intact	Quadriplegia and pseudobulbar palsy; eye movement preserved	Yes	Normal	Normal or minimally abnormal	Minimally or moderately reduced	Recovery unlikely; persistent quadriplegia with prolonged survival possible
Akinetic mutism	Present	Intact	Paucity of movement	Yes	Normal	Nonspecific slowing	Unknown	Recovery very unlikely (depends on cause)
Dementia	Present	Intact	Variable; limited	Yes	Normal	Nonspecific slowing	Variably reduced	Irreversible (ultimate outcome depends on cause)

* Determined by positron-emission or single-photon-emission computed tomography.

NOTE: EEG, electroencephalographic

SOURCE: Reprinted by permission of *The New England Journal of Medicine.* From The Multi-Society Task Force on PVS: Medical aspects of the persistent vegetative state. *N Engl J Med* 330: 1499,1572. Copyright (1994), Massachusetts Medical Society.

Brain Death

Traditionally, death has been described in clinical terms such as apnea, pulselessness, and unresponsiveness. Successive organ failure leads to cardiac arrest, and is rapidly followed by brain anoxia and death. Alternatively, complete cessation of brain stem function from direct injury such as trauma or hemorrhage, results in loss of respiratory drive and is quickly followed by anoxia and cardiac arrest. In both instances, the separate entities of brain and cardiac deaths are not temporally discernible. However, with the advent of modern resuscitative techniques and cardiopulmonary support in the intensive care unit (ICU), cessation of brain function became recognizable as a distinct entity that may precede cardiopulmonary arrest for a significant period of time, if other systemic organ functions are maintained.[5]

The imperative for a consensual definition of brain death was triggered mainly by developments in organ transplantation in the 1960s. Organ procurement from patients with absence of brain function not legally or medically defined as dead, made this procedure controversial, as transplanatation surgery was becoming technically feasible.[6–8] More significantly, it was also recognized that without a clear medical definition of brain death, a significant physical, emotional, and financial burden was imposed on irreversibly brain-damaged patients and their families, and hospital facilities were denied to other patients in need of finite medical resources.

In 1968, an ad hoc committee of the Harvard Medical School first published criteria to define irreversible coma as death.[9] Half a year later, the brain death committee at the University of Pittsburgh, School of Medicine, published its criteria, leading to the first hospital-approved brain-death policy in the United States at Presbyterian University Hospital in Pittsburgh.[10,11] In 1981, the medical consultants to the President's Commission for the Study of Ethical Problems in Medicine and Biomedical and Behavioral Research published guidelines on the determination of death based on neurologic criteria.[12] The American Bar and American Medical Associations, at a National Conference on Uniform State Laws, also agreed on the Uniform Determination of Death Act (UDDA), which has since become federal law. The UDDA concludes that an individual is dead if there is either irreversible cessation of circulatory and respiratory functions or irreversible cessation of all function of the entire brain, including the brain stem. These guidelines and statutes form the current medicolegal basis for the definition and certification of brain death.

BRAIN DEATH CRITERIA

Definitions of brain death have been proposed on the basis of cessation of (1) whole brain, (2) brain stem, or (3) cerebral functions. The guidelines published by the President's Commission require establishment of irreversible cessation of all brain function. Tests to confirm loss of both cerebral and brain stem functions are recommended in this guideline. In other criteria, such as those of the United Kingdom Conference of the Medical Royal Colleges and their Faculties, permanent cessation of all brain stem function constitutes brain death.[13] In this view, death of the brain stem results in an irreversible loss of capacity for consciousness, breathing, and vasomotor control, which are core physiologic functions of the brain.[14] This position is shared indirectly by many criteria which do not require examination of the cerebrum beyond clinical confirmation of absent cognition.[15] In support of using the brain stem criteria alone to diagnose brain death, Pallis analyzed reports on 1036 such patients who had brain stem death declared, but continued to be maintained on ventilators, and showed that asystole was the invariable outcome, occurring within hours to days after the diagnosis of brain death.[16]

Conversely, loss of cerebral function alone has not been accepted as equivalent to death. However, advocates support this view, known as the neocortical or "higher-brain" criterion, on an understanding of death that is based on the loss of "personhood" and/or "consciousness."[17,18] Although such a view would be in line with the concept, in many religions, of the departure of the spirit from the body, acceptance of such a consciousness-based standard would define some or all spontaneously breathing patients in a permanent vegetative state as dead. Emotionally, society has yet to accept the concept of a "breathing corpse." Other objections to cerebral criteria of death include an inability to ensure that loss of cerebral function is permanent. Furthermore, the fear that noncognitive patients may be declared dead using progressively less stringent criteria has been raised (i.e., the "slippery slope" argument). Anencephalic infants represent a special category of noncognitive patients for which the cerebral criteria may be relevant.[19] Since these infants lack cortical tissue entirely, they have never experienced cognition nor will they ever do so. This position has been legally supported for the purpose of kidney procurement and transplantation in Germany.[20]

EXCLUSION OF CONFOUNDING FACTORS

Prior to the examination of patients suspected of brain death, it is necessary to exclude the presence of confounding factors that may render this examination in-

TABLE 38-2
Guidelines for the Determination of Death[12]

A. Individual with irreversible cessation of circulatory and respiratory functions is dead

  1. Cessation recognized by appropriate clinical examination

  2. Irreversibility recognized by persistent cessation of functions during appropriate period of observation and/or trial of therapy

B. Individual with irreversible cessation of all functions of the entire brain, including the brainstem, is dead

  1. Cessation recognized when evaluation discloses findings of absent cerebral and brainstem functions

  2. Irreversibility recognized when cause of the coma is established and is sufficient to account for the loss of brain functions, the possibility of recovery of any brain function is excluded, and the cessation of all brain function persists for an appropriate period of observation and/or trial of therapy.

valid. These include the presence of shock or hypotension, profound hypothermia below 32°C, brain stem encephalitis, the Guillian-Barré syndrome, metabolic encephalopathies, and severe electrolyte derangements (e.g., hypophosphatemia).[21] A toxicologic screen to exclude drugs that may alter the result of neurologic examination, neuromuscular function, or electroencephalographic testing must also be performed. Such agents include opioids, barbiturates, benzodiazepines, alcohols, general anesthetics, neuromuscular blockers, methaqualone, mecloqualone, amitriptyline, meprobamate, and high-dose bretylium.[21]

Determination of a specific mechanism for suspected brain death is important. For example, severe head injury or a primary brain lesion that causes progressive clinical and radiological evidence of raised intracranial pressure leading to transtentorial herniation, would clearly define the circumstances in which brain death has occurred. Conversely, in the absence of a known cause for coma, a rigorous exclusion of reversible causes of global encephalopathy, as outlined above, must be sought before the examining physicians should proceed with the certification process.[22]

EXAMINATION CRITERIA AND METHODS

While the Harvard Criteria was prototypical in serving as a model for many subsequent criteria, a large number of different protocols have since been established by different authoritative groups in testing for brain death.[10,13,23,24] The President's Commission recognized that tests used for determining cessation of brain function "continue to change with the advent of new research and technologies" and offered advisory guidelines (Table 38-2) while encouraging "local, state, and national institutions and professional organizations to examine and publish their practices."[12]

Cessation of cerebral function is demonstrated by deep coma and cerebral unreceptivity and unresponsivity. This condition includes absence of spontaneous movement, decorticate or decerebrate posturing, seizures, or shivering. There is a lack of response to verbal stimuli and to noxious stimuli administered through a cranial nerve pathway. It is currently recognized that peripheral nervous system activity and simple or complex spinal cord reflexes may persist after established brain death.[25,26] Elevation and rotation of the shoulders mimicking decerebrate posturing, as well as asymmetric movements especially of the upper extremities, have been reported.[27] These phenomena are consistent with a definition of brain death that does not preclude spinal cord function below the level of the foramen magnum.[28]

Cessation of brain stem function is determined by the absence of pupillary light, corneal, oculocephalic, oculovestibular, cough, oropharyngeal, and respiratory (apnea) reflexes. The pupils must be nonreactive to light stimulation but need not be equal or dilated. It is important to exclude preexisting facial weakness as a cause for an absent corneal reflex.[29] Absence of response to painful stimulus to the face is tested by firm supraorbital pressure.

The oculocephalic reflex is tested by rapidly turning the head from side to side. Any eye movement indicates residual brain stem function. This test is omitted in patients with concurrent cervical spine injury. The oculovestibular reflex is tested by instilling 50 ml of ice water irrigated into each external auditory canal, cleared of cerumen, after elevating the patient's head to 30 degrees. Ocular motions in response to this powerful labyrinthine stimulus imply presence of brain stem function. This reflex may be altered by labyrinthine injury or disease, anticholinergics, anticonvulsants, tricyclic antidepressants, barbiturates, and other sedatives.

Pharyngeal reflexes, indicative of glossopharyngeal and vagal nerve function, are tested by inserting pharyngeal and endotracheal catheters. Any gagging or coughing indicates persistent brain stem function. Vagus nerve function is further tested by administering intravenous atropine in a dose of 0.04 mg/kg. Atropine would oppose the action of any underlying vagal tone that normally slows the heart rate. An increase in the pulse rate thus indicates baseline vagal activity that is inconsistent with brain stem death.

The apnea test is performed only if prior tests of brain stem reflexes are found to be absent since increased arterial carbon dioxide tension (Pa_{CO_2}) may increase intracranial pressure and the potential for further compromise of residual brain function. The test is performed by disconnection from mechanical ventilation and observing for spontaneous respiration after

TABLE 38-3
Confirmatory Tests for Brain Death

Evaluate neuronal function
   Electroencephalogram or cerebral function monitor
   Evoked potentials
   Biochemical tests of cerebrospinal fluid or jugular venous blood
Evaluate intracranial blood flow
   Contrast angiography, magnetic resonance or computed tomography imaging
   Radionuclide perfusion studies using technetium-HMPAO scintography
   Xenon-enhanced computed tomography
   Digital subtraction angiography/venography
   Ophthalmic artery blood flow
   Transcranial Doppler study
Miscellaneous (Optional)
   Intracranial pressure higher than systolic blood pressure
   Sustained cerebral perfusion pressure < 5 mmHg

SOURCE: Adapted from Powner DJ, et al: Controversies in brain death certification. In Shoemaker W, Ayres SM, Grenvik ANA, Holbrook PR (eds): *Textbook of Critical Care*, 2d ed. Boston, WB Saunders Company, 1995, chap. 173, pp 1580, with permission.

the Pa_{CO_2} is allowed to increase to levels greater than 60 mmHg for at least 30 s. This extremely powerful stimulus has no effect on the respiratory center in a nonfunctioning brain stem. As Pa_{CO_2} accumulates at a rate of 4 to 6 mmHg per min of apnea, the apneic test could last from 3 to 6 min, during which time hypoxemia must be avoided to prevent cardiac arrest or organ injury, especially in potential organ donors. This may be prevented by ventilating the patient with 100% oxygen for 5 min before the test and insufflating 4 to 6 liters/min of oxygen through the endotracheal tube while the patient is disconnected from the ventilator.[30] Conversely, in patients with known chronic respiratory failure, who are dependent on hypoxic stimulus for respiratory drive, the Pa_{O_2} must be less than 50 mmHg at the end of the apnea test. Arterial blood samples are drawn to document oxygen and carbon dioxide levels on completion of the test.

CONFIRMATORY TESTS AND THEIR LIMITATIONS

The EEG and cerebral blood flow studies are important confirmatory tests if specific evidence of death of the cerebrum is required. Table 38-3 lists tests that have been used in conjunction with the neurologic examination. These are broadly categorized as tests of neuronal function, which is valid only in the absence of the confounding factors discussed earlier, and tests for presence or absence of cerebral blood flow, which may be utilized if confounding factors are present. The clinical and technical limitations of each confirmatory test, however, must be understood.

Electrocerebral silence (ECS) recorded on EEG testing may be taken as a sign of brain death, if neurologic signs of cortical and brain stem functions are lacking, confounding factors are absent, and the ECS lasts for a distinct length of time of at least 30 min. Reversible and transient ECS is known to occur after drug overdose, profound hypothermia, circulatory arrest associated with intraoperatively induced hypothermia, head trauma, extracranial causes of circulatory arrest, metabolic encephalopathy, and encephalitis.[11] In such patients, persistence or return of cranial nerve function may occur.[31,32] Another limitation of the EEG is its failure to measure subcortical electrical activity. Recommendations for EEG recordings in suspected cerebral death have been published.[33-35] The most important recommendation is the use of high instrument sensitivity to differentiate ECS from low voltage output, and the need for continuous recognition and elimination of artifacts. Positive evoked potentials may be present despite electrocerebral silence on EEG testing, if cranial nerve function is preserved.[32] Absence of sensory evoked potentials must be interpreted cautiously in patients with primary brain stem dysfunction from hemorrhage or infarction, since cortical activity may still be present.[35] In both instances, a diagnosis of brain death should not be made.

Transcranial Doppler (TCD) ultrasonography can be used as an ancillary tool to support the diagnosis of brain death when blood flow is absent on attempted insonation of multiple intracranial arteries.[15] The technique, however, requires considerable expertise to perform and false positive results have been reported. Xenon and technetium radionuclide scans have been used to detect small amounts of cerebral blood flow at the bedside.[21] However, the posterior circulation is poorly visualized with these techniques and absence of detectable flow to the anterior circulation must be combined with a reliable clinical examination of absent brain stem function before brain death is diagnosed. Serial four-vessel angiography demonstrating absence of both carotid and vertebral blood flow to the brain is considered by some to be the definitive diagnostic test,[36] and is consistently seen in brain death in the presence of ECS on EEG, and absent cranial nerve function. Technical errors may make interpretation difficult and risk to viable brain tissue may occur due to bradycardia, hypotension, or transient anoxia inducible by the procedure. However, angiography showing persistent absence of four vessel flow may be reliably accepted as being diagnostic of brain death, even in the presence of drug intoxication, therapy, or hypothermia.[21]

UNIVERSITY OF PITTSBURGH
MEDICAL CENTER

DeSoto at O'Hara Streets
Pittsburgh, Pennsylvania 15213

CHECK LIST FOR CLINICAL DIAGNOSIS OF BRAIN DEATH

	CLINICAL EVALUATIONS #1	#2
CAUSE OF BRAIN DEATH _____		
Date of Exam:	_____	_____
Time of Exam:	_____	_____

I. ABSENCE OF CONFOUNDING FACTORS

	#1	#2
A. Systolic blood pressure > 90 mmHg	_____	_____
B. Temperature > 32°C	_____	_____
C. No CNS depressants (e.g., anesthetics, sedatives, narcotics, alcohol) or neuromuscular blocking agents	_____	_____
D. No uremia, meningoencephalitis, hepatic encephalopathy or other metabolic encephalopathies	_____	_____

II. ABSENCE OF CEREBRAL AND BRAINSTEM FUNCTION

	#1	#2
A. Unresponsiveness to painful stimuli, e.g., supraorbital pressure	_____	_____
B. No spontaneous muscular movements, posturing, or seizures	_____	_____
C. Pupils light-fixed	_____	_____
D. Absent corneal reflexes	_____	_____
E. Absent response to upper and lower airway stimulation, e.g., pharyngeal and endotracheal suctioning	_____	_____
F. Absent oculocephalic reflexes	_____	_____
G. Absent oculovestibular reflexes (irrigation of the ears with 50 ml of ice water)	_____	_____
H. No increase in heart rate after IV atrophine (2 mg)	_____	_____
1. Heart rate before atropine	_____	_____
2. Heart rate after atropine	_____	_____
I. Apnea (at $PaCO_2$ > 60 mmHg)	_____	_____
1. $PaCO_2$ at end of apnea test	_____	_____
2. PaO_2 at end of apnea test	_____	_____

III. CONFIRMATORY TESTS (See Guidelines in Section III)

A. An electroencephalogram demonstrating electrocerebral silence	_____
B. Cerebral arteriography showing absent intracranial circulation	_____

IV. COMMENTS: _____
_____
_____

CERTIFICATION OF DEATH

Having considered the above findings, we hereby certify the death of:

Date _____ Time of death _____
Physicians' Signatures _____ MD _____ MD
Names Printed _____ MD _____ MD

This doeument must be signed by two physicians licensed by the State of Pennsylvania.

Figure 38-1 University of Pittsburgh Brain Death Certification Form, with permission.

CERTIFICATION PROCESS

Brain death certification should be performed according to an individual institution's policy (Fig. 38-1). This should include a protocol detailing clinical and confirmatory tests, their frequency, and interval between tests. Two or more appropriately licensed physicians with experiences in brain death certification should perform the examination. The protocol should be adhered to rigidly, in order to minimize the possibility of death certification when brain function exists.[22] Transplant physicians are generally not involved in brain death certification of a potential organ donor to avoid conflicts of interest. Brain death certification is equivalent to the pronouncement of death, and the time documented for this certification is considered the time of death medically and legally. Certification of death is the physicians's duty. Seeking consent is inappropriate but the family must be informed of the

PUH GUIDELINES FOR THE DETERMINATION OF BRAIN DEATH

Introduction:

The clinical diagnosis of brain death in adults at Presbyterian University Hospital is made in accordance with standards recommended by the President's Commission for the Study of Ethical Problems in Medicine (JAMA 246 (19):2184–2186, 1981). The etiology of brain death must be well established using historical and adjunctive testing (e.g., CT scanning when indicated). The brain death evaluation should only be performed after all correctable abnormalities that might contribute to abnormal brain function (e.g., hypothermia, shock, hypoxemia) have been addressed. The patient should be observed for a reasonable period of time after he/she is first noted to be brain dead to the time that brain death is formally declared. The duration of observation is a matter of clinical judgement and depends on the nature and severity of injury as well as certainty of prognosis. Two clinical examinations at least two hours apart must be performed by two physicians licensed in Pennsylvania. Finally, the brain death <u>check list</u> must be filled out.

I. ABSENCE OF CONFOUNDING FACTORS

Before the clinical examination for brain death can be performed, systolic blood pressure (with or without vasopressors) must be at least 90 mmHg with evidence of adequate peripheral perfusion. The following conditions must be excluded before a clinical diagnosis of brain death can be made without confirmation of absent brain circulation: hypothermia (Temp. < 32°C), presence of CNS depressants in therapeutic or toxic concentrations (opiates, benzodiazepenes, phenothiazines, lithium, tricyclic antidepressants, barbiturates, glutethimide, methaqualone) alcohol level $\geq$ 100 mg%, or the presence of neuromuscular blockers. Brain death may be declared in patients with sedative levels in the subtherapeutic range or when alcohol is present at levels < 100 mg% without confirmation of absent circulation as long as the cause of brain death is not due to global brain ischemia/anoxia and sedative and alcohol are not present in combination. If uremia, hepatic encephalopathy, meningitis, encephalitis or other metabolic encephalopathies are present, an EEG must be obtained to confirm the clinical diagnosis of brain death.

*If there is clinical suspicion of the presence of sedative, alcohol or other CNS depressants, toxicological studies must be obtained to exclude their presence. The results of toxicological studies must be recorded in the comments section of the check list along with the time at which the sample was obtained.

II. THERE MUST BE DEMONSTRABLE EVIDENCE OF ABSENT CEREBRAL AND BRAINSTEM FUNCTION.

The clinical exam must demonstrate:

A. Cerebral unresponsivity and unreceptivity.

B. Absent brain stem reflexes, including a test for apnea.

    1. Apnea is confirmed by the absence of spontaneous breathing movements at a $PaCO_2$ above 60 torr at the end of the test. If the history suggests dependence on a hypoxic stimulus for ventilation (e.g., a COPD patient), the PaO_2 at the end of test must be less than 50 torr.

    2. Atropine test—heart rate changes less than five beats/min. after 2 mg atropine IV.

III. CONFIRMATORY TESTS

A. An EEG demonstrating electrocerebral silence is required for the diagnosis of brain death under the following circumstances:

    1. When at least one of the clinical examinations is not performed by a neurologist, neurosurgeon or critical care medicine physician.

    2. When apnea testing cannot be performed because of the potential for cardiac arrest due to hypoxemia.

    3. When the cause of death is uncertain, or is due to global ischemic/anoxic brain injury and the patient has been observed for less than 24 h.

    4. When uremia, hepatic encephalopathy or other metabolic encephalopathies are present.

B. A four vessel cerebral angiogram demonstrating absent intracranial circulation must be obtained when the brain death evaluation is confounded by hypothermia, the presence of CNS depressants, sedatives, alcohol, sedatives and alcohol in combination, or neuromuscular blocking agents as indicated in Section 1.

Figure 38-1 (*Continued*)

certification process. In cases which lie within a coroner's jurisdiction, permission is not required for death certification or termination of medical therapy, but consent of the coroner and the next of kin must be obtained for the removal of organs for transplantation.

CONTROVERSIES IN BRAIN DEATH DETERMINATION

Despite widespread acceptance of the present methodology in the definition and diagnosis of brain death, evidence shows that residual neuronal function may persist even when a patient has fulfilled whole-brain criteria. Such evidence includes continuing or inducible pituitary and/or hypothalamic hormone production, and maintenance of normal body temperature in some patients despite an absence of blood flow demonstrated with four-vessel angiography.[17,37] Spontaneous depolarizations may be detected by deeply placed electrodes despite an isoelectric cortical EEG.[38] Environmental responsiveness, as evidenced by an increase in blood pressure and pulse rate, has been documented in one study of 10 brain dead organ donors in response to surgical incision during organ procurement.[39] These effects are supposedly caused by stimulation of the extracranial component of the autonomic nervous system. Some have argued that such events imply an internal inconsistency between the conceptual definition and the clinical criteria used to make the diagnosis of brain death.[17] It is clear, however, that no criteria are sufficiently detailed for the purpose of documenting that all cellular function of the entire brain is absent before confirming brain death. Implied in the current clinical definition is the permanent loss of all integrated neuronal organ function but not necessarily death of all cells. The potential that residual cellular and tissue function may exist is recognized but not specifically sought.[15]

Management of the Heartbeating "Brain Dead" Organ Donor

IDENTIFICATION AND ASSESSMENT

Availability of donor organs is currently the single most important factor limiting organ transplantation in the United States. It has recently been reestimated that the potential pool of brain dead cadaveric organ donors is approximately 10,000 to 12,000 per year.[40,41] Since the major cause of death in organ donors is severe head injury (56 to 77 percent), followed by nontraumatic intracranial hemorrhages and brain tumors, the neurointensivist or neuroanesthesiologist should always be vigilant in recognizing potential organ donors in the ICU before loss of transplantable organs occurs due to unexpected cardiac arrest, hemodynamic instability, or infection.[42] Failure to discuss organ donation with grieving families has been cited as the most important obstacle to recovering organs for transplantation.[43] Certain states have now enacted "required request" legislation that compels hospitals to notify organ procurement agencies of all deaths in their institution for potential organ and/or tissue donation. The impact on increasing the ratio of actual to potential organ donors has however been disappointing.[44]

A thorough history, physical examination, and evaluation of laboratory values are all necessary for initial assessment of donor suitability. General exclusion criteria for organ donation exist but beyond these absolute contraindications, assessment of individual organ function and the impact of the patient's clinical course on individual organs determine their suitability for donation (Tables 38-4 and 38-5). The final arbitrament of individual organ viability is made at the time of procurement by direct inspection and, if necessary, biopsy by the transplantation team.

MAINTENANCE PHASE

After declaration of brain death, continuation of therapy is indicated if organs are to be removed for trans-

TABLE 38-4
Age Guidelines for Organ and Tissue Donation Used at the Pittsburgh Transplantation Institute

Organ/Tissue	Age
Heart	<60 y[a]
Heart-lungs	<60 y[a]
Lungs	<60 y[a]
Kidney	1 mo–75 y[a]
Liver	<75 y[a]
Pancreas	<65 y[a]
Intestine[b]	
Bone	15–65 y
Marrow	<75 y
Cornea	1–65 y
Skin	15–65 y
Heart valves	<55 y

[a] Donors beyond these age limits could be accepted on the basis of the individual organ function.

[b] No age limits have been set for intestinal donors. Intestines should be available from most organ donors and are always evaluated on an individual basis

SOURCE: From Marino IR, et al: Multiple organ procurement. In Shoemaker W, Ayres SM, Grenvik ANA, Holbrook PR (eds): *Textbook of Critical Care*, 2d ed. Boston, WB Saunders Company, 1995, chap. 178, p 1613, with permission.

plantation. Progressive hemodynamic instability, leading eventually to cardiac arrest, is inevitable after brain death, and may occur within hours to days. Although a clear explanation for cardiac decompensation is lacking, a significant contribution may be traced to events leading to brain death. In the course of rostral to caudal neurologic deterioration or direct injury to the brain stem, massive sympathetic discharge occurs in response to the development of raised intracranial pressure and medullary ischemia. A combination of severe systemic hypertension and excess of circulating catecholamines results in pathologic microinfarcts of the heart. The rapidity and severity of intracranial pressure elevation determine the degree of myocyte injury and myocardial depression after brain death.[45,46] After brain death, sympathetic outflow and circulating catecholamine levels fall dramatically, due to destruction of the pontine and medullary vasomotor structures. Hypotension will impair coronary perfusion and further contribute to myocardial injury.

The goals of medical therapy are aimed at improving posttransplantation allograft survial by (1) the early recognition and treatment of hemodynamic instability in the donor, (2) the maintenance of adequate end-organ perfusion and tissue homeostasis. A balanced and cohesive management approach is needed when multi-organ procurement is planned, since specific therapies, aimed at optimizing any particular organ function may be detrimental to the survival of other organs. For instance, vigorous fluid administration may benefit the kidneys but induce pulmonary edema and jeopardize function of the lungs.

TABLE 38-5
Contraindications to Organ Procurement

A. Systemic, absolute
  1. Severe trauma (to specific organ)
  2. Malignancy (except for primary CNS tumors)
  3. Active infections
    a. Systemic sepsis
    b. Active tuberculosis
    c. Viral encephalitis
    d. Guillian-Barré syndrome
    e. Active hepatitis, presence of hepatitis B surface antigen
    f. Human immunodeficiency virus carrier

B. Systemic, relative
  1. Severe hypotension or prolonged cardiac arrest
  2. Long-standing systemic diseases
    a. Hypertension
    b. Cardiac
    c. Peripheral vascular
    d. Diabetes mellitus

C. Organ specific
  1. Kidney
    a. Chronic renal disease
    b. Consistently elevated serum creatinine and blood urea nitrogen
  2. Liver
    a. Elevated serum aspartate aminotransferase (AST), serum alanine aminotransferase (ALT), bilirubin, prothrombin time
  3. Pancreas
    a. Diabetes mellitus
  4. Intestines
    a. Unstable hemodynamics,
    b. Dopamine requirements > 10 μg/kg per min
  5. Heart
    a. Systolic blood pressure < 90 mmHg
    b. Dopamine requirements > 10 μ/kg per min
    c. Significant coronary artery disease
    d. Severe cardiac hypertrophy, valvular defects, global myocardial dysfunction or segmental wall motion abnormalities (by transesophageal echocardiography)
  6. Heart-lung, or isolated single or double lung
    a. As in Section 5, a–d
    b. History of heavy smoking
    c. Chronic lung disease
    d. Pulmonary aspiration
    e. PaO_2/FiO_2 ratio < 250 mmHg
    f. Peak ariway pressure > 30 cmH$_2$O at 15 ml/kg tidal volume and 5 cmH$_2$O positive end-expiratory pressure

SOURCE: Adapted from Marino IR, et al: Multiple organ procurement. In Shoemaker W, Ayres SM, Grenvik ANA, Holbrook PR (eds): *Textbook of Critical Care,* 2d ed. Boston, WB Saunders Company, 1995, Chap. 178, pp 1610–1625, with permission.

GENERAL INTENSIVE CARE

The general intensive care of potential donors should continue after brain death has occurred. This includes the prevention of atelectasis and pneumonia by regular hyperinflation therapy and bronchial toilet, precautions against gastric aspiration by continual orogastric suctioning, prevention of decubitus ulcerations with regular repositioning and skin care, and removal and replacement of potentially contaminated intravascular catheters. Antibiotics are routinely administered in many centers although there is no evidence that this reduces infectious complications in the recipient.[42] Documented or suspected infections should, however, be treated with appropriate antibiotics. Caution should be exercised in obtaining proper blood and urine specimens for cultures since false-positive results can increase uncertainty in the care of organ donors and transplant recipients.

HEMODYNAMICS

The main hemodynamic problems encountered are hypotension and cardiac arrhythmias. Hypotension occurs as a result of loss of arterial and venous sympathetic tone, volume depletion secondary to diabetes insipidus (DI) and prior use of diuretics, or prior fluid restriction in the management of the primary brain injury. Myocardial depression further contributes to the effects of hypotension in reducing tissue perfusion.

Relative or absolute volume depletion is initially treated with aggressive intravenous fluid infusions using a combination of crystalloids and colloids. Ringer's lactate has been preferred as a crystalloid volume expander because of its lower sodium content compared to normal saline, as hypernatremia occurs commonly in the donor population. Excessive use of crystalloids has, however, been shown experimentally to lead to impaired oxygenation of the liver.[47] Blood may be transfused to maintain a hematocrit between 0.25 and 0.35. Transfusion of red blood cells has a beneficial effect on renal allograft function by modifying the immune response in recipients.[48] Volume repletion is guided by monitoring central venous pressure to a goal of 8 to 10 mmHg and systolic blood pressure above 90 mmHg.[49,50] Fluid replacement volumes up to 10 liters may be needed.[51]

Vasopressors are added if arterial hypotension persists despite achieving an adequate central venous pressure. Frequently, vasopressor infusion is initiated early to maintain an adequate arterial perfusion pressure while fluid resuscitation is in progress, and may be withdrawn gradually with improvement in mean arterial blood pressure. Dopamine hydrochloride is the agent of choice, because it augments cardiac contractility while preferentially dilating the renal and splanchnic vessels at levels below 10 μg/kg per min. Pure vasoconstrictors such as phenylephrine hydrochloride or norepinephrine bitartrate are contraindicated to avoid potential ischemic injury to the liver and kidneys. Excessive use of inotropes is clearly associated with an increased incidence of acute tubular necrosis and reduced renal allograft survival.[52,53] However, a stated correlation with poorer outcome in heart, lung, and liver recipients from donors requiring high levels of inotropic support remains unproved.[54,55] Furthermore, inotropic support may be inevitable in donors who have sustained significant myocardial injury in the events leading to brain death. Arginine vasopressin (AVP) also greatly potentiates the effects of catecholamines on pressor tone after brain death and has been used successfully in combination with low-dose epinephrine infusion to maintain prolonged hemodynamic stability and survival for up to 54 days after brain death. More importantly, laboratory indices of renal and hepatic functions using this regime were unchanged.[56]

The frequency of central diabetes insipidus (DI) after brain death ranges from 38 to 87 percent, and may occur hours to weeks after brain injury, when there is partial or complete destruction of the supraoptic nucleus or neurohypophysis.[42] Features suspicious of central DI include urine output greater than 4 ml/kg per h, urine specific gravity less than 1.005, hypernatremia greater than 145 mmol/liter, low urine osmolality, and an elevated serum osmolality of greater than 300 mmol/kg. Initial management should include hypotonic fluid repletion and guided correction of hypokalemia, hypomagnesemia, hypophosphatemia, and hypocalcemia. Of the various synthetic arginine vasopressin preparations used as replacement therapy for central DI, desmopressin or DDAVP (desamino-D-arginine vasopressin) is favored because of its high antidiuretic to vasopressor activity ratio (2000 : 1) and long duration of action.[57] Single intravenous doses of 0.5 to 2 μg may be administered every 8 to 12 h as indicated.[58] Continuous intravenous infusion of synthetic vasopressin may also be used as a rate of 0.5 to 1.0 U/h to titrate for an optimal urine output of 100 to 250 cc per h without the excessive vasopressor effects of intermittent boluses.

Supraventricular and ventricular tachyarrhythymias commonly occur in association with high levels of circulating catecholamines during brain stem ischemia. Beta-blockers have been used successfully to abolish the hypertensive response during experimental brain herniation.[46] Esmolol hydrochloride is an ideal agent in this setting, because its short duration of action allows discontinuation if severe myocardial depression develops. Bradyarrhythmias may also occur in association with the hypertensive response to brain herniation (Cushing's reflex). It is treated with isoproterenol hydrochloride, epinephrine, or temporary cardiac pacing. Atropine sulphate is ineffective because of the absence of underlying vagal tone.

Ten percent of all donors develop cardiopulmonary arrest during the maintenance phase.[59] Resuscitation based on established protocol should be initiated and organ procurement performed promptly where possible. Cardiopulmonary bypass or intraaortic balloon counterpulsation are options to support the circulation until organ procurement can take place.[60–62] If circulation cannot be restored within 15 min, organ recovery should not be considered.

VENTILATION AND OXYGENATION

The goals of mechanical ventilation in the organ donor are to achieve adequate tissue oxygenation, carbon dioxide elimination, and maintenance of normal acid-base balance. Inspired concentration of oxygen is titrated to achieve arterial oxygen saturation above 95%. For lung donors, hyperoxia is avoided to reduce absorption atelectasis and oxygen toxicity. Excessive positive end expiratory pressure is also avoided as it impedes venous return, impairs renal and hepatic perfusion, reduces cardiac output, and increases barotrauma to the lungs. Minute ventilation is titrated for a normal arterial pH measured at 37°C but not corrected for the donor's body temperature (i.e., alpha-stat pH regulation).[63] In the presence of metabolic acidosis, mild hyperventilation may be necessary to correct acidemia. However, excessive ventilatory requirements for this purpose may lead to raised mean intrathoracic pressure and further compromise cardiac output and end-organ perfusion. Severe metabolic acidosis should therefore be corrected with intravenous bicarbonate.

TEMPERATURE HOMEOSTATIS

Cessation of blood flow to the hypothalamus results in loss of temperature regulation (i.e., poikilothermy). Complications from hypothermia secondary to uncompensated heat loss include myocardial depression, cardiac arrhthymias, platelet dysfunction, renal tubular acidosis, and impaired oxygen molecule release from the oxyhemoglobin moiety. Brain death certification is also confounded. Delivery of heated humidified oxygen, warmed intravenous fluids, and warming blankets are used to maintain temperature at or above 35°C.

COAGULOPATHY

Disseminated intravascular coagulation (DIC) is present in up to 88 percent of patients with lethal head injury and in 25 to 65 percent of cadaveric donors.[64,65] Its etiology includes shock, sepsis, or thromboplastin release by the injured brain. Since the degree of end organ damage is variable, DIC is not considered an absolute contraindication to organ procurement. Correction with the appropriate blood component therapy is indicated to reduce the risk of severe operative blood loss and prolonged organ ischemia during procurement. Epsilon-aminocaproic acid should not be used because microvascular thrombosis may potentially be induced in donor organs, causing subsequent graft failure.[66]

ENDOCRINE ASPECTS

There are conflicting data regarding the benefit of exogenous hormonal replacement therapy for hemodynamic stability and maintenance of temperature homeostasis in organ donors. Depletion of circulating thyroid hormones, insulin, and cortisol have been observed in animal and human studies after brain death.[46,47] In an uncontrolled study by Novitzky and colleagues on cardiac donors, an improved hemodynamic profile and reduction in the severity of metabolic acidosis was found after treatment with repeated doses of triiodothyronine, cortisol, and insulin.[67] However, a later controlled study using triiodothyronine (T3) alone did not show a similar beneficial effect. Instead, metabolic acidosis during the period of T3 infusion was worsened.[68] Powner has also shown that the thyroid function profiles in donors before and after brain death were similar, consistent with a variant of the euthyroid sick syndrome, and not of hypothyroidism.[69] The euthyroid sick syndrome is commonly seen in patients with nonthyroidal critical illness and is characterized by low free thyroxine (fT4), normal free triiodothyronine (fT3), normal or high reverse T3 (rT3), and normal TSH levels. Measured levels of insulin and cortisol were also normal or high. Such hormonal assays are consistent with the existence of a functional hypothalamic-pituitary axis after brain death. This may be explained anatomically by blood supply to the anterior pituitary from the inferior hypophysial artery which arises extradurally from the internal carotid artery. The use of exogenous T3 may have a pharmacological effect independent of the actual physiologic status of the donor.[66] The current data therefore does not support the routine use of triiodothyronine or any other hormone replacement therapy, with the possible exception of steroid replacement therapy in patients with adrenal suppression from recent exogenous steroid therapy.

PROCUREMENT

Management of the donor in the operating room during organ procurement is based on continuation of principles adopted in the intensive care unit. Familiarity with the surgical technique and communication between members of the procurement team is important to anticipate and correct hemodynamic and respiratory perturbations in the course of operative manipulation. Routine monitoring of vital signs is continued during the intraoperative period. Pulmonary artery catheters are seldom necessary for assessment of volume status and have the potential to cause right-sided endocardial lesions.[70] The incidence of catheter-induced endocardial disruption detected by pathological examination is in the range of 20 to 30 percent. Intravenous pancuronium bromide

0.15 mg/kg is administered to abolish complex spinal reflex movements of the limbs and trunk to nociceptive stimuli, which may interfere with surgery or cause undue anxiety amongst operating room personnel.[25–27] A reflex hypertensive response to surgical stimulus also occurs and should be treated with short-acting vasodilator agents such as sodium nitroprusside, nitroglycerin, or isoflurane.

Operative techniques may differ between centers but, in general, are based on the principles of in situ core cooling of organs using chilled preservation solution at the time of circulatory arrest, followed by "no-touch" en bloc removal of the core cooled solid organs. These techniques minimize ischemic injury from surgically induced arterial vasospasm and reduce the risk of uneven flushing, cooling, and preservation of the donor organ.[71,72] For multiple organ procurement, an incision is made from the suprasternal notch to the symphysis. The abdominal contents are examined to ensure no penetrating wound, hematoma, or laceration is present in the intestinal tract. The supraceliac aorta, the aorta at the level of the inferior mesenteric artery, and the inferior mesenteric vein are isolated. The inferior mesenteric artery is then ligated and divided. The pleural spaces are opened wide after initial mediastinal dissection and inspection of the lungs. Following systemic heparinization, circulation is arrested by an infusion of cardioplegic solution into the root of the aorta. The distal aorta is ligated and cannulated. The aorta is cross clamped just proximal to the innominate artery and at the diaphragm. Infusion of preservation solutions for the lungs occurs via cannulation of the right and left pulmonary arteries. The kidneys and gastrointestinal organs are perfused via the distal aortic cannula and the inferior mesenteric vein. Outflow for the perfusate is provided by transection of the vena cava at the level of the diaphragm or near its abdominal bifurcation. Sequential removal of organs then proceeds, beginning with the heart and lungs, gastrointestinal organs, and kidney. Monitoring and hemodynamic support is discontinued after surgical occlusion of the proximal aorta and start of in situ flushing of organs. Ventilation of the lung, usually at four breaths per minute, is discontinued once the trachea has been transected. In the event of cardiac arrest, cardiopulmonary resuscitation is initiated while surgery progresses without delay. This surgical technique allows for isolation and infusion of cold preservation solution to organs within minutes.

Vegetative State

The term "persistent vegetative state" (PVS) was coined by Jennett and Plum in 1972 to describe the

TABLE 38-6
Diagnostic Criteria for the Persistent Vegetative State

1. Absence of awareness of self or environment; inability to interact with others

2. Absence of sustained, reproducible, purposeful, or voluntary behavioral responses to visual, auditory, tactile, or noxious stimuli

3. No evidence of language comprehension or expression

4. Intermittent wakefulness manifested by the presence of sleep-wake cycles.

5. Sufficiently preserved hypothalamic and brain stem autonomic functions to permit survival with medical and nursing care

6. Bowel and bladder incontinence

7. Variably preserved cranial-nerve reflexes (pupillary, oculocephalic, corneal, vestibulo-ocular, and gag) and spinal reflexes

SOURCE: Reprinted by permission of *The New England Journal of Medicine.* Adapted from The Multi-Society Task Force on PVS: Medical aspects of the persistent vegetative state. *N Engl J Med* 330: 1499,1572. Copyright (1994), Massachusetts Medical Society.

condition of patients with severe brain damage in whom coma has progressed to a state of wakefulness without detectable awareness.[73] This definition was accepted by the President's Commission for the Study of Ethical Problems in Medicine and Biomedical and Behavioral Research in 1983.[74] In 1989, the American Academy of Neurology published a position paper on the persistent vegetative state and addressed the issue of withdrawal of artificial hydration and nutrition in these patients.[75] More recently, a Multi-Society Task Force on PVS was established in 1991 to create a document summarizing the medical facts about the persistent vegetative state. The material in this section draws extensively from the task force report, which was published in 1994.[2] The vegetative state is a clinical condition of complete unawareness of self and the environment, accompanied by sleep-wake cycles with either complete or partial preservation of hypothalamic and brain stem autonomic functions.[2] The vegetative state may be transient, representing a stage in the recovery or deterioration from severe acute or chronic brain injury, degenerative and metabolic neurologic diseases, or developmental malformations of the nervous system. A vegetative state is defined as persistent when it has been present for at least a month.[2,73]

DIAGNOSTIC CRITERIA

The vegetative state can be diagnosed according to the criteria listed in Table 38-6. Its distinguishing feature is an irregular but cyclic state of circadian sleeping and waking unaccompanied by any behaviorally detectable expression of self-awareness, specific recognition of external stimuli, or consistent evidence of attention or intention or learned responses. Patients in a vegeta-

tive state have no sustained visual pursuit, consistent and reproducible visual fixation, or response to threatening gestures. In fact, the presence of sustained visual pursuit represents one of the first and most readily observable signs of transition from a vegetative state to a state of awareness.[2]

ETIOLOGY

The persistent vegetative state may be caused by traumatic or nontraumatic head injuries, degenerative or metabolic disorders, and developmental malformations (Table 38-7). Head trauma and hypoxic-ischemic encephalopathy are the most common acute causes of the vegetative state in adults and children. PVS occurs in up to 14 percent of patients in a prolonged traumatic coma, and in 12 percent of those in prolonged nontraumatic coma.[76,77]

In patients with degenerative diseases, awareness is initially retained even as progressive loss of intellect, memory, language, motor skills, and social behavior occurs. Superimposed metabolic encephalopathy from sepsis, malnutrition, dehydration, or seizures may result in temporary loss of awareness. Eventually, a persistent vegetative state evolves over a period of several months or years.[78]

Severe congenital malformations of the nervous system in infants and children may prevent the development of awareness or cognition. The diagnosis of the vegetative state is, however, not usually made before 3 months of age since higher cognitive functions are limited, and differentiation of voluntary from involuntary responses are unreliable.[79] Furthermore, immaturity of the developing brain and the ongoing influences of development on the potential for reorganization of structure and function renders a diagnosis of PVS problematic before the age of 3 months.[80] Exceptions would be the anencephalic or hydrancephalic infant, with minimal or no cerebral cortex.[2]

PATHOLOGIC FEATURES

The neuropathologic changes that characterize the persistent vegetative state are variable, depending on the length of survival and the presence or absence of other complicating diseases such as severe atherosclerotic disease. While there has been no systemic investigation of the neuropathologic changes in patients with PVS secondary to degenerative, metabolic, or developmental disorders, two major patterns have characterized most detailed reports on the neuropathology of a PVS due to acute traumatic or nontraumatic brain injury.

Extensive multifocal or diffused laminar cortical necrosis follows acute, global hypoxia and ischemia. There is invariably involvement of the hippocampus, as well as possible scattered small areas of infarction

TABLE 38-7
Common Causes of the Persistent Vegetative State

Acute Injuries
  Traumatic
    Motor vehicle accidents
    Gunshot wound or other form of direct cerebral injury
    Nonaccidental injury to children
    Birth injury
  Nontraumatic
    Hypoxic ischemic encephalopathy
    Cardiorespiratory arrest
    Perinatal asphyxia
    Pulmonary disease
    Prolonged hypotensive episode
    Near-drowning
    Suffocation or strangulation
    Cerebrovascular injury
    Cerebral hemorrhage
    Cerebral infarction
    Subarachnoid hemorrhage
    CNS infection
    Bacterial meningitis
    Viral meningoencephalitis
    Brain abscess
    CNS tumor
    CNS toxins or poisoning
Degenerative and metabolic disorders
  In adults
    Alzheimer's disease
    Multi-infarct dementia
    Pick's disease
    Creutzfeldt-Jakob disease
    Parkinson's disease
    Huntington's disease
  In children
    Ganglioside storage disease
    Adrenoleukodystrophy
    Neuronal ceroid lipofuscinosis
    Organic aciduria
    Mitochondrial encephalopathy
    Gray-matter degenerative disorders
Developmental malformations
  Anencephaly
  Hydranencephaly
  Lissencephaly
  Holoprosencephaly
  Encephalocele
  Schizencephaly
  Congenital hydrocephalus
  Severe microcephaly

SOURCE: Reprinted by permission of *The New England Journal of Medicine*. From The Multi-Society Task Force on PVS: Medical aspects of the persistent vegetative state. *N Engl J Med* 330: 1499,1572. Copyright (1994), Massachusetts Medical Society.

or neuronal loss in the deep forebrain nuclei, hypothalamus, brain stem, or thalamus.[81-84]

In acute trauma, a shearing force results in an extensive subcortical axonal injury that virtually isolates the cortex from other parts of the brain. Small primary brain stem injuries may accompany diffuse axonal injury, as may secondary damage to the brain stem from transtentorial herniation soon after the injury. In acute trauma accompanied by circulatory or respiratory failure, diffuse laminar necrosis may also be present.[85,86]

DIAGNOSTIC STUDIES

Neurodiagnostic tests, when used in conjunction with a clinical evaluation, may provide useful supportive data in the diagnosis and prognostication of PVS. In most patients, EEG shows diffuse generalized polymorphic delta or theta activity. Desynchronization is noted in the transition from wakefulness to sleep. Very low voltage EEG activity or persistent alpha activity may be seen in other patients. It is unusual to record an isoelectric EEG, epileptiform, or seizure activity. Clinical recovery from the vegetative state may be paralleled by diminished delta and theta activity and the reappearance of a reactive alpha rhythm.[2,87,88]

Somatosensory evoked responses are useful in the assessment of outcome in children and adults who are in a coma as a result of an acute neurologic injury. The bilateral absence of such responses one week after the insult is highly predictive of failure to regain consciousness, leading to death or survival in a vegetative state.[89,90] Absence of somatosensory evoked potentials after traumatic coma may, however, still lead to recovery with at least minimal cognitive activity.[91] Brain stem auditory evoked response is of limited value, and may be preserved even when the somatosensory evoked response is absent, and the outcome is either survival in a vegetative state or death.[2]

Computed tomographic or magnetic resonance imaging of patients in a persistent vegetative state often reveals diffuse or multifocal cerebral disease involving the gray and white matter. The results of neuroimaging studies do not confer any predictive value for progression to the vegetative state nor its recovery to consciousness. However, in the initial few months after a traumatic or nontraumatic brain injury, patients in a persistent vegetative state are more likely to recover consciousness, yet remain severely disabled, if serial neuroimaging scans are normal than if they are abnormal. More commonly, serial documentation of progressive brain atrophy reduces the likelihood of neurologic recovery.[2]

Cerebral metabolic studies using positron-emission tomographic (PET) studies have shown substantial reductions (50 to 60 percent) of the glucose metabolic rates in the cerebral cortex, basal ganglia, and cerebellum. The parieto-occipital and mesiofrontal regions had the most consistent reduction in metabolic activity.[92,93] In comparison with patients in the locked-in state, no overlap in metabolic impairment was noted. However, patients who regained consciousness after anoxic cerebral injuries also had lesser degrees of metabolic impairment. These studies therefore do not war-

TABLE 38-8
Glasgow Outcome Score

1. Death

2. Persistent Vegetative State

3. Severe disability (conscious but disabled)
   Dependent for daily support due to mental or physical disabilities or both. Include patients only able to maintain self-care within the room and house.

4. Moderate disability (disabled but independent)
   Ability to travel by public transport and can work in a sheltered environment. Disabilities include varying degrees of dysphasia, hemiparesis, ataxis, intellectual and memory deficits, and personality change.

5. Good recovery
   Resumption of normal life. May have minor neurologic and psychologic deficits.

SOURCE: Adapted from Jennet B, Bond M: Assessment of outcome after severe brain damage. A practical scale. *Lancet* 1:480–4; 1975, with permission.

rant the use of PET scanning for the purpose of prognostication. This is especially so in children and infants where normal cerebral metabolic activity is substantially lower than that reported in adults.[94]

Studies of cerebral blood flow using xenon-133 isotopes, PET scanning, or HM-PAO-single photon-emission computed tomography generally show a reduction of cerebral blood flow ranging from 10 to 50 percent of normal values. Acute measurements of cerebral blood flow immediately after an acute neurologic injury do not predict a vegetative outcome in either adults or children.[95–100]

In summary, neurodiagnostic tests provide useful supportive information when used in conjunction with a careful clinical evaluation, but can neither confirm the diagnosis of a vegetative state nor predict its potential for recovery of awareness.[101]

PROGNOSIS

The spectrum of recovery from the persistent vegetative state ranges in a continuum from recovery of consciousness to recovery of function. Consciousness is determined by evidence of awareness of self and the environment, consistent voluntary behavioral responses to visual and auditory stimuli, and interaction with others. Recovery of function is characterized by communication, the ability to learn and perform adaptive tasks, mobility, self care, and participation in recreational or vocational activities.[2] The Glasgow Outcome Scale, which classifies outcome in five categories is shown in Table 38-8.[103]

The prognosis for cognitive and functional recovery depends on the cause of the underlying brain disease. The Multi-Society Task Force on PVS reviewed data on 434 patients in previously reported series who were in a persistent vegetative state one month after severe head injury, and followed their recovery of consciousness and function over 12 months[2] (Table 38-9). Recovery of consciousness had occurred in 33 percent of patients after 3 months, 46 percent at 6 months, and 52 percent at 12 months. Of the 434 patients, 67 percent survived at one year; 15 percent remained in a persistent vegetative state, 28 percent had severe disability, 17 percent had moderate disability, and 7 percent had a good recovery.[2] Good recovery was associated with signs of improvement within 3 months after injury while a later recovery was almost invariably associated with severe disability. Almost all patients who recovered with moderate or severe disability showed signs of improvement within 6 months after injury. Recovery of consciousness after 12 months was exceedingly rare, occurring in only 7 of 434 patients. Increasing age, ventilatory dysfunction, lack of early motor reactivity, late-onset epilepsy, or the development of hydrocephalus may also indicate a poorer prognosis for recovery of awareness.[103–105] The prognosis for recovery of consciousness after a traumatic injury is slightly better in children than in adults.[2] Recovery of function was comparable to that in the adults but the degree of functional recovery was better for a similar duration of vegetative state.[107]

By comparison, recovery of consciousness after a nontraumatic injury was poor. In reviewing the data of 169 patients in a vegetative state 1 month after a nontraumatic injury, the Multi-Society Task Force on PVS found that only 11 percent had recovered consciousness 3 months after injury; 89 percent remained in a vegetative state or had died.[2] One year after injury, 15 percent of the 169 patients had recovered consciousness, 32 percent were in a persistent vegetative state, and 53 percent had died. Recovery of function in the 15 percent of those patients who regained consciousness was extremely poor and only one patient had a good recovery. Other reports have also shown that good functional recovery is only associated with early improvement.[88,107] Recovery from a vegetative state more than 6 months after nontraumatic injury is associated with moderate to severe disability. The prognosis for recovery from a vegetative state in young infants with birth injuries and perinatal asphyxia is more variable than in older infants and children. In general, children usually recover more function than adults.[2]

Patients in a vegetative state due to degenerative or metabolic disease have no possibility of recovery.[2] However, a transient and reversible deterioration in mental status must be considered before the vegetative state is labeled as persistent. This may be caused by a concurrent systemic illness, leading to encephalopathy in patients with few neuronal reserves. Infants and

TABLE 38-9
Probability of Recovery from PVS

	ADULTS[a]		CHILDREN[a]	
Outcome	Traumatic Injury ($n = 434$)[b]	Nontraumatic Injury ($n = 169$)[b]	Traumatic Injury ($n = 106$)[b]	Nontraumatic Injury ($n = 45$)[b]
Patients in PVS for 3 months[c]				
Death	35(27–43)	46(31–61)	14(1–27)	3(0–11)
PVS	30(22–28)	47(32–62)	30(13–47)	94(83–100)
Severe disability	19(12–26)	6(0–13)	24(8–40)	3(0–11)
Moderate disability or good recovery	16(10–22)	1(0–4)	32(15–49)	0
Patients in PVS for 6 months[d]				
Death	32(21–43)	28(12–44)	14(0–31)	0
PVS	52(40–64)	72(56–88)	54(30–78)	97(89–100)
Severe disability	12(4–20)	0	21(1–41)	3(0–11)
Moderate disability or good recovery	4(0–9)	0	11(0–26)	0

[a] Expressed as % of patients (99% confidence interval).

[b] Number of patients given in parentheses refer to the number of patients who were in a vegetative state one month after injury.

[c] Total of 218 adults with traumatic injuries, 77 adults with nontraumatic injuries, 50 children with traumatic injuries, and 31 children with nontraumatic injuries.

[d] Total of 123 adults with traumatic injuries, 50 adults with nontraumatic injuries, 28 children with traumatic injuries, and 30 children with nontraumatic injuries.

SOURCE: Reprinted by permission of *The New England Journal of Medicine.* From The Multi-Society Task Force on PVS: Medical aspects of the persistent vegetative state. *N Engl J Med* 330: 1499,1572. Copyright (1994), Massachusetts Medical Society.

children with brain malformations severe enough to cause a developmental vegetative state are unlikely to regain consciousness. Patients who are in a vegetative state at 3 months of age and show no evidence of consciousness by the age of 6 months are almost completely precluded from the potential for future improvement.[108] The anencephalic infant is also incapable of consciousness in the complete absence of the cerebral cortex.[109]

The Multi-Society Task Force on PVS has concluded that "a persistent vegetative state can be judged to be permanent 12 months after a traumatic injury in adults and children; recovery after this time is exceedingly rare and almost always involves severe disability. In adults and children with non-traumatic injuries, a persistent vegetative state can be considered to be permanent after three months; recovery does occur, but it is rare and at best associated with moderate or severe disability."[2]

The survivability of patients in PVS is related, in some degree, to the quality and intensity of the medical treatment and nursing care that they receive. In general, the severe neurologic injury necessary to produce the vegetative state in adults and children reduces the average life expectancy to approximately 2 to 5 years. Survival beyond 10 years is unusual. Infants and elderly patients have a shorter life expectancy than young or middle-aged adults.[2] Causes of death include pulmonary and urinary tract infections, multiorgan failure, sudden death of unknown etiology, respiratory failure, and other disease-related causes such as recurrent strokes or tumors.[81,105,110]

TREATMENT

Therapy aimed at reversing the persistent vegetative state has not been successful.[2] Although there are reports suggesting benefits with different modalities of therapy, their validity suffers from a lack of placebo-control or double-blindedness and insufficient details as to the quality of the recovered state reported. Such therapies have included use of dopamine agonists or dextroamphetamine; direct stimulation of the mesencephalic reticular formation, nonspecific thalamic nuclei, or dorsal columns; and use of coma sensory stimulation programs.[111-115]

In instances where a decision is made to fully support the patient at the current level of disability, initial therapy may need to be aggressive in order to stabilize cardiopulmonary function and treat multiorgan injuries associated with the primary event. Concurrently, a rigorous medical and nursing regime is instituted to prevent or forestall complications associated with states of severe brain damage. There should be consideration for an early tracheostomy to maintain airway patency and access for pulmonary toilet. Gastrostomy or jejunostomy catheters placed percutaneously or surgically to facilitate adequate nutrition and hydration can bypass the oropharyngeal route to reduce the risk for aspiration pneumonia. A regular bowel regime is necessary to prevent constipation and interruption in delivery of nutrients. Surveillance for pulmonary or urinary tract infections is maintained and treatment with antibiotics started when appropriate. Risks for pulmonary embolism are reduced with prophylactic anticoagulation therapy, pneumatic calf stockings, and regular monitoring for deep venous thrombosis by Doppler ultrasonography. Daily passive range of motion exercises and frequent repositioning to prevent contractures and skin care to prevent decubitus ulcers are also important aspects of nursing care.

Cessation of Therapy

Cessation of life-sustaining therapy encompasses a whole range of medical, ethical, religious, legal, and sociological issues of which a comprehensive discussion is beyond the scope of this chapter. This section focuses on the guiding principles relating to cessation of therapy, with particular emphasis on the patient in a persistent vegetative state and the critically ill intensive care patient. A practical description of terminal weaning is included, as is the special circumstance in which the patient or surrogate gives prior consent for his or her organs to be donated after death. The neurointensivist plays a vital role in communicating with the patient or his or her next-of-kin, and in orchestrating the process to ensure its medical appropriateness and the patient's dignity and comfort.

The ethical principles guiding doctor-patient relationships are (1) beneficence: acting to benefit patients by sustaining life, treating illness, and relieving pain; (2) nonmaleficence: refraining from harm; (3) autonomy: respecting the right of patients to medical self-determination; (4) disclosure: providing adequate and truthful information for competent patients to make medical decisions; and (5) social justice: allocating medical resources fairly and according to medical need.[116]

A decision to limit, withdraw, or withhold therapy must be consistent with the above principles. In the physicians' discussion with the patient, a full disclosure is made on the nature of the patient's condition. This discussion should include objective and reliable prognostic indicators of the severity of injury, the likelihood for recovery, and the degree of disability predicted. Then, the patient's life philosophy with regards to the level and intensity of medical intervention in the event of such a terminal, catastrophic, or severely incapacitating illness is carefully sought. In the likely event that the patient is comatose or is assessed to be no longer mentally competent, surrogates usually represent the patient's interest and previously expressed wishes. Ideally, such surrogates have been designated in advance, and hold durable powers of attorney for health care for the patient.[117] Proxy and instructional directives or living wills may be helpful in discerning patient's wishes although they are generally considered to be either too broadly, or too narrowly drawn.[117] When surrogates are not available, the patient's wishes may be sought from other individuals, who may have discussed this issue with the patient. They include the patient's primary physcians, clergy members, or critical care nurses who frequently may have explored these issues with the patient at the bedside. Referral to the hospital's biomedical ethics committee is useful in reviewing the medical decision process should difficulties arise, such as families' or surrogates' rejection of physicians' recommendations.[118,119]

Referral to judicial involvement for resolution of conflicts is generally not favored.[120] Most courts defer to the customary practices of a profession in determining whether a particular course of conduct is legally acceptable, and have taken the position that they are available to assist in the decision-making process, but that a rule requiring judicial involvement is unnecessary to protect the patient's well-being and may be cumbersome.[120]

After sufficient discussions with the family, level-of-care decisions may be made. Termination of therapy is made with the understanding that, first, everything possible was done for their loved ones and, second, when it became obvious that there was no reasonable possibility for survival, all unindicated forms of treatment were to be discontinued or gradually withdrawn to permit the patient to die in peace with dignity.[121] Such decisions must be carefully documented and communicated to all physicians, nurses, and paramedical personnel involved, and explicitly translated into what treatment forms should be administered or withheld, and individually tailored to each specific case. The guidelines at the University of Pittsburgh Health Center have been in existence since 1975, and were last modified in 1992.[120] Table 38-10 lists the individual classifications of treatment within these guidelines.

In the acute and critically ill neurologic patient whose lungs are mechanically ventilated, the provision of comfort measures and termination of therapy will include discontinuation of mechanical ventilation or "terminal weaning."[121] This takes place over several hours and many patients may die in this phase. Those who survive to the point of spontaneous breathing should be extubated, as this is more comforting to family, being a more natural state for death to occur. Patients who are prone to acute airway obstruction may need to remain intubated. Similarly, agonal breathing or gasping may be distressing to relatives who want their loved ones to die quietly without

TABLE 38-10
University of Pittsburgh Medical Centre Classification of Levels of Therapy in the ICU

Each situation is unique, detailed orders specific to each individual patient may be required. If detailed orders are not provided, to facilitate communication when therapy is to be limited, one of the following categories should be indicated:

1. All but cardiac resuscitation—Treated vigorously, including intubation, mechanical ventilation, and measures to prevent cardiac arrest. However, in the event of cardiac arrest in these patients despite every therapeutic effort, resuscitation should not be attempted and the patient is permitted to die. The possibility of unexpected cardiac arrest occurring as an iatrogenic complication should be discussed with the patient and/or family in advance and may be treated with full cardiopulmonary resuscitation.

2. Limited therapy—In general, no additional therapy is initiated except for hygienic care and for comfort. Should cardiac arrest occur, no resuscitative efforts are made. Therapy already initiated will be limited by specific written order only. Exceptions may occur—for example, it may be appropriate to initiate certain drug therapy in a patient who had decided in advance against intubation, dialysis, etc.

3. Comfort measures only—These patients will only receive nursing and hygienic care and medications appropriate to maintain comfort as ordered. Therapy (e.g., administration of narcotics) which is necessary for comfort may be utilized even if it contributes to cardiorespiratory depression. Therapies already initiated will be reviewed by the physician and discontinued if not related to comfort or hygiene.

"signs of suffering." Sedation in the form of intravenous morphine sulphate in 1- to 2-mg aliquot or as an incremental infusion is used to decrease reflex hypoxic responses. Such "comfort measures" are administered even at the risk of hastening death.[74,123] All other therapies unrelated to comfort and hygienic care are discontinued.

Limitation of treatment decisions on patients with a persistent vegetative state are made with an understanding of their prognosis and the improbability of recovery. In 1975, efforts by the family of Karen Ann Quinlan initiated a movement towards an ethical and legal consensus for families and other proxies to authorize the termination of all forms of life-sustaining medical treatment, including hydration and nutrition, for patients in a permanent vegetative state.[74,124] Currently, this position is supported by the President's Commission for the Study of Ethical Problems in Medicine and Biomedical and Behavioral Research (1983), the Hastings Center (1987), the American Academy of Neurology (1989), the American Medical Association (1990), and the United Kingdom Institute of Medical Ethics Working Party on the Ethics of Prolonging Life and Assisting Death (1991).[74,75,125,126] Specific clinical guidelines are available for physicians terminating treatment in adult patients in a per-

sistent vegetative state.[75,127–129] Since many of these patients are beyond the acute phase of illness and are no longer ventilator dependent, the process of dying may occur gradually and the families should be forewarned. When artificial nutrition and hydration are withdrawn, death usually occurs within 10 to 14 days due to dehydration and electrolyte imbalance.[130] Discontinuation of medications may also result in death from intercurrent acute infections or cardiac or renal disease.[2] By definition, the patient does not experience hunger, thirst, or discomfort. Physical manifestations of acute dehydration such as dryness of the skin and mucous membranes of the mouth and eyes may be prevented by appropriate nursing care and should not distress the family.[131]

TERMINAL WEANING OF THE NON-HEART-BEATING CADAVER DONOR (NHBCD) CANDIDATES

An increasing and ever-frustrating shortage of transplantable organs from brain dead heart-beating cadaver donors (HBCDs) has led to renewed interest in alternative sources, including living donors (kidneys), partial transplants (livers and lungs), ancephalic infants, and animals.[132–135] Historically, patients who have been declared dead by traditional cardiopulmonary, rather than neurologic criteria, served as a major source of transplantable kidneys although problems with warm ischemia limited their usefulness. These patients are also known as non-heart-beating-cadaver donors (NHBCDs). The problem of warm ischemia has been circumvented by recent procurement techniques with (1) in situ organ preservation immediately following uncontrolled cardiopulmonary arrest and (2) controlled immediate procurement from patients who have died after choosing to forgo life-sustaining treatment. Potential NHBCDs who fall into the latter category must be dependent on life-sustaining treatment such as mechanical ventilation or cardiac assist devices, so that stopping them would result in rapid and predictable death. The clinical spectrum would range from critically ill cognitive patients to severely brain-injured patients who are ventilator-dependent.[136]

To establish a formal protocol and set practice standards to deal with controlled procurement from NHBCDs, the University of Pittsburgh Medical Center established a comprehensive policy in April 1992.[137] Decision on comfort measures and cessation of therapy is made separately and prior to discussion of organ donation. Furthermore, the latter discussion must be initiated by the patient or family, and not by physicians or hospital staff. A fully informed consent process is specified, including its withdrawal at any time without prejudice. Removal of life-sustaining therapy occurs in the manner outlined above for critically ill intensive care patients, but takes place in the operating room. Narcotics and sedatives are used as indicated for patient comfort, irrespective of their effect on organ viability or timing of death. Organ procurement takes place only after the irreversible cessation of cardiopulmonary function, as specified by a pulse pressure of zero (as measured via femoral arterial catheter), and when the patient is apneic and unresponsive and has one of the following electrocardiographic criteria: (1) 2 min of ventricular fibrillation; (2) 2 min of electrical asystole (i.e., no complexes, agonal baseline drift only); or (3) 2 min of electromechanical dissociation.

If removal of life support does not lead to the death of the patient in a very short time or if organ ischemia is prolonged in the judgment of the transplant surgeon, organ procurement may be canceled and the patient returned to the intensive care unit. To avoid conflicts of interest, all physicians attending to the terminal weaning must have no clinical, research, or administrative responsibilities with the transplant service. In all cases rigorous documentation of discussions, clinical decisions, clinical course, and involvement of the hospital ethics consultation service are further safeguards under the protocol. The concept of NHBCDs has nevertheless raised important ethical, psychosocial, and public policy implications which have been discussed by a working group and summarized by Youngner and Arnold.[136]

Conclusion

The clinical and ethical responsibilities of the physician towards his or her patient involve implementing specific therapies within an overall treatment plan that will not only stabilize the patient acutely, but improve outcome, and ultimately lead to recovery with a level of disability that is compatible with the patient's life philosophy. Otherwise, indiscriminate and aggressive therapy will result in either a prolonged death process in the ICU, accompanied by pain and suffering, or worse, subject severely disabled patients and their families to an extended period of physical, emotional, and psychosocial burden.

When diagnoses of permanent vegetative state or brain death are made, these must be unmistakable and irrefutable, since they commit the patient's course towards definitive clinical end-points of irreversibility, and death, respectively. A methodical and rigid adherence to institutional protocols, based on established criteria, ensures that all possible errors will be prevented.

Beyond the physician's commitment to the dignity and comfort of each of his or her individual patients, lies a responsibility toward the critically ill community at large. For many, organ transplantation represents their last, but eminently curative, hope. Identification of potential organ donors, discussion of organ donation with bereaved relatives, and rational physiologic management of the cadaveric donor, ensure that even in death, others may be assured of a new lease on life.

References

1. Plum F, Posner JB: *The Diagnosis of Stupor and Coma*, 3d ed. Philadelphia, FA Davis, 1980.
2. The Multi-Society Task Force on PVS: Medical aspects of the persistent vegetative state. *N Engl J Med* 1994; 330:1499, 1572.
3. McCormick DA, Von Krosigk M: Corticothalamic activation modulates thalamic firing through glutamate "metabotropic" receptors. *Proc Natl Acad Sci USA* 1992; 89:2774.
4. Position Statement: Certain aspects of the care and management of profoundly and irreversibly paralyzed patients with retained consciousness and cognition: Report of the Ethics and Humanities Subcommittee of the American Academy of Neurology. *Neurology* 1993; 43:222.
5. Black PM: Brain death. *N Engl J Med* 1978; 299:338, 393.
6. Loisell DW: Transplantation: Existing legal constraints. In Wolstenholme G, O'Connor M (eds): *Ethics in Medical Progress: With Special Reference to Transplantation.* Boston, Little Brown, 1966:78–103.
7. Grenvik A: Brain death and organ transplantation, a 40-year review. *Opuscula Medica* 1992; 37:33.
8. Barnard CN: A human cardiac transplant; an interim report of a successful operation at Groote Schuur Hospital in Cape Town. *S Afr Med J* 1967; 41:1268.
9. Beecher H: A definition of irreversible coma. Special communication: Report of the Ad Hoc Committee of the Harvard Medical School to Examine the Definition of Brain Death. *JAMA* 1968; 205:337.
10. Wecht C, et al: Determination of death. Ad Hoc Committee on Human Tissues Transplantation Reports Criteria. *Bull of the Allegh County Med Soc* 1969; 25:29.
11. Powner DJ, et al: Brain death certification: A review. *Crit Care Med* 1977; 5:230.
12. President's Commission for the Study of Ethical Problems in Medicine and Biomedical and Behavioral Research: Guidelines for the determination of death. Report of the medical consultants on the diagnosis of death. *JAMA* 1981; 246:2184.
13. Diagnosis of brain death: Statement issued by the honorary secretary of the Conference of Medical Royal Colleges and their Faculties in the United Kingdom on 11 October 1976. *Br Med J* 1976; 2:1187.
14. Pallis C: From brain death to brain stem death. *Br Med J* 1982; 285:1487.
15. Powner DJ, et al: Controversies in brain death certification. In Shoemaker W, et al (eds): *Textbook of Critical Care*, 2d ed. Boston, WB Saunders Company, Chap. 173, 1995:1579–1583.
16. Pallis C: Prognostic significance of a dead brain stem. *Br Med J* 1983; 286:123.
17. Troug RD, Fackler JC: Rethinking brain death. *Crit Care Med* 1992; 20:1705.
18. Cranford RE, Smith DR: Consciousness: The most critical moral (constitutional) standard for human personhood. *Am J Law Med* 1987; 13:233.
19. Shinnar S, Arras J: Ethical issues in the use of anencephalic infants as organ donors. *Neurol Clin* 1989; 7:729.

20. Holzgreve W, et al: Kidney transplantation from anencephalic infants as organ sources. *JAMA* 1989; 261:1773.

21. Powner DJ: The diagnosis of brain death in the adult patient. *J Intensive Care Med* 1987; 2:181.

22. Jastremski M, et al: Problems in brain death determination. *Forensic Sci* 1978; 11:201.

23. Mohandas A, Chou SN: Brain death—a clinical and pathological study. *J Neurosurg* 1971; 35:211.

24. An appraisal of the criteria of cerebral death: A summary statement. A collaborative study. *JAMA* 1977; 237:982.

25. Ropper AH: Unusual spontaneous movements in brain dead patients. *Neurology* 1984; 34:1089.

26. Ivan LP: Spinal reflexes in cerebral death. *Neurology* 1973; 23:650.

27. Jorgensen EO: Spinal man after brain death. *Acta Neurochir* 1973; 28:259.

28. Powner DJ, et al: Decision making in brain death and vegetative states—multiple considerations. *Clin Crit Care Med* 1981; 2:239.

29. Grenvik A: Ethical dilemmas in organ donation and transplantation. *Crit Care Med* 1988; 16:1012.

30. Ropper AH, et al: Apnea testing in the diagnosis of brain death. *J Neurosurg* 1981; 55:942.

31. Jorgensen EO: EEG without detectable cortical activity and cranial nerve areflexia as parameters of brain death. *Electroencephalogr Clin Neurophysiol* 1974; 36:70.

32. Trojaborg W, Jorgensen EO: Evoked cortical potentials in patients with "isoelectric" EEGs. *Electroencephalogr Clin Neurophysiol* 1973; 35:301.

33. Jorgensen EO: Requirements for recording the EEG at high sensitivity in suspected brain death. *Electroencephalogr Clin Neurophysiol* 1974; 36:65.

34. Silverman D, et al: Irreversible coma associated with electrocerebral silence. *Neurology* 1970; 20:5255.

35. Black PM: Clinical problems in the use of brain death standards. *Arch Intern Med* 1983; 143:121.

36. Nau R, et al: Results of four technical investigations in fifty clinically brain dead patients. *Intensive Care Med* 1992; 18:82.

37. Sugimoto T, et al: Morphological and functional alterations of the hypothalamus-pituitary system in brain death with long term bodily living. *Acta Neurochir (Wien)* 1992; 115:31.

38. Pallis C: Brainstem death: The evolution of a concept. *Semin Thorac Cardiovas Surg* 1990; 2:135.

39. Wetzel RC, et al: Hemodynamic responses in brain dead organ donor patients. *Anesth Analg* 1985; 64:125.

40. Evans RW, et al: The potential supply of organ donors: An assessment of the efficiency of organ procurement efforts in the United States. *JAMA* 1992; 267:239.

41. Nathan HM, et al: Estimation and characterization of the potential renal organ donor pool in Pennsylvania. *Transplantation* 1991; 51:142.

42. Darby JM, et al: Approach to management of the heartbeating "brain dead" organ donor. *JAMA* 1989, 261:2222.

43. Gallup Organization: Attitudes and Options of the American Public towards Kidney Donation. Prepared for the National Kidney Foundation, Inc., Princeton, NJ, 1983.

44. Caplan AL, Welvang P: Are required request laws working? *Clin Transplant* 1989; 3:170.

45. Shivalkar B, et al: Variable effects of explosive or gradual increase of intracranial pressure on myocardial structure and function. *Circulation* 1993; 87:230.

46. Novitzky D, et al: Electrocardiographic, hemodynamic and endocrine changes occurring during experimental brain death in the Chacma baboon. *J Heart Transplant* 1984; 4:63.

47. Makisalo H, et al: Correction of hemorrhagic shock-induced liver hypoxia with whole blood, Ringer's solution or with hetastarch. *Res Exp Med* 1989; 189:397.

48. Jeekel J, et al: Beneficial effect of blood transfusion to the donor on kidney graft in man: A study in three centers. *Transplant Proc* 1983; 15:973.

49. Lucas BA, et al: Identification of donor factors predisposing to high discard rates of cadaver kidneys and increased graft loss within one year post transplantation: SEOPF 1977–1982. *Transplantation* 1987; 43:253.

50. Flanigan WJ, et al: Etiology and diagnosis of early post-transplantation oliguria. *AM J Surg* 1976; 132:808.

51. Randell T, et al: Peroperative fluid management of the brain-dead multiorgan donor. *Acta Anaesthesiol Scand* 1990; 34:592.

52. Whelchel D, et al: The effects of high-dose dopamine in cadaver donor management on delayed graft function and graft survival following renal transplantation. *Transplant Proc* 1986; 18:523.

53. Schneider A, et al: Effect of dopamine and pitressin on kidneys procured and harvested for transplantation. *Transplantation* 1986; 36:110.

54. Makowka L, et al: Analysis of donor criteria for the prediction of outcome in clinical liver transplantation. *Transplant Proc* 1987; 19:2378.

55. Trento A, et al: Early function of cardiac homografts: Relationship to hemodynamics in the donor and the length of the ischemic period. *Circulation* 1986; 74(Suppl 3):111.

56. Yosioka T, et al: Prolonged hemodynamic maintenance by the combined administration of vasopressin and epinephrine in brain death: A clinical study. *Neurosurgery* 1986; 18:565.

57. Richardson DW, Robinson AG: Desmopressin. *Ann Intern Med* 1985; 103:228.

58. Debelak L, et al: Arginine vasopressin versus desmopressin in the treatment of diabetes insipidus in the brain dead organ donor. *Transplantation Proc* 1990; 22:351.

59. Emery RW, et al: The cardiac donor: A six year experience. *Ann Thorac Surg* 1986; 41:356.

60. Link J, et al: Cardiopulmonary bypass in brain dead organ donors. *Lancet* 1993; 1:238.

61. Wheeldon DR, et al: Hemodynamic corrections in multiorgan donation. *Lancet* 1992; 339:1175.

62. Tisherman SA, et al: Cardiopulmonary-cerebral resuscitation: Advanced and prolonged life support with emergency cardiopulmonary bypass. *Acta Anaesthesiol Scand* 1990; 34(Suppl 94):63.

63. Swain JA: Hypothermia and blood pH: A review. *Arch Intern Med* 1988; 148:1643.

64. Kaufman HH, et al: Clinicopathologic correlations of disseminated intravascular coagulation in patients with severe head injury. *Neurosurgery* 1984; 15:34.

65. Gil-Vernet S, et al: Disseminated intravascular coagulation in multiorgan donors. *Transplant Proc* 1992; 24:33.

66. Robertson KM, Cook DR: Perioperative management of the multiorgan donor. *Anesth Analg* 1990; 70:546.

67. Novitzky D, et al: Hemodynamic and metabolic responses to hormonal therapy in brain-dead potential organ donors. *Transplantation* 1987; 43:852.

68. Randell T, Hockerstedt KAV: Triiodothyronine treatment in brain-dead multiorgan donors—a controlled study. *Transplantation* 1992; 54:736.

69. Powner DJ, et al: Hormonal changes in brain dead patients. *Crit Care Med* 1990; 18:702.

70. Rowley KM, et al: Right-sided infective endocarditis as a consequence of flow directed pulmonary artery catheterization. A clinicopathological study of 55 autopsied patients. *N Engl J Med* 1984; 311:1152.

71. Rosenthal JJ, et al: Principles of multiple organ procurement from cadaver donors. *Ann Surg* 1983; 198:617.

72. Starzl TE, et al: An improved technique for multiple organ harvesting. *Surg Gynecol Obstet* 1987; 165:343.

73. Jennett B, Plum F: Persistent vegetative state after brain damage: A syndrome in search of a name. *Lancet* 1972; 1:734.

74. President's Commission for the Study of Ethical Problems in Medicine and Biomedical and Behavioral Research: Deciding to forgo life-sustaining treatment: A report on the ethical, medical, and legal issues in treatment decisions. U.S. Government Printing Office, 1983.

75. Position of the American Academy of Neurology on certain aspects of the care and management of the persistent vegetative state patient: Adopted by the Executive Board, American Academy of Neurology, April 21, 1988, Cincinnati, Ohio. *Neurology* 1989; 39:125.

76. Levy DE, et al: Prognosis in nontraumatic coma. *Ann Intern Med* 1981; 94:293.

77. Levin HS, et al: Vegetative state after closed-head injury: A Traumatic Coma Data Bank Report. *Arch Neurol* 1991; 48:580.

78. Walsh TM, Leonard C: Persistent vegetative state: Extension of the syndrome to include chronic disorders. *Arch Neurol* 1985; 42:1045.

79. Coulter DL: Is the vegetative state recognizable in infants? *Med Ethics Physician* 1990; 5:13.

80. Ashwal S: The persistent vegetative state in children. In: Fukuyama Y, et al (eds): *Fetal and Perinatal Neurology.* Basel, S. Karger, 1992:357–366.

81. Dougherty JH Jr, et al: Hypoxic-ischemic brain injury and the vegetative state: Clinical and neuropathologic correlation. *Neurology* 1981; 31:991.

82. Ingvar DH, et al: Survival after severe cerebral anoxia with destruction of the cerebral cortex: The apallic syndrome. *Ann NY Acad Sci* 1978; 315:184.

83. Relkin NR, et al: Coma and the vegetative state associated with thalmic injury after cardiac arrest. *Ann Neurol* 1990; 28:221.

84. Kinney HC, et al: Neuropathological findings in the brain of Karen Ann Quinlan—the role of the thalamus in the persistent vegetative state. *N Engl J Med* 1994; 330:1469.

85. Strich SJ: Diffuse degeneration of the cerebral white matter in severe dementia following head injury. *J Neurol Neurosurg Psychiatry* 1956; 19:163.

86. Adams JH, et al: Diffuse axonal injury due to non missile head injury in humans: An analysis of 45 cases. *Ann Neurol* 1982; 12:557.

87. Chatrian E: Coma and brain death. In Daly DD, Pedley TA, (eds): *Current Practice of Clinical Electroencephalography,* 2d ed. New York, Raven Press, 1990:463.

88. Hansotia PL: Persistent vegetative state: Review and report of electrodiagnostic studies in eight cases. *Arch Neurol* 1985; 42:1948.

89. Frank LM, et al: Prediction of chronic vegetative states in children using evoked potentials. *Neurology* 1985; 35:931.

90. Judson JA, et al: Early prediction of outcome from cerebral trauma by somatosensory evoked potentials. *Crit Care Med* 1990; 18:363.

91. Zegers de Beyl D, Brunko E: Prediction of chronic vegetative state with somatosensory evoked potentials. *Neurology* 1986; 36:134.

92. DeVolder AG, et al: Brain glucose metabolism in postanoxic syndrome: Positron emission tomographic study. *Arch Neurol* 1990; 47:197.

93. Levy DE, et al: Differences in cerebral blood flow and glucose utilization in vegetative versus locked-in patients. *Ann Neurol* 1987; 22:673.

94. Chugani HT, et al: Positron emission tomography study of human brain functional development. *Ann Neurol* 1987; 22:487.

95. Ashwal S, et al: Xenon computed tomography measuring cerebral blood flow in the determination of brain death in children. *Ann Neurol* 1989; 25:539.

96. Jaggi JL, et al: Relationship of early cerebral blood flow and metabolism to outcome in acute head injury. *J Neurosurg* 1990; 72:176.

97. Muizelaar JP, et al: Cerebral blood flow and metabolism in severely head-injured children: Part 1: Relationship with GCS score, outcome, ICP, and PVI. *J Neurosurg* 1989; 71:63.

98. Ashwal S, et al: Prognostic implications of hyperglycemia and reduced cerebral blood flow in childhood near-drowning. *Neurology* 1990; 40:820.

99. Oder W, et al: HM-PAO-SPECT in persistent vegetative state after head injury: Prognostic indicator of the likelihood of recovery: *Intensive Care Med* 1991; 17:149.

100. Agardh CD, et al: Persistent vegetative state with high cerebral blood flow following profound hypoglycemia. *Ann Neurol* 1983; 14:482.

101. Shewmon DA, De Giorgio CM: Early prognosis in anoxic coma: reliability and rationale. *Neurol Clin* 1989; 7:823.

102. Jennett B, Bond M: Assessment of outcome after severe brain damage: A practical scale. *Lancet* 1975; 1:480.

103. Braakman R, et al: Prognosis of the posttraumatic vegetative state. *Acta Neurochir (Wien)* 1988; 95:49.

104. Sazbon L, et al: Prognosis for recovery from prolonged posttraumatic unawareness: logistic analysis. *J Neurol Neurosurg Psychiatry* 1991; 54:149.

105. Sazbon L, Groswasser Z: Medical complications and mortality of patients in the postcomatose unawareness (PC-U) state. *Acta Neurochir (Wien)* 1991; 112:110.

106. Kriel RL, et al: Pediatric closed head injury: Outcome following prolonged unconsciousness. *Arch Phys Med Rehabil* 1988; 69:678.

107. Falk RH: Physical and intellectual recovery following prolonged hypoxic coma. *Postgrad Med J* 1990; 66:384.

108. Ashwal S, et al: The persistent vegetative state in children: Report of the Child Neurology Society Ethics Committee. *Ann Neurol* 1992; 32:570.

109. The Medical Task Force on Anencephaly: The infant with anencephaly. *N Engl J Med* 1990; 322:669.

110. Higashi K, et al: Epidemiological survey on patients with a persistent vegetative state. *J Neurol Neurosurg Psychiatry* 1977; 40:876.

111. Haig AJ, Ruess JM: Recovery from vegetative state of six months' duration associated with Sinemet (levodopa/carbidopa). *Arch Phys Med Rehabil* 1990; 71:1081.

112. Tsubokawa T, et al: Deep brain stimulation in a persistent vegetative state: Follow-up results and criteria for selection of candidates. *Brain Inj* 1990; 4:315.

113. LeWinn EB, Dimancescu MD: Environmental deprivation and enrichment in coma. *Lancet* 1978; 2:156.

114. DeYoung S, Grass RB: Coma recovery program. *Rehabil Nurs* 1987; 12:121.

115. Pierce JP, et al: The effectiveness of coma arousal intervention. *Brain Inj* 1990; 4:191.

116. Luce JM: Ethical principles in critical care. *JAMA* 1990; 263:696.

117. Raffin TA: Value of the living will. *Chest* 1986; 90:444.

118. Rosner F: Hospital medical ethics committee: A review of their development. *JAMA* 1985; 255:2693.

119. Brennan TA: Ethics committees and decisions to limit care in the experience at the Massachusetts General Hospital. *JAMA* 1988; 260:803.

120. Meisel A, et al: Hospital guidelines for deciding about life-

sustaining treatment: Dealing with health "limbo." *Crit Care Med* 1986; 14:239.

121. Grenvik A: "Terminal weaning": Discontinuance of life-support therapy in the terminally ill patient. *Crit Care Med* 1983; 11:394.

122. Grenvik A, et al: Cessation of therapy in terminal illness and brain death. *Crit Care Med* 1978; 6:284.

123. Childress JF: Non-heart beating donors of organs: Are the distinctions between direct and indirect effects and between killing and letting die relevant and helpful? *Kennedy Inst Ethics J* 1993; 3:203.

124. Angell M: After Quinlan: The dilemma of the persistent vegetative state. *N Engl J Med* 1994; 330:1524.

125. Council on Scientific Affairs and Council on Ethical and Judicial Affairs: Persistent vegetative state and the decision to withdraw or withhold life support. *JAMA* 1990; 263:426.

126. Institute of Medical Ethics Working Party on the Ethics of Prolonging Life and Assisting Death: Withdrawal of life-support from patients in a persistent vegetative state. *Lancet* 1991; 337:96.

127. ANA Committee on Ethical Affairs: Persistent Vegetative State: Report of the American Neurological Association Committee on Ethical Affairs. *Ann Neurol* 1993; 33:386.

128. Cranford RE: Termination of treatment in the persistent vegetative state. *Semin Neurol* 1984; 4:36.

129. Bernat JL: Ethical issues in neurology. In Joynt RJ (ed): *Clinical Neurology*, vol. 1. Philadelphia, J. B. Lippincott, 1991:2–57.

130. Alfonso I, et al: Discontinuation of artificial hydration and nutrition in hopelessly vegetative children. *Ann Neurol* 1992; 32:454 (abstr).

131. Printz LA: Is withholding hydration a valid comfort measure in the terminally ill? *Geriatrics* 1988; 43:84.

132. Spital A, et al: The living kidney donor: Alive and well. *Arch Intern Med* 1986; 146:1993.

133. Singer PA, et al: Ethics of liver transplantation with living donors. *N Engl J Med* 1989; 321:620.

134. Anonymous: Anencephalic infants as sources of transplantable organs. *Hastings Cent Rep* 1988; 18(5):28.

135. Caplan AL: Is xenografting morally wrong? *Transplant Proc* 1992; 24:722.

136. Youngner SJ, Arnold RM: Ethical, psychosocial, and public policy implications of procuring organs from non-heart-beating cadaver donors. *JAMA* 1993; 269:2769.

137. DeVita MA, Snyder JV: Development of the University of Pittsburgh Medical Center Policy for the care of the terminally ill patients who may become organ donors after death following the removal of life support. *Kennedy Inst Ethics J* 1993; 3:131.

INDEX

The letter *f* or *t* following a page number indicates that either a figure or a table is being referenced.

ISBN 0-07-000966-X

90000>